Treatment of
Skin Disease
Comprehensive Therapeutic Strategies

Fifth Edition

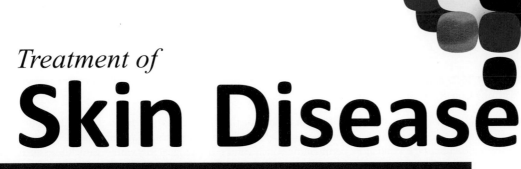

Treatment of
Skin Disease

Comprehensive Therapeutic Strategies

Fifth Edition

Mark G. Lebwohl, MD

Waldman Professor and Chairman
Kimberly and Eric J. Waldman Department of
Dermatology
Icahn School of Medicine at Mount Sinai
New York, NY, USA

Warren R. Heymann, MD

Professor of Medicine and Pediatrics
Head, Division of Dermatology
Cooper Medical School of Rowan University
Camden, NJ, USA;
Clinical Professor of Dermatology
Perelman School of Medicine at the University of
Pennsylvania
Philadelphia, PA, USA

John Berth-Jones, FRCP

Consultant Dermatologist
Department of Dermatology
University Hospital
Coventry, UK

Ian H. Coulson, BSc, MB, FRCP

Consultant Dermatologist
Dermatology Unit
Burnley General Hospital
Burnley, UK

For additional online content visit Expert Consult.com

online

ELSEVIER

ELSEVIER

© 2018, Elsevier Limited. All rights reserved.

First edition 2002
Second edition 2006
Third edition 2010
Fourth edition 2014

The right of Mark G. Lebwohl, Warren R. Heymann, John Berth-Jones, Ian H. Coulson to be identified as authors of this work has been asserted by them in accordance with the Copyright, Designs and Patents Act 1988.

No part of this publication may be reproduced or transmitted in any form or by any means, electronic or mechanical, including photocopying, recording, or any information storage and retrieval system, without permission in writing from the publisher. Details on how to seek permission, further information about the Publisher's permissions policies and our arrangements with organizations such as the Copyright Clearance Center and the Copyright Licensing Agency, can be found at our website: www.elsevier.com/permissions. This book and the individual contributions contained in it are protected under copyright by the Publisher (other than as may be noted herein).

The chapter entitled "Xeroderma Pigmentosum" is in the public domain.

Notices

Practitioners and researchers must always rely on their own experience and knowledge in evaluating and using any information, methods, compounds or experiments described herein. Because of rapid advances in the medical sciences, in particular, independent verification of diagnoses and drug dosages should be made. To the fullest extent of the law, no responsibility is assumed by Elsevier, authors, editors or contributors for any injury and/or damage to persons or property as a matter of products liability, negligence or otherwise, or from any use or operation of any methods, products, instructions, or ideas contained in the material herein.

 your source for books, journals and multimedia in the health sciences
www.elsevierhealth.com

  Working together to grow libraries in developing countries

www.elsevier.com • www.bookaid.org

The Publisher's policy is to use **paper manufactured from sustainable forests**

Content Strategists: Russell Gabbedy, Charlotta Kryhl
Content Development Specialists: Humayra Rahman Khan, Trinity Hutton
Project Manager: Srividhya Vidhyashankar
Content Coordinator: Joshua Mearns
Design: Christian J. Bilbow
Illustration Manager: Teresa McBryan
Marketing Manager: Kristin Koehler

ISBN: 978-0-7020-6912-3
Ebook ISBN: 978-0-7020-6913-0

Printed in China
Last digit is the print number: 9 8 7 6 5 4 3 2

Contents

---

† deceased

---

† deceased

Preface

Every four years, as we plan the next edition of *Treatment of Skin Disease*, the editors ask ourselves these questions: Do we need another edition? Has enough changed in the practice of dermatology to justify all the work needed for another edition? Thanks to extraordinary advances in our specialty, the answer has always been an emphatic *yes*.

The last four years has seen dramatic changes in the treatment of common dermatologic conditions like psoriasis and atopic dermatitis. Anti-IL-17 antibodies were only investigational four years ago, and now two, secukinumab and ixekizumab, are approved and a third antibody to the IL-17 receptor, brodalumab, has also been approved and is about to enter the market for psoriasis. Pure anti-IL-23 antibodies were only in experimental stages based on the earlier success of ustekinumab which blocks both IL-23 and IL-12. Guselkumab has now been released and tildrakizumab has completed phase III trials and will hopefully be approved in the coming months. Another anti-IL-23 antibody, risankizumab, is already in phase III trials and has very promising results in phase II, and other anti-IL-23 antibodies are already in development for psoriasis. Dupilumab, an anti-IL-4/IL-13 antibody has just been approved for moderate to severe atopic dermatitis, and crisaborole, a topical phosphodiesterase 4 inhibitor has been introduced for the treatment of mild to moderate atopic dermatitis. Tofacitinib, a janus kinase inhibitor, has shown substantial efficacy in psoriasis and atopic dermatitis, though regulators have not allowed approval for those diseases thus far. Because the drug is available for rheumatoid arthritis in the US, it has been used to treat other inflammatory skin diseases like alopecia areata and vitiligo with striking success.

Treatment of less common conditions has advanced as well. Four years ago, we were just beginning to use the first hedgehog inhibitor for catastrophic basal cell carcinomas. We now have a second oral hedgehog inhibitor, sonidegib. We also have many new uses for drugs introduced earlier. The best example is the approval of adalimumab for the treatment of hidradenitis. Dermatologists were only starting to prescribe omalizumab for chronic idiopathic urticaria, and that treatment, first approved for asthma, is now well established for chronic urticaria.

Advances in the treatment of rare diseases have been extraordinary as well. Sildenafil is now commonly used for lymphatic malformations, and topical rapamycin is commonly used for facial angiofibromas. In some countries, afamelanotide has been approved for the treatment of erythropoietic protoporphyria.

Off label uses of many old therapies have also been tried for many dermatologic diseases and are covered well in the updated versions of our chapters. Many of the drugs approved for adults are also being studied in children, and hopefully we will see many new therapy approvals for pediatric indications.

The commercial successes of multiple biologic, oral and topical therapies for dermatologic indications, has sparked a tremendous amount of research and innovation in our field. As we send this edition to the printer, new oral agents are being studied for inflammatory skin diseases. Both topical and oral janus kinase inhibitors including ruxolitinib, baricitinib, and tofacitinib are being studied for alopecia areata, vitiligo, psoriasis, and atopic dermatitis. Investigation of phosphodiesterase inhibitors for itch and for other inflammatory skin conditions are underway. Creams that change the bacterial flora of conditions like atopic dermatitis are also in development, and numerous biologic therapies like nemolizumab for itch and anti-IL-13 antibodies like lebrikizumab and tralokinumab are being studied for atopic dermatitis.

Every chapter of this new edition has been carefully revised and updated with the latest innovations. As you read on, it will become clear how profoundly the rapid pace of progress is impacting on the benefits we can offer our patients - this is such an exciting time to be practising dermatology.

Mark G. Lebwohl
Warren R. Heymann
John Berth-Jones
Ian H. Coulson
2017

List of Contributors

Anthony Abdullah, BSc (Hons), MBChB (Hons), FRCP, DTM&H
Consultant Dermatologist, Lead Clinician
The Birmingham Skin Centre
Sandwell and West Birmingham Hospitals
NHS Trust
Birmingham, UK

Michael Abrouk, BS
University of California San Francisco
Department of Dermatology
San Francisco, CA, USA

Tashmeeta Ahad, MA (Cantab), BM BCh, MRCP
Salford Royal NHS Foundation Trust
Manchester, UK

Imtiaz Ahmed, MBBS, FRCP
Consultant Dermatologist
Department of Dermatology
University Hospitals Coventry and
Warwickshire
Coventry, UK

Anwar Al Hammadi, MD, FRCPC, FAAD
Consultant and Head of Dermatology
Dubai Health Authority, UAE
Associate Professor of Dermatology, Dubai
Medical College
Dubai, UAE

Caroline Allen, MA, MBBS, MRCP
Dermatologist
Department of Dermatology
Churchill Hospital
Oxford, UK

Amer Ali Almohssen, MD
Rutgers New Jersey Medical School
Newark, NJ, USA

Wisam Alwan, MBBS, BSc, MRCP (Dermatology)
St. John's Institute of Dermatology, Guy's
and St. Thomas' Hospitals NHS Trust
London, UK

Mahreen Ameen, MBBS, MA, MSc, MRCP, MD
Consultant Dermatologist
Royal Free London NHS Foundation Trust
London, UK

Sadegh Amini, MD
Voluntary Assistant Professor
Department of Dermatology and
Cutaneous Surgery
University of Miami
Miller School of Medicine
Miami, FL, Dermatologist, Hollywood
Dermatology & Cosmetic Specialists
Doral, FL, USA

Bryan E. Anderson, MD
Professor of Dermatology
Penn State College of Medicine
Hershey Medical Center
Hershey, PA, USA

Grant J. Anhalt, MD
Professor of Dermatology and Pathology
Department of Dermatology
Johns Hopkins University School of
Medicine
Baltimore, MD, USA

Donald J. Baker, MD
Clinical Assistant Professor
Department of Medicine
Division of Dermatology
Cooper Medical School of Rowan University
Gibbsboro, NJ, USA

Harini Rajgopal Bala, MBBS, B.Pharm, MPH
Diploma of Dermatology
Skin and Cancer Foundation Inc
Melbourne, Australia

Julia Baltz, MD
Chief Resident
Dermatology
University of Massachusetts Medical School
Worcester, MA, USA

David Banach, MD, MPH
Assistant Professor of Medicine
University of Connecticut School of
Medicine
Farmington, CT USA

Cedric C. Banfield, FRCP
Consultant Dermatologist, NHS
Peterborough City Hospital
Peterborough, UK

Robert Baran, MD
Honorary Professor of Dermatology
University of Franche-Comté
Besançon
Nail Disease Center
Cannes, France

Ajoy Bardhan, MBBS BSc MRCP
University Hospitals Coventry and
Warwickshire NHS Trust
Coventry, UK

Melissa C. Barkham, MRCP
Consultant Dermatologist
Ashford and St. Peter's Hospital
St. Peter's Hospital,
Surrey, UK

Ysabel M. Bello, MD
Voluntary Assistant Professor
Department of Dermatology and Cutaneous
Surgery
University of Miami Miller School of Medicine
Miami, FL, USA

Emma Benton, FRCP
Consultant Dermatologist
St. John's Institute of Dermatology
Guy's and St. Thomas' NHS Trust
London, UK

Wilma F. Bergfeld, MD
Professor, Dermatology and Pathology
Cleveland Clinic
Cleveland, OH, USA

Eric Berkowitz, MD
Assistant Clinical Professor
Department of Medicine (Dermatology)
Albert Einstein College of Medicine
Bronx, NY, USA

Brian Berman, MD, PhD
Professor Emeritus, Dermatology and
Cutaneous Surgery
University of Miami Miller School of Medicine
Miami, FL, USA
Co-Director Center for Clinical and
Cosmetic Research
Aventura, FL, USA

Jeffrey D. Bernhard, MD, FRCP (Edin)
Professor Emeritus
University of Massachusetts Medical School
Worcester, MA, USA

Daniel Bernstein
The Mount Sinai Hospital
New York, NY, USA

John Berth-Jones, FRCP
Consultant Dermatologist
Department of Dermatology
University Hospital
Coventry, UK

Chinmoy Bhate, MD
Clinical Assistant Professor, Dermatology
and Pathology
Rutgers New Jersey Medical School
Newark, NJ, USA

Bhavnit K. Bhatia, MD
Henry Ford Hospital
Detroit, MI, USA

Jonathan E. Blume, MD
Clinical Instructor of Dermatology
Department of Dermatology
Columbia University College of Physicians
and Surgeons
New York, NY, USA

Nevianna Bordet, MBChB, FRCP
Consultant Dermatologist
Spire Cambridge Lea Hospital
Cambridge, UK

Catherine Borysiewicz, MA MBBS MRCP
Consultant Dermatologist
Dermatology Department
Imperial college healthcare NHS trust
London, UK

Gary J. Brauner, MD
Associate Clinical Professor of Dermatology
Icahn School of Medicine at Mount Sinai
New York, NY, USA

Robert T. Brodell, MD
Professor and Chair
Department of Dermatology
Professor and Interim Chair
Department of Pathology
University of Mississippi Medical Center
Jackson, MS, USA

Marc D. Brown, MD
Professor of Dermatology and Oncology
Division of Dermatologic Surgery
University of Rochester School of Medicine
Rochester, NY, USA

Robert M. Burd, MBChB, FRCP
Consultant Dermatologist
Department of Dermatology
Leicester Royal Infirmary
Leicester, UK

Anne E. Burdick, MD, MPH
Professor of Dermatology
Leprosy Program Director
Associate Dean for TeleHealth and Clinical
Outreach
University of Miami Miller School of
Medicine
Miami, FL, USA

Niraj Butala, MD
Rowan University
Department of Dermatology
Glassboro, NJ, USA

Jeffrey P. Callen, MAAD, FACR, FACP
Chief, Division of Dermatology
Department of Medicine
University of Louisville School of Medicine
Louisville, KY, USA

Ivan D. Camacho, MD
Private Practice
Voluntary Assistant Professor
Department of Dermatology and Cutaneous
Surgery
University of Miami
Miami, FL, USA

Helena Camasmie
Dermatology Department
Gaffree and Guinle University Hospital
Federal University of the State of Rio de
Janeiro
Rio de Janeiro, Brazil

Daniel Caplivski, MD
Director,
Travel Medicine Program
Associate Professor
Division of Infectious Diseases
Icahn School of Medicine at Mount Sinai
New York, NY, USA

Mitchell S. Cappell, MD, PhD
Chief, Division of Gastroenterology &
Hepatology
William Beaumont Hospital;
Professor of Medicine
Oakland University William Beaumont
School of Medicine
Royal Oak, MI, USA

Genevieve A. Casey, MBBS, FACD
Honorary Clinical Fellow
Oxford University Hospitals NHS
Foundation Trust
Oxford, UK

Lawrence S. Chan, MD
Professor of Dermatology
University of Illinois College of Medicine
Chicago, IL, USA

Loi-Yuen Chan, MBBS, MRCPI, Dip Derm
(London), FHKAM
Private Practice
Hong Kong, China

Jennifer K. Chen, MD
Clinical Assistant Professor, Dermatology
Stanford University School of Medicine
Redwood City, CA, USA

Chen "Mary" Chen
Dermatopathology
Mount Sinai Hospital
New York, NY, USA

Nicole Yi Zhen Chiang, MBChB (Hons) MRCP
(UK) MRCP (UK) (Derm)
Consultant Dermatologist
University Hospital of South Manchester &
Salford Royal Hospital
Salford, UK

Anthony J. Chiaravalloti, MD
University of Connecticut Health Center,
Department of Dermatology
Farmington, CT, USA

Fiona J. Child, BSc, MD, FRCP
Consultant Dermatologist
Skin Tumour Unit
St. John's Institute of Dermatology
Guy's and St. Thomas' NHS Foundation
Trust
London, UK

Anthony C. Chu, FRCP
Professor of Dermatologic Oncology
Buckingham University
Consultant Dermatologist
Imperial Health Care Trust
Hammersmith Hospital
London, UK

Timothy H. Clayton, FRCP (Edin), MBChB,
MRCPCH
Consultant Paediatric Dermatologist
Royal Manchester Children's Hospital
The Centre for Dermatology
Salford Royal Foundation NHS Trust
Manchester, UK

Steven R. Cohen, MD, MPH
Professor and Chief
Division of Dermatology
Albert Einstein College of Medicine
New York, NY, USA

Elizabeth A. Cooper, BSc, BESc
Clinical Research Manager
Mediprobe Research, Inc.
London, ON, Canada

Susan M. Cooper, MRCGP, FRCP, MD
Consultant Dermatologist
Oxford University Hospitals NHS
Foundation Trust
Oxford, UK

Nick Collier
Dermatology Department
Salford Royal Foundation Trust
Salford, UK

Christina M. Correnti, MD, MS
University of Maryland School of Medicine,
Department of Dermatology
Baltimore, MD, USA

Ian H. Coulson, BSc, MB, FRCP
Consultant Dermatologist
Dermatology Unit
Burnley General Hospital
Burnley, UK

M. Laurin Council, MD
Assistant Professor of Dermatology
Washington University
St. Louis, MO, USA

Shawn E. Cowper, MD
Associate Professor of Dermatology and
Pathology
Dermatopathology Service
Department of Dermatology
Yale University School of Medicine
New Haven, CT, USA

Nicholas M. Craven, BM, BCh, MA, FRCP
Consultant Dermatologist
Mid Cheshire Hospitals NHS Foundation
Trust
Crewe, Cheshire, UK

Daniel Creamer, BSc, MD, FRCP
Consultant Dermatologist
Department of Dermatology
King's College Hospital
London, UK

Ponciano D. Cruz Jr., MD
Distinguished Professor and Vice Chair
Department of Dermatology
The University of Texas Southwestern
Medical Center
Dallas, TX, USA

Carrie Ann R. Cusack, MD
Assistant Professor of Dermatology
Department of Dermatology
Drexel University College of Medicine
Philadelphia, PA, USA

Adam Daunton, BSc, MBChB, MRCP
Salford Royal Hospital NHS Foundation
Trust
Manchester, UK

Mark D. P. Davis, MD
Professor & Chair
Department of Dermatology
Mayo Clinic
Rochester, MN, USA

Robert S. Dawe, MBChB, MD, FRCP
Consultant Dermatologist & Honorary
Reader in Dermatology
Photobiology Unit
Department of Dermatology
Ninewells Hospital and Medical School
Dundee, UK

David P. D'Cruz, MD, FRCP
Consultant Rheumatologist
Louise Coote Lupus Unit
Guy's Hospital
London, UK

David de Berker, BA, MBBS, MRCP
Consultant Dermatologist and Honorary
Senior Lecturer
Bristol Dermatology Centre
Bristol Royal Infirmary Hospital
Bristol, UK

Danielle M. DeHoratius, MD
Clinical Associate
Department of Dermatology
Hospital of the University of Pennsylvania
Philadelphia, PA, USA

Min Deng, MD
Assistant Professor
Center for Dermatologic Surgery
West Virginia University School of Medicine
Morgantown, WV, USA

Seemal R. Desai, MD
Founder and Medical Director
Innovative Dermatology, PA
Clinical Assistant Professor
Department of Dermatology
University of Texas Southwestern Medical
Center
Dallas, Texas, USA

Georgina Devlin, BA (Hons)
Paediatric Dermatology Specialist Nurse
Salford Royal Foundation Trust
Manchester, UK

John J. DiGiovanna, MD
Senior Research Physician
DNA Repair Section
Laboratory of Cancer Biology and Genetics
Center for Cancer Research
National Cancer Institute
National Institutes of Health
Bethesda, MD, USA

Alexander Doctoroff, DO, MS
Clinical Assistant Professor of Dermatology
Columbia University Medical Center
New York, NY;
Medical Director and CEO
Metropolitan Dermatology
Clark, NJ, USA

Roni P. Dodiuk-Gad, MD
Vice Head - Dermatology Department
Emek Medical Center
Israel, Clinical Assistant Professor
Bruce Rappaport Faculty of Medicine
Technion - Institute of Technology
Israel, Research Fellow;
Division of Dermatology
Sunnybrook Health Sciences Centre
University of Toronto
Toronto, ON, Canada

Dawn Z. Eichenfield, MD, PhD
Departments of Medicine and Dermatology
University of California
San Diego School of Medicine
San Diego, CA, USA

Lawrence F. Eichenfield, MD
Professor of Dermatology and Pediatrics
Chief, Division of Pediatric Dermatology
Vice Chair, Department of Dermatology
University of California, San Diego and
Rady Children's Hospital
San Diego, CA, USA

Drore Eisen, MD, DDS
Dermatologists of Southwest Ohio
Cincinnati, OH, USA

Ure Eke, MBChB, MRCP
Consultant Dermatologist
University Hospitals Coventry and
Warwickshire NHS Trust
Coventry, UK

Dirk M. Elston, MD
Professor and Chairman
Department of Dermatology and
Dermatologic Surgery
Medical University of South Carolina
Charleston, SC, USA

Patrick O. M. Emanuel, MB, ChB
Dermatopathologist
Auckland District Health Board
Auckland, New Zealand

Clinton W. Enos, MD, MS
Eastern Virginia Medical School
Norfolk, VA

Shaheen H. Ensanyat, MS
The Tisch Cancer Institute
Mount Sinai School of Medicine
New York, NY, USA

Anna F. Falabella, MD, CWS
Voluntary Associate Professor
Department of Dermatology and Cutaneous
Surgery
University of Miami Miller School of Medicine
Miami, FL, USA

Aaron S. Farberg, MD
Department of Dermatology
Icahn School of Medicine at Mount Sinai
New York, NY, USA

Lawrence S. Feigenbaum, MD
Department of Dermatology
University of Texas Southwestern Medical
Center
Dallas, TX, USA

Kristen Heins Fernandez, MD
Assistant Professor
University of Missouri;
Chief of Dermatology
Harry S. Truman VA
Columbia, MO, USA

Nicole Fett, MD, MSCE
Associate Professor of Dermatology
Oregon Health and Science University
Portland, OR, USA

Andrew Y. Finlay, CBE, FRCP (Lond and Glasg)
Professor of Dermatology
School of Medicine
Cardiff University
Cardiff, UK

Bahar F. Firoz, MD MPH
Dermatologist
Dermatology Surgery Fellow
Derm Surgery Associates
Houston, TX, USA

Elnaz F. Firoz, BA
Dermatologist
Columbia University College of Physicians
and Surgeons
Short Hills, NJ, USA

James E. Fitzpatrick, MD
Professor of Dermatology and Pathology
(retired)
University of Colorado School of Medicine
Aurora, CO, USA

Amy E. Flischel, MD, FAAD
Clinical Assistant Professor of Dermatology
University of Illinois at Chicago College of
Medicine
Chicago, IL, USA

Kelly A. Foley, PhD
Medical Research Associate
Mediprobe Research, Inc.
London, ON, Canada

Derek Freedman, MD, FRCPI
Genitourinary Physician
GUIDE Clinic
St. James' Hospital
Dublin, Ireland

Georgina A. Fremlin, MBChB, MRCP
Dermatology Specialist Registrar
The Birmingham Skin Centre
Sandwell and West Birmingham Hospitals
NHS Trust Birmingham
Birmingham, UK

Richard Fried, MD, PhD
Clinical Director
Yardley Dermatology
Yardley Clinical Research Associates
Yardley, PA, USA

Philip Friedlander, MD, PhD
Assistant Professor of Medicine
Department of Hematology and Oncology
Department of Dermatology
The Tisch Cancer Institute
Mount Sinai School of Medicine
New York, NY, USA

Adam Friedman, MD
Assistant Professor of Medicine (Dermatology)
Assistant Professor of Physiology and Biophysics
Director of Dermatologic Research
Division of Dermatology
Montefiore-Einstein College of Medicine
Bronx, NY, USA

Amy K. Forrestel, MD
Dermatology / Internal Medicine
University of Pennsylvania
Philadelphia, PA, USA

Brian S. Fuchs, MPH, MD
Dermatologist
Department of Psychiatry
Mount Sinai School of Medicine
New York, NY, USA

Joanna E. Gach, MD, FRCP
Consultant Dermatologist
Department of Dermatology
University Hospital
Coventry, UK

Anjela Galan, MD
Associate Professor, Dermatology and Pathology Associate Director
Dermatopathology Fellowship and Training Program
Yale University School of Medicine
New Haven, CT, USA

Jaya Ganesh, MD
Associate Professor of Pediatrics
Cooper Medical School at Rowan University
Division Chief, Genetics
Cooper University Hospital
Camden, NJ, USA

Amit Garg, MD
Professor and Founding Chair
Department of Dermatology
Hofstra Northwell School of Medicine
SVP, Dermatology Service Line
Northwell Health
Hempstead, NY, USA

Lauren Geller, MD
The Mount Sinai Hospital
Department of Pediatrics
New York, NY, USA

Carlo M. Gelmetti, MD
Head, Unit of Pediatric Dermatology
Fondazione IRCCS Ca' Granda "Ospedale Maggiore Policlinico," Milan
Department of Pathophysiology and Transplantation, University of Milan
Milan, Italy

Elizabeth Ghazi, MD
Department of Dermatology
University of Pennsylvania, School of Medicine
Philadelphia, PA, USA

Sneha Ghunawat, MD, DNB
Department of Dermatology Venereology and Leprology
Maulana Azad Medical College
New Delhi, India

Leonard H. Goldberg, MD, FRCP
Medical Director and Chief of Surgery
Derm Surgery Associates PA
Clinical Professor in Dermatology
University of Texas Medical School;
Clinical Professor
Department of Dermatology
Weill Medical College of Cornell University;
Director
Procedural Dermatology Fellowship
The Methodist Hospital
Houston, TX, USA

Mark J. D. Goodfield, MD FRCP
Consultant Dermatologist
Department of Dermatology
Leeds General Infirmary
Leeds, UK

Marsha L. Gordon, MD
Professor and Vice Chairman
Department of Dermatology
Mount Sinai School of Medicine
New York, NY, USA

Asha Gowda, MS
University of Toledo College of Medicine
Toledo, OH, USA

Daniel A. Grabell, MD, MBA
Clinical Research Fellow
University of Texas Health Science Center at Houston McGovern Medical School
Department of Dermatology
Houston, TX, USA

Matthew Grant, MD
Assistant Professor of Medicine
Section of Infectious Diseases
Yale School of Medicine
New Haven, CT, USA

Clive E. H. Grattan, MA, MD, FRCP
Consultant Dermatologist
St. John's Institute of Dermatology, Guy's Hospital
London, UK

Malcolm W. Greaves, MD, PhD, FRCP
Emeritus Professor of Dermatology
Consultant Specialist in Dermatology and Allergy
Cutaneous Allergy Clinic
St. John's Institute of Dermatology
St. Thomas' Hospital
London, UK

Justin J. Green, MD
Assistant Professor of Medicine, Division of Dermatology
Cooper Medical School of Rowan University
Camden, NJ, USA

Christopher E. M. Griffiths, MD, FRCP, FMedSci
Foundation Professor of Dermatology
The University of Manchester, Manchester Academic Health Science Centre
The Dermatology Centre, Barnes Building
Salford Royal NHS Foundation Trust
Manchester, UK

Charles A. Gropper, MD
Associate Clinical Professor of Dermatology
Icahn School of Medicine at Mount Sinai
Clinical Affiliate Professor of Medicine
CUNY School of Medicine
Chief of Dermatology Saint Barnabas Hospital
New York, NY, USA

Anna L. Grossberg, MD
Assistant Professor, Departments of Dermatology and Pediatrics
The Johns Hopkins University School of Medicine
Baltimore, MD, USA

Aditya K. Gupta, MD, PhD, FAAD, FRCP(C)
Department of Medicine
University of Toronto
Toronto, ON, Canada
Director
Mediprobe Research, Inc.
London, ON, Canada

Ali S. Hadi, MD
Department of Dermatology
Icahn School of Medicine at Mount Sinai
New York, NY, USA

Suhail M. Hadi, MBchB, MPhil, FAAD
Associate Professor
Department of Dermatology
Icahn School of Medicine at Mount Sinai
New York, NY, USA

Iris A. Hagans, MD
Cooper University Healthcare
Camden, NJ, USA

Bethany R. Hairston, MD
Private Practice
The Dermatology Clinic
Columbus, MS, USA

Analisa Vincent Halpern, MD
Assistant Professor
Division of Dermatology
Department of Medicine
Cooper Medical of Rowan University
Camden, NJ, USA

Caroline Halverstam, MD
Assistant Professor and Director
Dermatology Section
Montefiore-Wakefield Medical Center
Division of Dermatology
Albert Einstein College of Medicine
Bronx, NY, USA

Natasha Harper
EB Clinical Fellow
Department of Dermatology
Solihull Hospital
Solihull, UK

Matthew J. Harries, PhD, FRCP
Consultant Dermatologist and Honorary
Senior Lecturer
The University of Manchester,
Salford Royal NHS Foundation Trust
Salford, Greater Manchester, UK

John Harris, MD, PhD
Associate Professor of Dermatology
University of Massachusetts Medical School
Worcester, MA, USA

Shannon Harrison, MBBS, MMed, FACD
Honorary Clinical Lecturer
Department of Medicine
University of Melbourne
Melbourne, Australia

Michael M. Hatch, MD
Texas Tech School of Medicine
Texas Tech University Health Sciences
Center
Lubbock, TX, USA

Adrian H. M. Heagerty, BSc, MD, FRCP
Consultant Dermatologist
Department of Dermatology
Solihull Hospital
West Midlands, UK

Adelaide A. Hebert, MD
Professor
Departments of Dermatology and
Pediatrics
The University of Texas Health Science
Center at Houston
Houston, TX, USA

Stephen E. Helms, MD
Professor, Department of Dermatology
University of Mississippi Medical Center
Jackson, MS, USA

Camile L. Hexsel, MD
Dermatologist
Mohs/Procedural Dermatology Fellow
DermSurgery Associates and the Methodist
Hospital
Houston, TX, USA;
Investigator
Brazilian Center for Studies in Dermatology
Porto Alegre, Brazil

Doris M. Hexsel, MD
Instructor
Department of Dermatology
Pontifícia Universidade Católica do Rio
Grande do Sul;
Investigator
Brazilian Center for Studies in Dermatology
Porto Alegre, Brazil

Warren R. Heymann, MD
Professor of Medicine and Pediatrics
Head, Division of Dermatology
Cooper Medical School of Rowan
University
Camden, NJ;
Clinical Professor of Dermatology
Perelman School of Medicine at the
University of Pennsylvania
Philadelphia, PA, USA

Elisabeth M. Higgins†, MA, FRCP
Consultant Dermatologist
Department of Dermatology
King's College Hospital
London, UK

Claire L. Higgins, BSc (Hons), MBBS (Hons), MPH
Skin and Cancer Foundation, Inc.
Melbourne, Australia

Whitney A. High, MD, JD, MEng
Associate Professor of Dermatology and
Pathology
Director of Dermatopathology
University of Colorado School of Medicine
Denver, CO, USA

Herbert Hönigsmann, MD
Professor of Dermatology
Emeritus Chairman
Department of Dermatology
Medical University of Vienna
Vienna, Austria

Marcelo G. Horenstein, MD
Director
Department of Pathology
The Dermatology Group
West Orange, NJ, USA

George J. Hruza, MD, MBA
Adjunct Professor of Dermatology
St. Louis University
St. Louis, MO;
Medical Director
Laser & Dermatologic Surgery Center
Chesterfield, MO, USA

Andrea Hui, MD
Dermatologist
Department of Dermatology
State University of New York Downstate
Medical Center
Brooklyn, NY, USA

Ran Huo, MD
Dermatologist
Department of Dermatology and Cutaneous
Surgery
University of Miami Miller School of
Medicine
Miami, FL, USA

Sally H. Ibbotson, BSc (Hons), MBChB (Hons);
MD with Commendation; FRCP
Professor of Photodermatology
University of Dundee
Ninewells Hospital & Medical School
Dundee, UK

Sherrif F. Ibrahim, MD, PhD
Associate Professor, Dermatology
Division of Dermatologic Surgery
University of Rochester Medical Center
Rochester, NY, USA

Andrew Ilchyshyn, MBChB, FRCP
Consultant Dermatologist
Department of Dermatology
University Hospitals Coventry and
Warwickshire NHS Trust
Coventry, UK

Dina Ismail, MBBS, BSc, MRCP
Dermatologist
Salford Royal NHS Foundation Trust
Manchester, UK

Stefania Jablonska, MD
Professor Emeritus of Dermatology
Medical University of Warsaw
Warsaw, Poland

Heidi T. Jacobe, MD, MCS
Associate Professor
Department of Dermatology
University of Texas Southwestern Medical Center
Dallas, TX, USA

William D. James, MD
Paul R. Gross Professor
Department of Dermatology
Hospital of the University of Pennsylvania
Philadelphia, PA, USA

Aysha Javed, MBChB, MRCP
Consultant Dermatologist
Countess of Chester Hospital
Cheshire, UK

Gregor B. E. Jemec, MD, DMSc
Professor of Dermatology
Department of Dermatology
Zealand University
Hospital Health Sciences Faculty
University of Copenhagen
Copenhagen, Denmark

Graham A. Johnston, MB, ChB, FRCP
Associate Professor
Department of Molecular and Cell Biology
University of Leicester;
Consultant Dermatologist
Department of Dermatology
Leicester Royal Infirmary
Leicester, UK

Stephen K. Jones, MD, FRCP
Emeritus Consultant Dermatologist
Clatterbridge Hospital
Wirral Teaching Hospital NHS Foundation
Trust
Wirral, UK

Jacqueline M. Junkins-Hopkins, MD
Senior Dermatologist
Dermpath Diagnostics
Ackerman Academy of Dermatopathology
New York, NY, USA

Jessica Kaffenberger, MD
Assistant Professor of Dermatology
The Ohio State University Medical Center
Columbus, OH, USA

Kelly R. Kane, MD
Dermatologist
Paolini Dermatology
Cape May Court House, NJ, USA

Antonios Kanelleas, MD, PhD
Consultant Dermatologist
1st Department of Dermatology and
Venereology
A. Sygros Hospital for Skin and Venereal
Diseases
University of Athens School of Medicine
Athens, Greece

† deceased

Ayşe Serap Karadağ
Associate Professor
Dermatology
Istanbul Medeniyet University
Cherry Hill, NJ, USA

Laura Karas
Center for Clinical Studies
Houston, TX, USA

Ruwani P. Katugampola, MD, FRCP
Consultant Dermatologist
Welsh Institute of Dermatology, University
Hospital of Wales
Cardiff, UK

Bruce E. Katz, MD
Clinical Professor
Icahn School of Medicine at Mount Sinai
Director, Juva Skin & Laser Center,
New York, NY, USA

Roselyn Kellen, MD
Department of Dermatology
Mount Sinai School of Medicine
New York, NY USA

Murtaza Khan, MBBS, MRCP
Dermatologist
Department of Dermatology
University Hospitals Coventry &
Warwickshire
Coventry, UK

Hooman Khorasani, MD
Chief
Division of Dermatologic & Cosmetic
Surgery
Department of Dermatology
Assistant Professor of Dermatology
Icahn School of Medicine at Mount Sinai;
Program Director
Micrographic Surgery & Dermatologic
Oncology Fellowship Program
Program Director Dermatologic Cosmetic
Surgery Fellowship Program
Icahn School of Medicine at Mount Sinai
New York, NY, USA

Ellen J. Kim, MD
Sandra J. Lazarus Professor of Dermatology
Perelman School of Medicine at the
University of Pennsylvania
Philadelphia, PA, USA

Hee J. Kim, MD
Department of Dermatology
Icahn School of Medicine at Mount Sinai
New York, NY, USA

Brian Kirby, MD, FRCPI
Consultant Dermatologist and Associate
Clinical Professor
St. Vincent's University Hospital and
University College Dublin
Dublin, Ireland

Joslyn S. Kirby, MD
Assistant Professor of Dermatology
Penn State College of Medicine
Hershey Medical Center
Hershey, PA, USA

Rachel S. Klein, MD
Dermatologist
Department of Dermatology
University of Pennsylvania
Philadelphia, PA, USA

Kate Kleydman, DO
Mohs/Procedural Dermatology Fellow
Department of Dermatology
Division of Mohs, Reconstructive &
Cosmetic Surgery
The Mount Sinai Medical Center
New York, NY, USA

Dimitra Koch, MD, MRCP (UK)
Consultant Dermatologist
Dorset County Hospital
Dorchester, Dorset, UK

John J. Kohorst, MD
Mayo Clinic
Rochester, MN, USA

John Y.M. Koo, MD, FAAD
Professor
Psoriasis and Skin Treatment Center
University of California San Francisco
San Francisco, CA, USA

Sandra A. Kopp, MD
Assistant Clinical Professor
Department of Dermatology
Mount Sinai School of Medicine
New York, NY, USA

Neil J. Korman, MD, PhD
Professor of Dermatology
University Hospitals Cleveland Medical Center
Cleveland, OH, USA

Carrie Kovarik, MD
Associate Professor of Dermatology and
Dermatopathology
Perelman School of Medicine at the
University of Pennsylvania
Philadelphia, PA, USA

Kenneth H. Kraemer, MD
Chief, DNA Repair Section
Laboratory of Cancer Biology and Genetics
Center for Cancer Research
National Cancer Institute
Bethesda, MD, USA

Bernice R. Krafchik, MBChB, FRCP(C)
Professor Emeritus
Pediatrics and Medicine
University of Toronto
Toronto, ON, Canada

Karthik Krishnamurthy, DO
Associate Professor, Division of Dermatology
Albert Einstein College of Medicine
Bronx, NY, USA;
Program Director, Dermatology Residency
Orange Park Medical Center
Orange Park, FL, USA

Knut Kvernebo, MD, PhD, FRCS
Professor of Cardiothoracic Surgery
Oslo University Hospital
Oslo University
Oslo, Norway

Charlene Lam, MD, MPH
Dermatologist
Penn State College of Medicine Hershey
Medical Center
Hershey, PA, USA

Peter C. Lambert, MD
Dermatology
Rutgers New Jersey Medical School
Newark, NJ, USA

James A. A. Langtry, MBBS, MRCP, FACMS
Consultant Dermatologist and
Dermatological Surgeon
Department of Dermatology
Royal Victoria Infirmary
Newcastle Upon Tyne, UK

Amir A. Larian, MD
Clinical Instructor
Department of Dermatology
Mount Sinai School of Medicine
New York, NY, USA

Cecilia A. Larocca, MD
Physician
Department of Dermatology
Boston University School of Medicine
Boston, MA, USA

E. Frances Lawlor, MD, FRCP (lond), FRCPI, DcH, DRCOG
St. John's Institute of Dermatology
The London Clinic
London, UK

Clifford M. Lawrence, MD, FRCP
Consultant Dermatologist
Royal Victoria Infirmary
Newcastle Upon Tyne, UK

Mark G. Lebwohl, MD
Waldman Professor of Dermatology
Department of Dermatology
The Mount Sinai Medical Center
New York, NY, USA

Oscar Lebwohl, MD
Richard and Rakia Hatch Professor of
Medicine
Columbia University Medical Center
New York, NY, USA

Julia S. Lehman, MD, FAAD
Associate Professor of Dermatology and
Laboratory Medicine and Pathology
Mayo Clinic
Rochester, MN, USA

Tabi A. Leslie, BSc, MBBS, FRCP
Consultant Dermatologist
Royal Free Hospital
London, UK

Stuart R. Lessin, MD
Medical Director
KGL Skin Study Center
Philadelphia, PA, USA

Jacob O. Levitt, MD
Professor, Vice Chairman, and Residency
Director
Department of Dermatology
The Mount Sinai Medical Center
New York, NY, USA

Fiona M. Lewis, MD, FRCP
Consultant Dermatologist
St. John's Institute of Dermatology, Guy's &
St. Thomas' NHS Trust
London, UK

Maryam Liaqat, MD
Cooper University Hospital
Camden, NJ, USA

Kristina J. Liu, MD
Director
Dermatology Simulation Education
Instructor
Harvard Medical School
Boston, MA, USA

Michael P. Loosemore, MD, FAAD
Staff Physician
Dermatologic and Mohs Micrographic
Surgery
Mission Hospital
Asheville, NC, USA

Thomas A. Luger, MD
Professor and Chairman
Department of Dermatology
University of Münster
Münster, Germany

Omar Lupi, MD, MSc, PhD
Professor of Dermatology
Federal University of the State of Rio de
Janeiro (UniRio);
Chairman and Titular Professor
Policlinica Geral do Rio de Janeiro (PGRJ)
Professor of Immunology
Federal University of Rio de Janeiro (UFRJ)
Rio de Janeiro, Brazil

Boris D. Lushniak, MD, MPH
Dean and Professor
University of Maryland
School of Public Health
College Park, MD, USA

Calum C. Lyon, MA, FRCP
Consultant Dermatologist
Department of Dermatology
York Hospital
York, UK

Andrea D. Maderal, MD
Assistant Professor
Department of Dermatology and Cutaneous
Surgery
University of Miami Miller School of
Medicine
Miami, FL, USA

Bassel H. Mahmoud, MD, PhD, FAAD
Associate Professor of Dermatology
University of Massachusetts
Worcester, MA, USA

Slawomir Majewski, MD
Head of the Department of Dermatology
and Venereology
Medical University of Warsaw
Warsaw, Poland

Richard B. Mallett, MB, FRCP
Consultant Dermatologist
Dermatology
Peterborough City Hospital
Peterborough, UK

Steven M. Manders, MD
Professor of Medicine and Pediatrics
Division of Dermatology
Cooper Medical School of Rowan University
Camden, NJ, USA

Ranon Mann, MD
Instructor of Medicine
Department of Dermatology
Albert Einstein College of Medicine
New York, NY, USA

Yasaman Mansouri, MD, MRCP
Dermatologist
Department of Dermatology
Heart of England NHS Foundation Trust
Solihull Hospital
Solihull, UK

David J. Margolis, MD, PhD
Professor of Dermatology
Professor of Epidemiology
Assistant Dean for Faculty Affairs
Perelman School of Medicine
University of Pennsylvania
Philadelphia, PA, USA

Orit Markowitz, MD
Director of Pigmented Lesions and Skin
Cancer
Associate Professor of Dermatology
Icahn School of Medicine at Mount Sinai
New York, NY, USA

Alexander Marsland, BSc (Hons), MBChB, FRCP
Consultant Dermatologist and Honorary
Senior Lecturer
Salford Royal Foundation Trust and
University of Manchester
Manchester, UK

Agustin Martin-Clavijo, MRCP
Dermatologist
Queen Elizabeth Hospital
Birmingham, UK

Daniela Martinez
Department of Dermatology
Unirio Hugg Gaffree and Guinle University
Hospital
Universidade Federal do Estado do Rio de
Janeiro(UNIRIO)
Tijuca, Rio de Janeiro, Brasil

Catalina Matiz, MD
Assistant Clinical Professor of Dermatology
and Pediatrics
Division of Pediatric and Adolescent
Dermatology
University of California, San Diego
and Rady Children's Hospital, San Diego
San Diego, CA, USA

Marcus Maurer, MD
Professor of Dermatology and Allergy
Director of Research
Dpt. of Dermatology and Allergy
Allergie-Centrum-Charité
Charité - Universitätsmedizin
Berlin, Germany

Kevin McKerrow, MB, ChB
Consultant Dermatologist
Skin Specialist Centre,
Auckland, New Zealand

Nekma Meah, MB ChB, MRCP (Derm)
Department of Dermatology
Royal Liverpool and Broadgreen University
Hospitals NHS Trust
Liverpool, UK

Giuseppe Micali, MD
Professor and Chairman
Dermatology Clinic
University of Catania
Catania, Italy

Robert G. Micheletti, MD
Assistant Professor
Dermatology and Medicine
University of Pennsylvania
Philadelphia, PA, USA

Leslie G. Millard, MD
Consultant Dermatologist
Hathersage, UK

James E. Miller, MBBS, BSc, PgDip
Dermatology Specialist Registrar
University Hospitals Leicester
Leicester, UK

Jillian W. Wong Millsop, MD, MS
University of California, Davis
Sacramento, CA, USA

Daniel Mimouni, MD
Associate Professor
Skin Cancer Unit - Director
Sackler School of Medicine, Tel Aviv
University
Tel Aviv, Israel;
Dermatology Department
Rabin Medical Center
Petah Tikva, Israel

Ginat W. Mirowski, DMD, MD, FAAD
Adjunct Associate Professor
Department of Oral Pathology, Medicine
Radiology
Indiana University School of Dentistry
Indianapolis, IN, USA

Sultan A. Mirza, MD
Mayo Clinic
Rochester, MN, USA

Sonja Molin, MD
Dermatologist
Department of Dermatology and Allergy
Ludwig Maximilian University
Munich, Germany

Adisbeth Morales-Burgos, MD
Assistant Professor
Department of Dermatology
University of Puerto Rico School of Medicine
San Juan, Puerto Rico

Warwick L. Morison, MBBS, MD, FRCP
Professor
Department of Dermatology
Johns Hopkins University School of Medicine
Baltimore, MD, USA

Cato Mørk, MD, PhD
Consultant Dermatologist
Akershus Dermatological Clinic
Lørenskog, Norway

Colin A. Morton, MBChB, FRCP(UK)
Consultant Dermatologist
Department of Dermatology, Stirling
Scotland, UK

Richard J. Motley, MA, MD, FRCP
Consultant in Dermatology and Cutaneous
Surgery
Welsh Institute of Dermatology
University Hospital of Wales
Cardiff, UK

Megan Mowbray, BSc (Hons), FRCP, MD
Consultant Dermatologist
Department of Dermatology
Queen Margaret Hospital
Dunfermline, UK

Eavan G. Muldoon, MBBCh, MD, MPH
Consultant in Infectious Diseases
Mater Misericordiae University Hospital
Eccles Street
Dublin, Ireland

Anna E. Muncaster, MBChB, FRCP
Consultant Dermatologist
Department of Dermatology
Rotherham General Hospital
Rotherham, UK

George J. Murakawa, MD, PhD
Clinical Professor
Department of Internal Medicine
Michigan State University
Somerset Skin Centre Troy,
MI, USA

Jenny E. Murase, MD
Associate Clinical Professor
University of California, San Francisco
San Francisco, CA, USA

Michele E. Murdoch, BSc, FRCP
Consultant Dermatologist
Department of Dermatology
Watford General Hospital
Watford, UK

Adam S. Nabatian, MD
Department of Dermatology
Mount Sinai School of Medicine
New York City, NY, USA

Mio Nakamura, MD
Psoriasis & Skin Treatment Center
Department of Dermatology
University of California San Francisco
San Francisco, CA, USA

Rajani Nalluri, MBBS, MRCPCH, DiPD
Dermatologist
Department of Dermatology
Northwestern Deanery
Manchester, UK

Zeena Y. Nawas, MD
University of Texas Health Science Center at
Houston
Center for Clinical Studies
Houston, TX, USA

Glen R. Needham, PhD
Associate Professor
Department of Entomology
Center for Life Sciences Education
The Ohio State University
Columbus, OH, USA

Glenn C. Newell, MD, FACP
Associate Professor of Medicine
Cooper Medical School at Rowan University
Camden, NJ, USA

Julia Newton-Bishop, MD, FRCP
Professor of Dermatology
University of Leeds
Leeds, UK

Adam V. Nguyen, MD
Department of Internal Medicine
(Preliminary)
McGovern Medical School at The University
of Texas Health Science Center at Houston
Houston, TX, USA

Rosemary L. Nixon, BSc (Hons), MPH, FACD,
FAFOEM
Adjunct Clinical Associate Professor
Monash University
Honorary Associate Professor
University of Melbourne;
Director
Occupational Dermatology Research and
Education Centre
Skin and Cancer Foundation
Carlton, Victoria, Australia

Jack C. O'Brien, BS
Department of Dermatology
University of Texas Southwestern Medical
Center
Dallas, TX, USA

Stephanie Ogden, PhD, MB ChB with honours
Consultant Dermatologist
Salford Royal NHS Foundation Trust
Manchester, UK

Suzanne M. Olbricht, MD
Associate Professor of Dermatology, Harvard
Medical School
Chief of Dermatology, Beth Israel Deaconess
Hospital
Boston, MA, USA

Sally Jane O'Shea, MB BCh BAO, BMedSc,
MRCPI, PhD
Consultant Dermatologist
South Infirmary-Victoria University Hospital
Cork, Ireland

Cindy E. Owen, MD
Assistant Professor
Division of Dermatology
University of Louisville
Louisville, KY, USA

Michael Pan, MD
Department of Dermatology, Mount Sinai
Health System
New York, NY, USA

Lisa Pappas-Taffer, MD
Assistant Professor of Clinical Dermatology
University of Pennsylvania
Philadelphia, PA, USA

Jennifer L. Parish, MD
Assistant Professor of Dermatology and
Cutaneous Biology
Sidney Kimmel Medical College at Thomas
Jefferson University
Philadelphia, PA, USA

Lawrence Charles Parish, MD, MD (Hon)
Clinical Professor of Dermatology and
Cutaneous Biology
Director of the Jefferson Center for
International Dermatology
Sidney Kimmel Medical College at Thomas
Jefferson University
Philadelphia, PA, USA

Michael Payette, MD, MBA, FAAD
Assistant Professor
Associate Program Director
Dermatology
University of Connecticut
Farmington, CT, USA

Gary L. Peck, MD
Dermatologist
Dermatologic Surgery Center of Washington
LLC
Chevy Chase, MD, USA

Sandra Pena, BA
Department of Dermatology
Wake Forest University School of Medicine
Winston Salem, USA

Jarad Peranteau, MD
Clinical Research Fellow - Dermatology
Center for Clinical Studies
Houston, TX, USA

Frederick A. Pereira, MD
Assistant Clinical Professor of Dermatology
Department of Dermatology
Mount Sinai School of Medicine
New York, NY, USA

William Perkins, MBBS, FRCP
Consultant Dermatologist
Oxford University Hospitals
Oxford, UK

Clifford S. Perlis, MD, MBe
Assistant Professor
Fox Chase Cancer Center
Philadelphia, PA, USA

Robert G. Phelps, MD
Professor of Dermatology
Department of Dermatology
Professor of Pathology
Department of Pathology
Mount Sinai School of Medicine
New York, NY, USA

Tania J. Phillips, MD, FRCPC
Professor of Dermatology
Boston University School of Medicine
Boston, MA, USA

Maureen B. Poh-Fitzpatrick, MD
Professor Emerita and Special Lecturer
(Dermatology)
Columbia University College of Physicians
and Surgeons
New York, NY, USA

Miriam Keltz Pomeranz, MD
Associate Professor
The Ronald O. Perelman Department of
Dermatology
New York University School of Medicine
New York, NY, USA

Samantha R. Pop
Cooper Medical School of Rowan University
Camden, NJ, USA

Pierluigi Porcu, MD
Associate Professor of Internal Medicine
Division of Hematology
The Ohio State University Comprehensive
Cancer Center
Arthur G. James Cancer Hospital and
Richard J. Solove Research Institute
Columbus, OH, USA

James B. Powell, BSc, MRCP (UK)
Dermatology Department
Hereford County Hospital
Wye Valley NHS Trust
Herefordshire, UK

Lori D. Prok, MD
Assistant Professor
Department of Dermatology
University of Colorado Denver
Aurora, CO, USA

Tia M. Pyle, MD
Division of Dermatology
Cooper University Hospital
Cooper Medical School of Rowan University
Camden, NJ, USA

Surod Qazaz
Department of Dermatology
University Hospital
Coventry, UK

Vikram Rajkomar, MBChB, MRCP (UK)
(Dermatology)
Consultant Dermatologist
Salford Royal NHS Foundation Trust
Manchester, UK

Rabia S. Rashid, MRCP
University Hospitals Coventry and
Warwickshire
Coventry, UK

Mehdi Rashighi, MD
Resident-Physician
University of Massachusetts Medical School
Worcester, MA, USA
Research Member
Center for Research & Training in Skin
Diseases and Leprosy
Tehran University of Medical Sciences
Tehran, Iran

Ravi Ratnavel, DM, FRCP
Consultant Dermatologist
Buckinghamshire Hospitals Trust
Buckinghamshire, UK

Christie G. Regula, MD
Dermatologist
Department of Dermatology
Penn State Milton S. Hershey Medical
Center
Hershey, PA, USA

Michael Renzi Jr., BS
Rowan University
Glassboro, NJ, USA

Jean Revuz, MD
Private Practice
Paris, France

Rachel V. Reynolds, MD
Assistant Professor of Dermatology
Program Director
Harvard Combined Dermatology Residency
Training Program
Beth Israel Deaconess Medical Center
Department of Dermatology
Boston, MA, USA

Elisabeth Richard, MD
Assistant Professor of Dermatology
Johns Hopkins University School of
Medicine
Baltimore, MD, USA

Gabriele Richard, MD, FACMG
Chief Medical Officer
GeneDx, Inc.
Gaithersburg, MD, USA

Darrell S. Rigel, MD
Clinical Professor of Dermatology
New York University Medical Center
New York, NY, USA

Wanda Sonia Robles, MBBS, MD, PhD
Consultant Dermatologist
Department of Dermatology
Barnet and Chase Farm Hospitals NHS Trust
Middlesex, UK

Megan Rogge, MD
Assistant Professor
Department of Dermatology
The University of Texas Health Science
Center at Houston
Houston, TX, USA

Alain H. Rook, MD
Professor of Dermatology and Director,
Cutaneous Lymphoma Program
Perelman School of Medicine, University of
Pennsylvania
Philadelphia, PA, USA

Jamie R. Manning, MD
Department of Dermatology
Albert Einstein College of Medicine
Bronx, NY, USA

Ted Rosen, MD
Professor of Dermatology
Department of Dermatology
Baylor College of Medicine
Houston, TX, USA

Misha Rosenbach, MD
Associate Professor, Dermatology & Internal
Medicine
University of Pennsylvania,
Perelman School of Medicine
Philadelphia, PA, USA

David Rosenfeld, MA, BS
University of Missouri
Columbia, MO, USA

Christopher Rowland Payne, MB, BS, MRCP
Consultant Dermatologist
The London Clinic
London, UK

Adam I. Rubin, MD
Assistant Professor of Dermatology
Pediatrics, and Pathology and Laboratory
Medicine
Hospital of the University of Pennsylvania
The Children's Hospital of Philadelphia
Perelman School of Medicine at the
University of Pennsylvania
Philadelphia, PA, USA

Courtney Rubin, MD, MBE
University of Pennsylvania
Philadelphia, PA, USA

Malcolm H. A. Rustin, BSc, MD, FRCP
Professor of Dermatology
Dermatology Department
The Royal Free NHS Foundation Trust
London, UK

Thomas Ruzicka, MD
Professor of Dermatology and Allergy
Department of Dermatology and Allergy
Ludwig Maximilian University
Munich, Germany

Sara Samimi, MD
Physician
Department of Dermatology
University of Pennsylvania
Philadelphia, PA, USA

Lawrence A. Schachner, MD
Professor, Chair Emeritus and Stiefel
Laboratories Chair
Director of the Division of Pediatric
Dermatology
Department of Dermatology & Cutaneous
Surgery
University of Miami Miller School of
Medicine
Miami, FL, USA

Noah Scheinfeld, MD, JD
Clinical Professor of Dermatology
Weill Cornell Medical College
New York, NY, USA

Bethanee J. Schlosser, MD, PhD
Associate Professor
Departments of Dermatology Northwestern
University
Chicago, IL, USA

Rhonda E. Schnur, MD, FACMG
Professor of Pediatrics, Division of Genetics
Cooper Medical School of Rowan University
Camden, NJ, USA;
Senior Clinical Scientist, GeneDx
Gaithersburg, MD, USA

**Robert A. Schwartz, MD, MPH, DSc (Hon),
FAAD, FRCP (Edin), FACP**
Professor & Head, Dermatology
Professor of Medicine
Professor of Pediatrics
Professor of Pathology
Visiting Professor
Rutgers School of Public Affairs and
Administration
Newark, NJ, USA

Matthew J. Scorer, BMBS
University Hospitals of Leicester
Leicester, UK

Bryan A. Selkin, MD
Dermatologist
Center for Dermatology and Cosmetic Laser
Surgery
Plano, TX, USA

Jamie Seymour, BSc (Hon), PhD
Associate Professor
School of Public Health and Tropical
Medicine
Faculty of Medicine, Health & Molecular
Sciences
James Cook University
Cairns, Queensland, Australia

Christine M. Shaver, MD
Drexel University College of Medicine
Philadelphia, PA, USA

Christopher R. Shea, MD
Eugene J. Van Scott Professor in
Dermatology
University of Chicago Medicine
Chicago, IL, USA

Neil H. Shear, MD, FRCPC
Professor of Medicine, Dermatology and
Clinical Pharmacology & Toxicology
University of Toronto, ON, Canada

Tang Ngee Shim, MB, BCh, MRCP (UK)
Dermatologist
Department of Dermatology
University Hospital
Coventry, UK

Hiroshi Shimizu, MD, PhD
Professor and Chairman
Department of Dermatology
Hokkaido University Graduate School of
Medicine
Sapporo, Japan

Julia Siegel, BA
University of Massachusetts Medical School
Worcester, MA, USA

Elisha Singer, MD
Dermatologist
Departments of Internal Medicine and
Dermatology
Northwestern University
Chicago, IL, USA

Maral Kibarian Skelsey, MD
Director of Dermatologic Surgery
Clinical Associate Professor
Department of Dermatology
Georgetown University Medical Center
Washington, DC, USA
Director, The Dermatologic Surgery Center
of Washington
Chevy Chase, MD, USA

Chris Sladden, MBBCh, FRCPC
Clinical Assistant Professor
Memorial University
St. John's Newfoundland, Canada

Michael Sladden, MAE, MRCP, FACD
Associate Professor of Dermatology
Department of Medicine
University of Tasmania
Launceston, Tasmania, Australia

Janellen Smith, MD
Professor
Department of Dermatology
University of California Irvine
Irvine, CA, USA

Joanne E. Smucker, MD
Department of Dermatology
Penn State/Hershey Medical Center
Hershey, PA, USA

Najwa Somani, MD, FRCPC
Department of Dermatology
Indiana University School of Medicine
Indianapolis, IN, USA

Lacy L. Sommer, MD
Assistant Professor of Medicine, Division of
Dermatology
Cooper Medical School of Rowan University
Camden, NJ, USA

Mary Sommerlad, BSc, MBBS, MRCP
Consultant Dermatologist
Homerton University Hospital
London, UK

Christine Soon, BM, MRCP
Consultant Dermatologist
Department of Dermatology
Northampton General Hospital
Northampton, UK

Jennifer A. Sopkovich, MD
Assistant Professor
Division of Dermatology
The Ohio State University Wexner Medical
Center
Columbus, OH, USA

Nicholas A. Soter, MD
Professor of Dermatology
Ronald O. Perelman Department of
Dermatology
New York University School of Medicine
New York, NY, USA

James M. Spencer, MD, MS
Professor of Clinical Dermatology
Department of Dermatology
Mount Sinai School of Medicine
New York, NY, USA

Richard C. D. Staughton, MA, MBBChir, FRCP
Consultant Dermatologist
Daniel Turner Clinic
Department of Dermatology
Chelsea and Westminster Hospital
London, UK

Jane C. Sterling, MBBChir, MA, FRCP, PhD
Consultant Dermatologist
Department of Dermatology
Addenbrooke's Hospital
Cambridge, UK

Cord Sunderkötter, MD
Chairman of the Department of
Dermatology
University Hospital of Münster
Münster, Germany

**Saleem M. Taibjee, MBBCh, BMedSci,
MRCPCH, DipRCPath**
Consultant Dermatologist
Dorset County Hospital
Dorchester, UK

Deborah Tamura, MS, RN, APNG
Research Nurse
DNA Repair Section
Laboratory of Cancer Biology and Genetics
Center for Cancer Research
National Cancer Institute
National Institutes of Health
Bethesda, MD, USA

Eunice Tan, MB, FRCP
Consultant Dermatologist
Norfolk and Norwich University Hospital
NHS Foundation Trust
Norwich, UK

**William Y-M. Tang, MBBS (HK), FRCP (Edin &
Glasg), Dip Derm (London), FHKAM (Medicine)**
Honorary Consultant Dermatologist
Department of Medicine & Geriatrics
Tuen Mun Hospital, Tuen Mun
Hong Kong, China

Lynsey Taylor, MB ChB, BSc (Hons), MRCP
Consultant Dermatologist
Department of Dermatology
Royal Infirmary of Edinburgh
Edinburgh, UK

Bruce H. Thiers, MD
Professor and Chairman Emeritus
Department of Dermatology and
Dermatologic Surgery
Medical University of South Carolina
Charleston, SC, USA

Lucy J. Thomas, MPharm, MBChB, MRCP (Derm)
Daniel Turner Dermatology Unit
Chelsea & Westminster Hospital
London, UK

Cody R. Thornton, MPH, MBA
Lieutenant Commander
U.S. Public Health Service
Acting Chief, International Response Policy
Branch
Office of the Assistant Secretary for
Preparedness and Response
U.S. Department of Health and Human
Services
Washington, DC, USA

Anne-Marie Tobin, MB, BSc, MRCPI
Consultant Dermatologist
Tallaght Hospital
Dublin, Ireland

Rochelle R. Torgerson, MD, PhD
Assistant Professor
Department of Dermatology
Mayo Clinic College of Medicine
Rochester, MN, USA

Antonella Tosti, MD
Fredric Brandt Endowed Professor
Department of Dermatology
Cutaneous Surgery, University of Miami
Miami, FL, USA

Fragkiski Tsatsou, MD, MSc, BSc
Dermatologist
Departments of Dermatology, Venereology,
Allergology and Immunology
Dessau Medical Center, Brandenburg
Medical School Theodore Fontane
Dessau, Germany

Yukiko Tsuji-Abe, MD, PhD
Dermatologist
Niigata City, Japan

William F. G. Tucker, MB, FRCP
Consultant Dermatologist
Private Practice
Worcester, UK

Stephen K. Tyring, MD, PhD, MBA
Clinical Professor
Department of Dermatology
University of Texas Medical School at
Houston
Houston, TX, USA

Jeremy Udkoff, MA, MAS
University of California, San Diego and
Rady Children's Hospital
San Diego, CA, USA

Robin H. Unger, MD
Assistant Professor
Department of Dermatology
Mt. Sinai Hospital
New York, NY, USA

Walter P. Unger, MD
Clinical Professor
Department of Dermatology
Mount Sinai School of Medicine
New York, NY, USA

Sarah Utz, MD
Icahn School of Medicine at Mount Sinai
New York, NY, USA

Martha C. Valbuena, MD
Consultant Dermatologist
Hospital Universitario Centro
Dermatológico Federico Lleras Acosta
Bogotá, Colombia

Peter van de Kerkhof, MD, PhD
Professor and Chairman
Department of Dermatology
Radboud University Nijmegen Medical Centre
Nijmegen, Netherlands

Abby S. Van Voorhees, MD
Chair, Program Director and Professor
Eastern Virginia Medical School Department
of Dermatology
Norfolk, VA, USA

Ramya Vangipuram, MD
Center for Clinical Studies
Houston, TX, USA

David Veitch, MBChB, BSc, MRCP
(Dermatology)
Leicester Royal Infirmary
Leicester, UK

Vanessa Venning, DM, FRCP
Consultant Dermatologist
Department of Dermatology
Churchill Hospital
Oxford, UK

Sarah G. Versteeg, MSc
Medical Research Associate
Mediprobe Research, Inc.
London, ON, Canada

Martha Viera, MD
Dermatologist
Department of Dermatology and Cutaneous
Surgery
University of Miami Miller School of
Medicine
Volunteer Faculty
Department of Dermatology
University of Miami
Miami, FL, USA

Carmela C. Vittorio, MD
Associate Professor
Department of Dermatology
Perelman School of Medicine
University of Pennsylvania
Philadelphia, PA, USA

Ruth Ann Vleugels, MD, MPH
Director, Autoimmune Skin Disease
Program
Brigham and Women's Hospital
Department of Dermatology
Associate Professor
Harvard Medical School Boston
Boston, MA, USA

Gorav N. Wali, MA (Hons), BMBCh, MRCP
Oxford University Hospitals
Oxford, UK

Joanna Wallengren, MD, PhD
Associate Professor
Department of Dermatology
Skane University Hospital
Lund, Sweden

Joy Wan, MD
Instructor
University of Pennsylvania
Philadelphia, PA, USA

Karolyn A. Wanat, MD
Assistant Professor of Dermatology and
Pathology
University of Iowa Hospitals and Clinics
Iowa City, IA, USA

Gabriele Weichert, MD, PhD
Medical Director
Skin Care West Medical and Surgical
Dermatology
Nanaimo, BC, Canada

Anja K. Weidmann, MBChB, MMedSci
Consultant Dermatologist
The Dermatology Centre
Stepping Hill Hospital
Stockport, UK

Jeffrey M. Weinberg, MD
Department of Dermatology
Mount Sinai St. Luke's
Mount Sinai Beth Israel
Associate Clinical Professor of Dermatology
Mount Sinai School of Medicine
New York, NY, USA

Victoria P. Werth, MD
Chief
Philadelphia Veterans Administration
Medical Center;
Professor
Department of Dermatology
University of Pennsylvania
Philadelphia, PA, USA

Lucile E. White, MD
Staff Dermatologist
The Methodist Hospital
Houston, TX, USA

Adam H. Wiener, DO
Dermatologist
Melbourne Dermatology Center
Melbourne, FL, USA

Jonathan K. Wilkin, MD
Dermatologist
Consultant, Wilkin Consulting LLC
Warner Robins, GA, USA

Nathaniel K. Wilkin, MD
Staff Dermatologist
Kaiser-Permanente Medical Center
Fresno, CA, USA

Jason Williams, BSc (Hons), MBChB (Hons),
MRCP
Consultant Dermatologist
Director
Contact Dermatitis Investigation Unit
Salford Royal Foundation Trust
Manchester, UK

Niall Wilson, BSc, MBChB, FRCP, FRCPI
Consultant Dermatologist
Royal Liverpool and Broadgreen University Hospital NHS Trust
Liverpool, UK

Karen Wiss, MD
Professor of Dermatology and Pediatrics
University of Massachusetts Medical School
Worcester, MA, USA

Joseph A. Witkowski†, MD, FACP
Emeritus Clinical Professor of Dermatology
University of Pennsylvania
Perelman School of Medicine
Philadelphia, PA, USA

Lauren E. Wiznia, MD
The Ronald O. Perelman Department of Dermatology
New York University School of Medicine
New York, NY, USA

Henry K. Wong, MD, PhD
Professor and Chairman
Department of Dermatology
University of Arkansas
College of Medicine
Little Rock, AR, USA

Junie Li Chun Wong, MBChB, MSc, MRCP
Dermatology Department
Royal Liverpool and Broadgreen
University Hospitals NHS Trust
Liverpool, UK

Andrew L. Wright, MB, FRCP
Hon Professor
University of Bradford
St. Luke's Hospital
Bradford, UK

Cooper C. Wriston, MD
Physician
Department of Dermatology
Mayo Clinic College of Medicine
Rochester, MN, USA

Benedict C. Wu, DO/PhD
Cell Biology
School of Osteopathic Medicine
Rowan University
Stratford, NJ, USA

Adam Wulkan, MD
Dermatologist
Department of Dermatology and Cutaneous Surgery
University of Miami Miller School of Medicine
Miami, FL, USA

Andrea L. Zaenglein, MD
Professor of Dermatology and Pediatrics
Penn State College of Medicine
Penn State/Hershey Medical Center
Hershey, PA, USA

Irshad Zaki, BMedSci (Hons), BMBS, FRCP
Consultant Dermatologist and Cutaneous Surgeon
Heart of England Foundation Trust
Solihull, UK

Joshua A. Zeichner, MD
Assistant Professor
Department of Dermatology
Mount Sinai School of Medicine
New York, NY, USA

Tian Hao Zhu, BA
Clinical Research Investigator
Psoriasis and Skin Treatment Center
Department of Dermatology
University of California
San Francisco
University of Southern California Keck School of Medicine
Los Angeles, CA, USA

John J. Zone, MD
Professor and Chairman
Department of Dermatology
University of Utah School of Medicine
Salt Lake City, UT, USA

Christos C. Zouboulis, MD, PhD
Departments of Dermatology, Venereology, Allergology and Immunology
Dessau Medical Center, Brandenburg Medical School Theodore Fontane
Dessau, Germany

Torstein Zuberbeir, MD
Department of Dermatology and Allergy
Allergy-centre-Charité
Charité-Universitätsmedizin Berlin
Charitéplatz, Berlin, Germany

†deceased

Acknowledgments

The editors want to acknowledge the constant, outstanding support they have received from Elsevier staff, particularly Trinity Hutton, Humayra Rahman Khan, Russell Gabbedy, Charlotta Kryhl, Joshua Mearns, and Srividhya Vidhyashankar. Many of the chapters were based on chapters written by authors of previous editions who created the excellent foundation on which our new chapters have been built. We must also thank our colleagues and residents who provided many of the clinical photos used in this edition and we offer a special thank you to Joe Bikowski, MD who gave us access to his spectular collection of clinical photographs.

Dedication

We thank our spouses Madeleine Lebwohl, Rhonda Schnur, Rebecca Berth-Jones and Susan Christopher-Coulson for their unwavering support of this endeavor.

Evidence Levels

Each therapy covered has been assigned a letter from A (most evidence) to E (least evidence), signifying the amount of published evidence available to support its use. The following criteria were used in making this classification.

A: DOUBLE-BLIND STUDY

At least one prospective randomized, double-blind, controlled trial without major design flaws (in the author's view).

B: CLINICAL TRIAL ≥20 SUBJECTS

Prospective clinical trials with 20 or more subjects; trials lacking adequate controls or another key facet of design that would normally be considered desirable (in the author's opinion).

C: CLINICAL TRIAL <20 SUBJECTS

Small trials with fewer than 20 subjects with significant design limitations, very large numbers of case reports (at least 20 cases in the literature), or retrospective analyses of data.

D: SERIES ≥5 SUBJECTS

Series of patients reported to respond (at least five cases in the literature).

E: ANECDOTAL CASE REPORTS

Individual case reports amounting to published experience of fewer than five cases.

Credits

PHOTOS

Chapter 2: Courtesy of Neil Fernandes, MD.

Chapter 14: With permission from Mayo Foundation for Medical Education and Research. All rights reserved.

Chapter 19: Courtesy of Dr Angana Mitra.

Chapter 29: With permission from Lebwohl MG. Atlas of the Skin and Systemic Disease. Churchill Livingstone: Elsevier, 1995. Courtesy of Fabio Barbosa, MD.

Chapter 30: Courtesy of Joseph Bikowski, MD.

Chapter 51: Courtesy of Tamara Lazic, MD.

Chapter 53: Courtesy of Dr Terence Casey.

Chapter 81: Courtesy of Fitzsimons Army Medical Center

Chapter 95: Courtesy of University Hospitals of Leicester NHS Trust, Department of Medical Illustration.

Chapter 118: Courtesy of Joseph Bikowski, MD.

Chapter 127: Courtesy of Joseph Bikowski, MD.

Chapter 128: Courtesy of Joseph Bikowski, MD.

Chapter 142: Courtesy of Yale Dermatology Residents Slide Collection.

Chapter 168: Reprinted from Cowper SE, Robin HS, Steinberg SM, Su LD, Leboit PE. Scleromyxedema-like cutaneous disease in renal dialysis patients. Lancet, 356(9234) 1000 to 1, 2000, with permission from Elsevier.

Chapter 214: Courtesy of Mark Lebwohl, MD.

Chapter 242: With permission from Tinea pedis. Busam Klaus J, ed. Dermatopathology: A Volume in the Series: Foundations in Diagnostic Pathology, 2nd edn. Philadelphia, PA: Elsevier, 2010.

TABLES

Chapter 31: Table 31.1, Adapted from Veale D, Ellison N, Werner TG, Dodhia R, Serfaty MA, Clarke A. Development of a cosmetic procedure screening questionnaire (COPSs) for body dysmorphic disorder. J Plast Reconstr Aesthet Surg 2012; 65: 530–2.

Chapter 259: Table 259.1, After Gupta AK. Cutis 1986; 37: 371–4 and Lotfolollhai L, et al. Tanaffos 2015; 14: 57–1.

BOXES

Chapter 195: Adapted from Setji TL, Brown AJ. Polycystic ovary syndrome: update on diagnosis and treatment. Am J Med 2014; 127: 912–9.

Chapter 207: Box 207.2, Modified from Schlosser BJ. Contact dermatitis of the vulva. Dermatol Clin 2010; 28: 697–706.

Chapter 207: Box 207.3, Modified from Schlosser BJ. Contact dermatitis of the vulva. Dermatol Clin 2010; 28, 697–706.

Chapter 259: Box 259.1, Modified from Decker A, et al. Skin Appendage Disord 2015; 1: 28–30.

1

Acanthosis nigricans

Lawrence S. Feigenbaum, Ponciano D. Cruz Jr.

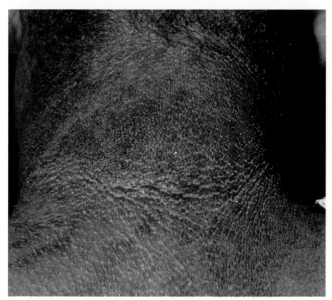

Acanthosis nigricans is characterized by hyperpigmented, verrucous or velvety plaques that usually appear on flexural surfaces and in intertriginous regions. It is most commonly seen in individuals with insulin resistance states, especially obesity, and less frequently in association with other metabolic disorders, genetic syndromes, drugs, and malignancy. Although hyperinsulinemia, hyperandrogenemia, circulating antiinsulin receptor antibodies, and activating mutations in fibroblast growth factor receptor (as found in both familial variants and syndromes associated with skeletal dysplasia such as Crouzon syndrome) have been implicated as causal factors, the precise pathogenesis is not yet known.

MANAGEMENT STRATEGY

The management of patients with acanthosis nigricans addresses the underlying cause, the identification of which requires a salient history, a targeted physical examination, focused diagnostic laboratory tests, and, occasionally, radiologic evaluation.

Relevant historical information includes age at onset, presence or absence of a family history, medications, transplant history, and presence or absence of symptoms related to hyperinsulinemia (with or without diabetes mellitus), hyperandrogenemia (with or without virilism), hypercortisolism, and internal malignancy (with or without weight loss).

Drugs reported in association with acanthosis nigricans include niacin, corticosteroids, estrogens, testosterone, insulin, aripiprazole, fusidic acid, protease inhibitors, triazinate, diethylstilbestrol, palifermin, and recombinant growth hormone. Acanthosis nigricans has also been associated with renal and lung transplantation.

Physical examination should document obesity, masculinization, lymphadenopathy, cushingoid features, and organomegaly. Initial laboratory screening should include fasting blood glucose and serum insulin tested concurrently to confirm or exclude insulin resistance (insulin value inappropriately high for the glucose level).

Because obesity is the most common cause of both insulin resistance and acanthosis nigricans, it is the likely cause of acanthosis nigricans in overweight patients with no historical suggestion of culprit drugs or evidence of malignancy.

Rare causes of insulin resistance and acanthosis nigricans include the type A and B syndromes, the former characterized by defective insulin receptors and manifesting typically in young girls with masculinized features, and the latter reported mostly in women with circulating antiinsulin receptor antibodies in association with autoimmune disorders such as lupus erythematosus. Other causes of insulin resistance and acanthosis nigricans are polycystic ovarian disease, HAIR-AN syndrome (hyperandrogenism, insulin resistance, and acanthosis nigricans), familial lipodystrophies, and various endocrinopathies.

The most commonly associated malignancy is gastric adenocarcinoma. Less frequent associations are endocrine, genitourinary, lung, and gastrointestinal carcinomas, and, even more rarely, melanoma and cutaneous T-cell lymphomas/Sézary syndrome. Malignant acanthosis nigricans may coexist with other cutaneous markers of internal malignancy, such as tripe palms, the sign of Leser–Trélat, florid cutaneous papillomatosis, and hyperkeratosis of the palms and soles (tylosis). If malignancy-associated acanthosis nigricans is suspected, the initial laboratory screen may include a complete blood count, stool test for occult blood, and chest and gastrointestinal radiographs, as well as gastrointestinal endoscopy. Pelvic and rectal examinations, pelvic ultrasonography, and other screening may be warranted.

In the absence of objective evidence for a specific cause, the acanthosis nigricans may be labeled as idiopathic, which may or may not be familial. Treatment of the underlying cause, if identified, often leads to resolution of the acanthosis nigricans. Otherwise, most published treatment modalities are symptomatic and/or cosmetic, and testimony to their efficacy has been anecdotal.

Specific Investigations

- Document obesity based on ideal body weight, height/weight, body mass index (BMI).
- Determine fasting blood glucose and insulin levels in parallel. Also consider ordering HbA_{1c}, alanine aminotransferase (ALT), and fasting lipoprotein profile in obese patients.
- Depending on historical clues, screen for other endocrine diseases.
- Consider malignancy; if suspected refer to appropriate specialist for the best diagnostic procedure.
- Consider drugs as a cause.
- Consider transplantation as a cause.
- Consider familial/genetic disorders as a cause.

Acanthosis nigricans: a practical approach to evaluation and management. Higgins S, Freemark M, Prose N. Dermatol Online J 2008; 14(9): 2.

A review of the pathogenesis, clinical features, and management of acanthosis nigricans.

An approach to acanthosis nigricans. Phiske M. Indian Dermatol Online J 2014; 5: 239.

A review of the prevalence, pathogenesis, types, and classifications of acanthosis nigricans. It also discusses the differential diagnosis, pertinent laboratory/radiologic investigations, and treatment options.

Prevalence and significance of acanthosis nigricans in an adult population. Hud J, Cohen J, Wagner J, Cruz P. Arch Dermatol 1992; 128: 941–4.

Up to 74% of obese adult patients seen at the Parkland Memorial Hospital Adult Obesity Clinic in Dallas, Texas, had acanthosis nigricans. The skin disorder predicted the existence of hyperinsulinemia.

Juvenile acanthosis nigricans. Sinha S, Schwartz RA. J Am Acad Dermatol 2007; 57: 502–8.

A review of the evaluation of children presenting with acanthosis nigricans.

Genes, growth factors and acanthosis nigricans. Torleyu D, Bellus G, Munro C. Br J Dermatol 2002; 147: 1096–101.

Craniosynostosis and skeletal dysplasia syndromes with acanthosis nigricans are associated with activating mutations in fibroblast growth factor receptors (FGR), particularly FGFR3.

Characterization of groups of hyperandrogenic women with acanthosis nigricans, impaired glucose tolerance and/or hyperinsulinemia. Dunaif A, Graf M, Mandeli J, Laumas V, Dobrjansky A. J Clin Endocrinol Metab 1987; 65: 499–507.

Among obese women with polycystic ovaries, 50% had acanthosis nigricans.

Malignant acanthosis nigricans: a review. Rigel D, Jacobe M. J Dermatol Surg Oncol 1980; 6: 923–7.

Gastric carcinoma was reported in 55% of 227 cases of acanthosis nigricans associated with an internal malignancy. Other intraabdominal malignancies accounted for 18% of cases, and the remaining 27% had extraabdominal sites of malignancy.

First-Line Therapy	
• Treat the underlying cause	D

Acanthosis nigricans: a cutaneous marker of tissue resistant to insulin. Rendon M, Cruz P, Sontheimer R, Bergstresser P. J Am Acad Dermatol 1989; 21: 461–9.

In a woman with systemic lupus erythematosus and the type B syndrome of insulin resistance, the acanthosis nigricans cleared after treatment with oral corticosteroids and subcutaneous injection of insulin. Her circulating antiinsulin antibodies also disappeared with treatment of the autoimmune disease.

Clearance of acanthosis nigricans associated with the HAIR-AN syndrome after partial pancreatectomy: an 11-year follow up. Pfeifer SL, Wilson RM, Gawkrodger DJ. Postgrad Med J 1999; 75: 421–2.

An obese woman with HAIR-AN syndrome was diagnosed a year later with insulinoma. One year after resection of the tumor the patient's virilism resolved, and 9 years after the surgery the acanthosis nigricans was much improved.

Acanthosis nigricans in association with congenital adrenal hyperplasia: resolution after treatment. Kurtoglu S, Atabek ME, Keskin M, Canöz O. Turk J Pediatr 2005; 47: 183–7.

A 3-day-old girl with the salt-wasting type of 21-hydroxylase–deficient congenital adrenal hyperplasia presented with acanthosis nigricans of both axillae. After corticosteroid and mineralocorticoid therapy for disease, the acanthosis nigricans resolved.

Second-Line Therapies	
• Topical trichloroacetic acid	C
• Topical adapalene	C
• Topical tretinoin +/– ammonium lactate	C
• Oral metformin	D
• Topical tazarotene	E
• Topical calcipotriol	E
• Topical glycolic acid	E

Using trichloroacetic acid in the treatment of acanthosis nigricans: a pilot study. Zayed A, Sobhi R, Abdel Halim D. J Dermatolog Treat 2012; 25: 223–5.

Topical 15% trichloroacetic acid as a superficial chemical peel weekly for 4 weeks led to less thickening and hyperpigmentation and improved overall appearance in six women studied.

The efficacy of topical 0.1% adapalene gel for use in the treatment of childhood acanthosis nigricans: a pilot study. Treesirichod A, Chaithirayanon S, Wongjitrat N, Wattanapan P. Indian J Dermatol 2015; 60: 103.

Topical 0.1% adapalene gel applied daily for 4 weeks led to less skin darkening in 16 patients with childhood acanthosis nigricans.

Topical therapy with tretinoin and ammonium lactate for acanthosis nigricans associated with obesity. Blobstein SH. Cutis 2003; 71: 33–4.

Five obese patients with acanthosis nigricans were successfully treated with 12% ammonium lactate cream twice daily and tretinoin 0.05% cream nightly to one side of the neck (the other side serving as control).

There was no mention of whether the obese patients lost weight during the treatment period, which could have contributed to the improvement.

Therapeutic approach in insulin resistance with acanthosis nigricans. Tankova T, Koev D, Dakovska L, Kirilov G. Int J Clin Pract 2002; 56: 578–81.

Five obese patients (two children and three adults with diabetes mellitus) were treated with metformin daily for 6 months, resulting in significant reduction in plasma insulin, body weight, and body fat mass. Both children and one adult showed improvement of acanthosis nigricans.

Acanthosis nigricans associated with primary hypogonadism: successful treatment with topical calcipotriol. Gregoriou S, Anyfandakis V, Kontoleon P, Christofidou E, Rigopoulos D, Kontochristopoulos G. J Dermatol Treat 2008; 19: 373–5.

Topical calcipotriol ointment 50 mcg/g applied twice daily for 8 weeks completely cleared a man's acanthosis nigricans without relapse after 6 months of observation.

Effective treatment by glycolic acid peeling for cutaneous manifestation of familial generalized acanthosis nigricans caused by FGFR3 mutation. Ichiyama S, Funasaka Y, Otsuka Y, Takayama R, Kawana S, Saeki H, et al. J Eur Acad Dermatol Venereol 2016; 30: 442–5.

Glycolic acid 35% to 70% peel performed on two patients every 2 weeks led to less hyperpigmentation and keratinization.

Evidence Levels: **A** Double-blind study **B** Clinical trial ≥ 20 subjects **C** Clinical trial < 20 subjects **D** Series ≥ 5 subjects **E** Anecdotal case reports

Continued peels every 2 to 5 months maintained improvement after 3 years.

Third-Line Therapies

• Oral isotretinoin	E
• Dietary fish oil	E
• Oral contraceptives	E
• Long-pulsed alexandrite laser	E
• Continuous wave carbon dioxide laser	E

Treatment of acanthosis nigricans with oral isotretinoin. Katz R. Arch Dermatol 1980; 116: 110–11.

An obese, hirsute, diabetic woman with acanthosis nigricans was treated with oral isotretinoin (2–3 mg/kg/day for 4 months), producing clearance of the skin problem, but long-term treatment was required to maintain clearance because the acanthosis nigricans recurred when the retinoid was discontinued. Side effects of isotretinoin may render long-term use impractical.

Acanthosis nigricans. Schwartz RA. J Am Acad Dermatol 1994; 31: 1.

A woman with lipodystrophic diabetes mellitus and acanthosis nigricans was treated with dietary fish oil supplementation, leading to improvement despite continued elevation of triglyceride levels.

Remission of acanthosis nigricans associated with polycystic ovarian disease and stromal luteoma. Andersen RN, Coleman SA, Fish SA. J Clin Endocrinol Metab 1974; 38: 347–55.

A girl with acanthosis nigricans and polycystic ovaries cleared completely after treatment with Ortho-Novum 2 mg/day.

Treatment of acanthosis nigricans of the axillae using a long-pulsed (5-msec) alexandrite laser. Rosenback A, Ram R. Dermatol Surg 2004; 30: 1158–60.

A woman with axillary acanthosis nigricans was treated with long-pulsed alexandrite laser (5 ms) on one axilla, with the other as an untreated control. The treated axilla showed significant improvement.

Acne keloidalis nuchae

William Perkins

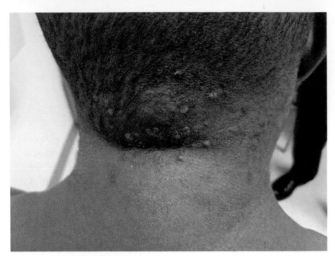

Courtesy of Neil Fernandes, MD.

Acne keloidalis nuchae (AKN) is an idiopathic chronic inflammatory process affecting the nape of the neck and the occipital scalp; it occurs predominantly in Afro-Caribbean males. Initial features consist of papules and pustules on the occiput and posterior neck, which subsequently coalesce into plaques of dense scar tissue with central scarring alopecia. Although the etiology is unknown, the histology of early cases shows evidence of acute and chronic folliculitis, with ruptured follicles, perifolliculitis, and a foreign body granulomatous response. Later cases may show similar features, but additionally there may be hypertrophic scar formation. Close shaving of the hair has been postulated as a cause for AKN, but even during the 1960s and 1970s, with the fashion for longer hair, AKN was still seen. Physical trauma due to collars rubbing and picking by patients has been suggested as a precipitant, but this has not been investigated in any systematic way. Whether folliculitis leading to ruptured follicles and the subsequent foreign body reaction or the development of ingrowing hairs is the primary event, the term *acne keloidalis* is a misnomer. Keloids at other sites or a family history of keloids are not features of AKN, and excision of the area does not result in keloid formation. Pseudofolliculitis barbae was associated with AKN in five of six cases in one series, but clinical or histologic evidence of superficial hair penetration is lacking. Lesions resembling AKN have been reported in those receiving long-term ciclosporin, and sarcoid papules may occasionally mimic the condition.

MANAGEMENT STRATEGY

A clear diagnosis is a prerequisite for the management of AKN. The presence of inflammatory papules, pustules, and hypertrophic scar formation on the occipital scalp and posterior neck in a black male is pathognomonic, but cases have been described in Caucasians and occasionally in females. Biopsy of the area is not usually required, but concerns about keloidal scarring should not inhibit obtaining histologic confirmation. Folliculitis secondary to bacterial infections, particularly staphylococcal, needs to be excluded. In staphylococcal folliculitis the pustules and papules tend to be more widely distributed across the scalp, especially over the crown. Culture will yield heavy growths of staphylococci, and the condition usually responds well to treatment with oral antibiotics, but may recur and require long-term treatment.

In view of the suggested associations with close-cropped hair and picking, it may be worthwhile inquiring about these factors. If present, these practices should be avoided.

Treatment depends on the stage of presentation. Unfortunately, the evidence base for many of the management recommendations is weak. Many patients will prefer no treatment or conservative treatment in the early stages of the disease. This is demonstrated by the fact that only 30% of patients identified in one survey had tried any treatment at all. Early disease with papules and pustules scattered across the posterior neck and occipital scalp may well be best managed by *topical antiseptics, antibiotics,* or *potent topical corticosteroids.*

With the development of hypertrophic scar formation, *topical or intralesional corticosteroids* may well be of benefit. Once scarring, alopecia, hypertrophic scars, and symptoms related to itch, pain, and discharging sinuses are present, treatment directed at the removal of the follicles from the affected area in their entirety is recommended.

Excisional surgery is the only treatment reported in any significant case series. The factors influencing the use of excision will be the severity of symptoms the patient is experiencing and the confidence the patient and surgeon have in the process of surgery. Scattered papules and pustules across the occipital scalp without confluent areas of hypertrophic scar formation and with only limited symptoms may lead patients to seek a more conservative treatment option.

Prioritization of the following treatments is not meant to be a strict hierarchy; for a well-developed case of AKN, the author's treatment of choice is excision. When this is not acceptable, some of the following nonsurgical approaches may be appropriate. Advice to *reduce the picking* (a consistently reported association) *and close cropping* of the hair is the first measure one should employ. This may be aided by the antiinflammatory effect of potent topical corticosteroids. In mild early cases, treatment with a topical antibiotic such as 1% *clindamycin* or *erythromycin* may be helpful. Oral antistaphylococcal antibiotics, such as *flucloxacillin,* may be helpful, but this is not a recommendation supported by trial evidence. A very good response to flucloxacillin or erythromycin in the early stages when no scarring is present may suggest staphylococcal folliculitis rather than AKN. Long-term oral *tetracycline* antibiotics may be of help in some cases of early disease. Limited hypertrophic scars may respond to intralesional *triamcinolone. Isotretinoin* has been used with success.

Specific Investigations

- Pustule swab
- Deep biopsy

Investigations are not particularly helpful in AKN, and even histology tends to be a by-product of excisional treatment. If the diagnosis is in doubt, a deep biopsy to below the level of the scar tissue and follicular bulbs will confirm the diagnosis. Folliculitis secondary to *Staphylococcus aureus* is worth excluding, largely based on clinical features such as the distribution and the lack of hypertrophic scar formation, but positive cultures from pustules may direct topical and systemic antibiotic therapy. Pustular

Evidence Levels: **A** Double-blind study   **B** Clinical trial ≥ 20 subjects   **C** Clinical trial < 20 subjects   **D** Series ≥ 5 subjects   **E** Anecdotal case reports

lesions of AKN may well grow *S. aureus*, but the response to treatment in the context of a simple bacterial folliculitis will be much greater than that seen in AKN.

First-Line Therapies

• Dissuade from picking and close hair cutting	E
• Topical clindamycin 1% twice daily	E
• Oral antistaphylococcal antibiotic flucloxacillin 250 mg four times daily	E
• Oral tetracycline (lymecycline 408 mg once daily)	E
• Topical corticosteroids–propionate ointment once daily	B

Pseudofolliculitis barbae. Chu T. Practitioner 1989; 233: 307–9.

In a limited open study, 1% topical clindamycin was anecdotally found to be effective for pseudofolliculitis and acne keloidalis.

An open label study of clobetasol propionate 0.05% and betamethasone valerate 0.12% foams in the treatment of mild to moderate acne keloidalis. Callender VD, Young CM, Haverstock CL, Carroll CL, Feldman SR. Cutis 2005; 75: 317–21.

Acne keloidalis is a form of scarring alopecia. Sperling LC, Homoky C, Pratt L, Sau P. Arch Dermatol 2000; 136: 479–84.

Medical treatment for early papular lesions includes intralesional injections of corticosteroids, topical steroids, and topical or oral antibiotics (usually tetracycline).

Second-Line Therapies

• 13-*cis*-retinoic acid 0.5 to 1 mg per kg daily	E
• Intralesional triamcinolone 10 to 40 mg per mL every 2 months	E

Folliculitis nuchae scleroticans – successful treatment with 13-*cis*-retinoic acid (isotretinoin). Stieler W, Senff H, Janner M Hautarzt 1988; 39: 739–42.

Oral therapy with 13-*cis*-retinoic acid (isotretinoin) in a 23-year-old white man resulted in a remarkable improvement within a few weeks.

If antibiotic treatment fails, oral isotretinoin may be helpful in selected cases. Once hypertrophic scarring has developed, treatment

with oral or topical antibiotics is less successful, and measures to control the formation of hypertrophic scar need to be employed. Potent topical corticosteroid creams may help, but intralesional injections of corticosteroids such as triamcinolone can reduce the bulk of the scar tissue. Despite these injections the process tends to continue and the treatment will need to be repeated at intervals.

Third-Line Therapies

• Excision to deep fat or fascia below follicles. Fusiform excision along posterior hairline where possible. Heal by second intention or primary closure as a staged procedure.	C

The surgical management of extensive cases of acne keloidalis nuchae. Gloster HM. Arch Dermatol 2000; 136: 1376–9.

Of 25 young African-Caribbean men with extensive AKN who underwent surgical excision of AKN, 20 underwent excision with layered closure in one stage. Four patients underwent two-stage excisions with layered closure. One patient underwent excision with second-intention healing. All rated the cosmetic result of surgery as good to excellent. No patient experienced complete recurrence of acne keloidalis; 15 patients developed tiny pustules and papules within the surgical scar; 5 developed hypertrophic scars, all of which were successfully treated with high-potency topical and intralesional corticosteroids. Extremely large lesions should be excised in several stages.

Surgical excision of acne keloidalis nuchae with secondary intention healing. Bajaj V, Langtry JA. Clin Exp Dermatol 2008; 33: 53–5.

Anesthesia can be achieved simply with either 0.5% or 1% lidocaine plus epinephrine (adrenaline) 1:200,000 or even 0.1% with epinephrine 1:1,000,000. The advantage of the latter is that it gives excellent longer-term control of bleeding, which can be a problem with large scalp excisions. The use of electrosurgical excision can thus be avoided, as this is associated with increased levels of postoperative pain and an increased risk of wound dehiscence.

Acknowledgment

With thanks to Neil Fernandez, MD for photograph.

3

Acne vulgaris

Fragkiski Tsatsou, Christos C. Zouboulis

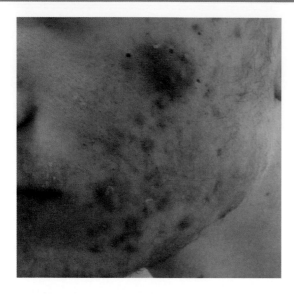

Acne vulgaris is a chronic inflammatory disorder of the pilosebaceous unit with a multifactorial pathogenesis.

MANAGEMENT STRATEGY

Treatment depends on the type and severity of acne lesions. Combination therapy is often appropriate to address the multifactorial pathophysiology.

In mild forms of acne, *topical therapy* is most appropriate. Topical therapy is first indicated in comedonal acne and mild-to-moderate papulopustular acne without scarring. Topical therapeutic agents and oral regimens or procedural therapies are optimally administered simultaneously as combination therapy for treatment of more severe forms of acne. Topical regimens are also used as maintenance therapy to suppress formation of microcomedones, the precursor stage of acne lesions. Topical agents include retinoids, antimicrobial and antibacterial agents, hormonal agents, or herbal remedies. Four to 12 weeks should be allowed for most topical treatments to work before altering the regimen.

Treatment of choice for **comedonal acne** is monotherapy with *topical retinoids* as initiation therapy, due to its usually mild-to-moderate severity. After successful treatment, topical retinoids are suitable for maintenance therapy. Topical retinoids are comedolytic—they act against macrocomedones and microcomedones—and have direct antiinflammatory effects. Retinoids approved for topical acne treatment include tretinoin, isotretinoin, adapalene, and tazarotene. Retinaldehyde is used in cosmetic preparations. All topical retinoids are effective as single agents in mild-to-moderate acne, but they can differ in speed of efficacy and tolerability at an individual level. Local adverse events may occur, including erythema, dryness, itching, and stinging. They typically resolve within the first few weeks of use; alternate-day dosing may be preferred if irritation persists.

Treatment of choice for **mild and moderate papulopustular acne without scarring** is a combination of *benzoyl peroxide* (BPO)

and *topical retinoids*, or *BPO* and *topical antibiotics*. Fixed-dose combination of BPO 2.5% with adapalene 0.1% or 0.3% and BPO 3% or 5% with clindamycin phosphate 1%, 1.2%, 3%, or 5% may increase the patient's adherence to treatment due to their once-daily-only application.

Topical antibiotics, mainly used for their role against *Propionibacterium acnes (P. acnes)*, also have antiinflammatory properties. Commonly prescribed topical antibiotics include clindamycin and erythromycin. They are effective, but are not recommended as monotherapy due to the possible induction of bacterial resistance. Instead, they should be combined with a topical retinoid or with BPO for faster lesion clearing and in order to reduce the likelihood of *P. acnes* resistance.

Azelaic acid 15% gel or 20% cream is a useful adjunctive topical acne treatment and can also be used in maintenance *therapy*, as well as to treat postinflammatory hyperpigmentation.

Topical dapsone 5% or 7.5% gel is recommended for inflammatory acne, particularly in adult females.

Topical adapalene, tretinoin, and benzoyl peroxide can be safely used in the management of preadolescent acne in children.

There is limited evidence to support recommendations for sulfur, nicotinamide, resorcinol, sodium sulfacetamide, aluminum chloride, and zinc in the treatment of acne.

For **moderate papulopustular acne with scarring** in males, *oral antibiotics* are the treatment of choice. They are also recommended in forms of inflammatory acne that are resistant to topical treatments. Although there is no correlation between the numbers of *P. acnes* and the severity of acne, the occurrence of antibiotic-resistant *P. acnes* correlates with poor clinical response. Second-generation tetracyclines (doxycycline, minocycline) have antiinflammatory properties, pharmacokinetic advantages over tetracycline, and are the agents of choice for papulopustular acne. Erythromycin use should be restricted due to increased risk of bacterial resistance. Although oral erythromycin and azithromycin can be effective in treating acne, their use should be limited to patients who cannot receive tetracyclines (i.e., pregnant women or children <8 years of age). Doxycycline is used at 100 or 200 mg daily in two equal doses. An initially higher dose of doxycycline or minocycline (4 weeks 100 mg daily, then 50 mg daily) is more effective than 50 mg daily over 12 weeks. Lower daily doses of bacterial subinhibitory concentrations of doxycycline are considered to promote bacterial resistance. Use of systemic antibiotics other than tetracyclines and macrolides is discouraged because there are limited data for their use. The administration of trimethoprim–sulfamethoxazole and trimethoprim alone should be restricted to patients who are unable to tolerate tetracyclines or in treatment-resistant patients.

Systemic antibiotic therapy of moderate papulopustular acne should be limited to the shortest possible duration. Concomitant topical therapy with BPO or a retinoid should be used to prevent antibiotic resistance and for maintenance therapy. Concurrent use of oral and topical antibiotics should be avoided. In acne relapse, the same antibiotic can be used if previously effective. BPO for 5 to 7 days could also be administered between antibiotic courses to avoid *P. acnes* resistance.

In **nodulocystic or conglobate acne**, *oral isotretinoin* is the treatment of choice. Systemic isotretinoin is the most effective antiacne drug available, especially in severe recalcitrant nodulocystic acne and in the prevention of acne scarring. Oral isotretinoin is also appropriate for the treatment of moderate treatment-resistant acne.

Current guidelines recommend 0.5 mg/kg/d for at least 4 months, being extended in recalcitrant cases, especially with severe involvement of the chest and back. The widely proposed cumulative dose of isotretinoin with respect to relapse of acne

Evidence Levels: **A** Double-blind study **B** Clinical trial ≥ 20 subjects **C** Clinical trial < 20 subjects **D** Series ≥ 5 subjects **E** Anecdotal case reports

is subject to controversy. Alternatively, isotretinoin can be initiated at a low dose of 10 mg/d and be gradually increased to the best tolerated dose. Intermittent dosing is not recommended for active treatment but can be administered during maintenance. Factors contributing to the need for longer treatment schedules include use of lower daily-dose regimens, presence of severe acne, extrafacial involvement, and prolonged history of the disease. In some patients only one course of oral isotretinoin leads to complete acne remission. Relapse is more likely in younger patients.

Isotretinoin treatment for acne can induce inflammatory flares of the disease during the first 3 to 4 weeks of treatment, occasionally leading to acne fulminans. Mild flares do not require modification of the oral dose and improve spontaneously. Severe episodes should be treated with addition of systemic *prednisolone* (30 mg/day), whereas dose reduction or discontinuation may only be required in individual cases.

The adverse event profile of oral isotretinoin includes characteristic dose-dependent mucocutaneous side effects (cheilitis, xerosis, dry mucosae, conjunctivitis, epistaxis), elevation of liver enzymes and/or serum lipids, arthralgia, myalgia, and rarely hyperostosis or extraskeletal calcification. Routine monitoring of liver function tests, serum cholesterol, and triglycerides at baseline and again until response to treatment is established is recommended. Low-dose long-term regimens (0.1–0.2 mg/kg daily) and a micronized isotretinoin formulation with similar efficacy are associated with a lower risk of adverse events.

The dose-independent teratogenic potential of isotretinoin with a high rate of spontaneous abortions and life-threatening congenital malformations demands the use of secure contraception when it is prescribed for females of fertile age. All patients treated with isotretinoin must adhere to the iPLEDGE risk management program. Contraception is recommended 1 month before initiation of treatment, during the entire period of drug administration, and over 3 months after regimen discontinuation. Oral isotretinoin is strictly contraindicated in pregnancy, during lactation, and in severe hepatic and renal dysfunction. Coadministration of vitamin A, tetracycline, and high doses of aspirin is contraindicated. Associated deterioration of preexisting depression, suicide, anxiety, bipolar disorder, psychosis, schizophrenia, and suicidal ideation have been reported during treatment and should be closely followed up, although a causal relationship has not been established.

Isotretinoin affects wound healing and could be associated with development of excessive tissue granulation after dermatologic procedures. It is suggested to delay elective surgical procedures, such as dermabrasion or laser resurfacing (e.g., with CO_2 or Er:YAG laser), for 6 to 12 months after treatment discontinuation. Tattoos, piercings, and epilation procedures should also be postponed.

For **acne fulminans,** a combination of an oral corticosteroid (e.g., prednisolone 30 mg/d for up to 4 weeks) and isotretinoin is indicated.

Infantile and **pediatric acne** may necessitate an alternative treatment. Topical adapalene, tretinoin, and BPO can be safely used in the management of acne in children of preadolescent age.

For **acne patients with adrenal hyperandrogenism,** a low-dose oral corticosteroid in combination with systemic retinoid is the treatment of choice.

Hormonal *antiandrogen* treatment of female acne is not a primary monotherapy and is largely reserved for female patients who present additional signs of peripheral hyperandrogenism or hyperandrogenemia. However, hormonal antiandrogens can be useful in females with acne tarda, in female patients with hormonally induced deterioration of acne (i.e., premenstrual flares), persistent acne recalcitrant to other treatments, an incidental need for contraception, and in order to provide contraceptive cover during systemic isotretinoin treatment.

Estrogen-containing combined oral contraceptives are effective and recommended in the treatment of inflammatory acne in females. Combination oral contraceptive pills (COCs) contain both an estrogen and a progestin component, where the progestin can be one of drospirenone, cyproterone acetate, chlormadinone acetate, or dienogest (the latter three not registered in the United States). Also, selective aldosterone antagonists (e.g., spironolactone 50–200 mg daily) are useful in the treatment of acne in selected females. Spironolactone is well tolerated overall and its side effects are dose related, including hyperkalemia, diuresis, menstrual irregularities, breast tenderness, fatigue, headache, and dizziness. It is contraindicated in pregnancy, and concomitant use of a COC is recommended.

Specific Investigations

None are required routinely.
- Consider microbiology to exclude gram-positive or gram-negative folliculitis.
- Consider endocrine workup if hyperandrogenemia is suspected.

First-Line Therapies

Comedonal acne
- Topical retinoids — B
- Dapsone gel with topical retinoid — B

Mild papulopustular acne
- Benzoyl peroxide with topical retinoid — A
- Benzoyl peroxide with topical antibiotic — A

Moderate papulopustular acne without scarring
- Benzoyl peroxide with topical retinoid — A
- Benzoyl peroxide with topical antibiotic — A

Moderate papulopustular acne with scarring
- For males use oral antibiotics (tetracyclines, macrolides) with benzoyl peroxide or topical retinoid — A
- For females use an oral antiandrogen contraceptive with benzoyl peroxide and topical antibiotic — A

Nodulocystic and/or conglobate acne
- Oral isotretinoin* — A

Acne fulminans
- Oral isotretinoin* with low-dose oral corticosteroids — C

* In women only under application of secure contraception.

Guidelines of care for the management of acne vulgaris. Zaenglein AL, Pathy AL, Schlosser BJ, Alikhan A, Baldwin HE, Berson DS, et al. J Am Acad Dermatol 2016; 74: 945–73.

An evidence-based guideline reviewing grading, topical, and systemic management of acne.

Treatment of acne in pregnancy. Chien AK, Qi J, Rainer B, Sachs DL, Helfrich YR. J Am Board Fam Med 2016; 29: 254–62.

A review on the safety profiles of common therapies used in pregnancy. Topical azelaic acid or BPO can be recommended as baseline therapy. A combination of topical erythromycin or clindamycin with BPO is recommended for inflammatory acne. Oral erythromycin or cephalexin is considered safe for moderate-to-severe inflammatory acne when used for a few weeks. A short course of oral prednisolone may be useful for treating fulminant nodular cystic acne after the first trimester.

Topical retinoids in acne – an evidence-based overview. Thielitz A, Naser MB, Fluhr JW, Zouboulis CC, Gollnick H. J Dtsch Dermatol Ges 2010; 8 (Suppl 1): S15–23.

A review on retinoids approved for topical acne treatment, their differences in efficacy and tolerability, and their adverse effects, according to evidence-based medicine (EBM) levels.

Efficacy and safety of once-daily dapsone gel, 7.5% for treatment of adolescents and adults with acne vulgaris: first of two identically designed, large, multicenter, randomized, vehicle-controlled trials. Stein Gold LF, Jaratt MT, Bucko AD, Grekin SK, Berlin JM, Bukhalo M, et al. J Drugs Dermatol 2016; 15: 553–61.

A 12-week, randomized, double-blind, vehicle-controlled, multicenter clinical trial of patients ≥12 years with moderate inflammatory acne, where dapsone gel 7.5% applied topically once daily was shown to be an effective, safe, and well-tolerated regimen. *Dapsone is a sulfone with antiinflammatory and antimicrobial properties. Dapsone gel delivers clinically effective doses of dapsone with minimal systemic absorption.*

Two randomized, double-blind, split-face studies to compare the irritation potential of two topical acne fixed combinations over a 21-day treatment period. Bhatia N, Bhatt V, Martin G, Pillai R. J Drugs Dermatol 2016; 15: 721–6.

Advances in formulation technology have provided new fixed combinations with higher concentrations of active ingredients and lower concentrations of potentially irritating ingredients without compromising efficacy. The tolerability of clindamycin–BPO 3.75% gel and adapalene 0.3%–BPO 2.5% gel was compared in healthy volunteers over 21 days, using a split-face methodology. Adverse events—stinging, erythema, dryness, scaling, burning, and itching—were twice as common with adapalene 0.3%–BPO 2.5% gel. Therefore clindamycin–BPO 3.75% gel is likely to be better tolerated than adapalene 0.3%–BP 2.5% gel in moderate-to-severe acne.

Effects of benzoyl peroxide 5% clindamycin combination gel versus adapalene 0.1% on quality of life in patients with mild to moderate acne vulgaris: a randomized single-blind study. Guerra-Tapia A. J Drugs Dermatol 2012; 11: 714–22.

The fixed-dose combination of BPO 5%/clindamycin 1% gel provided earlier improvement of quality of life than adapalene 0.1% gel. This could result from better efficacy and tolerability.

A randomized, single-blind comparison of topical clindamycin + benzoyl peroxide (Duac) and erythromycin + zinc acetate (Zineryt) in the treatment of mild to moderate facial acne vulgaris. Langner A, Sheehan-Dare R, Layton A. J Eur Acad Dermatol Venereol 2007; 21: 311–9.

Comparison of two combination treatments for facial acne: a ready-mixed, once-daily gel containing clindamycin phosphate (1%) plus benzoyl peroxide (5%) (CDP + BPO) and a twice-daily solution of erythromycin (4%) plus zinc acetate (1.2%) (ERY + Zn). Both regimens are effective, but CDP + BPO has an earlier onset of action that should improve compliance.

Study of the efficacy, tolerability, and safety of 2 fixed-dose combination BPO gels in the management of acne vulgaris. Zouboulis CC, Fischer TC, Wohlrab J, Barnard J, Alió AB. Cutis 2009; 84: 223–9.

Comparison of clindamycin 1%/benzoyl peroxide 5% gel with hydrating excipients (C/BPO HE) and adapalene 0.1%/BPO 2.5% gel. After 12 weeks of once-daily application, the treatments showed similar improvements of inflammatory and noninflammatory lesions, but C/BPO HE achieved better overall treatment success in less time with better tolerability and safety.

Clindamycin phosphate/tretinoin gel formulation in the treatment of acne vulgaris. Abdel-Naser MB, Zouboulis CC. Expert Opin Pharmacother 2008; 9: 2931–7.

Clindamycin phosphate 1.2% with tretinoin 0.025% fixed-dose combination gel is approved by the Food and Drug Administration (FDA) for treatment of acne in patients ≥12 years old. This formulation enhances effectiveness and minimizes irritation. The once-daily use, the rapid effect, and good tolerability have a positive impact on disease duration, compliance, and cost.

Making sense of the effects of the cumulative dose of isotretinoin in acne vulgaris. Rademaker M. Int J Dermatol 2016; 55: 518–23.

A study to determine the influence of daily and cumulative dosage on acne relapse. A chart review of 1453 patients, where daily and cumulative doses and duration were compared among patients who received one course and two or more courses, respectively. *Neither daily nor cumulative dosages influenced relapse of acne vulgaris in patients treated with varying doses of isotretinoin as long as treatment was continued for ≥2 months after the acne had completely resolved.*

Interrelationships between isotretinoin treatment and psychiatric disorders: depression, bipolar disorder, anxiety, psychosis and suicide risks. Ludot M, Mouchabac S, Ferreri F. World J Psychiatry 2015; 5: 222–7.

A literature review aiming to specify the link between isotretinoin and specific psychiatric disorders. *Many studies demonstrated an increased risk of depression, attempted suicide, and suicide. Several studies showed patients with bipolar disorder have an increased risk for symptom exacerbation. Few studies suggested a possible link between isotretinoin and psychosis.*

Hormonal antiandrogens in acne treatment. Zouboulis CC, Rabe T. J Dtsch Dermatol Ges 2010; 8 (Suppl 1): S60–74.

A review of the efficacy, classification, and mechanism of action of antiandrogens. Combinations of ethinyl estradiol with cyproterone acetate, chlormadinone acetate, dienogest, desogestrel, and drospirenone have shown the strongest anti-acne activity. Gestagens or estrogens as monotherapy, spironolactone, flutamide, gonadotropin-releasing hormone agonists, and inhibitors of peripheral androgen metabolism are not recommended.

Efficacy and safety of 3 mg drospirenone/20 mcg ethinylestradiol oral contraceptive administered in 24/4 regimen in the treatment of acne vulgaris: a randomized, double-blind, placebo-controlled trial. Koltun W, Lucky AW, Thiboutot D, Niknian M, Sampson-Landers C, Korner P, et al. Contraception 2008; 77: 249–56.

This nonandrogenic progestin-containing contraceptive with strong antiandrogenic activity (drospirenone 3 mg) but reduced concentration of ethinyl estradiol (20 μg) has been shown to be effective and may replace the classic cyproterone acetate/ethinyl estradiol and chlormadinone acetate/ethinyl estradiol oral contraceptives due to an improved side effect profile.

Evidence Levels: **A** Double-blind study **B** Clinical trial ≥ 20 subjects **C** Clinical trial < 20 subjects **D** Series ≥ 5 subjects **E** Anecdotal case reports

Efficacy of a combined oral contraceptive containing 0.030 mg ethinylestradiol/2 mg dienogest for the treatment of papulopustular acne in comparison with placebo and 0.035 mg ethinylestradiol/2 mg cyproterone acetate. Palombo-Kinne E, Schellschmidt I, Schumacher U, Gräser T. Contraception 2009; 79: 282–9.

A combined oral contraceptive containing the antiandrogen dienogest with ethinylestradiol proved superior to placebo and not inferior to one containing the potent antiandrogen cyproterone acetate and ethinylestradiol.

Second-Line Therapies

Comedonal acne

• Benzoyl peroxide (topical)	B
• Azelaic acid	B
• Superficial peels (lipohydroxy acid, salicylic acid)	B

Mild-to-moderate papulopustular acne

• Azelaic acid	A
• Benzoyl peroxide (topical)	C
• Topical retinoid	A
• Azelaic acid with topical clindamycin	A
• Azelaic acid with topical erythromycin	A
• Dapsone gel	A
• Dapsone gel with topical retinoid	A
• Dapsone gel with benzoyl peroxide (topical)	A
• Systemic antibiotic with adapalene	C
• Topical erythromycin with topical retinoid	C
• Oral zinc	C
• Photodynamic therapy	B
• Intense pulsed light (IPL)	B
• Photodynamic therapy with IPL	B
• Blue light	B
• Blue/red light combinations	C
• Red low-level laser therapy (LLLT)	B
• 1450-nm diode laser	C
• Topical cyproterone acetate	A
• Zileuton	C
• Topical copaiba essential oil gel	A
• Topical 5% tea tree oil gel	A
• Glycolic acid oil-in-water emulsion	A
• Chemical peels (α-hydroxy acid, glycolic acid, β-hydroxy acid, salicylic acid)	B
• Microdermabrasion	C

Nodulocystic and/or conglobate acne

• Oral antibiotic plus topical retinoid	C
• Oral antibiotic plus azelaic acid	C
• Oral antibiotic plus topical retinoid plus benzoyl peroxide	C

New and emerging treatments in dermatology: acne. Katsambas A, Dessinioti C. Dermatol Ther 2008; 21: 86–95.

An overview of the treatment of acne, including new therapies and future perspectives. Oral zinc sulfate and zinc gluconate have been used for the treatment of inflammatory acne vulgaris with conflicting results. Zinc acts via inhibition of polymorphonuclear cell chemotaxis and inhibition of growth of *P. acnes*. Its antiinflammatory activity could also be related to a decrease in tumor necrosis factor-α production, the modulation of the expression of integrins, and the inhibition of TLR2 surface expression by keratinocytes. Zinc salts have been used at a dosage of 30 to 150 mg

of elemental zinc daily for 3 months. Zinc gluconate does not induce bacterial resistance, has a favorable safety profile, and can be administered to pregnant women.

A multicenter, randomized, single-blind, parallel-group study comparing the efficacy and tolerability of benzoyl peroxide 3%/clindamycin 1% with azelaic acid 20% in the topical treatment of mild-to-moderate acne vulgaris. Schaller M, Sebastian M, Ress C, Seidel D, Hennig M. J Eur Acad Dermatol Venereol 2016; 30: 966–73.

A randomized, single-blind, parallel-group, multicenter study over 12 weeks, where clindamycin 1% + BPO demonstrated greater efficacy than azelaic acid 20% in the treatment of mild-to-moderate acne. *Azelaic acid has a predominant antibacterial action and possesses a modest comedolytic effect. Burning upon application is common. Systemic side effects are not likely to occur, making it safe for acne treatment during pregnancy and lactation.*

Zileuton, a new efficient and safe systemic antiacne drug. Zouboulis CC. Dermato-Endocrinology 2009; 1: 188–92.

In a multicenter study, zileuton, an oral 5-lipoxygenase inhibitor, showed a significant decrease in inflammatory lesions compared with placebo. Zileuton reduces the number of inflammatory lesions in moderate acne and inhibits the synthesis of sebaceous lipids. It appears to be safe and well tolerated.

Application of the essential oil from copaiba (*Copaifera langsdori Desf.*) for acne vulgaris: a double-blind, placebo-controlled clinical trial. Da Silva AG, Puziol Pde F, Leitao RN, Gomes TR, Scherer R, Martins ML, et al. Altern Med Rev 2012; 17: 69–75.

Treatment with 1.0% copaiba oil significantly reduced the surface area affected with acne. Copaiba oil resin is widely used in traditional medicine due to its antiinflammatory, healing, and antiseptic activities.

The efficacy of 5% topical tea tree oil gel in mild to moderate acne vulgaris: a randomized, double-blind placebo-controlled study. Enshaieh S, Jooya A, Siadat AH, Iraji F. Indian J Dermatol Venereol Leprol 2007; 73: 22–5.

This was found to be effective.

Nutritional clinical studies in dermatology. Liakou AI, Theodorakis MJ, Melnik BC, Pappas A, Zouboulis CC. J Drugs Dermatol 2013; 12: 1104–9.

The relationship between acne and diet, predominantly the role of high-glycemic-load diets and dairy consumption, has recently gained increased interest. The data on the relationship between nutrition and skin are until now controversial, and much more work is needed to be done to clarify possible etiologic correlations.

A 10% glycolic acid containing oil-in-water emulsion improves mild acne: a randomized double-blind placebo-controlled trial. Abels C, Kaszuba A, Michalak I, Werdier D, Knie U, Kaszuba A. J Cosmet Dermatol 2011; 10: 202–9.

Treatment was applied once daily in the evening in 120 patients with mild acne over 90 days and improved mild acne significantly after 45 days with good tolerability. α-Hydroxy acids exhibit comedolytic and antimicrobial properties.

Clinical evaluation of glycolic acid chemical peeling in patients with acne vulgaris: a randomized, double-blind, placebo-controlled, split-face comparative study. Kaminaka C, Uede M, Matsunaka H, Furukawa F, Yamomoto Y. Dermatol Surg 2014; 40: 314–22.

A prospective, randomized, double-blind, placebo-controlled, split-face clinical trial of 26 patients with moderate acne who were treated with 40% glycolic acid (pH 2.0) on half the face and placebo on the other half five times at 2-week intervals showed significant improvement of moderate acne in Asians.

Randomized trial comparing a chemical peel containing a lipophilic hydroxy acid derivative of salicylic acid with a salicylic acid peel in subjects with comedonal acne. Levesque A, Hamzavi I, Seite S, Rougier A, Bissonnette R. J Cosmet Dermatol 2011; 10: 174–82.

A split-face study. Twenty subjects received a total of six peels at 2-week intervals. There was no significant difference in response. Lipohydroxy acid is a lipophilic derivative of salicylic acid with comedolytic properties.

Photodynamic therapy for the treatment of different severity of acne: a systematic review. Keyal U, Bhatta AK, Wang XL. Photodiagnosis Photodyn Ther 2016; 14: 191–9.

Thirty-six clinical trials were selected, among which 24 trials were performed to see the effect of photodynamic therapy (PDT) in acne, whereas 12 trials compared the effect of PDT with light- or laser-alone therapy. Among 24 trials that used PDT only, 3 were clinical trials with control, 14 were clinical trials without control, 6 were randomized controlled trials (RCTs), and 1 was a retrospective study. PDT has been extensively studied and found to be safe and effective in acne. PDT can control inflammatory and noninflammatory acne lesions and can improve all acne lesions, ranging from mild to severe. More RCTs are needed to establish standard guidelines regarding concentrations and the incubation period of photosensitizers and optimal parameters of light sources.

Daylight photodynamic therapy with 1.5% 3-butenyl 5-aminolevulinate gel as a convenient, effective and safe therapy in acne treatment: a double-blind randomized controlled trial. Kwon HH, Moon KR, Park SY, Yoon JY, Suh DH, Lee JB. J Dermatol 2016; 43: 515–21. A study on the efficacy and safety of daylight PDT in acne treatment. The novel variant of 5-aminolevulinate (ALA)-ester, 1.5% 3-butenyl ALA-bu gel, was applied using daylight only as the potential visible light source. Forty-six acne patients were randomly assigned to either ALA-bu or vehicle application group in a double-blind fashion. Both groups applied the allocated gel to facial acne lesions every other day for 12 weeks. Daylight-PDT was effective, very well tolerated, and convenient for treating inflammatory acne lesions.

A randomized controlled study for the treatment of acne vulgaris using high-intensity 414 nm solid state diode arrays. Ash C, Harrison A, Drew S, Whittall R. J Cosmet Laser Ther 2015; 17: 170–6.

A randomized controlled study quantifying the efficacy of a blue light device as a self-treatment regimen. Forty-one adults with mild-to-moderate facial inflammatory acne achieved a reduction of inflammatory lesions after 12 weeks. Treatment was free of pain and side effects. *Blue light phototherapy using a narrowband light-emitting diode (LED) appears to be a safe and effective additional therapy for mild-to-moderate acne.*

Comparison of red and infrared low-level laser therapy in the treatment of acne vulgaris. Aziz-Jalali MH, Tabaie SM, Djavid GE. Indian J Dermatol 2012; 57: 128–30.

In this single-blind randomized study, two different wavelengths of LLLT (630 and 890 nm) were evaluated. Twenty-eight patients with mild-to-moderate acne vulgaris were treated with red LLLT (630 nm) and infrared LLLT (890 nm) on the right and left sides of the face, respectively, twice a week for 12 sessions. There was significant clinical improvement with 630 nm but not with 890 nm.

Treating acne scars in patients with Fitzpatrick skin types IV to VI using the 1450-nm diode laser. Semchyshyn N, Prodanovic E, Varade R. Cutis 2013; 92: 49–53.

A study assessing the efficacy and side effect profile of a 1450-nm diode laser for the treatment of acne scars in participants with Fitzpatrick skin types IV to VI. Findings show the nonablative 1450-nm diode laser is safe and effective in improving the appearance of atrophic acne scars in darker skin types. Postinflammatory hyperpigmentation was a common occurrence.

Combined autologous platelet-rich plasma with microneedling versus microneedling with distilled water in the treatment of atrophic acne scars: a concurrent split-face study. Asif M, Kanodia S, Singh K. J Cosmet Dermatol 2016; 15: 434-43.

Microneedling was performed on both face halves of 50 patients with atrophic acne scars. Intradermal injections plus platelet-rich plasma (PRP) was administered on the right face half, intradermal administration of distilled water on the left half. Three treatment sessions were given at a 1-month interval. PRP showed efficacy in the management of atrophic acne scars. It can be combined with microneedling to enhance the final clinical outcomes in comparison with microneedling alone.

The efficacy of topical cyproterone acetate alcohol lotion versus placebo in the treatment of the mild to moderate acne vulgaris: a double blind study. Iraji F, Momeni A, Naji SM, Siadat AH. Dermatol Online J 2006; 12: 26.

A trial with 86 female patients with mild-to-moderate acne vulgaris. The use of cyproterone acetate alcohol lotion is suggested as one of the main treatments for mild-to-moderate acne in female patients and as an adjuvant treatment for moderate-to-severe acne vulgaris.

Superficial chemical peels and microdermabrasion for acne vulgaris. Kempiak SJ, Uebelhoer N. Semin Cutan Med Surg 2008; 27: 212–20.

A description of the procedure steps and the complications in the office setting. The evaluation of patients before the procedure is discussed, as well as postpeel regimens. Comparative studies between the two most commonly used superficial peeling agents, glycolic and salicylic acid, are discussed.

Third-Line Therapies

Mild-to-moderate acne

• Chemical peels (α-hydroxy acid, glycolic acid, β-hydroxy acid, salicylic acid)	B
• Microdermabrasion	B

Acne sinuses and scars

• Intralesional steroids	C
• Medium-depth chemical peels (Jessner solution/ trichloroacetic acid (TCA), TCA, phenol)	B
• Dermabrasion ± platelet-rich plasma	B
• Radiofrequency	C
• Fractional laser resurfacing (ablative, nonablative)	B
• Surgical scar revision	C
• Injectable fillers	C

Evidence Levels: **A** Double-blind study **B** Clinical trial ≥ 20 subjects **C** Clinical trial < 20 subjects **D** Series ≥ 5 subjects **E** Anecdotal case reports

Trichloroacetic acid versus salicylic acid in the treatment of acne vulgaris in dark-skinned patients. Abdel Meguid AM, Elaziz Ahmed Attallah DA, Omar H. Dermatol Surg 2015; 41: 1398–404.

Comparison of efficacy of TCA 25% peels with salicylic acid 30% in 25 patients with acne vulgaris. Twenty-five percent TCA was applied to the right half of the face and 30% salicylic acid to the left half at 2-week intervals for 2 months. TCA is superior in treating comedonal lesions, whereas salicylic acid is better at treating inflammatory lesions with no statistical difference between the results.

Comparison of fractional microneedling radiofrequency and bipolar radiofrequency on acne and acne scar and investigation of mechanism: comparative randomized controlled clinical trial. Min S, Park SY, Yoon JY, Suh DH. Arch Dermatol Res 2015; 307: 897–904.

Fractional microneedling radiofrequency (FMR) is one of the promising methods in acne treatment. Moreover, bipolar radiofrequency (BR) generates heat, inducing neocollagenesis. Twenty subjects with mild-to-moderate acne and acne scars were treated in a split-face manner with FMR and BR in a prospective single-blind, randomized clinical trial over 12 weeks, receiving two treatment sessions 4 weeks apart. Both treatments showed no severe adverse events other than erythema. FMR showed superior efficacy in acne and acne scars compared with BR.

Treatment of acne scars by fractional bipolar radiofrequency energy. Gold MH, Biron JA. Cosmet Laser Ther 2012; 14: 172–8.

Fifteen patients with mild-to-moderate acne scars received three monthly treatments with a fractional bipolar RF device. Physician-assessed acne scar severity was significantly reduced at 1 month and 3 months. Adverse events were limited to transient erythema. Dryness, bruising, and crusting erosion were limited. Subject-assessed fine lines and wrinkles, brightness, tightness, acne scar texture, and pigmentation improved significantly.

Deep peeling using phenol versus percutaneous collagen induction combined with trichloroacetic acid 20% in atrophic postacne scars: a randomized controlled trial. Leheta TM, Abdel Hay RM, El Garem YF. J Dermatolog Treat 2014; 25: 130–6.

Deep peeling using phenol and percutaneous collagen induction (PCI) with TCA 20% were both effective in treating post-acne atrophic scars. Comparison of the degree of improvement in different types of scars within the same group after treatment revealed very highly significant improvement in the rolling scar type.

Treatment of acne vulgaris with salicylic acid chemical peel and pulsed dye laser: a split face, rater-blinded, randomized controlled trial. Lekakh O, Mahoney AM, Novice K, Kamalpour J, Sadeghian A, Mondo D, et al. J Lasers Med Sci 2015; 6: 167–70.

An evaluation of the safety and efficacy of concurrent use of salicylic acid peels with pulsed dye laser (PDL) versus salicylic acid peels alone in 19 patients with moderate-to-severe acne vulgaris. The adjunctive utilization of PDL to salicylic acid peel therapy can lead to better outcomes in acne management.

Comparison of two kinds of lasers in the treatment of acne scars. Reinholz M, Schwaiger H, Heppt MV, Poetschke J, Tietze J, Epple A, et al. Facial Plast Surg 2015; 31: 523–31.

A pilot study comparing the results of acne scars treated either with a fractional Er:YAG (erbium-doped yttrium-aluminum-garnet [Er:Y3Al5O1]) or a carbon dioxide (CO_2) laser at different wavelengths. Fourteen patients with severe scars on both cheeks were treated four times in a random split-face approach: on one side with Er:YAG laser and on the contralateral side with CO_2 laser following a standardized protocol. Treatment results displayed a higher efficacy of the fractional CO_2 laser compared with the Er:YAG laser.

Acne scars in ethnic skin treated with both nonablative fractional 1550 nm and ablative fractional CO_2 lasers: comparative retrospective analysis with recommended guidelines. Alajlan AM, Alsuwaidan SN. Lasers Surg Med 2011; 43: 787–91.

Eighty-two patients with skin phototype III–V were included; 45 were treated with nonablative fractional (NAF) 1550 nm laser and 37 with ablative fractional (AF) CO_2 laser. Both lasers were effective in treating acne scars with good patient satisfaction rate and high safety profiles. Transient postinflammatory hyperpigmentation was noted in both groups, but decreased with routine use of bleaching creams.

Acrodermatitis enteropathica

Joanna E. Gach

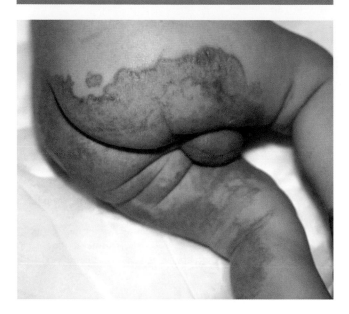

Acrodermatitis enteropathica (AE) OMIM 201100 is a rare, autosomal-recessive, inherited disorder of zinc deficiency. It is caused by mutations in the *SLC39A* gene located on 8q24.3, which encodes for *ZIP4* intestinal zinc transporter expressed in enterocytes that absorb dietary zinc from the small intestine. The estimated prevalence is 1 in 500,000 children worldwide, without apparent predilection for race or gender. AE manifests itself shortly after birth in a bottle-fed infant and sometime soon after weaning in a breast-fed infant. Zinc within breast milk is more bioavailable to infants than within bovine milk due to binding to a low-molecular-weight ligand secreted by the pancreas. Characteristic clinical signs are lesions in acral and periorificial sites; the first signs are eczematous, pink, scaly plaques that can become vesicular, bullous, pustular, or desquamative. They can resemble the severe diaper dermatitis of infancy. Angular cheilitis and paronychia can also be seen early. If left untreated, AE usually causes diarrhea, irritability, and alopecia, and skin lesions become secondarily infected with bacteria and *Candida albicans*. Impaired physical and mental development is seen in advanced disease. Appropriate supplementation of zinc in the infant's diet results in a rapid improvement.

The diagnosis of AE is applied only to *inherited* zinc deficiency; noninherited zinc deficiency is called *acquired zinc deficiency*. Transient neonatal zinc deficiency OMIM 608118, caused by mutations of the ZnT2/SLC30A2 in mothers, occurs in breast-fed, full-term infants due to low zinc concentrations in the mother's breast milk. Clinical symptoms identical to AE are alleviated with zinc supplementation to the infant, but not to the mother. Long-term therapy and management of zinc deficiency vary depending on the severity of the disorder.

MANAGEMENT STRATEGY

Chronic dermatitis in periorificial and acral areas should suggest the possibility of zinc deficiency, but establishing the diagnosis of AE may be difficult. The first step is laboratory determination of blood plasma or serum zinc levels. A blood sample needs to be drawn into a trace element–free bottle with a stainless steel needle. Avoid contact with rubber stoppers, as they contain zinc, avoid hemolysis, use zinc-free anticoagulants, and separate plasma or serum from cells within 45 minutes. Zinc levels will decrease in states of hypoalbuminemia because zinc binds albumin in the circulation. If the diagnosis of zinc deficiency has been confirmed, management becomes relatively simple: *oral zinc supplementation* produces dramatic resolution of the problem. High-dose supplementation will allow for increased paracellular zinc absorption despite the absence of a functional *ZIP4* zinc transporter.

The patient or his or her family must understand the need for life-long management of the disorder in terms of zinc supplementation and medical supervision. Discuss *foods rich in zinc, such as shellfish, nuts, and green leafy vegetables.* Bioavailability of zinc can be reduced by phytates, which naturally occur in plant fibers, and also with regular iron supplementation. With age and a more varied diet, the dose of daily zinc supplementation may be reduced. Zinc therapy should be monitored periodically with morning fasting specimen, full blood count, serum copper level, and stool examination for occult blood. Zinc supplementation has a theoretical risk of reducing copper absorption, leading to refractory microcytic anemia that will not respond to iron therapy until the serum copper level is normalized.

Specific Investigations

- Morning fasting blood plasma or serum zinc levels
- Urine zinc excretion
- Serum albumin and alkaline phosphatase
- Serum copper levels
- Genetic studies

The normal plasma zinc level is 70 to 110 µg/dL and in serum 80 to 120 µg/dL. Urinary zinc can be measured but is not definitive for diagnosis.

Homozygosity mapping places the acrodermatitis enteropathica gene on chromosomal regions 8q24.3. Wang K, Pugh EW, Griffen S, Doheny KF, Mostafa WZ, al-Aboosi MM, et al. Am J Hum Genet 2001; 68: 1055–70.

Identification of *SLC39A4*, a gene involved in acrodermatitis enteropathica. Küry S, Dréno B, Bézieau S, Giraudet S, Kharfi M, Kamoun R, et al. Nature Genet 2002; 31: 239–40.

Overview of inherited zinc deficiency in infants and children. Kambe T, Fukue K, Ishida R, Miyazaki S. J Nutr Sci Vitaminol 2015; 61 Suppl: S44–6.

Genetic causes and gene-nutrient interactions in mammalian zinc deficiencies: acrodermatitis enteropathica and transient neonatal zinc deficiency as examples. Kasana S, Din J, Maret W. J Trace Elem Med Biol 2015; 29: 47–62.

First-Line Therapy

- Oral zinc supplementation   A

Evidence Levels: **A** Double-blind study   **B** Clinical trial ≥ 20 subjects   **C** Clinical trial < 20 subjects   **D** Series ≥ 5 subjects   **E** Anecdotal case reports

In most cases, oral supplementation with two to three times the recommended daily allowance of zinc salts in doses of 30 to 55 mg of elemental Zn^{2+} will be sufficient to restore normal zinc status within days to a few weeks, depending on the degree of depletion. The dose of elemental zinc must be determined by the patient's blood or plasma zinc levels and by body weight. In AE, zinc replacement should begin at 2 to 3 mg/kg/day of elemental zinc. Serum or plasma zinc should be checked every 3 to 6 months, adjusting the zinc dosage accordingly. In patients with acquired or dietary zinc deficiency, treatment should begin at 0.5 to 1 mg/kg/day. Available forms of zinc supplementation include zinc sulfate, zinc acetate, zinc gluconate, and zinc propionate. *Dosage must be based on the amount of elemental zinc present in the preparation, which varies between compounds. For example, a standard 220-mg capsule of a commercial zinc preparation contains approximately 55 mg Zn^{2+}, which is an adequate daily dose for most deficient individuals. A commonly used preparation is Zincate, which is $ZnSO_4 \cdot 7H_2O$.*

A significant side effect of zinc supplementation is gastric irritation with nausea, vomiting, and gastric hemorrhage. Large accidental overdoses of zinc may cause fatal multisystem organ failure.

Zinc deficiency in acrodermatitis enteropathica: multiple dietary intolerance treated with synthetic diet. Barnes PM, Moynahan EJ. Proc Roy Soc Med 1973; 66: 327–9.

In 1973 Barnes and Moynahan were treating children with chronic, unresponsive AE-type acral dermatoses and having poor results. They then tried different medications, one of which was oral zinc. To their surprise, the patients receiving the zinc supplements cleared rapidly and completely.

Acrodermatitis enteropathica and an overview of zinc metabolism. Maverakis E, Fung MA, Lynch PJ, Draznin M, Michael DJ, Ruben B, et al. J Am Acad Dermatol 2007; 56: 116–24.

An excellent review of AE and other zinc deficiency disorders.

Zinc therapy in dermatology: a review. Gupta M, Mahajan VK, Mehta KS, Chauhan PS. Dermatol Res Pract 2014; 2014: 709152.

A detailed review of the use of zinc in over 20 dermatologic conditions.

Acknowledgment

We acknowledge Dr. Kenneth H. Neldner for his contribution to this chapter.

Actinic keratoses

Sherrif F. Ibrahim, Marc D. Brown

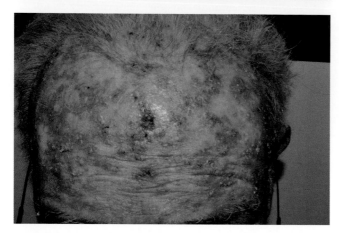

Actinic keratoses (AKs) are ill-defined, pink-to-skin–colored, scaly papules found on chronically sun-exposed areas in light-skinned individuals. They most frequently appear on the face, ears, balding scalp, extensor forearms, and dorsal hands. AKs are a strong predictor for the development of squamous cell carcinoma (SCC) and, to a lesser extent, basal cell carcinoma. Australians have the highest reported prevalence, which approaches 60%, and in the United States AKs are the second most common reason for visits to the dermatologist.

MANAGEMENT STRATEGY

Actinic keratoses are common dysplastic intraepidermal lesions that are considered precursors to SCC. Reports have varied as to the rates of progression to invasive SCC, from 0.025% to over 25% per year, and AKs are commonly located adjacent to SCC histologically. For these reasons, most practitioners advocate the treatment of AKs, because considerable morbidity and potential mortality can be associated with invasive disease. However, no randomized controlled studies have demonstrated a reduction in the frequency of SCC with treatment of AKs.

The diagnosis of AK is primarily clinical, and because of their superficial nature, a variety of effective management approaches exist. Biopsy of suspected AKs is typically not warranted; however, in patients with a history of multiple skin cancers, immunosuppressed patients, and lesions in high-risk areas such as the lip or ear, clinicians should have a low threshold for biopsy to rule out invasive SCC. Indications for biopsy include tenderness, rapid growth or thickening of lesions, bleeding, hyperkeratosis, and failure to respond to treatment.

Prevention of AKs through sun avoidance and diligent use of broad-spectrum sunscreens and blocking agents is an important aspect of management. This has been shown to prevent the development of new AKs and reduce the incidence of nonmelanoma skin cancers.

With cumulative sun exposure and advancing age, rates of AK development increase, necessitating either *ablative* or *topical treatment. Cryotherapy* with liquid nitrogen is by far the most commonly employed therapeutic modality because it can be performed quickly and effectively in the office setting. However, given the common appearance of AKs on a background of diffuse actinic damage, individual lesions may be poorly defined and involve large, confluent areas requiring field treatment with topical agents such as *5-fluorouracil* (5-FU) and *imiquimod*. The latter has recently been shown to have high rates of treatment success with durable results and has become an accepted first-line therapy with a newer 3.75% formulation recently introduced. The most recently approved topical agent, *ingenol mebutate*, is derived from the *Euphorbia peplus* plant and has efficacy for the field treatment of AKs. The advantages of topical approaches are that they are patient administered, non-invasive, carry little risk of scarring or pigmentary change, and can be used for anatomically difficult or cosmetically sensitive areas. However, these agents require adequate patient compliance and are often accompanied by prolonged erythema lasting several weeks. *Photodynamic therapy* (PDT) with aminolevulinic acid (ALA) or methyl aminolevulinate (MAL) has continued to become more widespread, given its proven therapeutic results and excellent cosmetic outcome. PDT offers a physician-administered approach to field treatment with shorter periods of inflammation and erythema than several topical agents, and thus many studies indicate higher patient satisfaction. Variations in the light dose, light source (including ambient daylight), sensitizing agent and its application time, and frequency of treatments may improve efficacy. Head-to-head trials of different treatment approaches are difficult to perform, as variations in treatment protocols make direct comparisons challenging. Recently there has been a continuing trend toward *combination therapy,* such as topical agents either before or after cryotherapy, or sequential use of multiple topical modalities with varying mechanisms of action. Other approaches such as *laser resurfacing, chemical peels,* and *dermabrasion* may be considered in certain situations when lesions have failed the aforementioned treatments or if severe photodamage is present. Finally, for recalcitrant or hyperkeratotic lesions, *curettage* or *excision* may be appropriate.

Specific Investigation

In selected cases:
- Biopsy

Actinic keratoses and the incidence of occult squamous cell carcinoma: a clinical–histopathologic correlation. Ehrig T, Cockerell C, Piacquadio D, Dromgoole S. Dermatol Surg 2006; 32: 1261–5.

A total of 271 clinically diagnosed AKs were biopsied. Clinical diagnosis was in agreement with histology 91% of the time, with about 1 in 25 lesions revealing invasive SCC.

Clinical recognition of actinic keratoses in a high-risk population: how good are we? Venna SS, Lee D, Stadecker MJ, Rogers GS. Arch Dermatol 2005; 141: 507–9.

Seventeen of 23 lesions (74%) with classic features of AK in patients with a history of previous skin cancer were confirmed histologically. Five lesions (22%) were shown to be SCC.

Actinic keratoses are typically diagnosed clinically. However, there should be a low threshold to biopsy tender, hyperkeratotic, large, or recalcitrant lesions to exclude malignancy.

First-Line Therapies	
• Sunscreens	A
• Cryosurgery	B
• Topical 5-FU	A
• Imiquimod	A
• Photodynamic therapy	A

A randomized controlled trial to assess sunscreen application and beta carotene supplementation in the prevention of solar keratoses. Darlington S, Williams G, Neale R, Frost C, Green A. Arch Dermatol 2003; 139: 451–5.

In this Australian study, 1621 adults were randomized to either daily use of sunscreen or application at their usual discretionary rate. There was a 24% reduction in AKs in the daily-use group.

Reduction of solar keratoses by regular sunscreen use. Thompson SC, Jolley D, Marks R. N Engl J Med 1993; 14: 1147–51.

In a 6-month randomized, placebo-controlled trial of 588 patients in Australia, SPF 17 sunscreen applied daily was found to both reduce the development of new AKs and increase the remission of existing AKs compared with a vehicle cream.

A prospective study of the use of cryosurgery for the treatment of actinic keratoses. Thai K, Fergin P, Freeman M, Vinciullo C, Francis D, Spelman L, et al. Int J Dermatol 2004; 43: 687–92.

In this prospective multicenter study, 90 patients with 421 AKs on the face and scalp were treated with cryotherapy with a single freeze–thaw cycle using different freeze times. The patients were reviewed 3 months later. Overall, the complete response (CR) rate was 67.2%, varying from 39% for freeze times less than 5 seconds to 83% for times longer than 20 seconds. The authors also found that hypopigmentation was present in 29% of CR lesions. Patients rated cosmetic outcomes as good to excellent for 94% of CR lesions.

Effect of a 1 week treatment with 0.5% topical fluorouracil on occurrence of actinic keratosis after cryosurgery. Jorizzo J, Weiss J, Furst K, VandePol C, Levy SF. Arch Dermatol 2004; 140: 813–16.

This study demonstrates that there is a role for the combination of therapeutic modalities in the treatment of AKs. In this prospective, double-blind, randomized controlled trial, 144 patients, each with at least five AKs on the face, were randomized to receive 1 week of treatment with 0.5% 5-FU cream daily for 7 days or placebo cream. Patients were then treated with single freeze–thaw cycle cryotherapy using liquid nitrogen, with a freeze time of 10 seconds. These patients were then followed up at 4 weeks and 6 months. The authors found that at 4 weeks, 16.7% of patients in the 5-FU group were completely clear of lesions, compared with 0% in the vehicle group ($p < 0.001$). At 6 months posttreatment, 30% of patients in the 5-FU group were clear of lesions, compared with 7.7% of patients in the vehicle group ($p < 0.001$).

Imiquimod 5% cream for the treatment of actinic keratosis: results from two phase III, randomized, double-blind, parallel group, vehicle-controlled trials. Lebwohl M, Dinehart S, Whiting D, Lee PK, Tawfik N, Jorizzo J, et al. J Am Acad Dermatol 2004; 50: 714–21.

In this report of two phase III double-blind, vehicle-controlled studies, 436 subjects at 24 centers in the United States were randomized to either 5% imiquimod or vehicle applied once daily,

2 days per week, for 16 weeks. The complete clearance rate for the treated arm was 45%, as opposed to 3.2% for the vehicle group. The median percent reduction in AK lesions was 83% for the treated group and 0% for the vehicle group, indicating that a reduced frequency of imiquimod application is quite effective.

Imiquimod 2.5% and 3.75% for the treatment of actinic keratoses: results of two placebo-controlled studies of daily application to the face and balding scalp for two 3-week cycles. Hanke CW, Beer KR, Stockfleth E, Wu J, Rosen T, Levy S. J Am Acad Dermatol 2010; 62: 573–81.

Imiquimod 2.5% and 3.75% for the treatment of actinic keratoses: results of two placebo-controlled studies of daily application to the face and balding scalp for two 2-week cycles. Swanson N, Abramovits A, Berman B, Kulp J, Rigel DS, Levy S. J Am Acad Dermatol 2010; 62: 582–90.

These two back-to-back reports demonstrate the efficacy and tolerability of lower-concentration formulations of imiquimod, as well as alternate dosing schedules. Interestingly, the results were essentially identical for two 3-week cycles as they were for two 2-week cycles, with the 3.75% strength imiquimod proving superior to the 2.5% in both studies and slightly less efficacious than previous studies that have investigated 5% imiquimod used twice weekly for 16 weeks.

A randomised study of topical 5% imiquimod vs. topical 5-fluorouracil vs. cryosurgery in immunocompetent patients with actinic keratoses: a comparison of clinical and histologic outcomes including 1-year follow-up. Krawtchenko N, Roewert-Huber J, Ulrich M, Mann I, Sterry W, Stockfleth E. Br J Dermatol 2007; 157 (Suppl 2): 34–40.

This study compared the baseline and 1-year follow-up rates of clinical clearance, histologic clearance, and cosmetic outcomes of imiquimod, 5-FU, and cryosurgery for the treatment of AKs. Patients were randomized to one of the three treatment groups. Clinical clearance was achieved in 68% of those treated with cryosurgery, 96% with 5-FU, and 85% with imiquimod. Histologic clearance rate was 32% for cryosurgery, 67% for 5-FU, and 73% for imiquimod. The 1-year sustained clearance rate was 28% for cryosurgery, 54% for 5-FU, and 73% for imiquimod. The patients treated with imiquimod were also judged to have superior cosmetic outcomes.

Guidelines on the use of photodynamic therapy for nonmelanoma skin cancer: an international consensus. Braathen LR, Szeimies R, Basset-Seguin N, Bissonnette R, Foley P, Pariser D, et al. J Am Acad Dermatol 2007; 56: 125–43.

This is a comprehensive evidence-based review and treatment recommendations for the use of PDT to treat nonmelanoma skin cancers, including AKs. The authors review each of the main clinical trials using PDT to treat AKs and conclude that PDT with MAL and ALA is highly effective, offering excellent cosmetic results, and should be considered as first-line therapy.

Intraindividual, right–left comparison of topical methyl aminolaevulinate–photodynamic therapy and cryotherapy in subjects with actinic keratoses: a multicentre, randomized controlled study. Morton C, Campbell S, Gupta G, Keohane S, Lear J, Zaki I, et al. Br J Dermatol 2006; 155: 1029–36.

In this 24-week study subjects received one treatment session of PDT to one side of their face and two cycles of freeze–thaw cryosurgery to the other. Of the 1501 lesions treated, PDT resulted in a higher rate of cure (87% vs. 76% reduction from baseline). Both subjects and investigators preferred PDT and also felt it had a better cosmetic outcome. Both treatment regimens were deemed safe and well tolerated.

Multicentre intraindividual randomized trial of topical methyl aminolaevulinate–photodynamic therapy vs. cryotherapy for multiple actinic keratoses on the extremities. Kaufmann R, Spelman L, Weightman W, Reifenberger J, Szeimies RM, Verhaeghe E, et al. Br J Dermatol 2008; 158: 994–9.

This was another intraindividual trial that treated one side of the body (nonface/scalp) with a single course of PDT and the other with cryotherapy. For the 1343 lesions treated, both treatment modalities had high efficacy rates at 24 weeks, although cryosurgery performed better (78% for PDT and 88% for cryosurgery). Investigator and patient assessment of cosmetic outcome was much higher for PDT than for cryosurgery (79% vs. 56% of lesions having "excellent cosmetic outcome" based on investigator evaluation, 50% vs. 22% based on patient evaluation).

Photodynamic therapy with aminolevulinic acid topical solution and visible blue light in the treatment of multiple actinic keratoses of the face and scalp: investigator-blinded, phase 3, multicenter trials. Piacquadio DJ, Chen DM, Farber HF, Fowler JF Jr, Glazer SD, Goodman JJ, et al. Arch Dermatol 2004; 140: 41–6.

In this randomized, placebo-controlled study 243 patients were randomized to receive vehicle or ALA followed by PDT within 14 to 18 hours. Clinical response rate was based on complete clearing of 75% of lesions measured at weeks 8 and 12. Of the PDT-treated group, 77% had a complete response by week 8 and 89% by week 12. This compared with 18% and 13% for the placebo group. Most patients experienced erythema and edema at the treated sites, which improved within 4 weeks of therapy. Stinging, burning, or pain occurred during the treatments, but resolved within 24 hours.

Results of an investigator-initiated single-blind split-face comparison of photodynamic therapy and 5% imiquimod cream for the treatment of actinic keratoses. Hadley J, Tristani-Firouzi P, Hull C, Florell S, Cotter M, Hadley M. Dermatol Surg 2012; 38: 722–7.

In this split-faced trial, 61 patients received 5% imiquimod twice weekly to half the face and two sessions of ALA-PDT to the other side of the face. No significant difference was noted with respect to partial or total clearance rate; however, ALA-PDT was superior when mean lesion reduction rate was evaluated.

Daylight photodynamic therapy with MAL cream for large-scale photodamaged skin based on the concept of 'actinic field damage': recommendations of an international expert group. Philipp-Dormston WG, Sanclemente G, Torezan L, Tretti Clementoni M, Le Pillouer-Prost A, Cartier H, et al. J Eur Acad Dermatol Venereol 2016; 30: 8–15.

A review of daylight PDT in both European and Australasian trials. Daylight MAL-PDT had a similar efficacy to conventional light source PDT at 3-month (lesion complete response rate of 89% vs. 93% in the Australian study and 70% vs. 74% in the European study, respectively) and 6-month follow-ups (97% maintenance of complete lesion response) in the treatment of AKs. Daylight PDT is not only efficacious, but also nearly pain free and easy to perform, and therefore results in high patient acceptance, especially for the treatment of areas of actinic field damage.

Network meta-analysis of the outcome 'participant complete clearance' in nonimmunosuppressed participants of eight interventions for actinic keratosis: a follow-up on a Cochrane review. Gupta AK, Paquet M. Br J Derm 2013; 169: 250–9.

In this thorough meta-analysis of eight common treatments for AKs, the authors conclude that 5% 5-FU was superior in achieving complete clearance. They comment on the inherent difficulty in comparing studies.

Second-Line Therapies	
• Topical adapalene	A
• Topical diclofenac	A
• Topical ingenol mebutate	A

Assessment of adapalene gel for the treatment of actinic keratoses and lentigines: a randomized trial. Kang S, Goldfarb MT, Weiss JS, Metz RD, Hamilton TA, Voorhees JJ, et al. J Am Acad Dermatol 2003; 49: 83–90.

In this prospective randomized, vehicle-controlled study 90 patients received either 0.1% adapalene gel, 0.3% adapalene gel, or vehicle gel, initially daily for 4 weeks, then twice daily for up to 9 months. Overall, 62% ($p < 0.01$) of those who received 0.1% adapalene gel and 66% ($p < 0.01$) of those who received 0.3% adapalene gel showed at least a moderate improvement of their AKs, compared with 34% of patients receiving a vehicle cream. Adapalene gel recipients reported a higher level of mild erythema, peeling, and dryness compared with control groups.

Three percent diclofenac in 2.5% hyaluronan gel in the treatment of actinic keratoses: a meta-analysis of the recent studies. Pirard D, Vereecken P, Melot C, Heenen M. Arch Dermatol Res 2005; 297: 185–9.

This meta-analysis pooled 364 patients from three studies that compared diclofenac with hyaluronan vehicle gel. Overall, patients treated with diclofenac had a significantly higher rate of complete clearance of lesions. They concluded that complete response rates were 39% with a mean treatment duration of 75 ± 21 days. Mild-to-moderate skin irritation was the major side effect of the treatment group.

Diclofenac sodium 3% gel for the management of actinic keratosis: 10+ years of cumulative evidence of efficacy and safety. Martin GM, Stockfleth E. J Drugs Dermatol 2012; 11: 600–8.

This comprehensive review draws from 17 publications beyond the initial phase III clinical trials that led to the approval of diclofenac sodium for the treatment of AKs. It discusses the data with regard to treatment efficacy, tolerability, and performance compared with other topical field agents, as well as its use in combination treatment strategies.

Ingenol mebutate gel for actinic keratosis. Lebwohl M, Swanson N, Anderson LL, Melgaard A, Xu Z, Berman B. N Engl J Med 2012; 366: 1010–19.

This multicenter, randomized, double-blind report investigated the use of 0.015% ingenol mebutate (IM) used once daily for 3 consecutive days for AKs on the face and scalp, as well as 0.05% IM used once daily for 2 consecutive days for AKs on the trunk and extremities. All analyses were conducted at day 57. The rate of complete clearance was 42% for the face/scalp group and 34% for the trunk/extremities group. Local skin reactions peaked between day 3 and day 8 and were mild to moderate in nature. Hypertrophic or hyperkeratotic lesions were excluded from the study.

Evidence Levels: **A** Double-blind study **B** Clinical trial ≥ 20 subjects **C** Clinical trial < 20 subjects **D** Series ≥ 5 subjects **E** Anecdotal case reports

Randomized, double-blind, double-dummy, vehicle-controlled study of ingenol mebutate gel 0.025% and 0.05% for actinic keratosis. Anderson L, Schmieder GJ, Werschler WP, Tschen EH, Ling MR, Stough DB, et al. J Am Acad Dermatol 2009; 60: 934–43.

A total of 222 patients from 22 U.S. centers with nonfacial AKs were randomized to receive vehicle for 3 days, 0.025% ingenol mebutate (IM) gel for 3 days, vehicle for 1 day followed by 0.05% IM gel for 2 days, or 0.05% IM gel for 3 days. Partial clearance rate (>75% reduction in baseline AKs), as well as complete clearance rate, was statistically significantly higher in all three treatment groups over baseline, and these results were dose dependent. Partial and complete clearance rates were 28%/20% for the 0.025% × 3 days group, 34%/24% for the 0.05% × 2 days group, and 43%/31% for the 0.05% × 3 days cohort. The most common local skin responses seen in all groups included erythema, scaling, crusting, swelling, erosion/ulceration, vesiculation, and pigmentary changes and were largely resolved by day 15. Patient satisfaction was high.

Third-Line Therapies	
• Curettage	E
• Excision	E
• Laser resurfacing	B
• Chemical peels	D
• Dermabrasion	D

Full face laser resurfacing: therapy and prophylaxis for actinic keratoses and nonmelanoma skin cancer. Iyer S, Friedli A, Bowes L, Kricorian G, Fitzpatrick RE. Lasers Surg Med 2004; 34: 114–19.

In this retrospective study of 24 patients with over 30 AKs on the face treated with full-face ultrapulse CO_2 laser or erbium (Er):YAG laser resurfacing, the authors found that 21 patients remained lesion free for at least 1 year.

Recurrence rates and long-term follow-up after laser resurfacing as a treatment for widespread actinic keratoses on the face and scalp. Ostertag JU, Quaedvlieg PJ, Neumann MH, Krekels GA. Dermatol Surg 2006; 32: 261–7.

A retrospective case-control study of 25 patients who underwent laser resurfacing for widespread AKs on the scalp and/or face. Forty-four percent had no recurrence in an average follow-up period of 39 months (range 7–70 months).

Nonablative fractional photothermolysis for facial actinic keratoses: 6-month follow-up with histologic evaluation. Katz TM, Goldberg LH, Marquez D, Kimyai-Asadi A, Polder KD, Landau JM, et al. J Am Acad Dermatol 2011; 65: 349–56.

In this study, 14 patients underwent five treatments of nonablative fractional resurfacing with 32% to 40% surface area coverage at 2- to 4-week intervals. Clinical images and biopsies were evaluated. Although clinical images had a reduced number of AKs, virtually all histologic specimens were positive for features of AK and/or SCC. It was concluded that fractional nonablative resurfacing was not adequate therapy for AKs.

A clinical comparison and long-term follow-up of topical 5-fluorouracil versus laser resurfacing in the treatment of widespread actinic keratoses. Ostertag JU, Quaedvlieg PJ, van der Geer S, Nelemans P, Christianen ME, Neumann MH, et al. Lasers Surg Med 2006; 38: 731–9.

A prospective randomized trial of 55 patients comparing 5-FU with Er:YAG laser resurfacing. At 3, 6, and 12 months there were significantly fewer recurrences in the laser group than in the 5-FU group. Side effects were more common in the group treated with laser resurfacing and included erythema and hypopigmentation.

Long-term efficacy and safety of Jessner's solution and 35% trichloroacetic acid vs. 5% fluorouracil in the treatment of widespread facial actinic keratoses. Witheiler DD, Lawrence N, Cox SE, Cruz C, Cockerell CJ, Freemen RG. Dermatol Surg 1997; 23: 191–6.

In this prospective study, 15 patients with severe facial AKs were treated on one side of the face with a single application of Jessner solution—a medium-depth chemical peel—and the other side with twice-daily applications of topical 5-FU 5% for 3 weeks. The authors found that both treatments resulted in a similar reduction of AKs at 12 months, with an increase in the number of AKs in both groups from 12 to 32 months. The authors concluded that both treatments were similarly efficacious in the treatment of AK and that retreatment for recurrences might be necessary after 12 months.

Dermabrasion for prophylaxis and treatment of actinic keratoses. Coleman WP, Yardborough JM, Mandy SH. Dermatol Surg 1996; 22: 17–21.

In this retrospective study, 23 patients who had undergone dermabrasion for facial AKs were followed for 2 to 5 years. The authors found that the benefits of dermabrasion diminished with time: 1 year postdermabrasion, 22 patients remained clear of AKs. Of 13 patients who were followed up for 5 years, 7 remained clear. The authors concluded that dermabrasion provided long term clearance of AKs in some patients.

Recalcitrant treatment-resistant AKs may be treated with physically destructive approaches that include curettage and surgical excision. Both techniques enable tissue to be obtained for histologic analysis. Surgical excision is particularly useful in lesions suspected of being SCC because this technique enables the clinician to treat the lesion and establish the diagnosis. Widespread, extensive AKs may benefit from field treatments of a destructive nature. These include ablative laser resurfacing, dermabrasion, and chemical peels.

Actinic prurigo

Robert S. Dawe, Martha C. Valbuena

(*Synonyms:* hereditary polymorphic light eruption of American Indians, Hutchinson summer prurigo, photodermatitis in North American Indians)

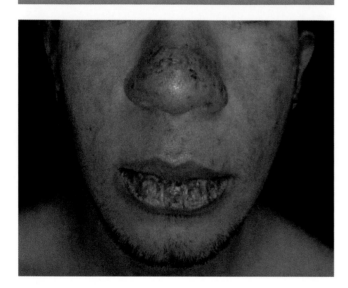

Actinic prurigo (AP) is a distinct photodermatosis, diagnosed on the basis of characteristic clinical features. It has a perennial nature, although it is worse in the sunnier months in countries with seasonal variation in sunlight exposure. Morphologically, it presents as a papular or mixed papular and vesicular (in Latin America, vesicles usually being a feature of eczematization or secondary infection) eruption during acute flares, persistent eroded nodules, and/or dermatitic patches (sometimes affecting covered sites), scarring, dorsal nose involvement, cheilitis, and conjunctivitis. Abnormal photosensitivity (to ultraviolet A [UVA], ultraviolet B [UVB]) is frequently severe, but when onset has been in childhood, the condition generally gradually improves (probably largely by learning to live with the condition), especially when presenting before the usual age of 10 years.

MANAGEMENT STRATEGY

Diagnosis is normally straightforward, but the differential diagnosis can include severe polymorphic light eruption and photoaggravated atopic dermatitis. Although differences between European and Amerindian forms of AP have been described, these are either closely related conditions or the same disease with some differences affected by population and environment. Phototesting and human leukocyte antigen (HLA) typing may sometimes be helpful in cases of diagnostic uncertainty. Possible coexisting conditions such as sunscreen allergic contact dermatitis or photocontact reactions should be considered, as their presence will affect the recommended treatments.

Once the diagnosis is established, initial treatment consists of advice on *sunlight avoidance* measures (behavioral, clothing, and topical sunscreen) and the use of potent or very potent *topical corticosteroids*. *Topical tacrolimus* can also be used, especially if prolonged treatment to the face is required. This approach alone is often insufficient, and many patients require the addition of a springtime course of narrowband (TL-01) UVB or psoralen-ultraviolet A (PUVA). When *phototherapy* is administered for this indication, only normally sunlight-exposed sites should be treated. It is helpful to apply a potent topical steroid to the treated areas immediately after each exposure to reduce the risk of AP flares.

In Scotland, systemic treatment is rarely required; it is more often necessary where the availability of phototherapy is limited and in countries with more intense year-round sunlight exposure. *Antimalarials* and *β-carotene* are sometimes tried, but it remains uncertain whether they are truly of value. *Thalidomide* is useful, but its value is restricted by teratogenicity and the risk of irreversible peripheral neuropathy. *Pentoxifylline* has anti–tumor necrosis factor (TNF)-α effects and, although listed as a third-line therapy here, may sometimes be worth considering before thalidomide because of its more attractive safety profile.

Specific Investigations

- Phototesting
- HLA typing
- Histopathology of cheilitis

Actinic prurigo—a specific photodermatosis? Addo HA, Frain-Bell W. Photodermatology 1984; 1: 119–28.

This study showed that almost 60% of AP patients have abnormal delayed erythema on monochromator phototesting.

Phototest abnormalities tend to be more severe in AP than in polymorphic light eruption.

Actinic prurigo among the Chimila Indians in Colombia: HLA studies. Bernal JE, Duran de Rueda MM, Ordonez CP, Duran C, de Brigard D. J Am Acad Dermatol 1990; 22: 1049–51.

In this population, the HLA class I antigen Cw4 was more frequent in AP patients than in controls.

HLA-DR4 may determine expression of actinic prurigo in British patients. Menage H du P, Vaughan RW, Baker CS, Page G, Proby CM, Breathnach SM, et al. J Invest Dermatol 1996; 106: 362–7.

Actinic prurigo and HLA-DR4. Dawe RS, Collins P, O'Sullivan A, Ferguson J. J Invest Dermatol 1997; 108: 233–4.

An even stronger association with the HLA class II antigen HLA-DR4 was shown and, more specifically, with HLA-DRB1*0407.

Association of HLA subtype DRB10407 in Colombian patients with actinic prurigo. Suárez A, Valbuena MC, Rey M, de Porras Quintana L. Photodermatol Photoimmunol Photomed 2006; 22: 55–8.

These associations are not a feature of polymorphic light eruption. The absence of HLA-DR4 can help to rule out the diagnosis of AP, whereas the presence of HLA-DRB1*0407 helps to rule in the diagnosis.

Actinic prurigo: clinical features and HLA associations in a Canadian Inuit population. Wiseman MC, Orr PH, MacDonald SM, Schroeder ML, Toole JW. J Am Acad Dermatol 2001; 44: 952–6.

No statistically significant association of AP with HLA-DR4 (frequent in the studied population) or HLA-DRB1*0407 was detected, and another HLA type (DRB1*14) was found more commonly than expected, although it was only present in 19 of 37 AP subjects. The authors acknowledge the possibility that they were studying a different condition from AP in other populations.

Actinic prurigo in Singaporean Chinese: a positive association with HLA-DRB1*03:01. Chen Q, Shen M, Heng YK, Theng TS, Tey HL, Ren EC, et al. Photochem Photobiol 2016; 92: 355–9.

In this population the strongest association was with HLA-DRB1*03:01, although it should be noted that although a strong association was compared with controls, only 6 of these 14 Chinese Singaporean patients diagnosed with AP had this HLA allele.

These findings suggest we should be cautious in attempting to use HLA typing as a diagnostic test, especially in populations in which strong HLA associations have not been confirmed. The diagnosis should still be based on the characteristic constellation of clinical features.

Actinic prurigo of the lower lip – review of the literature and report of five cases. Mounsdon T, Kratochvil F, Auclair P, Neale J, Lee L. Oral Surg Oral Med Oral Pathol 1988; 65: 327–32.

Follicular cheilitis – a distinctive histopathologic finding in actinic prurigo. Herrera-Geopfert R, Magana M. Am J Dermatopathol 1995; 17: 357–61.

Actinic prurigo cheilitis: clinicopathologic analysis and therapeutic results in 116 cases. Vega-Memije ME, Mosqueda-Taylor A, Irigoyen-Camacho ME, Hojyo-Tomoka MT, Dominguez-Soto L. Oral Surg Oral Med Oral Pathol Oral Radiol Endod 2002; 94: 83–91.

A "follicular cheilitis" has been reported to be characteristic of AP. Thirty-two of 116 patients attending a dermatology clinic in Mexico City had cheilitis as their sole manifestation of disease.

Lip histopathology may be helpful diagnostically, especially in patients presenting with cheilitis without cutaneous features at presentation. Where other typical features (skin, eyes) are present, it is arguable how much lip histopathology will contribute to diagnosis.

First-Line Therapies

* Sunlight avoidance – environmental, behavioral, clothing, topical sunscreen   C
* Potent/very potent topical corticosteroids   C
* Topical tacrolimus   E
* Narrowband (TL-01 lamp) UVB phototherapy   C

Topical photoprotection for hereditary polymorphic light eruption of American Indians. Fusaro RM, Johnson JA. J Am Acad Dermatol 1991; 24: 744–6.

The authors of this open study found 18 of 30 patients with hereditary polymorphic light eruption of American Indians (with described features indistinguishable from AP) to show "good to excellent results" with use of a broad-spectrum sunscreen.

Although broad-spectrum sunscreens are useful, advice on other sunlight avoidance measures, including appropriate clothing and behavioral avoidance, is equally important.

Actinic prurigo deterioration due to degradation of DermaGard window film. Kerr AC, Ferguson J. Br J Dermatol 2007; 157: 619–20.

Window films that reduce the transmission of UV rays can be used as a method of environmental photoprotection. This case report describes an exacerbation of AP explained by increased transmission through such a window film as it aged. Because the technology of such window films has matured, such degradation now might be less likely, but the possibility of it should be considered.

Treatment of actinic prurigo with intermittent short-course topical 0.05% clobetasol 17-propionate: a preliminary report. Lane PR, Moreland AA, Hogan DJ. Arch Dermatol 1990; 126: 1211–3.

Seven out of eight patients treated with intermittent 3- to 14-day courses of topical 0.05% clobetasol 17–propionate cream or ointment cleared or markedly improved. All had previously found less potent topical steroids ineffective.

Narrow-band UVB (TL-01) phototherapy: an effective preventative treatment for the photodermatoses. Collins P, Ferguson J. Br J Dermatol 1995; 132: 956–63.

Six patients with AP were included in this open study. All reported at least a sixfold increase in tolerable duration of sunlight exposure, which was sustained 4 months after treatment. In one patient whose phototesting (severely abnormal before treatment) was repeated after treatment, the test results normalized.

Actinic prurigo: treatment with tacrolimus. Favorable response in two pediatric patients. Vivoda JI, Mantero N, Jaime LJ, Rueda ML, Grees SA. Rev Arg Derm 2015; 96: 30–4.

These two girls showed a good response by 10 days of treatment with tacrolimus ointment.

Treatment of actinic prurigo with tacrolimus 0.1%. Gonzalez-Carrascosa Ballesteros M, De la Cueva DP, Hernanz Hermosa JM, Chavarria E. Med Cutan Ibero Lat Am 2006; 34: 233–6.

A 13-year-old boy with only facial involvement with AP was reported to respond rapidly to 0.1% tacrolimus ointment after topical corticosteroids (uncertain what strengths) had not worked.

Tacrolimus ointment can be helpful in treating facial AP, especially when there are concerns about topical corticosteroid adverse effects.

The quality of life of 790 patients with photodermatoses. Jong CT, Finlay AY, Pearse AD, Kerr AC, Ferguson J, Benton EC, et al. Br J Dermatol 2008; 159: 192–7.

Of the photodermatoses assessed in the British tertiary referral photodermatology centers participating in this study, AP was associated with the greatest health-related quality of life impairment. We do not know whether measuring health-related quality of life is useful in the day-to-day management of these patients, but important effects of AP on quality of life should be considered when planning treatments.

Second-Line Therapies

* Psoralen–UVA photochemotherapy   C
* Thalidomide   C

Treatment of actinic prurigo with PUVA: mechanism of action. Farr PM, Diffey BL. Br J Dermatol 1989; 120: 411–8.

Five patients were treated in this open study. Clinical improvement was accompanied by an increase of UVA minimal erythemal doses to within the normal range on phototesting. Corroboration that PUVA worked through a local effect was provided by before and after phototesting of areas kept covered during treatment. The UVA minimal erythema dose did not increase in these areas.

In the absence of any controlled study comparisons of PUVA and TL-01 phototherapy for this condition, PUVA should generally be reserved for those who fail to benefit from TL-01.

Thalidomide in the treatment of actinic prurigo. Londoño F. Int J Dermatol 1973; 12: 326–8.

Thirty-four patients were treated, with a starting dose of 300 mg thalidomide daily, gradually reducing to a minimum of 15 mg; 32 had good results while on the drug, but relapsed on stopping.

Thalidomide in actinic prurigo. Lovell CR, Hawk JL, Calnan CD, Magnus IA. Br J Dermatol 1983; 108: 467–71.

Of 14 patients treated with thalidomide (adult starting dose 100–200 mg daily), 13 (one could not tolerate the drug due to dizziness) reported improvement. This benefit was sustained in 11, of whom 8 required maintenance doses of between 50 mg weekly and 100 mg daily.

Includes a review of earlier open studies reporting the use of thalidomide in AP.

Third-Line Therapies

• β-Carotene	C
• Pentoxifylline	C
• Tetracycline and vitamin E	C
• Oral corticosteroids	E
• Azathioprine	E
• Chloroquine	E
• Ciclosporin eye drops	E

Hereditary polymorphic light eruption in American Indians: photoprotection and prevention of streptococcal pyoderma and glomerulonephritis. Fusaro RM, Johnson JA. JAMA 1980; 244: 1456–9.

Seventeen of 54 patients who participated in this open study were reported to have achieved complete photoprotection, and 16 "marked improvement." The plasma carotene level tended to be higher in those who benefited. The authors also comment on their use of dihydroxyacetone and lawsone cream, with apparent benefit.

The clinical features of the study patients were not reported, but the authors' introductory description of hereditary polymorphic light eruption suggests that they probably included AP.

Pentoxifylline in the treatment of actinic prurigo: a preliminary report of 10 patients. Torres-Alvarez B, Castanedo-Cazares JP, Moncada B. Dermatology 2004; 208: 198–201.

Clinical improvement was reported in all 10 participants in this 6-month open-label uncontrolled study.

Treatment of actinic prurigo in Chimila Indians. Duran MM, Ordonez CP, Prieto JC, Bernal J. Int J Dermatol 1996; 35: 413–16.

One group of eight patients was treated with tetracycline (1.5 g daily), and another eight with vitamin E (100 IU daily). On follow-up analysis comparing signs and itch, no difference was found between the groups. Both treatments were considered promising and the possibility of using a tetracycline–vitamin E combination therapy raised.

These treatments need further investigation, but may be worth considering if first-line therapies are inadequate and thalidomide is contraindicated or not tolerated.

The clinical features and management of actinic prurigo: a retrospective study. Lestarini D, Khoo LS, Goh CL. Photodermatol Photoimmunol Photomed 1999; 15: 183–7.

This is a review of the features and clinical course of 11 patients. Of three treated with systemic corticosteroids, one improved slightly. Intralesional steroids helped one. Three patients were treated with azathioprine: two appeared to benefit.

Actinic prurigo: clinico-pathologic correlation. Hojyo-Tomoka MT, Dominguez-Soto L, Vargasocamp F. Int J Dermatol 1978; 17: 706–10.

In this review, the authors comment that chloroquine "seems to give temporary relief" and also suggest that antihistamines and tranquilizers may be of some benefit.

Use of topical ciclosporin for conjunctival manifestations of actinic prurigo. McCoombes JA, Hirst LW, Green WR. Am J Ophthalmol 2000; 130: 830–1.

Topical ciclosporin in the treatment of ocular actinic prurigo. Ortiz-Castillo JV, Boto-De-Los-Bueis A, De-Lucas-Laguna R, Pastor-Nieto B, Peláez-Restrepo N, Fonseca-Sandomingo A. Arch Soc Esp Oftalmol 2006; 81: 661–4.

In these two case reports topical 2% ciclosporin eye drops were associated with improvement in chronic AP conjunctivitis.

Evidence Levels: **A** Double-blind study **B** Clinical trial ≥ 20 subjects **C** Clinical trial < 20 subjects **D** Series ≥ 5 subjects **E** Anecdotal case reports

7

Actinomycosis

Jonathan E. Blume, Daniel Caplivski

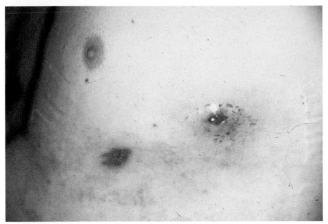

Actinomycosis is an indolent infection that may be difficult to recognize initially and is caused by an anaerobic, gram-positive rod that is a normal human commensal. Infections are usually the result of introduction of bacteria into a normally sterile space from the oropharynx, gastrointestinal tract, or vaginal tract. The organism may be difficult to recover in the microbiology laboratory because it grows slowly and is ideally cultured under anaerobic conditions. Microscopically, it has a similar appearance to *Nocardia* spp.; however, it does not retain the modified acid-fast stain, and the colonies may have a molar tooth appearance. Infections of the cervical region are typified by the slow induration of the skin at the angle of the jaw that progresses over several weeks or months. A mass may be palpable and, due to the slow progression and absence of systemic inflammatory symptoms, the infection can often be confused with other conditions such as malignancies. Patients may notice the discharge of small yellow grains known as *sulfur granules*. These are macroscopic colonies of the organism that may be cultured for confirmation, but their absence should not exclude the diagnosis from consideration.

MANAGEMENT STRATEGY

Actinomyces spp. are universally susceptible to penicillin. The severity of the illness will dictate whether the patient requires intravenous or oral formulations of the antibiotic, but the general principle is that prolonged treatments for 6 months or more are often required for cure. In patients who are penicillin allergic, the tetracycline class of antibiotics is a useful substitute. Surgical removal of the abscess may also be required in order to ensure complete resolution. Treatment failures are rare, but may be due to coinfecting organisms from the oropharynx. In order to treat these organisms, the combination of a β-lactam antibiotic with a β-lactamase inhibitor may be sufficient. Carbapenems such as imipenem, meropenem, or ertapenem are also effective.

Clinical review: actinomycosis. Wong VK, Turmezei TD, Weston VC. BMJ 2011; 343: d6099.

Susceptibility of pathogenic actinomycetes to antimicrobial compounds. Lerner PI. Antimicrob Agents Chemother 1974; 5: 302–9.

SPECIFIC INVESTIGATIONS

Diagnostic methods for human actinomycosis. Holmberg K. Microbiol Sci 1987; 4: 72–8.

An excellent review of the diagnosis of actinomycosis.

The most accurate way to diagnose actinomycosis is by culture—usually a difficult task—which requires thioglycolate or brain–heart-enriched agar at 37°C under anaerobic or microaerophilic conditions. "Molar-tooth" and "breadcrumb" colonies may take up to 3 weeks to grow. Unfortunately, definitive identification cannot be based on colony morphology and requires the measurement of physiologic and biochemical characteristics (e.g., sensitivity to oxygen, presence of preformed enzymes).

Because cultures of *Actinomyces* spp. are often unsuccessful, observation of "sulfur granules" on a peripheral smear or histology often helps make the diagnosis. The granules are bacterial colonies, which on hematoxylin and eosin staining have a basophilic central area surrounded by a zone of eosinophilic "clubs." Other typical histologic findings include extensive fibrosis, chronic granulation tissue, sinus tracts, and scattered microabscesses.

Immunofluorescent staining of *Actinomyces* spp. is available and can be used on clinical material, granules, and formalin-fixed tissues. The direct immunoperoxidase technique can specifically show *Actinomyces* spp. in formalin-fixed sections via light microscopy. These techniques, as well as gene sequencing (see later), are promising diagnostic modalities given the difficulty of culture and histologic identification.

Cervicofacial actinomycosis: diagnosis and management. Oostman O, Smego RA. Curr Infect Dis Resp 2005; 7: 170–4.

Culture isolation of *Actinomyces* spp. and microscopic visualization of gram-positive, nonacid-fast, thin, branching filaments remain the best methods of diagnosing cervicofacial actinomycosis.

Diagnosis of pelvic actinomycosis by 16S ribosomal RNA gene sequencing and its clinical significance. Woo PCY, Fung AMY, Lau SKP, Hon E, Yuen KY. Diagn Microbiol Infect Dis 2002; 43: 113–8.

Actinomyces odontolyticus was identified by rRNA gene sequencing. Because the 16 S ribosomal RNA gene is conserved within a species, it can be used to identify a specific species of bacteria.

Cervicofacial actinomycosis: CT and MR imaging findings in 7 patients. Park JK, Lee HK, Ha HK, Choi HY, Choi CG. AJNR Am J Neuroradiol 2003; 24: 331–3.

Findings on computed tomography (CT) and magnetic resonance imaging (MRI) may be helpful in distinguishing cervicofacial actinomycosis from malignant neoplasms, tuberculosis, and fungal infections.

First-Line Therapy

- Penicillin   C

Antimicrobial susceptibility testing of *Actinomyces* species with 12 antimicrobial agents. Smith AJ, Hall V, Thakker B, Gemmell CG. J Antimicrob Chemother 2005; 56: 407–9.

The authors tested the susceptibility of 87 strains of *Actinomyces* to 12 different antimicrobial agents. All isolates were susceptible to penicillin and amoxicillin.

Actinomycosis. Smego RA, Foglia G. Clin Infect Dis 1998; 26: 1255–63.

The authors recommend 2 months of oral penicillin V (2–4 g/day divided every 6 hours) or a tetracycline (e.g., oral doxycycline 100 mg twice daily) for mild cervicofacial disease. For more complicated infections, parenteral penicillin G (10–20 million U/day divided every 6 hours) for 4 to 6 weeks followed by 6 to 12 months of oral penicillin V (2–4 g/day divided every 6 hours) is suggested. Tetracycline, erythromycin, clindamycin, or cephalosporins are advocated for patients allergic to penicillin.

Actinomycosis and nocardiosis. A review of basic differences in therapy. Peabody JW, Seabury JH. Am J Med 1960; 28: 99–115.

The authors review the treatment of actinomycosis and state that penicillin is the drug of choice.

Second-Line Therapies	
• Amoxicillin	C
• Ceftriaxone	D
• Clindamycin	C
• Doxycycline	D
• Erythromycin	D
• Imipenem	C
• Minocycline	C
• Tetracycline	D

The use of oral amoxicillin for the treatment of actinomycosis: a clinical and in vitro study. Martin MV. Br Dent J 1984; 156: 252–4.

Ten patients with cervicofacial actinomycosis were cured in less than 6 weeks with a combination of amoxicillin (500 mg four times daily) and surgery.

Actinomycosis abscess of the thyroid gland. Cevera JJ, Butehorn HF, Shapiro J, Setzen G. Laryngoscope 2003; 113: 2108–11.

A 39-year-old woman who developed actinomycosis of the thyroid gland after tooth extraction was cured with thyroidectomy and 6 months of ceftriaxone (1 g intravenously every 12 hours).

Successful treatment of thoracic actinomycosis with ceftriaxone. Skoutelis A, Petrochilos J, Bassaris H. Clin Infect Dis 1994; 19: 161–2.

A 38-year-old patient with pulmonary actinomycosis was successfully treated with a 3-week course of daily ceftriaxone (2 g intravenously), followed by 3 months of daily oral ampicillin (no dose listed but typically given 500 mg orally every 6 hours).

Mandibular actinomycosis treated with oral clindamycin. Badgett JT, Adams G. Pediatr Infect Dis J 1987; 6: 221–2.

Clindamycin in the treatment of cervicofacial actinomycosis. deVries J, Bentley KC. Int J Clin Pharmacol 1974; 9: 46–8.

A 60-year-old man with cervicofacial actinomycosis that was resistant to penicillin and tetracycline responded fully to a 1-month course of clindamycin (150 mg four times a day).

Clindamycin in the treatment of serious anaerobic infections. Fass RJ, Scholand JF, Hodges GR, Saslaw S. Ann Intern Med 1973; 78: 853–9.

Four patients with cervicofacial actinomycosis and one with thoracic actinomycosis were successfully treated with a combination of intravenous (1.8–2.7 g/day) and oral (0.9–1.2 g/day) clindamycin.

Primary actinomycosis of the hand: a case report and literature review. Mert A, Bilir M, Bahar H, Torun M, Tabak F, Ozturk R, et al. Int J Infect Dis 2001; 5: 112–4.

A 35-year-old man with primary actinomycosis of the hand was cured with 1 month of intravenous ampicillin (12 g/day), followed by 11 months of oral doxycycline (200 mg/day).

Actinomycosis of the prostate. de Souza E, Katz DA, Dworzack DL, Longo G. J Urol 1985; 133: 290–1.

A case of acute prostatitis due to *Actinomyces* spp. was cured with long-term erythromycin (500 mg intravenously every 6 hours followed by 500 mg orally every 6 hours), chosen because of its excellent penetration into prostatic secretions.

Actinomycosis of the temporomandibular joint. Bradley P. Br J Oral Surg 1971; 9: 54–6.

A 58-year-old man with actinomycosis of the temporomandibular joint was cured with a 12-week course of erythromycin (500 mg six times a day).

Use of imipenem in the treatment of thoracic actinomycosis. Yew WW, Wong PC, Wong CF, Chau CH. Clin Infect Dis 1994; 19: 983–4.

Report of eight cases of pulmonary actinomycosis and their treatment with imipenem–cilastatin. Yew WW, Wong PC, Lee J, Fung SL, Wong CF, Chan CY. Monaldi Arch Chest Dis 1994; 54: 126–9.

Seven of eight patients with pulmonary actinomycosis were successfully treated with a 4-week course of parenteral imipenem–cilastatin (500 mg intravenously every 8 hours).

Cutaneous disseminated actinomycosis in a patient with acute lymphocytic leukemia. Takeda H, Mitsuhashi Y, Kondo S. J Dermatol 1998; 25: 37–40.

A patient with primary cutaneous disseminated actinomycosis was cured with a 3-month course of intravenous minocycline (2 mg/kg/day).

Antibiotic treatment of cervicofacial actinomycosis for patients allergic to penicillin: a clinical and in vitro study. Martin MV. Br J Oral Maxillofac Surg 1985; 23: 428–34.

Six patients with cervicofacial actinomycosis were cured with 8 to 16 weeks of oral minocycline (250 mg four times a day). There were no recurrences after 1 year.

Primary actinomycosis of the quadriceps. Langloh JT, Lauerman WC. J Pediatr Orthop 1987; 7: 222–3.

Surgical drainage followed by a 6-week course of oral tetracycline (500 mg orally every 6 hours) cured a case of actinomycosis of the quadriceps.

Comparative in vitro susceptibilities of 396 unusual anaerobic strains to tigecycline and eight other antimicrobial agents. Goldstein EJ, Citron DM, Merriam CV, Warren YA, Tyrrell KL, Fernandez HT. Antimicrob Agents Chemother 2006; 50: 3507–13.

Evidence Levels: **A** Double-blind study **B** Clinical trial ≥ 20 subjects **C** Clinical trial < 20 subjects **D** Series ≥ 5 subjects **E** Anecdotal case reports

Tigecycline (50 mg intravenously every 12 hours, with a 100-mg loading dose) had good in vitro activity against isolates of *Actinomyces* spp.

Third-Line Therapies	
• Ciprofloxacin	E
• Levofloxacin	E
• Rifampicin	E
• Hyperbaric oxygen	E

Treatment of recalcitrant actinomycosis with ciprofloxacin. Macfarlane DJ, Tucker LG, Kemp RJ. J Infect 1993; 27: 177–80.

Treatment of pulmonary actinomycosis with levofloxacin. Ferreira D de F, Amado J, Neves S, Taveira N, Carvalho A, Nogueira R. J Bras Pneumol 2008; 34: 245–8.

Treatment of pulmonary actinomycosis with rifampin. Morrone N, De Castro Pereira CA, Saito M, Dourado AM, Pereira Da Silva Mendes ES. G Ital Chemioter 1982; 29: 121–4.

Pulmonary actinomycosis. Rapid improvement with isoniazid and rifampin. King JW, White MC. Arch Intern Med 1981; 141: 1234–5.

Adjunctive hyperbaric oxygen therapy for actinomycotic lacrimal canaliculitis. Shauly Y, Nachum Z, Gdal-On M, Melamed Y, Miller B. Graefes Arch Clin Exp Ophthalmol 1993; 231: 429–31.

A 52-year-old patient with treatment-resistant lacrimal canaliculitis due to *A. israelii* was cured with hyperbaric oxygen.

Hyperbaric oxygen in the treatment of actinomycosis. Manheim SD, Voleti C, Ludwig A, Jacobson JH. J Am Med Assoc 1969; 210: 552–3.

After failing to respond to surgery and intravenous penicillin, a 63-year-old patient with perirectal actinomycosis was cured with hyperbaric oxygen.

Acute generalized exanthematous pustulosis

Aysha Javed, Ian H. Coulson

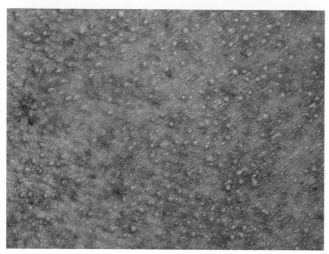

Acute generalized exanthematous pustulosis (AGEP) is characterized by the acute onset of numerous small, nonfollicular, sterile pustules arising on a diffuse erythematous base in a febrile patient with an accompanying blood neutrophilia. The majority of cases occurs in the context of drug ingestion (commonly within 24 hours). Rapid resolution after drug withdrawal is the usual outcome.

MANAGEMENT STRATEGY

Treatment of AGEP involves establishing the correct diagnosis coupled with the *withdrawal of any implicated medication* (Table 8.1). Pustular psoriasis is its main differential diagnosis. A comprehensive drug history and a personal or family history of psoriasis are therefore required.

Intraepidermal or subcorneal pustules in conjunction with a leukocytoclastic vasculitis, focal necrosis of keratinocytes, marked edema of the papillary dermis, and an infiltrate of eosinophils are histologic features that help distinguish AGEP from pustular psoriasis; biopsy is thus an integral facet of management.

Differentiation of AGEP from other inflammatory, toxic, or infectious conditions, such as Sneddon–Wilkinson disease (subcorneal pustular dermatosis) or, in severe cases, toxic epidermal necrolysis, is often readily apparent both clinically and histologically. The clinician should, however, be aware that erythema multiforme–like targetoid lesions, mucous membrane involvement, facial edema, purpura, and vesiculobullous lesions have all been documented in the context of AGEP.

Antibiotics (primarily penicillin or macrolide based) are the most frequently implicated medications. Numerous case reports have cited various other causative agents, including calcium channel blockers, nonsteroidal antiinflammatory drugs (NSAIDs), angiotensin-converting enzyme (ACE) inhibitors, and anticonvulsants (Table 8.1). Acute enterovirus infection, mycoplasma pneumonia, cytomegalovirus, parvovirus B19, spider bites, Chinese herbal compounds (ginkgo biloba), contrast media, and mercury exposure have also been reported as possible causes.

There is no specific therapy for AGEP. A skin swab establishes the sterile nature of the pustules, and drug withdrawal, if feasible, results in rapid spontaneous resolution. *Supportive therapy* is all that is required. A superficial desquamation often occurs during this time and may be treated with *simple emollients*. Several case reports cite the use of patch testing to confirm the causative medication. Only a single case report supports the use of *systemic corticosteroids* for this self-limiting condition.

Specific Investigations

- Detailed history
- Hematology
- Skin swab of pustule
- Microscopy, culture, Gram stain
- Skin biopsy

First-Line Therapy

- Drug withdrawal   **E**

Risk factors for acute generalized exanthematous pustulosis (AGEP) – results of a multinational case-control study (EuroSCAR). Sidoroff A, Dunant A, Viboud C. Br J Dermatol 2007; 157: 6.

A multinational case-control study (97 cases of AGEP and 1009 controls) that assessed the risk for different drugs causing severe cutaneous adverse reactions.

The most frequently implicated drugs were pristinamycin (a macrolide marketed in France), ampicillin/amoxicillin, quinolones, (hydroxy) chloroquine, antiinfective sulfonamides, terbinafine, and diltiazem. Infections and a personal or family history of psoriasis were not deemed to be significant risk factors for developing AGEP. Of note, the median treatment duration was 1 day for antibiotics and 11 days for all other associated drugs.

Acute generalized exanthematous pustulosis. Analysis of 63 cases. Roujeau JC, Bioulac-Sage P, Bourseau C, Guillaume JC, Bernard P, Lok C, et al. Arch Dermatol 1991; 127: 1333–8.

A thorough retrospective review of cases of AGEP. Almost 90% of cases were attributable to drugs, with 50% of reactions occurring within 24 hours of ingestion.

AGEP is distinct from pustular psoriasis based on histologic differences, drug induction in most cases, a more acute course of fever and pustulosis, blood neutrophilia, and rapid spontaneous healing (within 15 days).

Acute generalized exanthematous pustulosis. Manders SM, Heymann WR. Cutis 1994; 54: 194–6.

Two of the three cases reported in this series were attributable to penicillin. This succinct overview of AGEP also provides the reader with useful clinicopathologic features that may help distinguish AGEP from pustular psoriasis.

Table 8.1 Drugs and other substances reported to have caused AGEP

Drugs

Antibiotics
Penicillins: amoxicillin, ampicillin, bacampicillin, pipemidic acid, piperacillin, propicillin, tazobactam, meropenem
Macrolides: azithromycin, erythromycin
Quinolones: ciprofloxacin, norfloxacin, ofloxacin
Tetracyclines: doxycycline, minocycline
Cephalosporins: cefaclor, cefazolin, cefuroxime, cephalexin, cephradine
Aminoglycosides: gentamicin, isepamicin sulfate, streptomycin
Other antibiotics: chloramphenicol, clindamycin, cotrimoxazole, imipenem/cilastatin, lincomycin, metronidazole, nifuroxazide, sulfamethoxazole, teicoplanin, vancomycin, daptomycin, telavancin

NSAIDs
Celecoxib, etoricoxib, ibuprofen, naproxen, nimesulide, valdecoxib

ACE inhibitors
Captopril, enalapril

Calcium channel blockers
Nifedipine, nimodipine, diltiazem

Anticonvulsants
Carbamazepine, phenobarbital, phenytoin

Analgesia (opioid/nonopioid)
Acetaminophen, paracetamol, morphine, codeine, dextropropoxyphene

Antiplatelets
Aspirin, ticlopidine, clopidogrel

Benzodiazepines
Clobazam, nitrazepam, tetrazepam

Antimalarials
Chloroquine, hydroxychloroquine, proguanil, pyrimethamine

Antipsychotics
Clozapine, chlorpromazine

Antifungals
Amphotericin, fluconazole, itraconazole, nystatin, terbinafine

Antivirals
Lamivudine, lopinavir, ritonavir, zidovudine

Antituberculosis drugs
Isoniazid, rifampicin

Proton pump inhibitors
Lansoprazole, omeprazole

Immunosuppressants
Azathioprine

Antidepressants
Amoxapine, sertraline

Antihistamines
Clemastine, hydroxyzine

Beta agonists
Buphenine, fenoterol, nadolol

H2 receptor antagonists
Cimetidine, famotidine, ranitidine

Cholesterol-lowering medications
Simvastatin, pitavastatin, fenofibrate

Corticosteroids
Dexamethasone, methylprednisolone, prednisolone

Diuretics
Furosemide, hydrochlorothiazide

Antineoplastic drugs
Gefitinib, imatinib, vemurafenib

Other drugs
Acetazolamide, allopurinol, bleomycin, carbimazole, cytarabine, disulfiram, eperisone hydrochloride, eprazinone, fluindione, icodextrin, interferon, metamizole, pentoxifylline, piperazine, bamifylline, propafenone, alprostadil, pseudoephedrine, psoralen + UVA, quinidine, sulbutiamine, senna, sulfasalazine, terazosin, thalidomide, cadralazine, progestogens, dalteparin, carbutamide, bupropion hydrochloride, ranolazine

Other substances
Chromium picolinate
Diphenyl sulfone
Contrast agents iohexol and iopamidol
Mercury
Pneumococcal vaccine
Essential oil
Andrographis paniculata

Pustular eruption after drug exposure: is it pustular psoriasis or a pustular drug eruption? Spencer JM, Silvers DN, Grossman ME. Br J Dermatol 1994; 130: 514–9.

Another series highlighting the diagnostic challenge when confronted with a patient with pustulosis and fever. One of the four cases of AGEP occurred in a patient with known psoriasis who was given trimethoprim for a urinary tract infection. An awareness of the condition, eosinophils in the biopsy, and rapid resolution after drug withdrawal prevented unnecessary treatment for pustular psoriasis.

Generalized pustular psoriasis or drug-induced toxic pustuloderma? The use of patch testing. Whittam LR, Wakelin SH, Barker JNWN. Clin Exp Dermatol 2000; 25: 122–4.

Patch testing to a 1% and 5% amoxicillin preparation confirmed a type 4 hypersensitivity reaction in a patient with long-standing plaque psoriasis who developed a generalized pustular eruption when treated with amoxicillin for an episode of epididymoorchitis.

A systemic reaction to patch testing for the evaluation of acute generalized exanthematous pustulosis. Mashiah J, Brenner S. Arch Dermatol 2003; 139: 1181–3.

The authors report a generalized AGEP-like reaction caused by patch tests carried out to determine the drug eliciting AGEP.

Interestingly, negative results were obtained with the drug in question.

Second-Line Therapies	
• Corticosteroids	E
• Cyclosporin	E

Acute generalised exanthematous pustulosis. Criton S, Sofia B. Indian J Dermatol Venereol Leprol 2001; 67: 93–5.

A case report in which the authors claim that parenteral corticosteroids hastened the resolution of AGEP presumptively caused by benzyl penicillin.

Successful treatment of hydroxychloroquine-induced recalcitrant acute generalized exanthematous pustulosis with ciclosporin: case report and literature review. Yalcin B, Cakmak S, Yidirim B. Ann Dermatol. 2015; 27: 431–4.

A case report of a 67-year-old rheumatoid arthritis patient with recalcitrant AGEP secondary to hydroxychloroquine responding successfully to cyclosporin 4 mg/kg/day tapered over 2 months.

Allergic contact dermatitis and photoallergy

Harini Rajgopal Bala, Claire L. Higgins, Rosemary L. Nixon

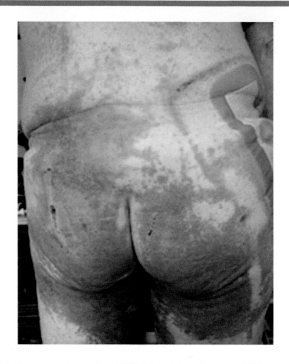

Allergic contact dermatitis (ACD) is a delayed or type IV hypersensitivity reaction, which generally manifests 24 to 48 hours after contact with an allergen to which the individual has previously been sensitized. The rash of acute ACD is characterized by pruritic papules and vesicles on an erythematous base. Lichenified plaques may occur in chronic disease. The rash is initially localized to the site of contact with the causative allergen, but may spread to other areas. This may occur due to a so-called *id reaction* (autoeczematization) or from transfer of the allergen, commonly from the hands to the face. Spread of the rash beyond the primary site is characteristic of ACD and may help to differentiate it clinically from irritant contact dermatitis.

The primary site may point toward the causative allergen: for example, involvement of the ears and neck in cases of ACD caused by nickel in earrings or necklaces; the hands in ACD caused by rubber glove accelerators; and the scalp, neck, and hairline in ACD caused by para-phenylenediamine or other intermediates in permanent hair dye. Infrequently, systemic contact dermatitis may occur when a previously sensitized individual is exposed to an allergen via the oral, intravenous, intramuscular, intraarticular, or inhalation route.

Determinants of whether sensitization will occur include the size and chemical nature of the allergen involved, the duration and concentration of skin contact with the allergen, and individual susceptibility, including skin integrity and likely genetic factors. Once an individual has been sensitized, ACD may be elicited through reexposure with only minute amounts of allergen.

Photoallergic contact dermatitis (PACD), or photoallergy, requires a substance to be activated by ultraviolet A (UVA) light (wavelength 320–400 nm) in order to become allergenic. The severity of the reaction does not correlate with the dose of photoallergen or UV. The two most common causes of PACD currently are organic UV absorbers in sunscreens, particularly octocrylene and benzophenone-3, and topical nonsteroidal antiinflammatory drugs (NSAIDs), such as ketoprofen and etofenamate. Other causes include antibiotics, such as fluoroquinolones and sulfonamide antibacterials, fragrances, and phenothiazines such as chlorpromazine and promethazine. Previously, halogenated salicylanilides in deodorant soaps, musk ambrette, and 6-methyl-coumarin in fragrances, quinidine, and some pesticides have been identified as important photoallergens.

Chronic actinic dermatitis (CAD) is a rare condition whereby individuals continue to develop dermatitis after removal of the photoallergen and may present with recurrent transient or persistent light reactions. CAD may occur after chronic ACD to sesquiterpene lactones, found in the *Compositae* group of plants, as well as fragrances, lichens, and NSAIDs, coupled with chronic UV radiation.

MANAGEMENT STRATEGY

The principal management strategy for both ACD and photoallergy is *identification* and *avoidance* of offending allergens and cross-reacting agents, education, and treatment. *Patch testing* is the gold standard for identifying skin allergens. From a public health perspective, ACD, and particularly occupational-related disease, represents a significant clinical, social, and economic burden. Allergen avoidance is therefore a priority and may occur at the manufacturing, workplace, or individual level—in some cases governed by legislation. For example, the European Nickel Directive restricts the nickel content of metal objects such as jewelry that contacts the skin. The addition of ferrous sulfate to cement in the European Union effectively reduces the available chromate through chemical reduction. Substitution of strong sensitizers in products by manufacturers is also important: the preservative methylisothiazolinone in baby wipes and toiletries is currently causing a major epidemic of ACD.

In the workplace, measures to reduce exposure to known allergens include substitution of common allergens, changing design processes to limit physical contact with chemicals, installation of appropriate ventilation to reduce airborne exposure to substances, and the use of personal protective equipment (PPE).

Gloves are a crucial part of PPE and must be appropriate for handling a particular chemical; for example, double nitrile gloves when working with acrylates. Cotton gloves may be worn underneath rubber or leather gloves to help prevent contact with rubber accelerators or chromate in cement, for example. This is particularly important when working in hot environments, where sweating and leaching of allergens may occur.

The initial treatment of ACD involves the general principles of eczema therapy, including avoidance of skin irritants such as wet work, soap, heat, and sweating. *Topical corticosteroids*, together with emollients, remain the most effective treatment to control an acute flare. The *topical calcineurin inhibitors tacrolimus and pimecrolimus* have also been shown to be effective. The use of *barrier creams* to prevent dermatitis has had limited success. Short courses of *oral corticosteroids*, such as prednisolone 25 to 50 mg daily for 1 week, are effective treatment in severe cases. *Oral antibiotics*, such as cephalosporins, erythromycin, flucloxacillin, or clindamycin, may be required if the dermatitis becomes secondarily infected. *Topical antibiotics* such as mupirocin or fusidic

Evidence Levels: **A** Double-blind study   **B** Clinical trial ≥ 20 subjects   **C** Clinical trial < 20 subjects   **D** Series ≥ 5 subjects   **E** Anecdotal case reports

acid may be helpful, particularly for the treatment of persistently cracked or fissured skin that becomes infected.

Once the cause of ACD has been identified, long-term treatments other than avoidance of the allergen(s) are usually not required, although recurrence may occur from inadvertent allergen exposure. In some cases, severe episodes of ACD may precipitate a recurring eczematous condition, termed *persistent postoccupational dermatitis*. It is believed that the longer an individual has severe ACD, the longer it will take for the condition to resolve once the cause is identified.

In adult patients with chronic ACD refractory to first-line treatment, short-term ultraviolet light therapy in the form of narrowband ultraviolet B (UVB) or psoralen plus UVA (PUVA) is suggested. *Alitretinoin* has a strong evidence base for treatment of chronic hand eczema, although not all patients studied had ACD. In fact many studies regarding the treatment of chronic hand eczema do not specify whether ACD was present. There is moderate evidence for efficacy of the *systemic immunosuppressant* cyclosporine. Azathioprine and methotrexate have less supporting evidence but traditionally have been considered helpful. *Acitretin* may be considered, particularly for hyperkeratotic palmar involvement.

In photoallergy, identification and avoidance of the photoallergen is the major treatment goal. If avoiding the causative allergen is not possible, sun-protective clothing and sunscreen are required. In the case of allergy to a chemical sunscreen agent, avoidance of the allergen or substitution with physical UV blockers such as zinc oxide or titanium dioxide is recommended.

Specific Investigations

- Patch testing to appropriately diluted allergens.
- Repeat open application test (ROAT) to determine whether a reaction is significant in individuals who develop weak (1+) positive reactions to an allergen.
- Photopatch testing if PACD is suspected: duplicate sets of allergens are applied, and after 48 hours one set is exposed to 5 J/cm^2 UVA; results are read after a further 48 hours.
- Phototesting (e.g., via monochromator) if CAD is suspected.

Allergic contact dermatitis. Paz Castanedo-Tardan M, Zug KA. In: Goldsmith L, Katz S, Gilchrest B, Paller A, Leffell D, Fitzpatrick T, et al, eds. Fitzpatrick's Dermatology in General Medicine. New York: McGraw Hill Medical, 2012; Chapter 13.

This chapter from a major dermatology text is an excellent place to start.

First-Line Therapies

Allergic contact dermatitis

Allergen avoidance and substitution	C
Skin care education	B
Personal protective equipment	D
Topical corticosteroids	B
Emollients and soap substitutes	C
Barrier creams	B
Calcineurin inhibitors (tacrolimus, pimecrolimus)	B
Prednisolone	D
Antibiotics – topical and systemic	D
Alitretinoin	A

Photoallergy

Allergen avoidance and substitution	C
Photoprotection	C
Sunscreens – physical UV blockers	E

Skin care education and individual counseling versus treatment as usual in healthcare workers with hand eczema: randomised clinical trial. Ibler KS, Jemec GBE, Diepgen TL, Gluud C, Hansen JL, Winkel P, et al. BMJ 2012; 345: e7822.

Two hundred and fifty-five health care workers with hand eczema were randomized to either an intervention group, comprising education in skin care, individual counseling based on patch and prick testing, and assessment of occupational and domestic exposures, or a control group. At the 5-month follow-up, hand eczema was significantly improved in the intervention group compared with the control group as measured both objectively and subjectively.

Determinants of epoxy allergy in the construction industry: a case–control study. Spee T, Timmerman JG, Rühl R, Kersting K, Heederik DJJ, Smit LAM. Contact Dermatitis 2016; 74: 259–66.

A case-control study compared 179 German epoxy workers with diagnosed ACD to epoxy (cases) with 151 epoxy workers without such an allergy (controls). ACD to epoxies was found to be associated with unusually high levels of exposure to the chemicals (OR 2.13) and with poor compliance with personal protection, including wearing short sleeves and trousers (OR 2.38), and incorrect glove use (OR 2.12).

The effect of a corticosteroid cream and a barrier-strengthening moisturizer in hand eczema. A double-blind, randomized, prospective, parallel group clinical trial. Lodén M, Wirén K, Smerud KT, Meland N, Hønnås H, Mørk G, et al. J Eur Acad Dermatol Venereol 2012; 26: 597–601.

Forty-four patients were randomized to either betamethasone 0.1% once daily with the use of a urea moisturizer in the evening or the use of betamethasone 0.1% twice daily. The trial concluded that twice-daily application of topical betamethasone was not superior to once-daily treatment and that once-daily treatment with an effective barrier cream had a greater response in patients with moderate eczema.

Tacrolimus 0.1% vs. mometasone furoate topical treatment in allergic contact hand eczema: a prospective randomized clinical study. Katsarou A, Makris M, Papagiannaki K, Lagogianni E, Tagka A, Kalogeromitros D. Eur J Dermatol 2012; 22: 192–6.

Thirty adults with chronic hand eczema and positive patch test reactions were randomized to either tacrolimus 0.1% ointment or mometasone furoate 0.1%. A significant difference was observed in both groups in all parameters between baseline and day 90 results. The results suggest tacrolimus is a favorable alternative therapy to topical corticosteroids with similar outcomes.

A phase 3, randomized, double-blind, placebo controlled study evaluating the efficacy and safety of alitretinoin (BAL4079) in the treatment of severe chronic hand eczema refractory to potent topical corticosteroid therapy. Fowler JF, Graff O, Hamedani AG. J Drugs Dermatol 2014; 13: 1198–204.

Five hundred and ninety-six participants were randomized to either a treatment arm, which administered 30 mg of alitretinoin, or placebo for 24 weeks. Patients were assessed every 4 weeks, with the primary end point being clear or almost clear of eczema at the end of the trial. Alitretinoin was shown to significantly improve severe chronic hand eczema.

New sunscreens confer improved protection for photosensitive patients in the blue light region. Moseley H, Cameron H, Macleod T, Clark C, Dawe R, Ferguson J. Br J Dermatol 2001; 145: 789–94.

Seven patients with known photosensitivity extending into the visible (blue) region at 430 ± 30 nm were tested with new reflectant sunscreens incorporating larger particle size zinc oxide and pigmentary-grade titanium dioxide as active ingredients. The mean photo protection factors at this wavelength were determined. The new sunscreens were found to provide protection for patients with sensitivity to visible light (blue light region), for example, those with CAD, compared with sunscreens using chemical UV absorbers and microfine particles, which scatter radiation.

Second-Line Therapies	
Allergic contact dermatitis	
• Ultraviolet light (PUVA, UVB)	B
• Azathioprine	C
• Cyclosporine	D
• Methotrexate	D
• Acitretin	E
• Low-nickel diet for nickel dermatitis	C

Local narrowband UVB phototherapy vs. local PUVA in the treatment of chronic hand eczema. Sezer E, Etikan I. Photodermatol Photoimmunol Photomed 2007; 23: 10–4.

Fifteen participants with chronic hand eczema of dry and dyshidrotic types were administered local narrowband UVB irradiation on one arm starting with 150 mJ/cm^2 with a 20% increase per session until a final dose of 2000 mJ/cm^2 was reached and local paint-PUVA using 0.1% 8-methoxypsoralen gel on the other hand three times a week over a 9-week period. The study found localized narrowband UVB therapy as effective as paint PUVA in patients with chronic hand eczema.

Azathioprine versus betamethasone for the treatment of Parthenium dermatitis: a randomized controlled study. Verma KK, Mahesh R, Srivastava P, Ranam M, Mukhopadhyaya AK. Indian J Dermatol Venereol Leprol 2008; 74: 453–7.

Fifty-five patients with contact dermatitis caused by airborne *Parthenium* were randomly assigned to azathioprine 100 mg daily or betamethasone 2 mg daily for 6 months in a double-blinded manner. Treatment effects appeared equal in each group; however, the group randomized to betamethasone appeared to have more adverse effects.

Oral cyclosporine inhibits the expression of contact hypersensitivity in man. Higgins EM, McLelland J, Friedmann PS, Matthews JN, Shuster S. J Dermatol Sci 1991; 2: 79–83.

The expression of delayed contact hypersensitivity was studied in six patients with chronic contact dermatitis treated with cyclosporine 5 mg/kg/day. Quantitative patch test reactions were diminished in all six; responses were reduced over the whole range of allergen concentrations. In addition, the clinical manifestations of ACD underwent complete resolution within 2 to 3 weeks of cyclosporine therapy.

Treatment of Parthenium dermatitis with methotrexate. Sharma VK, Bhat R, Sethuraman G, Manchanda Y. Contact Dermatitis 2007; 57: 118–9.

Sixteen patients with Parthenium dermatitis unresponsive to topical treatment were treated with methotrexate, topical corticosteroids, and sunscreen. Some improvement was observed, suggesting a role for methotrexate in this condition.

Open-label exploratory study of acitretin for the treatment of severe chronic hand dermatitis. Tan J, Maari C, Nigen S, Bolduc C, Bissonnette R. J Dermatolog Treat 2015; 26: 373–5.

In a pilot study, nine participants with severe chronic hand dermatitis were treated with 10 to 30 mg of acitretin daily for up to 24 weeks. Three patients withdrew from the study. In the remaining patients 33.3% achieved clear or almost clear on physician global assessment.

Systemic nickel allergy: oral desensitization and possible role of cytokines interleukins 2 and 10. Ricciardi L, Carni A, Loschiavo G, Gangemi S, Tigano V, Arena E, et al. Int J Immunopathol Pharmacol 2013; 26: 251–7.

Twenty-two participants with known systemic nickel allergy syndrome (SNAS) were initiated on an oral desensitization therapy associated with a low-nickel diet for 3 months. Patients' tolerability to nickel improved significantly, and 18 of 22 participants had a negative nickel oral challenge at the end of the treatment.

Third-Line Therapy	
Allergic contact dermatitis	
• Pentoxifylline	E

The effect of the topical application of different pentoxifylline concentrations on the patch test results of nickel-sensitive patients. Saricaoglu H, Baskan EB, Tunali S. Int J Dermatol 2004; 43: 315–6.

Twenty-two volunteers with nickel-induced contact dermatitis were pretreated with three concentrations of pentoxifylline and then patch tested to nickel. Though there was some evidence of suppressed patch test results, the decrease in patch test reactions was statistically insignificant.

Evidence Levels: A Double-blind study B Clinical trial ≥ 20 subjects C Clinical trial < 20 subjects D Series ≥ 5 subjects E Anecdotal case reports

10

Alopecia areata

John Berth-Jones

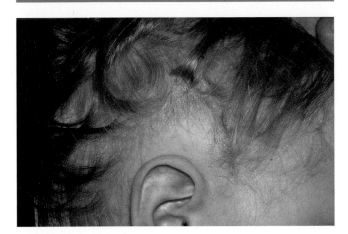

Alopecia areata (AA) is a T-lymphocyte–mediated autoimmune disease of the hair follicle. It is characterized by patchy hair loss developing in otherwise normal skin, with "exclamation mark" hairs around margins of expanding areas. Most cases are limited to one or more coin-sized patches, but in severe cases there may be complete baldness of the scalp (alopecia totalis, AT) or of the entire body (alopecia universalis, AU). The alopecia is noncicatrizing.

MANAGEMENT STRATEGY

Leaving AA untreated is a reasonable option for many patients. Spontaneous remission usually occurs within a few months, and no treatment has been shown to alter the long-term prognosis. Treatment can be time consuming, uncomfortable, and potentially toxic, and relapse after treatment may be difficult to cope with. Many patients are distressed, so psychologic support can be helpful, and careful "management of expectations" from treatment is important. Contact with other sufferers and support groups may also help.

The treatments listed as first line are the most consistently effective and safe; however, the response to any treatment is variable and depends largely on the extent and duration of the alopecia. This is one reason why the results of trials are often conflicting. Trials involving recent-onset patchy alopecia may have a high rate of spontaneous remission, whereas trials limited to severe long-standing disease that is resistant to treatment do not exclude efficacy in mild alopecia.

Intralesional corticosteroid injections are considered first-line treatment for adult patients when only one or two small patches of alopecia are present, but can be used on larger areas if patients can tolerate the discomfort. The author most frequently uses triamcinolone acetonide aqueous suspension (2.5–10 mg/mL) injected intradermally in multiple 0.05- to 0.1-mL doses and does not inject more than 20 mg in total at one visit. Treatment is repeated at intervals of 4 to 12 weeks. A concentration of 2.5 mg/mL can be used on the eyebrow area. The main side effect is pitting atrophy, which is usually transient.

Topical immunotherapy is the induction of contact allergy on the scalp. Contact sensitizers include dinitrochlorobenzene (DNCB;

now considered potentially carcinogenic and therefore no longer used), squaric acid dibutyl ester (SADBE; this has limited stability), and *diphencyprone* (DPCP, diphenylcyclopropenone). The latter compound combines efficacy and safety with a practical shelf life and has become the most widely used. Diphencyprone can initially be applied as 2% lotion to a small area (2–4 cm²) of scalp until the site of application becomes pruritic and erythematous. Treatment is then continued over a larger area with weekly applications of lower concentrations, typically ranging from 0.001% to 0.1%. The lowest concentration that maintains mild erythema or pruritus should be used. My patients usually have half of their scalp treated initially until a favorable result means treatment can then be extended to the contralateral scalp. This is one of the best-documented therapies for AA, and is the one most likely to be effective in extensive long-standing disease. However, the timing of the response is quite unpredictable, so the author treats patients for as long as they wish to continue. Relapse rates may be high. Side effects include regional lymphadenopathy and, rarely, generalized eczema or even an eruption resembling erythema multiforme. Vitiligo may develop, although this is usually confined to the treated areas. For this reason, sensitization therapy is best avoided in patients with pigmented skin types.

Topical corticosteroids have demonstrated efficacy in some studies of patchy AA, particularly those using potent steroids with occlusion. They are inexpensive and practical to use, and the main side effect is transient folliculitis. Results are variable, however, and they do not appear to be very effective in AT or AU.

Topical prostaglandin analogs have been reported as effective in treating the eyelashes of patients affected with AU.

Irritants, including *anthralin (dithranol)* and *retinoic acid*, are safe and practical to use, although the evidence for their efficacy is limited. For patients with dark hair, anthralin has the advantage of camouflaging a pale area of scalp by staining it brown. Application needs to be frequent and at a fairly high concentration, with the purpose of inducing significant irritation to be effective. Retinoic acid is more practical for use in patients with fair hair.

Topical minoxidil is a safe treatment, but most studies have failed to demonstrate a response of cosmetic value in most patients.

Systemic corticosteroids are effective in some cases if high doses are used. However, AT, AU, and ophiasiform AA do not respond well, and high relapse rates make this toxic treatment hard to justify. Given the level of emotional disturbance associated with alopecia, there is clearly a risk of encountering serious difficulty in withdrawing treatment. It is difficult to justify the use of potentially harmful modalities.

Less conventional treatments from which benefit has been reported are listed next as third line. Many patients find wigs an acceptable *camouflage*. Tattooing (dermatography) of the eyebrows may lead to a more socially acceptable image for some patients. Most recently, anecdotal reports of the oral Janus kinase (JAK) inhibitor, *tofacitinib*, have led to its off-label use for AT, AU, and ophiasiform AA.

The wide variety of treatments that have been investigated attest to the tantalizing nature of this disease, which can resolve spontaneously even after many years, yet currently continues to represent a therapeutic challenge.

Specific Investigations

No investigation is routinely required. However, in patients with symptoms or a family history of autoimmune disease, investigation may be indicated.
- Consider full blood count, thyroid function tests, serum B$_{12}$, and autoantibodies.

First-Line Therapies

- Intralesional steroids   A
- Topical clobetasol propionate   A
- Topical immunotherapy   B

Benefit of different concentrations of triamcinolone acetonide in alopecia areata: an intrasubject pilot study. Chu TW, Aljasser M, Albarbi A, Abahussein O, McElwee K, Shapiro J. J Am Acad Dermatol 2015; 73: 338–40.

Four patients each received six injections of saline and triamcinolone acetonide (TCA) 2.5, 5, and 10 mg/mL at 6-week intervals. All three concentrations yielded similar responses, and all were superior to the placebo.

Intralesional treatment of alopecia areata with triamcinolone acetonide by jet injector. Abell E, Munro DD. Br J Dermatol 1973; 88: 55–9.

A report of 84 patients treated with 0.1-mL needleless injections of triamcinolone acetonide 5 mg/mL and normal saline controls. After 6 weeks, regrowth was observed in 86% of patients treated with triamcinolone and 7% of controls. Mild transient atrophy was frequently observed.

Intralesional triamcinolone acetonide versus topical betamethasone valerate (BV) in management of localized alopecia areata. Devi M, Rashid A, Ghafoor R. J Coll Physicians Surg Pak 2015; 25: 860–2.

Two randomized groups of 113 patients received twice-daily 0.1% BV or injection, at baseline, of TCA 10 mg/mL. Regrowth was seen at 12 weeks in 74% of the intralesional group, versus 47% of the topical group ($p < 0.001$).

Clobetasol propionate, 0.05%, vs. hydrocortisone, 1%, for alopecia areata in children. Lenane P, Macarthur C, Parkin PC, Krafchik B, DeGroot J, Khambalia A, et al. JAMA Dermatol 2014; 150: 47–50.

A double-blinded study in a relatively responsive population. Creams were applied twice daily for two 6-week cycles (6 weeks on, 6 weeks off) over 24 weeks. Clobetasol yielded a significantly greater response.

Clobetasol propionate 0.05% under occlusion in the treatment of alopecia totalis/universalis. Tosti A, Piraccini B, Pazzaglia M, Vincenzi C. J Am Acad Dermatol 2003; 49: 96–8.

A refractory group of 28 patients with AT/AU of 3 to 12 years' duration who had not responded to immunotherapy were treated on half of their scalp with 2.5 g of clobetasol propionate ointment under plastic film on 6 nights per week for 6 months. Regrowth started at 6 to 14 weeks, and eight patients (28.5%) achieved >75% regrowth, which was then extended to the other side of the scalp. Eleven patients developed painful folliculitis, including five of the six who withdrew from the study. After a further 6 months' follow-up 18% of the 28 patients retained complete regrowth.

Diphencyprone in the treatment of alopecia areata. Happle R, Hausen BM, Weisner-Menzel L. Acta Derm Venereol 1983; 63: 49–52.

This study nicely illustrated the unilateral response observed when one side of the scalp is treated, which so convincingly establishes the efficacy of this treatment.

Topical immunotherapy with diphenylcyclopropenone in the treatment of chronic extensive alopecia areata. Sotiriadis D, Patsatsi A, Lazaridou E, Kastanis A, Vakirlis E, Chrysomallis F. Clin Exp Dermatol 2007; 32: 48–51.

In this prospective open clinical trial, 17 patients had either AT or AU and 24 had severe alopecia (>50% scalp involvement). After sensitization with DPCP 2% in acetone, progressively higher concentrations (from 0.001%–0.1%) were applied once a week for a period of 6 to 12 months. Of the 41 patients, 38 (16 with AT or AU and 22 with extensive AA) completed therapy. Significant hair regrowth was observed in five patients with AT or AU (31.25%) and ten patients with extensive alopecia (45.4%). These results were sustained in 66.6% of patients for a 12-month follow-up period.

Second-Line Therapies

- Anthralin/dithranol   B
- Retinoic acid   B
- Topical minoxidil   B
- Bimatoprost/latanoprost eye drops   B

Treatment of alopecia areata by anthralin-induced dermatitis. Plewig G, Braun-Falco O. Arch Dermatol 1979; 115: 1254–5.

In this study using 0.5% and 1.0% concentrations of anthralin, the mean time to response was 11 weeks and the mean time to cosmetic response was 23 weeks (range 8–60 weeks). Cosmetic response was achieved in 29% (11/38) of patients with <75% scalp hair loss and in 20% (6/30) of patients with >75% scalp hair loss. Approximately 75% of responders maintained adequate hair growth with continued treatment.

Topical tretinoin as an adjunctive therapy with intralesional triamcinolone acetonide for alopecia areata. Clinical experience in northern Saudi Arabia. Kubeyinje EP, C'Mathur M. Int J Dermatol 1997; 36: 320.

In this open study 58 patients with mainly patchy alopecia were treated with monthly triamcinolone injections; 28 patients also had daily application of 0.05% tretinoin cream. More than 90% regrowth was achieved in 66.7% of patients with triamcinolone alone and in 85.7% of patients with both treatments, which was statistically significant.

Comparative assessment of topical steroids, topical tretinoin (0.05%) and dithranol paste in alopecia areata. Das S, Ghorami RC, Chatterjee T, Banerjee G. Indian J Dermatol 2010; 55: 148–9.

This prospective study of 80 patients with AA concluded that there was a good response in 55% of patients treated with topical tretinoin, in comparison with 70% of patients treated with topical steroids and 35% of patients treated with dithranol.

Topical minoxidil solution (1% and 5%) in the treatment of alopecia areata. Fiedler-Weiss VC. J Am Acad Dermatol 1987; 16: 745–8.

Sixty-six patients with >75% scalp hair loss applied the treatments twice daily. Even in the high-dose group only 6% showed a cosmetically acceptable response. Occlusion of the treated area with white petrolatum at night was necessary to achieve maximum results.

Bimatoprost in the treatment of eyelash universalis alopecia areata. Vila OT, Camacho Martinez FM. Int J Trichology 2010; 2: 86–8.

Evidence Levels: **A** Double-blind study   **B** Clinical trial ≥ 20 subjects   **C** Clinical trial < 20 subjects   **D** Series ≥ 5 subjects   **E** Anecdotal case reports

In this retrospective study of 41 patients, 0.03% bimatoprost eye drops were applied to the eyelid margins once a day for 1 year. Complete regrowth of the eyelashes was noted in 24.3% of patients and moderate regrowth in 18.9% of subjects.

Latanoprost in the treatment of eyelash alopecia in alopecia areata universalis. Coronel-Perez IM, Rodriguez-Rey EM, Camacho-Martinez FM. J Eur Acad Dermatol Venereol 2010; 24: 481–5.

A 2-year prospective, nonblinded, nonrandomized, controlled study of 54 subjects with AAU and eyelash alopecia. The control group comprised 10 subjects who received injections of 0.5 mg/cm² of triamcinolone acetonide (TAC) in their eyebrows and 1 mg/cm² of TAC injections in affected scalp. The treatment group included 44 subjects who received the same treatment as the control group in scalp and eyebrows, but they also applied a drop of latanoprost 0.005% (50 µg/mL) ophthalmic solution to their eyelid margins every night. In the treatment group, there was complete regrowth in 17.5%, moderate regrowth in 27.5%, slight regrowth in 30%, and no response in 25%. No patients had cosmetically acceptable eyelash regrowth in the control group.

Lack of efficacy of topical latanoprost and bimatoprost ophthalmic solutions in promoting eyelash growth in patients with alopecia areata. Roseborough I, Lee H, Chwalek J, Stamper RL, Price VH. J Am Acad Dermatol 2009; 60: 705–6.

A controlled trial of 16 weeks' duration with 11 patients did not confirm any response.

Another small trial of similar design has also shown the same negative result.

Bimatoprost versus mometasone furoate in the treatment of scalp alopecia areata: a pilot study. Zaher H, Gawdat HI, Hegazy RA, Hassan M. Dermatology 2015; 230: 308–13.

A study on patchy AA of the scalp in which 30 adult subjects applied each treatment to separate patches of AA. The prostaglandin analog yielded superior regrowth.

Use of these prostaglandin (PGF$_{2\alpha}$) analogs has occasionally been associated with increased pigmentation of the iris and eyelid.

Bimatoprost (Latisse) is licensed in the United States as a "cosmetic" product used to thicken normal eyelash growth, an effect that may also be beneficial for patients with AA.

Third-Line Therapies

• PUVA	B
• Systemic corticosteroids	B
• Systemic cyclosporine	C
• Intralesional autologous platelet rich plasma	B
• Oral minoxidil	B
• Sulfasalazine	B
• Methotrexate	C
• Azathioprine	C
• Tofacitinib	E
• Inosiplex (inosine pranobex)	B
• Nitrogen mustard	C
• Dermatography	B
• Cryotherapy	B
• Pulsed infrared diode laser	C
• Excimer laser	C
• Topical bexarotene	C
• Topical azelaic acid	C
• Combination treatment of simvastatin and ezetimibe	C
• Diphencyprone with imiquimod	C

• Hydroxychloroquine	E
• Adalimumab	E
• Phenol	C
• Aromatherapy	B
• Onion juice	B
• Garlic gel with betamethasone valerate	B

Treatment of alopecia areata with three different PUVA modalities. Lassus A, Eskelinen A, Johansson E. Photodermatology 1984; 1: 141–4.

Seventy-six patients with severe AA were treated with local or oral 8-methoxypsoralen and local or whole-body UVA irradiation. In 43 cases (57%) a good-to-excellent result was obtained, with 20 to 40 treatments being sufficient in most cases. No particular treatment method was significantly superior. Patients with circumscribed or ophiasic alopecia responded better than patients with AT or AU. Disease duration, onset before the age of 20 years, and atopy were poor prognostic factors. During a follow-up period of 6 to 68 months, 22 patients had a relapse.

High-dose pulse corticosteroid therapy in the treatment of severe alopecia areata. Seiter S, Ugurel S, Tilgen W, Reinhold U. Dermatology 2001; 202: 230–4.

In this prospective open study 30 patients with >30% hair loss were treated with three courses of IV methylprednisolone (8 mg/kg) on 3 consecutive days at 4-week intervals. Twelve of 18 AA patients achieved >50% regrowth. None of the four patients with AT, five with AU, or three with ophiasic AA responded. Ten patients who responded retained the growth at 10 months.

Placebo-controlled oral pulse prednisolone therapy in alopecia areata. Kar BR, Handa S, Dogra S, Kumar B. J Am Acad Dermatol 2005; 53: 1100–1.

Forty-three patients were randomized to receive oral prednisolone 200 mg weekly (23) or placebo (20) for 3 months. All patients had more than 40% scalp hair loss, or more than 10 patches of AA, for more than 9 months. Eight of 23 in the treatment group showed more than 30% regrowth, compared with none in the placebo group. More than 60% regrowth occurred in only two patients, both within the treatment group. Side effects occurred in 55% of the treatment group, compared with 11% in the placebo group, although all were temporary.

Numerous reports of using systemic corticoids over the last 60 years in various doses and regimens indicate that high doses can be effective while treatment is continued. There is no convincing evidence of any change to the natural course of the disease when treatment is stopped.

Oral cyclosporine for the treatment of alopecia areata. Gupta AK, Ellis CN, Cooper KD, Nickoloff BJ, Ho VC, Chan LS, et al. J Am Acad Dermatol 1990; 22: 242–50.

Six patients with alopecia (two AA, one AT, and three AU) were treated with oral cyclosporine, 6 mg/kg/day, for 12 weeks. Hair regrowth in the scalp of all patients occurred within the second and fourth weeks of therapy, but cosmetically acceptable regrowth occurred in only three patients. In no case did this persist 3 months after stopping the drug.

A randomized, double-blind, placebo- and active-controlled, half head study to evaluate the effects of platelet-rich plasma on alopecia areata. Trink A, Sorbellini E, Bezzola P, Rodella L, Rezzani R, Ramot Y, et al. Br J Dermatol 2013; 169: 690–4.

A controlled study with 45 subjects. Platelet-rich plasma (PRP) was obtained by centrifugation of 36 mL peripheral blood and injected intralesionally on three occasions at monthly intervals.

PRP was significantly superior to no treatment, placebo, and triamcinolone acetonide in stimulating hair growth in assessments at 2, 6, and 12 months.

Evaluation of oral minoxidil in the treatment of alopecia areata. Fiedler-Weiss VC, Rumsfield J, Buys CM, West DP, Wendrow A. Arch Dermatol 1987; 123: 1488–90.

Sixty-five patients with severe AA were treated with oral minoxidil 5 mg twice daily. Cosmetic response was reported in 18% of patients. The drug was well tolerated at this dose, provided the recommended restriction on sodium intake (2 g daily) was observed. Higher sodium intake increased the risk of fluid retention.

Treatment of persistent alopecia areata with sulfasalazine. Rashidi T, Mahd AA. Int J Dermatol 2008; 47: 850–2.

An uncontrolled prospective trial of sulfasalazine in 39 patients with persistent AA demonstrated regrowth of more than 60% in 25.6% of patients and a moderate response in 30.7% of patients.

Long-term follow-up of the efficacy of methotrexate alone or in combination with low doses of oral corticosteroids in the treatment of alopecia areata totalis or universalis. Chartaux E, Joly P. Ann Dermatol Venereol 2010; 137: 507–13.

In a long-term follow-up study of methotrexate in 33 patients with AA, complete regrowth was achieved in 57% of patients who took 15 to 25 mg methotrexate a week and in 63% of patients who took 10 to 20 mg prednisone a day. Recurrence of AA occurred in 57% of responders after a decrease in the methotrexate dose or after stopping treatment.

Efficacy and tolerability of methotrexate in severe childhood alopecia areata. Royer M, Bodemer C, Vabres P, Pajot C, Barbarot S, Paul C, et al. Br J Dermatol 2011; 165: 407–10.

In this retrospective study of 14 children aged 8 to 18 with AA, 5 experienced a clinically relevant therapeutic response. The treatment was administered once weekly with a mean maximal dose of 18.9 mg weekly (0.38 mg/kg) and a mean duration of treatment of 14.2 months.

The authors have subsequently reported that response was maintained in two of the five responders at 6 and 4.3 years after treatment.

Could azathioprine be considered as a therapeutic alternative in the treatment of alopecia areata? A pilot study. Farshi S, Mansouri P, Safar F, Khiabanloo SR. Int J Dermatol 2010; 49: 1188–93.

A total of 20 patients with minimum 6 months, history of AA were included in this pilot study. Azathioprine was taken at a dose of 2 mg/kg of body weight. The mean regrowth was 52.3% and the mean hair loss before treatment was 72.7%, compared with 33.5% after 6 months of treatment.

Killing two birds with one stone: oral tofacitinib reverses alopecia universalis in a patient with plaque psoriasis. Craiglow BG, King BA. J Invest Dermatol 2014; 134: 2988–90.

A patient demonstrated improvement of both conditions, including complete regrowth of hair at all body sites at 8 months, on treatment with the JAK inhibitor, tofacitinib, 10 mg in the morning and 5 mg at night. The drug was well tolerated.

There is also a report of AA responding to baricitinib, another JAK inhibitor. This is a relatively novel class of immunosuppressants. Tofacitinib is used in the treatment of psoriasis. In that indication, topical application can be effective, and perhaps this might be developed into a safer approach for AA.

Inosiplex for treatment of alopecia areata: a randomized placebo-controlled study. Georgala S, Katoulis AC, Befon A, Georgala K, Stavropoulos PG. Acta Dermatol Venereol 2006; 86: 422–4.

In this double-blind trial 32 subjects were randomized to two groups of 16 subjects: oral inosiplex 50 mg/kg/day in five divided doses for 12 weeks or placebo. Patients had treatment-resistant disease for 11 to 34 months; 21 with AA, 9 with ophiasis, and 2 with AT. In the 15 treatment patients who completed the trial, 33% achieved full regrowth and 53% achieved more than 50% regrowth. None of the 14 placebo patients responded completely, and 28.5% achieved more than 50% regrowth. After a further 6 months, tapering to half-dose, there were no recurrences.

A parallel study of inosine pranobex, diphencyprone and both treatments combined in the treatment of alopecia totalis. Berth-Jones J, Hutchinson PE. Clin Exp Dermatol 1991; 16: 172–5.

Thirty-three subjects with AT were randomized into three groups and treated with inosine pranobex 50 mg/kg/day, topical DPCP, or both. There was no response to inosine pranobex in the 22 subjects who received this treatment. Only 2 of 22 patients responded to DPCP.

Treatment of alopecia areata with topical nitrogen mustard. Arrazola JM, Sendagorta E, Harto A, Ledo A. Int J Dermatol 1985; 9: 608–10.

Cosmetically acceptable hair regrowth was seen in 7 of 11 patients (including 2 of 6 with AT) after 4 to 8 weeks of self-treatment with mechlorethamine hydrochloride 0.2 mg/mL once daily. Two patients became sensitized and treatment was discontinued.

Topical nitrogen mustard in the treatment of alopecia areata: a bilateral comparison study. Bernardo O, Tang L, Lui H, Shapiro J. J Am Acad Dermatol 2003; 49: 291–4.

In this half-head controlled study 10 patients with AA for at least 1 year and >50% head involvement applied nitrogen mustard three times weekly for 16 weeks. A significant change was seen in only one patient, and another four did not complete the trial.

Dermatography as a new treatment for alopecia areata of the eyebrows. Van der Velden EM, Drost RHIM, Ijsselmuiden OE, Baruchin AM, Hulsebosch HJ. Int J Dermatol 1998; 37: 617–21.

Thirty-three patients with AA of the eyebrows were treated. The eyebrow areas were covered with a halftone pattern of tiny dots of color pigments, using a Van der Velden Derma-injector, without anesthesia. On average, two or three dermatography sessions of 1 hour each were required. The follow-up was 4 years. The results were excellent in 30 patients and good in 3 patients.

Effect of superficial hypothermic cryotherapy with liquid nitrogen on alopecia areata. Lei Y, Nie Y, Zhang JM, Liao DY, Li HY, Man MQ. Arch Dermatol 1991; 127: 1851–2.

Seventy-two patients with AA involving >25% of their scalp (disease duration 3 days–15 years) were treated with liquid nitrogen on a cotton swab for 2 to 3 seconds on a double freeze–thaw cycle. This was repeated weekly for 4 weeks. Forty comparable controls were treated with glacial acetic acid in a bland emollient vehicle three times a day for 4 weeks. More than 60% regrowth occurred in 70 (97.2%) of the active group, compared with 14 (35%) of the controls.

Use of the pulsed infrared diode laser (904 nm) in the treatment of alopecia areata. Waiz M, Saleh AZ, Hayani R, Jubory SO. J Cosmet Laser Ther 2006; 8: 27–30.

An open study of 16 patients with 34 patches of treatment-resistant alopecia, duration 12 months to 6 years. Patients were treated with four sessions of 904-nm pulsed diode laser once weekly. Seven patients had control patches. Regrowth occurred in 32 patches (94%) but not in the 7 control patches and was maintained for the 2 months of follow-up.

308-nm excimer laser for the treatment of alopecia areata. Al-Mutairi N. Dermatol Surg 2007; 33: 1483–7.

Eighteen patients with 42 patches of alopecia on the scalp and other sites for more than 6 months were treated twice weekly with the 308-nm excimer laser for 24 sessions. One patch in each patient was not treated; 41.5% of treated patches and 76.5% of scalp patches had cosmetically acceptable regrowth. No untreated patches regrew. Two patients relapsed at 6 months.

Phase I/II randomized bilateral half-head comparison of topical bexarotene 1% gel for alopecia areata. Talpur R, Vu J, Bassett R, Stevens V, Duvic M. J Am Acad Dermatol 2009; 61: 592–8.

In this bilateral half-head study, hair regrowth of at least 50% on treated sites was noticed in 11/42 (26%) patients treated with 1% bexarotene gel.

Comparison of azelaic acid and anthralin for the therapy of patchy alopecia areata: a pilot study. Sasmaz S, Arican O. Am J Clin Dermatol 2005; 6: 403–6.

Thirty-one subjects with patchy AA were randomized to apply either 20% azelaic acid (15 subjects) or 0.5% anthralin (16 subjects) for 12 consecutive weeks. In a subsequent 8-week follow-up period no cream was applied. A complete response was observed in 53.3% of cases in the azelaic acid group and in 56.2% of cases in the anthralin group.

Treatment of alopecia areata with simvastatin/ezetimibe. Latouf C, Jimenez JJ, Tosti A, Miteva M, Wikramanayake TC, Kittles C, et al. J Am Acad Dermatol 2015; 72: 359–61.

A series of 29 patients with AA were treated with simvastatin 40 mg and ezetimibe 10 mg daily. Nineteen completed 24 weeks treatment, and 14 of these were considered responders (20% hair regrowth). Five out of seven responders who discontinued the treatment relapsed, whereas five out of seven who continued for a further 24 weeks maintained the response.

Alopecia areata (AA) and treatment with simvastatin/ezetimibe: experience of 20 patients. Loi C, Starace M, Piraccini BM. J Am Acad Dermatol 2016; 74: e99–100.

No convincing response was observed in this study, which seems to have sampled a more severely affected population.

Possible advantage of imiquimod and diphenylcyclopropenone combined treatment versus diphenylcyclopropenone alone: an observational study of nonresponder patients with alopecia areata. Wasylyszn T, Borowska K. Australas J Dermatol 2016; doi:10.111/ajd.12478. [epub ahead of print]

A study with 20 subjects. A group receiving the combined therapy responded better than the group using DPCN alone.

Successful treatment of alopecia totalis with hydroxychloroquine: report of 2 cases. Stephan F, Habre M, Tomb R. J Am Acad Dermatol 2013; 68: 1048–9.

"Spectacular" and "excellent" results at 2 months and 5 months on 200 mg twice daily.

Hydroxychloroquine is ineffective in treatment of alopecia totalis and extensive alopecia areata: a case series of 8 patients. Nissen CV, Wulf HC. JAAD Case Rep 2016; 2: 117–8.

Sadly, these authors were unable to demonstrate any convincing response using 200 mg twice daily for 101 to 300 days.

Alopecia universalis successfully treated with adalimumab. Gorcey L, Gordon Spratt EA, Leger MC. JAMA Dermatol 2014; 150: 1341–4.

A patient improved within 2 weeks of starting treatment with adalimumab 40 mg subcutaneously every other week, relapsed on discontinuation, and improved again after resuming treatment.

Evaluation of utility of phenol in alopecia areata. Chikhalkar S, Jerajani H, Madke B. Int J Trichology 2013; 5: 179–84.

An open-label study on 50 patients with patchy hair loss. Three applications of 88% phenol were performed at 3-week intervals. Some regrowth was seen in 49 patients, with terminal hair in 20. Moderate improvement was observed in 78% of untreated patches. The treatment, which induced a mild-to-moderate burning sensation, frosting, and peeling, is believed to work as a result of the irritant reaction.

Randomized trial of aromatherapy. Successful treatment for alopecia areata. Hay IC, Jamieson M, Ormerod AD. Arch Dermatol 1998; 134: 1349–52.

The active group massaged essential oils (thyme, rosemary, lavender, and cedarwood) in a mixture of carrier oils (jojoba and grape seed) into their scalp daily. The control group used only carrier oils for their massage. Nineteen (44%) of 43 patients in the active group showed improvement, compared with 6 (15%) of 41 in the control group.

Perhaps the nicest-smelling treatment!

Onion juice (*Allium cepa L.*), a new topical treatment for alopecia areata. Sharquie KE, Al-Obaidi HK. J Dermatol 2002; 29: 343–6.

Sixty-two patients with patchy alopecia were randomized to either topical onion juice or tap water twice daily for 2 months. Mean duration of disease was 3 weeks and 2.7 weeks, respectively. Twenty-three of the 45 onion juice group completed the trial, with full regrowth occurring in 20 patients. In the tap water–treated group, hair regrowth occurred in 2 of 17 patients. Mild erythema occurred in 14 of the onion juice group.

Combination of topical garlic gel and betamethasone valerate cream in the treatment of localized alopecia areata: a double-blinded randomized controlled study. Hajheydari Z, Jamshidi M, Akbari J, Mohammadpour R. Indian J Dermatol Venereol Leprol 2007; 73: 29–32.

In this double-blinded randomized controlled trial, 40 patients were divided into two groups of garlic gel and placebo. Garlic gel was rubbed on the alopecia patches under dressing and left for 1 hour, twice daily for 3 months, in the garlic group. The same procedure was carried out in the control group with placebo gel. Both groups received topical corticosteroid (betamethasone cream 0.1% in isopropyl alcohol) twice daily. Good and moderate responses were observed in 19 (95%) patients in the group treated with garlic gel and 1 (5%) patient in the placebo group.

Undoubtedly the worst-smelling treatments!

Amyloidosis

William Y-M. Tang, Loi-Yuen Chan

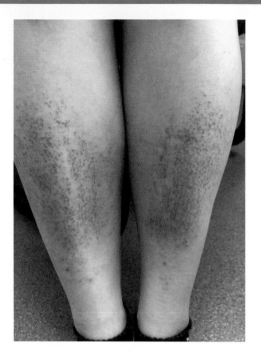

Amyloid is an altered, insoluble protein folded in β-pleated sheets that is deposited extracellularly. Amyloid can accumulate in one or many organs, thereby causing dysfunction. There is an increasing number (more than 28) of proteins identified to be amyloidogenic. The common amyloid entities are AL (amyloid light chain), AA (amyloid associate), ATTR (transthyretin), and β_2-microglobulin.

Systemic amyloidosis consists of primary systemic amyloidosis (AL amyloidosis), secondary systemic amyloidosis (AA amyloidosis), dialysis-associated amyloidosis (β_2-microglobulin), and senile systemic amyloidosis. Skin changes such as petechiae, ecchymoses, waxy papules and plaques, nail dystrophy, and, rarely, blisters may occur. Management of systemic amyloidosis is complex. Treatment of any skin lesions is dependent on treating the underlying systemic amyloidosis and is beyond the scope of this chapter.

Cutaneous amyloidosis may be primary or secondary. The latter refers to deposition of amyloid within skin tumors such as seborrhoeic keratosis, porokeratosis, pilomatricoma, and basal cell carcinoma and is detectable histologically. Primary localized cutaneous amyloidosis (PLCA) is characterized by the deposition of amyloid in the skin without involving any internal organ. It occurs more commonly in Southeast Asians, Chinese, Middle Easterners, and South Americans. There are three types of primary localized cutaneous amyloidosis: lichen amyloidosis, macular amyloidosis (keratinic amyloid in both types, derived from degenerated keratinocytes), and nodular amyloidosis (AL amyloid, derived from immunoglobulin light chains). *Biphasic amyloidosis* refers to the co-occurrence of macular and lichen amyloidosis in a patient.

Lichen amyloidosis (LA) (see Figure) is a persistent eruption of multiple red-brown hyperkeratotic papules often affecting extensor aspects of extremities, especially the pretibial surfaces. The male-to-female ratio varies among studies from 2:1 and 1:2. Apart from its cosmetic nuisance, marked itching can occur. Although familial cases of lichen amyloidosis have been reported, most are isolated cases without any association with systemic disease.

Macular amyloidosis (MA) is characterized by an eruption consisting of small, dusky-brown or grayish pigmented macules distributed symmetrically over the upper back and upper arm. It has a reticulated or rippled pattern. Itch is variable, and patients seek medical advice for esthetic issues.

Nodular amyloidosis is the rarest subtype of PLCA. It is characterized by single or multiple waxy, firm, brown or pink nodules involving the legs, head, trunk, arms, and genitalia. It is usually asymptomatic.

Both lichen and macular amyloidosis run a benign course. However, for primary localized cutaneous nodular amyloidosis (PLCNA), an estimated 7% risk of progression to systemic amyloidosis has been reported. Further, a case of PLCNA associated with CREST and Sjögren syndrome was also reported.

MANAGEMENT STRATEGY

Pruritus and unsightly presentation are common in localized cutaneous amyloidosis. Currently, effective treatment of cutaneous amyloidosis is lacking. *Antihistamines* and *topical corticosteroids* are commonly prescribed.

Phototherapy (ultraviolet B or PUVA) has been used to treat lichen amyloidosis successfully for relief of pruritus. Acitretin may be added for combined therapy. Laser treatments reported to be successful in treating cutaneous amyloidosis include carbon dioxide laser, pulsed dye laser (PDL), and neodymium:yttrium aluminum garnet (Nd:YAG) laser.

Dermabrasion has been successful in treating lichen and nodular amyloidosis. This improves cosmesis and alleviates pruritus, but brings accompanying procedural pain and possible skin atrophy. There is an anecdotal report that dermabrasion of lichen amyloidosis under tumescent anesthesia reduced procedural pain.

Other treatment choices include tacrolimus, transcutaneous electrical nerve stimulation (TENS), capsaicin, tocoretinate, and amitriptyline. Topical dimethyl sulfoxide (DMSO) also has been reported to benefit lichen and macular amyloidosis. However, a more recent study on 25 patients reported a lack of efficacy.

Specific Investigation

- Skin biopsy

All forms of amyloidosis have similar histologic findings. On light microscopy, amyloid is characteristically a pink, amorphous material. Special stains, such as Congo red and crystal violet, can highlight the amyloid deposit. Amyloid can be metachromatically stained red by crystal violet staining of an aqueous mount of the specimen. Congo red staining of amyloid shows apple-green birefringence under polarized light microscopy.

First-Line Therapies

• Sedating antihistamines	E
• Topical high-potency corticosteroids	E

Evidence Levels: **A** Double-blind study **B** Clinical trial ≥ 20 subjects **C** Clinical trial < 20 subjects **D** Series ≥ 5 subjects **E** Anecdotal case reports

Although there are no specific studies evaluating the efficacy of antihistamines and topical corticosteroids for treating cutaneous amyloidosis, they are considered first-line therapies. Sedating antihistamines and high-potency steroids help in the relief of pruritus and thinning of lesions.

Second-Line Therapies	
• Phototherapy/photochemotherapy	D
• Oral retinoids	D
• Laser	D
• Tacrolimus	E
• TENS	D
• Capsaicin	E
• Tocoretinate	D
• Amitriptyline	E

Thermosensitive lichen amyloidosis. Parsi K, Kossard S. Int J Dermatol 2004; 43: 925–8.

A 26-year old man with a 3-year history of lichen amyloidosis with lesions characteristically sparing areas with higher cutaneous temperatures. The clinical response to topical steroids and moisturizers was unsatisfactory. The patient received an average of three treatment sessions per week for a total of 55 sessions of narrowband ultraviolet B phototherapy over a 5-month period. This resulted in a marked improvement of pruritus and clearing of the amyloid deposit.

Successful treatment of lichen amyloidosis with combined bath PUVA photochemotherapy and oral acitretin. Grimmer J, Weiss T, Weber L, Meixner D, Scharffetter-Kochanek K. Clin Exp Dermatol 2007; 32: 39–42.

Two male patients with lichen amyloidosis over the extensor surfaces of the lower legs were treated with bath PUVA three to four times per week for 11 weeks, plus oral administration of acitretin 0.5 mg/kg/day for 7 months. There was almost complete resolution of skin lesions in both patients. No relapse was observed for 8 months after discontinuation of treatment.

Widespread biphasic amyloidosis: response to acitretin. Hernandez-Nunez A, Dauden E, Moreno de Vega MJ, Fraga J, Aragues M, Garcia-Diez A. Clin Exp Dermatol 2001; 26: 256–9.

A 73-year-old man with a 15-year history of biphasic amyloidosis was treated with acitretin 35 mg once daily (0.5 mg/kg/day). Pruritus resolved completely after 2 weeks of treatment. Acitretin was continued for 6 months and then stopped. There was no recurrence during the subsequent 6 months of follow-up.

Efficacy of different modes of fractional CO_2 laser in the treatment of primary cutaneous amyloidosis: a randomized clinical trial. Esmat SM, Fawzi MM, Gawdat HI, Ali HS, Sayed SS. Lasers Surg Med 2015; 47: 388–95.

Twenty-five patients with primary cutaneous amyloidosis (16 MA and 9 LA) were treated by fractional CO_2 laser using superficial ablation and deep rejuvenation to equal areas of randomly assigned lesions after the application of a topical anesthetic cream. Each patient received four sessions with 4-week intervals. Both modes yielded significant reduction of pigmentation, thickness, itching, and amyloid deposit. The superficial ablation was better tolerated by patients.

Successful treatment of lichen amyloidosis using a CO_2 surgical laser. Norisugi O, Yamakoshi T, Shimizu T. Dermatol Ther 2014; 27: 71–3.

Two male patients with LA on their legs not responding to topical corticosteroids were treated with CO_2 laser twice a month, using a setting of 10 to 15 W with a 0.12-second pulse duration, 0.36-second rest duration, and a 5-mm laser spot size. The papules gradually flattened, and there was marked reduction of the itching as assessed by the Visual Analog Scale (VAS) score. No complications of the treatment were noted.

A case of lichen amyloidosis treated with pulsed dye laser. Sawamura D, Sato-Matsumura KC, Shibaki A, Akiyama M, Kikuchi T, Shimizu H. J Eur Acad Dermatol Venereol 2005; 19: 262–3.

A 59-year-old man with lichen amyloidosis for 5 years was treated with two sessions of 585-nm PDL. The treatment parameters were 7-mm spot size and a fluence of 6.0 J/cm². Reassessment at 8 weeks showed great reduction of itch with decreasing size of papules, although complete clearance was not achieved. The improvement persisted for more than 15 months after treatment.

532-nm and 1064-nm Q-switched Nd:YAG laser therapy for reduction of pigmentation in macular amyloidosis patches. Ostovari N, Mohtasham N, Oadras MS, Malekzad F. J Eur Acad Dermatol Venereol 2008; 22: 442–6.

Twenty patients with histology-confirmed macular amyloidosis were treated with Q-switched Nd:YAG laser with 532 nm in a part of their plaques and with 1064 nm in another part of their plaques. Assessment of efficacy was done by colorimetric scores and digital photographs before laser therapy and 8 weeks after treatment. Both lasers were effective in reducing pigmentation, with the 532 nm more effective. Ninety percent of cases treated by 532 nm had good or very good response, and for the 1064 nm–treated patches, 60% of cases had a good or very good response.

Lichen amyloidosis improved by 0.1% topical tacrolimus. Castanedo-Cazares JP, Lepe V, Moncada B. Dermatology 2002; 205: 420–1.

One patient with lichen amyloidosis diagnosed clinically was treated with tacrolimus 0.1% ointment twice daily. Resolution of pruritus was noted after 2 weeks of therapy, and marked improvement of plaque thickness was observed after 2 months.

Transcutaneous electrical nerve stimulation for reduction of pruritus in macular amyloidosis and lichen simplex. Yüksek J, Sezer E, Aksu M, Erkokmaz U. J Dermatol 2011; 38: 546–52.

Eight patients with macular amyloidosis and eight with lichen simplex were treated with high-frequency TENS thrice weekly for 4 weeks, 30 minutes duration, to areas with most intense itching. All patients with macular amyloidosis and six (75%) with lichen simplex had relief of their pruritus.

Successful treatment of lichen amyloidosis using capsaicin 8% patch. Zeidler C, Metze D, Ständer S. J Eur Acad Dermatol Venereol 2016; 30(7): 1236–8.

Two male patients with long-standing lichen amyloidosis not responding to topical corticosteroid and systemic antihistamine were treated with an 8% capsaicin patch applied once directly over the itchy area for 60 minutes. Pruritus subsided totally the next day, and the improvement lasted for at least 2 to 3 months. The mechanism of action is due to capsaicin inducing regrowth of anatomically normal nerves and restoring normal neuronal function over the treated areas.

Clinical effect of tocoretinate on lichen and macular amyloidosis. Terao M, Nishida K, Murota H, Katayama I. J Dermatol 2011; 38: 179–84.

Tocoretinate is a synthetic esterified compound of retinoic acid and tocopherol that is used for treating skin ulcers and improving skin manifestations of scleroderma, morphea, and hypertrophic scars. Ten patients with lichen amyloidosis and macular amyloidosis were treated daily with topical tocoretinate ointment. The outcome was very good for four, good for two, moderate for two, and poor for two. Normalization of epidermal differentiation shown in vivo is thought to be beneficial in the treatment of amyloidosis.

Itch in familial lichen amyloidosis: effective treatment with amitriptyline in two cases. Yew YW, Tey HL. Dermatol Ther 2014; 27: 12–5.

Two Chinese male patients with lichen amyloidosis had extensive, pruritic, and hyperkeratotic papules affecting the shins. In both patients, the pruritus was not improved with potent topical steroids and oral antihistamines. Amitriptyline was started at a dose of 10 mg every other night, resulting in significant reduction of itch score and Dermatology Life Quality Index score assessed 3 weeks after commencement of treatment. Itch was well controlled at 8 months and 6 months, respectively. Side effects were minimal. However, the lesions of lichen amyloidosis remained unchanged. The action of amitriptyline may be related to inhibition of the reuptake of 5-HT and noradrenaline in the brainstem and spinal cord and the inhibition of voltage-dependent sodium and potassium channels in peripheral nerves.

Evidence Levels: **A** Double-blind study **B** Clinical trial ≥ 20 subjects **C** Clinical trial < 20 subjects **D** Series ≥ 5 subjects **E** Anecdotal case reports

Androgenetic alopecia

Walter P. Unger, Robin H. Unger

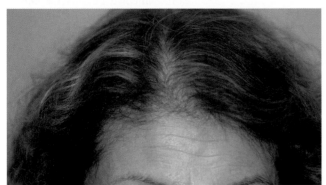

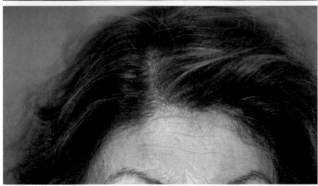

Androgenetic alopecia (AGA) is the most common type of hair loss affecting both men and women. The hair loss is secondary to the involution of hair follicles due to both genetic predisposition and hormonal influences. Other factors may cause telogen effluvium and thus accelerate the process, including those such as endocrine imbalances, nutritional deficiencies, general anesthesia, drug therapies, anabolic supplements, and seborrheic dermatitis. The main hormone implicated in male pattern baldness (MPB) is dihydrotestosterone (DHT), which induces miniaturization, shortens anagen duration, and prolongs telogen in genetically susceptible hair follicles. The primary cause of female pattern hair loss (FPHL) is still unclear. Although the pathogenesis in the hair follicles in FPHL is largely similar to MPB and DHT may have a significant role in FPHL in women with elevated levels of androgens, decreased intracutaneous synthesized estrogens, prolactin, and other factors may have a greater influence in the majority of patients with FPHL.

Specific Investigations

- Full blood count
- Ferritin
- Thyroid function tests
- Female androgen screen
- Trichoscopy
- Photographic documentation
- Scalp biopsy

Management begins with a thorough physical examination of the patient, relevant blood tests, and scalp biopsies where indicated. The use of dermoscopy (such as the FotoFinder system) in the evaluation of patients presenting with alopecia is especially helpful. Many other conditions (alopecia areata, frontal fibrosing alopecia, and lichen planopilaris) can mimic AGA or unmask an underlying patterned hair loss.

MPB is most commonly graded by the Hamilton–Norwood patterns and may affect up to 80% of Caucasian men by the age of 70 years. Patients presenting with early onset of MPB are particularly important to address with medical management. FPHL is also exceptionally common. Dawber found that 87% of premenopausal women had Ludwig type I to III loss. Women may also present with a pattern more similar to MPB—79% of women develop type II MPB after puberty, and that number increases to Hamilton type IV in 25% of women by age 50 years and 50% by age 60 years. FPHL has traditionally been graded by the Ludwig scale; however, a group of esteemed dermatologists have recently proposed a new FPHL Severity Index that combines measurements of hair shedding, midline hair density, and scalp trichoscopy criteria.

Towards a consensus on how to diagnose and quantify female pattern hair loss – The 'Female Pattern Hair Loss Severity Index (FPHL-SI).' Harries M, Tosti A, Bergfeld W, Blume-Peytavi U, Shapiro J, Lutz G, et al. Eur Acad of Dermatol and Venereol 2016; 30: 667–76.

The Ludwig scale has long been utilized to evaluate patients with FPHL, yet it is insufficient in many regards. Early-stage loss cannot be graded, and the scale is not precise enough to evaluate efficacy of treatments. Nine experts in the field have proposed a new scale to describe FPHL that can be used in clinical practice. It is a three-point scale with a maximum score of 20 that evaluates hair shedding, midline hair density, and scalp trichoscopy.

Imposters of androgenetic alopecia: diagnostic pearls for the hair restoration surgeon. Rogers N. Facial Plast Surg Clin North Am 2013; 21: 325–35.

This is a detailed review of the potential causes for hair loss, which may be mistakenly ascribed to AGA. The article discusses diagnostic tools, including trichoscopy and scalp biopsy, to determine the underlying etiology. This is particularly important for hair restoration surgeons, as it may lead to poor growth or future loss of transplanted hair.

MANAGEMENT STRATEGY

Medical treatment for AGA, if utilized appropriately in the early stages of loss, may reverse miniaturization and slow the future rate of loss. Topical *minoxidil* 5% has been proven to be an effective therapy for AGA, with minimal side effects. It is a biologic response modifier, and its active metabolite, minoxidil sulfate, opens potassium channels and growth factor production, thus increasing the duration of the anagen cycle and enlarging miniaturized follicles. The recommendation is twice-daily use, and the peak hair growth is seen between 26 and 52 weeks. Some clinical improvement is seen after 2 years of use in 40% to 60% of patients. The vertex has the best response; however, recent studies have proven that in a smaller percentage of patients the frontal area may also benefit from treatment. The bioavailability of sulfotransferase differs among patients and may account for the variable response rate. Continued use is necessary for long-term efficacy, and patients may experience a significant telogen effluvium 3 to 4 months after stopping treatment.

The second option for medical therapy in MPB is the use of 5-alpha-reductase inhibitors. *Finasteride* is a competitive inhibitor of type II 5-alpha-reductase, which at 1 mg/day achieves close to a 70% reduction in serum and scalp levels of DHT. The use of finasteride for 2 years prevents progression of the disease in 99% of patients and produces clinical improvement in 66%. Continued improvement has been shown to be related to the reentry of resting follicles into the anagen phase and anagen prolongation. If the drug is discontinued, return to baseline hair counts is seen within 1 year. The side effects of finasteride use in men include primarily decreased libido, erectile dysfunction, and decreased semen volume. Additional side effects that have been reported include gynecomastia, depression, and lowering of sperm count and motility. A meta-analysis performed in 2015 suggests that toxicity information and drug safety were not accurately presented in studies performed. *Dutasteride* blocks type I and II 5-alpha-reductase and is used as an off-label treatment for AGA by many practitioners. Studies have shown that a dose of 0.5 mg/day is more effective than finasteride for the treatment of AGA.

The only Food and Drug Administration (FDA)–approved treatment for FPHL is topical minoxidil; the 5% strength is now approved for once-daily use, which is easier with respect to compliance and more effective than the twice-daily 2% preparation. Clinical improvement may be seen in up to 80% of patients. It is contraindicated in pregnancy and may cause scalp pruritus, palpitations, or headaches in women with very low blood pressure, but is usually very well tolerated.

Women with FPHL may also benefit from the use of antiandrogens, although these have been shown to be most effective in women with clear endocrine disorders resulting in hyperandrogenism. Other than minoxidil, all medications are off-label use for FPH, including *cyproterone acetate, flutamide,* and *spironolactone.* Finasteride 1 to 5 mg daily has been used by many practitioners for the treatment of FPHL. Its efficacy has been debated and remains unproven in controlled studies. Furthermore there is no defined safety profile in women, and the increase in estrogen (due to conversion of testosterone to estradiol) may be of particular concern in patients with uterine fibroids, as well as a known personal or family history of breast/ovarian cancer.

Surgical treatment is an effective option for treatment in patients who have not responded to medical therapy or in whom the results have not provided a significant cosmetic improvement. Advances in *hair transplant surgery* have enabled surgeons to create a very natural and cosmetically significant increase in hair density even after one operation. The photos included show an example of the results that can typically be achieved after just one hair replacement surgery. Hair from the relatively permanent fringe may be harvested with either a single elliptical excision (strip) or utilizing follicular unit extraction (FUE). The latter method is becoming increasingly popular, whether via robot, manual punch, or motorized punch. Both methods have advantages and disadvantages, and a good surgeon should have all tools at their disposal. Grafts produced from a single-strip harvest have the distinct advantage of being taken from the center of the area, with the highest percentage of permanent hairs in the donor area, and the limited studies performed to date indicate the grafts from the strip have a higher survival rate than those obtained with FUE. An initial small study presented at the 2015 annual ISHRS international conference found that 14 months after surgery 547/890 grafts grew in the FUE study area (61.4%) compared with 765/890 follicles in the strip graft study area—a difference of 24.6%. Hopefully further refinements and studies will show improved results in FUE. Regardless of technique, the follicular units harvested are placed into small incisions created between existing hairs, and therefore it produces an excellent increase in density in both men and women with AGA.

Platelet-rich plasma (PRP) treatment for hair loss is still an unproven therapy, although limited studies, case reports, and anecdotal reports are very encouraging. It may be used adjunctively as part of hair transplant surgery or as a treatment on its own. Physicians who use PRP as a stand-alone treatment for AGA may also use microneedling or ACell powder to increase efficacy. Unfortunately, there is no consensus on the best method of treatment or on the efficacy of each technique.

Additional management strategies include camouflage aids. These include various tinted powders or sprays, tattooing of the scalp, hairpieces, or wigs. Hair extensions add density and length, but can produce permanent traction alopecia. *Hairthickening shampoos* and sprays may also help to temporarily increase the look of volume. *Low-level laser light* has some supporting evidence.

First-Line Therapies

• Topical minoxidil	A
• Finasteride	A
• Spironolactone	B

Androgenetic alopecia: an evidence-based treatment update. Varothai S, Bergfeld W. Am J Clin Dermatol 2014; 15: 217–30.

A thorough review of the treatment options for AGA grounded in evidence-based medicine. Studies of hair loss and growth are notoriously difficult to perform, and this leads to studies with limited patient populations or poor controls. The authors review studies of clinical relevance.

A single-centre, randomized, double-blind, placebo controlled clinical trial to investigate the efficacy and safety of minoxidil topical foam in frontotemporal and vertex androgenetic alopecia in men. Hillman K, Garcia-Bartels N, Kottner J, Stroux A, Canfield D, Blume-Peytavi U. Skin Pharmacol Physiol 2015; 28: 236–44.

Although the efficacy of 5% minoxidil in vertex and mid-scalp AGA has been proven in multiple studies, this is the first study to prove its efficacy in the frontotemporal area. Maximum improvement was seen at 16 weeks, but continued to 24 weeks in all regions. The cumulative nonvellus hair caliber showed the most significant increase from baseline. The subject self-assessment also revealed a significant improvement in scalp coverage in all areas. A follow-up study was published in September 2015, indicating that cosmetic effectiveness continued to 104 weeks without significant regional differences, although hair counts had returned to baseline.

A randomized, single-blind trial of 5% minoxidil foam once daily versus 2% minoxidil solution twice daily in the treatment of androgenetic alopecia in women. Blume-Peytavi U, Hillmann K, Dietz E, Canfield D, Garcia Bartels N. J Am Acad Dermatol 2011; 65: 1126–34.

A 6-month study involving 113 women with AGA demonstrated that once-daily 5% minoxidil foam is as effective for stimulating hair growth and caliber increase as twice-daily propylene glycol containing 2% topical minoxidil. Patients were more compliant with the once-daily 5% foam due to convenience of use and low levels of side effects.

Efficacy and safety of finasteride therapy for androgenetic alopecia: a systematic review. Mella JM, Perret MC, Manzotti M, Catalano HN, Guyatt G. Arch Dermatol 2010; 146:1141–50.

A meta-analysis of 12 studies (3927 male patients) revealed moderate-quality evidence suggesting that daily use of oral finasteride (1 mg or 5 mg) significantly increases hair count and improves patient and investigator assessment of hair appearance, while increasing the risk of sexual dysfunction. A Jadad score was used to assess the methodology of each study analyzed (through 2009).

Finasteride treatment of female pattern hair loss. Iorizzo M, Vincenzi C, Voudouris S, Piraccini BM, Tosti A. Arch Dermatol 2006; 142: 298–302.

Thirty-seven women with FPHL were treated with oral finasteride, 2.5 mg a day, while taking an oral contraceptive containing drospirenone and ethinyl estradiol. At 12 months' follow-up, 23 of the 37 patients were rated as improved using global photography (12 were slightly improved, 8 were moderately improved, and 3 were greatly improved). No improvement was recorded in 13 patients. One patient experienced worsening of the condition. There was a statistically significant increase in the hair density score in 12 patients. It was unclear whether the success was due to a higher dosage of finasteride than used in prior studies (2.5 mg instead of 1 mg) or to its association with the oral contraceptive containing drospirenone, which has an antiandrogenic effect.

Treatment of female pattern hair loss with oral anti-androgens. Sinclair R, Wewerinke M, Jolley D. Br J Dermatol 2005; 152: 466–73.

The results of this study of 80 women treated with either spironolactone or cyproterone acetate indicated a positive effect with treatment. In the treatment group 44% of women showed regrowth, 44% demonstrated no progression of hair loss, and 12% continued with progressive hair loss. Women with more severe baseline FPHL were more likely to be responders. This study did not compare results with a placebo group, nor were the investigators blinded. Spironolactone is generally used at 100 to 200 mg a day and cyproterone at 52 mg a day on days 5 to 15 of the menstrual cycle, with Estinyl 20 µg twice daily on days 5 to 24 of the menstrual cycle.

Second-Line Therapy

• Dutasteride	A

Long-term safety and efficacy of dutasteride in the treatment of male patients with androgenetic alopecia. Tsunemi T, Irisawa R, Yoshiie H, Brotherton B, Ito H, Tsuboi R, et al. J Dermatol 2016; 43: 1051–8.

This study aimed to determine long-term safety, tolerability, and efficacy of dutasteride 0.5 mg, an inhibitor of type 1 and 2 5-α-reductase, in Japanese male patients with AGA. *A multicenter, open-label, prospective outpatient study of 120 men given dutasteride 0.5 mg once daily for 52 weeks.* Nasopharyngitis, erectile dysfunction, and decreased libido were the most frequently reported adverse events, and most adverse events were mild. Drug-related adverse events were reported, with an incidence of 17%, none of which led to study withdrawal. Hair growth (mean target area hair count at week 52), hair restoration (mean target area hair width at week 52), and global appearance of hair (mean of the median score at week 52) improved from baseline during the study. Dutasteride exhibited long-term safety in this Japanese population.

Regenerative medicine and hair loss: how hair follicle culture has advanced our understanding of treatment options for androgenetic alopecia. Higgins CA, Christiano AM. Regen Med 2014; 9: 101–11.

A review of the current research being done on hair follicle culture. Growth modulators found to be effective in culturing hair follicles may lead to treatment options for AGA that were previously unexplored. The article also describes the current state of research in follicular stem cell implantation—a potential future treatment modality.

Third-Line Therapies

• Hair transplant surgery	A
• Lasers	C
• Platelet-rich plasma	C

Female hair restoration. Unger R. Facial Plast Surg Clin North Am 2013; 21: 407–19.

A detailed article describing the latest surgical techniques used in treating female hair loss. The article describes the treatment of women with AGA, as well as those with cicatricial or trauma-induced alopecia. Technical surgical pearls are explained. Most importantly, the article addresses the most significant aspects in the unique approach required for planning female hair restoration surgery.

Planning and organization. Unger WP. In: Unger WP, Shapiro R, Unger RH, Unger M, eds. Hair Transplantation, 5th edn. New York: Marcel Dekker, 2011; 106–52.

An in-depth review of the most important aspects in planning a successful hair transplant, including the nomenclature of scalp anatomic landmarks and determination of patient candidacy, in addition to surgical techniques and esthetic principles essential to achieving *long-term* esthetic results. Key background factors for surgical planning are highlighted in both women and men, with a particular emphasis on addressing the areas of future hair loss in younger patients.

Robotic hair restoration. Rose P, Nusbaum B. Dermatol Clin 2014; 32: 97–107.

The authors describe the use of robotic FUE. Included are challenges and benefits of this method of harvesting grafts, which are fairly similar to those with FUE performed with a manual or motorized punch. Challenges include the time necessary for extraction, the availability of only two punch sizes, and the requirement of shaving the donor area. The robot does allow physicians to include hair transplantation in their practice without a significant number of additional support staff; however, good results are still dependent on surgical planning and artistry in the recipient area.

Efficacy and safety of a low-level laser device in the treatment of male and female pattern hair loss: a multicenter, randomized, sham device-controlled, double-blind study. Jiminez J, Wikramanayake T, Bergfeld W, Hordinsky M, Hickman J, Hamblin M, et al. Am J Clin Dermatol 2014; 15: 115–27.

Multiple centers enrolled a total of 128 male and 141 female patients to evaluate an at-home low-level light therapy (LLLT) device with differing number of beams. The patients were randomly assigned to the device or the sham device in sealed packages and instructed to use them three times a week for 26 weeks. Terminal hair density was evaluated at baseline, 16 weeks, and 26 weeks, and a blinded independent evaluator looked at Canfield photographs to determine the change in hair counts. Meta-analyses were conducted and showed a significant mean terminal hair density increase at 26 weeks. Compared with the sham device, there was a statistically significant improvement from baseline.

The effect of platelet-rich plasma in hair regrowth: a randomized placebo-controlled trial. Gentile P, Garcovich S, Bielli A, Scioli MG, Orlandi A, Cervelli A. Stem Cells Transl Med 2015; 4: 1317–23.

This study is a randomized, half-head, placebo-controlled evaluation of PRP. Results were evaluated by a blinded evaluator using computerized trichograms. The main weakness in the study is that only 20 patients were enrolled. The results were evaluated after three treatments at 30-day intervals, and a mean increase of 33.6 hairs in the target area and a mean increase in total hair density of 45.9 hairs per cm^2 were found compared with baseline values. Biopsies were also evaluated and showed increased epidermis thickness and number of hair follicles, as well as increased Ki-67 indicating cell proliferation.

Evidence Levels: **A** Double-blind study **B** Clinical trial ≥ 20 subjects **C** Clinical trial < 20 subjects **D** Series ≥ 5 subjects **E** Anecdotal case reports

13

Angiolymphoid hyperplasia with eosinophilia

William Y.M. Tang, Loi Yuen Chan

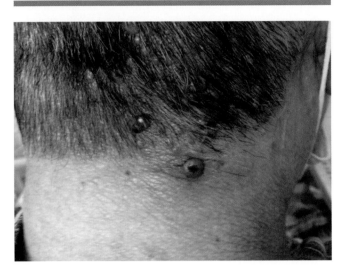

Angiolymphoid hyperplasia with eosinophilia (ALHE) was first described by Wells and Whimster in 1969. It is a benign vascular proliferation of unknown etiology with a characteristic component of epithelioid endothelial cells. It is an uncommon disease, so data on its natural course and treatment response are based on a small number of patients.

ALHE usually affects women in their third decade and presents as cutaneous papules or subcutaneous nodules, sometimes with inflammatory features on the head, neck, and periauricular region. Involvement elsewhere is rare. Approximately 20% of patients have blood eosinophilia. Although considered benign in nature, the etiology of ALHE is unknown, but neoplastic proliferation of vascular tissue, arteriovenous shunting, and reactive hyperplasia of vascular tissue secondary to trauma, infection, renin, or hyperestrogenic states have been proposed as causal factors. ALHE may cause symptoms such as disfigurement, bleeding, itch, and pain. It has been associated with various lymphoproliferative conditions, supporting the contention that it may represent a monoclonal T-cell process.

The differential diagnoses of ALHE include Kimura's disease, pyogenic granuloma, lymphocytoma cutis, insect bite, sarcoidosis, Kaposi sarcoma, and angiosarcoma. ALHE and Kimura's disease are generally regarded as separate clinicopathologic entities. Kimura's disease is a chronic inflammatory condition of unknown etiology often affecting young male Asians and typically presents as cervical lymphadenopathy and subcutaneous nodules in the head and neck region. However, coexistence of ALHE and Kimura's disease in the same patient has been reported.

MANAGEMENT STRATEGY

Treatment is usually required for ALHE, as spontaneous remission is rare. *Complete surgical excision* is preferred for persistent lesions.

Recurrence may occur if excision is incomplete. *Laser therapy and radiofrequency ablation* are alternative surgical options. *Cryotherapy,* inexpensive and easily available, is a conventional treatment, but reports on its efficacy are lacking. Other treatments reported effective include *topical and intralesional corticosteroids, propranolol, topical imiquimod, topical tacrolimus, isotretinoin, suplatast tosilate, intralesional interferon-α_{2b}, thalidomide, and photodynamic therapy.*

Specific Investigations

- Histopathology
- Imaging

Microscopically, ALHE is characterized by a proliferation of blood vessels of varying sizes lined by plump endothelial cells. These histiocytoid endothelial cells are enlarged, with abundant eosinophilic or clear cytoplasm and large vesicular nuclei. The cells are mostly cuboidal with occasional "hobnailing," which is related to the presence of cytoplasmic vacuoles in these cells, causing cytoplasmic protrusion into lumina. There is also an accompanying perivascular lymphocytic and eosinophilic infiltrate.

The location and extent of underlying vascular anomalies may be assessed by angiography, angiomagnetic resonance imaging, and angiocomputed tomography.

Due to its predominant occurrence in females, hyperestrogenic states may have a causative role in ALHE. However, successful treatment of ALHE using hormonal therapy has not yet been reported.

Angiolymphoid hyperplasia with eosinophilia associated with pregnancy: a case report and review of the literature. Zarrin-Khameh N, Spoden JE, Tran RM. Arch Pathol Lab Med 2005; 129: 1168–71.

The authors reported a 33-year-old woman who developed ALHE in her right ear during the second trimester of pregnancy. The lesion was completely excised. The authors also reviewed a total of five other ALHE cases associated with pregnancy. Lesions in some of these patients increased in size during pregnancy. One patient improved with cessation of oral contraceptive pills, whereas the lesions in another patient reduced in size by half during the postpartum period. Two patients had skin biopsy expressing a significant amount of estrogen and progesterone receptors but not in the uninvolved skin.

First-Line Therapies

• Surgery	D
• Laser therapy	D
• Corticosteroid, topical or intralesional	E

A refractory case of angiolymphoid hyperplasia with eosinophilia successfully treated by surgery. Baghestani S, Firooz A, Ghazisaidi MR. J Dermatolog Treat 2011; 22: 49–51.

The authors reported a 30-year-old woman with ALHE on her right ear successfully treated by surgery after several unsuccessful attempts with other conventional therapies, including cryotherapy, electrodesiccation, and intralesional plus oral corticosteroids.

Epidemiology and treatment of angiolymphoid hyperplasia with eosinophilia (ALHE): a systematic review. Adler BL, Krausz AE, Minuti A, Silverberg JI, Lev-Tov H. J Am Acad Dermatol 2016; 74: 506–12.

This report includes 416 studies detailing 908 patients. The authors concluded that surgical excision was the best option, albeit suboptimal. Pulsed dye lasers or other lasers may represent other reasonable therapeutic options.

Facial angiolymphoid hyperplasia with eosinophilia: sustained remission following treatment with carbon dioxide laser. Ali FR, Madan V. Clin Exp Dermatol 2016; 41: 96–8.

A 35-year-old woman presented with biopsy-proven ALHE lesions on her left temple, which had developed during pregnancy 5 years previously. Ablation with CO_2 laser (15W, 4-mm spot, 10,600 nm) was undertaken in three sessions over the course of 8 months, with an excellent clinical response. There was no recurrence after 30 months.

Angiolymphoid hyperplasia successfully treated with an ultralong pulsed dye laser. Angel CA, Lewis AT, Griffin T, Levy EJ, Benedetto AV. Dermatol Surg 2005; 31: 713–6.

A 72-year-old man with ALHE presented with a tender, enlarging lesion over the left posterior helix and mastoid region for 1 year not responding to intralesional steroids. He was successfully treated with two sessions of ultralong pulsed dye laser (PDL) (595 nm, 7-mm round spot, 3.0-ms pulse width, 15 J/cm²). There was no recurrence 3 years after treatment. The longer wavelength produces deeper penetration into dermal tissue and more uniform coagulation necrosis across the entire diameter of the targeted blood vessel.

Angiolymphoid hyperplasia with eosinophilia: successful treatment with the Nd:YAG laser. Kadurina MI, Dimitrov BG, Bojinova ST, Tonev SD. J Cosmet Laser Ther 2007; 9: 107–11.

This is the first review of Nd:YAG laser for treating ALHE. A 31-year-old woman presented with a rapidly enlarging, itchy, and bleeding tumor of ALHE affecting the right ear tragus and ear canal. The lesion was treated with 1064-nm Nd:YAG (6-mm round spot, two pulses of 7.0 ms with a 20-ms interpulse delay, fluence of 100–150 J/cm²). A total of five treatments were administered with an interval of 30 days between each procedure. The patient showed complete remission after 1-year follow-up.

Angiolymphoid hyperplasia with eosinophilia treated with vascular laser. Alcántara González J, Boixeda P, Truchuelo Díez MT, Pérez García B, Jaén Olasolo P. Lasers Med Sci 2011; 26: 285–90.

The sequential laser combines 595-nm PDL with 1064-nm Nd:YAG targeting structures at different dermal levels using two different wavelengths. Greater effectiveness and lower recurrence rates are possible with the Nd:YAG laser, which allows the destruction of deeper vessels than does PDL. Three patients with ALHE were treated with this sequential laser system. Complete resolution was observed in two of them 3 years after their last treatment; the other patient showed a marked improvement.

Second-Line Therapies	
• Propranolol	E
• Imiquimod	E
• Tacrolimus	E
• Isotretinoin	E
• Radiofrequency ablation and sclerotherapy	E

Propranolol: a novel treatment for angiolymphoid hyperplasia with eosinophilia. Horst C, Kapur N. Clin Exp Dermatol 2014; 39: 810–2.

A 32-year-old woman presented with multiple ALHE lesions in the left periauricular area and the vertex of her scalp. She was started on oral propranolol 40 mg daily. Within 6 weeks, several lesions had decreased in size, and all were less erythematous. Propranolol was subsequently stopped within a few months of initiating treatment. Propranolol targets the vascular proliferative element of ALHE. It is also effective in decreasing the vasculature of hemangiomas of infancy.

Angiolymphoid hyperplasia with eosinophilia treated successfully with imiquimod. Isohisa T, Masuda K, Nakai N, Takenaka H, Katoh N. Int J Dermatol 2014; 53: e43–4.

A 49-year-old woman with multiple ALHE lesions in her left postauricular area and external auditory canal was treated with 5% imiquimod cream five times per week. The pruritus improved markedly within 2 weeks. By 22 weeks of treatment, the small lesions had almost completely regressed. The authors suggested that topical imiquimod should be considered for treatment of ALHE because of its excellent cosmetic results and safety record, especially for those with multiple lesions. The underlying mechanism may be related to the immunomodulating and antiangiogenic effect of imiquimod.

Angiolymphoid hyperplasia with eosinophilia: efficacy of isotretinoin? El Sayed F, Dhaybi R, Ammoury A, Chababi M. Head Face Med 2006; 2: 32.

The authors report a 32-year-old man with multiple pruritic lesions of ALHE treated with isotretinoin 0.5 mg/kg/day for 1 year with complete resolution of one of the two scalp nodules. Two lesions on the cheeks and two in the preauricular region that decreased in size, but did not totally resolve, were surgically removed. The success of isotretinoin was due to its antiangiogenic properties via a reduction of vascular endothelial growth factor production by keratinocytes.

Angiolymphoid hyperplasia with eosinophilia treated with a novel combination technique of radiofrequency ablation and sclerotherapy. Khunger N, Pahwa M, Jain RK. Dermatol Surg 2010; 36: 422–5.

Three patients with ALHE were treated with radiofrequency ablation (RFA) after intralesional sclerotherapy with 3% polidocanol. Lesions were mostly treated with cutting plus coagulation mode with an intensity of 4 U. One to four sessions of treatment were required to achieve complete response. No recurrence was seen after a follow-up period of 6 months to 2 years. The synergistic effect is due to sclerosants treating the deeper vascular component while RFA ablates the lesion.

Third-Line Therapies	
• Suplatast tosilate	E
• Interferon-α_{2b}	E
• Thalidomide	E
• Photodynamic therapy	E

Angiolymphoid hyperplasia with eosinophilia on the leg successfully treated with T-helper cell 2 cytokine inhibitor suplatast tosilate. Bito T, Kabashima R, Sugita K, Tokura Y. J Dermatol 2011; 38: 300–2.

Suplatast tosilate is a Th2 cytokine inhibitor that inhibits T helper cell production of interleukin (IL)-4 and IL-5. This results in reduced eosinophil infiltration and suppression of IgE production in B cells. A 63-year-old man with ALHE on the right calf was treated with suplatast tosilate both orally and topically. The lesions dramatically improved after 4-week administration and completely disappeared 4 months after the beginning of the treatment. No recurrence was observed even 15 months later.

There is an earlier report on a 32-year-old man with ALHE successfully treated with suplatast tosilate 300 mg/day.

Evidence Levels: A Double-blind study   B Clinical trial ≥ 20 subjects   C Clinical trial < 20 subjects   D Series ≥ 5 subjects   E Anecdotal case reports

Angiolymphoid hyperplasia with eosinophilia responding to interferon-alpha 2B. Oguz O, Antonov M, Demirkesen C. J Eur Acad Dermatol Venereol 2007; 21: 1277–8.

Interferon-α is a potential treatment in benign angioproliferative disorders. Local intralesional injection of interferon-α$_{2b}$ was reported effective for a 27-year-old female with occipital lesions of ALHE. Recurrence of lesions 9 years later was noted, but this time the response to repeated interferon-α$_{2b}$ treatment was poor.

In another report (Shenefelt PD et al. Arch Dermatol 2000; 136: 837–9) intralesional interferon alfa-2a caused almost complete resolution of lesions in one patient. However, recurrence of lesions was noted within about 1 year of the last injection, and no response occurred with the second course of injection.

Successful management of refractory angiolymphoid hyperplasia with eosinophilia with thalidomide. Rongioletti F, Cecchi F, Pastorino C, Scaparro M. J Eur Acad Dermatol Venereol 2016; 30: 527–9.

A 58-year-old woman with multiple ALHE lesions on the occipital area unresponsive to oral propranolol, cryotherapy, topical and systemic steroids, and topical tacrolimus was put on thalidomide 50 mg twice a day for 2 months, then three times daily for 4 months, with progressive decolorization, flattening, and regression of the lesions. After 6 months of therapy, the lesions almost resolved; however, she developed neuropathy necessitating the discontinuation of thalidomide. No new lesions were noted at 3 months of follow-up. The action of thalidomide is considered to be due to its antiangiogenic, antiinflammatory, and antitumor effects.

Angiolymphoid hyperplasia with eosinophilia: good response to photodynamic therapy. Sotiriou E, Apalla Z, Patsatsi A, Panagiotidou DD, Ioannides D. Clin Exp Dermatol 2009; 34: e629–31.

Photodynamic therapy (PDT) causes suppression of tumor growth by damaging endothelial cells in the tumor neovasculature. A 60-year-old woman with multiple ALHE lesions on the forehead was treated with two sessions of aminolevulinic acid (ALA) PDT, with a 2-week interval. A 20% 5-ALA cream occluded from light for 4 hours, followed by exposure to red light (570–670 nm, dose 80 J/cm^2) from a noncoherent light source was used. Marked improvement, though not complete regression, was achieved 8 weeks after treatment and maintained at 4 months after treatment. The moderate response achieved in this study could be due to poor penetration of the photosensitizer to the deep part of the lesion.

Angular cheilitis

Jennifer K. Chen, Janellen Smith

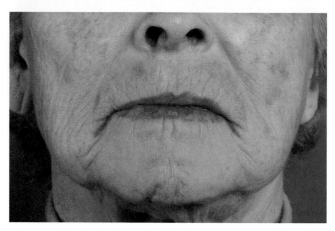

Angular cheilitis. With permission from Mayo Foundation for Medical Education and Research. All rights reserved.

Angular cheilitis is a chronic reactive inflammatory condition of the oral commissures characterized by atrophy, fissures, crusting, erythema, and scaling. The etiology is often multifactorial, and causes may be mechanical (intertrigo), infectious, nutritional, hormonal, or inflammatory. Angular cheilitis may be a sign of systemic disease (see later).

MANAGEMENT STRATEGY

Successful therapy is based on identifying and correcting any underlying condition(s). The presence of dentures, palatal erythema, and/or edema may suggest candidiasis and denture stomatitis. A pale, depapillated, atrophic tongue suggests iron deficiency. A tender depapillated tongue suggests folate or vitamin B_{12} deficiency. An eczematous dermatitis of the lower face suggests a staphylococcal infection (infectious eczematoid dermatitis). A history of allergic contact dermatitis may suggest an allergy.

Unilateral lesions are usually short lived and induced by mechanical factors. This has also been reported to be a manifestation of plasma cell cheilitis. Bilateral lesions tend to be chronic and caused by infection or nutritional deficiency and are more likely to be associated with an underlying disease process.

Maceration of the commissural epithelium and adjacent skin is a common, noninfectious cause of mechanical angular cheilitis. Trauma from dental flossing, habitual lip-licking, and excessive salivation all contribute. Periods of oral hydration and then dryness disrupt epithelial integrity, causing fissuring of the commissures. This provides an ideal environment for low-grade candidiasis and infectious eczematoid dermatitis. Other mechanical factors are ill-fitting dentures, loss of vertical dimension of the jaws, sagging skin folds, xerostomia, and perioral dermatitis.

Infectious and systemic causes must be investigated. Angular cheilitis is frequently present in patients with HIV disease, where 10% may have localized candidiasis. Highly active antiretroviral therapy (HAART) may decrease this incidence. Both *Candida albicans* and *Staphylococcus aureus* can colonize the fissures. Anemia, nutritional deficiencies, Down syndrome, acrodermatitis enteropathica, pemphigus vulgaris, diabetes mellitus, orofacial granulomatosis, and Crohn disease may be present.

Recurrence of angular cheilitis may be prevented by eliminating offending organisms from their reservoirs. Denture stomatitis, candidiasis, and nasal colonization by staphylococci should be investigated. *Topical imidazole creams* after meals and at bedtime may treat candidiasis, whereas *topical mupirocin* is valuable in treating staphylococcal colonization. Dentures should be removed from the mouth nightly and cleansed well before reinsertion in the morning. *New dentures* may restore facial contours, increasing the vertical dimension of the jaws and face. *Injection of fillers* into the commissures may alleviate causative mechanical factors.

Specific Investigations

- Culture or wet mount to evaluate for candidiasis
- Culture for bacteria
- For refractory or recurrent cases, laboratory evaluation should include a complete blood cell count; iron panel; vitamin B, folate, and zinc levels; glucose; hemoglobin A_{1c}; and HIV testing
- Patch testing

Angular cheilitis, part 1: local etiologies. Park KK, Brodell RT, Helms SE. Cutis 2011; 87: 289–95.

Angular cheilitis, part 2: nutritional, systemic, and drug-related causes and treatment. Park KK, Brodell RT, Helms SE. Cutis 2011; 88: 27–32.
 A discussion of the multifactorial nature and evaluation of angular cheilitis.

Epidemiology and etiology of denture stomatitis. Gendreau L, Loewy ZG. J Prosthodont 2011; 20: 251–60.

Angular cheilitis. Scully C, Bagan J-V, Eisen D, Porter S, Rogers RS III, eds. Dermatology of the Lips. Oxford: Isis Medical, 2000; 68–73.
 Excellent clinical photographs and summary.

Nickel-induced angular cheilitis due to orthodontic braces. Yesudian PD, Memon A. Contact Dermatitis 2003; 48: 287–8.

First-Line Therapies

Topical miconazole, ketoconazole, or nystatin cream two or three times daily for 2 to 3 weeks	D
Topical polymyxin B or mupirocin ointments	D
Remove dentures nightly and cleanse overnight with chlorhexidine 2% solution or sodium hypochlorite 0.02% solution. Rinse and air-dry before reinsertion. *Please note that chlorhexidine and nystatin inactivate each other and therefore should not be used together.*	D

Evidence Levels: A Double-blind study B Clinical trial ≥ 20 subjects C Clinical trial < 20 subjects D Series ≥ 5 subjects E Anecdotal case reports

Oral candidiasis and angular cheilitis. Sharon V, Fazel N. Dermatol Ther 2010; 23: 230–42.

An excellent review of topical and systemic therapy of candidiasis. The authors also recommend prophylaxis with chlorhexidine 0.12% mouthwash in recurrent cases.

Diseases of the lips. Rogers III, RS, Bekic M. Semin Cutan Med Surg 1997; 16: 325–36.

Discussion of the evaluation and treatment of angular cheilitis. Evren BA, Uludamar A, Iseri U, Ozkan YK. Arch Gerontol Geriatr 2011; 53: 252–7.

The association between socioeconomic status, oral hygiene practice, denture stomatitis, and oral status in elderly people living in different residential homes, is stressed.

Second-Line Therapies

• Systemic antifungal therapy (fluconazole)	E
• Amphotericin B cream	E

Oral candidiasis and angular cheilitis. Sharon V, Fazel N. Dermatol Ther 2010; 23: 230–42.

Reviews the treatment of candidiasis, highlighting challenges in the immunocompromised patient.

Third-Line Therapies

• Filler injections	E
• Prosthodontic evaluation and treatment	E
• Chewing gum with xylitol or chlorhexidine acetate and xylitol	B
• Gentian violet 0.5% solution twice daily	E
• Photodynamic therapy	E

Collagen implant in management of perleche (angular cheilosis). Chernosky ME. J Am Acad Dermatol 1985; 12: 493–6.

Soft tissue augmentation may be used to decrease the depth of the fold at the oral commissures, thus decreasing salivary stasis.

Prosthodontic management of angular cheilitis and persistent drooling: a case report. Lu DP. Compend Contin Educ Dent 2007; 28: 572–7.

The author describes a method to incorporate a cannula into the dental prosthesis to channel saliva toward the oropharynx, suitable for elderly or handicapped patients who suffer from chronic drooling and angular cheilitis.

The effects of medicated chewing gums on oral health in frail older people: a 1 year clinical trial. Simons D, Brailsford SR, Kidd EA, Beighton D. J Am Geriatr Soc 2002; 50: 1348–53.

A controlled, double-blind trial of 111 dentate patients in residential homes showed significant reductions in denture stomatitis and angular cheilitis in patients using chlorhexidine acetate/xylitol gums.

Oral candidiasis and angular cheilitis. Sharon V, Fazel N. Dermatol Ther 2010; 23: 230–42.

Gentian violet solution may be difficult to tolerate given the side effects of purple staining, skin irritation, and occasionally mucosal ulceration.

Antimicrobial photodynamic therapy to treat chemotherapy-induced oral lesions: report of three cases. Rocha BA, Filho MRM, Simoes A. Photodiagnosis Photodyn Ther 2016; 13: 350-2.

A case of angular cheilitis nonresponsive to nystatin alone responded within 48 hours to nystatin and miconazole 2% gel four times daily, in combination with photodynamic therapy with diode laser followed 2 days later by low-level laser therapy for improved wound healing and pain control.

Antiphospholipid syndrome

Julia S. Lehman, Mark D.P. Davis

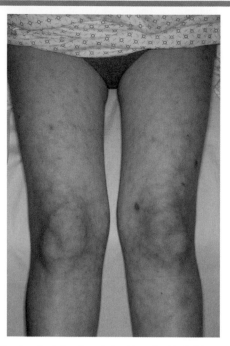

Fig. 15.1. Livedo reticularis, characterized by reticulated violaceous changes of the skin. This is a nonspecific skin finding that may be seen in patients with antiphospholipid antibody syndrome

Antiphospholipid syndrome (APS; Hughes syndrome) is characterized by the propensity for recurrent venous and arterial thrombosis in the presence of circulating antibodies against phospholipid-binding proteins. Diagnostic criteria for APS require that patients experience vascular thrombosis (venous or arterial) or pregnancy morbidity (e.g., three or more unexplained consecutive spontaneous abortions before the tenth week of gestation with exclusion of other causes) and harbor at least one serum antiphospholipid (aPL) antibody (i.e., lupus anticoagulant, anticardiolipin, anti-β_2-glycoprotein 1) on two or more occasions over a 12-week period. It is important that patients not be diagnosed with APS based on isolated laboratory test abnormalities, as no laboratory test for APS is entirely specific.

Although cutaneous manifestations of APS are not part of the diagnostic criteria, they may represent the initial presentation of APS. Cutaneous signs result from thromboocclusion of the cutaneous vasculature and may include livedo reticularis or racemosa, livedoid vasculopathy (atrophie blanche), superficial thrombophlebitis, or ulceration. Patients with Sneddon syndrome, a condition characterized by cerebrovascular disease in patients with livedo reticularis, may have persistently positive serum aPL. Whether Sneddon syndrome represents a subset of APS is controversial.

MANAGEMENT STRATEGY

In some cases, APS may represent a primary condition. However, a search for underlying causes or other contributing factors, such as infection, prothrombotic medications (such as oral contraceptives),

primary hematologic coagulopathies (e.g., factor V Leiden, prothrombin G20210A gene mutation), and connective tissue diseases (e.g., systemic lupus erythematosus [SLE]), is warranted. Patients should be offered subspecialty referral where available.

Because patients with APS are at increased risk for recurrent thromboembolism, the goal of therapy is thromboprophylaxis. Nonpharmacologic interventions include reduction of other prothrombotic risk factors, such as prolonged immobility and oral contraceptive use. Pharmaceutical interventions should be guided by the patient's age and comorbidities, pregnancy status, presence of correctable prothrombotic factors, and coagulation history. In patients with persistently elevated aPL antibodies but no history of thrombosis (thereby not meeting strict criteria for APS), *aspirin* has **not** been shown to be effective in preventing future thromboembolic events. In patients with definitive APS and a history of venous thromboembolism, the mainstay of treatment is long-term *warfarin* therapy. The optimal duration of warfarin therapy has not been established. Based on limited available data, indefinite treatment with warfarin appears to be associated with reduced rates of recurrent thromboembolism without an elevated risk for hemorrhagic complications, compared with treatment discontinuation after 6 months. Decisions regarding termination of warfarin therapy should be individualized. Long-term *heparin* use is discouraged because of the risk of heparin-induced osteopenia. Early reports of oral direct thrombin inhibitors (dabigatran) and factor Xa inhibitors (rivaroxaban, apixaban, edoxaban) are inconclusive; randomized clinical trials are ongoing.

Inferior vena cava filters may be required in patients with recurrent venous thromboembolism to prevent pulmonary embolism.

In patients with APS who have experienced arterial thromboembolism or have developed recurrent thrombosis despite achieving target international normalized ratio (INR) on warfarin, other treatment options must be pursued. These modalities, such as *rituximab, intravenous immunoglobulin,* and *plasmapheresis,* address circulating pathogenic antibodies directly rather than the resultant coagulopathy.

In patients with SLE and APS, *hydroxychloroquine* has been shown to reduce aPL antibody levels and to have intrinsic anticoagulative properties. Potential future APS therapies may include *mTOR inhibitors, factor Xa inhibitors, oral direct thrombin inhibitors,* and *statins.* Correction of reversible prothrombotic factors, such as oral contraceptive use and smoking, is advisable.

Warfarin is contraindicated in pregnancy, a particularly high-risk state for patients with APS. Women with APS should be treated with aspirin before conception, with the introduction of low-molecular-weight heparin thereafter.

In acute thrombosis, monitored intravenous *unfractionated heparin* or subcutaneous *low-molecular-weight heparin,* with or without subsequent initiation of *warfarin,* is standard therapy. Thrombolytic medications (e.g., *streptokinase, tissue plasminogen activator* [tPA]) or *percutaneous or surgical interventions* may be necessary in life- or limb-threatening thrombotic events. Catastrophic antiphospholipid syndrome (CAPS), the development of widespread thromboses with end-organ damage, requires intensive multidisciplinary interventions to halt disease progression and to reverse end-organ damage. *Plasma exchange* may have a role in the treatment of CAPS.

Specific Investigations

- Inquiry into history of thromboembolism, pregnancy morbidity, and medication use
- aPL antibodies (i.e., lupus anticoagulant, anticardiolipin IgG and IgM antibodies, anti-β_2-glycoprotein 1 antibodies)

Evidence Levels: **A** Double-blind study **B** Clinical trial ≥ 20 subjects **C** Clinical trial < 20 subjects **D** Series ≥ 5 subjects **E** Anecdotal case reports

Specific Investigations—cont'd

- Coagulopathy screen (i.e., INR, partial thromboplastin time [PTT], protein C, protein S, antithrombin III, prothrombin G20210A gene mutation, antiprothrombin antibodies, factor V Leiden, homocysteine level)
- Screening for underlying disease state (hematology, fasting blood glucose, fasting lipids, connective tissue serology, HIV testing, hepatitis serology) and other prothrombotic risk factors

International consensus statement on an update of the classification criteria for definite antiphospholipid syndrome (APS). Miyakis S, Lockshin MD, Atsumi T, Branch DW, Brey RL, Cervera R, et al. J Thromb Haemost 2006; 4: 295–306.

Consensus guidelines require a history of thromboembolism and documentation of elevated aPL antibodies on at least two occasions separated by at least 12 weeks for definitive diagnosis of APS.

Controversies and unresolved issues in antiphospholipid syndrome pathogenesis and management. Baker WF Jr, Bick RL, Fareed J. Hematol Oncol Clin North Am 2008; 22: 155–74.

Thorough investigation into underlying (and potentially correctable) conditions is recommended.

First-Line Therapies

• Observation (persistent aPL elevation but no thromboembolic events)	A
• Long-term warfarin, target INR 2.0 to 3.0	A
• Correction of reversible prothrombotic factors	B
• Long-term warfarin, target INR >3.0 (recurrent or arterial thrombosis)	B
• Low-molecular-weight heparin and low-dose aspirin (pregnancy)	B
• Heparin followed by warfarin (acute thrombosis)	C
• Hydroxychloroquine with low-dose aspirin (SLE)	D
• Thrombolytic therapy or percutaneous/surgical intervention (critical thrombosis)	E
• Reduction of prothrombotic risk factors, such as prolonged immobilization	E

Aspirin for primary thrombosis prevention in the antiphospholipid syndrome. Erkan D, Harrison MJ, Levy R, Peterson M, Petri M, Sammaritano L. Arthritis Rheum 2007; 56: 2382–91.

A randomized, double-blind, placebo-controlled trial of aspirin versus placebo in asymptomatic patients with persistently positive aPL antibodies found no benefit of aspirin in primary thromboprophylaxis.

A comparison of two intensities of warfarin for the prevention of recurrent thrombosis in patients with the antiphospholipid syndrome. Crowther MA, Ginsberg JS, Julian J, Denburg J, Hirsch J, Douketis J, et al. N Engl J Med 2003; 349: 113–8.

A randomized clinical trial of high-intensity warfarin vs. conventional antithrombotic therapy for the prevention of recurrent thrombosis in patients with the antiphospholipid syndrome. Finazzi G, Marchioli R, Brancaccio V, Schinco P, Wisloff F, Musial J, et al. Thromb Haemost 2005; 3: 848–53.

These two randomized, double-blind trials comparing high-intensity warfarin (target INR 3.0–4.0) and moderate-intensity warfarin (target INR 2.0–3.0) in patients with APS found no significant difference in preventing secondary thrombosis between the two treatment regimens.

A systematic review of secondary thromboprophylaxis in patients with antiphospholipid antibodies. Ruiz-Irastorza G, Hunt BJ, Khamashta MA. Arthritis Rheum 2007; 57: 1487–95.

In several cohort studies of patients with APS, INR at the time of recurrent thromboembolism on warfarin was <3.0 in 86%. The authors propose that the target INR should be >3.0 in patients with recurrent or arterial thrombosis.

Treatment of antiphospholipid antibody syndrome (APS) in pregnancy: a randomized pilot trial comparing low-molecular-weight heparin to unfractionated heparin. Stephenson MD, Ballen PJ, Tsang P, Purkiss S, Ensworth S, Houlihan E, et al. J Obstet Gynaecol Can 2004; 26: 729–34.

In a randomized trial, 28 women with APS received low-dose aspirin and either low-molecular-weight heparin or unfractionated heparin before conception or early in pregnancy. Pregnancy was successful in 9 of 13 (69%) women treated with low-molecular-weight heparin and low-dose aspirin and in 4 of 13 (31%) women treated with unfractionated heparin and low-dose aspirin.

In addition, the obstetrics literature tends to favor low-molecular-weight over unfractionated heparin because of its superior safety profile.

Second-Line Therapies

• Long-term low-molecular-weight heparin (recurrent thrombosis)	D
• Rituximab (SLE)	D
• Hydroxychloroquine (SLE)	E
• Intravenous immunoglobulin (IVIG) (in pregnancy)	E

Rituximab usage in systemic lupus erythematosus-associated antiphospholipid antibody syndrome: a single-center experience. Wang CR, Liu MF. Semin Arthritis Rheum 2016; 46(1): 102-8.

A series of six patients with APS treated with rituximab suffered no relapse of thrombosis with a mean follow-up period of over 3 years.

Evidence-based management of thrombosis in the antiphospholipid antibody syndrome. Petri M. Curr Rheum Rep 2003; 5: 370–3.

Hydroxychloroquine appears to reduce aPL antibody titers and the risk for recurrent thrombosis in patients with SLE.

An excellent evidence-based review of APS treatments.

A multicenter, placebo-controlled pilot study of intravenous immune globulin (IVIG) treatment of antiphospholipid syndrome during pregnancy. Branch DW, Peaceman AM, Druzin M, Silver RK, El-Sayed Y, Silver RM. Gen Obstet Gynecol 2000; 182: 122–7.

In this pilot study of 16 pregnant women with APS, patients were randomized to receive IVIG or placebo. All patients also received heparin and low-dose aspirin. A trend toward decreased fetal growth restriction was observed in the IVIG group compared with the placebo group, but differences were not statistically significant.

Intravenous immunoglobulins and antiphospholipid syndrome: how, when and why? A review of the literature. Tenti S, Cheleschi S, Guidelli GM, Galeazzi M, Fioravanti A. Autoimmun Rev 2016; 15: 226–35.

Results of this literature analysis indicate that the addition of IVIG to low-dose aspirin and low-molecular-weight heparin in the setting of obstetric APS is controversial.

Third-Line Therapies

• Plasma exchange (pregnancy)	D
• Placement of inferior vena cava (IVC) filter (medically refractory, recurrent venous thromboses)	D
• Statins (recurrent venous thromboses)	E
• IVIG (recurrent venous thromboses)	E
• Sirolimus (APS-related arterial vasculopathy)	E

Plasma exchange in the management of high risk pregnant patients with primary antiphospholipid syndrome. A report of 9 cases and a review of the literature. Ruffatti A, Marson P, Pengo V, Favaro M, Tonello M, Boralati M, et al. Autoimmunity Rev 2007; 6: 196–202.

Nine patients with APS and triple-positive aPL antibodies were treated with plasma exchange for secondary prophylaxis during pregnancy. The authors found that combined plasma exchange and IVIG therapy contributed to favorable pregnancy outcomes in high-risk patients.

Insertion of inferior vena cava filters in patients with the antiphospholipid syndrome. Zifman E, Rotman-Pikielny P, Berlin T, Levy Y. Semin Arthritis Rheum 2009; 38: 472–7.

Ten patients with APS who experienced recurrent thrombosis despite warfarin therapy received IVC filters. One patient had a documented pulmonary embolus (PE) after intervention, and two died suddenly of unknown causes (PE could not be excluded). The authors state that the results were suggestive of a protective effect of IVC filters in refractory APS.

A prospective open-label pilot study of fluvastatin on proinflammatory and prothrombotic biomarkers in antiphospholipid antibody positive patients. Erkan D, Willis R, Murthy VL, Bastra G, Vega J, Ruiz-Limon P, et al. Ann Rheum Dis 2014; 73: 1176–80.

This study showed that daily use of fluvastatin significantly reduced levels of proinflammatory and prothrombotic biomarkers in patients with positive aPL.

Though some small reports demonstrate benefit of IVIG when used as an additive therapy for secondary prophylaxis, large, well-designed studies are lacking.

The NF-κβ specific inhibitor DHMEQ prevents thrombus formation in a mouse model of antiphospholipid syndrome. Nishimura M, Nii T, Trimova G, Miura S, Umezawak K, Ushiyama A, et al. J Nephropathology 2013; 2: 114–21.

Catastrophic Antiphospholipid Syndrome

• Anticoagulation, systemic corticosteroids, and plasmapheresis or IVIG	D
• Eculizumab	E

Catastrophic antiphospholipid syndrome (CAPS): proposed guidelines for diagnosis and treatment. Asherson RA, Espinosa G, Cervera R, Font J, Carles Reverter J. J Clin Rheumatol 2002; 8: 157–65.

Based on experience from 130 cumulative cases of CAPS, the authors recommend heparin, systemic corticosteroids, and plasmapheresis in the treatment of CAPS.

Catastrophic antiphospholipid syndrome presenting with multiorgan failure and gangrenous lesions of the skin. Incalzi RA, Gemma A, Moro L, Antonelli M. Angiology 2008; 59: 517–8.

A 38-year-old woman with CAPS triggered by abrupt withdrawal of systemic corticosteroids recovered completely after treatment with immunosuppressive and antibiotic treatment combined with plasmapheresis.

Brief report: induction of sustained remission in recurrent catastrophic antiphospholipid syndrome via inhibition of terminal complement with eculizumab. Shapira I, Andrade D, Allen SL, Salmon JE. Arthritis Rheum 2012; 64: 2719–23.

First report of eculizumab's efficacy in CAPS. Larger studies are ongoing.

Evidence Levels: **A** Double-blind study **B** Clinical trial ≥ 20 subjects **C** Clinical trial < 20 subjects **D** Series ≥ 5 subjects **E** Anecdotal case reports

16

Aphthous stomatitis

Maryam Liaqat, Justin J. Green

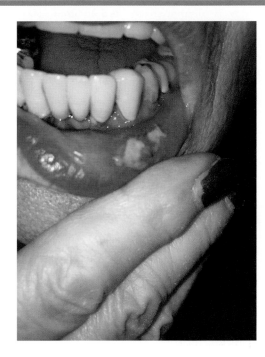

Recurrent aphthous stomatitis (RAS) is the most common cause of oral ulceration, affecting 5% to 25% of the population. It is characterized by the recurrence of one or more painful, shallow, sharply marginated ulcerations with a fibrinous base and surrounding erythematous halo on mobile oral mucosa. Three main types include minor, major, and herpetiform aphthae, which differ in size, duration, number, potential for scarring, and location of ulcerations. The etiology remains unclear; however, genetic predisposition (with at least 40% of patients having a positive family history), nutritional deficiencies, infections, hormonal alterations, immunodeficiency, and environmental agents have been implicated. It is important to differentiate aphthae from other causes of mucosal ulcers. The differential diagnosis would include viral and bacterial infections (herpes simplex virus [HSV], Epstein-Barr virus, cytomegalovirus, varicella zoster virus, Coxsackie virus, syphilis, gonorrhea, tuberculosis), erythema multiforme, lichen planus, autoimmune bullous diseases (pemphigus vulgaris and cicatricial pemphigoid), contact dermatitis, chronic ulcerative stomatitis, and trauma. Malignancy and systemic vasculitis must also be considered in lesions that are not self-resolving.

MANAGEMENT STRATEGY

The therapeutic approach to aphthae is dependent on the frequency of recurrence, duration, and severity of symptoms. In addition, underlying hematologic abnormalities, nutritional deficiencies, and medications should be considered as causative agents, as well as systemic disorders such as Crohns disease, Behcet disease, mouth and genital ulcers with inflamed cartilage syndrome (MAGIC syndrome), cyclic neutropenia, Sweet syndrome, reactive arthritis, HIV infection, and autoinflammatory syndromes such as periodic fever, aphthous stomatitis, pharyngitis, and cervical adenitis syndrome

(PFAPA syndrome). Stress is also thought to play a role in exacerbation of the disease. Unfortunately, because there is no curative treatment to date, the emphasis of treatment is on measures that may afford symptomatic relief and decrease occurrence, without causing significant adverse effects.

Topical corticosteroids are the mainstay of therapy. For milder disease, corticosteroids such as *fluocinonide* can be used. Superpotent corticosteroids such as *clobetasol* or *halobetasol* are appropriate for more severe episodes. Most practitioners suggest the use of topical therapy after meals. These can be applied in equal parts with an occlusive agents such as *Orabase* for better adherence. Drug delivery can be enhanced by cotton-tip applications for 30 seconds and avoidance of eating and drinking for 30 minutes after application. Initial concentrations of 3 to 10 mg/mL of *intralesional triamcinolone acetonide* are helpful for major aphthae. Repeat injections over 2- to 4-week intervals are suggested. *Dexamethasone elixir* 0.5 mg/5 mL three times daily used as a mouthwash or *beclomethasone dipropionate* aerosol spray can target ulcers on the soft palate or oropharynx. Elixirs can be combined with *sucralfate* or *Kaopectate* to improve adhesion to ulceration. When used for less than 3 weeks, systemic absorption and hypothalamic–pituitary–adrenal axis suppression are unlikely.

RAS that elicits severe pain may require intermittent *systemic corticosteroid therapy*. Prednisone 1 mg/kg (40–60 mg) daily can be given with a 2-week taper or as "burst therapy" for shorter periods. Concomitant therapy with topical corticosteroids may be helpful. *Thalidomide* 50 to 200 mg daily is the most effective steroid-sparing agent. It is also the only Food and Drug Administration (FDA)–approved treatment for major aphthae in HIV-positive patients. *Dapsone* 100 mg daily, *pentoxifylline* 400 mg three times daily, and *clofazimine* 100 mg daily may also lead to suppression of aphthae. Oral *rofecoxib* 50 mg on the first day and 25 to 50 mg per day on the following days or oral *tinidazole* 1 g per daily may have some benefit. *Antitumor necrosis factor (TNF)-α* therapies may be effective in recalcitrant cases. Those patients who require suppressive therapy but cannot tolerate the side effects of systemic agents can try medications such as *topical cyclosporine* rinse 500 mg/5 mL three times daily, or *interferon-α_{2a}* 1200 IU daily as a 1-minute rinse and swallow.

Application of *amlexanox 5% paste* four times daily has been shown to reduce aphthous ulcer healing time, and the application of amlexanox OraDisc four times daily to prodromal areas of the buccal mucosa has shown promise in the prevention of recurrent minor aphthous ulceration.

Lidocaine gel or spray, dyclonine, diphenhydramine (12.5/5 mL), or *benzocaine* are helpful for pain reduction. Patients must avoid desensitization of the entire oral vault, which may lead to self-induced trauma. A compounded *anesthetic mouthwash* (aluminum hydroxide–magnesium hydroxide, diphenhydramine, and lidocaine) has better mucosal adherence. Systemic *nonsteroidal antiinflammatory drugs* (NSAIDs), sucralfate suspension, 0.2% *chlorhexidine gluconate* mouthwash, triclosan, or *tetracycline* suspension (250 mg/5 mL) may provide pain relief and reduce healing time, although these are less effective than potent topical corticosteroids. Bioadhesives such as *carboxymethylcellulose* provide a protective film and may reduce healing time. Use of laser therapies, including CO_2 laser, Nd:YAG, and low-level light therapies in recurrent aphthous stomatitis, has also been shown to improve symptoms caused by consumption of food, beverages, and brushing of teeth.

Trigger avoidance can be useful. Predisposing factors include food (nuts, chocolate, tomatoes, citrus fruits, and spices), alcohol and carbonated beverages, trauma, menstruation, and stress. A *food diary* may be of value in identifying an offending agent. Certain medications, such as β-blockers, NSAIDs, and antioxidants, as well as sensitivity to sodium lauryl sulfate found in toothpaste, may contribute to the recurrence of aphthae. *Hormonal therapy* may alleviate RAS associated with menstruation. *Reassurance* of the benignity of this condition is paramount, and *relaxation techniques* or *biofeedback* can be discussed if stress is found to be a significant trigger.

Specific Investigations

- Complete blood count
- Vitamins B_1, B_2, B_6, and B_{12}; folate, zinc, and iron levels
- Culture/polymerase chain reaction of aphthae to exclude HSV
- Consider HIV testing

Aphthous ulcers. Messadi DV, Younai F. Dermatol Ther 2010; 23: 281–90.

Review article containing the summary of possible etiologies and clinical presentations of aphthae, differential diagnosis, and treatment options.

Oral mucosal disease: recurrent aphthous stomatitis. Scully C, Porter S. Br J Oral Maxillofac Surg 2008; 46: 198–206.

Review article highlighting possible etiologies and differential diagnosis of RAS. This article recommends checking complete blood count, folate, iron studies, and B_{12}, as well as excluding infections or systemic diseases that may include aphthae-like ulcerations, namely Behçet disease and HSV.

Haematological deficiencies in patients with recurrent aphthosis. Compilato D, Carroccio A, Calvino F, Di Fede G, Campisi G. J Eur Acad Dermatol Venerol 2010; 24: 667–73.

Thirty-two patients with RAS and 29 healthy controls were subjected to hematologic investigations. Deficiencies were noted in 56.2% of RAS patients and in 7% of controls. All patients with a negative family history of RAS showed complete remission after replacement therapy, whereas patients with a family history of RAS showed reduction in frequency and severity. The authors recommended that routine screening for serum iron, folic acid, and vitamin B_{12} deficiencies should be performed.

First-Line Therapies

• Vitamin and mineral deficiency replacement	A
• Topical corticosteroids	A
• Amlexanox 5% paste	A
• Intralesional corticosteroids	B
• Tetracycline suspension	A
• Antimicrobial mouth rinses	A
• Sucralfate	A
• Hydroxypropyl cellulose/carboxymethylcellulose	C
• Herbal supplements	D

Urban legends: recurrent aphthous stomatitis. Baccaglini L, Lalla RV, Bruce AJ, Sartori-Valinotti JC, Latortue MC, Carrozzo M, et al. Oral Dis 2011; 17: 755–70.

Review article examining several myths about aphthous ulcerations, with specific emphasis of literature review of treatments in the last 6 years. The authors concluded that low-dose topical tetracyclines and amlexanox showed possible benefit.

Topical corticosteroids in recurrent aphthous stomatitis. Systematic review. Quijano D, Rodriguez M. Acta Otorhinolaringol Esp 2008; 59: 298–307.

This is a systematic review of published literature evaluating the effectiveness of topical corticosteroids in treating RAS. The authors were able to show a trend toward reduced healing times and decreased pain but commented on the lack of high-quality experiments in the literature.

Efficacy and safety of dexamethasone ointment on recurrent aphthous ulceration. Lui C, Zhou Z, Lui G, Wang Q, Chen J, Wang L, et al. Am J Med 2012; 125: 292–301.

This study is a randomized, double-blind, placebo-controlled, parallel, multicenter clinical trial which showed that dexamethasone 0.1% ointment three times a day for 5 days safely reduced the size and duration of aphthae compared with placebo.

Amlexanox for the treatment of recurrent aphthous ulcers. Bell J. Clin Drug Investig 2005; 25: 555–6.

A review of four double-blind randomized controlled trials (RCTs) indicating that amlexanox 5% paste up to four times per day significantly reduced ulcer size compared with placebo.

Double-blind trial of tetracycline in recurrent aphthous ulceration. Graykowski EA, Kingman A. J Oral Pathol 1978; 7: 376–82.

A suspension of tetracycline 250 mg/5 mL was used four times daily in patients with RAS. The suspension was held in the mouth for 2 minutes and then swallowed. This study found that tetracycline therapy significantly reduced ulcer duration, size, and pain, but did not alter the recurrence rate.

Other studies using tetracycline or its derivatives (topically or orally) have drawn similar conclusions.

Chlorhexidine gluconate mouthwash in the management of minor aphthous ulceration: a double-blind, placebo-controlled cross-over trial. Hunter L, Addy M. Br Dent J 1987; 162: 106–10.

This crossover study included 38 patients who used 0.2% chlorhexidine gluconate mouthwash three times daily for 6 weeks. The total number of days with ulcers was significantly reduced, and the interval between successive ulcers was increased.

Gel and mouthwash formulations of 0.1% chlorhexidine have also been efficacious. Chlorhexidine mouthwash can stain teeth.

Effect of an antimicrobial mouth rinse on recurrent aphthous ulcerations. Meiller TF, Kutcher MJ, Overholser CD, Niehaus C, DePaola LG, Siegel MA. Oral Surg Oral Med Oral Pathol 1991; 72: 425–9.

A 6-month double-blind study compared Listerine antiseptic and a hydroalcoholic control used as a vigorous mouthwash twice daily. The duration of ulcers and pain severity were significantly reduced in the Listerine group. Both the Listerine group and the control group experienced a reduced incidence of ulcers.

Mouth rinses containing triclosan reduce the incidence of recurrent aphthous ulcers (RAU). Skaare AB, Herlofson BB, Barkvoll P. J Clin Periodontol 1996; 23: 778–81.

In a double-blind crossover study, 0.15% triclosan mouthwash caused a significant reduction in the number of ulcers during the experimental period. Compared with the 7.8% ethanol and triclosan formulation, the efficacy of the mouthwashes was reduced when propylene glycol or a higher concentration of ethanol (15.6%) was used as a solubilizing agent.

Evidence Levels: **A** Double-blind study **B** Clinical trial ≥ 20 subjects **C** Clinical trial < 20 subjects **D** Series ≥ 5 subjects **E** Anecdotal case reports

Sucralfate suspension as a treatment of recurrent aphthous stomatitis. Rattan J, Schneider M, Arber N, Gorsky M, Dayan D. J Intern Med 1994; 236: 341–3.

Sucralfate applied four times daily to ulcers was found to be superior to antacid (aluminum hydroxide and magnesium hydroxide) and placebo with regard to duration of pain, reduction in healing time, response to first treatment, and duration of remission. The 2-year prospective, randomized, double-blind, placebo-controlled, crossover trial included 21 patients unresponsive to conventional therapy.

A randomized, placebo-controlled, double-blind study of sucralfate applied four times daily to oral and genital ulcerations of Behçet disease resulted in reduced frequency, healing time, and pain in oral ulcerations, and reduced healing time and pain in genital ulcers.

Performance of a hydroxypropyl cellulose film former in normal and ulcerated mucosa. Rodu B, Russell CM. Oral Surg Oral Med Oral Pathol 1988; 65: 699–703.

Zilactin, which contains hydroxypropyl cellulose, led to pain relief after an acidic challenge followed by rechallenge.

Orabase, which contains carboxymethylcellulose, has been beneficial in trials when combined with topical corticosteroids, possibly due to its adhesive properties.

Efficacy and safety of topical herbal medicine treatment on recurrent aphthous stomatitis: a systemic review. Li CL, Huang HL, Wang WC, Li CL. Drug Des Devel Ther 2015; 10: 107–15.

Nine electronic databases in English and Chinese were evaluated for RCT, and clinical controlled trials were searched and narrowed to 13 trials with a total of 1515 patients included in the analysis. The authors concluded there is some benefit with regard to previously established RAS outcomes with fewer side effects. No single supplement recommendations were made by the authors.

Second-Line Therapies	
• Oral corticosteroids	A
• Colchicine	A
• Thalidomide	A
• Dapsone	A
• Zinc sulfate	A
• Low-level laser therapy	B
• Omega 3	B

Systemic interventions for recurrent aphthous stomatitis. Brocklehurst P, Tickle M, Glenny AM, Lewis MA, Pemberton MN, Taylor J, et al. Cochrane Database Syst Rev 2012; 9: CD005411.

Review article in which a total of 25 trials were included, 22 of which were placebo controlled and 8 made head-to-head comparisons with a total of 21 interventions that were reviewed. These included immunodulators including clofazimine, colchicine, prednisone vs. uncertain category including homeopathy, tetracycline, vitamin B_{12}, and propolis. The main conclusions were that no single treatment was found to be effective; therefore no recommendations regarding best systemic intervention for RAS were made. The reviewers' primary concern was the methodologic rigor of the trials and high risk of bias.

Systemic treatment in severe cases of recurrent aphthous stomatitis: an open trial. Mimura MA, Hirota SK, Sugaya NN, Sanches JA Jr, Migliari DA. Clinics 2009; 64: 193–8.

An open, 4-year clinical trial of 21 patients with RAS treated with thalidomide (100 mg/day), dapsone (100 mg/day), colchicine (1.5 mg/day), and pentoxifylline (400 mg three times a day). Thalidomide was the most efficient and well tolerated. Dapsone and colchicine provided good results; however, dapsone was not well tolerated. Pentoxifylline was mildly effective.

Comparison of colchicine versus prednisolone in recurrent aphthous stomatitis: a double-blind randomized clinical trial. Pakfetrat A, Mansourian A, Momen-Heravi F, Delavarian Z, Momen-Beitollahi J, Khalilzadeh O, et al. Clin Invest Med 2010; 33: E189–95.

In this double-blind RCT, 34 patients with RAS were split into two groups: prednisolone 5 mg daily or colchicine 0.5 mg daily for 3 months. Both medications were equally effective in reducing pain, recurrence, size, and number of aphthae, although colchicine had a higher rate of side effects.

Clinical, historic, and therapeutic features of aphthous stomatitis: literature review and open trial employing steroids. Vincent SD, Lilly GE. Oral Surg Oral Med Oral Pathol 1992; 74: 79–86.

"Burst therapy" with prednisone 40 mg once daily for 5 days, followed by 20 mg every other day for 1 week, in addition to topical triamcinolone acetonide 0.1% or 0.2% four times daily, led to complete or partial control of aphthae in 12 of 13 patients.

Effects of colchicine treatment on mean platelet volume and the inflammatory markers in recurrent aphthous stomatitis. Seçkin HY, Bütün I, Baş Y, Takcı Z, Kalkan G. J Dermatolog Treat 2016; 1–3.

RAS is associated with increased inflammatory markers. Fifteen male and 45 female RAS patients who were taking colchicine were investigated retrospectively. The whole blood parameters of the patients were observed before starting colchicine treatment and in the third month of colchicine treatment. It was determined that colchicine lowers the levels of neutrophil–lymphocyte ratio (NLR), white blood cell count, and red cell distribution width (RDW). Furthermore, no changes were seen on mean platelet volume, platelet–lymphocyte ratio, and hemoglobin.

Thalidomide for the treatment of oral aphthous ulcers in patients with human immunodeficiency virus infection. Jacobson JM, Greenspan JS, Spritzler J, Ketter N, Fahey JL, Jackson JB, et al. National Institute of Allergy and Infectious Diseases AIDS Clinical Trials Group. N Engl J Med 1997; 336: 1487–93.

Fifty-seven HIV-positive patients were included in this double-blind, randomized, placebo-controlled study of thalidomide 200 mg daily versus placebo as therapy for oral aphthous ulcers in HIV-infected patients. Sixteen of 29 patients in the thalidomide group (55%) had complete healing of their aphthous ulcers after 4 weeks, compared with only 2 of 28 patients in the placebo group (7%).

Refractory aphthous ulceration treated with thalidomide: a report of 10 years' clinical experience. Cheng S, Murphy R. Clin Exp Dermatol 2012; 37: 132–5.

Retrospective review of 15 patients treated with thalidomide after failing topical and oral steroids. Out of 15 patients, 14 showed improvement with thalidomide; however, 9 patients showed a decline in their nerve conduction study, independent of dose. Despite these findings only three patients stopped the medication, and the patient with the largest decline in nerve conduction (80%) opted to continue thalidomide rather than risk recurrence of the ulcers.

The therapeutic and prophylactic role of oral zinc sulfate in management of recurrent aphthous stomatitis (RAS) in comparison with dapsone. Sharquie KE, Najim RA, Al-Hayani RK, Al-Nuaimy AA, Maroof DM. Saudi Med J 2008; 29: 734–8.

In this double-blind placebo-controlled study of 45 patients with RAS, patients were treated with zinc sulfate 150 mg twice daily, dapsone 50 mg twice daily, and glucose 250 mg daily as placebo. Results showed that both zinc sulfate and dapsone had significant therapeutic effects in decreasing ulcer size. They concluded that zinc sulfate had much more rapid and sustained action.

Recurrent aphthous stomatitis and pain management with low-level laser therapy: a randomized controlled trial. Albrektson M, Hedstrom L, Bergh H. Oral Surg Oral Med Oral Pathol Oral Radiol 2014; 117: 590–4.

This study is a randomized, single-blinded, placebo-controlled trial conducted with low-level laser therapy (wavelength, 809 nm; power, 60 mW; pulse frequency, 1800 Hz; duration, 80 seconds per treatment; dose, 6.3 J/cm^2) in 40 patients with RAS. Improvement was assessed with visual analog scale (VAS) and patients' experience of eating, drinking, and brushing teeth. Compared with placebo there was a statistically significant decrease in VAS score, as well as the other symptoms noted.

Efficacy of omega-3 in treatment of recurrent aphthous stomatitis and improvement of quality of life: a randomized, double-blind, placebo-controlled study. El Khouli AM, El-Gendy EA. Oral Surg Oral Med Oral Pathol Oral Radiol Endod 2014; 117: 191–6.

A parallel-design, double-blind, placebo-controlled study was conducted on 50 participants divided into treatment to receive omega-3 (1 g three times daily) and control group for 6 months. Results indicated a significant reduction in the number of ulcer outbreaks, the average level of pain, and the duration of ulcer episodes per month starting in the third month of treatment.

Third-Line Therapies	
• Pentoxifylline	A
• Clofazimine	B
• Ascorbate (Vitamin C)	C
• Vitamin B$_{12}$	A
• Topical cyclosporine	D
• Oral interferon-α$_{2a}$	C
• CO$_2$ laser	D
• Penicillin G potassium troches	A
• TNF-α inhibitors	D
• Silver nitrate	B
• Montelukast	A

A randomized, double-blind, placebo-controlled trial of pentoxifylline for the treatment of recurrent aphthous stomatitis. Thornhill MH, Baccaglini L, Theaker E, Pemberton MN. Arch Dermatol 2007; 143: 463–70.

Twenty-six patients were randomized to pentoxifylline 400 mg three times daily or placebo. Patients taking pentoxifylline had less pain, smaller ulcers, fewer ulcers, and more ulcer-free days, but this was not statistically significant. However, smaller median ulcer size in the treatment group was statistically significant. Adverse events were common and included dizziness, headaches, gastrointestinal symptoms, and fatigue.

According to the study, patients taking the active drug stated that if it was shown to be effective in the treatment of aphthous ulcers, they would not want to use it because of the side effects.

Topical cyclosporine for oral mucosal disorders. Eisen D, Ellis CN. J Am Acad Dermatol 1990; 23: 1259–64.

Four of eight patients with severe aphthous stomatitis obtained nearly complete suppression of ulcers during an 8-week course of topical cyclosporine 500 mg/5 mL, swish and rinse three times daily.

Chronic recurrent aphthous stomatitis: oral treatment with low-dose interferon alpha. Hutchinson VA, Angenend JL, Mok WL, Cummins JM, Richards AB. Mol Biother 1990; 2: 160–4.

Oral administration of interferon-α$_2$ (1200 IU daily) resulted in remissions of aphthae within 2 weeks of initiating therapy compared with no improvement in the placebo group. The placebo group was then treated similarly with interferon-α$_2$ leading to complete remission of their aphthae.

Managing aphthous ulcers: laser treatment applied. Colvard M, Kuo P. J Am Dent Assoc 1991; 122: 51–3.

Pain alleviation was observed in 16 of 18 patients after CO$_2$ laser therapy of minor aphthae.

Evaluation of penicillin G potassium troches in the treatment of minor recurrent aphthous ulceration in a Chinese cohort: a randomized, double-blinded, placebo and no-treatment-controlled, multicenter clinical trial. Zhou Y, Chen Q, Meng W, Jiang L, Wang Z, Liu J, et al. Oral Surg Oral Med Oral Radiol Endod 2010; 109: 561–6.

A randomized double-blinded control trial in 258 nonpenicillin-allergic Chinese patients was performed with subjects split between placebo, treatment, and no-treatment groups. Patients treated with penicillin G potassium troches showed significant objective decreased ulcer size and subjective decrease in pain.

Efficacy and safety of TNF-α inhibitors in refractory primary complex aphthosis: a patient series and overview of the literature. Sand FL, Thomsen SF. J Dermatolog Treat 2013; 24: 444–6.

In this case series, a total of 18 patients were treated with etanercept, adalimumab, infliximab, or golimumab for frequent recurrent oral and genital aphthae or continuous aphthous stomatitis. Of these patients, 16 had complete or almost clearance of the aphthosis, whereas 5 had adverse reactions.

Treatment of recurrent aphthous stomatitis with clofazimine. de Abrue MA, Hirata CH, Pimentel DR, Weckx LL. Oral Surg Oral Med Oral Pathol Radiol Endod 2009; 108: 714–21.

In this randomized controlled partially blinded study, clofazimine (100 mg daily for 30 days, then 100 mg every other day) and colchicine (0.5 mg three times a day) were investigated for 6 months in the treatment of RAS. Patients taking clofazimine showed significant improvement to colchicine at the second, third, fifth, and sixth months of therapy.

The effect of ascorbate on minor recurrent aphthous stomatitis. Yasui K, Kurata T, Yashiro M, Tsuge M, Ohtsuki S, Morishima T. Acta Paediatr 2010; 99: 442–5.

In this study, 16 patients with minor RAS were given daily vitamin C (2000 mg/m^2) for 3 months. Treatment was then discontinued for 3 months and then restarted for another 3 months. Patients experienced a significant decrease in stomatitis during treatment months compared with months without treatment.

Evidence Levels: **A** Double-blind study **B** Clinical trial ≥ 20 subjects **C** Clinical trial < 20 subjects **D** Series ≥ 5 subjects **E** Anecdotal case reports

Effectiveness of vitamin B$_{12}$ in treating recurrent aphthous stomatitis: a randomized, double-blind, placebo-controlled trial. Volkov I, Rudoy I, Freud T, Sardal G, Naimer S, Peleg R, et al. J Am Board Fam Med 2009; 22: 9–16.

In this randomized, double-blind, placebo-controlled trial, 58 patients with RAS were split into treatment groups of 1000 µg of sublingual vitamin B$_{12}$ and placebo. No patients had baseline B$_{12}$ levels less than 150 pg/mL. The treatment group had significantly fewer outbreaks than the controls, regardless of baseline B$_{12}$ level.

Of note, there have also been several studies negating the benefits of vitamin replacement in the literature.

Silver nitrate cautery in aphthous stomatitis: a randomized controlled trial. Alidaee MR, Taheri A, Mansoori P, Ghodsi SZ. Br J Dermatol 2005; 153: 521–5.

Ninety-seven patients with painful minor aphthae were randomized to receive one stick application of silver nitrate cautery or placebo. After 1 day, a statistically significant reduction in severity of pain was shown. Silver nitrate did not prolong or shorten healing time examined after 7 days. No side effects were noted.

The authors note that the treatment is simple and cost effective for patients, with few recurrences.

Pilot study on recurrent aphthous stomatitis (RAS): a randomized placebo-controlled trial for the comparative therapeutic effects of systemic prednisone and systemic montelukast in subjects unresponsive to topical therapy. Femiano F, Buonaiuto C, Gombos F, Lanza A, Cirillo N. Oral Surg Oral Med Oral Pathol Oral Radiol Endod 2010; 109: 402–7.

In this double-blind, randomized, placebo-controlled trial of 60 patients with minor RAS, patients were split equally into treatment groups of prednisone 25 mg daily tapered over 2 months, 10 mg montelukast daily for 1 month, then every other day for the second month, and cellulose (placebo). Both interventions significantly reduced number of lesions and pain relief compared with placebo; however, prednisone was more effective than montelukast. This suggests montelukast may be a safer alternative to prednisone.

17

Atopic dermatitis

Jeremy Udkoff, Lawrence F. Eichenfield

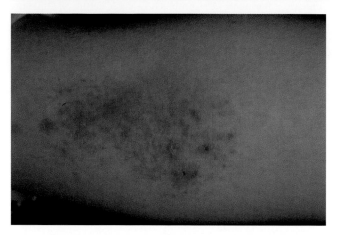

Atopic dermatitis (AD) is a chronic, relapsing, and intensely pruritic dermatosis that develops most commonly during early infancy and childhood and is, in most cases, associated with a personal or family history of atopy (allergic rhinitis, asthma, or eczema). It is frequently associated with abnormalities in skin barrier function and immune dysregulation. Skin involvement ranges from acute weeping and crusted areas of eczema to papular lesions or lichenified plaques.

MANAGEMENT STRATEGY

Successful AD therapy considers the patient's age and needs, the extent and localization of AD at presentation, and the overall disease course. Other factors to consider include previous response to treatment, disease persistence, frequency of flares, and susceptibility to and past history of infection (especially those due to *Staphylococcus aureus* and herpes simplex virus). The goals of management are to educate patients and caregivers about the disease, promote excellent skin care, reduce the degree and frequency of flares, monitor medication quality/quantity of use, and, if possible, modify the overall disease course and the atopic march.

Interventional education

Education concerning chronic disease management is a core part of therapy. Learning modalities beyond in-office disease education may be useful, including handouts, Internet-based written material, and instructional videos. Comprehensive multispecialty "eczema clinics" offer intensive education as a distinct component of long-term AD management. This model, with its longer appointments, focused educational curricula, patient support networks, and the ability to elicit patient and family feedback, parallels strategies shown to be effective for managing asthma, diabetes, and other chronic diseases. These methods empower patients and caregivers while improving both clinical and quality-of-life outcomes. Long-term comparative evaluations are required to examine the cost-effectiveness and suitability of these educational programs. Shared decision making—where therapeutic options and the rationales for recommending them, along with weighing the risks and benefits, are discussed with patients to arrive at therapeutic strategies—is an evolving method thought to improve patient outcomes (e.g., www.eczemacenter.org; www.nationaleczema.org; www.eczema.org).

Skin care

Excellent skin care remains a cornerstone of management. Emollients improve the xerosis and skin barrier dysfunction associated with AD and may improve pruritus and spare the use of prescription antiinflammatory medications. With little evidence to recommend the use of one emollient or moisturizer over another, patient and caregiver preference should be considered, with product selection based on the premise that "an emollient that is applied works better than one that remains on a shelf." Very occlusive ointments may not be tolerated during the summer months or in humid climates because of interference with the function of eccrine sweat ducts and the induction of folliculitis; in these situations, a cream may be a more practical choice. It is best to avoid preparations that contain topical sensitizers such as fragrance, neomycin, benzocaine, etc. Emollients and moisturizers should be applied after any topical pharmacologic therapies to allow active medications to penetrate the skin with full effect.

The value of *bathing* and the frequency with which it should be undertaken remain controversial, though most experts believe that daily bathing with application of emollients to follow is well tolerated and may be beneficial. The chief benefits of bathing include cleansing, debridement of infected eczema, improved penetration of topical therapies, and skin hydration (when postbath emollients are used to "lock in" moisture). Potential drawbacks of bathing are drying of the skin and disruption of the stratum corneum barrier during water evaporation when emollients are not used.

Fillagrin is a structural protein found in the stratum corneum. Loss of function mutations in the fillagrin gene can lead to increased transepidermal water loss and an increased risk of developing AD, as well as asthma, allergies, and herpes simplex virus infections. Recent data regarding transepidermal water loss suggest that the frequency of application of emollients or moisturizers may be more important than timing the application to coincide strictly with bathing (the traditional "soak and seal" approach); this finding remains to be confirmed in larger, more controlled studies.

Several *barrier repair products* thought to target and correct epidermal molecular deficiencies have been approved by the U.S. Food and Drug Administration (FDA) as 510(k) medical devices. However, there are limited comparative effectiveness or safety studies of these prescription devices and specially formulated emollients against traditional emollients or moisturizers for AD management.

Wet wraps are a useful tool in the intensive treatment of severe AD and/or disease that is refractory to standard topical therapies. They may increase skin hydration, serve as an effective mechanical barrier to scratching, and act as an occlusive layer that promotes penetration of topical corticosteroids into the skin, thereby increasing the amount of medication delivered to the most severely affected areas. Temporary systemic bioactivity of the corticosteroids and potential hypothermia are concerns. When wet wraps are overused or used incorrectly, maceration of the skin may occur. Because of these concerns, wet wraps should only be used under close supervision of a physician.

Evidence Levels: **A** Double-blind study **B** Clinical trial ≥ 20 subjects **C** Clinical trial < 20 subjects **D** Series ≥ 5 subjects **E** Anecdotal case reports

Topical therapies

Topical corticosteroids remain the first-line therapy for inflammation and pruritus associated with AD that is unresponsive to good skin care and moisturizers. Variations in corticosteroid-prescribing habits (e.g., quantity, frequency, and duration of therapy) are common even among dermatologists. Some clinicians start treatment with high-potency topical corticosteroid preparations in order to induce remission, followed by a relatively quick tapering down of potency as the dermatitis improves. Alternatively, other clinicians use short bursts of high-potency corticosteroids followed by moisturizers alone until relapse occurs. Another treatment regimen advocates more prolonged treatment with less potent steroid preparations. Weekend topical steroids to prevent flares have gained popularity. Drug-specific FDA indications and an expanding body of clinical trial data should help guide clinicians when educating and instructing patients on topical corticosteroid usage.

The *topical calcineurin inhibitors* (TCIs) tacrolimus and pimecrolimus have the important advantage of not being associated with skin atrophy. Current indications for TCI use are as "*second-line therapy* for the short-term and noncontinuous chronic treatment" of mild to moderate AD (pimecrolimus) or moderate to severe AD (tacrolimus) in nonimmunocompromised adults and children "who have failed to respond adequately to other topical prescription treatments for atopic dermatitis, or when those treatments are not advisable." Patients who are especially likely to benefit include those in whom the clinical course of AD is marked by steroid tachyphylaxis (versus simple noncompliance), disease persistence, and/or frequent flares, which would otherwise result in an almost continuous need for topical corticosteroid (TCS) treatment. TCIs may also be specifically indicated in sensitive thin skin areas, such as around the eye, face, neck, and genital area where local safety and systemic absorption are of special concern.

The safety and efficacy of tacrolimus and pimecrolimus have been studied in multiple short (6 weeks) and long-term (longer than 2 years) clinical trials. Data from these trials demonstrate that pimecrolimus reduces the number and severity of flares, extends the period between major flares, and reduces pruritus and other cutaneous signs associated with AD. Prospective studies spanning up to 10 years have investigated the clinical use of TCI in pediatric populations and have suggested that the use of TCI is not associated with systemic immunosuppression or an increased risk of skin cancer; nor does it appear to affect the delayed-type hypersensitivity response. In most countries, regulatory agencies do not recommend the use of TCI in patients under 2 years of age. Tacrolimus ointment 0.03% is indicated for adults and children aged 2 to 15 years, whereas tacrolimus ointment 0.1% is indicated only for adults.

"Proactive" treatment with intermittent TCS or TCI is recommended for disease maintenance for persistent or frequently flaring disease. Long-term, intermittent maintenance use of tacrolimus ointment in patients with stabilized AD has been shown to significantly increase the period between disease exacerbations and the total number of disease-free days compared with vehicle. Despite the frequency of use, the incidence of side effects in these studies was generally low and most commonly included transient application-site stinging.

Phosphodiesterase (PDE)-4 inhibitors are a new class of therapy for AD. Studies have shown the topical agent crisaborole to be an effective therapy for AD with a good short-term safety profile. However, future studies are required to elucidate crisaborole's long-term efficacy and safety.

Careful *supervision*, combined with appreciation of the risk–benefit profiles of moisturizers, barrier repair agents, topical corticosteroids, and TCIs, allows for individualized and optimized patient care. Treatment should be readily adjusted on an "as-needed" basis that takes advantage of available therapeutic modalities. For children with severe flares, this may mean using short-term bursts of mid- to high-potency topical steroids—with or without wet wraps—instead of relying on long-term use of less potent agents. Close re-examination of the patient at regular intervals to evaluate the efficacy and tolerability of local and systemic therapies is warranted. Once control of a flare is achieved, topical corticosteroids can be tapered to a lower-potency agent and/or from daily to intermittent (e.g., twice- or thrice-weekly) application. Transition to, or incorporation of, nonsteroid agents may also be considered. There is a positive risk-to-benefit ratio of proactive, scheduled (biweekly), topical antiinflammatory agents applied to frequently relapsing areas in preventing AD flares. During quiescent periods, therapy should shift to a less intense regimen with a focus on maintenance and proper skin care at its core. The use of TCIs or topical PDE-4 inhibitor monotherapy to control flare recurrence while limiting patients' extended exposure to corticosteroids is supported by some physicians.

Other treatment considerations

Total avoidance of environmental aeroallergens is almost impossible and may not significantly influence atopic dermatitis; however, *avoidance of known triggers* is a reasonable approach. Food allergy is more common in children with atopic dermatitis than without, and in a subset of individuals clinically relevant food allergy may exacerbate atopic dermatitis. U.S. national guidelines for food allergy recommend evaluation for milk, egg, peanut, wheat, and soy food allergies be considered in children less than 5 years old with moderate to severe AD if the child has a reliable history of an immediate reaction after ingestion of any of these foods, or the child has persistent AD in spite of optimized management and topical therapy. In addition, recent national guidelines recommend that children in the first year of life with severe AD and/or egg allergy have early evaluation with serum immunoglobulin E (IgE) or skin prick tests and also recommend early feeding of peanut as a method to decrease development of peanut allergy. Specific serum IgE and skin prick tests have high rates of false positives and poor predictive value for food allergy diagnosis, and severely restrictive diets based on positive tests rather than true allergy can be harmful. Thus positive IgE testing should be verified through controlled food trials or other means unless there is a reliable history of an immediate allergic reaction after ingestion of a specific food. Maternal dietary restrictions during pregnancy and lactation are not considered to have a significant role in development of AD and are generally not recommended.

Although they do not appear to have direct effects on the pruritus associated with AD, *sedating systemic antihistamines* such as hydroxyzine and diphenhydramine may be useful in improving sleep in flaring patients. This practice has not been evaluated rigorously in large, randomized, double-blind, placebo-controlled trials, and the drowsiness that may be associated with daytime use is a legitimate concern for school-age children. Second-generation, nonsedating antihistamines are less useful in managing AD, but may benefit patients with allergic triggers and, with chronic use, are suggested in some studies to reduce the rate of progression to other atopic disease (the atopic march). It is important to note that *topical antihistamines* are not recommended because of potential cutaneous sensitization.

Oral doxepin hydrochloride, a tricyclic antidepressant with anxiolytic effects, is a strong H_1- and H_2-receptor antagonist. It is typically used in doses of 10 to 75 mg orally at night or up to 75 mg twice daily in adult patients; it is not approved for use in children. As oral doxepin possesses a side effect profile that includes daytime sedation, hypotension, tolerance, and an increased risk of depression/suicide, it is generally reserved for severe cases of AD. Topical 5% doxepin cream has been reported to reduce pruritus; however, these topical formulations have also been associated with reports of allergic contact dermatitis and sedation.

Patients may have sudden exacerbations of AD due to overgrowth of *Staphylococcus aureus*— honey-colored crusting, folliculitis, and pyoderma are signs of overt infection. Topical and/or oral antibiotic therapy—typically of short duration to avoid the development of bacterial resistance—is indicated in these cases. Skin cultures and sensitivity testing should be considered before initiating treatment, as methicillin-resistant *S. aureus* (MRSA) may be an important pathogen in some patients. Recurrent, deep-seated *S. aureus* infections should raise the possibility of an immunodeficiency syndrome such as hyper-IgE syndrome or Dedicator of cytokinesis 8 (DOCK8) deficiency.

The addition of *antiseptics* to bath water, for example, diluted bleach baths ("like swimming in pool water"), may help reduce the number of local skin infections and the need for systemic antibiotics in AD patients with heavily colonized and/or superinfected skin. A bleach bath can be prepared by mixing one-quarter to one-half a cup of sodium hypochlorite 6% solution (chlorine liquid bleach) in a bathtub full of lukewarm water; the goal is to create a modified Dakin's-like solution with a final bleach concentration that approximates 0.005%. The patient may soak for 5 to 10 minutes, with or without a rinse of the skin with fresh water, pat dry, and then apply their topical therapy and/or emollient/moisturizer. Proprietary bath additives containing antiseptics are also available. For added convenience, newer formulations of bleachlike products are specially formulated and available as a body washes, sprays, or gels.

Eczema herpeticum may be easily misdiagnosed as bacterial superinfection and presents a serious risk in patients with widespread AD. Patients can present with multiple vesiculopustular lesions and painful "punched-out" erosions that fail to respond to oral antibiotics. Document herpes infection before treatment via culture and/or direct fluorescent antibody, and initiate *antiviral therapy* as soon as possible. Intravenous treatment is certainly indicated in cases of severe disseminated eczema herpeticum. Oral acyclovir (or equivalent dosage of another antiherpetic medication) may be useful in adults with herpes simplex confined to the skin; 400 mg three times daily for 10 days or 200 mg four times daily for 10 days usually provides a sufficient dosage.

Antifungal therapy has been shown to reduce the severity of AD lesions exacerbated by *Malassezia furfur*, particularly in the seborrheic areas of the skin and scalp. Patients with documented dermatophyte infection or IgE antibodies to *Malassezia* may benefit from a trial of topical or systemic antifungal therapy.

Due to a greater understanding of immunologic reaction patterns in the skin, gut, and airways there has been great interest in *probiotics*. As the findings to date on their utility in preventing or modifying AD are conflicting, the long-term significance of probiotics in the treatment of atopic dermatitis warrants further investigation.

Although the exact mechanism of action is unknown, *phototherapy* in AD is thought to suppress proinflammatory cytokines (such as IL-2 and IL-12) and induce T-cell apoptosis. Broadband ultraviolet (UV)B, broadband UVA, narrowband UVB (311 nm), UVA1 (340–400 nm), and combined UVA-B phototherapy have been reported to be useful for widespread or recalcitrant disease. Photochemotherapy with psoralen and UVA light may be indicated in severe cases. Multiple treatments are usually required to be effective, and this can be inconvenient for patients and their families, depending on location and accessibility to a suitable light source. Side effects can include skin pain, erythema, pruritus, and pigment changes. Likewise, UV radiation may increase the long-term risk of premature skin aging and cutaneous malignancies. Shielding and appropriate eye protection may help minimize unnecessary exposure.

Systemic therapies

Systemic corticosteroids are often prescribed in pediatric outpatient and emergency settings for AD exacerbations, though there are limited data surrounding their use. The temptation to use systemic corticosteroids can be great, given the dramatic clinical improvement that can occur. The propensity to flare with abrupt discontinuation of treatment and the well-known associated systemic side effect profile, however, suggest that systemic corticosteroids should be reserved for "crisis cases"—and, even then, used with the intent to bridge to another systemic agent or phototherapy.

Cyclosporine is a calcineurin inhibitor that blocks activation of T lymphocytes and reduces the transcription of cytokines, including IL-2, shown to be involved in the pathogenesis of AD. It may be used as a short-term treatment or as a bridge between other steroid-sparing alternatives. Cyclosporine is typically dosed at 2.5 to 5 mg/kg/day, and a response may be seen in 2 to 3 weeks. Alternatively, some experts prefer dosing cyclosporine microemulsion at 3 mg/kg/day in children, or 150 mg (low dose) or 300 mg (high dose) in adults, as the microemulsion offers more predictable absorption. Flares can occur after discontinuation of therapy; therefore gradual tapering or use of another immunosuppressive for maintenance therapy should be considered. The safety, efficacy, and risks of cyclosporine are well documented in both adults and children, and treatment with this agent is associated with reduced skin disease and an improved quality of life. Hypertension and renal toxicity, as well as concerns about malignancy, are limitations to long-term therapy. Continuous therapy beyond 1 year is not recommended, and it is unknown how many short courses may be given safely. Blood pressure, complete blood cell count, renal and hepatic function tests, magnesium, and uric acid should be monitored.

Azathioprine, a 6-mercaptopurine analog that inhibits purine synthesis and demonstrates cytotoxic and immunosuppressive properties, can be an effective monotherapy for AD. Marrow suppression and liver toxicity are major concerns; blood cell counts and liver function tests should be monitored closely. One in 300 individuals is homozygous for low metabolic activity alleles that correlate with higher risk of bone marrow suppression; azathioprine should be dosed according to thiopurine methyltransferase (TPMT) genotype/levels. Dosing in children and adults is generally 2.5 mg/kg/day in patients with normal TPMT activity and adjusted to lower doses for carriers of mutant alleles and/or definite intermediate TPMT levels (e.g., 1.0 mg/kg/day). Higher doses, up to 5 mg/kg/day, have been utilized in children. Very low or absent TPMT activity indicating homozygous TPMT mutations may be associated with life-threatening myelotoxicity. Drug hypersensitivity and gastrointestinal disturbances have been reported. An increased risk of malignancy is recognized with long-term use to prevent transplant rejection or manage inflammatory bowel disease.

Methotrexate is a folic acid analog that inhibits dihydrofolate reductase and interferes with DNA synthesis and lymphocyte proliferation leading to antiinflammatory effects; however, its greatest advantage may be that the relatively low doses used for skin disease appear less immunosuppressive than other AD systemic therapies. An open-label, prospective, 24-week trial of adults with AD demonstrated a response plateau at approximately 12 weeks with little additional improvement at doses greater than 15 mg weekly.

Alternatively, some experts dose methotrexate at 2.5 mg daily for 4 days per week. A retrospective review of children showed that AD was well controlled with effective dosing of 0.5 to 0.8 mg/kg/week (either as a single weekly dose or divided 3 or 4 days/week). There is a long history of methotrexate use in pediatric and adult inflammatory disease. Nausea and liver function abnormalities/hepatotoxicity may limit dosing. Pulmonary toxicity may be another potential concern. It is unclear what role folic acid supplementation plays in the treatment of AD with methotrexate.

Mycophenolate mofetil (MMF) has a good safety profile and represents a possible therapeutic alternative for severe, refractory AD. It is an inhibitor of inosine monophosphate dehydrogenase involved in de novo purine synthesis and has been used as an immunosuppressant in organ transplantation. Several adult studies have demonstrated efficacy at doses up to 2 g daily. A retrospective review of MMF as monotherapy in 14 pediatric AD patients showed it to be safe and effective at doses of 40 to 50 mg/kg/day in younger children (presumably due to increased surface area–to–volume ratios) and 30 to 40 mg/kg/day in adolescents, with maximal effect after 8 to 12 weeks of therapy. Patients should be monitored for leukopenia and anemia, and drug levels may be increased in the setting of renal insufficiency. MMF has been loosely linked to herpes retinitis, dose-related bone marrow suppression, and increased infection. Further prospective controlled studies are needed for this promising therapy.

Interferon-γ (IFN-γ) is well known to inhibit Th2-cell proliferation/function and to suppress IgE responses. Several adult AD studies have demonstrated efficacy with three-times-weekly high-dose ($150 \mu g/m^2$) and low-dose ($50 \mu g/m^2$) therapy. Disadvantages of therapy include flulike symptoms (which are especially common early in the treatment course), myelosuppression, neurotoxicity/confusion, hypotension, tachycardia, and high cost.

Systemic biologic therapies specifically developed and tested for atopic dermatitis are rapidly evolving. Dupilumab, an IL4 receptor alpha blocker that targets IL-4 and IL-13, has been shown to be efficacious in treating moderate to severe AD, with generally good safety data in phase II and III clinical trials.

Referral, quality of life issues, and educational resources

Referral to a pediatric dermatologist or an adult dermatologist/AD specialist may help with comprehensive management of skin care and barrier repair. Referral should be considered in patients with a diagnosis of moderate or severe AD, those who are unresponsive to standard treatments (including midpotency topical corticosteroids), those with persistent disease and/or frequent flares, those who have been hospitalized as a direct consequence of their AD, and those requiring systemic therapies for flares and/or maintenance. *Allergy testing* is not generally a first-line referral recommendation in the routine evaluation and treatment of uncomplicated AD. However, consultation with an allergist can be useful when proper skin care alone is not effective and/or when the clinical picture hints strongly at specific allergic triggers. Immunotherapy with aeroallergens has not been proven effective in the treatment of AD. Referral to immunology or gastroenterology is warranted if underlying systemic infections are frequent or when eosinophilic gastroenteritis/esophagitis becomes a concern in younger children with concomitant failure to thrive.

Emotional stress can exacerbate AD in some patients who may respond to frustration, anxiety, embarrassment, or other psychologically stressful events with a perceived increase in pruritus and subsequent scratching. This may be particularly important in the adolescent population, where even very mild skin disease may be considered "disfiguring." In some cases, patients may use scratching for secondary gain, and in others scratching has simply become habitual. *Relaxation, biofeedback,* and *behavioral modification* techniques may be helpful in such patients. *Psychosocial evaluation* and counseling should be considered in families where emotional triggers appear to function as obstacles to disease management, or where quality of life is clearly affected. *Therapeutic education* has been shown beneficial in managing AD and may be accomplished through extended in-office discussion, written handouts, eczema "school programs," and/or web resources, which include video training modules (e.g., www.eczemacenter.org). Families may also benefit from *support groups* such as the U.S. National Eczema Association (www.nationaleczema.org) and the UK National Eczema Society (www.eczema.org).

Hospitalization

Erythrodermic AD patients, those with suspected widespread superinfection, or those with severe recalcitrant disease may benefit from hospitalization. Removal from environmental or emotional stressors, intensive therapy, and caregiver education should be the goals. Hospitalization may be particularly useful in those patients being transitioned to systemic therapies and also provides an opportunity for coordinated care between multiple specialty services.

Specific Investigations

In selected cases only

- Skin biopsy: Especially in adult onset-AD and when cutaneous T-cell lymphoma is being considered as an alternative diagnosis
- Quantification of IgE, IgA, IgM, and IgG levels
- Specific serum IgE assays for food or environment allergens and oral food challenges
- Patch testing for allergic contact dermatitis: Allergic contact dermatitis may be both an alternative diagnosis and exacerbator of AD
- Bacterial cultures and sensitivities
- HIV enzyme-linked immunosorbent assay (ELISA) screening

Translating atopic dermatitis management guidelines into practice for primary care providers. Eichenfield LF, Boguniewicz M, Simpson EL, Russell JJ, Block JK, Feldman SR, et al. Pediatrics 2015; 136: 554–65.

This paper presents an overview of the strategy for diagnosis and management of AD in the pediatric population.

Guidelines of care for the management of atopic dermatitis: section 1. Diagnosis and assessment of atopic dermatitis. Eichenfield LF, Tom WL, Chamlin SL, Feldman SR, Hanifin JM, Simpson EL, et al. J Am Acad Dermatol 2014; 70: 338–51.

Guidelines of care for the management of atopic dermatitis: section 2. Management and treatment of atopic dermatitis with topical therapies. Eichenfield LF, Tom WL, Berger TG, Krol A, Paller AS, Schwarzenberger K, et al. J Am Acad Dermatol 2014; 71: 116–32.

Guidelines of care for the management of atopic dermatitis: section 3. Management and treatment with phototherapy and systemic agents. Sidbury R, Davis DM, Cohen DE, Cordoro KM, Berger TG, Bergman JN, et al. J Am Acad Dermatol 2014; 71: 327–49.

Guidelines of care for the management of atopic dermatitis: Section 4. Prevention of disease flares and use of adjunctive therapies and approaches. Sidbury R, Tom WL, Bergman JN, Cooper KD, Silverman RA, Berger TG, et al. J Am Acad Dermatol 2014; 71: 1218–33.

This comprehensive set of guidelines discusses the management of AD—from diagnosis to treatment and prevention— in both adult and pediatric populations.

Guidelines for the diagnosis and management of food allergy in the United States: report of the NIAID-sponsored expert panel. Boyce JA, Assaad A, Burks AW, Jones SM, Sampson HA, Wood RA et al. J Allergy Clin Immunol 2010; 126: S1–58.

This includes consensus definition for food allergy and discussion of comorbid conditions and IgE-mediated and non-IgE-mediated reactions to food.

Addendum guidelines for the prevention of peanut allergy in the United States: Report of the National Institute of Allergy and Infectious Diseases-Sponsored Expert Panel. Togias A, Cooper SF, Acebal ML, Assa'ad A, Baker JR Jr, Beck LA et al. Pediatr Dermatol 2017; 34: e1–21.

This paper presents guidelines for infants at various risk levels for the development of peanut allergy, including the highest-risk group, and infants with severe AD and/or egg allergy. Topics addressed include the definition of risk categories, appropriate use of testing (specific IgE measurement, skin prick tests, and oral food challenges), and the timing and approaches for introduction of peanut-containing foods.

Seborrheic dermatitis-like and atopic dermatitis-like eruptions in HIV-infected patients. Cockerell CJ. Clin Dermatol 1991; 9: 49–51.

Crusting and lichenification in the flexural areas or in a more widespread distribution, characteristic of an "AD-like" dermatitis, may represent advanced human immunodeficiency virus (HIV) infection.

First-Line Therapies

• Education	A
• Emollients*	A
• Topical corticosteroids	A
• Proactive therapy	A
• Wet wraps	B

*The choice of using an emollient or barrier repair cream should be made based on personal preference.

Age related, structured educational programmes for the management of atopic dermatitis in children and adolescents: multicentre, randomized controlled trial. Staab D, Diepgen T, Fartasch M, Kupfer J, Lob-Corzilius T, Ring J et al. Br Med J 2006; 332: 933–8.

A comparison of children with AD whose parents had received 6 weeks of intensive AD education versus those children whose parents received no education. The investigators taught age-appropriate interventions to the parents. Patients in the "treatment" group demonstrated significantly improved subjective quality-of-life scores and objective measures of eczema severity over the 12-month period.

Psychological and educational interventions for atopic eczema in children. Ersser SJ, Latter S, Sibley A, Satherley PA, Welbourne S. Cochrane Database Syst Rev 2007; 3:CD004054.

Emollients improve treatment results with topical corticosteroids in childhood atopic dermatitis: a randomized comparative study. Szczepanowska J, Reich A, Szepietowski JC. Pediatr Allergy Immunol 2008; 19: 614–8.

A randomized study of 52 patients aged 2 to 12 years found that the use of emollients can significantly improve xerosis and pruritus during corticosteroid treatment of AD and helped maintain clinical improvement after discontinuation of therapy.

Quantitative assessment of combination bathing and moisturizing regimens on skin hydration in atopic dermatitis. Chiang C, Eichenfield LF. Pediatr Dermatol 2009; 26: 273–8.

A crossover study in five pediatric patients with AD and five patients with healthy skin in whom objective parameters of cutaneous hydration status were assessed after various combinations of bathing and moisturizing regimens. This study found that bathing without moisturizer may compromise skin hydration. Bathing followed by moisturizer application provides modest hydration benefits, though less than that of simply applying moisturizer alone.

A pilot study of emollient therapy for the primary prevention of atopic dermatitis. Simpson EL, Chalmers JR, Hanifin JM, Thomas KS, Cork MJ, McLean WH, et al. J Allergy Clin Immunol 2014; 134: 818–23.

Emollient enhancement of the skin barrier from birth offers effective AD prevention, and early interventions to repair the epidermal barrier may be useful as a primary prevention of AD. In one study, neonates at high risk for developing AD were randomized to apply daily emollient or receive no intervention. At 6 months of age, 21.8% (12/55) of completed subjects in the emollient group developed AD, whereas 43.4% (23/53) of completed subjects in the control group developed AD. Thus there is evidence to suggest that primary prevention of AD may be achieved through daily emollient use in high-risk neonates.

Application of moisturizer to neonates prevents development of atopic dermatitis. Horimukai K, Morita K, Narita M, Kondo M, Kitazawa H, Nozaki M, et al. J Allergy Clin Immunol 2014; 134: 824–30.e6.

A Japanese study of 118 neonates reported similar results. The 59 subjects who received daily moisturizer for the first 32 weeks of life were 32% less likely to develop AD compared with no intervention.

Scoping systematic review of treatments for eczema. Nankervis H, Thomas KS, Delamere FM, Barbarot S, Rogers NK, Williams HC. NIHR Journals Library 2016; 4: 1–528.

A systematic review of 287 trials covering 92 different AD interventions.

Topical corticosteroids for atopic eczema: clinical and cost effectiveness of once-daily vs. more frequent use. Green C, Colquitt JL, Kirby J, Davidson P. Br J Dermatol 2005; 152: 130–41.

A systematic review found no clear differences in outcomes between once-daily and more frequent application of topical corticosteroids.

A systematic review of the safety of topical therapies for atopic dermatitis. Callen J, Chamlin S, Eichenfield LF, Ellis C, Girardi M, Goldfarb M et al. Br J Dermatol 2007; 156: 203–21.

This review of topical therapies for AD found that although some systemic exposure to topical steroids does occur, physiologic changes appear to be uncommon, and systemic complications are rare when medications are used properly.

Efficacy and safety of wet-wrap dressings in children with severe atopic dermatitis: influence of corticosteroid dilution. Wolkerstorfer A, Visser RL, De Waard van der Spek FB, Mulder PG, Oranje AP. Br J Dermatol 2000; 143: 999–1004.

In children with severe refractory AD, 5%, 10%, and 25% dilutions of fluticasone propionate 0.05% cream proved highly

Evidence Levels: **A** Double-blind study **B** Clinical trial ≥ 20 subjects **C** Clinical trial < 20 subjects **D** Series ≥ 5 subjects **E** Anecdotal case reports

efficacious, irrespective of dilution, when applied under wet-wrap dressings. Improvement occurred mainly during the first week, and the only significant adverse effect was folliculitis.

Wet dressing therapy in conjunction with topical corticosteroids is effective for rapid control of severe pediatric atopic dermatitis: experience with 218 patients over 30 years at Mayo Clinic. Dabade TS, Davis DM, Wetter DA, Hand JL, McEvoy MT, Pittelkow MR, et al. J Am Acad Dermatol 2012; 67: 100–6.

Intensive inpatient treatment (with wet dressings and topical corticosteroids) was highly effective in controlling severe and recalcitrant atopic dermatitis.

Second-Line Therapies

- Topical immunomodulators   A
- Against routine antimicrobial use   A
- Against routine antihistamines/anxiolytics use   A
- Avoidance of true IgE-mediated triggers   A
- Topical phosphodiesterase inhibitors   A*

*At the time of the writing of this chapter, this drug was not commercially available and was therefore listed as a second-line agent.

Efficacy and safety of crisaborole ointment, a novel, nonsteroidal phosphodiesterase 4 (PDE4) inhibitor for the topical treatment of atopic dermatitis (AD) in children and adults. Paller AS, Tom WL, Lebwohl MG, Blumenthal RL, Boguniewicz M, Call RS, et al. J Am Acad Dermatol 2016; 75: 494–503.e6.

Crisaborole's safety and efficacy were established through two phase III clinical trials. The studies included 1522 randomized patients; 1016 received crisaborole ointment and 506 received vehicle twice daily for 28 days. At the completion of the study, a statistically significant ≥2 grade improvement in Investigator's Static Global Assessment (ISGA) score ($p = 0.038$ for center 1 and $p < 0.001$ for center 2) was noted. In addition, there was a greater percentage of patients with clear or almost clear ISGA scores (51.7% and 40.6%) in the crisaborole groups than the vehicle groups (40.6% and 29.7, $p = 0.005$ and $p < 0.001$). A decrease in pruritus occurred by day eight in the crisaborole ointment group (pooled results from center 1 and 2, $p < 0.001$). Application site pain was the most common adverse effect, present in 4.4% of crisaborole-treated and 1.2% of vehicle-treated patients. However, 77.6% of patients had resolution of this symptom within 1 day of onset.

Efficacy and safety of pimecrolimus cream in the long-term management of atopic dermatitis in children. Sigurgeirsson B, Boznanski A, Todd G, Vertruyen A, Schuttelaar MA, Zhu X, et al. Pediatrics 2015; 135: 597–606.

This is a 5-year-long randomized control trial of pimecrolimus 1% cream compared with TCS. After 5 years, >85% of patients achieved overall and facial treatment success. In addition, safety of this treatment modality was demonstrated.

A meta-analysis of the efficacy and tolerability of proactive treatment with TCS versus TCI. Schmitt J, von Kobyletzki L, Svensson A, Apfelbacher C. Br J Dermatol 2011; 164: 415–28.

This meta-analysis suggests that topical fluticasone propionate (relative risk = 0.46) may be more efficacious in preventing disease flares than topical tacrolimus (relative risk = 0.78).

0.03% Tacrolimus ointment applied once or twice daily is more efficacious than 1% hydrocortisone acetate in children

with moderate to severe atopic dermatitis: results of a randomized double-blind controlled trial. Reitamo S, Harper J, Bos JD, Cambazard F, Bruijnzeel-Koomen C, Valk P, et al. European Tacrolimus Ointment Group. Br J Dermatol 2004; 150: 554–62.

This study involving 624 children aged 2 to 15 years with moderate-to-severe AD, demonstrated that tacrolimus 0.03% ointment applied once or twice daily resulted in a significantly greater reduction in modified Eczema Area and Severity Index (mEASI) scores than hydrocortisone acetate 1% ointment applied twice daily ($p < 0.001$).

Once- or twice-daily tacrolimus ointment 0.03% was significantly more effective than hydrocortisone acetate 1% in treating moderate to severe AD in children. Twice-daily application was particularly effective in patients with severe baseline disease compared with once-daily application.

Intermittent therapy for flare prevention and long-term disease control in stabilized atopic dermatitis: a randomized comparison of 3-times-weekly applications of tacrolimus ointment versus vehicle. Breneman D, Fleischer AB Jr, Abramovits W, Zeichner J, Gold MH, Kirsner RS, et al. J Am Acad Dermatol 2008; 58: 990–9.

A double-blind study in which 197 clinically clear patients with a history of moderate to severe AD were randomized to three-times-weekly topical tacrolimus or vehicle for 40 weeks; tacrolimus ointment was associated with significantly more flare-free days than vehicle and a significantly longer time until relapse.

Topical calcineurin inhibitors and malignancies in AD patients. Legendre L, Barnetche T, Mazereeuw-Hautier J, Meyer N, Murrell D, Paul C. J Am Acad Dermatol 2015; 72: 992–1002.

A systematic review of the long-term safety of topical corticosteroids and topical calcineurin inhibitors in pediatric AD patients.

Systematic review of published trials: long-term safety of topical corticosteroids and topical calcineurin inhibitors in pediatric patients with atopic dermatitis. Siegfried EC, Jaworski JC, Kaiser JD, Hebert AA. BMC Pediatr 2016; 16: 75.

A systematic review of the literature included multiple tacrolimus trials for pediatric AD.

The study included over 5800 patients and did not note any cases of lymphoma.

Long-term efficacy and tolerability of tacrolimus 0.03% ointment in infants: a 2-year open-label study. Mandelin JM, Rubins A, Remitz A, Cirule K, Dickinson J, Ho V, et al. Int J Dermatol 2012; 51: 104–10.

Tacrolimus 0.03% ointment was associated with substantial clinical improvement of AD in infants aged <2 years. Treatment tolerability was similar to that seen in older children.

Effects of cefuroxime axetil on *Staphylococcus aureus* colonization and superantigen production in atopic dermatitis. Boguniewicz M, Sampson H, Leung SB, Harbeck R, Leung DY. J Allergy Clin Immunol 2001; 108: 651–2.

***Staphylococcus aureus*: colonizing features and influence of an antibacterial treatment in adults with atopic dermatitis.** Bath-Hextall FJ, Birnie AJ, Ravenscroft JC, Williams HC. Br J Dermatol 2010; 163: 12–26.

Twenty-six studies involving 1229 participants were included. The authors failed to find any evidence that commonly used anti-staphylococcal interventions are clinically helpful in AD that is not clinically infected.

Children with atopic dermatitis appear less likely to be infected with community acquired methicillin-resistant *Staphylococcus aureus*: the San Diego experience. Matiz C, Tom WL, Eichenfield LF, Pong A, Friedlander SFF. Pediatr Dermatol 2011; 28: 6–11.

In this study, children with AD had a much lower rate of community-acquired MRSA infection compared with the general outpatient pediatric population. Clindamycin-inducible resistance was very low in both groups. Therefore first-line therapies such as cephalosporins may have a place for those patients with non-life-threatening mild infections who do not possess risk factors for MRSA, pending culture results.

An evidence-based review of the efficacy of antihistamines in relieving pruritus in atopic dermatitis. Klein PA, Clark RA. Arch Dermatol 1999; 135: 1522–5.

This review of 16 AD-associated antihistamine trials found that the majority of studies were flawed in terms of sample size or study design.

A double-blinded, randomized, placebo-controlled trial of cetirizine in preventing the onset of asthma in children with atopic dermatitis: 18 months' treatment and 18 months' posttreatment follow-up. Warner JO, ETAC Study Group. J Allergy Clin Immunol 2001; 108: 929–37.

Infants between 1 and 2 years of age with AD in this double-blinded trial were randomized to 0.25 mg/kg body weight cetirizine administered twice daily compared with placebo. After 18 months of treatment, follow-up continued for a further 18 months. Although there was no difference in the cumulative prevalence of asthma between active and placebo treatment in the intention-to-treat population ($p = 0.7$), cetirizine did appear to delay (and in some cases to prevent) the development of asthma in those patients sensitized to grass pollen and, to a lesser extent, house dust mites.

Management of sleep disturbance associated with atopic dermatitis. Kelsay K. J Allergy Clin Immunol 2006; 118: 198–201.

The author suggests an algorithm for clinicians treating sleep problems associated with AD.

New treatments for restoring impaired epidermal barrier permeability: skin barrier repair creams. Draelos ZD. Clin Dermatol 2012; 30: 345–8.

This article examines the formulation and effect of skin barrier creams.

Third-Line Therapies	
• Dupilumab	A*
• Dust mite reduction	A
• Timing of solid food introduction	A
• Phototherapy	B
• Azathioprine	B
• Cyclosporine	B
• Methotrexate	B
• Mycophenolate mofetil	C
• Interferon-γ	B
• Systemic corticosteroids	B

*At the time of the writing of this chapter, this drug was not commercially available but was added based on its merit in two phase III clinical trials.

Two phase 3 trials of dupilumab versus placebo in AD. Simpson EL, Bieber T, Guttman-Yassky E, Beck LA, Blauvelt A, Cork MJ, et al. New Eng J Med 2016; 375: 2335–48.

This two-center, double blind randomized controlled trial (RCT) compared dupilumab weekly and biweekly to placebo in 671 adults with moderate-to-severe AD not controlled by topical therapies. Dupilumab weekly and biweekly both resulted in an Investigator's Global Assessment (IGA) score reduction of 2 points or more in 36% of patients versus 10% in the placebo control group. Additionally, there was a significant improvement in AD severity observed in those receiving dupilumab compared with placebo based on a >75% change in EASI score ($p < 0.001$). Dupilumab therapy was also associated with a statistically significant improvement in other clinical end points, including reduction in pruritus, symptoms of anxiety and depression, and improvement in quality of life. Side effects more frequent in the dupilumab therapy groups than placebo included injection-site reactions (8%–19% versus 6%) and conjunctivitis (3%–5% versus ≤1%).

Prescribing practices for systemic agents in controlling pediatric AD. Totri CR, Eichenfield LF, Logan K, Proudfoot L, Schmitt J, Lara-Corrales I, et al. J Am Acad Dermatol 2017; 76: 281–5.

The TREAT survey included 133 dermatologists from the Society for Pediatric Dermatology. Of these participants, 86.5% used systemic treatments for severe pediatric AD. Cyclosporine (45.2%), methotrexate (29.6%), and mycophenolate mofetil (30.4%) were the most frequently preferred initial treatments. Factors that discouraged systemic therapy use included side effect profiles and suspected risks of long-term toxicities.

Double-blind controlled trial of effect of housedust-mite allergen avoidance on atopic dermatitis. Tan BB, Weald D, Strickland I, Friedmann PS. Lancet 1996; 347: 15–8.

Measures to reduce house dust mites using a combination of Gore-Tex bedcovers, benzyl tannate spray, and a high-filtration vacuum cleaner were compared with cotton bedcovers, water spray, and a conventional vacuum cleaner in the households of 48 children and adults with AD. Both active and placebo treatments caused significant reductions in house dust mite antigen concentrations. The severity of eczema decreased in both groups, but the active group showed significantly greater improvement.

Rice nightmare: kwashiorkor in 2 Philadelphia-area infants fed Rice Dream beverage. Katz KA, Mahlberg MJ, Honig PJ, Yan AC. J Am Acad Dermatol 2005; 52: S69–72.

Probiotics during pregnancy and breast-feeding might confer immunomodulatory protection against atopic disease in the infant. Rautava S, Kalliomäki M, Isolauri E. J Allergy Clin Immunol 2002; 109: 119–21.

Probiotic supplementation for the first 6 months of life fails to reduce the risk of atopic dermatitis and increases the risk of allergen sensitization in high-risk children: a randomized controlled trial. Taylor AL, Dunstan JA, Prescott SL. J Allergy Clin Immunol 2007; 119: 184–91.

Effects of early nutritional interventions on the development of atopic disease in infants and children: the role of maternal dietary restriction, breastfeeding, timing of introduction of complementary foods, and hydrolyzed formulas. Greer FR, Sicherer SH, Burks AW. Committee on Nutrition and Section on Allergy and Immunology. Pediatrics 2008; 121: 183–91.

The role of psoralen photochemotherapy (PUVA) in the treatment of severe atopic eczema in adolescents. Atherton DJ, Carabott F, Glover MT, Hawk JL. Br J Dermatol 1988; 118: 791–95.

Evidence Levels: A Double-blind study B Clinical trial ≥ 20 subjects C Clinical trial < 20 subjects D Series ≥ 5 subjects E Anecdotal case reports

Oral PUVA resulted in initial clearance of eczema in 14 of 15 children, 9 of whom achieved complete remission. This was associated with resumption of normal growth in children who were previously growing poorly.

Phototherapy for atopic eczema with narrow-band UVB. Grundmann-Kollmann M, Behrens S, Podda M, Peter RU, Kaufmann R, Kerscher M. J Am Acad Dermatol 1999; 40: 995–7.

Five patients with moderate to severe AD were treated with narrowband UVB for a cumulative dose of 9.2 J/cm² over a mean of 19 treatments. Narrowband UVB was effective after 3 weeks in all patients.

Half-side comparison study on the efficacy of 8-methoxy-psoralen bath-PUVA versus narrow-band ultraviolet B phototherapy in patients with severe chronic atopic dermatitis. Der-Petrossian M, Seeber A, Honigsmann H, Tanew A. Br J Dermatol 2000; 142: 39–43.

In this randomized, investigator-blinded study of 12 patients, half-side irradiation with threshold erythemogenic doses of 8-methoxypsoralen bath-PUVA and narrowband UVB was performed three times weekly for 6 weeks. The two modalities were equally effective in equierythemogenic doses.

Long-term efficacy of medium-dose UVA1 phototherapy in atopic dermatitis. Abeck D, Schmidt T, Fesq H, Strom K, Mempel M, Brockow K, et al. J Am Acad Dermatol 2000; 42: 254–7.

Thirty-two patients with acute exacerbated AD underwent medium-dose UVA1 therapy consisting of 15 treatments over 3 weeks (cumulative dose 750 J/cm²). There was a significant improvement in the skin condition at the end of the treatment period; this was still present 1 month later, but by 3 months the condition had returned to pretreatment levels.

Phototherapy in the management of atopic dermatitis: a systematic review. Meduri NB, Vandergriff T, Rasmussen H, Jacobe H. Photodermatol Photoimmunol Photomed 2007; 23: 106–12.

Azathioprine in severe adult atopic dermatitis: a double-blind, placebo-controlled, crossover trial. Berth-Jones J, Takwale A, Tan E, Barclay G, Agarwal S, Ahmed I, et al. Br J Dermatol 2002; 147: 324–30.

In this double-blind crossover trial, adult patients with severe AD were treated with azathioprine 2.5 mg/kg daily and placebo for 3 months each. There was a significant difference in favor of azathioprine in the improvement of the six area, six sign atopic dermatitis (SASSAD) sign score, decreasing by 26% during treatment with azathioprine versus 3% on placebo. Pruritus, sleep disturbance, and disruption of work/daytime activity all improved significantly on active treatment, but the difference in mean improvement between azathioprine and placebo was statistically significant only for disruption of work/daytime activity. The authors suggested that a longer period of treatment might have further improved the eczema. Gastrointestinal disturbances and deranged liver enzymes were common. Of the 37 patients enrolled, 12 prematurely terminated treatment with azathioprine and 4 with placebo.

A retrospective evaluation of azathioprine in severe childhood atopic eczema, using thiopurine methyltransferase levels to exclude patients at high risk of myelosuppression. Murphy LA, Atherton DJ. Br J Dermatol 2002; 147: 308–15.

Parallel-group randomized controlled trial of azathioprine in moderate to severe atopic eczema, using a thiopurine methyltransferase-based dose regimen. Meggitt SJ, Gray JC, Reynolds NJ. Br J Dermatol 2003; 149: 3.

There was again a significant improvement in sign score on azathioprine (39%) relative to placebo (24%). Pruritus and the physician's global assessment also improved significantly better in the azathioprine group. Six patients withdrew from azathioprine treatment because of nausea or hypersensitivity.

Efficacy and tolerability at 3 and 6 months following use of azathioprine for recalcitrant atopic dermatitis in children and young adults. Hon KL, Ching GK, Leung TF, Chow CM, Lee KK, Ng PC. J Dermatolog Treat 2009; 20: 141–5.

The clinical efficacy of azathioprine, and its hematologic and biochemical effects (serum IgE level, liver and renal function), were assessed at 3 months and 6 months in 17 patients with recalcitrant AD. Disease severity was evaluated with the scoring atopic dermatitis (SCORAD) score. Azathioprine reduced the severity of AD within 3 months in these children. Better efficacy was observed in females at 6 months. Mild transient elevation of glutamic-pyruvic transaminase was noted in one patient and mild elevation of serum bilirubin in two other patients.

Systemic treatment of pediatric atopic dermatitis with azathioprine and mycophenolate mofetil. Waxweiler WT, Agans R, Morrell DS. Pediatr Dermatol 2011; 28: 689–94.

Medical records of 28 pediatric patients with AD treated with either azathioprine (AZ) or mycophenolate mofetil (MM) were analyzed for laboratory values, TPMT levels, symptoms, infections, and other relevant data. Seventeen of 28 (61%) patients treated with AZ and 8 of 12 (66%) treated with MM reported significant improvement. Lower rates of laboratory abnormalities and side effects were seen with MM compared with AZ; however, similar rates of cutaneous infections were noted.

Oral azathioprine for recalcitrant pediatric atopic dermatitis: clinical response and thiopurine monitoring. Caufield M, Tom WL. J Am Acad Dermatol 2012; 68: 29–35.

This prospective study of 12 children with severe, recalcitrant AD who were treated with oral azathioprine showed that azathioprine can be of benefit in the treatment of recalcitrant pediatric AD. In addition, repeat assessment of TPMT activity (not thiopurine metabolite levels) may be helpful for evaluation of nonresponse or change in response to treatment.

Cyclosporine in the treatment of patients with atopic eczema – a systematic review and meta-analysis. Schmitt J, Schmitt N, Meurer M. J Eur Acad Dermatol Venereol 2007; 21: 606–19.

The authors conducted a systematic review of the effectiveness of systemic cyclosporine in patients with severe atopic eczema and included 15 studies comprising a total of 602 patients. In all studies analyzed, cyclosporine consistently decreased the severity of atopic eczema. Data from 12 of the 15 studies were pooled and showed a dose-related response with a mean decrease in disease severity of 22% (95% CI: 8%–36%) under low-dose cyclosporine (3 mg/kg) and 40% (95% CI: 29%–51%) at dosages ≥4 mg/kg after 2 weeks of treatment. After 6 to 8 weeks the relative effectiveness was 55% (95% CI: 48%–62%). Effectiveness of cyclosporine was similar in adults and children, but tolerability may be better in children.

Double-blind, controlled, crossover study of cyclosporine in adults with severe refractory atopic dermatitis. Sowden JM, Berth-Jones J, Ross J, Motley RJ, Marks R, Finlay AY, et al. Lancet 1991; 338: 137–40.

A multicenter, randomized, double-blind, controlled crossover clinical trial was conducted on 33 patients with severe refractory atopic dermatitis to determine the effects of cyclosporine (5 mg/kg/day) on their health-related quality of life. After treatment with cyclosporine, patients indicated significant improvement in quality of life; however, there was either no correlation or only a very poor correlation between the quality-of-life parameters and clinical measures of extent and activity of eczema. Twenty patients receiving cyclosporine reported adverse events, compared with eight taking placebo. Relapse was noted when cyclosporine was stopped; however, the mean scores for disease activity and extent of disease in these patients were less than their baseline values.

Cyclosporine greatly improves the quality of life of adults with severe atopic dermatitis. Salek MS, Finlay AY, Luscombe DK, Allen BR, Berth-Jones J, Camp RD, et al. Br J Dermatol 1993; 129: 422–30.

In this study, both sign score and quality of life improved rapidly on 5 mg/kg cyclosporine daily. Whereas the sign score deteriorated rapidly on stopping treatment, the improvement in quality of life was more persistent.

Cyclosporine in atopic dermatitis: time to relapse and effect of intermittent therapy. Granlund H, Erkko P, Sinisalo M, Reitamo S. Br J Dermatol 1994; 132: 106–12.

Forty-three patients with severe AD were treated with a 6-week course of cyclosporine 5 mg/kg daily and then retreated after a follow-up of 6 to 26 weeks (depending on the time to relapse) with an identical course of cyclosporine. A significant reduction in disease activity was observed after 2 weeks of cyclosporine treatment. After both treatment periods, approximately half of the patients relapsed after 2 weeks; after 6 weeks follow-up the relapse rates were 71% and 90%, respectively, for the two treatment periods. Notably, after the first treatment period, five patients did not relapse during the 26-week follow-up, and for the second treatment period two did not relapse. All of these seven patients were still in remission at 1 year.

Long-term efficacy and safety of cyclosporine in severe adult atopic dermatitis. Berth-Jones J, Graham-Brown RAC, Marks R, Camp RD, English JS, Freeman K, et al. Br J Dermatol 1997; 136: 76–81.

An open-label study of 100 patients over 48 weeks' duration. Improvements in sign score, itch, and sleep disturbance were maintained throughout treatment. Sixty-five subjects completed the trial, and only seven were withdrawn due to adverse events considered likely to have been related to treatment.

Cyclosporine in atopic dermatitis: review of the literature and outline of a Belgian consensus. Naeyaert JM, Lachapelle JM, Degreef H, de la Brassinne M, Heenen M, Lambert J. Dermatology 1999; 198: 145–52.

This excellent review summarizes all the major trials of cyclosporine for AD and gives practical recommendations for the clinician. These authors recommend that cyclosporine be reserved for adults with severe AD and only used in children with recalcitrant disease for short periods. A starting dosage of 2.5 mg/kg daily can be adjusted up after 2 weeks, depending on response, to a maximum dose of 5 mg/kg daily. Screening for gynecologic or prostate malignancy and skin biopsy to exclude cutaneous T-cell lymphoma, as well as close monitoring of renal function and blood pressure, are recommended.

An open-label, dose-ranging study of methotrexate for moderate-to-severe adult atopic eczema. Weatherhead SC, Wahie S, Reynolds NJ, Meggitt SJ. Br J Dermatol 2007; 156: 346–51.

This 24-week, open-label safety and efficacy study evaluated 12 adults with moderate to severe AD in a dose-ranging, prospective trial of methotrexate.

A randomized trial of methotrexate versus azathioprine for severe atopic eczema. Schram ME, Roekevisch E, Leeflang MM, Bos JD, Schmitt J, Spuls PI. J Allergy Clin Immunol 2011; 128: 353–9.

Forty-two patients were randomly assigned to receive either methotrexate or azathioprine for 12 weeks. Both treatments were found to be safe in the short term and achieved clinically relevant improvement with a 42% reduction in AD severity seen with methotrexate and 39% with azathioprine.

Treatment of atopic eczema with oral mycophenolate mofetil. Neuber K, Schwartz I, Itschert G, Dieck AT. Br J Dermatol 2000; 143: 385–91.

Ten patients with severe AD were treated with oral mycophenolate mofetil at an initial dose of 1 g/day during the first week and then 2 g daily for a further 11 weeks. Median scores for disease severity improved by 68% (100% in one patient, >75% in three patients, and >50% in the remainder).

Mycophenolate mofetil for severe childhood atopic dermatitis: experience in 14 patients. Heller M, Shin HT, Orlow SJ, Schaffer JV. Br J Dermatol 2007; 157: 127–32.

Enteric-coated mycophenolate sodium versus cyclosporin A as long-term treatment in adult patients with severe atopic dermatitis: a randomized controlled trial. Haeck IM, Knol MJ, Ten Berge O, van Velsen SG, de Bruin-Weller MS, Bruijnzeel-Koomen CA. J Am Acad Dermatol 2011; 64: 1074–84.

An observer-blinded, randomized controlled trial was conducted comparing enteric-coated mycophenolate sodium (EC-MPS) with cyclosporine A (CsA) as long-term treatment in adult patients with severe AD. This study showed that EC-MPS is as effective as CsA as maintenance therapy in patients with AD. However, clinical improvement with EC-MPS was delayed in comparison with CsA. Remission after stopping EC-MPS lasted longer compared with CsA.

Recombinant interferon gamma therapy for atopic dermatitis. Hanifin JM, Schneider LC, Leung DY, Ellis CN, Jaffe HS, Izu AE, et al. J Am Acad Dermatol 1993; 28: 189–97.

In this randomized, double-blind study, patients with moderate to severe AD received recombinant human IFN-γ (rIFN-γ, 50 μg/m^2) or placebo by daily subcutaneous injection for 12 weeks. Significant reductions in erythema, pruritus, and excoriation occurred in rIFN-γ-treated patients. Edema, papulation, induration, scaling, dryness, and lichenification showed greater improvement in the rIFN-γ group, but differences were not statistically significant.

Long-term effectiveness and safety of recombinant human interferon gamma therapy for atopic dermatitis despite unchanged serum IgE levels. Stevens SR, Hanifin JM, Hamilton T, Tofte SJ, Cooper KD. Arch Dermatol 1998; 134: 799–804.

The initial efficacy and adverse effects reported for rIFN-γ treatment of patients with AD were maintained after 2 years of long-term use.

Do some patients with atopic dermatitis require long term oral steroid therapy?. Sonenthal KR, Grammer LC, Patterson R. J Allergy Clin Immunol 1993; 91: 971–73.

Three patients with recalcitrant AD were successfully managed on oral corticosteroids.

Evidence Levels: **A** Double-blind study **B** Clinical trial ≥ 20 subjects **C** Clinical trial < 20 subjects **D** Series ≥ 5 subjects **E** Anecdotal case reports

18

Atypical fibroxanthoma

Min Deng, Warren Heymann

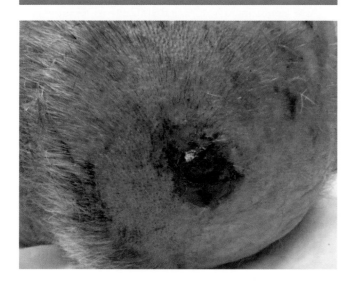

Atypical fibroxanthoma (AFX) is an uncommon cutaneous neoplasm arising from mesenchymal or fibrohistiocytic cells. AFX is found predominantly in sun-damaged skin, especially of the head and neck of elderly males, and comprises approximately 0.2% of all skin tumors. Rare cases have also been reported in children with xeroderma pigmentosum. Risk factors include male sex, ultraviolet (UV) exposure, history of radiation therapy, immunosuppression, and trauma. Clinically these lesions typically appear as rapidly growing, ulcerated, exophytic, dome-shaped nodules, usually <2 cm in diameter. Despite its severe cytologic atypia, it is considered a benign neoplasm. Care should be taken to distinguish these tumors from pleomorphic dermal sarcoma (PDS) and undifferentiated pleomorphic sarcoma (UPS).

The classification of fibrohistiocytic tumors is ambiguous and controversial. This has been compounded by the evolving nomenclature as understanding of the genetic and molecular basis of these tumors improved. Previously, fibrohistiocytic tumors encompassed the superficial AFX and its deep dermal/subcutaneous version, the malignant fibrous histiocytoma (MFH). Since 2002, the World Health Organization (WHO) has started dismantling the term MFH due to the heterogeneity of these tumors, most of which are better aligned under other classifications. The term MFH has been completely eliminated from the 2013 WHO classification of sarcomas.

In the current nomenclature, AFX is primarily a dermally based tumor that remains a diagnosis of exclusion by use of immunohistochemical stains. If invasion into subcutaneous tissue is observed, it is superficial and focal. The presence of extensive or deep subcutaneous tissue invasion, perineural invasion, lymphovascular invasion, or tumor necrosis in a tumor that otherwise resembles an AFX histologically is more appropriately classified as a pleomorphic dermal sarcoma, which carries a worse prognosis. *PDS* is a term newly proposed in 2012 by Dr. C.D. Fletcher, and therefore its adoption in the literature is included only in newer publications.

Although AFX and PDS likely represent a disease spectrum, this has not been conclusively proven. PDS is clinically indistinguishable from AFX, although reports suggest these tumors are typically larger on presentation (>2 cm). It similarly predominantly arises on sun-damaged skin of elderly men, especially on the scalp. Unlike AFX, PDS is associated with a recurrence rate of 29%, and estimates of metastasis are as high as 20%.

UPSs are a diagnosis of exclusion for sarcomas that do not fit into other categories, including AFX and PDS. When MFH was dismantled in 2002 many authors used UPS to describe what would now be considered PDS. Since the adoption of PDS in 2012, however, UPS should be limited to describing sarcomas arising from deeper tissues, often involving the extremities or retroperitoneum.

MANAGEMENT STRATEGY

Proper management relies on an adequate biopsy specimen that should include subcutaneous tissue to help distinguish between AFX and PDS. Because these are typically rapidly growing tumors, first-line management is aimed at complete eradication with surgery. Incomplete removal results in recurrences that typically manifest within a year postoperatively. In instances of incomplete removal of PDS, recurrence can manifest as satellite lesions that represent in-transit metastases.

Due to the rarity of these tumors, the lack of consensus for an excisional safety margin, and the overlap clinically with PDS, Mohs micrographic surgery with complete margin evaluation is preferable over wide local excision (WLE) for primary tumors, especially for tumors with substantial subcutaneous invasion. Recurrent tumors should be treated with Mohs micrographic surgery.

Although radiation and chemotherapy are often used as adjunctive therapies, local tumor control remains the first-line therapy. Because AFX and PDS are induced by radiation exposure, the utility of radiation therapy is unclear. There is also literature suggesting that radiation-induced sarcomas are less responsive to radiation therapy.

Specific Investigation

- Biopsy with adequate subcutaneous tissue

Diagnosis requires an adequate biopsy specimen with appropriate immunohistochemical stains (high-molecular-weight cytokeratins, S100, SMA, MelanA/MART1, EMA, CD34, and CD31) to exclude other spindle cell tumors, particularly squamous cell carcinoma, melanoma, angiosarcoma, and leiomyosarcoma. Biopsy and excision specimens should also evaluate for perineural invasion, lymphovascular invasion, and tumor necrosis to distinguish between AFX and PDS.

First-Line Therapy

- Mohs micrographic surgery   C

More than 2 decades of treating atypical fibroxanthoma at Mayo Clinic: what have we learned from 91 patients? Ang GC, Roenigk RK, Otley CC, Phillips PK, Weaver AL. Dermatol Surg 2009; 35: 765–72.

This is an updated retrospective chart review of 93 AFX tumors treated at the Mayo Clinic from 1980 to 2004. The average age at time of diagnosis was 71.7 years old. The majority of tumors (83.9%) were located on the face and scalp. The average clinical size was 1.5 cm, with immunosuppressed patients having slightly larger tumors (1.6 vs. 1.3 cm, $p = 0.10$). Treatment information was available for 88 cases. Sixty-six of 88 tumors (67%) were treated with Mohs micrographic surgery (MMS), 23/88 (26.1%) with WLE, 5 cases with electrodesiccation and curettage (ED&C), and 1 with shave excision. The authors report that based on their MMS experience, a 2-cm margin would be needed to clear 96.6% of AFX tumors. Tumors treated with MMS were larger than those treated with WLE (1.5 vs. 1.0 cm, $p = 0.02$). Of the 86 tumors with follow-up data, 2 recurred and both had been treated with WLE.

The median follow-up time for patients treated with MMS was shorter than those treated with WLE (4.5 years vs. 8.7 years); however, because recurrences typically occur within the first year postoperatively, this retrospective chart review suggests improved outcomes with MMS despite larger preoperative tumor size.

Clinical spectrum of atypical fibroxanthoma and undifferentiated pleomorphic sarcoma in solid organ transplant recipients: a collective experience. McCoppin HH, Christiansen D, Stasko T, Washington C, Martinez JC, Brown MD, Zwald FO. Dermatol Surg 2012; 38: 230–9.

This is a retrospective chart review of 17 cases of AFX and MFH/UPS in solid organ transplant recipients (renal, heart, liver, and lung transplants). Patients were younger on presentation (average age 62 for AFX, 65 for UPS/MFH) compared with immunocompetent patients. All patients were male and presented on average 10.5 years after transplantation. Fifteen of 17 (88%) presented on the head and neck, 1 on the shin, and 1 on the arm. Of the 8 AFX and UPS/MFH tumors treated with MMS, there were no recurrences or metastases. In contrast, two thirds of AFX and 2/2 UPS/MFH cases treated with surgical excision recurred or metastasized.

This is a small case series of immunosuppressed patients treated with either MMS or WLE. Although there was no information on tumor characteristics between patients treated with the two modalities or the initial surgical margins used to excise the primary tumor, this suggests a better outcome with MMS.

Second-Line Therapies	
• Wide local excision	C
• Radiation therapy	D
• Chemotherapy	B

Pleomorphic dermal sarcoma: adverse histologic features predict aggressive behavior and allow distinction from atypical fibroxanthoma. Miller K, Goodlad JR, Brenn T. Am J Surg Pathol 2012; 36: 1317–26.

This is an excellent retrospective chart review of histologically confirmed pleomorphic dermal sarcoma cases treated with WLE. The median age of patients at presentation was 81 years old, with a male-to-female ratio of 7:1. With the exception of one tumor, all presented on the head, with the majority presenting on the scalp. Tumors were large, with a median diameter of 2.5 cm and thickness of 1.15 cm. Local recurrence occurred in 28% of patients (three treated with ED&C and three with WLE) and metastasis in 10% of patients. The median time to recurrence was 10 months.

Atypical fibroxanthoma – histologic diagnosis, immunohistochemical markers, and concepts of therapy. Koch M, Freundl AJ, Agaimy A, Kiesewetter F, Junzel J, Cicha I, et al. Anticancer Res 2015; 35: 5717–35.

This is a case series of 18 patients with 21 AFX treated with WLE as well as a literature review of 2912 patients with 2939 AFX cited in the literature between 1962 and 2014. Follow-up data for 17 of the authors' 18 patients were available. The authors report a 25% (5/20) recurrence rate with WLE. Recurrences developed within 24 months after initial diagnosis. Recurrences were typically <1 cm from the site of the primary tumor or scar. One patient (5%) developed locoregional parotid metastasis. In their review of the published literature on AFX, approximately 80% (1031/1289) of tumors were treated with WLE and 17.2% (222/1289) treated with MMS. The recurrence rate was approximately 7.6% (113/1488) and similar between those treated with WLE and MMS. The metastatic rate was 2.75%.

The authors report a case series of 21 AFX treated with WLE, with a recurrence rate of 25% and metastatic rate of 5%. Although this is a good comprehensive review of the published case reports on AFX, the authors' conclusion that MMS is not superior to WLE based on published cases is premature, as there is no information on whether tumor parameters (size, depth, AFX vs. PDS) between those treated with WLE and MMS are similar. The authors do suggest that based on the close vicinity of recurrences, WLE for AFX tumors smaller than 2 cm should encompass a safety margin of at least 1 cm.

Radiation-associated undifferentiated pleomorphic sarcoma is associated with worse clinical outcomes than sporadic lesions. Dineen SP, Roland CL, Feig R, May C, Zhou S, Demicco E, et al. Ann Surg Oncol 2015; 22: 3913–20.

This is a retrospective chart review of 1068 patients with the diagnosis of UPS/MFH treated at a single institution from 1990 to 2012. Patients with sarcomas arising from bone were excluded. Of these cases, 55 (5.1%) were radiation induced and the rest were sporadic. The median latency period between radiation and the development of radiation-associated sarcoma (RAS) was 9.33 years (range 1–40 years). The median dose of radiation these patients received was 50 ± 5.2 Gy. Twenty-four percent of patients with RAS underwent repeat radiation therapy without reduction in the rate of local recurrence.

Although radiation is often used as an adjunctive therapy to local control, this study suggests that radiation-induced sarcomas are not responsive to this treatment modality.

Pleomorphic dermal sarcoma: a more aggressive neoplasm than previously estimated. Tardio JC, Pinedo F, Aramburu JA, Suarez-Massa D, Pampin A, Requena, L et al. J Cutan Pathol 2016; 434: 101–12.

In this retrospective chart review of 18 histologically confirmed PDS cases, the ratio of males to females was 1:1. All lesions occurred on the head, with half occurring on the scalp. All cases were treated with WLE and two cases also received adjuvant radiation therapy. Of the 15 patients with follow-up data, 3 (20%) developed local recurrence and 3 (20%) developed distant metastases. Of the patients with recurrences, half had evidence of incomplete resection. One patient developed pulmonary metastases 11 months after surgery despite negative surgical margins followed by adjuvant radiation therapy.

Pleomorphic dermal sarcoma. Adverse histologic features predict aggressive behavior and allow distinction from atypical fibroxanthoma. Miller K, Goodlad JR, Brenn T. Ann J Surg Pathol 2012; 36: 1317–26.

The authors report a case of PDS with multiple cutaneous metastases and radiologically enlarged lymph nodes that responded to adriamycin and ifosfamide without evidence of recurrence or further metastasis 79 months later.

Evidence Levels: A Double-blind study B Clinical trial ≥ 20 subjects C Clinical trial < 20 subjects D Series ≥ 5 subjects E Anecdotal case reports

Randomized phase II study of gemcitabine and docetaxel compared with gemcitabine alone in patients with metastatic soft tissue sarcomas: results of Sarcoma Alliance for Research through Collaboration Study 002. Maki RG, Wathen K, Patel SR, Priebat DA, Okuno SH, Samuels B, et al. J Clin Oncol. 2007; 25: 2755–63.

In this multicenter, open-label, phase II clinical trial of 122 patients with recurrent or progressive soft tissue sarcoma, patients were randomized to receive either gemcitabine alone or gemcitabine–docetaxel combination therapy. The combination therapy group achieved improved RECIST (Response Evaluation Criteria in Solid Tumors) partial response rate (16% vs. 8%). Within the subgroup of patients with MFH/UPS, 4 of 11 patients (31.6%) achieved partial response in the gemcitabine–docetaxel treatment arm compared with 2 of 8 (25%) in the gemcitabine-only arm. The median overall survival was also improved in the combination therapy arm (17.9 months vs. 11.5 months).

The standard of care for the majority of soft tissue sarcomas, including AFX and PDS, is local tumor control with surgery. Therefore there is no literature for systemic chemotherapy treatment of localized tumors limited to the skin. However, metastatic soft tissue sarcoma typically has a poor prognosis. In this phase II clinical trial, which included multiple types of metastatic soft tissue sarcoma, the combination of gemcitabine with docetaxel showed improved outcomes in tumor size and overall survival.

Third-Line Therapy	
• Electrodesiccation and curettage	D

Atypical fibroxanthoma: a case series and review of literature. Mahalingam S, Shah A, Stewart A. Auris Nasus Larynx 2015; 42: 469–71.

A case series of seven patients with AFX treated with ED&C (five) and local excision (two). At 2 years' follow-up, two of the five patients (40%) treated with ED&C had developed local recurrence. These patients subsequently underwent complete excision without further recurrences.

This case series, along with multiple other case series previously discussed, have all demonstrated a high recurrence rate when the primary tumor is inadequately removed.

Atypical nevi

Julia Newton-Bishop, Sally O'Shea

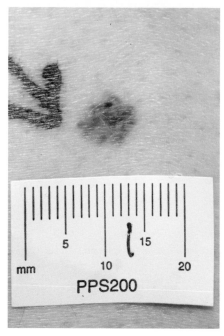

Courtesy of Dr Angana Mitra.

The term *atypical nevi* refers to clinically diagnosed lesions, defined as nevi that are more than 5 mm in diameter with an irregular or diffuse edge and variable color. Biologically such nevi are believed to be melanocytic neoplasms that result from more protracted proliferation (leading to a stromal reaction) than do banal benign melanocytic nevi. Histologically atypical nevi are characterized by elongated rete ridges, bridging of melanocytes between rete ridges, a predominance of single melanocytes over nested melanocytes, and a dermal inflammatory reaction with papillary dermal fibroplasia. Although these histologic changes are characteristic, there may be a lack of correlation between the clinical and histologic features, which has led to controversy which has largely been unhelpful. Suffice it to say that the entity remains an important one, which is clinically diagnosed, but characteristic histologic correlates are variably present in lesions that fulfill the clinical criteria.

We use the term *atypical nevi* to mean nevi that others might call dysplastic nevi. Atypical nevi may be considered more of a marker of patients at higher risk of melanoma than as frequent precursors of melanoma. The indication for excision is to exclude melanoma, not to make a diagnosis of an atypical nevus. There is no role for prophylactic excision except perhaps when a single atypical nevus appears in an individual who is older than the usual age for such nevi (over 50 years). It is important to note that two thirds of melanomas do not arise from previous nevi, so that removing all atypical nevi does not prevent melanoma even in patients who are genetically predisposed. It is mandatory to perform total-body skin examinations in patients at risk for melanoma, looking for the *ugly duckling nevus*, which stands out as different from that patient's typical *signature nevi*. The mnemonic ABCDE has been used as a clinical aid (*a*symmetry, *b*order irregularity, *c*olor variegation, *d*iameter >6 mm, and *e*volution or change in a lesion), but in practice most experts make the diagnosis based upon a global clinical examination. This is similar to a child who recognizes her written name without understanding the meaning of the individual letters.

Some authorities advocate grading atypical nevi as mild, moderate, or severe (NIH Consensus Conference: Diagnosis and treatment of early melanoma. JAMA 1992; 268: 1314–9). Others have argued that such grading has poor reproducibility, and therefore they do not grade the severity of the atypia. The majority of dermatopathologists prefer to grade the architectural and the cytologic atypia separately. It is not uncommon for severely atypical nevi to cause diagnostic difficulty. Histopathologists may report that such a lesion is of unknown malignant potential and recommend that the lesion best be treated as melanoma with a wide local excision as for melanoma.

It is common to have a single atypical nevus. In a mildly atypical nevus with a bland dermoscopic appearance, the risk of malignant change under the age of 50 is very small. Such nevi therefore should not be excised. It is then important to educate the patient how to monitor the lesion and to give that patient information booklets with photographs of atypical nevi and melanoma so that the patient knows what to look for. Merely asking the patient to "keep an eye out for change" is insufficient.

Where the atypical nevus shows more markedly atypical features, and especially in older individuals, the lesion should probably be excised. In such cases, taking a photograph and reviewing is rarely helpful, as one usually feels no less comfortable to leave alone on review than at first visit; the hypothesis is that if an atypical nevus is single, the patient's risk can be removed, or at least significantly reduced, by an excision of the lesion. If an atypical nevus causes concern, then it should be excised in its entirety rather than sampled incisionally. Although data have been published to suggest that there is a low rate of clinical recurrence after biopsy of benign moderately "dysplastic" nevi, sampling is risky as sample error may lead to histopathologic examination of a less atypical portion of the tumor. For the patient and the clinician, complete excision is a safer approach, as melanocyte pathology is difficult to interpret and the pathologist could make an error in this gray area—it is better to have excised the lesion completely in the face of ambiguity. Incisional biopsy may furthermore stimulate proliferation of residual melanocytes to lead to a clinically and histologically concerning lesion known as a *pseudomelanoma*; if there is enough clinical concern to sample such a nevus, an experienced clinician will be sampling a lesion with some clinically worrisome features, thereby supporting the argument that a complete excision is desirable.

Patients with increased numbers of banal nevi and/or multiple clinically atypical nevi are said to have the atypical mole syndrome and require different management. These patients have a melanoma risk that cannot be removed by excision of nevi. The key components of good treatment are:

- Taking a detailed family history to determine whether cases of melanoma have occurred in the family. Risk estimation is strongly modified by family history (see www.genomel.org).
- Education about monitoring of nevi.
- Follow-up/supervision in clinic for a period whose length is determined by risk estimation based upon family or personal history of melanoma and the clinical phenotype, as well as the patient's ability to discriminate change.
- Excision of atypical nevi where it is necessary to exclude melanoma.
- Education about ensuring sufficient sun protection without becoming vitamin D depleted. Sunburn avoidance is crucial in that sunburn is established to be associated with melanoma risk in multiple studies. Sunbathing, independently of sunburn, may also increase risk and so should be avoided in those with atypical moles.

Evidence Levels: **A** Double-blind study **B** Clinical trial ≥ 20 subjects **C** Clinical trial < 20 subjects **D** Series ≥ 5 subjects **E** Anecdotal case reports

MANAGEMENT STRATEGY

The strategy is essentially to excise clinically atypical nevi if there is a reasonable suspicion of malignancy while avoiding excessive numbers of procedures. The history of the lesion, the appearance to the naked eye, and the dermoscopic appearance are all important. Clinically atypical nevi that are behaving in an unusual fashion should prompt a decision to excise such lesions. Examples include a new atypical nevus over the age of 50 or a lesion that looks like an atypical nevus that has grown rapidly in the previous 6 months. Dermoscopy has been shown to increase diagnostic accuracy. Although anecdotal reports in the literature have utilized topical tretinoin, imiquimod, laser surgery, or cryosurgery, these modalities cannot be advocated for treating atypical nevi.

Treatment strategies for atypical nevi:

- Single nevi
  - Clinically assess
  - Reassure if banal but give photographic information about monitoring
  - If borderline consider photograph and review at 3 months
  - Excise if melanoma cannot be excluded after dermoscopy
  - Consider excision if nevus is new and/or the patient is over 50 years
- Multiple nevi
  - Excise nevi if melanoma cannot be excluded (not usually necessary)
  - Assess risk based upon history of change, clinical appearance, and family history
  - Consider genetic counseling if three or more cases of melanoma in the family, especially if those cases have multiple primaries or pancreatic cancer, or uveal melanoma, mesothelioma, or meningioma, which may indicate inherited *BAP1* mutations (see www.genomel.org)
  - Photograph atypical nevi at high magnification and with dermoscopy
  - Educate the patient and partner about self-examination
  - Educate the family about sun protection without becoming vitamin D deficient

SPECIFIC INVESTIGATIONS

The details of how to perform dermoscopy and the criteria for atypical nevi and melanoma are beyond the scope of this book, but there are increasing numbers of dermoscopy teaching sites on the intranet including www.genomel.org, and an Interaction Atlas of Dermoscopy CD from Medisave.

Handbook of Dermoscopy. Malvehy J, Puig S, Braun RP, Marghoob AA, Kopf AW. Andover, UK: Taylor & Francis, 2006.

Atlas of Dermoscopy. Marghoob AA, Malvehy J, Braun RP, eds. Boca Raton, FL: Informa Healthcare, 2012.

Color Atlas of Melanocytic Lesions of the Skin. Soyer HP, Argenziano G, Hofmann-Wellenhof R, Johr R, eds. Berlin: Springer Verlag, 2007.

Diagnostic Dermoscopy: The Illustrated Guide. Bowling J. Wiley-Blackwell, 2012.

Dermoscopy: The Essentials. Soyer HP, Argenziano G, Hofman-Wellenhof, Zalaudek I. Philadelphia: Elsevier Saunders, 2012.

Dermoscopy increases diagnostic accuracy. We have not highlighted recent literature relating to dermoscopy, as its use is now routine in clinical practice. In the UK, the NICE Melanoma Clinical Guideline recommends dermoscopy and dermoscopic photography in the assessment of all pigmented lesions suspicious for melanoma. [Macbeth F, Newton-Bishop J, O'Connell S, Hawkins JE. Melanoma: summary of NICE guidance. BMJ 2015; 351: h3708.] We have instead focused on published papers regarding excision because this is an area where there is current disagreement.

Diameter of dysplastic nevi is a more robust biomarker of increased melanoma risk than degree of histologic dysplasia: a case-control study. Xiong MY, Rabkin MS, Piepkorn MW, Barnhill RL, Argenyi, Z, Erickson L et al. J Am Acad Dermatol 2014; 71(6): 1257–8 e4.

In this study, 86 melanoma patients and their spouses had their most atypical nevus biopsied. Nine dermatopathologists, who were blinded to the source, were asked to evaluate the lesions. Interestingly the diameter of the lesion was associated with melanoma status in the person sampled. The degree of histologic dysplasia was however no more common in melanoma cases than controls in a multivariate analysis. Training of observers increased the concordance between them.

Selective use of sequential digital dermoscopy imaging allows a cost reduction in the melanoma detection process: a Belgian study of patients with a single or a small number of atypical nevi. Tromme I, Devleesschauwer B, Beutels P, Richez P, Praet N, Sacre L, et al. PLoS One 2014; 9(10): e109339.

In this retrospective study, dermoscopy and surgery for sufficiently atypical nevi were compared with dermoscopic imaging and possible delayed excision on review. In the dermoscopy and surgery group, 640 excisions were performed in 603 individuals, and the ratio of melanoma/nonmelanoma lesions excised was 1 to 8. In the dermoscopic imaging group, 111 excisions were carried out in 219 patients with a ratio of 1 melanoma to 2.5 nonmelanoma lesions overall.

This study is interesting and suggests an overall estimated cost difference per melanoma excised of 548 euros between the two groups, favoring the approach of dermoscopy imaging and delayed excision where appropriate. It is difficult to fully evaluate, however, as the two approaches were used in very different clinical settings. Dermoscopy and excision were carried out by 12 dermatologists in a mixture of private and public settings, whereas digital dermoscopy imaging with delayed excision was performed by 2 dermatologists in a specialist clinic.

The impact of multispectral digital skin lesion analysis on German dermatologist decisions to biopsy atypical pigmented lesions with clinical characteristics of melanoma. Winkelmann RR, Hauschild A, Tucker N, White R, Rigel DS. J Clin Aesthet Dermatol 2015; 8(10): 27–9.

This study of 41 dermatologists attending a conference examined whether or not multispectral digital skin lesion analysis (MSDSLA) could improve the diagnostic accuracy of atypical pigmented lesions. This handheld device produces a score of disorganization and the likelihood of melanoma/dysplastic nevi in <1 minute per lesion. The dermatologists first diagnosed 12 lesions based on dermoscopic images: these were a mixture of melanoma, melanoma in situ, and dysplastic nevi. Diagnoses were then made after additional MSDSLA information was given.

Using MSDSLA, the overall accuracy improved by 8% ($p < 0.001$) and the data suggested a potential reduction of 16% in the biopsy rate of dysplastic nevi ($p < 0.001$). In the future, larger studies on MSDSLA will be helpful to see how useful and cost effective it could be in clinical practice. A limitation is that the device cannot be used for thicker lesions (>2.5 mm).

Impact of guidance from a computer-aided multispectral digital skin lesion analysis device on decision to biopsy lesions clinically suggestive of melanoma. Rigel DS, Roy M, Yoo J, Cockerell CJ, Robinson JK, White R. Arch Dermatol 2012; 148(4): 541–3.

In this study, 179 dermatologists attending a conference were asked whether or not they would biopsy 24 lesions. They were first provided with dermoscopic images only and then asked again after MSDSLA information. The average true positive rate before and after MSDSLA was 69% and 94%, respectively, but the true negative rate decreased from 54% to 40% after MSDSLA. Although the addition of information from MelaFind led to an increase in sensitivity, there was a reduction in specificity. The number of lesions evaluated was small. It is not clear whether or not the dermatologists had a special interest in pigmented lesions, which could affect the results.

To excise or not: impact of MelaFind on German dermatologists' decisions to biopsy atypical lesions. Hauschild A, Chen SC, Weichenthal M, Blum A, King HC, Goldsmith J, et al. J Dtsch Dermatol Ges Deutsche 2014; 12(7): 606–14.

In this online survey, 101 dermatologists evaluated 130 lesions using dermoscopic images, 101 had additional information from MelaFind, a computerized imaging system, and 9 pigmented skin lesion experts used dermoscopic images alone. The lesions included dysplastic nevi and early melanomas (ranging from in situ to 1.2 mm thick). The average number of melanomas that would have been missed with and without MelaFind information was 14 and 20, respectively. Although there was less likelihood of missing a melanoma using MelaFind, the biopsy rate would probably increase: MelaFind alone had a sensitivity of 97% but a specificity of only 9%. This study focused on early melanomas, which may be more difficult to diagnose.

FIRST-LINE THERAPIES

Consensus statement: addressing the knowledge gap in clinical recommendations for management and complete excision of clinically atypical nevi/dysplastic nevi Pigmented Lesion Subcommittee consensus statement. Kim CC, Swetter SM, Curiel-Lewandrowski C, Grichnik JM, Grossman D, Halpern AC, et al. JAMA Dermatol 2015; 151(2): 212–8.

This consensus statement from the Pigmented Lesion Subcommittee of the Melanoma Prevention Working Group Party addressed the management of dysplastic nevi with positive surgical margins but without residual clinical pigmentation. The committee judged that lesions suspicious for melanoma should be completely excised with narrow margins, whereas clinically atypical nevi could be monitored clinically. Additional recommendations were as follows: If there are positive margins and there is still doubt that the lesion could be a melanoma, reexcision is advised. Reexcision of dysplastic nevi with positive margins is recommended if the clinical suspicion for melanoma is high, even if the histology shows low-grade dysplasia. If there is severe dysplasia and positive margins, the lesion should be reexcised with a 2- to 5-mm margin. No further excision is needed for mildly and moderately dysplastic nevi with clear histologic margins. Clinical observation is recommended for mildly dysplastic nevi with positive histologic margins but no residual clinical pigmentation. There is insufficient evidence for the management of moderately dysplastic lesions, but clinical observation may be appropriate. All biopsied sites should be monitored for recurrence, and patients should be counseled about how to do this.

Several studies have looked at the surgical approach to atypical pigmented lesions. Cheng et al performed a retrospective study of 607 melanocytic lesions that had been punch or shave biopsied and found that the rate of positive margins was comparable for each procedure. [Cheng R, Bialis RW, Chiu ST, Lawrence TJ, Lesesky EB. Punch biopsy vs. shave biopsy: a comparison of margin status of clinically atypical pigmented lesions. Br J Dermatol, 2015; **173**(3): 849–51.] However, positive margins were more likely with punch rather than shave biopsy when the trephine size was only 1 mm greater than the lesion. Lozeau et al performed a retrospective study of dysplastic nevi where a histopathologic diagnosis was provided without any grading of the degree of dysplasia. Two thirds of 17,024 nevi had positive margins, and of the 11% of cases where reexcision was advised, 80% had no residual melanocytic lesion; however, melanoma was diagnosed in 2% upon reexcision [Lozeau DF, Farber MJ, Lee JB. A nongrading histologic approach to Clark (dysplastic) nevi: a potential to decrease the excision rate. J Am Acad Dermatol 2016; 74: 68–74]. A study by Strazzula et al found positive margins in 42% of dysplastic nevi. Sixty-five per cent were reexcised: 18% had a residual atypical nevus and 2% were upgraded to severely dysplastic nevi. The authors suggest clinical monitoring of mild-to-moderately dysplastic nevi with positive histopathologic margins in view of the low yield on reexcision and the proposed low risk of malignant transformation [Strazzula L, Vedak P, Hoang MP, Sober A, Tsao H, Kroshinsky D. The utility of reexcising mildly and moderately dysplastic nevi: a retrospective analysis. J Am Acad Dermatol 2014; 71(6): 1071–6]. In Britain, the emphasis is on complete excision, with a 2-mm margin, as this provides the pathologist with the best information for diagnosis [Marsden JR, Newton-Bishop JA, Burrows L, Cook M, Corrie PG, Cox NH, et al. Revised U.K. guidelines for the management of cutaneous melanoma 2010. Br J Dermatol 2010; 163(2): 238–56]. The position of Strazzula et al to monitor these lesions clinically is held to be less feasible from an economic perspective: it is best to excise the lesion completely to minimize the risk of missing melanoma and to reduce the need for further clinical follow-up.

Management of dysplastic nevi: a 14-year follow-up survey assessing practice trends among US dermatologists. Winkelmann RR, Rigel DS. J Am Acad Dermatol 2015; 73(6): 1056–9.

In this follow-up survey, 78% of U.S. dermatologists in 2015 thought that patients with dysplastic nevi have an increased risk of melanoma compared with 59% in 2001. In spite of this, 69% aimed to completely excise dysplastic nevi in 2015 compared with 86% in 2001. In severely dysplastic nevi with positive margins, the vast majority of dermatologists would reexcise (98%), compared with 67% for moderate and 12% for mildly dysplastic nevi with positive margins. About half of dermatologists would not reexcise if the surgical margins were negative, but 39% would reexcise if the lesion was a severely dysplastic nevus (vs. 57% in 2001). The use of dermoscopy increased by 56% during the study interval.

The MPATH-Dx reporting schema for melanocytic proliferations and melanoma. Piepkorn MW, Barnhill RL, Elder DE,

Evidence Levels: **A** Double-blind study **B** Clinical trial ≥ 20 subjects **C** Clinical trial < 20 subjects **D** Series ≥ 5 subjects **E** Anecdotal case reports

Knezevich SR, Carney PA, Reisch LM, et al. J Am Acad Dermatol 2014; 70(1): 131–41.

The Melanocytic Pathology Assessment Tool and Hierarchy for Diagnosis (MPATH-Dx) reporting system was developed in an effort to standardize the histopathologic reporting of melanocytic lesions. This tool includes a management recommendation.

Three dermatopathologists designed this reporting system over the course of a year. They initially performed a blinded, independent review of 240 randomly chosen melanocytic lesions from a database. They subsequently met several times to jointly assess 279 lesions and to reach a consensus about the diagnosis. Seven diagnostic categories were described, ranging from benign melanocytic lesions to melanoma. A treatment recommendation was provided, based on the pathologists' suspicion of risk. This included options such as no further treatment or wide local excision. The reliability and feasibility in clinical practice will be explored in future studies.

Autoimmune progesterone dermatitis

Ian Coulson, Adam Daunton, Tashmeeta Ahadlan Coulson

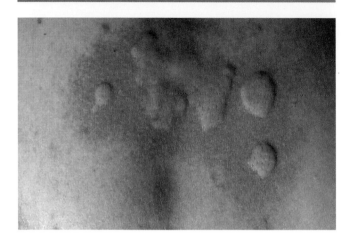

Autoimmune progesterone dermatitis is an uncommon cyclical pruritic dermatosis affecting women of childbearing age. The diagnosis is suggested by premenstrual flares and improvement during pregnancy. It can present in a variety of morphologies, including eczematous, vesicular, and papulovesicular, with urticarial and erythema multiforme–like lesions the commonest. Angioedema or anaphylaxis may accompany the skin eruptions. Hypersensitivity after exposure to exogenous progesterone, usually in the form of an oral contraceptive pill, has been implicated in some cases of autoimmune progesterone dermatitis. Endogenous progesterone may also serve as a trigger for autoimmune progesterone dermatitis in cases arising during menarche or pregnancy. The diagnosis is one of exclusion and is based upon the occurrence of cyclical premenstrual flares, the response to inhibition of ovulation, and the results of intradermal testing and hormone challenge.

MANAGEMENT STRATEGY

The mainstay of treatment is to *inhibit endogenous progesterone secretion* by suppressing ovulation. Classically, *conjugated estrogens* 0.625 to 1.25 mg daily in a 21-day cycle was a mainstay of therapy, but recently this treatment has been supplanted by gonadotropin-releasing hormone (GnRH) agonists. A transient worsening of the skin eruption is expected after initial treatment with GnRH agonists, with improvement thereafter. A major side effect of GnRH agonists is loss of bone density, which generally limits their use to 6 months of therapy. However, concomitant administration of osteoprotective agents may partly mitigate this risk and may allow longer treatment in carefully selected cases. Patients frequently require estrogen replacement while on GnRH agonist therapy.

The *antiestrogen tamoxifen*, 20 mg daily or 10 mg twice a day, exerts its effect by interfering with clinical estrogen sensitivity, possibly by competitive binding of the estrogen receptors.

Oral contraceptive pills have been implicated in triggering some cases of autoimmune progesterone dermatitis. However, in patients naïve to exogenous progesterone, inducing anovulation with oral contraceptive pills may be successful.

Mild cases of autoimmune progesterone dermatitis may be controlled with *short courses of systemic corticosteroids* before the luteal phase of the menstrual cycle. Very limited disease may respond to potent *topical corticosteroids and oral antihistamines*.

Danazol 200 mg twice daily for 1 to 2 days before menses and continued for 3 days thereafter may prevent the skin eruptions by inhibiting pituitary gonadotropins.

For severe, intractable cases, bilateral oophorectomy is curative.

Autoimmune estrogen dermatitis is a separate entity that can be difficult to distinguish clinically from autoimmune progesterone dermatitis. Intradermal testing that is positive to estrone and negative to progesterone clarifies the diagnosis. Autoimmune estrogen dermatitis responds to tamoxifen, progesterone, and oophorectomy.

The only alternative approach to the inhibition of endogenous progesterone production by suppressing ovulation is progesterone desensitization. This represents the only treatment option that preserves a patient's fertility, and it may be especially useful for patients undergoing in vitro fertilization (IVF) treatment, who are required to take high doses of exogenous progesterone.

There is wide variation between desensitization protocols. There is also a theoretical concern that desensitization treatment could aggravate latent autoimmunity in genetically predisposed women.

Specific Investigations

- Intradermal testing with progesterone
- Progesterone challenge (oral or intravaginal)
- Enzyme-linked immunosorbent assay (ELISA) and ELISpot testing

Different authors have advocated intradermal testing with progesterone in varying amounts and dilutions. One common method of intradermal testing is with 0.1 mL of aqueous progesterone suspension at 100 mg/mL diluted with normal saline to 0.1 mg/mL, 0.01 mg/mL, and 0.001 mg/mL, with normal saline serving as the control. There may be an immediate urticarial reaction within 30 minutes, or a delayed-type hypersensitivity reaction at 24 to 48 hours.

Progesterone challenge may also be attempted intramuscularly (medroxyprogesterone 10–20 mg) or orally (10 mg) in the first half of the menstrual cycle. Intramuscular skin testing with the depot form of medroxyprogesterone acetate is not advised because of the risk of severe systemic reactions.

ELISA and ELISpot testing can detect elevated levels of IFN-γ–producing peripheral blood mononuclear cells in response to progesterone.

If progesterone testing is negative, consider estrogen sensitivity. Intradermal testing with either estrone (0.1 mL at 1 mg/mL) or conjugated estrogen (0.1 mL of 1, 10, and 100 µg/mL) can be attempted. A positive reaction may be immediate or delayed for several hours and should persist for more than 24 hours.

The use of a progesterone pessary has recently been proposed as an effective tool in the diagnosis of autoimmune progesterone dermatitis.

Autoimmune progesterone dermatitis: update and insights.
Nguyen T, Ahmed R. Autoimmun Rev 2016; 15: 191–7.

A systematic review of the 89 cases published in English, examining diagnostic tests and treatment methods.

Evidence Levels: A Double-blind study   B Clinical trial ≥ 20 subjects   C Clinical trial < 20 subjects   D Series ≥ 5 subjects   E Anecdotal case reports

Sixty four of sixty seven patients who underwent an intradermal progesterone challenge experienced a positive response within 24 hours. All six patients who underwent an intramuscular challenge experienced a positive response. One patient was diagnosed after an intravaginal challenge. The remaining patients did not undergo a progesterone challenge.

Complete remission was attained in 4/86 (5%) patients without any intervention. Fourteen of eighty six (16%) patients eventually underwent bilateral oophorectomy after failure of other treatment modalities, and all subsequently attained complete remission. Of 7 patients who underwent desensitization therapy, 4/7 (57%) attained complete remission, and 1/47 (14%) attained partial control. Four of twelve (33%) attained complete remission on GnRH analogs, whereas 3/12 attained partial remission. Five of five patients treated with tamoxifen attained a partial remission. One of nineteen patients treated with conjugated estrogen/ethinyl estradiol attained a complete remission, and 8/19 attained a partial remission. Seven of nine patients treated with the combined oral contraceptive pill attained a partial remission.

The role of intradermal skin testing and patch testing in the diagnosis of autoimmune progesterone dermatitis. Stranahan D, Rausch D, Deng A, Gaspari A. Dermatitis 2006; 17: 39–42.

A case report and a detailed review of the various methods of performing intradermal progesterone testing, highlighting the need for standardization.

Progesterone sensitive interferon-γ-producing cells detected by ELISpot assay in autoimmune progesterone dermatitis. Cristaudo A, Bordignon V, Palamara F, De Rocco M, Pietravalle M, Picardo M. Clin Exp Dermatol 2007; 32: 439–41.

Describes the ELISpot technique of diagnosing autoimmune progesterone dermatitis.

Estrogen dermatitis. Kumar A, Georgouras KE. Australas J Dermatol 1999; 40: 96–8.

A case report comparing progesterone dermatitis and estrogen dermatitis, as well as useful information on the technique and interpretation of intradermal testing for both disorders.

Iatrogenic autoimmune progesterone dermatitis caused by 17 alpha-hydroxyprogesterone caproate for preterm labor prevention. Bandino JP, Thoppil J, Kennedy JS, Hivnor CM. Cutis 2011; 88: 241–3.

A 30-year-old woman, gravida 2, para 1, developed autoimmune progesterone dermatitis 4 days after her third injection of 17-α-hydroxyprogesterone caproate (17P), presenting as an urticarial exanthema. Direct immunofluorescence was negative. The injections were discontinued and lesions resolved within 7 days.

The use of progestational agents, most recently 17P, to reduce preterm labor for patients at risk may result in more cases of autoimmune progesterone dermatitis being recognized.

Recurrent anaphylaxis in menstruating women. Treatment with a luteinizing hormone-releasing hormone agonist – a preliminary report. Slater JE, Raphael G, Cutler GB, Loriaux DL, Meggs WJ, Kaliner M. Obstet Gynecol 1987; 70: 542–6.

A double-blind, placebo-controlled crossover study of four women with cyclic anaphylaxis associated with progesterone secretion. Two of the subjects experienced dramatic reduction in the severity and number of attacks while receiving an investigational luteinizing hormone-releasing agonist imbzl-D-his[6]-pro[9]-NEt-LHRH, 4 µg/kg/day for 4 months. Liaison with a gynecologic endocrinologist may help in the selection of an appropriate GnRH agonist and estrogen combination of therapies.

Autoimmune progesterone dermatitis: a diagnosis easily missed. Toms-Whittle L, John L, Griffiths D, Buckley D. Clin Exp Dermatol 2010; 36: 378–80.

Successful treatment with intranasal buserelin 150 µg thrice daily. Symptoms recurred after cessation of buserelin after the maximum licensed period of 6 months, and consideration is being given to continuing it off-license with osteoprophylaxis.

Autoimmune progesterone dermatitis. Cocuroccia B, Gisondi P, Gubinelli E, Girolomoni G. Gynecol Endocrinol 2006; 22: 54–6.

Treatment with tamoxifen 20 mg daily produced complete and durable clearing of the eruption after 3 months.

A case of autoimmune progesterone dermatitis in an adolescent female. Kakarla N, Zurawin RK. J Pediatr Adolesc Gynecol 2006; 19: 125–9.

A case report describing a patient with no prior exogenous hormone exposure who cleared on oral contraceptive therapy. For patients naïve to exogenous progesterone, an oral contraceptive pill is considered to be first-line therapy (the preparation used contained 30 µg of ethinyl estradiol and 0.15 mg of levonorgestrel).

Autoimmune progesterone dermatitis. Anderson RH. Cutis 1984; 33: 490–1.

A case successfully treated with prednisolone 20 mg/day for 10 days during menstruation. The dosage of prednisolone was reduced slowly over several cycles, and the patient was eventually managed on topical corticosteroids only.

Autoimmune progesterone dermatitis associated with infertility treatment. Jenkins J, Geng A, Robinson-Bostom L. J Am Acad Dermatol 2008; 58: 353–5.

Oral contraceptives and GnRH agonists were contraindicated in this patient undergoing treatment for infertility. The limited disease was well controlled with halobetasol propionate 0.05% cream.

Autoimmune progesterone dermatitis. Case report with histologic overlap of erythema multiforme and urticaria. Walling HW, Scupham RK. Int Soc Dermatol 2008; 47: 380–2.

Durable improvement on cetirizine 10 mg every morning and hydroxyzine 10 mg at bedtime taken on the days of the menstrual cycle previously associated with skin eruptions.

First-Line Therapies

• Gonadotropin-releasing hormone agonists	A
• Tamoxifen	D
• Oral contraceptive pill	E
• Oral corticosteroids	E
• Potent topical corticosteroids	E
• Antihistamines	E

Second-Line Therapies

• Conjugated estrogens	E
• Danazol	E
• Azathioprine	E
• Progesterone desensitization	D

Autoimmune progesterone anaphylaxis. Bemanian MH, Gharagozlu M, Farashahi MH, Nabavi M, Shirkhoda Z. Iran J Allergy Asthma Immunol 2007; 6: 97–9.

A case report of a patient with perimenstrual urticaria associated with angioedema and respiratory symptoms, all of which improved on conjugated estrogen 0.625 mg once daily.

Autoimmune progesterone dermatitis: effective prophylactic treatment with danazol. Shahar E, Bergman R, Pollack S. Int J Dermatol 1997; 36: 708–11.

Successful prophylactic treatment with danazol in two patients at a dose of 200 mg twice daily, starting 1 to 2 days before menstruation and continuing for 3 days thereafter.

Case 2. Diagnosis: erythema multiforme as a presentation of autoimmune progesterone dermatitis. Warin AP. Clin Exp Dermatol 2001; 26: 107–8.

Successful treatment with azathioprine 100 mg daily.

Autoimmune progesterone dermatitis: clinical presentation and management with progesterone desensitization for successful in vitro fertilization. Prieto-Garcia A, Sloane DE, Gargiulo AR, Feldweg AM, Castells M. Fertil Steril 2011; 95: 1121.e9–13.

Six patients with documented autoimmune progesterone dermatitis were desensitized by a rapid 8- or 10-step protocol, receiving escalating intravaginal progesterone suppositories. The initial dose of intravaginal progesterone was either 0.05 or 0.1 mg. The same dose was repeated for a total of two to three doses, before being increased by a factor of 10. This pattern was completed for a total of 8 to 10 doses. Intravaginal suppositories were administered every 20 minutes. One of the patients received an oral protocol. Four patients achieved desensitization. Three patients received successful IVF subsequently.

Iatrogenic autoimmune progesterone dermatitis treated with a novel intramuscular progesterone desensitization protocol. Hill JL, Carr TF. J Allergy Clin Immunol Pract 2013; 1: 537–8.

A single case of a patient desensitized with an intramuscular progesterone protocol.

Autoimmune progesterone dermatitis. Soloman M, Itsekson A, Lev-Sagie A. Curr Derm Rep 2013; 2: 258–63.

Authors' description of their own protocol for both diagnosis and desensitization. For desensitization, they suggest monthly intradermal progesterone injections, commencing with 0.04 mL of 50 mg/mL progesterone, doubled each month for a total of 3 months.

Third-Line Therapy

* Bilateral oophorectomy   E

Autoimmune progesterone dermatitis: treatment with oophorectomy. Medeiros S, Rodrigues-Alves R, Costa M, Afonso A, Rodrigues A, Cardosa J. Clin Exp Dermatol 2010; 35: e12–3.

Bilateral oophorectomy was curative in this case of autoimmune progesterone dermatitis that was unresponsive to oral corticosteroids and GnRH agonist.

Evidence Levels: A Double-blind study   B Clinical trial ≥ 20 subjects   C Clinical trial < 20 subjects   D Series ≥ 5 subjects   E Anecdotal case reports

21

Bacillary angiomatosis

Lucy J. Thomas, Richard C.D. Staughton

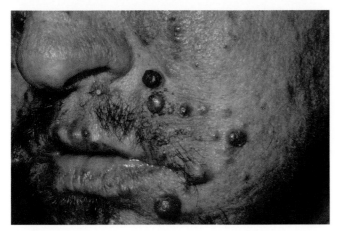

First described in 1983, bacillary angiomatosis (BA) is a vasculoproliferative disorder caused by the *intra*erythrocytic bacteria *Bartonella henselae* and *Bartonella quintana* (previously *Rochalimaea* spp.). It typically presents in profoundly immunocompromised patients (e.g., advanced HIV infection, posttransplant or during cytotoxic chemotherapy), although the incidence in patients receiving newer biologic therapies is unknown. Cutaneous lesions can be superficial, cherry-red, round papules with an eroded surface, similar to pyogenic granulomas; violaceous, lichenoid plaques; or deep subcutaneous nodules. Single lesions have been reported in immunocompetent patients at inoculation sites, whereas in the immunocompromised the entire body surface may be affected. Lesions can be mistaken for Kaposi sarcoma or in-transit metastatic amelanotic melanoma because of the highly vascular and erosive nature of the lesions. In advanced HIV deep fungal infection (e.g., cryptococcosis and histoplasmosis) should also be considered. Patients with extracutaneous disease may or may not have skin signs and can present with vomiting, abdominal pain, and deranged liver function (peliosis hepatis) or pancytopenia and splenomegaly (peliosis splenis). Fever, lymphadenopathy, night sweats, endocarditis, blindness, and anemia can also be present.

B. henselae is transmitted through a cat scratch or bite and can also result in a localized skin papule and regional lymphadenitis known as *cat scratch disease*. *B. quintana* is transmitted by the human body louse and also causes trench fever (fever, headache, dizziness, and shin pain). Localized cutaneous lesions virtually identical to BA and typically in immunocompetent individuals are seen in verruga peruana, which occurs in Peru, Ecuador, and Colombia due to *B. bacilliformis*, which is transmitted by sandflies. Preceding acute infection known as *Oroya fever/Carrion disease* results in massive hemolytic anemia with >85% mortality if untreated.

MANAGEMENT STRATEGY

Prompt diagnosis is essential to prevent dissemination, which can be fatal. Clinical suspicion should be aroused in the context of a low CD4 lymphocyte count (<100) or other immunosuppression, especially with a history of exposure to cats (>35% harbor *B. henselae*) or body lice (*B. quintana*). Treatment is determined by species, clinical course, and immunologic status.

The response of bacillary angiomatosis to antibiotic treatment is usually dramatic, in contrast to cat scratch disease. Due to antiinflammatory and antiangiogenic effects *erythromycin* is our first-line therapy at a dose of 500 mg four times daily, but *doxycycline* 100 mg twice daily is also consistently successful. In severe or complicated disease either of these drugs combined with rifampicin 300 mg twice daily has been advocated and intravenous treatment may be required. Treatment should be continued for 3 months where there is only skin disease and 4 months where there is bone/visceral involvement. Should relapse occur on these regimens, long-term prophylaxis with erythromycin or doxycycline may be indicated. However, in practice highly active antiretroviral therapy (HAART) should reverse the immunocompromised state, making long-term antibiotic therapy less necessary. The patient should be evaluated for parenchymal and osseous disease before treatment and warned that a Jarisch–Herxheimer reaction may occur after the first few doses of antibiotic.

In the case of verruga peruana oral rifampicin at a dose of 10 mg/kg/day for 2 to 3 weeks achieved a cure in over 93% of patients. Streptomycin (15–20 mg/kg/day for 2–3 weeks) has a reported cure rate of 56% and is therefore considered second line.

In the absence of randomized clinical trials, treatment is guided by anecdotal experience, retrospective cohort studies/case series, and microbiologic susceptibility data. A wide variety of therapeutic agents are mentioned in the literature, but there is a lack of correlation between the in vitro and in vivo drug susceptibility of *Bartonella* spp., which reduces the usefulness of laboratory data. The picture is clouded further by the different response of *Bartonella* spp. to drugs in each of the diseases it causes.

Specific Investigations

- Full blood count, liver function tests, HIV serology, and CD4 lymphocyte count
- Biopsy and Warthin–Starry stains/electron microscopy
- Prolonged culture of blood and biopsy tissue
- Polymerase chain reaction (PCR) of biopsy material
- Serology – indirect fluorescence assay

Multiple investigations are frequently required to confirm infection. Culture of the fastidious gram-negative rods of *Bartonella* spp. is extremely difficult, requiring special media and prolonged incubation of up to 45 days; it is invariably negative if antibiotics have been given. Skin biopsy is the essential diagnostic tool and shows a characteristic lobular proliferation of capillaries and venules with swollen endothelial cells containing clumps of bacteria. *Bartonella* spp. can also be visualized using the Warthin–Starry silver stains or electron microscopy and PCR can confirm the species. Reliance on serology in the immunosuppressed is hazardous, but the Centers for Disease Control (CDC) definition of a positive test is an indirect fluorescence assay (IFA) titer >1:64.

Bacillary angiomatosis and bacillary peliosis in patients infected with human immunodeficiency virus: clinical characteristics in a case–control study. Mohle-Boetani JC, Koehler JE, Berger TG, LeBoit PE, Kemper CA, Reingold AL, et al. Clin Infect Dis 1996; 22: 794–800.

Forty-two cases were compared with 84 matched controls and the distinguishing clinical characteristics were evaluated. Significant differences included the presence of anemia (hematocrit <0.36), raised alkaline phosphatase and aspartate aminotransferase levels, and a low CD4 lymphocyte count (median being 21/mm^3 compared with 186/mm^3 in controls). Clinical signs included fever, abdominal pain, and lymphadenopathy.

Bacillary angiomatosis in immunocompromised patients. Gasquet S, Maurin M, Brouqui P, Lepidi H, Raoult D. AIDS 1998; 12: 1793–803.

Diagnosis remains mainly based on histologic appearance. On hematoxylin and eosin stains the appearance can be highly variable and so Warthin–Starry stains are essential to visualize the bacillus and confirm the diagnosis.

Laboratory diagnosis of *Bartonella* infections. Agan BK, Dolan MJ. Clin Lab Med 2002; 22: 937–62.

Culture methods have improved, but are still prolonged. Serologic testing for *B. henselae* has become the cornerstone for diagnosis in the immunocompetent patient. Ideal antigens for enzyme immunoassays have yet to be clearly identified. PCR currently offers the ability to establish the diagnosis when other tests fail.

Culture of *Bartonella quintana* and *Bartonella henselae* from human samples: a 5-year experience (1993–1998). La Scola B, Raoult D. J Clin Microbiol 1999; 37: 1899–905.

In the large number of samples cultured, seven patients were diagnosed with bacillary angiomatosis. PCR was 100% sensitive in diagnosing these cases, in contrast to culture, which isolated *Bartonella* spp. from only three specimens. Serology was of no value, being positive in only one patient.

Rapid identification and differentiation of *Bartonella* species using a single step PCR assay. Jensen WA, Fall MZ, Rooney J, Kordick DL, Breitschwerdt EB. J Clin Microbiol 2000; 38: 1717–22.

The single-step assay described provided a simple and rapid means of identifying *Bartonella* spp.

First-Line Therapies	
• Erythromycin	C
• Doxycycline	C
• Rifampicin	C

Pathogenicity and treatment of *Bartonella* infections. Angelakis E, Raoult D. Int J Antimicrob Agents 2014; 44: 16–25.

An excellent review of existing data and treatment recommendations for all *Bartonella* infections based on pathogenicity. A table clearly summarizes the various organisms, disease manifestations, and current treatment regimens (including doses and durations).

Treatment outcomes of human bartonellosis: a systematic review and meta-analysis. Prutsky G, Domecq JP, Mori L, Bebko S, Matzumura M, Sabouni A, et al. Int J Infect Dis 2013; 17: e811–9.

This systematic review of treatment regimens for *B. henselae*, *B. quintana*, and *B. bacilliformis* identified only two randomized controlled trials analyzing the treatment of cat scratch disease and chronic bacteremia along with seven observational studies. With respect to BA they concluded that erythromycin might be better than other antibiotics but there was no statistically significant difference compared with doxycycline.

Molecular diagnosis of deep nodular bacillary angiomatosis and monitoring of therapeutic success. Schlupen E-M, Schirren CG, Hoegl L, Schaller M, Volkenandt M. Br J Dermatol 1997; 136: 747–51.

An HIV-positive man presented with a 10-month history of bacillary angiomatosis on his ankle and was treated with erythromycin 500 mg four times daily. The swabs became negative on PCR at 12 weeks, at which point treatment was successfully stopped.

Clarithromycin therapy for bacillary peliosis did not prevent bacillary angiomatosis. Mukunda BN, West BC, Shekar R. Clin Infect Dis 1998; 27: 658.

A patient with AIDS presented with bacillary peliosis and was initially treated for a presumed *Mycobacterium avium intracellulare* complex infection with clarithromycin, ciprofloxacin, and rifabutin. He continued to be febrile and represented 15 days later with bacillary angiomatosis. This swiftly responded to doxycycline, which was continued for 6 weeks.

AIDS commentary: bacillary angiomatosis and bacillary peliosis in patients infected with human immunodeficiency virus. Koehler JE, Tappero JW. Clin Infect Dis 1993; 17: 612–4.

This review article refers to 50 patients whose lesions and symptoms responded to erythromycin or doxycycline therapy.

Molecular epidemiology of *Bartonella* infections in patients with bacillary angiomatosis-peliosis. Koehler JE, Sanchez MA, Garrido CS, Whitfeld MJ, Chen FM, Berger TG, et al. N Engl J Med 1997; 337: 1876–83.

A case–control study of 49 patients (92% HIV positive) in whom macrolides, doxycycline, tetracycline, and rifampin were found to be effective. This was in contrast to patients treated with trimethoprim–sulfamethoxazole, ciprofloxacin, penicillins, and cephalosporins in whom *Bartonella* spp. could be isolated on PCR or culture.

Bacillary angiomatosis: presentation of six patients, some with unusual features. Schwartz RA, Nychay SG, Janniger CK, Lambert WC. Br J Dermatol 1997; 136: 60–5.

This article describes a variety of successful treatment regimens, including tetracycline and ciprofloxacin.

Although rifampicin has activity in vitro, its efficacy when used alone has not yet been established and so it is recommended in combination with either erythromycin or doxycycline for severely ill patients or where there is neurologic involvement (doxycycline has good central nervous system [CNS] penetration). Rifampicin monotherapy is, however, effective in the treatment of verruga peruana (B. bacilliformis).

Second-Line Therapies	
• Azithromycin	C
• Clarithromycin	C
• Streptomycin	D

MICs of 28 antibiotic compounds for 14 *Bartonella* (formerly *Rochalimaea*) isolates. Maurin M, Gasquet S, Ducco C, Raoult D. Antimicrob Agents Chemother 1995; 39: 2387–91.

The newer macrolides were highly effective in preventing bacterial growth with MIC 90s of 0.03 µg/mL for azithromycin and clarithromycin. Erythromycin, doxycycline, and rifampin all had MIC 90s of 0.25 µg/mL.

Evidence Levels: A Double-blind study   B Clinical trial ≥ 20 subjects   C Clinical trial < 20 subjects   D Series ≥ 5 subjects   E Anecdotal case reports

Recommendations for the treatment of human infections caused by *Bartonella* species. Rolain JM, Brouqui P, Koehler JE, Maguina C, Dolan MJ, Raoult D. Antimicrob Agents Chemother 2004; 48: 1921–33.

A good review article. Although erythromycin and azithromycin are the authors' first-line treatments for bacillary angiomatosis, their use has been based on case series and case reports rather than on controlled clinical trials.

Bartonellosis (Carrion's disease) in the modern era. Maguina C, Garcia PJ, Gotuzzo E, Cordero L, Spach DH. Clin Infect Dis 2001; 33: 772–9.

Case series of patients with verruga peruana who demonstrated a good response to treatment with rifampicin (80%) and streptomycin (56%).

Third-Line Therapies	
• Gentamicin	E
• Third- and fourth-generation cephalosporins	E

Lack of bactericidal effect of antibiotics except aminoglycosides on *Bartonella (Rochalimaea) henselae.* Musso D, Drancourt M, Raoult D. J Antimicrob Chemother 1995; 36: 101–8.

Aminoglycosides display in vitro bactericidal activity against *Bartonella* spp. and as such warrant further clinical investigation. For culture-positive *Bartonella* endocarditis, doxycycline for 6 weeks plus intravenous gentamicin for the first 14 days are recommended.

Bacillary angiomatosis in a pregnant patient with acquired immunodeficiency syndrome. Riley LE, Tuomala RE. Obstet Gynecol 1992; 79: 818–9.

A pregnant patient was treated with a third-generation cephalosporin, ceftizoxime. However, there are inadequate data to recommend use at present.

Balanitis

Tia M. Pyle, Warren R. Heymann

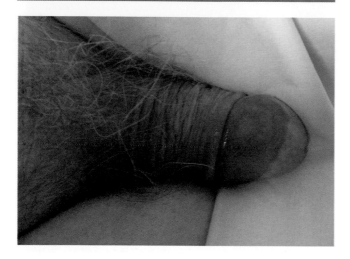

Balanitis is a general term for inflammation of the glans penis, which may also extend to the foreskin (prepuce). It may be seen in all age groups and occurs more frequently in the uncircumcised. Etiologies include inflammatory, infectious, and neoplastic disorders. All types of balanitis may be aggravated by poor hygiene, warmth, and friction. This chapter will focus on Zoon balanitis and balanitis xerotic obliterans (BXO, lichen sclerosus).

Balanitis plasmacellularis (Zoon balanitis interchangeably) represents a nonvenereal, nonspecific, chronic inflammation of the glans penis occasionally extending to the foreskin. The presentation is almost exclusively in uncircumcised men past the second decade of life. The shiny, red, sharply demarcated patch is often asymptomatic, though symptoms of pruritus, dysuria, and pain may be reported. The evaluation for Zoon balanitis should include thorough history and clinical workup to exclude genital herpes, secondary syphilis, and other etiologies of penile lesions. Zoon balanitis can also be associated with dermatoses of the genital area such as erosive lichen planus, lichen sclerosus, and penile psoriasis as a type of reaction pattern.

Other differentials (allergic contact dermatitis, erythroplasia of Queyrat or Bowen disease of the glans penis, and pemphigus vulgaris) should be ruled out. Biopsy demonstrates an atrophic epidermis with diamond-shaped keratinocytes overlying a predominately plasma cell–rich, bandlike infiltrate in the papillary dermis. Complications may include fissuring and pain, phimosis (inability to retract the foreskin due to agglutination/scarring), and stenosis or obstruction of the urethral meatus; surgical correction of sequelae may be necessary.

Lichen sclerosus (BXO) is treated similarly to Zoon (plasma cell) balanitis. Lichen sclerosus is also of unclear etiology, although an autoimmune pathogenesis associated with other conditions such as autoimmune thyroid disease, alopecia areata, and vitiligo may be involved. Histopathology confirms the diagnosis of BXO. This condition may be underrecognized in boys. It is important to identify the disorder and have continued follow-up because of the 4% to 5% lifetime risk of developing a squamous cell carcinoma.

MANAGEMENT STRATEGY

Evaluation of a patient with balanitis should include chief complaint, history of present illness, past medical and surgical history, medications, allergies, and review of systems. Specific information should be sought regarding sexual habits (number of encounters, gender, and symptomatology of sexual partners) and alleviating of exacerbating factors. To identify potential allergens and/or irritants, the patient's genital hygiene practices and the use of oral and topical agents (condoms, spermicides, sexual-enhancing products, lubricants, etc.) should be sought. A complete mucocutaneous examination, including extragenital sites, should be performed. The genital examination includes skin and soft tissue structures extending from the lower abdomen to the perianal skin/gluteal cleft. Examination findings should direct the acquisition of microbiologic studies (KOH preparation; bacterial, fungal, and viral cultures), biopsy (hematoxylin and eosin, direct immunofluorescence), and serologic studies. Treatment of balanitis is dictated by results of these investigations.

Patients with balanitis should be instructed about appropriate local hygiene care, including retraction of the foreskin before cleansing. The glans and shaft should be cleaned with plain water or normal saline twice daily and after sexual activity. Soap and topical products may be irritants or allergens and should be avoided. A bland emollient (plain white petrolatum or similar agent) applied twice daily will minimize friction and improve barrier function.

Medical therapy for balanitis is directed by etiology. Circumcision is indicated in refractory cases. Urethral meatotomy or meatoplasty, glans resurfacing, and other surgical procedures may be required for patients with significant anatomic distortion or compromised urinary function. Collaboration with urologic specialists is essential.

Specific Investigations

- KOH microscopy for fungi
- Tzanck smear or direct fluorescent antigen testing for herpes viruses
- Swab culture for bacteria, viruses, and fungi
- Biopsy for routine histopathology and direct immunofluorescence, if indicated
- Fasting blood glucose
- Urinalysis and urine glucose
- Serologic tests for syphilis, herpes virus, and human immunodeficiency virus
- Serologic tests for vesiculobullous diseases (systemic lupus erythematosus, pemphigus vulgaris, bullous pemphigoid, etc.)
- Patch testing

2013 European guideline for the management of balanoposthitis. Edwards S, Bunker C, Ziller F, van der Meijden W. Int J STD AIDS 2014; 25: 615–26.

Comprehensive review of the many causes of balanitis with specific recommendations for evaluation and management.

Zoon balanitis: a comprehensive review. Dayal S, Sahu P. Indian J Sex Transm Dis 2016; 37: 129–38.

A complete review of Zoon balanitis with history, differential diagnosis, and treatment.

Balanitis xerotica obliterans in children and adolescents: a literature review and clinical series. Celis S, Reed F, Murphy F, Adams S, Gillick J, Abdelhafeez A, et al. J Ped Urol 2014; 10: 34–9.

Evidence Levels: **A** Double-blind study **B** Clinical trial ≥ 20 subjects **C** Clinical trial < 20 subjects **D** Series ≥ 5 subjects **E** Anecdotal case reports

A literature review of the diagnosis, treatment, and management of children under the age of 18 who were diagnosed with balanitis xerotica obliterans.

Dermoscopy in plasma cell balanitis: its usefulness in diagnosis and follow-up. Corazza M, Virgili A, Minghetti S, Toni G, Borghi A. J Eur Acad Dermatol Venereol 2016; 30: 182–4.

A case report showing dermoscopy findings of a "rusty," spatterlike pattern with vascular prominence before treatment. Resolution revealed a rich vascular pattern after 3 months of twice-daily treatment with fusidic acid 2% and betamethasone valerate 0.1% cream-fixed combination (FA/BM). The "rusty" pattern persisted after treatment.

First-Line Therapies	
• Hygiene	B
• Emollients	B

Clinical features and management of recurrent balanitis: association with atopy and genital washing. Birley HD, Walker MM, Luzzi GA, Bell R, Taylor-Robinson D, Byrne M, et al. Genitourin Med 1993; 69: 400–3.

Forty-three patients with recurrent balanitis were evaluated. Thirty-one patients diagnosed with irritant contact dermatitis had a greater lifetime incidence of atopy and more frequent genital hygiene habit; 90% responded to conservative treatment, use of emollient creams, and restriction of soap use.

Second-Line Therapies	
• Topical antifungals	B
• Topical corticosteroids	A
• Circumcision	B

Candida balanitis: risk factors. Lisboa C, Santos A, Dias C, Azevedo F, Pina-Vaz C, Rodrigues A. J Eur Acad Dermatol Venereol 2010; 24: 820–6.

A prospective cross-sectional study of 478 men who attended a sexually transmitted diseases clinic revealed *Candida* balanitis in 18%, more than 40% of whom had a concomitant cause of balanitis. *Candida albicans* was the most common isolate. *Candida* colonization and infection were associated with age greater than 60 years and diabetes mellitus in males aged 40 years or older.

Comparison of the efficacy and safety of oral fluconazole and topical clotrimazole in patients with candida balanitis. Stary A, Soeltz-Szoets J, Ziegler C, Kinghorn G, Roy R. Sex Transm Infect 1996; 72: 98–102.

A randomized, open-label, parallel-group, multicenter study evaluating the efficacy of a single oral fluconazole dose of 150 mg compared with clotrimazole applied twice daily for 7 days in 157 men with candidal balanitis. The single 150-mg fluconazole dose was comparable in efficacy to 7 days of topical clotrimazole.

Lichen sclerosus: review of the literature and current recommendations for management. Pugliese JM, Morey AF, Peterson AC. J Urol 2007; 178: 2268–76.

Extensive review of the literature. Goals for treatment include symptomatic relief, prevention of scarring/anatomic distortion, and prevention of malignant transformation. An algorithmic approach to medical and surgical management of lichen sclerosus is provided with topical corticosteroids as first-line treatment.

Prevention of malignant transformation has not been assessed in the literature to date in the authors' opinion.

British Association of Dermatologists' guidelines for the management of lichen sclerosus 2010. Neill SM, Lewis FM, Tatnall FM, Cox NH. Br J Dermatol 2010; 163: 672–82.

Evidence-based recommendations for the evaluation and treatment of lichen sclerosus in men, women, and children. Topical corticosteroids are the treatment of choice. Testosterone is no longer recommended. Topical and systemic retinoids have not shown efficacy in uncomplicated lichen sclerosus, although they may be beneficial in recalcitrant cases. Surgery is only recommended when scarring and destruction have occurred. Circumcision is highly effective; recurrences and koebnerization have been documented.

Systematic review and meta-analysis of randomized controlled trials on topical interventions for genital lichen sclerosus. Chi C, Kirtschig G, Baldo M, Lewis F, Wang S, Wojnarowska F. J Am Acad Dermatol 2012; 67: 305–12.

Topical clobetasol propionate 0.05% applied for 3 months and mometasone furoate 0.05% applied for 5 weeks were both superior to placebo. Pimecrolimus 1% cream and clobetasol propionate 0.05% cream after 12 weeks of application were both effective at relieving pruritus and burning; there were no significant differences between clobetasol propionate and pimecrolimus. No evidence was found supporting the topical use of androgens and progesterone.

Conservative treatment of phimosis with fluticasone propionate 0.05%: a clinical study in 1185 boys. Zavras N, Christianakis E, Mpourikas D, Ereikat K. J Pediatr Urol 2009; 5: 181–5.

A prospective study of 1185 boys with suspected phimosis using fluticasone propionate cream 0.05% (class 5 corticosteroid) twice daily for 4 to 8 weeks yielded successful resolution (full retraction of foreskin) in 91.1%.

Plasma cell balanitis of Zoon: response to Trimovate cream. Tang A, David N, Horton LW. Int J STD AIDS 2001; 12: 75–8.

Ten patients with plasma cell balanitis treated with a topical mixture of oxytetracycline 3%, nystatin 100,000 U/g, and clobetasone butyrate 0.05% (Trimovate) for 3 to 12 weeks had complete resolution. Four required retreatment(s).

Lichen sclerosus of the male genitalia and urethra: surgical options and results in a multicenter international experience with 215 patients. Kulkarni S, Berbagli G, Kirpekar D, Mirri F, Lazzeri M. Eur Urol 2009; 55: 945–54.

A total of 215 males (age range 11–85 years) with lichen sclerosus limited to the foreskin and/or external urethral meatus underwent circumcision or urethral reconstructive surgery. Thirty-four patients with foreskin-limited lichen sclerosus underwent circumcision with 100% success rate and no recurrences at mean follow-up of 65 months. Urethral involvement required more extensive surgical intervention with lower rates of success.

Plasma cell balanitis: clinical and histopathological features – response to circumcision. Kumar B, Sharma R, Rajagopalan M, Radotra BD. Genitourin Med 1995; 71: 32–4.

Twenty-seven patients with plasma cell balanitis were cured with circumcision. There were no recurrences at 3-year follow-up.

Plasma cell balanitis: clinicopathologic study of 112 cases and treatment modalities. Kumar B, Narang T, Dass Radotra B, Gupta S. J Cutan Med Surg 2006; 10: 11–5.

A study of 112 males with plasma cell balanitis demonstrated complete resolution and no recurrence in the 85 who underwent circumcision. Twenty-two of 27 showed healing at 2 to 3 months with topical therapy (corticosteroids, corticosteroids–antifungal, or tacrolimus).

Third-Line Therapies	
• Topical tacrolimus	B
• Topical pimecrolimus	A/E
• Imiquimod	E
• CO_2 laser	C
• Erbium:YAG laser	B
• Photodynamic therapy	E
• Acitretin	A

Multicentre, phase II trial on the safety and efficacy of topical tacrolimus ointment for the treatment of lichen sclerosus. Hengge UR, Krause W, Hofmann H, Stadler R, Gross G, Meurer M, et al. Br J Dermatol 2006; 155: 1021–8.

Prospective, multicenter phase II study of tacrolimus 0.1% ointment in 84 patients (49 women, 32 men, 3 girls) with lichen sclerosus twice daily for 16 weeks demonstrated clearance of clinical disease in 43% and partial resolution in 34% at 24 weeks. Maximal response occurred at 10 to 24 weeks. No gender difference in response to therapy was noted.

Safety and tolerability of adjuvant topical tacrolimus treatment in boys with lichen sclerosus: a prospective phase 2 study. Ebert AK, Rosch WH, Vogt T. Eur Urol 2008; 54: 932–7.

Twenty boys with biopsy-confirmed lichen sclerosus underwent circumcision followed by topical tacrolimus 0.1% ointment twice daily for 3 weeks. All completed treatment without adverse side effects and no evidence of clinical disease at follow-up. Topical tacrolimus without circumcision was not evaluated.

Plasma cell balanitis of Zoon treated with topical tacrolimus 0.1%: report of 3 cases. Roe E, Dalmau J, Peramiquel L, Perez M, Lopez-Lozano HE, Alomar A. J Eur Acad Dermatol Venereol 2007; 21: 284–5.

Three patients with Zoon balanitis refractory to topical corticosteroids, antifungals, and antibacterials responded favorably to tacrolimus 0.1% ointment twice daily within 3 to 4 weeks.

Topical tacrolimus: an effective therapy for Zoon balanitis. Santos-Juanes J, Sanchez del Rio J, Galache C, Soto J. Arch Dermatol 2004; 140: 1538–9.

Complete remission was reported in three patients with Zoon balanitis after using topical tacrolimus 0.1% cream or ointment twice daily for 3 to 5 weeks. Mild irritation was noted in one patient.

Pimecrolimus 1% cream in non-specific inflammatory recurrent balanitis. Georgala S, Gregoriou S, Georgala C, Papaioannou D, Befon A, Kalogeromitros D, et al. Dermatology 2007; 215: 209–12.

A randomized controlled study of 26 men with nonspecific balanitis used pimecrolimus cream twice daily for 7 days. Seven of 11 men in the treatment group and 1 of 11 in the control group were free of all symptoms and lesions at day 14. As-needed use for 90 days showed good response.

Two cases of Zoon's balanitis treated with pimecrolimus 1% cream. Bardazzi F, Antonucci A, Savoia F, Balestri R. Int J Dermatol 2008; 47: 198–201.

Two cases of resistant Zoon balanitis were treated with topical pimecrolimus 1% cream twice daily for 2 months. One patient achieved complete clinical regression. One patient noted improvement with persistence of a hyperpigmented patch. Treatment was well tolerated. Neither relapsed at 9 to 10 months follow-up.

Although the use of calcineurin inhibitors appears to be effective for both BXO and Zoon balanitis, with continued use, surveillance for the development of squamous cell carcinoma (notably in BXO) is essential because of the theoretical possibility that these agents increase the risk of malignancy.

Zoon's balanitis treated with imiquimod 5% cream. Marconi B, Campanati A, Simonetti O, Savelli A, Conocchiari L, Santinelli A, et al. Eur J Dermatol 2010; 20: 134–5.

A case report of Zoon balanitis successfully treated with imiquimod 5% cream three times weekly for 12 weeks.

Ablative erbium:YAG laser treatment of idiopathic chronic inflammatory non-cicatricial balanoposthitis (Zoon's disease). A series of 20 patients with long-term outcome. Wollina U. J Cosmet Laser Ther 2010; 12: 120–3.

Ablative erbium:YAG laser treatment was used in 20 patients with Zoon balanitis with complete reepithelialization within 2 to 3 weeks in all patients.

Genital lichen sclerosus treated by carbon dioxide laser. Aynaud O, Plantier F. Eur J Dermatol 2010; 20: 387–8.

A report of four cases of penile lichen sclerosus successfully treated with CO_2 laser and a review of the literature on CO_2 laser treatment for genital lichen sclerosus.

Zoon's balanitis: presentation of 15 patients, five treated with a carbon dioxide laser. Retamar RA, Kien MC, Chouela EN. Int J Dermatol 2003; 42: 305–7.

Discussion of CO_2 laser treatment in five patients with Zoon balanitis with variable efficacy.

Zoon's balanitis successfully treated with photodynamic therapy: case report and literature review. Borgia F, Vaccaro M, Foti A, Giuffrida R, Cannavò S. Photodiagnosis Photodyn Ther 2016; 13: 347–9.

A patient with recalcitrant Zoon balanitis who refused circumcision was treated with 10% ALA in polyethylene glycol ointment under occlusion for 3 hours followed by diode red light at 630 nm at a distance of 50 mm from the skin surface for a total time of 8 minutes with a resulting light dose of 75 J/cm². Almost complete clearance was seen at 3 months' follow-up after a total of three treatments at 2-week intervals.

Acitretin for severe lichen sclerosus of male genitalia: a randomized, placebo controlled study. Ioannides D, Lazaridou E, Apalla Z, Sotiriou E, Gregoriou S, Rigopoulos D. J Urol. 2010; 183: 1395–9.

A randomized, double-blind, placebo-controlled study to evaluate the efficacy of a 35-mg daily dose of acitretin for 20 weeks compared with placebo in men with severe, recalcitrant lichen sclerosus. Of 49 patients completing the study, 24 of the 33 in the acitretin group had complete or partial resolution, whereas only 3 out of 16 in the control group responded. This study found acitretin to be safe and effective.

Evidence Levels: **A** Double-blind study **B** Clinical trial ≥ 20 subjects **C** Clinical trial < 20 subjects **D** Series ≥ 5 subjects **E** Anecdotal case reports

Basal cell carcinoma

James M. Spencer

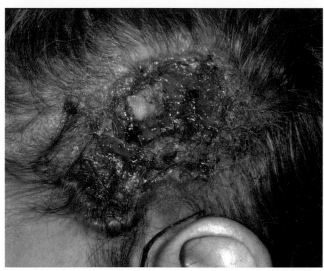

Basal cell carcinoma (BCC) is a slow-growing, rarely metastasizing but destructive malignancy, originating in the epidermis. It most commonly arises in areas chronically exposed to ultraviolet (UV) light, especially the head and neck.

MANAGEMENT STRATEGY

BCC slowly but relentlessly grows larger and deeper, and therefore therapeutic intervention is geared toward complete eradication of all malignant cells. Local recurrence is the consequence of inadequate therapy. Complete eradication is especially important because recurrent tumors are often larger and more aggressive than the original, incompletely treated primary tumor. The therapy chosen should achieve tumor eradication with the maximal preservation of function and the optimal cosmetic result. Most often, therapy uses destructive techniques such as *cryotherapy* or *curettage and electrodesiccation (C&D)*; more complex tumors may be treated by *excisional surgery, Mohs surgery*, or *radiation therapy*. The decision about which therapy to use is best made by considering four factors: tumor size, location, histology, and history (recurrent vs. primary). The clinician should consider each of these four factors and decide whether the patient is high risk or low risk for each to determine whether to use a simple or complex therapeutic strategy.

Most BCCs are discovered as primary tumors when they are still less than 1 cm in diameter. Generally tumors smaller than 1 cm on the face and 2 cm on the body are low risk.

Histologic growth pattern is a separate risk factor. The cytology of BCC does not vary: that is, all BCCs have well-differentiated, relatively monomorphic cell populations. However, the pattern of growth is variable and makes a large difference in choosing therapy. One must consider whether the tumor has a circumscribed or a diffuse growth pattern. BCC most typically exhibits a circumscribed, cohesive growth pattern known as *nodular*. Nodular BCCs may show partial differentiation toward other structures, such as cystic or keratotic, but these variants are without

therapeutic significance because the growth pattern is still nodular. Morpheaform, micronodular, infiltrating, and superficial BCCs are all variants that exhibit a diffuse growth pattern. These lesions are more likely to recur as a result of subclinical extension or more aggressive tumor behavior, or both. Unfortunately, all too often biopsy reports simply state "BCC," with no information about the growth pattern. Inadequately treated nodular BCC often recurs with a more aggressive diffuse growth pattern, such as infiltrating or micronodular.

Location is also an important variable to consider when choosing therapy. BCC tends to occur in chronically sun-exposed sites, especially the head and neck. Approximately 80% occur on the head and neck, and 25% occur on the nose. The central portion of the face, which has the highest incidence of BCC, contains the eyes, nose, and mouth, structures of functional and cosmetic importance highly vulnerable to the destructive effects of BCC, as well as the destructive effects of therapy directed against BCC. The center of the face extending onto the area around the ears defines a roughly H-shaped area known as the *H zone*. Tumors in this zone have the highest recurrence rate and thus deserve special therapeutic attention. This zone also contains the most vulnerable structures and has the highest rate of BCC occurrence. Tumors near the ear canal in the H zone are of special concern. Extension down the ear canal provides the tumor with access to the brain, and when there is evidence of ear canal invasion, particularly aggressive therapy is warranted.

Recurrent tumors are more difficult to treat than primary tumors and require more aggressive methods.

When confronted with a BCC, the clinician may wish to consider these four variables in the context of the individual patient. The patient's overall medical status, medical history, and age may influence the therapeutic decision-making.

Specific Investigation

- Biopsy with adequate dermal component

An adequate biopsy is critical in assessing the tumor. The tumor growth pattern is important information that is impossible to determine when only a superficial fragment is submitted to the laboratory. Deep shave, punch, incisional, or excisional biopsy can all give sufficient dermis for such an evaluation.

A number of noninvasive imaging technologies are being investigated to delineate tumor depth and extent preoperatively and thus guide treatment. These include confocal microscopy, infrared spectroscopy, and ultrasound, but these all remain experimental and are not part of routine care.

Rarely, a BCC may have been neglected and reached a size such that direct bony invasion has occurred. If this is strongly suspected, a preoperative computed tomography (CT) scan should be considered.

The possibility that patients with a BCC have an increased risk of developing subsequent internal malignancies has been suggested over the years and remains controversial. At present there is no recommendation for extraordinary evaluation for internal malignancies.

Basal cell carcinoma and risk of subsequent malignancies: a cancer registry-based study in southwest England. Bower CP, Lear JT, Bygrave S, Etherington D, Harvey I, Archer CB. J Am Acad Dermatol 2000; 42: 988–91.

A cohort of 13,961 patients diagnosed with BCC between 1981 and 1988 were followed for additional malignancies. There was a significant increased risk of subsequent melanoma, but no increased risk for internal malignancies.

Further complicating the relationship of BCC to other cancers is the argument that vitamin D provides chemoprevention for some visceral cancers. Specifically, it has been theorized that elevated levels of vitamin D lower the incidence of a variety of tumors, including breast, colon, and prostate cancers. Because vitamin D is manufactured in the skin after exposure to UVB, it has been suggested that those with high UVB exposure should have a higher incidence of BCC but a lower incidence of breast, colon, and prostate cancers, among others.

Are patients with skin cancer at lower risk of developing colorectal or breast cancer? Soerjomataram I, Louwman WJ, Lemmens VE, Coebergh JW, de Vries E. Am J Epidemiol 2008; 167: 1421–9.

Patients (*n* = 26,916) with skin cancer (*n* = 4089 squamous cell carcinoma, *n* = 19,319 BCC, and *n* = 3508 melanomas) from the Netherlands were identified during the years 1972 to 2002 and analyzed for their incidence of colorectal and breast cancers. Squamous cell carcinoma (SCC) and BCC of the head and neck only were associated with a lower incidence of colorectal cancer, but not breast cancer. Patients with melanoma had a higher incidence of breast cancer.

The effect of vitamin D on cancer incidence remains controversial.

First-Line Therapies

• Curettage and electrodesiccation	B
• Cryosurgery	B
• Excisional surgery	B
• Mohs micrographic surgery	B

Recurrence rates of treated basal cell carcinomas. Part 2: curettage–electrodesiccation. Silverman MK, Kopf AW, Grin CM, Bart RS, Levenstein MJ. J Dermatol Surg Oncol 1991; 17: 720–6.

This retrospective study of 2314 primary BCCs treated by C&D at a university dermatology clinic reports a 13.2% 5-year recurrence rate after C&D. Further analysis showed that size and location were important variables, with 5-year recurrence rates varying from 9.5% in low-risk locations to over 16.3% in high-risk sites. Similarly, 5-year recurrence rates ranged from 8.5% for tumors 0 to 5 mm in diameter to 19.8% for tumors 20 mm or more.

Long-term recurrence rates in previously untreated (primary) basal cell carcinoma: implications for patient follow-up. Rowe DE, Carroll RJ, Day CL. J Dermatol Surg Oncol 1989; 15: 315–28.

Reviewed literature since 1947 and reported a weighted average 5-year recurrence rate of 7.7% of primary BCCs treated with C&D.

Mohs surgery is the treatment of choice for recurrent (previously treated) basal cell carcinoma. Rowe DE, Carroll RJ, Day CL. J Dermatol Surg Oncol 1989; 15: 424–31.

Reports an almost 40% 5-year recurrence rate of recurrent tumors treated by C&D, emphasizing that this modality is not appropriate for recurrent tumors.

Extensive retrospective studies exist supporting the utility of this simple, rapid, and inexpensive method to treat BCC. However, prospective studies directly comparing C&D with other therapeutic modalities are lacking, and drawing conclusions from retrospective studies not controlled for size, histology, location, and history makes comparisons impossible.

Cryosurgery of basal cell carcinoma: a study of 358 patients. Bernardeau K, Derancourt C, Cambie M, Salmon-Ehr V, Morel M, Cavenelle F, et al. Ann Dermatol Venereol 2000; 127: 175–9.

A retrospective study of 395 BCCs in 358 patients reports a 5-year recurrence rate of 9%, which is in line with other reports, but that the use of a cryoprobe or other temperature-sensing device made no difference to outcome.

A systematic review of treatment modalities for primary basal cell carcinomas. Thissen MR, Neumann MH, Schouten LJ. Arch Dermatol 1999; 135: 1177–83.

Meta-analysis of published studies evaluating therapeutic methods for treating BCC. Inclusion criteria were prospective studies of at least 50 patients with primary BCC and at least 5 years' follow-up. Four studies of cryosurgery filled these criteria, with recurrence rates ranging from 0% to 20.4%.

Several large retrospective reports indicate a greater than 95% cure rate with cryotherapy. The authors of such series generally recommend two freeze–thaw cycles to maximize cell death and the use of a cryoprobe to assess tissue temperature achieved: −50°C is generally regarded as sufficiently cytotoxic.

Surgical margins for basal cell carcinoma. Wolf DJ, Zitelli JA. Arch Dermatol 1987; 123: 340–4.

Detailed histologic examination after excision with various margins revealed that for BCC <1 cm in diameter in low-risk areas, a surgical margin of 4 mm of normal-appearing skin around the tumor gave a 98% histologic cure rate.

Morpheaform basal-cell epitheliomas: a study of subclinical extensions in a series of 51 cases. Salasche SJ, Amonette RA. J Dermatol Surg Oncol 1981; 7: 387–94.

The average subclinical extension of morpheaform BCC is 7 mm, so a 4-mm margin would be inadequate.

Use the 4-mm margin for primary nodular BCC <1 cm in diameter. Larger tumors, diffuse growth pattern tumors, and recurrent tumors require larger margins or intraoperative histologic control.

Efficacy of curettage before excision in clearing surgical margins of nonmelanoma skin cancer. Chiller K, Passaro D, McCalmont T, Vin-Christian K. Arch Dermatol 2000; 136: 1327–32.

Preoperative curettage to better delineate surgical margins produced a statistically significant reduction in positive margins after surgical excision, suggesting the utility of curettage immediately before surgical excision.

Long-term recurrence rates in previously untreated (primary) basal cell carcinoma: implications for patient follow-up. Rowe DE, Carroll RJ, Day CL. J Dermatol Surg Oncol 1989; 15: 315–28.

Retrospective analysis of the literature since 1947 reports a weighted average 5-year recurrence rate of 1% when primary BCCs are treated using the Mohs technique.

Mohs surgery is the treatment of choice for recurrent (previously treated) basal cell carcinoma. Rowe DE, Carroll RJ, Day CL. J Dermatol Surg Oncol 1989; 15: 424–31.

Retrospective analysis of the literature since 1947 reports weighted average 5-year recurrence rate of 5.6% when recurrent BCCs are treated using the Mohs technique.

Both this and the previous study are retrospective rather than prospective, and thus direct comparison with other therapeutic modalities is difficult. However, it is most likely that the Mohs technique was used for higher-risk tumors, whereas simple methods such as C&D or cryosurgery are used for low-risk lesions, so the superior results utilizing the Mohs technique may be greater than these numbers would indicate.

Evidence Levels: A Double-blind study **B** Clinical trial ≥ 20 subjects **C** Clinical trial < 20 subjects **D** Series ≥ 5 subjects **E** Anecdotal case reports

Surgical excision versus Mohs micrographic surgery for basal cell carcinoma of the face: a randomized clinical trial with 10 year follow up. van Loo E, Mosterd K, Krekels GA, Roozeboom MH, Ostertag JU, Dirksen CD, et al. Eur J Cancer 2014; 50: 3011–20.

For many years, the evidence for the utility of Mohs surgery has consisted of retrospective case series. In a randomized prospective study 408 high-risk facial BCCs and 204 recurrent facial BCCs were submitted to conventional surgery or Mohs surgery. At 10-year follow-up, the recurrence rate for Mohs surgery was 4.4%, whereas for conventional surgery it was 12.2%. For recurrent facial BCC, Mohs surgery produced 3.9% recurrence rate versus 13.55% for conventional surgery. This study suggests Mohs surgery produced superior cure rates for both primary high-risk BCC and facial recurrent BCC.

Second-Line Therapy

• Radiation therapy	B

Basal cell carcinoma of the face: surgery or radiotherapy? Results of a randomized study. Avril MF, Auperin A, Margulis A, Gerbaulet A, Duvillard P, Benhamou E, et al. Br J Cancer 1997; 76: 100–6.

A randomized trial in which 347 primary BCCs <4 cm in size were assigned to surgical excision or radiotherapy (RT). The 4-year recurrence rate was 0.7% for surgical excision and 7.5% for RT. More significantly, cosmesis as judged by the patient and blinded judges was significantly better in the surgery group than in the RT group.

This is a significant result because RT is often recommended as an option for those patients who wish to avoid a scar.

Therapeutic ionizing radiation and the incidence of basal cell carcinoma and squamous cell carcinoma. The New Hampshire Skin Cancer Study Group. Lichter MD, Karagas MR, Mott LA, Spencer SK, Stukel TA, Greenberg ER. Arch Dermatol 2000; 136: 1007–11.

There is a statistically significant increased risk of the development of BCC in the exposure window after therapeutic RT. The development of subsequent tumors is a significant possible side effect.

Radiation therapy is an effective, albeit expensive and time-consuming, option for patients unable or unwilling to undergo surgery. Generally, 3000 to 5000 cGy are given in 6 to 20 fractionated doses, so therapy may take weeks. Cure rates have repeatedly been reported to be in excess of 90%. BCCs with perineural invasion have a very high local recurrence rate, and postoperative radiation is a wise precaution.

Third-Line Therapies

• Intralesional interferon	B
• Retinoids	D
• Topical imiquimod	A
• Photodynamic therapy	A
• Topical 5-fluorouracil	A
• CO$_2$ laser	D
• PEG–interleukin 2	D
• NSAIDs	D
• Ingenol mebutate	D
• Vismodegib	A
• Intralesional interleukin	D
• Systemic chemotherapy	D

Intralesional recombinant interferon beta-1a in the treatment of basal cell carcinoma: results of an open-label multicenter study. Kowalzick L, Rogozinski T, Wimheuer R, Pilz J, Manske U, Scholz A, et al. Eur J Dermatol 2002; 12: 558–61.

A total of 133 BCCs were treated with intralesional interferon-β_{1a}, 1 million units three times a week for 3 weeks. At 16 weeks' follow-up, 66.9% were clinically and biopsy clear. At 2-year follow-up, 4.5% of those that had cleared had recurred.

Alternative preparations of interferons have not been as successful as the α_{2a} preparation.

Treatment and prevention of basal cell carcinoma with oral isotretinoin. Peck GL, DiGiovanna JJ, Sarnoff DS, Gross EG, Butkus D, Olsen TG, et al. J Am Acad Dermatol 1988; 19: 176–85.

Twelve patients with multiple BCCs from varying causes were treated with high-dose oral isotretinoin (mean daily dosage 3.1 mg/kg/day) for a mean of 8 months. Of the 270 tumors monitored in these patients, only 8% underwent complete clinical and histologic regression.

Topical tretinoin treatment in basal cell carcinoma. Brenner S, Wolf R, Dascalu DI. J Dermatol Surg Oncol 1993; 19: 264–6.

Four lesions (single patient) were treated with 0.05% topical tretinoin twice a day for 3 weeks, followed by a 3-week rest, and a second treatment cycle. Short-term clinical and histologic evaluation showed initial clearance in all four lesions, but all four recurred within 9 months.

Topical treatment of basal cell carcinoma with tazarotene: a clinicopathological study on a large series of cases. Bianchi L, Orlandi A, Campione E, Angeloni C, Costanzo A, Spagnoli LG, et al. Br J Dermatol 2004; 151: 148–56.

A total of 154 small superficial and nodular BCCs were treated daily for 24 weeks with topical tazarotene. At the end of the treatment period, 70.8% of the lesions showed evidence of regression, but only 30.5% actually resolved clinically.

Retinoids, either systemically or topically, have not shown great efficacy in the treatment of BCC. However, retinoids definitely have an effective role in the chemoprevention of future BCCs in high-risk patients.

Imiquimod 5% cream for the treatment of superficial basal cell carcinoma: results from two phase III, randomized, vehicle-controlled studies. Geisse J, Caro I, Lindholm J, Golitz L, Stampone P, Owens M. J Am Acad Dermatol 2004; 50: 722–33.

This paper reports results of 724 subjects who applied the cream daily, 5 to 7 days a week for 6 weeks. Twelve weeks after the treatment period, the area of the tumor was excised and examined histologically. The excised area was tumor free in 82% of the five times a week group and 79% of the seven times a week group.

Open study of the efficacy and mechanism of action of topical imiquimod in basal cell carcinoma. Vidal D, Matias-Guiu X, Alomar A. Clin Exp Dermatol 2004; 29: 518–25.

Fifty-five BCCs measuring more than 8 mm in diameter with superficial, nodular, or infiltrative histologic growth patterns were treated daily, either three times a week for 8 weeks or five times a week for 5 weeks. Punch biopsies were taken 6 weeks after therapy, and patients were followed clinically for 2 years: 4/4 (100%) superficial BCCs, 7/8 (88%) nodular BCCs, and 30/43 (70%) infiltrating BCCs were tumor free after therapy.

This product upregulates interferons α and γ, and interleukin 12, among other cytokines. It seems to be reasonably effective for superficial BCCs, but less so for other histologic growth patterns.

Photodynamic therapy for the treatment of basal cell carcinoma. Wilson BD, Mang TS, Stoll H, Jones C, Cooper M, Dougherty TJ. Arch Dermatol 1992; 128: 1597–601.

A total of 151 BCCs in 37 patients were treated with Photofrin, a systemic photosensitizer that preferentially accumulates in tumors, followed by exposure to 630 nm laser light. Overall, complete response rate by clinical observation at 3 months was 88%.

These authors noted that failures tended to be in high-risk areas such as the nose and high-risk histologic variants (morpheaform). Photofrin is a systemic photosensitizer, and some degree of cutaneous and ocular photosensitivity may last up to 4 to 6 weeks. A variety of other systemic photosensitizers are currently under investigation.

Photodynamic therapy of multiple nonmelanoma skin cancers with verteporfin and red light-emitting diodes: two year results evaluating tumor response and cosmetic outcomes. Lui H, Hobbs L, Tope WD, Lee PK, Elmets C, Provost N, et al. Arch Dermatol 2004; 140: 26–32.

Fifty-four patients with 421 nonmelanoma skin cancers, including superficial BCC, nodular BCC, and SCC in situ, were treated with intravenous verteporfin followed by varying doses of red light. Treated areas were biopsied 6 months after treatment, and patients were followed clinically for 2 years. At the highest light dose, 93% of treated tumors were clear on biopsy, and 95% were clinically clear at 2-year follow-up.

Like Photofrin, verteporfin is an intravenous medication but has the advantage that patients are photosensitive for only 3 to 5 days.

Five year follow-up of a randomized prospective trial of topical methyl aminolevulinate photodynamic therapy vs. surgery for nodular basal cell carcinoma. Rhodes LE, de Rie MA, Leifsdottir R, Yu RC, Bachmann I, Goulden V, et al. Arch Dermatol 2007; 143: 1131–6.

Fifty-three nodular BCCs were treated with two to four sessions of mALA photodynamic therapy (PDT), and 52 nodular BCCs were treated by surgical excision. At 5-year follow-up there was a 14% recurrence rate in the PDT group versus 4% in the surgical excision group. However, the cosmetic outcome was rated higher in the PDT group than in the excision group.

Multiple sessions with topical mALA give a lower cure rate but a better cosmetic outcome than surgical excision.

Topical PDT with δ-aminolevulinic acid (ALA) and its methylated derivative (mALA) has become more popular and is commonly used in Europe. Surgical excision remains the gold standard to which other therapies must be compared. Comparison of different therapeutic modalities has been hard because few randomized prospective comparative trials have been performed. One such trial with 5-year follow-up has been completed comparing PDT with mALA to conventional surgical excision.

Treatment of basal cell carcinoma of the skin with 5-fluorouracil ointment. A 10 year follow-up study. Reymann F. Dermatologica 1979; 158: 368–72.

Ninety-five BCCs were treated with 5% 5-FU ointment. At 10-year follow-up there was a 21.4% recurrence rate.

Fluorouracil paste treatment of thin basal cell carcinomas. Epstein E. Arch Dermatol 1985; 121: 207–13.

Forty-four thin BCCs were treated with 25% 5-FU in petrolatum under occlusion for 3 weeks with weekly dressing changes. The 5-year recurrence rate was 21%.

These older papers suggested that topical 5-FU is not a good option for BCC. However, two more recent papers suggest this area may deserve a second look.

5% 5-fluorouracil cream for the treatment of small superficial basal cell carcinoma: efficacy, tolerability, cosmetic outcome, and patient satisfaction. Gross K, Kircik L, Kricorian G. Dermatol Surg 2007; 33: 433–9.

Thirty-one superficial BCCs were treated with 5% 5-FU BID for up to 12 weeks. Three weeks after stopping therapy the area of the tumor was excised, which revealed 90% of the treated lesions to be tumor free; 10% had residual tumor.

Can the carbon dioxide laser completely ablate basal cell carcinomas? A histologic study. Horlock N, Grobbelaar AO, Gault DT. Br J Plastic Surg 2000; 53: 286–93.

Use of the continuous-wave CO_2 laser to destroy BCCs was examined by postlaser excision and histologic check. Superficial BCCs of the trunk could be reliably ablated, but nodular and infiltrating (a diffuse growth pattern) could not reliably be treated by this method.

Effect of perilesional injections of PEG–interleukin-2 from one dose a week to four doses a week. Kaplan B, Moy RL. Dermatol Surg 2000; 26: 1037–40.

Intralesional injection of interleukin-2 (3000–120,000 IU in one to four weekly doses) in varying doses from one dose a week to four doses a week was given to eight patients with 12 BCCs. A complete response was seen in 8 of the 12 (66%) tumors.

PEP005 (ingenol mebutate) gel for the topical treatment of superficial basal cell carcinoma: results of a randomized phase IIa trial. Siller G, Rosen R, Freeman M, Welburn P, Katsamas J, Ogbourne SM. Australas J Dermatol 2010; 51: 99–105.

Application of 0.05% ingenol mebutate gel on days 1 and 2 resulted in the highest clearance both clinically and histologically. This study was designed to examine the safety and efficacy of topic ingenol mebutate. They report a favorable safety profile and 71% tumor clearance rate. Further studies are needed for optimal dosage to treat superficial BCC.

The pulsed dye laser for the treatment of basal cell carcinoma. Ballard CJ, Rivas MP, McLeod MP, Choudhary S, Elgart GW, Nouri K. Lasers Med Sci 2011; 26: 641–4.

Nine biopsy-proven BCCs, were treated with the PDL (585-nm wavelength, a single 450-μs pulse, 7-mm spot size, and 9.0 J/cm(2) energy) with a 4-mm border of normal skin were treated. A deep shave biopsy with histological examination occurred 4 weeks after the laser treatment. On histology, 5/9 (55.6%) sites demonstrated no evidence of BCC; however, 4/9 (44.4%) sites showed residual BCC

Pulsed dye laser as a novel non-surgical treatment for basal cell carcinomas: response and follow up 12–21 months after treatment. Konnikov N, Avram M, Jarell A, Tannous Z. Lasers Surg Med 2011; 43: 72–8.

Fourteen patients with 20 biopsy-proven BCCs on the trunk and extremities (8–35 mm in diameter) were treated with four consecutive PDL treatments at 3–4 week intervals. A 4-mm margin of clinically normal skin was also treated. Complete clinical response was seen with 19 of 20 treated BCCs, regardless of size and histologic subtype. All remaining 19 BCCs were followed between 12 and 21 months (median = 18 months) after the last PDL treatment. Of these 19 BCCs, only one recurred at 17 months follow up. The remaining 18 BCCs did not show any clinical signs of residual or recurrent tumor at 12–21 months follow-up.

Pulsed dye laser has emerged as a potential treatment for BCC. Treatment is not standardized, but most trials have utilized four

treatments at high fluence. Success rates in case series range from 90% to 65% clear for low-risk tumors with short follow-up generally under 2 years.

Hedgehog pathway inhibitor therapy for locally advanced and metastatic basal cell carcinoma: a systematic review and pooled analysis of interventional studies. Jacobsen AA, Aldahan AS, Hughes OB, Shah VV, Strasswimmer J. JAMA Dermatol 2016; 152: 816–24.

A review of 8 pooled articles included 744 total patients with 704 patients clinically evaluable. Sonidegib did not yield enough publications for a formal analysis. Objective response to vismodegib for locally advanced BCC had a weighted average of 64.7%; complete response averaged 31.1%. Objective response for metastatic BCC was 33.6% complete response averaged 3.9% Median duration of therapy was 35.8 weeks. Vismodegib was identified to have a significant, consistent effect on the median duration of therapy of locally advanced and metastatic BCC. While metastatic BCC responses are superior to any traditional approach, the response rate for laBCC might be considered in the context of other standard treatment options including surgery and radiation therapy.

A phase II, randomized, double-blind study of sonidegib in patients with advanced basal cell carcinoma. Dummer R, Guminski A, Gutzmer R, Dirix L, Lewis KD, Combemale P, et al. J Am Acad Dermatol 2016; 75: 113–25.

Mutations in the sonic hedgehog pathway have been shown to occur in 90% of BCCs. Essential to this pathway is the protein smoothened, and two inhibitors of this protein are now available. The first and best studied is vismodegib. In a meta-analysis of eight studies, pooled data showed locally advanced BCC had a 64.7% objective partial response, whereas 31.3% were completely clear. For metastatic BCC, there was a 33.6% objective partial response and a 3.9% complete clearance rate.

Sonidegib has less evidence for analysis. One paper examined two different doses in locally advanced and metastatic BCC. A dose of 200 mg was given to 79 patients with locally advanced and 13 with metastatic BCC. At this dose for locally advanced BCC, the objective partial response rate was 57.6% and the complete clearance rate was 4.5%. For metastatic BCC, there was a 7.7% objective partial response. At a dose of 800 mg per day, locally advanced BCC showed a 43.8% objective partial response and a 1.6% complete clearance rate. For metastatic BCC there was a 17.4% objective partial response rate.

Becker nevus

Michael P. Loosemore, Adisbeth Morales-Burgos, Elnaz F. Firoz, Bahar F. Firoz, Leonard H. Goldberg

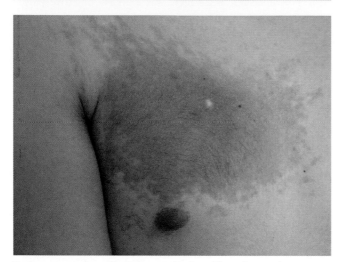

Becker nevus, also called *pigmented hairy epidermal nevus*, is a cutaneous hamartoma that may have increased epidermal (melanocyte), dermal (smooth muscle), and appendageal (hair follicle) components. Classically, Becker nevus is first noticed around puberty on the shoulders and chest in males, but may be congenital, involve any area of the body, and occur in women. The prevalence in postpubertal males is approximated to be 0.5%, or 1 in 200.

MANAGEMENT STRATEGY

Becker nevus is usually asymptomatic and may come to the attention of a physician for cosmetic or diagnostic purposes. It is important to examine the patient for developmental abnormalities that may accompany Becker nevus and occur within the spectrum of *Becker nevus syndrome,* one of several epidermal nevus syndromes. Reported associations include:

- Cutaneous
  - Acneiform eruptions
  - Hypohidrosis
  - Lichen planus
  - Localized lipoatrophy
  - Localized scleroderma
  - Polythelia (supernumerary nipples)
  - Psoriasiform dermatitis
  - Unilateral breast hypoplasia
  - Osteoma cutis
- Musculoskeletal
  - Limb asymmetry
  - Pectus excavatum or carinatum
  - Scoliosis, including other vertebral defects

Associations of Becker nevus with cutaneous malignancies have been reported. Both basal cell carcinoma and intraepithelial squamous cell carcinoma (Bowen disease) have been described separately in two young women without significant risk factors (i.e., photodamage, papillomavirus infection, arsenic exposure). Although melanoma has been described in patients with Becker nevus, the risk of malignant transformation of the nevus itself appears to be very low. Enhanced screening for melanoma is likely unnecessary.

Traditional *surgical* approaches to remove Becker nevus are either unsuccessful or result in significant scarring. *Laser* technology offers the clinician a means to reduce both the pigmentation and the hypertrichosis often seen in Becker nevus, and therefore may improve the cosmetic appearance of the lesion. Management of asymptomatic benign lesions should comprise diagnosis confirmation and fully evaluating for any associated pathology.

Becker's nevus syndrome revisited. Danarti R, König A, Salhi A, Bittar M, Happle R. J Am Acad Dermatol 2004; 51: 965–9.

A review of ipsilateral breast hypoplasia, other cutaneous anomalies, musculoskeletal abnormalities, and maxillofacial findings that may be observed in Becker nevus syndrome. The concept of paradominant inheritance is presented to explain occasional familial aggregation in this syndrome.

Becker nevus syndrome. Happle R, Koopman RJ. Am J Med Genet 1997; 68: 357–61.

Proposes term *Becker nevus syndrome* to describe association of Becker nevus with developmental defects such as unilateral breast hypoplasia and other cutaneous, muscular, or skeletal defects in 23 cases.

Becker's nevus and malignant melanoma. Fehr B, Panizzon RG, Schnyder UW. Dermatologica 1991; 182: 77–80.

Report of nine patients with Becker nevus and malignant melanoma. Five melanomas were on the same body site as the Becker nevus, but only one arose within the nevus itself.

A case of Becker's nevus with osteoma cutis. Park SB, Song BH, Park EJ, Kwon IH, Kim KH, Kim KJ. Ann Dermatol 2011; 23 (Suppl 2): S247–9.

An 18-year-old female was reported to have osteoma cutis accompanying her Becker nevus.

Specific Investigations

- The diagnosis of Becker nevus can be made on clinical examination. Although skin biopsy is diagnostic, it is often unnecessary. Familial Becker nevus has been regularly reported, so it is prudent to inquire about other family members, especially same-sex siblings.
- In some instances, differentiating between large congenital melanocytic nevus and Becker nevus may be difficult. Dermoscopy may help in equivocal cases. Reticulated pigment network, focal hypopigmentation, furrow hypopigmentation, hair follicles, perifollicular hypopigmentation, and vessels are the main dermoscopic features of Becker nevus.

Familial Becker's nevus. Fretzin DF, Whitney D. J Am Acad Dermatol 1985; 12: 589–90.

The first two published cases of familial Becker nevus.

Dermoscopic features of congenital melanocytic nevus and Becker nevus in an adult male population: an analysis with a 10-fold magnification. Ingordo V, Iannazzone SS, Cusano F, Naldi L. Dermatology 2006; 212: 354–60.

Assessed the use of optical dermoscopy with 10-fold magnification in differentiating between large congenital melanocytic nevus and Becker nevus.

First-Line Therapies

Treatment requested by patients can be divided into two components:
- Reduction of hyperpigmentation
- Removal of excess hair

Reduction of hyperpigmentation

• Erbium:YAG laser	C
• Long-pulse alexandrite laser	D
• Erbium-doped fiber laser (Fraxel)	D
• Q-switched ruby laser (QSRL)	D

Becker's naevus: a comparative study between erbium:YAG and Q-switched neodymium:YAG; clinical and histopathological findings. Trelles MA, Allones I, Moreno-Arias GA, Vélez M. Br J Dermatol 2005; 152: 308–13.

Twenty-two patients with Becker nevi were studied, 11 with each laser. Both erbium:YAG and Nd:YAG safely treated the lesions. For pigment removal, one pass with erbium:YAG was superior to three treatment sessions with Nd:YAG.

Treatment of Becker's nevi with a long-pulse alexandrite laser. Choi JE, Kim JW, Seo SH, Son SW, Ahn HH, Kye YC. Dermatol Surg 2009; 35: 1105–8.

Eleven Korean patients with Becker nevi and skin types III to V were treated with the 755-nm long-pulse alexandrite laser with a spot size of 15 to 18 mm, fluence of 20 to 25 J/cm^2, a pulse duration of 3 ms, and no cooling spray. Two patients had an excellent response, five good, and four a fair response. There was one case of partial hypertrophic scarring, and some patients had mild hypopigmentation; all outcomes were noted to be cosmetically acceptable.

Fractional resurfacing: a new therapeutic modality for Becker's nevus. Glaich AS, Goldberg LH, Dai T, Kunishige JH, Friedman PM. Arch Dermatol 2007; 143: 1488–90.

Two male patients with Becker nevi were treated with the 1550-nm wavelength erbium-doped fiber laser between 6 and 10 mJ at 4-week intervals and between five and six treatment sessions. Greater than 75% of the pigment had faded by 1 month in both patients. There was no improvement in hypertrichosis.

Q-switched ruby laser treatment of tattoos and benign pigmented skin lesions: a critical review. Raulin C, Schönermark MP, Greve B, Werner S. Ann Plast Surg 1998; 41: 555–65.

This review recommends 3 to 10 treatments at monthly intervals with Q-switched ruby laser at fluences between 7 and 20 J/cm^2 for hyperpigmentation. Although Q-switched ruby laser for long-term removal of associated hypertrichosis is not recommended, long-pulsed (755 nm) alexandrite laser has produced promising results.

The removal of cutaneous pigmented lesions with the Q-switched ruby laser and the Q-switched neodymium:yttrium-aluminum-garnet laser. A comparative study. Tse Y, Levine VJ, McClain SA, Ashinoff R. J Dermatol Surg Oncol 1994; 20: 795–800.

An area of Becker nevus was anesthetized and bisected, and each half treated with either Q-switched ruby laser or Q-switched (QS) Nd:YAG at 532 nm. Clinical lightening occurred in 63% and 43% of the lesion, respectively, at fluences of 8.4 and 2.8 J/cm^2. Q-switched ruby laser caused intraoperative pain, whereas QSNd:YAG caused postoperative discomfort.

Formation of fibrosis after nonablative and ablative fractional laser therapy. Wind BS, Meesters AA, Kroon MW, Beek JF, van der Veen JP, van der Wal AC, et al. Dermatol Surg 2012; 38: 437–42.

Eighteen patients with pigment disorders were randomized to either a nonablative 1550-nm fractional laser at 15 mJ/microbeam with 14% to 20% coverage (patients with erythema dyschromicum perstans and postinflammatory hyperpigmentation) or an ablative 10,600-nm fractional laser at 10 mJ/microbeam with 35% to 35% coverage (Becker nevi) and treated for three to five sessions. Biopsies were performed 3 months after the last treatment to assess fibrosis formation. Patients treated with nonablative fractional laser did not exhibit any fibrosis, whereas 50% of patients treated using ablative fractional laser showed fibrosis.

The ruby laser in the normal or long-pulsed mode has been

Reduction of hypertrichosis

• Normal mode ruby laser	D

used for laser epilation. A common side effect is hypopigmentation of adjacent skin, which can be used when treating hypertrichosis of a Becker nevus. Low-fluence hair removal has been reported to be effective as well, perhaps with fewer side effects.

Treatment of a Becker's nevus using a 694-nm long-pulsed ruby laser. Nanni CA, Alster TS. Dermatol Surg 1998; 24: 1032–4.

A single case report that showed reduction in pigmentation and a 90% reduction in hair growth after three treatments with the long-pulsed ruby laser. Improvement was maintained for 10 months.

Hypertrichosis in Becker's nevus: effective low-fluence hair removal. Lapidoth M, Adatto M, Cohen S, Ben-Amitai D, Halachmi S. Lasers Med Sci 2014; 29: 191–3.

Fifteen patients treated with low-fluence, 808- to 810-nm diode laser had decreased hair growth at 6 and 12 months, without adverse effects.

Second-Line Therapy

Reduction of hyperpigmentation

• Frequency-doubled QSNd:YAG	D

The Q-switched Nd:YAG laser operating at 532 nm has been shown to reduce pigmentation in Becker nevus, but does not

Reduction of excess hair

• Electrolysis	E

appear to be as successful as the ruby laser.

Electrolysis is a well-established method of epilation, but its use in removing hair from Becker nevus has not been described.

Third-Line Therapies

- Spironolactone   E
- Corrective camouflage   E

Congenital linear Becker's nevus, with underlying breast hypoplasia that spontaneously corrected during pregnancy: role of androgen receptors. Felton SJ, Al-Niaimi F, Thornton J, Lyon CC. J Clin Trials 2012; 2: 125.

The authors report a patient with congenital linear Becker nevus and breast hypoplasia. The Becker nevus was confirmed to have increased androgen receptors, and the breast hypoplasia improved when the patient became pregnant.

Becker's nevus with ipsilateral breast hypoplasia: improvement with spironolactone. Hoon Jung J, Chan Kim Y, Joon Park H, Woo Cinn Y. J Dermatol 2003; 30: 154–6.

The androgen receptor plays an important role in Becker nevus pathology, especially breast hypoplasia. This has been reported both to resolve during pregnancy and to improve with spironolactone treatment. Spironolactone, an antiandrogenic agent, was administered for the treatment of breast hypoplasia associated with Becker nevus in one case. After 1 month, breast enlargement was observed only in the hypoplastic breast.

Becker nevus is thought to be an androgen-dependent lesion, as it becomes more prominent after puberty, displays increased hairiness in males, and contains an increased number of androgen receptors and androgen-receptor messenger RNA compared with surrounding skin.

Corrective camouflage in pediatric dermatology. Tedeschi A, Dall'Oglio F, Micali G, Schwartz RA, Janniger CK. Cutis 2007; 79: 110–2.

Corrective camouflage using a variety of water-resistant and light to very opaque products was used in two patients with Becker nevi. Parents were satisfied with the cosmetic cover results. Corrective makeup may be a valid adjunctive therapy for patients undergoing long-term treatments or in whom conventional therapy is ineffective.

Evidence Levels: **A** Double-blind study **B** Clinical trial ≥ 20 subjects **C** Clinical trial < 20 subjects **D** Series ≥ 5 subjects **E** Anecdotal case reports

Bed bugs

25

Whitney A. High, Glen R. Needham

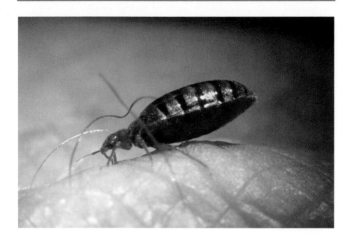

Human bed bugs (*Cimex lectularius*) are insects that require a blood meal to complete their life cycle, which is acquired by biting sleeping humans. The bite can elicit an allergic reaction, creating pruritic, erythematous papules that are often excoriated and even secondarily infected.

MANAGEMENT STRATEGY

Bed bug infestations have become more common with the eventual resistance and subsequent banning of the use of dichlorodiphenyltrichloroethane (DDT).

Most bed bugs bite just before dawn, lying in close proximity to the sleeping quarters. Although the bite of a bed bug is painless, an allergic reaction may ensue in some individuals, resulting in a skin lesion. Bed bug bites tends to occur on exposed surfaces, such as the extremities or head/neck. The insect will not typically venture beneath bedding or bed clothes. A linear arrangement to the bites is common.

The insect does not reside or lay eggs upon humans, and hence, treatment focuses upon *detection and eradication of the household infestation. Insecticides, growth-regulating agents, and destructive modalities* may be employed to kill adults, progeny, and eggs. Many authorities believe that safe and successful eradication requires professional assistance.

Use of insecticides in the United States is regulated by the Environmental Protection Agency. The extended residual effect of DDT resulted in environmental damage; ultimately its use was banned. Resistance, first to DDT, and later to malathion, may be an issue with its reemergence as a scourge. More recently, pyrethroids (e.g., deltamethrin) have been utilized in controlling bed bug infestations, but again, resistance has emerged.

There is great interest in the use of temperature extremes to eradicate infestations. *Steam* may be utilized to sterilize a mattress or similar materials for which insecticides are inappropriate, but a target temperature of 160°F to 180°F must be reached over the entirety of the surface.

Commercial *whole room/whole home heating*, using propane heaters and fans to develop convective cycles, exist. Most of these

systems achieve a target temperature of around 113°F, held for 15 to 60 minutes. Although this temperature is less than the thermal death point of bed bugs (118°F), such treatments are often successful, presumably due to powerful convection currents that desiccate the insects. Other comparatively simplistic measures, such as impermeable mattress covers, are also widely employed.

The manipulation of insect pheromones is gaining interest, as bed bugs use pheromones to aggregate for mating and to increase local humidity and avoid desiccation. Ergot blocking of this pheromone signaling, which may have disastrous effects upon a bed bug colony.

Treatment of bed bug bites among humans is directed at symptoms. Skin lesions are due to an allergic reaction to the saliva leaked during feeding. Sensitization is not universal, and some individuals will not react.

Symptomatic bed bug bites often produce an erythematous wheal, followed by a firm, reddish papule, sometimes with a small central hemorrhagic punctum. Papulonecrotic and bullous forms have been described. Bites are often pruritic and are usually present on surfaces exposed during sleep, such as the head, neck, arms, legs, and shoulders. Bites are treated in a symptomatic fashion, with *potent topical steroids* and *antihistamines.*

The position of the U.S. Centers for Disease Control and Prevention (CDC), and the bulk of other experts, is that, as of yet, there is no clear evidence of successful transmission of a bloodborne pathogen via bed bug bites. Additional laboratory testing beyond bacterial culture of superinfected bites is not recommended.

A widely recognized contributing factor to the "epidemic" of bed bugs is travel. Hotels and other shared lodging facilities, regardless of cleanliness or cost, may be infested, and it is possible to bring an infestation home after a stay in infested lodgings.

An inspection of lodging facilities upon check-in is important. Luggage should be kept closed, or even sealed in plastic bags, to then be left at the destination upon departing. Use of dressers and bureaus at a hotel is discouraged. Metal luggage stands are preferable to wooden ones.

The re-emergence of the bed bug as a nuisance pest: implications of resistance to the pyrethroid insecticides. Davies TG, Field LM, Williamson MS. Med Vet Entomol 2012; 26: 241–54.

Resistance of bed bugs to insecticides is contributing to its resurgence as a pest. Reports of increasing resistance to pyrethroids exist throughout the world. The authors of this review report deltamethrin resistance in colonies obtained from more than 20 cities in the United States.

Insecticide resistance among bed bugs may be mediated by genetic mutations on target proteins, by overexpression of detoxifying enzymes, or by thickening of the insect cuticle, with reduced insecticide penetration. The existence of multiple pathways of resistance bodes ominously for ever-increasing problems with eradication of infestations.

Acute illnesses associated with insecticides used to control bed bugs – seven states, 2003–2010. Centers for Disease Control and Prevention (CDC), MMWR 2011; 60: 1269–74.

Although subject to concerns of overreporting or underreporting, the CDC recently detailed 111 illnesses over the span of 2003 to 2010, including one fatality, that were attributed to excessive and/or inappropriate use of insecticides for bed bugs. The authors encourage persons with bed bug infestations to seek the services of a certified exterminator; strict adherence is necessary with regard to product instructions and warnings.

Use of consumer-grade, indoor "foggers" or "bombs" for bed bugs is discouraged by experts because often they only scatter the bed bugs over a larger area. Silica gel or diatomaceous earth may be used as a less toxic (but also less effective) alternative that kills via dehydration. There is no effective "repellant" for bed bugs.

Identification of the airborne aggregation pheromone of the common bed bug, *Cimex lectularius*. Siljander E, Gries R, Khaskin G, Gries G. J Chem Ecol 2008; 34: 708–18.

Adult males, virgin adult females, and juvenile bed bugs respond to an airborne aggregation pheromone. The authors suggest that purposeful manipulation of this aggregation pheromone might be useful for control devices, such as traps.

Bed bugs reproduce via traumatic insemination, and females have structural adaptations to deal with this insult, whereas males have no such adaptations. Young males secrete pheromones to discourage other adult males from destructive same-sex copulation, and this represents another avenue of potential susceptibility.

Bedbugs as vectors for drug-resistant bacteria. Lowe CF, Romney MG. Emerg Infect Dis 2011; 17: 1132–4. https://dx.doi.org/10.3201/eid1706.101978.

A recent report from Canada demonstrated that bed bugs may be capable of transmitting methicillin-resistant *Staphylococcus aureus* within an impoverished community.

Bedbugs. Kolb A, Needham GR, Neyman KM, High WA. Dermatol Ther 2009; 22: 347–52.

In this review article the authors instruct that, upon returning home, immediate inspection of luggage and other belongings aids in the discovery of bed bugs or eggs in the midst of transport. Unpacking in the garage and/or vacuuming the exterior, or even the interior, of bags, with immediate disposal of the vacuum bag itself in a sealed plastic bag, may be of benefit in preventing undesired translocation.

Specific Investigations

- Visualization of the bed bug by inspection, traps, or trained dogs
- Skin biopsy

The eggs, adults, and nymphal stages of the organism may be visualized with the human eye. Therefore when bed bug bites are suspected clinically, an appropriate starting point in investigation is simply careful inspection of sleeping quarters. Other techniques to detect infestation include simple taping of bed legs with sticky tape, placing bed posts in isolating devices or traps (either homemade or purchased), or trained dogs.

Visual inspection

Visual inspections should begin around the bed area. Adult bed bugs are 5 to 7 mm in length and vary in color from light brown to dark brown or even violaceous if they have recently fed. Nymphs are smaller and are often clearer in appearance, again unless having fed. Eggs are about 1 mm long, ovoid with an operculum, and are sticky, adhering to surfaces in small aggregates.

In addition to simply detecting the organism, there should be a search for fecal smears or flecks of blood upon the bed linens and upon the edges of the mattress and box springs. Bed bugs, even adults, may fit within extraordinarily narrow cracks and crevices in furniture and walls, behind peeling wallpaper, and even behind switch plates. If a credit card can be inserted into a crevice, then it may also host bed bugs!

Lastly, when populations of bed bugs are particularly dense, a pungent but sweet odor, likened to coriander or cut cilantro, may permeate an infested room or even an entire house.

Canine inspection

Dogs have been successfully trained to detect the odor of bed bugs. The training protocol of the commercial kennels is proprietary, and the exact odor the dogs are detecting is unknown.

Bed bug traps

Bed bugs are attracted to humans via a combination of heat, carbon dioxide exhalation, and perhaps other detectable scents, such as human body volatiles, such as aldehydes and sulcatone.

Using this information, two commercial bed bug trapping devices have been marketed, and plans to build a homemade trap (using a cat feeding bowl, dry ice, and a Thermos vessel) have been widely published.

The principle in all these devices is to attract bugs coupled with a "pitfall area" into which the bed bugs fall and cannot escape, or sticky material that entraps the organisms.

Other monitoring devices

A recently marketed device (Climbup Interceptor) consists of two nested plastic bowls, one inside the other, into which the feet of the bed may be placed. Bugs migrating either into the bed or away from the bed are entrapped between the bowls. Along these same lines, inverted duct tape may be placed, sticky side out, upon the legs of the bed to entrap bed bugs as they migrate across it.

Effectiveness of bed bug monitors for detecting and trapping bed bugs in apartments. Wang C, Tsai WT, Cooper R, White J. J Econ Entomol 2011; 104: 274–8.

A comparison was made of several bed bug monitoring devices, including the CDC3000, NightWatch, and a homemade dry ice trap, and a passive monitor (the Climbup Interceptor), without attractants, was used for estimating the bed bug numbers before and after placing active monitors. In occupied apartments, the relative effectiveness of the active monitors was as follows: dry ice trap > CDC3000 > NightWatch. In lightly infested apartments, the Interceptor (operated for 7 days) trapped a similar number of bed bugs as the dry ice trap (operated for 1 day) and trapped more bed bugs than CDC3000 and NightWatch (operated for 1 day). The authors concluded that all the monitors were effective tools in detecting early bed bug infestations and evaluating the results of bed bug control programs.

Ability of bed bug-detecting canines to locate live bed bugs and viable bed bug eggs. Pfiester M, Koehler PG, Pereira RM. J Econ Entomol 2008; 101: 1389–96.

The authors examined dogs trained to locate bed bugs by smell. Under test conditions they were able to discriminate bed bugs from other insects with a 97.5% positive indication rate (correct indication of bed bugs when present) and with zero false positives (incorrect indication of bed bugs when not present). They were able to discriminate live bed bugs and viable bed bug eggs from dead bed bugs, cast skins, and feces, with a 95% positive indication rate and a 3% false-positive rate on bed bug feces. In experimentally contrived "hotel rooms," canines were 98% accurate in locating live bed bugs.

Skin biopsy

The histology of bed bug bites is nonspecific and similar to that of many other insect and arthropod assault reactions and includes a perivascular infiltrate of lymphocytes, histiocytes, eosinophils, and mast cells within the upper dermis, perhaps with dermal edema and/or extravasated erythrocytes.

Bullous reactions to bedbug bites reflect cutaneous vasculitis. deShazo RD, Feldlaufer MF, Mihm MC Jr, Goddard J. Am J Med 2012; 125: 688–94.

The authors examined "severe" cutaneous reactions, termed *bullous or complex reactions*, to bed bug bites and concluded the phenomenon is not rare. Of 357 photographs of bed bug bites posted on the Internet, 6% were bullous. Histopathologic evaluation of bullous reactions showed a polymorphous picture with histologic evidence of an urticarial-like reaction early on that rapidly developed into a hybrid leukocytoclastic vasculitis, similar to the dermal vasculitis in patients with Churg–Strauss disease.

First-Line Therapies

- Identify and eradicate the infestation   **A**
- Control symptoms associated with the bites using antihistamines, topical steroids, and in rare cases oral steroids   **E**

Toxicity and potential utility of ivermectin and moxidectin as xenointoxicants against the common bed bug, *Cimex lectularius.* Sheele JM, Ridge GE. Parasitol Res 2016; 115: 3071–81. http://dx.doi.org/10.1007/s00436-016-5062-x.

In a controlled laboratory experiment, laboratory-reared bed bugs were exposed to varying concentrations of ivermectin and moxidectin using a feeding apparatus. Exposure to ivermectin, more than moxidectin, resulted in long-term sequelae among the insects to include reduced fecundity, feeding difficulty, and incomplete molting, but this was not a clinical trial.

Although interest in a xenotoxicant approach persists, the authors speculated that if ivermectin were used in such a schema, it might require a daily dose of 0.2 mg/kg for a 20-day period, and the safety of such a regimen in humans is not yet well established.

Behçet disease

Samantha R. Pop, Maryam Liaqat, Justin J. Green

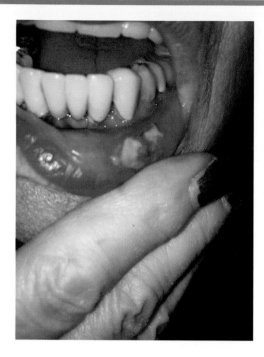

Behçet disease (BD) is a chronic inflammatory disorder leading to systemic vasculitis characterized by oral aphthae (at least three episodes in a 12-month period), plus two of the following: genital aphthae, cutaneous lesions (erythema nodosum, pustulosis, acneiform lesions, and pseudofolliculitis), uveitis or retinal vasculitis, or positive pathergy test. A strong correlation between BD and HLA-B51 is widely replicated in several studies. Arthritis, gastrointestinal, cardiac, and neurologic manifestations may also occur. Many regimens effective for recurrent aphthous stomatitis are used to treat the aphthae of BD (see chapter on aphthous stomatitis). Recently 32 different countries joined together to establish new international guidelines, and data from 2556 BD patients were used to create a new diagnostic scoring system. In 98% of the patients, oral aphthous ulcer was a feature.

MANAGEMENT STRATEGY

In the absence of multisystem disease, the severity and extent of the mucocutaneous manifestations direct the treatment strategy. First-line therapy for oral and genital aphthae is a *high-potency topical corticosteroid* in a gel or ointment formulation. Alternatively, *intralesional corticosteroids* (triamcinolone 5 mg/mL) can be used for major aphthae and severe minor aphthae. Other topical therapies accelerate healing or diminish the pain associated with oral aphthae. These include viscous *lidocaine* 2% to 5% applied directly to lesions, *amlexanox* 5% oral paste, *sucralfate, tetracycline suspension, topical pimecrolimus* cream, *and tacrolimus* 0.1% ointment.

Colchicine 0.6 mg three times daily combined with topical corticosteroid therapy is efficacious in mucocutaneous disease. *Dapsone* 100 to 200 mg daily is also effective, but requires more frequent laboratory follow-up. The newer agent, *apremilast* 30 mg twice a day, for oral lesions has been noted to be beneficial in reducing mean numbers of ulcers and associated pain.

Those patients who fail the more conservative approaches or have severe mucocutaneous disease may require aggressive therapy. *Thalidomide* 100 to 300 mg daily (pediatric dose varies from 1 mg/kg/week to 1 mg/kg daily) is more effective than low-dose *methotrexate* 7.5 to 20 mg/week for severe disease. *Prednisone* taper begun at 1 mg/kg daily can be used for severe mucocutaneous flares, but rebound is a possible complication.

Systemic *interferon (IFN)*-α_{2a} and *anti–tumor necrosis factor (TNF)*-α therapies may be best suited for those with severe mucocutaneous lesions and nonocular systemic manifestations. *Etanercept* 50 mg weekly by subcutaneous injection or *infliximab* 5 mg/kg in single or multiple intravenous infusions has been shown to be effective in patients with recalcitrant disease and may be used as monotherapy or as an adjunct to conventional immunosuppressive therapy. Notably, *infliximab* has demonstrated rapid therapeutic effect, which may be useful in patients with vision-threatening posterior uveitis. These patients should be screened for latent tuberculosis infection before initiating anti-TNF therapies. Patients with certain extracutaneous signs (e.g., uveitis, aneurysms) may warrant combination therapy with *prednisone* and an immunosuppressive agent such as *ciclosporin, azathioprine, chlorambucil,* or *cyclophosphamide.* Mucocutaneous disease alone rarely warrants this therapy; however, these agents have a beneficial effect on skin and mucous membrane lesions.

Specific Investigations

- Pathergy test optional
- Culture/polymerase chain reaction of aphthae to exclude herpes simplex virus
- Vitamins B_1, B_2, B_6, and B_{12}; folate, zinc, and iron levels
- Urinalysis
- HLA-B51
- Exclude inflammatory bowel disease

Behçet's syndrome: immunopathological and histopathological assessment of pathergy lesions is useful in diagnosis and follow-up. Jorizzo JL, Soloman AR, Cavallo T. Arch Pathol Lab Med 1985; 109: 747–51.

This method of pathergy testing may be more sensitive than standard techniques devoid of histologic study.

Behçet's disease and complex aphthosis. Ghate JV, Jorizzo JL. J Am Acad Dermatol 1999; 40: 1–18.

A review of investigations that should be carried out in a patient with complex aphthosis is presented.

Herpes simplex virus, nutritional deficiencies, neutropenia, lymphopenia, reactive arthritis, and inflammatory bowel disease may simulate the oral aphthae of BD.

Evaluation of current therapeutic strategies in Behçet's disease. Alexoudi I, Kapsimali V, Vaiopoulos A, Kanakis M, Vaiopoulos G. Clin Rheumatol 2011; 30: 157–63.

An excellent review and guide to treatment of all aspects of BD.

Interventions for the management of oral ulcers in Behçet's disease. Taylor J, Glenny AM, Walsh T, Brocklehurst P, Riley P, Gorodkin R, et al. Cochrane Database Syst Rev 2014; 9: CD011018.

In this review, 15 trials (n = 888 randomized participants) were included, 13 were placebo controlled, and 3 were head to head (2 trials had more than two treatment arms). According to the authors, due to the heterogeneity of trials, including trial design, choice of intervention, and choice and timing of outcome measures, it was not possible to carry out a meta-analysis.

Evidence Levels: **A** Double-blind study **B** Clinical trial ≥ 20 subjects **C** Clinical trial < 20 subjects **D** Series ≥ 5 subjects **E** Anecdotal case reports

First-Line Therapies

• Topical/intralesional corticosteroid	B
• Tacrolimus ointment	A
• Pimecrolimus cream	A
• Amlexanox 5% paste	A
• Sucralfate	A
• Tetracycline suspension	D
• Chlorhexidine gluconate	D
• Colchicine	A
• Zinc sulfate	A

Management of Behçet's disease: a systematic literature review for the European League Against Rheumatism evidence-based recommendations for the management of Behçet's disease. Hatemi G, Silman A, Bang D, Bodaghi B, Chamberlian AM, Gul A, et al. Ann Rheum Dis 2009; 68: 1528–34.

In this systematic literature review from 1966 to 2006, systemic medications for BD were analyzed for treating different aspects of the disease.

The use of sucralfate suspension in the treatment of oral and genital ulceration of Behçet disease: a randomized, placebo-controlled, double-blind study. Alpsoy E, Er H, Durusoy C, Yilmaz E. Arch Dermatol 1999; 135: 529–32.

In this study, 40 patients with BD were included in this randomized, double-blind study, which compared 5 mL sucralfate suspension with placebo suspension used as an oral rinse for 1 to 2 minutes after routine oral care and before bed. Results showed sucralfate significantly decreased the mean frequency, healing time, and pain of oral ulcers in comparison with baseline.

A double-blind trial of colchicine in Behçet's syndrome. Yurdakul S, Mat C, Tuzun Y, Ozyazgan Y, Hamuryudan V, Uysal O, et al. Arthritis Rheum 2001; 44: 2686–92.

A prospective, double-blind, controlled trial of 116 patients treated with colchicine vs. placebo. Therapy with colchicine 1 to 2 mg daily was effective for arthritis and erythema nodosum. Orogenital aphthae were more responsive to treatment in females.

Oral zinc sulfate in the treatment of Behçet's disease: a double blind cross-over study. Sharquie KE, Najim RA, Al-Dori WS, Al-Hayani RK. J Dermatol 2006; 33: 541–6.

In a prospective, randomized, double-blind, controlled trial, 27 patients with mucocutaneous and/or joint disease and 30 healthy subjects matched for age and gender were treated with zinc sulfate vs. placebo. Zinc sulfate 100 mg three times daily was found to be effective in reducing disease severity, and no adverse effects were reported.

Patients with ocular, neurologic, cardiac, or other systemic manifestations were excluded.

Pimecrolimus versus placebo in genital aphthous ulcers of Behçet's disease: a randomized double-blind controlled trial. Chams-Davatchi C, Barikbin B, Shahram F, Nadji A, Moghaddassi M, Yousefi M, et al. Int J Rheum Dis 2010; 13: 253–8.

This was a randomized, double-blind controlled trial of twice-daily topical pimecrolimus versus placebo in genital aphthous ulcers in patients with BD. There was a significant decrease in healing time with pimecrolimus and slight improvement of pain.

Second-Line Therapies

• Dapsone	A
• Thalidomide	A
• Methotrexate	E
• Systemic corticosteroid	B

Dapsone in Behçet's disease: a double-blind, placebo-controlled, cross-over study. Sharquie KE, Najim RA, Abu-Raghif AR. J Dermatol 2002; 29: 267–79.

Randomized, double-blind, placebo-controlled, crossover trial of 20 patients treated with either dapsone 100 mg daily or placebo. There was a significant reduction of orogenital ulcers and other cutaneous manifestations in the dapsone group.

Vitamin E 800 IU daily may reduce the hemolysis induced by dapsone. Other studies have confirmed the utility of dapsone for mucocutaneous BD.

Thalidomide in the treatment of the mucocutaneous lesions of Behçet syndrome: a randomized, double-blind, placebo-controlled trial. Hamuryudan V, Mat C, Saip S, Ozyazgan Y, Siva A, Yurdakul S, et al. Ann Intern Med 1998; 128: 443–50.

A randomized, double-blind, controlled trial of 96 males evaluated thalidomide 100 mg daily vs. 300 mg daily vs. placebo for 24 weeks. Both thalidomide dosages led to a significant suppression of oral ulcers at 4 weeks, and genital ulcers and follicular lesions at 8 weeks. Complete responses were observed in 11% of patients treated with thalidomide.

Low-dose weekly methotrexate for unusual neutrophilic vascular reactions: cutaneous polyarteritis nodosa and Behçet's disease. Jorizzo JL, White WL, Wise CM, Zanolli MD, Sherertz EF. J Am Acad Dermatol 1991; 24: 973–8.

Two female patients with oral and genital aphthae, pyoderma gangrenosum-like lesions, and cutaneous pustular vasculitic lesions cleared with methotrexate 15 to 20 mg/week.

Practical treatment recommendations for pharmacotherapy of Behçet's syndrome. Yazici H, Barnes CG, Drugs 1991; 42: 796–804.

Intravenous pulse methylprednisolone 1 g on 3 alternate days, or 1 mg/kg daily of prednisone for several weeks with subsequent taper, is recommended for severe or life-threatening major ulcerations.

Third-Line Therapies

• IFN-α_{2a}	A
• Isotretinoin	E
• Ciclosporin	A
• Azathioprine	A
• Cyclophosphamide	E
• Chlorambucil	D
• Minocycline	C
• Penicillin	B
• Prostaglandin E_1	D
• Rebamipide	A
• Etanercept	A
• Infliximab	D
• Adsorption apheresis	E
• Azithromycin	D
• Oral contraceptives	E
• Nicotine patch	D
• Mycophenolate sodium	C
• Lenalidomide	E
• Apremilast	A

Successful treatment of Behçet's disease with lenalidomide. Green J, Upjohn E, McMormack C, Zeldis J, Prince HM. Br J Dermatol 2008; 158: 197–8.

A case report of improvement of oral ulceration and lethargy in Behçet disease with lenalidomide (10 mg/day).

Of note the patient tolerated the medication well; however, the patient did develop a deep vein thrombosis, which can be independently associated with lenalidomide or BD.

Interferon alfa-2a in the treatment of Behçet disease: a randomized placebo-controlled and double-blind study. Alpsoy E, Durusoy C, Yilmaz E, Ozgurel Y, Ermis O, Yazar S, et al. Arch Dermatol 2002; 138: 467–71.

A randomized, double-blinded, placebo-controlled trial of 23 patients receiving interferon-α_{2a}, 6×10^6 IU, subcutaneously three times a week. After 3 months, 15 of 23 patients demonstrated improvement in oral, genital, and papulopustular lesions.

Interferon-alpha treatment of Behçet's disease. O'Duffy JD, Calamia K, Cohen S, Goronzy JJ, Herman D, Jorizzo J, et al. J Rheumatol 1998; 25: 1938–44.

Seven patients underwent daily subcutaneous injections of 3 million units of interferon-α_{2a}. This open trial reported a substantial reduction in mucocutaneous lesions and joint disease. Flulike symptoms, leukopenia, psoriasis, seizure, hyperthyroidism, and psychosis were side effects reported.

Systemic isotretinoin in the treatment of a Behçet's patient with arthritic symptoms and acne lesions. Akyol M, Dogan S, Kaptanoglu E, Ozcelik S. Clin Exp Rheumatol 2002; 20: S55.

A patient with oral ulcers, acne lesions, and arthritis was treated with 6 months of isotretinoin (total dosage 120 mg/kg). The patient experienced complete resolution of his acne and arthritis and reduced severity of oral ulcers, controlled with only topical treatment.

Double-masked trial of cyclosporine versus colchicine and long-term open study of cyclosporine in Behçet's disease. Masuda K, Nakajima A, Urayama A, Nakae K, Kogure M, Inaba G. Lancet 1989; 1: 1093–6.

Ciclosporin (10 mg/kg) was more effective than colchicine (1 mg/kg) in reducing the number and frequency of oral aphthae and cutaneous lesions (erythema nodosum–like, subcutaneous thrombophlebitis, and folliculitis-like lesions).

Several case reports and open studies corroborate these findings. Note higher doses of ciclosporin used in this study.

Cyclosporine in Behçet's disease: results in 16 patients after 24 months of therapy. Pacor ML, Biasi D, Lunardi C, Cortina P, Caramaschi P, Girelli D, et al. Clin Rheumatol 1994; 13: 224–7.

Sixteen subjects with BD received 5 mg/kg ciclosporin daily for 24 months. A marked improvement of the symptoms was observed after 3 months of therapy, and 14 out of 16 patients obtained a complete clinical remission. Two patients dropped out of the study because of anemia and renal dysfunction, which returned to normal when ciclosporin was withdrawn.

A controlled trial of azathioprine in Behçet's syndrome. Yazici H, Pazarli H, Barnes CG, Tüzün Y, Ozyazgan Y, Silman A, et al. N Engl J Med 1990; 322: 281–5.

A randomized, controlled, double-blind trial of azathioprine 2.5 mg/kg daily vs. placebo in patients with BD resulted in prevention and decreased frequency of ocular disease. The prevalence of oral ulcers and the incidence of genital ulcers were diminished in the azathioprine group.

High-dose cyclophosphamide without stem cell rescue for the treatment of refractory Behçet's disease. Henderson CF, Brodsky RA, Jones RJ, Levine SM. Semin Arthritis Rheum 2011; 41: 301–4.

In this case report, two patients with refractory BD were successfully treated with cyclophosphamide 200 mg/kg intravenously divided over 4 days with disease-free remission lasting 18 to 24 months. Both patients had a transient pancytopenia, and one suffered episodes of pneumonia and *Clostridium difficile* colitis.

Long-lasting remission of Behçet's disease after chlorambucil therapy. Abdalla MI, Bahgat NE. Br J Ophthalmol 1973; 57: 706–11.

Remission of aphthae was achieved in all seven patients treated with oral chlorambucil and corticosteroids, but only in a minority of patients treated with corticosteroids alone.

Streptococcal infection in the pathogenesis of Behçet's disease and clinical effects of minocycline on the disease symptoms. Kaneko F, Oyama N, Nishibu A. Yonsei Med J 1997; 38: 444–54.

In 11 patients treated with minocycline 100 mg daily the frequency of cutaneous symptoms was reduced by 10% for oral aphthae and by 100% for perifolliculitis.

Oral prostaglandin E1 as a therapeutic modality for leg ulcers in Behçet's disease. Takeuchi A, Hashimoto T. Int J Clin Pharm Res 1987; 7: 283–9.

In five patients, leg ulcers began to regranulate within 2 weeks of using oral prostaglandin E_1 15 to 30 µg daily.

Efficacy of rebamipide as adjunctive therapy in the treatment of recurrent oral aphthous ulcers in patients with Behçet's disease. Matsuda T, Ohno S, Hirohata S, Miyanaga Y, Ujihara H, Inaba G, et al. Drugs R&D 2003; 4: 19–28.

A multicenter, randomized, double-blind, placebo-controlled prospective study of rebamipide 300 mg/day plus usual therapy ($n = 19$) vs. placebo plus usual therapy ($n = 16$) showed moderate-to-marked improvement of oral aphthae and pain in 65% of the treatment group vs. 36% in the placebo group.

Rebamipide is not available in U.S. however is available in may countries world wide and other uses include treatment for recurrent aphthous ulcers.

Short-term trial of etanercept in Behçet's disease: a double blind, placebo controlled study. Melikoglu M, Fresko I, Mat C, Ozyazgan Y, Gogus F, Yurdakul S, et al. J Rheumatol 2005; 32: 98–105.

A randomized, double-blind, controlled trial of 40 BD patients who received either etanercept 25 mg or placebo subcutaneously twice a week for 4 weeks. Etanercept was found to be effective in suppressing oral ulcers, nodular lesions, and papulopustular lesions.

Infliximab treatment for ocular and extraocular manifestations of Behçet's disease. Accorinti M, Pirraglia MP, Paroli MP, Priori R, Conti F, Pivetti-Pezzi P. Jpn J Ophthalmol 2007; 51: 191–6.

Twelve patients with BD and uveitis refractory to conventional immunosuppressive therapy were given infliximab (5 mg/kg at 0 and 2 weeks, then monthly for 4–6 months and quarterly 1–2 months thereafter). After a median 15-month follow-up, 11 of the 12 showed a significant reduction in the number of ocular relapses, as well as fewer extraocular manifestations, resulting

Evidence Levels: A Double-blind study **B** Clinical trial ≥ 20 subjects **C** Clinical trial < 20 subjects **D** Series ≥ 5 subjects **E** Anecdotal case reports

in less systemic corticosteroid use. One patient stopped treatment after 2 months because of the development of pulmonary tuberculosis.

Anti-TNF agents for Behçet's disease: analysis of published data on 369 patients. Arida A, Fragiadaki K, Giavri E, Sfikakis P. Semin Arthritis Rheum 2011; 41: 61–70.

In this evidence-based review of the literature regarding anti-TNF agents in BD, the authors concluded that there is enough evidence to suggest that TNF blockade should be considered in patients with severe or resistant disease.

Treatment of Behçet's disease with granulocyte and monocyte adsorption apheresis. Kanekura T, Gushi A, Fukumaru S, Fukumaru S, Sakamoto R, Kawahara K, et al. J Am Acad Dermatol 2004; 51: S83–7.

A report of successful treatment of orogenital ulceration in two patients who underwent five and eight treatments each.

Clinical and immunologic effects of azithromycin in Behçet's disease. Mumcu G, Ergun T, Elbir Y, Eksioglu-Demiralp E, Yavuz S, Atalay T, et al. J Oral Pathol Med 2005; 34: 13–6.

In eight patients treated with azithromycin 500 mg three times per week for 4 weeks, faster healing times of preexisting oral ulcers, as well as complete resolution of folliculitic lesions, were observed.

Effect of prophylactic benzathine penicillin on mucocutaneous symptoms of Behçet's disease. Calguneri M, Ertenli I, Kiraz S, Erman M, Celik I. Dermatology 1996; 192: 125–8.

A prospective, randomized trial with 60 patients revealed statistically significant reduction in frequency and duration of oral aphthae and erythema nodosum–like lesions and the frequency of genital aphthae with the addition of benzathine penicillin 1.2 million units every 3 weeks to colchicine vs. colchicine monotherapy.

This study was apparently nonblinded and not placebo controlled.

Behçet's disease: remission of patient symptoms after oral contraceptive therapy. Oh SH, Kwon JY, Lee JH, Hand EC, Bang D. Clin Exp Dermatol 2009; 34: e88–90.

In this case report, a patient with BD had clearing of erythema nodosum and oral and genital ulcers with the administration of oral contraceptives. Upon discontinuation of the oral contraceptive the symptoms returned; however, with readministration the symptoms resolved.

Nicotine-patch therapy of mucocutaneous lesions of Behçet's disease: a case series. Ciancio G, Colina M, La Corte R, Lo Monaco A, De Leonardis F, Trotta F, et al. Rheumatology 2010; 49: 501–4.

This case report demonstrated improvement of mucocutaneous lesions with nicotine replacement in ex-smokers with BD.

This cannot be extrapolated to nonsmokers; however, it represents an interesting therapeutic consideration in those patients who are trying to quit smoking.

Mycophenolate sodium in the treatment of mucocutaneous Behçet's disease. Köse O, Simşek I, Pay S. Int J Dermatol 2011; 50: 895–6.

In this open, prospective trial mycophenolate sodium was effective in treating 10 patients with refractory mucocutaneous BD without major complications.

Apremilast for Behçet's syndrome—a phase 2, placebo-controlled study. Hatemi G, Melikoglu M, Tunc R, Korkmaz C, Turgut Ozturk B, Mat C, et al. N Engl J Med 2015; 372: 1510–18.

In this phase II, multicenter, placebo-controlled study, 111 patients received 30 mg of apremilast twice daily or placebo for 12 weeks followed by a 12-week extension phase in which the placebo group was switched to apremilast with a 28-day post-treatment observation phase. The mean number of ulcers per patient was significantly lower in the apremilast group than in the placebo group, and the mean reduction in pain from baseline was greater with apremilast than placebo.

This study was not long enough or large enough to assess long-term efficacy.

Apremilast, a phosphodiesterase-4 inhibitor, appears to be promising as an effective treatment of oral ulcers in BD.

Bioterrorism

*Cody R. Thornton, Boris D. Lushniak**

Bioterrorism is defined as the use of viruses, bacteria, fungi, or toxins from living organisms to produce death or disease in humans, animals, or plants. The diseases that are of greatest concern are smallpox, anthrax, tularemia, plague, the hemorrhagic fevers, and botulism (which has no cutaneous features and will not be further discussed here). Several of the conditions discussed, including smallpox, pneumonic plague, and viral hemorrhagic fevers, are contagious to caregivers, so appropriate care must be taken to prevent the further transmission of disease.

SMALLPOX

After a worldwide vaccination campaign, the last natural case occurred in Somalia in 1977, and by 1980 the World Health Assembly declared smallpox eradicated. The virus now remains stored in secure laboratory facilities in the United States and Russia.

Smallpox is a highly stable virus, spread by direct contact, short distance (6 feet) aerosol exposure, or, in rare cases, through fomites. The incubation period ranges from 7 to 19 days, followed by a prodrome of 2 to 4 days, which includes high fever (101–104°F), prostration, malaise, and myalgias. After the prodrome, an exanthem appears with a mostly centrifugal distribution. Lesions progress in a synchronous fashion from macule (day 0–1), to papule (day 2–3), to deep tense umbilicated vesicle (day 3–5), to deep round tense pustule (day 6–12), to crust formation (day 13–20), to crust separation (day 21–28), and resulting depressed scars. Complications of smallpox include sepsis and toxemia, encephalitis, and blindness.

The differential diagnosis for smallpox includes varicella and disseminated herpes simplex or zoster; molluscum contagiosum; erythema multiforme; pustular drug eruption; purpura fulminans; hand, foot, and mouth disease; and monkeypox. Varicella has a relatively benign prodrome, with more superficial lesions in a centripetal distribution with asynchronous evolution and crusting in 4 to 7 days.

Smallpox vaccination with the scarification technique using the live vaccinia virus can cause adverse reactions in those vaccinated as well as their close contacts. Contraindications to nonemergency vaccination include immunodeficiency states, immunomodulating medications, allergic reactions, pregnancy, cardiovascular diseases, and epidermal-disrupting diseases such as atopic dermatitis, pemphigus, or Darier disease in vaccine recipients or family members. Localized skin reactions include

a robust primary reaction at the site, autoinoculation or contact transmission of the vaccinia, and ocular vaccinia. Generalized skin reactions with systemic symptoms can also occur, including generalized vaccinia (distant site viremic spread), erythema multiforme major, progressive vaccinia (progressive necrosis at the site), and eczema vaccinatum (localized or systemic dissemination) as seen in those with atopic dermatitis or other skin diseases. Other adverse reactions of vaccination include post-vaccinial encephalopathy and encephalomyelitis and myopericarditis. A new-generation vaccine given by the subcutaneous route, a nonreplicating attenuated modified *vaccinia* ankara (Imvamune), has been investigated, and adverse reactions seem to be minimized and may be used in atopics. This new vaccine is stockpiled in the U.S. Strategic National Stockpile but would require investigational new drug or emergency use authorization protocols.

MANAGEMENT STRATEGY

The management of smallpox includes the recognition, diagnosis, and isolation of index cases; notification of public health authorities; *vaccination*; treatment; supportive care of the cases; and vaccination and isolation of those who were in contact with the cases. Although there is no specific treatment for smallpox, several investigational antiviral candidates are undergoing study for both treatment of disease and for adverse events associated with vaccination. *Vaccinia immune globulin* is also available from the CDC to treat specific adverse events. In an outbreak scenario a "ring vaccination" strategy, as used in the eradication program, would be used initially whereby the case would be vaccinated, as well as those exposed to the case and those exposed to the exposed, in an expanding ring fashion. Vaccination should be effective in limiting the disease if given within 3 to 4 days of exposure.

Specific Investigations

- Tzanck smear
- Direct fluorescent antibody testing for varicella zoster virus (VZV) and herpes simplex virus (HSV)
- Polymerase chain reaction (PCR) for VZV, vaccinia, variola, other orthopox viruses (monkeypox)
- Electron microscopy
- Orthopox virus culture
- Serology

Laboratory diagnosis to differentiate smallpox, vaccinia, and other vesicular/pustular illnesses. Besser JM, Crouch NA, Sullivan M. J Lab Clin Med 2003; 142; 246–51.

Patients who are at risk should have laboratory testing to include electron microscopy, PCR, orthopox virus culture, and variola serology performed at designated laboratories. Tzanck smears and real-time PCR assays for HSV and VZV can be performed at standard reference laboratories.

Cutaneous manifestations of category A bioweapons. Aquino LL, Wu JJ. J Am Acad Dermatol 2011; 65: 1213.e1–15.

Reviews the diagnosis and treatment of diseases caused by potential biowarfare agents that produce cutaneous manifestations and provides information regarding reporting and containment of possible bioterrorism-related diseases.

---

*The content of this publication is the sole responsibility of the authors and does not necessarily reflect the views, assertions, opinions, or policies of the Department of Health and Human Services, the Uniformed Services University of the Health Sciences, the Department of Defense, or the Departments of the Army, Navy, or Air Force. Mention of trade names, commercial products, or organizations does not imply endorsement by the U.S. government.

Clinical management of potential bioterrorism-related conditions. Adalja AA, Toner E, Inglesby TV. N Engl J Med 2015; 372: 954–62.

The purpose of this review is to highlight clinically useful issues and management of deliberate infection with several pathogens of greatest bioweapons concern. Because most of these conditions can occur naturally, suspicion for bioterrorism depends on clinicians being alert to unusual patterns, such as unexplained clusters of infection.

Development and experience with an algorithm to evaluate suspected smallpox cases in the United States, 2002–2004. Seward JF, Galil K, Damon I, Norton SA, Rotz L, Schmid S, et al. Clin Infect Dis 2004; 39: 1477–83.

Diagnostic criteria and a CDC algorithm to evaluate and manage suspected cases of smallpox. Three categories (i.e., low, moderate, or high risk of actually having smallpox) dictate subsequent diagnostic strategies. Specific variola laboratory testing is reserved for high-risk persons. An interactive version of the algorithm is available online at http://www.bt.cdc.gov/agent/smallpox/diagnosis/riskalgorithm/index.asp.

First-Line Therapies

Suspected cases

• Isolation—negative-pressure room	A
• Respiratory and contact isolation	A
• Vaccination of early-stage patients	A
• Maintenance of hydration and adequate nutrition	A

Vaccination reactions

• Vaccinia immune globulin	D
• Idoxuridine for corneal lesions	D
• Antivirals	E

Countermeasures and vaccination against terrorism using smallpox: pre-event and post-event smallpox vaccination and its contraindications. Sato H. Environ Health Prev Med 2011; 16: 281–9.

Core components of the public health management of a terrorist attack using smallpox are vaccination (ring vaccination and mass vaccination); adverse event monitoring; confirmed and suspected smallpox case management; contact management; identifying, tracing, and monitoring contacts; and quarantine.

Inactivation of poxviruses by upper-room UVC light in a simulated hospital room environment. McDevitt JJ, Milton DK, Rudnick SN, First MW. PLoS ONE 2008; 3: e3186.

A reduction in airborne *Vaccinia* concentrations can be obtained by combining UV light, upper-room 254-nm germicidal UVC, with air mixing using a conventional ceiling fan. Although the greatest risk for an aerosol attack with smallpox is during the winter, protective measures using UVC would be best suited during winter due to the increased survival at baseline and greater UVC susceptibility of *Vaccinia* under winter conditions.

Vaccinia virus infection after sexual contact with a military smallpox vaccinee. Morb Mortal Wkly Rep 2010; 59: 773–5.

Health care providers should consider vaccinia virus infection in the differentials of clinically compatible genital lesions (conjugal transfer vaccinia).

Progressive vaccinia in a military smallpox vaccinee: United States, 2009. MMWR Morb Mortal Wkly Rep 2009; 58: 532–6.

This report summarizes the patient's clinical course and medical management. This is the first confirmed case of progressive vaccinia in the United States since 1987. Therapy included imiquimod, VIG, oral and topical ST-246 (a smallpox drug candidate with antiorthopox activity inhibiting virus maturation), and oral CMX001 (a lipid conjugate of cidofovir) under emergency investigational new drug protocols.

Household transmission of vaccinia virus from contact with a military smallpox vaccinee: Illinois and Indiana, 2007. MMWR Morb Mortal Wkly Rep 2007; 56: 478–81.

This case highlights the need for clinicians to maintain a high index of suspicion when evaluating recently vaccinated patients and their family members with vesiculopustular rash. This is the first eczema vaccinatum case reported in the United States since 1988. Therapy included cidofovir, VIG, and oral ST-246 under emergency investigational new drug protocols.

A randomized, double-blind, dose-finding phase II study to evaluate immunogenicity and safety of the third generation smallpox vaccine candidate Imvamune. von Krempelhuber A, Vollmar J, Pokorny R, Rapp P, Wulff N, Petzold B, et al. Vaccine 2010; 28: 1209–16.

Imvamune is a modified *Vaccinia* ankara–based virus that is being developed as a safer third-generation smallpox vaccine, especially in those for whom traditional smallpox vaccines are contraindicated, such as the immunocompromised and those with eczema or dermatitis. Imvamune has displayed a favorable safety profile, with local reactions as the most frequent observation.

Smallpox vaccine, ACAM2000: sites and duration of viral shedding and effect of povidone iodine on scarification site shedding and immune response. Pittman PR, Garman PM, Kim SH, Schmader TJ, Nieding WJ, Pike JG, et al. Vaccine 2015; 33: 2990–6.

Counter to current dogma, this study showed that VACV continues to shed from the vaccination site after the scab separates. The use of povidone iodine in addition to a semipermeable dressing may reduce the rates of autoinoculation and contact transmission originating from the vaccination site in smallpox-vaccinated individuals.

Adverse events following smallpox vaccination with ACAM2000 in a military population. Beachkofsky TM, Carrizales SC, Bidinger JJ, Hrncir DE, Whittemore DE, Hivnor CM. Arch Dermatol 2010; 146: 656–61.

Presentation of the first confirmed case of generalized vaccinia after immunization with the second-generation smallpox vaccine ACAM2000. In addition, there is a description of seven cases of benign, acral, papulovesicular eruptions thought to be associated with ACAM2000 administration.

Clinical efficacy of intramuscular Vaccinia immune globulin: a literature review. Hopkins RJ, Lane JM. Clin Infect Dis 2004; 39: 819–26.

Vaccinia immune globulin (VIG) reduces the morbidity and mortality associated with progressive vaccinia (vaccinia necrosum) and eczema vaccinatum. Indications for treatment include generalized vaccinia, progressive vaccinia, eczema vaccinatum, and some accidental implantations. The use of intramuscular administration of VIG to prevent smallpox in contacts of patients with documented cases is also discussed.

Pregnancy discovered after smallpox vaccination: is vaccinia immune globulin appropriate? Napolitano PG, Ryan MA, Grabenstein JD. Am J Obstet Gynecol 2004; 191: 1863–7.

VIG is not approved for use in fetal vaccinia complications, and a risk of teratogenicity from mercury in the thimerosal preservative has been cited. Fetal vaccinia is a rare complication of smallpox vaccination during pregnancy, and although some have suggested that therapeutic treatment with VIG can prevent fetal vaccinia, VIG should only be given if a pregnant woman develops a condition in which VIG is indicated (e.g., eczema vaccinatum, progressive vaccinia, or serious generalized vaccinia).

A prospective study of the incidence of myocarditis/pericarditis and new onset cardiac symptoms following smallpox and influenza vaccination. Engler RJ, Nelson MR, Collins LC Jr, Spooner C, Hemann BA, Gibbs BT, et al. PLoS One 2015; 10: e0118283.

Passive surveillance significantly underestimates the true incidence of myocarditis/pericarditis after smallpox immunization. A postsmallpox incidence rate was more than 200 times higher than the presmallpox background population surveillance rate of myocarditis/pericarditis (RR 214, 95% CI 65–558). Active safety surveillance is needed to identify adverse events that are not well understood or previously recognized.

Traditional smallpox vaccination with reduced risk of inadvertent contact spread by administration of povidone iodine ointment. Hammarlund E, Lewis MW, Hanifin JM, Simpson EL, Carlson NE, Slifka MK. Vaccine 2008; 26: 430–9.

This ointment rapidly inactivated virus on the skin without reducing neutralizing antibody titers or antiviral T-cell responses. Moreover, there was no delay in healing/eschar separation after povidone iodine application.

Second-Line Therapies	
• Penicillinase-resistant antibiotics for secondary skin infection	D
• Local treatments—manage like a "burn patient"	C
• Idoxuridine (topical) treatment of corneal lesions	C
• Efficacy is probable in view of use in vaccinia (see earlier).	

Third-Line Therapies	
• Cidofovir plus VIG plus drug candidates ST-246 or CMX001 (see vaccination reactions)	D
• Cidofovir	E
• Cidofovir plus VIG	E
• Imvamune	E
• Brincidofovir	E

Severe eczema vaccinatum in a household contact of a smallpox vaccinee. Vora S, Damon I, Fulginiti V, Weber SG, Kahana M, Stein SL, et al. Clin Infect Dis 2008; 46: 1555–61.

A 28-month-old child with refractory atopic dermatitis developed severe eczema vaccinatum after exposure to his father, a U.S. military member who had recently received smallpox vaccine. In this first confirmed case of eczema vaccinatum in the United States related to smallpox vaccination since routine vaccination was discontinued in 1972, the child was treated with intravenous *Vaccinia* immune globulin, used for the first time in a pediatric patient, cidofovir, and ST-246, an investigational drug being studied for orthopoxvirus infection.

Cidofovir in the treatment of poxvirus infections. De Clercq E. Antiviral Res 2002; 55: 1–13.

Experimental use of cidofovir in poxvirus infections.

Cutaneous infections of mice with vaccinia or cowpox viruses and efficacy of cidofovir. Quenelle DC, Collins DJ, Kern ER. Antiviral Res 2004; 63: 33–40.

In hairless mice, 5% topical cidofovir was more effective than systemic treatment at reducing virus titers in skin, lung, kidney, and spleen.

Repeated high-dose (5 × 10(8) TCID50) toxicity study of a third generation smallpox vaccine (Imvamune) in New Zealand white rabbits. Tree JA, Hall G, Rees P, Vipond J, Funnell SG, Roberts AD. Hum Vaccin Immunother 2016; 12: 1795–801.

Subcutaneous injection of two high-doses of Imvamune to rabbits was well tolerated, producing only minor changes at the site of administration.

The efficacy and pharmacokinetics of brincidofovir for the treatment of lethal rabbitpox virus infection: a model of smallpox disease. Trost LC, Rose ML, Khouri J, Keilholz L, Long J, Godin SJ, et al. Antiviral Res 2015; 117: 115–21.

Observation of a dose-dependent increase in survival occurred in all brincidofovir (BCV)-treatment groups demonstrating the activity of BCV in the rabbitpox model of smallpox and the feasibility of scaling doses efficacious in the model to a proposed human dose and regimen for treatment of smallpox.

ANTHRAX

Anthrax is caused by spores from the gram-positive, nonmotile *Bacillus anthracis*. Farm workers or processors of wool, hair, or hides are at risk. After a livestock vaccination campaign in the 1950s, anthrax became a very rare disease in the United States, with only 409 cases (of which 18 were inhalational and the remainder cutaneous) described from 1951 to 2000. In 2001 anthrax spores were disseminated in a bioterrorist incident through the U.S. mail system resulting in 11 inhalational cases (5 deaths) and 11 cutaneous cases.

Cutaneous anthrax is the form most commonly encountered in naturally occurring cases. A nontender pruritic macule and then papule develops 1 to 12 days after skin exposure and inoculation of spores (see the figure). Within 48 hours this lesion develops into a vesicle or bulla, which then ruptures, forming a depressed, black, necrotic ulcer (black eschar) within an edematous, erythematous plaque. The greatest concern in a bioterrorist event would be inhalational anthrax, which can occur from 1 to over 40 days after exposure. The initial prodrome is a viral-like illness with myalgias, fatigue, and fever followed by hypoxia and dyspnea (with evidence of radiographic mediastinal widening) and respiratory failure. After the initial infection the spores produce toxins that do not respond to antibiotics. Historically inhalation anthrax resulted in a high fatality rate.

The diagnosis of any form of anthrax, especially in nonrural areas, requires a high index of suspicion and would mandate a notification of public health authorities. The varied differential diagnosis of cutaneous anthrax includes insect bite, brown recluse spider bite, tularemia, the *tache noir* of rickettsial diseases, ecthyma gangrenosum, staphylococcal or streptococcal ecthyma, cat scratch disease, orf, and other conditions with eschar or an ulceroglandular presentation.

MANAGEMENT STRATEGY

Universal precautions should be maintained in evaluating a patient with suspected cutaneous anthrax. *Ciprofloxacin* and *doxycycline* are the mainstays of therapy. The need for postexposure prophylaxis with antibiotics would be determined by public health officials based upon the epidemiologic investigation and the likelihood of exposure to spores. The duration of treatment and postexposure prophylaxis may be up to 60 days.

The vaccine, anthrax vaccine adsorbed (AVA), induces immunity to a protein in the toxins. The regimen consists of six injections at 0, 2, and 4 weeks, followed by doses at 6, 12, and 18 months plus annual boosters. Vaccination is only indicated for at-risk laboratory workers, select emergency responders, and military personnel. In combination with antibiotics, postexposure vaccination may be effective in preventing disease after exposure to *B. anthracis* spores.

Specific Investigations

- Culture and Gram stain of tissue, blood, or other fluids
- For cutaneous anthrax, use a Dacron or rayon swab (not cotton) to swab the vesicle, ulcer, or eschar edge
- Punch biopsy fixed in formalin from a papule or vesicular lesion and including adjacent skin
- Biopsies should be taken from both vesicle and eschar, if present
- A photograph, digital image, or diagram indicating the site of each biopsy in relation to the lesion
- Immunohistochemical assays
- Serology (available through CDC)
- PCR assay

Cutaneous manifestations of category A bioweapons. Aquino LL, Wu JJ. J Am Acad Dermatol 2011; 65: 1213.e1–15.

Reviews diagnosis, treatment, reporting, and containment of diseases caused by potential biowarfare agents that produce cutaneous manifestations.

Severe systemic *Bacillus anthracis* infection in an intravenous drug user. Veitch J, Kansara A, Bailey D, Kustos I. BMJ Case Rep 2014; 2014: pii: bcr2013201921.

Summarization of the steps in diagnosis and the management options, including extensive surgical debridement and a prolonged course of combination antibiotic therapy, in patients presenting with systemic *Bacillus anthracis* infection.

Anthrax infection. Sweeney DA, Hicks CW, Cui X, Li Y, Eichacker PQ. Am J Respir Crit Care Med 2011; 184: 1333–41.

Clues to anthrax infection include history of exposure to herbivore animal products, heroin use, or clustering of patients with similar respiratory symptoms suggesting a bioterrorist event. This review summarizes the microbiology, pathogenesis, diagnosis, and management of anthrax.

An overview of anthrax infection including the recently identified form of disease in injection drug users. Hicks CW, Sweeney DA, Cui X, Li Y, Eichacker PQ. Intensive Care Med 2012; 38: 1092–104.

Patients with gastrointestinal, inhalational, or injectional anthrax may have advanced infection at presentation that can be highly lethal. Once anthrax is suspected, the diagnosis can usually be made with Gram stain and culture from blood or tissue followed by confirmatory testing (e.g., PCR).

Application of r-PFE hyperimmune sera for concurrent detection of *Bacillus anthracis*, *Yersinia pestis* and staphylococcal enterotoxin B. Balakrishna K, Tuteja U, Murali HS, Batra HV. J Appl Microbiol 2014; 116: 1465–73.

Evaluate the potential of an intergeneric multidomain recombinant chimeric protein for the simultaneous detection of *Bacillus anthracis*, *Yersinia pestis*, and staphylococcal enterotoxin B.

First-Line Therapies

• Raxibacumab—human monoclonal antibody	D
• Ciprofloxacin	D
• Doxycycline	D

Oral antibiotics are used for cutaneous anthrax below the head and neck if systemic symptoms and malignant edema are absent. If they are present, intravenous antibiotics are used.

Anthrax prevention and treatment: utility of therapy combining antibiotic plus vaccine. Klinman DM, Yamamoto M, Tross D, Tomaru K. Expert Opin Biol Ther 2009; 9: 1477–86.

For the foreseeable future, vaccination will rely on first- and second-generation vaccines coadministered with immune adjuvants. Optimal postexposure treatment of immunologically naive individuals should include a combination of vaccine plus antibiotic therapy.

Raxibacumab [treatment of inhalation anthrax]. Mazumdar S. mAbs 2009; 1: 531–8.

Raxibacumab (ABthrax) is a human IgG1 monoclonal antibody against *Bacillus anthracis* and protective antigen approved through the U.S. Food and Drug Administration's (FDA) animal efficacy rule, better known as the *animal rule pathway*.

Second-Line Therapies

• Amoxicillin	D
• Penicillin	D
• Chloramphenicol	D
• Clindamycin	D
• Systemic corticosteroids for treatment of edema	E

Amoxicillin for postexposure inhalational anthrax in pediatrics: rationale for dosing recommendations. Alexander JJ, Colangelo PM, Cooper CK, Roberts R, Rodriguez WJ, Murphy MD. Pediatr Infect Dis J 2008; 27: 955–7.

Covers dosage considerations and dosing intervals for postexposure inhalational anthrax.

Third-Line Therapies

• Macrolides	E
• Aminoglycosides	E
• Chloroquine—experimental	E
• Combination MAb—experimental	E

Combinations of monoclonal antibodies to anthrax toxin manifest new properties in neutralization assays. Pohl MA, Rivera J, Nakouzi A, Chow SK, Casadevall A. Infect Immun 2013; 81: 1880–8.

Although no single MAb to LF provided significant toxin neutralization, LF-immunized mice were completely protected from infection with *B. anthracis* strain Sterne, which suggested that a polyclonal response is required for effective toxin neutralization. A combination of multiple MAbs may provide the most effective form of passive immunotherapy, with the caveat that these may demonstrate emergent properties with regard to protective efficacy.

A dual-purpose protein ligand for effective therapy and sensitive diagnosis of anthrax. Vuyisich M, Gnanakaran S, Lovchik JA, Lyons CR, Gupta G. Protein J 2008; 27: 292–302.

Article reports the design of a bivalent protein ligand with dual use in therapy and diagnosis of anthrax caused by *Bacillus anthracis*.

Prophylaxis	
• Vaccination	A
• Antibiotics	A

Use of anthrax vaccine in the U.S.: recommendations of the Advisory Committee on Immunization Practices (ACIP). Wright JG, Quinn CP, Shadomy S, Messonnier N. MMWR 2010; 59: 1–30.

This statement (1) provides updated information on anthrax epidemiology; (2) summarizes the evidence regarding the effectiveness and efficacy, immunogenicity, and safety of AVA; (3) provides recommendations for preevent and preexposure use of AVA; and (4) provides recommendations for postexposure use of AVA.

A short course of antibiotic treatment is effective in preventing death from experimental inhalational anthrax after discontinuing antibiotics. Vietri NJ, Purcell BK, Tobery SA, Rasmussen SL, Leffel EK, Twenhafel NA, et al. J Infect Dis 2009; 199: 336–41.

In the treatment of inhalational anthrax, the prolonged course of antibiotics required to achieve prophylaxis may not be necessary to prevent anthrax that results from the germination of retained spores after the discontinuation of antibiotics.

Comprehensive analysis and selection of anthrax vaccine adsorbed immune correlates of protection in rhesus macaques. Chen L, Schiffer JM, Dalton S, Sabourin CL, Niemuth NA, Plikaytis BD, et al. Vaccine Immunol 2014; 21: 1512–20.

The anti-PA IgG levels at the time of challenge (last) were the most accurate single measure for determining the probability of survival against inhalation anthrax in rhesus macaques completing a 3-i.m. priming series of AVA. In the absence of a last anti-PA IgG measurement concurrent with aerosol exposure, the month-7 anti-PA IgG and TNA responses to 3-i.m. priming are suitable alternative correlates of protection.

TULAREMIA

Tularemia is caused by the very infectious (as few as 10–50 organisms can cause disease) gram-negative coccobacillus *Francisella tularensis*, found in rodents, rabbits, and hares. Exposure can occur through insect bites (usually infected ticks or deerflies), handling of infected animal carcasses, eating or drinking contaminated food or water, or through inhalation. Symptoms can appear 1 to 14 days after exposure, and person-to-person transmission is not seen. Inhalational (pneumonic) tularemia would most likely be the chief concern in a bioterrorist event. It starts abruptly as a flulike illness or atypical pneumonia with fever, chills, headaches, sore throat, and myalgia. Pulmonary symptoms can include a dry cough and pleuritic chest

pain and, if untreated, can escalate to severe bronchopneumonia, hemoptysis, and respiratory failure, with marked hilar lymphadenitis.

Ulceroglandular tularemia presents with a painful papule at the site of inoculation. The papule progresses to a pustule and then to a tender ulcer with eschar formation. Regional lymph nodes become enlarged and tender (buboes), usually within a few days after the appearance of the papule. Oculoglandular tularemia presents with conjunctival ulcerations and purulent conjunctivitis, periorbital edema, and nodules of the conjunctivae, along with tender preauricular or cervical lymphadenopathy. Glandular tularemia is marked by lymphadenopathy with no ulcer formation. Oropharyngeal tularemia presents with gastrointestinal symptoms, stomatitis, and exudative pharyngitis or tonsillitis, sometimes with ulceration and pronounced cervical or retropharyngeal lymphadenopathy

The varied clinical manifestations of tularemia may show exanthems, which may be macular, papular, papulovesicular, pustular, or petechial, and are most prominent on the face and extremities. Erythema nodosum, erythema multiforme, and Sweet syndrome have also been described.

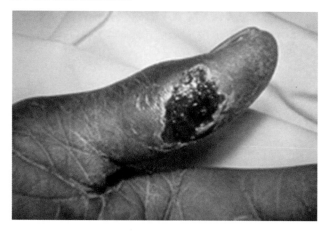

Although a high level of suspicion would be necessary, ulceroglandular or oculoglandular disease has a rather straightforward presentation. However, pneumonic tularemia has variable pulmonary symptoms.

MANAGEMENT STRATEGY

The organism can be cultured and detected in secretions, exudates, or biopsy specimens by direct fluorescent antibody or immunohistochemical techniques. Antigen detection assays, polymerase chain reaction (PCR), enzyme-linked immunoassays (ELISA), and other specialized techniques may be used. Serum antibody titers could be helpful, but not until 10 days into the disease course.

For severe disease, parenteral therapy is indicated. *Streptomycin* has been used successfully for many years for tularemia, but it is not widely available and has been replaced by gentamicin. Streptomycin is ototoxic and nephrotoxic to patients, and if administered to pregnant women can cause fetal hearing loss and kidney damage. Oral *ciprofloxacin* and *doxycycline* have proven effective in the treatment of tularemia. There is no vaccine currently available.

Specific Investigations
• Gram stain
• Culture
• Serology—agglutination and ELISA testing
• Direct fluorescent antibody and immunohistochemistry
• PCR

Ultrasound of lymph nodes. Clinical and laboratory findings of tularemia: a retrospective analysis. Koç S, Duygu F, Söğüt E, Gürbüzler L, Eyibilen A, Aladağ I. Kulak Burun Bogaz Ihtis Derg 2012; 22: 26–31.

Aims to define demographic characteristics and clinical and laboratory findings of the patients with tularemia and to assess the treatment outcomes. Tularemia should be differentiated from upper respiratory tract infections and cervical lymphadenopathy.

WHO guidelines on tularaemia. WHO/CDS/EPR. Geneva: World Health Organization, 2007.

This text provides comprehensive data about tularemia, epidemiology, clinical expression, laboratory diagnostics, and treatment considerations.

Evaluation of clinical and sonographic features in 55 children with tularemia. Oz F, Eksioglu A, Tanır G, Bayhan G, Metin Ö, Teke TA. Vector Borne Zoonotic Dis 2014; 14: 571–5.

Sonographic findings may be useful in the evaluation and staging of lymphadenopathy.

First-Line Therapies	
• Streptomycin	B
• Gentamicin	B
• Ciprofloxacin for uncomplicated disease	C

Second-Line Therapies	
• Doxycycline	D
• Chloramphenicol	D

Tularemia: current diagnosis and treatment options. Hepburn MJ, Simpson AJ. Expert Rev Anti Infect Ther 2008; 6: 231–40.

This review focuses on the utility of culture, PCR, and serologic testing for tularemia. In addition, it reviews the evidence to support different therapeutic options for tularemia, highlighting both the most effective supporting evidence for therapeutic recommendations and gaps in current knowledge.

Evaluation of tularaemia courses: a multicentre study from Turkey. Erdem H, Ozturk-Engin D, Yesilyurt M, Karabay O, Elaldi N, Celebi G, et al. Clin Microbiol Infect 2014; 20: O1042–51.

Cervical lymphadenomegaly was the most common clinical sign, and granulomatous inflammation of lymph nodes was the most common histopathologic finding. The most common complication of oropharyngeal tularemia was lymph node suppuration. Hence, the differential diagnosis of tuberculosis is an important concern for tularemia patients. The most commonly used antibiotics were streptomycin and doxycycline.

Tularemia in children: evaluation of clinical, laboratory and therapeutic features of 27 tularemia cases. Kaya A, Deveci K, Uysal IO, Güven AS, Demir M, Uysal EB, et al. Turk J Pediatr 2012; 54: 105–12.

Streptomycin should be the first-line antibiotic in the treatment of pediatric tularemia cases.

PLAGUE

Plague, caused by the gram-negative bacillus *Yersinia pestis*, is a disease of rodents and their fleas. Bubonic plague usually occurs after a bite and begins with fever and flulike symptoms. Then swollen, tender lymph nodes (buboes) develop near the site of the infected bite, most often in the cervical, axillary, femoral, or inguinal areas. Vesicles, pustules, eschars, or ulcerations can appear at the site of the bite. Without antibiotic treatment, secondary pneumonia or septicemia may follow. Highly contagious pneumonic plague can be primary and spread from person to person (or even cat to person) or may develop secondarily from bubonic or septicemic plague. One to 6 days after exposure, patients with pneumonic plague present with fever, headache, weakness, gastrointestinal symptoms, and rapidly developing pneumonia with dyspnea, chest pain, productive cough, and hemoptysis, and can progress to respiratory failure and sepsis.

MANAGEMENT STRATEGY

Early diagnosis mandates a high level of suspicion. Diagnostic tools include antigen detection, immunoassays, immunostaining, and PCR. Cultures and staining of sputum, blood, or lymph node aspirate will assist in the diagnosis. Cases should be reported immediately to public health authorities. Drainage and secretion precautions are indicated for buboes, and strict respiratory isolation and respiratory droplet precautions are mandatory for the first 48 hours of therapy of pneumonic plague. Postexposure prophylactic treatment of at-risk contacts is mandatory.

Streptomycin is the drug of choice for plague but has limited availability. It is ototoxic and nephrotoxic, and if administered to pregnant women can cause fetal hearing loss and kidney damage. *Gentamicin* is also used for plague and is favored in pregnancy. *Doxycycline, ciprofloxacin, and chloramphenicol* can also be used in treatment. All are highly effective if used early. Vaccines are not available.

Specific Investigations
• Gram stain and culture of sputum and fluid from buboes
• Serology
• PCR

Sentinel laboratory guidelines for suspected agent of bioterrorism: *Yersinia pestis*. American Society for Microbiology, Washington DC, 2009.

Comprehensive guide to *Yersinia pestis*.

Detection of *Yersinia pestis* using real-time PCR in patients with suspected bubonic plague. Riehm JM, Rahalison L, Scholz HC, Thoma B, Pfeffer M, Razanakoto LM, et al. Mol Cell Probes 2011; 25: 8–12.

The best real-time PCR assay was the 5′-nuclease assay targeting the plasminogen activator gene (*pla*), which was positive in 120 cases. In conclusion, the 5′-nuclease assay targeting *pla* can be recommended as a diagnostic tool for establishing a presumptive diagnosis when bubonic plague is clinically suspected.

Outbreak of human pneumonic plague with dog-to-human and possible human-to-human transmission—Colorado, June-July 2014. Runfola JK, House J, Miller L, Colton L, Hite D, Hawley A, et al. MMWR Morb Mortal Wkly Rep 2015; 64: 429–34.

This outbreak highlights (1) the need to consider plague in the differential diagnosis of ill domestic animals, including dogs, in areas where plague is endemic; (2) the limitations of automated diagnostic systems for identifying rare bacteria such as *Y. pestis*; and (3) the potential for milder plague illness in patients taking antimicrobial agents. Hospital laboratorians should be aware of the limitations of automated identification systems, and clinicians should suspect plague in patients with clinically compatible symptoms from whom *Pseudomonas luteola* is isolated.

Bioterrorism: class A agents and their potential presentations in immunocompromised patients. Richard JL, Grimes DE. Clin J Oncol Nurs 2008; 12: 295–302.

The variable signs and symptoms that may be present in immunocompromised patients with cancer are discussed with a focus on assessment and early recognition of an outbreak. The availability of vaccines and the implications for patients with cancer receiving these vaccines is also discussed.

First-Line Therapies

• Intramuscular streptomycin	**A**
• Intramuscular or intravenous gentamicin	**A**

In vitro efficacy of antibiotics commonly used to treat human plague against intracellular *Yersinia pestis*. Wendte JM, Ponnusamy D, Reiber D, Blair JL, Clinkenbeard KD. Antimicrob Agents Chemother 2011; 55: 3752–7.

Provides an understanding of the selection of antibiotics for prophylactic treatment in the case of a bioterrorism event with *Yersinia*.

Second-Line Therapies

• Doxycycline	**C**
• Ciprofloxacin	**C**

Third-Line Therapies

• Chloramphenicol	**D**
• Sulfonamides	**D**

Use of an in vitro pharmacodynamic model to derive a moxifloxacin regimen that optimizes kill of *Yersinia pestis* and prevents emergence of resistance. Louie A, Heine HS, VanScoy B, Eichas A, Files K, Fikes S, et al. Antimicrob Agents Chemother 2011; 55: 822–30.

The efficacies of simulated pharmacokinetic profiles for human 10-day clinical regimens of ampicillin, meropenem, moxifloxacin, ciprofloxacin, and gentamicin were compared with the gold standard, streptomycin.

VIRAL HEMORRHAGIC FEVERS

The viral hemorrhagic fevers are caused by viruses of four distinct families: arenaviruses, filoviruses, bunyaviruses, and flaviviruses.

They are all RNA viruses and are found in animal or insect hosts that can infect humans. In some cases human-to-human spread through bodily fluids is possible as in Ebola, Marburg, Lassa, and Crimean-Congo hemorrhagic fevers. The mode of transmission, clinical course, and mortality of these illnesses vary with the specific virus involved, but each is capable of causing a hemorrhagic fever syndrome. Symptoms include fever, fatigue, dizziness, myalgias, exhaustion, vomiting, diarrhea, and hemorrhagic manifestations, such as hemorrhagic or purpuric skin lesions, epistaxis, hematemesis, hemoptysis, blood in stools, multiple organ failure, hypotension, and shock.

MANAGEMENT STRATEGY

As a result of the outbreak of Ebola in West Africa from 2014 to 2015 there have been significant updates to the scientific literature, specifically on Ebola virus. However, many of the same foundational requirements for detection and case management remain, including a high index of suspicion for patients presenting with a febrile illness and hemorrhagic manifestations and strict infection control practices for provider safety. Atypical presentations are possible and include asymptomatic cases. Cases, even suspect ones, should be reported immediately to public health authorities. Because of the high risk to close contacts, including health care workers, strict *universal precautions, appropriate barrier protection, and isolation* should be instituted. Contacts of suspected cases must be closely monitored. Care depends largely on availability of appropriate resources and treatment facilities and still remains primarily supportive. Ribavirin may be effective in Lassa fever or hemorrhagic fever with renal syndrome. Diagnostic tests are only available through select federal labs. Vaccines are available only for yellow fever and Argentine hemorrhagic fever; nonlicensed vaccines are currently developed for Ebola.

Specific Investigations

- Antigen detection by antigen-capture ELISA
- IgM antibody detection by antibody-capture ELISA
- Reverse transcriptase PCR
- Viral isolation is of limited value because it requires a biosafety level 4 laboratory

Clinical presentation, biochemical, and haematological parameters and their association with outcome in patients with Ebola virus disease: an observational cohort study. Hunt L, Gupta-Wright A. Lancet Infect Dis 2015; 15: 1292–9.

Ebola virus disease (EVD) is associated with a high prevalence of hematologic and biochemical abnormalities, even in mild disease and in the absence of gastrointestinal symptoms. Clinical care that targets hypovolemia, electrolyte disturbance, and acute kidney injury is likely to reduce historically high case fatality rates.

Clinical illness and outcomes in patients with Ebola in Sierra Leone. Schieffelin JS, Shaffer JG, Goba A, Gbakie M, Gire SK, Colubri A, et al. N Engl J Med 2014; 371: 2092–100.

A study of 106 EVD-positive patients in Sierra Leone showed that the incubation period was estimated to be 6 to 12 days and the case fatality rate was 74%. Common findings at presentation included fever, headache, weakness, dizziness, diarrhea, abdominal pain, and vomiting. Clinical and laboratory factors at presentation that were associated with a fatal outcome included fever,

Evidence Levels: **A** Double-blind study **B** Clinical trial ≥ 20 subjects **C** Clinical trial < 20 subjects **D** Series ≥ 5 subjects **E** Anecdotal case reports

weakness, dizziness, diarrhea, and elevated levels of blood urea nitrogen, aspartate aminotransferase, and creatinine. Exploratory analyses indicated that patients under the age of 21 years had a lower case fatality rate than those over the age of 45 years, and patients presenting with fewer than 100,000 EBOV copies per milliliter had a lower case fatality rate than those with 10 million EBOV copies per milliliter or more.

Confronting Ebola as a sexually transmitted infection. Fischer WA 2nd, Wohl DA. Clin Infect Dis 2016; 62: 1272–6 .

Medical care of survivors must consider that Ebola virus persists in genital fluids and can be sexually transmitted, along with the potential for lingering virus in other body compartments to permit recrudescence of EVD. Authors provide a review of the epidemiology, pathophysiology, clinical presentation, diagnosis, treatment, and complications of HFRS.

Prognostic indicators for Ebola patient survival. Crowe SJ, Maenner MJ, Kuah S, Erickson BR, Coffee M, Knust B, et al. Emerg Infect Dis 2016; 22: 217–23.

Viral load in the first Ebola virus–positive blood sample was inversely associated with survival: 52 (87%) of 60 patients with a Ct of >24 survived and 20 (22%) of 91 with a Ct of <24 survived. Ct values may be useful for clinicians making treatment decisions or managing patient or family expectations.

First-Line Therapies	
• Supportive care (fluid replacement, electrolyte management)	A
• Intravenous ribavirin (Lassa)	C
• Renal replacement therapy	D
• Antibiotic treatment	C

Severe Ebola virus disease with vascular leakage and multi-organ failure: treatment of a patient in intensive care. Wolf T, Kann G. Lancet 2015; 385: 1428–35.

The effective treatment of vascular leakage and multiorgan failure by combination of ventilatory support, antibiotic treatment, and renal replacement therapy can sustain a patient with severe EVD until virologic remission. FX06 could potentially be a valuable agent in contribution to supportive therapy.

Review of the literature and proposed guidelines for the use of oral ribavirin as postexposure prophylaxis for Lassa fever. Bausch DG, Hadi CM, Khan SH, Lertora JJ. Clin Infect Dis 2010; 51: 1435–41.

Recommend oral ribavirin postexposure prophylaxis for Lassa fever exclusively for definitive high-risk exposures. These guidelines may also serve for exposure to other hemorrhagic fever viruses susceptible to ribavirin.

Second-Line Therapies	
• Convalescent plasma	B
• Ventilatory support (given appropriate infection control/ICU setting)	C
• Vaccine development	E

Protective monotherapy against lethal Ebola virus infection by a potently neutralizing antibody. Corti D, Misasi J, Mulangu S, Stanley DA, Kanekiyo M, Wollen S, et al. Science 2016; 351: 1339–42.

Monoclonal antibodies (mAbs) isolated from a survivor neutralize recent and previous outbreak variants of Ebola virus and mediate antibody-dependent, cell-mediated cytotoxicity in vitro. Strikingly, monotherapy with mAb114 protected macaques when given as late as 5 days after challenge. Treatment with a single human mAb suggests that a simplified therapeutic strategy for human Ebola infection may be possible.

Update: management of patients with suspected viral hemorrhagic fever – United States. MMRW 1995; 44; 475–9.

CDC guidelines for the management of suspected cases of viral hemorrhagic fever.

Efficacy and effectiveness of an rVSV-vectored vaccine in preventing Ebola virus disease: final results from the Guinea ring vaccination, open-label, cluster-randomised trial. Henao-Restrepo AM, Camacho A, Longini IM, Watson CH, Edmunds WJ, Egger M, et al. Lancet 2017; 389: 505–18.

Study results add weight to the interim assessment that rVSV-ZEBOV offers substantial protection against Ebola virus disease, with no cases among vaccinated individuals from day 10 after vaccination in both randomised and non-randomised clusters.

Discovery of an antibody for pan-ebolavirus therapy. Furuyama W, Marzi A. Sci Rep 2016; 6: 20514.

Report on the generation of an Ebola virus glycoprotein–specific monoclonal antibody that effectively inhibits cellular entry of representative isolates of all known Ebola virus species in vitro and shows its protective efficacy in mouse models of Ebola virus infections.

Bites and stings

Dirk M. Elston

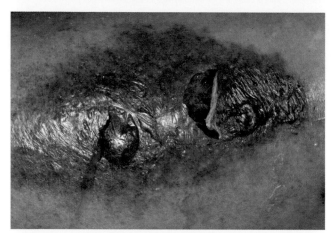

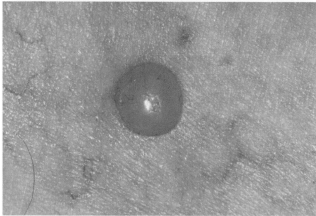

This chapter presents strategies for the prevention and management of bites and stings and their complications.

MANAGEMENT STRATEGY

Bite reactions

DEET is effective for prevention of bites from a broad range of arthropods. Picaridin is effective against mosquitoes. Permethrin can be used on fabric. A veterinarian should be consulted about flea infestation in pets. Antivenin is available for many arachnid toxins, but most respond to rest, ice, and elevation.

If prevention fails, second-line treatments aim to improve pruritus. *Topical antipruritics*, such as ¼% camphor and menthol, and *topical anesthetics*, such as pramoxine and lidocaine, can be helpful. For persistent bite reactions, topical or intralesional corticosteroids may be helpful.

Anaphylaxis

Individuals who experience anaphylaxis in response to stings should be referred to an allergist for *desensitization*. Rush desensitization is possible for those with life-threatening allergy. Patients with a history of anaphylaxis should also carry an *epinephrine autoinjector* (EpiPen).

Vectorborne disease

Most tickborne illness responds to *doxycycline*. For early Lyme disease, evidence suggests that a 10-day course is as effective as longer courses of antibiotic. Babesiosis responds to *clindamycin and quinine*, but *azithromycin* and *atovaquone* may be as effective with a lower incidence of side effects. *Atovaquone-proguanil* has been effective in refractory cases in immunocompromised patients.

Scorpion-related cardiomyopathy: clinical characteristics, pathophysiology, and treatment. Abroug F, Souheil E, Ouanes I, Dachraoui F, Fekih-Hassen M, Ouanes Besbes L. Clin Toxicol (Phila) 2015; 53: 511–8.

More than 1 million scorpion stings occur each year. Acute cardiogenic shock and pulmonary edema are the most severe complications, with a 0.27% lethality rate. Oxygen supplementation to maintain an oxygen saturation of 92% or more, continuous positive airway pressure, and dobutamine infusion improve outcomes.

Immunological aspects of the immune response induced by mosquito allergens. Cantillo JF, Fernández-Caldas E, Puerta L. Int Arch Allergy Immunol 2014; 165: 271–82.

The most common mosquito species implicated in allergic reactions belong to the genera *Aedes*, *Culex*, and *Anopheles*. Allergen-specific immunotherapy with mosquito extracts is capable of inducing a protective response with decreased production of immunoglobulin E (IgE) antibodies, increased IgG levels, and a reduction in the severity of both cutaneous and respiratory symptoms.

Anaphylaxis to insect stings. Golden DB. Immunol Allergy Clin North Am 2015; 35: 287–302.

Anaphylaxis to insect stings occurs in 3% of adults and can be fatal. The risk of a subsequent severe systemic reaction to a sting varies between 30% and 65% in adults with previous reactions, and serum tryptase level correlates with the risk. Venom immunotherapy is 75% to 98% effective in preventing anaphylaxis from stings.

Secondary cutaneous diphtheria due to the bite of a Thai centipede (*Scolopendra*). Jüngling C, Sadowski C, Glitsch M, Vandersee S. J Dtsch Dermatol Ges 2014; 12: 1043–4.

Secondary infection, including cutaneous diphtheria, can follow arthropod bites and stings.

Scorpion stings in pregnant women: an analysis of 11 cases and review of literature. Kaplanoglu M, Helvaci MR. Clin Exp Obstet Gynecol 2015; 42: 228–30.

Although local pain, hyperemia, swelling, and itching were common, pregnancy complications were not.

Cutaneous and systemic mastocytosis in children: a risk factor for anaphylaxis? Matito A, Carter M. Curr Allergy Asthma Rep 2015; 15: 22.

In contrast to adults, hymenoptera stings are an uncommon trigger of anaphylaxis in children with mastocytosis.

Unusual reactions to *Hymenoptera* stings: what should we keep in mind? Mingomataj EÇ, Bakiri AH, Ibranji A, Sturm GJ. Clin Rev Allergy Immunol 2014; 47: 91–9.

Hemodynamic compromise of vital organs with hypoxia and hypovolemia, together with evidence of IgE sensitization, are indications for venom immunotherapy.

Evidence Levels: A Double-blind study   B Clinical trial ≥ 20 subjects   C Clinical trial < 20 subjects   D Series ≥ 5 subjects   E Anecdotal case reports

Recognition, treatment, and prevention of anaphylaxis. Moore LE, Kemp AM, Kemp SF. Immunol Allergy Clin North Am 2015; 35: 363–74.

Reactions to medications, foods, and insect stings cause most episodes of anaphylaxis. Treatment involves prompt administration of epinephrine and supportive care.

Centipede venom: recent discoveries and current state of knowledge. Undheim EA, Fry BG, King GF. Toxins (Basel) 2015; 7: 679–704.

Centipede venom proteins are highly diverse, with 61 distinct venom protein and peptide families, with little overlap with other animal venoms.

Specific Investigations

- CBC and fibrin split products after brown recluse spider bite
- Rickettsial immunofluorescence and immunoperoxidase
- Lyme serologic tests
- ELISA, PCR, and immunofluorescence for virus such as West Nile, Dengue, and Chikungunya

PCR assays can also be used to identify biting insects too small for conventional identification

IgE typing, skin testing, and basophil activation testing can be used to confirm the cause of anaphylaxis.

Tryptase levels can be used to predict severe reactions and in forensic investigations to confirm death from anaphylaxis. Expression of Th1 and Th2 trafficking can be used to follow the course of immunotherapy.

Venom immunotherapy: an updated review. Antolín-Amérigo D, Moreno Aguilar C, Vega A, Alvarez-Mon M. Curr Allergy Asthma Rep 2014; 14: 449.

In patients with negative serum IgE and skin prick testing, basophil activation tests are promising to guide therapy.

Expression of Th1, Th2, lymphocyte trafficking and activation markers on CD4+ T-cells of *Hymenoptera* allergic subjects and after venom immunotherapy. Cabrera CM, Urra JM, Alfaya T, Roca Fde L, Feo-Brito F. Mol Immunol 2014; 62: 178–85.

A shift toward a Th1-type response characterized by an increase in IFN-γ levels is observed after venom immunotherapy.

New directions in diagnostic evaluation of insect allergy. Golden DB. Curr Opin Allergy Clin Immunol 2014; 14: 334–9.

Measurement of IgE to recombinant venom allergens can distinguish cross-sensitization from dual sensitization to honeybee and vespid venoms, helping to limit venom immunotherapy to a single venom.

Anaphylaxis to insect venom allergens: role of molecular diagnostics. Ollert M, Blank S. Curr Allergy Asthma Rep 2015; 15: 26.

Knowledge about the molecular composition of *Hymenoptera* venoms has increased and resulted in the ability to measure specific IgE in venom-allergic patients. Recombinant venom allergens are not available.

Advances in allergic skin disease, anaphylaxis, and hypersensitivity reactions to foods, drugs, and insects in 2014. Sicherer SH, Leung DY. J Allergy Clin Immunol 2015; 135: 357–67.

Baseline platelet-activating factor acetylhydrolase levels are promising as a marker to predict the severity of sting reactions.

First-Line Therapies

Prevention

DEET	A
Permethrin	A
Picaridin	B
Combinations of DEET and permethrin	A

Flea treatments for pets

Lufenuron	A
Fipronil	A
Imidacloprid	A

Anaphylaxis

Epinephrine	A
Immunotherapy	A

Spider bites

Rest, ice, and elevation	B
Tetracycline or triamcinolone for brown recluse bites	C
Antivenin for brown recluse bites	C
Antivenin for black widow and red-black spider bites	A

Scorpion stings

Antivenin for stings in Arizona	B
Prazosin for Indian red scorpion stings	A

Arthropod borne infections

Lyme borreliosis	
Tetracycline	A
Amoxicillin in children	A
Intravenous ceftriaxone	A
Rocky Mountain spotted fever	
Doxycycline	A
Human monocytic ehrlichiosis	
Human anaplasmosis	
Babesiosis	
Azithromycin and atovaquone	A
Quinine and clindamycin	A

Venom immunotherapy: an updated review. Antolín-Amérigo D, Moreno Aguilar C, Vega A, Alvarez-Mon M. Curr Allergy Asthma Rep 2014; 14: 449.

Venom immunotherapy is the most effective form of specific immunotherapy in use.

Mildly heated forceps: a useful instrument for easy and complete removal of ticks on the skin. Jang YH, Moon SY, Lee WJ, Lee SJ, Kim Do W. J Am Acad Dermatol 2014; 71: e199–200.

Heating of forceps has been used to enhance tick removal.

Mosquito repellents for travelers. Stanczyk NM, Behrens RH, Chen-Hussey V, Stewart SA, Logan JG. BMJ 2015; 350: h99.

Repellents have improved and provide sustained protection against insect bites and mosquitoborne disease.

Are we doing enough to promote the effective use of mosquito repellents? Webb CE. Med J Aust 2015; 202: 128–9.

Despite their wide availability, mosquito repellents are often not used.

Are topical insect repellents effective against malaria in endemic populations? A systematic review and meta-analysis. Wilson AL, Chen-Hussey V, Logan JG, Lindsay SW. Malar J 2014; 13: 446.

Meta-analysis suggests that although topical repellents provide individual protection against mosquito bites, their ability to provide effective sustained protection against malaria in endemic populations did not reach statistical significance, suggesting continued need for malaria prophylaxis in long-term travelers and the need for other effective strategies to control the disease.

Second-Line Therapies	
Repellents	
• Botanicals	C
• Novel pyrethroids	C
Relief of pruritus	
• Camphor and menthol	E
• Pramoxine	E
• Lidocaine	E
• Benzocaine	E
• Lidocaine/prilocaine	E
Treatment of bite and sting reactions	
• Superpotent and potent topical corticosteroids	E
• For young children: mild-to-moderate–strength topical corticosteroids	E
• Local ice	C
• Local heat	C
• New immunotherapy agents	B
• Omalizumab for patients with adverse reactions to immunotherapy	C
Indian red scorpion stings	
• Captopril	C
• Antivenin	D
Arthropodborne infections	
• Babesiosis	
• Atovaquone-proguanil in immunosuppressed patients	C

Insecticide-treated clothes for the control of vector-borne diseases: a review on effectiveness and safety. Banks SD, Murray N, Wilder-Smith A, Logan JG. Med Vet Entomol 2014; 28 (Suppl 1): 14–25.

New microencapsulation technologies may prolong the activity of insecticides on clothing. These can help to overcome reduction in efficacy as a result of washing, ultraviolet light exposure, and normal wear and tear.

Persistently high estimates of late night, indoor exposure to malaria vectors despite high coverage of insecticide treated nets. Bayoh MN, Walker ED, Kosgei J, Ombok M, Olang GB, Githeko AK, et al. Parasit Vectors 2014; 7: 380.

Despite the use of impregnated nets, indoor bites continue at a high rate, suggesting the need for better agents.

Developing a preventive immunization approach against insect bite hypersensitivity using recombinant allergens: a pilot study. Jonsdottir S, Hamza E, Janda J, Rhyner C, Meinke A, Marti E, et al. Vet Immunol Immunopathol 2015; 166: 8–21.

Recombinant allergens for immunotherapy have been used successfully in horses.

Treatment with a combination of omalizumab and specific immunotherapy for severe anaphylaxis after a wasp sting. Palgan K, Bartuzi Z, Gotz-Zbikowska M. Int J Immunopathol Pharmacol 2014; 27: 109–12.

Venom immunotherapy may provoke immediate anaphylaxis, which can lead to treatment withdrawal. The antiimmunoglobulin (Ig) E monoclonal antibody omalizumab proved useful to allow resumption of immunotherapy.

Third-Line Therapies	
Treatment of bites	
• Intralesional corticosteroids	E
• Enhanced penetration topical antihistamines	B
Repellents	
• Newer agents and botanicals	C
• New vaccines in development for vectorborne illness	C

Good performances but short lasting efficacy of Actellic 50 EC Indoor Residual Spraying (IRS) on malaria transmission in Benin, West Africa. Aïkpon R, Sèzonlin M, Tokponon F, Okè M, Oussou O, Oké-Agbo F, et al. Parasit Vectors 2014; 30: 256.

Pirimiphos methyl used for indoor residual spraying resulted in a significant reduction (94.25%) in bite rate and the entomologic inoculation rate (99.24% reduction).

A *Listeria monocytogenes*-based vaccine that secretes sand fly salivary protein LJM11 confers long-term protection against vector-transmitted *Leishmania major*. Abi Abdallah DS, Pavinski Bitar A, Oliveira F, Meneses C, Park JJ, Mendez S, et al. Infect Immun 2014; 82: 2736–45.

A sand fly salivary protein vaccine using an attenuated strain of *Listeria monocytogenes* shows promise for the prevention of leishmaniasis.

Ethosomes-based topical delivery system of antihistaminic drug for treatment of skin allergies. Goindi S, Dhatt B, Kaur A. J Microencapsul 2014; 31: 716–24.

An ethosome-based topical formulation of cetirizine dihydrochloride consisting of drug, phospholipon 90 G, and ethanol was effective in atopic dermatitis–related itching and could be of benefit for bite reactions.

Laboratory evaluation of citronella, picaridin, and DEET repellents against *Psorophora ciliata* and *Psorophora howardii*. Scott JM, Hossain T, Davidson C, Smith ML, Xue RD. J Am Mosq Control Assoc 2014; 30: 136–7.

Citronella-based repellents are less effective than standard chemical repellents.

Evidence Levels: **A** Double-blind study **B** Clinical trial ≥ 20 subjects **C** Clinical trial < 20 subjects **D** Series ≥ 5 subjects **E** Anecdotal case reports

Blastomycosis

Wanda Sonia Robles, Mahreen Ameen

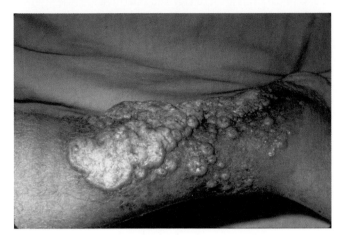

With permission from Lebwohl MG. Atlas of the Skin and Systemic Disease. Churchill Livingstone: Elsevier, 1995. Courtesy of Fabio Barbosa, MD.

Blastomycosis is a systemic, suppurative granulomatous infection caused by the thermally dimorphic fungus *Blastomyces dermatitidis*. It is acquired by inhalation of the conidia, which are transformed into the yeast form in the lungs. It is an endemic mycosis that is most prevalent in the North American continent, particularly in the states that border the Mississippi and Ohio rivers and the Great Lakes region. Cases have also been reported in Latin America, Africa, the Middle East, and India. Consequently, the term *North American blastomycosis* is now obsolete. Point-source epidemics have been reported in endemic regions relating to recreational activities in wooded areas along waterways.

Blastomycosis is associated with a spectrum of disease ranging from subclinical infection to an acute or chronic pneumonia. Most cases are restricted to the respiratory system, and many are asymptomatic. Extrapulmonary infection occurs in 25% to 40% of cases and most commonly affects the skin. Cutaneous manifestations range from papules to verrucous and ulcerative lesions. The bones, genitourinary system, and central nervous system (CNS) may also be involved. Dissemination occurs more frequently in the immunocompromised, such as organ transplant recipients and those with HIV infection. The immunocompromised are at high risk of CNS involvement and adult respiratory distress syndrome. Their prognosis is poor and therefore they require aggressive management. There are also rare reports of primary cutaneous blastomycosis acquired after accidental inoculation, and in some cases infection has been self-limiting.

MANAGEMENT STRATEGY

In the immunocompetent individual, acute pulmonary blastomycosis may be mild and self-limiting. However, all diagnosed cases are treated in order to prevent extrapulmonary dissemination. Itraconazole is the drug of choice for the treatment of non-CNS infection that is not life threatening. A loading dose of 200 mg three times daily for 3 days followed by 200 mg once or twice

daily for 6 to 12 months is recommended. Serum itraconazole levels should be measured 2 weeks after commencement of treatment. Ketoconazole (400–800 mg daily) and fluconazole (400–800 mg daily) are second-line agents, as they have lower efficacy against *Blastomyces*. In addition, long-term treatment with ketoconazole is associated with adverse effects. The new-generation azoles, voriconazole and posaconazole, have demonstrated activity against *B. dermatitidis* in in vitro and animal studies. There have been reports of the successful use of voriconazole in the treatment of CNS blastomycosis. Amphotericin B is the treatment of choice for those who fail on treatment with azoles, who have severe infection, the immunosuppressed, in pregnancy, and with CNS involvement. The experience to date has been largely with the use of amphotericin B deoxycholate. Liposomal amphotericin B is recommended for CNS infection, as it achieves higher CNS penetration and is better tolerated with prolonged therapy. This is also recommended for severe lung disease. After an initial response with amphotericin B, step-down therapy to an azole is common practice.

Specific Investigations

- Direct microscopy
- Culture
- Histopathology
- Chest radiography
- Bone scanning (radionuclide bone scan/computed tomography/magnetic resonance imaging [CT/MRI])
- Serology for HIV infection (where relevant)

Definitive diagnosis of blastomycosis is based on the identification of characteristic thick-walled, broad-based budding yeasts by direct examination of tissue or the isolation of *Blastomyces* in culture. Specimens for direct microscopy in 10% KOH can be skin scrapings, pus from skin lesions, sputum, and biopsy tissue from any lesion suspicious of infection. Successful culture of sputum, tissue biopsy specimens, cerebrospinal fluid, or urine produces a white mold at 25°C on Sabouraud agar and a brown wrinkled colony at 37°C on blood agar. Histopathology of infected tissues reveals a pyogranulomatous response without caseation and pseudoepitheliomatous hyperplasia. A *Blastomyces* antigen assay is available to test urine, blood, and other fluids, but it is not always specific. Antibody assays are nonspecific and insensitive.

Cutaneous inoculation blastomycosis. Gray NA, Baddour LM. Clin Infect Dis 2002; 34: e44–9.

This article reports a case in a male adult that resulted from inoculation after being struck by a projectile while performing yard work. It also reviews 21 previous published cases of cutaneous inoculation. Skin lesions were associated with lymphadenopathy or lymphangitis in 65% of cases. Organisms were recovered from skin lesions by direct microscopy or culture. Fifty percent of cases occurred after exposure in a clinical setting (laboratory or morgue). The median incubation period was only 2 weeks. One case was self-limiting, a further three were treated with surgery, and the remainder were successfully treated with the antifungals ketoconazole and itraconazole.

First-Line Therapies

• Itraconazole	B
• Amphotericin B	C

Blastomycosis. Castillo CG, Kauffman CA, Miceli MH. Infect Dis Clin North Am 2016; 30: 247–64.

This very good review advocates the use of itraconazole for either mild-to-moderate pulmonary or extrapulmonary infection and lipid formulation amphotericin B for cases of severe or life-threatening infection followed by step-down therapy with itraconazole.

Itraconazole therapy for blastomycosis and histoplasmosis. NIAID Mycoses Study Group; Dismukes WE, Badcher RW, Cloud JC, Kauffman CA, Chapman SW, George RB, et al. Am J Med 1992; 93: 489–97.

A prospective, nonrandomized, multicenter trial involving 48 patients with pulmonary or disseminated blastomycosis without CNS involvement. Patients were treated with itraconazole 200 to 400 mg/day for a median period of 6.2 months with a 90% cure rate (43/48). Treatment was very well tolerated, and there was no therapeutic advantage for patients treated with the higher dose.

Endemic blastomycosis in Mississippi: epidemiologic and clinical studies. Chapman SW, Lin AC, Hendricks KA, Nolan RL, Currier MM, Morris KR, et al. Semin Respir Infect 1997; 12: 219–28.

This was a review of 326 confirmed cases of blastomycosis from Mississippi. There was involvement of lungs (91.4%), skin (18.1%), bone (4.3%), genitourinary system (1.8%), and CNS (1.2%). Skin or bone disease was associated with multiorgan involvement. A successful outcome without relapse was noted in 86.5% of amphotericin B deoxycholate–treated patients and in 81.7% of ketoconazole-treated patients. The relapse rate for ketoconazole-treated patients was higher than for amphotericin B–treated patients (14% and 3.9%, respectively).

Blastomycosis of the central nervous system: a multicenter review of diagnosis and treatment in the modern era. Bariola JR, Perry P, Pappas PG, Proia L, Shealey W, Wright PW, et al. Clin Infect Dis 2010; 50: 797–804.

A retrospective study of 22 patients with CNS infection treated with either amphotericin B deoxycholate or a lipid formulation of amphotericin B followed by a prolonged course of oral azole therapy (voriconazole, fluconazole, or itraconazole).

The most favorable outcomes were achieved with initial treatment with a lipid formulation of amphotericin B followed by a prolonged course of oral voriconazole.

Second-Line Therapies	
• Ketoconazole	B
• Fluconazole	B
• Voriconazole	D
• Caspofungin	E
• Isavuconazole	E

Treatment of blastomycosis and histoplasmosis with ketoconazole. Results of a prospective randomized clinical trial. National Institute of Allergy and Infectious Diseases Mycoses Study Group; Dismukes WE, Cloud G, Bowles C. Ann Intern Med 1985; 103: 861–72.

This was a multicenter, prospective, randomized trial. Of 65 patients with blastomycosis treated for 6 months or more, high-dose ketoconazole (800 mg daily) was significantly more effective than low-dose ketoconazole (400 mg daily) (100% vs. 79% cure rate, *p* = 0.001). Adverse effects occurred in 60% of patients and were more common in those treated at higher doses. Therefore the study group recommended that treatment should commence at the lower dose.

Despite its efficacy, ketoconazole is now rarely used because of its associated adverse effects as well as the availability of better-tolerated azoles.

Treatment of blastomycosis with fluconazole: a pilot study. The National Institute of Allergy and Infectious Disease Mycoses Study Group; Pappas PG, Bradsher RW, Chapman SW, Kauffman CA, Dine A, Cloud GA, et al. Clin Infect Dis 1995; 20: 267–71.

A multicenter, randomized, open-label, pilot study compared two doses of fluconazole (200 and 400 mg daily) for the treatment of non–life-threatening blastomycosis. The analysis data included 23 patients who were treated for a minimum 6-month period. There was a successful outcome in 65% of patients (15/23) with no relapse at follow-up at 7 months. Of those who responded, 62% (8/15) had received 200 mg daily and 70% (7/10) received 400 mg daily.

The results of this study were disappointing. However, fluconazole has excellent CNS penetration and may therefore have a better role in the treatment of CNS infection, although there are no studies to support this.

Treatment of blastomycosis with higher doses of fluconazole. The National Institute of Allergy and Infectious Disease Mycoses Study Group; Pappas PG, Bradsher RW, Kauffman CA, Cloud GA, Thomas CJ, Campbell GD Jr, et al. Clin Infect Dis 1997; 25: 200–5.

This multicenter, randomized, open-label study investigated the efficacy of high-dose fluconazole (400–800 mg daily) for the treatment of non–life-threatening blastomycosis. There was an 87% cure rate (34/39) after a mean treatment period of 8.9 months.

This study demonstrates a much higher efficacy for fluconazole at doses of 400 to 800 mg daily.

The role of voriconazole in the treatment of central nervous system blastomycosis. Ta M, Flowers SA, Rogers PD. Ann Pharmacother 2009; 43: 1696–700.

Seven cases of CNS blastomycosis successfully treated sequentially with amphotericin B followed by voriconazole are described.

Animal and human studies indicate that high concentrations of voriconazole can be achieved in the cerebrospinal fluid (CSF) and brain tissue. The authors suggest that voriconazole may be considered an azole option for either follow-up therapy after liposomal amphotericin B therapy or as salvage therapy in patients intolerant of amphotericin B or other azoles.

Voriconazole use for endemic fungal infections. Hage CA, Bowyer S, Tarvin SE, Helper D, Kleiman MB, Joseph Wheat L. Clin Infect Dis 2010; 50: 85–92.

Eight patients with blastomycosis either improved or remained stable with voriconazole therapy, although two subsequently relapsed. In these cases voriconazole was used as salvage therapy, particularly in patients who demonstrated intolerance to other antifungal agents.

Treatment of chronic pulmonary blastomycosis with caspofungin. Mardini J, Nguyen B, Ghannoum M, Couture C, Lavergne V. J Med Microbiol 2011; 60: 1875–8.

This is a case report of chronic pulmonary blastomycosis successfully treated with caspofungin.

Evidence Levels: **A** Double-blind study **B** Clinical trial ≥ 20 subjects **C** Clinical trial < 20 subjects **D** Series ≥ 5 subjects **E** Anecdotal case reports

Echinocandins have not been recommended for the treatment of blastomycosis because of poor in vitro activity against Blastomyces dermatitidis and until now a lack of supporting clinical data.

Isavuconazole treatment of cryptococcosis and dimorphic mycoses. Thompson GR 3rd, Rendon A, Ribeiro Dos Santos R, Queiroz-Telles F, Ostrosky-Zeichner L, Azie N, et al. Clin Infect Dis. 2016; 63: 356–62.

An open-label, nonrandomized, phase III trial to evaluate efficacy and safety of isavuconazole in the management of invasive fungal infections.

Findings: well tolerated, clinical activity against endemic fungi, with safety profile similar to those observed in larger studies.

This drug is recommended as a valuable alternative to currently available agents.

GUIDELINES

Clinical practice guidelines for the management of blastomycosis: 2008 update by the Infectious Diseases Society of America. Infectious Diseases Society of America; Chapman SW, Dismukes WE, Proia LA, Bradsher RW, Pappas PG, Threlkeld MG, et al. Clin Infect Dis 2008; 46: 1801–12.

This updated evidence-based guideline replaces the previous guidelines published in 2000. Treatment is guided by the extent of infection, CNS involvement, and the immune state of the host. Previously, mild cases of pulmonary blastomycosis were managed conservatively, as they are sometimes self-limiting. However, with the advent and high efficacy of oral azoles, primarily itraconazole, most cases are now actively treated in order to prevent extrapulmonary spread and any risk of future reactivation.

- Itraconazole is the drug of choice for the treatment of mild-to-moderate pulmonary or disseminated infection. The recommended dose is an initial loading dose of 200 mg three times daily for 3 days, followed by 200 mg once or twice daily for 6 to 12 months. Serum levels should be measured after 2 weeks to ensure adequate drug exposure.
- Amphotericin B is the treatment of choice for those with severe pulmonary or disseminated infection and in the immunocompromised. Either the lipid formulation (3–5 mg/kg/day) or amphotericin deoxycholate (0.7–1 mg/kg/day) is given for 1 to 2 weeks or until improvement is noted. Itraconazole is then recommended as step-down therapy (loading dose and then 200 mg twice daily for 6–12 months, except in the immunocompromised, who require at least 12 months of treatment or until immunosuppression has been reversed).
- Liposomal amphotericin B at a dose of 5 mg/kg/day is the recommended treatment for CNS infection. Treatment should be given for 4 to 6 weeks followed by an oral azole (fluconazole 800 mg daily/itraconazole 200 mg two to three times daily/voriconazole 200–400 mg twice daily), which should be given for at least 12 months and until there is resolution of CSF abnormalities.
- Amphotericin B is the drug of choice for patients who have failed to respond to azole treatment.
- Amphotericin B is the only drug approved for the treatment of blastomycosis in pregnant women.

30

Blistering distal dactylitis

Irshad Zaki

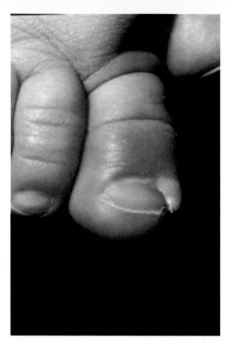

Courtesy of Joseph Bikowski, MD.

Blistering distal dactylitis (BDD) is a superficial, tender, blistering infection seen in childhood and the early teens. It is usually caused by group A β-hemolytic streptococci, although group B organisms, staphylococci, and more recently methicillin-resistant *Staphylococcus aureus* (MRSA) have also been implicated. The distal volar fat pads of the fingers are the most common site of infection, but involvement of the nail folds and toes can occasionally occur.

MANAGEMENT STRATEGY

BDD can cause considerable alarm to parents, as large tense blisters rapidly develop. Despite the absence of constitutional symptoms, patients usually seek help soon after the onset of the infection. The condition does not resolve spontaneously, but prompt treatment results in rapid improvement. *Blisters should be incised to release fluid*, which can vary from clear and watery to frank pus. Subsequent application of topical antibiotics can be helpful, but systemic treatment is usually also required. *Penicillin V* is the treatment of choice for streptococcal infection, but *erythromycin* is an effective alternative for patients allergic to penicillin. It is important to exclude MRSA or immunosuppression for resistant cases.

The differential diagnosis of the condition includes traumatic blisters, herpetic whitlow, staphylococcal bullous impetigo, and the Weber–Cockayne variant of epidermolysis bullosa.

Specific Investigations

- Gram stain of blister fluid
- Culture of blister fluid
- Swab of nasopharynx for bacteriology

A clinically recognizable streptococcal infection. Hays GC, Mullard JE. Paediatrics 1975; 56: 129–31.

First large series report describing 13 patients with BDD. Streptococci were found on culture of blister fluid in all cases, and gram-positive cocci were usually found on Gram staining. This report suggests a link with infection of the nasopharynx, but this has not been confirmed in other case reports.

Blistering distal dactylitis in an adult. Kollipara R, Downing C, Lee M, Guidry J, Robare-Stout S, Tyring S. J Cutan Med Surg 2015; 19: 397–9.

Although the majority of cases are in children over the age of 2, this has also been described in adults, particularly if immunosuppressed. Bacteriology should be considered for an isolated distal phalanx blister at any age.

First-Line Therapies

• Incision and drainage of blister	C
• Topical antibiotics	C
• Systemic penicillin	C

Is blistering distal dactylitis a variant of bullous impetigo? Scheinfeld NS. Clin Exp Dermatol 2007; 32: 314–6.

Good review of literature and treatment. Confirms the importance of incision and drainage, adequate dressings, and the need to consider *S. aureus* as a cause if penicillin is ineffective.

Second-Line Therapies

• Systemic erythromycin	D
• Intravenous vancomycin	D

Blistering distal dactylitis: a manifestation of group A beta-haemolytic streptococcal infection. Schneider JA, Parlette HL. Arch Dermatol 1982; 118: 879–80.

Short report of the authors' personal experience, suggesting that this is a relatively common problem. Systemic penicillin and erythromycin were both found to be effective. It is likely that many cases of BDD are wrongly diagnosed as bullous impetigo by clinicians not familiar with this disorder.

MRSA blistering distal dactylitis and review of reported cases. Fretzayas A, Moustaki M, Tsagris V, Brozou T, Nicolaidou P. Pediatr Dermatol 2011; 28: 433–5.

First report of BDD due to MRSA infection. This case highlights the importance of culture of blister fluid, as infection with this organism may increase in the future.

Evidence Levels: A Double-blind study B Clinical trial ≥ 20 subjects C Clinical trial < 20 subjects D Series ≥ 5 subjects E Anecdotal case reports

Third-Line Therapies	
• Amoxicillin/clavulanic acid	D
• Conservative measures for herpetic whitlow	D

A review and report of blistering distal dactylitis due to *Staphylococcus aureus* in two HIV-positive men. Scheinfeld N. Dermatol Online J 2007; 13: 8.

S. aureus was found to be the etiologic agent in two HIV-positive patients. The condition improved after treatment with a proprietary mixture of amoxicillin trihydrate and clavulanate potassium. The report highlights that blisters may not always be present and that BDD may present with erosions.

Coexistent infections on a child's distal phalanx: blistering dactylitis and herpetic whitlow. Ney AC, English JC 3rd, Greer KE. Cutis 2002; 69: 46–8.

Consider comorbidity if BDD does not respond to antibiotics.

31

Body dysmorphic disorder (dermatologic nondisease)

Synonyms: Dermatologic nondisease, Body dysmorphic disease, Dysmorphophobia.

Colin A. Morton

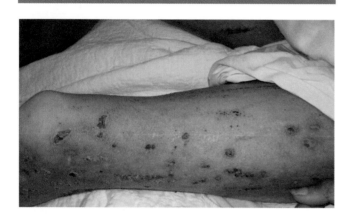

Body dysmorphic disorder (BDD) is an alteration in perception of body image that causes preoccupation with a minimal or imagined defect in appearance. The preoccupation can be markedly excessive, causing clinically significant emotional distress and impairment in social, occupational, or other important areas of functioning. Preoccupations commonly involve the face and head, with skin and hair being the most frequent areas of concern. However, any area of the body may be involved. Dermatologic preoccupations are distressing, time consuming, and difficult or impossible for patients to resist. Insight is typically poor, and alterations in perception are often to delusional proportion. Most patients have ideas of reference, thinking that others take special notice or mock them for their perceived defect. Repetitive behaviors are present in almost all patients, such as excessive checking or grooming, innumerable consultations with dermatologists and plastic surgeons, constant need for reference and reassurance, and skin manipulations. Risk of suicidal ideation and attempts are high, affecting approximately one quarter of BDD patients.

MANAGEMENT STRATEGY

BDD is common in dermatologic settings, with prevalence estimated at 11.9%. Recognition of these patients is extremely important because they typically have psychiatric comorbidities, diminished quality of life, and impairments in psychosocial and vocational function. They are usually poor candidates for cosmetic procedures. Dissatisfaction, anger, and even aggression directed toward the treating clinician have been reported.

Patients with BDD often have associated psychiatric disorders, including major depression, substance abuse and dependence, social phobia, and obsessive-compulsive disorder (OCD). Recent studies have suggested abnormal brain network organization with magnetic resonance (MR) imaging, which may provide some biologic basis for the characteristic distortions in self-perception. The majority of these patients also have a personality disorder. Appropriate psychiatric treatment can result in a generally favorable outcome.

Typical body areas of preoccupation include:

- Face. Preoccupation with facial itching and burning or obsessive preoccupation with imagined acne, scars, wrinkles, pigmentation, oiliness, redness, paleness, facial vessels, and facial hair are common. Preoccupation with the nose, ears, and pore size is reported. Despite the fact that others usually do not see these minimal or nonexistent flaws, patients can spend hours in front of mirrors, preventing them from working or socializing.
- Scalp. Dysesthesias (burning or itch) and obsession with imagined hair loss are common.
- Genital. Genital size, scrotal, perineal, and perianal burning, as well as vulvar redness and burning are common symptoms. Preoccupation with sexually transmitted disease or neoplastic process is common. Symptoms can be incapacitating.

Hallmarks and Flags for Diagnosis of Body Dysmorphic Disorder

Patients presenting with extreme concern that appears out of proportion to their chief complaint accompanied by a paucity of objective physical findings should raise suspicion that BDD may be present. Obsession, rumination, and extreme psychological distress are striking features. These patients usually report dissatisfaction with previous physicians and describe poor outcomes from past medical and surgical interventions. Skin picking and related behaviors such as excessive tanning, excessive grooming, and relentless need for reassurance are characteristic. Attempts to correct their perceptions are inevitably futile because their perceptual distortions and associated cognitions are deeply entrenched. It can be argued that the distorted perceptions are delusional, which, by definition, suggests that they are unresponsive to objective logic and persuasion. Patients often wear heavy makeup, hats, sunglasses, scarves, and other clothing to hide their imperfections and perceived ugliness.

Patients with BDD often make unusual and excessive requests for cosmetic procedures with the belief that the procedure will transform or fix their lives. Poor psychosocial functioning with difficulties in relationships, school, and work is almost always seen. Depression is frequently evident, and previous suicide attempts are not infrequent. Bear in mind that there have been instances of violent behavior toward treatment providers.

Clinical interactions and consultations with these patients are typically long, difficult, and emotionally draining. Regardless of the actual length of time spent with them, BDD patients often feel that they were not given adequate time and attention. As already stated, it is inadvisable to perform procedures on these patients because less than 10% will be satisfied with the results of medical or surgical interventions.

Serotonin selective reuptake inhibitors (SSRIs) and cognitive behavior psychotherapy remain the treatments of choice. Fluoxetine, fluvoxamine, and citalopram are the best-studied agents, but recent evidence suggests that all SSRIs are probably effective. Higher dosing regimens than those used for depression

Evidence Levels: **A** Double-blind study **B** Clinical trial ≥ 20 subjects **C** Clinical trial < 20 subjects **D** Series ≥ 5 subjects **E** Anecdotal case reports

Table 31.1 Screening questions

1. How much do you currently think about your skin?
2. On an average day, how many hours do you spend thinking about your skin? Please add up all the time that your feature is on your mind and make your best estimate.
3. Do you feel your skin is ugly or very unattractive?
4. How noticeable do you think your skin is?
5. Does your skin currently cause you a lot of distress?
6. How many times a day do you usually check your skin, either in a mirror or by feeling it with your fingers?
7. How often do you feel anxious about your skin in social situations? Does it lead to you avoiding social situations?
8. Has your skin had an effect on dating or on an existing relationship?
9. Has your skin interfered with your ability to work or study, or your role as a homemaker?

(Adapted from Veale D, Ellison N, Werner TG, Dodhia R, Serfaty MA, Clarke A. Development of a cosmetic procedure screening questionnaire (COPSs) for body dysmorphic disorder. J Plast Reconstr Aesthet Surg 2012; 65: 530–2.)

are usually required. For example, fluoxetine and citalopram should be titrated to 60 mg per day, and fluvoxamine should be increased to 300 mg per day at monthly intervals. Patients should receive a trial of 12 to 16 weeks before efficacy is assessed. If one agent fails, another should be substituted because some patients idiosyncratically respond more favorably to one agent over another. SSRIs appear to be more effective than antipsychotic agents despite the fact that BDD can involve severe distortions in self-perception to delusional proportion. Interestingly, only about 20% of patients will become free of their delusional thinking. However, the intrusiveness of the thoughts and distress will diminish sufficiently such that many patients will be able to resume some social and vocational functioning.

Cognitive behavior therapy (CBT) is a reality-based, in-the-present therapy that specifically focuses on the affected individual's cognitions and associated emotional experiences. The key elements are known as *exposure, response prevention, perceptual retraining*, and *cognitive restructuring*. Exposure consists of having patients expose the perceived defect in social and work situations. Response prevention techniques help patients avoid performance of their repetitive behaviors such as avoidance of others, excessive camouflage, picking, hyperventilating, etc. Perceptual retraining involves the development of a more holistic positive view of appearance. Cognitive restructuring helps patients challenge and eventually change their erroneous beliefs about their appearance. Ideally, treatment of BDD should encompass both CBT and an SSRI.

To initiate treatment or referral, suggest to the patient in a gentle manner that they may have a body image disorder called BDD. Convey your concern regarding the amount of their time being usurped by their preoccupation and their emotional distress. Psychiatric referral is preferable but often not feasible. Dermatologists are encouraged to align themselves, if possible, with mental health professionals who are experienced in treating this entity. Euphemisms for the psychiatric practitioner such as skin-emotion specialist may reduce the stigma of psychiatric referral and may increase patient acceptance. If referral is not possible, treating with an SSRI may be successful. If suicidal ideation or intent is present, immediate hospitalization is recommended.

Specific Investigations

- Assess for potential suicide risk; emergent referral and appropriate notification if active ideation or intent
- Assess for any evidence of physical or emotional abuse
- Assess for evidence of substance abuse

- Assess for concomitant underlying psychiatric disease (i.e., depression/anxiety/OCD/psychosis), and make an appropriate psychiatric referral
- Appropriately diagnose and acknowledge genuine skin disease (i.e., hair loss, acne, rosacea, psoriasis, eczema, keratosis pilaris, seborrheic keratoses, dyschromia) and offer legitimate therapies
- Investigate perceived skin changes appropriately to rule out atypical presentations of an underlying organic process if suspicion is present; perform bacterial, viral, fungal cultures, skin biopsy, serologies, and imaging studies when deemed appropriate

Depression, anxiety, anger, and somatic symptoms in patients with body dysmorphic disorder. Phillips KA, Siniscalchi JM, McElroy SL. Psychiatr Q 2004; 75: 309–20.

Seventy-five patients with BDD completed a symptom questionnaire assessing depression, anxiety, somatic/somatization, and anger-hostility. Compared with normal controls, BDD subjects had markedly elevated scores on all four scales, indicating severe distress and psychopathology. When treated with fluvoxamine, all symptoms significantly improved.

Quality of life for patients with body dysmorphic disorder. Phillips KA. J Nerv Ment Dis 2000; 188: 170–5.

This is the only published study looking at quality of life (QOL) in BDD patients. These patients were found to have a poorer mental health QOL than has been reported for patients with other severe illnesses such as type 2 diabetes, recent myocardial infarction, or depression. These findings highlight the dramatic impact of a nondisease.

Thirty-three cases of body dysmorphic disorder in children and adolescents. Albertini RS, Phillips KA. J Am Acad Child Adolesc Psychiatry 1999; 38: 453–9.

Thirty-three cases were examined. Onset was usually during adolescence but sometimes occurred in childhood. Earlier identification and treatment may avert unnecessary cosmetic and medical interventions as well as suicide.

Gender differences in body dysmorphic disorder. Phillips KA, Diaz S. J Nerv Ment Dis 1997; 185: 570–7.

This study looked at a large series of patients with DSM-IV–defined BDD and found that one quarter of patients had attempted suicide. Female patients with severe symptoms are at greater risk.

Suicide in dermatological patients. Cotterill JA, Cunliffe WJ. Br J Dermatol 1997; 137: 246–50.

Sixteen patients who had committed suicide are described. Most of these patients had acne or BDD. Females with facial complaints and men with facial scarring appeared more at risk for suicide. The authors relate these findings to the possible preventive benefits of early isotretinoin to prevent scarring in patients predisposed to BDD.

Diagnostic Aids

The Body Dysmorphic Disorder Symptom Scale: development and preliminary validation of a self-report scale of symptom specific dysfunction. Wilhelm S, Greenberg JL, Rosenfield E, Kasarskis I, Blashill AJ. Body Image 2016; 17: 82–7.

This report evaluates and compares the psychometric characteristics of the BDD-SS (Body Dysmorphic Disorder Symptom Scale) in relation to other measures of BDD, body image, and depression in 99 adult participants diagnosed with BDD.

First-Line Therapies	
• SSRIs	A
• Cognitive behavior therapy	B

Treating body dysmorphic disorder with medication: evidence, misconceptions, and a suggested approach. Phillips KA, Hollander E. Body Image 2008; 5: 13–27.

SSRIs are associated with improvement in core BDD symptoms, psychosocial functioning, QOL, suicidality, and other aspects of BDD.

Pharmacotherapy and psychotherapy for body dysmorphic disorder. Ipser JC, Sander C, Stein DJ. Cochrane Database Syst Rev. 2009; 1: CD005332.

Supports efficacy of SSRIs.

A randomized placebo-controlled trial of fluoxetine in body dysmorphic disorder. Phillips KA, Albertini RS, Rasmussen SA. Arch Gen Psychiatry 2002; 59: 381–8.

This is the only placebo-controlled BDD pharmacotherapy study. In the 74 patients studied, fluoxetine was significantly more effective than placebo, with a response rate of 53% versus 18%.

Pharmacotherapy relapse prevention in body dysmorphic disorder: a double-blind, placebo-controlled trial. Phillips KA, Keshaviah A, Dougherty DD, Stout RL, Menard W, Wilhelm S. Am J Psychiatry 2016; 173: 887–95.

One hundred BDD subjects treated with citalopram for 14 weeks with 81% response rate. Fifty-eight responders were treated with additional citalopram or placebo for 6 months. Placebo group was 40% versus 18% for citalopram. Study supports ongoing maintenance therapy.

An open label study of venlafaxine in body dysmorphic disorder. Allen A, Hadley SJ, Kaplan A, Simeon D, Friedberg J, Priday L, et al. CNS Spectr 2008; 13: 138–44.

Seventeen patients enrolled; 11 completed 12 to 16 weeks of venlafaxine at a minimum dose of 150 mg a day. All 11 patients significantly improved.

Clomipramine versus desipramine crossover trial in body dysmorphic disorder: selective efficacy of a serotonin reuptake inhibitor in imagined ugliness. Hollander E, Allen A, Kwon J, Mosovich S, Schmeidler J, Wong C. Arch Gen Psychiatry 1999; 56: 1033–9.

This double-blind, crossover study of 29 randomized patients found clomipramine (an SSRI) superior to desipramine (a non-SSRI tricyclic antidepressant).

Efficacy and safety of fluvoxamine in body dysmorphic disorder. Phillips KA, Dwight MM, McElroy SL. J Clin Psychiatry 1998; 59: 165–71.

Open-label study of fluvoxamine demonstrated good clinical response in 19 (63%) of 30 patients.

Delusionality and response to open-label fluvoxamine in body dysmorphic disorder. Phillips KA, McElroy SL, Dwight MM, Eisen JL, Rasmussen SA. J Clin Psychiatry 2001; 62: 87–91.

Thirty patients with BDD were treated with fluvoxamine for 16 weeks in this open-label trial. Sixty-three percent of treated patients significantly improved. Important to note that both delusional and nondelusional patients responded similarly.

Change in psychosocial functioning and quality of life of patients with body dysmorphic disorder treated with fluoxetine: a placebo-controlled study. Phillips KA, Rasmussen SA. Psychosomatics 2004; 45: 438–44.

This was a 12-week, placebo-controlled study of psychosocial functioning and mental health–related QOL in 60 patients. At baseline, the patients had impaired psychosocial functioning and markedly poor mental health–related QOL. Significant decrease in the severity of BDD was demonstrated along with improvement in functioning and QOL.

Modular cognitive behavioral therapy for body dysmorphic disorder: a randomized controlled trial. Wihelm S, Phillips KA, Didie E, Buhlmann U, Greenberg JL, Fama JM, et al. Behav Ther 2014; 34: 314–27.

Thirty-six adults treated with 22 sessions of modular CBT. Eighty-one percent achieved significant improvement in BDD symptoms, and high levels of satisfaction with treatment were reported.

Cognitive-behavioral body image therapy for body dysmorphic disorder. Rosen JC, Reiter J, Orosan P. J Consult Clin Psycho 1995; 63: 263–9.

Exposure and response prevention was effective in 77% of 27 women treated with cognitive behavior group therapy for 8 weeks. Subjects in the treatment group improved more than those in the no-treatment waiting-list control group.

Body dysmorphic disorder: a cognitive behavioral model and pilot randomized controlled trial. Veale D, Gournay K, Dryden W, Boocock A, Shah F, Wilson R, et al. Behav Res Ther 1996; 34: 717–29.

Nineteen patients randomly assigned to CBT or a waiting-list control group. There was significantly greater improvement in BDD symptoms in the CBT group.

Second-Line Therapy	
• Additional psychotropic agents and insight-oriented psychotherapy	D

Treating body dysmorphic disorder with medication: evidence, misconceptions, and a suggested approach. Phillips KA, Hollander E. Body Image 2008; 5: 13–27.

Excellent review of alternative and concomitant psychotropic medications, including clomipramine, venlafaxine, buspirone, and pimozide.

Evidence Levels: **A** Double-blind study **B** Clinical trial ≥ 20 subjects **C** Clinical trial < 20 subjects **D** Series ≥ 5 subjects **E** Anecdotal case reports

An open study of buspirone augmentation of serotonin-re-uptake inhibitors in body dysmorphic disorder. Phillips KA. Psychopharmacol Bull 1996; 32: 175–80.

Thirteen patients with DSM-IV BDD who had not responded or had responded only partially to an SSRI had buspirone added to the regimen. Six of these subjects (46%) improved. Three who decreased or discontinued buspirone experienced an increase in symptom severity.

Bowen disease and erythroplasia of Queyrat

Colin A. Morton

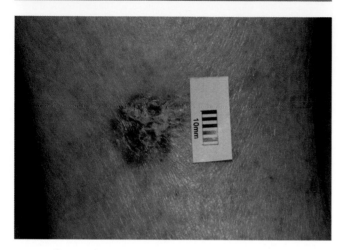

Bowen disease (in situ squamous cell carcinoma, in situ SCC) and erythroplasia of Queyrat (EQ) are forms of intraepidermal squamous cell carcinoma, with the latter located on the penis. The lesions typically present as well-demarcated, erythematous, hyperkeratotic plaques with an irregular border that are persistent and slowly enlarging. Plaques of EQ develop on the glans or inner aspect of the foreskin and can be smooth or scaly/warty. Risk factors for the development of Bowen disease and EQ vary according to the site of disease, but include sun exposure, HPV (human papilloma virus) infection, arsenic exposure, radiation exposure, and HIV or other forms of immunosuppression.

DIAGNOSIS

An initial diagnostic biopsy is recommended, especially for EQ and atypical presentations of Bowen, but many dermatologists will initiate treatment of typical Bowen disease on the basis of clinical diagnosis, aided by dermoscopy.

The specific dermoscopic criteria of Bowen's disease. Zalaudek I, Di Stefani A, Argenziano G. J Eur Acad Dermatol Venereol 2006; 20: 361–2. Dermoscopy can offer assistance in diagnosis with irregular clusters of coiled "glomerular vessels" together with a scaly surface characteristic, with small pigmented globules and/or homogeneous pigmentation present in pigmented variants.

MANAGEMENT STRATEGY

Therapy aims to cure disease by preventing progression to invasive SCC. SCC arises in only around 3% to 5% of typical Bowen disease but about 10% for EQ. Several treatment options are available, and evidence-based guidelines seek to balance efficacy, tolerability, and cosmesis as well as cost effectiveness. Partners of patients with EQ should be screened for other forms of intraepithelial neoplasia caused by HPV in the genital area.

British Association of Dermatologists' guidelines for the management of squamous cell carcinoma in situ (Bowen's disease) 2013. Morton CA, Birnie AJ, Eedy DJ. Br J Dermatol 2014; 170: 245–60.

Quality of evidence for reported treatments for Bowen disease and EQ was reviewed in detail. The strongest evidence was for topical photodynamic therapy (PDT), 5-fluorouracil, and imiquimod, as well as cryotherapy. Nonsurgical options are increasingly used and offer advantages for large/multiple lesions. Surgical excision and curettage remain in common use, although with lower-quality evidence available. Treatment tolerability is a greater challenge for patients with EQ, but with a similar choice of therapy as for Bowen disease.

Direct surgical excision can be considered if a lesion is small and well defined, especially if there is doubt over possible invasive SCC. Lesion ablation may also be achieved with electrodesiccation and curettage or cryotherapy. Mohs micrographic surgery (MMS) is the surgical treatment of choice in severe/recurrent cases of EQ and indicated for certain sites (e.g., digital Bowen disease) where tissue-sparing benefits are important. Laser and radiotherapy have a more limited evidence base, with poor healing reported after radiotherapy. Several treatment combinations are also reported in the literature, but so far lack a substantial evidence base.

First-Line Therapies

• Photodynamic therapy	A
• Cryotherapy	A
• Standard excision	B
• Electrodesiccation and curettage	B

Interventions for cutaneous Bowen's disease. Bath-Hextall FJ, Matin RN, Wilkinson D, Leonardi-Bee J. Cochrane Database Syst Rev 2013; 6: CD007281.

Review of interventions for SCC in situ by the Cochrane Skin Group identified nine randomized controlled trials (RCTs), but noted limited data for surgery and topical cream therapies. MAL-PDT was shown to be an effective treatment, more efficacious than cryotherapy, but equivalent to topical 5-fluoruracil, whereas ALA-PDT achieved a higher clearance rate compared with 5-fluorouracil, but with no difference in efficacy between 5-fluorouracil and cryotherapy.

Comparison of topical methyl aminolevulinate photodynamic therapy with cryotherapy or fluorouracil for treatment of squamous cell carcinoma in situ. Morton C, Horn M, Leman J, Tack B, Bedane C, Tjioe M, et al. Arch Dermatol 2006; 142: 729–35.

Complete response rates at 1 year were highest for methyl aminolevulinate PDT ($n = 96$) at 80% (two treatments spaced 1 week apart, with the methyl aminolevulinate applied for 3 hours before red light illumination) compared with cryotherapy ($n = 96$) at 67% (a minimum 20-second freeze/thaw cycle) and 5% 5-fluorouracil cream at 69% (4 weeks of treatment applied once a day for the first week then twice a day), although the three therapies were equivalent at 24 months. Cosmetic outcomes were best after methyl aminolevulinate PDT.

Given the smaller sample size of 30 lesions treated by 5-fluorouracil in this study where comparator was chosen by clinician's preference and more limited study data elsewhere, topical 5-fluorouracil has been overall considered a second-line therapy in this chapter.

Evidence Levels: **A** Double-blind study **B** Clinical trial ≥ 20 subjects **C** Clinical trial < 20 subjects **D** Series ≥ 5 subjects **E** Anecdotal case reports

European guidelines for photodynamic therapy. Part 1: treatment delivery and current indications – actinic keratoses, Bowen's disease, basal cell carcinoma. Morton CA, Szeimies RM, Sidoroff A, Braathen LR. J Eur Acad Dermatol Venereol 2013; 27: 536–44.

Review of the literature observing high efficacy (86% to 93%) of typical lesions of Bowen disease at 3 months after MAL-PDT with sustained clearance of 68% to 71%, equivalent to cryotherapy and topical 5-fluorouracil. PDT has been shown effective for large lesions over 3 cm in diameter, clearing 96%, as well as a tissue-sparing option for digital, subungual, and nipple lesions.

Methyl-aminolevulinate photodynamic therapy for the treatment of erythroplasia of Queyrat in 23 patients. Fai D, Romano I, Cassano N, Vena GA. J Dermatolog Treat 2012; 23: 330–2.

Nineteen patients obtained a complete clinical remission without any sign of recurrence over an average posttreatment period of 18 months, although local adverse reactions were common during treatment.

Bowen's disease involving the urethra. Yasuda M, Tamura A, Shimizu A, Takahashi A, Ishikawa O. J Dermatol 2005; 32: 210–3.

A case report highlighting the importance of early and definitive surgical treatment of EQ, recognizing the limited options when EQ extends to include the urethral meatus.

Comparison of cryotherapy with curettage in the treatment of Bowen's disease: a prospective study. Ahmed I, Berth-Jones J, Charles-Holmes S, O'Callaghan CJ, Ilchyshyn A. Br J Dermatol 2000; 143: 759–66.

Eighty lesions were randomized to two groups, cryotherapy ($n = 36$) or curettage ($n = 44$), and followed for a median of 2 years. Curettage produced comparable cure rates with more rapid healing, less pain, and fewer complications.

Second-Line Therapies

• 5-Fluorouracil	B
• Imiquimod 5%	B
• Mohs micrographic surgery	B

Topical treatment of Bowen's disease with 5-fluorouracil. Bargman H, Hochman J. J Cutan Med Surg 2003; 7: 101–5.

Only 2 of 26 biopsy-confirmed lesions recurred up to 10 years after treatment.

Imiquimod 5% cream monotherapy for cutaneous squamous cell carcinoma in situ (Bowen's disease): a randomized, double-blind, placebo-controlled trial. Patel GK, Goodwin R, Chawla M, Laidler P, Price PE, Finlay AY, et al. J Am Acad Dermatol 2006; 54: 1025–32.

Seventy-three percent of 31 patients achieved clinical remission with no recurrence at the 9-month follow-up.

Treatment of Bowen's disease with topical 5% imiquimod cream: retrospective study. Rosen T, Harting M, Gibson M. Dermatol Surg 2007; 33: 427–31.

Forty-two of 49 patients (86%) treated with 5% imiquimod cream once daily for a mean of 9 weeks achieved complete clinical remission at 1.5-year follow-up.

Erythroplasia of Queyrat treated with imiquimod 5% cream. Micali G, Nasca MR, De Pasquale R. J Am Acad Dermatol 2006; 55: 901–3.

Case report of an elderly man with EQ treated with 5% imiquimod with clinical and histologically confirmed cure.

Cutaneous squamous carcinoma in situ (Bowen's disease): treatment with Mohs micrographic surgery. Leibovitch I, Huilgol SC, Selva D, Richards S, Paver R. J Am Acad Dermatol 2005; 52: 997–1002.

A case series evaluating 270 cases of Bowen disease treated with MMS with 5-year follow-up demonstrating recurrence rates of approximately 6%. The majority of lesions treated were on the head and neck, and many were recurrent at the time of MMS.

Extensive Bowen's disease of the penile shaft treated with fresh tissue Mohs micrographic surgery in two separate operations. Moritz DL, Lynch WS. J Dermatol Surg Oncol 1991; 17: 374–8.

Third-Line Therapies

• Laser	C
• Radiotherapy	C

Bowen's disease treated by carbon dioxide laser. A series of 44 patients. Covadonga Martinez-Gonzalez M, del Pozo J, Paradela S, Fernández-Jorge B, Fernández-Torres R, Fonseca E. J Dermatolog Treat 2008; 19: 293–9.

A larger retrospective study that used a CO_2 laser in superpulsed mode ($2 W/cm^2$) to treat SCC in situ in 44 patients reported clearance after one treatment in 86% of patients, with all but one of the remaining lesions cleared after a total of two to four treatments.

Radiation therapy for Bowen's disease of the skin. Lukas VanderSpek LA, Pond GR, Wells W, Tsang RW. Int J Radiat Oncol Biol Phys 2005; 63: 505–10.

Forty-four cases of Bowen disease treated with radiation therapy were reviewed, demonstrating remission in 42 patients, with three recurrences at a mean follow-up period of 2.5 years. A broad range of radiation schedules were used and compared for efficacy and safety. These demonstrated no significant differences between low- to medium- and high-dose radiation schedules on disease remission or recurrence.

Bullous pemphigoid

Sandra Peña, Victoria P. Werth

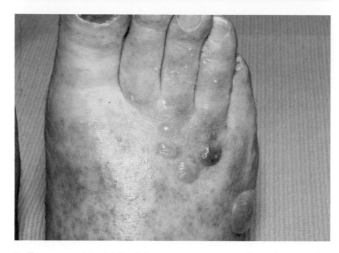

Bullous pemphigoid (BP) is an autoimmune subepidermal blistering disease that mainly affects elderly patients, although childhood cases do occur. Subepidermal blistering is mediated by activation of complement and release of tissue-destructive proteases after IgG autoantibody complex formation with hemidesmosomal antigens BPAg1 (BP230) and BPAg2 (BP180 or collagen XVII). IgE autoantibodies to BPAg2 have also been identified in the majority of patients and have been shown to be pathogenic. The clinical hallmarks of the eruption are tense bullae with either generalized or localized distribution; however, variants, including urticarial, vesicular, vegetative, erythrodermic, and nodularis, have been described. Pruritus associated with BP can be severe and adversely affect quality of life. Mucosal involvement with small blisters or erosions may exist in a minority of patients. Although there can be relapses and exacerbations, BP is generally self-limiting, with remission in most adults by 5 years, and more rapidly in children. Mortality can be high in patients with poor overall health and advanced age.

MANAGEMENT STRATEGY

The Cochrane Skin Group updated its review on the treatment of BP in 2011. The review focused on evidence from 10 randomized controlled trials (RCTs) to help guide physicians with treatment. Although the quality of evidence from the majority of the trials was limited by small sample size and lack of blinding, 2 of the 10 studies were large and included more than half of the participants in the review (Joly 2002, Joly 2009). The reviewers concluded that very potent topical steroids were effective and safe in the treatment of BP and that milder regimens are effective in moderate BP. Doses of prednisolone >0.75 mg/kg/day showed no added benefit over lower doses and had an increased incidence of adverse effects. The data also showed that topical clobetasol propionate 0.05% cream (40 g/day) was as effective as oral corticosteroids in controlling disease and associated with fewer side effects. These are the only recommendations with strong evidentiary support.

Patients with localized disease may be successfully treated with clobetasol propionate 0.05% or *intralesional corticosteroids*. Those with generalized disease in which topical therapy is not feasible can be treated with *prednisone*, 0.5 to 0.75 mg/kg/day, depending on disease severity and considering the overall health of the patient. The risks of both short- and long-term systemic corticosteroid therapy are well known and are heightened in the elderly patient population. Every effort should be made to find the minimum dosage of systemic corticosteroids required to suppress disease. With only a few exceptions, all elderly patients started on systemic corticosteroids should also start calcium, vitamin D, and bisphosphonate therapy. All patients on systemic corticosteroids should be screened for tuberculosis and have their blood pressure and serum glucose levels followed closely.

Tetracycline combined with *nicotinamide* can be used for patients unable to tolerate or who have contraindications to corticosteroids. If gastrointestinal side effects manifest, *minocycline* may be substituted. Tetracycline alone has also been used in one case with success.

Azathioprine is a second-line alternative that may be used alone or as a corticosteroid-sparing agent in more severe disease. Due to genetic polymorphisms in the expression of thiopurine methyltransferase (TPMT), the enzyme that metabolizes azathioprine, a TPMT level before initiating treatment may assist the physician in appropriate dosing. *Azathioprine* has a slow onset of action and should be started in conjunction with corticosteroids during the acute stage. Patients usually respond within 3 to 4 weeks of initiation. *Mycophenolate mofetil*, an immunosuppressant, is an effective corticosteroid-sparing agent in BP. It is generally well tolerated and does not carry the risk of liver toxicity seen with azathioprine. *Dapsone* is particularly useful when histologic examination reveals a predominance of neutrophils. *Methotrexate* is another corticosteroid-sparing agent that may be useful in BP. It is given in a weekly, low-dosage protocol in a similar manner to psoriasis therapy.

For severe and refractory BP, a variety of immunosuppressive and immunomodulatory therapies have demonstrated efficacy, including *intravenous immunoglobulin, chlorambucil, pulsed intravenous corticosteroids, cyclophosphamide, ciclosporin, etanercept, rituximab, daclizumab,* and *omalizumab.*

An international consensus on the definition of end points and a disease severity measure for studies in BP was recently published and should allow for better comparisons between studies in the future (**Definitions and outcome measures for bullous pemphigoid: recommendations by an international panel of experts.** Murrel DF, Daniel BS, Joly P, Borradori L, Amagai M, Hashimoto T, et al. J Am Acad Dermatol 2012; 66: 479–85).

Specific Investigations

- Evaluation of medications to rule out drug-induced cases
- Consider patient age and overall medical condition for therapeutic decision-making
- Biopsy of intact bulla for histologic examination with hematoxylin and eosin
- Biopsy of perilesional skin for direct immunofluorescence (sent in Michel's transport medium)
- Consider BP180 (BPAg2) ELISA or indirect immunofluorescence on blood or blister fluid sample
- Consider fasting glucose screening
- Consider screening for antiphospholipid antibodies

Evidence Levels: **A** Double-blind study **B** Clinical trial ≥ 20 subjects **C** Clinical trial < 20 subjects **D** Series ≥ 5 subjects **E** Anecdotal case reports

Drug-induced pemphigoid: bullous and cicatricial. Vassileva S. Clin Dermatol 1998; 16: 379–87.

Many drugs have been recognized to induce BP, including furosemide, bumetanide, spironolactone, phenacetin, penicillins, ibuprofen, D-penicillamine, captopril, fluoxetine, β-adrenergic blockers, terbinafine, gabapentin, risperidone, and PUVA.

Prediction of survival for patients with bullous pemphigoid: a prospective study. Joly P, Benichou J, Lok C, Hellot MF, Saiag P, Tancrede-Bohin E, et al. Arch Dermatol 2005; 141: 691–8.

The only prospective trial evaluating factors that influence survival in 341 BP patients found that increasing age and poor overall health were direct predictors of mortality. They showed that disease activity had no correlation with mortality.

Increased frequency of diabetes mellitus in patients with bullous pemphigoid: a case–control study. Chuang TY, Korkij W, Soltani K, Clayman J, Cook J. J Am Acad Dermatol 1984; 6: 1099–102.

The prevalence of diabetes mellitus before administration of systemic corticosteroids was significantly higher in patients with BP (20%) than in controls (2.5%).

Bullous pemphigoid and comorbidities: a case-control study in Portuguese patients. Teixeira VB, Cabral R, Brites MM, Vieira R, Figueiredo A. An Bras Dermatol 2014; 89: 274–8

The prevalence of at least one neurologic disease was significantly higher in BP cases before the diagnosis of BP compared with that of controls. Researchers did not find any significant associations between BP and malignancy or diabetes.

Antiphospholipid antibodies in patients with autoimmune blistering disease. Echigo T, Hasegawa M, Inaoki M, Yamazaki M, Sato S, Takehara K. J Am Acad Dermatol 2007; 57: 397–400.

A higher prevalence of antiphospholipid antibodies was detected in patients with autoimmune blistering diseases (pemphigus vulgaris, pemphigus foliaceous, bullous pemphigoid, cicatricial pemphigoid, and linear IgA disease) compared with normal controls. Of the 10 patients with an autoimmune blistering disease and positive antiphospholipid antibodies, 7 were found to have occult thromboembolism.

First-Line Therapies

• Clobetasol propionate 0.05%	B
• Systemic corticosteroids	B
• Tetracycline and nicotinamide	B
• Minocycline	C
• Tetracycline	E

A comparison of oral and topical corticosteroids in patients with bullous pemphigoid. Joly P, Roujeau JC, Benichou J, Picard C, Dreno B, Delaporte E, et al. N Engl J Med 2002; 346: 321–7.

A total of 341 patients were enrolled in a nonblinded, randomized, multicenter trial and were stratified by disease severity (moderate or extensive). Patients received either topical clobetasol (40 g/day) or oral prednisolone (0.5 mg/kg for moderate disease and 1 mg/kg for extensive disease). Topical corticosteroid therapy was found to be equal to oral corticosteroids in both survival and efficacy for moderate BP. Survival was higher in extensive disease with the use of topical steroids compared with oral corticosteroids.

A comparison of two regimens of topical corticosteroids in the treatment of patients with bullous pemphigoid: a multicenter randomized study. Joly P, Roujeau JC, Benichou J, Delaporte E, D'Incan M, Dreno B, et al. J Invest Dermatol 2009; 129: 1681–7.

This nonblinded, randomized study stratified 312 patients to moderate or extensive disease and compared treatment with clobetasol propionate cream in a mild regimen (10–30g/day for 4 months) to a standard regimen (40g/day with tapering over 12 months). The mild regimen was as effective as the standard regimen in both moderate and extensive disease. There was a 70% reduction in the cumulative dose of topical steroids with the mild regimen, and there were fewer adverse effects. The mild regimen reduced the risk of death or life-threatening side effects in patients with moderate BP.

Treatment of bullous pemphigoid with prednisolone only: 0.75 mg/kg/day versus 1.25 mg/kg/day. A multicenter randomized study. Morel P, Guillaume JC. Ann Dermatol Venereol 1984; 11: 925–8.

A randomized, prospective study of 50 patients found no difference in effectiveness with a higher dose of prednisolone compared with the lower dose.

Bullous pemphigoid in infants: characteristics, diagnosis and treatment. Schwieger-Briel A, Moellmann C, Mattulat B, Schauer F, Kiritsi D, Schmidt E, et al. Orphanet J Rare Dis 2014; 9:185.

A group of researchers studying a cohort of infantile BP patients developed the first treatment algorithm for BP in infants. They determined that all patients should be treated with mid- to high-potency topical steroids and those with moderate-to-severe disease should also be started on systemic steroids.

Nicotinamide and tetracycline therapy of bullous pemphigoid. Fivenson DP, Breneman DL, Rosen GB, Hersh CS, Cardone S, Mutasim D. Arch Dermatol 1994; 130: 753–8.

A randomized, open-label trial of 20 patients showed that the combination of nicotinamide (500 mg three times daily) and tetracycline (500 mg four times daily) was equally efficacious as systemic corticosteroids and resulted in less toxicity.

Minocycline as a therapeutic option in bullous pemphigoid. Loo WJ, Kirtschig G, Wojnarowska F. Clin Exp Dermatol 2001; 26: 376–9.

A retrospective analysis of 22 patients treated with adjuvant minocycline (50–100 mg daily) showed a major response in 6 six patients, a minor response in 11, and no response in 5.

Generalized bullous pemphigoid controlled by tetracycline therapy alone. Pereyo NG, Loretta SD. J Am Acad Dermatol 1995; 32: 138–9.

An 82-year-old woman with generalized BP responded completely to oral tetracycline (500 mg twice daily) within 2 weeks. The tetracycline was successfully tapered over 6 weeks.

Second-Line Therapies

• Azathioprine	B
• Mycophenolate mofetil	B
• Dapsone	C
• Methotrexate	C

Azathioprine in the treatment of bullous pemphigoid. Greaves MW, Burton JL, Marks J. Br Med J 1971; 1: 144–5.

Of 11 patients on long-term maintenance therapy with systemic corticosteroids, 9 remained symptom free on azathioprine alone and 2 were able to have a reduced dosage of prednisone.

Azathioprine plus prednisone in treatment of pemphigoid. Burton J, Harman R, Peachey R, Warin R. Br Med J 1978; 2: 1190–1.

A controlled trial of 25 patients comparing azathioprine (2.5 mg/kg daily) plus prednisone with prednisone alone showed that azathioprine greatly reduced the need for prednisone and improved outcome.

A comparison of oral methylprednisolone plus azathioprine or mycophenolate mofetil for the treatment of bullous pemphigoid. Beissert S, Werfel T, Frieling U, Böhm M, Sticherling M, Stadler R, et al. Arch Dermatol 2007; 143: 1536–42.

In this nonblinded, randomized controlled trial of 73 patients on methylprednisolone, 38 received azathioprine 2 mg/kg/day and 35 received mycophenolate mofetil 2 g/day. Both regimens were found to be equally effective, although faster remission and a lower cumulative dose of methylprednisolone was seen with azathioprine. Azathioprine was associated with more liver toxicity. Both treatment groups had 100% remission of lesions.

Dapsone as first line therapy for bullous pemphigoid. Venning VA, Millard PR, Wojnarowska F. Br J Dermatol 1989; 120: 83–92.

In an open trial of 13 patients placed on dapsone as initial treatment, 6 were completely controlled with dapsone (50–100 mg daily). Dapsone may be used as initial treatment for BP, particularly when there are contraindications to the use of corticosteroids or immunosuppressants.

Combined treatment with low-dose methotrexate and initial short-term superpotent topical steroids in bullous pemphigoid: an open, multicentre, retrospective study. Du-Thanh A, Merlet S, Maillard H, Bernard P, Joly P, Esteve E, et al. Br J Dermatol 2011; 165: 1337–43.

A retrospective review of 70 patients treated concurrently with superpotent topical steroids and low-dose methotrexate (5–15 mg/week) showed complete clinical remission in all patients. Seventy-six percent of patients showed sustained clinical remission on low-dose methotrexate with a mean treatment duration of 8 months. Twenty-four percent of patients experienced one or more side effects, primarily hematologic and gastrointestinal.

Low-dose methotrexate treatment in elderly patients with bullous pemphigoid. Paul MA, Jorizzo JL, Fleischer AB, White WL. J Am Acad Dermatol 1994; 31: 620–5.

In a retrospective chart review of 34 patients, 8 therapy-resistant patients received low-dose weekly methotrexate (average 5–10 mg) combined with oral prednisone. Patients receiving combination therapy required significantly lower doses of prednisone to control their disease at 1 month compared with baseline.

Low-dose oral pulse methotrexate as monotherapy in elderly patients with bullous pemphigoid. Heilborn JD, Ståhle-Bäckdahl M, Albertioni F, Vassilaki I, Peterson C, Stephansson E. J Am Acad Dermatol 1999; 40: 741–9.

In a prospective study of low-dose oral methotrexate (5–12.5 mg/week) in 11 elderly patients with generalized BP, every patient demonstrated a rapid decrease in disease activity within 4 to 30 days.

Third-Line Therapies	
• Intravenous immunoglobulin (IVIG)	C
• Chlorambucil + prednisolone	C
• Pulse intravenous corticosteroids	D
• Cyclophosphamide + pulse intravenous corticosteroids	E
• Cyclophosphamide	E
• Ciclosporin	E
• Etanercept	E
• Rituximab	E
• Daclizumab	E
• Omalizumab	E

Consensus statement on the use of intravenous immunoglobulin therapy in the treatment of autoimmune mucocutaneous blistering diseases. Ahmed AR, Dahl MV. Arch Dermatol 2003; 139: 1051–9.

In 27 of 32 cases of BP reported in the literature as unresponsive to conventional therapy, IVIG was of significant benefit and produced lasting clinical results with minimal adverse effects. General recommendations included dosing at 2 mg/kg per cycle with a cycle consisting of the total dose divided into three equal doses, given on 3 consecutive days. Before starting therapy, an IgA level should be obtained. A cycle should be given every 3 to 4 weeks, and a slow tapering is advised to prevent recurrences and sustain the obtained clinical benefit.

Chlorambucil as a steroid-sparing agent in bullous pemphigoid. Chave TA, Mortimer NJ, Shah DS, Hutchinson PE. Br J Dermatol 2004; 151: 1107–8.

In a retrospective study of 45 patients, 26 patients received prednisolone only and 19 received prednisolone and chlorambucil (0.1 mg/kg/day reduced after 2 weeks to 0.05 mg/kg/day, and after 1 month to 2 mg daily). Patients treated with chlorambucil had a shorter treatment course and reduced total steroid requirement.

High-dose methylprednisolone in the treatment of bullous pemphigoid. Siegel J, Eaglstein WH. Arch Dermatol 1984; 120: 1157–65.

Seven of eight hospitalized patients with active BP responded within 24 hours after receiving methylprednisolone pulse therapy (15 mg/kg intravenously over 1 hour daily for 3 days). Moderate doses of oral prednisone (0.4 mg/kg) were required for maintenance.

Severe bullous pemphigoid responsive to pulsed intravenous dexamethasone and oral cyclophosphamide. Dawe RS, Naidoo DK, Ferguson J. Br J Dermatol 1997; 137: 826–7.

Refractory BP in a 59-year-old woman with diabetes mellitus cleared with pulsed intravenous dexamethasone therapy (100 mg dexamethasone in 500 mL 5% dextrose infused over 4 hours on three consecutive days, monthly) and low-dose oral cyclophosphamide (50 mg/day between pulses).

Evidence Levels: **A** Double-blind study **B** Clinical trial ≥ 20 subjects **C** Clinical trial < 20 subjects **D** Series ≥ 5 subjects **E** Anecdotal case reports

Successful treatment of bullous pemphigoid with pulsed intravenous cyclophosphamide. Itoh T, Hosokawa H, Shirai Y, Horio T. Br J Dermatol 1996; 134: 931–3.

A 67-year-old man with refractory BP was reported to respond to monthly pulsed intravenous doses of cyclophosphamide (500–1000 mg) along with low-dose oral cyclophosphamide (50 mg/day).

Treatment of bullous pemphigoid with low-dose oral cyclophosphamide: a case series of 20 patients. Gual A, Iranzo P, Mascaro JM Jr. J Eur Acad Dermatol Venereol 2014; 28: 814–8.

A retrospective study assessing the efficacy and safety of low-dose oral cyclophosphamide in patients with moderate-to-severe BP found a marked therapeutic effect in 79% of patients. Additionally, of the patients to achieve complete resolution of BP, 73% did so on a low dose of cyclophosphamide.

Effects of cyclosporin on bullous pemphigoid and pemphigus. Thivolet J, Harthelemy H, Rigot-Muller G, Bendelac A. Lancet 1985; 1: 334–5.

Ciclosporin (6 mg/kg daily), adapted to obtain a plasma level of 80 to 180 µg/L, was successful in treating two patients with BP.

Treatment of coexisting bullous pemphigoid and psoriasis with the tumor necrosis factor antagonist etanercept. Yamauchi PS, Lowe NJ, Gindi V. J Am Acad Dermatol 2006; 54: S121–2.

A 64-year-old man with both psoriasis and bullous pemphigoid failed mycophenolate mofetil treatment and was started on prednisone 60 mg/day. To reduce rebound effect with steroid tapering, etanercept 50 mg/week was started. Bullae returned as the prednisone was tapered, so the dose of etanercept was increased to 50 mg twice weekly. At this dose, prednisone could be tapered and the psoriasis and BP remained in remission.

Rituximab for treatment-refractory pemphigus and pemphigoid: a case series of 17 patients. Kasperkiewicz M, Shimanovich I, Ludwig R, Rose C, Zillikens D, Schmidt E. J Am Acad Dermatol 2011: 65: 552–8.

Two patients with BP and five with mucous membrane pemphigoid (MMP) were treated with rituximab at a dose of 375 mg/m^2 weekly for four doses or twice with 1000 mg at a 2-week interval. One patient with MMP showed a complete remission off therapy, four patients (two patients with MMP, two patients with BP) showed a complete remission while on therapy, and two patients with MMP had a partial remission. Six of the seven patients were on concomitant immunosuppressive therapy.

Bullous and mucous membrane pemphigoid show a mixed response to rituximab: experience in seven patients. Lourari A, Herve C, Doffoel-Hantz V, Meyer N, Bulai-Livideanu C, Viraben R, et al. JEADV 2011; 25: 1230–42.

In a retrospective study of five patients with BP and two with MMP, all patients received four infusions of rituximab at a dose of 375 mg/m^2 weekly. One patient received an additional four doses at 11 months' follow-up due to relapse of disease. Four patients showed complete remission on therapy, and two patients showed partial remission. The median time to improvement was 4 months.

Daclizumab: a novel therapeutic option in severe bullous pemphigoid. Mockenhaupt M, Grosber M, Norganer J. Acta Dermatol Venereol 2005; 85: 65–6.

A 52-year-old with diffuse BP failed combination treatment with prednisolone 100 mg/day plus azathioprine 100 mg/day, ciclosporin 200 mg/day, and mycophenolate mofetil 2 g/day. The steroids were reduced to 5 mg/day secondary to glucose intolerance, so daclizumab was added at 1 mg/kg/day. The patient had six infusions and remained on prednisolone 5 mg/day and azathioprine 50 mg/day, with complete resolution of lesions at 2 weeks.

Daclizumab inhibits the IL-2 receptor and downstream T cell activation

Pathogenicity of IgE in autoimmunity: successful treatment of bullous pemphigoid with omalizumab. Fairley J, Baum C, Brandt D, Messingham K. J Allergy Clin Immunol 2009; 123: 704–5.

A 70-year-old woman with a 1-year history of BP showed poor control on prednisone 40 mg/day, azathioprine 150 mg/day, and minocycline 200 mg/day. Prednisone was discontinued and omalizumab 300 mg subcutaneously every 2 weeks for 16 weeks was initiated. By 16 weeks, affected body surface area decreased from 50% to 5%. The patient relapsed 4 months after discontinuing omalizumab therapy but lesions resolved once treatment was reinstituted. No side effects were reported.

Omalizumab therapy for bullous pemphigoid. Yu KK, Crew AB, Messingham KA, Fairley JA, Woodley DT. J Am Acad Dermatol 2014; 71: 468–74.

Researchers were able to demonstrate a therapeutic benefit in six patients treated with systemic omalizumab, an IgE monoclonal antibody. None of the patients had untoward side effects from omalizumab.

Successful management of severe infant bullous pemphigoid with omalizumab. Dufour C, Souillet AL, Chaneliere C, Jouen F, Bodemer C, Jullien D, et al. BJD 2012; 166: 1140–1.

A 5-month-old male infant with BP failed prednisolone 2.5 mg/kg daily and was subsequently treated with prednisolone 3 mg/kg daily, dapsone 2 mg/kg daily, azithromycin 10 mg/kg daily, three pulse doses of intravenous methylprednisolone 120 mg, and topical betamethasone 0.05% without control. He was then given omalizumab 100 mg subcutaneously and achieved disease control within 8 days. He received omalizumab injections every 2 weeks for 3 months, then monthly for 4 months. He remained in clinical remission after a 7-month follow-up period.

Burning mouth syndrome (glossodynia)

John J. Kohorst, Cooper C. Wriston, Rochelle R. Torgerson

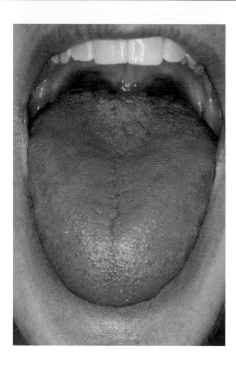

Primary burning mouth syndrome (BMS) is a rare, chronic, debilitating disease characterized by intraoral burning in the absence of systemic disease or identifiable abnormalities on physical examination and laboratory testing. Current evidence suggests that altered neurophysiology of the central or peripheral nervous system may play an etiopathogenic role. The diagnosis of primary BMS is a clinical diagnosis of exclusion. Various medical conditions and medications can induce oral burning, a condition referred to as *secondary BMS*.

MANAGEMENT STRATEGY

A detailed history and physical examination should be completed to identify all alternative or correctable causes of oral burning. Several associated factors may be simultaneously present requiring treatment. Correctable, associated factors may be local, systemic, or psychological.

Local factors

Local factors include xerostomia (age, medication, radiotherapy); direct irritation (oral care products, tobacco); mechanical trauma (rough dental restorations, poorly fitting dental prostheses); parafunctional habits (bruxism, tongue thrusting); microbial infection or colonization (candidiasis, herpetic, fusospirochetal);

geographic or fissured tongue; mucocutaneous diseases (lichen planus, pemphigus, pemphigoid); and allergic contact stomatitis (flavorings, food additives, dental materials).

Systemic factors

Systemic factors include deficiency states (iron, zinc, folate, cobalamin, thiamin, riboflavin, pyridoxine, ascorbic acid, magnesium); autoimmune disease (Sjögren syndrome); gastrointestinal disease (gastroesophageal reflux); neurologic disease (trigeminal neuralgia, acoustic neuroma, Parkinson disease, glossopharyngeal neuralgia); medication related (angiotensin-converting enzyme [ACE] inhibitors, angiotensin receptor blockers [ARBs], antidepressants, antihistamines, antiretrovirals, benzodiazepines, proton pump inhibitors [PPIs], anticonvulsants, radiochemotherapy); and endocrinopathies (hypothyroidism, diabetes).

Psychological factors

Psychological factors include anxiety (including cancerophobia), depression, adjustment disorder, and psychosocial stressors.

SPECIFIC INVESTIGATIONS

Laboratory evaluation and empiric treatment should be directed by the history and physical examination findings. If burning persists after eliminating or treating potential local, systemic, and psychological factors, a working diagnosis of primary BMS is adopted. Although consensus on treatment for primary BMS is lacking, many have found some degree of success with multimodal approaches resembling those used for the treatment of chronic, neuropathic pain.

Pathophysiology of primary burning mouth syndrome. Jaaskelainen SK. Clin Neurophysiol 2012; 123: 71–7.

A review of the evidence for neurophysiologic alterations in the peripheral or central nervous systems in the etiopathogenesis of BMS. A neurophysiologic evaluation is suggested to characterize the neuropathology in individual patients and target treatments.

Psychiatric comorbidity in patients with burning mouth syndrome. Bogetto F, Maina G, Ferro G, Carbone M, Gandolfo S. Psychosom Med 1998; 60: 378–85.

In a case-control study of 102 patients with BMS, 59.8% had concomitant psychiatric disorders.

Interventions for the treatment of burning mouth syndrome. Zakrzewska JM, Forssell H, Glenny AM. Cochrane Database Syst Rev 2005; CD002779.

In nine comparative trials identified for BMS, only α-lipoic acid, clonazepam, and cognitive behavior therapy were effective. Therapeutic efficacy for painkillers, hormones, and antidepressants was not found.

Clinical assessment and outcome in 70 patients with complaints of burning or sore mouth symptoms. Drage LA, Rogers RS, 3rd. Mayo Clin Proc 1999; 74: 223–8.

A burning or sore mouth was retrospectively associated with psychiatric disease (30%), xerostomia (24%), geographic tongue (24%), nutritional deficiency (21%), and allergic stomatitis (13%) in 70 patients.

Table 34.1 Specific investigations

History
Oral symptoms	Timing, quality, duration, location, alleviating/exacerbating factors
Medications	Efavirenz, clonazepam, fluoxetine, sertraline, venlafaxine, enalapril, captopril, lisinopril, candesartan, eprosartan, omeprazole, topiramate, hormone replacement therapy
Dental	Prostheses, recent procedures, dentifrices, topical medicaments
Parafunctional habits	Bruxism, tongue thrusting
Review of symptoms	Weakness, headache, fatigue, concentration, sleep disturbance, arthralgia

Physical examination
Oral	Complete oral examination, including head and neck (remove any dental prostheses)
Nodal	Adenopathy
Musculoskeletal	Temporomandibular joint

Table 34.2 Laboratory evaluation

Hematologic	Complete blood count, ferritin, serum folate, cobalamin (+ methylmalonic acid, homocysteine)
Metabolic	Serum thiamine, riboflavin, pyridoxine, zinc (+ alkaline phosphatase), magnesium
Endocrinologic	Glycosylated hemoglobin, thyrotropin (+ free thyroxine)
Immunologic	Antinuclear factor (+ Ro/SSA, La/SSB)
Dermatologic	Biopsy (+ direct immunofluorescence) if visible abnormality on oral examination
Microbiology testing	Herpes simplex (polymerase chain reaction [PCR]); varicella zoster (PCR); candidosis (swab from site of pain for direct examination and culture); human immunodeficiency virus screening

Table 34.3 Consultations

Otolaryngology	Nasopharyngoscopy
Gastroenterology	Esophagogastroduodenoscopy
Oral/maxillofacial	Periapical radiographs, magnetic resonance imaging
Mental health	Psychiatry consultation
Neurology	Neurologic examination, magnetic resonance imaging
Hypersensitivity testing	Epicutaneous patch testing (preservatives, oral flavors, metals, adhesives)

Burning mouth syndrome: an update. Lopez-Jornet P, Camacho-Alonso F, Andujar-Mateos P, Sánchez-Siles M, Gómez-Garcia F. Med Oral Patol Oral Cir Bucal 2010; 15: e562–8.

BMS is reviewed as a chronic orofacial pain disorder. Serotonin reuptake inhibitors, clonazepam, and capsaicin may be effective treatments.

Burning mouth syndrome. Torgerson RR. Dermatol Ther 2010; 23: 291–8.

Multiple possible etiologies of BMS, including neuropathic, exocrine dysfunction, taste disturbance, mucosal atrophy, and psychological illness, are reviewed. Recommendations for evaluation and management are given.

First-Line Therapies

• Acknowledge and validate patient symptoms and experience; reassure	E
• Avoid contact irritants (alcohol-based oral rinses, caustic mouthwashes, flavored dentifrices, acidic foods, carbonated beverages)	E
• Treat xerostomia (sialagogues, artificial oral lubricants)	D
• Discontinue or change causative medications (ACE inhibitor, ARB, selective serotonin reuptake inhibitor [SSRI], serotonin-norepinephrine reuptake inhibitor, benzodiazepine, nonnucleoside reverse-transcriptase inhibitor, PPI, anticonvulsant, anticholinergics)	E
• Replace thiamine, riboflavin, pyridoxine, folate, cobalamin, iron, zinc, ascorbic acid, magnesium	C
• Manage concomitant psychiatric illness	C
• Assess and address parafunctional habits (bruxism, tongue thrusting)	E
• Assess oral prostheses and dental work	C
• Imidazole/azole therapy (presence of functional pain)	C

Patients complaining of a burning mouth. Further experience in clinical assessment and management. Main DM, Basker RM. Br Dent J 1983; 154: 206–11.

A high rate of intraoral burning attributable to shortcomings in denture design.

Glossodynia from *Candida*-associated lesions, burning mouth syndrome, or mixed causes. Terai H, Shimahara M. Pain Med 2010; 11: 856–60.

Ninety-five glossodynia patients with no objective tongue findings were assessed for functional pain (significant increase in tongue pain while eating or no tongue pain at rest). Seventy-two (75.7%) of the patients with functional glossodynia improved with imidazole therapy (25 mg gel four times a day for 2–4 weeks).

Drug-induced burning mouth syndrome: a new etiologic diagnosis. Salort-Llorca C, Minguez-Serra MP, Silvestre FJ. Med Oral Patol Oral Cir Bucal 2008; 13: E167–70.

Antihypertensive medications that interact with the renin–angiotensin system are the most frequent cause of drug-associated BMS. Efavirenz, clonazepam, venlafaxine, fluoxetine, and sertraline were also associated.

Proton pump inhibitors. Scully C. Br Dent J 2010; 208: 147.

A case report of BMS-like symptoms that resolved after discontinuing omeprazole.

Topiramate-induced burning mouth syndrome. Friedman DI. Headache 2010; 50: 1383–5.

A case report of BMS that resolved after discontinuing topiramate. Symptoms recurred upon rechallenge.

Zinc deficiency may be a cause of burning mouth syndrome as zinc replacement therapy has therapeutic effects. Cho GS, Han MW, Lee B, Roh JL, Choi SH, Cho KJ, et al. J Oral Pathol Med 2010; 39: 722–7.

In a series of 276 patients with BMS, 55 zinc-deficient patients who received zinc supplementation reported a greater reduction of oral pain compared with patients without supplementation (p = 0.004).

Second-Line Therapies	
• Topical capsaicin	A
• Topical clonazepam	B
• Low-dose clonazepam	A
• Low-dose tricyclic antidepressant (doxepin)	C
• Paroxetine	D
• Milnacipran	D
• Low-dose pregabalin	E
• Duloxetine	E
• Low-dose olanzapine	E
• Cognitive behavioral therapy	B

Application of a capsaicin rinse in the treatment of burning mouth syndrome. Silvestre FJ, Silvestre-Rangil J, Tamarit-Santafé C, Bautista D. Med Oral Patol Oral Cir Bucal 2012; 17: e1–4.

A randomized, double-blind, crossover study of topical capsaicin rinse (0.02%) or placebo three times daily found reduced pain scores among capsaicin-treated, but not placebo-treated, patients with BMS.

Spice R, Hagen NA. Capsaicin in burning mouth syndrome: titration strategies. J Otolaryngol 2004; 33: 53–4.

Guidelines and recommendations for the use of capsaicin in BMS.

Topical clonazepam in stomatodynia: a randomised placebo-controlled study. Gremeau-Richard C, Woda A, Navez ML, Attal N, Bouhassira D, Gagnieu MC. Pain 2004; 108: 51–7.

Forty-eight patients with BMS received either "suck and spit" clonazepam (1 mg) or placebo three times daily for 14 days. Patients receiving topical clonazepam had a greater reduction in pain scores.

A double-blind study on clonazepam in patients with burning mouth syndrome. Heckmann SM, Kirchner E, Grushka M, Wichmann MG, Hummel T. Laryngoscope 2012; 122: 813–6.

Twenty patients with BMS received either clonazepam (0.5 mg) or placebo daily for 9 weeks. Clonazepam-treated patients had reduced pain scores.

Outcome predictors affecting the efficacy of clonazepam therapy for the management of burning mouth syndrome (BMS). Ko JY, Kim MJ, Lee SG, Kho HS. Arch Gerontol Geriatr 2012; 55: 755–61.

One hundred patients with BMS took clonazepam (0.5 mg) once or twice daily for 4 weeks. Patients with fewer psychological symptoms, higher initial pain scores, and the presence of xerostomia or taste disturbance experienced greater therapeutic efficacy.

A population-based study of the incidence of burning mouth syndrome. Kohorst JJ, Bruce AJ, Torgerson RR, Schenck LA, Davis MD. Mayo Clin Proc 2014: 1545–52.

Annual age- and sex-adjusted incidence of BMS of 11.4 per 100,000 person-years.

An open-label, noncomparative, dose escalation pilot study of the effect of paroxetine in treatment of burning mouth syndrome. Yamazaki Y, Hata H, Kitamori S, Onodera M, Kitagawa Y. Oral Surg Oral Med Oral Pathol Oral Radiol Endod 2009; 107: e6–11.

Out of 52 BMS patients, 42 (80.8%) responded to paroxetine (10–30 mg daily) over 12 weeks. Nineteen (70.4%) had a complete response by the end of the treatment period. The effects were dose dependent.

Milnacipran dose–effect study in patients with burning mouth syndrome. Kato Y, Sato T, Katagiri A, Umezaki Y, Takenoshita M, Yoshikawa T. Clin Neuropharmacol 2011; 34: 166–9.

An open-label, dose-escalation pilot study of milnacipran in 56 patients with BMS. The cumulative response rate was 67.9% and 50.8% for daily dosages of 90 mg and 60 mg, respectively.

Marked response of burning mouth syndrome to pregabalin treatment. Lopez V, Alonso V, Martí N, Calduch L, Jordá E. Clin Exp Dermatol 2009; 34: e449–50.

Report of one case of BMS responsive to pregabalin treatment (50 mg daily).

Gabapentin has little or no effect in the treatment of burning mouth syndrome: results of an open-label pilot study. Heckmann SM, Heckmann JG, Ungethüm A, Hujoel P, Hummel T. Eur J Neurol 2006; 13: e6–7.

A dose-escalation pilot study of gabapentin in BMS showed none to minimal benefit. Maximum titrated dose was 2400 mg daily.

Burning mouth syndrome responsive to duloxetine: a case report. Mignogna MD, Adamo D, Schiavone V, Ravel MG, Fortuna G. Pain Med 2011; 12: 466–9.

Report of one case of BMS responsive to duloxetine (60 mg daily).

Two cases of burning mouth syndrome treated with olanzapine. Ueda N, Kodama Y, Hori H, Umene W, Sugita A, Nakano H. Psychiatry Clin Neurosci 2008; 62: 359–61.

Two cases of BMS responsive to olanzapine treatment (2.5–5.0 mg daily).

Alpha lipoic acid in burning mouth syndrome: a randomized double-blind placebo-controlled trial. Cavalcanti DR, da Silveira FR. J Oral Pathol Med 2009; 38: 254–61.

Alpha-lipoic acid failed to provide a therapeutic benefit.

Cognitive therapy in the treatment of patients with resistant burning mouth syndrome: a controlled study. Bergdahl J, Anneroth G, Perris H. J Oral Pathol Med 1995; 24: 213–5.

A randomized trial in resistant BMS found cognitive therapy superior to an attention program.

Third-Line Therapies	
• Avoid contact allergens	E
• Group psychotherapy	B
• Low-level laser therapy (diode)	D

Burning mouth syndrome. Zakrzewska J, Buchanan JA. BMJ Clin Evid 2016. Pii; 1301.

A systematic review of benzodiazepines, benzydamine hydrochloride, cognitive behavior therapy, SSRIs, and tricyclic antidepressants for BMS treatment.

Evidence Levels: **A** Double-blind study **B** Clinical trial ≥ 20 subjects **C** Clinical trial < 20 subjects **D** Series ≥ 5 subjects **E** Anecdotal case reports

Type 3 burning mouth syndrome: psychological and allergic aspects. Lamey PJ, Lamb AB, Hughes A, Milligan KA, Forsyth A. J Oral Pathol Med 1994; 23: 216–9.

In 33 patients with BMS and intermittent symptoms at atypical sites, 65% were found to have positive patch tests to food flavorings or additives. Symptoms improved in 80% with allergen avoidance.

Group psychotherapy: an additional approach to burning mouth syndrome. Miziara ID, Filho BC, Oliveira D, Rodrigues dos Santos RM. J Psychosom Res 2009; 67: 443–8.

Forty-four patients with BMS were randomized to oral capsules (placebo) for 30 days or a psychological interview and weekly group psychotherapy for 3 months. Seventeen patients (70.8%) receiving group psychotherapy and eight patients (40%) receiving placebo capsules experienced some improvement in pain intensity.

The low level laser therapy in the management of neurological burning mouth syndrome. A pilot study. Romeo U, Del Vecchio A, Capocci M, Maggiore C, Ripari M. Ann Stomatol (Roma) 2010; 1: 14–8.

Twenty-five patients with BMS received twice-weekly treatment with low-level double diode laser therapy (λ = 650 and 910 nm, contemporarily; fluence = 0.53 J/cm^2; time = 15 minutes) to the sides of the tongue for 4 weeks. Seventeen patients (68%) experienced a reduction in pain scores.

Treatment of burning mouth syndrome with a low-level energy diode laser. Yang HW, Huang YF. Photomed Laser Surg 2011; 29: 123–5.

Seventeen patients with BMS received low-level energy diode laser therapy (λ = 800 nm; power = 3 W; 50-msec intermittent pulsing; frequency = 10 Hz) to the affected tongue surface between one and seven times. The average reduction in pain was 47.6%, and it persisted for up to 12 months.

Calcinosis cutis

Ian H. Coulson, Rajani Nalluri

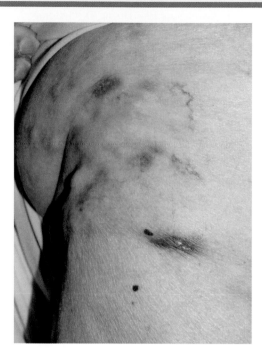

Calcinosis cutis is a rare disease of aberrant calcium deposition in the skin and subcutaneous tissue. There are four major types:

- Idiopathic: occurs without tissue injury or metabolic defect (e.g., idiopathic scrotal calcinosis)
- Dystrophic: (most common form) secondary to local tissue damage or alterations in collagen, elastin, or subcutaneous fat but normal calcium and phosphate levels (e.g., in autoimmune connective tissue diseases, posttrauma or infection)
- Metastatic: abnormal calcium and/or phosphate metabolism leading to precipitation of calcium salts in normal tissue (hyperparathyroidism, sarcoidosis, chronic kidney failure, malignant neoplasms)
- Iatrogenic: secondary to a treatment or procedure (such as extravasation of calcium or phosphate infusions)

Other rare variants of calcinosis cutis that have been described include calcinosis cutis circumscripta, calcinosis universalis, tumoral calcinosis, transplant-associated calcinosis cutis, and milia-like idiopathic calcinosis cutis (usually associated with Down syndrome). Firm white or yellow dermal lesions may ulcerate and extrude a gritty material. It most commonly involves the extensor aspect of joints, particularly the fingers, but can also involve large areas of the body. Stiffening of the skin can limit joint mobility and function, and fingertip lesions may be painful.

MANAGEMENT STRATEGY

The first step in management is to identify any underlying cause. Dystrophic calcification occurs in approximately 25% of patients with systemic sclerosis (SSc) and 10% to 40% of patients with juvenile dermatomyositis, but is rare in systemic lupus erythematosus.

Examination and investigations for connective tissue disease are therefore strongly recommended. Skin biopsy can help to distinguish cutaneous calcification from ossification.

Elevated interleukin-1 levels, along with interleukin-6, interleukin-1β, and tumor necrosis factor (TNF)-α, are found in patients with juvenile dermatomyositis. Mannose-binding lectin levels were significantly increased in SSc patients with calcinosis. It is positively associated with positive anticentromere, anti-PM/Scl, and anticardiolipin antibodies in SSc patients with calcinosis.

A number of malignancies have been implicated in causing metastatic calcification (e.g., leukemia and multiple myeloma). However, successful treatment of the underlying cause does not always have an impact on calcinosis cutis, which frequently requires other treatment modalities. There are no large studies for the treatment of calcinosis cutis, and most therapies are based on case reports or small case series.

Spontaneous extrusion of calcium salts may occur; this may need *surgical* encouragement. General measures to improve blood flow to extremities such as avoiding smoking, stress, and cold exposure are crucial. *Intralesional corticosteroids, aluminum hydroxide supplements, bisphosphonates, diltiazem, colchicine,* and *probenecid* have shown success, mostly in calcinosis associated with dermatomyositis. Low-dose *minocycline* has been reported to reduce the frequency of ulceration and inflammation associated with cutaneous calcinosis in patients with limited SSc. The mechanism of action may be mainly through inhibition of matrix metalloproteinases and antiinflammatory effects.

Warfarin has been advocated in both dermatomyositis and SSc-associated calcinosis for small calcified deposits. *Carbon dioxide laser vaporization, extracorporeal shock wave lithotripsy,* and *intravenous immunoglobulin* are recent approaches that have been tried in cutaneous calcinosis secondary to CREST syndrome. Surgical removal can be of benefit for larger lesions.

Specific Investigations

- Full blood count
- Urea and creatinine
- Serum calcium and phosphate
- Parathyroid hormone levels
- Vitamin D levels
- Serum electrophoresis
- Muscle enzymes: creatine kinase, lactate dehydrogenase (LDH), aldolase
- Connective tissue disease screen: antinuclear antibodies (ANAs) and other autoantibodies
- Skin biopsy
- Plain radiographs
- Bone scintigraphy
- Computed tomography (CT) and magnetic resonance imaging (MRI)

First-Line Therapies

No treatment/self-healing	E
Diltiazem	C
Aluminum hydroxide	D
Intralesional corticosteroid/oral prednisolone	E

Self-healing dystrophic calcinosis following trauma with transepidermal elimination. Pitt AE, Ethington JE, Troy JL. Cutis 1990; 45: 28–32.

A case of dystrophic calcinosis after trauma that resolved over 8 weeks with spontaneous transepidermal elimination.

Calcinosis cutis: part II. Treatment options. Reiter N, El-Shabrawi L, Leinweber B, Berghold A, Aberer E. J Am Acad Dermatol 2011; 65: 15–22.

Calcinosis cutis in dermatomyositis has been successfully treated with diltiazem (2–4 mg/kg/day), with lower doses being ineffective. Surgical excision or curettage is the treatment of choice in idiopathic calcinosis cutis, especially scrotal calcinosis. It is also effective for small, digital calcified skin lesions. A 16-year-old boy with morphea profunda developed small calcified deposits on both arms, his chest, and left thigh. He was treated with ceftriaxone 2 g/day intravenously for 20 days, and the calcification diminished within weeks.

A case of juvenile dermatomyositis with severe calcinosis and successful treatment with prednisone and diltiazem. Jiang X, Yi Q, Liu D, Wang S, Li L. Int J Dermatol 2011; 50: 74–7.

A 12-year-old boy with calcinosis secondary to juvenile dermatomyositis received diltiazem at a dose of 30 mg/day resulting in obvious softening and radiologic regression and functional improvement at 4 months.

Calcinosis cutis occurring in association with autoimmune connective tissue disease: the Mayo Clinic experience with 78 patients, 1996 to 2009. Balin SJ, Wetter DA, Andersen LK, Davis MD. Arch Dermatol 2012; 148: 455–62.

Nine of 17 patients with autoimmune connective tissue disorders showed partial response to treatment with diltiazem at the dose of <480 mg/day. This is recommended as first-line treatment. Eight patients were treated with colchicine (<1.2 g/day), resulting in one patient showing complete response and two patients showing partial response. Six patients received minocycline (200 mg/day). Only one patient showed partial response, two patients did not respond, and the response was unknown in three patients. Four patients were treated with warfarin with only one patient partially responding. Out of the 11 patients who received surgical excision alone, all 11 responded, with 8 having a complete response. Another 17 patients had surgical and medical treatment with complete response in 14 patients, partial response in 2 patients, and no response in 1 patient.

Large subcutaneous calcification in systemic lupus erythematosus: treatment with oral aluminium hydroxide administration followed by surgical excision. Park YM, Lee SJ, Kang H, Cho SH. J Korean Med Sci 1999; 14: 589–92.

A 22-year-old woman with systemic lupus erythematosus developed soft tissue calcification with ulceration, infection, and abscess formation. She was treated with aluminum hydroxide 600 mg three times a day with reduction in size and softening of the deposits after 9 months.

Calcinosis cutis in juvenile dermatomyositis responsive to aluminum hydroxide treatment. Nakagawa T, Takaiwa T. J Dermatol 1993; 20: 558–60.

A case of calcinosis cutis in juvenile dermatomyositis was successfully treated with oral aluminum hydroxide; near-complete clearance was observed after 8 months of therapy.

The use of these agents in patients with renal insufficiency may result in aluminum toxicity.

Localized calcinosis in juvenile dermatomyositis: successful treatment with intralesional corticosteroids injection. Al-Mayouf SM, Alsonbul A, Alismail K. Int J Rheum Dis 2010; 13: e26–8.

A 10-year-old boy with juvenile dermatomyositis had calcinosis of his left elbow. It was treated with Depo-Medrol 80 mg and Xylocaine 1% under ultrasound guidance with significant improvement.

Severe calcinosis cutis with cutaneous ulceration in juvenile dermatomyositis. Meher BK, Mishra P, Sivaraj P, Padhan P. Indian Pediatr 2014; 51: 925–7.

A 7-year-old girl with severe calcinosis cutis with ulceration improved, with healing of the ulcer and resolution of nodules, after 1 month of oral prednisolone (1mg/kg/day) and methotrexate (10 mg/week).

Second-Line Therapies	
• Bisphosphonates	D
• Probenecid	E
• Colchicine	E
• Minocycline	E

Dramatic improvement of subcutaneous calcinosis by intermittent, high-dose etidronate plus cimetidine in a patient with juvenile dermatomyositis. Wakabayashi T, Sasaki N, Chinen N, Suzuki Y. Case Rep Rheumatol 2015; 2015: Article ID 817592.

A 17-year-old boy with juvenile dermatomyositis and bilateral extensive lower limb calcinosis extending into the subcutaneous tissue and muscle showed marked improvement with intermittent 6 monthly high-dose etidronate (800 mg/day for 3 months) and cimetidine for over 5 years.

Effectiveness of the treatment with intravenous pamidronate in calcinosis in juvenile dermatomyositis. Marco Puche A, Calvo Penades I, Lopez Montesinos B. Clin Exp Rheumatol 2010; 28: 135–40.

Three children with juvenile dermatomyositis received treatment with intravenous pamidronate at 1 mg/kg/day on 3 consecutive days every 3 months. In all three cases calcinosis significantly decreased and even totally cleared in one of them.

Improvement of calcinosis using pamidronate in a patient with juvenile dermatomyositis. Martillotti J, Moote D, Zemel L. Pediatr Radiol 2014; 44: 115–8.

A 7-year-old girl with juvenile dermatomyositis developed severe calcinosis, despite an extensive medication regimen. Three administrations of intravenous pamidronate (1 mg/kg/dose every month for 3 months) produced significant improvement in calcinosis, pain, and function, leading to remission less than 1 year after induction of therapy.

Efficacy of probenecid for a patient with juvenile dermatomyositis complicated with calcinosis. Nakamura H, Kawakami A, Ida H, Ejima E, Origuchi T, Eguchi K. J Rheumatol 2006; 33:1691–3.

An 11-year-old boy with juvenile dermatomyositis developed calcinosis of both legs. Probenecid was used to reduce calcinosis, resulting in remarkable improvement of calcinosis accompanied by normalization of serum phosphorus level.

Treatment of cutaneous calcinosis in limited systemic sclerosis with minocycline. Robertson LP, Marshall RW, Hickling P. Ann Rheum Dis 2003; 62: 267–9.

In an open-label study, eight out of nine patients with limited cutaneous SSc prescribed minocycline 50 or 100 mg daily showed definite improvement. The frequency of ulceration and inflammation associated with the calcinosis deposits decreased with treatment. A reduction in calcinosis size was evident but less dramatic, with improvement occurring by 5 months. The mean duration of treatment was 3.5 years.

See also Balin et al. earlier regarding colchicine and minocycline.

Third-Line Therapies	
• Warfarin	D
• Ceftriaxone	E
• Rituximab	E
• Intravenous immunoglobulin	D
• Intravenous sodium thiosulfate	E
• Topical sodium thiosulfate	E
• Topical sodium metabisulfite	E
• Surgery	C
• Carbon dioxide laser	E
• Extracorporeal shock wave lithotripsy	D

Low dose warfarin treatment for calcinosis in patients with systemic sclerosis. Cukierman T, Elinav E, Korem M, Chajek-Shaul T. Ann Rheum Dis 2004; 63: 1341–3.

Three patients with disseminated subcutaneous calcinosis were treated with low doses of warfarin (1 mg/day) for 1 year. Two patients (relatively small lesions up to 2 cm in diameter) had complete resolution within 2 months. The other patient (larger and longer-standing lesions reaching up to 5 cm) did not respond to treatment. None of the patients showed a prolongation of prothrombin time, partial thromboplastin time, or an increased tendency for bleeding.

See also Reiter et al. earlier regarding ceftriaxone.

Rituximab-induced regression of CREST-related calcinosis. de Paula DR, Klem FB, Lorencetti PG, Muller C, Azevedo VF. Clin Rheumatol 2013; 32: 281–3.

A 54-year-old lady with limited cutaneous scleroderma and calcinosis in her hands had complete resolution 7 months after the first infusion of rituximab (four weekly infusions 375 mg/m^2).

Treatment of systemic sclerosis-associated calcinosis: a case report of rituximab-induced regression of CREST-related calcinosis and review of the literature. Daoussis D, Antonopoulos I, Liossis SN, Yiannopoulos G, Andonopoulos AP. Semin Arthritis Rheum 2012; 41: 822–9.

This patient with frequently ulcerating and painful extensive CREST-related calcinosis received two rituximab courses (consisting of four weekly infusions, 375 mg/m^2 each); calcinosis significantly improved and pain disappeared.

Intravenous immunoglobulin for treatment of dermatomyositis-associated dystrophic calcinosis. Galimberti F, Li Y, Fernandez AP. J Am Acad Dermatol 2015; 73: 174–6.

In a retrospective analysis of dermatomyositis-associated calcinosis in an institution, five out of eight patients showed clinical improvement of calcinosis after IV immunoglobulin (1–3 g/kg over 2 days monthly).

Calcinosis cutis associated with amyopathic dermatomyositis: response to intravenous immunoglobulin. Peñate Y, Guillermo N, Melwani P, Martel R, Hernández-Machín B, Borrego L. J Am Acad Dermatol 2009; 60: 1076–7.

A 55-year-old female with amyopathic dermatomyositis and progressive dystrophic calcinosis on the limbs with ulceration and pain failed to respond to various immunosuppressants and diltiazem. She had treatment with intravenous immunoglobulin (IVIG) (2 g/kg/month) at a dose of 0.4 g/day for 5 consecutive days, in combination with a reduced dose of prednisolone. After five courses of IVIG the dermal calcifications reduced, both clinically and radiologically, and became asymptomatic.

Successful treatment of severe iatrogenic calcinosis cutis with intravenous sodium thiosulfate in a child affected by T-acute lymphoblastic leukemia. Raffaella C, Annapaola C, Tullio I, Angelo R, Giuseppe L, Simone C. Pediatr Dermatol 2009; 26: 311–15.

A 5-year-old boy with T-cell acute lymphoblastic leukemia developed soft tissue calcification with motility impairment at sites of intravenous 10% calcium gluconate infusion. Treatment with intravenous sodium thiosulfate 435 mg/kg three times a week for 3 months resulted in massive reduction of soft tissue calcification and functional recovery of affected limbs.

Sodium thiosulfate for the treatment of calcinosis secondary to juvenile dermatomyositis. Pagnini I, Simonini G, Giani T, Marrani E, Moretti D, Vannucci G, et al. Clin Exp Rheumatol 2014; 32: 408–9.

There was successful use of sodium thiosulfate in a patient with juvenile dermatomyositis complicated by ulcerative skin disease and progressive calcinosis.

Dramatic diminution of a large calcification treated with topical sodium thiosulfate. Ratsimbazafy V, Bahans C, Guigonis V. Arthritis Rheum 2012; 64: 3826.

A 12-year-old boy with a large subcutaneous calcification on the left elbow showed significant reduction in the mass, both clinically and radiologically, after 6 months of once-daily application of sodium thiosulfate topically.

Topical sodium metabisulfite for the treatment of calcinosis cutis: a promising new therapy. Del Barrio-Díaz P, Moll-Manzur C, Álvarez-Veliz S, Vera-Kellet C. Br J Dermatol 2016; 175: 608–11.

Four female patients with calcinosis cutis showed decrease in size, erythema, and pain after 6 weeks of topical 25% sodium metabisulfite twice daily.

See also Reiter et al earlier regarding surgical excision.

Surgical debridement of painful fingertip calcinosis cutis in CREST syndrome. Saddic N, Miller JJ, Miller OF 3rd, Clarke JT. Arch Dermatol 2009; 145: 212–3.

A 58-year-old woman with CREST syndrome underwent 2-mm curettage. There was immediate pain relief, and 7 months after the procedure, calcinosis had not recurred.

See also Balin et al earlier. Surgical excision of large, discrete, and symptomatic lesions can be beneficial to patients.

A dystrophic calcinosis cutis case treated with CO$_2$ laser. Kutlubay Z, Yardimci G, Gokler G, Engin B. J Cosmet Laser Ther 2014; 16: 144–6.

A 12-year-old boy with 2- to 4-mm calcinosis on his right knee was treated with 8 to 10 passes with a CO$_2$ laser (Candela CO2RE) at a wavelength of 10.600 nm, in classical mode, 3- to 5-mm spot size, fluence of 5 mJ, and pulse duration of 0.104 ms. There was resolution and no recurrence after 3 months.

Therapy of calcinosis cutis using erbium-doped yttrium aluminum garnet laser treatment. Meissner M, Ochsendorf F, Kaufmann R. Dermatol Surg 2010; 36: 727–8.

Evidence Levels: A Double-blind study B Clinical trial ≥ 20 subjects C Clinical trial < 20 subjects D Series ≥ 5 subjects E Anecdotal case reports

Patients with subcutaneous nodules smaller than 2 cm in diameter were given local anesthesia, then the skin over the mass was opened using a focused erbium-doped yttrium aluminum garnet (Er:YAG) beam (5 J/cm^2, 5 mm diameter, 5 Hz). The chalky material was then removed with a swab or curette. Reepithelialization and cosmetic recovery were seen at 2 to 3 weeks and 14 weeks, respectively.

Treatment of calcinosis cutis by extracorporeal shock-wave lithotripsy. Sultan-Bichat N, Menard J, Perceau G, Staerman F, Bernard P, Reguiaï Z. J Am Acad Dermatol 2012; 66: 424–9.

A single center study, including eight consecutive patients (with 10 calcinosis cutis lesions) who underwent three extracorporeal shock wave lithotripsy sessions at 3-week intervals for 6 months. At the end of this treatment period the median area had decreased by more than 50% in three calcinosis cutis lesions, with pain scores decreasing significantly in five patients and analgesia consumption decreasing in three patients, with no difference in results according to the underlying causal disease.

Calciphylaxis

Alexander Doctoroff

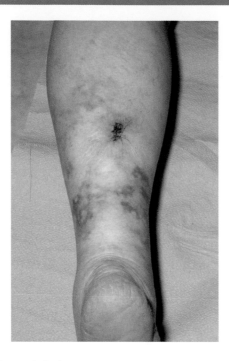

Calciphylaxis (calcific uremic arteriolopathy, uremic small-artery disease with medial calcification and intimal hyperplasia, vascular calcification–cutaneous necrosis syndrome, calcifying panniculitis) is a serious and often lethal condition affecting mostly patients with renal disease, although normorenal calciphylaxis is becoming increasingly recognized. Calciphylaxis may be considered the cutaneous equivalent of myocardial infarction. Medial calcification and subintimal fibrosis of arterioles result in arteriolar stenosis. This is followed by thrombotic occlusion and cutaneous necrosis. Calciphylaxis can present either with tender subcutaneous plaques or skin ulcers reflecting various stages of the progression of the disease process.

MANAGEMENT STRATEGY

Because calciphylaxis is a deadly disease with a mortality rate of up to 80%, early diagnosis via skin biopsy and aggressive treatment are essential.

Monitoring the patient's metabolic environment is of utmost importance. Hyperphosphatemia must be controlled with non–calcium-containing *phosphate binders*. Phosphorus-restricted diet should be introduced, and *vitamin D supplementation stopped*. *Discontinuation of warfarin* due to its proposed procoagulant effect is paramount. Aggressive *wound debridement* needs to be initiated without delay. Monitoring for infection and appropriate use of *antibiotics* are a mainstay of treatment, because most patient deaths occur from sepsis.

Intravenous sodium thiosulfate recently emerged as a promising new treatment for calciphylaxis. This medication is currently used as an antidote for the treatment of cyanide poisoning and prevention of toxicity in cancer therapies. The mechanism of action is believed to be chelation of calcium resulting in dissolution of calcium deposits. Additionally, sodium thiosulfate appears to act as an antioxidant, reducing damage from intravascular reactive oxygen species. The evidence in favor of sodium thiosulfate is limited to multiple case reports. Yet it appears to be safe and nontoxic and therefore deserves a trial as a first-line therapy for calciphylaxis.

Bisphosphonates are another group of medications that alone or in combination with sodium thiosulfate are emerging as an important part of calciphylaxis treatment. They are thought to inhibit local proinflammatory cytokines and decrease arterial calcification.

Cinacalcet may also be used for patients with elevated parathyroid hormone. This medication is believed to act by reducing serum parathyroid hormone and stabilizing calcium and phosphate levels. It is useful in patients with elevated parathyroid hormone levels. Parathyroid hormone should be monitored throughout treatment to minimize the risk of adynamic bone disease associated with cinacalcet therapy.

If the patient's calciphylaxis is uncovered at an early stage (indurated plaques without ulcerations), oral *prednisone* appears to be helpful.

The use of zero or *low-calcium dialysate* with induction of hypocalcemia and calcium shift into intravascular space appears to be a reasonable therapy. If *hyperbaric oxygen therapy* is available, it can be very helpful to some patients.

Parathyroidectomy, which improves calcium, phosphate, and parathyroid hormone levels, is a useful therapy for those patients with high parathyroid hormone levels. Despite being a subject of controversy, for many patients this surgery results in rapid healing of ulcerations. In many cases the use of cinacalcet avoids parathyroidectomy.

The treatment of calciphylaxis should be a multidisciplinary effort with internists, critical care specialists, nephrologists, dermatologists, infectionists, surgeons, and pain specialists being involved.

Specific Investigations

- Skin biopsy
- Serum parathyroid hormone, calcium, phosphate
- Bone scan
- Measurements of transcutaneous oxygen saturation
- X-ray or xeroradiography

Pathogenesis of calciphylaxis: Hans Selye to nuclear factor kappa-B. Weenig RH. J Am Acad Dermatol 2008; 58: 458–71.

Calciphylaxis from nonuremic causes: a systematic review. Nigwekar SU, Wolf M, Sterns RH, Hix JK. Clin J Am Soc Nephrol 2008; 3: 1139–43.

A review of 38 cases of cutaneous calciphylaxis in patients with normal renal function.

Associated conditions were malignancy, connective tissue disease, hyperparathyroidism, alcoholic cirrhosis, and thrombophilia (protein S and C deficiency). Recent use of steroids, anticoagulants, and weight loss has also been implicated.

First-Line Therapies

Debridement of necrotic tissue and aggressive wound care	C
Discontinuation of calcium and vitamin D supplementation	C
Decrease of serum phosphorus	C
Treatment of low serum albumin	C
Monitoring for infection	C

First-Line Therapies—cont'd

• Intravenous sodium thiosulfate	D
• Prednisone (for patients without ulcerations only)	C
• Pamidronate	E
• Cinacalcet	D

Calcium use increases risk of calciphylaxis: a case-control study. Zacharias JM, Fontaine B, Fine A. Perit Dial Int 1999; 19: 248–52.

Retrospective case-control study of eight patients suggests increased risk of calciphylaxis with calcium ingestion.

Risk factors and mortality associated with calciphylaxis in end-stage renal disease. Mazhar AR, Johnson RJ, Gillen D, Stivelman JC, Ryan MJ, Davis CL, et al. Kidney Int 2001; 60: 324–32.

Retrospective case-control study of 19 cases demonstrated female gender, hyperphosphatemia, high alkaline phosphatase, and low serum albumin to be risk factors for calciphylaxis.

Calciphylaxis: natural history, risk factor analysis, and outcome. Weenig RH, Sewell LD, Davis MD, McCarthy JT, Pittelkow MR. J Am Acad Dermatol 2007; 56: 569–79.

Retrospective case-control study of 64 cases showed that obesity, liver disease, systemic corticosteroid use, and elevated calcium–phosphate product and serum aluminum were risk factors for calciphylaxis.

The evolving pattern of calciphylaxis: therapeutic considerations. Llach F. Nephrol Dial Transplant 2001; 16: 448–51.

This and other reviews suggest aggressive lowering of serum phosphorus with non–calcium-containing phosphate binders (such as Renagel) and dietary control of calcium and phosphorus intake, as well as aggressive wound debridement and monitoring for infection. Six out of eight patients had significant improvement with zero calcium dialysate.

Sodium thiosulfate as first-line treatment for calciphylaxis. Ackermann F, Levy A, Daugas E, Schartz N, Riaux A, Derancourt C, et al. Arch Dermatol 2007; 143: 1336–7.

This is one of several case reports of successful calciphylaxis therapy with IV infusions of sodium thiosulfate (25 g IV infusions three times per week).

Calciphylaxis is usually nonulcerating: risk factors, outcome and therapy. Fine A, Zacharias J. Kidney Int 2002; 61: 2210–7.

Review of 36 patients who presented without ulcerations but with subcutaneous indurated plaques in the legs who demonstrated improvement from steroid therapy (prednisone 30–50 mg orally daily for 3–8 weeks) in 80% of cases. Contraindications to steroid therapy include ulceration anywhere (related to peripheral vascular disease [PVD] or calciphylaxis) or high risk of infection.

Proximal calciphylaxis treated with calcimimetic "cinacalcet." Mohammed IA, Sekar V, Bubtana AJ, Mitra S, Hutchison AJ. Nephr Dial Transpl 2008; 23: 387–9.

A case report of successful calciphylaxis treatment with 30 mg/day of cinacalcet. *Doses from 30 mg to 120 mg/day have been used in other cases.*

Rapid improvement of calciphylaxis after intravenous pamidronate therapy in a patient with chronic renal failure. Monney P, Nguyen QV, Perroud H, Descombes E. Nephrol Dial Transplant 2004; 19: 2130–2.

Five intravenous doses of 30 mg pamidronate resulted in healing of ulcerations in a patient whose clinical condition was worsening despite other medical therapy. When 6 weeks after discharge calciphylaxis returned, an additional 30 mg pamidronate dose aborted the recurrence.

Multiintervention management of calciphylaxis: a report of 7 cases. Baldwin C, Farah M, Leung M, Taylor P, Werb R, Kiaii M, et al. Am J of Kidney Dis 2011; 58: 988–91.

Various combinations of intravenous sodium thiosulfate (12.5–25 g IV three times a week), oxygen therapy (given through a face mask or hyperbaric chamber), and cinacalcet resolved calciphylaxis in six out of seven patients.

Second-Line Therapies

• Parathyroidectomy (for patients with elevated parathyroid hormone)	C
• Hyperbaric oxygen therapy	D
• Low-calcium dialysate	D
• Vitamin K supplementation in patients who are deficient	E
• Tissue plasminogen activator	E

Calciphylaxis: a syndrome of skin necrosis and acral gangrene in chronic renal failure. Hafner J, Keusch G, Wahl C, Berg G. Vasa 1998; 27: 137–43.

Meta-analysis of all case reports of calciphylaxis from 1936 to 1996 revealed that 70% of patients who were parathyroidectomized survived compared with 43% of those who did not receive the operation. *This study did not stratify patients into those with and without hyperparathyroidism.*

Hyperbaric oxygen in the treatment of calciphylaxis: a case series. Podymow T, Wherrett C, Burns KD. Nephrol Dial Transplant 2001; 16: 2176.

In this retrospective study, two out of five patients with calciphylaxis had complete resolution of their ulcers with hyperbaric oxygen therapy.

Successful treatment of severe calciphylaxis in a hemodialysis patient using low-calcium dialysate and medical parathyroidectomy: case report and literature review. Wang HY, Yu CC, Huang CC. Ren Fail 2004; 26: 77–82.

This is one of several case reports of successful calciphylaxis treatment with low-calcium dialysis.

Skin necrosis and protein C deficiency associated with vitamin K depletion in a patient with renal failure. Soundararajan R, Leehey DJ, Yu AW, Miller JB. Am J Med 1992; 93: 467–70.

Vitamin K replacement resulted in reversal of calciphylaxis in a vitamin K–deficient patient.

Low-dose tissue plasminogen activator for calciphylaxis. Sewell LD, Weenig RH, Davis MD, McEvoy MT, Pittelkow MR. Arch Dermatol 2004; 140: 1045–8.

Tissue plasminogen activator (tPA; alteplase) in a 10-mg intravenous daily dose for 14 days, followed by warfarin anticoagulation resulted in eventual healing of ulcerations.

- Maggot therapy and pentoxifylline   E
- Ozone therapy   E
- Cryofiltration apheresis   E

Painful ulcers in calciphylaxis – combined treatment with maggot therapy and oral pentoxifylline. Tittelbach J, Graefe T, Wollina UJ. Dermatolog Treat 2001; 12: 211–4.

Maggot therapy and 800 mg/day of oral pentoxifylline were successful in healing ulcers over a 6-month period.

Ozone therapy in a dialyzed patient with calcific uremic arteriolopathy. Biedunkiewicz B, Tylicki L, Lichodziejewska-Niemierko M, Liberek T, Rutkowski B. Kidney Int 2003; 64: 367–8.

Fifteen sessions of treatment with ozonated autohemotherapy with ozone concentration of 50 to 70 μg/mL over 3 weeks, accompanied by local wound lavage with ozonated water, led to healing of necrotic areas.

Intensive tandem cryofiltration apheresis and hemodialysis to treat a patient with severe calciphylaxis, cryoglobulinemia, and end-stage renal disease. Siami GA, Siami FS. ASAIO J 1999; 45: 229–33.

This is a report on tandem cryofiltration apheresis (CFA) and hemodialysis (HD) in a critically ill patient with type II mixed cryoglobulinemia, hepatitis C virus infection, calciphylaxis, and end-stage renal disease. The patient received 18 tandem CFA/HD treatments and 4 extra HD treatments in 1 month. His plasma cryoglobulin level dropped, and his calciphylaxis also improved.

Evidence Levels: **A** Double-blind study   **B** Clinical trial ≥ 20 subjects   **C** Clinical trial < 20 subjects   **D** Series ≥ 5 subjects   **E** Anecdotal case reports

Capillaritis (pigmented purpuric dermatoses)

Cord Sunderkötter, Thomas A. Luger

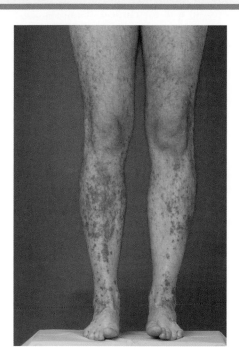

Capillaritis (a generic term for the various pigmented purpuric dermatoses) presents with the common feature of petechial macules or plaques and is characterized histologically by erythrocyte extravasation and perivascular infiltration with T lymphocytes. Lesions develop a characteristic brown-to-orange color due to hemosiderin deposits in macrophages. These conditions may also present with additional, distinctive, and sometimes overlapping, morphologic patterns, which have given rise to several descriptive or eponymous names: papules in pigmented purpuric lichenoid dermatosis (of Gougerot and Blum) or in the rarely described granulomatous pigmented purpura (non-necrotizing granulomata with concomitant lymphocytic infiltrate); eczematous spongiosis with pruritus in eczematoid-like purpura; annular forms with telangiectases and central clearing in purpura annularis telangiectodes (Majocchi disease); and often solitary, ochre-golden plaques or patches with bandlike infiltrates, including a grenz zone in lichen aureus. Sites of predilection are mostly both lower extremities. A form of unilateral linear capillaritis or involvement of other areas of the skin is rare. Pigmented purpuric dermatoses also occur in children, albeit less frequently than in adults.

The etiology of capillaritis, including these variants, is not known. The reason for extravasation of erythrocytes is not an inflammatory fibrinoid necrosis of vessels (no vasculitis). Possible pathophysiologic factors that can be addressed therapeutically are a cell-mediated immune response, increased venous pressure, increased vascular permeability, or vascular fragility due to subtle defects in the extracellular matrix.

MANAGEMENT STRATEGY

Diagnostic hallmarks are the yellow-brown or orange patches with superimposed pinpoint cayenne pepper spots, which represent petechiae and persist with diascopy. The main differential diagnosis is leukocytoclastic or small vessel vasculitis. The discerning criterion is the lack of a palpable infiltrate in capillaritis, but there are courses or variants of small vessel vasculitis with petechial maculae only. Thus biopsies are warranted when in doubt.

In the differential diagnosis, allergic contact dermatitis may be purpuric or hemorrhagic (e.g., in response to textile or azo dyes), mimicking capillaritis. Thrombocytopenia, hypergammaglobulinemic purpura of Waldenström, and the pigmented purpuric dermatitis–like variant of mycosis fungoides also need to be excluded. Capillaritis has a benign course and therefore must be differentiated from these more serious diseases.

Usually there is no need for treatment unless the patient has pruritus or suffers from cosmetic disfigurement. Detection and avoidance of possible eliciting agents should always be attempted. Reported causes include:

- Drugs (14% in one series), for example, acetaminophen, acetylsalicylic acid, bromine-containing drugs, carbamazepine, furosemide, interferon-α, nonsteroidal antiinflammatory drugs (NSAIDs), raloxifene (selective estrogen receptor modulator), thiamine, or sildenafil.

  As a rule, drug-induced capillaritis is more generalized and does not usually present with epidermal involvement or lichenoid infiltrate; its onset is around 10 days after intake of the suspected drug.
- Dietary supplements or ingredients; reported triggers include creatine or Coca-Cola and apple-cherry fruit spritzer, as well as ingredients of an energy drink (vitamin B complex, caffeine, taurine).
- Chronic infections such as viral hepatitis B or C (though relation is questionable) or odontogenic infections.

When the etiology remains obscure, therapy has to be empirical. However, immunohistochemical analyses have suggested a cell-mediated immune response, so treatment with *local corticosteroids, calcineurin inhibitors, or psoralen plus UVA* (PUVA) may be rational. Increased venous pressure (particularly in the legs) or exercise are not direct causes, but can aggravate capillaritis. In these cases compression stockings may be helpful.

There is some evidence for increased vascular permeability or vascular fragility due to subtle defects in the extracellular matrix. This may explain reported responses to *bioflavonoids* (which may be due to inhibition of elastase and hyaluronase and of leukocyte activation), *ascorbic acid* (antioxidant effects and perhaps reduction of vascular permeability), and *calcium dobesilate* (reduction of microvascular permeability in part by antioxidant properties).

Specific Investigations

- Careful drug history
- Look for signs of chronic infection or rheumatoid arthritis
- Exclude chronic venous insufficiency and purpuric contact eczema (e.g., by modified patch test performed at the site of skin lesions to look after a petechial reaction to azo dyes, for example)
- Dermoscopy
- Hematology (complete blood count)
- C-reactive protein
- Immunoglobulins, protein electrophoresis
- Histology
- In granulomatous variant: triglycerides and cholesterol

Purpura simplex (inflammatory purpura without vasculitis): a clinicopathologic study of 174 cases. Ratnam KV, Su WP, Peters MS. J Am Acad Dermatol 1991; 25: 642–7.

A retrospective review of 174 cases. A correlation between purpuric reaction and drugs was observed in 14%. Of the 87 patients who were followed up, 67% appeared to eventually have clearing of lesions.

Pigmented purpuric dermatosis: clinicopathologic characterization in a pediatric series. Coulombe J, Jean SE, Hatami A, Powell J, Marcoux D, Kokta V, et al. Pediatr Dermatol 2015; 32: 358–62.

A retrospective chart review of 17 children. Pigmented purpuric dermatosis resolved in 13 cases with a median duration <1 year in 5 of them without treatment; those cases treated with topical corticosteroids improved in 75%, those with narrowband ultraviolet B in 100%. No associated disease or drug exposure was found.

Granulomatous pigmented purpuric dermatosis: report of a case with atypical clinical presentation including dermoscopic findings. MacKenzie AI, Biswas A. Am J Dermatopathol 2015; 37: 311–4.

Granulomatous pigmented purpuric dermatosis is rare and affects the distal extremities of mainly Far East Asian patients. There was an association with hyperlipidemia or other associated systemic derangements.

Progression of pigmented purpura-like eruptions to mycosis fungoides: report of three cases. Barnhill RL, Braverman IM. J Am Acad Dermatol 1988; 19: 25–31.

Initial eruptions, resembling pigmented purpuric dermatitis both clinically and histologically, developed into histologically definite mycosis fungoides in follow-up period averaging 8.4 years.

Exclusion or diagnosis of mycosis fungoides may require repeated biopsies. In capillaritis small cerebriform lymphocytes exhibiting epidermotropism should be absent.

Drug-induced purpura simplex: clinical and histologic characteristics. Pang BK, Su D, Ratnam KV. Ann Acad Med Singapore 1993; 22: 870–2.

A prospective study of 183 patients with purpura simplex was carried out. Of these, 27 cases were confirmed to be drug induced, as the purpura cleared within 4 months of withdrawal of medications. NSAIDs, diuretics, meprobamate, and ampicillin were the most common offenders.

Acetaminophen-induced progressive pigmentary purpura (Schamberg's disease). Abeck D, Gross GE, Kuwert C, Steinkraus V, Mensing H, Ring J. J Am Acad Dermatol 1992; 27: 123–4.

Pigmented purpura dermatosis and viral hepatitis: a case-control study. Ehsani AH, Ghodsi SZ, Nourmohammad-Pour P, Aghazadeh N, Damavandi MR. Australas J Dermatol 2013; 54: 225–7.

A prospective case-control study with 60 PPD patients and 230 randomly selected controls. The prevalence of HBS Ag in PPD patients and the controls was 3% and 4.3%, respectively, and the prevalence of HCV was 1.7% vs. 1.3%. Thus direct involvement of HBV or HCV in pathogenesis of PPD is not certain.

Chronic pigmented purpura associated with odontogenic infection. Satoh T, Yokozeki H, Nishioka K. J Am Acad Dermatol 2002; 46: 942–4.

Appearance of purpuric spots in five patients ceased after treatment for periodontitis, pulpitis, or both.

Capillaritis associated with interferon-alfa treatment of chronic hepatitis C infection. Gupta G, Holmes SC, Spence E, Mills PR. J Am Acad Dermatol 2000; 43: 937–8.

Pigmented purpuric dermatosis after taking a dietary supplement. Unal E, Ergül G. Cutan Ocul Toxicol 2015; 10: 1–3.

Dermoscopy of pigmented purpuric dermatoses (lichen aureus): a useful tool for clinical diagnosis. Zaballos P, Puig S, Malvehy J. Arch Dermatol 2004; 140: 1290–1.

Dermatoscopy is a useful aid in diagnosis. In lichen aureus, in which the lichenoid tissue reaction is condensed, it shows coppery-red to brownish diffuse coloration of the background (likely caused by the dermal infiltrate and extravascular or intracellular hemosiderin), as well as a partial network of interconnected pigmented lines (hyperpigmentation of the basal layer and pigment released into the dermis); round to oval red dots, globules, or patches (these could reflect dilated vessels and extravasated erythrocytes); and gray dots (probably accumulation of hemosiderin-containing macrophages). It is likely that these criteria also apply for other forms of capillaritis with different accentuations.

Cutaneous symptoms of various vasculitides. Sunderkötter C, Pappelbaum KI, Ehrchen J. Hautarzt 2015; 66: 589–98.

Careful clinical examination allows the differentiation of capillaritis from small vessel vasculitis or similar conditions.

First-Line Therapies

• Oral bioflavonoids and ascorbic acid	C
• Local corticosteroids initially in cases of pruritus/ eczematoid or itching purpura	D
• Narrowband UVB or PUVA	D
• Calcium dobesilate	D
• Compression stocking when aggravated by increased venous pressure	E

Early treatment with rutoside and ascorbic acid is highly effective for progressive pigmented purpuric dermatosis. Schober SM, Peitsch WK, Bonsmann G, Metze D, Thomas K, Goerge T, et al. J Dtsch Dermatol Ges 2014; 12: 1112–9.

A retrospective review of 35 patients treated with 1000 mg ascorbic acid and 2 × 50 mg rutoside (a form of bioflavonoid, often available without a prescription). The mean treatment duration was 8.2 months. 71.4% of the participants experienced complete clearance and 20.0% an improvement of more than 50%; 9 (25.1%) relapsed after discontinuation, and in 7 treatment was successfully reinitiated. Only 3 participants reported mild adverse effects. Participants with shorter disease duration showed better and faster therapeutic success and lower risk of recurrence.

Treatment of progressive pigmented purpura with oral bioflavonoids and ascorbic acid: an open pilot study in 3 patients. Reinhold U, Seiter S, Ugurel S, Tilgen W. J Am Acad Dermatol 1999; 41: 207–8.

First report on this treatment; complete clearance of skin lesions after 4 weeks of treatment.

We recommend rutoside (50 mg twice a day) and ascorbic acid (500 mg twice daily) as our therapy of choice because it is

Evidence Levels: A Double-blind study **B** Clinical trial ≥ 20 subjects **C** Clinical trial < 20 subjects **D** Series ≥ 5 subjects **E** Anecdotal case reports

efficacious, especially in early disease and because it has fewer potential side effects than UV light or topical corticosteroids.

Capillaritis: a manifestation of rheumatoid disease. Wilkinson SM, Smith AG, Davis M, Dawes PT. Clin Rheumatol 1993; 12: 53–6.

Seven cases of capillaritis were described in patients with rheumatoid arthritis. In the majority, the rash and itch resolved spontaneously with the use of a topical corticosteroid.

PUVA therapy in lichen aureus. Ling TC, Goulden V, Goodfield MJ. J Am Acad Dermatol 2001; 45: 145–6.

One case of lichen aureus that responded dramatically to photochemotherapy (PUVA).

Treatment of pigmented purpuric dermatoses with narrow-band UVB: a report of six cases. Fathy H, Abdelgaber S. J Eur Acad Dermatol Venereol 2011; 25: 603–6.

Successful treatment was achieved in all six patients after 24 to 28 treatments and maintenance of 9 treatments. Two patients who showed flare of their lesions were efficiently controlled with a further 14 treatments.

Calcium dobesilate (Cd) in pigmented purpuric dermatosis (PPD): a pilot evaluation. Agrawal SK, Gandhi V, Bhattacharya SN. J Dermatol 2004; 31: 98–103.

Nine male patients (seven with Schamberg disease and one each with lichenoid dermatosis of Gougerot and Blum and lichen aureus) were given calcium dobesilate 500 mg twice daily for 2 weeks initially, and then 500 mg once daily for 3 months. No new lesions occurred within 2 weeks, and itching ceased in all patients. The improvement of existing lesions 1 year after cessation of therapy was moderate in 11.11% and mild in 66.67% of cases; 22.22% did not show any improvement.

Second-Line Therapies

• Pentoxifylline	E
• Topical calcineurin inhibitors	E
• Advanced fluorescence technology (AFT) of broadband pulsed light	D

Successful treatment of Schamberg's disease with pentoxifylline. Kano Y, Hirayama K, Orihara M, Shiohara T. J Am Acad Dermatol 1997; 36: 827–30.

Three patients with Schamberg disease were treated with pentoxifylline 300 mg daily for 8 weeks. A significant response was observed within 2 to 3 weeks. One patient had recurrence after discontinuation, but promptly responded to resumption of therapy.

Resolution of lichen aureus in a 10-year-old child after topical pimecrolimus. Böhm M, Bonsmann G, Luger TA. Br J Dermatol 2004; 150: 519–20.

A 10-year-old boy with lichen aureus resistant to topical corticosteroids for 4 months. A significant improvement was observed within 3 weeks with pimecrolimus cream twice daily.

Unlike topical corticosteroids, topical immunomodulators do not cause fragility of blood vessels, which is an advantage when treating this group of diseases thought to be caused by vascular fragility and permeability.

Treatment of Schamberg's disease with advanced fluorescence technology. Manolakos DA, Weiss J, Glick B, Weiss KD, Weiss E. J Drugs Dermatol 2012; 11: 528–9.

Favorable treatment of five patients with Schamberg disease using advanced fluorescence technology (AFT) pulsed light, a broadband pulsed light platform device used for nonablative treatment of photodamaged skin.

Third-Line Therapies

• Colchicine	E
• Cyclosporine	E
• Methotrexate	E

The authors would recommend neither cyclosporine A nor methotrexate because of the severity of possible adverse events or side effects and because of the benign nature of capillaritis.

Benefit of colchicine in the treatment of Schamberg's disease. Geller M. Ann Allergy Asthma Immunol 2000; 85: 246.

Purpura pigmentosa chronica successfully treated with oral cyclosporin A. Okada K, Ishikawa O, Miyachi Y. Br J Dermatol 1996; 134: 180–1.

Purpura annularis telangiectodes of Majocchi: case report and review of the literature. Hoesly FJ, Huerter CJ, Shehan JM. Int J Dermatol 2009; 48: 1129–33.

A solitary case report on the efficacy of methotrexate.

Cat scratch disease

Adam H. Wiener, Bryan A. Selkin,
George J. Murakawa

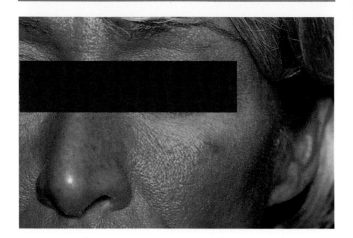

Cat scratch disease (CSD) is a benign, usually self-limited disease caused by *Bartonella henselae* (formerly *Rochalimaea henselae*), a gram-negative pleomorphic rod. The primary lesion consists of a 0.5- to 1-cm papule or pustule, which may undergo ulceration, and adjacent unilateral lymphadenopathy is the hallmark of the disease. Systemic symptoms and complications include low-grade fever, malaise, nonspecific exanthem, hepatosplenomegaly, lytic bone lesions, oculoglandular syndrome of Parinaud (granulomatous conjunctivitis and preauricular adenopathy), and encephalopathy.

MANAGEMENT STRATEGY

No clear guidelines for the treatment of CSD exist. As there is a paucity of data showing a clear benefit of antimicrobial therapy in the treatment of patients with mild to moderate CSD, these patients should be managed with *conservative, symptomatic treatment*. The lymphadenopathy associated with CSD is self-limited and resolves in 2 to 4 months; therefore most patients can be managed with *observation* until involution of the node.

For patients with systemic symptoms and/or complications, antibiotic therapy should be instituted. *Azithromycin* (500 mg on day 1, followed by 250 mg on days 2–5) is the only antibiotic that has been shown in a double-blind, placebo-controlled evaluation to be beneficial to immunocompetent patients with CSD. In a retrospective analysis of 202 patients with CSD who had been on at least 3 days of antimicrobial therapy, only four antibiotics (*rifampin, ciprofloxacin, gentamicin,* and *trimethoprim–sulfamethoxazole*) provided clinical benefit. Presumably, it is the paucity of organisms and the host inflammatory response that result in the poor efficacy of antibiotics.

In immunosuppressed patients, infection with the CSD bacillus can produce a spectrum of disease, from classic CSD to bacillary angiomatosis (BA), peliosis, or septicemia (see chapter on bacillary angiomatosis). Antimicrobial treatment for such patients is beneficial and clearly indicated. Lesions and symptoms respond rapidly to *erythromycin* 500 mg four times daily or *doxycycline* 100 mg twice daily. Other antimicrobials used to successfully treat BA in immunocompromised patients include *tetracycline, minocycline, azithromycin,* and *trimethoprim–sulfamethoxazole*. A Jarisch–Herxheimer reaction frequently occurs after the first dose. Patients with AIDS should be maintained on lifelong antimicrobial therapy.

Of note, *B. henselae* has rarely been isolated from patients with CSD; however, patients who are immunosuppressed may be culture positive. A single dose of oral antibiotics will rapidly sterilize blood and lesional cultures.

Specific Investigations

- Histopathology
- Culture
- Serology
- Polymerase chain reaction (PCR)–based techniques

The agent of bacillary angiomatosis. Relman DA, Loutit JS, Schmidt TM, Falkow S, Tompkins LS. N Engl J Med 1990; 323: 153–80.

PCR was used to amplify, clone, and sequence a portion of eubacterial *16S rRNA* gene directly from tissue infected with the presumed agent of BA. Subsequent analysis of this sequence and study of infected tissues from other patients suggested that BA is caused by a rickettsia-like organism closely related to *Rochalimaea quintana*.

Bartonella-associated infections. Spach DH, Koehler JE. Infect Dis Clin North Am 1998; 12: 137–55.

Findings on lymph node biopsy specimens from immunocompetent patients with CSD depend on the stage of the infection. Early in the course, lymphoid hyperplasia and arteriolar proliferation are prominent. Subsequently, granulomas appear. Late in the disease, multiple stellate microabscesses are prominent. Warthin–Starry stains may show clumps of pleomorphic bacilli.

Evaluation of sensitivity, specificity and cross-reactivity in *Bartonella henselae* **serology.** Vermeulen MJ, Verbakel H, Notermans DW, Reimerink JH, Peeters MF. J Med Microbiol 2010; 59: 743–5.

The combined use of (Houston strain) IFA, IgM, and IgG improves sensitivity with significant reduction of specificity. As falsely diagnosing CSD can have a major impact for the patient, we believe that IgG results must be interpreted with caution.

Cat-scratch disease. Midani S, Ayoub EM, Anderson B. Adv Pediatr 1996; 43: 397–422.

PCR is a powerful tool for the detection of *B. henselae* but is not widely available. Using PCR, *B. henselae* can be detected in aspirates from lymph nodes or cutaneous lesions within 1 to 2 days. Currently, serologic and PCR-based analyses are considered definitive.

Detection by immunofluorescence assay of *Bartonella henselae* **in lymph nodes from patients with cat scratch disease.** Rolain JM, Gouriet F, Enea M, Aboud M, Raoult D. Clin Diagn Lab Immunol 2003; 10: 686–91.

Immunofluorescence detection in lymph node smears using a specific monoclonal antibody directed against *B. henselae* and a commercial serology assay (IFA) compared with PCR detection showed high specificity in diagnosis of *B. henselae*, especially when associated with histologic analysis and conventional bacterial culture.

Evidence Levels: **A** Double-blind study   **B** Clinical trial ≥ 20 subjects   **C** Clinical trial < 20 subjects   **D** Series ≥ 5 subjects   **E** Anecdotal case reports

The use of *Bartonella henselae*-specific age dependent IgG and IgM in diagnostic models to discriminate diseased from non-diseased in cat scratch disease serology. Herremans M, Vermeulen MJ, Van de Kassteele J, Bakker J, Schellekens JF, Koopmans MP. J Microbiol Methods 2007; 71: 107–13.

The use of diagnostic models using the combination of both the enzyme-linked immunosorbent assay (ELISA) IgM and the IgG results combined with a correcting age factor can be useful in serodiagnosis of CSD.

First-Line Therapy

• Observation only	C

Bartonellosis. Murakawa GJ, Berger T. In: Freedberg IM, Eisen AZ, Wolff K, Austen KF, Goldsmith LA, Katz SI, et al, eds. Dermatology in General Medicine. 5th edn. New York: McGraw-Hill, 1999; 2249–56.

In the majority of patients with CSD, conservative management with careful observation over several months is sufficient. Spontaneous involution of lymphadenopathy should occur over 6 months.

Second-Line Therapy

• Azithromycin	A

Prospective randomized double blind placebo-controlled evaluation of azithromycin for treatment of cat-scratch disease. Bass JW, Freitas BC, Freitas AD, Sisler CL, Chan DS, Vincent JM, et al. Pediatr Infect Dis J 1998; 17: 447–52.

Seven of 14 azithromycin-treated patients (500 mg on day 1, followed by 250 mg on days 2–5) showed an 80% reduction in initial lymph node volume compared with 1 of 15 placebo-treated controls during the first 30 days of observation.

This is the only controlled clinical trial of an antibiotic for the therapy of CSD; the use of all other antibiotics is based on anecdotal reports.

Third-Line Therapies

• Erythromycin	C
• Doxycycline	C
• Rifampin	C
• Ciprofloxacin	C
• Gentamicin	C
• Trimethoprim–sulfamethoxazole	C
• Surgical intervention	C

Immunocompetent individuals

Antibiotic therapy for cat-scratch disease: clinical study of therapeutic outcome in 268 patients and a review of the literature. Margileth AM. Pediatr Infect Dis J 1992; 11: 474–8.

In 60 patients with CSD with systemic symptoms, one of four antibiotics was effective at least 72% of the time. Patients who received rifampin (10–20 mg/kg daily for 7–14 days), ciprofloxacin (20–30 mg/kg daily for 7–14 days), gentamicin (5 mg/kg daily intravenously in divided doses every 8 hours for at least 3 days), or trimethoprim–sulfamethoxazole (6–8 mg/kg of trimethoprim

component two to three times daily for 7 days) had a shorter mean duration of posttreatment illness than those who received either no antibiotics or antibiotics thought to be ineffective.

Antimicrobial susceptibility of *Rochalimaea quintana, Rochalimaea vinsonii,* and the newly recognized *Rochalimaea henselae.* Maurin M, Raoult D. J Antimicrob Chemother 1993; 32: 587–94.

In vitro testing revealed β-lactam drugs to be ineffective, tetracyclines to be intermediate, and erythromycin and rifampin to be most effective against *Rochalimaea* spp.

Hepatosplenic cat-scratch disease in children: selected clinical features and treatment. Arisoy ES, Correa AG, Wagner ML, Kaplan SL. Clin Infect Dis 1999; 28: 78–84.

Sixteen children with hepatosplenic CSD treated with rifampin (15–20 mg/kg daily), either alone or in combination with gentamicin (7.5 mg/kg daily) or trimethoprim–sulfamethoxazole (10–12 mg/kg daily), showed clinical improvement within 1 to 5 days.

Successful treatment of cat-scratch disease with ciprofloxacin. Holley HP. JAMA 1991; 265: 1563–5.

Five patients treated with oral ciprofloxacin, 500 mg twice daily, had a dramatic improvement in symptoms within a few days, with no relapse during follow-up.

It should be noted that quinolones are not recommended for children or adolescents because of concerns about arthropathy. Moreover, in vitro studies show only intermediate efficacy for ciprofloxacin.

Cat-scratch disease of the head and neck in a pediatric population: surgical indications and outcomes. Munson PD, Boyce TG, Salomao DR, Orvidas LJ. Otolaryngol Head Neck Surg 2008; 139: 358–63.

In children, failure of medical therapy in cases that presented as persistent lymphadenopathy often were accompanied by violaceous skin changes, extreme tenderness to palpation, and even chronic drainage. In this subgroup of patients the benefit of surgical intervention and concurrent tissue examination outweighed the risk.

Molecular epidemiology of *Bartonella* infections in patients with bacillary angiomatosis-peliosis. Koehler JE, Sanchez MA, Garrido CS, Whitfeld MJ, Chen FM, Berger TG, et al. N Engl J Med 1997; 337: 1876–83.

Treatment with macrolide antibiotics (e.g., erythromycin or clarithromycin) is protective for patients with *Bartonella* spp. infection.

Cat scratch disease, bacillary angiomatosis, and other infections due to *Rochalimaea.* Adal KA, Cockerell CJ, Petri WA. N Engl J Med 1994; 330: 1509–15.

For the treatment of BA, bacillary peliosis hepatitis, and *Rochalimaea* spp. bacteremic syndrome, erythromycin 500 mg four times daily is the drug of choice on the basis of an excellent clinical response in virtually all patients treated to date.

Cutaneous vascular lesions and disseminated cat-scratch disease in patients with the acquired immunodeficiency syndrome (AIDS) and AIDS-related complex. Koehler JE, LeBoit PE, Egbert BM, Berger GT. Ann Intern Med 1988; 109: 449–55.

Erythromycin (500 mg four times daily), rifampin, and doxycycline (100 mg twice daily) were effective in the treatment of angiomatous skin nodules in three patients with HIV infection.

Cellulite

Bruce E. Katz, Doris M. Hexsel, Camile L. Hexsel

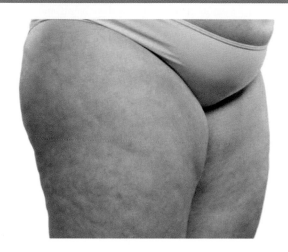

Cellulite consists of surface relief alterations resulting in depressions and raised areas and thus an irregular appearance, such as an orange peel, cottage cheese, or mattresslike appearance of the skin, located mainly on the thighs and buttocks but also on the arms, abdomen, legs, and other areas. Depressed lesions are due to the presence of fibrous septa that pull the skin surface down; raised areas result from the projection of underlying fat to the skin surface as shown on anatomic and imaging studies. Women are most frequently affected by this condition; this is due to the structure and anatomy of the subcutaneous septa compared with their structure in men. In addition, cellulite is aggravated by progressive skin laxity or flaccidity, localized fat deposition, and obesity. Furthermore, other factors have been implicated in the pathogenesis of cellulite, such as hormonal, biochemical, inflammatory, and circulatory factors.

Subcision: a treatment for cellulite. Hexsel DM, Mazzuco R. Int J Dermatol 2000; 39: 539–44.

Based on clinical assessment of pre and post-treatment standardized photographs on 232 patients, subcision was shown to be efficacious in the treatment of high-grade cellulite. Targeted specifically for the treatment of major cellulite depressions on the skin surface of patients with cellulite through three action mechanisms: sectioning the connective tissue septa responsible for the depressions; provoking the formation of new connective tissue.

MANAGEMENT STRATEGY

Specific treatments:

- Subcision, which treats the subcutaneous septae that pulls the skin down and addresses specifically cellulite depressions
- Devices that target the dermis and thus improve flaccidity and projection of fat and devices that target localized fat
- Weight control to a normal body mass index (BMI)
- Oral treatment
- Topical treatment

The diagnosis is clinical. No imaging studies are required in clinical practice.

Specific Investigations

- Physical examination: patient in standing position with relaxed gluteus muscles. Determine morphologic characteristics of cellulite on each patient, which will help guide treatment option selection:
  - Presence and depth of cellulite depressions
  - Presence of localized fat and obesity
  - Presence of flaccidity and fat herniation
- Pretreatment and posttreatment photographs (relaxed gluteus muscles)
- Validated photonumeric scale: cellulite severity scale (CSS), for objective assessment of cellulite before and after different treatments
- Preoperative investigations for subcision: prothrombin time (PT), partial thromboplastin time (PTT), and international normalization ratio (INR); history of coagulation disorders; use of medications that alter blood coagulation

---

A validated photonumeric cellulite severity scale. Hexsel DM, Dal'forno T, Hexsel CL. J Eur Acad Dermatol Venereol 2009; 23: 523–8.

A new photonumeric severity quantitative and qualitative scale was developed and validated; five key morphologic aspects of cellulite were identified for comparison. Each item was graded from 0 to 3, allowing final classification of cellulite as mild, moderate, and severe, according to the sum of the scores of the CSS.

Side-by-side comparison of areas with and without cellulite depressions using magnetic resonance imaging. Hexsel DM, Abreu M, Rodrigues TC, Soirefmann M, do Prado DZ, Gamboa MM. Dermatol Surg 2009; 35: 1471–7.

Thirty female patients with cellulite depressions on the buttocks had underlying fibrous septa, which were thicker, ramified, and perpendicular to the skin surface.

First-Line Therapies

Subcision	B
Laser, light sources, devices	B
Radiofrequency devices	B

Magnetic resonance imaging of cellulite depressed lesions successfully treated by subcision. Hexsel D, Dal Forno T, Hexsel C, Schilling-Souza J, Naspolini Bastos F, Siega C. Dermatol Surg 2016; 42: 693–6.

The authors present a 7-month follow-up of cellulite-depressed lesions treated with subcision, showing a considerable reduction in the number and depth of the treated lesions, and thus an evident reduction in CSS grading in the two assessed patients (from severe to moderate). Using magnetic resonance imaging, the authors demonstrated that the subdermal portion of the septum underlying the treated lesion was absent after subcision. This finding suggests that subcision produces long-lasting anatomic alterations in the subcutaneous tissue and positive outcomes in depressed lesions of cellulite.

Evidence Levels: **A** Double-blind study   **B** Clinical trial ≥ 20 subjects   **C** Clinical trial < 20 subjects   **D** Series ≥ 5 subjects   **E** Anecdotal case reports

Treatment of cellulite using a 1440-nm pulsed laser with one-year follow-up. DiBernardo BE. Aesthet Surg J 2011; 31: 328–41.

Ten women with cellulite on their thighs received a single treatment with a 1440 nm pulsed laser delivered through a cannula. Mean skin thickness (as shown by ultrasound) and skin elasticity increased. Subjective physician evaluations indicated improvement in the appearance of cellulite.

Quantitative and qualitative evaluation of efficacy of a 1440 nm Nd:YAG laser with novel bi-directional optical fiber in the treatment of cellulite as measured by 3-dimensional surface imaging. Katz BE. J Drugs Dermatol 2013; 12: 1224–30.

Fifteen women with cellulite were treated with 1440 nm pulsed laser with side-firing fiber. There was improvement in cellulite in 68% of subjects on photographic evaluation by two independent observers, revealing good-to-excellent results by physician evaluation, and significant improvement in 65% of subjects assessed by three-dimensional surface imaging.

Multicenter pivotal study of vacuum-assisted precise tissue release for the treatment of cellulite. Kaminer MS, Coleman III WP, Weiss RA, Robinson DM, Coleman IV WP, Hornfeldt C. Derm Surg 2015; 41: 336–47.

Fifty-five women with moderate-to-severe cellulite underwent one treatment with a vacuum-assisted precise tissue release device. Assessments by subject photographs, cellulite severity scales, GAIS (Global Aesthetic Improvement Scale), and subject satisfaction showed significant improvements lasting up to 1 year.

Reduction in thigh circumference and improvement in the appearance of cellulite with dual-wavelength, low-level laser energy and massage. Gold MH, Khatri KA, Hails K, Weiss RA, Fournier N. J Cosmet Laser Ther 2011; 13: 13–20.

In this controlled, open-label, multicenter study, 83 subjects with mild-to-moderate cellulite received eight treatments with a device comprising a low-level, dual-wavelength diode laser (650 nm and 915 nm, to target fat), combined with heat induction and mechanical massage by suction (Smoothshapes), in one leg, with the untreated contralateral thigh serving as a control. The maximum reduction in thigh circumference of the treated areas (−0.82 cm) occurred in the upper thigh at 1 month. There was subjective clinical improvement of the appearance of cellulite when comparing pretreatment and posttreatment photographs.

A single center, randomized, comparative, prospective clinical study to determine the efficacy of the VelaSmooth system versus the Triactive system for the treatment of cellulite. Nootheti PK, Magpantay A, Yosowitz G, Calderon S, Goldman MP. Lasers Surg Med 2006; 38: 908–12.

Twenty female patients were treated twice weekly for 6 weeks with randomization to VelaSmooth on one side and TriActive on the other side. Velasmooth combines infrared light (680–1550 nm) with bipolar radiofrequency and mechanical massage by vacuum suction. Triactive has six diode lasers (808/810 nm) combined with mechanical massage, suction, and localized cooling. In both treatment groups, 25% of the patients had improvement in the appearance of cellulite, with average percentage improvement in roughness for the VelaSmooth versus TriActive of 7% and 25%, respectively. There was a perceived change grade of cellulite; 75% of subjects showed improvement in the VelaSmooth leg, whereas 55% of subjects showed improvement in the TriActive leg. There was no statistically significant difference (p > 0.05) in all variables between the two treatment arms.

Cellulite treatment using a novel combination radiofrequency, infrared light, and mechanical tissue manipulation device. Alster TS, Tanzi EL. J Cosmet Laser Ther 2005; 7: 81–5.

Twenty adult women with moderate bilateral thigh and buttock cellulite received eight biweekly treatments to a randomly selected side with a combined bipolar radiofrequency (RF), infrared (IR) light, and mechanical suction–based massage device (Velasmooth), applied at 20 W RF, 20 W IR (700–1500 nm) light, and 200 millibar vacuum (750 mm Hg negative pressure). Clinical improvement scores of photographs were made independently by two blinded physicians and averaged approximately 50% after the series of treatments. Circumferential thigh measurements were reduced by 0.84 cm on the treated side.

A prospective clinical study to evaluate the efficacy and safety of cellulite treatment using the combination of optical and RF energies for subcutaneous tissue heating. Sadick NS, Mulholland RS. J Cosmet Laser Ther 2004; 6: 187–90.

Thirty-five females with cellulite on the thighs and/or buttocks were treated with the VelaSmooth device with 8 to 16 treatments twice weekly. Based on physician assessment using pretreatment and posttreatment photographs, all patients showed some level of improvement in skin texture and cellulite. The mean decrease in thigh circumference was 0.8 inches.

The effectiveness of anticellulite treatment using tripolar radiofrequency monitored by classic and high-frequency ultrasound. Mlosek RK, Woźniak W, Malinowska S, Lewandowski M, Nowicki A. J Eur Acad Dermatol Venereol 2012; 26: 696–703.

In this randomized controlled study, 28 women with cellulite grade I to III underwent eight treatments with RF; 17 women were in the placebo group, in which the treatments were performed without emitting RF. The treatment began with 110 J/cm², increased by 10 to 20 J/cm² in subsequent procedures. Cellulite was reduced in 89.3% of the women who underwent RF treatment, based on the Nürnberger–Müller scale. In the placebo group, no statistically significant changes were observed.

A multicenter study of cellulite treatment with a variable emission radio frequency system. Van der Lugt C, Romero C, Ancona D, Al-Zarouni M, Perera J, Trelles MA. Dermatol Ther 2009; 22: 74–84.

The buttocks of 50 patients were treated with bipolar RF technology (ThermaLipo) at 6 J/cm². Twelve weekly sessions were given for 12 minutes on each buttock, with the treatment end point of 42°C external skin temperature. Based on the photography at baseline and at the 2-month assessment, the blinded independent clinicians' objective assessment of the cellulite appearance demonstrated that results were apparent in 66% of patients.

Unipolar radiofrequency treatment to improve the appearance of cellulite. Alexiades-Armenakas M, Dover JS, Arndt KA. J Cosmet Laser Ther 2008; 10: 148–53.

In this randomized, blinded, split-design study, 10 individuals with clinically observable excess of subcutaneous fat and cellulite (grades II–IV) on the thighs received up to six unilateral treatments (number of treatments at the investigator's discretion and resulted in a mean of 4.22 and range of 3 to 6 treatments) at 2-week intervals with unipolar RF (Accent). The untreated side of the thigh served as control. The results were assessed by two blinded investigators by using photographs and the authors' cellulite grading scale. A novel quantitative four-point cellulite grading system was applied. All participants responded to treatment. The blinded evaluations of photographs using the cellulite grading scale demonstrated the following improvements in mean grading scores for the treated leg versus the control leg: 11.2% in dimple density, 10.7% in dimple distribution, 2.5% in dimple depth, and 8±2.8% mean score improvement.

Second-Line Therapies

- Topical retinol, caffeine, and ruscogenin **B**
- Occluded topical caffeine with extracts of green tea, black pepper seed, citrus, ginger, and cinnamon **B**
- Topical retinol **C**
- Topical caffeine **B**
- Topical phosphatidylcholine gel and light-emitting diode (LED) **C**

A double-blind evaluation of the activity of an anticellulite product containing retinol, caffeine, and ruscogenin by a combination of several noninvasive methods. Bertin C, Zunino H, Pittet JC, Beau P, Pineau P, Massonneau M, et al. J Cosmet Sci 2001; 52: 199–210.

A placebo-controlled, double-blind study (n = 46) evaluated a topical anticellulite product that combined *retinol* microcapsules, *caffeine, asiatic centella,* l-*carnitine, esculoside,* and *ruscogenin.* The product was more effective than placebo in reducing cellulite appearance: decrease of the "orange peel" effect and increase in cutaneous microcirculation.

A two-center, double blinded, randomized trial testing the tolerability and efficacy of a novel therapeutic agent for cellulite reduction. Rao J, Gold MH, Goldman MP. J Cosmet Dermatol 2005; 4: 93–102.

This placebo-controlled study (n = 34 women with moderate degree of cellulite) assessed a cream containing a combination of caffeine, green tea extract, black pepper seed extract, citrus extract, ginger root extract, cinnamon bark extract, and capsicum annum resin under occlusion with bioceramic-coated neoprene shorts. The average measured decrease in thigh circumference was 1.9 cm with active product versus 1.3 cm with placebo. Upon review of the prestudy and poststudy photographs, dermatologists noted greater improvement in the treated group in 68% of subjects.

Topical retinol improves cellulite. Kligman AM, Pagnoni A, Stoudmayer T. J Dermatol Treat 1999; 10: 119–25.

This placebo-controlled study (n = 19) demonstrated improvement in cellulite on the side treated with topical *retinol 0.3%* on the thighs for 6 months in 63.1% of the patients compared with the untreated side by clinical dermatologic evaluation.

Parallel placebo-controlled clinical study of a mixture of herbs sold as a remedy for cellulite. Lis-Balchin M. Phytother Res 1999; 13: 627–9.

This placebo-controlled clinical trial study showed lack of effect of the topical combination product Cellasene.

Evaluation of the effects of caffeine in the microcirculation and edema on thighs and buttocks using the orthogonal polarization spectral imaging and clinical parameters. Lupi O, Semenovitch IJ, Treu C, Bottino D, Bouskela E. J Cosmet Dermatol 2007; 6: 102–7.

This controlled clinical study investigated 7% caffeine solution (n = 134). There was a reduction of 2.1 cm in the thigh circumference in >80% of women. No specific measurement of effect on the appearance of cellulite was assessed.

The effectiveness and safety of topical PhotoActif phosphatidylcholine-based anticellulite gel and LED (red and near-infrared) light on grade II–III thigh cellulite: a randomized, double-blinded study. Sasaki GH, Oberg K, Tucker B, Gaston M. J Cosmet Laser Ther 2007; 9: 87–96.

In this placebo-controlled, double-blinded study, nine subjects with grade II–III thigh cellulite were randomly treated twice daily with a phosphatidylcholine-based anticellulite gel on one thigh. Twice weekly, each thigh was exposed for a 15-minute treatment with LED array (660 nm and 950 nm) for 24 treatments. At the end of 3 months, eight out of nine thighs treated with the combination were downgraded to a lower cellulite grade by clinical examination, digital photography, and pinch test assessment. At the 18-month evaluation period for the eight responsive thighs, five thighs had reverted back to their original cellulite grading.

Third-Line Treatments

Cellulite treatment: a myth or reality: a prospective randomized, controlled trial of two therapies, Endermologie and aminophylline cream. Collis N, Elliot LA, Sharpe C, Sharpe DT. Plast Reconstr Surg 1999; 104: 1110–4. Discussion 1115–7.

This randomized, controlled trial assessed the efficacy of aminophylline cream and Endermologie (n = 52). Neither of these two treatments was effective.

Evidence Levels: **A** Double-blind study **B** Clinical trial ≥ 20 subjects **C** Clinical trial < 20 subjects **D** Series ≥ 5 subjects **E** Anecdotal case reports

40

Cellulitis and erysipelas

Adrian H.M. Heagerty, Natasha Harper

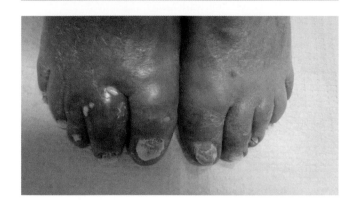

Eron Classification System

Class I — There are no signs of systemic toxicity and the person has no uncontrolled comorbidities.

Class II — The person is either systemically unwell or systemically well but with a comorbidity (e.g., peripheral arterial disease, chronic venous insufficiency, or morbid obesity), which may complicate or delay resolution of infection.

Class III — The person has significant systemic upset such as acute confusion, tachycardia, tachypnea, hypotension, or unstable comorbidities that may interfere with a response to treatment, or a limb-threatening infection due to vascular compromise.

Class IV — The person has sepsis syndrome or a severe life-threatening infection such as necrotizing fasciitis.

Cellulitis is strictly an acute, subacute, or chronic infection of the subcutaneous tissues, whereas erysipelas is an infection of the dermis and superficial subcutis. Infection of the more superficial layers gives rise to superficial edema and inflammation, with the consequent development of a palpable, often advancing, edge. In the literature, these infections, along with abscesses and wound infections with significant skin involvement, are now sometimes grouped together and referred to as *acute bacterial skin and skin-structure infection (ABSSSI)*. The causative organism is usually regarded as *Streptococcus*, though many organisms have been isolated, including *Staphylococcus*, *Haemophilus influenzae*, and more rarely, *Aeromonas hydrophilia* and *Pseudomonas aeruginosa*, as well as fungi and gram-negative rods. Fulminating and necrotic cellulitis and fasciitis may occur rarely, usually in relation to immunosuppression or atypical organisms. These are rare, but necrotizing fasciitis may have a mortality of up to 50%.

MANAGEMENT STRATEGY

The management of cellulitis and erysipelas should initially be directed to assessment of systemic features of sepsis, which may suggest that admission to hospital and/or intravenous antibiotics is required, trying to identify the organism responsible for the infection when indicated, and then directing appropriate antimicrobial therapy. Any underlying and predisposing condition should be identified and treated to prevent subsequent recurrence.

The distinction between purulent and nonpurulent cases is an important one as the therapeutic strategy is different. The cause of purulent cellulitis (where there is purulent discharge or pustules present) is much more likely to be *Staphylococcus*, and possibly methicillin-resistant *Staphylococcus aureus* (MRSA), whereas most cases of nonpurulent cellulitis will be caused by *Streptococcus*.

Clinical knowledge summaries provided by the National Institute for Health and Care Excellence suggest that the Eron Classification System should be used for the assessment of the patient with cellulitis, although this is more likely to be used in the primary care setting.

Uncomplicated cellulitis and erysipelas may be managed without admission if the patient does not exhibit signs of systemic toxicity (i.e., Eron Classification I). In such cases *oral broad-spectrum antibiotics*, chosen to cover group A streptococci and staphylococci, may be sufficient. The drug of choice is *oral penicillin V (phenoxymethylpenicillin) and/or flucloxacillin* (especially when there is a suspicion of possible staphylococcal involvement). Many local antibiotics guidelines in the UK recommend *flucloxacillin* alone as the first-line treatment, as when given in high doses it is effective against *Streptococcus* as well as *Staphylococcus*. *Clarithromycin* is used if the patient has a known penicillin allergy. Some authorities have recommended the use of *clindamycin* rather than a macrolide because of apparent increased tissue penetration, but this may be associated with an increased incidence of *Clostridium difficile* superinfection. Further, although most group A β-hemolytic streptococci are sensitive to this, increasing numbers of MRSA are displaying resistance to clindamycin, and widespread use may exacerbate this resistance. The incidence of MRSA as the causative organism in ABSSSI is increasing, especially in the United States. It is therefore important to take a swab when the condition is purulent and to consider MRSA as a possible cause of treatment failure. Immunocompromised patients, those with signs of systemic toxicity, and otherwise debilitated patients (Eron Classification II–IV) should be treated with *intravenous antimicrobials*. First line is usually *penicillin G (benzylpenicillin) and/or flucloxacillin*, depending on local guidelines. A wide range of antibiotics may be used second line such as *ciprofloxacin, vancomycin, teicoplanin, imipenem/cilastatin, daptomycin, linezolid*, or even new agents such as *oritavancin*. Some patients may be safely treated on an outpatient basis (outpatient parenteral antimicrobial therapy). If there is evidence of head and neck disease or sinus infection, *amoxicillin combined with clavulanic acid* should be considered to cover *H. influenzae* infection.

Sites of entry for infection should be sought, such as excoriations in eczema or after trauma, and these should be treated. Perhaps the commonest condition that is not identified and treated is toe web tinea pedis, which provides a portal of entry for infection. Lymphedema can be associated with recurrence of cellulitis and so should be treated effectively.

The use of long-term antibiotics for the prevention of recurrent cellulitis has produced some conflicting evidence, but the PATCH I and II trials concluded that antibiotic prophylaxis reduces cellulitis recurrence by nearly a third.

- Blood cultures—not routinely done in uncomplicated patients due to low yield
- Swabs of any purulent exudate, pustules, or wounds
- ASO titer/anti-DNase B
- Cultures of aspirates
- Skin scrapings for mycology

Blood cultures may be positive and significant in only about 10% to 25% of cases but should be taken if there is any evidence of systemic toxicity or if staphylococcal involvement is suspected. Swabs of wounds, pus, and broken skin may be helpful, but surface swabs of unbroken skin provide little or no useful information. If available, aspirate of bullae may yield positive cultures. Slightly better rates for isolation than those of needle aspirates have been achieved with punch skin biopsies.

If there is doubt regarding the presence of an abscess, ultrasound should be performed as this has therapeutic implications.

Rising titers of streptococcal antibodies (ASO titer and anti-DNase B) may be helpful but are more commonly of value retrospectively.

In the case of cellulitis or erysipelas of the lower leg, skin scrapings from toe webs should be taken for mycologic examination. Facial erysipelas should warrant sinus radiographs to exclude underlying sinusitis. Crepitus should prompt the clinician to the presence of either clostridia or non–spore-forming anaerobes, either alone or mixed with other bacteria such as *Pseudomonas*, *Escherichia coli*, or *Klebsiella* spp.

Cellulitis: a review. Raff AB, Kroshinsky D JAMA 2016; 316: 325–37.

A review article from 2016 advises that nonpurulent cellulitis without systemic toxicity should be treated with antistreptococcal agents

Current and future trends in antibiotic therapy of acute bacterial skin and skin-structure infections. Russo A, Concia E, Cristini F, De Rosa FG, Esposito S, Menichetti F, et al. Clin Microbiol Infect 2016; 22 (Suppl 2): S27–36.

New terminology—ABSSSI. The new classification includes cellulitis, erysipelas, major skin abscesses, and wound infection with a considerable extension of skin involvement, clearly referring to a severe subset of skin infections.

Blood cultures in the evaluation of uncomplicated cellulitis. Bauer S, Aubert CE, Richli M, Chuard C. Eur J Intern Med 2016; 36: 50–6.

Blood cultures are no longer recommended in uncomplicated cellulitis due to poor yield.

Methicillin-resistant *S. aureus* infections among patients in the emergency department. Moran GJ, Krishnadasan A, Gorwitz RJ, Fosheim GE, McDougal LK, Carey RB, et al. N Engl J Med 2006; 355: 666–74.

A study of 422 patients in the United States who presented with purulent skin and soft tissue infections found that swabs showed 59% had MRSA, 17% had methicillin-sensitive *S. aureus*, and 2.9% had β-hemolytic *Streptococcus*. This demonstrates the importance of swabs in such cases.

Costs and consequences associated with misdiagnosed lower extremity cellulitis. Weng QY, Raff AB, Cohen JM, Gunasekera N, Okhovat JP, Vedak P, et al. JAMA Dermatol 2016. 2017; 153: 141–6.

Misdiagnosis of lower extremity cellulitis is common and may lead to unnecessary patient morbidity and considerable health care spending.

First-Line Therapies

• Penicillin G	B
• Penicillin G with flucloxacillin	B
• Penicillin V	B
• High-dose flucloxacillin	A
• Amoxicillin with clavulanic acid	B
• Ceftriaxone	A
• Roxithromycin	B

Interventions for cellulitis and erysipelas. Kilburn SA, Featherstone P, Higgins B, Brindle R. Cochrane Database Syst Rev. 2010; 16: CD004299.

A Cochrane review in 2010 could not recommend any particular antibiotic regimen for cellulitis and erysipelas due to the large variation in treatment regimens studied.

The course, costs and complications of oral versus intravenous penicillin therapy of erysipelas. Jorup-Ronstrum C, Britton S, Gavlevik A, Gunnarsson K, Redman AC. Infection 1984; 12: 390–4.

In this study of 60 patients there appeared to be no appreciable benefit from intravenous rather than oral therapy with penicillin for erysipelas, and so oral therapy is recommended if there are no associated complications with the infection.

Management and morbidity of cellulitis of the leg. Cox NH, Colver GB, Paterson WD. J R Soc Med 1998; 91: 634–7.

A case note review of 92 patients admitted for inpatient care for ascending cellulitis of the leg revealed a portal of entry, most commonly minor injury. The mean hospital stay was 10 days. Bacteriology was seldom helpful, but group G streptococci were the most frequently identified pathogens. Benzylpenicillin was used in 43 cases (46%). The authors emphasize the need for benzylpenicillin, treatment of tinea pedis, and retrospective diagnosis of streptococcal infection by serology.

Skin concentrations of phenoxymethylpenicillin in patients with erysipelas. Sjoblom AC, Bruchfeld J, Eriksson B, Jorup-Rönström C, Karkk1n K, Malmborg AS, et al. Infection 1992; 20: 30–3.

Tissue and serum blood levels were measured in 45 patients with erysipelas after oral penicillin (phenoxymethylpenicillin); the minimal inhibitory concentrations were exceeded for streptococci isolated, supporting the role of oral therapy.

A randomized comparative study of once-daily ceftriaxone and 6-hourly flucloxacillin in the treatment of moderate to severe cellulitis. Clinical efficacy, safety and pharmacoeconomic implications. Vinen J, Hudson B, Chan B, Vinen J, Hudson B, Chan B, et al. Clin Drug Invest 1996; 12: 221–5.

A randomized comparative study in 58 patients with cellulitis; intravenous ceftriaxone cured 92%, but intravenous flucloxacillin cured only 64% after 4 to 6 days.

Roxithromycin versus penicillin in the treatment of erysipelas in adults: a comparative study. Bernard P, Plantin P, Roger H, Sassolas B, Villaret E, Legrain V, et al. Br J Dermatol 1992; 127: 155–9.

Evidence Levels: **A** Double-blind study   **B** Clinical trial ≥ 20 subjects   **C** Clinical trial < 20 subjects   **D** Series ≥ 5 subjects   **E** Anecdotal case reports

This prospective randomized multicenter trial compared oral roxithromycin with intravenous benzylpenicillin. Overall efficacy was similar.

Amoxicillin combined with clavulanic acid for the treatment of soft tissue infections in children. Fleischer GR, Wilmott CM, Capos JM. Antimicrob Agents Chemother 1983; 24: 679–81.

Amoxicillin with clavulanic acid was compared with cefaclor in children with impetigo and cellulitis due to staphylococci, streptococci, and *Haemophilus* spp. There was a 100% response to therapy with the combination, compared with 90% with the cephalosporin; the incidence of relapse and reinfection and side effects was small but greater with the combination therapy.

Nurse-led management of uncomplicated cellulitis in the community: evaluation of a protocol incorporating intravenous ceftriaxone. Seaton RA, Bell E, Gourlay Y, Semple L. J Antimicrob Chemother 2005; 55: 764–7.

The safety and efficacy of a nurse-led outpatient parenteral antibiotic therapy service for cellulitis were examined in 114 patients and 230 historical controls. No alteration in outcomes, complications, or readmission rates was seen compared with the earlier physician-supervised outpatient treatment. Treatment duration was reduced from 4 to 3 days.

Prospective evaluation of the management of moderate to severe cellulitis with parenteral antibiotics at a pediatric day treatment centre. Gouin S, Chevalier I, Gautier M, Lamarre V. Paediatr Child Health 2008; 44: 214–8.

The clinical outcomes of 92 children receiving outpatient treatment in a day treatment center were examined prospectively; after a mean of 2.5 days of intravenous therapy, 73 patients (79.3%) were switched to oral agents and discharged from the day treatment center. There were no relapses in this group.

Oral flucloxacillin and phenoxymethylpenicillin versus flucloxacillin alone for the emergency department outpatient treatment of cellulitis: study protocol for a randomised controlled trial. Quirke M, Wakai A, Gilligan P, O'Sullivan R. Trials 2013; 14: 164.

There are no studies comparing oral flucloxacillin alone or in combination with phenoxymethylpenicillin for cellulitis, but a trial is planned in Ireland.

Second-Line Therapies	
• Ciprofloxacin	B
• Teicoplanin	B
• Imipenem/cilastatin	B
• Linezolid	A
• Daptomycin	A
• Vancomycin	A
• Oritavancin	A

Comparative efficacy of antibiotics for the treatment of acute bacterial skin and skin structure infections (ABSSSI): a systematic review and network meta-analysis. Thom H, Thompson JC, Scott DA, Halfpenny N, Sulham K, Corey GR. Curr Med Res Opin 2015; 31: 1539–51.

This meta-analysis of 52 trials concluded that there is equivalence of clinical efficacy between vancomycin, daptomycin, linezolid, and the novel antimicrobial agent, oritavancin. However, they noted the heterogeneity of the available evidence and the need for further research.

Ciprofloxacin for soft tissue infections. Wood MJ, Logan MN. J Antimicrob Chemother 1986; 18: 159–64.

Twenty-one patients with cellulitis or other soft tissue infection were treated with oral ciprofloxacin; 19 were clinically cured or improved, and 1 was withdrawn from the study because of nausea and vomiting. Nine of the original 18 bacterial isolates were eradicated, but the majority of failures were due to staphylococci and streptococci.

Teicoplanin in the treatment of skin and soft tissue infections. Turpin PJ, Taylor GP, Logan MN, Wood MJ. J Antimicrob Chemother 1988; 21: 117–22.

Twenty-four patients with cellulitis or other soft tissue infection were treated with once-daily teicoplanin, resulting in clinical cure or improvement without severe adverse reactions but with a rise in the plasma platelet count.

Twice daily intramuscular imipenem/cilastatin in the treatment of skin and soft tissue infections. Sexton DJ, Wlodaver CG, Tobey LE, Yangco BG, Graziani AL, MacGregor RR. Chemotherapy 1991; 37: 26–30.

Of 102 patients enrolled in this study with mild to moderately severe skin and soft tissue infections, 74 were evaluable, with 20 having cellulitis, 23 wound infections, and 31 abscesses. Imipenem/cilastatin was given intramuscularly using doses of 500 or 750 mg 12-hourly. In this study there was no assessment by type of infection, but 82% were cured and 16% improved. Eight patients reported minor side effects.

Randomized comparison of linezolid (PNU-100766) versus oxacillin-dicloxacillin for treatment of complicated skin and soft tissue infections. Stevens DL, Smith LG, Bruss JB, McConnell-Martin MA, Duvall SE, Todd WM, et al. Antimicrob Agents Chemother 2000; 12: 3408–13.

Eight hundred twenty-six hospitalized adult patients were randomized to receive linezolid (600 mg intravenously) every 12 hours or oxacillin (2 g intravenously) every 6 hours; after sufficient clinical improvement, patients were switched to the respective oral agents (linezolid 600 mg orally every 12 hours or dicloxacillin 500 mg orally every 6 hours). The clinical cure rates were 88.6% and 85.8%, respectively.

Third-Line Therapies	
• Prednisolone as an adjunct to antibiotics	A
• Granulocyte colony-stimulating factor	A
• Hyperbaric oxygen	E

Antibiotic and prednisolone therapy of erysipelas: a randomized, double blind, placebo-controlled study. Bergkvist PI, Sjobeck K. Scand J Infect Dis 1997; 29: 377–82.

Although prednisolone may predispose to infection, its use in combination with intravenous antibiotics reduced the median time to cure by 1 day (5 vs. 6 days); at the 90th centile healing time was 10 days vs. 14.6 days, and median hospital stay was reduced from 6 to 5 days. The relapse rate within 3 weeks was approximately the same in both groups.

Randomized placebo controlled trial of granulocyte-colony stimulating factor in diabetic foot infection. Gough A, Clapperton M, Rolando N, Foster A, Philpott-Howard J, Edmonds ME. Lancet 1997; 350: 855–9.

This randomized controlled trial compared the ability of granulocyte-colony stimulating factor (G-CSF) to improve clinical outcome in the treatment of cellulitis in diabetes mellitus, using resolution as the end point. G-CSF stimulates the neutrophil response, which is impaired in diabetes mellitus but is important for defense against infection. The risk is principally that of high white cell counts, which may predispose to coronary and cerebral vascular events.

Cellulitis owing to *Aeromonas hydrophilia*: treatment with hyperbaric oxygen. Mathur MN, Patrick WG, Unsworth IP, Bennett FM. Aust NZ J Surg 1995; 65: 367–9.

This case report of *Aeromonas hydrophilia* cellulitis, unresponsive to antibiotics and surgical debridement, responded to hyperbaric oxygen therapy. Although there are few objective reports of similar treatment in streptococcal necrotizing fasciitis, it has been suggested that in all types of necrotizing fasciitis hyperbaric oxygen reduces mortality.

Prophylaxis	
• Low-dose oral penicillin	A
• Intramuscular weekly penicillin	C
• Treatment of predisposing factors	E

Prophylactic antibiotics in erysipelas. Duvanel T, Merot Y, Saurat JH. Lancet 1985; 1: 1401.

Sixteen patients who received weekly intramuscular penicillin as prophylaxis were followed and assessed at 2 years. On cessation of prophylaxis the risk of recurrence rapidly returned to the nontreatment/no prophylaxis level.

Cellulitis and erysipelas. Morris A. Clin Evid 2004; 12: 2268–74.

Although there is a consensus that successful treatment of predisposing factors such as leg edema, tinea pedis, and traumatic wounds reduces the risk of developing cellulitis, there are no randomized controlled trials or observational studies to support this.

Prophylactic antibiotics for the prevention of cellulitis (erysipelas) of the leg: results of the UK Dermatology Clinical Trials Network's PATCH II trial. UK Dermatology Clinical Trials Network's PATCH Trial Team. Br J Dermatol 2012; 166: 169–78.

A double-blind, randomized controlled trial examining whether prophylactic antibiotics prescribed after an episode of cellulitis of the leg can prevent further episodes. A total of 123 patients were recruited and randomized between low-dose oral phenoxymethyl penicillin and placebo for 6 months. Recurrence rates were 20% on penicillin vs. 33% on placebo ($p = 0.08$).

Prophylactic antibiotics to prevent cellulitis of the leg: economic analysis of the PATCII I & II trials. Mason JM, Thomas KS, Crook AM, Foster KA, Chalmers JR, Nunn AJ, et al. PLoS One 2014; 9: e82694.

Economic analysis of the PATCH trials concluded that after a first episode or recurrent cellulitis of the leg, prophylactic low-dose penicillin is a low-cost intervention that is medically effective and cost effective at preventing subsequent attacks.

Antibiotic prophylaxis for preventing recurrent cellulitis: a systematic review and meta-analysis. Oh CC, Ko HC, Lee HY, Safdar N, Maki DG, Chlebicki MP. J Infect 2014; 69: 26.

This meta-analysis concluded that antibiotic prophylaxis can prevent recurrent cellulitis but that further research is needed to establish indication, choice of drug, and dosage regimens.

Evidence Levels: A Double-blind study   B Clinical trial ≥ 20 subjects   C Clinical trial < 20 subjects   D Series ≥ 5 subjects   E Anecdotal case reports

41

Chancroid

Iris A. Hagans, Glenn C. Newell

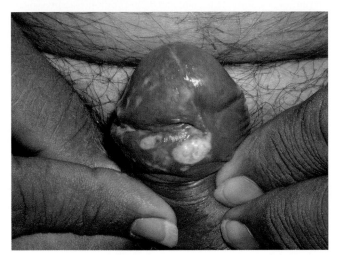

Chancroid is a genital ulcer disease caused by the gram-negative facultative anaerobic coccobacillus *Haemophilus ducreyi*. It is common in many parts of the world, including Africa, the Caribbean basin, and Southwest Asia. The incidence is decreasing worldwide; however, outbreaks in developed countries can be seen after travelers return from high-risk areas after having unprotected sex. Chancroid is typically a painful, ragged, deep genital ulcer 3 to 20 mm in diameter without induration. There may be surrounding erythema, and the base is often covered with a yellow-gray exudate. The lesion may be single, but can be multiple as a result of autoinoculation (kissing lesions), and non-genital lesions have been noted. Painful lymphadenitis occurs in 30% to 60% of patients, and approximately one quarter of patients with lymphadenopathy may develop a suppurative bubo. Of note, uncircumcised men may have a higher risk of infection and may take longer to cure.

DIAGNOSIS AND MANAGEMENT STRATEGY

Diagnosis on clinical criteria alone is difficult. The painful ulcer of chancroid can easily be confused with genital herpes or secondarily infected syphilis. A presumptive diagnosis of chancroid can be made with one or more painful genital ulcers, with or without a bubo, with negative laboratory tests for herpes simplex virus (HSV) and syphilis. Coinfection with either of these diseases occurs in as many as 10% of patients.

A definitive diagnosis may be made by culturing the exudates from the ulcer base or by aspiration of a bubo. Gram stain of the ulcer base in chancroid may show gram-negative coccobacilli in a "school of fish" appearance. Special culture media should be used, and the specimen should be handled by laboratories familiar with *H. ducreyi*. It should be noted that sensitivity of culture as shown by DNA amplification techniques can be as low as 75%. The newer nucleic acid amplification tests (NAATs) show higher positivity rates than culture and do not depend on live bacteria, making the test especially useful. However, only few laboratories have established NAATs for the diagnosis of chancroid. Polymerase chain reaction testing has the advantage of simultaneous testing of *H. ducreyi* along with *T. pallidum* and HSV.

Concurrent HIV infection can alter the manifestations of chancroid. HIV prolongs the incubation period of *H. ducreyi* and can increase the number of genital ulcers. With HIV coinfection, ulcers tend to heal poorly and non-genital ulcers are frequently found. Recent research shows that this may be more strongly correlated with coinfection with HSV rather than HIV. Treatment guidelines for patients coinfected with HIV are the same as for those without HIV, but closer follow-up and a potentially longer course of therapy may be recommended, as there are increased treatment failures with HIV coinfection. Additionally, chancroid has been noted to increase the susceptibility to HIV, probably by disrupting mucosal integrity. Patients should be tested for HIV at the time of chancroid diagnosis and should be retested for HIV 3 months after the diagnosis of chancroid if initial testing was negative.

A recent study found that many skin lesions diagnosed as yaws were instead *Haemophilus ducreyi* infections. These lesions are often not sexually transmitted and can be found in children as well as adults (see later under Special Considerations).

Specific Investigations

- Gram stain of ulcer base or bubo aspirate
- Culture of ulcer base or bubo aspirate
- NAATs
- Syphilis serology
- HIV serology

First-Line Therapies

• Azithromycin 1 g orally (one dose)	A
• Ceftriaxone 250 mg intramuscularly (one dose)	A

European guideline for the management of chancroid. Kemp M, Christensen JJ, Lautenschlager S, Vall-Mayans M, Moi H. Int J STD AIDS 2011; 22: 241–4.

A comprehensive review of chancroid diagnosis and management. The authors cite an unblinded prospective study that found that ceftriaxone versus azithromycin in doses noted earlier were equally efficacious.

UK National Guideline for the management of chancroid. O'Farrell N, Lazaro N. Int J STD AIDS 2014; 25: 975–83.

Thorough guidelines confirming prior management choices are presented as well as an epidemiology update. The prevalence of chancroid, even in endemic countries, is decreasing, and HSV is now the most common cause of ulcerative genital lesions worldwide.

Second-Line Therapies

• Ciprofloxacin 500 mg twice a day for 3 days	B
• Erythromycin 500 mg orally four times a day for 7 days	B
• Granulated thiamphenicol 5.0 g orally (one dose)	B

A randomized, double-blind, placebo-controlled trial of single dose ciprofloxacin versus erythromycin for the treatment of chancroid in Nairobi, Kenya. Malonza IM, Tyndall MW, Ndinya-Achola JO, Maclean I, Omar S, MacDonald KS, et al. J Infect Dis 1999; 180: 1886–93.

This clinical trial compared single-dose therapy with ciprofloxacin to a 7-day course of erythromycin for the treatment of chancroid. Cure rates of 92% and 91% were reported with ciprofloxacin and erythromycin, respectively, for the 111 participants with chancroid. Failure rates were attributed to ulcer etiologies of HSV or syphilis.

A comparative study of a single-dose treatment of chancroid using thiamphenicol versus azithromycin. Junior WB, Di Chiacchio NG, Di Chiacchio N, Romiti R, Criado PR, Velho PE, Braz J. Infect Dis 2009; 13: 218–20.

For 54 patients with chancroid, cure rates with single-dose treatment were 73% with azithromycin and 89% with thiamphenicol. HIV seropositivity was found to be associated with treatment failure ($p = 0.001$). The treatment failed in all HIV-positive patients treated with azithromycin ($p = 0.002$), and this drug should be avoided in these coinfected patients. In the view of the authors, thiamphenicol is the most indicated single-dose regimen for chancroid treatment.

SPECIAL CONSIDERATIONS: EVACUATION OF BUBOES AND UNUSUAL MANIFESTATIONS

Incision and drainage versus aspiration of fluctuant buboes in the emergency department during an epidemic of chancroid. Ernst AA, Marvez-Valls E, Martin DH. Sex Transms Dis 1995; 22: 217–20.

Evacuation of buboes has historically been recommended to prevent fistula formation, and needle aspiration was previously the procedure of choice. This study compared incision and drainage with packing to needle aspiration of suppurative buboes during an epidemic in Louisiana. No difference in cure rate was seen; however, aspirated buboes required reaspiration in 6/15 patients. As such, the authors recommended considering incision and drainage as an alternative to needle aspiration.

***Haemophilus ducreyi*: from sexually transmitted infection to skin ulcer pathogen.** Lewis DA, Mitjà O. Curr Opin Infect Dis 2016; 29: 52–7.

The authors of this review discuss recent investigations discerning yaws from chancroid as the culprit for chronic skin ulceration in endemic countries. They suggest that chancroid be considered in the evaluation of chronic limb ulceration.

Evidence Levels: **A** Double-blind study **B** Clinical trial ≥ 20 subjects **C** Clinical trial < 20 subjects **D** Series ≥ 5 subjects **E** Anecdotal case reports

42

Chilblains

Antonios Kanelleas, John Berth-Jones

Chilblains (also called *perniosis*) are localized, inflammatory, erythematous lesions that are caused by exposure to cold ambient temperatures above freezing point. High humidity and wind, which exacerbate conductive heat loss, also play a significant part. They are thought to be caused by a persistent vasoconstriction of the deep cutaneous arterioles with accompanying dilatation of the small superficial vessels. The onset is usually in the autumn or winter. Chilblains are more common in temperate climates, when winters get rather cold and damp and people are not used to these conditions. Lesions occur acutely as single or multiple erythematous or dusky swellings that may occasionally ulcerate or blister. They are usually accompanied by pruritus or a burning sensation. Sites of predilection are the fingers, toes, heels, lower legs, thighs, nose, and ears. A specific subset occurs on the thighs of patients wearing tight-fitting, poorly insulating trousers (e.g., as worn by young horsewomen). Perniosis can also be a manifestation of eating disorders (anorexia nervosa, poor nutrition) and systemic diseases (lupus erythematosus and hematologic malignancies).

MANAGEMENT STRATEGY

Appropriate investigation to exclude myeloproliferative disorders, connective tissue diseases, and eating disorders is sometimes required. Particularly in children, chilblains have been linked with cold-sensitive dysproteinemia. In elderly patients and those with ulcerative lesions, peripheral vascular insufficiency must be excluded. The condition must be distinguished from chilblain lupus erythematosus (LE). The latter is a form of cutaneous LE manifesting with lesions resembling chilblains. Lesions develop in cold weather but tend to persist and ulcerate. Chilblain LE may be accompanied by discoid LE. Up to 20% of patients with chilblain LE will develop systemic LE.

For cold-induced perniosis with no underlying pathology, the most important aspect of management is *prophylaxis*. This will be achieved through the use of *warm clothing and warm, properly insulated housing*. Avoidance of exposure in cold weather is, obviously, equally important. Once chilblains occur, they usually run a self-limiting course over a period of a few weeks. Treatment

includes *rest in a warm environment and possibly topical antipruritics*, if needed. *Vasodilator calcium channel blockers* (nifedipine 20–60 mg daily, diltiazem 60–120 mg three times daily) have been shown to be an effective therapy and preventative measure in patients with idiopathic acral perniosis and in those patients with perniosis associated with low body weight. *Pentoxifylline* provides a safe alternative approach. A range of topical vasodilators and other treatments have been deployed with a largely anecdotal evidence base.

Specific Investigations

Investigation is not routinely required in typical cases, but consider:
- Full blood count
- Autoimmune profile
- Cryoglobulins
- Cold agglutinins
- Cryofibrinogen
- Vascular assessment in elderly patients
- Histology and immunofluorescence

Chilblain lupus erythematosus – a review of literature. Hedrich CM, Fiebig B, Hauck FH, Sallmann S, Hahn G, Pfeiffer C, et al. Clin Rheumatol 2008; 27: 949–54.

This article reviews the clinical presentation, pathogenesis, diagnosis, and management of chilblain lupus erythematosus.

Pernio. A possible association with chronic myelomonocytic leukaemia. Kelly JW, Dowling JP. Arch Dermatol 1985; 121: 1048–52.

A series of four elderly men has been described in whom perniosis preceded the onset of chronic myelomonocytic leukemia.

Anorexia nervosa associated with acromegaloid features, onset of acrocyanosis and Raynaud's phenomenon and worsening of chilblains. Rustin MH, Foreman JC, Dowd PM. J Roy Soc Med 1990; 83: 495–6.

Two patients are reported who developed severe perniosis in association with anorexia nervosa.

Perniosis in association with anorexia nervosa. White KP, Rothe MJ, Milanese A, Grant-Kels JM. Paediatr Dermatol 1994; 11: 1–5.

Celiac disease presenting with chilblains in an adolescent girl. St Clair NE, Kim CC, Semrin G, Woodward AL, Liang MG, Glickman JN, et al. Pediatr Dermatol 2006; 23: 451–4.

This is a case report of an adolescent girl in whom chilblains were the main presenting sign of celiac disease. A gluten-free diet resulted in both weight gain and resolution of chilblains.

Childhood pernio and cryoproteins. Weston WL, Morelli JG. Pediatr Dermatol 2000; 17: 97–9.

A 10-year retrospective study of a pediatric clinic identified eight patients with perniosis, four of whom had cryoglobulins or cold agglutinins and two had positive rheumatoid factor.

First-Line Therapies

• Conservative management	C
• Avoidance of further cold injury	E
• Calcium channel blockers	C
• Topical corticosteroids	E

Clinical characteristics, etiologic associations, laboratory findings, treatment, and proposal of diagnostic criteria of pernio (chilblains) in a series of 104 patients at Mayo Clinic, 2000 to 2011. Cappel JA, Wetter DA. Mayo Clin Proc 2014; 89: 207–15.

Conservative treatments (e.g., warming, drying, and smoking cessation) provided complete response in 23 (82%) of the 28 patients for whom follow-up data were available.

The treatment of chilblains with nifedipine: the results of a pilot study, a double blind placebo-controlled randomized study and a long term open trial. Rustin MH, Newton JA, Smith NP, Dowd PM. Br J Dermatol 1989; 120: 267–75.

Ten patients with severe recurrent acral perniosis were treated with 20 mg of nifedipine retard or placebo in a double-blind crossover trial for 12 weeks total. No patients developed new lesions while on treatment, and 70% were clear after a mean of 8 days. In the open study, 34 patients received up to 60 mg of nifedipine retard for 2 months; this was shown to be effective in reducing the healing time and symptoms of lesions.

Diltiazem vs. nifedipine in chilblains: a clinical trial. Patra AK, Das AL, Ramadasan P. Indian J Dermatol Venereol Leprol 2003; 69: 209–11.

The authors compared two groups of patients with chilblains. Group A (12 patients) was treated with diltiazem 60 mg three times daily and group B (24 patients) with nifedipine 10 mg three times daily until complete relief and then 20 mg twice daily for maintenance. They concluded that nifedipine has greater efficacy than diltiazem (80%–90% of patients from group B showed relief by the fourteenth day of treatment).

Corticosteroid therapy for pernio. Gaynor S. J Am Acad Dermatol 1983; 8: 13.

This author reports successful treatment of patients with perniosis using topical corticosteroids (0.025% fluocinolone cream) under occlusion nightly.

Topical corticosteroids are frequently used for the treatment of chilblains, but their use is not based on controlled trials.

Second-Line Therapies

• Topical nitroglycerine	C
• Pentoxifylline	A
• Topical 2% hexyl nicotinate cream	E
• Minoxidil 5% lotion	E
• Acidified nitrate cream	E
• Tamoxifen	E

Topical nitroglycerine in perniosis/chilblains. Verma P. Skinmed 2015; 13: 176–7.

An uncontrolled study on 0.2% nitroglycerine ointment. Eighteen of 22 patients had regression of lesions within a week.

Treatment of primary perniosis with oral pentoxifylline (a double-blind placebo-controlled randomized therapeutic trial). Al-Sudany NK. Dermatol Ther 2016; 29: 263–8.

Pentoxifylline 400 mg three times daily for 3 weeks proved superior to placebo in a double-blind trial undertaken in Iraq.

Chilblains. Dowd PM, Blackwell V. In: Lebwohl M, Heymann W, Berth-Jones J, Coulson I, eds. Treatment of Skin Disease: Comprehensive Therapeutic Strategies, 2nd edn. Chicago: Mosby, 2006; 39–40.

These authors reported use of 2% hexyl nicotinate in aqueous cream preparation and minoxidil 5% lotion applied three times a day in patients with chilblains and Raynaud phenomenon and acidified nitrite cream (3% salicylic acid and 3% potassium nitrate) three times daily in patients with chilblains intolerant of calcium channel blockers. Low-dose (5 mg daily) tamoxifen proved useful in anorexia-associated perniosis.

Third-Line Therapies

• Salbutamol sulfate ointment	E
• Nonsteroidal antiinflammatory drugs	E
• Prednisolone	E
• Hydroxychloroquine	E
• Intense pulsed light	E

Anon: http://www.drdo.gov.in/drdo/labs/INMAS/collaboration/brochure.htm. **Accessed 5/4/16.** The use of 0.5% salbutamol sulfate ointment has been proposed by the Defence Research and Development Organization (DRDO) of India for the prevention of cold injuries after pilot studies on soldiers and workers residing in high altitudes.

Treatment of perniosis with oral pentoxifylline in comparison with oral prednisolone plus topical clobetasol ointment in Iraqi patients. Noaimi AA, Fadheel BM. Saudi Med J 2008; 29: 1762–4.

Forty patients with chilblains were randomly divided into two equal groups. Group A received oral prednisolone 0.5 mg/kg/day in two doses and topical clobetasol ointment for 2 weeks. Patients in group B received pentoxifylline tablets 400 mg three times daily for 2 weeks. In group B, 5 of 9 patients (55.5%) who completed the study showed a significant improvement, compared with 3 of 11 patients (27.2%) in group A.

Major cluster of chilblain cases in a cold dry Western Australian winter. Larkins N, Murray KJ. J Paediatr Child Health 2013; 49: 144–7.

Thirty-two patients with perniosis are described. Most received some form of treatment including nonsteroidal antiinflammatory drugs, prednisolone, or nifedipine, but most improved spontaneously with warmer weather or responded to cold protection advice.

Successful treatment of perniosis with hydroxychloroquine. Yang X, Perez OA, English JC 3rd. J Drugs Dermatol 2010; 9: 1242–6.

In this retrospective study hydroxychloroquine improved symptoms in four out of five patients with perniosis.

Pernio of the hips in young girls wearing tight-fitting jeans with a low waistband. Weismann K, Grønhøj Larsen F. Acta Dermatol Venereol 2006; 86: 558–9.

Two adolescent girls from Denmark developed chilblains on their right hips. This was attributed to exposure to cold associated with wearing tight-fitting jeans with a low waistband that left uncovered the upper part of the hip region. Both were treated with intense pulsed light (555–950 nm), 14 J/cm². After three monthly treatments, the redness was reduced.

Evidence Levels: A Double-blind study B Clinical trial ≥ 20 subjects C Clinical trial < 20 subjects D Series ≥ 5 subjects E Anecdotal case reports

43

Chondrodermatitis nodularis helicis chronicus

Clifford Lawrence

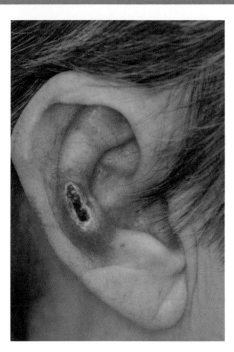

Chondrodermatitis is a benign condition; the chief indication for treatment is pain causing sleep disturbance. Painless areas of chondrodermatitis can be ignored or managed conservatively. Lesions on the helix are easier to treat surgically than antihelix lesions and are easier to cure. A pressure-relieving cushion is a good first-choice alternative to surgery for antihelix lesions.

MANAGEMENT STRATEGY

Chondrodermatitis usually occurs on the lateral portion of the ear on the preferred sleeping side. It is generally caused by the weight of the head crushing the ear against the pillow during sleep. Ear injury or surgery may leave an irregular cartilage edge that becomes a focus for sleep-related pressure. The most protuberant part of the ear is affected; generally this is the helix in men and the antihelix in women. People who can only adopt one sleeping position due to arthritis, etc., are particularly vulnerable. The incidence increases with age because ear cartilage becomes less flexible with time. Patients should be reassured that it is not skin cancer, advised to use a soft pillow that is still compressible when the head is resting on it, and to change their sleeping position. Conservative or medical treatment, such as *lidocaine (lignocaine) gel*, a potent *topical corticosteroid, self-adhesive foam dressing,* or *a pressure-relieving cushion* can be tried in all patients. If sleep is not disturbed, there is really no need for any further intervention unless cosmesis is a concern.

Numerous surgical strategies have been described to treat chondrodermatitis, and most work to some degree; it is tempting to suggest that some techniques make the ear so painful that the subject is forced to adapt his or her sleeping position until the lesion resolves spontaneously. Most authors believe that the principle of surgical treatment is *excision* of the affected area of cartilage without the need for skin or ulcer excision. Other destructive therapies have been advocated but tend to be less effective. Antihelix lesions respond so well to cartilage excision that many recommend surgery as a first-line treatment.

Specific Investigations

- None required.
- Biopsy is only necessary if surgery is indicated or there is doubt about the diagnosis. Lesions managed conservatively do not require biopsy

First-Line Therapies

• Reassurance that chondrodermatitis is not a cancer	B
• Conservative management	B
• Topical corticosteroids	B
• Intralesional corticosteroids	B
• 0.2% topical nitroglycerin	C

Treatment of chondrodermatitis nodularis helicis and conventional wisdom? Beck MH. Br J Dermatol 1985; 113: 504–5.

Topical corticosteroids (betamethasone valerate cream 0.025%) used twice a day for 6 weeks and intralesional triamcinolone (0.2–0.5 mL or 10 mg/mL) are effective will improve symptoms and aid healing in almost 25% of patients.

Intralesional triamcinolone for chondrodermatitis nodularis: a follow-up study of 60 patients. Cox NH, Denham PF. Br J Dermatol 2002; 146: 712–3.

A retrospective analysis of 60 patients with chondrodermatitis nodularis helicis (CNH) treated with 0.1 mL intralesional triamcinolone acetonide 10 mg/mL or triamcinolone hexacetonide 5 mg/mL showed good response on 43% of helix and 31% of antihelix lesions.

The usefulness of 0.2% topical nitroglycerin for chondrodermatitis nodularis helicis. Sanz-Motilva V, Martorell-Calatayud A, Gutiérrez García-Rodrigo C, Hueso-Gabriel L, Garcia-Melgares ML, Pelufo-Enguix C, et al. Actas Dermosifiliogr 2015; 106: 555–61.

Ninety-three percent of 29 patients treated showed clinical improvement with a mean follow-up of 5.9 months. There were fewer side effects using the 0.2% preparation compared with the original 2% ointment.

Reassurance that this is not a tumor puts the patient's mind at rest. In many instances the symptoms are mild and can be tolerated without any major intervention. Initially, conservative therapy should be tried. Recommend a 6-week course of a potent topical steroid with a change in sleeping position and a soft pillow that can still be further compressed when the head is resting on it.

Second-Line Therapies

• Helix lesions – excision of cartilage without skin excision	B
• Antihelix lesions – pressure-relieving cushion or device	B

The treatment of chondrodermatitis nodularis with cartilage removal alone. Lawrence CM. Arch Dermatol 1991; 127: 530–5.

Cartilage excision without skin removal resulted in cure rates of 84% for helix and 75% for antihelix lesions. Local anesthesia with lidocaine and epinephrine (adrenaline) reduced bleeding and improved the visibility without ear skin necrosis. On the helix, the skin was reflected back from a helix rim incision to expose the cartilage. On the antihelix, a medially based skin flap was raised to expose cartilage. After exposed cartilage excision, all remaining cartilage edges were left smooth and gently shelving up to the uninvolved cartilage to prevent recurrences that may develop on rough or protuberant cartilage edges. Cartilage excision alone is not disfiguring, and further cartilage edges can be removed if recurrences occur.

Treatment of chondrodermatitis nodularis with removal of the underlying cartilage alone: retrospective analysis of experience in 37 lesions. de Ru JA, Lohuis PJ, Saleh HA, Vuyk HD. J Laryngol Otol 2002; 116: 677–81.

Most otolaryngologists treat patients with chondrodermatitis nodularis by wedge excision. This can leave the patient with an asymmetric deformed ear. The authors described their results after changing to removal of cartilage alone. In a mean follow-up of 30 months, all 34 patients remained symptom free, and only 1 required revisional surgery.

Twelve years' experience of simplified surgical treatment of chondrodermatitis nodularis by cartilage trimming and sutureless skin closure. Hussain W, Chalmers RJ. Br J Dermatol 2009; 160: 116–8.

After skin incision, mosquito forceps were used to "nibble" away fragments of cartilage to leave a smooth cartilage contour without the need for full exposure of the cartilage edge. Skin nodules or ulcers are not excised but are left to resolve spontaneously. Tape strips were used for skin closure. Thirty-two of 34 (94%) patients with chondrodermatitis, 7 on the antihelix and 27 on the helix, showed no discomfort or clinical recurrence 4 months after this procedure.

Chondrodermatitis nodularis chronica helicis et antihelicis. Munnoch DA, Herbert KJ, Morris AM. Br J Plast Surg 1996; 49: 473–6.

Fifty-four chondrodermatitis lesions (36 helix, 18 antihelix), including 23 recurrent after previous surgery, were treated by minimal skin excision combined with extensive cartilage resection. There were no recurrences and minimal postoperative deformity.

Narrow elliptical skin excision and cartilage shaving for chondrodermatitis nodularis. Rex J, Ribera M, Bielsa I, Mangas C, Xifra A, Ferrándiz C. Dermatol Surg 2006; 32: 400–4.

A narrow elliptical excision of the papule followed by a slice of the underlying cartilage was taken and trimmed carefully to remove any cartilage spikes. Good cosmetic results were obtained in all 74 patients retrospectively analyzed. The recurrence rate ranged from 10% for helical and 37% for antihelical lesions after a median follow-up of 54 and 50 months, respectively.

Modified surgical excision for the treatment of chondrodermatitis nodularis. Ormond P, Collins P. Dermatol Surg 2004; 30(2 Pt 1): 208–10.

Excision of the cartilage alone is therapeutically and cosmetically effective. To simplify the surgical procedure, a narrow ellipse of skin over the nodule was excised and cold steel dissection of the adjacent skin replaced by hydrodissection to create a plane of cleavage between the skin and cartilage. These two refinements

maintained the clinical and cosmetic efficacy and simplified the surgical technique.

All of these techniques are based on removal of damaged cartilage and avoidance of leaving irregular cartilage margins, as these may act as a focus for recurrence. Treatment outcome is operator dependent. Skin excision can be included if this makes the procedure easier to perform, but this is not required for surgical success.

Auricular pressure relieving cushions for chondrodermatitis nodularis helicis. Allen DL, Swinson PA, Arnstein PM. J Maxillofac Prosthet Tech 1998; 2: 5–10.

Thirty-five of 46 patients treated in this way had complete resolution of their symptoms.

Effective treatment of chondrodermatitis nodularis chronica helicis using a conservative approach. Moncrieff M, Sassoon EM. Br J Dermatol 2004; 150: 892–4.

A simple-to-construct ear cushion design was used, made up of a bath sponge with the center removed and held in place with a head band. Thirteen out of 15 patients followed for 1 month responded.

The bath sponge pressure-relieving device is commercially available (CNH ear protector, Delasco).

Management of chondrodermatitis nodularis chronica helicis using a "doughnut pillow." Sanu A, Koppana R, Snow DG. J Laryngol Otol 2007; 121: 1096–8.

Patients used a doughnut-shaped pillow made of a modern orthopedic "memory foam." This distributes the weight of the recumbent head more evenly and is designed to relieve the pressure on the affected ear. Thirteen of 23 (56%) patients treated remained pain free after a 1-year follow-up.

Management of chondrodermatitis nodularis helicis by auricular pressure-relieving device: a retrospective study. Belgi A, Logan RA. Br J Dermatol 2007; 157(Suppl 1): 68.

Seventy-eight patients with CNH used a custom-made ear pressure–relieving device designed and built by the local maxillofacial technicians. Forty-eight patients responded to a questionnaire examining the outcome. Only 7 found it helpful (15%). Twenty reported no benefit (42%) and 20 some benefit (42%).

Management of chondrodermatitis helicis by protective padding: a series of 12 cases and a review of the literature. Timoney N, Davison PM. Br J Plast Surg 2002; 55: 387–9.

Fourteen patients with CNH were prospectively enrolled and used protective padding of the ear at night. Most patients were rapidly relieved of their symptoms, although healing was frequently prolonged.

Chondrodermatitis nodularis chronica helicis: a conservative therapeutic approach by decompression. Kuen-Spiegl M, Ratzinger G, Sepp N, Fritsch P. J Dtsch Dermatol Ges 2011; 9: 292–6.

Using a self-made bandage of foam plastic applied during the night, 11 out of 12 patients reported substantial reduction of pain within the first month and were pain free after an average of 1.75 months.

Self-adhering foam: a simple method for pressure relief during sleep in patients with chondrodermatitis nodularis helicis. Travelute CR. Dermatol Surg 2013; 39: 317–9.

An inexpensive method using a self-adhering foam sponge (Reston Foam 3M, St Paul, MN) placed on the back of the ear and

Evidence Levels: **A** Double-blind study **B** Clinical trial ≥ 20 subjects **C** Clinical trial < 20 subjects **D** Series ≥ 5 subjects **E** Anecdotal case reports

used nightly for several months described as effective for helix and antihelix lesions.

Various types of ear cushions are described. They all share the same aim, that is, to transfer the weight of the sleeping head from the ear to the surrounding scalp. Authors report a wide range of benefit with between 15% and 80% of patients not requiring surgery. In the hands of this writer the results are generally disappointing. This technique can be helpful for patients in whom surgery has been unsuccessful and in antihelix lesions in frail patients with thin skin who are unable to adapt their sleeping position. In these circumstances postsurgical recurrences are more common.

Third-Line Therapies	
• Curettage	B
• Incision and cartilage curettage	E
• CO_2 laser ablation	C
• Punch and graft	B

Chondrodermatitis nodularis chronica helicis treated with curettage and electrocauterization: follow-up of a 15-year material. Kromann N, Hoyer H, Reymann F. Acta Derm Venereol 1983; 63: 85–7.

One hundred forty-two cases of chondrodermatitis were principally treated by curettage followed by electrocauterization. Seventy-eight patients were reexamined after an average interval of 7.1 years. This simple surgical technique produced a relapse rate of 31%.

The surgical management of chondrodermatitis nodularis chronica helicis. Coldiron BM. J Dermatol Surg Oncol 1991; 17: 902–4.

An ellipse of skin is removed around the ulcerated area. The central necrotic or damaged cartilage is removed using a curette and the skin edges sutured. A series is not reported.

Chondrodermatitis nodularis chronica helicis. Successful treatment with the carbon dioxide laser. Taylor MB. J Dermatol Surg Oncol 1991; 17: 862–4.

The CO_2 laser was used to vaporize the cutaneous nodules and involved cartilage. The wounds were allowed to heal with only minimal care using hydrogen peroxide cleansing and applications of topical antibiotic ointment. Twelve lesions have been treated with no recurrences after 2 to 15 months.

The punch and graft technique: a novel method of surgical treatment for chondrodermatitis nodularis helicis. Rajan N, Langtry JA. Br J Dermatol 2007; 157: 744–7.

Twenty-three lesions (15 helix, 3 antihelix, 5 not recorded) were treated by punch removal of the nodule and underlying cartilage. The small defect was closed with a full-thickness skin graft taken from behind the ear using the same punch.

This novel "punch and graft" technique eschews all the dogma about the need to just remove cartilage and leave smooth cartilage margins but still produces a cure rate of 83%.

Cryotherapy has been advocated, but there are no published outcomes.

44

Chromoblastomycosis

Wanda Sonia Robles, Mahreen Ameen

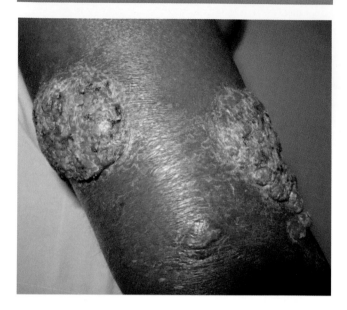

Chromoblastomycosis is a chronic fungal infection of cutaneous and subcutaneous tissues endemic in Central and South America, Africa, Australia, and Japan. It is caused by the traumatic implantation of pigmented (dematiaceous) fungi, which produce characteristic thick-walled sclerotic bodies (also known as *muriform* or *Medlar bodies*) in infected tissues. The most common etiologic agents are *Fonsecaea pedrosoi*, *Phialophora verrucosa*, and *Cladophialophora carrionii*. Clinically, chromoblastomycosis presents as plaques, nodules, or warty, exophytic lesions, which most commonly affect the feet and lower legs. Lesions are slow growing and over years extend centripetally leaving central areas of scarring. Disease is usually localized but can spread through autoinoculation or lymphatic dissemination, producing metastatic lesions away from the primary site. Complications include ulceration, secondary bacterial infection, and lymphedema. Rarely, malignant transformation (squamous cell carcinoma) in chronic lesions and systemic involvement have been reported.

MANAGEMENT STRATEGY

Chromoblastomycosis is a difficult-to-treat deep mycosis that is characterized by low cure rates and high rates of relapse, particularly in chronic and extensive disease. Studies report highly variable rates of clinical and mycologic cure, ranging from 15% to 80%. The choice of treatment and outcome depend on the etiologic agent, the extent of the lesions, clinical topography, and the presence of complications (dermal fibrosis and edema may reduce tissue antifungal drug levels). *F. pedrosoi* is the most common etiologic agent, but has the lowest sensitivity to the major systemic antifungal agents. *C. carrionii* and *P. verrucosa* are much more sensitive and have been found to respond more favorably to treatment.

Surgical excision may be successful for small and localized lesions. It is performed with wide surgical margins and is usually accompanied by chemotherapy in order to reduce the risk of recurrence. Curettage and electrodesiccation is not recommended because it may promote lymphatic spread. Other physical modalities include cryosurgery using liquid nitrogen, as well as thermotherapy (applying local heat to produce controlled temperatures ranging from 42°C to 45°C that inhibit fungal growth) using a variety of methods, including benzene pocket warmers and pocket handkerchief–type warmers. Cryosurgery and thermotherapy have the advantage that they are relatively inexpensive treatment options.

There are no comparative trials of antifungal chemotherapy for chromoblastomycosis. Itraconazole (100–400 mg daily) and terbinafine (250–500 mg daily) are considered first-line treatments, with both drugs having shown high in vitro activity against the causative agents of chromoblastomycosis. They are typically given for long periods at high doses. Dual therapy with itraconazole and terbinafine is recommended if it is affordable and tolerated. It is not uncommon for more than one treatment modality to be used, such as oral antifungals combined with surgery, cryotherapy, or thermotherapy. For example, itraconazole and/or terbinafine combined with cryosurgery is advocated for extensive disease. The antifungal is given first until there is a maximum reduction in lesion size, which usually requires 6 to 12 months of chemotherapy. The lesions then require several treatments with cryosurgery.

Of the other antifungal agents, ketoconazole is not recommended for treating chromoblastomycosis, as it cannot be given at high doses for long treatment periods because of its toxicity profile. Despite a few cases in the early literature reporting successful treatment with fluconazole, it, too, is not recommended as in vitro studies have shown that it has little activity against black fungi. Flucytosine (converted into 5-fluorouracil in fungal cells) was an early treatment that demonstrated some degree of efficacy. It is associated with a high risk of developing resistance, but this can be overcome if it is used in combination with another antifungal. It is also hepatotoxic and myelotoxic, requiring regular monitoring of serum levels. With the emergence of newer antifungals it is rarely used now except for resistant cases. Amphotericin B monotherapy is ineffective, and even in combination with other antifungals results are generally poor. However, amphotericin B and flucytosine dual therapy has demonstrated efficacy, with in vitro studies having demonstrated synergistic activity between the two drugs. The new second-generation triazoles such as posaconazole and voriconazole are promising drugs in the management of deep cutaneous mycoses, but experience to date is limited by their prohibitively high costs in endemic settings.

Specific Investigations

- Direct microscopy
- Culture
- Histopathology

A positive direct examination of scrapings in 10% potassium hydroxide will demonstrate the thick-walled, brown sclerotic cells that are pathognomonic of chromoblastomycosis, irrespective of the causative species. Specimens are more likely to yield a positive result if they include the "black dots" visible on the surface of the lesion. Culture enables the identification of the causative agent. It is a slow-growing fungus, and culture may be inconclusive due to poor morphologic differentiation. Polymerase chain reaction (PCR) has been developed for the identification of *Fonsecaea* and *C. carrionii*. Serologic tests such as enzyme-linked immunosorbent assay (ELISA) can be useful in evaluating therapy response, but like PCR, they are not widely available in most endemic settings. A biopsy demonstrates the typical sclerotic bodies in a granulomatous lesion with transepithelial elimination.

First-Line Therapies	
● Itraconazole	B
● Terbinafine	B
● Posaconazole	D

Treating chromoblastomycosis with systemic antifungals. Bonifaz A, Paredes-Solis V, Saul A. Expert Opin Pharmacother 2004; 5: 247–54.

A review article highlighting the difficulties in treating this condition. The authors state that the best results for therapy have been obtained with combination and high-dose itraconazole and terbinafine for a minimum treatment period of 6 to 12 months.

Chromoblastomycosis. López Martínez R, Méndez Tovar LJ. Clin Dermatol 2007; 25: 188–94.

A comprehensive review article. Itraconazole is considered the treatment of choice in combination with surgery in some cases.

Chromoblastomycosis: an overview of clinical manifestations, diagnosis and treatment. Queiroz-Telles F, Esterre P, Perez-Blanco M, Vitale RG, Salgado CG, Bonifaz A. Med Mycol 2009; 47: 3–15.

The authors state that there is no treatment of choice but rather several treatment options: they suggest that physical therapies should augment chemotherapy and that systemic combination therapies may increase cure rate but may be associated with a higher risk of adverse effects.

Chromoblastomycosis: clinical and mycologic experience of 51 cases. Bonifaz A, Carrasco-Gerard E, Saúl A. Mycoses 2001; 44: 1–7.

This is a study of 51 cases diagnosed over a 17-year period in a tertiary referral center in Mexico. Ninety percent of the cases were caused by F. pedrosoi. The overall cure rate for all treatment modalities was 31%, and a further 57% showed clinical improvement. For large lesions, itraconazole proved to be the most effective treatment, and cryosurgery for small lesions. Itraconazole combined with cryosurgery was also effective.

Subcutaneous mycoses. Queiroz-Telles F, McGinnis MR, Salkin I, Graybill JR. Infect Dis Clin North Am 2003; 17: 59–85.

In this study from Brazil, 30 patients with chromoblastomycosis due mainly to F. pedrosoi were treated with itraconazole 200 to 400 mg daily depending on the clinical severity. Nineteen patients (63%) achieved clinical and mycologic cure after 12 months of treatment (range 5–31 months). Treatment success depended on lesion size and extent.

This is the largest case series of itraconazole monotherapy for chromoblastomycosis.

Pulse itraconazole 400 mg daily in the treatment of chromoblastomycosis. Ungpakorn R, Reangchainam S. Clin Exp Dermatol 2006; 31: 245–7.

In this small study, six cases of F. pedrosoi infection in Thailand were treated with pulse itraconazole, 400 mg daily, for 1 week each month. All achieved clinical and mycologic cure. Four patients were cured after 12 pulses of treatment, and one after 15 pulses of treatment. The remaining patient required 20 pulses of itraconazole as well as cryosurgery. Disease severity and duration

did not appear to be predictive of treatment response. This study demonstrated that the monthly pulse regimen is well tolerated and as effective as the conventional continuous 200- to 400-mg daily regimen for the treatment of F. pedrosoi. The authors recommend that treatment is continued until absence of organisms is proven by histology and tissue culture. Given that the total drug dosage is reduced, there is a marked reduction in cost of therapy by 50% to 75%. They also claim that pulse therapy is associated with higher compliance, although therapy duration remains long.

The cost of long-term itraconazole therapy is expensive in endemic settings, making this an important and relevant study.

Chromoblastomycosis: a clinical and molecular study of 18 cases in Rio de Janeiro, Brazil. Mouchalouat Mde F, Gutierrez Galhardo MC, Zancopé-Oliveira RM, Monteiro Fialho PC, de Oliveira Coelho JM, Silva Tavares PM, et al. Int J Dermatol 2011; 50: 981–6.

The vast majority of these cases were caused by F. pedrosoi, and disease duration varied from 4 months to 32 years. Systemic treatment included either itraconazole monotherapy 200 to 400 mg daily (n = 6) or itraconazole 200 to 400 mg daily combined with fluconazole 200 mg daily (n = 5), which was given for 12 to 60 months. There was an 80% cure rate and no relapse after 2 years of follow-up.

This study demonstrated good tolerability to combination azole therapy, which was given for more severe disease forms that also responded well to drug therapy, suggesting that there may be a role for fluconazole in combination with itraconazole.

Treatment of chromomycosis with terbinafine: preliminary results of an open pilot study. Esterre P, Inzan CK, Ramarcel ER, Andriantsimahavandy A, Ratsioharana M, Pecarrere JL, et al. Br J Dermatol 1996; 134: 33–6.

A multicenter study from Madagascar. Of 43 patients treated, 36 (F. pedrosoi, n = 29; C. carrionii, n = 7) could be completely evaluated. Approximately one third of the patients had been resistant to previous treatment with thiabendazole. Oral terbinafine 500 mg daily was given for 6 to 12 months. Within 2 to 4 months of commencement of treatment, there was a marked clinical improvement with resolution of secondary bacterial infection, edema, and elephantiasis. There was mycologic cure in 83% (24/29) of patients infected with F. pedrosoi at 12 months. Of those infected with C. carrionii, there was cure in one and clinical improvement in a further three. Total cure was observed even in imidazole-refractory patients or those with chronic disease present for over 10 years. There was a mild transient rise of hepatic enzymes in some patients, but no serious adverse effects were reported.

Treatment of chromoblastomycosis with terbinafine: experience with four cases. Bonifaz A, Saúl A, Paredes-Solis V, Araiza J, Fierro-Arias L. J Dermatolog Treat 2005; 16: 47–51.

Four cases from Mexico (F. pedrosoi, n = 3; P. verrucosa, n = 1) were treated with oral terbinafine 500 mg daily. Three cases achieved clinical and mycologic cure after a mean treatment period of 7 months. Treatment was well tolerated with no abnormalities of liver enzymes.

Treatment of chromoblastomycosis with terbinafine: a report of four cases. Xibao Z, Changxing L, Quan L, Yuqing H. J Dermatolog Treat 2005; 16: 121–4.

Four cases from China (C. carrionii, n = 2; F. pedrosoi, n = 2) treated with terbinafine 500 mg daily for the first month followed by 250 mg daily were cured after 4 to 8 months of therapy without evidence of relapse at follow-up 6 months later. The total dosage of terbinafine ranged from 37.5 g to 60 g.

Alternate week and combination itraconazole and terbinafine therapy for chromoblastomycosis caused by *Fonsecaea pedrosoi* in Brazil. Gupta AK, Taborda PR, Sanzovo AD. Med Mycol 2002; 40: 529–34.

Four patients with long-standing disease refractory to standard therapies were treated with alternate week and combination therapy with itraconazole (200–400 mg daily) and terbinafine (250–1000 mg daily). Combination therapy proved to be more effective and was well tolerated.

The authors suggest that combination therapy with itraconazole and terbinafine may be synergistic, with in vitro studies having already demonstrated this against other fungi. Larger studies are required to evaluate combination therapy with itraconazole and terbinafine. However, it must be noted that both drugs are expensive in endemic settings.

Posaconazole treatment of refractory eumycetoma and chromoblastomycosis. Negroni R, Tobon A, Bustamante B, Shikanai-Yasuda MA, Patino H, Restrepo A. Rev Inst Med Trop Sao Paulo 2005; 47: 339–46.

Cure was achieved in five of six patients with chromoblastomycosis refractory to standard antifungal therapies. They were treated with posaconazole 800 mg in divided doses. The maximum treatment period was for 34 months. Treatment was very well tolerated.

This new triazole demonstrates high efficacy and tolerability, but its use in most endemic settings is currently restricted due to its high cost.

Chromoblastomycosis: a neglected tropical disease. Queiroz-Telles F. Rev Inst Med Trop Sao Paulo 2015; 57 (Suppl 19): 46–50.

Itraconazole, either as monotherapy or associated with other drugs or with physical methods, is the mainstay of treatment. More recently photodynamic therapy has been successfully used in combination with antifungals.

Second-Line Therapies

• Cryotherapy	B
• Surgical excision	D
• Thermotherapy	D

Treatment of chromoblastomycosis with itraconazole, cryosurgery, and a combination of both. Bonifaz A, Martinez-Soto E, Carrasco-Gerard E, Peniche J. Int J Dermatol 1997; 36: 542–7.

This study included 12 patients assigned to three different groups. Group 1, with small lesions, was treated with itraconazole 300 mg/day. Group 2, also with small lesions, was treated with one or more sessions of cryosurgery. Group 3, with large lesions, started treatment with itraconazole 300 mg/day until reduction of lesions was achieved, followed by one or more sessions of cryosurgery. The results showed complete clinical and mycologic cure in two out of four patients in both groups 1 and 3. All four patients in group 2 achieved complete cure.

Although the case numbers were small, this study suggests that cryosurgery is a more suitable treatment option than antifungal therapy for small lesions.

Treatment of chromomycosis by cryosurgery with liquid nitrogen: 15 years' experience. Castro LG, Pimentel ER, Lacaz CS. Int J Dermatol 2003; 42: 408–12.

This retrospective study included 22 patients with *F. pedrosoi*. Small lesions were frozen in a single session, whereas larger lesions were frozen in small parts. The average number of cryosurgery treatments that each patient received was 6.7 (range 1–22

sessions). Nine patients (40.9%) were considered cured (clinically disease-free period of at least 3 years), and eight patients (36.4%) were under observation (clinically disease-free but fewer than 3 years of follow-up). The rest failed to clear with treatment.

This study suggests high efficacy for cryosurgery therapy. This study, as well as others, suggests that cryosurgery is a useful and inexpensive option for small lesions.

Successful treatment of chromoblastomycosis with topical heat therapy. Tagami H, Ginoza M, Imaizumi S, Urano-Suehisa S. J Am Acad Dermatol 1984; 10: 615–9.

Four cases (*F. pedrosoi* isolated from three) were treated with topical application of tolerable heat from pocket warmers. Three patients responded after 2, 3, and 6 months of treatment. The fourth patient who received treatment in an irregular manner cleared only after a 12-month period.

Third-Line Therapies

• Flucytosine	C
• Amphotericin B	D
• Voriconazole	E
• Posaconazole	E

Six years experience in treatment of chromomycosis with 5-fluorocytosine. Lopez CF, Alvarenga RJ, Cisalpino EO, Resende MA, Oliveira LG. Int J Dermatol 1978; 17: 414–8.

Twenty-three patients with chromoblastomycosis were treated with oral flucytosine for 2 to 67 months. Sixteen patients achieved clinical and mycologic cure (59%). However, seven patients developed resistance, and they failed to respond with subsequent treatment with amphotericin B, calciferol, or thiabendazole. Resistance appeared to occur particularly in those with long-standing lesions or widespread involvement.

A case of chromoblastomycosis with an unusual clinical manifestation caused by *Phialophora verrucosa* on an unexposed area: treatment with a combination of amphotericin B and 5-flucytosine. Park SG, Oh SH, Suh SB, Lee KH, Chung KY. Br J Dermatol 2005; 152: 560–4.

This case from Korea was treated with liposomal amphotericin monotherapy for 3 months, which had some effect. The addition of 5-flucytosine 4 g daily resulted in marked clinical improvement after only 1 month. Amphotericin was then discontinued, and dual therapy with 5-flucytosine and itraconazole 200 mg daily was given for 12 months until mycologic cure.

This case illustrates the low efficacy of amphotericin B monotherapy, and the synergistic activity in combination with 5-flucytosine. 5-Flucytosine is renally excreted, and therefore careful monitoring is required when it is used with other nephrotoxic drugs. Despite the toxicity of both drugs, this combination has been advocated by some mycologists as a very useful alternative to azoles.

Extensive chromoblastomycosis caused by *Fonsecaea pedrosoi* successfully treated with a combination of amphotericin B and itraconazole. Paniz-Mondolfi AE, Colella MT, Negrín DC, Aranzazu N, Oliver M, Reyes-Jaimes O, et al. Med Mycol 2008; 46: 179–84.

This report describes a case of extensive disease affecting the whole of the right lower limb of 22 years' duration that had failed 15 years of previous therapy consisting of ketoconazole and fluconazole. The patient then achieved clinical and mycologic cure with amphotericin (cumulative dose of 2150 mg) in combination with itraconazole 100 mg twice daily for approximately 3 months followed by a further 1 year of itraconazole 100 mg daily.

Extensive long-standing chromomycosis due to *Fonsecaea pedrosoi*: three cases with relevant improvement under voriconazole therapy. Criado PR, Careta MF, Valente NY, Martins JE, Rivitti EA, Spina R, et al. J Dermatolog Treat 2011; 22: 167–74.

Three patients with long-standing (10, 20, and 21 years) and extensive disease refractory to previous therapy with itraconazole and terbinafine were treated with voriconazole 200 mg twice daily for 12 months. Clinical response was evident after 30 to 50 days, but at the end of treatment despite significant clinical improvement, none of the patients achieved cure. All patients showed elevations of serum gamma-glutamyl transpeptidase during the treatment without clinical relevance, and a single patient developed visual abnormalities and tremors requiring dose reduction.

This is the first report of the use of voriconazole for chromoblastomycosis. The partial response may be attributed to the severity of the disease. The report suggests that voriconazole represents an option for extensive disease refractory to conventional treatment.

Photodynamic therapy combined with terbinafine against chromoblastomycosis and the effect of PDT on *Fonsecaea monophora* in vitro. Hu Y, Huang X, Lu S, Hamblin MR, Mylonakis E, Zhang J, et al. Mycopathologia 2015; 179: 103–9.

Report of one case of refractory chromoblastomycosis treated with nine sessions of photodynamic therapy in combination with terbinafine. The lesions were improved after two sessions of ALA-PDT treatment, each including nine times, at an interval of 1 week, combined with terbinafine 250 mg/day oral, and clinical improvement could be observed.

Successful sequential treatment with itraconazole and ALA-PDT for chromoblastomycosis because of *Alternaria alternata*. Liu ZH, Xia XJ. Dermatol Ther 2014; 27: 357–60.

Case report of chromoblastomycosis due to *Alternaria alternata* successfully treated with systemic antifungals and subsequent 5 ALA-PDT.

Photodynamic antifungal therapy against chromoblastomycosis. Lyon JP, Pedroso e Silva Azevedo Cde M, Moreira LM, de Lima CJ, de Resende MA. Mycopathologia 2011; 172: 293–7.

Report of the use of methylene blue as photosensitizer and a light-emitting diode as light source in the treatment of chromoblastomycosis.

Chronic actinic dermatitis

Sally H. Ibbotson, Robert S. Dawe

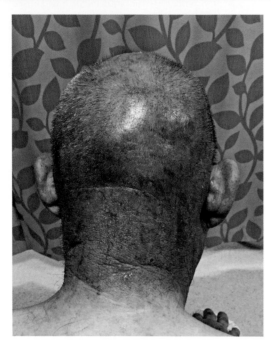

Chronic actinic dermatitis (CAD) is a chronic dermatitis mainly involving photoexposed sites, which is associated with objective evidence of abnormal photosensitivity. The photosensitivity is usually broadband although predominantly involving the ultraviolet B (UVB) waveband and often extending into the ultraviolet A (UVA) and even visible wavebands. The condition is considered to have an immunological basis, and no specific genetic susceptibility has been identified. Typically CAD affects elderly males, although in younger patients it is reported particularly in association with atopic dermatitis. Indeed, most cases arise on the background of a dermatitis, such as atopic, seborrhoeic, or contact allergic dermatitis. In fact, in more than 75% of cases of CAD, patch testing is positive, confirming the association with contact allergic dermatitis. Patient and clinician may not be aware of the link with sunlight because of perennial symptoms and covered site involvement, leading to delays in diagnosis.

MANAGEMENT STRATEGY

Thus the essential first step of management is accurate diagnosis and exclusion of other conditions, such as photoaggravated eczema, and reversible causes, particularly drug-induced photosensitivity. Phototesting is essential, and the gold standard investigation is monochromator phototesting, allowing accurate definition of wavelengths involved (action spectrum) and the degree of photosensitivity.

Photoprotection is essential, with emphasis on *environmental and behavioral measures* (use of window film to prevent all ultraviolet (UV) transmission and double-envelope compact fluorescent

lamps or light-emitting diodes [LEDs] for those with severe photosensitivity; seeking out the shade and avoiding sunlight in the middle of the day), *clothing choices* (tightly woven and dark colors if visible wavelengths are involved), and high SPF fragrance-free sunscreens. Patient education to reduce exposure to *contact allergens* is also essential, as contact allergy tends to persist indefinitely, whereas photosensitivity can resolve over time.

Active disease should be treated with *emollients* and *topical corticosteroids*. With severe flares or erythroderma, admission to hospital may be required in order to allow the patient to be nursed behind photoprotective screens. *Systemic corticosteroids* may be required for acute flares and then tapered over weeks. *Desensitization with photo(chemo)therapy* may be possible, although patients are usually too UVB sensitive to be able to tolerate UVB phototherapy, and thus, psoralen-UVA (PUVA) may be more effective and better tolerated. If these measures are inadequate for disease control, systemic immunosuppression may be needed.

Specific Investigations

- Phototesting (with UVB, UVA, and visible light from monochromator or broadband sources)
- Provocation testing (with solar simulator or other broadband source)
- Patch and photopatch tests
- Consider concomitant disease

The construction and development of a grating monochromator and its application to the study of the reaction of the skin to light. MacKenzie LA, Frain-Bell W. Br J Dermatol 1973; 89: 251–64.

Phototesting using an irradiation monochromator, if available, should be performed.

False-negative monochromator phototesting in chronic actinic dermatitis. Kerr AC, Dawe RS, Lowe G, Ferguson J. Br J Dermatol 2010; 162: 1406–8.

A case of false-negative monochromator phototesting in a patient with chronic actinic dermatitis taking prednisolone. Ferguson J, Ibbotson SH. Br J Dermatol 2012; 167: 214–5.

If testing shows severe photosensitivity despite topical corticosteroid therapy, this can allow the diagnosis to be made, but topical corticosteroid therapy or even low-dose oral prednisolone (10 mg/day) can lead to misleading false-negative testing.

Chronic actinic dermatitis in the elderly: recognition and treatment. Dawe RS. Drugs Aging 2005; 22: 201–7.

Phototesting is required to diagnose CAD. This review gives guidance on testing where specialized facilities are not available.

A preliminary investigation into the effect of exposure of photosensitive individuals to light from compact fluorescent lamps. Eadie E, Ferguson J, Moseley H. Br J Dermatol 2009; 160: 659–64.

Energy-saving lamps and their impact on photosensitive and normal individuals. Fenton L, Ferguson J, Ibbotson S, Moseley H. Br J Dermatol 2013; 169: 910–5.

Tungsten lamp and chronic actinic dermatitis. Hu SC, Lan CE. Australas J Dermatol 2017; 58: e14–6.

Evidence Levels: **A** Double-blind study **B** Clinical trial ≥ 20 subjects **C** Clinical trial < 20 subjects **D** Series ≥ 5 subjects **E** Anecdotal case reports

Is photodynamic diagnostic flexible ureterorenoscopy suitable for a patient presenting with chronic actinic dermatitis? Valentine R, Kata S, Ibbotson S, Nabi G, Moseley H. Photoderm Photoimmunol Photomed 2015; 31: 279–81.

Be aware that patients with CAD may be at risk from exposure to UV radiation from compact fluorescent ("energy saving") lamps. Indeed, patients with CAD who have severe broadband photosensitivity, including visible light sensitivity (such as visible light through window glass and exposure to a bright "ordinary" tungsten source used for ear cleaning), may be at risk from exposure to a wide range of artificial light sources, and this should be investigated and considered in management approaches.

Contact allergic sensitivity to plants and the photosensitivity dermatitis and actinic reticuloid syndrome. Frain-Bell W, Johnson BE. Br J Dermatol 1979; 101: 503–12.

Contact and photocontact sensitization in chronic actinic dermatitis: sesquiterpene lactone mix is an important allergen. Menagé H du P, Ross JS, Norris PG, Hawk JLM, White IR. Br J Dermatol 1995; 132: 543–7.

A European multicenter photopatch test study. European Multicenter Photopatch Test Study (EMCPPTS) Taskforce. Br J Dermatol 2012; 166: 1002–9.

Photopatch testing: recommendations for a European photopatch test baseline series. Goncalo M, Ferguson J, Bonevalle A, Bruynzeel DP, Gimenez-Amau A, Goossens A, et al. Contact Dermatitis 2013; 68: 239–43.

Contact and/or photocontact allergy is common in CAD. Standard allergens, including fragrances, plants, and sunscreens, must be considered. Patch and photopatch testing, repeated at intervals as indicated by history, are essential investigations in order not to "miss" new allergens or photoallergens. Because many CAD patients are abnormally sensitive to the UVA sources used for photopatch testing, this technique may be difficult to undertake and interpret. However, photopatch testing with suberythemal UVA doses should be undertaken where possible.

Contact and photocontact sensitization in chronic actinic dermatitis: a changing picture. Chew AL, Bashir SJ, Hawk JLM, Palmer R, White I, McFadden JP. Contact Dermatitis 2010; 62: 42–6.

Be aware of changing allergen patterns with alteration in exposure over time. Para-phenylenediamine reactions in CAD may have increased.

Chronic actinic dermatitis in Asian skin: a Singaporean experience. Tan AW, Lim KS, Chong WS. Photoderm Photoimmunol Photomed 2011; 27: 172–5.

Three of 26 Singaporean patients with CAD were positive for HIV.

Other case series have found even greater proportions of CAD patients to have HIV. This does not prove a cause-and-effect relationship, but the possible association should be considered.

Sunlight exposure behavior and vitamin D status in photosensitive patients: longitudinal comparative study with healthy individuals at UK latitude. Rhodes LE, Webb AR, Berry JL, Felton SJ, Marjanovic EJ, Wilkinson JD, et al. Br J Dermatol 2014; 171: 1478–86.

Photosensitive patients are at higher risk of vitamin D insufficiency/deficiency, and we therefore need to be vigilant about vitamin D status in patients with CAD.

First-Line Therapies

• Photoprotective measures	C
• Avoidance of relevant contact allergens	C
• Topical corticosteroids	C
• Topical emollients	C

Photodermatoses: environmentally induced conditions with high psychological impact. Rizwan M, Reddick CL, Bundy C, Unsworth R, Richards HL, Rhodes LE. Photochem Photobiol Sci 2013; 12: 182–9.

Depression, anxiety, and dermatology life quality index scores were assessed in 185 of 260 adult patients with photosensitivity diseases who returned questionnaires. Twenty-three percent showed evidence of anxiety and 7.9% depression, and particular risk factors were facial involvement and duration of photosensitivity. This study showed high levels of psychological comorbidity in patients with photosensitivity diseases.

Chronic actinic dermatitis: a retrospective analysis of 44 cases referred to an Australian photobiology clinic. Yap LM, Foley P, Crouch R, Baker C. Australas J Dermatol 2003; 44: 256–62.

Restriction of sunshine and allergen exposure, along with sunscreens and topical corticosteroids, gave relief in 36% of CAD patients. The remainder also required oral immunosuppressants or phototherapy.

Photosensitivity dermatitis/actinic reticuloid syndrome in an Irish population: a review and some unusual features. Healy E, Rogers S. Acta Derm Venereol 1995; 75: 72–4.

Of nine CAD patients treated with sunscreens, emollients, topical corticosteroids, and antigen avoidance, six responded well, two achieved complete remission, and four were controlled on topical corticosteroids alone, although five also required oral corticosteroids initially.

Protection against ultraviolet radiation by commercial summer clothing: need for standardised testing and labeling. Gambichler T, Rotterdam S, Altmeyer P, Hoffmann K. BMC Dermatol 2001; 1: 6.

Summer clothing textiles ($n = 236$) were investigated spectrophotometrically for their ultraviolet protection factors (UPF). Over 70% of wool and polyester, but less than 30% of cotton, linen, and viscose fabrics, had UPFs over 30.

New advances in protection against solar ultraviolet radiation in textiles for summer clothing. Aguilera J, de Galvez MV, Sanchez-Roldan C, Herrera-Ceballos E. Photochem Photobiol 2014; 90: 1199–206.

Some clothing, such as normal shirts, may offer very little protection against ultraviolet radiation (UVR), and information about UVR protection levels should be included in textile labeling.

Dosimetric investigation of the solar erythemal UV radiation protection provided by beards and moustaches. Parisi AV, Turnbull DJ, Downs N, Smith D. Radiat Prot Dosimetry 2012; 150: 278–82.

Some protection from UVR is provided by facial hair, with the ultraviolet protection factor ranging from 2 to 21. However, protection levels may not be high, particularly at the higher solar zenith angle; thus beards and moustaches should not be considered reliable means of photoprotection in CAD.

Second-Line Therapies	
• Azathioprine	A
• cyclosporine	E
• Mycophenolate	E
• Hydroxycarbamide	E
• PUVA	D
• UVB	D
• Topical calcineurin inhibitors	B

Chronic actinic dermatitis. Paek SY, Lim HW. Dermatol Clin 2014; 32: 355–61.

If conservative management of CAD with photoprotection and topical therapies is insufficient, systemic immunosuppressants, such as glucocorticoids, azathioprine, cyclosporine, or mycophenolate mofetil, may be effective.

Azathioprine treatment in chronic actinic dermatitis: a double-blind controlled trial with monitoring of exposure to ultraviolet radiation. Murphy GM, Maurice PD, Norris PG, Morris RW, Hawk JL. Br J Dermatol 1989; 121: 639–46.

Five of eight patients with CAD treated in this randomized trial had complete clinical disease remission within 6 months of azathioprine (150 mg/day) commencement. No useful clinical response was seen in 10 patients treated with placebo. It is not known whether azathioprine causes objective improvement in photosensitivity.

Azathioprine in dermatology: a survey of current practice in the UK. Tan BB, Gawkrodger DJ, English JSC. Br J Dermatol 1997; 136: 351–5.

A questionnaire survey of 253 UK dermatologists demonstrated that 68% use azathioprine in CAD, 66% alone, and the others as a steroid-sparing agent. Most used 100 mg daily, with only 13% prescribing it by body weight. CAD had the highest proportion of perceived efficacy (62%) of all disorders treated with azathioprine.

Severe chronic actinic dermatitis treated with cyclosporine: 2 cases. Paquet P, Piérard GE. Ann Dermatol Venereol 2001; 128: 42–5.

Two patients with CAD unresponsive to high-dose oral steroids responded well to oral cyclosporine without significant adverse effects. One was in remission for 3 years after stopping cyclosporine.

Chronic actinic dermatitis treated with mycophenolate mofetil. Thomson MA, Stewart DG, Lewis HM. Br J Dermatol 2005; 152: 784–6.

Two patients with CAD who had failed to respond to topical steroids, prednisolone, PUVA, azathioprine, and cyclosporine were treated with mycophenolate mofetil, resulting in clearance over weeks, without adverse effects.

Chronic actinic dermatitis (photosensitivity dermatitis/actinic reticuloid syndrome): beneficial effect from hydroxyurea. Gramvussakis S, George SA. Br J Dermatol 2000; 143: 1340.

Hydroxycarbamide (previously called hydroxyurea) at 500 to 1000 mg/day induced remission of CAD in one patient.

PUVA therapy of chronic actinic dermatitis. Hindson C, Spiro J, Downey A. Br J Dermatol 1985; 113: 157–60.

Four patients with severe CAD were treated twice weekly with PUVA, with starting UVA doses of 0.25 J/cm^2 and increases of 0.25 to 1 J/cm^2 up to a maximum 10 J/cm^2. Topical steroids were applied immediately after each of the first six exposures. All patients responded well and remained controlled on twice-monthly treatments of 10 J/cm^2.

Chronic actinic dermatitis: two patients with successful management using narrowband ultraviolet B phototherapy with systemic steroids. Khaled A, Kerkeni N, Baccouche D, Zeglaoui F, Kamoun M, Mohamed R. EDP Sciences 2011; 66: 453–7.

Two patients were successfully treated with narrowband UVB under cover of systemic corticosteroid therapy.

Actinic reticuloid. A clinical photobiologic, histopathologic, and follow-up study of 16 patients. Toonstra J, Henquet CJ, van Weelden H, van der Putte SC, van Vloten WA. J Am Acad Dermatol 1989; 21: 205–14.

Fifteen CAD patients were treated with broadband UVB phototherapy five times a week, starting at a 10% minimal erythema dose, with gradual increments as tolerated. Thirteen improved well clinically, with increased sunlight tolerance. Discontinuation of therapy was followed by gradual relapse.

Treatment with topical tacrolimus favors chronic actinic dermatitis: a clinical and immunopathological study. Ma Y, Lu Z. J Dermatolog Treat 2010; 21: 171–7.

Forty patients with CAD were treated with topical tacrolimus 0.1%, and skin biopsies were performed pretreatment and posttreatment in 15 patients. Clinical efficacy was seen in 25 (63%), with significant downregulation of Langerhans/dendritic cell function.

Erythrodermic chronic actinic dermatitis responding only to topical tacrolimus. Evans AV, Palmer RA, Hawk JLM. Photodermatol Photoimmunol Photomed 2004; 20: 59–61.

An erythrodermic patient with CAD resistant to oral immunosuppressants and phototherapy responded well to topical tacrolimus.

Successful treatment of chronic actinic dermatitis with topical pimecrolimus. Larangeira de Almeida H. Int J Dermatol 2005; 44: 343–4.

Pimecrolimus can be considered an alternative therapy.

No comparative studies have been reported. Potent topical corticosteroids should generally be favored over topical calcineurin inhibitors, but these newer topical immunomodulators are appropriate to consider for those with inadequate responses to topical corticosteroids.

Third-Line Therapies	
• Hydroxychloroquine	D
• Etretinate	E
• Danazol	E
• Thalidomide	E
• Interferon	E
• Infliximab	E

Chronic actinic dermatitis. An analysis of 51 patients evaluated in the United States and Japan. Lim HW, Morison WL, Kamide R, Buchness MR, Harris R, Soter NA. Arch Dermatol 1994; 130: 1284–9.

Evidence Levels: **A** Double-blind study **B** Clinical trial ≥ 20 subjects **C** Clinical trial < 20 subjects **D** Series ≥ 5 subjects **E** Anecdotal case reports

Photoprotection and topical corticosteroids were useful in 51 patients with CAD. Azathioprine (50–200 mg/day) was also commonly helpful. PUVA and oral corticosteroids were beneficial in 7 patients, cyclosporine in 4, and etretinate in 2. Hydroxychloroquine (200 mg once or twice daily) achieved partial/good responses in 9 patients.

Chronic actinic dermatitis responding to danazol. Humbert P, Drobacheff C, Vigan M, Quencez E, Laurent R, Agache P. Br J Dermatol 1991; 124: 195–7.

A patient with CAD with low α_1-antitrypsin levels responded dramatically to danazol (600 mg/day for 3 weeks), relapsed on stopping, improved on restarting, and remained controlled 18 months later while still on the drug. Danazol raises low serum α_1-antitrypsin and protease inhibitor levels, and a protease–antiprotease imbalance has been said to cause abnormal inflammatory responses in several dermatoses.

Recalcitrant chronic actinic dermatitis treated with low-dose thalidomide. Safa G, Pieto-Le Corvaisier C, Hervagault B. J Am Acad Dermatol 2005; 52: E6.

A patient with CAD resistant to PUVA, azathioprine, cyclosporine, and hydroxychloroquine responded dramatically to thalidomide (100 mg/day reduced to 50 mg twice weekly) over 5 months without adverse effect.

Actinic reticuloid: treatment with recombinant interferon alpha-2b. Trevisi P, Farina P, Borda G, Passarini B, Bonelli U. G Ital Dermatol Venereol 1993; 128: 327–31.

Natural α-interferon in chronic actinic dermatitis. Report of a case. Parodi A, Gallo R, Guarrera M, Rebora A. Acta Derm Venereol 1995; 75: 80.

In one patient with CAD in whom cyclosporine had to be discontinued because of hypertension, natural α-interferon (3 MU three times per week) was effective.

Successful therapy of chronic actinic dermatitis with infliximab. Schopf RE, Poblete-Gutiérrez P. Exp Dermatol 2009; 18: 302 (abstract at 36th Annual Meeting of Arbeitsgemeinschaft Dermatologische Forschung, Heidelberg, 2009).

Infliximab infusions were associated with marked improvement in one patient who had not shown useful response to previous therapies, including topical corticosteroids, PUVA, and cyclosporine.

Coccidioidomycosis

Mahreen Ameen, Wanda Sonia Robles

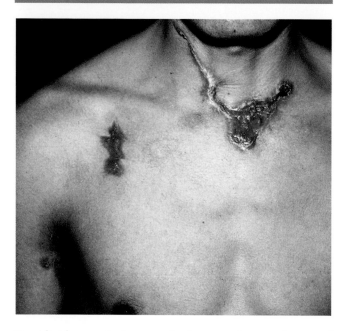

Coccidioidomycosis is an endemic systemic mycosis caused by inhalation of dimorphic fungi of the genus *Coccidioides* (*C. immitis* and *C. posadasii*). It is endemic in desert regions of the Southwestern United States and Central and South America. Primary pulmonary disease is usually subacute and self-limiting. The immunocompromised are particularly susceptible to chronic pulmonary disease. One percent progress to disseminated disease, and again those with impaired cell-mediated immunity are at greater risk of this. Coccidioidomycosis is an opportunistic infection with advanced HIV infection and CD4 counts less than 250. Solid organ transplant recipients, patients with hematologic malignancies, and those on long-term immunosuppressants, including corticosteroids and tumor necrosis factor-alpha (TNF-α) antagonists, are also at risk. Extrapulmonary hematogenous dissemination can affect almost any organ but most frequently involves the skin, lymph nodes, skeletal system, and meninges. Dissemination to the skin can give rise to ulcerative and verrucous lesions with a predilection for the nasolabial area. Subcutaneous abscesses, sinus tracts, and fistulae can develop as a **result of coccidioidal infection in neighboring lymph nodes, bones, or joints.** Other dermatologic manifestations include erythema nodosum and erythema multiforme associated with primary pulmonary infection. Primary infection of the skin is rare.

Dermatologists should be aware that the combination of atypical skin lesions, pulmonary infiltrates, and a history of travel to endemic areas of the disease may represent disseminated infection with coccidioidomycosis.

MANAGEMENT STRATEGY

Treatment depends on disease extent and predisposing factors. Those with primary pulmonary infection and no risk factors require only periodic assessments up to 2 years to ensure that the infection is self-limiting. Some clinicians, however, prefer to treat with oral azoles to prevent any risk of progression, although there are no trial data to support this. Antifungal therapy is indicated for severe or chronic pneumonia or progressive or disseminated infection. Fluconazole (400–800 mg daily) and itraconazole (200–600 mg daily) are the initial choice of therapy for most chronic pulmonary and disseminated infections. Ketoconazole (400 mg daily) shows comparable efficacy to the other azoles, but is associated with a higher risk of adverse effects with long-term use. Parenteral amphotericin B (AmB deoxycholate 0.5–1.5 mg/kg/day or lipid formulations of AmB 2.0–5.0 mg/kg/day) is recommended for those with severely acute infection with respiratory failure, those with rapidly progressive and disseminated infection, women during pregnancy, and those who fail azole therapy. Published reports of its use, however, are still limited to small numbers of patients treated in open-label, nonrandomized studies. There have been no clinical trials assessing the efficacy of lipid formulations of amphotericin B. Newly available antifungals that may be used for refractory infection include the triazoles, posaconazole and voriconazole, with in vitro studies having demonstrated their efficacy. However, there have been no comparative studies as yet evaluating their efficacy against the established azoles used for treating coccidioidomycosis. There are early reports too of the successful use of caspofungin, an echinocandin, although results of in vitro susceptibility studies have varied widely.

In addition to drug therapy, surgery is sometimes indicated for the removal of focal infection such as pulmonary cavities, focal osseous infection, or the debridement of soft tissue. Long-term prophylaxis with azoles is indicated for the immunocompromised, and meningeal infection requires lifelong azole therapy in order to prevent recurrence. Recovery from infection confers lifelong immunity and provides the rationale for the ongoing development of a possible vaccine.

Treatment considerations in pulmonary coccidioidomycosis. Hartmann CA, Aye WT, Blair JE. Expert Rev Respir Med 2016; 10: 1079–91.

This review discusses current literature regarding medical treatment options, including the various triazoles and amphotericin B products. In addition, it discusses uncomplicated and complicated pulmonary infections and their sequelae and the approach to managing coccidioidomycosis in certain patient populations, such as pregnant women, transplant recipients, HIV-infected individuals, and recipients of TNF-α inhibitors.

Specific Investigations

- Direct microscopy
- Culture
- Serologic tests
- Imaging studies (chest and bone radiography)
- Serology for HIV/AIDS infection (where relevant)

The characteristic globular spherules may be seen in potassium hydroxide mounts of infected material: sputum, cerebrospinal fluid, or pus. Culture is the definitive method of establishing the diagnosis. *Coccidioides* spp. grow rapidly on most media within 5 days. In the mycelial form, the fungus is highly infectious, so cultures should be handled with care. Serologic tests are useful and can be used to assess response to therapy.

Evidence Levels: **A** Double-blind study **B** Clinical trial ≥ 20 subjects **C** Clinical trial < 20 subjects **D** Series ≥ 5 subjects **E** Anecdotal case reports

First Line Therapies

- Fluconazole   A
- Itraconazole   A

Fluconazole therapy for coccidioidal meningitis. The NIAID Mycoses Study Group. Galgiani JN, Catanzaro A, Cloud GA, Higgs J, Friedman BA, Larsen RA, et al. Ann Intern Med 1993; 119: 28–35.

Uncontrolled clinical trial that included 50 patients with coccidioidal meningitis. Forty-seven patients were evaluated. Twenty-five had received no previous treatment, and nine were HIV positive. Thirty-seven of 47 patients (79%) responded to treatment. Response rates were similar in patients who had or had not received previous therapy.

Fluconazole demonstrates efficacy in the treatment of coccidioidal meningitis.

Comparison of oral fluconazole and itraconazole for progressive, nonmeningeal coccidioidomycosis. A randomized, double-blind trial. Galgiani JN, Catanzaro A, Cloud GA, Johnson RH, Williams PL, Mirels LF, et al. Ann Intern Med 2000; 133: 676–86.

In this randomized, double-blind, placebo-controlled trial, 198 patients with pulmonary and nonmeningeal infection were treated with either fluconazole 400 mg daily or itraconazole 200 mg twice daily. Overall efficacy rates at 12 months were similar (itraconazole 63%; fluconazole 50%; $p = 0.8$). However, the response rate was higher in patients with bone disease treated with itraconazole (52% vs. 26%; $p = 0.05$). The rates of relapse were comparable (itraconazole, 18%; fluconazole, 28%; $p > 0.2$). Both drugs were well tolerated.

This is the first prospective, randomized trial comparing two different azole drugs for the treatment of an endemic mycosis. The results demonstrate that both itraconazole and fluconazole are effective therapies for nonmeningeal coccidioidomycosis.

Second-Line Therapies

- Amphotericin B   D
- Ketoconazole   B

Amphotericin B and coccidioidomycosis. Johnson RH, Einstein HE. Ann N Y Acad Sci 2007; 1111: 434–41.

This article provides a comprehensive review of the use of amphotericin B in the treatment of coccidioidomycosis. The availability of effective azoles and triazoles mean that amphotericins are only used now for widely disseminated infection, in cases of azole intolerance, or when there are contraindications to azoles, such as pregnancy.

Given that all studies to date of amphotericin use for coccidioidomycosis are limited by small numbers, this review article provides a detailed assessment of current indications for its use.

Ketoconazole therapy of progressive coccidioidomycosis. Comparison of 400- and 800-mg doses and observations at higher doses. Galgiani JN, Stevens DA, Graybill JR, Dismukes WE, Cloud GA. Am J Med 1988; 84: 603–10.

A randomized clinical trial involving 112 patients with progressive pulmonary, skeletal, or soft tissue infections. Success rate was similar for the two groups (23.2% vs. 32.1% for low- and high-dose therapy). Side effects were significantly higher with high-dose therapy (66% vs. 38%). Relapse rates were higher with high-dose therapy (52% vs. 11%), although it depended also on the organs involved. The study concluded there is little or no benefit with high-dose ketoconazole for nonmeningeal infection.

Third-Line Therapies

- Posaconazole   B
- Voriconazole   C
- Caspofungin   D
- Adjunctive interferon-γ immunotherapy   E

Safety, tolerance, and efficacy of posaconazole therapy in patients with nonmeningeal disseminated or chronic pulmonary coccidioidomycosis. Catanzaro A, Cloud GA, Stevens DA, Levine BE, Williams PL, Johnson RH, et al. Clin Infect Dis 2007; 45: 562–8.

In this multicenter trial, 20 patients with chronic pulmonary or nonmeningeal disseminated coccidioidomycosis were treated with posaconazole 400 mg daily for up to 6 months (median 173 days). Seventeen (85%) patients had a satisfactory response to treatment (≥50% reduction in the Mycoses Study Group score from baseline). No serious adverse effects were reported. Paired baseline and end-of-treatment culture results for *Coccidioides* species were available for four patients, all of whom converted from being positive to being negative for *Coccidioides* species. Relapse was experienced by three of nine patients who did not receive antifungal therapy during the follow-up period.

Posaconazole therapy for chronic refractory coccidioidomycosis. Stevens DA, Rendon A, Gaona-Flores V, Catanzaro A, Anstead GM, Pedicone L, et al. Chest 2007; 132: 952–8.

This was an open-label multinational study, which included 15 patients with pulmonary ($n = 7$) and disseminated ($n = 8$) disease that was refractory to previous therapy, which included amphotericin B with and without an azole. They were treated with posaconazole 800 mg daily in divided doses for 34 to 365 days (median 306 days). Seventy-three percent of patients (11/15) responded to treatment, with cure in four patients. Treatment was very well tolerated.

Treatment of refractory coccidioidomycosis with voriconazole or posaconazole. Kim MM, Vikram HR, Kusne S, Seville MT, Blair JE. Clin Infect Dis 2011; 53: 1060–6.

This was a retrospective study of all cases treated with either voriconazole ($n = 21$) or posaconazole ($n = 16$) in a single center. There was a 67% and 75% improvement after a median duration of 6 and 17 months of treatment with voriconazole and posaconazole, respectively.

The authors concluded that voriconazole and posaconazole are reasonable, but not infallible, options for salvage treatment of refractory coccidioidomycosis.

Use of the echinocandins (caspofungin) in the treatment of disseminated coccidioidomycosis in a renal transplant recipient. Antony S. Clin Infect Dis 2004; 39: 879–80.

Caspofungin monotherapy was successfully used to treat this case of disseminated infection without meningeal involvement.

Treatment of pediatric refractory coccidioidomycosis with combination voriconazole and caspofungin: a retrospective case series. Levy ER, McCarty JM, Shane AL, Weintrub PS. Clin Infect Dis 2013; 56: 1573–8.

A retrospective review of nine pediatric patients treated with combination voriconazole and caspofungin salvage therapy for refractory coccidioidomycosis after failing conventional therapy consisting of a triazole, amphotericin B, or a combination of both. Eight of the nine patients achieved remission.

Two cases illustrating successful adjunctive interferon-γ immunotherapy in refractory disseminated coccidioidomycosis. Duplessis CA, Tilley D, Bavaro M, Hale B, Holland SM. J Infect 2011; 63: 223–8.

The authors report two cases of refractory coccidioidomycosis, which demonstrated improved responses with adjunctive interferon (IFN)-γ.

IFN-γ augments the antifungal activity of effector immune cells against a variety of fungi. Adjunctive immunotherapy given with chemotherapy has the potential to improve host immune responses and facilitate complete eradication of pathogens.

CURRENT GUIDELINES

Coccidioidomycosis. Infectious Diseases Society of America. Galgiani JN, Ampel NM, Blair JE, Catanzaro A, Johnson RH, Stevens DA, et al. Clin Infect Dis 2005; 41: 1217–23.

These guidelines replace the 2005 guidelines and have expanded recommendations for diagnosing and managing early coccidioidal infections, which are the most common clinical presentation, as well as the management of coccidioidal meningitis. Management of coccidioidomycosis in specific at-risk groups such as those with HIV, solid organ transplants, and pregnancy are also specifically addressed. The 2005 guidelines were notable for replacing amphotericin B with fluconazole and itraconazole as first-line therapy for most chronic and disseminated forms of infection. Recommended dosages of these commonly used azoles are fluconazole 400 to 800 mg daily and itraconazole 400 to 600 mg daily.

Evidence Levels: **A** Double-blind study **B** Clinical trial ≥ 20 subjects **C** Clinical trial < 20 subjects **D** Series ≥ 5 subjects **E** Anecdotal case reports

47

Confluent and reticulated papillomatosis

Dina Ismail, Noah Scheinfelt, Ian Coulson

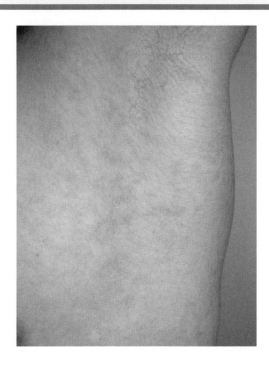

Synonyms: Gougerot-Carteaud syndrome; papillomatose pigmentée innominée; papillomatose pigmentée confluente et reticule; reticulated and confluent papillomatosis of Gougerot and Carteaud

Confluent and reticulated papillomatosis (CARP) is a rare disorder of epidermal keratinization presenting mainly in young adults, with equal sex incidence. A number of etiologic factors have been proposed, including an abnormal host immune response to *Malassezia furfur* colonization. Bacterial colonization may also play a role, although no species has been consistently isolated. Most cases are sporadic, but several familial cases have been reported. The role of metabolic and endocrine abnormalities has also been proposed.

Typically lesions begin as erythematous, hyperkeratotic, flat-topped papules that coalesce to form confluent plaques with a reticular brown pattern peripherally on the chest, trunk, and back simulating tinea versicolor or acanthosis nigricans.

MANAGEMENT STRATEGY

In asymptomatic patients, no treatment is an option. Mild topical steroids can be prescribed to manage any associated pruritus, in addition to soap avoidance and emollients. Spontaneous remissions and exacerbations may be encountered.

Randomized controlled trials for therapies are lacking. Treatment advice stems from retrospective analyses, case series, and reports. Diagnostic criteria have also been proposed.

A wide range of antibiotics and topical agents have been effective; however, recurrence rate is high, and repeat treatment is often needed. Topical and oral antifungals are usually not effective. *Minocycline* is regarded as first-line therapy at a dose of 50 to 200 mg daily for a minimum of 6 weeks. Other macrolide antibiotics found to be effective include *clarithromycin* (500 mg daily for 5 weeks), *azithromycin* (500 mg daily for 1 to 4 weeks), *erythromycin* (1000 mg daily for 6 weeks), and *roxithromycin* (300 mg daily for 8 weeks). Alternative antibiotics include *doxycycline* (200 mg daily for 3 months), *amoxicillin* (250 mg 3 times daily for 3 months), *fusidic acid* (1000 mg daily for 4 weeks), *cefdinir* (300 mg daily for 3 days), and topical *mupirocin* 2% ointment for 1 month.

Topical therapies are also an option, either used as a single agent or adjunct to systemic treatment. Both topical *tazarotene* (0.1%) gel and *tretinoin* of various strengths (0.1%, 0.01%, and 0.25%) for 6 to 8 weeks have been reported as effective in case reports. *Tacrolimus* 0.1% ointment used twice daily for 3 months achieved clinical improvement. Topical vitamin D analogs have also been used.

Oral retinoids at both high and low doses have been reported as effective in case reports but are usually reserved for patients with recalcitrant CARP in view of the associated side effect profile.

Specific Investigations

- Mycology
- Biopsy
- None required

CARP is a clinical diagnosis that should be suspected in young patients with classical findings and absence of fungal hyphae on potassium hydroxide preparation (KOH) to rule out tinea versicolor. If clinical features remain unclear, a biopsy can be taken to identify the histologic features suggestive of CARP. These include focal parakeratosis, acanthosis, papillomatosis, and superficial perivascular lymphocytic infiltrate.

First-Line Treatments

Minocycline	C
Do nothing	E

Confluent and reticulated papillomatosis: response to minocycline. Montemarano AD, Hengge M, Sau P, Welch M. J Am Acad Dermatol 1996; 34: 253–6.

An uncontrolled study of nine patients diagnosed with CARP receiving minocycline 50 mg twice a day for 6 weeks. All patients except two had a 90% to 100% response to therapy over an average follow-up period of 11 months. Recurrence was noted in three patients, all of whom responded to retreatment with minocycline.

Confluent and reticulate papillomatosis (Gougerot-Carteaud syndrome): a minocycline-responsive dermatosis without evidence for yeast in pathogenesis. A study of 39 patients and a proposal of diagnostic criteria. Davis MD, Weenig RH, Camilleri MJ. Br J Dermatol 2006; 154: 287–93.

A retrospective review of 39 CARP cases. Minocycline was prescribed for 22 patients. The majority received 100 mg twice daily for 1 to 3 months. Complete clearing of skin eruption was achieved in 14 of 18 (78%), and 4 (22%) showed a partial response. Recurrence occurred in six cases after stopping treatment, mean time 8 months. The authors also propose a useful diagnostic criterion for CARP, which includes excellent response to minocycline.

Clinicopathological and diagnostic characterisation of Confluent and Reticulate Papillomatosis of Gougerot and Carteaud: a retrospective study in a South-East Asian population. Huang W, Ong G, Chong WS. Am J Clin Dermatol 2015; 16: 131–6.

A retrospective review of 29 patients who failed antifungal treatment for CARP. Good or complete clearance was achieved in 100% (11) of patients on minocycline. Three patients had received doxycycline and achieved clearance. Four patients experienced recurrence (mean time 19.4 months), which was cleared with repeat treatment. Patients treated with topical antifungals, retinoids, and salicylic acid failed to respond.

A clinical analysis of 20 patients with confluent and reticulate papillomatosis. Zeng YP, Ma DL, Qu T, Liu YH, Jin HZ, Sun QN, et al. J Clin Dermatol 2011; 40: 206–9.

Minocycline was prescribed for 10 patients, 8 (80%) of whom had complete clearing of the skin eruption (2 cases relapsed after stopping the drug) and 2 (20%) had no response.

Confluent and reticulated papillomatosis: successful treatment with minocycline. Fung MA, Frieden IJ, LeBoit PE, Berger TG, Epstein E, Kay D, et al. Arch Dermatol 1996; 132: 1400–1.

Eight patients treated with minocycline. Seven achieved complete clearance, and one improved. Three patients developed recurrence.

Several other case series from around the world indicate a high initial response rate to minocycline.

Chronology of confluent and reticulated papillomatosis: spontaneous regression in a case after long-term follow-up may imply transient nature of the condition. Sakiyama T, Amagi M, Ohyama M. J Dermatol 2015; 42: 335–6.

A 50-year-old male patient with IgA nephropathy failed topical ketoconazole and refused oral medications. The cutaneous manifestation repeated a cycle of improvement and exacerbation for about 2 years and 3 months and then finally started to improve.

Second-Line Treatments	
• Azithromycin	E
• Doxycycline	E
• Clarithromycin	E
• Erythromycin	E
• Roxithromycin	E
• Oral fusidic acid	E
• Cefdinir	E
• Amoxicillin	E
• Topical retinoids	E
• Topical tacrolimus	E
• Vitamin D analogs	E
• Topical mupirocin	E

For patients in whom minocycline is contraindicated or show no response, other macrolide antibiotics have been used with success. Topical therapies are also an option used as a single agent or adjunct to oral treatments.

Confluent and reticulate papillomatosis: successful treatment with azithromycin. Raja Babu KK, Snehal S, Sudha Vani D. Br J Dermatol 2000; 142: 1252–3.

Seventeen-year-old male patient initially treated with a course of topical antifungal treatment (1% clotrimazole) and keratolytic with no improvement. Azithromycin 500 mg daily for 7 days was initiated. Total regression was noted within 4 weeks. Recurrence after 5 months successfully treated in 3 weeks with a repeat course. No further recurrence noted at 3 months.

Treatment of confluent and reticulated papillomatosis with azithromycin. Gruber F, Zamolo G, Saftic M, Peharda V, Kastelan M. Clin Exp Dermatol 1998; 23: 191.

Eighteen-year-old patient treated with azithromycin 500 mg daily for 7 days. Complete clearance achieved by 4 weeks with no recurrence. A 15-year-old girl initially treated with clotrimazole 1% cream for 2 weeks without improvement. The patient was then given azithromycin 500 mg daily for 1 week, which cleared the eruption.

Several other single-case reports confirm the efficacy of azithromycin 500 mg daily for 7 days as the usual regimen.

Confluent and reticulated papillomatosis accompanied by obesity: three cases. Demirseren DD, Emre S, Akoğlu G, Kılınç F, Yavuz SO, Metin A. 2014. Turk J Dermatol 2014; 3: 166–9.

Three obese female patients in their 20s were treated with doxycycline 100 mg day for 2 months. Two patients developed recurrence.

Confluent and reticulated papillomatosis (Gougerot-Carteaud syndrome) in 2 brothers. Acikgoz G, Huseynov S, Ozmen I, Ozturk Meral A, Gamsizkan M, Caliskan E. Acta Dermato Venerologica Croatica 2014; 22: 57–9.

Two brothers treated with doxycycline 100 mg/day and topical tretinoin cream. After 3 months a marked improvement was noted.

Updated diagnostic criteria for confluent and reticulated papillomatosis: a case report. Jo S, Park HS, Cho S, Yoon HY. Ann Dermatol 2014; 26: 409–10.

A patient was treated with doxycycline 100 mg twice per day for 2 months with complete resolution. Initially treated with oral itraconazole with no response.

Other similar single reports exist; typically 100 mg daily is exhibited for 2 to 3 months.

Confluent and reticulated papillomatosis (Gougerot-Carteaud syndrome) case successfully treated with oral doxycycline and calcipotriol ointment combination. Acikgoz G, Toklu S, Calickan E, Tunca M, Gamsizkan M. Gazi Med J 2015; 26: 112–4.

A female patient failed treatment with topical antifungals. Instead she was treated with doxycycline 100 mg per day for 2 months and topical calcipotriol 0.005% ointment. She required retreatment for 2 months with complete resolution and no recurrence at 6-month follow-up.

Six cases of confluent and reticulated papillomatosis alleviated by various antibiotics. Jang HS, Oh CK, Cha JH, Cho SH, Kwon KS. J Am Acad Dermatol 2001; 44: 652–5.

CARP lesions cleared in 1 patient treated with oral minocycline 100 mg daily for 8 weeks. The eruption recurred after 8 months but cleared with a repeat course. Two patients were treated with oral fusidic acid 1000 mg daily for 4 weeks. Despite clearing the eruption, one patient relapsed after 2 years and required a repeat course. Cutaneous lesions cleared in a 14-year-old girl with clarithromycin 500 mg daily for 5 weeks. In another, clearance was achieved with oral erythromycin 1000 mg daily for 6 weeks. Azithromycin 500 mg daily 3 times per week for 3 weeks treated a CARP eruption of 5 years' duration in a 24-year-old man.

A case of confluent and reticulated papillomatosis that successfully responded to roxithromycin. Ito S, Hatamochi A, Yamazakis S. J Dermatol 2006; 33: 71–2.

A 28-year-old Japanese man was started on oral minocycline 200 mg daily with no improvement after 3 months. The antibiotic was changed to oral roxithromycin 300 mg daily. The eruption almost completely disappeared after 8 weeks of treatment.

Two cases of confluent and reticulate papillomatosis: successful treatments of 1 case with cefdinir and another with minocycline. Yamamoto A, Okubo Y, Oshima H, Oh-i T, Koga M. J Dermatol 2000; 27: 598–603.

Twenty-four-year-old male patient treated with 300 mg per day of cefdinir for 3 days with improvement. Repeat course of cefdinir needed due to recurrence. Eruption cleared after 2 weeks with no reemergence at 16 months.

Confluent and reticulated papillomatosis successfully treated with amoxicillin. Davis RF, Harman KE. Br J Dermatol 2007; 156: 583–4.

A pregnant female patient treated with amoxicillin 250 mg three times per day for a respiratory infection and incidentally noticed improvement of CARP. Eruption recurrence at 3 months was treated with further 1-month course of amoxicillin with complete clearance at 3 weeks.

Response of confluent and reticulate papillomatosis of Gougerot and Carteaud to topical tretinoin. Schwartzberg JB, Schwartzberg HA. Cutis 2000; 66: 291–3.

Three patients treated successfully with topical retinoids. Two brothers were treated with tretinoin 0.025% gel once daily with marked improvement or clearance at 7 to 8 weeks. Topical tretinoin 0.01% gel once daily was used by the third patient. There was a marked improvement after 6 weeks and complete resolution in 10 weeks.

Confluent and reticulated papillomatosis: response to tazarotene. Bowman PH, Davis LS. J Am Acad Dermatol 2003; 48: S80–1.

Treatment with 0.1% tazarotene gel was initiated twice daily. A noticeable decrease in pigmentation and plaques occurred in 1 week, and within 2 months the eruption had completely resolved. There was no recurrence at 9 months.

Confluent and reticulated papillomatosis (Gougerot-Carteaud): report of a case successfully treated with tazarotene. Gallo L, Ayala F, Lembo S, Mansueto G. G Ital Dermatol Venereol 2006; 141: 529–32.

Eleven-year-old girl was treated with tazarotene 0.05% gel twice daily, and within 2 months the lesions had completely regressed.

Tacrolimus in confluent and reticulated papillomatosis of Gougerot Carteaud. Tirado-Sanchez A, Ponce-Olivera RM. Int J Dermatol 2013; 52: 513–4.

Eighteen-year-old female patient developed CARP recurrence after completion of minocycline treatment. She was retreated with tacrolimus 0.1% ointment for 3 months twice per day

with good response and control of recurrence 2 months after withdrawal.

Confluent and reticulated papillomatosis: treatment with topical calcipotriol. Gulec AT, Seckin D. Br J Dermatol 1999; 14: 1150–1.

A 34-year-old female patient treated with topical calcipotriol ointment (50 mcg/g) twice daily at a dose of less than 100 g per week. Complete response noted in 4 weeks and no recurrence at 11-month follow-up.

Confluent and reticulated papillomatosis: response to topical calcipotriol. Kürkçüoğlu N, Çelebi CR. Dermatology 1995; 191: 341–2.

Twenty-five-year-old patient started on calcipotriol ointment 50 mcg/g twice daily. Clearance of lesions noted after 1 month of treatment.

Confluent and reticulated papillomatosis (Gougerot-Carteaud) successfully treated with topical tacalcitol. Ginarte M, Fabeiro JM, Toribio J. J Dermatolog Treat 2002; 13: 27–30.

Fourteen-year-old patient with CARP and *Malassezia furfur* infection eliminated with antifungal, but skin eruption remained. She was treated with topical tacalcitol twice daily for 6 weeks without relapse after 8 months, follow-up.

Calcipotriol treatment of confluent and reticulated papillomatosis (Gougerot-Carteaud syndrome). Carrozzo AM, Gatti S, Ferranti G, Primavera G, Vidolin AP, Nini G. J Eur Acad Dermatol Venereol 2000; 14: 131–3.

Topical calcipotriol 0.005% ointment was used twice per day for 3 weeks with marked improvement.

Two different therapeutic choices in confluent and reticulated papillomatosis. Patrone P, Trotter D, Stinco G. G Ital Dermatol Venereol 2004; 139: 499–503.

Remission achieved with calcipotriol ointment 0.005% applied twice daily for a period of 3 months. No known recurrence occurred in either.

Successful treatment of confluent and reticulated papillomatosis with topical mupirocin. Gonul M, Cakmak SK, Soylu S, Kilic A, Gul U, Ergul G. J Eur Acad Dermatol Venereol 2008; 22: 1140–2.

Nineteen-year-old patient treated with mupirocin 2% ointment for 1 month with improvement in CARP lesions.

Gougerot-Carteaud syndrome treated with 13-cis-retinoic acid. Carlin N, Marcus LS, Carlin R. J Clin Aesthet Dermatol 2010; 3: 56–7.

Case report of patient treated with daily isotretinoin 1 mg/kg for 20 weeks with excellent response after CARP recurrence after minocycline treatment.

Confluent and reticulated papillomatosis: favourable response to low-dose isotretinoin. Erkek, E, Ayva S, Atasoy P, Emeksiz MC. J Eur Acad Dermatol Venereol 2009; 23: 1342–3.

Forty-eight-year-old female patient treated with isotretinoin 20 mg (0.25 mg/kg) on alternate days. Favorable response was witnessed within 4 weeks, and treatment was terminated at the eighth week when the patient was virtually free of cutaneous lesions. The patient also experienced alleviation of pruritus.

Confluent and reticulated papillomatosis: response to high dose oral isotretinoin therapy and reassessment of

epidemiologic data. Lee MP, Stiller MJ, McClain SA, Shupack JL, Cohen DE. J Am Acad Dermatol 1991; 31: 327–31.

Confluent and reticulated papillomatosis: response to isotretinoin. Hodge JA, Ray MC. J Am Acad Dermatol 1991; 24: 654.

Two patients with confluent and reticulated papillomatosis: response to oral isotretinoin and 10% lactic acid lotion. Solomon BA, Laude TA. J Am Acad Dermatol 1996; 35: 645–6.

These are single reports of oral isotretinoin used at 0.5 to 1 mg/kg/day for up to 4 months with remission in most.

Confluent and reticulated papillomatosis. Treatment with etretinate. Baalbaki SA, Malak JA, al-Khars MA. Arch Dermatol 1993; 129: 961–3.

Reported response of CARP to etretinate (0.25–0.4 mg/kg per day for 1 month) in five adult men who had been previously treated with ketoconazole without success.

Evidence Levels: **A** Double-blind study **B** Clinical trial ≥ 20 subjects **C** Clinical trial < 20 subjects **D** Series ≥ 5 subjects **E** Anecdotal case reports

Cryopyrin-associated periodic syndromes (CAPS)

Alexander Marsland

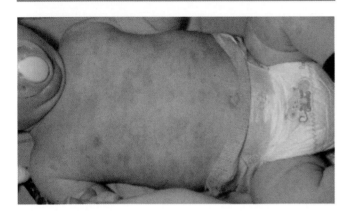

Cryopyrin-associated periodic syndrome (CAPS) is a rare genetic condition characterized by urticarial rashes, fever, fatigue, articular involvement, and inflammation, which, if left untreated, may result in the long term in irreversible end organ damage. It encompasses a spectrum of conditions previously thought to be separate entities before inflammasome genetics were better understood at a molecular level. These conditions are familial cold autoinflammatory syndrome (FCAS), Muckle–Wells syndrome (MWS), and chronic infantile neurological cutaneous and articular syndrome (CINCA), and their overlaps (FCAS-MWS and MWS-CINCA).

CAPS is caused by gain-of-function mutations in *NLRP3*, leading to a persistently active inflammatory state. This leads to rashes, conjunctivitis, and articular involvement that are typically triggered by cold exposure. Patients who have more severe involvement may also have sensorineural hearing loss, visual loss, chronic meningitis, and amyloidosis. Treatment of CAPS aims to suppress this inflammatory state, thus reducing symptoms, improving functionality, and preventing end organ damage.

MANAGEMENT STRATEGY

Early diagnosis and aggressive treatment of CAPS are essential in suppressing inflammatory symptoms and preventing end organ damage. Early CAPS-specific symptoms may be reversible if treatment is commenced expediently. Some manifestations of severe disease such as bone deformities and bony overgrowth may be irreversible.

Symptoms may be present from birth or, in milder forms, may not become apparent until childhood or even early adulthood. Diagnosis is complicated by the fact that, even if molecular genetic analysis of *NLRP3* is available, gain-of-function mutations cannot always be demonstrated; thus expert referral may be indicated to confirm diagnosis on clinical grounds. A model proposed for the diagnosis of CAPS includes one mandatory criterion (raised C-reactive protein [CRP] or

serum amyloid A [SAA]) plus at least two of six CAPS-typical symptoms (urticarial rash, cold/stress-triggered episodes, sensorineural hearing loss, musculoskeletal symptoms, chronic aseptic meningitis, and skeletal signs such as frontal bossing or epiphyseal overgrowth).

CAPS is best managed by a multidisciplinary team in a tertiary center with expertise in autoinflammatory disease (AID), where there is access to genetic counseling and psychosocial support. Patients should also have appropriate access to adjunct therapies such as hearing aids, orthotic aids, and physiotherapy. The mainstay of medical management is with drugs that block interleukin 1 (IL-1). Once a diagnosis has been made, it is important to commence this treatment as soon as possible to prevent complications. During symptomatic flares, short courses of nonsteroidal antiinflammatory drugs (NSAIDs) or oral corticosteroids may be used as adjunct therapy. During flares/inflammatory episodes in patients whose symptoms are normally controlled, infections and other causes of inflammation unrelated directly to CAPS itself must also be considered.

Three IL-1 blockers are currently used to treat CAPS: anakinra, canakinumab, and rilonacept. All are administered as subcutaneous injections. Anakinra is a recombinant IL-1 receptor antagonist that is usually given daily; canakinumab is a human monoclonal antibody targeted at IL-1 beta that has a much longer half-life and is usually given every 8 weeks; and rilonacept, usually administered weekly, is a fusion protein consisting of the binding domains of IL-1 receptor and its accessory protein linked to the Fc portion of human IgG1. All three drugs currently have U.S. Food and Drug Administration (FDA) approval for use in CAPS, whereas European Medicines Agency (EMA) approval only currently exists (January 2017) for anakinra and canakinumab.

Side effects associated with IL-1 blockers include injection-site reactions and an increased propensity to infections such as upper and lower respiratory tract infections, gastroenteritis, sinusitis, and ear infections. Headaches and arthralgia, both symptoms of severe CAPS, may also be side effects associated with IL-1 blockers. Vaccinations with killed vaccines are recommended, as with other biologics, due to the immunosuppressive action of IL-1 blockers.

Anakinra is given at a starting dose of 100 mg daily (adults) or 0.5 to 2 mg/kg/day (children). Some patients require higher doses, however: adults may need treatment during flares of 100 mg twice daily, and doses as high as 8 mg/kg/day have been reported to be required in some children.

Canakinumab is started at 150 mg every 8 weeks (adults) or 2 mg/kg every 8 weeks (children), but some patients require dose escalation to 600 mg every 8 weeks (adults) or up to 8 mg/kg every 8 weeks (children).

Rilonacept has been used at 160 mg weekly or 2.2 mg/kg in adults and children with MWS and FCAS. It is FDA approved for patients with MWS and FCAS 12 years and older. The marketing authorization holder voluntarily withdrew the European marketing authorization in 2012, citing commercial reasons.

Specific Investigations

- CRP and SAA to demonstrate raised inflammatory state in diagnosis and monitor treatment efficacy
- Genetic testing for *NRLP3* mutations to confirm diagnosis (although mutations may not be apparent in some patients due to mosaicism)

Monitoring

- Full general physical examination, including ophthalmologic examination
- Audiologic testing
- Urinalysis for protein

- Growth monitoring in children
- Laboratory evidence of inflammatory activity with CRP and SAA
- Quality of life using a validated tool such as Dermatology Life Quality Index (DLQI) or Children's Dermatology Life Quality Index (CDLQI)
- Disease activity using a validated tool such as MWS-DAS or AIDAI
- End organ damage using scoring system such as autoinflammatory disease damage index (ADDI)

In patients with severe disease consider

- Cognitive testing
- Radiologic imaging of brain, inner ear, and bones
- Lumbar puncture for investigation of aseptic meningitis

First-Line Therapies

• Anakinra	B
• Canakinumab	A
• Rilonacept	A

Recommendations for the management of autoinflammatory diseases. ter Haar NM, Oswald M, Jeyaratnam J, Anton J, Barron KS, Brogan PA, et al. Ann Rheum Dis 2015; 74: 1636–44.

Guidelines for treatment of autoinflammatory diseases, including CAPS, developed by an international consensus committee after a systematic literature review.

Efficacy and safety of anakinra therapy in pediatric and adult patients with the autoinflammatory Muckle-Wells syndrome. Kuemmerle-Deschner JB, Tyrrell PN, Koetter I, Wittkowski H, Bialkowski A, Tzaribachev N, et al. Arthritis Rheum 2011; 63: 840–9.

Observational study of 12 patients (5 children and 7 adults) with severe MWS showed excellent responses in all patients within 2 weeks, with sustained improvement over the observational period of 5 to 14 months (median 11 months). Improvement in hearing loss was seen in two patients.

Sustained response and prevention of damage progression in patients with neonatal-onset multisystem inflammatory disease treated with anakinra: a cohort study to determine 3- and 5-year outcomes. Sibley CH, Plass N, Snow J, Wiggs EA, Brewer CC, King KA, et al. Arthritis Rheum 2012; 64: 2375–86.

Observational study of 26 patients (adults and children) with CINCA receiving anakinra over 3 to 5 years. Dose escalation was described in some patients. Damage progression in eye, ear, and CNS was prevented, but bony lesions progressed.

Long-term safety profile of anakinra in patients with severe cryopyrin-associated periodic syndromes. Kullenberg T, Löfqvist M, Leinonen M, Goldbach-Mansky R, Olivecrona H. Rheumatology (Oxford, England) 2016; 55: 1499–1506.

Prospective open-label study of 43 patients with severe CAPS treated for up to 5 years, in which 14 patients experienced 24 serious adverse events, such as pneumonia and gastroenteritis, all of which resolved during the study period and did not result

in discontinuation of the drug. Continued anakinra treatment during infective episodes did not appear to complicate their course and prevented complications of CAPS.

Anakinra use during pregnancy in patients with cryopyrin-associated periodic syndromes (CAPS). Chang Z, Spong CY, Jesus AA, Davis MA, Plass N, Stone DL, et al. Arthritis Rheumatol 2014; 66: 3227–32.

Observational study of nine women who had 1 to 4 pregnancies (total 24) while on anakinra for all forms of CAPS. There were no serious complications of pregnancy or preterm births reported. A twin pregnancy in which dose escalation occurred resulted in the demise of one twin (who carried the CAPS mutation) due to renal agenesis.

Use of canakinumab in the cryopyrin-associated periodic syndrome. Lachmann HJ, Kone-Paut I, Kuemmerle-Deschner JB, Leslie KS, Hachulla E, Quartier P, et al. N Engl J Med 2009; 360: 2416–25.

Randomized, double-blind, placebo-controlled withdrawal study after an open run-in period demonstrated 34 of 35 patients aged 4 to 75 years with CAPS associated with an *NLRP3* mutation had complete response to treatment. Disease flares occurred in 13 of 16 patients receiving placebo, whereas all 15 patients who received canakinumab remained in remission during the withdrawal phase of the study.

Real-life effectiveness of canakinumab in cryopyrin-associated periodic syndrome. Kuemmerle-Deschner JB, Hofer F, Endres T, Kortus-Goetze B, Blank N, Weissbarth-Riedel E, et al. Rheumatology (Oxford) 2016; 55: 689–96.

Observational study of 68 patients (27 children, 41 adults) with all types of CAPS who had received canakinumab with a median follow-up of 28 months. Seventy-two percent of patients achieved complete remission, and 53% achieved this with a standard dose alone. Overall, updosing was more frequent in children and a complete response more frequent in less severely affected patients.

Efficacy and safety of rilonacept (interleukin-1 Trap) in patients with cryopyrin-associated periodic syndromes: results from two sequential placebo-controlled studies. Hoffman HM, Throne ML, Amar NJ, Sebai M, Kivitz AJ, Kavanaugh A, et al. Arthritis Rheum 2008; 58: 2443–52.

Forty-seven patients with *NLRP3* mutations and symptoms of CAPS underwent a 6-week trial of weekly 160-mg rilonacept injections versus placebo in a randomized double-blinded trial. A second study followed, which consisted of 9 weeks of single-blind treatment. Eighty-seven percent of patients who received rilonacept achieved at least 50% reduction in key symptom score versus 8% who received placebo.

Long-term efficacy and safety profile of rilonacept in the treatment of cryopyrin-associated periodic syndromes: results of a 72-week open-label extension study. Hoffman HM, Throne ML, Amar NJ, Cartwright RC, Kivitz AJ, Soo Y, et al. Clin Ther 2012; 34: 2091–103.

A total of 101 patients were studied, including 44 of the 47 patients who were involved in the phase III studies described earlier. All had *NLRP3* gene mutations. The improvements seen after 6 weeks of treatment with rilonacept were shown to be present in the observation period of up to 96 weeks after treatment, with persistence of normalization of biomarkers seen for up to 48 weeks after treatment.

Evidence Levels: A Double-blind study B Clinical trial ≥ 20 subjects C Clinical trial < 20 subjects D Series ≥ 5 subjects E Anecdotal case reports

SECOND-LINE THERAPY

Some patients show symptomatic improvement with nonsteroidal antiinflammatory drugs (NSAIDs) and oral corticosteroids as adjunct therapy (in association with IL-1 blockers described earlier). Monotherapy with NSAIDs and oral corticosteroids was used before the advent of IL-1 blockers with limited success; due to the potential disease-modifying ability of IL-1 blockers and the lack of evidence for corticosteroids/NSAIDs (and long-term side effect profile of corticosteroids), this is not recommended.

Second-Line Therapies	
• NSAIDs	D
• Oral corticosteroids	D

Treatment of autoinflammatory diseases: results from the Eurofever Registry and a literature review. Ter Haar N, Lachmann H, Özen S, Woo P, Uziel Y, Modesto C, et al. Ann Rheum Dis 2013; 72: 678–85.

Analysis of 94 patients with CAPS on the Eurofever Registry found that NSAIDs and corticosteroids were beneficial in 19/24 and 25/36 patients already receiving IL-1 blockers. Four patients receiving NSAIDs alone showed partial response, and one was reported to have complete response. One patient had partial response to corticosteroids alone. Two patients had partial response to NSAIDs and corticosteroids.

Cryptococcosis

Wanda Sonia Robles, Mahreen Ameen

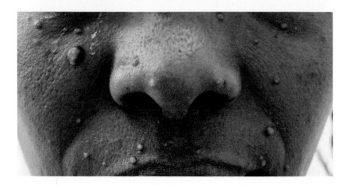

Cryptococcosis is a systemic mycosis acquired by the respiratory route with the primary focus of infection in the lungs. It is caused by yeasts associated with avian feces of which there are two species: *Cryptococcus neoformans* and *C. gattii*. *C. neoformans* occurs worldwide, and *C. gattii* is restricted mainly to subtropical regions and usually affects immunocompetent hosts. Pulmonary infection is often asymptomatic and self-limiting. Hematogenous dissemination typically involves the central nervous system (CNS), causing meningitis. Dissemination to the skin occurs in 10% to 15% of cases and produces a variety of lesions, including flesh-colored or erythematous papules and nodules. In the immunocompromised individual, molluscum contagiosum–like and acneiform lesions occur, particularly affecting the face. Cryptococcal cellulitis with necrotizing vasculitis can mimic bacterial cellulitis and occurs more commonly in the immunocompromised patient.

With the global emergence of AIDS, the incidence of cryptococcosis is increasing, and it represents the most common invasive mycosis in advanced HIV infection. With HIV coinfection, the disease is characteristically widespread, affecting the lungs, meninges, skin, bone marrow, and genitourinary tract, including the prostate. In the era of highly active antiretroviral therapy (HAART), the overall survival after cryptococcosis has dramatically improved: immune restoration and low serum cryptococcal antigen titers are associated with lower cryptococcosis relapse rates. However, a subset of HIV-infected individuals commenced on HAART is at risk of immune reconstitution inflammatory syndrome (IRIS)–associated cryptococcosis that can be severe. Other immunosuppressed patients also at risk of cryptococcosis include solid organ transplant recipients, those with hematologic malignancies, and those on long-term immunosuppressive therapy, including corticosteroids and anti–tumor necrosis factor-α therapies. There are also increased reports of infections associated with biologic therapies.

MANAGEMENT STRATEGY

Cryptococcal infection left untreated is fatal. Treatment depends on disease extent and predisposing factors, particularly AIDS or any other immunosuppressive state. The recommended treatment in the immunocompetent individual with symptomatic nonmeningeal infection is fluconazole 200 to 400 mg daily for

3 to 6 months. An alternative is itraconazole 200 to 400 mg daily for 6 to 12 months. More severe nonmeningeal infection is treated with amphotericin B (AmB) 0.5 to 1.0 mg/kg daily for 6 to 10 weeks. Meningeal infection in the immunocompetent or non-HIV immunocompromised is treated with AmB 0.7 to 1.0 mg/kg daily plus 5-flucytosine 100 mg/kg daily for 2 weeks followed by fluconazole 400 mg daily for a minimum of 10 weeks (up to 6 to 12 months depending on the clinical status of the patient).

Cryptococcal disease with HIV always requires treatment. For nondisseminated infection, fluconazole (200–400 mg daily) is given or itraconazole (200–400 mg daily) as an alternative. More severe infection is treated with a combination of fluconazole (400 mg daily) and flucytosine (100–150 mg daily) for 10 weeks followed by fluconazole maintenance therapy (200 mg daily). Cryptococcal meningitis with HIV is treated with AmB (0.7–1.0 mg/kg daily) and flucytosine (100 mg/kg daily) for a 2- to 10-week induction period followed by fluconazole maintenance therapy, or alternatively with fluconazole (400–800 mg daily) and flucytosine (100–150 mg/kg daily) for 6 weeks. The lipid formulation of AmB can be used instead in those with impaired renal function. There is now trial data suggesting that it is safe to discontinue maintenance therapy in patients treated for cryptococcal meningitis receiving HAART, provided the CD4 count increases to an excess of 100 cells/μL.

The extended-spectrum azoles (posaconazole and voriconazole) may have a role in salvage situations. The echinocandins have no in vivo activity against *Cryptococcus* species.

Dexamethasone as adjunctive therapy did not reduce mortality in HIV-associated cryptococcal meningitis.

Specific Investigations

- Direct microscopy
- Culture
- Cryptococcal antigen test (by latex agglutination or enzyme-linked immunosorbent assay [ELISA])
- Histology (Mayer mucicarmine and Masson–Fontana silver stains used to identify *C. neoformans*)
- Pulmonary and brain imaging studies
- Serology for HIV

India ink examination of cerebrospinal fluid (CSF), pus, skin scrapings, and other fluids may demonstrate the yeast. Culture of skin, CSF, blood, sputum, urine, or bone marrow enables confirmation. The cryptococcal antigen test (on CSF, blood, and urine) is sensitive and specific, and it can be used after therapy response. In tissue specimens, *C. neoformans* is difficult to visualize with routine hematoxylin and eosin stains, requiring the use of special stains.

Cryptococcal disease and HIV infection. Waters L, Nelson M. Expert Opin Pharmacother 2005; 6: 2633–44.

This article reviews the epidemiology, clinical features, and management of cryptococcal disease in HIV-infected patients. It focuses particularly on current guidelines and future developments in antifungal therapy.

Adjunctive dexamethasone in HIV-associated cryptococcal meningitis. Beardsley J, Wolbers M, Kibengo FM, Ggayi AB, Kamali A, Cuc NT, et al. N Engl J Med 2016; 374: 542–54.

A double-blind, randomized, placebo-controlled trial. This trial was stopped for safety reasons and after enrollment of 451 patients. Mortality was reported as 47% in the dexamethasone group and 41% in the placebo group by 10 weeks. The study

Evidence Levels: **A** Double-blind study   **B** Clinical trial ≥ 20 subjects   **C** Clinical trial < 20 subjects   **D** Series ≥ 5 subjects   **E** Anecdotal case reports

concluded that dexamethasone did not reduce mortality among patients with HIV-associated cryptococcal meningitis. It was indeed associated with more adverse events and disability was than placebo.

First-Line Therapies	
● Amphotericin	B
● Amphotericin B plus flucytosine	B
● Fluconazole	B

Treatment of cryptococcosis in the setting of HIV coinfection. Khawcharoenporn T, Apisarnthanarak A, Mundy LM. Expert Rev Anti Infect Ther 2007; 5: 1019–30.

This review discusses evidence-based treatment algorithms that exist for the use of antifungal drugs, as well as the importance of maintaining normal intracranial pressure in HIV-infected hosts with cryptococcal meningitis. The suggest that further studies are required for the management of refractory infection, cryptococcosis-related immune reconstitution syndrome, and the role of adjuvant therapies. Primary and secondary prevention strategies remain at the crux of global control strategies for cryptococcal disease.

Epidemiology and management of cryptococcal meningitis: developments and challenges. Pukkila-Worley R, Mylonakis E. Expert Opin Pharmacother 2008; 9: 551–60.

This article examines developments in the management of cryptococcal meningitis, including new antifungal agents and new strategies for controlling elevated intracranial pressure.

Cryptococcosis in human immunodeficiency virus-negative patients in the era of effective azole therapy. Pappas PG, Perfect JR, Cloud GA, Larsen RA, Pankey GA, Lancaster DJ, et al. Clin Infect Dis 2001; 33: 690–9.

A multicenter case study of HIV-negative patients with cryptococcosis from 1990 to 1996. Of 306 patients, there were 109 with pulmonary involvement and 157 with CNS involvement. Patients with pulmonary disease were usually treated with fluconazole (63%), and patients with CNS disease usually received AmB (92%). Two thirds of these patients also received fluconazole for consolidation therapy. Therapy was reported as successful in 74% of patients. The mortality attributable to cryptococcosis was 12%.

Clinical and epidemiological features of 123 cases of cryptococcosis in Mato Grosso do Sul, Brazil. Lindenberg Ade S, Chang MR, Paniago AM, Lazéra Mdos S, Moncada PM, Bonfim GF, et al. Rev Inst Med Trop Sao Paulo 2008; 50: 75–8.

In this study, 84.5% (104/123) of patients had HIV infection, 4.9% (6/123) had other predisposing conditions, and 10.6% (13/123) were immunocompetent. There was CNS involvement in 83.7% (103/123); 89.6% were infected with *C. neoformans* and 10.4% with *C. gattii*. For treatment AmB was the drug of choice in 86% (106/123), followed by fluconazole in 60% (57/123).

This cohort of patients typifies features of this infection found in other study cohorts.

Combination antifungal therapies for HIV-associated cryptococcal meningitis: a randomised trial. Brouwer AE, Rajanuwong A, Chierakul W, Griffin GE, Larsen RA, White NJ, et al. Lancet 2004; 363: 1764–7.

This controlled trial assessed the fungicidal activity of combinations of AmB, flucytosine, and fluconazole for the treatment of cryptococcal meningitis. Sixty-four patients with a first episode of HIV-associated cryptococcal meningitis were randomized to initial treatment with AmB (0.7 mg/kg daily); AmB plus flucytosine (100 mg/kg daily); AmB plus fluconazole (400 mg daily); or triple therapy with AmB, flucytosine, and fluconazole. Results demonstrated that clearance of cryptococci from the CSF was exponential and significantly faster with AmB and flucytosine dual therapy than with any other drug combination.

Primary cutaneous cryptococcosis in Brazil: report of 11 cases in immunocompetent and immunosuppressed patients. Marques SA, Bastazini Jr I, Martins AL, Barreto JA, Barbieri D'Elia MP, Lastória JC, et al. Int J Dermatol 2012; 51: 780–4.

Eleven cases confirmed by culture had atypical clinical features with infiltrative and tumoral lesions. All cases responded to fluconazole 400 mg daily.

Primary cutaneous infection is very rare and is often, but not always, associated with underlying immunosuppression.

Cutaneous cryptococcosis in solid organ transplant recipients. Sun HY, Alexander BD, Lortholary O, Dromer F, Forrest GN, Lyon GM, et al. Med Mycol 2010; 48: 785–91.

Fluconazole and lipid formulations of AmB were used to treat localized and disseminated disease, respectively. The outcomes in both groups were comparable.

This study described cutaneous cryptococcosis representing disseminated infection in transplant recipients with preferential involvement of the extremities.

Successful use of amphotericin B lipid complex in the treatment of cryptococcosis. Baddour LM, Perfect JR, Ostrosky-Zeichner L. Clin Infect Dis 2005; 40: S409–13.

The efficacy and renal safety of AmB lipid complex (ABLC) were assessed in 106 patients, 83 (78%) of whom had CNS infection. Twenty-seven received concomitant azole therapy. Sixty-six percent of evaluable patients (67/101) achieved clinical response (cured or improved). Response rates with and without CNS infection were 65% (51/78) and 70% (16/23), respectively, and for patients with HIV infection it was 58% (30/52). A mean serum creatinine level decrease of 0.02 mg/dL occurred. ABLC was an effective treatment for cryptococcal infection in immunocompromised patients.

High-dose amphotericin B with flucytosine for the treatment of cryptococcal meningitis in HIV-infected patients: a randomized trial. Bicanic T, Wood R, Meintjes G, Rebe K, Brouwer A, Loyse A, et al. Clin Infect Dis 2008; 47: 123–30.

In this study from South Africa, 64 HIV-seropositive, antiretroviral therapy–naive patients with a first episode of cryptococcal meningitis were randomized to receive either AmB 0.7 mg/kg/day plus flucytosine 25 mg/kg four times daily (*n* = 30) or AmB 1 mg/kg daily plus flucytosine 25 mg/kg four times daily (*n* = 34). Both regimens were given for 2 weeks followed by oral fluconazole. The primary outcome measure was early fungicidal activity determined by CSF cryptococcal cultures. Early fungicidal activity was significantly greater for the first regimen. The 10-week mortality rate was 24%, with no difference between groups.

Second-Line Therapies	
● Itraconazole	B
● Flucytosine plus fluconazole	C
● Voriconazole	B

The efficacy of fluconazole 600 mg/day versus itraconazole 600 mg/day as consolidation therapy of cryptococcal meningitis in AIDS patients. Mootsikapun P, Chetchotisakd P, Anunnatsiri S, Choksawadphinyo K. J Med Assoc Thai 2003; 86: 293–8.

In this trial, HIV-infected patients with primary cryptococcal meningitis who had been treated with AmB for 2 weeks were randomized to receive either fluconazole 600 mg daily or itraconazole 600 mg daily for 10 weeks. The results demonstrated equal efficacy of both of these regimens. In addition, the results suggested that the higher-dose regimens may be superior to treatment regimens using lower doses of these medications.

Voriconazole treatment for less-common, emerging, or refractory fungal infections. Perfect JR, Marr KA, Walsh TJ, Greenberg RN, DuPont B, de la Torre-Cisneros J, et al. Clin Infect Dis 2003; 36: 1122–31.

A multicenter, controlled clinical trial to assess the efficacy, tolerability, and safety of voriconazole as salvage treatment for patients with refractory and intolerant-to-treatment fungal infections, as well as primary treatment for patients with infections for which there is no approved treatment. The efficacy rate for voriconazole in the treatment of cryptococcosis was 38.9%. Voriconazole was reported to be well tolerated, and discontinuation of treatment was observed in less than 10% of patients.

Third-Line Therapies

Recombinant interferon-gamma 1b as adjunctive therapy for AIDS-related acute cryptococcal meningitis. Pappas PG, Bustamante B, Ticona E, Hamill RJ, Johnson PC, Reboli A, et al. J Infect Dis 2004; 189: 2185–91.

This was a phase II, double-blind, placebo-controlled study to evaluate the safety and antifungal activity of adjuvant recombinant interferon (rIFN)-gamma 1b in patients with AIDS and acute cryptococcal meningitis. Patients received 100 or 200 µg of rIFN-gamma 1b or placebo thrice weekly for 10 weeks, plus standard therapy with AmB, with or without flucytosine, followed by fluconazole. Among 75 patients, 2-week culture conversion occurred in 13% of placebo recipients, 36% of rIFN-gamma 1b (100 µg) recipients, and 32% of rIFN-gamma 1b (200 µg) recipients. There was improved combined mycologic and clinical success in rIFN-gamma 1b recipients (26% vs. 8%; $p = 0.078$), and therapy was well tolerated.

This study suggests a role for adjuvant therapies.

GUIDELINES

Clinical practice guidelines for the management of cryptococcal disease: 2010 update by the Infectious Diseases Society of America. Perfect JR, Dismukes WE, Dromer F, Goldman DL, Graybill JR, Hamill RJ, et al. Clin Infect Dis 2010; 50: 291–322.

These updated guidelines emphasize that control of host immunity, the site of infection, antifungal drug toxicity, and underlying disease are still the most critical factors for the successful management of cryptococcosis. The management strategy for cryptococcal disease is organized under four major headings with additional subdivisions: treatment of meningoencephalitis (in HIV-infected individuals, transplant recipients, and others); treatment of non-meningeal cryptococcosis (pulmonary and extrapulmonary sites); complications during treatment (including IRIS and relapse); and cryptococcosis in special clinical situations (pregnancy, children, resource-limited regions, and *C. gattii* infections).

The recommended treatment for immunosuppressed and immunocompetent patients with mild to moderate nonmeningeal cryptococcosis is fluconazole 400 mg daily for 6 to 12 months. The treatment of choice for patients with HIV infection and cryptococcal meningitis is induction therapy with parenteral AmB 0.7 to 1.0 mg/kg daily plus oral flucytosine 100 mg/kg daily for 2 weeks, followed by fluconazole 400 mg daily for a minimum period of 8 weeks. Amphotericin B in lipid formulations can be used for patients with renal impairment. It is recommended that all HIV-infected individuals receive prophylaxis against cryptococcosis and that this be continued for life. Fluconazole 200 mg daily is given or itraconazole 200 mg twice daily in those unable to tolerate fluconazole.

50

Cutaneous candidiasis and chronic mucocutaneous candidiasis

Caroline Halverstam, Steven R. Cohen

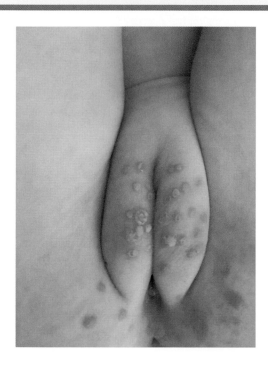

CUTANEOUS CANDIDIASIS

Cutaneous candidiasis is typically caused by *Candida albicans*, which exists as normal flora of human skin as well as in the gastrointestinal and genitourinary systems. Overgrowth of *Candida* species is suppressed by normal bacterial flora. Other *Candida* species occasionally cause mucocutaneous infections, the second most common being *Candida tropicalis*. Under certain conditions, these *Candida* species overgrow and become pathogens. Warmth and moisture of the intertriginous skin (axilla, inguinal folds, abdominal creases, inframammary creases), an increased skin pH, and the administration of antibiotics can disrupt the normal bacterial flora, allowing *Candida* to proliferate. Clinically, candidiasis presents as scaly erythematous patches with satellite papules and pustules. The diagnosis is made either microscopically, with a potassium hydroxide (KOH) preparation revealing spores and pseudohyphae, or by culture.

MANAGEMENT STRATEGY

Topical antifungal agents include, but are not limited to, polyenes, azoles, allylamines, and ciclopirox olamines. Most studies

required therapy twice daily for 4 weeks to ensure complete clearance in all patients. Notably, microscopic cure was often present before complete clinical clearance.

Topical corticosteroids are a source of controversy. Although the addition of corticosteroids to local antifungal therapy may reduce local inflammation in acute candidiasis, their use should be limited to 1 or 2 days because of their immunosuppressant properties.

Systemic therapy may be appropriate for cutaneous infections in immunosuppressed patients, in the setting of extensive disease not responding to topical therapy, or in patients noncompliant with topical therapy. Fluconazole 150 mg weekly appears to be as efficacious as fluconazole 50 mg daily. As in topical therapy, microscopic cure often precedes complete clinical clearance. Since 2013, the Food and Drug Administration (FDA) has removed the indication for oral ketoconazole to be used in *Candida* and dermatophyte infections due to the risk of severe hepatotoxicity and adrenal insufficiency.

Specific Investigations
• KOH
• Culture

First-Line Therapies	
• Topical antifungal	A
• Topical antifungal combined with topical corticosteroids	A

The efficacy and safety of sertaconazole cream in diaper dermatitis. Bonifaz A, Tiredo-Sanchez A, Graniel MJ, Mena C, Valencia A, Ponce-Olivera RM. Mycopathologia 2013; 175: 249–54.

Twenty-seven patients with a clinical and mycologic diagnosis of candida diaper dermatitis were treated twice daily for 2 weeks with sertaconazole. Eighty-nine percent of patients showed a clinical and mycologic cure by the end of 4 weeks (2 weeks after treatment ended).

A multicenter, open-label study to assess the safety and efficacy of ciclopirox topical suspension 0.77% in the treatment of diaper dermatitis due to *Candida albicans*. Gallup E, Plott T. J Drugs Dermatol 2005; 4: 29–34.

A multicenter, open-label study that included 44 male and female subjects aged 6 to 29 months with diaper dermatitis due to *C. albicans*. The study medication was applied topically to the affected area twice daily for 1 week. The results showed a statistically significant improvement in both the rate of mycologic cure and the reduction of severity score.

Topical treatment of dermatophytosis and cutaneous candidiasis with flutrimazole 1% cream: double-blind randomized comparative trial with ketoconazole 2% cream. Del Palacio A, Cuetara S, Perez A, Garau M, Calvo T, Sánchez-Alor G. Mycoses 1999; 42: 649–55.

A double-blind, randomized study in which the efficacy and tolerance of flutrimazole 1% cream was compared with ketoconazole 2% cream, applied once daily for 4 weeks, in 60 patients with culture-proven dermatophytosis (47 patients) or cutaneous candidiasis (13 patients). The results of this study showed that flutrimazole 1% cream is as safe and effective as ketoconazole 2% cream for *Candida* and dermatophyte skin infections.

Naftifine cream in the treatment of cutaneous candidiasis. Zaias N, Astorga E, Cordero CN, Day RM, de Espinoza ZD, DeGryse R, et al. Cutis 1988; 42: 238–40.

In a double-blind, parallel-group clinical trial, 60 patients with cutaneous candidiasis were randomly assigned to receive naftifine cream 1% or its vehicle twice a day for 3 weeks. Two weeks after the end of therapy, 77% of the naftifine-treated patients were mycologically cured (negative results on KOH preparations and culture) and had no clinically apparent disease, compared with only 3% of patients treated with vehicle alone.

A comparison of nystatin cream with nystatin/triamcinolone acetonide combination cream in the treatment of candidal inflammation of the flexures. Beveridge GW, Fairburn E, Finn OA, Scott OL, Stewart TW, Summerly R. Curr Med Res Opin 1977; 4: 584–7.

In a multicenter, double-blind trial, 31 patients with bilateral candidal lesions of the flexures were treated for 14 days with nystatin cream on one side and with a combination of nystatin and triamcinolone acetonide cream on the other side. Both treatments proved equally effective in terms of mycologic cure rate and clinical improvement. There was a weak trend by both patients and physicians to favor the combination preparation because symptoms resolved more rapidly.

Second-Line Therapy	
• Systemic azoles	B

Prospective aetiological study of diaper dermatitis in the elderly. Foureur N, Vanzo B, Meaume S, Senet P. Br J Dermatol 2006; 155: 941–6.

Of 46 patients, all over 85 years of age with dermatitis of the diaper area, 24 were identified as candidiasis. Of these, 8 (33%) were cured after 1 month of topical bifonazole therapy, 3 (12.5%) improved, and 13 (54%) were cured after the addition of oral fluconazole 100 mg once daily for 1 month. Although topical antifungal drugs represent the first line of treatment for diaper dermatitis in the elderly, more than half the patients in this study required an oral antifungal to achieve a complete cure.

A comparison of the efficacy of oral fluconazole, 150 mg/week versus 50 mg/day, in the treatment of tinea corporis, tinea cruris, tinea pedis, and cutaneous candidosis. Nozickova M, Koudelkova V, Kulikova Z, Malina L, Urbanowski S, Silny W. Int J Dermatol 1998; 37: 703–5.

Patients received either fluconazole 150 mg/week or 50 mg/day until clinically cured or for a maximum of 4 weeks. Of the patients in this study with candidiasis, 10 of 11 patients receiving fluconazole 150 mg weekly had a positive response (microscopic cure with marked clinical improvement) and 12 of 13 taking fluconazole 50 mg daily had a positive response. Thus weekly treatment was determined to be equivalent to daily dosing.

Clinical trials and double-blind studies of oral antifungals for cutaneous candidiasis are sparse.

Third-Line Therapies	
• Lavender oil	E
• Topical mupirocin	C

Antifungal activity of *Lavandula angustifolia* essential oil against *Candida albicans* yeast and mycelial form. D'Auria FD, Tecca M, Strippoli V, Salvatore G, Battinelli L, Mazzanti G. Med Mycol 2005; 43: 391–6.

The antifungal activity of the essential oil of *Lavandula angustifolia* (lavender oil) and its main components, linalool and linalyl acetate, was studied. Lavender oil showed both fungistatic and fungicidal activity against *C. albicans* strains.

Perianal candidosis: a comparative study with mupirocin and nystatin. De Wet PM, Rode H, Van Dyk A, Millar AJ. Int J Dermatol 1999; 38: 618–22.

This clinical trial compared the efficacy and clinical outcome of 2% mupirocin in a polyethylene glycol base and nystatin cream for the treatment of diaper candidiasis. Eradication of all *Candida* organisms was achieved within 2 to 6 days (mean 2.6 days) in 10 patients receiving topical mupirocin therapy (three to four times daily or with each diaper change). The 10 patients who received topical nystatin cream successfully cleared within 5 days (mean 2.8 days). Although both agents eradicated *Candida*, a major difference was the marked response of the diaper dermatitis to mupirocin, presumably due to its well-documented bacteriocidal effects. The authors conclude that mupirocin is an excellent antifungal agent and a superior therapy for diaper dermatitis because of its polymicrobial toxicity.

CHRONIC MUCOCUTANEOUS CANDIDIASIS

Chronic mucocutaneous candidiasis (CMC) is a heterogeneous group of disorders with progressive and recurrent infections of the skin, nails, and mucosal surfaces caused by *C. albicans*. The clinical presentation in patients with CMC can range from recurrent or recalcitrant thrush with a mild rash and dystrophic nails to severe, generalized, crusted plaques. Affected individuals have a defect in T-cell–mediated immunity; specifically, Th17 cells have been implicated. CMC typically presents in childhood. Half of those affected are identified as having autoimmune polyendocrinopathy candidiasis and ectodermal dystrophy (APECED). APECED is caused by mutations in the *AIRE* gene, which plays a key role in immunotolerance. It is characterized by hypoparathyroidism, hypothyroidism, and adrenal or gonadal failure. *Candida* susceptibility in APECED is attributed to autoantibodies directed against IL-17 and IL-22. Malabsorption, gastric cell atrophy, or autoimmune hepatitis occurs in about a third of patients. Alopecia, vitiligo, dental enamel dysplasia, and keratitis are frequent associations.

Other subtypes of CMC include autosomal-dominant CMC with or without thyroid disease and autosomal-recessive, isolated CMC. Recently, mutations in the *STAT1* gene were found to underlie autosomal-dominant CMC and lead to defective Th1 and Th17 responses. Thymoma has been also associated with rare cases of IL-17 and IL-22 autoantibody-positive CMC.

MANAGEMENT STRATEGY

Once the etiology of the symptoms is confirmed with a positive culture for *C. albicans*, a workup should be done to test for immunodeficiency. Patients should also be tested for endocrine dysfunction characteristic of APECED. If clinical suspicion for APECED is high, genetic analysis for the *AIRE* gene can be performed. An association of CMC with abnormalities in iron metabolism or thymoma has also been reported in adult patients,

Evidence Levels: **A** Double-blind study   **B** Clinical trial ≥ 20 subjects   **C** Clinical trial < 20 subjects   **D** Series ≥ 5 subjects   **E** Anecdotal case reports

so iron and radiologic studies may be warranted in HIV-negative patients with adult-onset CMC.

Treatment usually begins with an oral azole, most commonly fluconazole 100 to 200 mg/day. Intermittent use is often advocated to prevent resistance. However, resistance in CMC patients to first-line drugs is frequent, and alternative options include second-generation azoles such as voriconazole and posaconazole, as well as echinocandins such as caspofungin and micafungin. Ketoconazole should be avoided because of the risk of hepatotoxicity and adrenal insufficiency. Amphotericin B can be administered orally with variable response but minimal side effects. Due to toxicity, intravenous amphotericin B should generally be limited to short treatment courses with a transition to alternative therapies. Relapse after withdrawal of these agents is the rule because the inherent immune defect remains. Therapeutic strategies that augment the immune response can be very beneficial, including transfer factor (orally or parenterally) or high-dose cimetidine.

Special Investigations

- Complete blood count with differential
- HIV antibody test
- Thyroid-stimulating hormone
- Fasting blood glucose
- Plasma cortisol level
- Parathyroid hormone
- Serum calcium
- Serum iron and ferritin
- Chest x-ray or computed tomography (CT) scan if thymoma suspected
- Genetic testing for *AIRE* gene if suspicious for APECED

Chronic mucocutaneous candidiasis in APECED or thymoma patients correlates with autoimmunity to Th17-associated cytokines. Kisand K, Boe Wolff AS, Podkrajsek KT, Tserel L, Link M, Kisand KV, et al. J Exp Med 2010; 207: 299–308.

Patients with APECED were found to have severely reduced IL-17F and IL-22 responses to *C. albicans* antigens.

STAT1 mutations in autosomal dominant chronic mucocutaneous candidiasis. van der Veerdonk FL, Plantinga TS, Hoischen A, Smeekens SP, Joosten LA, Gilissen C, et al. N Engl J Med 2011; 365: 54–61.

DNA sequencing identified missense mutations in *STAT1*.

First-Line Therapy

Systemic azole antimycotics	C

Fluconazole in the management of patients with chronic mucocutaneous candidiasis. Hay RJ, Clayton YM. Br J Dermatol 1988; 119: 683–4.

Eight patients with CMC (five idiopathic cases, three APECED cases) and oral candidiasis were treated with 50 mg of fluconazole daily for up to 4 weeks. Clinical and mycologic remissions were achieved in all patients after a mean of 10 days. Three patients relapsed within 4 months (mean 56 days), but all responded to fluconazole 50 mg daily for 3 days. The authors suggest intermittent oral antifungal therapy as the most appropriate method to manage patients with oral candidiasis in CMC after induction of remission.

Itraconazole in the treatment of two young brothers with chronic mucocutaneous candidiasis. Tosti A, Piraccini BM, Vincenzi C. Pediatr Dermatol 1997; 14: 146–8.

Two children with CMC involving the mouth and nails were successfully treated with itraconazole 200 mg/day for 2 months. A rapid cure rate of both infections was observed. No relapses of oral or nail candidiasis were identified at a follow-up examination more than a year later. The drug was very well tolerated.

Voriconazole: a broad spectrum triazole for the treatment of serious and invasive fungal infections. Maschmeyer G, Haas A. Future Microbiol 2006; 1: 365–85.

This is an excellent review of voriconazole (a second-generation triazole) for treating life-threatening fungal infections. Voriconazole can be given intravenously (6 mg/kg every 12 hours for two doses and then 4 mg/kg every 12 hours for maintenance dosing) or orally (200 mg every 12 hours for individuals over 40 kg and 100 mg every 12 hours for individuals less than 40 kg). It is effective for fluconazole-susceptible and fluconazole-resistant candidiasis.

Although transient visual disturbances, liver enzyme abnormalities, skin cancers, and skin rashes are reported, these rarely lead to discontinuation of treatment.

Successful treatment of chronic mucocutaneous candidiasis caused by azole-resistant *Candida albicans* with posaconazole. Firinu D, Massidda O, Lorrai MM, Serusi L, Peralta M, Barca MP, et al. Clin Dev Immunol 2011: 4. Article ID 283239.

A 39-year-old female patient with familial CMC who developed candidiasis that was resistant to multiple antifungal drugs was successfully treated with amphotericin B. She was treated with amphotericin B 50 mg/day intravenously for 2 weeks followed by posaconazole 400 mg twice daily. After 2 months the dose was reduced to 200 mg/day without a relapse in symptoms. When posaconazole was discontinued, a relapse of oral candidiasis occurred after 2 weeks. She was thereafter maintained successfully on cycles of posaconazole 200 mg, three times per day, for a month with a 15-day discontinuation.

Second-Line Therapies

Echinocandins	E
Oral amphotericin B	E
Intravenous amphotericin B	D

Activity of amphotericin B, anidulafungin, caspofungin, micafungin, posaconazole, and voriconazole against *Candida albicans* with decreased susceptibility to fluconazole from APECED patients on long-term azole treatment of chronic mucocutaneous candidiasis. Rautemaa R, Richardson M, Pfaller MA, Perheentupa J, Saxen H. Diagn Microbiol Infect Dis 2008; 62: 182–5.

Forty-three isolates of *C. albicans* were taken from 23 patients with APECED and tested for resistance to various antifungals. Isolates were divided into two groups: fluconazole-susceptible dose-dependent and fluconazole-susceptible groups. All isolates were highly susceptible to amphotericin B and echinocandins. Posaconazole and voriconazole were active against all isolates, but more active in the fluconazole-susceptible group, suggesting a possibility that patients may develop some cross-resistance to these drugs when they take fluconazole.

Successful treatment of azole-resistant chronic mucocutaneous candidiasis with caspofungin. Jayasinghe M, Schmidt S, Walker B, Rocken M, Schaller M. Acta Derm Venereol 2006; 86: 563–4.

An 18-year-old woman with CMC developed severe symptoms from an azole-resistant strain of *C. albicans* after 3 years of treatment with fluconazole. After a 70-mg loading dose of intravenous caspofungin on the first day, the regimen was adjusted to 50-mg infusions four to seven times per week for almost 12 months. Clinical improvement of oral and cutaneous candidiasis was sustained during a follow-up period of 12 months. The treatment was well tolerated; the only side effect was a temporary elevation of hepatic enzyme levels that did not necessitate discontinuation of therapy.

Prolonged oral treatment of chronic mucocutaneous candidiasis with amphotericin B. Montes LF, Cooper MD, Bradford LG, Lauderdale RO, Taylor CD. Arch Dermatol 1971; 104: 45–56.

Amphotericin B was given orally to four patients with CMC in doses of 1000 to 1800 mg/day. One patient had complete clearance of extensive candidal granulomas after 6 months of treatment; one patient had a slower but excellent response. Two other patients had minimal or no response; of these, one was hypothyroid and the other had a thymoma. Of note, the serum levels were significantly higher in the first two patients than in the latter two. In all four patients the oral amphotericin B was free of side effects both clinically and in laboratory studies.

Chronic mucocutaneous candidiasis treated with amphotericin B. Case report. Waweru HW, Owili DM. East Afr Med J 1983; 60: 588–91.

A 5-year-old girl with CMC was treated with intravenous amphotericin B at a dose of 1 mg/kg every other day for a cumulative dose of 200 mg. The crusts and plaques completely cleared, but with residual atrophy, hypopigmentation, and scarring alopecia. She remained free of recurrence for 2 years.

Third-Line Therapies	
• Transfer factor	C
• Cimetidine and zinc sulfate	E

Case report: successful treatment with cimetidine and zinc sulphate in chronic mucocutaneous candidiasis. Polizzi B, Origgi L, Zuccaro G, Matti P, Scorza R. Am J Med Sci 1996; 311: 189–90.

The clinical efficacy of high-dose cimetidine, 400 mg, three times daily, and zinc sulfate, 200 mg daily (subsequently adjusted to maintain blood zinc levels at the upper normal range), was evaluated in a patient with CMC for 16 months. An impressive reduction in infectious events was correlated with an increased CD4 (helper/inducer) cell count.

Transfer factor in chronic mucocutaneous candidiasis. Masi M, De Vinci C, Baricrdi OR. Biotherapy 1996; 9: 97–103.

Fifteen patients with CMC were treated with an in vitro–produced transfer factor (TF) specific for *C. albicans* antigens and/or with TF extracted from pooled buffy coats of blood donors: 400 million cell equivalent (CEU) per week for the first 2 weeks, followed by 100 million CEU per week for 6 to 12 months. All but one patient experienced significant improvement during treatment with specific TF.

Evidence Levels: **A** Double-blind study   **B** Clinical trial ≥ 20 subjects   **C** Clinical trial < 20 subjects   **D** Series ≥ 5 subjects   **E** Anecdotal case reports

51

Cutaneous larva migrans

Georgina A. Fremlin, Anthony Abdullah

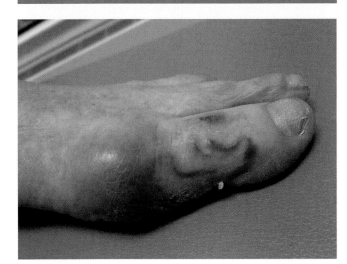

Courtesy of Tamara Lazic, MD.

Hookworm-related cutaneous larva migrans (Hr-CLM) is a disease caused by percutaneous penetration and migration of animal hookworm larvae in the human skin, most commonly *Ancylostoma braziliense, Ancylostoma caninum, Uncinaria stenocephala*, and *Bunostonum phlebotomum*. People at risk are the inhabitants and returning travelers from tropical and subtropical countries and children playing in sandpits. Incubation period can vary between a few days and 7 months after exposure to contaminated soil or sand. The clinical picture is that of characteristic "creeping eruption" with serpiginous, papular, vesiculobullous, and erythematous lesions due to the presence of moving parasites. The common sites involved are the feet, buttocks, and thighs. Rare complications include pulmonary eosinophilic infiltrates, hookworm folliculitis, and oral mucosal lesions.

MANAGEMENT STRATEGY

Hr-CLM is self-limiting: most lesions resolve within 2 to 8 weeks because the human is a "dead-end host." However, the lesions are extremely pruritic, can be extensive, and can significantly reduce the quality of life, so treatment is often required.

The systemic treatment normally used by the authors for patients over the age of 2 years is oral *albendazole* 400 mg daily for 3 days. An alternative is *ivermectin* given as a single dose of 12 mg orally (or 200 µg/kg) for adults and children older than 5 years or more than 15 kg in weight. Topical treatment usually takes the form of *thiabendazole* in a suitable lipophilic vehicle.

SPECIFIC INVESTIGATIONS

Clinical appearance is characteristic. Peripheral eosinophilia and raised serum IgE may be seen.

First-Line Therapies	
• Systemic albendazole	B
• Systemic ivermectin	B

One-week therapy with oral albendazole in hookworm-related cutaneous larva migrans: a retrospective study on 78 patients. Veraldi S, Bottini S, Rizzitelli G, Persico MC. J Dermatolog Treat 2012; 23: 189–91.

Seventy-eight patients with multiple and/or extensive lesions of Hr-CLM were treated with albendazole 400 mg/day for 1 week. Cure rate was 100% at 3 months' follow-up. The disappearance of pruritus was reported after 2 to 3 days and skin lesions after 5 to 7 days of therapy. The authors concluded that this regimen was very effective and had no severe side effects.

Cutaneous larva migrans: clinical features and management of 44 cases presenting in the returning traveler. Blackwell V, Vega-Lopez F. Br J Dermatol 2001; 145: 434–7.

Thirty-one patients received oral albendazole 400 mg daily for 3 to 5 days, and 24 were cured (77%). Five patients received 10% thiabendazole cream topically for 10 days, and 4 were cured (80%). There were no reported side effects. Four patients needed no treatment.

A randomized trial of ivermectin versus albendazole for the treatment of cutaneous larva migrans. Caumes E, Carriere J, Datry A, Gaxotte P, Danis M, Gentilini M. Am J Trop Med Hyg 1993; 49: 641–4.

A comparison of efficacy between oral ivermectin (12 mg) and oral albendazole (400 mg). Twenty-one patients were randomly assigned to receive ivermectin (*n* = 10) or albendazole (*n* = 11). All patients who received ivermectin responded and none relapsed (cure rate 100%). All except one patient in the group receiving albendazole responded, but 5 relapsed after a mean of 11 days (cure rate 46%; *p* = 0.017). No major adverse effects were observed. The authors suggest that a single dose of ivermectin is more effective than a single dose of albendazole.

Hookworm-related cutaneous larva migrans in Northern Brazil: resolution of clinical pathology after a single dose of ivermectin. Schuster A, Lesshafft H, Reichert F, Talhari S, de Oliveira SG, Ignatius R, et al. Clin Infect Dis 2013; 57: 1155–7.

Ninety-two patients, median age 9.5 years, were treated with a single dose of 200 µg/kg ivermectin. All responded clinically. Two weeks after treatment there was a significant reduction in complex tracts, and at 4 weeks all complex tracts had disappeared with marked symptomatic improvement.

The efficacy of single dose ivermectin in the treatment of hookworm related cutaneous larva migrans varies depending on the clinical presentation. Vanhaecke C, Perignon A, Monsel G, Regnier S, Bricaire S, Caumes E. J Eur Acad Dermatol Venereol 2014; 28: 655–7.

Sixty-two travelers with Hr-CLM and creeping dermatitis were treated with a single 200-µg/kg ivermectin dose. Six of these patients had additional hookworm folliculitis. Ivermectin was well tolerated in all patients. Fifty-nine patients (95%) completed responded with one dose. 98% response rate in those with only creeping dermatitis was achieved and 66% (4/6) in the 6 patients presenting with additional hookworm folliculitis (*p* = 0.02). Of the two travelers that failed treatment, 2, 1 responded after a second dose of ivermectin and 1 needed two doses of ivermectin and

5 days of oral albendazole (400 mg BID). The non–hookworm folliculitis cases responded after a second dose of ivermectin.

Treatment of 18 children with scabies or cutaneous larva migrans using ivermectin. Del Mar Saez-De-Ocariz M, McKinster CD, Orozco-Covarrubias L, Tamayo-Sánchez L, Ruiz-Maldonado R. Clin Exp Dermatol 2002; 27: 264–7.

A report of 18 children aged 14 months to 17 years, of whom 7 had Hr-CLM. All 7 were cured with a single dose of 150 to 200 µg/kg ivermectin, with no significant adverse effects. In the authors' experience ivermectin is a safe and effective alternative treatment for cutaneous parasitosis in children.

Second-Line Therapy	
• Topical thiabendazole in a lipophilic vehicle	D

Efficacy and tolerability of thiabendazole in a lipophilic vehicle for cutaneous larva migrans. Chatel G, Scolari C, Gulletta M, Casalini C, Carosi G. Arch Dermatol 2000; 136: 1174–5.

Six patients were treated twice daily for 5 days with topical applications of 15% thiabendazole ointment in a lipophilic vehicle of base fat cream (24 g) and dimethyl sulfoxide gel (35 g). The ointment was prepared by crushing the tablets of thiabendazole in the lipophilic base. All patients experienced a clinical resolution within a median of 48 hours. No adverse effects and no recurrence had occurred in any patient at 3 months' follow-up.

Treatment with topical thiabendazole ointment at 10% to 15% concentration in a hydrophilic vehicle has shown 98% efficacy within a median of 10 days of treatment.

Third-Line Therapies	
• Topical albendazole	E
• Cryotherapy	E

Efficacy of albendazole ointment on cutaneous larva migrans in 2 young children. Caumes E. Clin Infect Dis 2004; 38: 1647–8.

Two 2-year-old patients were treated with a 10% albendazole ointment, prepared by crushing three 400-mg tablets of albendazole in 12 g of petroleum jelly. Treatment was applied three times daily for 10 days. The cutaneous lesions disappeared within a week. One patient had recurrence at 3 months, and the lesion disappeared within a week after repeated treatment. The author suggests that albendazole ointment is a safe and effective treatment for Hr-CLM in children.

A case of cutaneous larva migrans presenting in a pregnant patient. Kudrewicz K, Crittenden KN, Himes A. Dermatol Online J 2014; 20(10): 25526012.

Cryotherapy with liquid nitrogen resulted in complete resolution of her lesion and symptoms. Oral anthelmintic agents are contraindicated in pregnancy.

Evidence Levels: **A** Double-blind study **B** Clinical trial ≥ 20 subjects **C** Clinical trial < 20 subjects **D** Series ≥ 5 subjects **E** Anecdotal case reports

52

Cutaneous polyarteritis nodosa

Cindy E. Owen, Jeffrey P. Callen

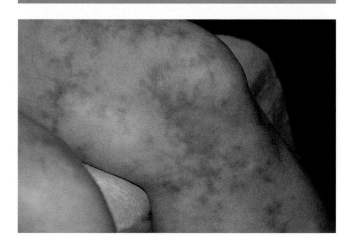

Polyarteritis nodosa (PAN) is a necrotizing vasculitis that involves small or medium-sized arterioles. Classic PAN is characterized by fever, weight loss, cutaneous ulcers, livedo reticularis, myalgias and weakness, arthralgias or arthritis, neuropathy, abdominal pain, ischemic bowel, testicular pain, hypertension, and renal failure. Microscopic polyarteritis (MPA) involves the same-sized vessels as well as smaller vessels and manifests clinically as a glomerulonephritis and a pulmonary capillaritis with alveolar hemorrhage. Patients with MPA may develop small-vessel vasculitis (palpable purpura), livedo reticularis with or without nodules, and/or ulcerations of the skin. Cutaneous PAN (cPAN), sometimes termed *benign cutaneous polyarteritis*, is characterized by livedo reticularis, nodules, and ulceration, usually of the leg; it has been postulated to be a localized necrotizing arteritis that does not affect internal organs and runs a chronic but benign course. Many reports, however, have linked cPAN to inflammatory bowel disease, hairy cell leukemia, streptococcal upper respiratory infection, or hepatitis B or C infection. Occasional reports have linked cPAN to antiphospholipid antibodies, cryoproteins, or antineutrophil cytoplasmic antibodies (pANCA or atypical ANCA more commonly than cANCA). One recent report has demonstrated that interleukin-6 is elevated in roughly 40% of patients. A mutation in the *CERC1* gene leading to deficiency in the ADA2 protein has been identified in some patients with early cPAN and early-onset vasculopathy. Cases of cPAN have occurred in patients treated with propylthiouracil and minocycline. cPAN appears to be more prevalent in children. Although it is generally benign, there have been reports of associated neuropathy, as well as visceral involvement.

MANAGEMENT STRATEGY

cPAN causes pain and discomfort and may ulcerate, thereby causing disability. Therapy may include local measures, for example, *gradient pressure stockings*, or *systemic therapies*, including *systemic corticosteroids, methotrexate, azathioprine, pentoxifylline*, and *intravenous immunoglobulin (IVIG)*. Most of the reports are anecdotes or small case series.

Treatment is often indicated for underlying and associated conditions.

Specific Investigations

- Skin biopsy
- Serology for hepatitis B and C, assessment for tuberculosis, antistreptolysin O antibody titers, antineutrophil cytoplasmic antibodies, antiphospholipid antibodies, and cryoproteins
- Assessment for systemic involvement
- Assessment for inflammatory bowel disease
- Assessment for hairy cell leukemia
- Assessment for drugs that have been linked to cPAN
- In cases with early onset, measurement of ADA2 levels

Cutaneous periarteritis nodosa: a clinicopathological study of 79 cases. Daoud MS, Hutton KP, Gibson LE. Br J Dermatol 1997; 136: 706–13.

This analysis attempted to identify features that may distinguish those cases likely to have a prolonged course. Most patients (60%) had no associated medical condition. The disease course was prolonged but benign, and systemic PAN did not develop in any patient. The ulcerative form of disease was more prolonged and frequently associated with neuropathy. Therapy was varied, and the patients with nonulcerative disease responded better than those with ulcers. Corticosteroids, azathioprine, pentoxifylline, and hydroxychloroquine appeared effective in individual patients.

High titer of phosphatidylserine–prothrombin complex antibodies in patients with cutaneous polyarteritis nodosa. Kawakami T, Yamazaki M, Mizoguchi M, Soma Y. Arthritis Rheum 2007; 57: 1507–13.

Antiphosphatidylserine–prothrombin complex and/or anticardiolipin antibodies were positive in all 16 cPAN patients tested compared with none in the control group.

Epidemiological, clinical and laboratory profiles of cutaneous polyarteritis nodosa patients: report of 22 cases and literature review. Criado PR, Marques GF, Morita TC, Freire de Carvalho J. Autoimmun Rev 2016; 15: 558–63.

cPAN was more prevalent in women (77%) with a mean age at time of diagnosis of 39.4 years (range from 9–61 years). The clinical manifestations in decreasing order of frequency were ulcers, livedo racemose, subcutaneous nodules, atrophie blanche lesions, and purpura. Lower limbs were affected in all cases, but trunk and upper limbs were affected at equal frequency of 27%. No cases of cPAN progressed to systemic PAN. Symptoms reported were pain (64%) and paresthesias (30%). Twenty-three percent were diagnosed with mononeuritis multiplex. The most common infectious agent in this study was *Mycobacterium tuberculosis*.

Tuberculosis testing should be performed in endemic areas in patients with cPAN.

Polyarteritis-like vasculitis in association with minocycline use: a single center case series. Kermani T, Ham E, Camilleri M, Warrington K. Semin Arthritis Rheum 2012; 42: 213–21.

Nine cases occurring in the context of minocycline use. Four had isolated cutaneous disease. All had positive pANCA. Minocycline was discontinued, and six patients required immunosuppressive therapy.

Vasculitic conditions mimicking cPAN have also been reported with isotretinoin and amphetamines.

First-Line Therapies

- Local measures (i.e., support stockings, local wound care)   E
- Nonsteroidal antiinflammatory drugs, penicillin (if antecedent streptococcal infection), systemic corticosteroids   E
- Immunosuppressants: azathioprine, methotrexate, mycophenolate mofetil, mizoribine   E

Low-dose weekly methotrexate for unusual neutrophilic vascular reactions: cutaneous polyarteritis nodosa and Behçet's disease. Jorizzo JL, White WL, Wise CM, Zanolli MD, Sherertz EF. J Am Acad Dermatol 1991; 24: 973–8.

Three patients responded dramatically.

Use of mizoribine in two patients with recalcitrant cutaneous polyarteritis nodosa. Kawakami T, Soma Y. J Am Acad Dermatol 2011; 64: 1213–4.

This antimetabolite/immunosuppressive agent is not available in the United States but has been regularly used in Japan for PAN and cPAN.

Ulcerative cutaneous polyarteritis nodosa treated with mycophenolate mofetil and pentoxifylline. Kluger N, Guillot B, Bessis D. J Dermatolog Treat 2011; 22: 175–7.

This single case report combines a second-line and a third-line therapy.

Second-Line Therapies

- Intravenous immunoglobulin   E
- Pentoxifylline   E

Intravenous immunoglobulins as treatment of severe cutaneous polyarteritis nodosa. Marie I, Miranda S, Girszyn N, Soubrane JC, Vandhuick T, Levesque H. Intern Med J 2012; 42: 459–62.

Three patients with refractory cPAN resulting in painful ulcers involving the lower limbs and causing toe necrosis were treated with IVIG 1 g/kg/day for 2 days monthly. After the second infusion, skin signs dramatically improved and completely healed after the third infusion.

Successful treatment of cutaneous PAN with pentoxifylline. Calderon MJ, Landa N, Aguirre A, Diaz-Perez JL. Br J Dermatol 1993; 12: 706–8.

A patient who failed to respond to aspirin and penicillin was treated with pentoxifylline. Withdrawal of the pentoxifylline resulted in a relapse that again responded to therapy.

Third-Line Therapies

- Tamoxifen   E
- Infliximab   E
- Etanercept   D
- Rituximab   E
- Tonsillectomy   D
- Warfarin   E

Estrogen-sensitive cutaneous polyarteritis nodosa: response to tamoxifen. Cvancara JL, Meffert JJ, Elston DM. J Am Acad Dermatol 1998; 39: 643–6.

Tamoxifen, an antiestrogenic agent, at a dose of 10 to 20 mg daily, led to control of disease in a patient who seemed to worsen with conjugated estrogen therapy. Relapse occurred within 5 days of interruption of the therapy and rapidly responded with reinitiation of the tamoxifen.

Successful response to infliximab in a patient with undifferentiated spondyloarthropathy coexisting with polyarteritis nodosa-like cutaneous vasculitis. Garcia-Porrua C, Gonzalez-Gay MA. Clin Exp Rheumatol 2003; 21: S138.

Remission induced by infliximab in a childhood polyarteritis nodosa refractory to convention immunosuppression and rituximab. Campanilho-Marques R, Ramos F. Joint Bone Spine 2014; 81: 267.

A 13-year-old boy responded to infliximab after failing prednisolone, methotrexate, cyclophosphamide, and rituximab.

Successful treatment of childhood cutaneous polyarteritis nodosa with infliximab. Vega Gutierrez J, Rodriguez Prieto MA, Garcia Ruiz JM. J Eur Acad Dermatol Venereol 2007; 21: 570–1.

A single case responding to infliximab.

A case of refractory cutaneous polyarteritis nodosa in a patient with hepatitis B carrier status successfully treated with tumor necrosis alpha blockade. Zoshima T, Matsumura M, Suzuki Y, Kakuchi Y, Mizushima I, Fujii H, et al. Mod Rheumatol. 2013; 23: 1029–33.

A case successfully treated with etanercept. The authors review five similar cases of response to this drug.

Young male patient diagnosed with cutaneous polyarteritis nodosa successfully treated with etanercept. Valor L, Monteagudo I, de la Torre I, Fernández CG, Montoro M, Longo JL, et al. Mod Rheumatol 2014; 24: 688–9.

A 7-year-old boy responded to etanercept after failing high-dose corticosteroids and cyclophosphamide.

Rituximab in refractory cutaneous polyarteritis. Krishnan S, Bhakuni DS, Kartik S. Int J Rheum Dis 2012; 15: e127.

A 34-year-old woman with cPAN refractory to prednisolone and cyclophosphamide developed digital gangrene of two fingers and was treated with rituximab (two courses) with complete healing of ulcers in 4 weeks. She had no recurrence over 6 months of follow-up on prednisolone and azathioprine.

Cutaneous polyarteritis nodosa: therapy and clinical course in four cases. Misago N, Mochizuki Y, Sekiyama-Kodera H, Shirotani M, Suzuki K, Inokuchi A, et al. J Dermatol 2001; 28: 719–27.

Two cases resolved after tonsillectomy. The authors proposed that chronic streptococcal disease might be responsible for cPAN.

Use of warfarin therapy at a target international normalized ratio of 3.0 for cutaneous polyarteritis nodosa. Kawakami T, Soma Y. J Am Acad Dermatol 2010; 63: 602–6.

Three patients with antiphosphatidylserine–prothrombin complex antibodies resolved on sustained warfarin therapy.

Evidence Levels: **A** Double-blind study   **B** Clinical trial ≥ 20 subjects   **C** Clinical trial < 20 subjects   **D** Series ≥ 5 subjects   **E** Anecdotal case reports

53

Darier disease

Genevieve A. Casey, Susan M. Cooper

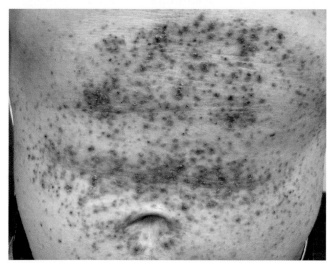

Courtesy of Dr Terence Casey.

Darier disease is a dominantly inherited condition, with an incidence 1:25,000 to 1:100,000, that is characterized by persistent greasy, hyperkeratotic papules. The disease is caused by mutations in the *ATP2A2* gene that encodes sarcoplasmic/endoplasmic reticulum calcium–ATPase type 2 (SERCA2).

MANAGEMENT STRATEGY

The warty, keratotic papules, which usually appear before the age of 20 years, can be malodorous, irritate, and look unsightly. The flexures can be a particular problem, as plaques here are frequently hypertrophic and may smell unpleasant. Initial treatment is aimed at controlling irritation. *Simple emollients, soap substitutes,* and *topical corticosteroid creams* are helpful. Keeping the skin cool by wearing comfortable cotton clothing helps. Sunscreen is recommended for those with a history of photoaggravation.

In mild disease or linear disease reflecting a genetic mosaicism, *topical retinoids* may be sufficient. These include topical isotretinoin (0.05%), tretinoin cream (0.05%), adapalene gel (0.1%), and tazarotene gel (0.1% short contact for 15 minutes). Treatment is applied on alternate days to begin with, increasing to once daily if possible, as irritation is common. The addition of a topical corticosteroid (alternating with the retinoid) may alleviate some of the side effects. Superinfection with viruses and bacteria is frequent, so combined corticosteroid/antibiotic preparations are logical.

In more extensive disease, an *oral retinoid* is required. Acitretin (10–25 mg daily and can be gradually increased), isotretinoin (0.5–1.0 mg/kg daily), and alitretinoin (30 mg daily) are effective. Teratogenicity is a problem, and pregnancy is contraindicated for 2 years after stopping treatment with acitretin and 1 month after isotretinoin or alitretinoin. For this reason, isotretinoin or alitretinoin is preferred in women of childbearing age. Treatment may be given either long term or as intermittent short courses.

The rare vesiculobullous form of the disease may respond to *prednisolone.* Hypertrophic flexural disease unresponsive to retinoids may require a surgical approach with *laser, electrosurgery, debridement, or excision.* Recurrence is a problem.

Oral lithium exacerbates the disease and should be avoided if possible.

Specific Investigations

- Skin biopsy. The characteristic finding is focal, suprabasal, acantholytic dyskeratosis.
- Skin swab/scraping for bacterial, viral, and fungal culture

Darier-White disease: a review of the clinical features in 163 patients. Burge SM, Wilkinson JD. J Am Acad Dermatol 1992; 27: 40–50.

Fourteen percent of patients in this series had herpes simplex complicating their disease.

Painful blisters arising in a patient with Darier disease are usually due to secondary infection with Staphylococcus aureus *or herpes simplex.*

First-Line Therapies

• Cool cotton clothing	E
• Emollients	D
• Topical corticosteroids	D
• Topical retinoids	D

Darier's disease. Cooper SM, Burge SM. Am J Clin Dermatol 2003; 4: 97–105.

A detailed review of the management of Darier disease.

Genetic counseling can be helpful, and written information is often appreciated.

Topical isotretinoin in Darier's disease. Burge SM, Buxton PK. Br J Dermatol 1995; 133: 924–8.

Six of 11 patients improved with 0.05% isotretinoin applied to a test patch. Erythema, burning, and irritation were common.

Successful treatment of Darier's disease with adapalene gel. Abe M, Inoue C, Yokoyama Y, Ishikawa O. Pediatr Dermatol 2011; 28: 197–8.

Adapalene gel 0.1% applied for 2 months to the abdomen of a 12-year-old boy resulted in dramatic improvement.

Second-Line Therapies

• Oral retinoids	B
• Topical 5-fluorouracil 5%	E
• Topical tacrolimus 0.03%, 0.1%	E
• Topical diclofenac sodium 3%	E

Clinical and ultrastructural effects of acitretin in Darier's disease. Lauharanta J, Kanerva L, Turjanmaa K, Geiger JM. Acta Dermatol Venereol 1988; 68: 492–8.

Thirteen patients treated with acitretin starting at 30 mg daily for 16 weeks showed some improvement, but side effects included itching (5 patients) and hair loss (2 patients).

Isotretinoin treatment of Darier's disease. Dicken CH, Bauer EA, Hazen PG, Krueger GG, Marks Jr JG, McGuire JS, et al. J Am Acad Dermatol 1982; 6: 721–6.

This multicenter open study assessed the effect of short and longer courses of treatment. The starting dose was 0.5 mg/kg, but longer courses were adjusted according to symptoms. Isotretinoin was effective but did not give long-term remission. Some patients were maintained on alternate-day or alternate-week regimens.

Successful treatment with oral alitretinoin in women of childbearing potential with Darier's disease. Zamiri M, Munro CS. Br J Dermatol 2013; 169: 709–10.

Two women were treated with 30 mg daily, with improvement after 4 to 6 weeks. Relapse occurred upon stopping, and treatment was continued in one patient for 18 months.

A case of Darier's disease successfully treated with topical tacrolimus. Rubegni P, Poggiali S, Sbano P, Risulo M, Fimiani M. J Eur Acad Dermatol Venereol 2006; 20: 84–7.

Topical tacrolimus 0.1% ointment to the face and neck resulted in complete remission after 6 weeks, with no relapse 1 year later using maintenance therapy of 0.03%.

Improvement of Darier disease with diclofenac sodium 3% gel. Millan-Parrilla F, Rodrigo-Nicolas B, Moles-Poveda P, Armengot-Carbo M, Quecedo-Estebanez E, Gimeno-Carpio E. J Am Acad Dermatol 2014; 70: e89–90.

Third-Line Therapies	
• Cyclosporine	E
• Oral prednisolone (vesiculobullous)	E
• Laser (CO_2, erbium:YAG, pulse-dye)	E
• Photodynamic therapy	D
• Botulinum toxin	E
• Electron beam radiation	E
• Dermabrasion	E
• Debridement	E
• Excision	E

Darier's disease: severe eczematization successfully treated with cyclosporine. Shahidullah H, Humphreys F, Beveridge GW. Br J Dermatol 1994; 131: 713–6.

Cyclosporine may be helpful in widespread eczematized Darier disease but had no effect on the underlying disease.

Vulval Darier's disease treated successfully with cyclosporine. Stewart LC, Yell J. J Obstet Gynaecol 2008; 28: 108–9.

A previously therapy-resistant case was treated with cyclosporine (initial dose 5 mg/kg) for 6 months with good response and was subsequently maintained on acitretin.

Vesiculobullous Darier's disease responsive to oral prednisolone. Speight EL. Br J Dermatol 1998; 139: 934–5.

A patient with the vesiculobullous form of the disease responded to a short course of oral prednisolone.

Prednisolone may also be useful in the eczematized form.

Extensive recalcitrant Darier disease successfully treated with laser ablation. Brown VL, Kelly SE, Burge SM, Walker NPJ. Br J Dermatol 2010; 162: 227–8.

Trunk, limbs and scalp were treated under general anaesthetic every 2 months with CO_2 laser. Wounds healed within 33 weeks, and the patient remained disease free in some areas for 9 years.

Darier-White disease treated with fractional CO_2 laser in two cases. Raszewska-Famielec M, Dudra-Jastrzebska M, Borzecki A, Chodorowska G. Dermatol Ther 2015; 24: 254–57.

Three sessions of fractional CO_2 laser resurfacing with 0.8- to 1-mm density every 6 weeks resulted in removal of papular lesions. Topical anesthetic (5% EMLA) cream was used. Some recurrence was observed after 6 months.

Efficacy of erbium:YAG laser ablation in Darier disease and Hailey-Hailey disease. Beier C, Kaufmann R. Arch Dermatol 1999; 135: 423–7.

Disease cleared in two patients, but follow-up was less than 2 years.

Successful treatment of Darier disease with the flash-lamp-pumped pulse-dye laser. Roos S, Karsai S, Ockenfel HM, Raulin C. Arch Dermatol 2008; 144: 1073–5.

Submammary disease improved at 8 weeks post treatment, with no progression at 15 months.

Treatment of Darier's disease with photodynamic therapy. Exadaktylou D, Kurwa HA, Calonje E, Barlow RJ. Br J Dermatol 2003; 149: 606–10.

Six patients received photodynamic therapy with topical 5-aminolevulinic acid as a photosensitizer. One patient could not tolerate the treatment, but five experienced sustained improvement, with initial inflammatory response lasting 2 to 3 weeks.

Botulinum toxin type A: an alternative symptomatic management of Darier's disease. Kontochristopoulos G, Katsavou AN, Kalogirou O, Agelidis S, Zakopoulou N. Dermatol Surg 2007; 33: 882–3.

Submammary disease was treated with botulinum toxin as adjuvant therapy: 100 U were injected, with improvement sustained for 4 months. Reduced sweating may alleviate maceration and reduce bacterial colonization.

Treatment of recalcitrant Darier's disease with electron beam therapy. Kittridge A, Wahlgren C, Fuhrer R, Zirwas M, Patton T. Dermatol Ther 2010; 23: 302–4.

Electron beam radiation therapy to the inframammary folds resulted in initial severe local dermatitis, followed by complete resolution sustained for 18 months.

The surgical treatment of hypertrophic Darier's disease. Wheeland RG, Gilmore WA. J Dermatol Surg Oncol 1985; 11: 420–3.

Recalcitrant hypertrophic lesions were debrided under local anesthesia. Symptomatic and cosmetic improvement was maintained for 2 years.

54

Decubitus ulcers

*Joseph A. Witkowski,[†] Lawrence Charles Parish,
Ayse Serap Karadag, Jennifer L. Parish*

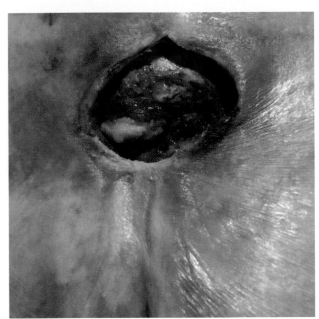

The decubitus ulcer represents a defect in the skin that can extend through the subcutaneous tissue and muscle layer onto the underlying bone.

MANAGEMENT STRATEGY

Prevention

A patient in an ordinary bed who is at risk of developing a decubitus ulcer should be repositioned at frequent intervals; however, the correct timing for turning has never been established. The regularity is determined by the level of risk of developing an ulcer and the duration of blanchable erythema. Pillows and foam wedges are used to maintain position and to keep bony prominences apart. Completely immobile patients should have their heels raised from the bed by a pillow or boot and not be placed on their trochanters, unless a specialized bed is used. To avoid the latter, use a 30-degree position from the horizontal lying on the side. The head of the bed should not be raised more than 30 degrees from the horizontal for an extended period. The concept of repositioning every 2 hours is arbitrary and varies from country to country, even facility to facility.

Where possible, use lifting devices or draw sheets to reposition or to transfer patients. Finally, when appropriate, the patient should be placed on a pressure-reducing device such as a foam, alternating air, gel, or water mattress.

A patient sitting in a wheelchair should be repositioned frequently, perhaps every hour, and be taught to shift weight every

[†] deceased

15 minutes. A pressure-reducing device made of foam, gel, air, or a combination of each is indicated. Unfortunately, even in paraplegics, the exact time interval for repositioning has never been accurately determined.

Theoretically, decubitus ulcers should be preventable, but despite these measures, many simply are not. If they are associated with immobility, sustained pressure, and the loss of pain sensibility, these problems can and should be addressed. In practice, successful prevention is often foiled by our limited understanding of the pathogenesis, as well as by complicating comorbidities. There is also some evidence that many deep ulcers are initiated by multiple microthromboses of deep tissues. This indicates that dehydration, along with any factor that might increase blood coagulability, should be addressed.

Management

The management of skin lesions caused by pressure is based on four principles:

- Elimination of relative/sustained pressure
- Removal of necrotic debris
- Maintenance of a moist wound environment
- Correction of the underlying contributing factors

The patient should not lie on the ulcer. A patient who is at risk for developing additional ulcers and can assume a variety of positions without lying on the ulcer should be placed on a *static support surface (i.e., air, foam, or water)*. If the patient cannot assume various positions without lying on the ulcer or bottoms out while on a static surface, or if the ulcer does not heal after 2 to 4 weeks of optimal care, place the patient on *a dynamic support surface* when possible—that is, *an alternating air overlay on the mattress, a low-air-loss bed, or an air-fluidized bed*. If a patient has large deep ulcers (stage III or IV) on multiple sleep surfaces or has excess moisture on intact skin, use a low-air-loss bed or an air-fluidized bed. A patient with an ulcer on the sitting surface should not sit, if possible.

Removal of Necrotic Debris

Surgical debridement is indicated for infected ulcers with necrotic debris and eschars other than those on the heel; however, the extent of tissue needing to be removed is highly variable. An eschar on the heel should be excised only if it is fluctuant, draining, or surrounded by cellulitis and if the patient is septic.

Major debridement is performed in the operating room, but serial sharp debridement can be performed at the bedside. The use of *systemic antimicrobials* should be considered to prevent bacteremia during significant debridement. A *bone biopsy* is recommended while debriding ulcers when bone is exposed and for nonhealing deep ulcers (stage III or IV) after 2 to 4 weeks of optimal therapy.

Other ulcers can be *debrided by the use of saline wet-to-dry gauze* every 4 to 6 hours, by the use of saline in a 35-mL syringe with an attached 19-gauge angiocatheter, or by whirlpool use. The use of enzymes should be reserved for ulcers that are not clinically infected. *Autolytic debridement* is indicated for noninfected ulcers that are not likely to become infected.

Debridement can also be indicated for staging of the ulcer. This assumes that staging is a requisite for treating the patient.

Maintenance of a Moist Wound Environment

The choice of a synthetic dressing depends on the presence of infection, amount of exudate, status of the periulcer skin, and amount of pain experienced by the patient. *Saline dressings and alginates* are indicated for infected ulcers. *Synthetic dressings (i.e., films)* are used on ulcers with minimal exudate, *hydrocolloid wafers* for moderate exudate, and *foam wafers* and *alginates* for ulcers with a large amount of exudate. Ulcers with fragile or dermatitic periulcer skin should be covered with *hydrogel wafers* or *nonadherent foam wafers*. All occlusive dressings relieve pain, when present, but the hydrogel wafers are best for this purpose.

Correction of the Underlying Contributing Factors

Attention to the medical status is important; diabetes mellitus, nutritional conditions (malnutrition, hypoproteinemia, anemia), peripheral vascular disease, cardiac disease, malignancy, mental health problems, and even Alzheimer disease may prevent any ulcer healing. Unfortunately, even the best medical care may not permit healing.

General Measures

Treatment of the decubitus ulcer can be simplified and made more effective if the following recommendations are considered:

- Saline should be used to clean most pressure lesions; soap and disinfectants are too irritating for more than occasional use. Scrubbing may prove too irritating, so gentle washing is indicated.
- When ulcers are not infected, synthetic dressings should be changed only if they become dislodged or wound fluid escapes from under the dressing.
- Periulcer skin must be kept dry not only to avoid maceration but also to permit the dressing to adhere to the skin.
- To obliterate dead space, *fill deep ulcers loosely with a hydrocolloid, a hydrogel wound filler, or an alginate rope* before applying a synthetic dressing. This same material should be placed under the edge of the ulcer when undermining is present. Bleeding after serial surgical debridement can often be controlled with an alginate dressing. Moistening with saline can loosen an alginate dressing that adheres to granulation tissue.
- A clean ulcer failing to show signs of healing and revealing inflammatory signs of erythema, edema, and warmth; purulent discharge and persistent excessive exudate; discoloring or darkening of granulation tissue, giving off a foul odor; and presenting with heightened local pain should be treated with antibacterial agents, such as *1% silver sulfadiazine, cadexomer iodine, triple antibiotic, or retapamulin*, for 2 weeks to reduce the bacterial burden. However, topical antimicrobials may create the risk of resistant bacterial strains emerging. Metronidazole would be the exception, as the odor of an infected ulcer can often be eliminated by applying *metronidazole gel* to the ulcer bed. Increased bacterial burden may impede healing before clinical signs of infection become apparent. *Systemic antimicrobial agents* are indicated for patients with bacteremia, sepsis, advancing cellulitis, or osteomyelitis.
- Although most synthetic dressings relieve pain, treatment for moderate to severe pain can include *topical anesthetics (lidocaine), nonsteroidal antiinflammatory drugs (NSAIDs), opiates, antidepressants, and sedatives.*

Blanchable Erythema and Nonblanchable Erythema

Blanchable and nonblanchable erythema represent the initial development of the decubitus ulcer. The early lesions of nonblanchable erythema are bright red; later, they become dark red to purple. Both can be treated with *adherent synthetic dressings* to protect the lesion from friction and shear, *topical corticosteroids*, or *zinc oxide paste*. The bright red lesion can also be treated with 2% *nitroglycerin ointment*; 0.5 to 1 cm of the ointment is applied over the lesion and covered with an impermeable plastic wrap (such as Saran Wrap) for 12 hours daily.

Decubitus Dermatitis

Decubitus dermatitis is treated with topical corticosteroids, Vaseline gauze, or a hydrogel wafer. Large bullae may be debrided before applying the dressing.

Superficial and Deep Ulcers

Superficial and deep ulcers without necrotic debris are treated with *saline wet-to-dry gauze* or an *adherent synthetic dressing*. Deep ulcers should be loosely filled with a *synthetic wound filler* before applying a synthetic dressing. The deep ulcer with necrotic debris requires debridement and is then treated as a clean ulcer.

Enzymatic debridement or the use of an *antimetabolite* can help manage the eschar. Covering the lesion with an adhesive occlusive dressing for several days after scarification will often soften the eschar before excision is undertaken. The firmly adherent dry eschar that is not attached to underlying bone can often be separated from the surrounding skin with 5% *5-fluorouracil cream*. After scarification and application of zinc oxide paste to protect the surrounding skin, 5-fluorouracil is applied to the eschar, including its margin, and then covered with an impermeable plastic wrap. Application is repeated every 8 hours. When separation occurs, it can be excised.

Underlying Contributing Factors

Management of anemia, malnutrition, diabetes mellitus, hydration, and incontinence is essential. The patient should be ingesting approximately *30 to 35 calories/kg daily* and *1.25 to 1.50 g protein/kg daily*. *Ascorbic acid* 500 mg twice daily may enhance healing.

Specific Investigations

- Categorize patient
- Stage decubitus ulcer
- Total protein, serum albumin, and daily calorie intake
- Complete blood count
- Care for comorbid disorders

Clinical observation is the key to making the diagnosis. Cutaneous biopsies will not be helpful, although biopsies for aerobic and anaerobic bacteriology cultures could be useful if infection is suspected. Bacterial testing and analysis with thorough swabbing may only provide a portion of the necessary information. In clinical practice, infection, defined as a number of bacteria greater than 10^5 CFU/g of tissue, is of only limited relevance.

Evidence Levels: **A** Double-blind study **B** Clinical trial ≥ 20 subjects **C** Clinical trial < 20 subjects **D** Series ≥ 5 subjects **E** Anecdotal case reports

Categories of Patients

Patients at risk need to be considered in terms of the underlying disease process:

- Spinal cord injury in an otherwise healthy person
- Neurologic disease with no medical disease but a devastating condition, such as multiple sclerosis or a cerebral vascular accident compromising the body integrity
- Debilitation with a multitude of medical diseases affecting the patient (e.g., arteriosclerosis, diabetes mellitus, Parkinson disease, Alzheimer disease, malignancy, malnutrition, and peripheral vascular disease)
- Surgical procedures requiring lengthy positioning on the operating table for cardiovascular or orthopedic procedures

Grading or Evaluation

Grading or evaluation can be accomplished by dermatologic observation and staging. Bear in mind that ulcer staging is arbitrary and does not reflect the dynamics of ulcer formation.

Dermatologic Observation

Observe for:

- Blanchable erythema
- Nonblanchable erythema
- Decubitus dermatitis
- Superficial ulcer
- Deep ulcer
- Eschar
- Necrosis
- Gangrene

Staging

Stages are as follows:

- Stage I: nonblanchable erythema of intact skin
- Stage II: partial-thickness skin loss involving the epidermis and/or dermis
- Stage III: full-thickness skin loss with damage to the subcutaneous tissue that may extend down to, but not through, the underlying fascia
- Stage IV: full-thickness skin loss with extensive destruction, tissue necrosis, or damage to muscle, bone, or supporting structures
- Unstageable: full-thickness tissue loss, base of the ulcer being covered by slough and/or eschar, where the true depth of ulcer cannot be classified

Most superficial ulcers do not progress to stage II and IV ulcers. The concept of staging need not be thought of as a progression.

Accumulating evidence suggests that a number of ulcers (most stage III and IV) may initially originate in the deep tissue compartment and progress outward to the dermis and epidermis (inside-out theory).

Pathophysiology

Pathophysiology of acute wound healing. Li J, Chen J, Kirsner R. Clin Dermatol 2007; 25: 9–18.

Dilemmas about the decubitus ulcer: skin-fold ulcerations and apposition lesions. Parish LC, Lowthian PT. Exp Rev Dermatol 2008; 3: 287–91.

Decubitus ulcers continue to have an uncertain etiology.

Histology

Pressure ulcer tissue histology: an appraisal of current knowledge. Edsberg LE. Ostomy Wound Manage 2007; 53: 40–9.

Risk Assessment Tools

Predictive validity of pressure ulcer risk assessment tools for elderly: a meta-analysis. Park SH, Lee YS, Kwon YM. West J Nurs Res 2016; 38: 459–83.

Typical screening tools (Braden, Norton, and Waterlow scales) utilized for pressure ulcer risk are limited with regard to their validity and accuracy among older adults because of heterogeneity throughout studies.

25 years of pressure ulcers. Parish LC, Sibbald RG. Adv Skin Wound Care 2012; 25: 57–8.

Role of staging may provide more confusion than merit.

Pressure ulcer staging - revisited. Spear M. Plast Surg Nurs 2013; 33: 192–4.

The European Pressure Ulcer Advisory Panel developed a staging system in 1998 that is composed of four stages: Grade 1 to Grade 4. The classification system most popularly adopted and used is the one presented in 1989 by the National Pressure Ulcer Advisory Panel (NPUAP). This classification system has been updated and revised. A new stage, suspected deep tissue injury, was incorporated in 2007.

Factors Predicting Pressure Ulcers

Nutritional parameters predicting pressure ulcers and short-term mortality. Montalcini T, Moraca M, Ferro Y, Romeo S, Serra S, Raso MG, et al. J Transl Med 2015; 13: 305.

Lower hemoglobin and albumin were inversely related to pressure ulcers, where patients with lower albumin showed notably higher short-term mortality than patients with higher serum albumin.

Factors predicting the development of pressure ulcers in an at-risk population who receive standardized preventive care. Demarre L, Verhaeghe S, Van Hecke A, Clays E, Grypdonck M, Beeckman D. J Adv Nurs 2015; 71: 391–403.

Pressure ulcers in category II to IV were significantly related to nonblanchable erythema, urogenital disorders, and higher body temperature. Predictive factors having to do with superficial pressure ulcers were admittance to an internal medicine ward, incontinence-associated dermatitis, nonblanchable erythema, and a lower Braden score. Incontinence-associated dermatitis was greatly related to superficial sacral pressure ulcers.

Risk factors associated with pressure ulcer development in critically ill traumatic spinal cord injury patients. Wilczweski P, Grimm D, Gianakis A, Gill B, Sarver W, McNett M. J Trauma Nurs 2012; 19: 5–10.

Clinical variables associated with pressure ulcers were fecal management systems, incontinence, acidosis, support surfaces, steroids, and additional equipment, with hypotension as the strongest predictor of pressure ulcers in 94 spinal cord injury patients.

Predicting pressure ulcer development in clinical practice: evaluation of Braden scale scores and nutrition parameters. Miller N, Frankenfield D, Lehman E, Maguire M, Schirm V. J Wound Ostomy Continence Nurs 2016; 43: 133–9.

Patients admitted who showed signs of infection, trauma, gastrointestinal, urologic/renal, and neurologic diagnoses were associated with hospital-related pressure ulcer occurrences, whereas cardiovascular, respiratory, and hematology/oncologic diagnoses were not. A higher body mass index (BMI) may protect against the presence of hospital-associated pressure ulcers by cushioning pressure points over the sacrum.

Treatment

Revised National Pressure Ulcer Advisory Panel Pressure Injury Staging System: Revised Pressure Injury Staging System. Edsberg LE, Black JM, Goldberg M, McNichol L, Moore L, Sieggreen M. J Wound Ostomy Continence Nurs 2016; 43: 585–97.

In a consensus conference that involved 24 stakeholder organizations from various disciplines, it was unanimously agreed that pressure ulcers are largely preventable but not always avoidable.

Pressure ulcer treatment strategies: a systematic comparative effectiveness review. Smith ME, Totten A, Hickam DH, Fu R, Wasson N, Rahman B, et al. Ann Intern Med 2013; 159: 39–50.

Moderate-strength evidence shows that the use of air-fluidized beds, protein supplementation, radiant heat dressings, and electrical stimulation improved the healing of pressure ulcers in adults.

First-Line Therapies	
• Elimination of pressure	C
• Pressure-reducing and pressure-relieving devices	C
• Palliative care	B
• Removal of necrotic debris	C
• Maintenance of a moist wound environment	C
• Synthetic dressings	B
• Topical antibacterials	B
• Cleansing	C
• Nutrition	C
• Dietary supplements	C

Eliminating Pressure and Relieving Devices

An Investigation of Geriatric Nursing Problems in Hospital. Norton D, McClaren R, Exton-Smith AN. London: Churchill Livingstone, 1975; 238.

Patients who developed fewer pressure sores were those who were turned every 2 to 3 hours.

This is based on a book published in 1916!

Shearing force as a factor in decubitus ulcers in paraplegics. Reichel SM. JAMA 1958; 166: 762–3.

As a result of shear, blood vessels in the sacral area become twisted and distorted, and the tissue may become ischemic and necrotic.

Drawsheets for prevention of decubitus ulcer. Witkowski JA, Parish LC. N Engl J Med 1981; 305: 1594.

Use of draw sheets reduces the incidence of friction burns.

Prevention of pressure ulcers among people with spinal cord injury: a systematic review. Groah SL, Schladen M, Pineda CG, Hsieh CH. PM&R 2015; 7: 613–36.

The evidence indicates staying away from the 90-degree lateral position due to high pressures and pressure ulcer risk over the trochanters. While sitting, pressures are linearly redistributed from the sitting area during recline and tilt; however, reclining has an increased risk of shear forces on this skin.

A randomized controlled clinical trial of repositioning, using the 30° tilt, for the prevention of pressure ulcers. Moore Z, Cowman S, Conroy RM. J Clin Nurs 2011; 20: 2633–44.

Older adults at risk of pressure ulcers should be repositioned every 3 hours throughout the night. Use of the 30-degree tilt minimizes the occurrence of pressure ulcers compared with usual care.

Repositioning for treating pressure ulcers. Moore ZE, Cowman S. Cochrane Database Syst Rev 2015; 1: CD006898.

Randomized trials that assess the impact of repositioning patients on the healing rates of pressure ulcers currently exist. The limited data derived from one economic evaluation suggest it remains undetermined as to whether repositioning every 3 hours using the 30-degree tilt is less expensive in terms of nursing time and more effective than standard care involving repositioning every 6 hours using a 90-degree tilt.

Palliative Care

Pressure ulceration and palliative care: prevention, treatment, policy and outcomes. Stephen-Haynes J. Int J Palliat Nurs 2012; 18: 9–16.

Nurses working in palliative care need to be aware of pressure ulcer development and to possess knowledge related to preventing and managing pressure ulceration.

How to reduce hospital-acquired pressure ulcers on a neuroscience unit with a skin and wound assessment team. McGuinness J, Persaud-Roberts S, Marra S, Ramos J, Toscano D, Policastro L, et al. Surg Neurol Int 2012; 3: 138.

Several changes were implemented in order to reduce hospital-acquired pressure ulcers; turning patients every 1 to 2 hours, repositioning, specialty beds, and skin and wound teams that consisted of one or two expert nursing assistants/nurses who made rounds for all patients in the unit at least once a week.

Debridement

Collagenase in the treatment of dermal and decubitus ulcers. Rao DB, Sane PG, Georgiev EL. J Am Geriatr Soc 1975; 23: 22–30.

Enzymes can be used alone or in combination with other forms of debridement.

Debridement of cutaneous ulcer: medical and surgical aspects. Witkowski JA, Parish LC. Clin Dermatol 1991; 9: 585–93.

Debridement can be accomplished by cold steel cutting, by chemical application, or by autohemolytic destruction under an occlusive dressing.

Maggot debridement therapy: a systematic review. Shi E, Shofler D. Br J Community Nurs 2014; Suppl Wound Care: S6–13.

Maggot debridement therapy, as unappetizing as it may be, promotes wound healing through debridement, disinfection, and growth-promoting activity. It may be utilized for the debridement of nonhealing necrotic skin and soft tissue wounds, especially pressure ulcers, and diabetic foot ulcers.

The role of surgical debridement in healing of diabetic foot ulcers. Gordon KA, Lebrun EA, Tomic-Canic M, Kirsner RS. Skinmed 2012; 10: 24–6.

Evidence to support debridement in enhancing healing is scarce, and there are insufficient data to support debridement for venous ulcers and pressure ulcers.

Cleansing

Cleansing the traumatic wound by high pressure syringe irrigation. Stevenson TR, Thacker JG, Rodeheaver GT, Bacchetta C, Edgerton MT, Edlich RF. J Am Coll Emerg Phys 1976; 5: 17–21.

Cleansing provides enough force to remove bacteria and other debris and loosen eschar.

Wound cleansing for pressure ulcers. Moore ZE, Cowman S. Cochrane Database Syst Rev 2013; 3: CD004983.

Studies that used saline spray containing aloe vera, silver chloride, and decyl glucoside; isotonic saline solution; and pulsatile lavage, water, and sham (the lavage flow was directed into a wash basin positioned adjacent to the wound and not visible to the participants).

There currently is no promising trial evidence to advocate for the use of a specific wound cleansing solution or technique for pressure ulcers.

Wound cleansing, topical antiseptics and wound healing. Atiyeh BS, Dibo SA, Hayek SN. Int Wound J 2009; 6: 420–30.

Wound cleansers, povidone-iodine, chlorhexidine, alcohol, acetate, hydrogen peroxide, boric acid, silver nitrate, silver sulfadiazine, and sodium hypochlorite may affect normal human cells and may be antimitotic, adversely affecting normal tissue repair. Negative outcomes may occur with repeated and excessive wound treatment with antiseptics without proper indications; however, when applied at the appropriate times and concentrations, some classes of antiseptics may function as a tool for the clinician to steer the wound bed in specific directions.

Antimicrobial Agents

Topical metronidazole for odor control in pressure ulcers. Lyvers E, Elliott DP. Consult Pharm 2015; 30: 523–6.

When metronidazole was applied to the wound two or three times daily, 0.75% and 1% creams, gels, lotions, and intravenous solutions of metronidazole were effective with nearly complete odor resolution in 2 to 7 days. Although there was the risk for systemic absorption, almost no systemic adverse events were reported in the literature. Monitoring is still required, as nausea, gastrointestinal distress, and neural toxicities from long-term use are still possible.

Which medical device and/or which local treatment are to be used, as of 2012, in patients with infected pressure sore? Developing French guidelines for clinical practice. Arzt H, Fromantin I, Ribinik P, Barrois B, Colin D, Michel JM, et al. Ann Phys Rehabil Med 2012; 55: 498–507.

The studies do not indicate that one particular topical product is better than another for wound cleaning. Local antimicrobial treatment may be applied when there are indications of local infection. Systemic antimicrobial treatment should be used when general medical signs of infection exist. The draining of exudates and pus is ensured by alginate dressings, carboxymethyl cellulose (CMC) fiber, draining, or irrigoabsorbent compresses covered, if possible, by a nonocclusive dressing until the signs of infection regress.

Bacteriology of pressure ulcers in individuals with spinal cord injury: what we know and what we should know. Dana AN, Bauman WA. J Spinal Cord Med 2015; 38: 147–60.

Staphylococcus aureus, Proteus mirabilis, Pseudomonas aeruginosa, and *Enterococcus fecalis* were the organisms most frequently identified in pressure ulcers.

Nutrition

A nutritional formula enriched with arginine, zinc, and antioxidants for the healing of pressure ulcers: a randomized trial. Cereda E, Klersy C, Serioli M, Crespi A, D'Andrea F; OligoElement Sore Trial Study Group. Ann Intern Med 2015; 162: 167–74.

Supplementation with arginine, zinc, and antioxidants within a high-calorie, high-protein formula may improve pressure ulcer healing with a 20% higher reduction in pressure ulcer area after 8 weeks of intervention.

The role of nutrition for pressure ulcer management: National Pressure Ulcer Advisory Panel, European Pressure Ulcer Advisory Panel, and Pan Pacific Pressure Injury Alliance white paper. Posthauer ME, Banks M, Dorner B, Schols JM. Adv Skin Wound Care 2015; 28: 175–88.

Adults who are underweight or who have experienced notable unintended weight loss may require additional energy intake. Provide fortified foods and/or high-calorie, high-protein oral nutritional supplements between meals if nutritional requirements remain deficient by dietary intake means. Consider enteral or parenteral nutritional support when oral intake is inadequate.

Synthetic Dressing

Successful treatment of unstageable pressure ulcers by using advanced wound dressing. Sunarti S. Med Indones 2015; 47: 251–2.

The stages of healing are cleaning, granulation, and epithelialization. Alginate dressing, dextranomer dressing, hydrofiber dressing, flax dressing, silver-supplemented dressing, or enzyme-supplemented dressing are the proposed dressings for the cleaning phase, whereas for the granulation phase, alginate dressing, hydrocolloid dressing, flax dressing, polyurethane foam dressing, or tender wet dressing should be utilized. For the epithelization phase, hydrofiber dressing, hydrocolloid dressing, hydrogel dressing, flax dressing, and semipermeable dressing may be used.

Using transparent polyurethane film and hydrocolloid dressings to prevent pressure ulcers. Dutra RA, Salomé GM, Alves JR, Pereira VO, Miranda FD, Vallim VB, et al. Wound Care 2015; 24: 268, 270–1, 273–5.

The transparent polyurethane film (8.7%) performed better and was more effective than the hydrocolloid dressing (15%) in preventing pressure ulcer development, as evidenced in 160 patients.

Hydrogel dressing for treating pressure ulcers. Dumville JC, Stubbs N, Keogh SJ, Walker RM, Liu Z. Cochrane Database Syst Rev 2015; 2: CD011226.

It is not explicit if hydrogel dressings are more or less effective than other treatments in healing pressure ulcers or if different hydrogels have contrasting effects. Most trials that have been performed in this area are very small and poorly reported, so the risk of bias is uncertain.

Dressings and topical agents for preventing pressure ulcers. Moore ZE, Webster J. Cochrane Database Syst Rev 2013; 8: CD009362.

Although the occurrence of pressure ulcers was reduced when dressings were employed to protect the skin, results were compromised by the low quality of the included trials. These trials contained considerable risk of bias and clinical heterogeneity (variations in population and intervention techniques); consequently, results should be interpreted as inconclusive.

Third-Line Therapies	
• Nitroglycerin ointment	D
• Becaplermin gel	A
• 5-Fluorouracil cream	D
• Hyperbaric oxygen	E
• Honey	B
• Platelet-rich plasma	B
• Electrical stimulation	C
• Negative pressure wound therapy	C
• Surgical management	D

Hyperbaric oxygen therapy for chronic wounds. Kranke P, Bennett MH, Martyn-St James M, Schnabel A, Debus S. Cochrane Database Syst Rev 2012; 4: CD004123.

There are no satisfactory studies available to prove that hyperbaric oxygen is useful in decubitus or arterial ulcers.

Nonpharmacologic interventions to heal pressure ulcers in older patients: an overview of systematic reviews (the SENATOR-ONTOP series). Vélez-Díaz-Pallarés M, Lozano-Montoya I, Abraha I, Cherubini A, Soiza RL, O'Mahony D, et al. J Am Med Dir Assoc 2015; 16: 448–69.

The most frequent interventions investigated in these trials were support surfaces (13 studies), nutrition (8), and electrotherapy (6). The evidence grade is too low or insufficient to support the utilization of any support surface, nutrition intervention, multicomponent interventions, repositioning, or other adjunctive therapy (ultrasound, negative pressure, laser, electromagnetic, light, shock wave, hydrotherapy, radiofrequency, or vibration therapy) to increase the rates of pressure ulcers healing in older patients. Electrotherapy may demonstrate some beneficial effect in the treatment of pressure ulcers, although the quality of evidence is low.

Honey as a topical treatment for wounds. Jull AB, Cullum N, Dumville JC, Westby MJ, Deshpande S, Walker N. Cochrane Database Syst Rev 2015; 3: CD005083.

Honey has become in vogue for healing partial-thickness burns more quickly than conventional treatment (which included polyurethane film, paraffin gauze, soframycin-impregnated gauze, sterile linen, and leaving the burns exposed) and healing infected postoperative wounds more quickly than antiseptics and gauze, but the evidence remains unconvincing.

Role of local application of autologous platelet-rich plasma in the management of pressure ulcers in spinal cord injury patients. Singh R, Rohilla RK, Dhayal RK, Sen R, Sehgal PK. Spinal Cord 2014; 52: 809–16.

Using local applications of platelet-rich plasma (PRP) may be deemed a promising alternative to standard saline dressings in 25 grade IV spinal cord injury patients with pressure ulcers healing.

Negative pressure wound therapy for treating pressure ulcers. Dumville JC, Webster J, Evans D, Land L. Cochrane Database Syst Rev 2015; 5: CD011334.

There is currently no rigorous randomized controlled trial (RCT) evidence available regarding the effects of negative pressure wound therapy (NPWT) compared with alternatives for the treatment of pressure ulcers.

Phototherapy for treating pressure ulcers. Chen C, Hou WH, Chan ES, Yeh ML, Lo HL. Cochrane Database Syst Rev 2014; 7: CD009224.

Trials compared the use of phototherapy with standard care only (six trials) or sham phototherapy (one trial). Among five studies reporting the rate of change in ulcer area, three studies found no statistically remarkable difference between the two groups. These are very uncertain as to the effects of phototherapy in treating pressure ulcers. The quality of evidence is very low due to the unclear risk of bias and small number of trials available for analysis.

Electromagnetic therapy for treating pressure ulcers. Aziz Z, Bell-Syer SE. Cochrane Database Syst Rev 2015; 9: CD002930.

There is no strong evidence indicating benefits of using electromagnetic therapy (EMT) to treat pressure ulcers; however, the possibility of a beneficial or harmful effect cannot be eliminated, because there were only two included trials, both with methodological limitations and small numbers of participants.

A review of the surgical management of heel pressure ulcers in the 21st century. Bosanquet DC, Wright AM, White RD, Williams IM. Int Wound J 2016; 13: 9–16.

Surgical interventions, such as simple debridement, partial or total calcanectomy, arterial revascularization in the context of coexisting peripheral vascular disease, or using free tissue flaps may be the only means of encountering successful healing in stage IV pressure ulcers. Amputation may be necessary for failed surgical intervention or as a definitive first-line procedure in certain high-risk or poor-prognosis patient groups.

Evidence Levels: **A** Double-blind study **B** Clinical trial ≥ 20 subjects **C** Clinical trial < 20 subjects **D** Series ≥ 5 subjects **E** Anecdotal case reports

55

Delusions of parasitosis

Mio Nakamura, Jillian W. Wong Millsop, John Y.M. Koo

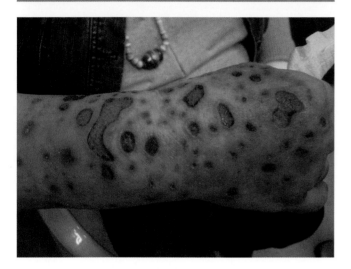

Delusions of parasitosis is a form of delusional disorder, somatic type (also known as a *monosymptomatic hypochondriacal psychosis*), in which patients have cutaneous dysesthesia that causes them to pick at their skin continuously in order to "extract" an organism or "foreign body" they believe is present in their skin. The cutaneous findings that result from these attempts to dig out the suspected parasites range from normal skin to excoriations, picker's nodules, and frank ulcerations. Patients develop elaborate and complex delusional ideations associated with their condition, and their fixed beliefs cannot be argued with reason. These patients often collect "samples" in bottles, Ziploc bags, jars, or slides of what is often lint, hair, debris, dead skin, and even common insects found in the home, using these specimens to provide "evidence" to physicians of the alleged underlying cause of their condition. Many of these patients can also have tactile hallucinatory experiences that are compatible with their delusion. The most characteristic hallucinatory symptom they may experience is formication, which manifests as sensations of cutaneous crawling, biting, or stinging. Many also complain of pruritus.

The condition has a bimodal age distribution, occurring in younger adults (men and women) and the elderly (mostly women). There can be secondary psychopathologies in delusions of parasitosis, such as depression and anxiety; these can be severe enough to cause the patient to commit suicide.

MANAGEMENT STRATEGY

First, it is imperative that the dermatologist carry out a detailed medical history to exclude a frank skin condition (e.g., scabies incognito) or other possible organic conditions, such as substance abuse (e.g., cocaine), neurologic (e.g., multiple sclerosis), endocrine (e.g., diabetes mellitus), hematologic/oncologic (e.g., lymphoma), nutritional (e.g., B_{12} or folate deficiency), infectious (e.g., Human Immunodeficiency Virus), cardiovascular

(e.g., congestive heart failure), or renal (e.g., uremic pruritus) disorders. The condition can also develop after the patient, relative, or pet has had a true parasitic infection, and so ruling out the presence of a real infestation is warranted. Importantly, when patients do *not* know the reason why they are itching, the clinician should consider a diagnosis other than delusions of parasitosis because patients with delusions typically "know" that a particular infestation is causing their symptoms.

Second, a thorough physical examination should be performed, including examining various "specimens" that the patient may bring to the dermatologist's office. These specimens can be observed under the microscope, which will demonstrate to the patient that his or her concerns are being taken seriously. One should not make any comments that may reinforce their delusional ideation, such as a statement that an organism responsible for the condition was found; this may ultimately render the patient more difficult to deal with by making him or her even more firmly fixated on the erroneous beliefs. On the other hand, by definition, rational argument or trying to talk a patient out of a delusion is both not possible (if the patient has a real delusion) and counterproductive. Dermatologists can acknowledge the patient's sensations and suffering as real and that they will do everything they can to help.

It is also important for the dermatologist to treat secondary skin changes in these patients. By doing so, the dermatologist will help to forge a therapeutic alliance with the patient. Dermatologists should consider soothing baths and topical agents such as steroid–anesthetic combinations or creams with menthol.

The most effective way to reverse delusional ideation is to start the patient on an *antipsychotic medication*. If this is described as an antipsychotic agent, however, few patients will accept the treatment. On the other hand, if this option is offered in a neutral way, emphasizing possible symptom reduction, such as reduced crawling, biting, or stinging sensations, while avoiding discussing pathophysiology or the mechanism of action of these medications, patients may be willing to accept.

The medication traditionally used to treat delusions of parasitosis is pimozide, a neuroleptic. This medication generally works very well, whether patients have classic delusions of parasitosis or formication without delusions. The starting dose of pimozide is deliberately kept low at 0.5 to 1 mg/day to minimize risks of side effects. The dose is gradually increased until the optimal clinical response is attained, as evidenced by reduced formication, mental preoccupation, and agitation. The dose of pimozide can be increased by as little as 0.5- to 1-mg increments and as slowly as on a biweekly to monthly basis until significant clinical response is noted, which is usually evident at a dose of 3 to 5 mg daily. It is very rare that a patient will require a dose of more than 5 mg daily, and the use of more than 10 mg daily is almost unheard of in the treatment of delusions of parasitosis. Once the patient reaches a stable, well-tolerated dose and agitation, mental preoccupation, and symptoms of formication have subsided, this dose should be maintained for a few months. During this time, if the patient continues to experience improvement, the dosage of pimozide can then be gradually reduced by as little as 1 mg every 2 to 4 weeks until the minimum necessary dosage is determined or the patient is slowly tapered off the pimozide altogether.

If the clinical state deteriorates again in the future with a new episode of a delusional belief system and formication, the patient can be restarted on pimozide and again treated on a time-limited fashion to control the particular episode. Most patients can be treated on an episodic basis and can be tapered off pimozide after several months, but some require long-term low-dose maintenance treatment.

Because pimozide blocks dopaminergic receptors, there is the possibility that extrapyramidal side effects such as stiffness in the muscles or akathisia, an inner sensation of restlessness, may develop. Acute dystonic reaction and tardive dyskinesia are other potential adverse consequences associated with pimozide, although with the relatively low dosages used to treat delusions of parasitosis, these side effects are rarely encountered. If they do develop, however, they can usually be controlled with anticholinergic agents such as benztropine (Cogentin) 1 to 2 mg up to four times a day as needed, or diphenhydramine (Benadryl) 25 mg four times a day as needed for stiffness or restlessness. Akathisia and pseudoparkinsonian side effects are not a reason for discontinuing treatment with pimozide provided they are kept under control with one of these agents.

Because pimozide can theoretically prolong the QT interval or cause ventricular arrhythmias, it is advisable to consider checking electrocardiograms (ECGs) pretreatment and, periodically, during treatment, especially in older patients or those with a history of cardiac arrhythmia. It should be noted that in most cases, the risk of ECG abnormalities, including prolongation of the QT interval, is minimal with doses at or less than 5 mg daily, provided that they are not elderly and have no history of arrhythmia. Caution must also be exercised in prescribing pimozide for those with hepatic or renal dysfunction.

Atypical antipsychotics, such as *risperidone* and *olanzapine*, have also been used successfully to treat patients with delusions of parasitosis. Atypical antipsychotics block more $5\text{-}HT_2$ (serotonin) receptors than D_2 receptors. Serotonin has been shown to be a key player in some states of psychosis, most cases of obsessive-compulsive disorder, and self-mutilation, which can all potentially manifest in patients with delusions of parasitosis. Thus atypical antipsychotics, by blocking both serotonin and dopaminergic receptors, are thought theoretically to be an effective choice for treating this condition. Furthermore, the burden of side effects with atypical antipsychotics may be reduced compared with that of older typical antipsychotics. Having the patient agree to go on risperidone or olanzapine, however, may be more difficult than pimozide, because pimozide's primary indication is Tourette syndrome, whereas the primary indication for risperidone and olanzapine is schizophrenia, with the latter indication being unacceptable to most patients with delusions of parasitosis.

Nevertheless, over the past several years, clinicians have reported many successful cases using atypical antipsychotics. It is usually advisable to start at low doses and titrate upward as needed. (For example, for risperidone, start from 0.5 mg once to twice daily up to the usual maximum dose of 5 mg daily.) To date, however, there have been no randomized, double-blind, placebo-controlled trials comparing the efficacy of pimozide with the atypical antipsychotics, and most of the medical literature on atypical antipsychotics is limited to case reports.

At any point, if feasible, it may be beneficial to try to refer the patient to a psychiatrist. However, many of these patients cannot be managed by psychiatrists because of their refusal to believe their condition is psychiatric in nature. Therefore, a dermatologist willing to use antipsychotic medications is likely to be the only way that most of these patients can receive the treatment they need. At the same time, the most difficult aspect of managing patients with delusions of parasitosis is trying to obtain their cooperation in taking the medication. This difficulty arises as a result of the difference between the patients' belief system and the physician's understanding of the patient's experience. Even with all the interpersonal skillfulness as described earlier, patients may be reluctant to take a psychotropic medication. It may be helpful to emphasize to them that these medications have worked well with patients with similar symptoms and that, in light of their suffering, they have nothing to lose by trying the medication with the spirit of "trial and error" as long as the patient is adequately supervised for safety. Even though managing psychotic patients in dermatologic settings has many challenges, when a dermatologist manages to connect with at least some of these patients and dramatically reverse their very miserable situation, these patients often turn out to be the most grateful patients one can have in a dermatologist's career.

Specific Investigations

These additional tests may be considered, depending on the patient's clinical presentation:
- Complete blood count
- Complete metabolic panel, including liver function tests
- Thyroid function tests
- Serum B_{12}, ferritin
- ECG before initiation of pimozide and periodically while on pimozide, if indicated
- Drug screen

Clinical, epidemiologic, histopathologic and molecular features of an unexplained dermopathy. Pearson ML, Selby JV, Katz KA, Cantrell V, Braden CR, Parise ME, et al. PLoS ONE 2012; 7: e29908.

This is a study by Kaiser Permanente Northern California that was funded by the Centers for Disease Control of 115 patients with self-reported fibers, threads, granules, and other solid substances coming out of their skin. The study included collection of epidemiologic data, clinical evaluations, and analysis of solid materials. The final conclusion of the study was that the patients studied appeared to have a psychiatric disorder consistent with delusions of parasitosis.

Contemporary Diagnosis and Management in Advanced Psychodermatology. Nguyen CM, Beroukhim K, Danesh MJ, Koo JYM. Longboat Key: Handbooks in Health Care, 2015.

This is a comprehensive handbook on psychodermatology, including diagnosis and management of patients with delusions of parasitosis.

Delusions of parasitosis: ethical and clinical considerations. Fabbro S, Aultman JM, Mostow N. J Am Acad Dermatol 2013; 69: 156–9.

A case is presented that demonstrates the dermatologist's dilemma when treating patients with primary psychiatric disease. There is a discussion on the best clinical and ethical action, using principle- and narrative-based approaches in ethical reasoning.

Delusional infestation is typically comorbid with other psychiatric diagnoses: review of 54 patients receiving psychiatric evaluation at Mayo Clinic. Hylwa SA, Foster AA, Bury JE, Davis MD, Pittelkow MR, Bostwick JM. Psychosomatics 2012; 53: 258–65.

This retrospective study found that 74% of patients with delusional infestation have multiple coexisting or underlying psychiatric disorders. Therefore evaluation by a psychiatrist, when possible, is advised for all patients with delusional infestation.

Diffuse pruritic lesions in a 37-year-old man after sleeping in an abandoned building. Dunn J, Murphy MB, Fox KM. Am J Psychiatry 2007; 164: 1166–72.

Evidence Levels: **A** Double-blind study **B** Clinical trial ≥ 20 subjects **C** Clinical trial < 20 subjects **D** Series ≥ 5 subjects **E** Anecdotal case reports

This is an excellent case presentation of a patient with delusions of parasitosis and contains a thorough discussion of the differential diagnosis.

First-Line Therapy

• Pimozide	**B**

Pimozide in dermatologic practice: a comprehensive review. Lorenzo CR, Koo J. Am J Clin Dermatol 2004; 5: 339–49.

This article reviews the utility of pimozide in dermatologic conditions.

Delusional parasitosis: a dermatologic, psychiatric, and pharmacologic approach. Driscoll MS, Rothe MJ, Grant-Kels JM, Hale MS. J Am Acad Dermatol 1993; 29: 1023–33.

Pimozide is suggested as the first line of therapy for this psychodermatologic condition. Relapse often occurs upon discontinuation of the drug.

Neurotropic and psychotropic drugs in dermatology. Tennyson H, Levine N. Dermatol Clin 2001; 19: 179–97.

This is a review article discussing the use of psychotropic drugs for psychodermatologic conditions such as delusions of parasitosis.

Second-Line Therapies

• Risperidone	**D**
• Olanzapine	**D**
• Quetiapine	**E**
• Aripiprazole	**E**
• Ziprasidone	**E**
• Trifluoperazine	**E**
• Haloperidol	**E**
• Sulpiride	**E**
• Fluphenazine	**E**
• Flupenthixol	**E**
• Promazine	**E**

Second-generation antipsychotics in primary and secondary delusional parasitosis: outcome and efficacy. Freudenmann RW, Lepping P. J Clin Psychopharmacol 2008; 28: 500–8.

The first retrospective case-based analysis of 63 cases from 434 available publications to determine the efficacy and outcome of second-generation antipsychotic agents. It was found that risperidone and olanzapine were the most frequently used of these agents, with full or partial remission in 69% and 72% of cases, respectively.

Therapeutic update: use of risperidone for the treatment of monosymptomatic hypochondriacal psychosis. Elmer KB, George RM, Peterson K. J Am Acad Dermatol 2000; 43: 683–6.

The authors discuss risperidone as being highly effective for delusions of parasitosis while avoiding the negative long-term side effects of pimozide (as discussed earlier).

Primary delusional parasitosis treated with olanzapine. Freudenmann RW, Schönfeldt-Lecuona C, Lepping P. Int Psychogeriatr 2007; 19: 1161–8.

A case report of an elderly woman with delusions of parasitosis successfully and safely treated with olanzapine monotherapy. The authors also present a review of all articles that report the use of atypical antipsychotics for delusions of parasitosis.

Aripiprazole as a viable alternative for treating delusions of parasitosis. Ladizinski B, Busse KL, Bhutani T, Koo JY. J Drugs Dermatol 2010; 9: 1531–2.

A case report of using aripiprazole as a safe and effective treatment for delusions of parasitosis.

Ziprasidone in the treatment of delusional parasitosis. Contreras-Ferrer P, de Paz NM, Cejas-Mendez MR, Rodriguez-Martin M, Souto R, Bustiduy MG. Case Rep Dermatol 2012; 4: 150–3.

This is a case report of successful treatment of delusions of parasitosis with pimozide and ziprasidone.

Promazine in the treatment of delusional parasitosis. Cubala WJ, Jakuszkowiak-Wojten K, Burkiewicz A, Wrońska A. Psychiatria Danubina 2011; 23: 198–9.

This case report demonstrates efficacy and safety of promazine in an elderly patient with delusions of parasitosis.

Antipsychotic treatment of primary delusional parasitosis: systematic review. Lepping P, Russell I, Freudenmann RW. Br J Psychiatry 2007; 191: 198–205.

This article is a systematic review of the use of typical and atypical antipsychotics in patients with delusions of parasitosis. Analyses showed that both typical and atypical antipsychotics were effective in the majority of patients. Particularly effective antipsychotics resulting in full or partial remission were pimozide, trifluoperazine, haloperidol, sulpiride, fluphenazine, and flupenthixol.

Dermatitis artefacta

Tian Hao Zhu, Jillian W. Wong Millsop, John Y.M. Koo

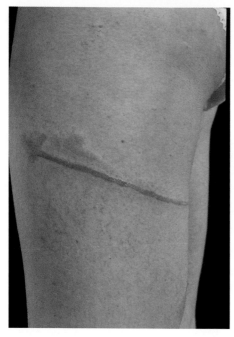

Dermatitis artefacta (DA), also known as *factitious dermatitis,* is a rare psychiatric condition in which patients self-induce a variety of skin lesions. The motive for creating the lesions is often a conscious or unconscious psychological need to seek attention or medical care, possibly due to childhood feelings of abandonment or neglect. Currently the disorder is found to occur in a 4-to-1 ratio of female-to-male patients with the average age at presentation of 12.5 years. Recent studies suggest that a large proportion of patients with dermatitis artefacta may also have comorbid generalized anxiety, major depression, or borderline personality disorder.

The method used to inflict the lesions is typically more elaborate than simple excoriations. The appearance of the lesions depends on the manner in which they are created and can range from minor cuts to large areas of trauma but is usually characterized by abnormally shaped superficial erosions surrounded by normal-looking skin within easily reachable areas. Chemical or thermal burns, injection of foreign materials, circulatory occlusion, and tampering with old lesions, such as existing scars or prior surgical incision sites, are some common methods of self-injury. More serious wounds can result in abscesses, gangrene, or even life-threatening infection.

Interestingly, when the patient is asked about the manner in which the skin condition evolved, he or she will invariably deny responsibility for the injury and is often vague, generally unmoved, and cannot provide sufficient detail, a unique aspect of the illness termed the *hollow history.*

MANAGEMENT STRATEGY

It is important to first rule out malingering as the etiology of the skin lesions. If the skin lesions are created deliberately for secondary gain, such as to obtain disability or insurance benefits, the case is no longer considered psychiatrically based. Rather, it is now considered a criminal act and may eventually need to be dealt with legally. On the other hand, if the lesions are created without underlying material or personal gain, then the condition is considered an illness, and medical/psychiatric intervention is warranted.

Most treatment for dermatitis artefacta is symptomatic and supportive. *Protective dressings,* such as an Unna boot, may be used to occlude the involved areas and protect against further self-injurious behavior.

Antidepressant medications, such as *selective serotonin reuptake inhibitors (SSRIs),* may be helpful for patients with dermatitis artefacta who have primary or secondary depression. If there is clinical evidence of a psychotic process, *pimozide* could be considered. There have also been recent case reports of patients responding to the atypical antipsychotic *olanzapine* when other modes of therapy, including antidepressants and other antipsychotics, have failed.

Importantly, physicians should be aware that patients presenting with dermatitis artefacta have a psychiatric illness, and the skin lesions are often an appeal for help. However, suggesting that the illness is psychiatrically based often has a negative effect on patient rapport. Direct confrontation should be avoided, if possible, and instead, *a supportive environment* and a *stable physician–patient therapeutic alliance* should be fostered, often initially through short (so as not to "burn out" the dermatologist) but frequent (so as to satisfy the patient) office visits. The clinician should be nonjudgmental; empathize with the patient's pain, discomfort, and restrictions imposed by the skin lesions; and potentially explore possible stressors in the patient's life.

In the case of an adolescent, the clinician should encourage the parents to become involved in identifying psychosocial stressors and helping to modify the patient's environment to meet his or her needs. Certain parents may be resistant to their child's diagnosis and can become angry and critical toward the clinician, so great discretion is recommended. If there is intense antagonism ("power struggle") between the adolescent patient and the parents, it may be advisable to see the patient alone, without the parents, to optimize the possibility of developing therapeutic rapport with the patient. Once the patient establishes trust in the physician by means of a stable relationship, the physician may help the patient recognize the psychosocial impact of the disorder and *recommend consultation with a psychiatrist* or *psychotherapy.* However, this approach should be attempted only if the clinician feels that the therapeutic rapport is strong enough to achieve possibility of success rather than being misinterpreted negatively and defensively by the patient.

Most patients with dermatitis artefacta will have a chronic waxing and waning course of disease. Thus even when the condition is under control, the physician should still follow the patient at regular intervals to ensure that the self-destructive behavior does not relapse. *Regular visits,* whether or not lesions are present, will help the patient feel cared for and diminish the need for self-mutilation as a call for help.

Specific Investigations

- Rule out malingering
- Rule out any organic dermatologic disease
- Assess for associated psychiatric disorders (e.g., depression)

Evidence Levels: A Double-blind study B Clinical trial ≥ 20 subjects C Clinical trial < 20 subjects D Series ≥ 5 subjects E Anecdotal case reports

Factitious Dermatitis

Contemporary Diagnosis and Management in Advanced Psychodermatology. Nguyen C, Beroukhim K, Danesh M, Koo J. 2015; 21–2.

This handbook is an up-to-date review of the diagnosis and treatment of dermatitis artefacta.

Self-induced skin lesions: a review of dermatitis artefacta. Gattu S, Rashid RM, Khachemoune A. Cutis 2009; 84: 247–51.

This article is an up-to-date review of dermatitis artefacta.

Cutaneous manifestations of psychiatric disease that commonly present to the dermatologist – diagnosis and treatment. Koblenzer CS. Int J Psychiatry Med 1992; 22: 47–63.

This article describes common dermatologic presentations of psychopathology, including dermatitis artefacta.

Dermatitis artefacta in pediatric patients: experience at the National Institute of Pediatrics. Saez-de-Ocariz M, Orozco-Covarrubias L, Mora-Magaña I, Duran-McKinster C, Tamayo-Sanchez L, Gutierrez-Castrellon P, et al. Pediatr Dermatol 2004; 21: 205–11.

In this study, the incidence of dermatitis artefacta was 1:23,000. It is considered rare in children; 12 of the 29 patients reported had an associated chronic illness, and 7 exhibited mild mental retardation.

Diagnostic clues to dermatitis artefacta. Joe EK, Li VW, Magro CM, Arndt KA, Bowers KE. Cutis 1999; 63: 209–14.

The clinical and histopathologic features, diagnostic aids, approach to therapy, and prognosis for dermatitis artefacta are discussed in this case report.

First-Line Therapies

• Occlusive dressings	D
• Psychotropic agents	D
• Psychotherapy (even if only supportive)	D
• Management of secondary cutaneous complications	D

Self-inflicted skin diseases. A retrospective analysis of 57 patients with dermatitis artefacta seen in a dermatology department. Nielsen K, Jeppesen M, Simmelsgaard L, Rasmussen M, Thestrup-Pedersen K. Acta Derm Venereol 2005; 85: 512–5.

This retrospective analysis of 57 patients reported the following findings: when self-infliction was suggested as the potential cause of illness to patients ($n = 30$), only one patient agreed to see a psychiatrist, and two thirds denied self-infliction or discontinued treatment. Ten patients had a psychiatric diagnosis. The most common subjective complaints were "pain" (59%) and "itching" (37%). The three most common lesion types were skin ulcers (72%), excoriations (46%), and erythema (30%). Of the 57 patients, 61% were treated with anxiolytic or antidepressant medications. In 32 patients, occlusive dressings were administered, and the lesions showed improvement except in two cases.

Training future dermatologists in psychodermatology. Van Moffaert M. Gen Hosp Psychiatry 1986; 8: 115–8.

Palliative dermatologic measures such as occlusive bandages, ointments, or placebo drugs, as well as hospitalization that includes bathing and massaging by nurses, can have a therapeutic impact on the psychiatric problem by symbolizing the medical attention and care the patient with dermatitis artefacta is craving.

Dermatitis artefacta. Clinical features and approach to treatment. Koblenzer CS. Am J Clin Dermatol 2000; 1: 47–55.

A good review article.

The current management of delusional parasitosis and dermatitis artefacta. Koblenzer CS. Skin Therapy Lett 2010; 15: 1–3.

This article briefly reviews treatment for dermatitis artefacta, including the use of aripiprazole.

Second-Line Therapy

• Olanzapine	D

Treatment of self-mutilation with olanzapine. Garnis-Jones S, Collins S, Rosenthal D. J Cutan Med Surg 2000; 4: 161–3.

Three patients were successfully treated with low-dose olanzapine when multiple other therapies (including antidepressants and other antipsychotics) failed.

Dermatitis herpetiformis

John J. Zone

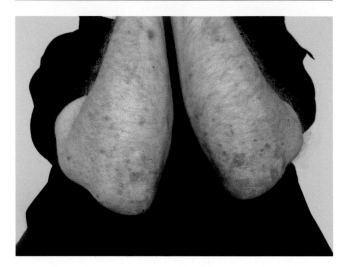

Dermatitis herpetiformis (DH) is a cutaneous manifestation of celiac disease. Rare exceptions have been reported, especially in the Japanese population. More than 85% of patients have an associated celiac disease that spans the spectrum of intestinal histologic severity. Both the skin disease and intestinal inflammation respond to dietary gluten restriction independent of the severity of the intestinal inflammation. The skin disease also presents with a spectrum of severity, ranging from minimal pruritic papules on the elbows and knees to severe, intensely pruritic vesicular lesions over multiple extensor surfaces. The prevalence of DH is approximately 10 to 39 per 100,000 persons in the Caucasian population. One in six patients diagnosed with celiac disease has DH. DH is distinguished from other bullous diseases by characteristic histologic, immunologic, and associated gastrointestinal findings. Histologically, vesicle formation at the dermal-epidermal junction and infiltration of dermal papillary tips with neutrophils occurs in two thirds of the cases, but other cases may show only nonspecific inflammatory findings. Direct immunofluorescence shows granular or fibrillar IgA localized in the dermal papillary tips or along the basement membrane of perilesional skin.

MANAGEMENT STRATEGY

The course of DH depends on the therapeutic choices that are made at the time of diagnosis. If patients choose a strict gluten-free diet and adopt a conscientious change in eating habits, they are likely to have a long-term remission. Associated intestinal symptoms are also minimized. Relapses are usually associated with dietary indiscretions. Elevated levels of IgA antibodies to tissue transglutaminase are characteristic of celiac disease, correlate with the degree of intestinal inflammation, and decrease with gluten restriction. Elevated levels of IgA epidermal transglutaminase antibodies are characteristic of DH and are responsible for the diagnostic IgA deposits in skin. If medical therapy with dapsone or sulfapyridine is chosen, the cutaneous lesions can be well controlled. However, attention must be paid to potential side effects of medications. Intestinal symptoms, if present, will continue. Occasionally, some patients (10%–20%) will enjoy a spontaneous remission without medication or dietary restriction. The reason for such remission is unclear.

Dapsone is the drug of choice for DH and is currently the only drug approved by the U.S. Food and Drug Administration (FDA) for use in this disease. Initial treatment with dapsone 25 mg daily will improve pruritus within 24 to 48 hours and the papulovesicular lesions within 1 week in adults. The skin disease recurs within 24 to 72 hours if dapsone is discontinued. Correspondingly smaller doses (0.5–1 mg/kg) should be used in children. Maintenance therapy is then adjusted on a weekly basis to maintain adequate suppression of symptoms. The average maintenance dose is 0.5 to 1.0 mg/kg daily. Despite adequate dapsone dosages, outbreaks of facial and scalp lesions are common. The most common cause of poor response to dapsone therapy is incorrect diagnosis.

Adherence to a gluten-free diet (GFD) improves clinical symptoms in patients with DH. The advantages of gluten restriction include a reduction of dapsone dosage and its attendant complications, improvement of gastrointestinal symptoms (which range from cramping pain to overt diarrhea), and a therapy aimed at the cause rather than the symptoms of the disease. The increased risk of lymphoma incident to DH and celiac disease is also reduced with a GFD, but not with dapsone. Dapsone improves the cutaneous lesions but has no effect on intestinal disease. Strict adherence to a GFD is challenging, and reintroduction of gluten can exacerbate symptoms. Extremely rare patients will not respond to gluten restriction. In the author's opinion, a useful therapeutic strategy is the initial control of DH symptoms with dapsone coincident with a GFD, with subsequent monthly tapering of dapsone as gluten restriction gradually improves the cutaneous symptoms. Oats have been found to be nontoxic in most patients with DH and may broaden the dietary options. Recently gluten-free foods have become more available, and patient support groups offer extensive information.

Sulfapyridine is an alternative choice in patients who are intolerant to dapsone and has been shown to result in significant therapeutic efficacy. Sulfapyridine is started at 500 mg three times a day and is usually increased to a maximum maintenance dose of 1.5 g three times a day. Sulfapyridine is not commercially available in the United States and must be compounded. Sulfasalazine can be used as a substitute. It is metabolized by intestinal bacteria to sulfapyridine and 5-amino salicylate. Recommended doses are 500 to 1000 mg twice daily.

Other agents that have been reported to have a therapeutic benefit in DH include *nicotinamide, tetracycline* (or a combination of the two), *heparin, ciclosporin, azathioprine, mycophenolate, colchicine,* and *systemic corticosteroids.* Rituximab has recently been shown to be effective for both DH and the underlying celiac disease. *Topical corticosteroid application* is generally inadequate when used alone to control DH symptoms. However, potent corticosteroids in gel form applied frequently may provide relief for occasional lesions that develop on otherwise adequate dapsone or GFD therapy. This allows patients to treat lesions without increasing the dosage of dapsone.

Specific Investigations

- Biopsy for histology and direct immunofluorescence
- Complete blood count and liver function tests
- Glucose-6-phosphate dehydrogenase levels
- IgA tissue transglutaminase antibodies
- IgA epidermal transglutaminase antibodies

Evidence Levels: **A** Double-blind study   **B** Clinical trial ≥ 20 subjects   **C** Clinical trial < 20 subjects   **D** Series ≥ 5 subjects   **E** Anecdotal case reports

Dermatitis herpetiformis: a cutaneous manifestation of coeliac disease. Collin P, Salmi TT, Hervn K, Kaukinen K, Reunala T. Ann Med 2016; 8: 1–25.

DH is a manifestation of celiac disease in virtually all cases. Not all cases have abnormal IgA TG2 antibodies or abnormal small intestinal biopsies, but nearly all cases respond slowly to dietary gluten restriction. Five percent of first-degree relatives of DH patients will have celiac disease if tested.

Deposition of granular IgA relative to clinical lesions in dermatitis herpetiformis. Zone JJ, Meyer LJ, Petersen MJ. Arch Dermatol 1996; 132: 912–8.

It is accepted that granular IgA deposition in perilesional, clinically normal-appearing skin is the most reliable diagnostic criterion for DH. Although the combination of characteristic clinical and pathologic features is highly suggestive of DH, the diagnosis should not be made without the identification of granular IgA in dermal papillae. If direct immunofluorescence is negative and histology is suggestive of DH, a repeat biopsy for direct immunofluorescence is recommended.

First-Line Therapies

• Dapsone	B
• Gluten-free diet	B

Suggested guidelines for patient monitoring: hepatic and hematologic toxicity attributable to systemic dermatologic drugs. Wolverton SE, Remlinger K. Dermatol Clin 2007; 25: 195–205.

Dapsone may produce a drug hypersensitivity syndrome with liver toxicity in the first 3 to 12 weeks. Monitoring of the aspartate transaminase (AST), alanine transaminase (ALT), and eosinophil count is indicated. Hepatocellular toxicity may also occur in a dose-related fashion, especially with doses greater than 2 mg/kg. AST and ALT should be monitored when the dosage is increased. There are three main hematologic toxicities of dapsone: hemolysis, methoglobinemia, and agranulocytosis. Methoglobinemia is usually mild and not problematic unless the patient has underlying cardiopulmonary problems. Agranulocytosis is rare and usually occurs in the first 3 to 12 weeks of therapy. Symptoms demanding attention include pharyngitis, fever, and oral ulcerations. Virtually all patients have at least some degree of hemolysis, and a fall of the hemoglobin of 1 to 3 g/dL is to be expected. A compensatory reticulocytosis occurs and may be monitored with a reticulocyte count. Hemolysis may be severe in patients with glucose-6-phosphate dehydrogenase deficiency. Glucose-6-phosphate dehydrogenase levels should be evaluated in blacks and those of Southern Mediterranean origin before the initiation of therapy to avoid potentially catastrophic hemolytic anemia.

Complete blood count and liver function tests should be checked every 2 to 3 weeks for the first 3 months and then every 3 to 6 months thereafter.

Celiac disease and the gluten-free diet: consequences and recommendations for improvement. Theethira TG, Dennis M. Dig Dis 2015; 33: 175–82.

GFD is the cornerstone of treatment for celiac disease and dermatitis herpetiformis. This review addresses the improvements in nutrition in celiac patients on a GFD and also potential problems that may develop on a GFD with deficiencies of fiber, iron, and trace minerals. They also review the issue of weight gain in celiac patients adhering to a GFD because of the high caloric content of commercially available gluten-free foods.

The GFD is complex, and patients need comprehensive nutrition education from a skilled dietitian. Patient support groups frequently provide answers to specific dietary questions.

A long-term gluten-free diet as an alternative treatment in severe forms of dermatitis herpetiformis. Nino M, Ciacci C, Delfino M. J Dermatolog Treat 2007; 18: 10–2.

This study evaluated the efficacy of treating severe skin manifestations of DH with a GFD alone and compared the results to treatment with GFD and dapsone. Eighty-seven percent of patients on GFD alone had complete remission in 18 months (67% of severe patients). A total of 89% of patients on diet and dapsone had remission of skin disease (70% of severe patients), and 11% were improved.

Second-Line Therapies

• Sulfapyridine and sulfasalazine	E
• Elemental diet	C

Management of dermatitis herpetiformis. Cardones AR, Hall RP. Immunol Allergy Clin North Am 2012; 32: 275–81.

Sulfapyridine is not readily available in the United States but can be prescribed through compounding pharmacies. Sulfasalazine, which is more readily available, is metabolized to 5-amino-salicylic acid and sulfapyridine. Patients have been reported to respond to sulfasalazine, 2 to 4 g/day administered twice daily.

The effect of elemental diet with and without gluten on disease activity in dermatitis herpetiformis. Kadunce DP, McMurry MP, Avots-Avotins A, Chandler JP, Meyer LJ, Zone JJ. J Invest Dermatol 1991; 97: 175–82.

In severe refractory cases of DH elemental diet therapy is effective and produces dramatic clinical improvement within 2 to 4 weeks. It involves the ingestion of amino acid and carbohydrate alone and is commercially available as Vivonex. It produces rapid healing of the intestine and relief of cutaneous symptoms but was designed for tube feeding and is considered unpalatable by many.

In this author's experience, elemental diet containing short-chain polypeptides is less effective.

Third-Line Therapies

• Tetracycline and nicotinamide	E
• Heparin	E
• Ciclosporin	E
• Colchicine	E
• Systemic corticosteroids	E
• Rituximab	E

Dermatitis herpetiformis effectively treated with heparin, tetracycline and nicotinamide. Shah SAA, Ormerond AD. Clin Exp Dermatol 2000; 25: 204–5.

This is a case report of a patient with severe DH who was intolerant to dapsone and sulfapyridine. The DH lesions resolved with a combination treatment consisting of subcutaneous low-dose heparin, nicotinamide 1.5 g daily in divided doses, and tetracycline 2 g daily. The patient was, however, on a GFD.

A rare case of dermatitis herpetiformis requiring parenteral heparin for long-term control. Tan CC, Sale JE, Brammer C, Irons RP, Freeman JG. Dermatology 1996; 192: 185–6.

A patient with severe DH who was intolerant of dapsone and sulfapyridine was treated with parenteral heparin, with complete resolution of her skin lesions within 1 week of therapy. This treatment is not practical for long-term management.

Efficacy of ciclosporin in two patients with dermatitis herpetiformis resistant to conventional therapy. Stenveld HJ, Starink TM, van Joost T, Stoof TJ. J Am Acad Dermatol 1993; 28: 1014–5.

Two patients with severe DH who were intolerant and/or unresponsive to conventional therapy were treated with ciclosporin (5–7 mg/kg daily) with resolution of skin lesions.

Treatment of dermatitis herpetiformis with colchicine. Silver DN, Juhlin EA, Berczeller PH, McSorley J. Arch Dermatol 1980; 116: 1373–84.

Oral colchicine resulted in a significant improvement of skin lesions in three of four patients with DH. The authors suggest that colchicine may be used when dapsone or sulfapyridine is contraindicated.

Rituximab treatment for recalcitrant dermatitis herpetiformis. Albers LN, Zone JJ, Stoff BK, Feldman RJ. JAMA Dermatol. 2017; 153: 315–8.

A single patient with refractory DH had a complete clinical response to rituximab 1000 mg on days 1 and 15 with a remission that was documented by normalization of IgA antibody levels to both tissue and epidermal transglutaminase.

Evidence Levels: **A** Double-blind study **B** Clinical trial ≥ 20 subjects **C** Clinical trial < 20 subjects **D** Series ≥ 5 subjects **E** Anecdotal case reports

58

Dermatofibrosarcoma protuberans

Daniel Bernstein, Kate Kleydman, Hooman Khorasani

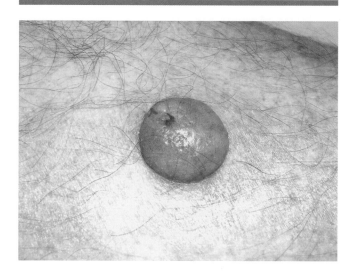

Dermatofibrosarcoma protuberans (DFSP) is a rare, low-grade, soft tissue, undifferentiated, CD34-positive, factor XIII–negative, mesenchymal tumor that arises in the dermis and characteristically invades deeper underlying soft tissue. It is associated with a high risk for local recurrence and widespread subclinical extension. The incidence of DFSP is 0.1% of all cancers and 1.8% of all soft tissue sarcomas. It occurs most often in adults aged 20 to 50 years; pediatric and infantile cases, particularly when congenital, are rare. The tumor most commonly involves the trunk (50%–60%) or upper limbs (25%). Head and neck sites account for an additional 10% to 15% of DFSP cases and may not always be completely resectable. If left untreated, the tumor often grows slowly, invading surrounding tissue and neurovascular bundles. Although DFSP can be locally destructive, the tumor rarely metastasizes.

MANAGEMENT STRATEGY

Surgical excision remains the mainstay of treatment for DFSP. Because DFSP commonly has an infiltrating growth pattern that extends far beyond the clinical margins, a wide excision is recommended, with margins of 2 to 3 cm or more beyond clinically identifiable tumor, down to and including fascia. Despite treatment with wide local excision, local recurrence rates vary significantly in the literature from 10% to 80%. Tumor size and location help determine the appropriate surgical procedure because generous margins are not always practical, particularly for tumors of acral location. The prognosis of DFSP has been investigated, and reduced recurrence-free survival was found to be most associated with acral tumors, whereas overall survival was reduced in cases with metastasis.

Because these neoplasms have a high tendency for local recurrence after surgical excision, a superior cure rate (an overall average recurrence rate of 1.3% among 463 cases reported) and tissue conservation are seen when Mohs micrographic surgery (MMS) is used; thus, *Mohs micrographic surgery* may be considered the treatment of choice. Mohs surgery with continuous histologic margin control requires less tissue removal, allows complete margin assessment, has low recurrence rates, and is rapidly emerging as a first-line treatment modality for this condition. A recent systematic review of the literature found that despite a lack of randomized prospective evidence, margin control via MMS has tended to produce superior results compared with conventional surgery. Alternatively, some dermatologic surgeons have adopted modified Mohs techniques, or so-called *slow Mohs*, by using rush paraffin sections instead of a fresh tissue technique.

Cytogenetically, DFSP is characterized by a t(17;22)(22;q13) aberration with fusion of the collagen type 1α (COL1A1) gene on chromosome 17 with the platelet-derived growth factor-β *(PDGFB)* gene on chromosome 22, which renders these tumors responsive to targeted therapy with tyrosine kinase inhibitors, such as *imatinib mesylate*. Originally approved for the treatment of chronic myelogenous leukemia, imatinib mesylate has been found to have significant therapeutic value in the treatment of DFSP. In 2006 the Food and Drug Administration (FDA) granted approval for imatinib mesylate *(Gleevec)* as a single agent for the treatment of adult patients with unresectable, recurrent, and/or metastatic DFSP at a recommended oral dose of 800 mg/day. Before starting imatinib therapy, cytogenetic studies to confirm *PDGFB* gene rearrangement may help predict clinical response, and it is recommended that all cases be evaluated before treatment is started.

Neoadjuvant imatinib therapy for DFSP has also been proposed in recent studies. It has been used as a preoperative therapy agent in locally advanced or recurrent DFSPs. This therapeutic strategy may decrease tumor load, promote tumor cell apoptosis, and subsequently reduce the extent of surgery.

Adjuvant radiotherapy, administered either before or after surgery, significantly reduces the risk of local recurrence in patients who have or who are likely to have close or positive margins. This appears to be true for radiation alone or postoperatively for margin-positive disease (primary or recurrent).

DFSP is a radioresponsive tumor, and radiation to doses of 50 to 60 Gy should be considered. Radiation is not recommended in younger patients (under the age of 50 because of increased risk of radiodermatitis and scarring) or in patients with a previous history of radiation therapy. Radiation is also contraindicated in patients with connective tissue diseases or genetic conditions predisposing to skin cancer (e.g., patients with Gorlin syndrome or xeroderma pigmentosum). Combined conservation resection and postoperative radiation should also be considered for situations where adequate wide excision alone would result in major cosmetic or functional morbidity.

Specific Investigations

- Skin biopsy
- Genetic studies

Dermatofibrosarcoma protuberans is a unique fibrohistiocytic tumor expressing CD34. Aiba S, Tabata N, Ishii H, Ootani H, Tagami H. Br J Dermatol 1992; 127: 79–84.

DFSP can be misdiagnosed as a keloid. Histopathology may help differentiate the two, but expression of CD34 by tumor cells occurs only in DFSP. CD34 expression by the tumor cells can be an extremely useful marker in establishing a definitive diagnosis of DFSP.

Stromelysin-3 (ST3) expression in the differential diagnosis of dermatofibroma (DF) and dermatofibrosarcoma protuberans: comparison with factor XIIIa and CD34. Kim HJ, Lee JY, Kim SH, Seo YJ, Lee JH, Park JK, et al. Br J Dermatol 2007; 157: 319–24.

Recent studies demonstrated that dermatofibromas (DFs) expressed ST3, whereas DFSPs were only rarely ST3 positive. ST3 staining might be more reliable than factor XIIIa staining in differential diagnosis of DF and DFSP.

First-Line Therapies	
• Mohs micrographic surgery	B
• Wide local excision	C

Dermatofibrosarcoma protuberans: a report on 29 patients treated by Mohs micrographic surgery (MMS) with long-term follow-up and review of the literature. Snow SN, Gordon EM, Larson PO, Bagheri MM, Bentz ML, Sable DB. Cancer 2004; 101: 28–38.

A retrospective review of a series of 29 patients with DFSP and, in an accompanying update of the medical literature, 136 patients with DFSP underwent MMS with over 5 years of follow-up. There were no regional and/or distant metastases. However, late recurrences beyond the usual recommended 5-year follow-up may occur.

Dermatofibrosarcoma protuberans: wide local excision vs. Mohs micrographic surgery. Paradisi A, Abeni D, Rusciani A, Cigna E, Wolter M, Scuderi N, et al. Cancer Treat Rev 2008; 34: 728–36.

The records of 79 patients with DFSP who underwent wide local excision (WLE; $n = 38$) or MMS ($n = 41$) between 1990 and 2005 were reviewed retrospectively. Five of the 38 WLE patients (follow-up = 4.8 years) had recurrences (13.2%, 95% confidence interval (CI): 4.4%–28.1%) as opposed to none (95% CI: 0%–8.6%) of the 41 MMS patients (follow-up = 5.4 years).

Outcomes in 11 patients with dermatofibrosarcoma protuberans treated with Mohs micrographic surgery. Galimberti G, Montaño AP, Kowalczuk A, Ferrario D, Galimberti R. Int J Dermatol 2012; 51: 89–93.

A retrospective chart review carried out for patients treated with MMS during a 6-year period. MMS with continuous histologic margin control allows for maximum tissue preservation and low recurrence rates and is rapidly emerging as a first-line treatment modality for this condition.

Dermatofibrosarcoma protuberans: 35 patients treated with Mohs micrographic surgery using paraffin sections. Tan WP, Barlow RJ, Robson A, Kurwa HA, McKenna J, Mallipeddi R. Br J Dermatol 2011; 164: 363–6.

A case review of 35 patients with DFSP treated with "slow" MMS using paraffin-embedded sections. Seventeen patients required one horizontal layer to clear their tumor, 10 patients needed two, and 8 patients needed three layers or more. Tumor persistence has not been observed in any of our patients after a median follow-up duration of 29.5 months.

Current treatment options in dermatofibrosarcoma protuberans. Lemm D, Mügge LO, Mentzel T, Höffken K. J Cancer Res Clin Oncol 2009; 135:653–65.

A literature review of DFSP to review modalities of diagnosis, including CD34 positivity and the unique molecular translocation involving chromosomes 17 and 22 t(17;22)(22;q13), in addition to an investigation of outcomes based on treatment. Although surgical excision remains the mainstay of treatment, MMS has been found to yield improved margin control and is associated with reduced recurrence rates. Adjuvant therapy with radiation or imatinib may be necessary in selected patients, especially when unresectable tumors are being addressed. Chemotherapy seems to be of little or no benefit.

Dermatofibrosarcoma protuberans treated with wide local excision and followed at a cancer hospital: prognostic significance of clinicopathologic variables. Erdem O, Wyatt AJ, Lin E, Wang X, Prieto VG. Am J Dermatopathol 2012; 34: 24–34.

A retrospective review of 122 patients with DFSP, including multivariate analysis of recurrence rates and overall survival, when comparing various methods of surgical excision. Whereas reduced recurrence-free survival was found to be most associated with acral location, overall survival was only decreased in cases of metastatic disease.

Surgical treatment of Darier-Ferrand dermatofibrosarcoma: a systematic review. Pallure V, Dupin N, Guillot B; Association for Recommendations in Dermatology. Dermatol Surg. 2013; 39: 1417–33.

A systematic literature review of DFSP to establish a consensus for lateral margin control. Despite a general lack of formal evidence, margins over 3 cm had decreased recurrence rates compared with margins less than 3 cm; MMS tended to yield the best clinical results. Patients should be followed for a minimum of 10 years postoperatively, and ideally indefinitely, to monitor for recurrences.

Mohs micrographic surgery for dermatofibrosarcoma protuberans (DFSP): a single-center series of 76 patients treated by frozen-section Mohs micrographic surgery with a review of the literature. Loghdey MS, Varma S, Rajpara SM, Al-Rawi H, Perks G, Perkins W. J Plast Reconstr Aesthet Surg 2014; 67: 1315–21.

A retrospective review of 76 cases in addition to a literature review of DFSP to review outcomes when comparing various excision margins. Clearance of tumor required varying margins of tissue, but the asymmetric nature of DFSP seems most suited for procedures that ensure complete margin control. These conclusions support the use of MMS, which is correlated with reduced recurrence rates. Furthermore, positive or narrow margins may be considered for adjuvant radiation or imatinib therapy.

Second-Line Therapies	
• Imatinib mesylate (Gleevec)	B
• Radiation	B

Treatment of advanced dermatofibrosarcoma protuberans with imatinib mesylate with or without surgical resection. Rutkowski P, Dębiec-Rychter M, Nowecki Z, Michej W, Symonides M, Ptaszynski K, et al. J Eur Acad Dermatol Venereol 2011; 25: 264–70.

Data of 15 patients with locally advanced/initially inoperable and/or metastatic DFSP treated with imatinib 400 to 800 mg

Evidence Levels: **A** Double-blind study **B** Clinical trial ≥ 20 subjects **C** Clinical trial < 20 subjects **D** Series ≥ 5 subjects **E** Anecdotal case reports

daily were analyzed. A 2-year progression-free survival rate was 60%, and a 2-year overall survival rate was 78%.

Using imatinib as neoadjuvant therapy in dermatofibrosarcoma protuberans: potential pluses and minuses. Johnson-Jahangir H, Sherman W, Ratner D. J Natl Compr Cancer Netw 2010; 8: 881–5.

Neoadjuvant imatinib mesylate therapy has been shown to reduce preoperative tumor size and lessen surgical morbidity associated with the removal of residual DFSP. Use of neoadjuvant imatinib before surgery, however, requires appropriate patient selection and careful weighing of the potential risks and benefits of this treatment.

Imatinib mesylate as a preoperative therapy in dermatofibrosarcoma: results of a multicenter phase II study on 25 patients. Kérob D, Porcher R, Vérola O, Dalle S, Maubec E, Aubin F, et al. Clin Cancer Res 2010; 16: 3288–95.

Twenty-five adults suffering from primary or recurrent DFSP were included in a phase II multicenter study. Percentage of clinical response was defined to a 2-month preoperative daily administration of 600 mg of imatinib mesylate before WLE. A clinical response was achieved in nine (36%) patients (95% CI: 18.9–57.5). The median relative tumoral decrease was 20.0% (range, −12.5–100).

Apart from expected grade II or III side effects, one grade III neutropenia, one grade III maculopapular rash, and one grade IV transient transaminitis were observed.

Radiation in management of patients with dermatofibrosarcoma protuberans. Suit H, Spiro I, Mankin HJ, Efird J, Rosenberg AE. J Clin Oncol 1996; 14: 2365–9.

The outcome of treatment of 18 patients with DFSP by radiation alone and radiation and surgery was assessed. Local control was realized in the three patients treated by radiation alone, with follow-up periods of at least 9 years. Among 15 patients treated by radiation and surgery, there have been three local failures.

Dermatofibrosarcoma protuberans: treatment results of 35 cases. Sun LM, Wang CJ, Huang CC, Leung SW, Chen HC, Fang FM, et al. Radiother Oncol 2000; 57: 175–81.

A retrospective study examined 35 consecutive patients, over a 10-year period, with pathologically proved DFSP who received surgery with or without radiation therapy. Adjuvant radiation therapy was given to 11 patients, with a dose ranging from 46 to 68 Gy (1 preoperative, 10 postoperative). At a median follow-up of 50 months, there were 11 patients (9 patients without radiation therapy) who developed local failure. After all patients underwent excision with or without radiation, 10 achieved disease control.

Dermatomyositis

Ruth Ann Vleugels, Jeffrey P. Callen

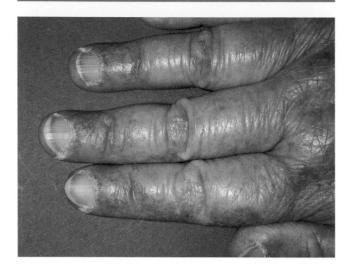

Dermatomyositis (DM) is an idiopathic inflammatory myopathy characterized by cutaneous disease, including a heliotrope eruption, Gottron papules, photodistributed erythema and poikiloderma, and/or periungual changes. Patients with cutaneous lesions of DM often have weakness of the proximal muscles; elevated enzymes such as creatine kinase or aldolase; or abnormal electromyogram, magnetic resonance imaging, or muscle biopsy findings. Some, however, have cutaneous disease that either precedes the onset of demonstrable muscle disease or occurs in its absence (clinically amyopathic DM). In addition, many patients have persistent cutaneous manifestations long after their muscle disease is adequately controlled. DM in children and adolescents may be complicated by calcinosis, particularly when treatment is delayed. Adults with DM have an increased risk of having or developing a malignancy, usually within the first 3 years after diagnosis.

MANAGEMENT STRATEGY

Before treatment the patient should be thoroughly evaluated to assess the severity of both skin and muscle disease; the presence of systemic involvement such as pulmonary, cardiac, or gastrointestinal involvement; and the presence of malignancy.

The goal of management is to *reverse the weakness, prevent contractures,* and allow the patient to return to normal functional status. The *prevention or treatment of calcinosis* is usually an issue in the management of children and adolescents but may occur in adults as well. Patients with cutaneous disease are troubled by intense *pruritus, photosensitivity, and the appearance of their skin* and may therefore require treatment even when the muscle disease has been effectively managed or is absent.

For the myopathy, systemic *corticosteroids, most often in conjunction with an immunosuppressive agent,* is standard treatment. Most patients respond to this strategy, but for those who do not, *high-dose* intravenous immune globulin (IVIG) may be of benefit. Patients with cutaneous disease are photosensitive and are treated with *sunscreens, photoprotective clothing, behavior modification, topical corticosteroids, and occasionally topical calcineurin*

inhibitors, *oral antimalarials*, and often an *immunosuppressive agent. High-dose IVIG* may also be used for recalcitrant cutaneous disease. Ultimately, the therapeutic goal is to provide relief from the cutaneous inflammation and associated symptoms utilizing a combination of topical and/or systemic medications selected after considering a patient's comorbidities.

One of the problems with many of the reports published to date regarding therapeutic options for cutaneous DM is the lack of the use of a validated measure to assess the activity of skin disease and response to therapy. To this end, three such measures have been developed: the Cutaneous Dermatomyositis Area and Severity Index (CDASI) (Arch Dermatol Res 2008; 300: 3–9, and Br J Dermatol 2012; 162: 669–73), the Dermatomyositis Skin Severity Index (DSSI) (Br J Dermatol 2008; 158: 345–50), and a cutaneous assessment tool in juvenile dermatomyositis (Arthritis Rheum 2008; 59: 352–6). Unfortunately, none of these measures has routinely been used in studies investigating therapeutic interventions for DM; however, the tools are being utilized more frequently and will ideally become incorporated as standard practice in the future as a means to assess cutaneous disease response.

Specific Investigations

- A thorough evaluation to exclude other causes of myopathy
- Malignancy evaluation, including computed tomography (CT) scans of chest, abdomen, and pelvis; transvaginal pelvic ultrasound; stool occult blood testing and age-appropriate endoscopy; Papanicolaou smear; mammography; complete blood count; comprehensive metabolic panel; CA-125; CA 19-9; urinalysis; and full physical examination
- Serum creatine kinase and aldolase
- Electromyogram, magnetic resonance imaging, or ultrasound of muscle
- Muscle biopsy
- Assessment for the presence of systemic involvement (e.g., pulmonary, esophageal, and cardiac)
- Myositis-specific antibodies

Treatment

Scalp involvement in dermatomyositis. Often overlooked or misdiagnosed. Kasteler JS, Callen JP. JAMA 1994; 272: 1939–41.

Skin lesions in patients with DM, particularly those of the scalp, are often confused with psoriasis or seborrheic dermatitis. Additionally, DM skin disease may simulate cutaneous lupus erythematosus or lichen planus.

Influence of age on characteristics of polymyositis and dermatomyositis in adults. Marie I, Hatron PY, Levesque H, Hachulla E, Hellot MF, Michon-Pasturel U, et al. Medicine (Baltimore) 1999; 78: 139–47.

This group compared characteristics of younger versus older adults and found that the incidence of malignancy was much higher in the older population, resulting in a poorer prognosis for this subset of patients.

Frequency of specific cancer types in dermatomyositis and polymyositis: a population-based study. Hill CL, Zhang Y, Sigurgeirsson B, Pukkala E, Mellemkjaer L, Airio A, et al. Lancet 2001; 357: 96–100.

Evidence Levels: A Double-blind study **B** Clinical trial ≥ 20 subjects **C** Clinical trial < 20 subjects **D** Series ≥ 5 subjects **E** Anecdotal case reports

This study demonstrated that malignancies of the ovaries, pancreas, stomach, colon and rectum, and non-Hodgkin lymphoma were overrepresented in patients with DM. The malignancy risk decreased with each passing year after DM diagnosis and approached background levels at 3 years.

Malignancy evaluations should be directed by abnormalities found on history, physical findings, or routine laboratory testing. The initial search should include CT scans of the chest, abdomen, and pelvis in most patients, and these scans should be repeated annually for at least 3 years. Malignancy screening should also include annual physical examinations.

Positron emission tomography (PET)-CT scanning is under evaluation in dermatomyositis.

A new approach to the classification of idiopathic inflammatory myopathy: myositis-specific autoantibodies define useful homogeneous patient groups. Love LA, Leff RL, Fraser DD, Targoff IN, Dalakas M, Plotz PH, et al. Medicine (Baltimore) 1991; 70: 360–74.

This study compared the usefulness of myositis-specific autoantibodies (antiaminoacyl-tRNA synthetases, antisignal recognition particle [anti-SRP], and anti-Mi-2) to the standard clinical categories (polymyositis, DM, overlap myositis, cancer-associated myositis, and inclusion body myositis) in predicting clinical signs and symptoms and prognosis in 212 adult patients. Compared with those without these antibodies, patients with antiaminoacyl-tRNA synthetase autoantibodies ($n = 47$) had significantly more frequent arthritis, fever, interstitial lung disease, and "mechanic's hands"; higher mean prednisone dose at survey; higher proportion of patients receiving cytotoxic drugs; and higher death rates. Those with anti-SRP antibodies ($n = 7$) had more frequent palpitations, myalgias, severe refractory disease, and higher death rates. Patients with anti-Mi-2 antibodies ($n = 10$) had increased "V-sign" and "shawl-sign" rashes and cuticular overgrowth, as well as a good response to therapy. These findings suggest that myositis-specific autoantibody status is a more useful guide than clinical group in assessing patients with myositis.

Currently only the antiaminoacyl-tRNA synthetase autoantibodies are frequently incorporated into clinical practice.

A novel dermato-pulmonary syndrome associated with MDA-5 antibodies: report of 2 cases and review of the literature. Chaisson NF, Park J, Orbai AM, Casciola-Rosen L, Fiorentino D, Danoff S, et al. Medicine (Baltimore) 2012; 91: 220–8.

This work describes the clinical features typically associated with a novel autoantibody termed *melanoma differentiation-associated protein 5 (MDA-5)*, including interstitial lung disease that can be rapidly progressive, arthritis, and a characteristic cutaneous phenotype, including ulcerations in Gottron papules; Gottron sign; and along the lateral nailfold, painful palmar papules, and prominent alopecia (this phenotype was first described in 2011 by Fiortentino et al. The mucocutaneous and systemic phenotype of dermatomyositis patients with antibodies to MDA5 (CADM-140): a retrospective study. J Am Acad Dermatol 2011; 65: 25–34). Most patients with the MDA-5 antibody have clinically amyopathic DM. Although this entity was first recognized in Asian populations, it has since been described in other populations as well.

Most patients with cancer-associated dermatomyositis have antibodies to nuclear matrix protein NXP-2 or transcription intermediary factor 1-γ. Fiorentino DF, Chung LS, Christopher-Stone L, Zaba L, Li S, Mammen AL, et al. Arthritis Rheum 2013; 65: 2954–62.

In two large DM cohorts, reactivity against either transcription intermediary factor-1γ (TIF-1γ) or NXP-2 identified 83% of patients with cancer-associated DM. In these cohorts, malignancy was associated with older age, male sex, and antibodies to either TIF-1γ or NXP-2 on multivariate analysis (OR 3.78).

The MDA-5 and TIF-1-gamma autoantibodies are largely considered investigational at present and are not routinely available in commercial laboratories. They are currently available through two laboratories in the United States (Johns Hopkins and Oklahoma Medical Research Foundation Myositis Testing Laboratory). These autoantibodies seem to define distinct clinical subsets and therefore may be useful in predicting patient outcomes in DM. The primary purpose of these autoantibodies is not in making a diagnosis of dermatomyositis but to potentially help prognosticate and alter screening practices for patients with DM in the future.

Interstitial lung disease in classic and skin-predominant dermatomyositis: a retrospective study with screening recommendations. Morganroth PA, Kreider ME, Okawa J, Taylor L, Werth VP. Arch Dermatol 2010; 146: 729–38.

In this retrospective cohort study, 23% of patients had interstitial lung disease (ILD) based on CT findings, and all of these had a reduced diffusion capacity (DLCO) on pulmonary function tests as well. Prevalence of ILD was not statistically different between patients with and without muscle disease. The authors conclude that serial DLCO testing is reasonable in all patients with DM to screen for pulmonary involvement.

Incidence of dermatomyositis and clinically amyopathic dermatomyositis: a population-based study in Olmstead County, Minnesota. Bendewald MJ, Wetter DA, Li X, Davis MD. Arch Dermatol 2010; 146: 26–30.

This retrospective population-based study found an overall age- and sex-adjusted incidence of dermatomyositis, including all subtypes, to be 9.63 (95% CI: 6.09–13.17) per 1 million persons, whereas the incidence of clinically amyopathic dermatomyositis was 2.08 (95% CI: 0.39–3.77) per 1 million persons. Twenty percent of the dermatomyositis cases were amyopathic in this population.

This epidemiologic study supports other data demonstrating that 20% to 30% of adult DM patients lack muscle involvement.

First-Line Therapies

For cutaneous disease

• Sunscreens	E
• Topical corticosteroids	E
• Antimalarials – hydroxychloroquine (HCQ) or chloroquine (CQ)	D
• Combination antimalarial therapy (quinacrine plus either HCQ or CQ)	E
• Methotrexate	D

For muscle disease

• Systemic corticosteroids	B
• Immunosuppressive agents – methotrexate, mycophenolate mofetil, azathioprine	A

The use of pulse corticosteroid therapy for juvenile dermatomyositis. Paller AS. Pediatr Dermatol 1996; 13: 347–8.

This report notes that pulse administration of systemic corticosteroids might result in less toxicity, and further that this therapy aids in the prevention of calcinosis.

Cutaneous lesions of dermatomyositis are improved by hydroxychloroquine. Woo TY, Callen JP, Voorhees JJ, Bickers D, Hanno R. J Am Acad Dermatol 1984; 10: 592–600.

Seven patients with cutaneous lesions of DM that had not responded to therapy with corticosteroids and/or immunosuppressive agents were treated with hydroxychloroquine 200 mg once or twice daily in an open study. The response to the addition of hydroxychloroquine was good in all patients, and three had total resolution of their skin lesions. In two patients the corticosteroid dosage could be tapered. Therapy with hydroxychloroquine did not appear to have any beneficial effect on the myositis.

Combination antimalarials in the treatment of cutaneous dermatomyositis: a retrospective study. Ang GC, Werth VP. Arch Dermatol 2005; 141: 855–9.

In this retrospective analysis, 7 of 17 patients experienced at least near clearance of cutaneous symptoms with the use of antimalarial therapy alone: 4 of them required combination therapy (hydroxychloroquine sulfate 200 mg once or twice daily + quinacrine hydrochloride 100 mg daily; or chloroquine phosphate 250 mg daily + quinacrine 100 mg daily), and 3 of them responded well to antimalarial monotherapy. The median time required to efficacy was 3 months.

When considering combination antimalarial agents as a therapeutic option, it is critical to use quinacrine in addition to either hydroxychloroquine or chloroquine, given that quinacrine lacks ocular toxicity. Hydroxychloroquine and chloroquine both have ocular toxicity and should not be given concurrently.

Adverse cutaneous reactions to hydroxychloroquine are more common in patients with dermatomyositis than in patients with cutaneous lupus erythematosus. Pelle MT, Callen JP. Arch Dermatol 2002; 138: 1231–3.

In this case-control study, 31% of patients with dermatomyositis developed a cutaneous reaction to hydroxychloroquine, compared with 2.5% of those with cutaneous lupus.

Given the fact that hydroxychloroquine is utilized as a first-line therapy for cutaneous DM, awareness of the increased risk of cutaneous reactions in approximately one third of DM patients is critical, as this can lead to worsening of the cutaneous DM and warrants cessation of hydroxychloroquine. A pretreatment warning is helpful in order to allow patients to alert the clinician to the development of a cutaneous reaction.

Second-Line Therapies

For cutaneous disease

- Topical calcineurin inhibitors
  (tacrolimus or pimecrolimus)   D
- Mycophenolate mofetil   D
- IVIG   A

For muscle disease

- Other immunosuppressive agents –
  cyclophosphamide, chlorambucil,
  cyclosporine, tacrolimus   D
- IVIG   A
- Rituximab   A

Topical tacrolimus 0.1% ointment for refractory skin disease in dermatomyositis: a pilot study. Hollar CB, Jorizzo JL. J Dermatol Treat 2004; 15: 35–9.

This open-label study of six patients with cutaneous DM treated with topical tacrolimus noted a very good to excellent response in two patients, a moderate response in one, and essentially no response in three.

This agent is worthy of a trial but does not seem to be highly effective.

Low-dose methotrexate administered weekly is an effective corticosteroid-sparing agent for the treatment of the cutaneous manifestations of dermatomyositis. Kasteler JS, Callen JP. J Am Acad Dermatol 1997; 36: 67–71.

The records of 13 patients who received oral methotrexate in doses ranging from 2.5 to 30 mg weekly were reviewed. Their skin lesions had not been completely responsive to sunscreens, topical corticosteroids, oral prednisone, oral antimalarial therapy, or, in 1 patient each, chlorambucil and azathioprine. Four of these 13 patients had complete clearance of cutaneous manifestations, and another 4 had almost complete clearance. In the remaining 5 patients, methotrexate induced moderate clearing of their cutaneous lesions. In all patients, the addition of methotrexate allowed a reduction in or discontinuation of other therapies, including prednisone.

Mycophenolate mofetil as an effective corticosteroid-sparing therapy for recalcitrant dermatomyositis. Edge JC, Outland JD, Dempsey JR, Callen JP. Arch Dermatol 2006; 142: 65–9.

Mycophenolate mofetil in dermatomyositis: is it safe? Rowin J, Amato AA, Deisher N, Cursio J, Meriggioli MN. Neurology 2006; 66: 1245–7.

These two open-label studies suggest that in 60% to 75% of patients with myositis, mycophenolate mofetil 1 to 1.5 g twice daily is an effective steroid-sparing agent for skin and muscle disease. Toxicity was noted in these relatively small case series, including an Epstein–Barr virus–associated lymphoma of the central nervous system in the former study, which resolved upon cessation of therapy, and opportunistic infections in the latter study, one of which was fatal.

This agent appears to be useful in some patients with refractory DM yet needs careful monitoring for the development of infection and potentially neoplasia.

A controlled trial of high-dose intravenous immune globulin infusions as treatment for dermatomyositis. Dalakas MC, Illa I, Dambrosia JM. N Engl J Med 1993; 329: 1993–2000.

These authors conducted a double-blind, placebo-controlled trial of IVIG in 15 patients with biopsy-proven treatment-resistant DM. The patients continued to receive prednisone (mean daily dose 25 mg) and were randomly assigned to receive one infusion of immunoglobulin (2 g/kg body weight) or placebo monthly for 3 months, with the option of crossing over to the alternative therapy for 3 more months. The 8 patients assigned to immunoglobulin showed a significant improvement in scores of muscle strength ($p < 0.018$) and neuromuscular symptoms ($p < 0.035$), whereas the 7 patients assigned to placebo did not. With crossovers, a total of 12 patients received immunoglobulin. Of these, 9 with severe disabilities showed a major improvement to near-normal function. Of 11 placebo-treated patients, none had a major improvement, 3 had a mild improvement, 3 had no change in their condition, and the condition of 5 worsened. Skin disease also responded in the treated patients, with 8 of 12 demonstrating "marked clearance" of cutaneous disease as assessed through clinical photographs.

Intravenous immunoglobulin for refractory cutaneous dermatomyositis: a retrospective analysis from an academic medical center. Femia AN, Eastham AB, Lam C, Merola JF, Qureshi AA, Vleugels RA. J Am Acad Dermatol 2013; 69: 654–7.

Clinical efficacy of intravenous immunoglobulins for the treatment of dermatomyositis skin lesions without muscle disease. Bounfour T, Bouaziz JD, Bezier M, Cordoliani F, Saussine A, Petit A, et al. J Eur Acad Dermatol Venereol 2014; 28: 1150–7.

Since the time of the small randomized controlled trial by Dalakas et al., two retrospective studies investigated the role of IVIG specifically in refractory cutaneous DM. The first study (Femia et al.) included 13 patients who received IVIG to specifically treat cutaneous DM. All patients, except 2, had previously been treated with various systemic immunosuppressive and immunomodulatory therapies, photoprotection, and topical agents. The validated CDASI was utilized when available to determine treatment response, in addition to review of clinical photography. All 13 patients demonstrated improvement on IVIG, with a complete clinical response noted in 8 patients. IVIG allowed for discontinuation of all concurrent immunosuppressive medications except in 2 patients.

A second retrospective study (Bounfour et al.) of 27 patients treated with IVIG for refractory cutaneous DM also found promising results. Utilizing clinical examination and photography, 19 of 27 patients were determined to have a major response to therapy, 4 demonstrated a partial response, and 4 had no response.

Chlorambucil. An effective corticosteroid-sparing agent for patients with recalcitrant dermatomyositis. Sinoway PA, Callen JP. Arthritis Rheum 1993; 36: 319–24.

Five patients with recalcitrant DM were treated with oral chlorambucil, 4 mg daily, after discontinuation of another immunosuppressive agent. Beneficial effects were noted within 4 to 6 weeks in all five patients, and corticosteroids were eventually discontinued in four. The chlorambucil was stopped after 13 to 30 months of treatment in four patients, and their disease remained in remission. Minimal chlorambucil toxicity was noted, consisting of leukopenia in two patients.

Although chlorambucil was effective, its potential for subsequent malignancy makes it a less desirable choice.

Cyclosporine A and intravenous immunoglobulin treatment in polymyositis/dermatomyositis. Danieli MG, Malcangi G, Palmieri C, Logullo F, Salvi A, Piani M, et al. Ann Rheum Dis 2002; 61: 37–41.

This is a retrospective review of 20 patients, including 12 with DM. It suggests that combining prednisone, cyclosporine, and IVIG was the most useful regimen.

A pilot trial of rituximab in the treatment of patients with dermatomyositis. Chung L, Genovese MC, Fiorentino DF. Arch Dermatol 2007; 143: 763–7.

In this open-label pilot study with seven evaluable patients who received 1-g infusions administered 2 weeks apart, only three had partial response of their muscle disease. Skin disease using the validated DSSI did not demonstrate notable improvement over the study period.

Rituximab in the treatment of refractory adult and juvenile dermatomyositis (DM) and adult polymyositis (PM): a randomized, placebo-phase trial (the RIM Study). Oddis CV, Reed AM, Aggarwal R, Ascherman DP, Barohn RJ, Feldman BM, et al. Arthritis Rheum 2013; 65: 314.

This multicenter randomized controlled trial of 200 participants, including 76 with DM, 48 with juvenile DM, and 76 with polymyositis, randomized participants to either a "rituximab early" arm, receiving drug at weeks 0 and 1 and placebo at weeks 8 and 9, or a "rituximab late" arm, receiving placebo at weeks 0 and 1 and rituximab at weeks 8 and 9. The primary end point, time to achieve improvement based on specifically defined muscle parameters, was not met, nor were the secondary end points, which were also based on muscle involvement. Despite this, 83% of patients met the definition of improvement (DOI) by week 44. In addition, a steroid-sparing effect of rituximab was noted in both groups. The authors propose that the trial design, particularly the short placebo phase of 8 weeks, may have reduced the ability to detect differences between the groups given the median time to DOI from rituximab. Of note, a validated DM skin index was not used in the rituximab for inflammatory myopathy (RIM Study).

Although design concerns with the RIM Study make recommendations regarding the use of rituximab in DM challenging, it is used for refractory muscle disease. At this time, however, there is little data to support the use of rituximab for cutaneous dermatomyositis specifically.

Third-Line Therapies	
• Dapsone for cutaneous disease	E
• Thalidomide for cutaneous disease	E
• Antiestrogen medication for cutaneous disease	E
• Diltiazem for calcinosis	D
• Total body irradiation	D
• Rituximab for cutaneous disease	D
• Leflunomide	E
• Sirolimus	E
• Tocilizumab	E
• Anakinra	D
• Sifalimumab	D
• Tofacitinib, ruxolitinib (JAK inhibitors)	D, E
• Stem cell transplantation	D

Calcinosis cutis occurring in association with autoimmune connective tissue disease: the Mayo Clinic experience with 78 patients, 1996 to 2009. Balin SJ, Wetter DA, Andersen LK, Davis MD. Arch Dermatol 2012; 148: 455–62.

This retrospective study found that DM and systemic sclerosis were the most common autoimmune connective tissue diseases associated with calcinosis cutis. Therapy with diltiazem resulted in partial benefit in 9 of 17 patients. Of 28 patients who had surgical excision of one or more lesions, 22 noted complete response, 5 had partial response, and 1 patient did not respond.

A wide variety of agents have been used in the treatment of DM-associated calcinosis, although none is uniformly effective.

Open-label trial of anti-TNF-alpha in dermato- and polymyositis treated concomitantly with methotrexate. Hengstman GJ, De Bleecker JL, Feist E, Vissing J, Denton CP, Manoussakis MN, et al. Eur Neurol 2008; 59: 159–63.

Although case series and reports have suggested that anti–tumor necrosis factor alpha (TNF-α) agents may be useful in DM, this open-label trial found differing results. The trial was terminated prematurely due to low rate of patient enrollment, as well as poor responses in many patients. The authors conclude that TNF antagonists do not have a place in the therapeutic armamentarium of dermatomyositis.

A randomized, pilot trial of etanercept in dermatomyositis. Amato A. Ann Neurol 2011; 70: 427–36.

In this randomized double-blind placebo-controlled trial of 16 participants with DM on prednisone (11 randomized to etanercept arm 50 mg subcutaneously weekly for 52 weeks and 5 to placebo arm), a steroid-sparing effect was demonstrated in 5 patients in the treatment arm. There was no statistically significant difference in skin disease response assessed by CDASI between the groups. In addition, cutaneous disease worsened in five etanercept-treated patients.

In addition to the potential worsening of muscle disease in patients with DM treated with anti-TNF-α therapy, reports of TNF inhibitor-associated DM have been reported. For these reasons, anti-TNF therapy is utilized with caution in patients with DM, and some experts suggest that the use of these agents in DM should occur only in the setting of approved clinical trials.

Improvement in dermatomyositis rash associated with the use of antiestrogen medication. Sereda D, Werth VP. Arch Dermatol 2006; 142: 70–2.

In this report, two women experienced improvement in their DM-associated skin eruptions while taking antiestrogen medication, either tamoxifen, a selective estrogen receptor modulator, or anastrozole, an aromatase inhibitor. When tamoxifen therapy was discontinued after 4 years of use in the first patient, her cutaneous DM worsened and remained difficult to control with conventional immunosuppressive agents

This observation offers a novel approach to consider for women with DM; however, no further reports of either medication have appeared in the literature.

Rapamycin (sirolimus) as a steroid-sparing agent in dermatomyositis. Nadiminti U, Arbiser JL. J Am Acad Dermatol 2005; 52: 17–9.

A single case of dermatomyositis that was recalcitrant to prior therapies responded to this antirejection agent 5 mg/day for 2 weeks, then 2 mg/day. Both muscle disease and skin manifestations were noted to improve.

Anakinra treatment in patients with refractory inflammatory myopathies and possible predictive response biomarkers: a mechanistic study with 12 months of follow-up. Zong M, Dorph C, Dastmalchi M, Alexanderson H, Pieper J, Amoudruz P, et al. Ann Rheum Dis 2014; 73: 913–20.

An open-label trial of 15 patients with refractory myositis, 4 of whom had DM, received anakinra for a 12-month period. Three of the four DM patients had improvement in their cutaneous disease, but no validated skin index was used.

Remission of recalcitrant dermatomyositis treated with ruxolitinib. Hournung T, Janzen V, Heidgen FJ, Wolf D, Bieber T, Wenzel J. N Engl J Med 2014; 371: 2537–8.

A case of refractory DM was incidentally noted to have complete resolution of both muscle weakness and cutaneous disease based on CDASI scores after being treated with ruxolitinib, a JAK 1 and 2 selective inhibitor, for concurrent myelofibrosis. The patient was able to discontinue systemic corticosteroids, mycophenolate mofetil, and IVIG while taking ruxolitinib.

Future studies or observations of this and other JAK inhibitors might add another agent to our therapeutic armamentarium for DM.

Efficacy of allogeneic mesenchymal stem cell transplantation in patients with drug-resistant polymyositis and dermatomyositis. Wang D, Zhang H, Cao M, Tang Y, Liang J, Feng X. J Ann Rheum Dis 2011; 70: 1285–8.

An open study of 10 patients with refractory DM ($n = 4$) or polymyositis who underwent stem cell transplantation (SCT) noted recurrence of disease in 3 patients and death in 2 patients. The remaining patients had improvement in muscle disease, pulmonary disease, and chronic cutaneous ulcers.

Other reports of patients with adult and juvenile DM have noted improvement in both skin disease and calcinosis after SCT in severe cases. Given infection risks, SCT is considered only in highly refractory cases at this time.

Evidence Levels: **A** Double-blind study **B** Clinical trial ≥ 20 subjects **C** Clinical trial < 20 subjects **D** Series ≥ 5 subjects **E** Anecdotal case reports

Diaper dermatitis

Catalina Matiz, Lawrence F. Eichenfield

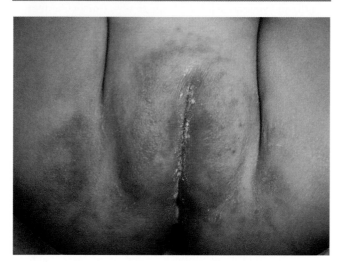

Diaper (napkin) dermatitis encompasses a broad set of conditions, although the most common form is irritant contact dermatitis. Irritant diaper dermatitis usually presents as erythema and mild scaling on the convex surfaces of the inner upper thigh, lower abdomen, and buttock areas, classically sparing the inguinal folds where the skin is not in contact with irritants. It usually presents as early as a few days after birth to as late as several years of age, whereas diaper use in older disabled and geriatric patients may be identical in pathogenesis and physical findings. Many other dermatoses such as psoriasis, seborrheic dermatitis, allergic contact dermatitis, acrodermatitis enteropathica, infections (*Candida*, *Staphylococcus*, and *Streptococcus*), and Langerhans cell histiocytosis can affect the diaper area and may need to be excluded.

MANAGEMENT STRATEGY

Irritant diaper dermatitis is triggered by irritants present in the area covered by the diaper, which acts as an occlusive surface. Moisture from urine and feces increases the friction coefficient of the skin, causing frictional damage. Skin integrity is further compromised by the increased pH from urine and fecal enzymes and the physical erosive effects of these activated enzymes. The reduction in skin barrier function and increase in pH contribute to the increased susceptibility to infections with microorganisms such as *C. albicans*, which further increases the severity of diaper dermatitis. Therefore management should aim at preventing overhydration and frictional damage in the diaper area.

Frequent diaper changes, particularly after defecation, reduce moisture and prevent the build-up of irritants. This is therefore one of the most important steps in the management of diaper dermatitis. Disposable diapers containing superabsorbent gelling materials and breathable backsheets are preferred to those without. Cloth diapers should be avoided, as they have been shown to be associated with an increased incidence of irritant diaper dermatitis compared with disposable diapers.

The skin in the area may be cleaned with water alone, with mild soap, or with commercial wipes. Optimally, wipes should not contain fragrance, isothiazolinones, iodopropyl butylcarbamate, or alcohol. Rubbing of the area can cause damage to the skin and should be avoided.

A *barrier cream* may be applied at every diaper change. This can provide a barrier between the skin and irritants in order to reduce friction and contact with stool and urine.

A *low-potency topical steroid* such as hydrocortisone 1% ointment can be used in more severe cases of diaper dermatitis, but must be used sparingly to avoid skin atrophy and systemic absorption. High-potency steroids should be avoided in diaper dermatitis, including the use of compound formulations containing potent steroids and antimicrobial agents.

Topical antifungal preparations are recommended for use in proven or suspected cases of *C. albicans* infection.

Specific Investigations

- Inquiry about recent antibiotic usage (predisposing to *Candida*)

  In selected cases:
- KOH preparation, fungal and bacterial cultures
- Serum zinc and biotin levels
- Skin biopsy
- Patch testing

Diaper dermatitis: clinical characteristics and differential diagnosis. Coughlin CC, Eichenfield LF, Frieden IJ. Pediatr Dermatol 2014; 31(Suppl 1):19–24.

This article characterizes three subgroups: skin conditions caused by the presence of the diaper, eruptions exacerbated by the diaper, and rashes present regardless of the presence of the diaper. Those caused by the presence of the diaper include irritant diaper dermatitis and its different presentations, as well as allergic contact dermatitis. The conditions exacerbated by the diaper include infectious causes (yeast and bacteria), seborrheic dermatitis, and psoriasis. The third group includes infantile hemangiomas, Langerhans cell histiocytosis, zinc deficiency, Kawasaki disease, and Coxsackie virus.

Potential allergens in disposable diaper wipes, topical diaper preparations and disposable diapers: under-recognized etiology of pediatric perineal dermatitis. Yu J, Treat J, Chaney K, Brod B. Dermatitis 2016; 27: 110–8.

Botanical extracts, which include members of the Compositae family, were the top potential allergens in both diaper wipes and topical preparations. Others identified include tocopherol, fragrances, propylene glycol, parabens, iodopropynyl butylcarbamate, and lanolin.

Patch test series for allergic perineal dermatitis in the diapered infant. Yu J, Treat J, Brod B. Dermatitis 2017; 28: 70–5.

Two suggested allergen panels for evaluation of perineal dermatitis in children.

The role of allergic contact dermatitis in diaper dermatitis. Smith WJ, Jacob SE. Pediatr Dermatol 2009; 26: 369–70.

Allergens to consider include many chemicals added to diapers, as well as preservatives in baby wipes. For example, sorbitan sesquioleate, fragrances, and disperse dye have been increasingly reported to cause contact dermatitis in the diaper area. Cyclohexl thiopthalimide and mercaptobenzothiazole, which are rubber additives, tend to cause "lucky Luke" dermatitis, a pattern that resembles a cowboy's holster due to elastic bands coming into contact with the skin. The authors suggest patch testing in diaper dermatitis that fails to improve despite treatment.

First-Line Therapies

• Water-repellant barrier cream	A
• Frequent changing of diapers	B
• Superabsorbent disposable diapers	A

Modern diaper performance: construction, materials, and safety review. Dey S, Kenneally D, Odio M, Hatzopoulos I. Int J Dermatol 2016; 55(Suppl 1): 18–20.

Typical modern diapers do not contain concerning ingredients such as latex and disperse dyes, but use spandex and pigments with a favorable safety profile. Today's disposable diapers are designed with layers and liners for optimal urine and feces absorption.

Prevention, diagnosis, and management of diaper dermatitis. Nield LS, Kamat D. Clin Pediatr (Philadelphia) 2007; 46: 480–6.

Differential diagnoses, prevention, and management strategies of diaper dermatitis in a stepwise, tabular format. The key prevention strategy is to keep the area dry. This can be accomplished by using superabsorbent disposable diapers, frequent diaper changes, eliminating irritants (e.g., avoiding baby wipes that contain fragrance and alcohol), using a water-impermeable topical barrier, and allowing for daily diaper-free time.

Diaper dermatitis and advances in diaper technology. Odio M, Friedlander SF. Curr Opin Pediatr 2000; 12: 342–6.

Absorbent gelling materials (AGM) have been proved to reduce skin overhydration and reduce the frequency and severity of diaper dermatitis compared with cellulose-only disposable diapers. In a study with nearly 4000 children, a temporal association between the introduction of AGM and a reduction in the incidence of severe diaper dermatitis was found. Polymeric covers or films, commonly known as *breathable backsheets*, allow moisture vapor to flow out of the diaper and significantly reduce overhydration in the area. The inner lining of diapers designed to deliver a petrolatum-based formulation to the skin continuously during use has been shown to be associated with a statistically significant and sustained reduction in the severity of diaper dermatitis.

Clinical approaches to skin cleansing of the diaper area: practice and challenges. Coughlin CC, Frieden IJ, Eichenfield LF. Pediatr Dermatol 2014; 31(Suppl 1): 1–4.

The authors very nicely review important factors in diaper area care, including skin pH, the local microbiome, irritant and allergic potential of certain products, and application of topical agents. The use of wet wipes is concluded to be a widespread practice, which is well tolerated and effective in several populations, including preterm infants.

Second-Line Therapies

• 1% hydrocortisone ointment	D
• Topical antifungal agent (miconazole, clotrimazole, nystatin, ketoconazole)	A

A prospective 2-year assessment of miconazole resistance in *Candida* spp. with repeated treatment with 0.25% miconazole nitrate ointment in neonates and infants with moderate to severe diaper dermatitis complicated by cutaneous candidiasis. Blanco D, van Rossem K. Pediatr Dermatol 2013; 30: 717–24.

This multicenter, open-label, long-term, phase IV study investigated the potential resistance of *Candida* spp. to repeated topical use of 0.25% miconazole nitrate in infants age 15 months and younger with moderate to severe diaper dermatitis complicated with cutaneous candidiasis. Results of the study showed that about half of the patients achieved clinical cure, 45.8% achieved a mycologic cure, and 29.2% achieved an overall cure (clinical and mycologic). The treatment with 0.25% miconazole nitrate ointment was effective and generally well tolerated. There was no evidence of resistance to miconazole in candida.

Efficacy and safety of two different antifungal pastes in infants with diaper dermatitis: a randomized, controlled study. Hoeger PH, Stark S, Jost G. J Eur Acad Dermatol Venereol 2010; 24: 1094–8.

This double-blinded, multicenter trial compared 1% clotrimazole versus nystatin with 20% zinc oxide for the treatment of diaper dermatitis complicated by *Candida* infection. Clotrimazole was superior to nystatin in symptom reduction. Both clotrimazole and nystatin had microbiologic cure rates of 100%, and both were safe and well tolerated.

Absorption and efficacy of miconazole nitrate 0.25% ointment in infants with diaper dermatitis. Eichenfield LF, Bogen ML. J Drugs Dermatol 2007; 6: 522–6.

Twenty-four infants with moderate to severe diaper dermatitis were evaluated for relative safety from systemic absorption of topical miconazole. Nineteen received 0.25% miconazole nitrate ointment, and five received 2% miconazole nitrate cream for 7 days. Blood concentrations in the 0.25% miconazole nitrate treatment group were undetectable in 83% and minimal in 17%, thereby demonstrating its safety as a treatment for diaper dermatitis.

Pediatricians who prescribe clotrimazole-betamethasone dipropionate (Lotrisone) often utilize it in inappropriate settings regardless of their knowledge of the drug's potency. Railan D, Wilson JK, Feldman SR, Fleischer AB. Dermatol Online J 2002; 8: 3.

High-potency topical corticosteroids can cause skin atrophy and systemic absorption. Products combining antibiotics with high-potency corticosteroids should be avoided in the diaper area.

Third-Line Therapies

• Continuous administration of petrolatum and zinc oxide by disposable diaper	A
• Oral antifungal agent	E

Skin benefits from continuous topical administration of a zinc oxide/petrolatum formulation by a novel disposable diaper. Baldwin S, Odio MR, Haines SL, O'Connor RJ, Englehart JS, Lane AT. J Eur Acad Dermatol Venereol 2001; 1: 5–11.

A double-blind, randomized trial comparing regular diapers to diapers designed to continuously deliver zinc oxide and

Evidence Levels: A Double-blind study B Clinical trial ≥ 20 subjects C Clinical trial < 20 subjects D Series ≥ 5 subjects E Anecdotal case reports

petrolatum in 268 infants over a 4-week period. The ointment formulation was effectively transferred to the skin, and a significant reduction in skin erythema and rash was observed in the treatment group compared with controls.

Contact dermatitis. Friedlander SF. Pediatr Rev 1998; 19: 166–71.

Some diaper dermatitis persists despite first- and second-line therapies. In these recalcitrant cases oral Mycostatin may be beneficial. In addition, an evaluation of the mother for infections of the nipples or genital tract should be considered, as continuous reinoculation of the infant is possible. If positive, a short course of oral fluconazole (5–7 days) can help eradicate the infection.

Discoid (Nummular) eczema

Ian H. Coulson

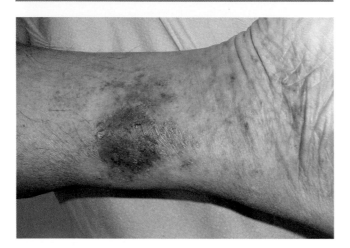

Discoid eczema comprises relatively well-defined, usually multiple, coin-sized plaques. In the acute stages they often weep or ooze; in the chronic phase lesions are discrete, hyperkeratotic, or lichenified. Itching is usual. It primarily affects the limbs (especially the legs), sometimes the trunk, and rarely the face or flexures.

MANAGEMENT STRATEGY

Discoid eczema (nummular dermatitis) has many causes. It is usually idiopathic in older patients, but similar lesions may occur due to contact allergic reactions, as a pattern of hand and foot eczema, in atopic dermatitis (AD), as an "id" eruption related to venous eczema, or locally (e.g., after trauma, insect bite reactions, "halo eczema" around melanocytic nevi). Discoid eczema has been reported as a manifestation of drug reaction to gold, tumor necrosis factor (TNF) antagonists, interferon, and retinoids. Comparisons among studies may be limited if the site(s) and etiology are not stated or represent a mixed spectrum.

There are few publications on the pathophysiology of discoid eczema to inform treatment. An association with dry skin (xerosis) is documented, and discoid lesions may appear during treatment with isotretinoin (which reduces sebum secretion). However, dry skin is not consistently present, and the morphology of discoid eczema differs from that of xerosis or asteatotic eczema.

One study suggested that patients with discoid eczema have a degree of xerosis similar to that of age-matched controls but have stronger delayed hypersensitivity to allergens that permeate the skin as a result of scratching. A link with atopy has been proposed, but serum IgE levels are generally normal.

Occult infections (e.g., dental abscess) and infections causing dry skin (e.g., leprosy) have rarely been linked with discoid eczema. *Helicobacter pylori* has been implicated, but the evidence is weak.

It is difficult to provide specific therapeutic strategies because of the various different causes and the paucity of pertinent publications; most reports are retrospective from individual departments or are anecdotal, rather than formal, trials. The main therapeutic issues are:

- Other disorders may need to be excluded, especially mycoses, psoriasis, Bowen disease, mycosis fungoides, and sarcoidosis.
- A medication and alcohol history should be taken.
- Patch testing may be useful; metals and medicaments (such as fusidic acid, lanolin, neomycin, and cetostearyl alcohol) are most implicated.
- The management of discoid eczema is generally similar to that of other eczemas; *emollients* appear to be helpful due to the link with dry skin.
- The mainstay of treatment is *topical corticosteroids*. Severe itch in discoid eczema usually dictates that strong agents are applied; this is safe because the individual lesions are small, rarely affect thin skin sites such as the face or flexures, and usually respond to this approach. Chronic lichenified lesions may respond better to steroid-impregnated tapes or by using a potent steroid with hydrocolloid dressing or paste bandage occlusion.
- *Calcineurin antagonists* have been used successfully both as monotherapy and in combination with topical steroids, but trials specifically looking at efficacy in discoid eczema exclusively, rather than atopic eczema generally, are lacking.
- If weeping is present, the use of soaks (with, e.g., 1 in 10,000 *potassium permanganate* solution) will help dry lesions up and prevent lesions from sticking to clothes or dressings.
- Secondary impetiginization, particularly in the exudative phase, is common, and combining a *topical antibiotic or antiseptic,* or the use of an *oral antistaphylococcal antibiotic,* helps.
- *Tar*-based treatments and impregnated bandages to minimize the effects of scratching may help.
- *Sedating antihistamines* before retiring will help nocturnal scratching and minimize excoriation.
- *Systemic immunosuppressive therapies* are usually not required.

Newer drugs such as *biological agents* (dupilumab) and small molecules such as *apremilast* and *topical PDE 4 antagonists* show efficacy in atopic eczema, but specific reports relating to discoid eczema are lacking to date.

Specific Investigations

- None usually required, except to exclude differential diagnoses
- Consider medications as a cause
- Consider mycology
- Consider patch testing
- Bacteriology if secondary infection likely
- Consider occult infections in resistant cases

Pityriasis rosea and discoid eczema: dose related reactions to treatment with gold. Wilkinson SM, Smith AG, Davis MJ, Mattey D, Dawes PT. Ann Rheum Dis 1992; 51: 881–4.

Discoid eczematous lesions occur in up to 30% of patients on gold therapy and may be dose related.

Severe, generalized nummular eczema secondary to interferon alpha-2b plus ribavirin combination therapy in a patient with chronic hepatitis C virus infection. Moore MM, Elpern J, Carter DJ. Arch Dermatol 2004; 140: 215–7.

Evidence Levels: **A** Double-blind study **B** Clinical trial ≥ 20 subjects **C** Clinical trial < 20 subjects **D** Series ≥ 5 subjects **E** Anecdotal case reports

Cutaneous disease and alcohol misuse. Higgins EM, du Vivier AW. Br Med Bull 1994; 50: 85–98.

Documents a strong link between discoid eczema and alcohol consumption.

Patch testing in discoid eczema. Fleming C, Parry E, Forsyth A, Kemmett D. Contact Dermatitis 1997; 36: 261–4.

Retrospective study of persistent and severe discoid eczema; 24 of 48 cases were positive (16 relevant) to rubber chemicals, formaldehyde, neomycin, chromate, and nickel.

Patch testing in discoid eczema. Khurana S, Jain VK, Aggarwal K, Gupta S. J Dermatol 2002; 29: 763–7.

Positive tests in 28 of 50 patients with relatively chronic discoid eczema, mainly to dichromate, nickel, cobalt, and fragrance. However, 44% had a purely hand-and-foot pattern and only 12% a trunk and limb distribution.

Challenge with metal salts. (II). Various types of eczema. Veien NK, Hattel T, Justesen O, Nørholm A. Contact Dermatitis 1983; 9: 407–10.

Patch testing can be helpful. Larger series suggest a 50% positive test rate, with clinical relevance in many. However, these are based on testing patients with chronic or therapy-resistant discoid eczema (i.e., a selected, potentially unrepresentative group); most reports are anecdotal. Implicated agents include chromate, nickel, mercury, thimerosal, rubber chemicals, formaldehyde, neomycin, fragrances, aloe, ethylene diamine, cyanoacrylate glue, textile dyes, and epoxy resin. Oral metal challenge tests rarely induce flares of discoid eczema. Irritants may also cause discoid eczema.

Dental infection associated with nummular eczema as an overlooked focal infection. Tanaka T, Satoh T, Yokozeki H. J Dermatol 2009; 36: 462–5.

Thirteen cases of extensive discoid eczema with moderate to severe odontogenic infections detected by panoramic x-ray screening test. In 11 patients, skin lesions partially or completely improved after the dental treatment.

First-Line Therapies

• Topical corticosteroids ± antibacterial agents	C
• Emollients	C
• Tar-based preparations	C
• Oral antibiotics	C
• Oral antihistamines	C
• Topical doxepin	A

Most of these are standard treatments for discoid eczema; however, in terms of evidence grading, most studies include a variety of different eczemas, few specifically identify results for discoid eczema, and no comparative trials have been identified.

Successful treatment of therapy-resistant atopic dermatitis with clobetasol propionate and a hydrocolloid occlusive dressing. Volden G. Acta Derm Venereol 1992; 176: 126–8.

Nummular AD lesions cleared rapidly.

Topical corticosteroids are the usual first-line therapy. Trial evidence is limited to pharmaceutically sponsored studies that are not specific to discoid eczema.

Nummular eczema. A review, follow-up and analysis of a series of 325 cases. Cowan MA. Acta Derm Venereol 1961; 41: 453–60.

Tar preparations were the main treatment. Recurrent crops of lesions occurred in 25% of cases, and relapse occurred when treatment was discontinued in 53% of patients, presumably representing the natural history of the disease, but possibly reflecting the limitations of therapy available at the time (other options were hydrocortisone or superficial x-ray therapy).

Tar preparations, historically used in the treatment of discoid eczema, have been largely superseded by potent topical corticosteroids as first-line therapy.

The antipruritic effect of 5% doxepin cream in patients with eczematous dermatitis. Drake LA, Millikan LE. Arch Dermatol 1995; 131: 1403–8.

Significant improvement in itch after 1 day, not at 7 days.

Studies suggest that doxepin has a short-term effect on itch only.

The use of antibacterial agents (e.g., clioquinol) or antibiotics is based on the fact that lesions are often moist and crusted. Secondary staphylococcal infection, as in AD, may aggravate the eczematous process.

Occlusion over a topical corticosteroid has been reported to lead to lesion clearance in previously therapy-resistant patients with discoid lesions due to AD; soaking in water for 20 minutes before treatment application has been recommended for a range of eczemas.

As with other itchy dermatoses, sedating antihistamines may help symptoms; the increase in mast cells in lesions provides the rationale for this approach. However, histamine itself has not been shown to be important.

Second-Line Therapies

• Phototherapy (broadband or narrowband UVB, 311 nm)	E
• Photochemotherapy (psoralen plus UVA, PUVA)	E
• Topical immune modulators	E
• Ciclosporin	E
• Intralesional corticosteroid injection	E
• Oral corticosteroids	E

Formal trials of these treatments in discoid eczema are lacking, and therefore the evidence gradings are weak; however, all are useful in AD or other dermatitis (see gradings in Atopic dermatitis, Chapter 17) and are therefore likely to be effective in discoid eczema. Personal experience is that narrowband UVB or ciclosporin is useful if required.

Photochemotherapy beyond psoriasis. Honig B, Morison WL, Karp D. J Am Acad Dermatol 1994; 31: 775–90.

Review article. Nothing specific to discoid eczema, but several eczemas respond to PUVA.

Half-side comparison study on the efficacy of 8-methoxypsoralen bath–PUVA versus narrow-band ultraviolet B phototherapy in patients with severe chronic atopic dermatitis. Der-Petrossian M, Seeber A, Honigsmann H, Tanew A. Br J Dermatol 2000; 142: 39–43.

Both were equivalent (at equi-erythemogenic doses) in AD.

Phototherapies also reduce staphylococci and superantigens and therefore may improve eczema with weeping and infection.

Antimicrobial effects of phototherapy and photochemotherapy in vivo and in vitro. Yoshimura M, Namura S, Akamatsu H, Horio T. Br J Dermatol 1996; 135: 528–32.

Antimicrobial effects are apparent after a single exposure.

Suppressive effect of ultraviolet (UVB and PUVA) radiation on superantigen production by *Staphylococcus aureus*. Yoshimura-Mishima M, Namura S, Akamatsu H, Horio T. J Dermatol Sci 1999; 19: 31–6.

Hand dermatitis: a review of clinical features, therapeutic options, and long-term outcomes. Warshaw E, Lee G, Storrs FJ. Am J Contact Dermat 2003; 14: 119–37.

One review recommends topical tacrolimus or pimecrolimus for nummular hand dermatitis. No evaluable evidence presented.

Long-term efficacy and safety of ciclosporin in severe adult atopic dermatitis. Berth-Jones J, Graham-Brown RA, Marks R, Camp RD, English JS, Freeman K, et al. Br J Dermatol 1997; 136: 76–81.

An open study of 100 patients with AD, with mostly good responses.

Side effects (drug interactions, hypertension, nephrotoxicity) limit ciclosporin therapy in older patients with discoid eczema, compared with AD. It is possibly useful for intermittent short-term treatment.

Oral corticosteroids are generally unnecessary. Intralesional corticosteroid injection is impractical, except in patients who have a small number of persistent thickened lesions.

Third-Line Therapies	
• Azathioprine	E
• Methotrexate	C
• Mycophenolate mofetil	E
• Hypnosis	D
• Relaxation therapy	D

As for second-line therapies, formal trials of these treatments in discoid eczema are lacking, and therefore the evidence gradings are weak; however, all are useful in AD or other dermatitis (see gradings in atopic dermatitis, Chapter 17) and are therefore likely to be effective in discoid eczema.

Azathioprine in dermatologic practice. An overview with special emphasis on its use in nonbullous inflammatory dermatoses. Scerri L. Adv Exp Med Biol 1999; 445: 343–8.

Documents the efficacy of azathioprine in AD and pompholyx.

Azathioprine in dermatology: a survey of current practice in the UK. Tan BB, Lear JT, Gawkrodger DJ, English JSC. Br J Dermatol 1997; 136: 351–5.

A questionnaire to 248 dermatologists showed that none was using azathioprine for discoid eczema.

Azathioprine is used in the treatment of several dermatoses, including various eczemas. It is likely to be beneficial in discoid eczema, although a study of azathioprine prescribing by UK dermatologists did not identify this as a current indication.

Methotrexate is a safe and effective treatment for pediatric discoid (nummular) eczema: a case series of 25 children. Roberts H, Orchard D. Australas J Dermatol 2010; 51: 128–30.

Sixteen out of 25 children completely cleared their eczema after an average of 10.5 months of methotrexate at a dose of 5 to 10 mg a week. A further three patients responded well but incompletely. Treatment was well tolerated, so it should be considered for recalcitrant or disabling disease.

Hypnosis in dermatology. Shenefelt PD. Arch Dermatol 2000; 136: 393–9.

Hypnosis as a complementary therapy may improve lesions or itch in discoid eczema.

Treatment of atopic dermatitis: a comparison of psychological and dermatologic approaches to relapse prevention. Ehlers A, Stangier U, Gieler J. Consult Clin Psychol 1995; 63: 624–35.

Although this study related to adults with atopic eczema, it may be applicable to discoid eczema too. Relaxation therapy produced a sustained benefit over a year and significantly reduced topical steroid use.

Evidence Levels: **A** Double-blind study **B** Clinical trial ≥ 20 subjects **C** Clinical trial < 20 subjects **D** Series ≥ 5 subjects **E** Anecdotal case reports

Discoid lupus erythematosus

Bruce H. Thiers

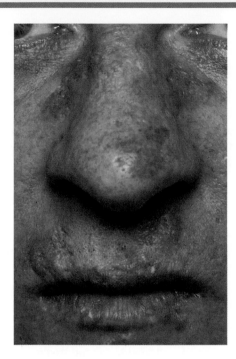

Discoid lupus erythematosus (DLE) is the most common form of chronic cutaneous lupus erythematosus (CCLE). Lesions predominate in sun-exposed areas, especially the face, scalp, upper chest, upper back, and extensor arms. Early lesions consist of sharply demarcated, erythematous, often hyperpigmented, hyperkeratotic papules and small plaques with adherent scale. The individual lesions spread peripherally, resulting in atrophy and central scarring, which may be associated with alopecia, telangiectasia, and depigmentation.

MANAGEMENT STRATEGY

The lesions of DLE are quite characteristic, especially in their later stages. When the diagnosis is in doubt, a skin biopsy should be performed. The histologic findings are usually diagnostic, although direct immunofluorescence examination can be obtained in questionable cases. A complete history and physical examination should be performed, looking for signs of systemic disease. Laboratory examinations to be obtained include a complete blood count with differential, erythrocyte sedimentation rate, serum chemistry profile, and urinalysis. Serum should be screened for antinuclear antibodies (ANAs) and Ro(SSA)/La(SSB) antibodies. It should be emphasized that although, as mentioned earlier, DLE is the most common form of CCLE, most patients do not have systemic involvement. Risk factors for systemic disease include widespread skin lesions, anemia or leukopenia, and a positive ANA, especially when the titer is high. Despite the relative infrequency of internal involvement, aggressive treatment of DLE is warranted because the scarring

from the disease can be devastating. The characteristic "carpet tack" scale associated with lesions indicates follicular involvement, and the disease can result in permanent scarring alopecia. Moreover, the depigmentation in fully evolved lesions can be disfiguring, especially in dark-skinned individuals. The goal of therapy is to halt the inflammatory process quickly and effectively to prevent these changes. The predominance of lesions in exposed areas emphasizes the urgency for prompt effective therapy.

Patients should be counseled on the role of ultraviolet (UV) light in the provocation of skin lesions, and a program of sun avoidance and sunscreen use should be instituted. Corticosteroids, either topical or intralesional, are the cornerstone of initial therapy for patients with limited involvement. Hydroxychloroquine and other antimalarial drugs appear to afford a measure of photoprotection and are often quite effective, although their onset of action is relatively slow. Systemic retinoids are useful, especially for hyperkeratotic lesions. Cytotoxic agents are generally reserved for refractory cases. The role of thalidomide and its analog, lenalidomide, in the treatment of DLE is evolving.

Specific Investigations

- Autoantibody studies
- Indicators of systemic disease

Cutaneous lupus erythematosus: an update on pathogenesis, diagnosis and treatment. Hejazi EZ, Werth VP. Am J Clin Dermatol 2016; 17: 135–46.

This article reviews the three recognized subtypes of cutaneous lupus erythematosus, including the acute, subacute, and chronic forms, as well as the nonspecific cutaneous manifestations of the disease. Diagnostic strategies that encompass histopathology, immunopathology, serology, and other laboratory studies are discussed, and an overview of treatment is provided.

First-Line Therapies

• Sunscreens	B
• Topical or intralesional corticosteroids	B
• Topical calcineurin inhibitors	B

A multicenter photoprovocation study to identify potential biomarkers by global peptide profiling in cutaneous lupus erythematosus. Calderon C, Zucht HD, Kuhn A, Wozniacka A, Szepietowski JC, Nyberg F, et al. Lupus 2015; 24: 1406–20.

Cutaneous lupus erythematosus can be precipitated and aggravated by exposure to UV light. Attempts have been made to identify biomarkers for predicting photosensitivity. Recommendation for use of a broad-spectrum sunscreen that includes protection against both UVB (sun protection factor 15 or higher) and UVA (e.g., containing oxybenzone, avobenzone, or ecamsule) is an essential disease management strategy.

Efficacy of tacrolimus 0.1% ointment in cutaneous lupus erythematosus: a multicenter, randomized, double-blind, vehicle controlled trial. Kuhn A, Gensch K, Haust M, Schneider SW, Bonsmann G, Gaebelein-Wissing N, et al. J Am Acad Dermatol 2011; 65: 54–64.

Effectiveness of topical calcineurin inhibitors as monotherapy or in combination with hydroxychloroquine in cutaneous lupus erythematosus. Avgerinou G, Papafragkaki DK, Nasiopoulou A, Arapaki A, Katsambas A, Stavropoulos PG. J Eur Acad Dermatol Venereol 2012; 26: 762–7.

The macrolactam immunosuppressive agents, tacrolimus and pimecrolimus, have been reported to be effective in the topical treatment of lesions of DLE, although most reports have consisted of uncontrolled case studies. These trials confirm that they may provide at least temporary benefit for patients with acute, edematous, nonhyperkeratotic lesions, particularly when cutaneous atrophy, either disease or treatment related, is a concern. Hypertrophic lesions may not respond well to calcineurin inhibitors or to other topical therapies, presumably because of limited penetration. Topical calcineurin inhibitors can also be used in combination with systemic therapy (e.g., hydroxychloroquine).

Second-Line Therapies

• Antimalarial drugs	B
• Systemic retinoids	B

Updated recommendations on the use of hydroxychloroquine in dermatologic practice. Anthony P. Fernandez. J Am Acad Dermatol 2017; 76:1176-1182.

Recommendations on Screening for Chloroquine and Hydroxychloroquine Retinopathy (2016 Revision). Marmor MF, Kellner U, Lai TY, Melles RB, Mieler WF, American Academy of Ophthalmology. Ophthalmology 2016; 123: 1386-94.

Long-term response to hydroxychloroquine in patients with discoid lupus erythematosus. Wahie S, Meggitt SJ. Br J Dermatol 2013; 169: 653–9.

The effect of increasing the dose of hydroxychloroquine (HCQ) in patients with refractory cutaneous lupus erythematosus (CLE): an open-label prospective pilot study. Chasset F, Arnaud L, Costedoat-Chalumeau N, Zahr N, Bessis D, Francés C. J Am Acad Dermatol 2016; 74: 693–9.

Influence of smoking on the efficacy of antimalarials in cutaneous lupus: a meta-analysis of the literature. Chasset F, Francés C, Barete S, Amoura Z, Arnaud L. J Am Acad Dermatol 2015; 72: 634–9.

Antimalarial drugs are favored for long-term treatment of DLE and are effective in many patients for whom topical therapy alone is unsuccessful or impractical, although in some series the long-term response rate is <50%. In most patients, 6 weeks of treatment is needed before they begin to exert their effect. Hydroxychloroquine (200 mg once or twice daily) is most often used, chloroquine (250–500 mg daily) being reserved for unresponsive patients. Quinacrine was widely used in the past but has become increasingly difficult to obtain. Baseline lupus severity may predict response to hydroxychloroquine, whereas the deleterious role of cigarette smoking on the efficacy of antimalarial drugs is controversial. Treatment failure may be associated with subtherapeutic blood concentrations of the drug, which may be managed by increasing the daily dose of hydroxychloroquine to reach blood concentrations >750 ng/mL.

Drugs for discoid lupus erythematosus. Jessop S, Whitelaw DA, Delamere FM. Cochrane Database Syst Rev 2009; 4: CD002954.

Oral retinoids, either isotretinoin (1 mg/kg/d in two divided doses) or acitretin (25–50 mg daily in one or two divided doses), are useful in the treatment of DLE, particularly the hypertrophic variety. Their teratogenic effects must be respected, especially because patients with DLE are often women of childbearing age. The long-term adverse effects of retinoids, including hypertriglyceridemia and possible bony abnormalities, must also be considered in constructing a treatment plan. As with other treatments for DLE, the disease occasionally flares, even with continued treatment.

Third-Line Therapies

• Cytotoxic agents	D
• Immune response–modifying agents	D
• Topical salbutamol	B

Treatment of cutaneous lupus erythematosus: current practice variations. Reich A, Werth VP, Furukawa F, Kuhn A, Szczęch J, Samotij D, et al. Lupus 2016; 25: 964-72.

Evidence-based data to support the efficacy of drugs commonly used to treat DLE is lacking, with few randomized, controlled trials. Case reports have claimed efficacy for a variety of systemic drugs with diverse mechanisms of action, including antibiotics (e.g., sulfasalazine, dapsone) and biologic agents (e.g., etanercept, infliximab, rituximab), as well as older and newer immune-response modifiers (e.g., clofazimine, apremilast, fumaric acid esters). Immunosuppressive drugs (e.g., azathioprine, methotrexate, mycophenolate mofetil) have also been used in patients with disease refractory to conventional treatment, as has the pulsed dye laser.

Thalidomide and lenalidomide for the treatment of refractory dermatologic conditions. Nahmias Z, Nambudiri VE, Vleugels RA. J Am Acad Dermatol 2016; 75: 210-2.

Lenalidomide treatment of cutaneous lupus erythematosus: the Mayo Clinic experience. Kindle SA, Wetter DA, Davis MD, Pittelkow MR, Sciallis GF. Int J Dermatol 2016; 55: e431-9.

Lenalidomide for refractory chronic and subacute cutaneous lupus erythematosus. Fennira F, Chasset F, Soubrier M, Cordel N, Petit A, Francès C. J Am Acad Dermatol 2016; 74: 1248-51.

Thalidomide (20 - 100 mg daily) has been used in the treatment of patients with cutaneous lupus erythematosus refractory to other modalities. The response is variable but may be quite favorable. It must be emphasized that the disease typically affects young women of childbearing age; thus the teratogenic potential of the drug should not be ignored. Sensory neuropathy and thromboembolic events are other potential complications of thalidomide administration. Some reports suggest that lenalidomide, an analog of thalidomide, may be a viable alternative, despite its similar adverse event profile.

A randomized controlled trial of R-salbutamol for topical treatment of discoid lupus erythematosus. Jemec GB, Ullman S, Goodfield M, Bygum A, Olesen AB, Berth-Jones J, et al. Br J Dermatol 2009; 161: 1365–70.

Salbutamol has antiinflammatory properties, and although not yet commercially developed, this study demonstrated promising results from a 0.5% cream applied twice daily for 8 weeks.

Evidence Levels: **A** Double-blind study **B** Clinical trial ≥ 20 subjects **C** Clinical trial < 20 subjects **D** Series ≥ 5 subjects **E** Anecdotal case reports

63

Dissecting cellulitis of the scalp

Vikram Rajkomar, Matt Harries

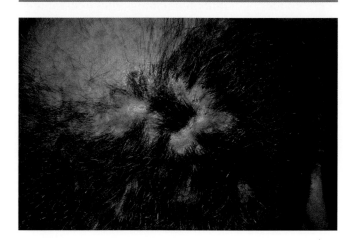

Dissecting cellulitis *(perifolliculitis capitis abscedens et suffodiens)* is a rare inflammatory disease of the scalp characterized by multiple fluctuant nodules and abscesses over the vertex and occipital region associated with interconnecting sinus tract formation and purulent discharge. Dissecting cellulitis of the scalp (DCS) follows a progressive relapsing course eventually resulting in permanent hair loss and hypertrophic scarring. The condition predominantly affects men aged 20 to 40 and is more common in those of African descent. Dissecting cellulitis may occur in association with hidradenitis suppurativa (HS) and acne conglobata to form the "follicular occlusion triad." The suggested common pathogenic mechanism is of follicular occlusion triggering a folliculitis with neutrophilic or granulomatous inflammation in the dermis and subcutis, leading to formation of sinus tracts, abscesses, and progressive fibrosis. An abnormal host response to (possibly commensal) bacteria may also be a factor in disease development.

MANAGEMENT STRATEGY

Dissecting cellulitis is characterized by a chronic, progressive course with temporary improvement on treatment followed by relapses when treatment is discontinued. There are no large therapeutic clinical trials, and recommendations for therapy are based on case reports or case series. Inflammatory tinea capitis and the very rare complication of squamous cell carcinoma should be excluded. Although no specific pathogenic organisms have been isolated, swabs should be obtained for bacteriology and the antibiotic sensitivity of organisms reviewed.

In mild cases or when disease is limited, *improved scalp hygiene* and the use of *antiseptics, topical antibiotics, intralesional corticosteroid injections,* and *aspiration of fluctuant lesions* may be adequate. At an early stage, *systemic antibiotics* such as

tetracyclines reduce inflammation and can control disease. In more severe cases a *combination of systemic antibiotics such as clindamycin with rifampicin, with or without corticosteroids,* may be effective. However, recognition that *oral isotretinoin* can provide sustained remission has led many to now regard it as first-line therapy in DCS. Oral *zinc sulfate* has received anecdotal reports of benefit when used long term. Recent reports highlight success with anti–tumor necrosis factor (TNF) therapy in those unresponsive to standard treatment. *Alitretinoin* and *photodynamic therapy* are new additions to the therapeutic armamentarium.

In those unresponsive to medical therapy a surgical approach may be considered. *X-ray epilation* of affected areas has largely been superseded by *laser epilation* techniques. The most resistant cases may require *surgical excision and skin grafting.*

Specific Investigations

- Swabs for bacteriology
- Scrapings and plucked hairs for mycology
- Scalp biopsy for histology and fungal culture

Inflammatory tinea capitis (kerion) mimicking dissecting cellulitis. Sperling LC, Major MC. Int J Dermatol 1991; 30: 190–2.

Two cases of inflammatory tinea capitis mimicking DCS are reported. If initial mycology is negative, consider biopsy for histology and fungal culture.

Squamous cell carcinoma arising in dissecting perifolliculitis of the scalp. Curry SS, Gaither DH, King LE. J Am Acad Dermatol 1981; 4: 673–8.

The rare complication of squamous cell carcinoma arising in DCS is presented.

First-Line Therapy

• Isotretinoin (oral)	**D**

Dissecting cellulitis of the scalp: response to isotretinoin. Scerri L, Williams HC, Allen BR. Br J Dermatol 1996; 134: 1105–8.

Three patients with DCS showed a sustained response to isotretinoin. The authors recommend isotretinoin initially at 1 mg/kg daily and maintained at 0.75 mg/kg daily for at least 4 months after clinical remission is achieved.

Dissecting cellulitis of the scalp: a retrospective study of 7 cases confirming the efficacy of oral isotretinoin. Koudoukpo C, Abdennader S, Cavelier-Balloy B, Gasnier C, Yédomon H. Ann Dermatol Venereol 2014; 141: 500–6.

Dissecting cellulitis of the scalp: a retrospective study of 51 patients and review of literature. Badaoui A, Reygagne P, Cavelier-Balloy B, Pinquier L, Deschamps L, Crickx B, et al. Br J Dermatol 2016; 174: 421–3.

A retrospective analysis of 51 patients with DCS treated from 1996 to 2013. Thirty-five patients received treatment with isotretinoin at 0.5 to 0.8 mg/kg/day with complete remission being achieved in 92%.

Second-Line Therapies	
• Systemic antibiotics	D
• Intralesional corticosteroid injection	D
• Incision and drainage	D
• Topical antibiotic/retinoid	E
• Systemic corticosteroids	E
• Oral zinc	E

Dissecting cellulitis of the scalp responding to oral quinolones. Greenblatt DT, Sheth N, Teixeira F. Clin Exp Dermatol 2008; 33: 99–100.

Dissecting cellulitis (perifolliculitis capitis abscedens et suffodiens): a comprehensive review focusing on new treatments and findings of the last decade with commentary comparing the therapies and causes of dissecting cellulitis to hidradenitis suppurativa. Scheinfeld N. Dermatol Online J 2014; 20: 22692.

Various treatment strategies for DCS are reviewed. Oral antibiotics and oral isotretinoin, either as monotherapy or in combination, represent the mainstay of treatment. Addition of intralesional corticosteroids or incision and drainage may improve local control. Reported antibiotic regimens include rifampicin 300 mg BID and clindamycin 300 mg BID, tetracyclines (e.g., doxycycline 100–200 mg/day), ciprofloxacin 250 to 500 mg BID, and trimethoprim-sulfamethoxazole 960 mg BID. Responses and relapse rates are variable and depend on the regimen chosen.

Perifolliculitis capitis abscedens et suffodiens successfully controlled with topical isotretinoin. Karpouzis A, Giatromanolaki A, Sivridis E, Kouskoukis C. Eur J Dermatol 2003; 13: 192–5.

A case of DCS controlled with topical isotretinoin and clindamycin gel.

Perifolliculitis capitis: successful control with alternate day corticosteroids. Adrian RM, Arndt KA. Ann Plast Surg 1980; 4: 166–9.

Successful control of DCS was achieved using high-dose oral prednisolone and maintained with alternate-day 5 mg prednisolone for 2 years.

Successful treatment of dissecting cellulitis and acne conglobata with oral zinc. Kobayashi H, Aiba S, Tagami H. Br J Dermatol 1999; 141: 1136–8.

A patient with DCS and acne conglobata responded to oral zinc sulfate 135 mg three times a day for 12 weeks followed by a reduced maintenance dose.

Third-Line Therapies	
• Excision and grafting	E
• Laser epilation	E
• Radiotherapy epilation	E
• Dapsone	E
• PDT	E
• Alitretinoin	E
• Infliximab/adalimumab	E

Dissecting cellulitis of the scalp. Williams CN, Cohen M, Ronan SG, Lewandowski CA. Plast Reconstruct Surg 1986; 77: 378–82.

Four patients with extensive scalp disease responded to wide excision and split-thickness skin grafting.

Dissecting cellulitis treated with the long-pulsed Nd:YAG laser. Krasner BD, Hamzavi FH, Murakawa GJ, Hamzavi IH. Dermatol Surg 2006; 32: 1039–44.

Four patients achieved sustained improvement at 1 year, with some regrowth of hair at treated sites.

Use of an 800-nm pulsed-diode laser in the treatment of recalcitrant dissecting cellulitis of the scalp. Boyd AS, Binhlam JQ. Arch Dermatol 2002; 138: 1291–3.

Complete clearance of recalcitrant disease after four monthly treatments, with remission maintained at 6 months.

Modern external beam radiation therapy for refractory dissecting cellulitis of the scalp. Chinnalayan P, Tena LB, Brenner MJ, Welsh JS. Br J Dermatol 2005; 152: 777–9.

Rapid improvement in four cases treated with electron beam therapy. No relapses reported after 4- to 13-year follow-up.

Successful treatment of recalcitrant dissecting cellulitis of the scalp with ALA-PDT: case report and literature review. Liu Y, Ma Y, Xiang LH. Photodiagnosis Photodyn Ther 2013; 10: 410–3.

The authors report complete response using ALA-PDT weekly for 6 weeks in recalcitrant DCS. Remission was maintained at 5 months' follow-up.

Successful treatment with alitretinoin of dissecting cellulitis of the scalp in keratitis-ichthyosis-deafness syndrome. Prasad SC, Bygum A. Acta Derm Venereol 2013; 93: 473–4.

Alitretinoin was given at 10 mg daily for 2 months followed by 20 mg daily in a patient with DCS and keratitis, ichthyosis, deafness (KID) syndrome. Significant improvement was noted after 5 months of therapy.

Perifolliculitis capitis abscedens et suffodiens successfully controlled with infliximab. Brandt HRC, Malheiros APR, Teixeira MG, Machado MCR. Br J Dermatol 2008; 159: 506–7.

Sustained response to infliximab given 8 weekly for 12 months in a case of DCS refractory to antibiotics and isotretinoin.

Three cases of dissecting cellulitis of the scalp treated with adalimumab. Navarini AA, Trüeb RM. Arch Dermatol 2010; 146: 517–20.

Rapid improvement with adalimumab, but relapse occurred on stopping treatment due to persistent underlying structural disease. The authors suggest continuous therapy or surgical excision of involved areas to prevent recurrence.

Evidence Levels: **A** Double-blind study **B** Clinical trial ≥ 20 subjects **C** Clinical trial < 20 subjects **D** Series ≥ 5 subjects **E** Anecdotal case reports

Drug eruptions

Roni P. Dodiuk-Gad, Neil H. Shear

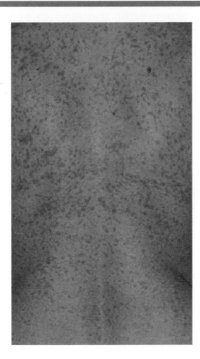

Drug eruptions are among the most frequent adverse reactions in patients receiving drug therapy. They have a wide spectrum of clinical manifestations, are caused by various drugs, and result from varied pathophysiologic mechanisms. Hence, their diagnosis and management are challenging. Drug eruptions can range from a mild, simple eruption involving only the skin to severe complex eruptions with systemic involvement, such as toxic epidermal necrolysis. Systemic involvement should be explored even in a mild cutaneous eruption due to a drug because the severity of skin manifestation does not necessarily mirror the severity of the systemic involvement. The image shows a widespread eruption of erythematous macules and papules coalescent into ill-defined plaques on the trunk—maculopapular morphology of cutaneous drug eruption. This can be localized to the skin with no systemic involvement (simple drug eruption) or be associated with systemic involvement (complex drug eruption).

MANAGEMENT STRATEGY

The following is the authors' protocol to approach a patient with a drug eruption: **4Ds**. **D**iagnosis of the adverse event is based on three key clinical elements: 1) Appearance: the morphology of the drug eruption based on four main categories of the primary lesion: maculopapular, urticarial, bullous, and pustular. 2) Systemic signs that differentiate between a simple reaction involving only the skin and a complex reaction that comprises systemic involvement in addition to the skin. Systemic involvement is evaluated by assessing the patient's symptoms such as fever, facial edema, malaise, chills, dyspnea, cough, palpitations, nausea, vomiting, diarrhea, sore throat, and arthralgia and a basic laboratory screen, which includes a full blood count, liver and renal function tests, and urine analysis. 3) Histology: histopathology and, if relevant, direct immunofluorescence studies of skin biopsies to confirm the clinical impression and to distinguish between a drug eruption and other skin diseases. In addition, it is valuable to use validated diagnostic criteria of specific types of drug eruptions, if available. Currently, only acute generalized exanthematous pustulosis (AGEP) and drug reaction with eosinophilia and systemic symptoms (DRESS) have published validated diagnostic criteria.

Differential diagnosis

Establishing a differential diagnosis that takes into account all possible diagnoses is essential.

Drug exposure (timing)

All medications, regardless of route of administration, must be considered, particularly new drugs taken in the 8 weeks before the drug eruption. Assessment of the lag period, the time between initiation of the drug and onset of the cutaneous reaction, is essential in view of the different lag times for different drug eruptions. A recommended method for drug exposure analysis is to chart a timeline in order to visualize the chronology and facilitate comprehension of the event.

Determine probabilities

An important step in assessing a drug eruption is to establish whether there is a causal relationship between the suspected drug and the clinical event. The following methods are helpful: 1) Patient history: the patient should be questioned about previous drug eruptions and whether dechallenge with the drug improved the eruption. 2) Analysis of the literature: PubMed (http://www.ncbi.nlm.nih.gov/pubmed/) and Litt's D.E.R.M. Drug Eruptions and Reactions Manual and database (http://www.drugeruptiondata.com/). 3) In vitro and in vivo diagnostic assessments, including human leukocyte antigen (HLA) genetic tests. An important progress in the underlying mechanisms of several types of drug eruptions has been achieved by the discovery of an association between a specific HLA allele, a drug, an ethnic background, and a drug eruption. These tests are best utilized as genetic screening before drug prescription. However, they may serve as a simple, safe, and reliable method for establishing causality in specific cases of drug eruptions such as toxic epidermal necrolysis and DRESS induced by specific drugs such as carbamazepine and allopurinol. Other in vitro tests may include lymphocyte transformation test and basophil activation test. Patch test is an important in vivo test that may be used in assessment of a drug eruption. Caution should always be exercised regarding false-positive and false-negative results of these in vitro and in vivo tests, and no test should be used as justification for rechallenge.

After the diagnosis of a drug eruption, the physician must provide the patient with clear information on the drug eruption, the name of the offending drug, potential cross-reacting drugs, and drugs that can be safely taken as an alternative to the offending drug. In cases of complex reactions, it is also necessary to explain to the patient the possible long-term medical complications, to provide him or her with information on medical follow-up and support groups, and to conduct family counseling because the predisposition may be genetic. The physician must also report the event to the patient's health care provider, the manufacturer, and regulatory agencies.

Specific Investigations

- Determination of the morphology of the primary lesion based on four main categories: maculopapular, urticarial, bullous, and pustular
- Assessment of systemic involvement based on patient's vital signs and symptoms
- Assessment of systemic involvement based on basic laboratory screen: full blood count, liver and renal function tests, and urine analysis
- Skin biopsy for histopathology and, if relevant, direct immunofluorescence studies
- Usage of validated diagnostic criteria, if available
- Establishment of a differential diagnosis that takes into account all possible diagnoses
- Drug exposure analysis: determination of the lag period and creation of a timeline
- Determination of probabilities for the associations between the suspected drug and the clinical event according to the patient's history, literature, and in vitro and in vivo diagnostic assessments, including HLA genetic tests

---

Phenotype standardization for immune-mediated drug-induced skin injury. Pirmohamed M, Friedmann PS, Molokhia M, Loke YK, Smith C, Phillips E, et al. Clin Pharmacol Ther 2011; 89: 896–901.

A drug-induced skin injury (DISI) expert working group comprising participants with varied expertise defined the minimum phenotypic criteria for selected forms of DISI (SJS/TEN, AGEP, and DRESS). In addition, an algorithm to aid appropriate clinical categorization of patients with DISI is presented.

Acute generalized exanthematous pustulosis (AGEP)—a clinical reaction pattern. Sidoroff A, Halevy S, Bavinck JN, Vaillant L, Roujeau JC. J Cutan Pathol 2001; 28: 113–19.

An algorithm for validating cases of AGEP is presented in this manuscript.

Variability in the clinical pattern of cutaneous side-effects of drugs with systemic symptoms: does a DRESS syndrome really exist? Kardaun SH, Sidoroff A, Valeyrie-Allanore L, Halevy S, Davidovici BB, Mockenhaupt M, et al. Br J Dermatol 2007; 156: 609–11.

Scoring system for classifying DRESS cases is presented in this manuscript.

The lymphocyte transformation test in the diagnosis of drug hypersensitivity. Pichler WJ, Tilch J. Allergy 2004; 59: 809–20.

The lymphocyte transformation test (LTT) measures the proliferation of T cells to a drug in vitro. The main advantage of this test is its applicability with many different drugs in different immune reactions. Its main disadvantages are that the test is technically demanding and with limited sensitivity.

A multicentre study to determine the value and safety of drug patch tests for the three main classes of severe cutaneous adverse drug reactions. Barbaud A, Collet E, Milpied B, Assier H, Staumont D, Avenel-Audran M, et al. Toxidermies group of the French Society of Dermatology. Br J Dermatol 2013; 168: 555–62.

In a multicenter study, patch tests were conducted on patients referred for AGEP, DRESS, and SJS/TEN. It was found that patch tests are useful and safe for identifying severe cutaneous drug eruptions, and the value of patch tests depended on the type of drug and the type of drug eruption. Testing for all possible agents is recommended in order to identify responsible products that are normally not suspected.

HLA associations and clinical implications in T-cell mediated drug hypersensitivity reactions: an updated review. Cheng CY, Su SC, Chen CH, Chen WL, Deng ST, Chung WH. J Immunol Res 2014; 2014: 565320.

Recent advances in pharmacogenetic studies show strong genetic associations between HLA alleles and susceptibility to drug hypersensitivity. This review summarizes the literature on recent progress in pharmacogenetic studies and clinical application of pharmacogenetic screening.

Various associations between a specific HLA and drug hypersensitivity were found. The following are the current most important associations related to severe cutaneous adverse drug reactions: HLA-B*1502 and carbamazepine-induced SJS/TEN in Asians, HLA-A*31:01 and carbamazepine-induced DRESS in both Caucasians and Asians, HLA-B*5701 and abacavir hypersensitivity in Caucasians, and HLA-B*5801 and allopurinol-induced SJS/TEN or DRESS in both Caucasians and Asians.

First-Line Therapies

- Discontinue the offending drug — D
- Supportive care — E
- Simple drug eruption (involving only the skin): oral antihistamines and topical corticosteroids — E
- Complex drug eruption (systemic involvement in addition to the skin): specific treatments based on the type of the drug eruption — E

Clinical practice. Exanthematous drug eruptions. Stern RS. N Engl J Med 2012; 366: 2492–501.

Identifying and discontinuing the causative drug are the most important steps in management of a drug eruption. In simple drug eruptions, symptomatic treatment with antihistamines and potent topical glucocorticoids may be helpful. A decision can be made to continue the drug and offer symptomatic treatment if the drug is of paramount importance, but the risk:benefit ratio of this option has to be carefully weighed, and the evolution of the eruption must be meticulously monitored. In cases of complex drug eruptions, it is always essential to discontinue the drug.

Second-Line Therapies

- Cyclosporine — B
- Intravenous immunoglobulin G — E
- TNF inhibitors — E
- Mucous membrane treatment — E
- Skin treatment — E
- Pain control — E

Open trial of cyclosporine treatment for Stevens-Johnson syndrome and toxic epidermal necrolysis. Valeyrie-Allanore L, Wolkenstein P, Brochard L, Ortonne N, Maitre B, Revuz J, et al. Br J Derm 2010; 163: 847–53.

Evidence Levels: A Double-blind study B Clinical trial ≥ 20 subjects C Clinical trial < 20 subjects D Series ≥ 5 subjects E Anecdotal case reports

Death rate and progression of detachment appeared lower than expected in 29 patients with a diagnosis of SJS or TEN who received cyclosporine (3 mg/kg/day for 10 days and tapered over a month).

Stevens-Johnson syndrome and toxic epidermal necrolysis: an update. Dodiuk-Gad RP, Chung WH, Valeyrie-Allanore L, Shear NH. Am J Clin Dermatol 2015; 16: 475–93.

This review summarizes up-to-date insights on SJS/TEN and describes a protocol for assessment and treatment.

Management of drug reaction with eosinophilia and systemic symptoms (DRESS). Descamps V, Ben Saïd B, Sassolas B, Truchetet F, Avenel-Audran M, Girardin P, et al. Groupe Toxidermies de la Société française de dermatologie. Ann Dermatol Venereol 2010; 137: 703–8.

This manuscript describes the management protocol for DRESS based on the consensus of experts from the French Society of Dermatology. A decisional tree of treatment options is proposed, based on the severity of visceral manifestations.

Other Therapies	
• Counsel the patient and family	E
• Report the event to the patient's health care provider, the manufacturer, and regulatory agencies	E

Eosinophilic fasciitis

Jamie R. Manning, Shaheen H. Ensanyat, Amir A. Larian, Brian S. Fuchs, Marsha L. Gordon

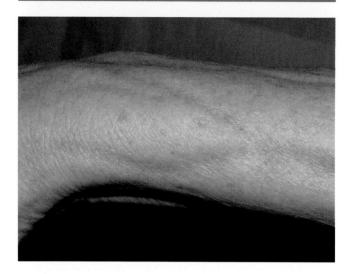

Eosinophilic fasciitis (EF), also known as *Shulman syndrome*, is a rare fibrosing disorder characterized by the rapid onset of symmetric induration of the extremities. The trunk and neck can be affected, with typical sparing of the hands, feet, and face. Clinically, the progression of EF is marked by edema and erythema followed by dimpling of the skin and a *peau d'orange* appearance evolving into woody induration and stiffness of the limbs. Depressions over superficial veins produce the "gutter" or "groove" sign. Laboratory investigations often reveal hypergammaglobulinemia, an elevated erythrocyte sedimentation rate, and peripheral blood eosinophilia but are not essential in securing a diagnosis, given their transient levels. Histologically, EF presents with severe fascial thickening associated with an inflammatory infiltrate composed of plasma cells, eosinophils, histiocytes, and lymphocytes that can ultimately lead to dermal sclerosis. Although the etiology remains unknown, vigorous physical activity and infection have been reported before the onset of EF in many cases, presumably triggering an aberrant immune response.

MANAGEMENT STRATEGY

Whether a distinct entity or variant of scleroderma, EF is differentiated by the relative absence of sclerodactyly, Raynaud phenomenon, and serologic markers. Unlike scleroderma, patients with EF typically demonstrate a more rapid onset with normal nail fold capillaries, infrequent visceral involvement, and response to corticosteroid therapy. Although organ involvement is not prominent in EF, rare cases have reported significant proteinuria, possibly representing an underestimated systemic feature. EF must also be distinguished from the eosinophilia–myalgia syndrome, which is characterized by diffuse muscle pain and weakness, polyneuropathy, respiratory and pulmonary problems, and most notably a history of contaminated L-tryptophan ingestion.

EF has been reported in association with hematologic disorders, including aplastic anemia, hemolytic anemia, thrombocytopenia,

leukemias, and lymphomas. In addition, EF has to a lesser extent been linked to administration of simvastatin or exposure to trichloroethylene; these should be checked for in the patient history.

Clinical and laboratory findings help identify EF; however, diagnosis can only be confirmed with histopathologic examination from a full-thickness skin-to-muscle biopsy, which characteristically reveals deep dermal fibrosis and fascial thickening with inflammatory infiltration of lymphocytes, plasma cells, and eosinophils. Magnetic resonance imaging (MRI), ultrasound and positron emission tomography/computed tomography (PET/CT) are useful noninvasive tools for establishing the diagnosis, choosing the optimal biopsy site, and monitoring the effectiveness of treatment. On MRI, findings typically show high signal intensity of the deep and superficial fasciae on T_1, T_2, and short tau inversion recovery (STIR) imaging with enhancement after intravenous contrast administration.

Although spontaneous remission of EF has been reported, treatment can help prevent the progression of flexion contractures and limited mobility. Clinical response is usually defined as marked improvement in skin thickening, as fibrosed tissue becomes softer and looser, allowing for increased range of motion. Serum aldolase levels have been proposed as a useful indicator of disease activity.

There is substantial agreement among published reports that moderate- to high-dose corticosteroids serve as the first-line treatment for EF with *prednisone* as the standard agent, initially at 40 to 60 mg daily. A clinical response usually is noted within the first few weeks, and the dosage is then tapered slowly over several months to an alternate-day regimen. In steroid-refractory patients, the addition of *hydroxychloroquine* at 200 to 400 mg daily has also been effective both in combination and as monotherapy.

In patients with partial or no response to corticosteroids, immunosuppressive drugs are frequently introduced as a second-line treatment. *Ciclosporin* at 3.7 mg/kg daily tapered to 2.5 mg/kg daily has been successful within 1 month at improving clinical symptoms with no relapse after a year. *Methotrexate* at 15 to 20 mg/week in conjunction with prednisone has also been commonly used with a favorable response.

Cimetidine at 400 mg every 6 to 12 hours has shown reported success in some cases. *Pulsed methylprednisolone* 1 g daily for 5 days combined with ciclosporin 150 mg twice daily is another regimen that has led to remission for patients in need of more aggressive therapy. *Infliximab*, D-*penicillamine, ketotifen, chloroquine, psoralen and ultraviolet light (PUVA), azathioprine, griseofulvin, dapsone,* and *sulfasalazine* have all been reported to have beneficial effects.

Specific Investigations

- Complete blood count
- Serum aldolase
- MRI
- Ultrasound
- Fludeoxyglucose (FDG) PET/CT
- History to exclude tryptophan, simvastatin, or trichloroethylene ingestion
- Infection

Eosinophilic fasciitis. Sibrack LA, Mazur EM, Hoffman R, Bollet AJ. Clin Rheum Dis 1982; 8: 443–54.

Peripheral eosinophilia is typically present during active disease, except in those patients who have an associated aplastic marrow. The eosinophilia is often transient and may precede the clinical diagnosis.

Evidence Levels: A Double-blind study **B** Clinical trial ≥ 20 subjects **C** Clinical trial < 20 subjects **D** Series ≥ 5 subjects **E** Anecdotal case reports

The use of an elevated aldolase in diagnosing and managing eosinophilic fasciitis. Nashel J, Steen V. Clin Rheumatol 2015; 34: 1481–4.

In this retrospective review of 15 patients, the aldolase level was the last parameter to normalize and the first to rise during a flare compared with eosinophilia and inflammatory markers.

Eosinophilic fasciitis: spectrum of MRI findings. Moulton SJ, Kransdorf MJ, Ginsburg WW, Abril A, Persellin S. AJR Am J Roentgenol 2005; 184: 975–8.

In this case series of six patients with histologically proven EF, MRI revealed characteristic findings, including thickening, signal abnormalities, and contrast enhancement of the superficial and, to a lesser extent, deep muscle fasciae.

Ultrasound assessment of subcutaneous compressibility: a potential adjunctive diagnostic tool in eosinophilic fasciitis. Kissin EY, Garg A, Grayson PC, Dubreuil M, Vradii D, York M, et al. J Clin Rheumatol 2013; 19: 382–5.

A cross-sectional study of 12 patients with EF revealed a significant reduction in subcutaneous compressibility quantified by ultrasound.

Usefulness of FDG PET/CT in the diagnosis of eosinophilic fasciitis. Kim HJ, Lee SW, Kim GJ, Lee JH. Clin Nucl Med 2014; 39: 801–2.

In one case report, increased uptake of FDG on PET/CT along the superficial and deep fasciae suggested FDG PET/CT may be a noninvasive tool to illustrate more detailed anatomic involvement of the disease, especially if MRI is contraindicated.

Eosinophilic fasciitis associated with tryptophan ingestion: a manifestation of eosinophilia myalgia syndrome. Gordon ML, Lebwohl MG, Phelps RG, Cohen SR, Fleischmajer R. Arch Dermatol 1991; 127: 217–20.

Ingestion of contaminated tryptophan is associated with a very similar clinical entity called *eosinophilia–myalgia syndrome.*

Although the eosinophilia–myalgia syndrome is now mostly of historical significance, a new case was reported in 2011.

Eosinophilic fasciitis associated with *Mycoplasma arginini* infection. Silló P, Pintér D, Ostorházi E, Mazán M, Wikonkál N, Pónyai K, et al. J Clin Microbiol 2012; 50: 1113–7.

A 23-year-old male and former bodybuilder with a history of consuming anabolic steroids was diagnosed with EF in conjunction with *Mycoplasma arginini* infection, suggesting a potential pathogenic association.

Eosinophilic fasciitis. A pathologic study of twenty cases. Barnes L, Rodnan GP, Medsger TA, Short D. Am J Pathol 1979; 96: 493–517.

Deep fascia and subcutaneous tissue are infiltrated with lymphocytes, plasma cells, histiocytes, and eosinophils early in the course of the disease. Sclerosis of the dermis with increased collagen occurs later in the course of the disease.

Analysis of leukemia inhibitory factor, type 1 and type 2 cytokine production in patients with eosinophilic fasciitis. Viallard JF, Taupin JL, Leng B, Pellegrin JL, Moreau JF. J Rheumatol 2001; 28: 75–80.

Peripheral blood mononuclear cells in patients with EF have increased capacity to produce type 2 cytokines such as interleukin-5 (IL-5) and IL-10. Elevations in type 1 (interferon gamma [IFN-γ] and IL-2) and leukemia inhibitor factor cytokines in the same patients may suggest a compensatory response.

First-Line Therapies

• Systemic corticosteroids and methotrexate	B
• Systemic corticosteroids	B
• Pulsed methylprednisolone	D
• Prednisone and D-penicillamine	C

Epidemiology and treatment of eosinophilic fasciitis: an analysis of 63 patients from 3 tertiary care centers. Wright NA, Mazori DR, Patel M, Merola JF, Femia AN, Vleugels RA. JAMA Dermatol 2016; 152: 97–9.

A retrospective chart review of 63 EF patients revealed that complete response was more likely in those treated with a combination of corticosteroids and methotrexate (64%), compared with corticosteroid monotherapy (30%), other treatment combinations (29%), and without steroids (17%).

Eosinophilic fasciitis: clinical spectrum and therapeutic response in 52 cases. Lakhanpal S, Ginsburg WW, Michet CJ, Doyle JA, Moore SB. Semin Arthritis Rheum 1988; 17: 221–31.

Of the 52 patients, 34 were treated with prednisone (40–60 mg/daily). The remaining 18 were treated with hydroxychloroquine, colchicine, D-penicillamine, or no medication. Twenty of the 34 patients treated with prednisone had a partial response, and 5 had complete resolution. Eight of the 9 patients who had a poor response were treated with the addition of hydroxychloroquine (200–400 mg/daily). Two responded completely, 2 had an improvement of over 50%, and 3 were lost to follow-up. Eight patients also responded to treatment with hydroxychloroquine alone. Relapses occurred in some patients.

Eosinophilic fasciitis (Shulman disease): new insights into the therapeutic management from a series of 34 patients. Lebeaux D, Francés C, Barete S, Wechsler B, Dubourg O, Renoux J, et al. Rheumatology (Oxford) 2012; 51: 557–61.

Prednisone served as a first-line therapy for all patients. Before treatment initiation, 15 patients received methylprednisolone pulses (MPPs), which reduced the need for an immunosuppressive drug and increased the probability of complete remission. After treatment initiation, 12 patients received methotrexate as a second-line therapy. A poor outcome was present in 10 patients and was associated with a diagnosis time delay of more than 6 months and a lack of MPPs at treatment initiation. Overall, complete remission was achieved in 69% of patients.

Severe eosinophilic fasciitis: comparison of treatment with D-penicillamine plus corticosteroids vs. corticosteroids alone. Mendoza FA, Bai R, Kebede AG, Jimenez SA. Scand J Rheumatol 2015; 73: 1010.

A prospective, nonrandomized, open-label trial of 16 patients with a clinicohistopathologic diagnosis of severe EF revealed that the combination treatment of D-penicillamine plus corticosteroids was more efficacious than corticosteroids alone. Proteinuria was the most common adverse event reported in both groups.

Four prolonged cases of eosinophilic fasciitis in children. Hui-Yuen J, Lauren C, Garzon M, Starr AJ, Imundo LF. Arthritis Rheumatol 2014; 66: S85.

Four pediatric patients with EF confirmed the efficacy of corticosteroids as a first-line therapy. All patients required either methotrexate or mycophenolate mofetil, and three required both, suggesting a more severe course within the pediatric population.

Second-Line Therapies

• Hydroxychloroquine	C
• Ciclosporin	E
• Methotrexate	D
• Cimetidine	C

Eosinophilic rheumatic disorders. Clauw DJ, Crofford LJ. Rheum Clin North Am 1995; 21: 231–46.

Hydroxychloroquine at a dose of 200 to 400 mg daily can be used either alone or in combination with corticosteroids.

Eosinophilic fasciitis successfully treated with ciclosporin. Bukiej A, Dropiński J, Dyduch G, Szczeklik A. Clin Rheumatol 2005; 24: 634–6.

Case report of a 45-year-old female unresponsive to treatment with prednisolone followed by cimetidine, who experienced clinical remission after a regimen of ciclosporin at 5 mg/kg daily for 4 weeks tapered to 2.5 mg/kg daily.

Eosinophilic fasciitis: clinical characteristics and response to methotrexate. Berianu F, Cohen MD, Abril A, Ginsburg WW. Rheum Dis 2015; 18: 91–8.

Sixteen patients with biopsy-proven EF were treated with methotrexate after a course of either prednisone alone or in combination with azathioprine or hydroxychloroquine. Clinical response was noted within 6 months of therapy.

The fasciitis–panniculitis syndromes. Clinical and pathologic features. Naschitz JE, Boss JH, Misselevich I, Yeshurun D, Rosner I. Medicine 1996; 75: 6–16.

Complete and partial remission on cimetidine 400 mg twice daily occurred in nine and five patients, respectively. Only three did not respond to cimetidine monotherapy.

Third-Line Therapies

• PUVA	E
• Extracorporeal photochemotherapy	E
• D-penicillamine	E
• Azathioprine	E
• Chloroquine	E
• Sulfasalazine	E
• Surgery	E
• Infliximab	E
• Hydroxyzine	E
• Rituximab	E
• Dapsone	E
• Combination UVA1–retinoid–corticosteroid	E
• Mycophenolate mofetil	E
• Tocilizumab	E

Eosinophilic fasciitis treated with psoralen–ultraviolet A bath photochemotherapy. Schiener R, Behrens-Williams SC, Gottlober P, Pillekamp H, Peter RU, Kerscher M. Br J Dermatol 2000; 142: 804–7.

PUVA had promising results within 6 months without side effects in a 56-year-old patient.

Extracorporeal photochemotherapy in the treatment of eosinophilic fasciitis. Romano C, Rubegni P, De Aloe G, Stanghellini E, D'Ascenzo G, Andreassi L, et al. J Eur Acad Dermatol Venereol 2003; 17: 10–3.

Three patients were treated with extracorporeal photochemotherapy. After 1 year of therapy two patients showed a considerable improvement in clinical parameters.

D-penicillamine in the treatment of eosinophilic fasciitis: case reports and review of the literature. Manzini CU, Sebastiani M, Giuggioli D, Manfredi A, Colaci M, Cesinaro AM, et al. Clin Rheumatol 2012; 31: 183–7.

Three patients, two of them refractory to previous steroid therapy, were successfully treated with D-penicillamine.

Eosinophilic fasciitis with late onset arthritis responsive to sulfasalazine. Jones AC, Doherty M. J Rheumatol 1993; 20: 750–1.

In this patient there was a complete response to 2 g/day of sulfasalazine within 3 months.

Surgical management of eosinophilic fasciitis of the upper extremity. Suzuki G, Itoh Y, Horiuchi Y. J Hand Surg 1997; 22: 405–7.

All four patients experienced improved mobility a few weeks after fasciectomy with follow-up oral prednisolone.

Infliximab may be effective in the treatment of steroid-resistant eosinophilic fasciitis: report of three cases. Khanna D, Agrawal H, Clements PJ. Rheumatology (Oxford) 2010; 49: 1184–8.

Three patients refractory to initial treatment with prednisone (60 mg/daily), two of whom also received methotrexate (20 mg/week), noticed clinical improvement within 8 weeks of starting infliximab therapy (3 mg/kg every 8 weeks), leading ultimately to drug-free remission.

Eosinophilic fasciitis successfully treated with oral hydroxyzine: a new therapeutic use of an old drug? Uckun A, Sipahi T, Akgun D, Oksal A. Eur J Pediatr 2002; 161: 118–9.

Case report of a 3-year-old boy with biopsy-proven EF successfully treated with oral hydroxyzine (2 mg/kg/day) for 15 days.

Severe aplastic anemia associated with eosinophilic fasciitis: report of 4 cases and review of the literature. de Masson A, Bouaziz JD, Peffault de Latour R, Benhamou Y, Moluçon-Chabrot C, Bay JO, et al. Medicine 2013; 92: 69–81.

In a case series of four EF patients with severe aplastic anemia refractory to standard treatment regimens, one patient had significant improvement in his cutaneous and hematologic symptoms with rituximab infusion.

Dapsone treatment for eosinophilic fasciitis. Smith LC, Cox NH. Arch Dermatol 2008; 144: 845–7.

Report of a 38-year-old woman with minimal improvement from oral steroids and intolerance to ciclosporin who was started on dapsone, with marked clinical improvement.

Eosinophilic fasciitis and combined UVA1-retinoid-corticosteroid treatment: two case reports. Weber HO, Schaller M, Metzler G, Rocken M, Berneburg M. Acta Derm Venereol 2008; 88: 304–6.

Two patients treated with UVA1 phototherapy (60 J/cm^2) three to five times per week, isotretinoin 20 mg daily, and prednisone showed marked improvement within 2 to 3 weeks.

Eosinophilic fasciitis in a pediatric patient. Loupasakis K, Derk CT. J Clin Rheumatol 2010; 16: 129–31.

A 9-year-old boy was successfully treated with early high-dose corticosteroids followed by mycophenolate mofetil (900 mg twice daily) with nearly complete resolution after 2 years.

Efficacy of tocilizumab in the treatment of eosinophilic fasciitis: report of one case. Espinoza F, Jorgensen C, Pers YM. Joint Bone Spine 2015; 82: 460–1.

Report of one case of biopsy-proven EF, refractory to high-dose corticosteroids and methotrexate, found to have an excellent response to a humanized monoclonal antibody targeting the IL-6 receptor, tocilizumab.

Epidermal nevi

Jeffrey M. Weinberg

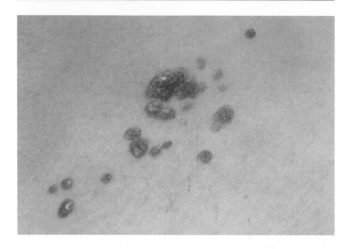

Epidermal nevi are congenital hamartomas of embryonal ecto-dermal origin classified on the basis of their major component. The components may be sebaceous, apocrine, eccrine, follicular, or keratinocytic. An estimated one third of individuals with epidermal nevi have involvement of other organ systems. In these cases, the condition is termed *epidermal nevus syndrome.*

The most common epidermal nevi are verrucous epidermal nevi, which are best treated with an ablative procedure using either surgical or laser technology. Inflammatory epidermal nevi may respond to topical or systemic therapy.

The pluripotential stem cell in the embryonic ectoderm can develop into any of the cell types found within the epidermis and skin adnexae. Therefore many potential nevi may develop from these cell types. Epidermal nevi may be classified according to the predominant cell type. However, there may be different cell populations or overlap between different areas within the same nevus.

The focus of this chapter will be on nevi derived from keratino-cytes. Of these, the verrucous epidermal nevus (VEN) is the most common. Other forms include an inflammatory linear verrucous epidermal nevus (ILVEN), an acantholytic or Darier-like nevus, an epidermolytic form, and linear porokeratosis. Very rarely an epidermal nevus may be associated with other birth defects, and a number of epidermal nevus syndromes have been described.

VEN may be localized, segmental, and rarely systematized. The individual lesions are verrucous papules, which may be pink, brown, or gray. These may develop as a result of mosaicism, and, if there is gonadal mosaicism, epidermal nevi may be transmitted to future offspring.

There are very rare case reports of malignant change within epidermal nevi, including squamous cell carcinoma and basal cell carcinoma.

MANAGEMENT STRATEGY

The major focus of therapy is improved cosmesis. A possible role for the dermis in the development of epidermal nevi is suggested by the difficulty experienced in ablating these lesions surgically without destroying the underlying dermis. *Surgical management* of these lesions presents challenges. Superficial treatments, which remove only the epidermis, have a high recurrence rate, whereas excision or more aggressive ablative procedures may produce unacceptable scarring. *Laser* technology provides the surgeon with more precise tools to maximize efficacy while minimizing scarring. Alternatively, for very widespread lesions, a variety of *topical regimens,* as well as *systemic retinoids,* have been reported to produce some benefit.

ILVEN presents in early childhood as a pruritic, erythematous, linear plaque. It shares many features with psoriasis, and certain cases respond to antipsoriatic therapies such as *topical vitamin D analogs, corticosteroids,* and *dithranol.* This has led some authors to suggest that this condition is a nevoid form of psoriasis. Epidermolytic and acantholytic nevi are more likely to respond to treatment with *retinoids.*

Specific Investigations

- Skin biopsy
- X-ray, imaging studies (magnetic resonance imaging [MRI], computed tomography [CT] scans), and ophthalmologic examinations

---

An epidermal nevus can most often be diagnosed solely on the clinical presentation and distribution of the lesion. A skin biopsy can be used both to confirm the diagnosis if necessary and to determine the predominant cell type and the presence of inflammatory changes, acantholysis, or dysplasia. This can be helpful in determining which therapeutic modality is most likely to succeed. If histopathology demonstrates an epidermolytic nevus, the individual should be counseled that there is a possibility that the mutation could be transmitted to offspring, with the risk that their children may have generalized cutaneous involvement. Biopsy can also indicate the rare occurrence of squamous or basal cell carcinoma, which can develop in epidermal nevi.

Epidermal nevus syndromes refer to the association of epidermal nevi with extracutaneous manifestations involving the central nervous system, eyes, or bones. The evaluation for systemic involvement should be based on the clinical extent of the epidermal nevi and the presence of any extracutaneous signs and symptoms.

Generalized epidermolytic hyperkeratosis in two unrelated children from parents with localized linear form, and prenatal diagnosis. Chassaing N, Kanitakis J, Sportich S, Cordier-Alex MP, Titeux M, Calvas P, et al. J Invest Dermatol 2006; 126: 2715–7.

The authors report two unrelated children with epidermolytic hyperkeratosis, both born to a parent affected with epidermolytic epidermal nevi (EEN); prenatal diagnosis in two successive pregnancies of one of the patients with EEN is described.

Squamous cell carcinoma arising in a verrucous epidermal naevus. Ichikawa T, Saiki M, Kaneko M, Saida T. Dermatology 1996; 193: 135–8.

A case report of a squamous cell carcinoma arising in a 74-year-old man with an epidermal nevus, plus a review of the literature, which revealed 18 previous reports of malignant change in epidermal nevi.

Basal cell carcinoma developing in verrucous epidermal nevus. De D, Kanwar AJ, Radotra BD. Indian J Dermatol Venereol Leprol 2007; 73: 127–8.

Evidence Levels: **A** Double-blind study   **B** Clinical trial ≥ 20 subjects   **C** Clinical trial < 20 subjects   **D** Series ≥ 5 subjects   **E** Anecdotal case reports

A 58-year-old farmer with a hyperpigmented, soft verrucous plaque on the right temporoparietal region since birth presented with an ulcer of 8 months' duration. A diagnosis of basal cell carcinoma (BCC) arising in a verrucous epidermal nevus was made. Biopsy was consistent with BCC.

Epidermal nevus syndromes. Sugarman JL. Semin Cutan Med Surg 2007; 26: 221–30.

Several subsets with characteristic features have been delineated, including the nevus sebaceous syndrome, Proteus syndrome, CHILD syndrome, Becker nevus syndrome, nevus comedonicus syndrome, and phakomatosis pigmentokeratotica.

Epidermal nevus syndromes: clinical findings in 35 patients. Vidaurri-de la Cruz H, Tamayo-Sanchez L, Duran-McKinster C, de la Luz Orozco-Covarrubias M, Ruiz-Maldonado R. Pediatr Dermatol 2004; 21: 432–9.

Of patients with epidermal nevi, 10% to 18% may have disorders of the eye, skeletal, and nervous systems.

Does inflammatory linear verrucous epidermal nevus represent a segmental type 1/type 2 mosaic of psoriasis? Hofer T. Dermatology 2006; 212: 103–7.

The author hypothesizes that inflammatory linear verrucous eruption besides nevoid psoriasis/linear psoriasis represents a further segmental type 1/type 2 mosaic of psoriasis, which, if a (verrucous) epidermal nevus exists, shows a high affinity of occurrence in close context to such a nevus. Heritability is thought to be possible.

Papular epidermal nevus with skyline basal cell layer (PENS): three new cases and review of the literature. Luna PC, Pannizardi AA, Martin CI, Vigovich F, Casas JG, Larralde M. Pediatr Dermatol 2016; 33: 296–300.

Papular epidermal nevus with skyline basal cell layer (PENS) is a recently described type of epidermal nevus with characteristic histopathologic findings. The authors note that cases of Blaschkoid distribution, associated extracutaneous manifestations, and familial cases have been reported. The probability of having extracutaneous manifestations is 6.3 times greater in those with more than four lesions. Therefore these patients require closer follow-up.

VERRUCOUS EPIDERMAL NEVI

First-Line Therapies	
• Excision under local anesthetic	D
• Shave or curettage under local anesthetic	D
• Cryotherapy	C

Comparison of treatment modalities for epidermal nevus: a case report and review. Fox BJ, Lapins NA. J Dermatol Surg Oncol 1983; 9: 879–85.

A case report of treatment for a VEN. Review of the treatment modalities then available indicated that surgical excision was only suitable for small lesions; superficial dermabrasion often led to recurrence, and, if performed more deeply, could result in hypertrophic scarring. Similar considerations applied to cryosurgery.

Epidermal nevus: surgical treatment by partial-thickness skin excision. Dellon AL, Luethke R, Wong L, Barnett N. Ann Plast Surg 1992; 28: 292–6.

A case report of treatment of a systematized epidermal nevus by partial-thickness skin excision. This cleared the nevus but led to extensive hypertrophic and keloidal scarring.

For small VEN, excision can be performed with an acceptable cosmetic result. In these cases, this approach is the treatment of choice. However, for larger lesions, or for those in cosmetically sensitive sites, excision may not be appropriate. For larger lesions, shave excision can be performed but often leads to recurrence. Cryotherapy can be used as a destructive method for these lesions, but recurrence is frequent. All these procedures have the benefit of being cost effective and easily performed.

Treatment of verrucous epidermal nevus: experience with 71 cases. Lapidoth M, Israeli H, Ben Amitai D, Halachmi S. Dermatology. 2013; 226: 342–6.

Of the 71 cases reviewed, 62 responded well to cryotherapy alone, and 9 facial VEN required CO_2 laser treatment. Small VEN required relatively few treatments (mean 3.4). Larger lesions required more treatments (mean 7.4) and did not respond as well.

Assessment of cryotherapy for the treatment of verrucous epidermal nevi. Panagiotopoulos A, Chasapi V, Nikolaou V, Stavropoulos PG, Kafouros K, Petridis A, et al. Acta Derm Venereol 2009; 89: 292–4.

Nine patients with VEN and two with extensive unilateral epidermal nevus were treated with cryosurgery. Ten patients had their nevi treated successfully in two to five sessions, in which two cycles of open spray technique were used, 10 to 15 seconds each, depending on the size and extent of the nevus. The authors reported that the cosmetic result was excellent, with no scarring. One patient showed a relapse within 8 months after the treatment. The authors noted postoperative healing times from 10 to 20 days.

Second-Line Therapies	
• Laser ablation	B
• Dermabrasion	E
• Ruby laser	E
• Erbium:YAG laser	C

Epidermal nevi treated by carbon dioxide laser vaporization: a series of 25 patients. Paradela S, Del Pozo J, Fernández-Jorge B, Lozano J, Martínez-González C, Fonseca E. J Dermatol Treat 2007; 18: 169–74.

A total of 25 patients were treated with the CO_2 laser in the superpulsed mode. Good results were achieved in 92% of patients with soft, flattened nevi but in only 33% of patients with keratotic nevi. The authors concluded that the CO_2 laser in the superpulsed mode is an effective and safe treatment for VEN and provides fewer recurrences than other laser therapies. They noted that the main determining factor for the cosmetic result is thickness of the nevus.

Laser therapy of verrucous epidermal naevi. Hohenleutner U, Landthaler M. Clin Exp Dermatol 1993; 18: 124–7.

A series of 43 patients (41 with VEN and two with ILVEN) were treated with either the argon laser or the CO_2 laser. Soft, papillomatous lesions responded well to the argon laser, whereas hard keratotic nevi did not. A better response was seen with the CO_2 laser, but there was a tendency to hypertrophic scarring.

Er:YAG laser treatment of verrucous epidermal nevi. Park JH, Hwang ES, Kim SN, Kye YC. Dermatol Surg 2004; 30: 378–81.

Twenty patients with VEN were treated with the erbium:YAG laser. After a single treatment, successful elimination of the VEN was observed in 15 patients. Five patients (25%) showed a relapse within the first year after treatment.

Successful treatment of dark-colored epidermal nevus with ruby laser. Baba T, Narumi H, Hanada K, Hashimoto I. J Dermatol 1995; 22: 567–70.

Five darkly pigmented epidermal nevi were successfully cleared after one to four treatments with a ruby laser in the normal mode. Two patients subsequently had hypopigmentation at the treatment site.

A resurfacing procedure, either mechanically by dermabrading or with laser technology using either the erbium:YAG or the CO_2 laser, can produce very acceptable results. However, both these techniques are operator dependent, and in the case of laser therapy, access to expensive equipment is necessary. Darkly pigmented nevi may be treated using pigmented lesion lasers such as the ruby laser.

Third-Line Therapies	
• Systemic retinoids	D
• Topical retinoids plus 5-fluorouracil	E
• Photodynamic therapy	E

A case of verrucous epidermal naevus successfully treated with acitretin. Taskapan O, Dogan B, Baloglu H, Harmanyeri Y. Acta Derm Venereol 1998; 78: 475–6.

Report of a case of VEN in a 20-year-old patient who responded to acitretin 75 mg daily. The nevus started to recur 6 weeks after cessation of therapy.

Topical tretinoin and 5-fluorouracil in the treatment of linear verrucous epidermal nevus. Kim JJ, Chang MW, Shwayder T. J Am Acad Dermatol 2000; 43: 129–32.

In a 7-year-old boy with an extensive facial epidermal nevus there was significant improvement using a combination of topical tretinoin 0.1% cream and 5-fluorouracil.

Verrucous epidermal nevus successfully treated with photodynamic therapy. Sim JH, Kang Y, Kim YC. Eur J Dermatol 2010; 20: 814–5.

A 9-year-old girl presented with asymptomatic linear papillomatous and hyperkeratotic papules on the right thigh that developed at birth. She had no history of previous therapy. Treatment with methyl-aminolevulinate–photodynamic therapy (MAL-PDT) was performed. After four treatment sessions, the lesion was almost completely resolved, with mild residual hyperpigmentation. After 3 months of follow-up, the authors reported that the cosmetic and clinical response was excellent and the patient was very satisfied. After 5 months of follow-up, no recurrence had been observed.

Systemic retinoids have been shown to reduce hyperkeratosis in very extensive and cosmetically troublesome lesions. However, long-term use is required if the benefit is to be maintained. The topical combination of tretinoin and 5-fluorouracil has also been reported to achieve a significant improvement. Photodynamic therapy has been recently reported in the treatment of VEN.

INFLAMMATORY/DYSPLASTIC EPIDERMAL NEVI

First-Line Therapy	
• Topical corticosteroids	D

Successful treatment of inflammatory linear verrucous epidermal nevus with tacrolimus and fluocinonide. Mutasim DF. J Cutan Med Surg 2006; 10: 45–7.

Successful treatment of ILVEN with potent topical steroid and tacrolimus ointments.

Nevi that have inflammatory, epidermolytic, acantholytic, or dysplastic features may respond more effectively to medical therapy than to surgical treatment. ILVEN is a relatively rare entity that presents during childhood and can be difficult to treat. Topical corticosteroids are often used as first-line therapy, but the response is variable. There is little clinical data on the use of topical corticosteroids, and their use appears to be empirical rather than evidence based; nevertheless, they are relatively cheap and safe.

Second-Line Therapy	
• Topical calcipotriol/tacalcitol	D
• Topical retinoids	E
• Systemic retinoids	E
• Topical dithranol	E

Topical calcipotriol for the treatment of inflammatory linear verrucous epidermal nevus. Zvulunov A, Grunwald MH, Halvy S. Arch Dermatol 1997; 133: 567–8.

A report on the use of calcipotriol in the treatment of an ILVEN.

Successful therapy of an ILVEN in a 7-year-old girl with calcipotriol. Bohm I, Bieber T, Bauer R. Hautarzt 1999; 50: 812–4.

A report on the successful use of calcipotriol 0.005% ointment in the treatment of an ILVEN. After 8 weeks of therapy the ILVEN had almost cleared. There was no relapse 25 weeks after treatment was discontinued.

Acitretin treatment of a systematized inflammatory linear verrucous epidermal naevus. Renner R, Rytter M, Sticherling M. Acta Derm Venereol 2005; 85: 348–50.

In this case treatment with oral acitretin was initiated at a dose of 25 mg daily but had to be reduced to 20 mg daily because of increasing erythema on the face and left leg after 3 days of therapy. The dose was slowly increased to 30 mg daily. After 2 weeks at this level, the erythema had almost entirely resolved, and the hyperkeratosis was distinctly reduced. After 8 weeks on this dose the inflammatory and hyperkeratotic lesions had almost disappeared.

Dithranol in the treatment of inflammatory linear verrucous epidermal nevus. De Mare S, van de Kerkhof PC, Happle R. Acta Derm Venereol 1989; 69: 77–80.

Evidence Levels: **A** Double-blind study **B** Clinical trial ≥ 20 subjects **C** Clinical trial < 20 subjects **D** Series ≥ 5 subjects **E** Anecdotal case reports

Treatment with dithranol resulted in complete relief from pruritus and clearing of all linear lesions, except for a small verrucous band on the shin.

Third-Line Therapies	
• Pulsed-dye laser	E
• CO₂ laser	E
• Surgical excision	D
• Etanercept	E
• Photodynamic therapy	E

Pulsed dye laser for inflammatory linear verrucous epidermal nevus. Sidwell RU, Syed S, Harper JI. Br J Dermatol 2001; 144: 1267–9.

Three cases of ILVEN in children ranging in age from 2 to 8 years were treated successfully with the pulsed-dye laser. The authors surmise that the destruction of capillaries by the laser reduces the release of inflammatory mediators.

Carbon dioxide laser therapy for an inflammatory linear verrucous epidermal nevus: a case report. Ulkur E, Celikoz B, Yuksel F, Karagoz H. Aesthet Plast Surg 2004; 28: 428–30.

A case of ILVEN was treated with the CO_2 laser. All symptoms, including erythema, excoriation, granulation, and pruritus, disappeared, and a pale pigmentation remained.

Full-thickness surgical excision for the treatment of inflammatory linear verrucous epidermal nevus. Lee BJ, Mancini AJ, Renucci J, Paller AS, Bauer BS. Ann Plast Surg 2001; 47: 285–92.

The authors report four patients with extensive ILVEN treated successfully with full-thickness surgical excision.

Successful treatment of a widespread inflammatory verrucous epidermal nevus with etanercept. Bogle MA, Sobell JM, Dover JS. Arch Dermatol 2006; 142: 401–2.

A 55-year-old woman diagnosed with widespread inflammatory epidermal verrucous nevi was presented. She had a history of multiple therapies, including emollients, topical and intramuscular steroids, topical lactic acid, pimecrolimus cream, and isotretinoin.

The authors initiated subcutaneous etanercept therapy at a dose of 25 mg twice weekly. After 1 month, the patient experienced good initial improvement in pruritus and erythema. The etanercept was increased to 50 mg twice weekly, which provided nearly 50% improvement over 3 months. She continued treatment at this dose for a total of 6 months and achieved almost complete resolution of pruritus and a significant improvement in roughness and erythema. The dose was then reduced to 25 mg twice weekly, and disease activity remained quiescent at follow-up.

Inflammatory linear verrucous epidermal nevus successfully treated with methyl-aminolevulinate photodynamic therapy. Parera E, Gallardo F, Toll A, Gil I, Sánchez-Schmidt J, Pujol R. Dermatol Surg 2010; 36: 253–6.

The authors report a 67-year-old man with ILVEN who had failed multiple modalities. Treatment with MAL-PDT was performed. Almost complete resolution of the lesions after three PDT sessions (once a week) was observed. Pruritus completely disappeared, although small prurigo-like papules remained at the periphery of the lesion. No recurrence was observed after a follow-up period of 15 months.

Epidermodysplasia verruciformis

Slawomir Majewski, Stefania Jablonska

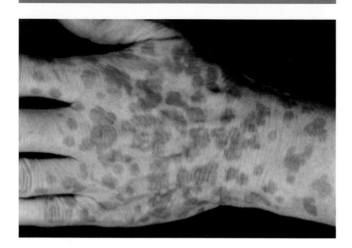

Epidermodysplasia verruciformis (EV) is a rare genetic disease characterized by an impaired immune response to human papillomavirus (HPV) and HPV-associated cutaneous oncogenesis. The disease is characterized by chronic infection with potentially oncogenic HPV types 5 and 8 as well as nononcogenic types. Flat warts and pityriasis versicolor–like lesions begin to appear in early childhood and become widespread. In the fourth and fifth decades 50% to 70% of patients begin to develop multiple cutaneous malignancies, mainly squamous cell carcinomas. It has been established that EV is mostly associated with mutations of two genes located on chromosome 17: *EVER1/TCM6* and *EVER2/TCM8*, coding transmembrane proteins located in the endoplasmic reticulum and involved in zinc transportation. However, about 25% of EV cases are not associated with these gene mutations.

A new and important problem is the occurrence of the EV phenotype in immunosuppressed individuals, which has been called *acquired epidermodysplasia verruciformis*. This EV-like syndrome has been described in patients with HIV infection, organ transplantation, Hodgkin disease, common variable immunodeficiency, systemic lupus erythematosus, immunoglobulin M deficiency, adult T-cell leukemia, some cases of graft-versus-host reaction, and others. Two varieties of acquired EV are described: a generalized verrucosis associated with large common warts mainly of HPV-3 type (sometimes referred to as *benign EV*) and a variety associated with diverse HPVs of types not usually related to EV.

The high risk of malignant transformation in genetic EV seems to be reduced in the acquired variety.

MANAGEMENT STRATEGY

No compound acts directly on HPV, and no therapy produces a complete and sustained clearing of both benign wartlike and keratotic lesions associated with oncogenic EV HPVs. A most important aspect of the management of EV is protection from ultraviolet radiation, which is a cancer cofactor. Light-avoiding behavior and topical sunblock creams (sun protection factor >50) are indicated. Other cancer cofactors (radiotherapy, immunosuppressants) must be avoided. Premalignant and troublesome benign lesions can be treated by a variety of destructive techniques: surgical (cryotherapy, shave excision, curettage, laser, full excision) or chemical (trichloroacetic acid, 5% 5-fluorouracil).

For more widespread lesions, with signs of premalignancy or malignancy, agents that modify keratinization are indicated, such as oral or topical retinoids, vitamin D_3 analogs, interferons, and imiquimod. Photodynamic therapy (PDT) can be useful for early malignancy. Larger malignancies can necessitate skin autografts.

Specific Investigations

- Family history and examination of other family members
- Skin biopsy
- HPV typing to identify potentially oncogenic and nononcogenic HPV types
- Evaluation of immune status and the presence of factors producing or enhancing immunosuppression: HIV, congenital and acquired immunodeficiency syndromes, iatrogenic immunosuppression

---

Common variable immunodeficiency syndrome associated with epidermodysplasia verruciformis. Vu J, Wallace GR, Singh R, Diwan H, Prieto V, Rady P. Am J Clin Dermatol 2007; 8: 307–10.

Generalized verrucosis: a review of the associated diseases, evaluation, and treatments. Sri JC, Dubina MI, Kao GF, Rady PL, Tyring SK, Gaspari AA. J Am Acad Dermatol 2012; 66: 2292–311.

Generalized verrucosis and distinct diseases (including EV) associated with generalized warts are defined. The indications for histopathologic examination, HPV typing, and other laboratory tests, as well as potential treatment options, are discussed.

Acquired epidermodysplasia verruciformis: a comprehensive review and proposal for treatment. Zampetti A, Giurdanella F, Manco S, Linder D, Gnarra M, Guerriero G, et al. Derm Surg 2013; 39: 974–9.

The treatment of acquired EV is not standardized, and several approaches have been described in the literature. Better results have been reported with combination procedures (e.g., photodynamic therapy and retinoids).

Deleterious effect of radiation therapy on epidermodysplasia verruciformis patients. de Oliveira WR, da Cruz Silva LL, Neto CF, Tyring S. J Cutan Med Surg 2015; 19: 416–21. Radiotherapy might be associated with progression of squamous cell carcinomas in EV patients, and it is recommended that this method of treatment be avoided in this patient population.

First-Line Therapies

Sun avoidance/protection	E
Cryotherapy with liquid nitrogen	E
Topical retinoic acid 0.05% to 0.1% for benign, flat, cosmetically troublesome lesions	E
Shave excision of flat lesions	E
Surgical excision of malignant lesions	E

Evidence Levels: **A** Double-blind study **B** Clinical trial ≥ 20 subjects **C** Clinical trial < 20 subjects **D** Series ≥ 5 subjects **E** Anecdotal case reports

Second-Line Therapies

• Interferon-α with retinoids (acitretin)	E
• Systemic isotretinoin	E
• Imiquimod 5% cream	E
• Topical 15% glycolic acid lotion	C
• Topical ingenol mebutate 0.015% gel	E
• Topical squaric acid dibutylester 2% solution (SADBE)	E
• Oral zinc sulfate	E
• Highly active antiretroviral therapy (HAART) in HIV-positive patients	E

Treatment of epidermodysplasia verruciformis with a combination of acitretin and interferon alfa-2a. Anadolu R, Oskay T, Erdem C, Boyvat A, Terzi E. J Am Acad Dermatol 2001; 45: 296–9.

A patient treated with oral acitretin 50 mg daily and systemic interferon-α_{2a}, 3 MU subcutaneously three times weekly for 6 months. Improvement was followed by relapse after discontinuation of treatment, and the same regimen was reintroduced. The interferon was then discontinued after 4 months and the acitretin reduced to 25 mg for 3 months, then stopped. Improvement was maintained during the subsequent 12-month follow-up. Used as monotherapy, interferon-α has only a slight effect and is not recommended.

Systemic low-dose isotretinoin maintains remission status in epidermodysplasia verruciformis. Rallis E, Papatheodorou G, Bimpakis E, Buutanska D, Menounos P, Papadakis P. J Eur Acad Dermatol Venereol 2008; 22: 523–5.

In this case isotretinoin 0.8 mg/kg/day for 6 months produced complete clearance, with relapse 4 months after discontinuation of medication. Maintenance treatment with 20 mg/day resulted in sustained remission. EV in this case was associated with HPV-3—that is, a more benign variant responsive to therapy.

Treatment of a patient with epidermodysplasia verruciformis carrying novel EVER2 mutation with imiquimod. Berthelot C, Dickerson MC, Rady P, He Q, Niroomand F, Tyring SK, et al. J Am Acad Dermatol 2007; 56: 882–6.

Acquired epidermodysplasia verruciformis syndrome in HIV-infected pediatric patients: prospective treatment trial with topical glycolic acid and human papillomavirus genotype characterization. Moore RL, de Schaetzen V, Joseph M, Lee IA, Miller-Monthrope Y, Phelps BR, et al. Arch Dermatol 2012; 148: 128–30.

Topical 15% glycolic acid lotion had a good effect in HIV-infected children; the therapy was regarded as safe and efficacious.

Treatment of imiquimod resistant epidermodysplasia verruciformis with ingenol mebutate. Kim C, Hashemi P, Caglia M, Shulman K. J Drugs Dermatol 2016; 15: 350–2. A patient with EV failed to respond to a 6-week course of 5% imiquimod on the forehead and was subsequently successfully treated with a 3-day course of 0.015% ingenol mebutate gel.

Epidermodysplasia verruciformis: successful treatment with squaric acid dibutylester. Kehdy J, Erickson C, Rady P, Tyring S, Gaspari AA. Cutis 2015; 96: 114–8. A case of 25-year history of refractory EV that was successfully treated with topical SADBE contact sensitizer agent. SADBE is used over the years for the treatment of a variety skin diseases, including alopecia areata and refractory cutaneous warts.

Efficacy of oral zinc therapy in epidermodysplasia verruciformis with squamous cell carcinoma. Sharma S, Barman KD, Sarkar R, Manjhi M, Kumar Garg V. Ind Derm Online J 2014; 5: 55–8.

A 24-year-old patient with EV was treated with oral zinc sulfate (550 mg/kg/day) with a satisfactory result (clearance of wartlike lesions on the face and upper and lower extremities by 30%–40%). The squamous cell carcinoma of the right hand was removed surgically.

Epidermodysplasia verruciformis in human immunodeficiency virus-infected patients: a marker of human papillomavirus-related disorders not affected by antiretroviral therapy. Jacobelli S, Laude H, Carlotti A, Rozenberg F, Deleuze J, Morini JP, et al. Arch Dermatol 2011; 147: 590–6.

Although there is no evidence-based therapy for acquired EV in HIV-positive patients, symptomatic treatments for HPV-induced lesions combined with HAART therapy could be partially effective. In most cases this therapy failed, although there was some improvement due to diminished viral load and increased CD4 cell count.

Third-Line Therapies

• Photodynamic therapy	E
• CO$_2$ laser for malignant and premalignant lesions	E
• Skin autografts	E

Photodynamic therapy for human papillomavirus-related diseases in dermatology. Szeimies RM. Med Laser Appl 2003; 18: 107–16.

Topical PDT using 20% 5-aminolevulinic acid was reported to yield excellent results in a case of EV associated with HPV-5, -8, -36, and other strains. Twelve months after PDT the lesions started to reappear but resolved after repeated treatments. The authors suggest annually repeated PDT is safe and will control EV lesions.

CO$_2$ laser treatment of warts in immunosuppressed patients. Lauchli S, Kempf W, Dragieva G, Burg G, Hafner J. Dermatology 2003; 206: 148–52.

Alternative therapies for recalcitrant HPV-induced cutaneous warts in EV may include CO$_2$ laser or neodymium laser. Laser therapy of recalcitrant warts proved to be efficacious in both immunosuppressed and immunocompetent individuals.

Skin autografts in epidermodysplasia verruciformis: human papillomavirus-associated cutaneous changes need over 20 years for malignant conversion. Majewski S, Jablonska S. Cancer Res 1997; 57: 4214–6.

For very widespread, constantly developing new lesions not responding to any therapy, the only effective method is removal of the most involved skin area (usually on the forehead) and its replacement with skin from nonexposed inner aspects of the arms.

Epidermolysis bullosa

Anna F. Falabella, Ysabel M. Bello, Lawrence A. Schachner

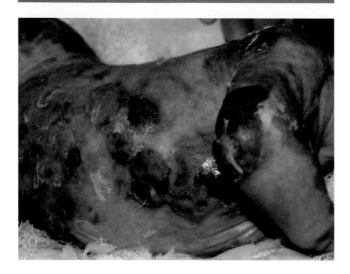

Epidermolysis bullosa (EB) is a complex group of mechanobullous disorders characterized by painful blister formation as a result of minor trauma to the skin. With the exception of the acquisita type, EB is an inherited disorder. The classification system for hereditary EB was updated in June 2014 and includes four major types according to the level of blister formation: simplex or intraepidermal ("epidermolytic"), junctional or intralamina lucida ("lamina lucidolytic"), dystrophic or sublamina densa ("dermolytic"), and Kindler syndrome or mixed. The disease can involve the skin, mucosae, and internal organs. The severity of EB ranges from mild to severe, and skin involvement can be localized or generalized.

In addition to the four major types of EB, there are several dozen subtypes, resulting from more than 1000 documented mutations on at least 18 structural genes. The genetic variability of EB results in a wide variety of clinical presentations, extracutaneous manifestations, degree of morbidity, and risk for early mortality.

MANAGEMENT STRATEGY

The management of inherited EB has classically been supportive: avoidance of trauma, blister management, wound management, treatment of infections, and nutritional support. More recent efforts have been directed at identifying and treating the underlying cause of disease with the goal of improving wound healing and preventing new wound formation.

Avoidance of trauma to intact skin is important but difficult. Sewing foam pads into the lining of clothing is helpful, especially over the elbows, knees, and other pressure points. Blister management involves *puncturing new blisters* with a sterile needle to avoid extension of the blister. The punctured area should be covered with a *topical antibiotic and a nonadherent dressing.*

Wound management comprises assessing the location and characteristics of the wound, *cleansing with low-toxicity solutions* (e.g., saline, water), *gentle debridement* of eschar/slough if present, and covering the wound with an appropriate nonadherent dressing. Wounds need to be evaluated and treated on a daily basis. In general, it is beneficial to soak wounds in a bathtub for 5 to 10 minutes. This facilitates cleansing and nontraumatic removal of dressings. Use of *low-concentration acetic acid or bleach* in the bath water may also help control bacterial load in wounds.

Minimizing trauma to wounds is vital. *Mepilex* is a nonadherent, absorbent polyurethane foam pad that can be applied, removed, and reapplied to wounds with little discomfort, no trauma to the wound bed or surrounding skin, and no disruption of wound healing. Other nonadherent dressings, such as *white petrolatum–impregnated gauzes, hydrogels, and foams,* can be used and held in place with soft, roller gauze bandages or elastic tube dressings.

A variety of *skin grafts* have been used to treat the wounds of EB, including split-thickness skin grafts, allogeneic and autogeneic cultured keratinocytes, and cryopreserved acellular human dermis. A study using intradermal injections of allogeneic fibroblasts demonstrated therapeutic potential in patients with recessive dystrophic epidermolysis bullosa (RDEB). Several trials have reported impressive results with *Apligraf*, a bilayered, tissue-engineered skin derived from neonatal foreskin. An allogeneic composite cultured skin *(OrCel)* has been approved by the U.S. Food and Drug Administration to treat hands and donor sites in patients with RDEB. More recently, amniotic membranes have been used to treat patients with EB with chronic nonhealing wounds.

Avoidance of wound infection is also critical to promote more rapid healing and to avoid overwhelming infections and sepsis, which are associated with an increased mortality rate. *Topical antibiotics* are routinely used but should be rotated monthly to avoid the development of resistant organisms. Cutaneous infections unresponsive to topical measures need to be treated with *systemic antibiotics,* but the chronic use of systemic antibiotics is not recommended as a preventive measure.

Common nutritional problems in patients with EB include chewing and swallowing difficulties, malnutrition, constipation, and vitamin and mineral deficiencies. Avoidance of malnutrition depends on *active and continuous nutritional support.* Early nutritional supplementation can promote better childhood growth rates and promote healing of skin lesions. In patients who develop esophageal strictures, balloon dilation is sometimes needed. *Daily multivitamin trace elements and zinc supplementation* is recommended. Anemia may be profound in EB, and *oral iron replacement* is mandatory for patients with iron deficiency. *Erythropoietin* has been recommended if the iron level is <500 mU/mL. Some have recommended intravenous iron therapy for patients resistant to oral replacement. Albumin should be monitored to assess the patient's nutritional status. If necessary, *protein supplements* can be added to the diet. Severe malnutrition can be treated with enteral feeding via gastrostomy tube if necessary.

Systemic therapies, such as *psoralens in combination with UVA irradiation, corticosteroids, vitamin E, cyclosporine, antimalarials, retinoids, phenytoin, tetracycline, trimethoprim–sulfamethoxazole, and cyproheptadine,* have been used to treat EB, but their efficacy is unproven.

Current therapies are focused on gene-, protein-, and cell-based techniques. There have been improvements in genetic manipulation of keratinocytes ex vivo and of graft techniques in vivo. Gene transfer of epidermal stem cells in combination with tissue engineering procedures is promising.

Evidence Levels: A Double-blind study B Clinical trial ≥ 20 subjects C Clinical trial < 20 subjects D Series ≥ 5 subjects E Anecdotal case reports

Specific Investigations

- Skin biopsy for transmission electron microscopy
- Skin biopsy for immunofluorescence antigenic mapping
- Mutational analysis

The classification of inherited epidermolysis bullosa (EB): report of the Third International Consensus Meeting on Diagnosis and Classification of EB. Fine J-D, Eady RAJ, Bauer EA, Bauer JW, Heagerty A, Bruckner-Tuderman L, et al. J Am Acad Dermatol 2008; 58: 931–50.

Both transmission electron microscopy (EM) and immunofluorescence have been successfully employed to diagnose EB. EM is likely to play a decreasing role in the diagnosis because there are only a few highly proficient EM laboratories, although it has an important place in research because it permits visualization and assessment of keratin filaments, hemidesmosomes, and anchoring fibrils. Immunofluorescence antigen mapping is relatively inexpensive and simple to perform, requiring immunofluorescence transport media. It can reveal the level of the split by defining its location relative to proteins expressed at various levels of the basement membrane zone. Mutational analysis remains a superb research tool that lets us determine the mode of inheritance, the precise site, and the type of molecular mutation. However, it is not considered the first-line diagnostic test.

First-Line Therapies

• Sterile dressing and topical antibiotics	B
• Nutritional support	C

Best practice guidelines for skin and wound care in epidermolysis bullosa. International consensus. Denyer J, Pillay E. DEBRA, 2012. www.woundsinternational.com/media/issues/623/files/content_10609.pdf.

Wound care is the cornerstone of treatment for patients with EB. This document was developed to help care for these patients. Skin and wound management must be tailored to suit both the type of EB and the specific characteristics of the wound. EB is a life-long disorder that requires specialist intervention and considerations to minimize complications and improve quality of life.

Management of epidermolysis bullosa in infants and children. Bello YM, Falabella AF, Schachner LA. Clin Dermatol 2003; 21: 278–82.

Open or only partially healed erosions are best covered with polymyxin, bacitracin, or silver sulfadiazine and then covered with either petrolatum-impregnated gauze or nonadherent synthetic dressing. Such dressings are usually changed daily. Mupirocin may be substituted for those infected sites unresponsive to milder antibiotics but is best avoided for routine use because of the potential for development of resistance.

The challenges of meeting nutritional requirements in children and adults with epidermolysis bullosa: proceedings of a multidisciplinary team study day. Hubbard L, Haynes L, Sklar M, Martinez AE, Mellerio JE. Clin Exp Dermatol 2011; 36: 579–83.

This is a report of a study day held in London on March 3, 2010, to discuss measures with which to meet the nutritional requirements of patients with EB. Members of national and international multidisciplinary teams (MDTs) caring for patients with EB attended this event. The study day focused on four challenging aspects of management intimately associated with nutritional status in EB necessitating close cooperation between MDT members: iron-deficiency anemia, gastrostomy placement and feeding, muscle mass and mobility, and dental health.

The study day provided a unique forum for dietitians, doctors, nurses, physiotherapists, psychologists, psychotherapists, dentists, dental hygienists, and occupational therapists to share knowledge and debate problems common to all who strive to promote best practice in this rare and complex group of conditions.

Second-Line Therapies

• Skin grafts	C
• Cultured keratinocytes	C
• Keratin gel	C
• Fibroblast cell therapy	D
• Amniotic cell membrane	D

Punch grafting of chronic ulcers in patients with laminin-332-deficient, non-Herlitz junctional epidermolysis bullosa. Yuen WY, Huizinga J, Jonkman MF. J Am Acad Dermatol 2012; 68: 93–7.

Four patients with laminin-332-deficient JEB-nH were treated with punch grafting. Over a 10-year period, 23 ulcers were treated using punch grafting without any complications or adverse effects. The ulcers had on average persisted 6 years before treatment. Healing rate after punch grafting was 70% (*n* = 16), with a mean healing time of 2 months. Thirty percent (*n* = 7) of the treated ulcers did not completely heal, but did show improvement. The recurrence rate after 3 months was 13% (*n* = 2) and was a result of renewed blistering. Punch grafting can be used as a first-line treatment in small persistent ulcers in patients with JEB-nH.

Tissue-engineered skin (Apligraf) in the healing of patients with epidermolysis bullosa wounds. Falabella AF, Valencia IC, Eaglstein WH, Schachner LA. Arch Dermatol 2000; 135: 1219–22.

An open-label uncontrolled study of 15 patients with 69 acute wounds and 9 chronic wounds who were treated with tissue-engineered skin; a week later, 79% of the wounds were healed. The patients and their families considered that healing with the tissue-engineered skin was faster and less painful and that quality of life was improved, compared with healing with conventional dressings.

Apligraf in the treatment of severe mitten deformity associated with recessive dystrophic epidermolysis bullosa. Fivenson DP, Scherschum L, Cohen LV. Plast Reconstruct Surg 2003; 112: 584–8.

Five patients with RDEB were treated for mitten deformity with a bioengineered skin equivalent. These patients exhibited increased range of motion and have maintained web space separation for more than 12 months, improving the quality of their life.

Keratin gel in the management of epidermolysis bullosa. Denyer J, Marsh C, Kirsner RS. J Wound Care 2015; 24: 446–50.

In this pilot study, keratin gel (keratin-rich hydrogels extracted from sheep wool) was introduced into the management of different types of EB wounds, maintaining other aspects of their care. This treatment reported faster healing and was found to be effective in 6 of 10 patients and ineffective in 2 and caused itching leading to discontinuation in 2 other patients.

Amniotic membrane grafting in patients with epidermolysis bullosa with chronic wounds. Lo V, Lara-Corrales I, Stuparich A, Pope E. J Am Acad Dermatol 2010; 62: 1038–44.

A retrospective chart review of two patients with EB who were treated with amniotic membranes revealed the potential usefulness of amniotic membrane grafting in promoting healing of chronic wounds in patients with EB.

Third-Line Therapies	
• Bone marrow transplantation	E
• Tetracycline	C
• Phenytoin (ineffective)	A
• Trimethoprim–sulfamethoxazole	D
• Cyproheptadine	C
• Isotretinoin	C
• Gene therapy	E
• Granulocyte colony-stimulating factor	C

Bone marrow transplantation for recessive dystrophic epidermolysis bullosa. Wagner JE, Ishida-Yamamoto A, McGrath JA, Hordinsky M, Keene DR, Woodley DT, et al. N Engl J Med 2010; 363: 629–39.

Seven children with RDEB were treated with immunomyeloablative chemotherapy and allogeneic stem-cell transplantation. One patient died of cardiomyopathy before transplantation. Of the remaining six patients, one had severe regimen-related cutaneous toxicity, with all having improved wound healing and a reduction in blister formation between 30 and 130 days after transplantation. Increased collagen type VII (C7) deposition was observed at the dermal–epidermal junction in five of the six recipients, albeit without normalization of anchoring fibrils. Five recipients were alive 130 to 799 days after transplantation; one died at 183 days as a consequence of graft rejection and infection. The six recipients had substantial proportions of donor cells in the skin, and none had detectable anti-C7 antibodies.

Allogeneic blood and bone marrow cells for the treatment of severe epidermolysis bullosa: repair of the extracellular matrix. Tolar J, Wagner JE. Lancet 2013 5; 382: 1214–23.

Several trials have demonstrated that protein replacement therapy by allogeneic blood and marrow transplantation can attenuate the mucocutaneous manifestations of epidermolysis bullosa and improve patients' quality of life. Further studies are needed to explore these therapies.

Treatment of epidermolysis bullosa simplex with tetracycline. Veien NK, Buus SK. Arch Dermatol 2000; 136: 424–5.

A number of patients using tetracycline were observed over a 7-year period. The article reports an increase in bulla formation during the summer months, but healing was more rapid and less painful while patients took the tetracycline.

Tetracycline and epidermolysis bullosa simplex: a double-blind, placebo-controlled, crossover randomized clinical trial. Weiner M, Stein A, Cash S, de Leoz J, Fine JD. Br J Dermatol 2004; 150: 613–4.

Six of 12 patients completed at least the first arm: 4 experienced a reduction in the total number of EB lesions; 2 experienced an increased number of lesions after 4 months of active therapy (oral tetracycline administered 1000 mg every morning and 500 mg every evening). The risk of tetracycline-induced dental discoloration in children needs to be balanced against the severity and chronicity of the symptoms.

A systematic review of randomized controlled trials of treatment for inherited forms of epidermolysis bullosa. Langan SM, Williams HC. Clin Exp Dermatol 2009; 34: 20–5.

There are five randomized double-blind placebo-controlled trial crossover studies for inherited epidermolysis bullosa. Two studies reported the use of oral tetracycline, but the beneficial effect is unclear. Another two randomized controlled trials (RCTs) assessed the use of aluminum chloride hexahydrate solution 20% and bufexamac cream 5% in EB reporting no benefit over placebo. In an RCT of 36 patients, phenytoin failed to show any difference compared with placebo.

The efficacy of trimethoprim in wound healing of patients with epidermolysis bullosa: a feasibility trial. Lara-Corrales I, Parkin PC, Stephens D, Hamilton J, Koren G, Weinstein M, et al. J Am Acad Dermatol 2012; 66: 264–70.

Ten patients with RDEB were treated with trimethoprim (TMP). The study assessed lesion counts, quality of life, and emergence of antibiotic resistance. All patients showed improved wound healing on TMP, but primary and secondary outcome measures did not achieve statistical significance. This proof-of-concept study demonstrates the potential efficacy of TMP in improving wound healing in RDEB and provides useful information for further prospective studies.

Chemoprevention of squamous cell carcinoma in recessive dystrophic epidermolysis bullosa: results of a phase I trial of systemic isotretinoin. Fine JD, Johnson LB, Weiner M, Stein A, Suchindran C. J Am Acad Dermatol 2004; 50: 563–71.

Patients with RDEB are at high risk of developing squamous cell carcinoma (SCC). An initial study on 20 patients aged 15 years or older who were treated with isotretinoin 0.5 mg/kg/day for 8 months reported that isotretinoin may be safely used. However, a chemoprevention effect has yet to be proven.

Correction of junctional epidermolysis bullosa by transplantation of genetically modified epidermal stem cells. Mavillo F, Pellegrini G, Ferrari S, Di Nunzio F, Di Iorio E, et al. Nature Med 2006; 12: 1397–402.

Ex vivo transduction of autologous epidermal stem cells with a normal copy of the defective gene, followed by reconstitution of the patient's skin with epithelial sheets that were grown from these genetically corrected cells, kept the epidermis firmly adherent and stable for the duration of follow-up (1 year).

Risk of squamous cell carcinoma in junctional epidermolysis bullosa, non-Herlitz type: report of 7 cases and a review of the literature. Yuen WY, Jonkman MF. J Am Acad Dermatol 2011; 65: 780–9.

SCC is the most severe complication and most common cause of death in patients with RDEB. The SCCs have a high recurrence rate and follow an aggressive course that results in death in one of five patients. It is recommended that annual checks of all JEB patients for SCC start at 25 years of age.

Systemic granulocyte colony-stimulating factor (G-CSF) enhances wound healing in dystrophic epidermolysis bullosa (DEB): results of a pilot trial. Fine JD, Manes B, Frangoul H. J Am Acad Dermatol 2015; 73: 56–61.

Seven patients with DEB were treated daily with subcutaneous G-CSF daily (10 µg/kg/dose) for 6 days with reduction in lesional size and blister/erosion count. However, small patient number is a limitation of this pilot study but could be considered an option when conventional therapies fail; new prospective studies are needed.

Evidence Levels: **A** Double-blind study **B** Clinical trial ≥ 20 subjects **C** Clinical trial < 20 subjects **D** Series ≥ 5 subjects **E** Anecdotal case reports

69

Epidermolysis bullosa acquisita

Lawrence S. Chan

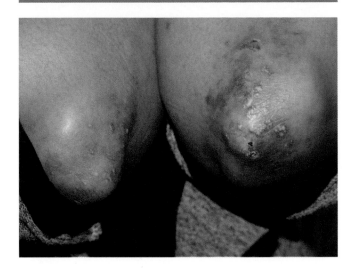

Epidermolysis bullosa acquisita is a relatively rare, chronic, autoimmune blistering disease affecting the skin and mucous membranes. The disorder predominantly affects elderly patients, and the skin lesions occur commonly at trauma-prone skin areas (in the noninflammatory mechanobullous scarring subset) or widespread skin areas (in the generalized inflammatory non-scarring subset). Although IgG (or rarely IgA) class autoantibodies targeting the skin basement membrane component type VII collagen (anchoring fibrils) are major contributing factors, minor physical trauma also plays an important role in the blister development.

MANAGEMENT STRATEGY

Epidermolysis bullosa acquisita, particularly the noninflammatory mechanobullous subset, is characteristically very refractory to conventional medical therapies. For an immune-mediated blistering disease associated with autoantibodies that target skin components, the obviously logical approach is to suppress the immune responses, thereby reducing the production and effect of the autoantibodies to their target skin component type VII collagen Unfortunately, currently there is no target-specific medication available. Thus the presently available non–target-specific immunosuppressive medications not only suppress the immune responses against type VII collagen but also reduce the patient's immune defense to pathogens, leading to a relative immunodeficiency. Therefore when treating patients with this disease, every effort should be made to use antiinflammatory instead of immunosuppressant agents, to use the lowest possible doses of immunosuppressant for the shortest time frame, and to replace immunosuppressants with antiinflammatory medications whenever feasible. A commonly used start-up regimen consists of *systemic corticosteroid combined with either mycophenolate mofetil or dapsone or both* as a corticosteroid-sparing agent. For adult patients

without major medical problems, a combination of oral prednisone (1 mg/kg daily), mycophenolate mofetil (1–2 g daily), and dapsone (100–200 mg daily) can be initiated. Because of its rarity, well-controlled clinical trials have not been performed for epidermolysis bullosa acquisita. The following therapeutic guidelines are derived mainly from case reports of small groups or single patients.

Other medications have also been reported to be beneficial for this disease. *Colchicine* (1–2 mg daily) has shown significant improvement for the disease. *Ciclosporin* (5–9 mg/kg daily) has been reported to be beneficial in reducing blister formation and speeding up healing. *Intravenous immunoglobulin (IVIG)* treatment (400 mg/kg daily) has also been determined to reduce new blister formation and facilitate healing. In addition, *extracorporeal photochemotherapy* has been used successfully in some patients. Most recently, a monoclonal antibody against B-cell–specific target CD20, *rituximab* (usual dose 375 mg/m^2 body surface area, multiple doses), has been reported to be effective in several cases. Due to its high cost the physician may encounter difficulty obtaining insurance company approval for the use of rituximab.

In addition, patients with this disease should be educated to *avoid physical trauma* as much as possible. Activities such as vigorous rubbing of their skin and the use of harsh soaps and hot water should also be eliminated. Patients should be informed to *care for open wounds promptly* and to recognize local skin infection and *seek medical attention when infection occurs.*

Specific Investigations

- Skin biopsy and serum for direct and indirect immunofluorescence, respectively, to detect in vivo bound and circulating IgG (or IgA, IgM) class skin basement membrane–specific autoantibodies
- Serum for enzyme-linked immunosorbent assay (ELISA) to detect IgG (or IgA, IgM) class type VII collagen-specific autoantibodies
- Gastrointestinal workup for possible inflammatory bowel disease

Epidermolysis bullosa acquisita: ultrastructural and immunologic studies. Yaoita H, Briggaman RA, Lawley TJ, Provost TT, Katz SI. J Invest Dermatol 1981; 76: 288–92.

Identification of the skin basement-membrane autoantigen in epidermolysis bullosa acquisita. Woodley DT, Briggaman RA, O'Keefe EJ, Inman AO, Queen LL, Gammon WR. N Engl J Med 1984; 310: 1007–13.

Direct immunofluorescence detects IgG deposits linearly at the dermoepidermal junction in all patients. Indirect immunofluorescence detects IgG circulating autoantibodies bound to the dermal side of salt-separated normal skin substrate in about 50% of patients with this disease.

Development of an ELISA for rapid detection of antitype VII collagen autoantibodies in epidermolysis bullosa acquisita. Chen M, Chan LS, Cai X, O'Toole EA, Sample JC, Woodley DT. J Invest Dermatol 1997; 108: 68–72.

ELISA using eukaryotically expressed recombinant protein of the noncollagenous (NC1) domain of type VII collagen is the most sensitive and specific method for detecting IgG class circulating autoantibodies in patients with this disease.

The use of biochip immunofluorescence microscopy for the serological diagnosis of epidermolysis bullosa acquisita. Marzano AV, Cozzani E, Biasin M, Russo I, Alaibac M. Arch Dermatol Res 2016; 308: 273–6.

A new biochip technology has been reported to be useful in the initial screening circulating autoantibodies to type VII collagen.

IgA-mediated epidermolysis bullosa acquisita: two cases and review of the literature. Vodegel RM, de Jong MC, Pas HH, Jonkman MF. J Am Acad Dermatol 2002; 47: 919–25.

In rare cases, IgA class rather than IgG class autoantibodies were found to target the type VII collagen, resulting in a clinical phenotype indistinguishable from the classic IgG-mediated disease. However, IgA-mediated disease has a lesser tendency to form scar and is more responsive to dapsone treatment.

IgM-type epidermolysis bullosa acquisita. Omland SH, Gniadecki R. Br J Dermatol 2015; 173: 1566–8.

This is a very rare case where the targeting autoantibodies appear to be the IgM class.

Epidermolysis bullosa acquisita and inflammatory bowel disease. Raab B, Fretzin DF, Bronson DM, Scott MJ, Roenigk Jr HH, Medenica M. JAMA 1983; 250: 1746–8.

Inflammatory bowel disease, particularly Crohn disease, is strongly associated with epidermolysis bullosa acquisita. All patients should be questioned for symptoms of inflammatory bowel disease. If symptoms are present, a comprehensive gastrointestinal workup is indicated.

The epidermolysis bullosa acquisita antigen (type VII collagen) is present in human colon and patients with Crohn's disease have autoantibodies to type VII collagen. Chen M, O'Toole EA, Sanghavi J, Mahmud N, Kelleher D, Weir D, et al. J Invest Dermatol 2002; 118: 1059–64.

The presence of type VII collagen in the gut and autoantibodies to type VII collagen in patients with inflammatory bowel disease without skin manifestations supports a link between the gut and the skin.

Black patients of African descent and HLA-DRB1*15:03 frequency overrepresented in epidermolysis bullosa acquisita. Zumelzu C, Le Roux-Villet C, Loiseau P, Busson M, Heller M, Aucouturier F, et al. J Invest Dermatol 2011; 131: 2386–93.

This study reported that a higher percentage of patients affected by epidermolysis bullosa acquisita are black patients of African descent and that the human leukocyte antigen HLA-DRB1*15:03 allele seems to contribute to this disease development.

Congenital epidermolysis bullosa acquisita: vertical transfer of maternal autoantibody from mother to infant. Abrams ML, Smidt A, Benjamin L, Chen M, Woodley D, Mancini AJ. Arch Dermatol 2011; 147: 337–41.

Although epidermolysis bullosa acquisita rarely occurs in children, it has never been reported in an infant until now. This case, which occurred in an infant, should raise the awareness of maternally transferred epidermolysis bullosa acquisita by physicians when they encounter blistering disease in a neonate.

Physicians need to recognize the possibility of maternal transfer of autoantibodies and the transient nature of the blisters (with no need for systemic treatment). This case of passive transfer of disease further demonstrates the pathogenic role of the autoantibodies, as was illustrated in an animal model of epidermolysis bullosa acquisita.

First-Line Therapies	
• Systemic corticosteroids	D
• Mycophenolate mofetil	E
• Dapsone	D

Epidermolysis bullosa acquisita – a pemphigoid-like disease. Gammon WR, Briggaman RA, Woodley DT, Heald PW, Wheeler Jr CE. J Am Acad Dermatol 1984; 11: 820–32.

Five patients with the generalized inflammatory subset of disease responded at least partially to prednisone (40–120 mg daily), with or without the addition of azathioprine 100 mg daily.

Childhood IgA-mediated epidermolysis bullosa acquisita responding to mycophenolate mofetil as a corticosteroid-sparing agent. Tran MM, Anhalt GJ, Barrett T, Cohen BA. J Am Acad Dermatol 2006; 54: 734–6.

Mycophenolate mofetil (700 mg/day) was added to the regimen of prednisolone (25 mg/day) and dapsone (25 mg/day) when the disease flared upon reduction of prednisolone dose in this 2-year-old patient affected by an IgA-mediated epidermolysis bullosa acquisita. With the addition of mycophenolate mofetil, the systemic corticosteroid was totally tapered off over a 9-month period. This case illustrates the usefulness of mycophenolate mofetil in childhood-onset disease.

Mycophenolate mofetil in epidermolysis bullosa acquisita. Kowalzick L, Suckow S, Zuiegler H, Waldmann T, Pönnighaus JM, Gläser V. Dermatology 2003; 207: 332–4.

Mycophenolate mofetil (1 g twice daily) was used successfully in conjunction with plasmapheresis as a corticosteroid-sparing agent in one patient with epidermolysis bullosa acquisita not controlled by azathioprine (150 mg daily) and prednisolone (60 mg daily). The clinical improvement was associated with a reduction in autoantibody titers.

Bullous pemphigoid and epidermolysis bullosa acquisita: presentation, prognosis, and immunotherapy in 11 children. Edwards S, Wakelin SH, Wojnarowska F, Marsden RA, Kirtschig G, Bhogal B, et al. Pediatr Dermatol 1998; 15: 184–90.

A survey of five childhood-onset cases showed good clinical responses to combined corticosteroids and dapsone, as well as a good long-term prognosis.

Epidermolysis bullosa acquisita responsive to dapsone therapy. Hughes AP, Callen JP. J Cutan Med Surg 2001; 5: 397–9.

One patient who failed to respond to prednisone (40 mg daily) plus tetracycline and niacinamide achieved complete control of blistering activities after 2 months on dapsone 150 mg daily.

Second-Line Therapies	
• Intravenous immunoglobulin	D
• Colchicine	D
• Ciclosporin	D

Severe, refractory epidermolysis bullosa acquisita complicated by an oesophageal stricture responding to intravenous immune globulin. Harman KE, Whittam LR, Wakelin SH, Black MM. Br J Dermatol 1998; 139: 1126–7.

Evidence Levels: **A** Double-blind study **B** Clinical trial ≥ 20 subjects **C** Clinical trial < 20 subjects **D** Series ≥ 5 subjects **E** Anecdotal case reports

The patient had the noninflammatory mechanobullous subset of disease and esophageal stricture and was refractory to prednisone (up to 80 mg daily), dapsone (100 mg daily), cyclophosphamide (150 mg daily), and azathioprine (3 mg/kg daily). The patient was treated with courses of IVIG (0.4 g/kg daily) on 5 consecutive days at 4- to 6-week intervals as a monotherapy, resulting in a dramatic fall in the circulating titers of anti–basement membrane IgG autoantibodies, reduction of new blister formation, and disappearance of dysphagia. However, not all patients reported in the literature responded to this treatment. The major disadvantage of this regimen is the high cost.

Treatment of epidermolysis bullosa acquisita with intravenous immunoglobulin in patients non-responsive to conventional therapy: clinical outcome and post-treatment long-term follow-up. Ahmed AR, Gürcan HM. J Eur Acad Dermatol Venereol 2012; 26: 1074–83.

In this report the authors examined 10 epidermolysis bullosa acquisita patients (mean age 57.4 years), who received 16 to 31 cycles (2 g/kg/cycle) of IVIG (mean 23.1 cycles) for 30 to 52 months (mean 38.8 months), with all other medications tapered off in 5 to 9 months (mean 7.2 months) and IVIG as monotherapy thereafter. All treated patients had satisfactory improvement. At the time of follow-up occurring 29 to 123 months post treatment (mean 53.9 months) they revealed no disease recurrence. No serious side effects were noted.

Colchicine for epidermolysis bullosa acquisita. Cunningham BB, Kirchmann TT, Woodley DT. J Am Acad Dermatol 1996; 34: 781–4.

Four patients with the noninflammatory mechanobullous subset of disease, some refractory to prednisone treatment, were treated with oral colchicine (1–2 mg daily), with or without the addition of cyclophosphamide (50 mg daily). In all patients there was substantial clinical improvement in the reduction of skin fragility and spontaneous blister formation. An initial dose of 0.4 to 0.6 mg daily is recommended, with an increase by 0.6 mg daily each week until diarrhea develops. The patients are instructed to take the highest tolerable doses. Other than diarrhea, the long-term administration of colchicine (up to 4 years) was well tolerated. The side effect of diarrhea, however, makes it questionably suitable for those patients who have associated inflammatory bowel disease.

Oral cyclosporine in the treatment of inflammatory and noninflammatory cases. A clinical and immunopathologic analysis. Gupta AK, Ellis CN, Nickoloff BJ, Goldfarb MT, Ho VC, Rocher LL, et al. Arch Dermatol 1990; 126: 339–50.

Two patients with epidermolysis bullosa acquisita (subset not defined) were treated with oral ciclosporin (6 mg/kg daily) for a total of 8 weeks. These patients experienced a gradual reduction in the frequency of new blister and erosion formation. The known renal toxicity of ciclosporin makes it questionable as a suitable long-term regimen and warranted only as a last-resort measure.

Third-Line Therapies	
• Rituximab	D
• Minocycline	E

Successful adjuvant treatment of recalcitrant epidermolysis bullosa acquisita with anti-CD20 antibody rituximab. Schmidt E, Benoit S, Brocker E-B, Zillikens D, Goebeler M. Arch Dermatol 2006; 142: 147–50.

The patient, who had both skin and oral mucosal involvement, was not controlled with prednisolone (up to 250 mg/day), dapsone (150 mg/day), and subsequently azathioprine (up to 175 mg/day) and colchicine (2.5 mg/day). The regimen was changed to rituximab weekly infusion (375 mg/m² body surface area) for 4 consecutive weeks, with continuous use of azathioprine (175 mg/day) and colchicine (2.5 mg/day) and reducing doses of prednisolone. The patient's lesions completely healed in 11 weeks post–rituximab infusion, allowing the tapering of systemic steroid, colchicine, and azathioprine. Fourteen weeks after the discontinuation of colchicine and prednisolone, the patient remained in clinical remission. No complication was reported except an event of deep vein thrombosis.

A successful therapeutic trial of rituximab in the treatment of a patient with recalcitrant, high-titer epidermolysis bullosa acquisita. Crichlow SM, Mortimer NJ, Harman KE. Br J Dermatol 2006; 156: 194–6.

A patient with both oral mucosal and skin lesions and a high titer of IgG autoantibodies to skin basement membrane zone (indirect immunofluorescence titer up to 1:3200) was treated with conventional therapeutic agents (prednisolone up to 60 mg/day, mycophenolate mofetil 2 g/day, and subsequently IVIG infusions (2 g/kg body weight/month)) without much success. Moreover, the patient could not tolerate azathioprine (due to liver toxicity) or ciclosporin (due to nephrotoxicity and hypertension). In the meantime, the patient's conditions were worsening, with increasing autoantibody titer and involvement of the esophagus. Therefore weekly rituximab infusions (375 mg/m² body surface area) were then given to the patient along with mycophenolate mofetil (2 g/day) and prednisolone (30 mg/day). The patient had slow but progressive improvement of the lesions, and all were healed 5 months after starting rituximab. One year after the rituximab treatment the patient was still in partial remission, suffering only occasional trauma-induced blisters, and the autoantibody titer fell to 1:10.

Epidermolysis bullosa acquisita following bullous pemphigoid, successfully treated with anti-CD20 monoclonal antibody rituximab. Wallet-Faber N, Franck N, Matteux F, Mateus C, Gilbert D, Carlotti A, et al. Dermatology 2007; 215: 252–5.

An interesting patient who initially developed bullous pemphigoid but who upon subsequent flare manifested a generalized skin and mucosal (oral and genital) blistering disease that was confirmed as epidermolysis bullosa acquisita by target antigen identification. The initial success of treatment (combined prednisone 1.5 mg/kg/day and azathioprine 100 mg/day) did not last long, as the reduction of prednisone resulted in rapid worsening of the condition, further complicated by a life-threatening *Legionella pneumonophila* infection. Furthermore, the patient could not tolerate mycophenolate mofetil. Therefore rituximab (375 mg/m² body surface area) was initiated on a weekly interval for 4 consecutive weeks, resulting in dramatic improvement of the patient's condition. At 10 months' follow-up post rituximab initiation the patient had only a few visible blisters.

Treatment-resistant classical epidermolysis bullosa acquisita responding to rituximab. Sadler E, Schafleitner B, Lanschuetzer C, Laimer M, Pohla-Gubo G, Hametner R, et al. Br J Dermatol 2007; 157: 417–9.

A patient with both skin and multiple mucosal (oral, esophageal, and laryngeal) lesions who failed to respond to multiple conventional immunosuppressive medications subsequently responded to rituximab. Over a 6-year period the patient failed to show complete clinical response to methylprednisolone (up to 5 mg/kg/day), azathioprine (up to 2.5 mg/kg body weight), ciclosporin (up to 9 mg/kg/day), mycophenolate mofetil (up to 30 mg/kg/day), cyclophosphamide (500 mg/m² body surface area IV, followed by 1 mg/kg/day orally), colchicine (up to 1.5 mg/day), IVIG (up to 2.5 g/kg body weight/cycle), gold (1 mg/kg/week IV, followed by IM and oral preparations), and daclizumab (1 mg/kg body weight, six infusions over 3 weeks). Therefore a regimen of a reduced dose of rituximab (144 mg/m² infusion per week for 5 weeks) along with azathioprine (2 mg/kg/day) was given; the patient tolerated the treatment without any side effects or infections. A remarkable improvement was noticed 4 weeks after the initiation of rituximab treatment, and all medications were subsequently discontinued. Two years after all medications were tapered, the patient's disease activity remained at a very low level.

Clinical response of severe mechanobullous epidermolysis bullosa acquisita to combined treatment with immunoadsorption and rituximab (anti-CD20 monoclonal antibodies). Niedermeier A, Eming R, Pfutze M, Neumann CR, Happel C, Reich K, et al. Arch Dermatol 2007; 143: 192–8.

Two patients affected by the mechanobullous type of epidermolysis bullosa acquisita were treated with combined immunoadsorption (daily treatment for 8 consecutive days) and rituximab (375 mg/m² body surface area/week for a total of 4 weeks). Mycophenolate mofetil (1–3 g/day) was given continuously during this period. In both patients treatment with multiple medications, including ciclosporin, azathioprine, dapsone, dexamethasone pulse, and cyclophosphamide pulse, was unsuccessful. One patient achieved near-complete clinical resolution, but the other could only obtain stable disease status. This report illustrates the treatment-resistant nature of this disease.

Inflammatory epidermolysis bullosa acquisita effectively treated with minocycline. Kawase K, Oshitani Y, Mizutani Y, Shu E, Fujine E, Selshima M. Acta Derm Venereol 2014; 94: 615–6.

In this report, a patient with generalized inflammatory subtype of the disease was effectively controlled with an antibiotic that has antiinflammatory function.

Evidence Levels: **A** Double-blind study **B** Clinical trial ≥ 20 subjects **C** Clinical trial < 20 subjects **D** Series ≥ 5 subjects **E** Anecdotal case reports

Erosive pustular dermatosis

Bhavnit K. Bhatia, Jenny E. Murase

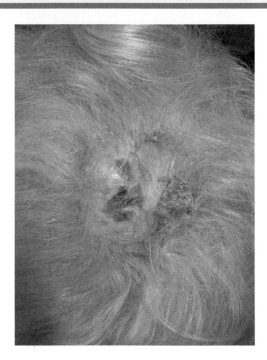

Erosive pustular dermatosis (EPD) is a rare condition characterized by pustular, erosive, and crusted lesions in areas of alopecia that tend to be atrophic, actinically damaged, or subject to local iatrogenic or external trauma. The condition primarily affects the elderly and is located on the scalp but has also been rarely documented to occur on the legs. EPD lesions tend to be chronic, progressive, and difficult to treat. Laboratory and histopathologic findings are not diagnostic.

MANAGEMENT STRATEGY

Traditionally, *potent topical corticosteroids* have been used in EPD with a generally positive but variable response within a few months of use. Due to steroid-related cutaneous atrophy and residual scarring, *tacrolimus 0.1% ointment, calcipotriol cream, oral zinc,* and *photodynamic therapy* (PDT) have been introduced as alternative therapies. A series has shown *dapsone 5% gel* to be effective in resolving EPD, and *oral dapsone* was shown to be successful in one case report. *Retinoids and oral corticosteroids* have also shown some promise when used in conjunction with topical antibiotics, topical corticosteroids, topical tacrolimus, oral dapsone, and oral zinc therapy. Topical and systemic antibiotics and antifungals are essentially ineffective.

First-Line Therapy

• High-potency topical corticosteroids	D

Chronic atrophic erosive dermatosis of the scalp and extremities: a recharacterization of erosive pustular dermatosis. Patton D, Lynch PJ, Fung MA, Fazel N. J Am Acad Dermatol 2007; 57: 421–7.

Topical steroids, predominantly in the form of clobetasol, successfully treated 10 of 11 patients, with the last patient responding to topical tacrolimus. Nine of the 11 had scalp EPD, and all but 1 patient were elderly.

Erosive pustular dermatosis of the scalp. Pye RJ, Peachey RD, Burton JL. Br J Dermatol 1979; 100: 559–66.

Six case reports are presented in the first description of erosive pustular dermatosis of the scalp (EPDS) in the literature. Five of the six cases were resolved after use of potent topical steroids, specifically 0.025% triamcinolone with 0.75% halquinol, 0.01% betamethasone valerate with neomycin, and 0.05% clobetasol propionate, often used with neomycin or nystatin.

Three series and 23 case reports exist for high-potency topical corticosteroids in the literature.

Second-Line Therapies

• Photodynamic therapy	D
• Topical 5% dapsone gel	E
• Topical 0.1% tacrolimus ointment	E

Aminolevulinic acid photodynamic therapy in the treatment of erosive pustular dermatosis of the scalp: a case series. Yang CS, Kuhn H, Cohen LM, Kroumpouzos G. JAMA Dermatol 2016; 152: 694–7.

Eight patients with EPDS underwent curettage followed by aminolevulinic acid photodynamic therapy 1 to 2 weeks later, with complete resolution of lesions in six patients. The remaining two patients had complete resolution after a second cycle of curettage and PDT.

One case series and two case reports for PDT exist in the literature. Although this case series shows good results after PDT, the literature also notes that PDT is a risk factor for developing EPD.

Erosive pustular dermatosis of the scalp: a review with a focus on dapsone therapy. Broussard KC, Berger TG, Rosenblum M, Murase JE. J Am Acad Dermatol 2012; 66: 680–6.

In the first of four cases, a patient had previously failed clobetasol foam, fluocinonide solution, topical salicylic acid, and ultraviolet (UV) phototherapy. Seventeen weeks of up to 200 mg topical dapsone therapy achieved resolution. In the second patient, 3 months of fluocinolone solution yielded no results, but switching to dapsone 5% gel for 3 months achieved full resolution. In the third patient, topical dapsone applied twice daily resolved crusting within 3 months. The last patient had failed courses of oral prednisone, cephalexin, minocycline, doxycycline, silver sulfadiazine cream, topical tacrolimus, topical betamethasone dipropionate, intralesional triamcinolone, and wound care with silver-impregnated dressings. A side-by-side trial of clobetasol ointment and topical 5% dapsone gel determined dapsone to be more efficacious, resolving all lesions in just over 4 weeks.

Erosive pustular dermatosis of the scalp: treatment with topical tacrolimus. Laffitte E, Kaya G, Piguet V, Saurat JH. Arch Dermatol 2003; 139: 712–4.

In two patients, topical 0.1% tacrolimus ointment resulted in marked improvement within 2 weeks, with complete resolution and recovery of skin atrophy within 6 to 8 months. In the second patient, 0.05% retinaldehyde cream was added but was stopped after 1 week of use due to lesion relapse.

Thirteen case reports exist for topical tacrolimus ointment in the literature, two in conjunction with oral steroids and two as maintenance therapy after successful short-term treatment with topical steroids.

Erosive pustular dermatosis of the scalp after photodynamic therapy. López V, López I, Ramos V, Ricart JM. Dermatol Online J 2012; 18: 13.

A patient was treated with mometasone furoate cream twice daily for 1 week, followed by tacrolimus ointment twice daily for 1 month, with scarring alopecia, but no signs of recurrence at 4-month follow-up.

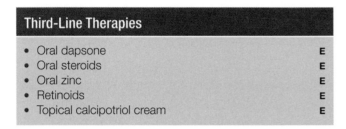

Third-Line Therapies	
• Oral dapsone	E
• Oral steroids	E
• Oral zinc	E
• Retinoids	E
• Topical calcipotriol cream	E

Disseminated erosive pustular dermatosis also involving the mucosa: successful treatment with oral dapsone. Feramisco JD, George T, Schulz SE, Ma HL, Metze D, Steinhoff M. Acta Derm Venereol 2012; 92: 91–2.

A patient presented after failing antifungal creams, antiseptic solutions, and oral antibiotics and experiencing only mild improvement with a combination of antiseptic solution, potent glucocorticoids, oral zinc replacement, and oral fluconazole. She was started on oral dapsone 50 mg twice a day for 1 week, then 50 mg three times a day, along with vitamin C 1000 mg daily. Significant improvement was observed in a few days and complete pustule resolution in 6 weeks.

Erosive pustular dermatosis of the scalp successfully treated with oral prednisone and topical tacrolimus. Zahdi MR, Seidel GB, Soares VC, Freitas CF, Mulinari-Brenner FA. An Bras Dermatol 2013; 88: 796–8.

The patient initially experienced significant improvement with prednisone 40 mg daily; however, the patient had increased purulent discharge when tapered. When prednisone was restarted with 0.1% topical tacrolimus, lesions healed completely after 10 weeks, and prednisone was successfully tapered.

Erosive pustular dermatosis of the scalp: an uncommon condition typical of elderly patients. Vaccaro M, Guarneri C, Barbuzza O, Guarneri B. J Am Geriatr Soc 2008; 56: 761–2.

An EPDS patient was treated with 16 mg/day (with progressive tapering) oral methylprednisolone, 200 mg/day oral zinc sulfate, and 0.05% clobetasol propionate foam, achieving complete resolution after 2 months.

Nine cases for oral steroids have been reported, three in combination with zinc and topical steroids and two in combination with topical tacrolimus.

Erosive pustular dermatosis of the scalp successfully treated with oral zinc sulfate. Ikeda M, Arata J, Isaka H. Br J Dermatol 1982; 106: 742–3.

A patient's pustules disappeared after 90 mg zinc sulfate daily for 5 days. The dose was increased to 180 mg daily thereafter, and the patient remained pustule free.

Six cases for oral zinc exist, five in combination with topical steroids, and two in combination with both oral and topical steroids.

Erosive pustular dermatosis of the scalp responding to acitretin. Darwich E, Muñoz-Santos C, Mascaró JM Jr. Arch Dermatol 2011; 147: 252–3.

After failing minocycline, betamethasone 17-valerate, and fusidic acid cream, a patient was started on acitretin 50 mg daily and topical 0.1% tacrolimus ointment. Tacrolimus was discontinued after 10 days due to burning. The lesions were completely healed after 3 months.

Four cases for retinoids are in the literature, one with worsening of erosions and three with good results when combined with combinations of the following: zinc, topical steroids, tacrolimus, antibiotics, topical antiseptics, oral dapsone.

Erosive pustular dermatosis of the scalp successfully treated with calcipotriol cream. Boffa MJ. Br J Dermatol 2003; 148: 593–5.

In a patient with significant skin atrophy, topical steroids were avoided and EPDS was treated with calcipotriol, first once daily and then twice daily. Calcipotriol was discontinued 2 months later after complete resolution, and some hair regrowth was seen at visits 3 and 9 months post treatment.

Evidence Levels: **A** Double-blind study **B** Clinical trial ≥ 20 subjects **C** Clinical trial < 20 subjects **D** Series ≥ 5 subjects **E** Anecdotal case reports

71

Erythema annulare centrifugum

Christie G. Regula, Bryan E. Anderson

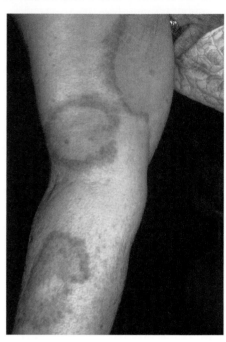

Erythema annulare centrifugum (EAC) is a gyrate erythema characterized by minimally pruritic, polycyclic, erythematous patches or plaques that may expand up to 2 to 3 mm/day and clear centrally. There are two forms: the far more common superficial form has trailing scale at the inner borders of the erythema, whereas the deep form has erythematous induration with minimal to no scale. EAC has a mean duration of 2.8 years, and treatment is often difficult. EAC has been seen to persist for decades.

MANAGEMENT STRATEGY

EAC represents a hypersensitivity reaction to a myriad of conditions; therefore a search for and treatment of an underlying disease is the primary management strategy. Most often an underlying cause is not found.

A concurrent skin infection is the most common underlying association. Fungal, bacterial, viral, mycobacterial, and parasitic pathogens have been reported. Typically, the infection is cutaneous and is at a distant location from the EAC eruption. Dermatophytosis is implicated in up to 48%. Thus the skin, especially the feet, groin, and nails, should be carefully examined for tinea. Anecdotal reports of other associated skin infections include molluscum contagiosum, herpesvirus infection, and *Phthirus pubis* infestation. Less commonly the infection is internal and intestinal *Giardia* or *Candida*. Latent Epstein–Barr virus infection, human immunodeficiency virus (HIV) infection, chronic viral hepatitis, appendicitis, tonsillitis, secondary syphilis, urinary tract *Escherichia coli*, and nematode infestations have

been anecdotally reported. Although EAC is typically associated with an active infection, it has also been reported to occur after reactivation of herpes zoster virus in corresponding dermatomes.

Rarely, EAC may be associated with either benign or malignant hematologic and solid neoplasms. This paraneoplastic erythema annulare centrifugum eruption (PEACE) is thought to result from hypersensitivity to tumor proteins released by these neoplasms. However, in the absence of strong clinical suspicion, an extensive search for malignancy is not recommended. Should neoplasia be identified, EAC activity correlates with tumor response to treatment.

Medications may be associated with EAC—anecdotal reports include acetazolamide, amitriptyline, ampicillin, chloroquine, cimetidine, cyclopenthiazide, cotrimoxazole, etizolam, finasteride, gold, hydrochlorothiazide, hydroxychloroquine, ibuprofen, iron, neutradonna (aluminum silicate and belladonna), oxprenolol, pegylated interferon-α-2a plus ribavirin, piroxicam, rituximab, salicylates, spironolactone, thiacetazone, and ustekinumab. Early reports of antimalarials as a cause of EAC may be debated: what was considered EAC in these reports may actually have been unrecognized forms of subacute cutaneous lupus erythematosus. EAC may also be caused by hypersensitivity to other ingested agents, such as blue cheese *Penicillium*.

Other conditions associated with EAC include thyroid disease, liver disease, hypereosinophilic syndrome, sarcoidosis, surgical trauma, linear IgA dermatosis, and autoimmune disease such as relapsing polychondritis, rheumatoid arthritis, pemphigus vulgaris, hemolytic anemia, polyglandular autoimmune disease, autoimmune hepatitis, and pregnancy. One form of EAC, described as *autoimmune progesterone dermatitis* (see Chapter 20), can be reproduced by intradermal and patch testing to progesterone and may involve Th1-type cytokines. Another form of EAC may occur annually and seasonally over 2 to 40 years and may be associated with hereditary lactate dehydrogenase deficiency. EAC may even be familial: there has been one report involving identical twins. Rarely, EAC may be a form of contact dermatitis: there is a single report of contact-induced EAC attributed to a hypersensitivity reaction from topical nickel and cobalt exposure.

Once the underlying condition is treated, EAC usually resolves spontaneously. Frequently, however, the cause is elusive, and treatment becomes empiric and temporizing. Spontaneous remission is also possible, making assessments of therapy difficult. *Topical steroids* may provide symptomatic relief and may improve its appearance. In one report of EAC with unknown etiology, all lesions cleared with *topical calcipotriol* treatment. *Topical tacrolimus* can be helpful as well. In another case, EAC remitted after the patient was treated with *oral metronidazole* given for rosacea. A trial of empiric antimicrobials may be helpful to eradicate an underlying, clinically undetected infection—a case series has shown significant improvement with *oral erythromycin* treatment. If these more conservative treatments fail, the patient's perceived need for treatment should be reassessed. Stronger treatments may be more harmful than the condition itself. Systemic glucocorticoids can usually suppress EAC, but it commonly recurs after the course is completed, and they cannot be routinely recommended. If EAC is very disabling to the patient, other *systemic immunomodulators* may need to be considered. One patient responded very well to *etanercept* therapy.

EAC should be distinguished from the following clinical mimickers: tinea corporis, granuloma annulare, sarcoidosis, mycosis fungoides, psoriasis, pityriasis rosea, tinea versicolor, cutaneous lupus, annular erythema of Sjögren syndrome, granuloma faciale, necrolytic migratory erythema, bullous pemphigoid, secondary syphilis, Hansen disease, annular urticarial and fixed drug reactions, hypereosinophilic dermatitis, annular erythema of infancy, and other reactive erythemas such as erythema multiforme, erythema gyratum repens, erythema migrans, and erythema marginatum. Such clinical possibilities are ruled out by routine histologic examination.

Specific Investigations

- Biopsy for histologic examination
  - Superficial type: focal spongiosis, superficial perivascular lymphocytic infiltrate
  - Deep type: superficial and deep perivascular lymphohistiocytic infiltrate
- Full skin examination for potential skin infections
- Potassium hydroxide (KOH) test or culture of suspected EAC lesion and any sites of potential dermatophyte infection
- Wood light examination
- Consider intradermal trichophyton or candidal skin injection and tuberculin test to test for underlying infection
- Review medication list
- Systemic workup: complete blood count (CBC), liver function tests (LFTs), urinalysis (UA), chest x-ray (CXR) initial screen; if warranted, antinuclear antibodies (ANAs), thyroid-stimulating hormone (TSH), HIV, syphilis serology, malignancy workup including serum protein electrophoresis/urine protein electrophoresis (SPEP/UPEP) with immunofixation

Gyrate erythema. White Jr JW. Dermatol Clin 1985; 3: 129–39.

Allergic confirmation that some cases of erythema annulare centrifugum are dermatophytids. Jillson OF. Arch Dermatol Syphilol 1954; 70: 54–8.

Erythema annulare centrifugum and intestinal *Candida albicans* infection – coincidence or connection? Schmid MH, Wollenber A, Sander CA, Beiber T. Acta Derm Venereol 1997; 77: 93–4.

Intradermal trichophyton and candidal skin injection tests may demonstrate a local cutaneous hypersensitivity. These tests may help confirm this reaction pattern and support a trial of empiric antifungals despite an inability to locate the site of a pathogen.

Erythema annulare centrifugum: a review of 24 cases with special reference to its association with underlying disease. Mahood JM. Clin Exp Dermatol 1983; 8: 383–7.

A basic workup for internal disease may include a CBC, LFTs, UA, and chest radiograph.

Erythema annulare centrifugum: results of a clinicopathologic study of 73 patients. Weyers W, Diaz-Cascajo C, Weyers I. Am J Dermatopathol 2003; 25: 451–62.

Clinicopathologic analysis of 66 cases of erythema annulare centrifugum. Kim KJ, Chang SE, Choi JH, Sng KJ, Moon KC, Koh JK. J Dermatol 2002; 29: 61–7.

Erythema annulare centrifugum in a HIV-positive patient. Gonzalez-Vela MC, Gonzalez-Lopez MA, Val-Bernal JF, Echevarria S, Arce F, Fernandez-Llaca H. Int J Dermatol 2006; 45: 1423–5.

Unusual huge erythema annulare centrifugum presentation of second syphilis. Liu ZH, Chen JF. QJM 2014; 107: 231–2.

Erythema annulare centrifugum induced by generalized *Phthirus pubis* infestation. Bessis D, Chraibi H, Guillot B, Guilhou J. Br J Dermatol 2003; 149: 1291.

Erythema annulare centrifugum. A case due to tuberculosis. Burkhart CG. Int J Dermatol 1982; 21: 538–9.

Erythema annulare centrifugum and *Escherichia coli* urinary infection. Borbujo J, de Miguel C, Lopez A, de Lucas R, Casado M. Lancet 1996; 347: 897–8.

Erythema annulare centrifugum following herpes zoster infection: Wolf's isotopic response? Lee HW, Lee DK, Rhee DY, Chang SE, Choi JH, Moon KC, et al. Br J Dermatol 2005; 153: 1241–3.

Erythema annulare centrifugum revealing chronic lymphocytic leukemia. Stokkermans-Dubois J, Beylot-Barry M, Vergier B, Bouabdallah K, Doutre MS. Br J Dermatol 2007; 157: 1045–7.

Erythema annulare centrifugum as the presenting sign of breast carcinoma. Panasiti V, Devirgiliis V, Curzio M, Rossi M, Roberti V, Bottoni U, et al. J Eur Acad Derm Venereol 2008; 23: 318–20.

Erythema annulare centrifugum as presenting sign of activation of breast cancer. Topal IO, Topal Y, Sargan A, Duman H, Gungor S, Goncu OE, et al. An Bras Dermatol 2015; 90: 925–7.

Erythema annulare centrifugum associated with ovarian cancer. Batycka-Baran A, Zychowska M, Baran W, Szepietowski JC, Maj J. Acat Derm Venereol 2015; 95: 1032–3.

Erythema annulare centrifugum associated with mantle B-cell non-Hodgkin's lymphoma. Carlesimo M, Fidanza L, Mari E, Pranteda G, Cacchi C, Veggia B, et al. Acta Derm Venereol 2009; 89: 319–20.

Erythema annulare centrifugum: a rare skin finding of autoimmune hepatitis. Aygun C, Kocaman O, Gurbuz Y, Celebi A, Senturk O, Hulagu S. Gastroenterol Res 2010; 3: 96–8.

Pemphigus vulgaris presenting as erythema annulare centrifugum. Aguilar-Duran S, Deroide F, Mee J, Rustin M. Clin Exp Dermtol 2015; 40: 466–7.

Erythema annulare centrifugum as the presenting sign of the hypereosinophilic syndrome: observations on therapy. Shelley WB, Shelley ED. Cutis 1985; 35: 53–5.

Erythema annulare centrifugum-like mycosis fungoides. Ceyhan AM, Akkaya VB, Chen W. Bircan Aust J Dermatol 2010; 52: e11–3.

Erythema annulare centrifugum following pancreaticobiliary surgery. Thami GP, Sachdeva A, Kaur S, Mohan H, Kanwar AJ. J Dermatol 2002; 29: 347–9.

Linear IgA dermatosis presenting with erythema annulare centrifugum lesions: report of three cases in adults. Dippel E, Orfanos CE, Zouboulis CHC. J Eur Acad Dermatol Venereol 2000; 15: 167–70.

Erythema annulare centrifugum and relapsing polychondritis. Dippel E, Orfanos CE, Zouboulis C. Ann Dermatol Venereol 2000; 127: 735–9.

236

Erythema annulare centrifugum in a patient with polyglandular autoimmune disease type 1. Garty B. Cutis 1998; 62: 231–2.

Pregnancy as a possible etiologic factor in erythema annulare centrifugum. Dogan G. Am J Clin Dermatol 2009; 10: 33–5.

Autoimmune progesterone dermatitis manifested as erythema annulare centrifugum: confirmation of progesterone sensitivity by in vitro interferon-gamma release. Halevy S, Cohen AD, Lunenfeld E, Grossman N. J Am Acad Dermatol 2002; 47: 311–3.

Contact erythema annulare centrifugum. Sambucety PS, Agapito PG, Preto MAR. Contact Dermatitis 2006; 55: 309–10.

First-Line Therapies

• Treatment of underlying condition	E
• Discontinue potential causative medications	E
• Topical corticosteroids	E
• Ultraviolet light therapy	E
• Oral erythromycin	D

Erythromycin as a safe and effective treatment option for erythema annulare centrifugum. Chuang FC, Lin SH, Wu WM. Indian J Dermatol 2015; 60: 519.

Case series of eight subjects with erythema annulare centrifugum. Subjects were given erythromycin stearate 1000 mg per day for 2 weeks. All subjects showed reduction in lesion size and erythema at 2 weeks. Upon completion of treatment course, three patients had recurrent disease. Retreatment with erythromycin was effective.

Erythema annulare centrifugum caused by Aldactone. Carsuzaa F, Pierre C, Dubegny M. Ann Dermatol Venereol 1987; 114: 375–6.

Ampicillin-induced erythema annulare centrifugum. Gupta HL, Sapra SM. J Indian Med Assoc 1975; 65: 307–8.

Erythema annulare centrifugum secondary to treatment with finasteride. Al Hammadi A, Asai Y, Patt MI, Sasseville D. J Drugs Dermatol 2007; 6: 460–3.

Erythema annulare centrifugum: an unusual case due to hydroxychloroquine sulfate. Hudson LD. Cutis 1985; 36: 129–30.

Erythema annulare centrifugum-like eruption associated with pegylated interferon treatment for hepatitis C. Naccarato M, Yoong D, Solomon R, Ostrowski M. Dermatol Reports 2013; 29: 5.

EAC has been associated with numerous medications. Elimination of the suspected agent may be curative.

Erythema annulare centrifugum. A case due to hypersensitivity to blue cheese *Penicillium*. Shelley WB. Arch Dermatol 1964; 90: 54–8.

Erythema annulare centrifugum and Hodgkin's disease: association with disease activity. Leimert JT, Corder MP, Skibba CA, Gingrich RD. Arch Intern Med 1979; 139: 486–7.

Erythema annulare centrifugum responding to natural ultraviolet light. Coronel-Perez IM, Morillo-Andújar M. Actas Dermosifiliogr 2010; 101: 177–8.

Two patients, ages 22 and 27 years, each with more than 8 years of EAC, failed treatment with topical corticosteroids. After years of sunlight avoidance, one patient cleared, and the other had significant improvement with summer sunlight exposure.

Second-Line Therapies

• Empiric antimicrobials	E
• Topical or systemic antipruritics	E
• Topical tacrolimus	E

Annular erythema responding to tacrolimus ointment. Rao NG, Pariser RJ. J Drugs Dermatol 2003; 2: 421–4.

Two patients with annular erythema of unclear etiology treated selected lesions with topical tacrolimus 0.1% ointment twice daily. Those lesions that were treated resolved within 2 to 6 weeks, whereas other untreated lesions did not respond until they, too, were treated with tacrolimus.

This suggests that tacrolimus, and not spontaneous remission, was responsible for the improvement.

Third-Line Therapies

• Systemic corticosteroids	E
• Immunomodulatory agents	E
• Topical calcipotriol	E
• Metronidazole	E

Erythema annulare centrifugum. Seidel DR, Burgdorf WHC. In: Demis DJ, et al., eds. Clinical Dermatology. Lippincott Williams & Wilkins, Philadelphia, 1999; Ch 7–5: 1–4.

Calcipotriol for erythema annulare centrifugum. Gnaiadecki R. Br J Dermatol 2002; 146: 317–9.

A 73-year-old woman had EAC of unknown cause that was resistant to topical and systemic steroids, antifungals, and psoralen and ultraviolet light (PUVA) treatment. It cleared completely after 3 months of topical, once-daily calcipotriol.

Erythema annulare centrifugum successfully treated with metronidazole. De Aloe G, Rubegni P, Risulo M, Sbano P, Poggiali S, Fimiani M. Clin Exp Dermatol 2005; 30: 583–4.

A 38-year-old man with EAC failed oral antibiotics and antifungals, as well as topical calcipotriol. Only systemic steroids provided temporary improvement of his skin lesions. Because the patient had rosacea, oral metronidazole 400 mg daily was prescribed for 6 weeks, with resolution of EAC.

A novel therapeutic approach to erythema annulare centrifugum. Minni J, Sarro R. J Am Acad Dermatol 2006; 54: S134–5.

In a personal communication, one patient with extensive EAC was reported to clear with etanercept 25 mg twice-weekly injections. After 4 weeks of treatment the patient was 95% clear, and complete remission was achieved after continued therapy. After 6 months the treatment was discontinued and EAC recurred. The lesions responded again to a repeat treatment regimen.

72

Erythema dyschromicum perstans

Christine Soon, John Berth-Jones

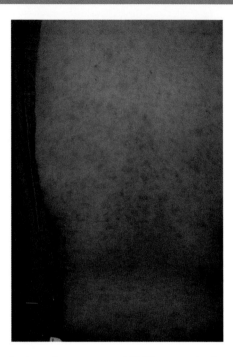

Erythema dyschromicum perstans (EDP) is an acquired, generalized dermal hypermelanosis of unknown etiology. Clinically it presents as asymptomatic, ashen-gray-blue macules of varying sizes, most commonly on the trunk and proximal extremities. Variable components include erythema and papulation. It has been reported most frequently in dark-skinned Latin American people, although all racial groups can be affected. EDP has similarities to lichen planus pigmentosus and the "ashy dermatosis" of Ramirez, although the precise relationship of these conditions remains uncertain.

MANAGEMENT STRATEGY

Histology reveals vacuolar degeneration of the basal layer associated with pigmentary incontinence. Dermal vessels are surrounded with an infiltrate of lymphocytes and histiocytes, and many melanophages are present.

EDP may need to be differentiated from the late stage of pinta. Dark-field examination and serologic tests for syphilis should be carried out to exclude this treponematosis in suspected cases. Idiopathic eruptive macular pigmentation is a similar condition. Histology demonstrates that the pigment is located in the basal layer of the epidermis, and the lichenoid inflammation characteristic of EDP is not present.

Although EDP may persist for many years, there have been reports of spontaneous resolution. *Camouflage creams* can be helpful. Treatment is otherwise based on anecdotal evidence. Treatments that are reportedly ineffective include sun protection, peeling lotions, antibiotics, topical hydroquinone, topical corticosteroid therapy, antimalarials, and griseofulvin.

THERAPY

• No therapy	D
• Topical corticosteroid	E
• Antihistamines	E
• Topical tacrolimus	E
• Isotretinoin	E
• Dapsone 100 mg/day for 3 months	D
• Oral corticosteroid therapy	E
• Clofazimine 100 mg/day for 3 months	E

Erythema dyschromicum perstans in children: a report of 14 cases. Torrelo A, Zaballos P, Colmenero I, Mediero IG, de Prada I, Zambrano A. J Eur Acad Dermatol Venereol 2005; 19: 422–6.

No treatment was used. In six of these cases the eruption cleared or improved during follow-up ranging from 1 to 5 years.

Erythema dyschromicum perstans: identical to ashy dermatosis or not? Numata T, Harada K, Tsuboi R, Mitsuhashi Y. Case Rep Dermatol 2015; 7: 146–50.

In this case the erythema responded to a topical steroid and the pruritus responded to an antihistamine.

Erythema dyschromicum perstans: response to topical tacrolimus. Mahajan VK, Chauhan PS, Mehta KS, Sharma AL. Indian J Dermatol 2015; 60: 525.

Two cases cleared within 2 to 3 months using 0.1% tacrolimus ointment twice daily.

Erythema dyschromicum perstans response to isotretinoin. Wang F, Zhao YK, Wang Z, Liu JH, Luo DQ. JAMA Dermatol 2016; 152: 841–2.

A 41-year-old man with EDP demonstrated 90% improvement within 4 months of isotretinoin (20 mg daily). Periodic recurrences responded to doses as low as 10 mg daily during 7 years of follow-up.

Erythema dyschromicum perstans in phototype II women: three unusual clinical cases studied with electron microscopy. Persechino S, Caperchi C, Cortesi G, Persechino F, Raffa S, Pulcini F, et al. Eur J Dermatol 2011; 21: 261–2.

Three cases demonstrated marked decrease in pigmentation on treatment with dapsone 100 mg daily for 3 months.

Erythema dyschromicum perstans: a case report and review. Osswald SS, Proffer LH, Sartori CR. Cutis 2001; 68: 25–8.

One case of EDP with active inflammatory areas responded to 3 weeks of oral corticosteroid therapy. The authors do not state the dose.

Involvement of cell adhesion and activation molecules in the pathogenesis of erythema dyschromicum perstans (ashy dermatitis). The effect of clofazimine therapy. Baranda L, Torres-Alvarez B, Cortes-Franco R, Moncada B, Potales-Perez DP, Gonzalez-Amaro R. Arch Dermatol 1997; 133: 325–9.

A prospective clinical and immunohistochemical study indicating that clofazimine reduces the inflammatory response in EDP. Four out of six patients treated with clofazimine 100 mg/day showed marked improvement after 3 months of treatment.

Evidence Levels: **A** Double-blind study **B** Clinical trial ≥ 20 subjects **C** Clinical trial < 20 subjects **D** Series ≥ 5 subjects **E** Anecdotal case reports

73

Erythema elevatum diutinum

Tashmeeta Ahad, Emma Benton, Ian Coulson

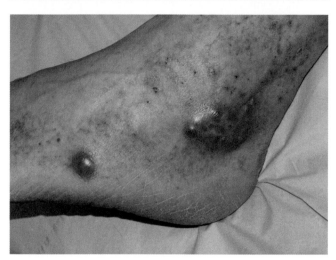

Erythema elevatum diutinum (EED) is a rare neutrophilic dermatosis consisting of violaceous, brown or red papules, plaques, nodules, and occasionally vesicobullous lesions over the extensor surfaces of the joints and buttocks, genitalia, trunk, and face. Early lesions tend to be soft and erythematous, whereas advanced lesions tend to be nodular and firm, secondary to fibrosis. EED is thought to be a form of immune complex–mediated leukocytoclastic vasculitis, although its etiology remains unclear. Infections (including HIV and streptococcal), hematologic abnormalities, autoimmune diseases, and other conditions have been associated.

MANAGEMENT STRATEGY

EED is a chronic disease; there are only a few well-documented instances of spontaneous long-term resolution.

EED has been reported in association with diseases such as HIV, hematologic disorders, inflammatory bowel disease, celiac disease, verrucous carcinoma, systemic lupus erythematosus, primary Sjögren syndrome, ophthalmic disorders (peripheral keratitis), and pulmonary lymphoepithelioma-like carcinoma (possibly as part of a paraneoplastic syndrome), and evidence of these should be sought. Drug-induced EED may result from interferon-β, erythropoietin, antituberculosis chemotherapy, and cisplatin exposure.

After management of any underlying disease, *dapsone* 100 mg daily remains the initial treatment of choice. The response may be partial and dose dependent. In other patients both intralesional and systemic corticosteroids (prednisolone 30–40 mg daily) have produced favorable responses.

Sulfonamides (sulfamethoxypyridazine 500 mg once daily and sulfapyridine 0.5–1 g three times daily), *nicotinamide/niacinamide* 100 mg three times daily, *colchicine* 0.5 mg twice daily with 0.5 mg three times daily for 3 to 4 days to abate minor disease flares, and *chloroquine* 300 mg daily have produced resolution of lesions.

Differential diagnoses of early lesions of EED include extrafacial granuloma faciale, Sweet syndrome, rheumatoid neutrophilic dermatitis or palisaded neutrophilic, and granulomatous dermatitis, and advanced lesions include rheumatoid nodules and multicentric reticulohistiocytosis.

> ### Specific Investigations
> - Full blood count
> - Full metabolic panel
> - Immunoglobulins and serum electrophoresis/ immunofixation electrophoresis
> - Antinuclear antibody (ANA)
> - Antineutrophil cytoplasmic antibodies (ANCA)
> - Anti-nDNA antibody
> - Antiphospholipid antibodies
> - Celiac disease screen
> - Hepatitis B and C serology
> - HIV test
> - Chest radiograph
> - Urinalysis
> - Histology
> - Skin biopsy

Erythema elevatum diutinum: clinical, histopathologic, and immunohistochemical characteristics of six patients. Wahl CE, Bouldin MB, Gibson LE. Am J Dermatopathol 2005; 27: 397–400.

The vascular endothelium of EED stains positive for CD31, CD34, VEGF, and factor VIII, and negative for factor XIIIa, TGFβ, and LANA. This pattern does not distinguish it from similar-appearing lesions. Therefore the chronic and recurrent nature of EED is the primary means of distinguishing it from entities that are clinically and histologically similar.

Erythema elevatum diutinum and IgA paraproteinaemia: 'a preclinical iceberg'. Chowdhury MMU, Inaloz HS, Motley RJ, Knight AG. Int J Dermatol 2002; 41: 368–70.

The technique of immunofixation electrophoresis is more sensitive than immunoelectrophoresis. This uses a combination of zone electrophoresis and immunoprecipitation with specific antisera to detect monoclonal immunoglobulins or light chains at very low concentrations in serum and urine. This is useful in EED because patients may have associated paraproteinemias which, in some cases, may undergo malignant transformation.

The authors note that in monoclonal disorders there is extensive asymptomatic tumor proliferation and possible malignant transformation in 20% of patients during long-term follow-up. It was recommended that there should be lengthy follow-up and monitoring for patients with both EED and IgA paraproteinemia because of the risk of progression to IgA myeloma.

Is IgA antineutrophil cytoplasmic antibody a marker for patients with erythema elevatum diutinum? A further three cases demonstrating this association. Crichlow SM, Alexandroff AB, Simpson RC, Saldanha G, Walker S, Harman KE. Br J Dermatol 2011; 164: 675–7.

Two studies evaluating the prevalence of ANCAs in EED. IgA ANCAs were present in all patients with EED.

Erythema elevatum diutinum and HIV infection: a report of five cases. Muratori S, Carrera C, Gorani A, Alessi E. Br J Dermatol 1999; 141: 335–8.

The largest case series of patients with EED and HIV infection. Streptococcal infection seemed to trigger exacerbations in four of five patients. EED can stimulate Kaposi sarcoma and bacillary angiomatosis, which may be particularly confusing in the context of an HIV-seropositive patient. Histopathologic confirmation of the diagnosis is therefore advocated.

Erythema elevatum diutinum associated with peripheral ulcerative keratitis. Vaiyavatjamai P, Wattanakrai P. J Eur Acad Dermatol Venereol 2011; 25: 741–2.

Progressive keratolysis with pseudopterygium associated with erythema elevatum diutinum. Lekhanont K, Patarakittam T, Mantachote K, Waiyawatjamai P, Vongthongsri A. Ophthalmology 2011; 118: 927–33.

Erythema elevatum diutinum with verrucous carcinoma: a rare association. Nair SR, Viswanath V, Sonavane AD, Doshi AC, Parab MG, Torsekar RG. Indian J Dermatol Venereol Leprol 2010; 76: 420–2.

Erythema elevatum diutinum as a paraneoplastic syndrome in a patient with pulmonary lymphoepithelioma-like carcinoma. Liu T-C, Chen I-S, Lin T-K, Lee JY-Y, Kirn D, Tsao C-J. Lung Cancer 2009; 63: 151–3.

Erythema elevatum diutinum presenting with a giant annular pattern. Di Giacomo TB, Marinho RT, Nico MMS. Int J Dermatol 2009; 48: 290–2.

Erythema elevatum diutinum associated with pyoderma gangrenosum in an HIV-positive patient. Maksimovic L, Duriez P, Lascaux-Cametz A-S, Andre C, Bagot M, Revuz J, et al. Ann Dermatol Venereol 2010; 137: 386–90.

Erythema elevatum diutinum in systemic lupus erythematosus. Chan Y, Mok CC, Tang WYM. Rheumatol Int 2011; 31: 259–62.

These citations indicate the range of pathologies associated with EED.

First-Line Therapies

• Dapsone	D
• Dapsone plus antiretrovirals in HIV-associated disease	E
• Dapsone plus another agent (e.g., corticosteroids, antibiotics)	D

Erythema elevatum diutinum: a review of presentation and treatment. Momen SE, Jorizzo J, Al-Niaimi F. J Eur Acad Dermatol Venereol 2014; 28: 1594–602.

Dapsone is considered to be the main mode of treatment for EED as per multiple case series and case reports. No randomized controlled trials have evaluated treatment. This review of the literature between 1977 and 2012 identified 66 reported cases of EED treated with dapsone, including 59 treated with dapsone monotherapy. Eighty percent (n = 47) of patients on dapsone monotherapy showed a reduction in lesion size or complete resolution. Dapsone was also found to improve extracutaneous manifestations of EED, such as arthralgia (n = 10).

Eleven out of 13 HIV-positive patients treated with dapsone showed a good clinical response.

Dapsone is often ineffective for fibrotic nodular advanced EED, in which case other agents such as corticosteroids, colchicine, or sulfonamide may be added.

Effective dapsone treatment doses ranged from 50 to 300 mg daily. It has been suggested that effectiveness may be dose dependent. A usual dose of 100 mg daily is used, and a lower dose (25–50 mg) may be administered at the start of treatment and titrated up depending on patient tolerance and response to therapy.

Other treatments have shown variable results. Oral glucocorticoids used alone or in conjunction with dapsone may improve EED. Sulfonamide antibiotics were used in nine cases, and clinical improvement was observed in three cases. Antibiotics such as clarithromycin, erythromycin, and penicillin were used in three patients in combination with excision (n = 2) and dapsone (n = 1) with variable results.

Dapsone may be ineffective once nodules appear; treatment of associated concomitant conditions is often beneficial to EED outcome.

Alternative procedure to allow continuation of dapsone therapy despite serious adverse reaction in a case of dapsone-sensitive erythema elevatum diutinum. Seneschal J, Guillet S, Ezzedine K, Taïeb A, Milpied B. Dermatology (Basel) 2012; 224: 115–9.

This patient responded well to dapsone but developed hypersensitivity reaction with DRESS, confirmed in vitro by the presence of circulating dapsone-specific T cells. As treatment alternatives to dapsone are limited, it is recommended that dapsone hypersensitivity syndrome is confirmed using interferon assay and modified lymphocyte transformation tests. After confirmation, a dapsone tolerance induction protocol may be administered over a period of days in order to obtain tolerance, thus allowing continuation of dapsone.

Nodular lesions of erythema elevatum diutinum in patients infected with the human immunodeficiency virus. LeBoit PE, Cockerell CJ. J Am Acad Dermatol 1993; 28: 919–22.

A clinicopathologic study of four patients with HIV infection who had unusual nodular lesions of EED. None of the patients responded to treatment with oral dapsone, and the authors commented that this observed lack of response may reflect the preponderance of fibrosis rather than neutrophils in these advanced lesions.

Second-Line Therapies

• Sulfonamides	D
• Colchicine	D
• Oral steroids	D
• Niacinamide and tetracycline	E
• Chloroquine	E
• Methotrexate	E
• Dapsone with ciclosporin	E

Erythema elevatum diutinum: a case successfully treated with colchicine. Henriksson R, Hofer PA, Hörnqvist R. Clin Exp Dermatol 1989; 14: 451–3.

A case report of a 68-year-old man with EED refractory to treatment with oral dapsone who responded well to treatment with colchicine 0.5 mg twice daily over 6 weeks. Minor flares were abated temporarily, increasing colchicine to 0.5 mg three times a day for 3 to 4 days, without provoking diarrhea.

Evidence Levels: A Double-blind study B Clinical trial ≥ 20 subjects C Clinical trial < 20 subjects D Series ≥ 5 subjects E Anecdotal case reports

Erythema elevatum diutinum treated with niacinamide and tetracycline. Kohler IK, Lorincz AL. Arch Dermatol 1980; 116: 693–5.

A 60-year-old woman with EED that cleared completely after 4 weeks of treatment with oral niacinamide 100 mg three times daily and oral tetracycline hydrochloride 250 mg four times daily. After this, oral niacinamide alone was sufficient for disease suppression.

Successful combination therapy with dapsone and cyclosporine for erythema elevatum diutinum with unusual appearance. Takahashi H, Fukami Y, Honma M, Ishida-Yamamoto A, Iizuka H. J Dermatol 2012; 39: 486–7.

In this case of EED with an unusual distribution on the soles, fingers, trunk, and feet accompanied with ulcerations, the patient initially failed to respond to oral dapsone 75 mg daily but improved with the addition of ciclosporin 4 mg/kg/day.

Third-Line Therapies

• Topical dapsone 5%	E
• Localized surgical excision (nodular EED)	E
• Cyclophosphamide	E
• Plasma exchange ± thalidomide	E
• Reduction in ciclosporin dose	E
• Transdermal nicotine patches	E
• Methylprednisolone	E
• Colectomy	E
• Gluten-free diet	E
• Phenformin	E

Novel use of topical dapsone 5% gel for erythema elevatum diutinum: safer and effective. Frieling GW, William NL, Lim SJ. J Drugs Dermatol 2013; 12: 481–4.

This case report showed some improvement in erythema and flattening of lesions of EED using dapsone 5% gel for 1 week before start of oral dapsone therapy.

Other topical treatments, including topical corticosteroids and intralesional steroid injections, have shown variable results in a few case reports.

Successful surgical treatment of advanced erythema elevatum diutinum. Rinard JR, Mahabir RC, Greene JF, Grothaus P. Can J Plast Surg 2010; 18: 28–30.

In this case report, a patient with late-stage nodular EED in whom medical treatment was contraindicated was treated with continued surgical excisions of recurrent nodules with symptomatic relief.

Fibrotic nodules often respond poorly to dapsone; surgical excision may help.

Erythema elevatum diutinum in a patient with relapsing polychondritis. Bernard P, Bedane C, Delrous JL, Catanzano G, Bonnetblanc JM. J Am Acad Dermatol 1992; 26: 312–5.

A 69-year-old man with a history of relapsing polychondritis developed EED, which responded to treatment with oral cyclophosphamide 100 mg daily and prednisolone 20 mg daily. Cyclophosphamide was discontinued after 2 months, and the prednisolone was subsequently tapered to 15 mg daily.

Erythema elevatum diutinum associated with IgA paraproteinemia successfully controlled with intermittent plasma exchange. Chow RK, Benny WB, Coupe RL, Dodd WA, Ongley RC. Arch Dermatol 1996; 132: 1360–4.

Intermittent plasma exchange has been reported to successfully control EED associated with IgA paraproteinemia.

Case of erythema elevatum diutinum associated with IgA paraproteinemia successfully controlled with thalidomide and plasma exchange. Manni E, Cervadoro E, Papineschi F. Ther Apher Dial 2015; 19: 195.

An 83-year-old woman with EED treated with dapsone for a year was found to have an IgA kappa paraproteinemia consistent with monoclonal gammopathy of undetermined significance and commenced on treatment with plasma exchange, three-weekly sessions down to one-weekly sessions. Commenced thalidomide on week 13, with 200 mg/day and 100 mg/day alternatively and plasma exchange reduced to one exchange every 2 weeks. Thalidomide was then continued as monotherapy followed by treatment regimen with periods of plasma exchange ± thalidomide, which led to improvement of skin lesions and stabilization of raised IgA values.

Erythema elevatum diutinum after liver transplantation: disappearance of the lesions associated with a reduction in cyclosporine dosage. Hernández-Cano N, De Lucas R, Lázaro TE, Mayor M, Burón I, Casado M. Pediatr Dermatol 1998; 15: 411–2.

Lesions of EED resolved after a reduction in ciclosporin dosage in a 10-year-old patient who had previously received a cadaveric hepatic allograft because of Alagille disease.

Erythema elevatum diutinum manifesting as a penile ulcer. Yoshii N, Kanekura T, Higashi Y, Oyama K, Azagami K, Kanzaki T. Clin Exp Dermatol 2007; 32: 211–3.

A 74-year-old man developed EED. The lesions on his limbs responded well to the nicotine patches that released 6.25 mg nicotine applied every 24 hours. The penile lesions remained recalcitrant to the nicotine patches as well as dapsone, requiring treatment with methylprednisolone (40 mg/day).

Erythema elevatum diutinum: an unusual association with ulcerative colitis. Buahene K, Hudson M, Mowat A, Smart L, Ormerod AD. Clin Exp Dermatol 1991; 16: 204–6.

A 58-year-old woman developed EED during severe acute exacerbation of ulcerative colitis, which resolved after a colectomy.

Erythema elevatum diutinum in association with coeliac disease. Tasanen K, Raudasoja R, Kallioinen M, Ranki A. Br J Dermatol 1997; 136: 624–7.

A 47-year-old woman who presented with typical EED in whom previously undiagnosed celiac disease was found. Treatment with dapsone was partially effective, but complete healing of the EED lesions was achieved only after the introduction of a strict gluten-free diet. Maintenance treatment with a gluten-free diet only was required.

Erythema elevatum diutinum: cutaneous vasculitis, impaired clot lysis, and response to phenformin. Schumacher HR, Carroll E, Taylor F, Shelley WB, Wood MG. J Rheumatol 1977; 4: 103–12.

A variety of treatments were tried with no success in this case report, but phenformin 50 mg three times daily produced marked improvement for periods of 11 and 16 months on two occasions.

Phenformin is a biguanide antidiabetic drug that has been withdrawn in many countries due to high risk of lactic acidosis.

Erythema multiforme

Jean Revuz

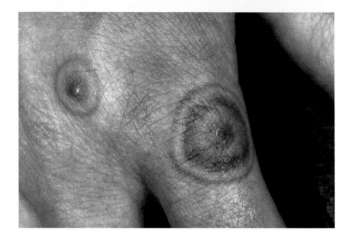

Erythema multiforme (EM) is a distinct cutaneous reaction pattern to a variety of stimuli, predominantly herpes simplex virus (HSV) infection, occurring predominantly in young adults. It usually runs a self-limiting course but has a tendency to recur. It is defined by the presence of "typical" three-zone target lesions, with a predominantly acral distribution. The presence of mucosal involvement at more than one site distinguishes EM major from EM minor. A specific variant has mucosal lesions only, without skin involvement. EM major can be distinguished from Stevens–Johnson syndrome, which lacks typical targetlike lesions and acral location but, instead, irregular macule or atypical targets and a truncal location. EM is frequently misdiagnosed in cases of urticarial and common rashes and more rarely in cases of cutaneous lupus, vasculitis, erythema annulare, and drug eruption.

MANAGEMENT STRATEGY

In 30% to 50% of cases the etiology of EM is unknown. The most commonly recognized precipitant is HSV infection, both types I and II. HSV-specific DNA has been isolated from lesional tissue in 60% to 70% of cases. HSV particles are found in the circulating precursors of epidermal Langerhans cells. A variety of other viral infections (orf, zoster varicella virus [VZV], Epstein–Barr virus [EBV], cytomegalovirus [CMV], HIV, hepatitis B vaccination), bacterial infections (mainly *Mycoplasma pneumoniae*), and fungal infections (mainly histoplasmosis) have been implicated. An extensive list of drugs has been reported to trigger EM, but most cases, if not all, are the result of confusion with Stevens–Johnson syndrome. Rare cases are attributed to contact allergy.

Acute episodes of EM need only *symptomatic treatment* in most cases. Recurrent EM, which may severely affect quality of life, has a well-recognized *preventive treatment* in case of HSV infection but may be highly recalcitrant when no cause is identified. A persistent continuous variety of EM has been reported; several patients had antidesmoplakin antibodies, the significance of which is debated: epiphenomena or defining a variety of pemphigus?

There are no double-blind or open trials of treatments for acute episodes of EM. Most cases, particularly EM minor, run a self-limiting course. Symptomatic measures include *oral antihistamines* and *mild- to moderate-potency topical corticosteroids* to reduce pruritus. Underlying conditions, mainly *Mycoplasma pneumoniae* infection, should be treated. Recurrent EM (>6 attacks per year) may respond to long-term *aciclovir*. In aciclovir resistant cases a variety of other therapies can be helpful (see later).

Mucosal manifestations of EM are a source of morbidity and occur in up to 70% of cases. The most common sites affected are the buccal mucosa and lips. Symptomatic measures include *mouthwashes*, a *soft diet*, *topical anesthetics* (lidocaine gel, benzocaine lozenges, or 0.15% benzydamine hydrochloride), and *topical corticosteroids* (e.g., 0.1% triamcinolone acetonide paste). Budesonide or beclomethasone inhalers (one puff three to four times daily) provide an alternative method of delivering local corticosteroid to the inflamed mucosal surfaces. Short courses of high-dose *oral prednisolone* may be needed for severe oral disease. Strict eye care to reduce secondary infection and scarring includes *saline washes* for removal of crusts, *local antibiotics*, and frequent *debridement of tarsal and bulbar conjunctival adherences*.

Specific Investigation

- Histology/immunofluorescence

EM is a clinical diagnosis. Histology, with direct immunofluorescence, can be useful in atypical cases to exclude other bullous diseases that present with oral manifestations, such as pemphigus vulgaris or cicatricial pemphigoid.

Investigations directed at determining the underlying trigger factors include culture or serologic testing for HSV or other infections, especially *M. pneumoniae*, as indicated by clinical findings.

First-Line Therapy

- Antivirals (aciclovir, valaciclovir, ganciclovir)   **A**

Recurrent erythema multiforme: clinical features and treatment in a large series of patients. Schofield JK, Tatnall FM, Leigh IM. Br J Dermatol 1993; 128: 542–5.

A review of 65 patients with recurrent EM: 71% had episodes triggered by HSV infection. Treatment with standard doses of aciclovir for HSV was relatively disappointing; continuous aciclovir 400 mg twice daily for 6 months was more effective, with remission in some responders. Some patients responded to dapsone, antimalarials, azathioprine (10 of 11), and human immunoglobulin.

A double-blind, placebo-controlled trial of continuous aciclovir therapy in recurrent erythema multiforme. Tatnall FM, Schofield JK, Leigh IM. Br J Dermatol 1995; 132: 267–70.

Aciclovir 400 mg twice daily for 6 months suppressed EM in 7 of 11 patients (including 1 with apparently idiopathic EM). Two patients went into complete remission.

A therapeutic trial of aciclovir is justified even when clinical evidence of HSV is lacking. aciclovir 400 mg twice daily can be administered for 6 months to 2 years because it has a good long-term safety profile. It is ineffective in an acute episode once the herpetic lesion or EM eruption has developed. Recurrence is usual after stopping the drug.

Recurrent erythema multiforme unresponsive to aciclovir prophylaxis and responsive to valaciclovir continuous therapy.

Evidence Levels: A Double-blind study   B Clinical trial ≥ 20 subjects   C Clinical trial < 20 subjects   D Series ≥ 5 subjects   E Anecdotal case reports

Kerob D, Assier-Bonnet H, Esnault-Gelly P, Blanc F, Saiag P. Arch Dermatol 1998; 134: 876–7.

A reduced response to aciclovir may be due to the low oral bioavailability of the drug, and one of the second-generation antivirals, such as valaciclovir (500 mg daily) or famciclovir (250 mg twice daily), may need to be substituted.

Recurrent erythema multiforme: clinical characteristics, etiologic associations, and treatment in a series of 48 patients at Mayo Clinic, 2000 to 2007. Wetter DA, Davis MD. J Am Acad Dermatol 2010; 62: 45–53.

Of 48 patients HSV was responsible in 11 (23%); the cause remained unknown in 28 (58%). Systemic corticosteroids were used in most patients. Sixteen of 33 patients receiving continuous antiviral treatment had either partial or complete disease suppression. Mycophenolate mofetil provided partial or complete response in 6 of 8 patients.

Erythema multiforme major associated with CMV infection in an immunocompetent patient. Vitiello M, Echeverria B, Elgart G, Kerdel F. J Cutan Med Surg 2011; 15: 115–7.

Ganciclovir was used successfully.

Second-Line Therapies

• Dapsone	C
• Azathioprine	C
• Thalidomide	B
• Potassium iodide	C

Oral EM

• Topical corticosteroid	B
• Levamisole	B
• Systemic corticosteroid	D

Dapsone-responsive persistent erythema multiforme. Mahendran R, Grant JW, Norris PG. Dermatology 2000; 200: 281–2.

Dapsone 100 mg daily was effective in controlling EM in a patient with ovarian malignancy.

Characteristics of the oral lesions in patients with cutaneous recurrent erythema multiforme. Farthing PM, Maragou P, Coates M, Tatnall F, Leigh IM, Williams DM. J Oral Pathol Med 1995; 24: 9–13.

In this series of 82 patients with typical cutaneous EM, 70% had oral mucosal involvement. Five patients with resistant disease were controlled with azathioprine 100 to 150 mg daily.

Azathioprine therapy in the management of persistent erythema multiforme. Jones RR. Br J Dermatol 1981; 105: 465–7.

Azathioprine 100 to 150 mg daily was effective in two patients and permitted reduction of the corticosteroid dosage.

Treatment by thalidomide of chronic multiforme erythema: its recurrent and continuous variants. A retrospective study of 26 patients. Cherouati K, Claudy A, Souteyrand P, Cambazard F, Vaillant L, Moulin G, et al. Ann Dermatol Venereol 1996; 123: 375–7 (in French).

Thalidomide reduces the duration of episodes of recurrent EM by 11 days on average; it is dramatically effective in the exceptional

continuous variant. Remission can be maintained with low-dose (25–50 mg daily) thalidomide.

Potassium iodide in erythema nodosum and other erythematous dermatoses. Horio T, Danno K, Okamoto H, Miyachi Y, Imamura S. J Am Acad Dermatol 1983; 9: 77–81.

Fourteen of 16 subjects with EM (6 related to HSV infection) responded within 1 week to 300 mg potassium iodide three times daily. Gastrointestinal and cutaneous side effects can occur with this treatment.

Erythema multiforme – response to corticosteroid. Ting HC, Adam BA. Dermatologica 1984; 169: 175–8.

Thirteen patients with EM minor treated with systemic corticosteroids were compared with 12 treated without. Apart from a shorter duration of fever, the corticosteroid-treated group did not respond better than the noncorticosteroid-treated group.

There is no reason to treat EM minor with steroids. This drug may still be useful in EM major.

Open preliminary clinical trial of clobetasol propionate ointment in adhesive paste for treatment of chronic oral vesiculoerosive diseases. Lozada-Nur F, Huang MZ, Zhou GA. Oral Surg Oral Med Oral Pathol 1991; 71: 283–7.

Clobetasol propionate 0.05% ointment mixed 1:1 with Orabase paste two to three times daily was helpful in four patients with chronic oral EM.

Erythema multiforme: diagnosis, clinical manifestations and treatment in a retrospective study of 22 patients. Sanchis JM, Bagán JV, Gavaldá C, Murillo J, Diaz JM. J Oral Pathol Med 2010; 39: 747–52.

Systemic corticosteroids are effective in controlling the outbreaks; their use as maintenance therapy is not clearly indicated.

Prednisone and azathioprine in the treatment of patients with vesiculoerosive oral diseases. Lozada F. Oral Surg Oral Med Oral Pathol 1981; 52: 257–63.

In this open trial, two patients with oral EM required lower doses of prednisolone (15–20 mg on alternate days) when treated simultaneously with azathioprine (50 mg daily).

Recurrent oral erythema multiforme. Clinical experience with 11 patients. Bean SF, Quezada RK. JAMA 1983; 249: 2810–2.

In this retrospective study, patients with severe recurrent oral EM involvement were treated with prednisolone 40 to 60 mg daily, subsequently tapered over 2 to 3 weeks. This reduced the time taken for oral erosions to heal but did not influence recurrences.

Some authorities, however, believe that use of corticosteroids in EM increases the frequency and chronicity of attacks.

Third-Line Therapies

• Antimalarials	D
• Human immunoglobulin	D
• Interferon-α	E
• Rituximab	D
• Tamoxifen	E
• Zinc sulfate	E
• Cimetidine	E
• Ciclosporin	E
• Pulsed methylprednisolone	E

Recurrent erythema multiforme: clinical features and treatment in a large series of patients. Schofield JK, Tatnall FM, Leigh IM. Br J Dermatol 1993; 128: 542–5.

The use of normal human immunoglobulins and antimalarials was reported in a few patients in this study. Intramuscular human immunoglobulin 750 g once a month caused suppression of EM in 11 of 13 patients. One responder remained in remission after therapy was discontinued. There was a 50% success rate with antimalarials (both hydroxychloroquine and mepacrine) used in four patients.

Recurrent erythema multiforme and chronic hepatitis C: efficacy of interferon alpha. Dumas V, Thieulent N, Souillet AL, Jullien D, Faure M, Claudy A. Br J Dermatol 2000; 142: 1248–9.

One patient with recurrent EM and hepatitis C virus infection responded to two courses of interferon-alpha (IFN-α) (9 MU weekly for 6 and 8 months, respectively).

Severe erythema multiforme responding to interferon alfa. Geraminejad P, Walling HW, Voigt MD, Stone MS. J Am Acad Dermatol 2006; 54: S18–21.

A patient with recurrent EM associated with hepatitis C had been in complete remission for 6 years after treatment with IFN-α. A new recurrence was successfully treated with IFN-α in the absence of recurring hepatitis C virus infection.

Interferon may be a first-line treatment for patients with hepatitis C.

Rituximab, a new treatment for difficult to treat chronic erythema multiforme major. Five cases. Hirsch G, Ingen-Housz-Oro S, Fite C, Valeyrie-Allanore L, Ortonne N, Buffard V, et al. J Eur Acad Dermatol Venereol 2016; 30:1140–3.

Chronic continuous or relapsing EM resistant to several drugs, including aciclovir corticosteroids, and thalidomide; four patients had antidesmoplakin antibodies; four had complete remission.

Progesterone-induced erythema multiforme. Wojnarowska F, Greaves MW, Peachey RD, Drury PL, Besser GM. J Roy Soc Med 1985; 78: 407–8.

EM linked to the luteal phase of the menstrual cycle was controlled with tamoxifen.

Topical treatment of recurrent herpes simplex and postherpetic erythema multiforme with low concentrations of zinc sulphate solution. Brody I. Br J Dermatol 1981; 104: 191–4.

Treatment of the skin at the site of the herpetic infection with zinc sulfate solution prevented relapse of postherpetic EM over a 2-year period of observation in one patient. For the skin, 0.025% to 0.05% and for the oral mucous membrane 0.01% to 0.025% zinc sulfate solution was used.

Cimetidine prevents recurrent erythema multiforme major resulting from herpes simplex virus infection. Kurkcuoglu N, Alli N. J Am Acad Dermatol 1989; 21: 814–5.

EM resistant to aciclovir responded to cimetidine 400 mg three times daily in one patient.

Ciclosporin therapy for bullous erythema multiforme. Wilkel CS, McDonald CJ. Arch Dermatol 1990; 126: 397–8.

High-dose ciclosporin (5–10 mg/kg daily) suppressed an atypical bullous eruption with histologic features of EM. The use of ciclosporin permitted tapering of the corticosteroid dosage.

Evidence Levels: **A** Double-blind study **B** Clinical trial ≥ 20 subjects **C** Clinical trial < 20 subjects **D** Series ≥ 5 subjects **E** Anecdotal case reports

75

Erythema nodosum

Amy Forrestel, Misha Rosenbach

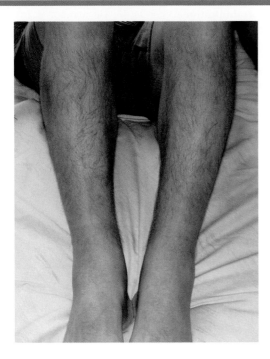

Erythema nodosum (EN) is a septal panniculitis that presents as tender, erythematous nodules and plaques classically located on the extensor surfaces of the lower extremities. EN is generally viewed as a cutaneous reactive process that can be seen as an isolated, idiopathic condition or, more commonly, as a secondary sign of another systemic disease (listed later). Individual lesions frequently resolve within 2 to 6 weeks, but persistent lesions and intermittent recurrent disease are not uncommon. EN is often accompanied by systemic symptoms such as fever, fatigue, arthritis, cough, and gastrointestinal complaints.

MANAGEMENT STRATEGIES

Management of EN first requires investigation for an underlying etiology, which should include detailed history and review of systems and a targeted evaluation. Numerous etiologies have been implicated, including chronic inflammatory states, infections, reactions to medications or hormones, and malignancies. Even after extensive evaluation, many cases are classified as idiopathic.

Many infectious agents have been associated with erythema nodosum. Bacterial and protozoan causes include *Streptococcus* (most common), *Mycoplasma pneumonia*, *Chlamydia pneumonia*, *Chlamydia trachomatis*, *Yersinia enterocolitica*, *Salmonella enteritidis*, *Giardia lamblia*, *Shigella*, *Klebsiella* spp., tuberculosis, brucellosis, psittacosis, cat scratch disease, chancroid, tularemia, rickettsiosis, leptospirosis, and *Campylobacter*. Viral causes include hepatitis B, hepatitis C, Human immunodeficiency virus (HIV), and herpes simplex virus (HSV). Fungal infections include blastomycosis, sporotrichosis, coccidioidomycosis, histoplasmosis, nocardiosis, and fungal kerions.

Chronic inflammatory conditions associated with EN include sarcoidosis (most common), inflammatory bowel disease (IBD), Behçet disease, Sweet syndrome, pyoderma faciale, and diverticulitis.

Associated medications include oral contraceptives (most common) and other female hormone therapies, antibiotics (in particular the penicillins and sulfonamides), iodides, bromides, quinolones, lidocaine injections, aromatase inhibitors, all-trans retinoic acid, propylthiouracil, granulocyte colony-stimulating factor, echinacea supplements, glatiramer acetate, valproate, nonsteroidal antiinflammatory drugs (NSAIDs), thalidomide, and dapsone. Targeted chemotherapeutic agents such as BRAF and MEK inhibitors have been recently described to cause an EN-like panniculitis. Multiple vaccines have been suggested as well, albeit in very small numbers—and the health benefits of vaccines outweigh the rare potential for this type of reaction.

Malignancies such as leukemias, lymphomas, myelodysplastic syndrome, and parathyroid carcinoma have been implicated.

Skin biopsy is generally not necessary if the history and physical signs are suggestive of EN. Biopsies are typically performed in atypical cases, persistent or treatment-refractory cases, or cases where there is a broad differential diagnosis and a biopsy may help exclude alternative etiologies. If a biopsy is done, the pathology classically demonstrates inflammation in the septae between fat lobules of the subcutis. The type of inflammation may vary between acute and chronic inflammation, including multinucleated giant cells ("Meischer granulomas"). Other findings can include fibrosis, increased thickness of the intralobular septae, and radial arrays of macrophages around blood vessels. A biopsy is usually helpful in ruling out other forms of panniculitis, and if an infectious cause is in the differential diagnosis, tissue may be sent for culture and stains.

If identified, treatment or elimination of an underlying trigger will often lead to spontaneous remission of EN. This is the primary treatment strategy and should be emphasized in all cases; if there is an EN-triggering disease, it should be treated, and if there is an EN-associated medication, it should be discontinued. Direct EN treatment consists primarily of bed rest, leg elevation, compression, NSAIDs, and potassium iodide. Of the NSAIDs, naproxen and indomethacin have the most evidence and experience. A reasonable starting dose of indomethacin is 50 mg three times daily. Note that NSAIDs have also been reported as potential EN-inducing drugs, and in such cases treatment with NSAIDs is not advised. Potassium iodide is generally well tolerated, effective, and nonimmunosuppressive but may not be widely available. Typical dosing is with a supersaturated solution of potassium iodide (SSKI) starting at 1 to 2 drops three times daily and gradually titrating up to 5 drops (often dissolved in orange juice to increase tolerability of taste) taken three times per day. Side effects include hypothyroidism and hyperkalemia; rarely, concentrated iodide can induce a neutrophilic eruption (iododerma). Thyroid-stimulating hormone (TSH) should be monitored monthly while on treatment.

In patients who fail these treatments, alternative treatments can be considered. Prednisone is very effective and may be used in particularly refractory, widespread, or very symptomatic patients to gain rapid control. Infection and malignancy should be ruled out before initiation. Colchicine, hydroxychloroquine, dapsone, and some immunomodulatory and immunosuppressive agents have anecdotal reports of efficacy, as described later.

- Complete blood count (with differential), erythrocyte sedimentation rate (ESR), C-reactive protein (CRP)
- Antistreptolysin O (ASO) titer or Anti-Deoxyribonuclease B (Anti-DNase B) titre, throat culture
- Urinalysis and urine pregnancy test
- Chest radiograph
- Purified protein derivative (PPD) standard tuberculosis skin test or interferon gamma release assay
- Skin biopsy

Erythema nodosum: a review. Soderstrom RM, Krull EA. Cutis 1978; 21: 806–10.

Streptococcal infection was the most common etiology, and sarcoidosis is the most common disease associated with EN.

All patients should have a chest radiograph, ASO titer, throat culture, and PPD/testing for latent tuberculosis.

Erythema nodosum: an evaluation of 100 cases. Mert A, Kumbasar H, Ozaras R, Erten S, Tasli L, Tabak F, et al. Clin Exp Rheumatol 2007; 25: 563–70.

The results showed a 6:1 female predominance; 53% idiopathic and 11% streptococcal infections, 10% tuberculosis, 10% sarcoidosis, 6% Behçet, 5% drug reactions, 3% IBD, and 2% pregnancy.

First-Line Therapies

• NSAIDs	E
• Potassium iodide	B

Suppression of erythema nodosum by indomethacin. Ubogy Z, Persellin RH. Acta Derm Venereol 1982; 62: 265–7.

Three patients with EN secondary to streptococcal pharyngitis refractory to erythromycin, penicillin, and aspirin improved with indomethacin 100 to 150 mg for 2 weeks.

Chronic erythema nodosum treated with indomethacin. Barr WG, Robinson JA. Ann Intern Med 1981; 95: 659.

Idiopathic EN in a 32-year-old woman refractory to aspirin resolved with indomethacin 25 mg three times daily for 1 month.

Control of chronic erythema nodosum with naproxen. Lehman CW. Cutis 1980; 26: 66–7.

A 28-year-old woman with recurrent EN refractory to phenylbutazone and aspirin was treated with naproxen 250 mg orally twice daily for 1 month, with cessation of symptoms within 96 hours and clearing in 14 days. Relapsed with therapy cessation but recleared when naproxen restarted.

Potassium iodide in erythema nodosum and other erythematous dermatoses. Horio T, Danno K, Okamoto H, Miyachi Y, Imamura S. J Am Acad Dermatol 1983; 9: 77–81.

Twelve of 16 patients treated with potassium iodide improved within a few days, with complete resolution in 10 to 14 days. Six had recurrent attacks, with resolution upon repeat dosing with potassium iodide. Better outcomes were obtained with earlier treatment initiation.

Potassium iodide may be a reasonable choice for those patients who cannot tolerate NSAIDs or corticosteroids.

Treatment of erythema nodosum and nodular vasculitis with potassium iodide. Schultz EJ, Whiting DA. Br J Dermatol 1976; 94: 75–8.

Twenty-four of 28 patients with EN improved within 48 hours and resolved within 2 weeks with 300 to 900 mg daily of potassium iodide.

Potassium iodide in dermatology. A 19th century drug for the 21st century: uses, pharmacology, adverse effects, and contraindications. Sterling JB, Heymann WR. J Am Acad Dermatol 2000; 43: 691–7.

An excellent review article.

Second-Line Therapies

• Colchicine	D
• Hydroxychloroquine	E
• Prednisone	E

Traitement de l'erythème noueux par la colchicine. De Coninck P, Baclet JL, Di Bernardo C, Büschges B, Plouvier B. Presse Med 1984; 13: 680.

Five women were treated with colchicine (2 mg daily for 3 days, then 1 mg daily for 2–4 weeks) and improved within 72 hours. None recurred after treatment cessation.

Erythema nodosum treated with colchicine. Wallace S. JAMA 1967; 202: 144.

One patient with EN was successfully treated with colchicine.

Hydroxychloroquine in the treatment of chronic erythema nodosum. Alloway JA, Franks LK. Br J Dermatol 1995; 132: 661–70.

A 38-year-old woman with a 24-year history of EN with almost monthly flares refractory to aspirin and indomethacin was treated with hydroxychloroquine 200 mg orally twice daily. Within 3 months she had a dramatic reduction in lesions and remained stable for at least 6 months.

Hydroxychloroquine and chronic erythema nodosum. Jarrett P, Goodfield MJD. Br J Dermatol 1996; 134: 373.

A 52-year-old with idiopathic EN refractory to NSAIDs and prednisone improved with hydroxychloroquine 200 mg orally twice a day and prednisone 15 mg four times a day for 8 weeks. Prednisone was stopped, and 8 weeks later the hydroxychloroquine dose was cut by half, but the patient experienced a flare, and the original dose was restarted. After 3 more months the hydroxychloroquine was stopped, although intermittent dosing was required.

Third-Line Therapies

• Dapsone	E
• Extracorporeal monocyte granulocytapheresis	E
• Erythromycin	E
• Mycophenolate mofetil	E
• Etanercept	E
• Adalimumab	E
• Infliximab	E
• Prophylactic penicillin	E
• Vitamin B_{12} (if levels low)	E
• Tetracycline	E

Acne fulminans and erythema nodosum during isotretinoin therapy responding to dapsone. Tan B, Lear J, Smith A. Clin Exp Dermatol 1997; 22: 26–7.

Acne fulminans and EN that occurred in a patient 3 weeks after starting isotretinoin responded to dapsone without oral prednisone.

Extracorporeal monocyte granulocytapheresis was effective for a patient of erythema nodosum concomitant with ulcerative colitis. Fukunaga K, Sawada K, Fukuda Y, Matoba Y, Natsuaki M, Ohnishi K, et al. Ther Apher Dial 2003; 7: 122–6.

A patient with ulcerative colitis and EN refractory to high-dose corticosteroids improved after monocyte granulocytapheresis once a week for 5 weeks. He was also on 5-aminosalicylic acid.

Severe erythema nodosum due to Behçet's disease responsive to erythromycin. Kaya TI, Tursen U, Baz K, Ikizoglu G, Dusmez D. J Dermatol Treat 2003; 14: 124–7.

A patient with refractory Behçet disease and EN responded to coincidental treatment with erythromycin for erythrasma.

Use of mycophenolate mofetil in erythema nodosum. Boyd AS. J Am Acad Dermatol 2002; 47: 968–9.

A patient taking estrogen replacement with EN refractory to discontinuing hormone therapy and azathioprine cleared with mycophenolate mofetil 750 mg twice a day and remained clear after a slow taper.

Dermatologic manifestations of Crohn disease in children: response to infliximab. Kugathasan S, Miranda A, Nocton J, Drolet BA, Raasch C, Binion DG. J Pediatr Gastroenterol Nutr 2003; 37: 150–4.

One child with Crohn disease and resistant EN cleared with infliximab 5 mg/kg and was maintained on 6-mercaptopurine.

Treatment of chronic erythema nodosum with infliximab. Clayton TH, Walker BP, Stables GI. Clin Exp Dermatol 2006; 31: 823–4.

A 26-year-old woman with IBD and EN improved with infliximab.

Etanercept treatment of erythema nodosum. Boyd AS. Skinmed 2007; 6: 197–9.

One patient with a 5-year history of recalcitrant EN was treated with etanercept 25 mg subcutaneously twice. She was clear after 4 months. After 6 months the etanercept dose was reduced to 25 mg subcutaneously weekly.

Prophylaxis of recurrent erythema nodosum with penicillin. Bhalla M, Thami GP. Dermatology 2007; 215: 363–4.

Three patients with recurrent EN were cleared with monthly doses of intramuscular benzathine penicillin 2.4 million units. One patient had high ASO titers, and the other two had idiopathic biopsy-proven EN. All patients remained clear at 6 months.

Refractory chronic erythema nodosum successfully treated with adalimumab. Ortego-Centeno N, Callejas-Rubio JL, Sanchez-Cano D, Caballero-Morales T. J Eur Acad Dermatol Venereol 2007; 21: 408–10.

A 79-year-old patient with chronic recalcitrant EN cleared with adalimumab 40 mg subcutaneously every 2 weeks and was clear after 7 months of follow-up.

Adalimumab for the treatment of Japanese patients with intestinal Behçet's disease. Tanida S, Inoue N, Kobayashi K, Naganuma M, Hirai F, Iizuka B, et al. Clin Gastroenterol Hepatol 2015; 13: 940–8.e3.

Twenty patients with active intestinal Behçet's disease refractory to corticosteroids and/or immunomodulator therapies were given 160 mg adalimumab, 80 mg 2 weeks later, then 40 mg every other week for 52 weeks. Eighty-eight percent of the patients with EN cleared.

Successful treatment of chronic erythema nodosum with vitamin B_{12}. Volkov I, Rudoy I, Press Y. J Am Board Fam Pract 2005; 18: 567–9.

One patient had EN resolve after being treated for a low serum B_{12} level with twice-weekly injections of 1000 μg of B_{12}.

Response of recalcitrant erythema nodosum to tetracyclines. Davis MD. J Am Acad Dermatol 2011; 64: 1211–2.

One patient with a renal transplant and recalcitrant EN resolved after 1 month of minocycline 100 mg twice daily. Minocycline was discontinued because of hyperpigmentation. EN recurred within a week and resolved again with tetracycline 500 mg twice a day.

Role of tetracycline in recalcitrant erythema nodosum. Rohatgi S, Basavaraj KH, Ashwini PK, Kanthraj GR. Indian Dermatol Online J 2014; 5: 314–5.

A 40-year-old male with chronic recurrent EN cleared after 2 weeks of tetracycline 500 mg four times daily. The patient was switched to doxycycline and the EN recurred, so tetracycline was restarted with sustained complete regression for 6 months.

Erythrasma

Melissa C. Barkham

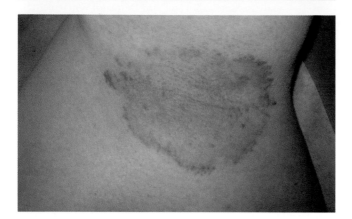

In its most typical form, erythrasma is characterized by well-defined, reddish-brown, flexural plaques that show fine scaling and no tendency to central clearing. It may also present with maceration of the toe webs.

The responsible organism, *Corynebacterium minutissimum*, is an inhabitant of normal human skin. Factors that predispose to clinically apparent infection include diabetes mellitus, obesity, Human Immunodeficiency Virus (HIV), old age, and a humid environment.

MANAGEMENT STRATEGY

Erythrasma is often a trivial infection, but therapy may be requested because of the cosmetic appearance or because of pruritus. Coinfection with dermatophyte fungi or *Candida albicans* is common and may influence the choice of treatment.

Fusidic acid cream is the topical treatment of choice where no concomitant yeast or fungal infection is found. It is both effective and well tolerated.

Topical imidazoles (miconazole, clotrimazole, bifonazole) are well tolerated and also effective against concomitant fungal or yeast infection.

When the disease is extensive or when compliance with topical therapy is unlikely, oral antibiotics such as *single-dose clarithromycin or oral erythromycin* should be considered.

A combination of oral and topical treatment may be required for stubborn infections, particularly of the toe webs.

Specific Investigations

- Examination under Wood light
- Potassium hydroxide (KOH) preparation of skin scrapings

Rapid confirmation of the diagnosis is achieved by examination of the skin under Wood (long-wave ultraviolet) light. The characteristic coral-red fluorescence observed is due to the production of coproporphyrin III by the organism. Fluorescence may not be seen if

the patient has bathed immediately before examination. Culture is unreliable because the organism does not always grow satisfactorily. Microscopy of skin scrapings is performed to seek evidence of concomitant infection, such as the presence of fungal hyphae or yeasts.

First-Line Therapies

• Fusidic acid cream	A
• Miconazole cream	B
• Clotrimazole cream	D
• Clindamycin lotion or solution	E
• Bifonazole cream	E

A comparison between the effectiveness of erythromycin, single dose clarithromycin and topical fusidic acid in the treatment of erythrasma. Avci O, Tanyildizi T, Kusku E. J Dermatolog Treatment 2013; 24: 70–4.

One hundred fifty-one patients were included in this study. Around two thirds of them had toe web infections. A complete response (defined as no fluorescence) was observed in 30/31 patients treated with 2% fusidic acid cream twice daily for 14 days in this double-blind, placebo-controlled trial. The response was superior to oral clarithromycin (20/30), oral erythromycin (16/30), placebo cream (4/30), and placebo tablets (1/30). The authors acknowledged the limitations of the grading system of fluorescence used to assess response. They mention that the higher efficacy of fusidic acid cream over oral antibiotics might well be due to the removal of coproporphyrin III from the stratum corneum during topical applications. Despite the apparent efficacy of fusidic acid cream alone, they supported the opinion of previous authors who have recommended a combination of oral and topical treatment for extensive or stubborn toe web infections.

A clinical double-blind trial of topical miconazole and clotrimazole against superficial fungal infections and erythrasma. Clayton YM, Knight AG. Clin Exp Dermatol 1976; 1: 225–32.

This was a comparison of the two preparations in dermatophyte infection, but 11 patients with erythrasma were also studied: 6 treated with miconazole, 5 with clotrimazole, both twice daily. All patients in both groups were free of infection at 4 weeks.

Topical treatment for erythrasma. Cochran RJ, Rosen T, Landers T. Int J Dermatol 1981; 20: 562–4.

Two cases cleared with two or three times daily application of 2% aqueous clindamycin solution for 1 week. No recurrence was noted 6 weeks later.

Bifonazole – an antifungal and antibacterial agent with excellent in vitro activity against *Corynebacterium minutissimum* – an in vitro study of erythrasma. Nenoff P, Herrmann J, Kruger C, Tchernev G, Becker N. Mycoses 2012; 55: 338.

Bifonazole exhibits very good in vitro activity against *Corynebacterium* spp. This cream is available over the counter for the treatment of dermatophyte infection of the toe webs. Because coinfections are common, it may be efficient at treating both.

Second-Line Therapies

• Single-dose clarithromycin	B
• Erythromycin	C

Evidence Levels: **A** Double-blind study **B** Clinical trial ≥ 20 subjects **C** Clinical trial < 20 subjects **D** Series ≥ 5 subjects **E** Anecdotal case reports

Erythrasma treated with single-dose clarithromycin. Wharton JR, Wilson PL, Kincannon JM. Arch Dermatol 1998; 134: 671–2.

Three patients treated with a single 1-g dose of clarithromycin showed no sign of residual disease at 2 weeks. Compliance is likely to be good with this regimen.

Systemic or local treatment of erythrasma? A comparison between erythromycin tablets and Fucidin cream in general practice. Hamann K, Thorn P. Scand J Prim Health Care 1991; 9: 35–9.

This double-blind trial compared 14 days' treatment with erythromycin 500 mg twice daily, 2% fusidic acid cream twice daily, and placebo. Four weeks after treatment 18 of 21 patients with erythromycin and 23 of 25 with fusidic acid cream were cured. Both were better than placebo.

Antibiotic susceptibility of *Corynebacterium minutissimum* isolated from lesions of Turkish patients with erythrasma. Turk BG, Turkmen M, Aytimur D. J Am Acad Dermatol 2011; 65: 1230–1.

This laboratory-based study examined antibiotic susceptibility in *C. minutissimum* isolates. Interestingly, it demonstrated high levels of antibiotic resistance to erythromycin and high levels of susceptibility to fusidic acid and amoxicillin clavulanate.

Erythroderma

Tang Ngee Shim, John Berth-Jones

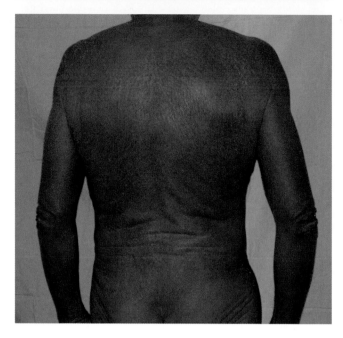

Erythroderma (exfoliative dermatitis) is defined as inflammation of at least 90% of the body surface, characterized by generalized erythema and a variable degree of scaling or desquamation. Erythroderma is commonly the result of generalization of a preexisting chronic dermatosis or a systemic disease (see Table 77.1). These include genodermatoses and congenital disorders such as severe ichthyoses and ichthyosiform erythrodermas; severe cases of dermatoses such as psoriasis and atopic, seborrheic, or contact allergic dermatitis; cutaneous T-cell lymphoma (CTCL); allergic reactions to drugs (see Table 77.2); and internal malignancies (especially lymphoma and other lymphoreticular malignancies). Some cases develop without any apparent trigger, and erythroderma remains "idiopathic" in up to 25% of the cases.

MANAGEMENT STRATEGY

Erythroderma, especially when fulminant, is a life-threatening state of skin failure that demonstrates vividly that the skin is as vital to life as any internal organ. The dangers arise from the loss of an effective barrier to entry of bacteria, from the loss of thermoregulation, from increased fluid loss through evaporation or exudation, from loss of protein due to the increased proliferative and metabolic activity that accompanies uncontrolled desquamation, and from the risk of high-output cardiac failure. All these hazards are greatest in the very young and the elderly. Many patients who are otherwise healthy can tolerate a chronic or permanently erythrodermic state. By contrast, very young and elderly patients with fulminant disease may develop septicemia and die within a matter of hours.

Many aspects of the management of a patient with erythroderma are similar, regardless of the etiology, and it is often necessary to treat a case without knowing the cause. However, for optimal longer term management it is vital to establish a more precise diagnosis whenever possible. In many cases there has been preexisting skin disease and the diagnosis may be quite clear from the history, but when erythroderma arises de novo, establishing the cause can be difficult or impossible. A comprehensive drug history should include all over-the-counter and herbal remedies such as St. John wort. Severe pruritus may suggest atopic eczema or lymphoma. Although physical examination may be entirely nonspecific, there may be clues such as bullae, indicating the presence of bullous pemphigoid or pemphigus foliaceus. Severe scaling is suggestive of psoriasis. Pityriasis rubra pilaris shows islands of uninvolved skin within erythrodermic regions with "orange" palmoplantar keratoderma and follicular keratotic plugs on the knees, elbows, and dorsal aspects of the hands and toes. Sparing of the flexures ("deck-chair sign") may suggest papuloerythroderma of Ofuji. Lymphadenopathy is often present but is more often reactive than malignant.

Histology of the skin is often nonspecific and rarely pathognomonic. Occasionally, however, the presence of atypical large lymphocytes will point to a diagnosis of CTCL, or there may be features suggestive of psoriasis, a lichenoid reaction, or pityriasis rubra pilaris. Repeated or multiple biopsies are sometimes helpful. Immunofluorescence for immunoglobulin deposition should be performed if an immunobullous disease is suspected.

Patients with acute onset of erythroderma are usually best managed in a hospital because frequent observations and intensive supportive care are required, and bed rest may be highly therapeutic. All unnecessary medications should be discontinued. Good skin care is essential. Frequent applications of abundant quantities of bland emollients such as petrolatum are required to soothe the skin, and these help to partially restore the barrier. Oatmeal baths and wet dressings to weeping or crusted sites should be followed by application of bland emollients and low-potency topical corticosteroids. Careful attention must be paid to body temperature, hydration, and nutrition.

The use of more active pharmaceutical intervention requires careful consideration. Some patients with erythroderma have multiple drug allergies. Immunosuppressive drugs may be considered to be contraindicated if malignancy is suspected (particularly cutaneous lymphoma). Topical treatments may be far more irritating than expected, and systemic absorption will be greater than usual. *Prophylactic antibiotics* such as *erythromycin* are often given orally. *Corticosteroids* are often applied topically. *Antihistamines* are often prescribed but act largely as sedatives.

If a diagnosis can be established, withdrawal of a causal drug or specific treatment for an underlying dermatosis, combined with the supportive measures described earlier, will usually produce a rapid improvement in the erythroderma. When a firm diagnosis cannot be made, treatment may have to be directed at the most likely cause, based on the clinical and histologic features.

Specific Investigations

- Hematology
- Urea and electrolytes
- Liver function tests
- Blood cultures
- Monitoring of temperature and vital signs
- Nasal and skin swabs
- Skin biopsy
- T-cell receptor analysis
- Lymph node biopsy
- Screening for connective tissue disease
- Immunodeficiency screen
- Potassium hydroxide preparation and fungal culture

Evidence Levels: **A** Double-blind study **B** Clinical trial ≥ 20 subjects **C** Clinical trial < 20 subjects **D** Series ≥ 5 subjects **E** Anecdotal case reports

Table 77.1 Cutaneous diseases that may present with or develop into erythroderma

Atopic dermatitis	Lichen planus
Bullous pemphigoid	Lupus erythematosus
Contact allergic dermatitis	Papuloerythroderma of Ofuji
Congenital ichthyoses	Pemphigus foliaceus
Cutaneous T-cell lymphoma	Pityriasis rubra pilaris
Dermatomyositis	Psoriasis
Dermatophytosis	Reiter syndrome
Graft-versus-host disease	Sarcoid
Hailey–Hailey disease	Seborrheic dermatitis
Human immunodeficiency virus	Scabies
Ichthyoses	Stasis dermatitis with autosensitization

Table 77.2 Examples of drugs that may induce erythroderma

Allopurinol	Isosorbide dinitrate
Amiodarone	Lamotrigine
Antimalarials	Lithium
Aspirin	Minocycline
Aztreonam	Nifedipine
Bupropion	Omeprazole
Carbamazepine	Penicillins
Cephalosporins	Phenothiazines
Cimetidine	Phenytoin
Codeine phosphate	Quinidine
Diaminodiphenyl sulfone (dapsone)	St John's wort (Hypericum)
Diltiazem	Sulfonamides
Diphenylhydantoin (phenytoin)	Sulfonylureas
Gentamicin	Terbinafine
Imatinib	Thiazides
Indinavir	Trimethoprim
Isoniazid	Vancomycin

Diagnosing erythrodermic cutaneous T-cell lymphoma. Russell-Jones R. Br J Dermatol 2005; 153: 1–5.

A very useful review with an algorithm to help differentiate between erythroderma due to CTCL and "reactive" causes of erythroderma. The author proposed three key procedures to determine the correct diagnosis for patients with chronic erythroderma of unknown etiology: biopsy of lesional skin, analysis of peripheral blood, and lymph node biopsy. Each sample should be analyzed for morphology, immunophenotype, and the presence of a T-cell clone.

Survival outcomes and prognostic factors in mycosis fungoides/Sézary syndrome: validation of the revised International Society for Cutaneous Lymphomas/European Organisation for Research and Treatment of Cancer staging proposal. Agar NS, Wedgeworth E, Crichton S, Mitchell TJ, Cox M, Ferreira S, et al. J Clin Oncol 2010; 28: 4730–9.

A significant difference in survival and progression was noted for patients with early-stage disease having patches alone (T1a/T2a) compared with those having patches and plaques (T1b/T2b).

Erythrodermic bullous pemphigoid. Amato L, Gallerani I, Mei S, Pestelli E, Caproni M, Fabbri P. Int J Derm 2001; 40: 343–6.

Two cases of bullous pemphigoid presented with exfoliative erythroderma. Both were treated with oral prednisolone with complete clinical resolution.

A case of erythrodermic dermatomyositis associated with gastric cancer. Kim SW, Kang YS, Park SH, Lee UH, Park HS, Jang SJ. Ann Dermatol 2009; 21: 435–9.

Subacute cutaneous lupus erythematosus presenting as erythroderma. Kalavala M, Shah V, Blackford S. Clin Exp Dermatol 2007; 32: 388–90.

Erythroderma is occasionally a presentation of dermatomyositis or lupus.

Idiopathic erythroderma: a follow-up study of 28 patients. Sigurdsson V, Toonstra J, van Vloten WA. Dermatology 1997; 194: 98–101.

During the median follow-up of 33 months, 35% of the patients went into remission and 52% improved. Three patients, all females, had persistent erythroderma. Two of these progressed to CTCL (one to Sézary syndrome and one to mycosis fungoides).

Interleukin-36γ (IL-1F9) identifies psoriasis among patients with erythroderma. Braegelmann J, D'Erme AM, Akmal S, Maier J, Braegelmann C, Wenzel J. Acta Derm Venereol 2016; 96: 386–7.

A retrospective review of histologic features seen in a series of 46 cases of erythroderma and a relatively specific stain to identify psoriasis.

Inherited ichthyoses: a review of the histology of the skin. Scheimberg I, Harper JI, Malone M, Lake BD. Pediatr Pathol Laboratory Med 1996; 16: 359–78.

A review of the histologic features in 46 cases of congenital ichthyosis. Features of bullous ichthyosiform erythroderma, Netherton syndrome, and neutral lipid storage disease can be recognized on routine hematoxylin and eosin staining. Electron microscopy, frozen sections, and other diagnostic techniques may also be required.

Early skin biopsy is helpful for the diagnosis and management of neonatal and infantile erythrodermas. Leclerc-Mercier S, Bodemer C, Bourdon-Lanoy E, Larousserie F, Hovnanian A, Brousse N, et al. J Cutan Pathol 2010; 37: 249–55.

Skin biopsy can be helpful to investigate early erythroderma of infancy, particularly in immunodeficiency and Netherton syndrome.

Use of the frozen section "jelly roll" technique to aid in the diagnosis of bullous congenital ichthyosiform erythroderma (epidermolytic hyperkeratosis). Galler B, Bowen C, Arnold J, Kobayashi T, Dalton SR. J Cutan Pathol 2016; 43: 434–7.

A neonate was initially diagnosed by histologic examination of detached skin (blister roof).

Congenital erythrodermic psoriasis: case report and literature review. Salleras M, Sanchez-Regana M, Umbert P. Pediatr Dermatol 1995; 12: 231–4.

A girl suffered from erythroderma, palmoplantar hyperkeratosis, and scalp desquamation since birth. A skin biopsy at 1 year of age showed features of psoriasis. She was successfully treated with acitretin at the age of 4 years. Plaque psoriasis developed at the age of 7 years.

Erythroderma due to dermatophyte. Gupta R, Khera V. Acta Dermatol Venereol 2001; 81: 70.

Dermatophytosis rarely presents as erythroderma. In this case the presence of multiple mycelia without spores in KOH preparation confirmed the clinical suspicion of dermatophytosis. The scaling and erythema completely cleared with oral fluconazole 150 mg daily and miconazole nitrate cream 2% topically.

Erythroderma as the initial presentation of the acquired immunodeficiency syndrome. Janniger CK, Gascon PM, Schwartz RA, Hennessey NP, Lambert WC. Dermatologica 1999; 183: 143–5.

Erythroderma can be the presenting feature of HIV infection.

First-Line Therapies

• Bed rest in a hospital	C
• Emollients	C

Second-Line Therapies

• Topical corticosteroids	C
• Psoralen and UVA (PUVA)	C
• Systemic corticosteroids	C
• PUVA with retinoid	E

Cushing's syndrome caused by short-term topical glucocorticoid use for erythrodermic psoriasis and development of adrenocortical insufficiency after glucocorticoid withdrawal. Durmazlar SP, Oktay B, Eren C, Eskioglu F. Eur J Dermatol 2009; 19: 169–70.

Salicylism from topical salicylates: review of the literature. Brubacher JR, Hoffman RS. J Toxicol Clin Toxicol 1996; 34: 431–6.

Hypercalcemia caused by vitamin D3 analogs in psoriasis treatment. Braun GS, Witt M, Mayer V, Schmid H. Int J Dermatol 2007; 46: 1315–7.

Low but detectable serum levels of tacrolimus seen with the use of very dilute, extemporaneously compounded formulations of tacrolimus ointment in the treatment of patients with Netherton syndrome. Shah KN, Yan AC. Arch Dermatol 2006; 142: 1362–3.

These reports illustrate the potential for unexpected toxicity due to systemic absorption of topical medications through erythrodermic skin. Care should be exercised with the use and quantities of topical medication.

Ofuji's papuloerythroderma: a study of 17 cases. Bech-Thomson N, Thomsen K. Clin Exp Dermatol 1998; 23: 79–83.

This retrospective study reviewed the clinical, laboratory, and histologic features; treatment methods; and disease course in 17 patients with papuloerythroderma. Psoralen photochemotherapy (PUVA) and oral prednisolone 10 to 20 mg daily given in combination or alone were effective, and a combination of UVB phototherapy and topical steroids was also successful.

Treatment of papuloerythroderma of Ofuji with Re-PUVA: a case report and review of the therapy. Mutluer S, Yerebakan O, Alpsoy E, Ciftcioglu MA, Yilmaz E. J Eur Acad Dermatol Venereol 2004; 18: 480–3.

A 60-year-old man with papuloerythroderma of Ofuji responded to retinoid plus PUVA (Re-PUVA).

A dermatitis–eosinophilia syndrome. Treatment with methylprednisolone pulse therapy. Dahl MV, Swanson DL, Jacob HS. Arch Dermatol 1984; 120: 1595–7.

A case of persistent erythroderma after a wasp sting despite intensive topical therapy and oral corticosteroids. Pulsed methylprednisolone, 2 g intravenously, repeated after a week, cleared the erythroderma.

Toxic shock syndrome responsive to steroids. Vergis N, Gorard DA. J Med Case Rep 2007; 1: 5.

Toxic shock syndrome should be considered in the differential diagnosis of unexplained fever, erythroderma, and features of septic shock. Systemic steroids can be lifesaving.

Third-Line Therapies

• Ciclosporin	B
• Cytotoxic drugs/antimetabolites	C
• Systemic retinoids	C
• Extracorporeal photochemotherapy	C
• UVA1 phototherapy	C
• Topical calcipotriol	E
• Topical tacrolimus	D
• Erythromycin	E
• Photopheresis and interferon	C
• Ustekinumab	E
• Brodalumab	D
• Infliximab	C
• Etanercept	C
• Alemtuzumab	E
• Daclizumab	E
• Bexarotene	D

Management of erythrodermic psoriasis with low-dose ciclosporin. Studio Italiano Multicentrico nella Psoriasi (SIMPSO). 1993; 187: 30–7.

In this open-label, multicenter study of 33 patients with erythrodermic psoriasis, ciclosporin (initial mean dose 4.2 mg/kg/day) was slowly tapered after remission by 0.5 mg/kg every 2 weeks. Sixty-seven percent achieved complete remission, and 27% had significant improvement at 2 to 4 months.

Papuloerythroderma of Ofuji responding to treatment with ciclosporin. Sommer S, Henderson CA. Clin Exp Dermatol 2000; 25: 293–5.

A patient with papuloerythroderma of Ofuji responded to systemic steroids, but remission was not maintained on reduction of the dose. Ciclosporin was added, which led to rapid clearing of the skin, and remission was maintained after discontinuation of treatment.

Psoriatic erythroderma and bullous pemphigoid treated successfully with acitretin and azathioprine. Roeder C, Driesch PV. Eur J Dermatol 1999; 9: 537–9.

A 59-year-old man with severe psoriasis who developed bullous pemphigoid was successfully treated with acitretin and azathioprine, avoiding the use of systemic corticosteroids.

Evidence Levels: **A** Double-blind study   **B** Clinical trial ≥ 20 subjects   **C** Clinical trial < 20 subjects   **D** Series ≥ 5 subjects   **E** Anecdotal case reports

Methotrexate in psoriasis: 26 years' experience with low-dose long-term treatment. Haustein UF, Rytter M. J Eur Acad Dermatol Venereol 2000; 14: 382–8.

A retrospective review of 36 patients with erythrodermic psoriasis treated with methotrexate at varying dosages (initial dose 7.5–40 mg/week, maintenance dose 7.5–15 mg/week). Response to therapy noted within 1 to 4 weeks of onset.

Systemic methotrexate treatment in childhood psoriasis: further experience in 24 children from India. Kaur I, Dogra S, De D, Kanwar AJ. Pediatr Dermatol 2008; 25: 184–8.

Twenty-two children showed >75% reduction in Psoriasis Area and Severity Index (PASI). This retrospective study supports the use of methotrexate in severe childhood psoriasis under expert supervision and laboratory monitoring.

An appraisal of acitretin therapy in children with inherited disorders of keratinization. Lacour M, Mehta-Nikhar B, Atherton DJ, Harper JI. Br J Dermatol 1996; 134: 1023–9.

A review of the use of acitretin and etretinate in 46 children with severe ichthyoses and erythrodermas. Acitretin therapy is safe and effective, provided the minimal effective dose is maintained and that side effects are carefully monitored.

Treatment of classic pityriasis rubra pilaris. Dicken CH. J Am Acad Dermatol 1994; 31: 997–9.

A retrospective review of 75 cases. Retinoids offer the best chance of complete clearing. Methotrexate should be considered if retinoids fail or are contraindicated.

Treatment of refractory adult-onset pityriasis rubra pilaris with TNF-alpha antagonists: a case series. Garcovich S, Di Giampetruzzi AR, Antonelli G, Garcovich A, Didona B. J Eur Acad Dermatol Venereol 2010; 24: 881–4.

Pityriasis rubra pilaris is a rare inflammatory dermatosis with frequent clinical presentation as erythroderma. Seven patients with resistance or contraindication to conventional systemic treatment (six were erythrodermic) received a single course of infliximab or etanercept therapy, alone or in combination with low-dose acitretin (>0.25 mg/kg/daily). Six patients achieved complete remission after a single course of anti–TNF-α therapy.

Evidence-based practice of photopheresis 1987 to 2001: a report of a workshop of the British Photodermatology Group and the UK Skin Lymphoma Group. McKeena KE, Whittaker S, Rhodes LE, Taylor P, Lloyd J, Ibbotson S, et al. Br J Dermatol 2006; 154: 7–20.

Extracorporeal photopheresis in Sézary syndrome: hematologic parameters as predictors of response. Evans AV, Wood BP, Scarisbrick JJ, Fraser-Andrews EA, Chinn S, Dean A, et al. Blood 2001; 98: 1298–301.

Twenty-three patients with Sézary syndrome who received monthly (up to 1 year) extracorporeal photopheresis (ECP) as the sole therapy showed that 57% achieved a reduction in erythema of more than 25% from baseline.

U.K. consensus statement on the use of extracorporeal photopheresis for treatment of cutaneous T-cell lymphoma and chronic graft-versus-host disease. Scarisbrick JJ, Taylor P, Hlltick U, Makar Y, Douglas K, Berlin G, et al. Br J Dermatol 2008; 158: 659–78.

The literature supports ECP as an effective therapy in CTCL and chronic graft-versus-host disease (GVHD).

Treatment of severe erythrodermic acute graft-versus-host disease with photochemotherapy. Kunz M, Wilhelm S, Freund M, Zimmermann R, Gross G. Br J Dermatol 2001; 144: 901–22.

A 34-year-old man with grade IV GVHD who failed three different high-dose immunosuppressive agents responded to photochemotherapy.

The benefit of PUVA treatment for acute GVHD is well known, but successful treatment of severe GVHD is less common.

"High-dose" UVA1 therapy of widespread plaque-type, nodular, and erythrodermic mycosis fungoides. Zane C, Leali C, Airó P, De Panfilis G, Pinton PC. J Am Acad Dermatol 2001; 44: 629–33.

In a series of 13 patients, 11 showed complete clinical and histologic response to 100 J/cm² UVA1 daily until remission. Nonirradiated control lesions did not improve. Serious short-term side effects were not recorded. "High-dose" UVA1 seems at least as effective as PUVA in the treatment of cutaneous mycosis fungoides.

Bullous congenital ichthyosiform erythroderma: safe and effective topical treatment with calcipotriol ointment in a child. Bogenrieder T, Landthaler M, Stolz W. Acta Venereol 2002; 83: 52–5.

A report of the safe and long-term (over 3 years) use of topical calcipotriol ointment in a 9-year-old boy with a keratinization disorder.

Successful treatment of Netherton's syndrome with topical calcipotriol. Godic A, Dragos V. Eur J Dermatol 2004; 14: 115–7.

Efficacy and safety of tacrolimus 0.03% ointment in a 1-month-old "red baby": a case report. Leonardi S, Rotolo N, Marchese G, La Rosa M. Allergy Asthma Proc 2006; 27: 523–6.

Erythrodermic chronic actinic dermatitis responding to topical tacrolimus. Evans AV, Palmer RA, Hawk JL. Photodermatol Photoimmunol Photomed 2004; 20: 59–61.

A 55-year-old man with erythrodermic chronic actinic dermatitis failed standard topical and systemic treatments but responded to topical tacrolimus ointment 0.1%.

Successful treatment of bullous congenital ichthyosiform erythroderma with erythromycin. Freyhaus K, Kaiser HW, Proelss J, Tüting T, Bieber T, Wenzel J. Dermatol 2007; 215: 81–3.

This patient failed to respond to acitretin 30 mg daily. Erythromycin 500 mg twice daily was instituted, and marked clinical improvement was observed within 1 month.

Combination therapy with extracorporeal photopheresis, interferon-alpha, PUVA and topical corticosteroids in the management of Sézary syndrome. Brooken N, Weiss C, Utikal J, Felcht M, Goerdt S, Klemke CD. J Dtsch Dermatol Ges 2010; 428–38.

Twelve Sézary patients were retrospectively analyzed to evaluate the combination therapy of ECP, interferon-α, PUVA, and topical corticosteroids. All Sézary patients had erythroderma, generalized lymphadenopathy, and circulating Sézary cells (>1000/μL) in the peripheral blood at the time of diagnosis. Four patients achieved a partial remission and one a stable disease.

Efficacy and safety of biologics in erythrodermic psoriasis: a multicenter, retrospective study. Viguier M, Pagés C, Aubin F,

Delaporte E, Descamps V, Lok C, et al. Br J Dermatol 2012; 167: 417–23.

This study addresses the efficacy and safety of biologics (infliximab, adalimumab, etanercept, ustekinumab, and efalizumab) in 28 patients. Overall 42% of patients with erythrodermic psoriasis reached a 75% improvement of skin severity 10 to 14 weeks after starting biologics. Safety is mostly affected by infectious complications with skin origin.

Erythrodermic psoriasis improved by ustekinumab: a report of two cases. Kim YS, Kim HJ, Lee S, Park YL. Ann Dermatol 2016; 28: 121–2.

Sustained responses are reported in two refractory cases.

Efficacy and safety of brodalumab in patients with generalized pustular psoriasis and psoriatic erythroderma: results from a 52-week, open-label study. Yamasaki K, Nakagawa H, Kubo Y, Ootaki K. Br J Dermatol 2017; 176: 741–51.

Improvement or remission was observed in 18 cases of psoriatic erythroderma over the course of this 52-week study.

Infliximab as sole or combined therapy, induces rapid clearing of erythrodermic psoriasis. Takahashi MDF, Castro LG, Romiti R. Br J Dermatol 2007; 157: 828–31.

This is an open-label, single-center study of seven patients with erythrodermic psoriasis. One patient was treated with infliximab 5 mg/kg at week 0, 4, and 6 and methotrexate 15 mg/week. Four patients were treated with infliximab (same regimen as before) and acitretin 0.3 to 0.6 mg/kg. All five patients reported excellent outcome at week 6 after the third infusion.

Treatment of erythrodermic psoriasis with etanercept. Esposito M, Mazzotta A. Br J Dermatol 2006; 155: 156–9.

An open-label study of 10 patients with erythrodermic psoriasis. Etanercept was administered as a 25-mg subcutaneous injection twice weekly; 6 achieved PASI 75 and 2 achieved PASI 50 at week 24. These improvements were noted as early as week 12 of the study.

Alemtuzumab for relapsed and refractory erythrodermic cutaneous T-cell lymphoma: a single institution experience from the Robert H Lurie Comprehensive Cancer Center. Querfeld C, Mehta N, Rosen ST, Guitart J, Rademaker A, Gerami P, et al. Leuk Lymphoma 2009; 50: 1969–76.

This is an open-label clinical trial on the use of alemtuzumab in 19 advanced and heavily pretreated erythrodermic cutaneous T-cell lymphomas.

Novel treatment of Sézary-like syndrome due to adult T-cell leukemia/lymphoma with daclizumab (humanized antiinterleukin-2 receptor alpha antibody). Osborne GE, Pagliuca A, Ho A, du Vivier AW. Br J Dermatol 2006; 15: 617–20.

A patient with erythrodermic T-cell leukemia/lymphoma resistant to multiple therapies developed a rapid and sustained complete response to daclizumab, which suggests significant activity of anti-IL-2 receptor-α antibody in this disease process.

The treatment of cutaneous T-cell lymphoma with a novel retinoid. Heald P. Clin Lymphoma 2000; 1: S45–9.

Four patients with erythrodermic CTCL were treated with high-dose oral bexarotene, and all showed rapid (within 2 weeks) improvement of erythroderma.

Bexarotene therapy for mycosis fungoides and Sézary syndrome. Abbott RA, Whittaker SJ, Morris SL, Russell-Jones R, Hung T, Bashir SJ, et al. Br J Dermatol 2009; 160: 1299–307.

This retrospective study of 66 patients demonstrates that bexarotene is well tolerated in most patients and responses are well seen in almost half of patients with all disease stages. Two patients with erythroderma achieved complete response with bexarotene (one subsequently received reduced-intensity stem cell transplant and the other remains on bexarotene).

Evidence Levels: A Double-blind study B Clinical trial ≥ 20 subjects C Clinical trial < 20 subjects D Series ≥ 5 subjects E Anecdotal case reports

78

Erythrokeratodermas

Gabriele Richard

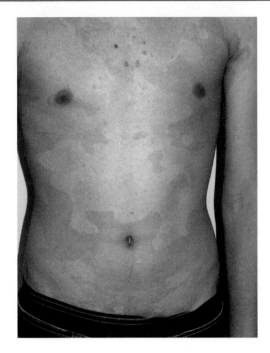

Erythrokeratodermas are a clinically and genetically heterogeneous group of rare inherited disorders of cornification characterized by two distinct morphologic features: localized hyperkeratosis and erythema. The hallmark of erythrokeratodermia variabilis (EKV) is the seemingly independent occurrence of transient, figurate erythema and hyperkeratosis, which can be localized or generalized. Progressive symmetric erythrokeratoderma (PSEK) is characterized by fixed, slowly progressive, symmetric, and well-defined hyperkeratotic plaques with underlying erythema, predominantly on the extensor surface of the extremities, on the trunk, and on the face. EKV and PSEK have been observed within the same family, and the same disease-causing *GJB4* (connexin 30.3) mutation has been reported in patients with EKV and PSEK. These findings indicate that a subset of PSEK cases belong to the clinical spectrum of EKV, and the name *erythrokeratodermia variabilis et progressiva (EKVP)* has been suggested. However, many other PSEK cases do not have identifiable connexin gene mutations and likely represent a heterogeneous group of other disorders that remain to be better defined on a clinical and molecular level.

MANAGEMENT STRATEGY

Erythrokeratodermas are heritable, chronic disorders that often require lifelong treatment. Management depends on the severity and extent of hyperkeratosis, which may vary over time and from patient to patient. The spectrum may range from fixed hyperkeratotic plaques over the knees and elbows to generalized hyperkeratosis with accentuated skin markings and peeling, or thickened plates with a spiny, hystrix-like appearance.

The *topical management* of erythrokeratodermas remains a therapeutic cornerstone, although it can be disappointing in some cases. Topical treatment of patients with mild, localized hyperkeratosis is symptomatic and focuses on hydration, lubrication, and keratolysis. Whereas in some patients *emollients* such as petrolatum twice daily may suffice, most patients require topical treatment with *keratolytic agents*. Lactic acid (6%–12%) and urea applied once or twice daily in combination with emollients are effective, although their use may be limited, especially in children, because of irritation. Other α-hydroxy acids, salicylic acid (3%–6%), propylene glycol, glycolic acid (11%), topical vitamin D analogs (calcipotriol), or combinations of these are alternative treatment options. Topical treatment with *retinoids* and derivatives has been successful in some patients (especially with EKV) but ineffective in others. Regimens with newer synthetic retinoids, such as short-contact topical tazarotene therapy combined with moisturizers, seem promising in EKV. In addition, avoidance of trauma to the skin, such as sudden temperature changes, friction, and mechanical irritation, may be beneficial.

Systemic retinoids are the treatment of choice in erythrokeratodermas with extensive or generalized skin involvement. Although they are highly effective in EKV, the therapeutic response in PSEK is less satisfactory. As is the case for other disorders of cornification, the effects of acitretin or etretinate are superior to those of systemic isotretinoin. It seems advantageous to start at low doses of acitretin for 3 to 6 weeks and then to gradually increase the dose until the desired therapeutic effect is achieved. The minimal effective maintenance dose for patients with EKV is usually lower than for patients with PSEK. Both morphologic components respond well to retinoid treatment, resulting in rapid and dramatic improvement or clearing of the hyperkeratosis and significant moderation of the erythema. In some patients with EKV the erythematous component may be completely suppressed. Nevertheless, the use of retinoids should always be considered carefully, as chronic therapy is required to achieve continuing results, and long-term side effects, especially in children, may ensue. In some cases, intermittent cycles of systemic retinoid treatment may be considered to balance between beneficial therapeutic and adverse effects. Anecdotally, *PUVA therapy* alone or combined with acitretin (Re-PUVA) has been beneficial in the treatment of PSEK. Few patients have been reported with clearing of skin lesions under oral treatment with low-dose vitamin A or a polyaromatic retinoid (arotinoid ethylester).

The variable erythema in EKV often results in cosmetic concerns, which can be limited by masking uncovered skin with makeup and camouflage. Serious discomfort due to burning and pruritus, which may accompany the variable erythema in some patients, can be therapeutically challenging. If systemic aromatic retinoid therapy alone fails to reduce or suppress erythema and the associated burning and itching sensations, symptomatic relief has been achieved in anecdotal cases with systemic therapy using sedating H_1-antihistamines.

Specific Investigations

- Family history
- Histopathology

Connexin disorders of the skin. Richard G. Clin Dermatol 2005; 23: 23–32.

Summary of the clinical features and molecular genetics of EKV and other connexin disorders. The review discusses the spectrum and mechanism of disease-causing missense mutations in the connexin genes *GJB3* and *GJB4*, which encode the gap junction proteins β-3 (connexin-31, Cx31) and β-4 (connexin-30.3, Cx30.3) associated with EKV. It also describes the mutation spectrum in other epidermal connexin genes, including *GJB2* (Cx26), *GJB6* (Cx30), and *GJA1* (Cx43).

The missense mutation G12D in connexin 30.3 can cause both erythrokeratodermia variabilis of Mendes da Costa and progressive symmetric erythrokeratodermia of Gottron. Van Steensel MAM, Oranje AP, van der Schroeff JG, Wagner A, van Geel M. Am J Med Genet Part A 2008; 149A: 657–61.

Mutation analysis in two patients with PSEK and three patients with EKV revealed the same G12D mutation in *GJB4* (Cx30.3). All five Dutch patients shared the same haplotype over 2 Mb across the disease locus, indicating that G12D might be a Dutch founder mutation, which may manifest with features of either EKV or PSEK. Systemic treatment of an adult male patient with features of PSEK with 20 to 40 mg etretinate during the wintertime reportedly resulted in satisfactory symptomatic relief. The name *erythrokeratodermia variabilis et progressiva* was proposed to indicate the clinical variability of this disorder.

Dominant de novo mutations in GJA1 cause erythrokeratodermia variabilis et progressiva, without features of oculodentodigital dysplasia. Boyden LM, Craiglow BG, Zhou J, Hu R, Loring EC, Morel KD, et al. J Invest Dermatol 2015; 135: 1540–7.

Three unrelated patients with features of EKVP as well as enlarged, porcelain-white lunulae were reported to have a pathogenic missense variant in the *GJA1* gene encoding connexin 43 (Cx43), the most widely expressed gap junction protein, which is coexpressed with *GJB3* and *GJB4* in human epidermis. In contrast, the vast majority of pathogenic sequence variants in *GJA1* cause the multisystem disorder oculodentodigital dysplasia (ODDD), which very rarely may include palmoplantar keratoderma.

Evidence for the absence of mutations at GJB3, GJB4 and LOR in progressive symmetric erythrokeratodermia. Wei S, Zhou Y, Zhang TD, Huang ZM, Zhang XB, Zhu HL, et al. Clin Exp Dermatol 2011; 36: 399–405.

None of 25 patients with PSEK was found to have a pathogenic mutation in the connexin genes *GJB3* (Cx31) and *GJB4* (Cx30.3) and the *loricrin* gene, suggesting that in the majority of cases PSEK is a disorder distinct from EKV and of currently unknown molecular cause.

First-Line Therapies	
• Emollients	E
• Topical keratolytics	E
• Topical retinoids	E
• Topical calcipotriol	E

Erythrokeratodermia variabilis successfully treated with topical tazarotene. Yoo S, Simzar S, Han K, Takahashi S, Cotliar R. Pediatr Dermatol 2006; 23: 382–5.

Topical short-contact (15 minutes) treatment with tazarotene (0.05% gel) once a day followed by the application of a topical corticosteroid (fluocinolone oil) on moist skin and hydrophilic ointments resulted in complete remission of hyperkeratotic plaques and erythematous patches in a 16-month-old child with EKV within 1 month. Emollients were continued during quiescent periods, and the aforementioned regimen during flares.

Tazarotene is a topical, receptor-selective retinoid.

Erythrokeratodermia variabilis. Report of 3 clinical cases and evaluation of the topical retinoic acid treatment. Lacerda E, Costa MH, de Brito Caldeira J. Med Cutan Ibero Lat Am 1975; 3: 281–7.

Topical retinoic acid (0.1% cream) treatment of three patients with EKV substantially reduced hyperkeratosis. Discontinuation resulted in prompt relapse.

Progressive symmetrische erythrokeratodermie Darier-Gottron. Ott H, Lehmann S, Poblete-Guitierrez P, Frank J. Hautarzt 2004; 10: 994–6.

A 5-year-old boy with PSEK and severe palmoplantar keratoderma leading to flexural contractures on both hands was treated with topical steroids of various strength and urea without lasting improvement. Topical tretinoin 0.03% cream combined with hydrophilic ointments as well as physical therapy resulted in significant and lasting skin improvement and regression of contractures after a few weeks.

Erythrokeratodermia variabilis. Case report and review of the literature. Knipe RC, Flowers FP, Johnson FR Jr, DeBusk FL, Ramos-Caro FA. Pediatr Dermatol 1995; 12: 21–3.

Topical treatment with 0.025% triamcinolone cream and retinoic acid 0.05% cream, each for 4 to 6 weeks, was ineffective in a 5-month-old boy with EKV.

Progressive symmetric erythrokeratoderma: report of an Indian family. Gupta LK, Saini P, Khare AK, Mittal A. Int J Dermatol 2014; 53: e317–9.

The proband of a multigenerational family with a clinical diagnosis of PSEK showed no appreciable improvement when treated with topical emollients, urea, and salicylic acid ointment, nor with acitretin 25 mg/d for 3 months.

Progressive symmetric erythrokeratoderma – response to topical calcipotriol. Bilgin I, Bozdağ KE, Uysal S, Ermete M. J Dermatol Case Rep. 2011; 5: 50–2.

A female with symmetrically distributed, reddish-brown, hyperkeratotic plaques in flexural regions and palmoplantar keratoderma was diagnosed with PSEK and treated with 0.5 mg/kg/day isotretinoin for 2 months without improvement. Topical calcipotriol ointment applied twice daily yielded marked improvement of hyperkeratosis within 2 weeks.

Second-Line Therapies	
• Acitretin	C
• Isotretinoin	E

Clinical and genetic heterogeneity of erythrokeratodermia variabilis. Common JEA, O'Toole EA, Leigh IM, Thomas A, Griffiths WAD, Venning V, et al. J Invest Dermatol 2005; 125: 920–7.

Four of six EKV patients had a reportedly good to excellent response to oral acitretin when treated with 0.125 to 0.25 mg/kg/day. Two of these patients cleared completely, one on 20 mg acitretin daily. The remaining patients had residual hyperkeratosis, especially on the legs.

Erythrokeratodermia variabilis caused by a recessive mutation in GJB3. Fuchs-Telem D, Pessach Y, Mevorah B, Shirazi I, Sarig O, Sprecher E. Clin Exp Dermatol 2011; 36: 406–11.

Evidence Levels: **A** Double-blind study **B** Clinical trial ≥ 20 subjects **C** Clinical trial < 20 subjects **D** Series ≥ 5 subjects **E** Anecdotal case reports

Third report of a consanguineous family with EKV due to an autosomal-recessive mutation in *GJB3* (Cx31). A 14-year-old boy with EKV showed dramatic improvement followed by complete resolution of hyperkeratosis with low-dose treatment (25 mg four times a week) with acitretin. The migratory erythematous patches, however, remained.

Erythrokeratodermia variabilis. Hunzeker CM, Soldano AC, Levis WR. Dermatol Online J 2008; 14: 13.

A 51-year-old woman with EKV was treated with acitretin 25 mg/day. After 4 months, near complete clearance of hyperkeratotic plaques and erythematous patches was achieved except for hyperpigmentation, and no appreciable side effects were observed.

Erythrokeratoderma variabilis responding to low-dose isotretinoin. Singh N. Pediatr Dermatol 2010; 27: 111–3.

Low-dose treatment with oral isotretinoin at a dose of 0.5 mg/kg body weight per day along with topical emollients yielded remarkable improvement of hyperkeratotic plaques and erythema in a 2-year-old boy with EKV. No significant side effects were observed during continued treatment over the next 6 months. The author concludes that low-dose therapy with isotretinoin is better tolerated, has fewer side effects, and is cheaper compared with high-dose therapy.

Both low-dose arotinoid ethylester and acitretin are effective in the treatment of familial erythrokeratodermia variabilis. Zhang L, Hong Y, Zheng S, Huo W, Qi R, Geng L, et al. Dermatol Ther 2014; 27: 240–3.

Two siblings clinically diagnosed with EKV reached clearing of skin lesions within 2 weeks/2 months with systemic therapy with either 0.03 mg/day arotinoid ethylester or 30 mg acitretin/day, respectively, and remained symptom free with reduced dosage for up to 6 to 12 months. Upon cessation of systemic treatment, relapse occurred after 3 or 6 months, respectively.

Erythrokeratodermia variabilis with adult onset: report of a sporadic case unresponsive to systemic retinoids. Erbagci Z, Tuncel AA, Deniz H. J Dermatol Treat 2006; 17: 187–9.

An unusual case with onset of fixed erythrokeratoderma at 23 years of age. Topical steroids, topical PUVA for 3 months, and keratolytics (10% salicylic acid) did not yield satisfactory results. Subsequent systemic isotretinoin (0.7 mg/kg/day) combined with topical ointments containing 20% urea did not show improvement after 3 months. Acitretin (0.5 mg/kg/day) for 5 months also did not achieve a significant therapeutic response. However, sedating oral H_1-antihistamines were beneficial for relief of pruritus.

Third-Line Therapies	
• PUVA	E
• H_1-antihistamines	E

Erythrokeratodermia variabilis: successful treatment with retinoid plus psoralen and ultraviolet A therapy. Yüksek J, Sezer E, Köseoglu D, Marcoç F, Yildiz H. Jpn Dermatol Assoc J 2010; 725–7.

A female with EKV was first treated with 10 mg/day acitretin. After 1 week, PUVA therapy was added with 0.5 J/cm^2 UVA twice weekly, with incremental increases by 0.5 J/cm^2 UVA up to a cumulative dose of 129 J/cm^2. A significant improvement of hyperkeratosis and erythema was achieved after 3 months; then PUVA was stopped, and acitretin was continued for up to 9 months. Dry lips were the only side effects observed. Follow-up after discontinued Re-PUVA was not reported.

Gottron's erythroderma congenitalis progressiva symmetrica. Levi L, Beneggi M, Crippa D, Sala GP. Hautarzt 1982; 33: 605–8.

In one family with PSEK an adult patient was treated with an aromatic retinoid for 8 weeks, whereas her child received PUVA therapy for a total of 63 J/cm^2 UVA. Both treatments were effective and reduced hyperkeratosis, but PUVA achieved superior results.

Erythrokeratodermia variabilis: case report and review of literature. Papadavid E, Koumantaki E, Dawber RPR. J Eur Acad Dermatol Venereol 1998; 11: 180–3.

A good therapeutic response to systemic etretinate with an initial dosage of 25 mg/day and a maintenance dosage of 10 mg/day. Regular use of an oral H_1-antihistamine was helpful in controlling the pruritus associated with the erythematous component of EKV.

Erythromelalgia

Cato Mørk, Knut Kvernebo

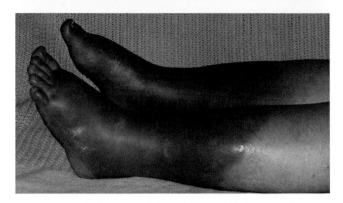

Erythromelalgia (*erythros* – redness; *melos* – extremity; *algos* – pain) is an uncommon neurovascular disorder characterized by redness, increased skin temperature, and pain that usually occurs in the extremities. Pain is aggravated by warming and relieved by cooling. Symptoms and findings are usually intermittent and often missing during examination. Between attacks acrocyanosis, perniosis, and Raynaud phenomenon may occur. Severity of symptoms varies from mild discomfort (most common) to disabling pain and gangrene. The diagnosis is often missed in cases with mild symptoms, whereas severe erythromelalgia is a rare condition.

Erythromelalgia can be a primary condition, or secondary to a primary microvascular event, or due to a primary autonomic nervous dysfunction. Regardless of etiology, the final common pathway of the pathogenesis includes maldistribution of skin perfusion with increased deep plexus thermoregulatory perfusion and a relative lack of papillary nutritive perfusion with a corresponding degree of skin hypoxia.

Some erythromelalgia patients have a family history with genetic variants within the *SCN9A* gene encoding for the $Na_v1.7$, a voltage-gated sodium channel located on nerve endings. These mutations substantially alter an individual's perception of pain secondary to detection and transmission of noxious stimuli by the peripheral nervous system. The genetic variants within this gene can also cause other diseases.

MANAGEMENT STRATEGY

Before beginning a treatment regimen, the patient's condition should be classified according to whether it is primary or secondary, the etiology (for secondary cases), and its severity. Erythromelalgia may be secondary to underlying diseases, such as myeloproliferative, connective tissue, cardiovascular, infectious, and neurologic diseases, diabetes mellitus, vasculitis, and neoplasia. If present, a primary condition should be optimally treated. There are many reports of remission after treatment of myeloproliferative disorders. Drug-induced erythromelalgia has been reported secondary to substances that may alter vasomotor tone, such as calcium channel blockers, bromocriptine, norepinephrine (noradrenaline), pergolide, ticlopidine, ciclosporin, iodine contrast, and mushroom and mercury poisoning.

All patients benefit from local *skin cooling* (applying cold towels or wet sand, walking on cold floors or even in the snow, air-conditioned rooms, or immersion in cooled water) and from elevation of the affected limb. Aggressive cooling may cause injury and worsen the erythromelalgia. Comfortable shoes to relieve pressure over the soles can help. Aggravating factors such as warmth, exercise, dependency of the extremity, tight shoes and gloves, and alcohol intake in some cases should be avoided.

No single medication or other treatment modality has been found to be universally helpful. Spontaneous remissions have occurred without treatment. There is a marked variation in therapeutic responses. Few controlled clinical trials have been published. The main reason may be the low prevalence, the heterogeneity of patients, and the lack of laboratory diagnostic methods.

Analgesics, including opiate analgesics, often have limited effect. Numerous drugs have been used with varying success. A few patients become free of symptoms with *acetylsalicylic acid*. Case reports or series of patients have shown beneficial effect with *vasodilators* (prostaglandin E_1/prostacyclin or analogs, sodium nitroprusside, naftidrofuryl, calcium channel blockers). Other drugs that may be of benefit are *sodium channel blockers*, *antidepressants*, and *anticonvulsants*.

Numerous treatment alternatives based on case reports have been presented in the literature, such as topical *amitriptyline/ketamine, lidocaine, capsaicin, midodrine*, and *nitroglycerin*. Anecdotally, *ketanserin, methysergide, pizotifen, β-blockers, cyproheptadine* or other *antihistamines, carbamazepine, clonazepam, corticosteroids* or other *immunosuppressants, pentoxifylline, phenoxybenzamine, opiates, prazosin*, and *pregabalin* have been presented as effective. *Hyperbaric oxygen* treatment, *spinal cord stimulation, thalamic stimulation*, and *epidural blocks* have also been proposed. *Sympathectomy* has been beneficial in some patients and in other patients caused worsening of symptoms. Treatment modalities such as *hypnosis, biofeedback*, and learning to avoid triggers can be beneficial for coping with pain. A survey of members of The Erythromelalgia Association (TEA, www.erythromelalgia.org) shows that more than 50 therapeutic regimens have been tried out. TEA is a nonprofit organization that may be helpful in providing information, awareness, and support.

Specific Investigations

- Full blood count with white cell differential count
- Serum chemistry, including blood sugar
- Antinuclear antibody and relevant rheumatologic tests
- Skin biopsy may be considered

Nonspecific capillary proliferation and vasculopathy indicate skin hypoxia in erythromelalgia. Kalgaard OM, Clausen OP, Mellbye OJ, Hovig T, Kvernebo K. Arch Dermatol 2011; 147: 309–14.

Platelet-mediated erythromelalgic, cerebral, ocular and coronary microvascular ischemic and thrombotic manifestations in patients with essential thrombocythemia and polycythemia vera: a distinct aspirin-responsive and Coumadin-resistant arterial thrombophilia. Michiels JJ, Berneman Z, Schroyens W, Koudstaal PJ, Lindemans J, Neumann HA, et al. Platelets 2006; 17: 528–44.

Erythromelalgia—a thrombotic complication in chronic myeloproliferative disorders. Tarach JS, Nowicka-Tarach BM, Matuszek B, Nowakowski A. Med Sci Monit 2000; 6: 204–8.

Evidence Levels: **A** Double-blind study **B** Clinical trial ≥ 20 subjects **C** Clinical trial < 20 subjects **D** Series ≥ 5 subjects **E** Anecdotal case reports

Erythromelalgia is seen secondary to platelet aggregation and peripheral microvascular occlusion in myeloproliferative disorders and, untreated, may progress to painful acrocyanosis and even peripheral gangrene. Remission is observed after treatment of the myeloproliferative disorder.

First-Line Therapies	
• Treatment of underlying disease	C
• Aspirin	D
• Prostaglandins/prostacyclin or oral analogs	A

Treatment of secondary erythromelalgia addresses treatment of the accompanying diseases, conditions, and elimination of pharmacologic substances. A beneficial effect on the symptoms of erythromelalgia after successful treatment or elimination of the primary condition indicates a causal relationship.

Aspirin-responsive, migraine-like transient cerebral and ocular ischemic attacks and erythromelalgia in JAK2-positive essential thrombocythemia and polycythemia vera. Michiels JJ, Berneman Z, Gadisseur A, Lam KH, De Raeve H, Schroyens W. Acta Hematol 2015; 133:56–63.

Aspirin 250 to 500 mg daily or less may completely abolish the symptoms in erythromelalgia secondary to myeloproliferative conditions. The response is probably due to the antiplatelet effect. A reduction of platelet numbers by cytostatic treatment may also lead to relief.

The Erythromelalgia Association Survey 2003. www.erythromelalgia.org.

In a survey, 128 respondents had used aspirin (80–250 mg daily): 4 reported complete, 17 moderate, and 22 minimal relief; 78 had no improvement; and 6 reported worsening of their symptoms.

Aspirin should be tried in all patients with erythromelalgia without contraindications to its use.

Erythromelalgia—a condition caused by microvascular arteriovenous shunting. Kvernebo K. Vasa 1998; 27: 3–39.

Based on the hypothesis of arteriovenous shunting, prostaglandin E_1 (PGE_1) and prostacyclin were tried as an intravenous infusion to enhance nutritive skin perfusion in severe erythromelalgia. In 9 of 10 patients, PGE_1 given as a continuous infusion for 3 days, starting with 6 ng/kg/min, then 10 ng/kg/min, and finally 12 ng/kg/min, induced remission from 3 months to 2 years. Two children were cured (observation time after treatment >25 years).

Prostacyclin reduces symptoms and sympathetic dysfunction in erythromelalgia in a double-blind randomized pilot study. Kalgaard OM, Mørk C, Kvernebo K. Acta Derm Venereol 2003; 83: 442–4.

Significant reduction in symptoms and sympathetic dysfunction were demonstrated in eight patients treated with prostacyclin infusion compared with four patients with placebo infusion.

The prostaglandin E1 analog misoprostol reduces symptoms and microvascular arteriovenous shunting in erythromelalgia—a double-blind, crossover, placebo-compared study. Mørk C, Salerud EG, Asker CL, Kvernebo K. J Invest Dermatol 2004; 122: 587–93.

Oral misoprostol (0.4–0.8 mg/day) reduced symptoms significantly more than placebo. Misoprostol is recommended as a first-line treatment, although many patients do not respond.

Second-Line Therapies	
• Sodium channel blockers (lidocaine, mexiletine, bupivacaine, XEN402)	C, D
• Gabapentin	D
• Antidepressants (venlafaxine, sertraline)	D
• Sodium nitroprusside	D

Treatment of Na$_v$1.7-mediated pain in inherited erythromelalgia using novel sodium channel blocker. Goldberg YP, Price N, Namdari R, Cohen CJ, Lamers MH, Winters C, et al. Pain. 2012; 153: 80–5.

An exploratory, randomized, double-blind, two-period, crossover pilot study was conducted in four *SCN9A* mutation-proven inherited erythromelalgia patients using the orally administered Na$_v$1.7 antagonist XEN402 400 mg twice daily or placebo for 2 days, separated by a 2-day washout period. Alleviation of erythromelalgia-associated pain was demonstrated. The result is interesting, but XEN402 is not commercially available.

Mexiletine as a treatment for primary erythromelalgia: normalization of biophysical properties of mutant L858F NaV 1.7 sodium channels. Gregg R, Cox JJ, Bennett DL, Wood JN, Werdehausen R. Br J Pharmacol 2014; 171: 2255–63.

Mexiletine has a normalizing effect on the pathologic gating properties of the L858F gain-of-function mutation in NaV 1.7.

Lidocaine patch for pain of erythromelalgia: follow-up of 34 patients. Davis MD, Sandroni P. Arch Dermatol 2005; 141: 1320–1.

Anesthetic agents (lidocaine, bupivacaine, mexiletine) that block the sodium channels may be used topically, intravenously, orally, epidurally, or intrathecally. A 90% reduction in pain was demonstrated with lidocaine IV infusion, but hospitalization is required. A 5% lidocaine patch for 12 hours/day was found helpful as first-line and adjunctive treatment of severely affected patients with erythromelalgia. Sixteen patients had no improvement, but 18 patients had a 5% to 90% improvement in pain score.

Pediatric erythromelalgia: a retrospective review of 32 cases evaluated at Mayo Clinic over a 37-year period. Cook-Norris RH, Tollefson MM, Cruz-Inigo AD, Sandroni P, Davis MDP, Davis DMR. J Am Acad Dermatol 2012; 66: 416–23.

Earlier treatment with gabapentin (2/6) and antidepressants (4/10) was reported very or somewhat helpful.

Treatment of familial erythromelalgia with venlafaxine. Firmin D, Roduedas AM, Greco M, Morvan C, Legoupil D, Fleuret C, et al. J Eur Acad Dermatol Venereol 2007; 21: 836–7.

Venlafaxine helped the mother. She had two sons with erythromelalgia—the drug did not help one son, and the other son discontinued the medication after 1 week because of a stomachache and vertigo.

Erythromelalgia—a condition caused by microvascular arteriovenous shunting. Kvernebo K. Vasa 1998; 27: 3–39.

Sodium nitroprusside intravenously for 7 days in increasing doses (1, 3, and 5 µg/kg/min) was successful in two patients with severe acute-onset erythromelalgia. The effect was accompanied by normalization of skin perfusion and transcutaneous oximetry.

Third-Line Therapies

Other therapies

- Oral: calcium channel blockers, magnesium, pregabalin,
- Topical: amitriptyline/ketamine, midodrine, capsaicin   **C**

Erythromelalgia: new theories and new therapies. Cohen JS. J Am Acad Dermatol 2000; 43: 841–7.

Various calcium channel blockers may be helpful in about 25% of patients with erythromelalgia (*n* = 43). As they can cause or exacerbate symptoms, they should be used with caution and with the use of short-acting drugs initially.

They are frequently used, but documentation for beneficial effect is sparse (6 of 14 patients). Their mechanism of action may be smooth muscle relaxation and reduced vascular responses elicited by β_2-adrenoceptors.

High-dose oral magnesium treatment of chronic, intractable erythromelalgia. Cohen JS. Ann Pharmacother 2002; 36: 255–60.

Magnesium is a naturally occurring calcium channel blocker. Eight of 13 patients reported improvement, 4 no response, and 1 deterioration using magnesium in various doses (up to 1000 mg/day) and forms.

Erythromelalgia. Davis MD, Rooke T. Curr Treat Options Cardiovasc Med 2006; 8: 153–65.

A review paper.

Response of primary erythromelalgia to pregabalin therapy. Kalava K, Roberts C, Adair JD, Raman V. J Clin Rheumatol 2013; 19: 284–5.

Using pregabalin at a dose of 100 mg three times a day, improvement was noted within 6 weeks in a 14-year-old girl.

Topical amitriptyline combined with ketamine for the treatment of erythromelalgia: a retrospective study of 36 patients at Mayo Clinic. Potrucha TJ, Weiss WT, Warndahl RA, Rho RH, Sandroni P, Davis MD, et al. J Drugs Dermatol 2013; 12: 308–10.

The authors reported 75% improvement in pain with topical application of a compounded amitriptyline–ketamine formulation. The medication was well tolerated.

Topically applied midodrine, 0.2%, an α1-agonist, for the treatment of erythromelalgia. Davies MD, Morr CS, Warndahl RA, Sandroni P. JAMA Dermatol 2015; 151: 1025–6.

Eleven of 12 improved, with only 2 of 12 having adverse reactions (one gastrointestinal discomfort, and the other displaying an increase in blood pressure).

The use of capsaicin cream in a case of erythromelalgia. Muhiddin KA, Gallen IW, Harries S, Pearce VR. Postgrad Med J 1994; 70: 841–3.

A 68-year-old woman with erythromelalgia responded to a twice-daily application of capsaicin cream 0.025% within 48 hours.

Evidence Levels: **A** Double-blind study   **B** Clinical trial ≥ 20 subjects   **C** Clinical trial < 20 subjects   **D** Series ≥ 5 subjects   **E** Anecdotal case reports

Erythropoietic protoporphyria

Maureen B. Poh-Fitzpatrick

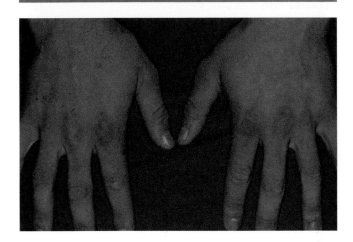

In this metabolic disorder, a genetically determined deficiency of ferrochelatase enzyme activity in bone marrow erythroid cells causes abnormally high protoporphyrin levels in erythrocytes, plasma, liver, bile, and feces. Protoporphyrin is a photoactive intermediary of heme synthesis. In the skin, its exposure to long-wave ultraviolet (UV) or visible light radiation can elicit oxygen-dependent acute cutaneous phototoxicity. Protoporphyrin undergoes hepatobiliary excretion, facilitating cholelithiasis. Protoporphyrin hepatotoxicity may develop and progress to irreversible liver failure. Hypochromic microcytic anemia, when present, is typically mild and rarely requires treatment. A rare phenotypically similar disorder (X-linked dominant protoporphyria), arising from gain-of-function mutations in the erythroid-specific 5-aminolevulinic acid synthase gene, has a larger ratio of excess erythrocyte zinc-protoporphyrin to metal-free protoporphyrin than does erythropoietic protoporphyria. It is amenable to the same therapies.

MANAGEMENT STRATEGY

Protoporphyric photosensitivity typically requires *sun avoidance* (lifestyle changes, protective clothing, physical barriers), which may lead to vitamin D deficiency. *Topical sunscreens* containing *titanium dioxide, zinc oxide, iron oxide,* or *dihydroxyacetone* block or filter long-wave UV and visible-light spectra, but offer limited relief. Epidermal melanization and hyperplasia achieved with *ultraviolet B (UVB)* or *psoralen plus ultraviolet A (PUVA) phototherapy,* or an *α-melanocyte–stimulating hormone analog (afamelanotide),* can increase sunlight tolerance. Oral agents believed to photoprotect by quenching excited oxygen species include *β-carotene, cysteine, vitamin E, vitamin C, flavonoids,* and possibly *pyridoxine. Antihistamines* may attenuate phototoxic flaring. Gallstones are managed *surgically.* Exacerbators of protoporphyrin-induced hepatotoxicity (alcohol, cholestatic drugs, dietary carbohydrate restriction) are best avoided. *Vaccination* against hepatitis A and B is recommended. Deteriorating liver function

is only sporadically reversible by *enteric sorbents (cholestyramine, activated charcoal)* that interrupt enterohepatic porphyrin circulation, *bile acids* (to stimulate biliary protoporphyrin secretion), *blood transfusion or exchange, hematin infusion, glucose loading* (to retard endogenous porphyrinogenesis), *iron* (to increase protoporphyrin conversion to heme), or various combinations thereof. *Cimetidine* is postulated to inhibit porphyrinogenesis. End-stage liver disease warrants *liver transplantation,* aided by measures to reduce preoperative, intraoperative, and postoperative porphyrin levels *(exchange transfusion, hematin infusion, plasmapheresis, vitamin E).* Operating room lamps should be filtered to exclude wavelengths damaging to porphyrin-photosensitized skin and internal organs. *Hematopoietic cell transplantation* has been curative in highly selected cases and is optimal prevention for protoporphyric hepatopathy in native or transplanted livers.

Specific Investigations

- Porphyrin analyses in erythrocytes (including metal-free: zinc protoporphyrin ratio), serum or plasma, urine, feces
- Hematologic profile, iron studies if anemic
- Liver function profile, liver imaging, liver biopsy as clinically indicated
- Mutation analysis (for diagnostic confirmation and family counseling)
- Vitamin D assessment, bone density scan

Liver failure occurs in <5% of all cases. Because urine is typically free of excess porphyrins in uncomplicated protoporphyria, surveillance for coproporphyrinuria may identify patients with asymptomatic hepatic dysfunction.

Erythropoietic protoporphyria. Lecha M, Puy H, Deybach JC. Orphanet J Rare Dis 2009; 4: 19.

A comprehensive review of protoporphyria.

First-Line Therapies

• Topical sunscreens, physical barriers	C
• β-Carotene	B
• Afamelanotide	A
• Vitamin D and calcium	D

Efficiency of opaque photoprotective agents in the visible light range. Kaye ET, Levin JA, Blank IH, Arndt KA, Anderson RR. Arch Dermatol 1991; 127: 351–5.

Efficacy and cosmetic quality of sunscreens containing zinc oxide, titanium dioxide, and iron oxide.

Erythropoietic protoporphyria: IV. Protection from sunlight. Fusaro RM, Runge WJ. Br Med J 1970; 1: 730–1.

Seven patients had prolonged sunlight tolerance after applying a 3% dihydroxyacetone and 0.13% lawsone skin cream causing brown coloration of the stratum corneum.

Beta-carotene therapy for erythropoietic protoporphyria and other photosensitivity diseases. Mathews-Roth MM, Pathak MA, Fitzpatrick TB, Harber LH, Kass EH. Arch Dermatol 1977; 113: 1229–32.

Of 133 patients with protoporphyria, 84% had a threefold increase in sunlight tolerance after ingesting pharmaceutical-grade β-carotene now available without prescription (Lumitene,

Tischcon). Doses producing serum levels of ~800 µg/dL (children: 30–120 mg/day, adults: 120–300 mg/day, in two to three doses with meals) should be started 4 to 6 weeks before seasonal symptoms are anticipated. Efficacy varies and is often nil. Contraindicated in smokers due to increased lung cancer among heavy smokers treated with β-carotene in cancer prevention trials.

Long-term observational study of afamelanotide in 115 patients with erythropoietic protoporphyria. Biolcati G, Marchesini E, Sorge F, Barbieri L, Schneider-Yin X, Minder EI. Br J Dermatol 2015; 172: 1601–12.

Afamelanotide for erythropoietic protoporphyria. Langendonk JG, Balwani M, Anderson KE, Bonkovsky HL, Anstey AV, Bissell DM, et al. N Engl J Med 2015; 373: 48–59.

Afamelanotide increases skin melanization and may have other beneficial effects. Clinical trials of a subcutaneously implantable form have involved ~300 protoporphyria patients worldwide. It is available by prescription in Europe and pending Food and Drug Administration (FDA) approval in the United States.

Bone mineral density and vitamin D levels in erythropoietic protoporphyria. Allo G, del Carmen Garrido-Astray M, Méndez M, De Salamanca RE, Martínez G, Hawkins F. Endocrine 2013; 44: 803–7.

Nine of 10 protoporphyria patients had low vitamin D levels, and 8 had low bone mineral density. Monitoring of serum vitamin D levels and supplementation with vitamin D and calcium are recommended.

Second-Line Therapies	
• Phototherapy (UVB, PUVA)	D

Narrow-band (TL-01) UVB phototherapy: an effective preventative treatment for the photodermatoses. Collins P, Ferguson J. Br J Dermatol 1995; 132: 956–63.

Six patients with protoporphyria had increased sunlight tolerance after serial narrowband UVB treatments.

Photo(chemo)therapy and general management of erythropoietic protoporphyria. Roelandts R. Dermatology 1995; 190: 330–1.

PUVA can increase sun tolerance; other treatments are reviewed.

Third-Line Therapies	
• Cysteine	A
• Antihistamines	D
• Vitamin E	D
• Vitamin C	A
• Pyridoxine	E
• Flavonoids	E
• Iron	D
• Cholestyramine, activated charcoal	D
• Blood transfusion or exchange	D
• Hematin infusion	D
• Plasmapheresis	D
• Bile acids	D
• Liver transplantation	B
• Hematopoietic cell transplantation	D

Long-term treatment of erythropoietic protoporphyria with cysteine. Mathews-Roth MM, Rosner B. Photodermatol Photoimmunol Photomed 2002; 18: 307–9.

Forty-seven patients received placebo for 1 month, then cysteine 500 mg twice daily in this phase III 3-year trial. Patient history forms and light exposure diaries were kept; some patients were phototested. Cysteine significantly increased light tolerance subjectively and objectively.

Inhibition of photosensitivity in erythropoietic protoporphyria with terfenadine. Farr PM, Diffey BL, Matthews JNS. Br J Dermatol 1990; 122: 809–15.

Terfenadine 60 to 120 mg twice daily for 48 days significantly reduced the flare surrounding, but not the erythema within, blue light phototest sites on seven subjects, compared with pretreatment reactions.

Antihistamines have not provided much relief in clinical practice.

Cimetidine reduces erythrocyte protoporphyrin in erythropoietic protoporphyria. Yamamoto S, Hirano Y, Horie Y. Am J Gastroenterol 1993; 88: 1465–6.

This H_2 receptor antagonist (800 mg four times daily orally) was given to a patient with protoporphyric liver disease. Erythrocyte protoporphyrin fell from 16,000 µg/dL to 11,000 µg/dL during treatment. Inhibition of heme synthesis by cimetidine was postulated.

Only three porphyrin measurements were obtained: before and immediately after 2 weeks of cimetidine and 2 weeks after discontinuation.

Novel Treatment Using Cimetidine for Erythropoietic Protoporphyria in Children. Briefly reported improved photosensitivity, erythrocyte protoporphyrins and hepatic transaminases after cimetidine treatment of 3 children calls for confirmatory studies. (Tu JH, Sheu SL, Teng JM. JAMA Dermatol 2016; 152: 1258–61).

A case of erythropoietic protoporphyria with liver cirrhosis suggesting a therapeutic value of supplementation with alpha-tocopherol. Komatsu H, Ishii K, Imamura K, Maruyama K, Yonei Y, Masuda H, et al. Hepatol Res 2000; 18: 298–309.

A patient with severe protoporphyric hepatopathy received intravenous vitamin E 500 IU/day. Erythrocyte protoporphyrin decreased significantly, and liver function improved. Sixteen weeks later, full clinical and biochemical recovery was noted.

Vitamin E has been used sporadically in protoporphyria, usually as adjunctive therapy.

A double-blind, placebo-controlled, crossover trial of oral vitamin C in erythropoietic protoporphyria. Boffa MJ, Ead RD, Reed P, Weinkove C. Photodermatol Photoimmunol Photomed 1996; 12: 27–30.

Vitamin C 1 g/day orally for 4 weeks was subjectively assessed by 9 of 12 patients to be associated with less photosensitivity than placebo, but the data did not reach significance.

Antioxidants such as vitamins C and E are postulated to quench porphyrin-generated oxyradicals in vivo.

Relief of the photosensitivity of erythropoietic protoporphyria by pyridoxine. Ross JB, Moss MA. J Am Acad Dermatol 1990; 22: 340–2.

Two patients given oral pyridoxine dosages varying from 100 mg to 1 g/day reported increased sunlight tolerance.

Treatment of erythropoietic protoporphyria with hydroxyethylrutosides. Schoemaker JH, Bousema MT, Zijlstra H, van der Horst FA. Dermatology 1995; 191: 36–8.

Evidence Levels: **A** Double-blind study **B** Clinical trial ≥ 20 subjects **C** Clinical trial < 20 subjects **D** Series ≥ 5 subjects **E** Anecdotal case reports

A flavonoid mixture was ingested by a patient for 3 months, during which time phototesting and subjective assessment indicated reduced photosensitivity.

Iron therapy for hepatic dysfunction in erythropoietic protoporphyria. Gordeuk VR, Brittenham GM, Hawkins CW, Mukhtar H, Bickers DR. Ann Intern Med 1986; 105: 27–31.

Carbonyl iron 400 to 4000 mg/day orally was given for 15 weeks to a patient with protoporphyria, iron-deficiency anemia, and liver dysfunction. Erythrocyte porphyrin fell, photosensitivity improved, and liver function normalized.

In the same case, oral ferrous sulfate 300 mg/day was given when liver function and porphyrin levels worsened again. Liver function again normalized and remained stable for several years.

Symptomatic response of erythropoietic protoporphyria to iron supplementation. Holme SA, Thomas CL, Whatley SD, Bentley AV, Badminton MN. J Am Acad Dermatol 2007; 56: 1070–2.

A patient reported greater sunlight tolerance while taking oral ferrous sulfate 200 mg twice daily.

Erythropoietic protoporphyria and iron therapy. McClements BM, Bingham A, Callendar ME, Trimble ER. Br J Dermatol 1990; 122: 423–4.

Oral ferrous fumarate 580 mg/day was followed by florid photosensitivity in a patient previously tolerant of iron supplements. Abnormal liver enzymes improved and erythrocyte protoporphyrin diminished after iron discontinuation.

In ferrochelatase-deficient protoporphyria patients, ALAS2 expression is enhanced and erythrocytic protoporphyrin concentration correlates with iron availability. Barman-Aksözen J, Minder EI, Schubiger C, Biolcati G, Schneider-Yin X. Blood Cells Mol Dis 2015; 54: 71–7.

It is been postulated that mild iron deficiency may limit protoporphyrin excess in erythropoietic protoporphyria and that iron should be repleted only when symptoms of iron deficiency are incapacitating.

Iron supplementation in protoporphyria is contentious, as patients have been both better and worse after iron. Fortunately, the mild iron-deficiency anemia is usually asymptomatic.

Fecal protoporphyrin excretion in erythropoietic protoporphyria: effect of cholestyramine and bile acid feeding. McCullough AJ, Barron D, Mullen KD, Petrelli M, Mukhtar H, Bickers DR. Gastroenterology 1988; 94: 177–81.

Ingesting cholestyramine 12 g daily, but not bile acids 300 to 900 mg, increased fecal protoporphyrin excretion threefold in one patient with hepatic dysfunction. Liver function and photosensitivity improved after 1 year of cholestyramine.

Bile acid ingestion has been reported to be associated with improved liver function and erythrocyte porphyrin levels in another patient who eventually succumbed to liver failure. Efficacy remains uncertain, but bile acids in conjunction with an enteric sorbent in selected cases are rational therapy.

Liver failure in protoporphyria: long-term treatment with oral charcoal. Gorchein A, Foster GR. Hepatology 1999; 29: 995–6.

A patient with deteriorating hepatic function given activated charcoal 10 to 12.5 g orally four times a day for 2 years exhibited improved liver function, and blood porphyrin and photosensitivity diminished. Other treatments included blood transfusions, vitamin supplements, amiloride, ranitidine, and lactulose, so it is difficult to assess their relative merits.

Liver disease in erythropoietic protoporphyria: insights and implications for management. Anstey AV, Hift RJ. Gut 2007; 56: 1009–18.

A detailed review of the pathogenesis of protoporphryic hepatopathy and recommendations for its monitoring and treatment.

Liver transplantation for erythropoietic protoporphyria liver disease. Mcguire BM, Bonkovsky HL, Carithers RL, Chung RT, Goldstein LI, Lake JR, et al. Liver Transpl 2005; 11: 1590–6.

Experience with 20 patients receiving liver transplants in the United States from 1999 to 2004 is reviewed, including preoperative use of hematin, with or without plasmapheresis.

Liver transplantation for erythropoietic protoporphyria in Europe. Wahlin S, Stal P, Adam R, Karam V, Porte R, Seehofer D, et al. Liver Transpl 2011; 17: 1021–6.

A comparable European review of 35 liver transplants performed from 1983 to 2008. Hematopoietic stem cell transplantation was performed for three patients to prevent graft loss due to disease recurrence. Offering curative stem cell transplantation to patients at high risk for liver failure to forestall transplantation is suggested.

Perioperative measures during liver transplantation for erythropoietic protoporphyria. Meerman L, Verwer R, Sloof MJH, van Hattum J, Beukeveld GJ, Kleibeuker JH, et al. Transplantation 1994; 57: 155–8.

Protocols for exchange transfusion and shielding of operating room lamps.

The value of intravenous heme-albumin and plasmapheresis in reducing postoperative complications of orthotopic liver transplantation for erythropoietic protoporphyria. Reichheld JH, Katz E, Banner BF, Szymanski IO, Saltzman JR, Bonkovsky HL. Transplantation 1999; 67: 922–8.

Three months of heme infusions (4 g daily to weekly), a high-carbohydrate diet (300 mg/day), intravenous glucose, ursodeoxycholic acid (900 mg/day orally), and cholestyramine (10 g thrice daily orally) initially improved severe liver dysfunction in a patient who then deteriorated and required urgent transplantation. Intensive heme infusions (daily for 18 days), plasmapheresis (exchanges of 1–1.5 × total plasma volume performed 12 times over 19 days), and blood transfusions (14 units packed cells over 19 days) reduced blood porphyrins before successful transplantation was performed in an illumination-filtered environment to exclude 300- to 480-nm wavelengths.

A barrage of medical therapy is typical in protoporphyric crises, when it is rational to consider any treatments that might reverse deterioration or contribute to successful transplantation. Subsequently, recurrent liver dysfunction was again successfully managed with heme-albumin and plasmapheresis (Do KD, Banner BF, Katz E, Szymanski IO, Bonkovsky HL. Transplantation 2002; 73: 469–7).

Treatment of recurrent allograft dysfunction with intravenous hematin after liver transplantation for erythropoietic protoporphyria. Dellon ES, Szczepiorkowski ZM, Dzik WH, Graeme-Cook F, Ades A, Bloomer JR, et al. Transplantation 2002; 73: 911–5.

Hematin given intermittently for 2 years after protoporphyric hepatopathy recurred 700 days after transplantation was well tolerated and aided the achievement and maintenance of disease remission in the allograft.

Erythropoietic protoporphyria: altered phenotype after bone marrow transplantation for myelogenous leukemia in a patient heteroallelic for ferrochelatase gene mutations. Poh-Fitzpatrick MB, Wang X, Anderson K, Bloomer JR, Bolwell B, Lichten AE. J Am Acad Dermatol 2002; 46: 861–6.

A symptomatic woman harboring two ferrochelatase gene mutations developed leukemia. Bone marrow transplantation from a mildly affected sibling with only one mutation and minimally elevated blood porphyrin resulted in marked reduction of the recipient's protoporphyrin levels and cutaneous photosensitivity, as well as leukemia remission.

Sequential liver and bone marrow transplantation for treatment of erythropoietic protoporphyria. Rand ER, Bunin ER, Cochran W, Ruchelli E, Olthoff KM, Bloomer JR. Pediatrics 2006; 118: e1896–9.

Bone marrow transplanted 6 months after a liver transplant corrected the severe phenotype of a 14-year-old boy and halted further protoporphyrin-induced liver graft damage.

Curative bone marrow transplantation in erythropoietic protoporphyria after reversal of severe cholestasis. Wahlin S, Aschan J, Björnstedt M, Broomé U, Harper P. J Hepatol 2007; 46: 174–9.

Eighty days of medical management normalized liver biochemistry and improved histology in a man who then received a bone marrow transplant. Ten months later, liver and porphyrin tests were normal; no photosensitivity was reported.

Evidence Levels: **A** Double-blind study **B** Clinical trial ≥ 20 subjects **C** Clinical trial < 20 subjects **D** Series ≥ 5 subjects **E** Anecdotal case reports

81

Extramammary Paget disease

Lori D. Prok, James E. Fitzpatrick

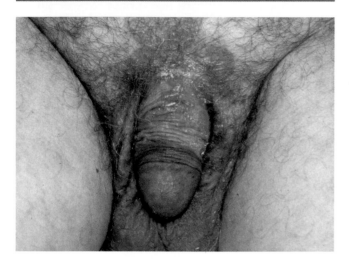

Courtesy of Fitzsimons Army Medical Center

Extramammary Paget disease (EMPD) was first described by Crocker in 1889, when he noted skin lesions affecting the penis and scrotum of a male patient that were identical to the nipple disease described by Paget in 1874. Although an uncommon malignancy, EMPD should be included in the clinical differential diagnosis of any chronic dermatitis of the groin or perineum. EMPD most commonly affects postmenopausal Caucasian women but can also be seen in men and all ethnicities. It typically presents as chronic, often sharply demarcated, erythematous scaling plaques on apocrine gland-bearing skin, including the genitalia, axillae, umbilicus, and external auditory canal. Pruritus is the most common presenting symptom. Primary EMPD results from epidermal infiltration of neoplastic glandular cells that share histologic and immunoperoxidase features of cells of apocrine origin. Recent evidence supports the role of Toker cells (clear cells found in 10% of normal nipples and recently identified in tissue of the milk line and the vulva) as the probable pathologic cell of origin. Secondary EMPD accounts for approximately 25% of cases and is the result of direct cutaneous extension of an underlying adenocarcinoma, most commonly of the genitourinary system or from the anal canal.

MANAGEMENT STRATEGY

Clinical suspicion of EMPD should prompt an immediate skin biopsy. Histologically, neoplastic cells are characterized by pale vacuolated cytoplasm and large pleomorphic nuclei, which can be seen infiltrating all levels of the epidermis. Extension into adnexal structures is common. In addition to hematoxylin and eosin (H&E) studies, the diagnosis is confirmed by utilizing a panel of immunoperoxidase studies that might include carcinoembryonic antigen (CEA), epithelial membrane antigen, CK7, gross cystic disease fluid protein-15, and/or Ber-EP4 to differentiate EMPD

from pagetoid variants of squamous cell carcinoma in situ and melanoma in situ. Recent studies have also demonstrated that HER2/neu overexpression is useful, both in helping to establish a diagnosis of EMPD and in identifying invasive cases that might be responsive to trastuzumab. The biopsy also establishes whether there is extension into the dermis, which is useful in identifying the subset of patients who should be considered for sentinel lymph node biopsy.

A full-body skin examination and lymph node evaluation should be performed in all patients with EMPD. Patients should then have appropriate evaluation for underlying malignancy, including age- and gender-appropriate screening (Papanicolaou smear, fecal occult blood, colonoscopy, cystoscopy, and prostate-specific antigen). Additional investigations (imaging, colposcopy, etc.) are guided by screening results and the anatomic location of cutaneous lesions.

EMPD is treated locally with *surgical excision,* with adjuvant therapies in selected cases. *Mohs micrographic surgery* is the preferred technique, offering the most reliable margin control, maximal tissue preservation, and lowest recurrence rates. However, this technique is still limited by noncontiguous tumor spread and the high likelihood of EMPD involving clinically normal-appearing skin.

Specific Investigations

- Skin biopsy
- Full-body skin examination and lymph node evaluation
- Cancer screening appropriate for age and gender (Papanicolaou smear, fecal occult blood, colonoscopy, cystoscopy, and prostate-specific antigen)
- Sentinel lymph node biopsy in patients with dermal and/or lymphatic extension

Extramammary Paget's disease: treatment, prognostic factors and outcome in 76 patients. Hatta N, Yamada M, Hirano T, Fujimoto A, Morita R. Br J Dermatol 2008; 158: 313–8.

Retrospective review of 76 patients with EMPD. Surgical margin was not correlated with local recurrence. Seventeen percent developed systemic metastases; 10 patients died. Nodules in the primary tumor, clinical lymph node swelling, elevated CEA levels, depth of tumor invasion, and lymph node metastasis were significant prognostic factors. Depth of tumor invasion and CEA level were associated with reduced survival.

Usefulness of sentinel lymph node biopsy for the detection of metastasis in the early stages of extramammary Paget's disease. Kusatake K, Harada Y, Mizumoto K, Kaneko S, Niihara H, Chinuki Y, et al. Eur J Dermatol 2015; 25: 156–61.

Eighteen patients with primary EMPD were enrolled in this prospective study. Nine of the 18 patients had histologic evidence of dermal extension of tumor cells. Of the patients with dermal extension of the tumor, 3/9 (33%) had a positive sentinel lymph node biopsy, and none of the patients with intraepidermal involvement only had a positive sentinel lymph node biopsy. The authors conclude that sentinel lymph node biopsy is useful to detect lymph node metastasis.

First-Line Therapies

Wide local excision, with or without lymph node dissection	B
Frozen section–guided wide local excision	B
Mohs micrographic surgery	B

Indications for lymph node dissection in the treatment of EMPD. Tsutsumida A, Yamamoto Y, Minakawa H, Yoshida T, Kokubu I, Sugihara T. Dermatol Surg 2003; 29: 21–4.

A prospective study of 34 patients with genital or perineal EMPD treated with wide local excision. Patients with clinical or histologic evidence of metastatic disease underwent lymph node dissection. No patients with carcinoma in situ or microscopic papillary dermal invasion had lymph node metastasis; all had 100% 5-year survival. Tumor invasion into the reticular dermis correlated with 33% 5-year survival. Tumor invasion into the subcutaneous tissue correlated with 100% lymph node metastasis and death.

Clinicopathological study of invasive extramammary Paget's disease: subgroup comparison according to invasion depth. Shiomi T, Noguchi T, Nakayama H, Yoshida Y, Yamamoto O, Hayashi N, et al. J Eur Acad Dermatol Venereol 2013; 27: 589–92.

Retrospective review of 51 surgical specimens of primary invasive EMPD. Cases were divided into subgroups according to invasion depth: dermal invasion ≤1 mm (minimal invasion) and dermal invasion >1 mm in depth. Lymph node metastases were detected in two (7.7%) of 26 patients with minimal invasion and nodal metastases in 22/25 (88%) of patients with invasion >1 mm in depth. The authors conclude there is evidence to suggest that a cut-off depth of 1 mm of invasion is useful in staging patients for prognosis and treatment.

Frozen section-guided wide local excision in the treatment of penoscrotal EMPD. Zhu Y, Ye D, Chen Z, Zhang SL, Qin XJ. BJU Int 2007; 100: 1282–7.

Retrospective review of 38 patients with primary penoscrotal EMPD who received wide local excision with intraoperative frozen-section analysis. Thirty-two percent had positive frozen-section margins and required immediate extended excision. Forty percent of patients had positive surgical margins after traditional wide local excision with 2-cm margins. At a mean follow-up of 33 months 16% of patients had recurrent disease, and four patients had systemic involvement.

Comparison of Mohs micrographic surgery and wide excision for EMPD. O'Connor W, Lim K, Zalla M. Dermatol Surg 2003; 29: 723–7.

Retrospective review of 95 patients at the Mayo Clinic comparing tumor recurrence in patients treated with Mohs micrographic surgery (8%) and those with wide local excision (22%). Surgeons used intraoperative staining with CK7.

Second-Line Therapies	
• Photodynamic therapy	B
• Radiation therapy	B
• Systemic chemotherapy	B
• Topical imiquimod	B

Photodynamic therapy with M-ALA as nonsurgical treatment option in patients with primary extramammary Paget's disease. Fontanelli R, Papadia A. Martinelli F, Lorusso D, Grijuela B, Merola M, et al. Gynecol Oncol 2013; 130: 90–4.

Prospective study of 32 women with vulvar EMPD who were treated with aminolevulinic-acid methyl-ester photodynamic therapy (M-ALA PD). Patients received at least three cycles and were then evaluated as to whether they would receive additional therapy. After three cycles, 3 patients had a complete response (9%), 25 patients (78%) had a partial response, and the remaining 4 patients (13%) had stable disease. The authors concluded that M-ALA PD, although not usually curative, is useful to control EMPD and preserve cosmetic and/or functional anatomy.

Radiation therapy for extramammary Paget's disease: treatment outcomes and prognostic factors. Hata M, Koike I, Wada H, Miyagi E, Kasuya T, Kaizu H, et al. Ann Oncol 2014; 25: 291–7.

Retrospective review of the outcomes of 41 patients with EMPD, including 15 patients with regional lymph node metastases. Total doses of 46 to 80.2 Gy (median = 60 Gy) were utilized with a median of 33 fractions. The local progression-free and disease-free rates were 82% and 46% at 5 years. Five patients (12%) died because of tumor progression. The authors conclude that radiation therapy is effective and safe, with this being a curative option for patients who are inoperable.

Combination chemotherapy for metastatic extramammary Paget disease. Oashi K, Tsutsumida A, Namikawa K, Tanaka R, Omata W, Yamamoto Y, et al. Br J Dermatol 2014; 170: 1354–7.

The authors studied seven patients with metastatic EMPD who were treated with combination chemotherapy composed of epirubicin, mitomycin C, and vincristine on day 1 followed by carboplatin on day 2 and 5-fluorouracil on days 2 to 6. All seven patients had at least a partial response or shrinkage in tumor size; however, there were no complete responses. The 1-year survival rate was 43%. The authors concluded that this combination chemotherapy may be a treatment option for patients with metastatic EMPD.

Combination chemotherapy of low-dose 5-fluorouracil and cisplatin for advanced extramammary Paget's disease. Tokuda Y, Arakura F, Uhara H. Int J Clin Oncol 2015; 29: 194–7.

Retrospective study of 22 patients with advanced (metastatic) EMPD who were treated with combination chemotherapy consisting of infusions of 5-fluorouracil and cisplatin. The overall survival rate ranges were 5 to 51 months, with 13 of 22 patients demonstrating a complete or partial response to therapy. Three of the 22 patients demonstrated progressive disease. The authors concluded that this is a relatively effective treatment option of advanced EMPD.

Usefulness of docetaxel as first-line chemotherapy for metastatic extramammary Paget's disease. Yoshino K, Fujisawa Y, Kiyohara Y, Kadono T, Murata Y, Uhara H, et al. J Dermatol 2016; 43: 633–7.

Retrospective multicenter analysis of 13 patients with metastatic EMPD who were treated with docetaxel with average number of treatment cycles of 9.1 (one treatment per month). Seven patients (58%) demonstrated a partial response, 3 patients had stable disease (25%), and 2 patients (17%) had progressive disease. The authors concluded that docetaxel is a promising treatment for metastatic EMPD but that a prospective clinical trial is needed to confirm these findings.

Effects of imiquimod on vulvar Paget's disease: a systematic review of the literature. Machida H, Moenini A, Roman LD, Matsuo K. Gynecol Oncol 2015; 139: 165–71.

This is a systematic review of the literature for cases of vulvar Paget disease treated with topical imiquimod that included 63 cases of untreated and recurrent EMPD. The treatment regimens were highly variable, but the most common regimen was topical application three or four times per week and a median treatment duration of 4 months. A complete response at 6 months

Evidence Levels: **A** Double-blind study **B** Clinical trial ≥ 20 subjects **C** Clinical trial < 20 subjects **D** Series ≥ 5 subjects **E** Anecdotal case reports

was present in 35 of 63 (72%) of the patients. Of the complete responders, 3 of 35 women had a disease recurrence.

Treatment of extramammary Paget disease of the vulva with imiquimod: a retrospective, multicenter study by the German Colposcopy Network. Luyten A, Sörgel P, Clad A, Gieseking F, Maass-Poppenhusen K, Lellé RJ, et al. J Am Acad Dermatol 2014; 70: 644–50.

Retrospective multicenter analysis of 21 women with first-time or recurrent vulvar EMPD treated with topical imiquimod. The dose and duration varied from patient to patient; however, the mean duration of treatment exceeded 16 weeks. Eleven of 21 patients (52%) had a complete response, 6 of 21 (29%) had a partial response, with the remaining 4 patients having stable disease. The authors concluded that topical imiquimod is a useful treatment option for recurrent EMPD to avoid extensive mutilating surgical procedures.

Third-Line Therapies

- Androgen receptor antagonist   E
- Intralesional interferon-α_{2b} E
- Topical 5-fluorouracil and retinoic acid   E
- Trastuzumab   E

Androgen-deprivation regimen for multiple bone metastases of EMPD. Yoneyama K, Kamada N, Kinoshita K. Br J Dermatol 2005; 153: 853–5.

Case report of EMPD with multiple bone metastases successfully suppressed with antiandrogen bicalutamide and LH-RH agonist leuprorelin. Tumor markers decreased and bone scintigraphy evidence of metastasis disappeared within 2 months. When tumor markers rose at day 70, other antiandrogens and systemic chemotherapy failed, and the patient ultimately died 14 months after the start of antiandrogen therapy. The authors postulate that the rapid development of resistance to the androgen-deprivation therapy suggests that mutation or amplification in the androgen receptor gene occurred in this case, as seen in cases of prostate cancer.

Intralesional interferon alfa-2b as neoadjuvant treatment for perianal EMPD. Panasiti V, Bottoni U, Devirgilis V, Mancini M, Rossi M, Curzio M, et al. J Eur Acad Dermatol Venereol 2008; 22: 522–3.

Report of a patient with perianal EMPD who, after refusing surgical excision, was treated with intralesional IFN-α_{2b} at a dose of 1 million IU three times per week for 3 weeks. At 7 weeks the tumor had decreased in diameter, and surgical resection was performed. Patient had no clinical disease at 108 months' follow-up.

EMPD resistant to surgery and imiquimod monotherapy but responsive to imiquimod combination topical chemotherapy with 5-fluorouracil and retinoic acid: a case report. Ye J, Rhew D, Yip F, Edelstein L. Cutis 2006; 7: 245–50.

Report of a patient with EMPD (recurrent after surgery and resistant to topical imiquimod alone) that resolved after treatment with a combination of imiquimod and topical 5-fluorouracil and retinoic acid.

Metastatic extramammary Paget's disease of scrotum responds completely to single agent trastuzumab in a hemodialysis patient: case reports, molecular profiling and brief review of the literature. Barth P, Dulaimi Al-Saleem E, Edwards KW, Millis SZ, Wong Y-N, Geynisman DM. Case Rep Oncol Med 2015; 2015: 895151.

Case report of metastatic EMPD with Her2/neu overexpression that was treated with trastuzumab as a single agent. The patient had a complete response. The authors note that this option is only available in the 30% to 40% of EMPD that overexpress Her2/neu.

Fabry disease

Jaya Ganesh, Rhonda E. Schnur, Fiona Child

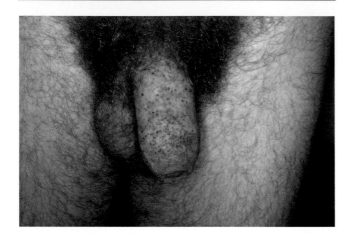

Fabry disease (or Anderson–Fabry disease, OMIM 301500) is a progressive, X-linked lysosomal storage disorder caused by the deficiency or absence of the enzyme α-galactosidase A (GLA). This results in the accumulation of globotriaosylceramide (Gb3) and related glycosphingolipids within lysosomes. Systemic manifestations of Fabry disease include renal dysfunction, cardiomyopathy and arrhythmias, cerebrovascular complications, corneal and lenticular opacities, tinnitus and hearing loss, gastrointestinal disturbances, pulmonary disease, osteopenia, and depression. Causes of death include end-stage renal disease (ESRD), cardiac disease, or stroke. Males are more severely affected, but female carriers may exhibit symptoms depending on the pattern of X-chromosome inactivation (lionization).

Cutaneous features include angiokeratoma, hypohidrosis (53% males and 28% females), telangiectasia (23% males and 9% females), and lymphedema (16% males and 6% females).

Diffuse angiokeratomas are a characteristic cutaneous manifestation of Fabry disease and should alert the clinician to the possibility of the diagnosis. They typically cluster symmetrically around the umbilicus, hips, back, thighs, buttocks, penis, and scrotum (bathing trunk distribution); increase in number and size over time; and may correlate with the severity of the systemic manifestations of disease. Diffuse angiokeratomas may also be seen in other lysosomal storage diseases including fucosidosis, sialidosis, aspartylglucosaminuria, and β-galactosidase deficiency. Acroparesthesia produces episodic burning, severe pain, and a constant tingling of the palms and soles. Pain crises result from glycolipid accumulation in the autonomic nervous system and vascular endothelium. A similar mechanism underlies Fabry-associated hypohidrosis.

MANAGEMENT STRATEGY

Comprehensive medical therapy for Fabry disease requires a multidisciplinary approach that includes a combination of *enzyme replacement therapy* and *conventional medical treatment*.

Angiokeratomas due to Fabry disease are typically asymptomatic; when indicated they can be treated with *surgical excision, electrocoagulation,* and *cryosurgery* and do not require targeted therapy. Various *lasers* have been utilized, including the CO_2, argon, copper vapor, and flashlamp–pumped-dye lasers. Copper vapor lasers are superior to argon because of their wavelength specificity for hemoglobin. However, the flashlamp–pumped-dye laser may produce less pain and bleeding and pigmentary change.

Neuropathic pain and acroparesthesias may benefit from avoidance of triggers, including physical exertion and temperature changes. *Diphenylhydantoin, carbamazepine, gabapentin, topiramate,* and *tricyclic antidepressants* are used for analgesia. Nonsteroidal antiinflammatory drugs (NSAIDs) are generally ineffective, and narcotics should be avoided if possible.

Used in conjunction with ERT, angiotensin-converting enzyme inhibitors and angiotensin receptor blockers may reduce proteinuria and stabilize glomerular filtration rate (GFR). Peritoneal dialysis, hemodialysis, and renal transplantation are utilized for patients with renal failure.

Gastrointestinal complications, including delayed gastric emptying and dyspepsia, have been treated with metoclopramide, pancrelipase, loperamide, and H_2 blockers. Hearing aids assist in moderate hearing loss, whereas profound deafness requires cochlear implantation. Aspirin or clopidogrel is recommended for cardiovascular disease prophylaxis. Conventional treatments are also utilized in the management of cardiovascular symptoms in Fabry disease.

Two human enzyme products have been utilized in ERT: *agalsidase-β (Fabrazyme, Sanofi-Genzyme Corporation)* and *agalsidase-α (Replagal, Shire Genetic Therapies)*. Both were approved by the European Agency for Evaluation of Medical Products in 2001, but only agalsidase-β is approved by the Food and Drug Administration (FDA) for use in the United States. The enzymes are administered intravenously biweekly at a dose of 0.2 mg/kg for agalsidase-α and 1.0 mg/kg for agalsidase-β. No clear difference in clinical effect between the two preparations was demonstrated in a randomized, controlled, prospective study.

ERT stabilizes or slows progression of renal and cardiac disease, reduces neuropathic pain, stabilizes hearing loss, and improves sweat function and quality of life. Patients treated with ERT have a slowing of progression to "major" clinical events (ESRD, myocardial infarction, stroke, or death). In a recent analysis of 969 male and 442 female patients enrolled in the longitudinal Fabry Registry, patients with more advanced disease before initiating ERT were at a significantly higher risk of sustaining a severe Fabry-related clinical event compared with those who had milder disease and earlier institution of ERT. ERT has been associated with immunogenicity leading to antibody-mediated infusion reactions that may also reduce its efficacy.

New, improved, and more effective treatment approaches are actively being studied. A promising therapeutic strategy involves small molecules called *active site-specific chaperones* that may be useful with certain types of mutations. In Fabry disease, missense mutations can cause misfolding of the mutant GLA enzyme and retention of the misfolded enzyme in the endoplasmic reticulum. The retained enzyme is then degraded rather than being trafficked to the appropriate location in the cell, the lysosome. Chaperones are orally active molecules that selectively bind to the misfolded enzyme, promote correct folding, and aid in delivery to lysosomes. Some mutant forms of the enzyme are more amenable to targeting and are responsive to migalastat (*1-deoxygalactonojirimycin [DGJ], Amicus Therapeutics, NJ, USA]*). Migalastat is an orally administered molecular chaperone that was assigned orphan drug status by the FDA in 2004. It is administered orally on alternate days. In a cohort of 67 patients, 75% had mutations deemed responsive to migalastat. In that group, improvements included the arrest of decline in GFR, left ventricular mass index, and gastrointestinal symptoms.

Substrate reduction therapy is an alternative investigative approach that involves inhibiting the production of Gb3 that accumulates as a result of GLA deficiency. A glucosylceramide synthase inhibitor slows the rate of Gb3 synthesis, thus decreasing storage within the lysosomes. Eliglustat tartrate (Genz 112638) is an immunosugar analog under investigation as a glucosylceramide synthase inhibitor for treating Gaucher disease and other lysosomal storage disorders including Fabry disease.

Fabry disease has now been added to the list of disorders screened for by newborn screening panels in some states in the United States.

Specific Investigations

Diagnostic workup

- Obtain family history
- Enzyme analysis (quantitation in plasma and white blood cells [WBCs], cultured cells, blood spot filter paper screening) (most definitive method in males, not reliable for females)
- *GLA* molecular DNA analysis (nearly 100% sensitivity in affected males; most reliable method for females)
- Preimplantation genetic diagnosis or prenatal diagnosis via amniocentesis or chorionic venous sampling (enzymatic and/or molecular assay)

Systemic workup (male and female)

- Renal function studies including urinalysis and assessment of 24-hour microalbuminuria and creatinine clearance
- Cardiac evaluation with electrocardiogram, echocardiography, 24-hour Holter monitoring, and cardiac magnetic resonance imaging (MRI)
- Dermatology evaluation
- Urine GB3, LysoGB3 (Fabry-associated lysosphingolipid) levels in blood
- Audiology
- Fundoscopy and slit-lamp examination
- Neurologic evaluation with surveillance MRI
- Pulmonary function studies
- Gastrointestinal examination with endoscopy as indicated

Angiokeratoma: decision making aid for the diagnosis of Fabry disease. Zampetti A, Orteu CH, Antuzzi D, Bongiorno MR, Manco S, Gnarra M, et al. and the Interdisciplinary Study Group on Fabry Disease. Br J Dermatol 2012; 166: 712–20.

This article proposes an algorithm for the diagnosis of Fabry disease and reviews clinical and histologic features of angiokeratomas in detail. The algorithm uses personal and family history, the number and distribution of angiokeratomas, skin biopsy, dermoscopy (to detect more subtle lesions), electron microscopy, and genetic studies as sequential tools in the diagnostic process.

Treatment of Fabry disease: current and emerging strategies. Rozenfeld P, Neumann PM. Curr Pharm Biotechnol 2011; 12: 916–22.

This is an excellent overview of therapeutic options, including new treatments such as chaperone therapy.

Fabry disease and the skin: data from FOS, the Fabry Outcome Survey. Orteu CH, Jansen T, Lidove O, Jaussaud R, Hughes DA, Pintos-Morell G, et al. Br J Dermatol 2007; 157: 331–37.

The Fabry Outcome Survey (FOS), a multicenter European database, was used to capture longitudinal multicenter data on patients with Fabry disease. This paper discusses the dermatologic manifestations present in that cohort.

A case of multiple angiomas without any angiokeratomas in a female heterozygote with Fabry disease. Mirceva V, Hein R, Ring J, Möhrenschlager M. Australas J Dermatol 2010; 51: 36.

Case report wherein multiple angiomas were the only visible cutaneous manifestation of Fabry disease in an oligosymptomatic female.

Fabry disease. Germain DP. Orphanet J Rare Dis 2010; 5: 30.

This is a very comprehensive overview of the clinical characteristics of Fabry disease, current treatment modalities, and therapies on the horizon.

Fabry disease: a review of current management strategies. Mehta A, Beck M, Eyeskens F, Feliciani C, Kantola I, Ramaswami U, et al. Q J Med 2010; 103: 641–59.

This review, written by a panel of experts with extensive clinical experience in Fabry disease, summarizes the recent literature and registry data to aid in providing therapy recommendations.

Human Gene Mutation Database: 2008 update. Stenson PD, Mort M, Ball EV, Howells K, Phillips AD, Thomas NST, et al. Genome Med 2009; 1: 13. http://www.hgmd.org. The Institute of Medical Genetics, Cardiff, United Kingdom, 2011. Accessed Sept 5, 2016.

Over 800 mutations in the *GLA* gene have been identified, including missense and loss of function mutations. Mutation information is used for diagnosis, particularly in female heterozygotes, prenatal testing, and partial correlation with clinical phenotype. Mutation specificity also has major implications for pharmacogenomic management, for example, for the potential use of chaperone therapy in patients with missense mutations that cause protein misfolding.

Fabry disease. Mehta A, Hughes DA. In: Pagon RA, Adam MP, Ardinger HH, Wallace SE, Amemiya A, Bean LJH, et al, eds. GeneReviews, Seattle, WA: University of Washington.

This easily accessed, frequently updated database provides a comprehensive review of the clinical, biochemical, and molecular aspects of Fabry disease, with links to information about diagnostic testing and patient resources.

Fabry disease in infancy and early childhood: a systematic literature review. Laney DA, Peck DS, Atherton AM, Manwaring LP, Christensen KM, Shankar SP, et al. Genet Med 2015; 17: 323–30.

The authors performed a systematic retrospective analysis of 120 peer-reviewed publications and case reports about the pediatric Fabry population. Forty-one individual patients younger than 5 years of age were identified. Acroparesthesia was the most common clinical symptom, reported in nine patients. Other symptoms in very young children included heat sensitivity and gastrointestinal disease, especially recurrent abdominal pain and diarrhea. Importantly, renal damage, including foot process effacement, was noted to occur even before there was clinically evident proteinuria.

First-Line Therapies

• Enzyme replacement therapy	A
• Laser therapy	E
• Intense pulsed light	E
• Surgical excision	E
• Diphenylhydantoin	B
• Cryotherapy	E

Enzyme replacement therapy for Anderson–Fabry disease. El Dib RP, Pastores GM. Cochrane Database Syst Rev 2010; 5: CD006663.

This Cochrane review summarizes the available evidence with regard to five randomized-controlled clinical trials (representing 23 publications) involving agalsidase-α and agalsidase-β. The authors concluded that ERT can modify disease course in treated patients with Fabry disease, improving neuropathic pain, cardiac morphology, and renal function. There is also a positive influence on quality of life. Treatment is generally well tolerated, although neutralizing antibodies may affect clinical outcome. Longer-term effects on morbidity and mortality remain to be established.

Response of women with Fabry disease to enzyme-replacement therapy: comparison with men, using data from the FOS – the Fabry Outcome Survey. Hughes DA, Barba Romero MÁ, Hollak CE, Giugliani R, Deegan PB. Mol Genet Metab 2011; 103: 207–14.

Data were obtained from the Fabry Outcome Survey of 78 affected women and 172 men. Clinical outcomes studied included cardiac structure and function, renal function, quality of life, pain, and a variety of other clinical features and quantifiable measures. Both sexes responded to agalsidase-α similarly. Anhidrosis improved, whereas angiokeratomas did not.

Agalsidase beta treatment is associated with improved quality of life in patients with Fabry disease: findings from the Fabry registry. Watt T, Burlina A, Cazzorla C, Shonfeld D, Banikazemi M, Hopkin RJ, et al. Genet Med 2010; 12: 703–12.

Seventy-one men and 59 women treated with agalsidase-β had baseline and posttreatment quality of life measurements. Health-related quality of life improved in both sexes, although the effect was more pronounced in men.

Four-year prospective clinical trial of agalsidase alfa in children with Fabry disease. Schiffmann R, Martin RA, Reimschisel T, Johnson K, Castaneda V, Lien YH, et al. J Pediatr 2010; 156: 832–7.

Seventeen of the 24 children who initially completed the 6-month open-label agalsidase-α study enrolled in this 3.5-year extension study. Pain severity and Gb3 levels were reduced, and heart rate variability improved. Kidney function and left ventricular mass remained stable.

Risk factors for severe clinical events in male and female patients with Fabry disease treated with agalsidase beta enzyme replacement therapy: data from the Fabry Registry. Hopkin RJ, Cabrera G, Charrow J, Lemay R, Martins AM, Mauer M, et al. Mol Genet Metab 2016; 119: 151–9.

This article provides an in-depth review of risk factors for developing severe clinical events in a large cohort of patients treated with ERT, highlighting the need for multidisciplinary care and adjuvant therapies.

Angiokeratomas in Fabry's disease and Fordyce's disease: successful treatment with copper vapor laser. Lapins J, Emtestam L, Marcusson JA. Acta Derm Venereol 1993; 73: 133–5.

Angiokeratomas in two treated subjects were undetected at 3-month follow-up; treated skin was smooth, with minimal pigmentary alteration.

Successful treatment of angiokeratoma with potassium titanyl phosphate laser. Gorse SJ, James W, Murison MSC. Br J Dermatol 2004; 150: 620–1.

Excellent results using this laser were seen in two subjects with angiokeratomas.

Angiokeratomas of Fabry successfully treated with intense pulsed light. Morais P, Santos AL, Baudrier T, Mota AV, Oliveira JP, Azevedo F. J Cosmet Laser Ther 2008; 10: 218–22.

There was almost complete clearance of angiokeratomas in one severely affected subject without recurrence at 12-month follow-up.

Fabry disease: recognition and management of cutaneous manifestations. Mohrenschlager M, Braun-Falco M, Ring J, Abech D. Am J Clin Dermatol 2003; 4: 189–96.

Review article about current laser treatments for the angiokeratomas of Fabry disease, including variable pulse width 532-nm neodymium:yttrium-aluminum-garnet (Nd:YAG) laser, 578-nm copper vapor laser, and flashlamp–pulsed-dye laser.

Intravenous infusion of phenytoin relieves neuropathic pain: a randomized, double-blinded, placebo-controlled, crossover study. McCleane GJ. Anesth Analg 1999; 89: 985–8.

This study evaluated 20 patients with acute flare-ups of neuropathic pain. Phenytoin reduced burning sensation, shooting pain, sensitivity, numbness, and overall pain.

Second-Line Therapies

• Gabapentin	D
• Carbamazepine	D

Use of gabapentin to reduce chronic neuropathic pain in Fabry disease. Ries M, Mengel E, Kutschke G, Kim KS, Birklein F, Krummenauer F, et al. J Inherit Metab Dis 2003; 26: 413–4.

Six patients with Fabry disease experienced less pain than at baseline with few side effects after 4 weeks of treatment.

Carbamazepine in Fabry's disease: effective analgesia with dose-dependent exacerbation of autonomic dysfunction. Filling-Katz MR, Merrick HF, Fink JK, Miles RB, Sokol J, Barton NW. Neurology 1989; 39: 598–600.

Five of seven patients had moderate to complete relief of pain based upon self-assessment. Complications included exacerbation of preexisting autonomic dysfunction, ileus, urinary retention, and gastrointestinal disturbance.

Third-Line and Future Therapies

• Site-specific molecular chaperone therapy (migalastat)	A
• Substrate reduction therapy (eliglustat tartrate, Genz 112638)	
• Gene replacement therapy	
• Renal transplantation/hemodialysis	C

Evidence Levels: **A** Double-blind study **B** Clinical trial ≥ 20 subjects **C** Clinical trial < 20 subjects **D** Series ≥ 5 subjects **E** Anecdotal case reports

Co-administration with the pharmacological chaperone AT1001 increases recombinant human α-galactosidase A tissue uptake and improves substrate reduction in Fabry mice. Benjamin ER, Khanna R, Schilling A, Flanagan JJ, Pellegrino LJ, Brignol N, et al. Mol Ther 2012; 20: 717–26.

This study evaluated the efficacy of combined ERT and chaperone therapy. Coincubation of Fabry fibroblasts with recombinant human α-galactosidase A (rhα-Gal A) and AT1001 (1-deoxygalactonojirimycin, migalastat hydrochloride) resulted in up to fourfold higher levels of cellular α-Gal A and approximately 30% greater Gb3 reduction compared with ERT alone. In rats, AT1001 increased the circulating half-life of rhα-Gal A by >2.5-fold, and in GLA knockout mice resulted in up to fivefold higher α-Gal A levels and fourfold greater GL-3 reduction.

Treatment of Fabry's disease with the pharmacologic chaperone migalastat. Germain DP, Hughes DA, Nicholls K, Bichet DG, Wilcox WR, Feliciani C, et al. New Eng J Med 2016; 375: 545–55.

Sixty-seven patients with Fabry disease who had never received ERT or had not received ERT within 6 months before enrollment were randomized to 6 months of treatment with migalastat or placebo followed by an open-label migalastat for 6 to 12 months plus an additional year. All patients were genotyped, and 50 patients had mutant enzyme suitable for targeting by migalastat. Beneficial effects were observed in annualized rates of change in GFRs, reduction in left ventricular mass index (a significant predictor of adverse cardiac events), and improvement in gastrointestinal symptoms that are frequently debilitating. None of the migalastat-treated patients progressed to end-stage kidney disease, had strokes, or had cardiac-related mortality during the study.

Kidney transplant outcomes in patients with Fabry disease. Shah T, Gill J, Malhotra N, Takemoto SK, Bunnapradist S. Transplantation 2009; 87: 280–5.

This study evaluated 197 renal transplant recipients with Fabry disease and ESRD from 1987 to 2007. Rates of graft loss and death were compared with renal transplant recipients with other (non-Fabry) causes of ESRD, as well as a 10:1 matched cohort of transplant recipients with other causes of ESRD. Patients with Fabry disease had a superior graft survival and similar patient survival compared with other (non-Fabry) ESRD patients. However, they had a higher risk of death compared with a matched cohort.

Flushing

Jennifer A. Sopkovich, Jonathan K. Wilkin

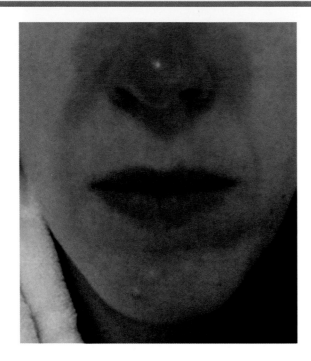

Flushing is a transient reddening of the face and frequently other areas, including the neck, upper chest, pinna, and epigastric area. Flushing is the visible sign of a generalized increase in cutaneous blood flow despite the limited distribution of the erythema.

MANAGEMENT STRATEGY

The initial step in the management of a patient with a flushing disorder is to make a specific diagnosis. The first algorithmic step is to distinguish between autonomic neural-mediated flushing, in which eccrine sweating occurs at the time of the flushing ("wet flushing"), and direct vasodilator-mediated flushing, in which there is no accompanying eccrine sweating ("dry flushing"). The dry flushing reactions are further divided into those with prominent dysesthesia and those without.

Dry flushing without dysesthesia is due to circulating vasodilators, either exogenous or endogenous. Exogenous vasodilators are almost always elicited from the patient's history. A diary listing all foods, beverages, medications, activities, etc., can help pinpoint the inciting agent. Avoidance of the vasodilator agent is the treatment of choice. However, there are some exceptions where antiflushing treatment is initiated and the vasodilator is continued, such as niacin (nicotinic acid) therapy for hyperlipidemia and tamoxifen for breast cancer.

Endogenous circulating vasodilator agents, typically from underlying neoplasias, are suggested by both multiple stimuli that provoke flushing and prominent associated features (e.g., itching, urticaria, hypertension, sweating, and diarrhea). Prominent features associated with flushing can occur with cholinergic urticaria,

cholinergic erythema, anxiety reactions, intolerance to foods, menopausal flushing, the dumping syndrome, diabetes mellitus, pancreatic cholera, medullary carcinoma of the thyroid, pheochromocytoma, multiple endocrine neoplasia syndromes II and III, mastocytosis, and carcinoid syndrome.

Specific Investigations

- 5-Hydroxyindoleacetic acid urine
- Histamine urine
- Serotonin blood/platelet
- Histamine plasma
- Tryptase serum

The red face: flushing disorders. Wilkin JK. Clin Dermatol 1993; 11: 211–23.

It is important to establish a diagnosis of flushing and rule out other causes of red face such as photosensitivity, lupus erythematosus, seborrhea, and other conditions before proceeding with a flushing workup and treatment. This review describes the three types of blushing, including the type that responds to a low-dose, long-acting nonselective β-blocker (nadolol 40 mg every morning). The use of aspirin to block niacin-induced flushing and amitriptyline to treat facial dysesthesia is described.

Red face revisited: flushing. İkizoğlu G. Clin Dermatol 2014; 32: 800–8.

This article reviews the differential diagnosis for facial flushing, including common benign disorders and uncommon but serious diseases. Medication-induced flushing is also discussed.

Influence of a serotonin- and dopamine-rich diet on platelet serotonin content and urinary excretion of biogenic amines and their metabolites. Kema IP, Schellings AM, Meiborg G, Hoppenbrouwers CJ, Muskiet FA. Clin Chem 1992; 38: 1730–6.

No diet restrictions are necessary during workup of catecholamine-secreting tumors. Avoidance of serotonin-containing foods is recommended before urinary 5-Hydroxyindoleacetic acid (5-HIAA) collection in the workup of carcinoid. Platelet serotonin is more sensitive and is not affected by diet.

The quantitative 24-hour urinary 5-HIAA level is useful in the follow-up of carcinoid tumors with a high serotonin production rate. It is also useful initially for diagnosis but only when it is positive during a low-serotonin diet. If the urinary 5-HIAA level is not elevated in a patient with flushing and other features characteristic of carcinoid, the platelet or blood serotonin level should be obtained.

Mastocytosis: the puzzling clinical spectrum and challenging diagnostic aspects of an enigmatic disease. Gülen T, Hägglund H, Dahlén B, Nilsson G. J Intern Med 2016; 279: 211–28.

Facial flushing is a chief complaint in mastocytosis. Attacks may include flushing, palpitations, dizziness, and hypotension. Serum tryptase levels are the first step in diagnosis.

Comparison of clinical trials with sildenafil, vardenafil and tadalafil in erectile dysfunction. Doggrell SA. Expert Opin Pharmacother 2005; 6: 75–84.

Flushing was identified as an adverse effect in the clinical trials of each of these selective phosphodiesterase-5 (PDE-5) inhibitors.

Facial flushing response to alcohol and the risk of esophageal squamous cell carcinoma: a comprehensive systematic review and meta-analysis. Andrici J, Hu SX, Eslick GD. Cancer Epidemiol 2016: 40: 31–8.

The alcohol-induced facial flushing response, common among East Asians, is associated with an increased risk of esophageal squamous cell carcinoma in moderate to heavy drinkers.

Heat urticaria: a revision of published cases with an update on classification and management. Pezzolo E, Peroni A, Gisondi P, Girolomoni G. Br J Dermatol 2016; 175: 473–8.

Heat urticaria, which presents as wheals immediately after heat exposure, may also be associated with flushing and other systemic symptoms.

Scombroid fish poisoning, Pennsylvania, 1998. Centers for Disease Control and Prevention. MMWR Morb Mortal Wkly Rep 2000; 49: 398–400.

Four adults in Pennsylvania had facial flushing, nausea, diarrhea, sweating, headache, metallic taste, and burning sensations in the mouth after eating tuna. Scombroid fish poisoning has been associated primarily with the consumption of tuna, mahi-mahi, and bluefish.

First-Line Therapies	
• Ice chips	B
• Aspirin	B
• Hormone replacement	A
• Brimonidine	A

Oral thermal-induced flushing in erythematotelangiectatic rosacea. Wilkin J. J Invest Dermatol 1981; 76: 15–8.

It is heat, not caffeine, that causes the flushing from drinking hot coffee and tea.

Sucking on ice chips can abort mild menopausal, thermal, or spicy food–induced flushing.

Aspirin blocks nicotinic acid-induced flushing. Wilkin JK, Wilkin O, Kapp R, Donachie R, Chernosky ME, Buckner J. Clin Pharmacol Ther 1982; 31: 478–82.

Aspirin and other cyclooxygenase inhibitors (nonsteroidals) block prostaglandin-mediated flushing without reducing the lipid-lowering effect of niacin.

A substantial number of patients taking niacin are taking a nonsteroidal agent. Patients should be instructed to change time of dosing to 1 hour before niacin.

Aspirin attenuation of alcohol-induced flushing and intoxication in Oriental and Occidental subjects. Truitt EB, Gaynor CR, Mehl DL. Alcohol 1987; 1: 595–9.

Eight Oriental and three Occidental subjects sensitive to alcohol manifested as facial flushing had markedly reduced flushing after 0.64 g of aspirin 1 hour before alcohol consumption.

Combined versus sequential hormonal replacement therapy: a double-blind, placebo-controlled study on quality of life-related outcome measures. Bech P, Munk-Jensen N, Obel EB, Ulrich LG, Eiken P, Nielsen SP. Psychother Psychosom 1998; 67: 259–65.

Hormone replacement therapy (HRT) was superior to placebo for many symptoms, including hot flashes in early postmenopausal women.

Although effective for controlling hot flashes, HRT has associated risks and is contraindicated for many women.

Brimonidine gel 0.33% rapidly improves patient-reported outcomes by controlling facial erythema of rosacea: a randomized, double-blind, vehicle-controlled study. Layton AM, Schaller M, Homey B, Hofmann MA, Bewley AP, Lehmann P, et al. J Eur Acad Dermatol Venereol 2015; 29: 2405–10.

Brimonidine gel, an alpha-2 adrenergic agonist, is approved for the topical treatment of erythema associated with rosacea. Once-daily application significantly improves persistent facial erythema of rosacea.

Dermatological adverse events associated with topical brimonidine gel 0.33% in subjects with erythema of rosacea: a retrospective review of clinical studies. Holmes AD, Waite KA, Chen MC, Palaniswamy K, Wiser TH, Draelos ZD, et al. J Clin Aesthet Dermatol 2015; 8: 29–35.

A retrospective review of adverse events associated with topical brimonidine demonstrated flushing and erythema as the most commonly reported side effects. These events were described as uncommon and transient.

Second-Line Therapies	
• H_1 and H_2 antihistamines	C
• Clonidine	A
• Selective serotonin reuptake inhibitors	A
• Serotonin–norepinephrine reuptake inhibitors	A

Histamine receptor antagonism of intolerance to alcohol in the Oriental population. Miller NS, Goodwin DW, Jones FC, Pardo MP, Anand MM, Gabrielli WF, et al. J Nerv Mental Dis 1987; 175: 661–7.

Seventeen subjects received placebo, diphenhydramine 50 mg, and cimetidine 300 mg, singly and in combination, 1 hour before drinking ethanol. Cimetidine given alone blocked the flushing significantly more than diphenhydramine alone or placebo but less than the combined antihistamines.

Patients should be screened for alcohol abuse and warned about gastritis and sedation before combination pretreatment consisting of cimetidine and a nonsteroidal is prescribed.

Primary care for survivors of breast cancer. Burstein HJ, Winer EP. N Engl J Med 2000; 343: 1086–94.

A variety of nonestrogenic agents, including selective serotonin reuptake inhibitors, selective serotonin and norepinephrine reuptake inhibitors, and clonidine, are noted to ameliorate hot flushes in breast cancer survivors.

Clonidine patches are frequently associated with contact dermatitis, so the author favors oral clonidine.

Nonhormonal therapies for menopausal hot-flashes. Nelson HD, Vesco KK, Haney E, Fu R, Nedrow A, Miller J, et al. JAMA 2006; 295: 2057–71.

In a review of published randomized controlled trials, there was evidence for the effectiveness of selective serotonin reuptake inhibitors, serotonin–norepinephrine reuptake inhibitors, clonidine, and gabapentin in controlling menopausal hot flashes. However, the efficacy of these nonhormonal treatments was less than that of estrogen.

Treatment strategies for reducing the burden of meno-pause-associated vasomotor symptoms. Umland EM. J Manag Care Pharm 2008; 14: S14–9.

Vasomotor symptoms are reported to be the most bothersome symptoms during menopause. Nonpharmacologic modalities, including relaxation techniques, avoiding overheating, weight loss, exercise, and smoking cessation, may reduce these symptoms.

Third-Line Therapies	
• Somatostatin analogs	E
• Excision for carcinoid tumors	D
• Sympathectomy for severe, refractory blushing	B
• β-Blockers	D
• Topical oxymetazoline	E
• Botulinum toxin	D
• Pulsed dye laser	D
• Ibuprofen gel	B

Treatment of type II gastric carcinoid tumors with soma-tostatin analogs. Tomassetti P, Migliori M, Caletti GC, Fusaroli P, Corinaldesi R, Gullo L. N Engl J Med 2000; 343: 551–4.

This is a report of three patients with multiple type II gastric carcinoids treated with lanreotide or octreotide acetate. In all three patients there was a reduction in size and number of the carcinoid tumors after 6 months of somatostatin analog treatment and complete disappearance of tumors after 1 year. A report of regression of a type III gastric carcinoid with octreotide is also cited.

Management of facial blushing. Licht PB, Pilegaard HK. Thorac Surg Clin 2008; 18: 223–8.

Blushing, specifically facial redness due to emotion and social stress, is discussed in this article. Thorascopic sympathectomy is a surgical treatment option for facial blushing that fails medical management.

Carvedilol for the treatment of refractory facial flushing and persistent erythema of rosacea. Hsu CC, Lee JY. Arch Dermatol 2011; 147: 1258–60.

Although there is a lack of objective laboratory evidence for the direct effects β-blockers have on cutaneous blood vessels during episodes of flushing, fewer symptoms have been observed in patients taking β-blockers. Low-dose carvedilol may be an effective treatment for severe rosacea flushing with less risk of hypotension than traditional β-blockers.

Symptomatic treatment of idiopathic and rosacea-associated cutaneous flushing with propranolol. Craige H, Cohen JB. J Am Acad Dermatol 2005; 53: 881–4.

Eight of nine patients experienced diminished symptoms and flushing episodes while taking various doses of propranolol.

Side effects must be monitored such as hypotension, bradycardia, dizziness, fatigue, somnolence, and sexual dysfunction.

Successful treatment of the erythema and flushing of rosacea using a topically applied selective alpha 1-adrenergic receptor agonist, oxymetazoline. Shanler SD, Ondo AL. Arch Dermatol 2007; 143: 1369–71.

Two patients with treatment-resistant erythrotelangiectatic rosacea experienced improvement in erythema, decrease of erythematous flares (flushing), and symptomatic relief of burning and stinging with once-daily topical oxymetazoline, without rebound flares or tachyphylaxis.

Topical oxymetazoline hydrochloride 1% cream was approved by the FDA in January 2017.

Impact of intradermal abobotulinumtoxinA on facial erythema of rosacea. Bloom BS, Payongayong L, Mourin A, Goldberg DJ. Dermatol Surg 2015; 41: S9–16.

Botulinum toxin injections were both safe and effective at treating the erythema of rosacea.

Idiopathic flushing with dysesthesia: treatment with the 585 nm pulsed dye laser. Fogelman JP, Stevenson ML, Ashinoff R, Soter NA. J Clin Aesthet Dermatol 2015; 8: 36–41.

The 585-nm pulsed dye laser was effective in decreasing dysesthesia symptoms and flushing episodes in patients suffering from idiopathic flushing.

Topical ibuprofen inhibits blushing during embarrassment and facial flushing during aerobic exercise in people with a fear of blushing. Drummond PD, Minosora K, Little G, Keay W. Eur Neuropsychopharmacol 2013; 23: 1747–53.

In this trial 30 subjects applied ibuprofen gel to a small patch on one cheek and the other cheek was used as a control.

Phytoestrogens for vasomotor menopausal symptoms. Lethaby A, Marjoribanks J, Kronenberg F, Roberts H, Eden J, Brown J, et al. Cochrane Database Syst Rev 2007; 4: CD001395.

The current evidence indicates no clinically meaningful effect for phytoestrogens.

Evidence Levels: **A** Double-blind study   **B** Clinical trial ≥ 20 subjects   **C** Clinical trial < 20 subjects   **D** Series ≥ 5 subjects   **E** Anecdotal case reports

Follicular mucinosis

Mary Sommerlad, Malcolm Rustin

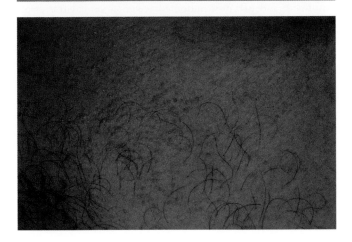

- Consider investigations to rule out lymphoma or other underlying disorders, depending on the presenting clinical features (general examination, plain radiology, and computed tomography [CT] scans)

The cutaneous mucinoses. Truhan AP, Roenigk HH. J Am Acad Dermatol 1986; 14: 1–18.

Follicular mucinosis: a clinicopathologic, histochemical, immunohistochemical and molecular study comparing the primary benign form and the mycosis fungoides-associated follicular mucinosis. Rongioletti F, De Lucchi D, Meyes D, Mora M, Rebora A, Zupo S, et al. J Cutan Pathol 2010; 37: 15–9.

Two excellent reviews of the follicular mucinosis literature, including histopathology and investigation.

Pediatric follicular mucinosis: presentation, histopathology, molecular genetics, treatment and outcomes over an 11-year period at the Mayo Clinic. Alikhan A, Griffin J, Nguyen N, Davis D, Gibson L. Pediatr Dermatol 2013; 30: 192–8.

A review of the clinical and histopathologic findings as well as the treatment and clinical outcomes in children with follicular mucinosis with and without mycosis fungoides.

Follicular mucinosis is characterized histologically by mucinous degeneration of the follicular outer root sheaths and sebaceous glands with an inflammatory infiltrate composed of lymphocytes, histiocytes, and eosinophils. Lesions consist of erythematous, scaly, and infiltrated plaques with follicular papules or prominent follicular orifices and alopecia (alopecia mucinosa). Benign follicular mucinosis tends to affect younger patients (under 40 years), with fewer lesions, usually situated on the head and neck. Although lesions may resolve spontaneously within 2 years, a more generalized form, with lesions on the trunk and extremities, may run a chronic relapsing course over many years. Follicular mucinosis is associated with lymphoma, particularly mycosis fungoides, in 15% to 30% of cases. It is still unclear whether follicular mucinosis is a transitional state evolving into mycosis fungoides in these cases. No single clinical or histologic feature predicts which patients will have a benign course, although those found to have mycosis fungoides rarely had initial lesions on the head and neck. Associated lymphoma tends (not invariably) to be associated with age over 30 years, a wider distribution of lesions, and possibly systemic features such as night sweats, weight loss, or lymphadenopathy.

MANAGEMENT STRATEGY

There is no standard therapy, and because spontaneous resolution occurs in the benign forms, *observation* alone is certainly justified, particularly in the younger patient with limited disease. However, the need for *follow-up and evaluation to exclude lymphoma* must be emphasized. Follicular mucinosis associated with mycosis fungoides or other neoplastic or inflammatory disorders is managed by treating the underlying associated condition.

Specific Investigations

- Skin biopsy
- Immunohistochemistry and T-cell gene receptor analysis may be helpful adjuncts

First-Line Therapies

- Topical and intralesional corticosteroids	**D**
- Dapsone	**E**
- Mepacrine	**E**
- Tetracycline	**E**

Follicular mucinosis: a study of 47 patients. Emmerson RW. Br J Dermatol 1969; 81: 395–413.

Topical or intralesional corticosteroids improved surface eczematous change in 8 of 22 patients with benign disease whose lesions resolved spontaneously, independently of treatment, within 2 years. Six of 10 patients with benign chronic disease of more than 2 years' duration showed slight improvement with topical or intralesional corticosteroids.

Neonatal follicular mucinosis. Dalle S, Marrou K, Balme B, Thomas L. Br J Dermatol 2007; 157: 609–10.

A solitary pink plaque on the occipital scalp of a 21-day-old newborn responded to mild-potency topical corticosteroid with resolution within 2 months.

Urticaria-like follicular mucinosis responding to dapsone. Al Harthi F, Kudwah A, Ajlan A, Nuaim A, Shehri F. Acta Derm Venereol 2003; 83: 389–90.

Itchy urticaria-like papules on the face, chest, and back of a 25-year-old man for 2 years responded to dapsone 100 mg daily long term after previously failing to respond to oral prednisolone. Attempts to reduce the dosage resulted in recurrence.

Atypical follicular mucinosis controlled with mepacrine. Sonnex TS, Ryan T, Dawber RPR. Br J Dermatol 1981; 105: 83–4.

Facial lesions in a 39-year-old man responded to mepacrine 100 mg twice daily. Lesions redeveloped on cessation of therapy.

A case of follicular mucinosis treated successfully with minocycline. Yotsumoto S, Uchimiya H, Kanzaki T. Br J Dermatol 2000; 142: 841–2.

A 36-year-old man presented with itchy papular lesions on his head, neck, and chest. After histologic confirmation of the diagnosis, indomethacin was tried (no time specified) but was not effective. Minocycline 100 mg daily for 6 weeks induced complete remission.

Follicular mucinosis: clinical, histologic and molecular remission with minocycline. Parker S, Murad M. J Am Acad Dermatol 2010; 62: 139–41.

A 28-year-old man with follicular mucinosis and a clonal rearrangement of the T-cell receptor gamma chain gene treated with minocycline 100 mg twice daily for 1 year had clinical, histologic, and molecular remission.

Second-Line Therapies			
• Isotretinoin	E	• Photodynamic therapy	E
• Psoralen and UVA (PUVA)	E	• Hydroxychloroquine	D
• UVA1	E	• Topical tacrolimus	E
• Indomethacin	E	• Topical pimecrolimus	E
• Interferon	E	• Topical bexarotene	E
• Systemic corticosteroids	E	• Topical imiquimod 5%	E
• Superficial radiotherapy	D		

Follicular mucinosis presenting as an acneiform eruption: report of four cases. Wittenberg GP, Gibson LE, Pittelkow MR, el-Azhary RA. J Am Acad Dermatol 1998; 38: 849–51.

Two women under 40 years of age had acneiform facial lesions. One had reduced numbers and size of lesions after tretinoin gel 0.01% daily and oral pentoxifylline 400 mg three times daily, followed 2 years later by isotretinoin 40 mg daily. The second significantly improved after isotretinoin 40 mg daily and intermittent clobetasol cream.

Follicular mucinosis treated with PUVA. Kenicer KJA, Lakshmipathi T. Br J Dermatol 1982; 107: 48–9.

A 79-year-old woman with facial, truncal, and limb papules with no evidence of systemic disease failed to respond to topical corticosteroids and localized radiotherapy (100 Gy over 5 days). After 98 sessions of psoralen and ultraviolet A (PUVA) over 5 months (total dose 45.4 J/cm^2) she remained disease free.

Treatment of idiopathic mucinosis follicularis with UVA1 cold light phototherapy. Von Kobyletzki G, Kreuter JA, Nordmeier R, Stücker M, Altmeyer P. Dermatology 2000; 201: 76–7.

A 26-year-old Caucasian woman with itchy follicular papules on the trunk for 7 months was diagnosed histologically and started on potent corticosteroids with no success. A ultraviolet A1 (UVA1) cold light source (340–530 nm) was used five times a week for 3 weeks and induced remission that had been sustained at 3 months.

Follicular mucinosis: response to indomethacin. Kodama H, Umemura S, Nohara N. J Dermatol 1988; 15: 72–5.

Plaques and papules on the face and back of a 48-year-old man with no signs of cutaneous lymphoma were unresponsive to topical corticosteroids, UVA, or dapsone. Topical indomethacin 1% in white petrolatum was applied until the lesions disappeared. Oral indomethacin 75 mg daily reduced untreated lesions but was not tolerated. The patient was lesion free 5 years later.

Successful treatment of recalcitrant primary follicular mucinosis with indomethacin and low-dose intralesional interferon alpha. Kim KR, Lee JY, Kim MK, Yoon TY. Ann Dermatol 2009; 21: 285–7.

A 52-year-old woman with plaques on both cheeks failed to respond to minocycline, dapsone, topical steroids, and methotrexate. A remarkable improvement was achieved with indomethacin 25 mg twice daily and intralesional corticosteroid administration after 3 months. Intralesional steroids were discontinued, and half-dose indomethacin maintained remission for a further 4 months until lack of availability led to its discontinuation. A rebound flare was controlled with intralesional interferon alpha-2a 3 × 10^6 biweekly for 5 weeks with subsequent increase in the injection interval to four times a week. Complete remission was achieved after 6 months with no recurrence 4 months later.

Acneiform follicular mucinosis. Passaro EMC, Silveira MT, Valente NYS. Clin Exp Dermatol 2004; 29: 396–8.

A 36-year-old man presented with a 1-year history of acneiform follicular mucinosis and was commenced on 40 mg prednisolone for 20 days. His symptoms improved quickly, and the prednisolone was weaned off by day 48. He had been clear for 7 months at the time of writing.

Alopecia mucinosa: a follow-up study. Coskey RJ, Mehregan AH. Arch Dermatol 1970; 102: 193–4.

Patients with one or two facial lesions were given superficial x-ray therapy in a weekly dose of 7.5 Gy for 4 weeks (three cases) or a combination of x-ray therapy and topical corticosteroid cream (six cases). In all cases lesions resolved.

Primary follicular mucinosis: excellent response to treatment with photodynamic therapy. Fernandez-Guarino M, Harto Castano A, Cariilo R. J Eur Acad Dermatol Venereol 2008; 22: 393–404.

A 74-year-old woman with a 4-year history of recalcitrant facial plaques cleared with one session of photodynamic therapy (topical methyl-aminolevulinic acid, red light source, 630 nm, 37 J/cm^2, 7.5 minutes). She had previously been recalcitrant to topical corticosteroids, narrowband ultraviolet B (UVB), and sulfone. She remained clinically clear 9 months post treatment.

Treatment of so-called idiopathic follicular mucinosis with hydroxychloroquine. Schneider SW, Metze D, Bonsmann G. Br J Dermatol 2010; 163: 420–3.

Six patients were treated with hydroxychloroquine 200 mg three times daily for 10 days with subsequent adjustment for weight, usually to 200 mg twice daily. All patients demonstrated clinical improvement within 6 weeks and complete remission within 2 to 5 months with full hair regrowth. Individual patients were observed for 3 to 23 years, and no relapses were seen.

Follicular mucinosis treated with topical 0.1% tacrolimus ointment. Kluk J, Krassilnik N, McBride S. Clin Exp Dermatol 2014; 39: 227–8.

A 36-year-old man treated with topical 0.1% tacrolimus ointment twice daily for lesions affecting the central forehead, upper cheeks, chin, and neck. Dramatic improvement was observed at 10 days. Topical 0.1% tacrolimus ointment was then tapered over 4 weeks, and remission has been maintained at 1 year.

A case of follicular mucinosis treated successfully with pimecrolimus. Gorpelioglu C, Sarifakioglu E, Bayrak R. Clin Exp Dermatol 2008; 34: 86–7.

A 24-year-old man applied topical 1% pimecrolimus twice daily to a plaque on his chin after lack of response to local corticosteroids. Complete remission was achieved within 1 month, and treatment was discontinued. He remained clear at 7 months' follow-up.

A case of idiopathic follicular mucinosis treated with bexarotene gel. Heyl J, Mehregan D, Kado J, Campbell M. Int J Dermatol 2014; 53: 838–41.

A 34-year-old man who had treatment failure with clobetasol 0.05% ointment and narrow-band UVB applied topical bexarotene gel twice daily to affected areas on the shins for 6 weeks and then reduced to once daily due to local erythema (known side effect of bexarotene). Complete hair regrowth on shins at 26 weeks.

Treatment of primary follicular mucinosis with imiquimod 5% cream. Alonso de Celada R, Feito Rodriguez F, Noguero Morel L, Beato Merino M, De Lucas Laguna R. Pediatr Dermatol 2014; 31: 406–8.

A 10-year-old child who had treatment failure with clobetasol propionate applied topical imiquimod 5% daily for 8 weeks, achieving full resolution. Complete remission persists after 3 years of follow-up.

Folliculitis

Chen "Mary" Chen, Robert G. Phelps

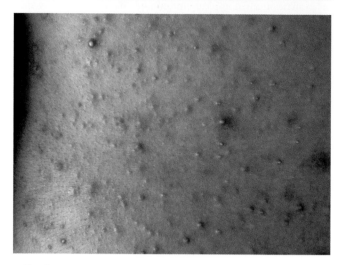

Folliculitis is defined as the inflammation of the pilosebaceous unit. When inflammation is limited to the superficial portion of the follicle, it clinically presents with erythematous papules and pustules. Deeper inflammation manifests with furuncles and abscesses. Etiologic factors include both infectious and noninfectious agents. Bacterial pathogens are the predominant causes of infectious folliculitis; these include gram-positive *Staphylococcus aureus* and gram-negative *Pseudomonas*. Herpes and molluscum cause viral folliculitis, and *Candida* and *Pityrosporum* cause fungal folliculitis. Parasitic folliculitis may be due to *Demodex*, scabies, or larva migrans.

Diagnosis is achieved through identification of the infectious agent, as well as thorough history and physical examination. There should be a high index of suspicion for gram-negative folliculitis in acne patients treated with long-term antibiotics. Exposure to contaminated water in pools or Jacuzzis can lead to folliculitis by *Pseudomonas aeruginosa*. *Pityrosporum* folliculitis, favoring the upper trunk, is more commonly found in hot and humid climates. *Demodex* folliculitis can be seen in rosacea-like lesions on the face with periorificial accentuation. This is common among young pubescent patients but may also be associated with human immunodeficiency virus (HIV) infection or leukemia. Immunocompromised patients, most notably with HIV infection, develop not only widespread folliculocentric lesions caused by bacteria, viruses, or parasites but also a characteristic sterile eosinophilic pustular folliculitis, which is paradoxically related to both immune suppression and reconstitution.

Noninfectious folliculitis may be associated with mechanical factors (friction, occlusion, or trauma), including epilation. Cutting oils and coal tar can cause irritant folliculitis, and sun exposure causes actinic folliculitis. Other associations include rheumatologic disorders (Behçet disease, Reiter syndrome, systemic lupus erythematosus, rheumatoid arthritis, and mixed connective tissue disease), inflammatory bowel disease, lymphoproliferative disease, and pregnancy. Perforating folliculitis is not only associated with diabetes mellitus and renal failure but also with tumor necrosis factor alpha (TNFα) inhibitors (infliximab). Agents responsible for drug-induced folliculitis include epidermal growth factor receptor (EGFR) inhibitors, TNFα inhibitors, trastuzumab, sorafenib, lithium, halogens, and corticosteroids.

MANAGEMENT STRATEGY

Infectious folliculitis is best managed with an optimally directed antimicrobial regimen. Therapeutic options include *antiseptics and topical or systemic antibiotics*. Early coverage for *Staphylococcus aureus* (MRSA) in high-risk populations and areas should be considered. Eosinophilic folliculitis may resolve with topical agents. EGFR inhibitor–induced folliculitis responds well to *tetracyclines*. Noninfectious folliculitis will improve when the precipitant is removed, although the improvement may be delayed for weeks to months. Intramuscular immunoglobulin and photodynamic therapy have been suggested as novel treatment options for refractory folliculitis.

Specific Investigations

- Clinical history, including medication usage, concurrent diseases, sun exposure, and family history
- Bacterial, fungal, or viral culture and polymerase chain reaction (PCR) methods with drug sensitivity testing
- Gram stain, Tzanck smear, potassium hydroxide (KOH) preparation
- Tissue biopsy for histologic examination with microorganism stains
- Complete blood count, workup for immunodeficiencies, blood chemistries, renal function test, HIV status
- Nasal culture in chronic bacterial cases

First-Line Therapies

Topical therapy

Mupirocin, clindamycin, and retapamulin for *S. aureus*	A
Mupirocin for eradication of *S. aureus* colonization of the nares	A
Daily chlorhexidine or tea tree oil soap body wash for recurrent *Staphylococcus* spp.	B
Selenium sulfide shampoo or propylene glycol for *Pityrosporum* spp.	C
Permethrin, ivermectin, or metronidazole for *Demodex* spp.	D
Corticosteroid or tacrolimus for eosinophilic pustular folliculitis	C, D

Oral therapy

Dicloxacillin or cephalexin for methicillin-sensitive *S. aureus* (MSSA)	B
Trimethoprim/sulfamethoxazole, clindamycin, doxycycline, or linezolid for *MRSA*	B
Ciprofloxacin for *Pseudomonas*	C
Ampicillin, trimethoprim/sulfamethoxazole, or ciprofloxacin for gram-negative bacteria	B
Itraconazole or fluconazole for *Pityrosporum* spp.	A
Acyclovir, valacyclovir, or famciclovir for herpes	A
Ivermectin and metronidazole (combination therapy) for *Demodex* spp.	A
Indomethacin or cyclosporin for eosinophilic pustular folliculitis	C
Tetracycline for EGFR inhibitor–induced folliculitis	B

Evidence Levels: A Double-blind study B Clinical trial ≥ 20 subjects C Clinical trial < 20 subjects D Series ≥ 5 subjects E Anecdotal case reports

Facial bacterial infections: folliculitis. Laureano AC, Schwartz RA, Cohen PJ. Clin Dermatol 2014; 32: 711–4.

Dicloxacillin (250–500 mg four times per day) or cephalexin (250–500 mg four times per day) for 7 to 10 days is usually sufficient in eradicating conventional facial folliculitis.

Topical retapamulin ointment, 1%, versus sodium fusidate ointment, 2%, for impetigo: a randomized, observer-blinded, noninferiority study. Oranje AP, Chosidow O, Sacchidanand S, Todd G, Singh K, Scangarella N, et al. Dermatology 2007; 215: 331–40.

Retapamulin was equally efficacious with sodium fusidate in the topical treatment of superficial skin infections.

Practice guidelines for the diagnosis and management of skin and soft tissue infections: 2014 update by the Infectious Diseases Society of America. Infectious Diseases Society of America, Stevens DL, Bisno AL, Chambers HF, Dellinger EP, Goldstein EJ, Gorbach SL, et al. Clin Infect Dis July 15, 2014; 59(2): e10–52.

The expert panel's recommendations include a decolonization regimen of 5 days of topical mupirocin and daily chlorhexidine body washes plus daily decontamination of personal items to prevent recurrences.

Demodex mites: facts and controversies. Elston DM. Clin Dermatol. 2010; 28: 502–4.

Topical permethrin 5% cream, oral ivermectin, and oral metronidazole are reasonable treatments.

Recalcitrant papulopustular rosacea in an immunocompetent patient responding to combination therapy with oral ivermectin and topical permethrin. Kallen KJ, Davis CL, Billings SD, Mousdicas N. Cutis 2007; 80: 149–51.

Resolution of the folliculitis was noted with treatment combination of 5% permethrin and ivermectin.

Successful treatment of eosinophilic pustular folliculitis with topical tacrolimus 0.1% ointment. Ng SS, Tay YK. Dermatol Online J 2012; 18: 10.

Folliculitis in a patient showed improvement with twice-daily application of 0.1% tacrolimus ointment for 2 weeks. Complete resolution was noted after 1 month.

Community-acquired methicillin-resistant *Staphylococcus aureus* skin infections: implications for patients and practitioners. Cohen PR. Am J Clin Dermatol 2007; 8: 259–70.

A 10- to 14-day course of oral trimethoprim/sulfamethoxazole (1–2 tablets twice daily), clindamycin (300–450 mg four times per day), or doxycycline (100 mg twice daily) is most useful.

Treatment of methicillin-resistant *staphylococcus aureus* (MRSA) soft tissue infections: an overview. Morgan M. Injury, Int. J. Care Injured 2011; 42: S11–7.

Suggested antimicrobials for folliculitis include cotrimoxazole, clindamycin, doxycycline, linezolid, rifampicin, and fusidic acid.

Folliculitis: recognition and management. Luelmo-Aguilar J, Santandreu MS. Am J Clin Dermatol 2004; 5: 301–10.

Pseudomonas folliculitis can resolves within 7 to 10 days with good skin hygiene and avoidance of contaminated water. Oral ciprofloxacin (250–750 mg twice daily) can be used for severe cases or immunocompromised patients.

Short-term treatment of pityrosporum folliculitis: a double blind placebo-controlled study. Parsad D, Saini R, Negi KS. J Eur Acad Dermatol Venereol 1998; 11: 188–90.

A randomized trial showed remarkable response to itraconazole (200 mg per day for 7 days) compared with placebo in 26 patients after 5 weeks.

Evidence-based Danish guidelines for the treatment of *Malassezia*-related skin diseases. Hald M, Arendrup MC, Svejgaard EL, Lindskov R, Foged EK, Saunte DM. Acta Derm Venereol 2015; 95: 12–9.

Despite the greater evidence for efficacy of itraconazole, oral fluconazole is still more used due to its more favorable side effect profile and lower risk for drug interactions.

Evaluation of the efficacy of oral ivermectin in comparison with ivermectin-metronidazole combined therapy in the treatment of ocular and skin lesions of *Demodex folliculorum*. Salem DA, El-Shazly A, Nabih N, El-Bayoumy Y, Saleh S. Int J Infect Dis 2013; 17: e343.

In this trial of 120 patients with skin lesions and blepharitis, combination therapy with oral ivermectin and oral metronidazole was more effective for reducing mite counts than oral ivermectin monotherapy.

Therapeutic effectiveness of various treatments for eosinophilic pustular folliculitis. Fukamachi S, Kabashima K, Sugita K, Kobayashi M, Tokura Y. Acta Derm Venereol 2009; 89: 155–9.

Oral cyclosporin was highly effective, as was indomethacin, in alleviating the folliculitis of 11 patients.

Folliculitis induced by epidermal growth factor receptor (EGFR) inhibitors, preventive and curative efficacy of tetracyclines in the management and incidence rates according to the type of EGFR inhibitor administered. Bachet JP, Peuvrel L, Bachmeyer C, Reguiai Z, Gourraud PA, Bouché O, et al. Oncologist 2012; 17: 555–68.

A tetracycline (doxycycline 200 mg/day) should be prophylactically prescribed together with an EGFR inhibitor to prevent folliculitis.

Second-Line Therapies	
Antimicrobial therapies	
• Topical fusidic acid for *S. aureus*	A
• Topical benzoyl peroxide washes and bleach baths for recurrent *Staphylococcus*	B
• Oral tigecycline and vancomycin for MRSA	A
Other treatment modalities	
• Intramuscular immunoglobulin	B
• Photodynamic therapy	D

High usage of topical fusidic acid and rapid clonal expansion of fusidic acid-resistant *Staphylococcus aureus*: a cautionary tale. Williamson DA, Monecke S, Heffernan H, Ritchie SR, Roberts SA, Upton A, et al. Clin Infect Dis 2014; 59: 1451.

Topical fusidic acid was once a first-line treatment option, but increasing resistance of *S. aureus* to fusidic acid has been observed, and the drug is not as readily available in the United States.

Efficacy and safety of tigecycline compared with vancomycin or linezolid for treatment of serious infections with methicillin-resistant *Staphylococcus aureus* or vancomycin-resistant *Enterococci*: a Phase III, multicenter, double-blind,

randomized study. Florescu I, Beuran M, Dimov R, Razbadauskas A, Bochan M, Fichev G, et al. J Antimicrob Chemother 2008; 62(Suppl 1): i17–28.

Tigecycline and vancomycin showed similar clinical cure rates in patients with skin and skin structure infections caused by MRSA.

Intramuscular immunoglobulin for recalcitrant suppurative diseases of the skin: a retrospective review of 63 cases. Goo B, Chung HJ, Chung WG, Chung KY. Br J Dermatol 2007; 157: 563–8.

Intramuscular human immunoglobulin injections reduced the severity and the appearance of new lesions in patients with intractable suppurative skin diseases, including folliculitis.

Topical methyl aminolevulinate photodynamic therapy for the treatment of folliculitis. Horn M, Wolf P. Photodermatol Photoimmunol Photomed 2007; 23: 145–7.

Six of seven patients with recalcitrant folliculitis had significant reduction in inflammation with one session of methyl aminolevulinate photodynamic therapy.

Evidence Levels: **A** Double-blind study **B** Clinical trial ≥ 20 subjects **C** Clinical trial < 20 subjects **D** Series ≥ 5 subjects **E** Anecdotal case reports

86

Folliculitis decalvans

Nekma Meah, Matthew Harries

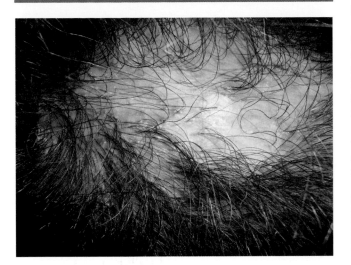

Folliculitis decalvans (FD) is a rare, neutrophilic, inflammatory scalp condition presenting as single or multiple areas of alopecia associated with pustule formation, erythema, and increased scale with "tufted" hair follicles evident at the edge of the scarring hair loss patch. Folliculitis decalvans can involve any areas of the scalp, although the vertex and occiput are most commonly affected and nonscalp involvement is uncommon. Folliculitis decalvans tends to run a chronic, progressive course. Multivariate analysis from one large retrospective case series suggests that onset at <25 years of age and presence of pustules are independently associated with severe disease.

The condition can occur in either sex but has a predilection for adult men. Frequent isolation of *Staphylococcus aureus* from lesional skin and observed improvement with anti-staphylococcal therapy has implicated this bacterium in disease development, perhaps through an abnormal host response in genetically susceptible individuals. However, recent identification of non-staphylococcal bacterial biofilms deeper in lesional hair follicles may suggest alternative microbial factors contributing to disease activity.

MANAGEMENT STRATEGY

The main aim of treatment in FD is to arrest the inflammatory process and prevent extension of alopecia. Initial investigations should exclude other conditions known to mimic FD (e.g., tinea capitis). A bacteriology swab from lesional skin is advised to determine culture and sensitivity as bacterial resistance is common. Nasal staphylococcal eradication should also be considered in confirmed carriers.

There are no reported randomized controlled trials for treatment in FD. Efficacy data are available from case reports, case series, and small studies only. *Systemic antibiotics* remain the mainstay of initial therapy, although relapses are common on stopping treatment. The combination of oral *rifampicin and clindamycin* administered as a 10-week course has been shown to reduce activity and induce remission and as such is regarded

by many as the most effective treatment for FD. *Rifampicin* monotherapy is not advised due to the risk of developing drug resistance.

Dapsone at a dose of 75 to 100 mg may also produce a satisfactory outcome, with low-dose maintenance therapy required to sustain remission. Oral *isotretinoin* is another potentially effective treatment reported to have lower relapse rates than antibiotics on treatment cessation. *Oral zinc sulfate,* as monotherapy or combined with *fusidic acid,* is also suggested in FD.

Topical, intralesional, and *oral corticosteroids* are adjunctive therapies that can temporarily suppress inflammation, although side effects preclude long-term use. Topical *tacrolimus ointment, photodynamic therapy,* and *human immunoglobulin therapy* may also be effective. More recently, the anti-TNF agents *adalimumab* and *infliximab* have been successfully used in patients with severe recalcitrant disease.

In those unresponsive to medical therapy surgical interventions, such as *scalp excision, laser epilation* or superficial *radiotherapy* may be considered to permanently epilate the scalp, thereby removing the inflammatory focus of the condition.

Specific Investigations

- Scalp skin swab for bacteriology
- Nasal swab for bacteriology
- Scrapings and plucked hairs for mycology
- Scalp biopsy
- Consider immunodeficiency screen

How not to get scar(r)ed: a guide to diagnosis in primary cicatricial alopecias. Harries MJ, Trueb R, Messenger A, Tosti A, Chaudhry I, Sinclair R, et al. Br J Dermatol 2009; 160: 482–501.

A systematic approach is presented to accurately diagnose scarring alopecias, including FD.

Tinea capitis mimicking folliculitis decalvans. Tangjaturonrusamee C, Piraccini BM, Vincenzi C, Starace M, Tosti A. Mycoses 2011; 54: 87–8.

A case of tinea capitis caused by *Microsporum canis* mimicking FD.

Folliculitis decalvans and cellular immunity – 2 brothers with oral candidiasis. Shitara A, Igareshi R, Morohashi M. Jpn J Dermatol 1974; 28: 133.

Severe FD in two siblings who also had chronic oral candidiasis; defective cell-mediated immunity was demonstrated.

First-Line Therapies

Topical antibiotics	
• Fusidic acid, clindamycin, erythromycin, mupirocin	E
Systemic antibiotics	
• Rifampicin and clindamycin	C
• Tetracycline antibiotics, flucloxacillin, and third-generation cephalosporins	C
• Azithromycin	D

Management of primary cicatricial alopecias: options for treatment. Harries MJ, Sinclair RD, MacDonald-Hull S, Whiting DA, Griffiths CE, Paus R. Br J Dermatol 2008; 159: 1–22.

A thorough evidence-based review on the range of treatment options for primary cicatricial alopecias.

Folliculitis decalvans: a multicentre review of 82 patients. Vañó-Galván S, Molina-Ruiz AM, Fernández-Crehuet P, Rodrigues-Barata AR, Arias-Santiago S, Serrano-Falcón C, et al. J Eur Acad Dermatol Venereol 2015; 29: 1750–7.

A retrospective review of 82 patients with FD. Ninety percent to 100% of patients on either oral doxycycline 100 mg daily, azithromycin 500 mg three times a daily, or combination of clindamycin and rifampicin demonstrated improvement.

Effective treatment of folliculitis decalvans using selected antimicrobial agents. Sillani C, Bin Z, Ying Z, Zeming C, Jian Y, Xingqi Z. Int J Trichology 2010; 2: 20–3.

Thirteen patients with mild to moderate FD. Minocycline 100 mg twice daily as monotherapy was effective in six patients, with a further three patients responding to minocycline and rifampicin in combination.

Folliculitis decalvans including tufted folliculitis: clinical, histological and therapeutic findings. Powell JJ, Dawber RPR, Gatter K. Br J Dermatol 1999; 140: 328–33.

Eighteen patients with folliculitis decalvans were treated with oral rifampicin 300 mg twice daily and oral clindamycin 300 mg twice daily combination for 10 weeks. All patients reported improvement during treatment, with 10 patients achieving a lasting remission.

Second-Line Therapies	
• Fusidic acid and oral zinc sulfate	E
• Dapsone	E
• Systemic/intralesional corticosteroids	D
• Isotretinoin	D

Folliculitis decalvans. Long-lasting response to combined therapy with fusidic acid and zinc. Abeck D, Korting HC, Braun-Falco O. Acta Derm Venereol 1992; 72: 143–5.

Three patients responded to oral fusidic acid (500 mg three times a day) and topical fusidic acid cream for 3 weeks combined with oral zinc sulfate 200 mg twice a day for 6 months and once a day thereafter. Disease relapse coincided with stopping zinc sulfate.

Dapsone treatment of folliculitis decalvans. Paquet P, Pierard GE. Ann Dermatol Venereol 2004; 131: 195–7.

Two patients treated with dapsone 75 to 100 mg daily showed clinical response 1 to 2 months into treatment. A maintenance dose of 25 mg daily resulted in sustained remission.

Retrospective review of folliculitis decalvans in 23 patients with course and treatment analysis of long-standing cases. Bunagan MJ, Banka N, Shapiro J. J Cutan Med Surg 2015; 19: 45–9

The combination of oral tetracycline, intralesional triamcinolone every 4 to 6 weeks, and clobetasol lotion resulted in remission in 7 out of 10 patients on this regimen.

Oral isotretinoin as the most effective treatment in folliculitis decalvans: a retrospective comparison of different treatment regimens in 28 patients. Tietze JK, Heppt MV, von Preußen A, Wolf U, Ruzicka T, Wolff H, et al. J Eur Acad Dermatol Venereol 2015; 29: 1816–21.

Nine of 10 patients receiving oral isotretinoin (0.2–0.5 mg/kg daily for 5–7 months followed by 10 mg daily two to three times a week) achieved complete remission. Three patients required low-dose isotretinoin long term.

Third-Line Therapies	
• Surgical excision	E
• Shaving of scalp	E
• Superficial radiotherapy	E
• Laser epilation	E
• Oral L-tyrosine	E
• Tacrolimus 0.1% ointment	E
• Keratolytics and tar shampoo	E
• Anti–TNF-α therapy	E
• Immunoglobulin therapy	E
• Photodynamic therapy	C

Tufted hair folliculitis. Tong AK, Baden HP. J Am Acad Dermatol 1989; 21: 1096–9.

Tufted folliculitis successfully treated by surgical excision.

Treatment of folliculitis decalvans using intensity-modulated radiation via tomotherapy. Elsayad K, Kriz J, Haverkamp U, Plachouri KM, Jeskowiak A, Sunderkötter C, et al. Strahlenther Onkol 2015; 191: 883–8.

A case of recalcitrant FD responding to 11 Gy delivered in two radiation series.

Nd:YAG laser treatment of recalcitrant folliculitis decalvans. Parlette EC, Kroeger N, Ross EV. Dermatol Surg 2004; 30: 1152–4.

Remission achieved with laser epilation in a patient with Fitzpatrick skin type VI.

Treatment of folliculitis decalvans with tacrolimus ointment. Bastida J, Valeron-Almazan P, Santana-Molina N, Medina-Gil C. Int J Dermatol 2012; 51: 216–20.

Tacrolimus 0.1% ointment applied twice daily in four patients with recalcitrant disease. A favorable outcome was achieved in all four cases.

Successful use of infliximab in a patient with recalcitrant folliculitis decalvans. Mihaljevic N, von den Driesch P. J Dtsch Dermatol Ges 2012; 10: 589–92.

Treatment with infliximab (5 mg/kg) resulted in rapid remission in a patient with treatment-resistant FD. No relapse occurred in the 12-month follow-up period.

Therapy-resistant folliculitis decalvans and lichen planopilaris successfully treated with adalimumab. Kreutzer K, Effendy I. J Dtsch Dermatol Ges 2014; 12: 74–6.

Two patients with FD responded well to adalimumab 40 mg administered fortnightly. Marked improvement was noted after 8 to 12 weeks.

Intramuscular immunoglobulin for recalcitrant suppurative diseases of the skin: a retrospective review of 63 cases. Goo B, Chung HJ, Chung WG, Chung KY. Br J Dermatol 2007; 157: 563–8.

Three patients with FD were rated to a have a "good response" after intramuscular human immunoglobulin administered once a month.

Intravenous human immunoglobulin for treatment of folliculitis decalvans. Ismail N, Ralph N, Murphy G. J Dermatol Treat 2015; 26: 471–2.

Evidence Levels: **A** Double-blind study **B** Clinical trial ≥ 20 subjects **C** Clinical trial < 20 subjects **D** Series ≥ 5 subjects **E** Anecdotal case reports

Intravenous human immunoglobulin (2 g/kg for the first month, followed by 1 g/kg for the second to fourth months) resulted in clinical improvement.

Treatment of folliculitis decalvans with photodynamic therapy: results in 10 patients. Miguel-Gomez L, Vano-Galvan S, Perez-Garcia B, Carrillo-Gijon R, Jaen-Olasolo P. J Am Acad Dermatol 2015; 72: 1085–7.

Prospective study of topical photodynamic therapy delivered every 4 weeks. Nine patients (90%) achieved clinical improvement at 16 weeks.

Fox–Fordyce disease

Ian Coulson

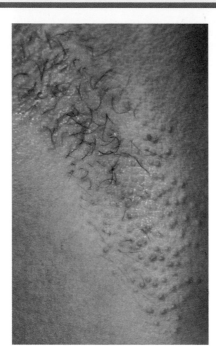

Obliteration of the follicular infundibulum with keratin in the apocrine gland–bearing skin is the cause of this rare, paroxysmally intensely itchy condition. Apocrine sweat retention and rupture of the gland duct under periods of apocrine sudomotor stimulation, particularly emotional stress, results in the development of an itchy, spongiotic intraepidermal vesicle. It mainly affects women between the ages of 13 and 35 years but has rarely been reported before puberty, after menopause, and in men. Itchy, dome-shaped, flesh-colored or keratotic papules that develop peripubertally in the apocrine areas of the axillae, pubic, periumbilical, and periareolar skin characterize this condition. Sparsity of axillary hair and hypohidrosis is usual, although rarely it can be exacerbated by hyperhidrosis. Improvement in pregnancy and during the administration of the oral contraceptive pill has led to speculation regarding an endocrine etiology, but this has been unsubstantiated by blood sex hormone investigations. Very few reports in twins and within families suggest a possible genetic component. It can occur after laser hair removal and has been reported in Turner syndrome.

MANAGEMENT STRATEGY

There are no controlled trials of any agents in Fox–Fordyce disease (FFD).

Topical and intralesional corticosteroids are frequently tried and may be of limited benefit, but atrophy in the axillary area will limit their potency and duration of use. Topical *tretinoin and adapalene* have been reported to reduce itch, but alternation with a mild corticosteroid may be needed to reduce retinoid irritancy. *Clindamycin* lotion may be of help. The *oral contraceptive pill (OCP)* may bring relief to some women. Oral *isotretinoin* may give temporary help. *Electrocautery* and *excision* of the periareolar skin may offer permanent solutions. A recent report advocates an ingenious method of removal of the apocrine glands using a microliposuction cannula. There is a single report of axillary disease responding to intralesional botulinum toxin injection.

Specific Investigation

- Biopsy

Fox–Fordyce disease: diagnosis by transverse histologic sections. Stashower ME, Krivda SJ, Turiansky GW. J Am Acad Dermatol 2000; 42: 89–91.

Transverse sectioning demonstrates the follicular plugging and infundibular spongiosis more readily than conventional sections.

Patterns histopathologic of Fox–Fordyce disease. Böer A. Am J Dermatopathol 2004; 26: 482–92.

An exhaustive review of the subtleties of the dermatopathology of Fox–Fordyce disease.

Dilation of apocrine glands. A forgotten but helpful histopathological clue to the diagnosis of axillary Fox-Fordyce disease. Macarenco RS, Garces S JC. Am J Dermatopathol 2009; 31: 393–7.

Apocrine gland dilation may be used as a low-power magnification clue, which should be followed by a search for further histologic changes to confirm or rule out the diagnosis.

Clinicopathological study of Fox-Fordyce disease. Kao PH, Hsu CK, Lee JY. J Dermatol 2009; 36: 485–90.

Focal spongiosis in the upper infundibulum with perifollicular fibrosis and lymphohistiocytic infiltrate were consistent features in their case series.

Axillary perifollicular xanthomatosis resembling Fox–Fordyce disease. Kossard S, Dwyer P. Australas J Dermatol 2004; 45: 146–8.

Fox-Fordyce-like disease following laser hair removal appearing on all treated areas. Helou J, Maatouk I, Moutran R, Obeid G. Lasers Med Sci 2013; 28: 1205–7.

The most recent of reports highlighting that laser epilation in several anatomic sites may induce FFD.

Perifollicular xanthomatosis as a key histologic finding in Fox–Fordyce disease. Mataix J, Silvestre JF, Niveiro M, Lucas A, Pérez-Crespo M. Actas Dermosifiliogr 2008; 99: 145–8.

There are occasional conditions to consider in the differential diagnosis! There is even controversy as to whether perifollicular xanthomatosis is part of the spectrum of this disorder.

First-Line Therapies

• Topical and intralesional corticosteroids	D
• Topical clindamycin	E
• Oral contraceptive pill	D
• Topical retinoids	D
• Ultraviolet B (UVB)	D
• Topical pimecrolimus and tacrolimus	D

Evidence Levels: A Double-blind study B Clinical trial ≥ 20 subjects C Clinical trial < 20 subjects D Series ≥ 5 subjects E Anecdotal case reports

A new treatment of Fox–Fordyce disease. Helfamn RJ. South Med J 1962; 55: 681–4.

A single report of successful symptom relief of axillary lesions with 10 mg/mL triamcinolone diluted with an equal volume of 1% lidocaine to four sites on nine occasions over 3 months.

Fox–Fordyce disease – successful treatment with topical clindamycin in alcoholic propylene glycol solution. Feldmann R, Masouye I, Chavaz P, Saurat JH. Dermatology 1992; 184: 310–3.

A single report of FFD in the axillary, pubic, and inguinal areas responding to 1% clindamycin in an alcoholic propylene glycol solution within 1 month (clindamycin 10 mg/mL; propylene glycol 50 mg/mL; isopropyl alcohol 0.5 mg/mL; water). Nine months later the treatment was stopped, and no recurrence was observed. The authors speculate that the keratolytic effect of propylene glycol may have been responsible for the therapeutic effect.

Fox–Fordyce disease. Treatment with an oral contraceptive. Kronthal HI, Pomeranz JR, Sitomer G. Arch Dermatol 1965; 91: 243–5.

Two female patients responded to a high-estrogen-dose combined OCP, norethynodrel, and mestranol.

Fox–Fordyce disease. Control with tretinoin cream. Giacobetti R, Caro WA, Roenigk HH Jr. Arch Dermatol 1979; 115: 1365–6.

A single report of 0.1% tretinoin cream applied to the axillae on alternate nights resulting in reduction of itch and regrowth of hair. Local retinoid irritation was controlled with 1% hydrocortisone cream.

Fox-Fordyce disease: response to adapalene 0.1%. Kassuga LE, Medrado MM, Chevrand NS, Salles Sde A, Vilar EG. An Bras Dermatol 2012; 87: 329–31.

0.1% adapalene cream produced satisfactory improvement of the signs and symptoms of a single patient with FFD. In acne, this product is less irritating than tretinoin, so it may be a more tolerable topical retinoid option.

Treatment of Fox–Fordyce disease. Pinkus H. JAMA 1973; 223: 924.

Erythemogenic doses of UVB (once weekly for 4–6 weeks) produced long-lasting relief to several patients.

Pimecrolimus is effective in Fox–Fordyce disease. Pock L, Svrcková M, Macháčková R, Hercogová J. Int J Dermatol 2006; 45: 1134–5.

A series of three patients who benefited from topical pimecrolimus.

Clinical effects of topical tacrolimus on Fox-Fordyce disease. Kaya Erdoğan H, Bulur I, Kaya Z. Case Rep Dermatol Med 2015: 205418.

Two case reports, one with a successful response in terms of itch, from twice-daily 0.1% tacrolimus ointment applied for 3 months.

The treatment of Fox–Fordyce disease. Shelley WB. JAMA 1972; 222: 1069.

A concise review of the therapies available to that date. The master of dermatologic therapy admits that sometimes all fails and that relief may only come at menopause!

Second-Line Therapies	
• Oral isotretinoin	E
• Electrocautery	D
• Excision	D
• Apocrine gland removal using microliposuction	E
• Botulinum toxin	E

Fox–Fordyce disease in a male patient – response to oral retinoid treatment. Effendy I, Ossowski B, Happle R. Clin Exp Dermatol 1994; 19: 67–9.

Oral treatment with isotretinoin (30 mg daily for 8 weeks and then 15 mg daily for 2 months) resulted in temporary relief. Relapse occurred 3 months after discontinuation.

Fox–Fordyce disease in the postmenopausal period treated successfully with electrocoagulation. Pasricha JS, Nayyar KC. Dermatologica 1973; 147: 271–3.

Electrocoagulation to a level of 3 to 4 mm under local anesthetic produced a permanent resolution of symptoms in the axillae of two patients.

Surgical treatment of areolar hidradenitis suppurativa and Fox–Fordyce disease. Chavoin J-P, Charasson T, Barnard J-D. Ann Chir Plast Esthet 1994; 39: 233–8.

A simple technique involving dermal detachment of the areola, excision of the underlying apocrine glands, and reattachment of the areola with good cosmetic results.

This treatment has not proved beneficial long term.

Axillary Fox–Fordyce disease treated with liposuction-assisted curettage. Chae KM, Marschall MA, Marschall SF. Arch Dermatol 2002; 138: 452–4.

A novel technique of curettage removal of the apocrine glands using a small liposuction cannula with symptom relief, great cosmesis, and a follow-up at publication of 8 months. A liposuction cannula was introduced through a stab incision in the axilla and, with the aperture of the cannula turned up toward the underside of the dermis, the deeper dermis was curetted to create inflammation and subsequent fibrosis. The same technique can be used to treat axillary hyperhidrosis.

Successful treatment of refractory pruritic Fox-Fordyce disease with botulinum toxin type A. González-Ramos J, Alonso-Pacheco ML, Goiburú-Chenú B, Mayor-IbargurenA, Herranz-Pinto P. Br J Dermatol 2016; 174: 458–9.

A single case report of a woman receiving 100 U of Botox to each axilla; itching completely abated and papules partially regressed, and the response was sustained over 8 months of follow-up after a single treatment.

Furunculosis

Charles A. Gropper, Karthik Krishnamurthy

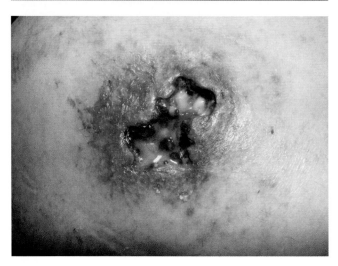

Furunculosis, commonly referred to as *boils,* is a deep infection of the pilosebaceous unit. Lesions may occur on any hair-bearing surface, including the nares. When many hair follicles are involved, the term *carbuncle* is used. These large, suppurative lesions are usually very tender and may have multiple draining sites.

MANAGEMENT STRATEGY

The infectious agent most commonly implicated is *Staphylococcus aureus;* methicillin-resistant strains of *S. aureus* (MRSA) are now recognized as the dominant isolate overall. In recent years, the designations of community-acquired MRSA (CA-MRSA) versus hospital-acquired MRSA (HA-MRSA) have become blurred due to a convergence in both antibiotic susceptibility profiles and risk of sequelae. Delay in diagnosis and appropriate therapy can lead to systemic involvement, including rare reports of epidural abscess, bacterial endocarditis, and pulmonary infection.

Other culprits such as group A beta-hemolytic *Streptococcus* and gram-negative bacteria should remain in the differential diagnosis. In addition, *Mycobacterium* spp., especially *M. fortuitum,* have been implicated in nonresponsive furunculosis in patients using footbaths in beauty salons.

Nasal, pharyngeal, axillary, perineal, and rectal pathogen carriage is implicated in recurrent disease. In rare cases, patients with impaired neutrophil function and immunodeficiency syndromes, such as common variable immunodeficiency and hyper-IgE syndrome, also present with recurrent furunculosis.

Isolated lesions should be *incised and drained.* Multiple, mostly observational, studies indicate high postsurgical cure rates (85%–90%) whether or not an active antibiotic is used. Therefore according to the Centers for Disease Control (2006) and Infectious Diseases Society of America (2011), empiric antibiotics should be reserved for those with

- Severe or extensive disease (e.g., involving multiple sites of infection)
- Rapid progression in presence of associated cellulitis
- Signs and symptoms of systemic illness
- Associated comorbidities/immunosuppression (diabetes mellitus, human immunodeficiency virus, neoplasm)
- Extremes of age
- Abscess in area difficult to drain completely (e.g., face, hand, and genitalia)
- Associated septic phlebitis
- Lack of response to incision and drainage alone

Swabs of any purulent discharge should be collected for bacterial culture; antibiotic therapy may be redirected based on sensitivities and clinical scenario. Acid-fast staining and culture may be warranted if a temporal relationship to a pedicure is noted. Currently, antibiotics carrying a Food and Drug Administration (FDA) indication for use against MRSA include *linezolid, ceftaroline* ("advanced"-generation cephalosporin), *telavancin* (similar to vancomycin), *tigecycline* (derivative of minocycline), and *teicoplanin.* These are mainly reserved for complicated infections requiring hospitalization. Other antibiotics with anti-MRSA activity include *trimethoprim/sulfamethoxazole (TMP-SX), daptomycin, vancomycin, doxycycline, minocycline, clindamycin, rifampin,* and *quinupristin–dalfopristin.* Evidence of nasal carriage of staphylococci should be sought in those with recurrent disease and eradicated with either *oral rifampicin (not as monotherapy)* or *nasal mupirocin or fusidic acid.*

Specific Investigations

- Culture and sensitivity of purulent drainage
- Acid-fast stain and culture (if indicated)
- Moistened nasal swab for culture (if recurrent)
- Neutrophil count and immunoglobulin levels (if relevant and/or recurrent)

First-Line Therapy

- Surgery: incision and drainage   **A**

Randomized, double-blind, placebo-controlled trial of cephalexin for treatment of uncomplicated skin abscesses in a population at risk for community-acquired methicillin-resistant *Staphylococcus aureus* infection. Rajendran PM, Young D, Maurer T, Chambers H, Perdreau-Remington F, Ro P, et al. Antimicrob Agents Chemother 2007; 51: 4044–8.

Randomized, double-blind trial of 166 outpatient subjects comparing placebo to cephalexin at 500 mg orally four times daily for 7 days after incision and drainage of skin and soft tissue abscesses. The primary outcome was clinical cure or failure 7 days after incision and drainage. Of the isolates tested 87.8% were MRSA. Clinical cure rates were 90.5% (95% confidence interval [CI], 0.82–0.96) in the 84 placebo recipients and 84.1% (95% CI, 0.74–0.91) in the 82 cephalexin recipients (difference in the two proportions, 0.0006; 95% CI, −0.0461–0.0472; $p = 0.25$). Provides strong evidence that antibiotics may be unnecessary after surgical drainage of uncomplicated skin and soft tissue abscesses caused by community strains of MRSA.

Evidence Levels: **A** Double-blind study   **B** Clinical trial ≥ 20 subjects   **C** Clinical trial < 20 subjects   **D** Series ≥ 5 subjects   **E** Anecdotal case reports

Second-Line Therapies

- Doxycycline or minocycline   B
- Trimethoprim/sulfamethoxazole   B
- Clindamycin   B
- Linezolid   B

Adjunctive for patients meeting criteria listed in the "Management Strategy" section.

Clinical practice guidelines by the Infectious Diseases Society of America for the treatment of methicillin-resistant *Staphylococcus aureus* infections in adults and children: executive summary. Liu C, Bayer A, Cosgrove SE, Daum RS, Fridkin SK, Gorwitz RJ, et al. Clin Infect Dis 2011; 52: 285–92.

Oral antibiotics that may be used as empiric therapy for CA-MRSA include TMP-SMX, doxycycline (or minocycline), clindamycin, and linezolid. Several observational studies and one small randomized trial suggest that TMP-SMX, doxycycline, and minocycline are effective for such infections. Clindamycin is effective in children with CA-MRSA skin and soft tissue infection (SSTI). Linezolid is FDA-approved for SSTI but is not superior to less expensive alternatives.

Tetracyclines as an oral treatment option for patients with community onset skin and soft tissue infections caused by methicillin-resistant *Staphylococcus aureus*. Ruhe JJ, Menon A. Antimicrob Agents Chemother 2007; 51: 3298–303.

Retrospective study of 276 outpatients. The median percentage of patients infected with MRSA strains that were susceptible to tetracycline was 95%. A total of 225 patients (80%) underwent incision and drainage. Doxycycline or minocycline was administered in 90 episodes (32%); the other 192 SSTI were treated with beta-lactams. Receipt of beta-lactam antibiotics was associated with treatment failure.

Prevalence, severity, and treatment of community-acquired methicillin-resistant *Staphylococcus aureus* (CA-MRSA) skin and soft tissue infections in 10 medical clinics in Texas: a South Texas Ambulatory Research Network (STARNet) study. Forcade NA, Parchman ML, Jorgensen JH, Du LC, Nyren NR, Treviño LB, et al. J Am Board Fam Med 2011; 24: 543–50.

Ten primary care clinics took part in this prospective, community-based study. Overall, 73 of 119 (61%) patients presenting with SSTIs meeting eligibility requirements had CA-MRSA. Most received incision and drainage plus an antibiotic (64%). Antibiotic monotherapy was frequently prescribed: TMP-SMX (78%), clindamycin (4%), doxycycline (2%), and mupirocin (2%). The rest received TMP-SMX in combination with other antibiotics. Isolates were 93% susceptible to clindamycin and 100% susceptible to TMP-SMX, doxycycline, vancomycin, and linezolid.

Trimethoprim-sulfamethoxazole or clindamycin for treatment of community-acquired methicillin-resistant *Staphylococcus aureus* skin and soft tissue infections. Hyun DY, Mason EO, Forbes A, Kaplan SL. Pediatr Infect Dis J 2009; 28: 57–9.

A retrospective study of 508 patients who had MRSA isolated either from surgically obtained drainage or from spontaneous drainage of the infection site; 215 patients were prescribed oral TMP-SMX therapy, and 200 were prescribed oral clindamycin. No significant differences were observed in the percentage who returned because of worsening or incomplete resolution. Most of the patients had incision and drainage (94% of TMP–SMX patients, 86% of clindamycin patients) so results may more likely reflect improvement from incision and drainage than antibiotic choice.

Third-Line Therapies/Prevention

- Topical nadifloxacin   B
- Nasal mupirocin   B
- Bleach bath   E
- Colonization with less pathogenic staphylococci   E
- Retapamulin   E
- Fusidic acid   B

Efficacy and safety of nadifloxacin for bacterial skin infections: results from clinical and postmarketing studies. Narayanan V, Motlekar S, Kadhe G, Bhagat S. Dermatol Ther 2014; 4: 233–48.

A total of 272 subjects were enrolled in the study, and subjects were randomly assigned to one of the three treatment groups: 92 in the nadifloxacin group, 90 in the mupirocin group, and 90 in the framycetin group. A significant reduction in the mean scores for bacterial infection symptoms in the nadifloxacin groups was observed compared with the mupirocin, framycetin, and fusidic acid groups. No adverse events (AEs) were reported in the clinical studies.

Randomized controlled trial of chlorhexidine gluconate for washing, intranasal mupirocin, and rifampin and doxycycline versus no treatment for the eradication of methicillin-resistant *Staphylococcus aureus* colonization. Simor AE, Phillips E, McGeer A, Konvalinka A, Loeb M, Devlin HR, et al. Clin Infect Dis 2007; 44: 178–85.

Treatment with this regimen for 7 days was safe and effective in eradicating MRSA colonization in hospitalized patients for at least 3 months.

Hypochlorite killing of community-associated methicillin-resistant *Staphylococcus aureus*. Fisher RG, Chain RL, Hair PS, Cunnion KM. Pediatr Infect Dis J 2008; 27: 934–5.

In vitro study of hypochlorite (bleach) against CA-MRSA. Maximal killing was found after 5 minutes in 2.5 µL/mL bleach. A 2.5-µL/mL bleach solution is approximately equivalent to one-half cup of bleach in one-quarter tub of water. In vivo studies will be required to show clinical effectiveness.

Recurrent staphylococcal infection in families. Steele R. Arch Dermatol 1980; 116: 189–90.

Fifteen of 17 families inoculated with less pathogenic strains of *S. aureus* remained disease free at 6 months, whereas only 4 of the 15 control families had no recurrences.

In vitro activity of retapamulin against *Staphylococcus aureus* isolates resistant to fusidic acid and mupirocin. Woodford N, Afzal-Shah M, Warner M, Livermore DM. J Antimicrob Chemother 2008; 766–8.

Retapamulin inhibited 99.9% of all *S. aureus* isolates. Further in vivo studies are indicated to assess efficacy in the treatment of furunculosis.

Treatment and prevention of recurrent staphylococcal furunculosis: clinical and bacteriologic follow-up. Hedstrom SA. Scand J Infect Dis 1985; 17: 55–8.

Sodium fusidate ointment was used twice daily for a month as prophylaxis for nasal furunculosis with cessation of furuncles in 10 of 20 cases. Controls took antibiotics systemically, and 3 of 20 had no furuncles. After a year, those who used topical therapy had fewer recurrent lesions.

89

Condyloma acuminata

Brian Berman, Sadegh Amini, Andrea Maderal

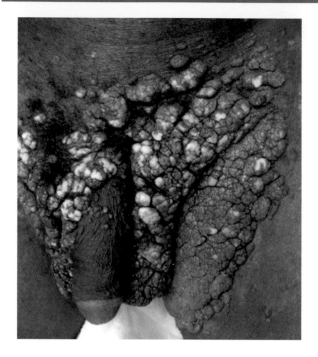

External anogenital warts develop on the skin and mucosal surfaces of the genitalia and perianal areas. They are caused by the human papillomavirus (HPV), sexually transmitted in approximately 65% of cases, with at least 40 of the more than 100 types identified capable of infecting the genital tract. Condyloma acuminata (CA), the classic form of anogenital warts, are frequently associated with "benign" HPV types 6 and 11 (up to 95%) but may also be caused by oncogenic HPV types such as 16, 18, 31, 33, and 35.

MANAGEMENT STRATEGY

Most cases are asymptomatic; however, they can be disfiguring; lead to physical discomfort; induce psychological suffering, guilt, and anger; and severely affect quality of life. Untreated genital warts may increase in size or number, remain unchanged, or resolve spontaneously.

Current treatments focus on stimulation of the host's immune response to enhance virus recognition. Treatments are categorized as either patient applied (i.e., *podofilox, imiquimod, and sinecatechin*) or provider administered. Podofilox (podophyllotoxin) is applied twice daily for 3 days and then no treatment for 4 days for four to six cycles, if necessary.

Imiquimod 5%, 3.75%, or 2.5% cream stimulates the host's immune response. Imiquimod 5% is applied overnight and washed off 6 to 10 hours after application, three times a week, until clearance of the warts or a maximum of 16 weeks. Imiquimod 3.75% is applied nightly for up to 8 weeks.

Sinecatechin 15% ointment extract of green tea from *Camellia sinensis* contains epigallocatechin gallate, exhibiting antiviral, antitumor, and immunostimulatory properties. It is applied three times a day until clearance of the warts or a maximum of 16 weeks.

Provider-administered therapies are either topically applied or surgical. Topical modalities include *podophyllin resin, podofilox (podophyllotoxin), bichloroacetic acid (BCA), trichloroacetic acid (TCA), intralesional bleomycin, and ingenol mebutate*. Surgical treatments include *cryotherapy, surgical removal* either by tangential shave using a cold knife or tangential scissor excisions, *curettage* with or without *electrosurgery*, and *lasers* (CO_2 and pulsed dye laser, PDL). *Intralesional interferon-α and bleomycin* are also effective therapies. *Podophyllin* resin is applied for 1 to 6 hours and is less effective on dry areas such as the penile shaft, scrotum, and labia majora.

The safety of podofilox, imiquimod, and sinecatechin (all category C) during pregnancy has not been established. Both TCA and BCA 80% to 90% solutions are applied weekly as needed.

Cryotherapy causes thermolysis and necrosis of keratinocytes hosting HPV. Liquid nitrogen either with cryospray or cryoprobe usually requires one to two freeze–thaw cycles per session for two to three sessions. However, HPV deoxyribonucleic acid (DNA) is detectable up to 1 cm from the wart periphery, and recurrence rates are up to 40%.

Surgery and *CO_2 lasers* are useful for treating extensive giant (i.e., Buschke–Lowenstein tumor) intraurethral and recalcitrant warts.

Recombinant HPV quadrivalent (6–11–16–18) vaccine is safe and efficacious in decreasing the incidence of persistent anogenital warts and cervical cancer by 90% and, within 6 years of introduction, has shown a 64% decrease in prevalence of those HPV types in females 14 to 19 years of age. A 9-valent HPV vaccine was also recently approved.

Estimates of clearance and recurrence rates with various therapies are difficult due to differences in method of analysis, patient population, and duration of follow-up. No available therapy can be guaranteed to clear genital warts without any recurrence. Combination therapy using an immunomodulator after physical ablative therapy reduces recurrence rates; however, the possibility of additive adverse events should be considered.

Specific Investigations

- Papanicolaou (Pap) smear
- HPV typing (not standard of care)
- Biopsy
- Acetic acid 3% to 5% (not recommended)

Evaluation of human papillomavirus testing in primary screening for cervical abnormalities: comparison of sensitivity, specificity, and frequency of referral. Kulasingam SL, Hughes JP, Kiviat NB, Mao C, Weiss NS, Kuypers JM, et al. JAMA 2002; 288: 1749–57.

HPV DNA testing has higher sensitivity but lower specificity than thin-layer Pap screening. In some settings (i.e., long or haphazard screening intervals), HPV DNA screening may be an alternative to cytology-based screening in women of reproductive age.

Evidence-based treatment and prevention of external genital warts in female pediatric and adolescent patients. Thornsberry L, English JC. J Pediatr Adolesc Gynecol 2012; 25: 150–4.

The diagnosis of anogenital warts is generally clinical. HPV DNA typing and 3% to 5% acetic acid testing to reveal subclinical lesions are not recommended. Anoscopy and/or speculum examination are useful for evaluation of the anal canal, vagina, or cervix. A biopsy is not indicated for typical condylomas but must

Evidence Levels: A Double-blind study   B Clinical trial ≥ 20 subjects   C Clinical trial < 20 subjects   D Series ≥ 5 subjects   E Anecdotal case reports

be performed for atypical-looking and recalcitrant lesions or in immunocompromised patients.

First-Line Therapies

- Imiquimod (5%, 3.75%)   **A**
- Podofilox (podophyllotoxin)   **A**
- Sinecatechin extract of green tea   **A**
- Cryotherapy   **A**
- Podophyllin   **B**

Imiquimod, a patient-applied immune response modifier for treatment of external genital warts. Beutner KR, Tyring SK, Trofatter KF Jr, Douglas JM Jr, Spruance S, Owens ML, et al. Antimicrob Agents Chemother 1998; 42: 789–94.

A multicenter, double-blind, vehicle-controlled, trial (n = 279) evaluated daily application of imiquimod for 16 weeks. At week 16, 52% of 5% imiquimod-treated patients, 14% of 1% imiquimod, and 4% of vehicle-treated patients cleared the warts ($p < 0.0001$). Recurrence rate after a complete response was 19% with 5% imiquimod.

Imiquimod cream 2.5% and 3.75% applied once daily to treat external genital warts in men. Rosen T, Nelson A, Ault K. Cutis 2015; 96: 277–82.

Two multicenter, randomized, double-blind, placebo-controlled studies evaluated 447 patients randomized to imiquimod cream 3.75% or 2.5% or placebo once daily until complete clearance or maximum of 8 weeks. Complete clearance at end of study period was 18.6% in the 3.75% imiquimod group and 14.3% in the 2.5% imiquimod group. Both groups were significantly superior to placebo in one study.

Human papillomavirus (HPV) viral load and HPV type in the clinical outcome of HIV-positive patients treated with imiquimod for anogenital warts and anal intraepithelial neoplasia. Sanclemente G, Herrera S, Tyring SK, Rady PL, Zuleta JJ, Correa LA, et al. J Eur Acad Dermatol Venereol 2007; 21: 1054–60.

Imiquimod 5% was evaluated in 37 HIV-positive males with anogenital warts or anal intraepithelial neoplasia (AIN). Imiquimod was applied three times per week for at least 8 hours overnight for 16 weeks. At week 20, 46% of patients cleared 100%, whereas 14 patients had >50% clearance. Recurrences occurred in 29% of patients who cleared 100%. Clearance was independent of patient's CD4 count, wart location, HIV viral load, or HPV viral load.

A multicenter, randomised, double-blind, placebo controlled study of cryotherapy versus cryotherapy and podophyllotoxin cream as treatment for external anogenital warts. Gilson RJ, Ross J, Maw R, Rowen D, Sonnex C, Lacey CJ. Sex Transm Infect 2009; 85: 514–9.

Patients (n = 140) received cryotherapy plus podophyllotoxin or cryotherapy alone. Podophyllotoxin cream or placebo was applied twice daily for 3 days per week for up to 4 weeks, with weekly cryotherapy continued to week 12 if required. Complete clearance rates with the combination versus cryotherapy alone were 60.0% and 45.7%, respectively (no statistical difference). At week 24 both groups had similar clearance rates, with new and recurrent lesions in 16.7% and 18.8% of patients, respectively.

Safety and efficacy of 0.5% podofilox gel in the treatment of anogenital warts. Tyring S, Edwards L, Cherry LK, Ramsdell WM, Kotner S, Greenberg MD, et al. Arch Dermatol 1998; 134: 33–8.

In a double-blind, multicenter, vehicle-controlled trial, 326 patients applied podofilox twice daily for 3 consecutive days followed by a 4-day treatment-free period (one treatment cycle). Treatment was repeated by the patient until all study warts had cleared, for a minimum of two and maximum of eight cycles. At week 8, 88.4% of warts in the vehicle-treated group and 35.9% in the podofilox-treated group remained ($p = 0.001$).

Efficacy, safety and tolerability of green tea catechins in the treatment of external anogenital warts: a systematic review and meta-analysis. Tzellos TG, Sardeli C, Lallas A, Papazisis G, Chourdakis M, Kouvelas D. J Eur Acad Dermatol Venereol 2011; 25: 345–53.

Three double-blind studies (n = 1247) evaluated sinecatechin ointment, obtaining complete clearance ranging from 52.6% to 64.6%. Recurrence ranged from 5.9% to 10.6%.

Sinecatechin ointment is applied three times a day for up to 16 weeks.

A single-blinded randomized controlled study to assess the efficacy of twice daily application of sinecatechins 1% ointment when used sequentially with cryotherapy in the treatment of external genital warts. On SC, Linkner RV, Haddican M, Yaroshinsky A, Gagliotti M, Singer G, et al. J Drugs Dermatol 2014; 13: 1400–5.

Single-blinded, randomized controlled trial of 42 subjects treated with cryotherapy alone versus cryotherapy with sinecatechin 15% ointment twice daily for up to 16 weeks. There was a reduction in the number of lesions in the combination group compared with cryotherapy alone (–5 lesions vs. –2.1 lesions, $p = 0.07$).

Treatment of external genital warts: a randomized clinical trial comparing podophyllin, cryotherapy, and electrodesiccation. Stone KM, Becker TM, Hadgu A, Kraus SJ. Genitourin Med 1990; 66: 16–9.

All treatments were provided weekly until clearance or until a total of six treatments had been administered. Patients were instructed to wash off the podophyllin 2 hours after the first treatment; this interval was lengthened by 2 hours to a maximum of 12 hours with each successive treatment. After evaluating 450 patients, complete clearance was observed in 41% of podophyllin-treated, 79% of cryotherapy-treated, and 94% of electrodesiccation-treated patients. The 3-month clearance rates were 17%, 55%, and 71%, respectively.

Cryotherapy is safe to use during pregnancy. Podophyllin, however, has been demonstrated to have severe systemic toxicity and should not be used in pregnant women.

Second-Line Therapies

- Surgical excision (with cold knife or scissors)   **B**
- Lasers (CO_2 and PDL)   **B**
- Loop electrosurgical excisional procedure   **B**
- Electrodesiccation (see also earlier)   **B**
- Trichloroacetic acid (see also earlier)   **B**

Comparison of podophyllin application with simple surgical excision in clearance and recurrence of perianal condyloma acuminata. Jensen SL. Lancet 1985; 2: 1146–8.

Patients (n = 60) randomly received podophyllin applied for 6 hours weekly for 6 weeks or surgery. Clearance rate was 76.6% and 93.3%, respectively. At 3 months, the cumulative recurrence rates were 43% and 18%, respectively.

Human papilloma virus type and recurrence rate after surgical clearance of anal condylomata acuminata. D'Ambrogio A, Yerly S, Sahli R, Bouzourene H, Demartines N, Cotton M, et al. Sex Transm Dis 2009; 36: 536–40.

Patients (n = 140) with anal canal condylomas had surgery followed by cauterization. Recurrence rate was 25% after day 120 of follow-up. HPV type 11 was statistically associated with higher recurrence rates.

CO(2) laser therapy versus cryotherapy in treatment of genital warts; a randomized controlled trial (RCT). Azizjalali M, Ghaffarpour G, Mousavifard B. Iran J Microbiol 2012; 4: 187–90.

Patients (n = 160) with genital warts were treated with CO_2 laser or cryotherapy. Complete clearance was achieved in 95% treated by CO_2 laser and 46.2% treated with cryotherapy ($p <$ 0.001). Laser therapy was associated with less recurrence compared with cryotherapy (0.05% vs. 0.18%).

Treatment of genital warts in males by pulsed dye laser. Badawi A, Shokeir HA, Salem AM, Soliman M, Fawzy S, Samy N, et al. J Cosmet Laser Ther 2006; 8: 92–5.

Patients (n = 174) with 550 uncomplicated anogenital warts underwent flashlamp-pumped PDL. Complete resolution was achieved in 96% of lesions, with a recurrence rate of 5%.

Treating vaginal and external anogenital condylomas with electrosurgery vs. CO_2 laser ablation. Ferenczy A, Behelak Y, Haber G, Wright TC Jr, Richart RM. J Gynecol Surg 1995; 148: 9–12.

In 208 patients, the efficacy and adverse effects of loop electrosurgical excision procedure (LEEP) were similar to those associated with laser ablation. LEEP adverse events included bleeding and scarring.

Scarring of the penis can result in dysfunction; therefore most physicians prefer CO_2 laser ablation or cryotherapy for penile warts.

Treatment of external genital warts comparing cryotherapy and trichloroacetic acid. Abdullah AN, Walzman M, Wade A. Sex Transm Dis 1993; 20: 344–5.

In this trial (n = 86), complete clearance was 86% with cryotherapy versus 70% with 95% TCA after up to six treatments. Application site reactions developed in 30% of the TCA-treated patients.

Third-Line Therapies

• Intralesional interferon-α	A
• Interferon-β gel	A
• Oral isotretinoin	B
• Intralesional fluorouracil/epinephrine gel	A
• Cidofovir	B
• aminolevulinic acid (ALA)–photodynamic therapy	B
• Intralesional bleomycin	C
• Ingenol mebutate	C

Natural interferon alfa for treatment of condyloma acuminata. Friedman-Kien AE, Eron LJ, Conant M, Growdon W, Badiak H, Bradstreet PW, et al. JAMA 1988; 259: 533–8.

In this double-blind, placebo-controlled trial, complete clearance was 62% (with intralesional interferon-α injections twice weekly for up to 8 weeks) versus 21% (placebo).

Combinations of interferon with cryosurgery, podophyllin, or laser ablation have been promising.

Treatment of condylomata acuminata with oral isotretinoin. Tsambaos D, Georgiou S, Monastirli A, Sakkis T, Sagriotis A, Goerz G. J Urol 1997; 158: 1810–2.

Oral isotretinoin 1 mg/kg daily during a 3-month period achieved complete response in 39.6% of 56 male patients with history of refractory condyloma acuminata. Oral isotretinoin may be considered an effective alternative treatment for immature and small condyloma acuminata.

Topical cidofovir (HPMPC) is an effective adjuvant to surgical treatment of anogenital condylomata acuminata. Coremans G, Margaritis V, Snoeck R, Wyndaele J, De Clercq E, Geboes K. Dis Colon Rectum 2003; 46: 1103–8.

Patients were treated with repetitive electrocoagulations (n = 27) (control) or cidofovir (n = 20) 1% cream applied to warts daily for 5 hours for 5 consecutive days per week, repeated weekly for up to 18 weeks or until complete clearance. Complete and partial responses with cidofovir were 32% and 60%, respectively. Fewer patients had remaining lesions after cidofovir. Recurrence rates were 3.7% and 55%, respectively.

Combined surgery and cidofovir is an effective treatment for genital warts in HIV-infected patients. Orlando G, Fasolo MM, Beretta R, Merli S, Cargnel A. AIDS 2002; 16: 447–50.

Seventy-four HIV-positive patients received electrocautery or cidofovir 1% gel applied 5 days per week for up to 6 weeks or electrocautery plus cidofovir for 5 days per week for 2 weeks within 1 month of cautery. Complete response was achieved in 93.1%, 76.2%, and 100% of patients, respectively (p = 0.033). After 6 months the recurrence rates were 73.68%, 35.24%, and 27.27% (p = 0.018).

Evaluation of photodynamic therapy using topical aminolevulinic acid hydrochloride in the treatment of condylomata acuminata: a comparative, randomized clinical trial. Liang J, Lu XN, Tang H, Zhang Z, Fan J, Xu JH. Photodermatol Photoimmunol Photomed 2009; 25: 293–7.

In a trial 91 patients received ALA–PDT or CO_2 laser. Complete response was 95.93% and 100%, respectively (p > 0.05). At week 12 of follow-up, 9.38% and 17.39% had recurrent lesions (p < 0.05). Adverse reactions were 8.82% and 100%, respectively (p < 0.05).

Preliminary study of intralesional bleomycin injection for the treatment of genital warts. Lee JY, Kim CW, Kim SS. Ann Dermatol 2015; 27: 239–41.

Fifteen patients with a total of 164 refractory genital warts were treated with intralesional bleomycin 1.5 mg/mL every 2 weeks until clearance. Clearance was achieved in 73.3%.

Ingenol mebutate gel is effective against anogenital warts – a case series in 17 patients. Schopf RE. J Eur Acad Dermatol Venereol 2016; 30: 1041–3.

The patients were treated with one to three applications with complete response in 16/17 patients.

Evidence Levels: **A** Double-blind study **B** Clinical trial ≥ 20 subjects **C** Clinical trial < 20 subjects **D** Series ≥ 5 subjects **E** Anecdotal case reports

Geographic tongue

90

Jennifer K. Chen, Janellen Smith

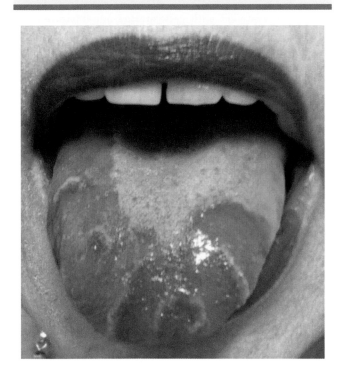

Geographic tongue is a reactive mucosal inflammatory condition characterized by arcuate or annular alternating hypertrophic or atrophic filiform papillae producing a geographic pattern. Synonyms include *benign migratory glossitis* and *glossitis areata migrans*. Geographic tongue may be an asymptomatic incidental finding. Similar changes may occur in oral sites other than the tongue (geographic stomatitis or benign migratory stomatitis).

MANAGEMENT STRATEGY

Geographic tongue is a common glossitis that affects 2% of the population. There is no racial predilection, and the condition may be seen in patients of all ages, more often children than adults. If asymptomatic, no treatment is necessary other than reassurance that the condition is benign and usually not a sign of systemic illness. Geographic tongue often will remit spontaneously but may persist for years. Occasionally, patients may complain of a burning discomfort, particularly in atrophic areas. Effective therapy can be challenging.

Geographic tongue has been associated with psoriasis (especially pustular psoriasis); reactive arthritis; pityriasis rubra pilaris; atopic diathesis; Down syndrome; nutritional deficiency; diabetes; hormonal changes; and medications including lithium, oral contraceptives, and vascular endothelial growth factor or multikinase inhibitors such as bevacizumab, sunitinib, and sorafenib. The clinician should also consider acute or chronic atrophic candidiasis.

For symptomatic patients, measures that may be considered include the avoidance of hot, spicy, or acidic foods; gentle brushing of the tongue; avoidance of harsh antibacterial mouthwashes, chewing gum, and breath mints; and soothing rinses with saline solutions. Occasionally, the topical application of *fluorinated corticosteroids* or *diphenhydramine elixir* after meals and at bedtime may be recommended. *Topical anesthetic rinses or gels* provide temporary relief. *Antiyeast treatments* may be palliative.

Specific Investigations

- Culture for candidiasis
- If symptomatic, consider complete blood cell count, iron panel, vitamin B, folate, and zinc levels; glucose; and hemoglobin A_{1c}
- No investigation necessary in asymptomatic patients

Geographic stomatitis: a critical review. Hume WJ. J Dent 1975; 3: 25–43.

The topic and the differential diagnosis are carefully reviewed.

Culture of the tongue for yeast organisms may help direct therapy. Some patients require reassurance that they do not have a systemic illness. Screening for diabetes mellitus or nutritional deficiency (vitamin B, folate, zinc, or iron) would be reasonable to exclude systemic associations.

First-Line Therapies

- Avoidance of spicy food, mouthwashes, chewing gum, and breath mints   **D**
- Topical corticosteroids (e.g., fluocinonide 0.05% gel, dexamethasone elixir)   **C**
- Topical antihistamines (e.g., diphenhydramine elixir 12.5 mg/5 mL diluted 1:4 with water)   **C**
- Antiyeast therapy   **E**

Symptomatic benign migratory glossitis: report of two cases and literature review. Sigal MJ, Mock D. Pediatr Dent 1992; 14: 392–6.

Management with topical corticosteroids and topical antihistamines is discussed.

Common tongue conditions in primary care. Reamy BV, Derby R, Bunt CW. Am Fam Physician 2010; 81: 627–34.

Glossitis and other tongue disorders. Byrd JA, Bruce AJ, Rogers RS III. Dermatol Clin 2003; 21: 123–34.

A review of geographic and other tongue disorders.

Painful geographic tongue (benign migratory glossitis) in a child. Menni S, Boccardi D, Crosti C. J Eur Acad Dermatol Venereol 2004; 18: 737–8.

The authors report a case of painful geographic tongue in a child in whom the only acceptable treatment was mometasone furoate cream. Treatment can be challenging in children because of the unpleasant taste of creams and difficulty with using mouthwashes.

Prevalence of fungi in cases of geographic tongue and fissured tongue. Dudko A, Kurnatowska AJ, Kurnatowski P. Ann Parasitol 2013; 59: 113–7.

In this case series, fungal cultures most commonly grew *Candida* species, which were more sensitive to nystatin than miconazole. The prevalence of fungi was highest in those who do not brush the tongue.

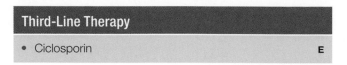

Second-Line Therapies

• Topical anesthetics	**C**
• Topical tretinoin	**E**
• Discontinue dentifrices and other oral flavoring agents	**D**
• Topical tacrolimus	**E**

The treatment of geographic tongue with topical Retin-A solution. Helfman RJ. Cutis 1979; 24: 179–80.

The use of topical Retin-A solution is described in three cases.

Anecdotally we have found that tretinoin gel is longer acting and better tolerated by patients.

Geographic tongue treated with topical tacrolimus. Ishibashi M, Tojo G, Watanabe M, Tamabuchi T, Masu T, Aiba S. J Dermatol Case Rep 2010; 4: 57–9.

Topical tacrolimus 0.1% ointment twice daily for 2 weeks cleared symptoms in two cases.

Third-Line Therapy

• Ciclosporin	**E**

Successful treatment with cyclosporine administration for persistent benign migratory glossitis. Abe M, Sogabe Y, Syuto T, Ishibuchi H, Yokoyama Y, Ishikawa O. J Dermatol 2007; 34: 340–3.

A patient with a 5-year history of refractory pain responded to ciclosporin 3 mg/kg/day for 2 months and then 1.5 mg/kg/day maintenance.

Evidence Levels: **A** Double-blind study **B** Clinical trial ≥ 20 subjects **C** Clinical trial < 20 subjects **D** Series ≥ 5 subjects **E** Anecdotal case reports

91

Gianotti–Crosti syndrome

Carlo Gelmetti

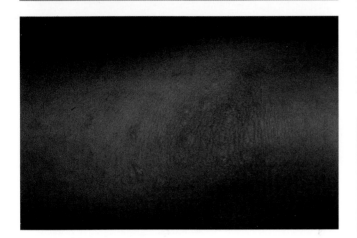

Gianotti–Crosti syndrome (GCS) was described in 1955 by Ferdinando Gianotti as a disease characterized by an exanthematic papular rash symmetrically distributed on the face, buttocks, and extremities. The disease had mild constitutional symptoms and a quite long but benign course. The term is now used to include all eruptive acrolocated dermatoses characterized by papular or papulovesicular lesions caused by microorganisms or vaccines. The first association was with hepatitis B (HBV); today, Epstein–Barr virus (EBV) is the etiology most frequently reported in the literature. As the number of immunizations increases and more combinations will be available, an increasing number of postimmunization cases are expected.

Synonyms include papular acrodermatitis of childhood, infantile papular acrodermatitis, and papulovesicular acrolocated syndrome.

MANAGEMENT STRATEGY

The diagnosis of GCS is clinical. Like other viral exanthems, it mainly affects children of preschool age. The typical eruption consists of monomorphic, lentil-sized lesions symmetrically distributed on the face, buttocks, and limbs. The lesions are papular or papulovesicular, sometimes edematous, and rarely purpuric. They may coalesce over the elbows and knees. A transient rash may be noted on the trunk in the early stage. Mucous membranes are not affected. In the eruptive phase, the Koebner phenomenon may be elicited. The eruption develops within a week, typically beginning on the thighs and buttocks, then involving the extensor aspects of the arms, and finally the face. Lesions vary in color from rose to red-brown. The pruritus is usually mild, and excoriation is rare. The lesions fade usually in 3 to 4 weeks with mild desquamation, and relapse is exceptional. Inguinal and axillary lymphadenopathy is common.

In cases associated with HBV, the hepatitis begins at the same time as, or 1 to 2 weeks after the onset of, GCS. The liver is usually enlarged but not tender; jaundice is exceptional. There are high levels of liver enzymes, and the viral markers become detectable depending on the duration of infection. Complications are rare, although some patients developed chronic hepatitis. Abnormalities in the peripheral blood are inconsistent; the erythrocyte sedimentation rate is not raised.

In HBV-negative cases, hepatomegaly and liver function abnormalities, if present, are mild, probably because some viruses that are able to provoke GCS are considered minor hepatitic viruses.

There is no specific recommended treatment for GCS. However, when itching is disturbing, oral antihistamines or topical antipruritics can be used. Although corticosteroids are sometimes used, their benefit is not established, because corticosteroids could prolong or delay the recovery of the disease.

In cases associated with HBV, the hepatitis can be treated with interferon-α_{2b} or pegylated interferon, with or without nucleoside analogs such as adefovir, entecavir, telbivudine, tenofovir, and lamivudine, with the last having been approved for children. It is important to investigate and treat other members of the family who may be carriers of HBV or may benefit from vaccination.

Specific Investigations

- Liver enzymes
- Viral serology for EBV, hepatitis B, hepatitis A, cytomegalovirus (CMV)
- Total IgE (paper radioimmunosorbent test [PRIST]) and specific IgE (radioallergosorbent test [RAST] or immuno solid-phase allergen chip [ISAC])

Other possible causes include coxsackievirus, adenovirus, enterovirus, human herpesvirus 6, reovirus, varicella, roseola, rotavirus, respiratory syncytial virus, Lyme borreliosis, *Mycoplasma pneumoniae*, meningococcal infection, etc., and immunization.

Gianotti–Crosti syndrome associated with transfusion acquired hepatitis B virus infection in a patient of sickle cell anemia. Pise GA, Vetrichevvel TP, Agarwal KK, Thappa DM. Indian J Dermatol Venereol Leprol 2007; 73: 123–4.

A 9-year-old boy presented with GCS. Liver function tests showed indirect hyperbilirubinemia and mildly elevated liver enzymes. HBsAg was detected. The patient was managed with antihistamines, and skin lesions cleared in 2 weeks.

Gianotti–Crosti syndrome in a child following hepatitis B virus vaccination. Karakas M, Durdu M, Tuncer I, Cevlik F. J Dermatol 2007; 34: 117–20.

A 5-year-old boy presented with a 1-month history of GCS. The lesions had appeared 3 weeks after a first dose of HBV recombinant vaccine.

Gianotti-Crosti syndrome and erythema nodosum: two distinct entities or two manifestations of the same infection? Bassi A, Venturini E, Montagnani C, de Martino M, Galli L. J Pediatr 2016; 172: 217.

An 18-month-old boy was referred for evaluation of a widespread "itchy" rash consistent with GCS. In addition, nodules characteristic for erythema nodosum appeared 3 days after the skin eruption and increased in size over the subsequent days.

Gianotti-Crosti syndrome as presenting sign of cytomegalovirus infection: a case report and a critical appraisal of its possible cytomegalovirus etiology. Drago F, Javor S, Ciccarese G, Parodi A. J Clin Virol 2016; 78: 120–2.

In this case of a 3-year-old girl, GCS was related to CMV primary infection and may be considered the presenting sign of the infection.

Gianotti-Crosti syndrome following immunization in an 18 months old child. Babu TA, Arivazhahan A. Indian Dermatol Online J 2015; 6: 413–5.

A rare case of GCS following diphtheria, pertussis, and tetanus (DPT) and oral polio immunization in an 18-month-old child is reported along with a review of similar vaccine-induced GCS cases reported in the literature.

Gianotti–Crosti syndrome. Brandt O, Abeck D, Gianotti R, Burgdorf W. J Am Acad Dermatol 2006; 54: 136–45.

EBV is now the most common cause of GCS. Other viruses have been connected with GCS, including Hepatitis A Virus (HVA); CMV; HHV6; coxsackie A16, B4, and B5; rotavirus; Parvovirus B19 (parvo B19); respiratory syncytial virus; mumps virus; and parainfluenza virus types 1 and 2. Human Immunodeficiency Virus (HIV) also appears capable of triggering GCS. The association between various immunizations and GCS has long been known. Despite the proven connection between HBV and GCS, immunization against HBV only rarely causes GCS.

Atypical Gianotti-Crosti syndrome in two HIV and hepatitis B coinfected adults. Cocciolone R, Morey A, Panasiuk P, Whitfeld MJ. Australas J Dermatol 2011; 52: 32–6.

Atypical GCS in two unrelated adult male patients with coexistent hepatitis B and HIV infection are described. Immunoperoxidase studies suggested the presence of HBsAg within the vessels of both lesional and perilesional skin, providing further support for the proposed immune-mediated pathogenesis.

Gianotti–Crosti syndrome and allergic background. Ricci G, Patrizi A, Neri I, Specchia F, Tosti G, Masi M. Acta Dermatol Venereol 2003; 83: 202–5.

In 29 children affected by GCS and 59 age- and sex-matched controls, the presence of atopic dermatitis (24.1%) was significantly higher ($p < 0.005$) than in the control group (6.8%).

First-Line Therapies

Systemic antihistamines	E
Systemic corticosteroids	E
Topical corticosteroids	E
Topical antiseptics	E

Topical antipruritics	E
Zinc shake lotions	E
Systemic steroids	E
Systemic antibiotics	E
Ribavirin	E
Emollients	E
Vitamin C	E
Interferon-α	B
Nucleoside analogs	B
Hepatitis B vaccine	B

Acute disseminated erythematous papulovesicular skin lesions in a 7-year-old child: a quiz. Diagnosis: vesicular Gianotti-Crosti syndrome. Linke M, Géraud C, Schneider SW, Goerdt S, Utikal J. Acta Derm Venereol 2011; 91: 491–4.

A 7-year-old girl presented with cutaneous lesions consistent with GCS in addition to tense blisters on the hands and feet. Oral corticosteroids and antihistamines were administered, and an antiseptic cream was applied topically. The skin lesions subsided within a week without relapse.

Recurrent Gianotti-Crosti syndrome. Metelitsa AI, Fiorillo L. J Am Acad Dermatol 2011; 65: 876–7.

A 2-year-old boy presented with GCS. Two weeks after onset of the eruption, he was immunized with influenza vaccination and new lesions appeared at the immunization site. Investigations revealed a positive urine culture for CMV and positive IgM for EBV. He was treated with hydrocortisone cream, and the eruption resolved. Twelve months later, he presented with a similar eruption at the site of influenza vaccination. Because GCS is a mild and self-limiting disease, further vaccinations are not contraindicated.

Efficacy of ribavirin in a case of long lasting and disabling Gianotti-Crosti syndrome. Zawar V, Chuh A. J Dermatol Case Rep 2008; 2: 63–6.

A 6-year-old girl presented with a history of a pruritic rash consistent with GCS after a febrile illness with common cold symptoms. Remission was not achieved despite several medications: topical emollients, topical and systemic corticosteroids, topical and systemic antibiotics, and oral histamines. A course of oral ribavirin at a dose of 300 mg daily for 5 days led to dramatic remission 5 days later.

92

Gonorrhea

Ted Rosen

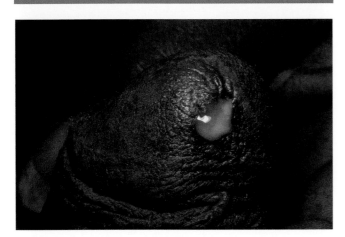

Gonorrhea is a common and potentially severe sexually transmitted disease caused by the gram-negative aerobic diplococcus *Neisseria gonorrhoeae*. This organism primarily infects the mucous membranes of the urethra, endocervix, rectum, and pharynx. The disease can also become disseminated, causing petechial or acral pustular skin lesions, tenosynovitis, arthralgia, true septic arthritis, perihepatitis, and less commonly endocarditis or meningitis.

MANAGEMENT STRATEGY

Individuals with gonorrhea should be treated as promptly as possible (1) to prevent regional infection such as epididymitis or pelvic inflammatory disease leading to infertility or ectopic pregnancy; (2) to prevent disseminated gonococcal infection, which occurs in about 1% to 3% of cases; and (3) to stop transmission to sexual partners. Prompt management has become especially important due to a resurgence in incidence of gonococcal disease in the United States and increasing multidrug antimicrobial resistance worldwide.

Gonococcal urethritis is typically characterized by mucopurulent to frankly purulent discharge along with a burning sensation during urination. Dysuria may be the only symptom.

Gonococcal cervicitis is characterized by a mucopurulent or purulent endocervical exudate. However, a cervical discharge is not specific for a gonococcal infection, and gonococcal infection of the cervix is often asymptomatic.

Pharyngeal infection is asymptomatic in more than 90% of cases, but when symptomatic it presents as a pharyngitis of variable severity.

Rectal infection is prevalent in homosexual men, causing anal discharge and pain. In women, rectal infection results from spread through vaginal secretions and does not necessarily imply anal intercourse.

Patients infected with *N. gonorrhoeae* are often coinfected with *Chlamydia trachomatis* and should be treated with *azithromycin* to cover this organism, with or without diagnostic evidence of chlamydial disease. Patients with gonorrhea have engaged in unprotected intercourse and, therefore, always should be tested for both syphilis and HIV.

Patients should be instructed to return for evaluation if symptoms persist or recur after therapy and to abstain from sexual intercourse until they and their sexual partners are cured. Because reinfection is so common, the Centers for Disease Control (CDC) recommends that all patients with known gonorrhea return for retesting 3 months posttreatment. A test of cure 3 to 4 weeks posttreatment is no longer recommended.

Antimicrobial resistance is a real threat, and treatment options for gonococcal disease are increasingly limited. To abate further spread of resistant strains of *N. gonorrhoeae*, physicians should strongly encourage patient referral of any sexual partner within the preceding 60 days for evaluation and treatment and obtain culture(s) to evaluate individual antimicrobial susceptibility in any patient whose symptoms do not resolve with initial treatment.

Specific Investigations

Men
- Microscopic examination of gram-stained urethral secretions
- Culture on Thayer–Martin medium
- Nonculture test based upon immunodiagnostics, as available

Women
- Culture on Thayer–Martin medium
- Nonculture test based upon immunodiagnostics, as available

Male urethritis with and without discharge. A clinical and microbiological study. Janier M, Lassau F, Casin I, Grillot P, Scieux C, Zavaro A, et al. Sex Transm Dis 1995; 22: 244–52.

N. gonorrhoeae was found in 21% of patients with urethral discharge and in no patient without discharge. Treatment for *N. gonorrhoeae* in patients without discharge in the absence of proven contact with an infected patient is not recommended.

Sexually transmitted diseases treatment guidelines, 2015. Workowski KA, Bolan GA; Centers for Disease Control and Prevention. MMWR Recomm Rep 2015; 64: 1–137.

Because of its high specificity (>99%) and sensitivity (>95%), a Gram stain of a male urethral specimen that demonstrates polymorphonuclear leukocytes with intracellular gram-negative diplococci can be considered diagnostic for infection with *N. gonorrhoeae* in symptomatic men. Culture is the most widely available option for diagnosis in asymptomatic men, in women, and in nongenital sites (rectum and pharynx). Nonculture tests cannot provide antimicrobial susceptibility results, but can rapidly and accurately confirm a clinical diagnosis.

Screening tests to detect *Chlamydia trachomatis* and *Neisseria gonorrhoeae* infections – 2002. Johnson RE, Newhall WJ, Papp JR, Knapp JS, Black CM, Gift TL, et al. MMWR Recomm Rep 2002; 51: 1–38.

Nonculture tests called *nucleic acid hybridization tests* and *nucleic acid amplification tests (NAATs)* have been developed. Commercial NAATs differ in their amplification methods and their target nucleic acid sequences. The majority of commercial NAATs have been cleared by the Food and Drug Administration (FDA) to detect *C. trachomatis* and *N. gonorrhoeae* in endocervical swabs and urethral swabs from men. The sensitivity of NAATs might be less when using urine than when using an endocervical swab. Testing of rectal and oropharyngeal specimens with NAATs is not recommended.

First-Line Therapies for Uncomplicated Gonorrhea of the Cervix, Urethra, Rectum, Pharynx, and Conjunctiva
• Ceftriaxone 250 mg intramuscularly in a single dose + azithromycin 1 g orally   **B**
• Only if ceftriaxone is NOT immediately available: cefixime 400 mg orally in a single dose + azithromycin 1 g orally   **B**

Second-Line Therapies (No Advantage over First-Line Therapies)
• Ceftizoxime 500 mg intramuscularly as a single dose + azithromycin 1 g orally   **B**
• Cefoxitin 2 g intramuscularly with probenecid 1 g orally + azithromycin 1 g orally   **B**
• Cefotaxime 500 mg intramuscularly as a single dose + azithromycin 1 g orally   **B**

Oral cefixime versus intramuscular ceftriaxone in patients with uncomplicated gonococcal infections. Portilla I, Lutz B, Montalvo M, Mogabgab J. Sex Transm Dis 1992; 19: 94–8.

The only current CDC-recommended options for treating *N. gonorrhoeae* infections are cephalosporins. The 400-mg dose of cefixime cured 97% of uncomplicated urogenital and anorectal gonococcal infections. The advantage of cefixime is that it can be administered orally. However, cefixime is no longer a reliable first-line therapy (see next citation).

Sexually transmitted diseases treatment guidelines, 2015. Workowski KA, Bolan GA; Centers for Disease Control and Prevention. MMWR Recomm Rep 2015; 64: 1–137.

The minimum concentrations of cefixime needed to inhibit in vitro growth of the *N. gonorrhoeae* strains circulating in the United States and many other countries have progressively increased since 2006. This suggests that the effectiveness of cefixime might be waning. In addition, treatment failures with cefixime (or other similar oral cephalosporins) have been reported in Asia, Europe, South Africa, and Canada. As a result, the CDC no longer recommends the routine use of cefixime as a first-line regimen for treatment of gonorrhea at any anatomic site in the United States. Ceftriaxone in a single injection of 250 mg is a safe, effective dose for uncomplicated gonococcal infection at all anatomic sites. However, ceftriaxone failures have also been rarely reported. Consequently, only one regimen, dual treatment with ceftriaxone and azithromycin, is currently recommended for gonorrhea treatment at all anatomic sites in adults. *All patients with gonorrhea should also be treated with azithromycin to (1) treat possible coinfection with* Chlamydia trachomatis *and (2) gain additive microcidal effects for* N. gonorrhoeae.

First *Neisseria gonorrhoeae* strain with resistance to cefixime causing gonorrhoea treatment failure in Austria, 2011. Unemo M, Golparian D, Stary A, Eigentler A. Euro Surveill 2011; 16: 1–3.

Globally the susceptibility of *N. gonorrhoeae* to antimicrobial therapy, including first-line treatment options ceftriaxone and cefixime, is decreasing.

UK national guideline for the management of gonorrhoea in adults, 2011. Bignell C, Fitzgerald M, Guideline Development Group, British Association for Sexual Health and HIV UK. Int J STD AIDS 2011; 22: 541–7.

Three cases of cefixime failure were reported in the UK in 2011. First-line treatment for gonococcal infection in the UK is now ceftriaxone 500 mg intramuscularly plus azithromycin 1 g orally with test of cure recommended in all cases. Cefixime is only advised when intramuscular injection is contraindicated, refused by the patient, or immediately unavailable.

***Neisseria gonorrhoeae* with high-level resistance to azithromycin: case report of the first isolate identified in the United States.** Katz AR, Komeya AY, Soge OO, Kiaha MI, Lee MV, Wasserman GM, et al. CID 2012; 54: 841–3.

Eight isolates with reduced susceptibility to azithromycin were identified in Hawaii followed by laboratory documentation of the first isolate with high-level azithromycin resistance in California. Previously, strains with high-level resistance had been documented in Argentina, Scotland, England, Wales, and Ireland.

Spectinomycin resistance in *Neisseria* spp. due to mutations in IGSrRNA. Galimand M, Gerbaud G, Courvalin P. Antimicrob Agents Chemother 2000; 44: 1365–6.

It is rare for a patient to be infected with a spectinomycin-resistant strain, but spectinomycin is expensive and must be injected. Spectinomycin is useful for patients who cannot tolerate cephalosporins and quinolones.

Pfizer discontinued U.S.-based distribution of spectinomycin in November 2005.

Update to CDC's sexually transmitted diseases treatment guidelines 2006: fluoroquinolones no longer recommended for treatment of gonococcal infections. Centers for Disease Control and Prevention MMWR Morb Mortal Wkly Rep 2007; 56: 332–6.

Due to the increasing resistance, the CDC no longer recommends the use of fluoroquinolones for patients who acquired their infection in the United States, Asia, or the Pacific Islands. Recent data suggest that resistant strains comprise about 13% of all American-acquired isolates. Fluoroquinolones remain off the recommended treatment list for gonorrhea 10 years later.

Surveillance of antibiotic resistance in *Neisseria gonorrhoeae* in the WHO Western Pacific and South East Asian Regions, 2009. WHO Western Pacific and South East Asian Gonococcal Antimicrobial Surveillance Programmes. Commun Dis Intell 2011; 35: 2–7.

Recent data from China, Hong Kong, Japan, and elsewhere in Asia also demonstrate a very high rate of fluoroquinolone resistance. Australia and New Zealand are experiencing 35% to 45% of isolates being quinolone resistant.

Annual report of the Australian Gonococcal Surveillance Programme, 2010. Australian Gonococcal Surveillance Programme. Commun Dis Intell 2011; 35: 229–36.

Penicillin has been removed from the standard treatment regimen in Australia because of nationwide isolate resistance (up to 44% in some regions). However, in remote areas of Australia with extremely high disease rates, treatment with penicillin often remains effective. The same is also true in other industrialized countries.

Evidence Levels: **A** Double-blind study   **B** Clinical trial ≥ 20 subjects   **C** Clinical trial < 20 subjects   **D** Series ≥ 5 subjects   **E** Anecdotal case reports

Cephalosporin resistant *Neisseria gonorrhoeae*: time to consider gentamicin? Ross JD, Lewis DA. Sex Transm Infect 2012; 88: 6–8.

Studies of efficacy of gentamicin from the 1970s and 1980s demonstrated cure rates of 65% to 100% with no report of adverse reactions.

***Neisseria gonorrhoeae* antimicrobial susceptibility surveillance— The Gonococcal Isolate Surveillance Project, 27 sites, United States, 2014.** Kirkcaldy RD, Harvey A, Papp JR, Del Rio C, Soge OO, Holmes KK, et al. MMWR Surveill Summ 2016; 65: 1–19.

This is the first report to present comprehensive surveillance data from the U.S. Gonococcal Isolate Surveillance Project (GISP) and summarize gonococcal susceptibility over time, as well as underscore the public health implications of emerging cephalosporin resistance. Antimicrobial susceptibility patterns vary by geographic region within the United States and by sex of sex partner. For example, the percentage of isolates resistant to tetracycline, ciprofloxacin, penicillin, or all three antimicrobials was greater in isolates from men who have sex with men than from men who exclusively have sex with women. Because dual therapy with ceftriaxone plus azithromycin is the only recommended gonorrhea treatment, increases in azithromycin and cephalosporin minimal inhibitory concentrations are cause for concern that resistance to these antimicrobial agents might be emerging. Reduced azithromycin susceptibility (defined as minimum inhibitory concentration ≥2.0 µg/mL) increased from 0.6% in 2013 to 2.5% in 2014. It is unclear whether increases in the percentage of isolates with reduced susceptibility to azithromycin mark the beginning of an adverse trend.

SPECIAL CONSIDERATIONS

Pharyngeal infection

Treating uncomplicated *Neisseria gonorrhoeae* infections: is the anatomic site of infection important? Moran JS. Sex Transm Dis 1995; 22: 39–47.

Pharyngeal infection is more difficult to cure. A cephalosporin regimen is the best choice, as it is likely to cure at least 80% of pharyngeal infections. Spectinomycin is unreliable (i.e., only 52% effective).

Azithromycin may increase efficacy for pharyngeal infection when using oral cephalosporins.

Disseminated gonococcal infection

Hospitalization is recommended for initial therapy. The experts recommend ceftriaxone 1 g intramuscularly or intravenously every 24 hours as the initial regimen, plus azithromycin 1 g orally as a single dose. The provider can switch to an oral agent guided by antimicrobial susceptibility testing 24 to 48 hours after substantial clinical improvement, for a total treatment course of at least 7 days. Acceptable alternative therapies include cefotaxime or ceftizoxime, with both drugs given in a dosage of 1 g intravenously every 8 hours, along with a single dose of azithromycin (1 g).

Pregnancy

Treatment of gonorrhoea in pregnancy. Cavenee MR, Farris JR, Spalding TR, Barnes DL, Castaneda YS, Wendel GD Jr. Obstet Gynecol 1993; 81: 33–8.

A randomized study on 250 cases comparing ceftriaxone 250 mg intramuscularly, spectinomycin 2 g intramuscularly, and amoxicillin 3 g orally with probenecid 1 g showed efficacy was 95%, 95%, and 89%, respectively. There was no increase in congenital malformations. Ceftriaxone and spectinomycin are the best choices. Pregnant women should not be treated with quinolones or tetracyclines. (Comment: Because spectinomycin is no longer available in the United States, ceftriaxone is the default drug of choice and is recommended, along with azithromycin, at standard doses enumerated earlier.)

Pregnant women who cannot tolerate a cephalosporin should receive azithromycin 2 g in a single dose.

Ophthalmia neonatorum

To prevent gonococcal ophthalmia neonatorum, a prophylactic agent should be instilled into both eyes of all newborn infants; this procedure is, in fact, required by law in most states. Prophylaxis consists of erythromycin (0.5%) ophthalmic ointment in each eye in a single application at birth. Ocular prophylaxis is warranted because it can prevent sight-threatening gonococcal ophthalmia, has an excellent safety record, is easy to administer, and is inexpensive. Gonococcal ophthalmia is strongly suggested when typical gram-negative diplococci are identified in conjunctival exudate, justifying presumptive treatment after appropriate cultures have been obtained. The recommended regimen is ceftriaxone 25 to 50 mg/kg IV or IM in a single dose, not to exceed 125 mg. Local treatment, with or without systemic antibiotics, is inappropriate.

Men who have sex with men

Gonorrhea screening among men who have sex with men: value of multiple anatomic site testing, San Diego, California, 1997–2003. Gunn RA, O'Brien CJ, Lee MA, Gilchick RA. Sex Transm Dis 2008; 35: 845–8.

This population should be screened annually for gonorrhea infection at the urethral, pharyngeal, and rectal sites.

(Comment: The CDC also now recommends annual screening for N. gonorrhoeae infection for all sexually active women aged <25 years and for older women at increased risk for infection (e.g., those who have a new sex partner, more than one sex partner, a sex partner with concurrent partners, or a sex partner who has an STI). Additional risk factors for gonorrhea include inconsistent condom use among persons who are not in mutually monogamous relationships, previous or coexisting sexually transmitted infections, and exchanging sex for money or drugs. Individuals who fall into those categories should also be screened annually.)

Treatment failure

Patients with suspected treatment failure or persons infected with a strain found to demonstrate in vitro resistance should consult an infectious disease specialist, where the use of gentamicin or gemifloxacin may be entertained. Patients should be retreated with at least 250 mg of ceftriaxone IM or IV and ensure partner treatment. The situation should be promptly reported to public health agencies.

93

Graft-versus-host disease

Robert G. Micheletti

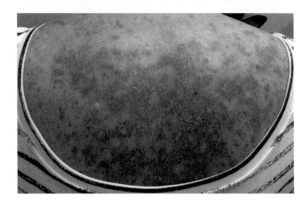

Graft-versus-host disease (GVHD) is the most significant source of morbidity and mortality among survivors of allogeneic hematopoietic stem cell transplantation, occurring in 30% to 70% of transplant recipients. Affecting the skin, liver, gastrointestinal tract, and other organs, it occurs when donor immune cells (the graft) recognize the transplant recipient (host) as foreign, resulting in inflammation and end organ damage. Of the organs involved, the skin is the most common and most severely affected.

MANAGEMENT STRATEGY

The risk, timing, presentation, and treatment of GVHD depend on many factors, including the type of transplant, the degree of HLA mismatch, donor and recipient sex, the intensity of pretransplant conditioning, and the GVHD prophylactic regimen used. Evolution of transplant strategies, such as reduced-intensity conditioning, increasing age of some transplant recipients, novel prophylaxis and treatment regimens, and donor lymphocyte infusion, together with improved recognition of overlap phenomena and late-onset acute GVHD, have blurred the classic understanding of a temporally defined disease. Acute and chronic GVHD are best differentiated on the basis of clinical manifestations, because features of either may occur at any time posttransplant. Atypical manifestations, particularly of chronic GVHD, can mimic other dermatologic diseases and present a diagnostic dilemma; input of a dermatologist and skin biopsy, when appropriate, can help shape diagnosis and management.

Initial management of GVHD includes adjustment of GVHD prophylaxis. Optimization of organ-specific supportive care and *topical therapies* may be sufficient for mild cutaneous GVHD, whereas in more severe disease, maximizing topical care can minimize the need for systemic immunosuppression and related side effects. For moderate or severe GVHD, *systemic corticosteroids* are first-line therapy, but in many cases GVHD becomes steroid refractory or dependent. Evidence for second- and third-line therapies is derived from small trials or series and is frequently contradictory. The optimal approach in patients

with steroid-refractory acute or chronic GVHD is therefore not known. Commonly used agents with reported activity and adequate safety profiles include *calcineurin inhibitors, extracorporeal photopheresis, mycophenolate mofetil, mTOR inhibitors, ruxolitinib* (increasingly), and several others. Additional skin-directed therapies such as *narrowband UVB and PUVA phototherapy* can benefit some patients.

Future work to identify effective therapies, using standardized criteria, is needed. In addition to aiding diagnosis and optimizing skin-directed therapies, dermatologists can play an important role in assessment of response, severity scoring, and research.

ACUTE GVHD

Specific Investigations

- Skin biopsy
- Medication history
- Liver function tests
- Complete blood count
- Serum chemistry
- Biomarker panel (investigational)
- Consider viral testing (e.g., cytomegalovirus)
- Consider colonoscopy/endoscopy

Clinical differentiation of acute cutaneous graft-versus-host disease from drug hypersensitivity reactions. Byun HJ, Yang JI, Kim BK, Cho KH. J Am Acad Dermatol 2011; 65:726–32.

Cutaneous manifestations of acute GVHD are generally nonspecific. However, a morbilliform eruption involving the face (including pinnae), palms, and soles is suggestive of acute GVHD (aGVHD), as is the presence of diarrhea or hyperbilirubinemia, typically developing within 2 to 3 days of rash onset. Absence of these findings favors a diagnosis of drug hypersensitivity reaction but does not rule out GVHD.

Quantitative analysis of eosinophils in acute graft-versus-host disease compared with drug hypersensitivity reactions. Weaver J, Bergfeld WF. Am J Dermatopathol 2010; 32: 31–4.

Interface dermatitis with basilar vacuolization and dyskeratotic keratinocytes with satellite cell necrosis are characteristic but nonspecific histologic findings of GVHD. Only significant tissue eosinophilia (≥16 eosinophils per 10 high-powered fields) safely excludes aGVHD in favor of drug hypersensitivity reaction. Therefore the decision to diagnose and treat aGVHD should not depend on skin biopsy findings.

ST2 as a marker for risk of therapy-resistant graft-versus-host disease and death. Vander Lugt MT, Braun TM, Hanash S, Ritz J, Ho VT, Antin JH, et al. N Engl J Med 2013; 369: 529–39.

Serum biomarkers to help diagnose and predict the severity and outcome of GVHD are under investigation but are not yet available for clinical use. Suppression of tumorigenicity 2 (ST2), a member of the interleukin-1 receptor family, is one such marker, which predicts the risk for treatment-refractory GVHD and nonrelapse mortality after bone marrow transplantation.

First-Line Therapies

• Topical corticosteroids	D
• Systemic corticosteroids (methylprednisolone 1–2 mg/kg/day)	A

Evidence Levels: **A** Double-blind study **B** Clinical trial ≥ 20 subjects **C** Clinical trial < 20 subjects **D** Series ≥ 5 subjects **E** Anecdotal case reports

Topical corticosteroids, along with sensitive skin care measures and optimization of prophylactic medications (e.g., ciclosporin, tacrolimus, methotrexate), may be sufficient therapy for mild cutaneous grade I aGVHD (defined as cutaneous GVHD involving ≤50% body surface area [BSA] without liver or gastrointestinal [GI] involvement).

Effectiveness and safety of lower dose prednisone for initial treatment of acute graft-versus-host disease: a randomized controlled trial. Mielcarek M, Furlong T, Storer BE, Green ML, McDonald GB, Carpenter PA, et al. Haematologica 2015; 10: 842–8.

For patients with grade II or higher aGVHD (skin involvement >50% BSA or with any liver or GI involvement), systemic corticosteroids are the mainstay of initial therapy, typically 2 mg/kg/day prednisone equivalent in divided doses, followed by gradual taper. A randomized controlled trial comparing standard vs. lower dose (0.5–1 mg/kg/day) glucocorticoids showed that initial treatment of aGVHD with lower-dose prednisone may be sufficient.

Second-Line Therapies

- Mycophenolate mofetil **B**
- Extracorporeal photopheresis **B**
- Etanercept **B**
- Calcineurin inhibitors (tacrolimus, ciclosporin)å **B**
- mTOR inhibitors (sirolimus) **B**

First- and second-line systemic treatment of acute graft-versus-host disease: recommendations of the American Society of Blood and Marrow Transplantation. Martin PJ, Rizzo JD, Wingard JR, Ballen K, Curtin PT, Cutler C, et al. Biol Blood Marrow Transpl 2012; 18: 1150–63.

In this review of primary and secondary treatments for aGVHD, evidence for second-line therapies is derived from small trials or series and is frequently contradictory. The optimal approach in patients with steroid-refractory aGVHD is not known.

Etanercept, mycophenolate, denileukin, or pentostatin plus corticosteroids for acute graft-versus-host disease: a randomized phase 2 trial from the Blood and Marrow Transplant Clinical Trials Network. Alousi AM, Weisdorf DJ, Logan BR, Bolaños-Meade J, Carter S, Difronzo N, et al. Blood 2009; 114: 511–7.

In this randomized phase II trial, the addition of mycophenolate to systemic corticosteroids resulted in higher complete response and overall survival rates and fewer infectious complications than did prednisone combined with etanercept, pentostatin, or denileukin diftitox.

Phase 3 clinical trial of steroids/mycophenolate mofetil vs. steroids/placebo as therapy for acute GVHD: BMT CTN 0802. Bolaños-Meade J, Logan BR, Alousi AM, Antin JH, Barowski K, Carter SL, et al. Blood 2014; 124: 3221–7.

Although mycophenolate mofetil appears to be more effective than other second-line agents for aGVHD and is commonly used for this purpose, its actual efficacy appears to be limited. This phase III randomized, double-blind trial was ended early for futility after showing no benefit to therapy with glucocorticoids plus mycophenolate versus glucocorticoids alone.

Etanercept plus methylprednisolone as initial therapy for acute graft-versus-host disease. Levine JE, Paczesny S, Mineishi S, Braun T, Choi SW, Hutchinson RJ, et al. Blood 2008; 111: 2470–5.

A regimen of etanercept plus corticosteroids was more likely to achieve complete response (69% vs. 33%) and 100-day survival (82% vs. 66%) than were steroids alone.

Sirolimus for treatment of steroid-refractory acute graft-versus-host disease. Hoda D, Pidala J, Salgado-Vila N, Kim J, Perkins J, Bookout R, et al. Bone Marrow Transplant 2010; 45: 1347–51.

Sirolimus was initiated in 34 patients with steroid-refractory aGVHD. The overall response rate was 76%, with 44% achieving complete response. Complications included myelosuppression and hemolytic uremic syndrome.

Extracorporeal photopheresis versus anticytokine therapy as a second-line treatment for steroid-refractory acute GVHD: a multicenter comparative analysis. Jagasia M, Greinix H, Robin M, Das-Gupta E, Jacobs R, Savani BN. Biol Blood Marrow Transplant 2013; 19: 1129–33.

A retrospective analysis of 98 patients with steroid-refractory aGVHD receiving photopheresis revealed superior complete response rates (54% vs. 20%) and survival compared with those receiving anticytokine therapy (etanercept or inolimomab). The safety profile of extracorporeal photopheresis was excellent.

Third-Line Therapies

- Pentostatin **B**
- Anti-CD52 antibody (alemtuzumab) **B**
- Ruxolitinib **C**
- Infliximab **B**
- Interleukin-2 receptor antibodies (basiliximab) **B**
- Mesenchymal stem cells **A**
- Methotrexate **B**
- Tocilizumab **C**
- Antithymocyte globulin **B**
- Denileukin diftitox **B**
- PUVA **B**
- Narrowband UVB **C**

Diagnosis and management of acute graft-versus-host disease. Dignan FL, Clark A, Amrolia P, Cornish J, Jackson G, Mahendra P, et al. Br J Haematol 2012; 158: 30–45.

Evidence-based guidelines for aGVHD are reviewed. Pentostatin, alemtuzumab, mesenchymal stem cells, and MTX are among third-line therapies used after second-line agents have failed or in the context of clinical trials. Most such drugs have limited or negative/conflicting data.

Other agents with a possible therapeutic role in steroid-refractory aGVHD include ruxolitinib, tocilizumab, antithymocyte globulin, and others.

Ruxolitinib in corticosteroid-refractory graft-versus-host disease after allogeneic stem cell transplantation: a multicenter survey. Zeiser R, Burchert A, Lengerke C, Verbeek M, Maas-Bauer K, Metzelder SK, et al. Leukemia 2015; 29: 2062–8.

Treatment with the Jak 1/2 inhibitor ruxolitinib resulted in an 82% response rate, including 25 complete responses, among 54 patients with steroid-refractory aGVHD. This class of medication is the subject of growing interest for treatment of both acute and chronic GVHD.

A phase III study of infliximab and corticosteroids for the initial treatment of acute graft-versus-host disease. Couriel DR, Saliba R, de Lima M, Giralt S, Andersson B, Khouri I, et al. Biol Blood Marrow Transplant 2009; 15: 1555–62.

Although several case series demonstrated benefit from infliximab, this trial's 63 patients with grade II to IV aGVHD had no benefit from initial therapy with combination steroids and infliximab compared with methylprednisolone alone.

Basiliximab for the treatment of steroid-refractory acute graft-versus-host disease after unmanipulated HLA-mismatched/haploidentical hematopoietic stem cell transplantation. Wang JZ, Liu KY, Xu LP, Liu DH, Han W, Chen H, et al. Transplant Proc 2011; 43: 1928–33.

The chimeric IL-2 receptor antagonist basiliximab yielded a therapeutic response in 46/53 patients with steroid-refractory aGVHD.

The mesenchymal stromal cells dilemma—does a negative phase III trial of random donor mesenchymal stromal cells in steroid-resistant graft-versus-host disease represent a death knell or a bump in the road? Galipeau J. Cytotherapy 2013; 15: 2–8.

Despite promising results of a phase II study, a phase III trial of mesenchymal stromal cells failed to meet its primary end points for treatment of both new-onset and steroid-refractory aGVHD.

Narrowband ultraviolet B phototherapy for treatment of steroid-refractory and steroid-dependent acute graft-versus-host disease. Feldstein JV, Bolaños-Meade J, Anders VL, Abuav R. J Am Acad Dermatol 2011; 65: 733–8.

Of 14 patients with skin-predominant steroid-refractory or dependent aGVHD, 11 had a complete or partial response, suggesting narrowband ultraviolet B phototherapy is a potentially effective and low-risk skin-directed therapy for selected patients with aGVHD.

CHRONIC GVHD

Specific Investigations

- Skin biopsy
- Liver function tests
- Complete blood count
- Quality-of-life assessment
- Range of motion/physical therapy evaluation
- Pulmonary function tests
- Schirmer test
- Evaluation of other organs (ocular, oral, genital, gastrointestinal, musculoskeletal)

National Institutes of Health consensus development project on criteria for clinical trials in chronic graft-versus-host disease: I. Diagnosis and staging working group report. Filipovich AH, Weisdorf D, Pavletic S, Socie G, Wingard JR, Lee SJ, et al. Biol Blood Marrow Transplant 2005; 11: 945–56.

Cutaneous signs that are considered diagnostic of chronic GVHD (cGVHD) include poikiloderma; lichen planus–like lesions; and lichen sclerosis–like, morphea-like, and sclerotic features. Standardization of response criteria, staging, and grading are detailed.

Atypical manifestations of graft-versus-host disease. Cornejo CM, Kim EJ, Rosenbach M, Micheletti RG. J Am Acad Dermatol 2015; 72: 690–5.

Numerous common and atypical manifestations of GVHD may be seen. Biopsy or additional investigations may help confirm a diagnosis of cGVHD in patients without diagnostic features.

First-Line Therapies

• Systemic corticosteroids	A
• Systemic corticosteroid and calcineurin inhibitor	C

Organ-specific management and supportive care in chronic graft-versus-host disease. Dignan FL, Scarisbrick JJ, Cornish J, Clark A, Amrolia P, Jackson G, et al. Br J Haematol 2012; 158: 62–78.

The choice of initial therapy depends on disease severity, organ involvement, and other factors. Organ-specific supportive care (e.g., emollients, sun protection) and a multidisciplinary approach can be beneficial.

Diagnosis and management of chronic graft-versus-host disease. Dignan FL, Amrolia P, Clark A, Cornish J, Jackson G, Mahendra P, et al. Br J Haematol 2012; 158: 46–61.

For those with moderate or severe cGVHD, corticosteroids are first-line systemic therapy, usually beginning at a daily dose of 1 mg/kg prednisone tapered slowly based on clinical response. There are no randomized studies comparing standard to higher or lower steroid doses. Optimization of topical steroids and other skin-directed therapies may enable dose reduction in those with skin-limited cGVHD.

Therapy for chronic graft-versus-host disease: a randomized trial comparing cyclosporine plus prednisone versus prednisone alone. Koc S, Leisenring W, Flowers ME, Anasetti C, Deeg HJ, Nash RA, et al. Blood 2002; 100: 48–51.

Initial treatment with prednisone plus ciclosporin may reduce some steroid-related toxicities compared with treatment with prednisone alone, but there is no difference in mortality or time at which therapy can be discontinued. Randomized trials of other agents for the initial treatment of cGVHD have failed to show benefit compared with prednisone alone.

Second-Line Therapies

• Calcineurin inhibitors (tacrolimus, ciclosporin)	C
• Extracorporeal photopheresis	B
• Mycophenolate mofetil	C
• mTOR inhibitors (sirolimus, everolimus)	C
• Rituximab	B
• Imatinib	C
• UVB, narrowband UVB	C
• PUVA, UVA1	C

Consensus conference on clinical practice in chronic GVHD: second-line treatment of chronic graft-versus-host disease. Wolff D, Schleuning M, von Harsdorf S, Bacher U, Gerbitz A, Stadler M, et al. Biol Blood Marrow Transplant 2011; 17: 1–17.

Additional therapy is warranted for those with cGVHD that progresses despite 1 mg/kg/day prednisone for 2 weeks, fails to respond after 4 to 6 weeks of therapy, or flares with attempts to taper below 0.5 mg/kg/day. Initial second-line therapy should include agents with documented activity and adequate safety profiles, such as calcineurin inhibitors, extracorporeal photopheresis, mycophenolate mofetil, mTOR inhibitors, imatinib, or rituximab. Unfortunately, without available predictors of response, "trial and error" is the only way to determine efficacy of a particular agent or combination regimen for a given patient.

Extracorporeal photopheresis for the treatment of acute and chronic graft-versus-host disease in adults and children: best practice recommendations from an Italian Society of Hemapheresis and Cell Manipulation (SIdEM) and Italian Group for Bone Marrow Transplantation (GITMO) consensus process. Pierelli L, Perseghin P, Marchetti M, Messina C, Perotti C, Mazzoni A, et al. Transfusion 2013; 53: 2340–52.

Among 735 patients with steroid-resistant or dependent cGVHD included for review, photopheresis resulted in a response rate of 50% to 65% (complete response 30%–35%). Approximately 25% to 35% of patients were able to taper steroid use significantly.

Efficacy of mycophenolate mofetil in the treatment of chronic graft-versus-host disease. Lopez F, Parker P, Nademanee A, Rodriquez R, Al-Kadhimi Z, Bhatia R, et al. Biol Blood Marrow Transplant 2005; 11: 307–13.

Eighteen of 24 (75%) patients receiving mycophenolate mofetil as second-line therapy responded to treatment, and 14 of 22 (64%) patients on prednisone were able to taper the dose of steroids. Complications included gastrointestinal side effects, hematologic toxicities, and infectious episodes.

Therapy of sclerodermatous chronic graft-versus-host disease with mammalian target of rapamycin inhibitors. Jedlickova Z, Burlakova I, Bug G, Baurmann H, Schwerdtfeger R, Schleuning M. Biol Blood Marrow Transplant 2011; 17: 657–63.

Thirty-four patients with severe scleroderma-like cGVHD had an overall response rate of 76% to sirolimus or everolimus. Hyperlipidemia, poor wound healing, cytopenias, infections, and thrombotic microangiopathy were seen in a minority.

A randomized phase II crossover study of imatinib or rituximab for cutaneous sclerosis after hematopoietic cell transplantation. Arai S, Pidala J, Pusic I, Chai X, Jaglowski S, Khera N, et al. Clin Cancer Res 2016; 22: 319–27.

In a randomized phase II study of patients with steroid-refractory sclerotic cGVHD, 9 of 35 (26%) patients receiving imatinib and 10 of 37 (27%) patients receiving rituximab had quantitative improvements in skin sclerosis or joint range of motion. The response rates in this study were somewhat lower than reported previously for these agents and likely reflect increased stringency of response criteria, as well as the refractory nature of sclerotic cGVHD in general.

Graft-versus-host disease: part II. Management of cutaneous graft-versus-host disease. Hymes SR, Alousi AM, Cowen EW. J Am Acad Dermatol 2012; 66: 535.

PUVA, PUVA bath, UVB, narrowband (NB)-UVB, and UVA1 have all shown efficacy for cGVHD in small series. UVB and NB-UVB may work best for lichen planus–like manifestations, whereas PUVA and UVA1 penetrate more deeply and are better suited for scleroderma-like disease.

Third-Line Therapies	
Systemic	
• Ruxolitinib	C
• Pulse corticosteroids	C
• Interleukin-2	C
• Pentostatin	B
• Low-dose methotrexate	C
• Thalidomide	B
• Hydroxychloroquine	C
• Infliximab	C
• Etanercept	C
• Alefacept	C
• Alemtuzumab	C
• Cyclophosphamide	C
• Etretinate / isotretinoin / acitretin	C
• Clofazimine	C
• Thoracoabdominal irradiation	C
• Mesenchymal stromal cell therapy	C
Oral GVHD	
• Topical corticosteroids	C
• Topical calcineurin inhibitors	C
• Intraoral PUVA	C
• Oral UVB	C

Ruxolitinib in corticosteroid-refractory graft-versus-host disease after allogeneic stem cell transplantation: a multicenter survey. Zeiser R, Burchert A, Lengerke C, Verbeek M, Maas-Bauer K, Metzelder SK, et al. Leukemia 2015; 29:2062–8.

In a multicenter retrospective study, 35 of 41 (85%) patients with steroid-refractory cGVHD responded to the JAK1/2 inhibitor ruxolitinib. Complications included cytopenias and cytomegalovirus reactivation.

Interleukin-2 and regulatory T cells in graft-versus-host disease. Koreth J, Matsuoka K, Kim HT, McDonough SM, Bindra B, Alyea EP 3rd, et al. N Engl J Med 2011; 365: 2055–66.

Low-dose IL-2 stimulates T-regulatory cell expansion. Of 23 patients in this phase I study, 12 had a partial response and 11 had stable disease.

Phase II study of pentostatin in patients with corticosteroid-refractory chronic graft-versus-host disease. Jacobsohn DA, Chen AR, Zahurak M, Piantadosi S, Anders V, Bolaños-Meade J, et al. J Clin Oncol 2007; 25: 4255–61.

Fifty-eight heavily pretreated patients (median four prior regimens) with cGVHD were given pentostatin 4 mg/m² every 2 weeks for 12 doses. The overall response rate was 32 of 58 (55%), with major improvements seen in 31 patients. Survival was 70% at 2 years, with infectious complications predominant.

Granuloma annulare

Andrew Ilchyshyn, Ajoy Bardhan

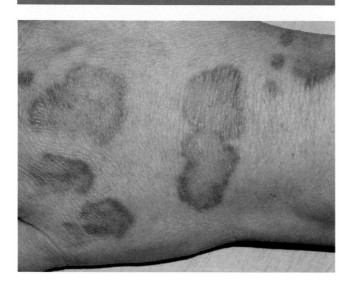

Granuloma annulare (GA) is a self-limiting inflammatory skin disease. Most commonly, it is characterized by smooth, skin-colored to pink or violaceous arciform and annular beaded plaques localized to the distal extremities. Other variants include generalized, perforating, and subcutaneous forms of GA. Histology shows palisading granulomas with a central core of necrobiotic collagen surrounded by a lymphohistiocytic infiltrate.

The etiology and pathogenesis are unclear. An association with diabetes mellitus is controversial, with conflicting evidence in the literature. Concomitant dyslipidemias, autoimmune thyroiditis, viral infection (hepatitis B and C and human immunodeficiency virus (HIV)), and malignancies (lymphoma and solid organ neoplasms) have also rarely been reported.

MANAGEMENT STRATEGY

The localized variety of GA is often diagnosed clinically, but a skin biopsy may be required to confirm the diagnosis of less common varieties. Once the diagnosis is made, it is prudent to exclude diabetes mellitus. Other disease associations, mentioned earlier, are rare.

The majority of cases of GA are asymptomatic and self-limiting; therefore the need for treatment should be considered carefully. In many cases reassurance that the disease is benign and will resolve spontaneously is sufficient. Painful or unsightly lesions may justify active treatment, but the evidence to support the efficacy of reported treatments is poor.

Localized GA may be treated with topical or intralesional steroids. Clobetasol propionate (Dermovate) lotion under occlusion with a hydrocolloid dressing, changed weekly, can be used for up to 6 weeks. Alternatively, intralesional triamcinolone injections may be used at intervals of 6 to 8 weeks. Cryotherapy using liquid nitrogen can be repeated every 3 to 4 weeks as required. Treatment of refractory lesions includes photodynamic therapy, ultraviolet A1 phototherapy (UVA1), intralesional interferon, and laser therapy; large, tumid lesions may require excision.

Generalized GA may be persistent, and its unsightly appearance causes patients to seek active treatment. Both UVA and psoralen and ultraviolet A (PUVA) may be used, but relapses can occur. Isotretinoin and dapsone have been associated with improvement or clearance of generalized GA. Topical tacrolimus and pimecrolimus have been used, with greater success in generalized disease than in the localized variety. Other reported treatments for this condition include laser, fumaric acid esters, hydroxychloroquine, methotrexate, chlorambucil, ciclosporin, hydroxyurea, doxycycline, pulsed triple-antibiotic therapy, systemic steroids, adalimumab, infliximab, anthralin, vitamin E, allopurinol, nicotinamide, pentoxifylline, and defibrotide.

Specific Investigation

- Check glycated hemoglobin (HbA1c)

Unlike necrobiosis lipoidica, in which there is a strong association with diabetes mellitus, the relationship between GA and diabetes is unclear. However, a simple check of HbA1c to exclude undiagnosed diabetes may be sensible.

Carbohydrate tolerance in patients with granuloma annulare. Study of fifty-two cases. Haim S, Friedman-Birnbaum R, Haimn Shafrir A, Ravina A. Br J Dermatol 1973; 88: 447–51.

In a study of 39 patients with localized GA the incidence of abnormal carbohydrate tolerance was 23% and similar to that of a control population, compared with an incidence of 77% in 13 patients with generalized disease.

Absence of carbohydrate intolerance in patients with granuloma annulare. Gannon TF, Lynch PJ. J Am Acad Dermatol 1994; 30: 662–3.

In a study of 23 patients in which 13 patients had localized lesions and 10 patients had generalized disease, glycosylated hemoglobin levels were found to be normal.

Localised granuloma annulare is associated with insulin-dependent diabetes mellitus. Muhlemann MF, Williams DR. Br J Dermatol 1984; 111: 325–9.

This retrospective study looked at 557 insulin-dependent diabetics and found that 16 patients had GA, significantly more than the 0.9 cases that might have been expected.

LOCALIZED GRANULOMA ANNULARE

First-Line Therapies

• Intralesional corticosteroids	B
• Cryotherapy	B
• Topical corticosteroid	E

Granuloma annulare and necrobiosis lipoidica treated by jet injector. Sparrow G, Abell E. Br J Dermatol 1975; 93: 85–9.

In this study of 45 patients with GA, intralesional triamcinolone produced a complete response in 68% of patients after three treatments carried out at 6- and 8-week intervals. About half of the patients suffered recurrences, which responded to retreatment.

Successful outcome of cryosurgery in patients with granuloma annulare. Blume-Peytavi U, Zouboulis CH, Jacobi H, Scholz A, Bisson S, Orfanos CE. Br J Dermatol 1994; 130: 494–7.

In a study of 31 patients with GA, 22 patients were treated with liquid nitrogen and 9 with nitrous oxide. After a single freeze – thaw cycle 81% of lesions were cleared. Four cases had persistent atrophic scars where large lesions had been treated with liquid nitrogen.

It should be possible to prevent cryoatrophy by avoiding freeze–thaw cycles of more than 10 seconds and taking care not to overlap treatment areas.

Granuloma annulare of childhood successfully treated with potent topical corticosteroids previously unresponsive to tacrolimus ointment 0.1%: report of three cases. Rallis E, Stavropoulou E, Korfitis C. Clin Exp Dermatol 2009; 34: e475–6.

Twice-daily application of clobetasol propionate 0.05% or mometasone furoate 0.1% without occlusion for 2 to 3 weeks led to complete remission of localized GA in three children aged between 7 and 10.

Successful treatment of chronic skin diseases with clobetasol propionate and a hydrocolloid occlusive dressing. Volden G. Acta Derm Venereol 1992; 72: 69–71.

One of three cases of GA showed a complete response after 4 weeks of treatment with clobetasol propionate under occlusion.

This treatment has the advantage of being painless, but evidence for its efficacy is not strong.

Second-Line Therapies	
• Pulsed dye laser	C
• 308-nm excimer laser	E
• Topical photodynamic therapy	D
• Topical imiquimod	E
• Topical dapsone	E
• Topical tacrolimus	E
• Topical pimecrolimus	E
• Scarification	E
• Surgery	E
• UVA1	E
• Intralesional Interferon	E
• Pulsed monthly rifampicin, ofloxacin, and minocycline	D

Treatment of granuloma annulare with the 595 nm pulsed dye laser (PDL), a multicenter retrospective study with long-term follow-up. Passeron T, Fusade T, Vabres P, Bousquet-Rouaud R, Collet-Vilette A-M, Dahan S, et al. J Eur Acad Dermatol Venereol 2013; 27: 785–8.

In this study, five patients with localized and eight with generalized GA were treated with three sessions of pulsed-dye laser. A significant response was seen only in the localized forms.

Granuloma annulare treated with excimer laser. Bronfenbrener R, Ragi J, Milgraum S. J Clin Aesthet Dermatol 2012; 5: 43–5.

A 73-year-old woman with a greater than 40-year history of generalized GA underwent treatment with excimer laser therapy on the dorsum of her hands. The regimen comprised fluence of 300 mJ/cm² with five doses per treatment session. After 15 treatment sessions, there was complete resolution, with no recurrence at treated sites at 6 months' follow-up.

Photodynamic therapy for granuloma annulare: more than a shot in the dark. Weisenseel P Kuznetsov AV, Molin S, Ruzicka T, Berking C, Prinz JC. Dermatology 2008; 217: 329–32.

Seven patients with GA were treated with three sessions of photodynamic therapy with topical aminolevulinic acid (ALA-PDT) with an interval of 2 to 4 weeks between each session. In two patients, GA cleared completely, in two the skin lesions improved markedly, and in three no response was observed.

A retrospective analysis of real-life practice of off-label photodynamic therapy using methyl aminolevulinate (MAL-PDT) in 20 Italian dermatology departments. Part 1: inflammatory and esthetic indications. Calzavara-Pinton PG, Rossi MT, Aronson E, Sala R, Arpaia N, Burtica EC. J Photochem Photobiol Sci 2013; 12: 148–57.

Nine out of 13 patients with GA showed improvement.

Successful treatment of granuloma annulare with imiquimod cream 5%: a report of four cases. Badavanis G, Monastirli A, Pasmatzi E, Tsambaos D. Acta Derm Venereol 2005; 85: 547–8.

Four patients with multiple lesions of GA treated with imiquimod cream once daily. The majority of lesions cleared within 12 weeks of treatment with no recurrence observed at 18 months' follow-up.

Granuloma annulare: dramatically altered appearance after application of 5% imiquimod cream. Stephenson S, Nedorost S. Pediatr Dermatol 2008; 25: 138–9.

GA *worsened* in a child after accidental application of imiquimod used to treat adjacent plane warts.

Management of periocular granuloma annulare using topical dapsone. Kassardjian M, Patel M, Shitabata P, Horowitz D. J Clin Aesthet Dermatol 2015; 8: 48–51.

A 41-year-old male with arciform GA of the right upper eyelid and lateral canthus was treated with dapsone 5% gel applied twice daily, with significant improvement seen at 3 weeks.

Periorbital granuloma annulare successfully treated with tacrolimus 0.1% ointment. Gomez-Moyano E, Vera-Casaño A, Martinez S, Sanz A. Int J Dermatol 2014; 53: e156–7.

Scarification treatment of granuloma annulare. Wilkin JK, DuComb D, Castrow FF. Arch Dermatol 1982; 118: 68–9.

Two patients successfully treated by scarification once weekly for 8 weeks and at 3-weekly intervals thereafter, using the point of a 19G injection needle drawn across the lesions to produce capillary bleeding.

Surgical pearl: surgical treatment of tumour sized granuloma annulare of the fingers. Shelley WB, Shelley ED. J Am Acad Dermatol 1997; 37: 473–4.

A case report of nodular GA treated with shave excision, allowing the wound to heal by secondary intention.

Multiple localized granuloma annulare: ultraviolet A1 phototherapy. Frigerio E, Franchi C, Garutti C, Spadino S, Altomare GF. Clin Exp Dermatol 2007; 32: 762–4.

Four patients responded to high-dose UVA1, starting with 60 J/cm² on day 1, followed by fixed daily doses of 100 J/cm², five times weekly for 3 weeks.

Treatment of granuloma annulare by local injections with low dose recombinant human interferon gamma. Weiss JM, Muchenberger S, Schöpf E, Simon JC. J Am Acad Dermatol 1998; 39: 117–9.

Three patients achieved clearance of localized GA treated with intralesional interferon-γ 2.5 × 10⁵ IU on 7 consecutive days and continued three times weekly for a further 2 weeks.

Granuloma annulare treated with rifampin, ofloxacin, and minocycline combination therapy. Marcus DV, Mahmoud BH, Hamzavi IH. Arch Dermatol 2009; 145: 787–9.

Six patients with localized GA achieved complete clearance after 3 to 5 months' combination therapy with rifampin 600 mg, ofloxacin 400 mg, and minocycline 100 mg administered monthly.

GENERALIZED (DISSEMINATED) GRANULOMA ANNULARE

First-Line Therapies	
• UVA1	B
• PUVA	C
• Narrowband-ultraviolet B (NB-UVB)	D
• Isotretinoin	C
• Oral dapsone	C
• Topical tacrolimus	E
• Topical photodynamic therapy	E

UVA1 phototherapy for disseminated granuloma annulare. Schnopp C, Tzaneva S, Mempel M, Schulmeister K, Abeck D, Tanew A. Photodermatol Photoimmunol Photomed 2005; 21: 68–71.

Twenty patients with disseminated GA underwent phototherapy with UVA1 340 to 400 nm, which provided good or excellent results in half of them and satisfactory responses in the majority. Discontinuation of treatment was followed by early recurrence.

Psoralen and ultraviolet A in the treatment of granuloma annulare. Browne F, Turner D, Goulden V. Photodermatol Photoimmunol Photomed 2011; 27: 81–4.

A retrospective study of 33 patients treated with twice-weekly PUVA, showing clearance in 50% of patients, a further 16% with good improvement, 25% with moderate benefit, and 9% with poor outcome. Seventy-nine percent remained in remission at 6 months, but only 32% remained in remission at 12 months.

Clearance of generalized papular umbilicated granuloma annulare in a child with bath PUVA therapy. Batchelor R, Clark S. Pediatr Dermatol 2006; 23: 72–4.

GA cleared with bath PUVA.

NB-UVB phototherapy for generalized granuloma annulare. Pavlovsky M, Samuelov L, Sprecher E, Matz H. Dermatol Ther 2016; 29: 152–4.

A retrospective study of 13 patients with generalized GA treated with NB-UVB phototherapy showed 54% of patients had a complete or partial response to treatment.

Generalized granuloma annulare in a patient with type 2 diabetes mellitus: successful treatment with isotretinoin. Sahin M, Türel-Ermertcan A, Oztürkcan S, Türkdogan P. J Eur Acad Dermatol Venereol 2006; 20: 111–4.

A case of generalized granuloma annulare with myelodysplastic syndrome: successful treatment with systemic isotretinoin and topical pimecrolimus 1% cream combination. Baskan EB, Turan A, Tunali S. J Eur Acad Dermatol Venereol 2007; 21: 693–5.

A man with generalized GA achieved full remission after 4 months of treatment with isotretinoin 0.5 mg/kg/day and topical pimecrolimus 1% cream twice daily.

There are several case reports in which isotretinoin has been successfully employed at doses of 0.5 to 1 mg/kg/day for generalized disease.

The response of generalised granuloma annulare to dapsone. Czarnecki DB, Gin D. Acta Derm Venereol 1986; 66: 82–4.

Six patients with generalized GA treated with dapsone 100 mg daily showed a complete response, with five clearing within 8 weeks and four remaining clear for 20 months after stopping treatment.

Efficacy of dapsone on disseminated granuloma annulare: a case report and review of the literature. Martín-Sáez E, Fernández-Guarino M, Carrillo-Gijón R, Muñoz-Zato E, Jaén-Olasolo P. Actas Dermosifilogr 2008; 99: 64–8.

A patient showed improvement taking 100 mg dapsone daily, with improvement noted at 2 months and clearance at 15 months. No recurrence was noted several months after discontinuation of treatment.

Successful treatment of disseminated granuloma annulare with topical tacrolimus. Jain S, Stephens CJM. Br J Dermatol 2004; 150: 1042–3.

Four patients were treated with twice- daily application of 0.1% tacrolimus ointment. At 6 weeks, two patients showed clearance, and the remaining two patients showed significant improvement. There was no recurrence or deterioration noted 6 weeks after discontinuation of treatment.

Generalized granuloma annulare treated with methylaminolevulinate photodynamic therapy. Piaserico S, Zattra E, Linder D, Peserico A. Dermatology 2009; 218: 282–4.

Three patients with persistent generalized GA responded to MAL-PDT.

Second-Line Therapies	
• Topical corticosteroids	E
• Systemic corticosteroids	E
• Topical pimecrolimus	E
• Hydroxychloroquine	D
• Fumaric acid esters	C
• Chlorambucil	D
• Doxycycline	E
• Allopurinol	E
• Nicotinamide	E
• Pentoxifylline	E
• Oral calcitriol	E
• Monthly rifampicin, ofloxacin, and minocycline	D
• Ciclosporin	E
• Methotrexate	E
• Hydroxyurea	E
• Defibrotide	E
• Anthralin	E
• Adalimumab	D
• Infliximab	E
• Etanercept	E
• Laser (Neodymium-doped Yttrium Aluminium Garnet, Nd:YAG)	E
• Oral vitamin E and leukotriene inhibitor	E
• Topical vitamin E	E

Evidence Levels: **A** Double-blind study **B** Clinical trial ≥ 20 subjects **C** Clinical trial < 20 subjects **D** Series ≥ 5 subjects **E** Anecdotal case reports

A contact dermatitis reaction to clobetasol propionate cream associated with resolution of recalcitrant, generalised granuloma annulare. Agarwal S, Berth-Jones J. J Dermatol Treat 2000; 11: 279–82.

A patient cleared of disseminated GA by topical clobetasol; however, the patient developed contact sensitization to the medication, raising the possibility that this reaction may also have played a therapeutic role.

Granuloma annulare, generalised. Larralde J. Arch Dermatol 1963; 87: 777–8.

A case report describing the use of systemic steroids in generalized GA.

Systemic corticosteroids may exacerbate preexisting diabetes.

Pimecrolimus 1% cream in the treatment of disseminated granuloma annulare. Rigopoulos D, Prantsidis A, Christofidou E, Ioannides D, Gregoriou S, Katsambas A. Br J Dermatol 2005; 152: 1364–5.

An adult improved with twice-daily treatment for 3 months.

Antimalarials for control of disseminated granuloma annulare in children. Simon M, Van Den Driesch P. J Am Acad Dermatol 1994; 31: 1064–5.

Six children achieved complete clearance within 6 weeks of treatment with 3 to 6 mg/kg/day hydroxychloroquine and remained clear for 2.5 years of follow-up.

Treatment of generalized granuloma annulare with hydroxychloroquine. Cannistraci C, Lesnoni La Parola I, Falchi M, Picardo M. Dermatology 2005; 211: 167–8.

Four patients out of nine achieved complete remission when treated with hydroxychloroquine for 4 months with the following reducing regimen: 9 mg/kg/day for 2 months, 6 mg/kg/day for month 3, and 2 mg/kg/day for month 4. One child was treated with 50% of the dose delineated.

Therapy of noninfectious granulomatous skin diseases with fumaric acid esters. Breuer K, Gutzmer R, Völker B, Kapp A, Werfel T. Br J Dermatol 2005; 152: 1290–5.

Thirteen patients with generalized GA were treated with Fumaderm, with gradual uptitration of dose, as tolerated. Eight patients experienced improvement of disease. Treatment courses were between 3 and greater than 14 months.

Treatment of disseminated granuloma annulare recalcitrant to topical therapy: a retrospective 10 year analysis with comparison of photochemotherapy alone versus photochemotherapy plus oral fumaric acid esters. Wollina U, Langner D. J Eur Acad Dermatol Venereol 2011; 26: 1319–21.

A retrospective study comparing PUVA alone with oral PUVA plus fumaric acid esters showed a better complete or almost complete clearance rate with a combination of PUVA and fumaric acid esters. In addition these patients needed a lower total UVA dosage to achieve this effect.

There are a number of small series of patients demonstrating the efficacy of fumaric acid esters in the management of disseminated GA using the dose regimen used in psoriasis.

Low dose chlorambucil in the treatment of generalised granuloma annulare. Kossard S, Winkelmann RK. Dermatologica 1979; 158: 443–50.

Six patients were treated with chlorambucil 2 mg twice daily. Five showed a marked improvement by 12 weeks.

Chlorambucil should only be considered in refractory cases of GA and only for a maximum of 12 weeks.

Generalized granuloma annulare: response to doxycycline. Duarte AF, Mota A, Pereira MA, Baudrier T, Azevedo F. J Eur Acad Dermatol Venereol 2009; 23: 84–5.

A woman with GA achieved almost complete resolution after treatment with doxycycline 100 mg/day for 10 weeks.

Treatment of disseminated granuloma annulare with allopurinol: case report. Mazzatenta C, Ghilardi A, Grazzini M. Dermatol Ther 2010; 23(Suppl 1): S24–7.

Allopurinol 300 mg twice daily is an alternative treatment in therapy-resistant patients with disseminated GA.

Response of generalized granuloma annulare to high dose niacinamide. Ma A, Medenica M. Arch Dermatol 1983; 119: 836–9.

A patient with generalized GA experienced resolution of her lesions after 6 months of treatment with niacinamide 1500 mg/day.

Generalised granuloma annulare successfully treated with pentoxifylline. Rubel DM, Wood G, Rosen R, Jopp-McKay A. Australas J Dermatol 1993; 34: 103–8.

A man with generalized GA showed dramatic clearing of papules after 4 weeks of treatment with pentoxifylline 400 mg three times a day.

Granuloma annulare responsive to oral calcitriol. Boyd AS. Int J Dermatol 2012; 51: 120–2.

One patient described improvement in pruritus at 1 month, and improvement in appearance was noted at 3 months with 0.25 μg oral calcitriol daily.

Monthly rifampicin, ofloxacin, and minocycline therapy for generalized and localized granuloma annulare. Garg S, Baveja S. Indian J Dermatol Venereol Leprol 2015; 81: 35–9.

Five patients with generalized disease and one patient with localized disease were treated with monthly pulses of rifampicin 600 mg, ofloxacin 400 mg, and minocycline 100 mg until clearance of lesions was achieved. Courses lasted between 4 and 8 months, with no recurrence seen in follow-up of between 9 and 18 months.

Disseminated granuloma annulare: efficacy of cyclosporine therapy. Spadino S, Altomare A, Cainelli C, Franchi C, Frigerio E, Garutti C, et al. Int J Immunopathol Pharmacol 2006; 19: 433–8.

Four patients treated with ciclosporin 4 mg/kg/day achieved complete clearance within 3 weeks, with no relapses during the following 12 months.

Cyclosporine for the treatment of granuloma annulare. Fiallo P. Br J Dermatol 1998; 138: 369–70.

Two patients treated with ciclosporin 3 mg/kg/day showed flattening and clearance of lesions within a month. Treatment was tapered and discontinued after 2 further months, with no recurrence noted at 12 months.

Successful treatment of disseminated granuloma annulare with methotrexate. Plotner AN, Mutasim DF. Br J Dermatol 2010; 163: 1123–4.

A patient experienced a resolution of the majority of lesions with methotrexate 15 mg weekly and daily folic acid supplementation for 6 weeks. Discontinuation of methotrexate upon two occasions for surgical procedures resulted in a recurrence of disease within 1 month.

Treatment of recalcitrant disseminated granuloma annulare with hydroxyurea. Hall CS, Zone JJ, Hull CM. J Am Acad Dermatol 2008; 58: 525.

Two patients with recalcitrant disseminated GA responded to hydroxyurea 500 mg three times per week for up to 2 months. Subsequently the dose was decreased to 500 mg two times a day.

There would need to be a strong indication for the use of hydroxyurea given the potential risk of toxicity.

A case of disseminated granuloma annulare treated with defibrotide: complete clinical remission and progressive hair darkening. Rubegni P, Sbano R, Fimiani M. Br J Dermatol 2003; 149: 437–8.

A man with generalized GA and deep vein thrombosis showed improvement in his skin disease within 30 days of starting treatment with defibrotide. His generalized GA subsequently cleared completely after 90 days.

Treatment of disseminated granuloma annulare with anthralin. Jantke ME, Bertsch H-P, Schön MP, Fuchs T. Hautarzt 2011; 62: 935–9.

Two cases demonstrated significant improvement after treatment with anthralin.

Treatment of recalcitrant granuloma annulare (GA) with adalimumab: a single-center, observational study. Min MS, Lebwohl M. J Am Acad Dermatol 2016; 74: 127–33.

Seven patients with generalized granuloma annulare were administered adalimumab 80 mg subcutaneously, followed by 40 mg every other week, 1 week after initiation. Patients were asked to return in 1 and 3 months. Adalimumab was either discontinued with disease clearance or patient wish or escalated to weekly injections if minimal improvement was noted after 3 months. In cases in which lesions recurred after discontinuing adalimumab, patients were permitted to restart therapy. All seven patients experienced clearance, with two requiring weekly injections. Three patients maintained remission at 40 months after discontinuation of treatment.

Disseminated granuloma annulare: a cutaneous adverse effect of anti-TNF agents. Ratnarathorn M, Raychaudhuri S, Naguwa S. Indian J Dermatol 2011; 56: 752–4.

A woman developed GA after receiving adalimumab for rheumatoid arthritis. There was clearance of the GA on stopping adalimumab, but this recurred when treatment was switched to etanercept.

Antitumor necrosis factor-α treatment with infliximab for disseminated granuloma annulare. Murdaca G, Colombo BM, Barabino G, Caiti M, Cagnati P, Puppo F. Am J Clin Dermatol 2010; 11: 437–9.

A 62-year-old female patient was administered infliximab intravenously at a dosage of 5 mg/kg at weeks 0, 2, and 6 and thereafter at monthly intervals for 10 additional months. Most of the GA lesions improved within 8 weeks and slowly resolved within 10 months of treatment.

Rapid improvement of recalcitrant disseminated granuloma annulare upon treatment with the tumor necrosis factor-α inhibitor, infliximab. Hertl MS, Haendle I, Schuler G, Hertl M. Br J Dermatol 2005; 152: 552–5.

A 59-year-old woman with type 1 diabetes and a 4-year history of recalcitrant generalized granuloma annulare was administered infliximab at 5 mg/kg/day at weeks 0, 2, and 6 and thereafter at a monthly interval for an additional 4 months. The majority of disease cleared within 4 to 6 weeks. New lesions were not seen in follow-up to 16 months.

Conflicting evidence emerges with reports of inefficacy as well as efficacy with regard to etanercept.

Resolving granuloma annulare with etanercept. Shupack J, Siu K. Arch Dermatol 2006; 142: 394–5.

A case report of improvement in generalized granuloma annulare after 12 weeks of treatment.

Failure of etanercept therapy in disseminated granuloma annulare. Kreuter A, Altmeyer P, Gambichler T. Arch Dermatol 2006; 142: 1236–7.

A case series of four patients in which two patients showed no improvement and two patients displayed more extensive disease after 12 weeks of treatment. Administered dosing was either 25 mg twice weekly or 50 mg twice weekly.

Fractional photothermolysis for the treatment of granuloma annulare: a case report. Karsai S, Hammes S, Rütten A, Raulin C. Lasers Surg Med 2008; 40: 319–22.

Remission of four lesions after two to three treatment sessions with a 1440 nm Nd:YAG laser.

Treatment of disseminated granuloma annulare with a 5-lipoxygenase inhibitor and vitamin E. Smith KJ, Norwood C, Skelton H. Br J Dermatol 2002; 146: 667–70.

Three patients were treated with vitamin E 400 IU daily and zileuton 2400 mg daily. All responded within 3 months with complete clinical clearing.

Disseminated granuloma annulare: therapy with vitamin E topically. Burg G. Dermatology 1992; 184: 308–9.

A patient with disseminated GA was successfully treated with topical vitamin E twice daily for 2 weeks.

Treatment of co-existing viral infection or malignancy

GA manifesting as a paraneoplastic phenomenon or associated with diabetes and viral infection has been reported to improve or clear with treatment of the coexisting pathology.

Disseminated granuloma annulare as a presentation of acquired immunodeficiency syndrome (AIDS). McGregor JM, McGibbon DH. Clin Exp Dermatol 1992; 17: 60–2.

Treatment with zidovudine was associated with resolution of cutaneous lesions.

Generalized granuloma annulare associated with chronic hepatitis B virus infection. Ma H, Zhu W, Yue X. J Eur Acad Dermatol Venereol 2006; 20: 186–9.

Generalized GA resolved after 3 months of treatment with interferon-α.

Generalized granuloma annulare associated with gastrointestinal stromal tumour: case report and review of clinical features and management. Chiu MLS, Tang MBY. Clin Exp Dermatol 2008; 33: 469–71.

Extensive generalized GA cleared 1 month after surgical excision of gastrointestinal stromal tumor.

Generalized granuloma annulare with open comedones in photoexposed areas. Bhushan P, Aggarwal A, Yadav R, Baliyan V. Clin Exp Dermatol 2011; 36: 495–8.

Patient with a background of diabetes mellitus was commenced upon metformin and glimepiride, resulting in a rapid improvement of granuloma annulare.

Evidence Levels: **A** Double-blind study **B** Clinical trial ≥ 20 subjects **C** Clinical trial < 20 subjects **D** Series ≥ 5 subjects **E** Anecdotal case reports

95

Granuloma faciale

Nevianna Bordet

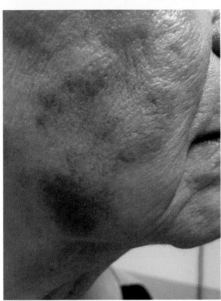

Courtesy of University Hospitals of Leicester NHS Trust, Department of Medical Illustration.

Granuloma faciale is a rare, benign, chronic inflammatory dermatosis caused by a localized form of cutaneous vasculitis. It presents primarily in middle-aged Caucasian males, usually as a single lesion on the face. Multiple lesions occur in up to a third of patients, and there are isolated reports of similar conditions affecting the eye and upper airways. Extensive involvement of the nose can mimic rhinophyma.

Lesions are red-brown, violaceous, or flesh-colored plaques or nodules with accentuation of follicular openings. Clinical diagnosis is difficult. Differential diagnosis includes sarcoid, lupus, lymphocytoma cutis, persistent insect bite reactions, and lymphoma. The histologic differential diagnosis includes erythema elevatum diutinum and angiolymphoid hyperplasia with eosinophilia.

MANAGEMENT STRATEGY

Granuloma faciale is a chronic condition, and spontaneous remission is unusual. Lesions are usually asymptomatic, but treatment is needed to reduce disfigurement. It is notoriously resistant to treatment and, because of the rarity of the condition, there are no formal trials of therapy. Treatment modalities can be divided into destructive techniques and antiinflammatory approaches. The optimal treatment depends on the size, site, and thickness of the lesions. For isolated or small numbers of lesions *intralesional steroid* or destructive treatments such as *cryotherapy, laser,* or surgical *excision* can be used. For multiple or widespread lesions systemic treatment, such as *dapsone* or *clofazimine*, can be considered. In the last few years, there have been increasing numbers of case reports of successful treatment with topical calcineurin inhibitors for isolated or multiple lesions.

Cosmetic camouflage can be helpful for some patients with flatter lesions.

Specific Investigations

- Skin biopsy
- Hematology (full blood count)
- Dermoscopy

Histologic findings include a dense eosinophilic and neutrophilic infiltrate, often perivascular, affecting the upper and sometimes deep dermis. The epidermis is spared, and there is a Grenz zone. Telangiectasia is common. Vasculitis with leukocytoclasis is reported. Dermal fibrosis is often seen.

Granuloma faciale: a clinicopathologic study of 66 patients. Ortonne N, Wechsler J, Bagot M, Grosshans E, Cribier B. J Am Acad Dermatol 2005; 53: 1002–9.

Peripheral blood eosinophilia is sometimes found.

Dermoscopic patterns of common facial inflammatory skin disease. Lallas A, Argenziano G, Apalla Z, Gourhant JY, Zaballos P, Di Lernia V, et al. J Eur Acad Dermatol Venereol 2014; 28: 609–14.

Dermoscopy is increasingly used to aid diagnosis in granuloma faciale. Follicle abnormalities such as dilated follicular openings, perifollicular whitish halo, follicular keratotic plugs, and linear slightly arborizing vessels in a parallel arrangement are the most commonly described dermoscopic criteria.

First-Line Therapies

• Corticosteroids	D
• Calcineurin inhibitors	D
• Cryotherapy	D
• Laser therapy	D
• 5-Fluorouracil	E

Granuloma faciale treated with intradermal dexamethasone. Arundell FD, Burdick KH. Arch Dermatol 1960; 82: 437–8.

This paper reports response to dexamethasone, but triamcinolone acetonide and triamcinolone hexacetonide have also been used. Patients should be warned of the risk of skin atrophy and pigment change.

Granuloma faciale: is it a new indication for pimecrolimus? A case report. Eetam I, Ertekin B, Unal I, Alper S. J Dermatol Treat 2006; 17: 238–40.

A case report of a lesion on the central face showing "dramatic recovery" after pimecrolimus cream 1% twice daily for 2 months.

Granuloma faciale: treatment with topical tacrolimus. Marcoval J, Moreno A, Bordas X, Peyri J. J Am Acad Dermatol 2006; 55: S110–1.

This and other papers describe response to topical tacrolimus, sometimes within a few months. In some patients lesions had previously failed to respond to other therapies. Remission for up to 2 years is described.

Assessment of the efficacy of cryosurgery in the treatment of granuloma faciale. Panagiotopoulos A, Anyfantakis V, Rallis E, Chasapi V, Stavropoulos P, Boubouka C, et al. Br J Dermatol 2006; 154: 357–60.

Nine patients were treated with either spray or closed probe cryotherapy. The open-spray technique was given as one or two freeze–thaw cycles of 20 to 30 seconds. The cryoprobe was given as one to three freeze–thaw cycles of 15 to 20 seconds. Patients were retreated after 1 and 3 months. All were clear of disease activity at 6 months. One patient developed severe inflammatory reaction with blistering. Two had hypopigmentation, but this resolved in 4 months. There was no recurrence within 2 to 4 years' follow-up.

Granuloma faciale: successful treatment of nine cases with a combination of cryotherapy and intralesional corticosteroid injection. Dowlati B, Firooz A, Dowlati Y. Int J Dermatol 1997; 36: 548–51.

Cryotherapy for 20 to 30 seconds was followed by triamcinolone acetonide 5 mg/mL intralesionally. Lesions cleared completely in all nine cases.

Granuloma faciale treated with pulsed-dye laser: a case series. Cheung S-T, Lanigan SW. Clin Exp Dermatol 2005; 30: 373–5.

Four patients who had all failed with cryotherapy were treated with pulsed-dye laser at 595 nm. In two patients the lesions resolved. Nasal lesions, especially flatter ones, seem to respond better to treatment.

Reports of granuloma faciale responding to argon laser and KTP laser are described in the literature, but the pulsed-dye laser is the type most frequently reported as achieving improvement.

Carbon dioxide laser treatment of granuloma faciale. Wheeland RG, Ashley JR, Smith DA, Ellis DL, Wheeland DN. J Dermatol Surg Oncol 1984; 10: 730–3.

A single treatment resulted in healing with no discernible scar. There was no recurrence at 1 year.

Rhinophyma-like granuloma faciale successfully treated with carbon dioxide laser. Bakkour W, Madan V. Br J Dermatol 2014; 170: 474–5.

A patient who failed to respond to topical and intralesional steroids as well as 150 mg dapsone showed an excellent response with no recurrence at 18 months.

A handful of other case reports show benefit with carbon dioxide laser.

Treatment of laser resistant granuloma faciale with intralesional triamcinolone acetonide and 5-fluorouracil combination therapy. Norris DL, Apikian M, Goodman GJ. J Cutan Aesthet Surg 2015; 8: 111–3.

Case report of one patient who failed to respond to topical tacrolimus and pulsed-dye laser achieving "an excellent response" with intralesional 0.8 mL 5-fluorouracil 50 mg/1 mL combined with 0.2 mL triamcinolone acetonide 10 mg/mL. No more than 2 mL per treatment should be used according to the authors.

Second-Line Therapies

- Dapsone   E
- Surgery   E

On the efficacy of dapsone in granuloma faciale. Van de Kerkhof PCM. Acta Derm Venereol 1994; 74: 61–2.

A 4-cm plaque showed "impressive improvement" with dapsone 200 mg daily. Dapsone needs careful monitoring, and many patients would not tolerate 200 mg daily.

Many authors mention dapsone as a treatment that has been tried but failed.

Granuloma faciale treated with topical dapsone: a case report. Babalola O, Zhang J, Kristjansson A, Whitaker-Worth D, McCusker M. Dermtol Online J 2014; 20: 25148282.

Twice-daily topical dapsone 5% gel was used successfully to treat a single patient who had failed with intralesional steroid injections, potent topical steroids, and a 6-month trial of doxycycline 20 mg twice daily. Near-complete resolution was achieved at 9 months with no recurrence at 18 months.

Recurrent facial plaques following full-thickness grafting. Phillips DK, Hymes SR. Arch Dermatol 1994; 130: 1436–7.

Although surgery is mentioned in many papers, recurrence can occur even after full-thickness excision and grafting.

Third-Line Therapies

- Clofazimine   E
- Topical PUVA   E

Granuloma faciale mimicking rhinophyma: response to clofazimine. Gomez-de la Fuente E, del Rio R, Guerra A, Rodriguez-Peralto JL, Iglesias L. Acta Derm Venereol 2000; 80: 144.

A patient with a 10-year history of histologically proven disease on the nose was treated with 300 mg clofazimine once daily for 5 months, with "remarkable improvement." Two similar reports are cited.

Granuloma faciale: treatment with topical psoralen and UVA. Hudson LD. J Am Acad Dermatol 1983; 8: 559.

A 62-year-old man with a 1-month history of biopsy-proven granuloma faciale affecting the nasal alae responded to 24 J UVA given over 10 weeks, showing a very marked improvement with no evidence of residual lesion at 6 months.

There are old reports of treatment with intralesional gold and bismuth, radiotherapy, oral colchicine, isoniazid, potassium arsenite, testosterone, and antimalarials, but within the past 30 years there have been no reports of successful response to these agents.

ACKNOWLEDGMENTS

With thanks to Dr. Susan E. Handfield-Jones as a previous contributor to this chapter.

Evidence Levels: **A** Double-blind study   **B** Clinical trial ≥ 20 subjects   **C** Clinical trial < 20 subjects   **D** Series ≥ 5 subjects   **E** Anecdotal case reports

96

Granuloma inguinale

Ted Rosen

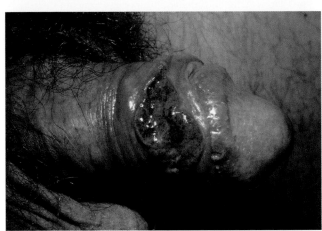

Granuloma inguinale, or donovanosis, is an infection causing granulomatous and destructive ulceration of genital, inguinal, and perineal skin. Cervical lesions are rare, but may clinically mimic carcinoma. Extragenital lesions occur in about 6% of cases. This disorder is extremely rare in Western Europe and the United States, but is still endemic or epidemic in India, South Africa, Brazil, Papua New Guinea, and rarely among aborigines in Australia. The causative organism is *Klebsiella granulomatis*, an intracellular gram-negative bacillus.

The disease presents with a subcutaneous granuloma or nodule that develops into characteristically painless, progressive ulcerative lesions without regional lymphadenopathy. Most often lesions are ulcerogranulomatous, highly vascular (i.e., a beefy red appearance), and friable (bleed easily on contact).

MANAGEMENT STRATEGY

Patients with donovanosis should be treated to prevent the gradual worsening of the disease leading to genital deformity or (very rarely) life-threatening disseminated infection, to prevent transmission, and to prevent the risk of concomitant transmission of human immunodeficiency virus (HIV) infection.

In the absence of evidence from randomized placebo-controlled trials, antibiotic treatment of donovanosis is based on the results of local clinical experience and individual case reports, typically involving relatively small numbers of patients.

The U.S. Centers for Disease Control and Prevention (CDC) (2015) currently recommends *azithromycin*, with many alternative regimens (e.g., *doxycycline, ciprofloxacin, erythromycin, trimethoprim–sulfamethoxazole*). Azithromycin is also recommended in the 2016 European Guideline on donovanosis. The addition of an aminoglycoside, such as *gentamicin*, is recommended by the CDC if lesions do not respond within the first few days.

Therapy should be continued until all lesions have healed completely. This typically starts at the outside margins and progresses inward. Despite seemingly effective initial therapy, a relapse can occur 6 to 18 months later. *Surgical excision* may be necessary for extensive disease that is unresponsive to antibiotic therapy. It should be noted that squamous cell carcinoma has been reported concurrent with active donovanosis, complicating long-standing cases, and even developing at sites of healed lesions.

Sexual partners of patients who have granuloma inguinale should be examined and treated if they had sexual contact with the patient during the 60 days preceding the onset of symptoms in the patient or have clinical signs and symptoms of the disease.

Specific Investigations

- Tissue smear or biopsy with Wright or Giemsa stains
- Screen for other sexually transmitted infections (e.g., HIV, syphilis)
- Culture (not readily available)
- Polymerase chain reaction (PCR) (not readily available)

Genital ulcer disease: accuracy of clinical diagnosis and strategies to improve control in Durban, South Africa. O'Farrell N, Hoosen AA, Coetzee KD, Van den Ende J. Genitourin Med 1994; 70: 7–11.

The clinical diagnostic accuracy for donovanosis was relatively high (63% in men, 83% in women). Donovanosis ulcers bled on touch and were not usually associated with inguinal lymphadenopathy.

Donovanosis. Hart G. Clin Infect Dis 1997; 25: 24–32.

Confirmation involves demonstration of typical intracellular Donovan bodies within large mononuclear cells visualized in smears prepared from lesions or biopsy specimens. The large mononuclear cells are 25 to 90 μm in diameter with a vesicular or pyknotic nucleus.

Sexually transmitted disease surveillance 2010. Centers for Disease Control and Prevention. U.S. Department of Health and Human Services, Atlanta; 2011.

Cases are confirmed by demonstration of intracytoplasmic Donovan bodies in Wright- or Giemsa-stained smears or biopsies of granulation tissue in a clinically compatible case (one or more painless or minimally painful granulomatous lesions in the anogenital area).

A colorimetric detection system for *Calymmatobacterium granulomatis*. Carter JS, Kemp DJ. Sex Transm Infect 2000; 76: 134–6.

A PCR test that could be used by well-equipped laboratories; largely a research tool.

Squamous cell carcinoma complicating donovanosis not a thing of the past! Sethi S, Sarkar R, Garg V, Agarwal S. Int J STD AIDS 2014; 25: 894–7.

A reminder that squamous cell carcinoma has been associated with active and even with healed donovanosis.

First-Line Therapy

- Azithromycin   **B**

Donovanosis: treatment with azithromycin. Bowden FJ, Savage J. Int J STD AIDS 1998; 9: 61.

An Australian report of over 100 patients treated with azithromycin with no primary treatment failures. Regimens employed were 500 mg orally daily for 7 days or 1 g orally weekly for 4 weeks. The

1996 to 1997 edition of the Australian Antibiotic Guidelines lists azithromycin as the first-line agent for donovanosis. The drug is listed as a B1 agent in pregnancy, meaning that it can be used for the treatment of antenatal patients with the disease.

2016 European guideline on donovanosis. O'Farrell N, Moi H. Int J STD AIDS 2016; 27: 605–7.

Azithromycin 1 g orally weekly or 500 mg orally daily until complete healing is achieved is recommended as first-line therapy. Second-line therapeutic recommendations parallel those enumerated by the CDC (see the next citation).

Centers for Disease Control and Prevention Sexually Transmitted Diseases Treatment Guidelines, 2015. Workowski KA. Clin Infect Dis 2015; 61(Suppl 8): S759–62.

The treatment of choice is azithromycin 1 g orally once per week or 500 mg daily for at least 3 weeks and until all lesions have completely healed. Alternative (second-line) therapies include doxycycline 100 mg orally twice a day for at least 3 weeks and until all lesions have completely healed, ciprofloxacin 750 mg orally twice a day for at least 3 weeks and until all lesions have completely healed, erythromycin base 500 mg orally four times a day for at least 3 weeks and until all lesions have completely healed, and trimethoprim–sulfamethoxazole one double-strength (160 mg/800 mg) tablet orally twice a day for at least 3 weeks and until all lesions have completely healed.

Second-Line Therapies

• Doxycycline	C
• Erythromycin	C
• Trimethoprim–sulfamethoxazole	B
• Ciprofloxacin	C

Clinico-epidemiologic features of granuloma inguinale in the era of acquired immune deficiency syndrome. Jamkhedkar PP, Hira SK, Shroff HJ, Lanjewar DN. Sex Transm Dis 1998; 25: 196–200.

Fifty patients (21 HIV positive and 29 HIV negative) treated with erythromycin 2 g orally daily. Healing took longer in the seropositive group (mean 25.7 vs. 16.8 days).

Granuloma inguinale. Rosen T, Tschen JA, Ramsdell W, Moore J, Markham B. J Am Acad Dermatol 1984; 11: 433–7.

Twenty patients were safely and effectively treated with trimethoprim–sulfamethoxazole. It has been used extensively in India with consistently good results.

Third-Line Therapies

• Ceftriaxone	C
• Gentamicin	C
• Surgical treatment	E
• Norfloxacin	C
• Trovafloxacin	C
• Ampicillin	C
• Chloramphenicol	C
• Thiamphenicol	C

Ceftriaxone in the treatment of chronic donovanosis in Central Australia. Merianos A, Gilles M, Chuah J. Genitourin Med 1994; 70: 84–9.

Eight women and four men treated with daily injections of 1 g ceftriaxone diluted in 2 mL of 1% lidocaine. Clinical improvement was dramatic in most lesions, and four patients healed completely without recurrence after a total 7 to 10 g of ceftriaxone.

1998 guidelines for treatment of sexually transmitted diseases. Centers for Disease Control and Prevention. MMWR Recomm Rep 1998; 47: 1–116.

The CDC recommends the addition of gentamicin (1 mg/kg IV every 8 hours) if lesions do not respond within the first few days of therapy.

Surgical treatment of granuloma inguinale. Bozbora A, Erbil Y, Berber E, Ozarmagan S. Br J Dermatol 1998; 138: 1079–81.

Fistulas and abscesses unresponsive to antibiotics may require surgical treatment.

Treatment of donovanosis with norfloxacin. Ramanan CR, Sarma PSA, Ghorpade A, Das M. Int J Dermatol 1990; 29: 298–9.

Ten patients treated with oral norfloxacin 400 mg twice daily showed complete healing in 2 to 11 days.

Trovafloxacin for the treatment of chronic granuloma inguinale. Hsu SL, Chia JK. Sex Transm Infect 2001; 77: 137.

One patient had complete resolution of lesions after 2 months of trovafloxacin 200 mg daily after previously failing doxycycline, ampicillin, erythromycin, trimethoprim–sulfamethoxazole, ceftriaxone, gentamicin, and chloramphenicol.

The diagnosis and treatment of donovanosis (granuloma inguinale). Richens J. Genitourin Med 1991; 67: 441–52.

Ampicillin is unreliable and not recommended as first-line therapy.

Donovanosis in Papua New Guinea. Maddocks I, Anders EM, Dennis E. Br J Vener Dis 1976; 52: 190–6.

Fifty cases treated with chloramphenicol 500 mg four times daily. Forty-three had complete or near-complete clinical and bacteriologic healing.

Chloramphenicol is effective, but risk of aplastic anemia limits its use to life-threatening disease.

Donovanosis treated with thiamphenicol. Belda W, Velho PE, Arnone M, Romitti R. Braz J Infect Dis 2007; 11: 388–9.

Ten patients with donovanosis of the penis treated with thiamphenicol 2.5 g orally on day 1 followed by 1 g daily for the next 14 days. Eight, including two HIV-positive patients, had healing of their lesions without recurrence.

Thiamphenicol is advantageous over chloramphenicol because of its once-daily administration and lack of reports of serious marrow toxicity.

SPECIAL CONSIDERATIONS

Pregnancy: Pregnant and lactating women should be treated with erythromycin with consideration for the addition of a parenteral aminoglycoside. Azithromycin may also be safe and effective. Doxycycline should be avoided in the second and third trimester of pregnancy because of the risk for discoloration of teeth and bones, but is compatible with breastfeeding. Ciprofloxacin presents a low risk to the fetus during pregnancy, but sulfonamides are associated with rare but serious kernicterus in those

Evidence Levels: **A** Double-blind study **B** Clinical trial ≥ 20 subjects **C** Clinical trial < 20 subjects **D** Series ≥ 5 subjects **E** Anecdotal case reports

with G6PD deficiency and should be avoided in the third trimester and during breastfeeding.

HIV infection: Patients often require prolonged antibiotic treatment after the regimens cited earlier. The addition of gentamicin should be strongly considered.

Children: Children should be treated with a short course of azithromycin dosed at 20 mg/kg. Infants born to mothers with donovanosis should be treated prophylactically with 3 days of azithromycin dosed at 20 mg/kg once daily.

Granulomatous cheilitis

Charlene Lam, Bryan E. Anderson

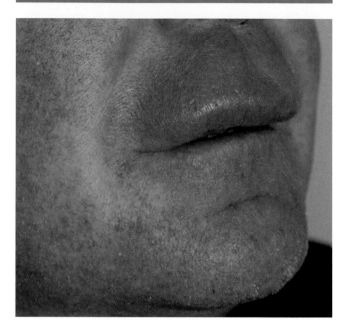

Granulomatous cheilitis is characterized by painless swelling of one or both lips, with histologic evidence of noncaseating granulomatous inflammation. Granulomatous cheilitis exists along the spectrum of orofacial granulomatosis, which encompasses localized disease (granulomatous cheilitis, Miescher cheilitis) to multisystem disease (Melkersson–Rosenthal syndrome). Melkersson–Rosenthal syndrome describes the triad of recurrent orofacial edema, recurrent facial nerve palsy, and lingua plicata (fissured tongue). Many investigators consider isolated granulomatous cheilitis to be a monosymptomatic form of Melkersson–Rosenthal syndrome.

MANAGEMENT STRATEGY

The treatment of granulomatous cheilitis is very challenging. Because the etiology is unknown, a variety of therapeutic strategies with varying degrees of success have been attempted. No randomized clinical trials or comparative studies have been performed. Given the waxing-and-waning nature of the condition, treatment outcomes are difficult to assess. Spontaneous remissions of granulomatous cheilitis rarely occur, further confounding assessment of therapies. Furthermore, a recent retrospective study demonstrated long-term treatment with topical medications and/or combination therapy may be required.

The aim of treatment is to prevent permanent labial deformity. Conservative measures for acute granulomatous cheilitis involve symptomatic relief, including *cold compresses* and *oral antihistamine*s to reduce erythema and *ointment*s to protect against fissuring of the lips. Initial therapy frequently includes *corticosteroids*, either topical, intralesional, or systemic. Initial topical therapy may include either triamcinolone or clobetasol (compounded into Orabase). Intralesional steroids may be used in doses ranging from 10 to 40 mg/kg. Nerve blocks may reduce patient discomfort in cases where large volumes at low concentrations are needed. Although short courses of prednisone will frequently improve tissue swelling, flares are often noted on cessation.

Clofazimine has been reported to treat granulomatous cheilitis successfully. Response to therapy has been variable. Possible side effects include transient orange-pink discoloration of the skin, nausea, and vomiting. Fatal enteropathy may occur but only at higher doses than those recommended for granulomatous cheilitis treatment. *Thalidomide* can also be considered, especially in refractory cases. Patients must be monitored for the development of peripheral neuropathy and warned of its teratogenicity. Monotherapy with *metronidazole, tetracyclines, azithromycin, hydroxychloroquine, or sulfasalazine*, although less well substantiated, may be attempted. These medications may be used with corticosteroids. The addition of *minocycline* 100 mg twice daily or *tetracycline* 500 mg daily may prevent rebound after prednisone discontinuation. The value of *dapsone* and topical *tacrolimus* in the treatment of granulomatous cheilitis is unclear. Biologics, including *infliximab* and *adalimumab*, have also been successful treatments.

Granulomatous cheilitis may become persistent. Patients who suffer from permanent esthetic deformity or functional impairment may benefit from cheiloplasty. Surgical intervention should be performed only when more conservative approaches have failed and when inflammation is quiescent. An important consideration for Melkersson–Rosenthal syndrome patients undergoing anesthesia for surgical intervention or any surgical procedures is the risk of urticarial reaction due to anesthetic triggers during the procedure. In the past, remission was maintained with the use of postoperative corticosteroid injections. More recent reports, however, have described long remissions after surgery, with no additional treatment needed.

Granulomatous cheilitis has characteristics that are associated with several conditions that may require evaluation, including Crohn disease, sarcoidosis, infections (tuberculosis, leprosy, deep fungal, Human Immunodeficiency Virus (HIV), and syphilis), acquired or hereditary angioedema, cheilitis glandularis, and leukemic infiltrates. It is also important to rule out any provocative cause such as odontogenic infections or allergenic sensitizers. Orofacial granulomatosis is associated with Crohn disease, especially in children, and may precede gastrointestinal symptoms. The signs and symptoms of Crohn disease may be minimal, necessitating a complete physical examination and continued observation and surveillance of the patient.

Initial biopsies of granulomatous cheilitis may reveal dilated lymphatic channels, nonspecific inflammatory infiltrates, and edema. In the later stages, the classic noncaseating granulomas are found. Absence of granulomata on biopsy does *not* exclude the diagnosis of granulomatous cheilitis. Granulomatous cheilitis is primarily a clinical diagnosis.

Specific Investigations

- Biopsy for histopathologic examination: polarization and stains/cultures for fungi and acid-fast bacilli
- Complete blood count and chemistry profile, including serum calcium
- Angiotensin-converting enzyme level
- Chest radiograph
- C1-esterase inhibitor; C1-esterase inhibitor functional assays; C1, C2, and C4 levels
- Consultation with dental professional if odontogenic infection suspected
- Consultation with gastroenterologist if there are any gastrointestinal complaints
- Standard patch testing (metal, bakery, dental, and other specialized patch series may be required) and food allergy testing to determine whether an allergen is causative

Evidence Levels: **A** Double-blind study **B** Clinical trial ≥ 20 subjects **C** Clinical trial < 20 subjects **D** Series ≥ 5 subjects **E** Anecdotal case reports

Orofacial granulomatosis. Miest R, Bruce A, Rogers RS. Clin Dermatol 2016; 34: 505–13.

This article reviews orofacial granulomatosis and provocative factors and discusses possible etiologies and differential diagnoses.

A comprehensive review of current treatments for granulomatous cheilitis. Banks T, Gada S. Br J Dermatol 2012; 166: 934–7.

Characteristics of patients with orofacial granulomatosis. McCartan BE, Healy CM, McCreary CE, Flint SR, Rogers S, Toner ME. Oral Dis 2011; 17: 696–704.

The largest review of clinical and laboratory findings in 119 patients with orofacial granulomatosis. Mean age of 28, with an equal male-to-female ratio. Almost all patients had clinical evidence of lip and/or facial swelling. Over 50% of biopsies showed granulomatous inflammation.

Melkersson–Rosenthal syndrome: a review of 36 patients. Greene RM, Rogers RS III. J Am Acad Dermatol 1989; 21: 1263–70.

Cheilitis granulomatosa. van der Waal RIF, Schulten EAJM, van de Scheur MR, Wauters IM, Starink TM, van der Waal I. J Eur Acad Dermatol Venereol 2001; 15: 519–23.

Cheilitis granulomatosa: overview of 13 patients with long-term follow-up: results of management. van der Waal RIF, Schulten AJM, van der Meij E, van de Scheur MR, Starink TM, van der Waal I. Int J Dermatol 2002; 41: 225–9.

Orofacial granulomatosis: clinical features and long-term outcome of therapy. Al Johani KA, Moles DR, Hodgson TA, Porter SR, Fedele S. J Am Acad Dermatol 2010; 62: 611–20.

Anesthetic management of patients with Melkersson–Rosenthal syndrome. Tekin M, Kati I. J Anesth 2008; 22: 294–6.

Is orofacial granulomatosis in children a feature of Crohn's disease? Khouri JM, Bohane TD, Say AS. Acta Paediatr 2005; 94: 501–4.

Re: Melkersson–Rosenthal syndrome as an early manifestation of Crohn's disease. Narbutt P, Dziki A. Colorectal Dis 2005; 7: 420–1.

Orofacial granulomatosis in a patient with Crohn's disease. van der Scheur MR, van der Waal RI, Völker-Dieben JH, Klinkeberg-Knol ED, Starink TM, van der Waal I. J Am Acad Dermatol 2003; 49: 952.

Cheilitis granulomatosa and Melkersson–Rosenthal syndrome: evaluation of gastrointestinal involvement and therapeutic regimens in 14 patients. Ratzinger G, Sepp N, Vogetseder W, Tilg H. J Eur Acad Dermatol Venereol 2007; 21: 1065–70.

Orofacial granulomatosis as the initial presentation of Crohn's disease in an adolescent. Bogenrieder T, Lehn N, Landthaler M, Stolz W. Dermatology 2003; 206: 273–8.

Cutaneous Crohn's disease mimicking Melkersson–Rosenthal syndrome: treatment with methotrexate. Tonkovic-Capin V, Galbraith SS, Rogers III RS, Binion DG, Yancey K. J Eur Acad Dermatol Venereol 2006; 20: 449–52.

Asymptomatic granulomatous vulvitis and granulomatous cheilitis in childhood: the need for Crohn disease workup. Nabatian AS, Shah KN, Iofel E, Rosenberg S, Javidian P, Pappert A, et al. J Pediatr Gastroenterol Nutr 2011; 53: 100–1.

Orofacial granulomatosis: three case reports illustrating the spectrum of disease and overlap with Crohn's disease. Smith VM, Murphy R. Clin Exp Dermatol 2013; 38: 33–5.

These articles highlight the possibility of Crohn disease presenting with, or subsequent to, the diagnosis of granulomatous cheilitis. Narbutt et al. notes that although the treatment of granulomatous cheilitis can be mostly cosmetic, Crohn disease is a systemic illness with multiple potential complications.

Though there are many similar clinical and histologic features between oral Crohn disease and orofacial granulomatosis, its relationship is controversial. Some contend that adolescent granulomatous cheilitis is a predictor of future Crohn disease. It is unknown what percentage of patients with granulomatous cheilitis will develop Crohn disease, but it may be prudent to discuss this issue with granulomatous cheilitis patients.

Melkersson–Rosenthal syndrome and cheilitis granulomatosa. A clinicopathologic study of thirty-three patients with special reference to their oral lesions. Worsaae N, Christensen KC, Schiødt M, Reibel J. Oral Surg Oral Med Oral Pathol 1982; 54: 404–13.

The elimination of odontogenic infections led to inactivity of orofacial edema in 11 of 18 patients.

The Melkersson–Rosenthal syndrome and food additive hypersensitivity. McKenna KE, Welsh MY, Burrows D. Br J Dermatol 1994; 131: 921–2.

Contact hypersensitivity in patients with orofacial granulomatosis. Armstrong DKB, Biagonia P, Lamey PJ, Burrows D. Am J Contact Dermatol 1997; 1: 35–8.

Ten of 48 patients showed positive reactions to an oral battery on standard patch testing. Of these 10, 7 showed an improvement on an elimination diet. In most cases this was not a complete result.

Patch testing for food-associated allergies in orofacial granulomatosis. Fitzpatrick L, Healy CM, McCartan BE, Flint SR, McCreary CE, Rogers S. J Oral Pathol Med 2011; 40: 10–3.

Orofacial granulomatosis associated with hypersensitivity to dental amalgam. Tomka M, Machovcova A, Pelclova D, Petanova J, Arenbergerova M, Prochazkova J. Oral Surg Oral Med Oral Pathol 2011; 112: 335–41.

First-Line Therapies

• Intralesional corticosteroids ± topical immunomodulators	C
• Oral corticosteroids	C

Long-term effectiveness of intralesional triamcinolone acetonide therapy in orofacial granulomatosis: an observational cohort study. Fedele S, Fung PPL, Bamashmous N, Petrie A, Porter S. Brit J Dermatol 2014; 170: 794–801.

This is the first retrospective observational cohort (*n* = 22) study demonstrating the long-term effectiveness of intralesional triamcinolone acetonide 40 mg/mL. Doses of 0.1 mL were injected into four equally distanced sites (left labial corner and next to median line, right corner and next to median line) per lip once a week for 3 weeks (one treatment course). The majority (14/22) of the patients were treated with one course and did not experience recurrence. There were no adverse effects.

Clinical behavior and long-term therapeutic response in orofacial granulomatosis patients treated with intralesional triamcinolone acetonide injections alone or in combination with topical pimecrolimus 1%. Mignogna MD, Pollio A, Leuci S, Ruoppo E, Fortuna G. J Oral Pathol Med 2013; 42: 763–81.

Triamcinolone acetonide 40 mg/mL diluted to 2:1 with saline (25 mg/mL) weekly was injected every 2 weeks for a maximum of 3 months (six sessions). The majority (11/19) responded. The eight partial responders who were then administered topical pimecrolimus 1% twice daily achieved clinical remission.

Effectiveness of small-volume, intralesional, delayed-release triamcinolone injections in orofacial granulomatosis: a pilot study. Mignogna MD, Fedele S, Lo Russo L, Adamo D, Satriano RA. J Am Acad Dermatol; 2004; 51: 265–8.

In this pilot study, triamcinolone 40 mg/mL, with each injection amounting to 0.1 mL, was used weekly for two to three sessions. The needle was injected between the prolabium and labia mucosa and directed to the oral mucosa to avoid atrophy and hypopigmentation of the labial skin.

With the growing evidence demonstrating the safety and efficacy of high-concentration, low volumes of intralesional steroids, the necessity of nerve blocks for low-concentration, large volumes of intralesional steroids is limited.

Melkersson–Rosenthal syndrome and orofacial granulomatosis. Rogers RS III. Dermatol Clin 1996; 14: 371–9.

Oral prednisone 1 to 1.5 mg/kg daily tapered over 3 to 6 weeks may be effective for more severe and symptomatic episodes of granulomatous cheilitis.

Second-Line Therapies	
• Clofazimine	C
• Biologics, including infliximab, adalimumab	C
• Azithromycin/roxithromycin	D
• Minocycline/tetracycline ± oral corticosteroids	E
• Metronidazole ± intralesional corticosteroids	E
• Mycophenolate mofetil ± topical corticosteroids	E

Clofazimine as elective treatment for granulomatous cheilitis. Fernandez-Freire LF, Gotarredona AS, Wittel JB, Ruis AP, Cabrera R, Ortoga MN, et al. J Drugs Dermatol 2005; 4: 374–7.

Three patients with granulomatous cheilitis treated with clofazimine 200 to 300 mg daily for 3 to 6 months obtained regression. Side effects included hyperpigmentation of the skin and elevation of liver enzymes.

Cheilitis granulomatosa Miescher: treatment with clofazimine and review of the literature. Ridder GJ, Fradis M, Löhle E. Ann Otol Rhinol Laryngol 2001; 110: 964–7.

A 15-year-old girl's granulomatous cheilitis was treated with clofazimine 100 mg daily. Regression was noted after 30 days of treatment. Thereafter, 100 mg of clofazimine three times a week was given for 3 months. Her lip eventually returned to normal size. Follow-up for 6 years revealed no recurrence.

This article reviews several case reports and a case series of clofazimine therapy and discusses the great variability in response to therapy.

Melkersson–Rosenthal syndrome: clinical, pathologic, and therapeutic considerations. Sussman GL, Yang WH, Steinberg S. Ann Allergy 1992; 69: 187–94.

Clofazimine 100 mg four times weekly for 3 to 11 months was used to treat 10 patients with granulomatous cheilitis/Melkersson–Rosenthal syndrome. Complete remission occurred in 5, partial clinical responses occurred in 3, and 2 patients had no clinical response.

Other studies have reported efficacy with a regimen consisting of clofazimine 100 mg daily for 10 days, followed by 200 to 400 mg weekly for 3 to 6 months.

Experience with anti-TNF-α therapy for orofacial granulomatosis. Elliot T, Campbell H, Esudier M, Poate T, Nunes C, Lomer M, et al. J Oral Pathol Med 2011; 40: 14–9.

A retrospective review of 14 patients treated with infliximab and adalimumab for orofacial granulomatosis with and without Crohn disease. Short-term remission was achieved with infliximab in 10 of the patients. Of those patients, 8 and 4 of them remained responsive at 1 and 2 years, respectively. Two of the patients who failed infliximab responded to adalimumab.

Treatment of granulomatous cheilitis with infliximab. Barry O, Barry J, Langan S, Murphy M, Fitzgibbon J. Arch Dermatol 2005; 141: 1081–3.

A 24-year-old woman with recalcitrant granulomatous cheilitis was treated with infliximab. In order to reduce the risk of infusion reactions, hydrocortisone (200 mg) was administered intravenously before treatment. The patient had restoration of normal lip architecture. Infliximab infusions were continued to maintain remission.

Melkersson–Rosenthal syndrome: a form of pseudoangioedema. Kakimoto C, Sparks C, White AA. Ann Allergy Asthma Immunol 2007; 99: 185–9.

A 19-year-old woman with recalcitrant granulomatous cheilitis was treated with infliximab infusions. The patient improved after the second infusion and had complete resolution after the third. Because adverse effects developed, therapy was changed to adalimumab (40 mg subcutaneously weekly), with no evidence of relapse noted.

Successful treatment of granulomatous cheilitis with adalimumab. Ruiz Villaverde R, Sanchez Cano D. Int J Dermatol 2012; 51: 118–20.

A 46-year-old woman with recalcitrant granulomatous cheilitis was treated with adalimumab at 80 mg SC for the first week, 40 mg the second week, and then every 2 weeks. After the third dose, clinical improvement was noticed, and no relapse occurred after completing 6 months of treatment.

Orofacial granulomatosis responding to weekly azithromycin pulse therapy. Yadav S, Dogra S, De D, Saikia UN. JAMA Dermatol 2015; 151: 219–20.

A case series of five patients with idiopathic orofacial granulomatosis on azithromycin 500 mg PO daily for 3 consecutive days

Evidence Levels: **A** Double-blind study **B** Clinical trial ≥ 20 subjects **C** Clinical trial < 20 subjects **D** Series ≥ 5 subjects **E** Anecdotal case reports

weekly demonstrated improvement after 1 month and significant improvement in 3 months.

Granulomatous cheilitis successfully treated with roxithromycin. Inui S, Itami S, Katayama I. J Dermatol 2008; 35: 244–5.

A 37-year-old man with granulomatous cheilitis was treated with 300 mg/day of roxithromycin. Swelling resolved in 6 weeks. Roxithromycin was tapered, and remission was achieved at 1 year of follow-up.

Successful treatment of granulomatous cheilitis with roxithromycin. Ishiguro E, Hatamochi A, Hamasaki Y, Ishikawa S, Yamazaki S. J Dermatol 2008; 35: 598–600.

A 13-year-old male with granulomatous cheilitis treated with roxithromycin 150 mg/day. No relapse was noticed after 6 months of follow-up.

Melkersson–Rosenthal syndrome in childhood: successful management with combination steroid and minocycline therapy. Stein SL, Mancini AJ. J Am Acad Dermatol 1999; 41: 746–8.

Two children with Melkersson–Rosenthal syndrome were treated successfully with minocycline and prednisone.

Tetracyclines would usually be contraindicated until the permanent dentition has erupted.

Minocycline in granulomatous cheilitis: experience with 6 cases. Veller Fornasa C, Catalano P, Peserico A. Dermatology 1992; 185: 220.

Six case reports of patients with granulomatous cheilitis treated with minocycline after failing other oral therapies (steroids, clofazimine, hydroxychloroquine, and surgery). Only one of the six patients responded to minocycline. The sole responder was later found to have chronic granulomatous disease.

Treatment and follow-up of persistent granulomatous cheilitis with intralesional steroid and metronidazole. Coskun B, Saral Y, Cicek D, Akpolat N. J Dermatol Treat 2004; 15: 333–5.

Cheilitis granulomatosa treated with metronidazole. Miralles J, Barnadas MA, de Moragas JM. Dermatology 1995; 191: 252–3.

A 30-year-old woman with monosymptomatic Melkersson–Rosenthal syndrome was successfully treated with metronidazole 750 to 1000 mg daily for an 8-month tapering course.

Metronidazole has also been useful in two patients with granulomatous cheilitis associated with Crohn disease. Treatment failures are also reported.

Orofacial granulomatosis successfully treated with mycophenolate mofetil. Antonyan AS, Pena-Robichaux V, McHargue CA. J Am Acad Dermatol 2014; 70: 137–9.

A 59-year-old woman with orofacial granulomatosis was successfully treated with mycophenolate mofetil 500 mg twice a day (BID) with significant improvement after 1 month and near-complete remission after 6 months of therapy.

Third-Line Therapies

• Cheiloplasty ± postoperative intralesional corticosteroids	C
• Thalidomide	E
• Hydroxychloroquine	E

Plastic surgical solutions for Melkersson–Rosenthal syndrome: facial liposuction and cheiloplasty procedures. Tan O, Atik B, Calka O. Ann Plast Surg 2006; 56: 268–73.

This article discusses surgical procedures in four patients, including reduction cheiloplasty consisting of mucosa, submucosa, and tangential muscle resection; crescent-shaped commissuroplasty; and facial liposuction. Mean follow-up duration was 13.7 months. No postoperative steroids were given, and there was no evidence of relapse in the follow-up period.

Cheilitis granulomatosa: successful treatment with combined local triamcinolone injections and surgery. Krutchkoff D, James R. Arch Dermatol 1978; 114: 1203–6.

A man with granulomatous cheilitis was treated with triamcinolone injections, followed by upper and lower cheiloplasty. Four months later, repeat cheiloplasty of the upper lip revealed granulomas were more numerous and larger than those observed initially. Postoperative corticosteroid injections maintained remission. The authors recommend postoperative corticosteroid injections to prevent exaggerated recurrences.

Long-term results after surgical reduction cheiloplasty in patients with Melkersson–Rosenthal syndrome and cheilitis granulomatosa. Ellitsgaad N, Andersson AP, Worsaaae N, Medgyesi S. Ann Plast Surg 1993; 31: 413–20.

A reduction cheiloplasty was performed on 13 patients. All were satisfied with their results, despite postoperative disease activity in six patients.

Lip reduction cheiloplasty for Miescher's granulomatous macrocheilitis (cheilitis granulomatosa) in childhood. Oliver DW, Scott MJL. Clin Exp Dermatol 2002; 27: 129–31.

Lip reduction cheiloplasty provided successful treatment of granulomatous cheilitis in an 11-year-old boy, suggesting surgery can be safely undertaken in young children.

Treatment of Miescher's cheilitis granulomatosa in Melkersson–Rosenthal syndrome. Camacho F, Garcia-Bravo B, Carrizosa A. J Eur Acad Dermatol Venereol 2001; 15: 546–9.

The authors conclude the best treatment for resistant granulomatous cheilitis is surgery with immediate injection of triamcinolone, followed by a course of oral tetracycline.

Successful treatment of granulomatous cheilitis with thalidomide. Thomas P, Walchner M, Ghoreschi K, Rocken M. Arch Dermatol 2003; 139: 136–8.

A 39-year-old woman was treated with thalidomide 100 mg daily for 6 months. Lip swelling almost completely resolved. Thalidomide was reduced to 100 mg every other day for 2 months and then stopped. One year later, the patient's condition was stable with no signs of relapse.

Baseline and follow-up neurologic assessments need to be done with thalidomide.

Thalidomide in treatment of refractory orofacial granulomatosis. Eustace K, Clowry J, Kirby B, Lally A. Br J Dermatol 2014; 171: 423–5.

Cheilitis granulomatosa: report of six cases and review of the literature. Allen CM, Camisa C, Hamzeh S, Stephens L. J Am Acad Dermatol 1990; 23: 444–50.

Hydroxychloroquine 200 to 400 mg daily has been reported to be efficacious in granulomatous cheilitis. Chloroquine therapy has not been successful in Melkersson–Rosenthal syndrome.

Hailey–Hailey disease

Anthony J. Chiaravalloti, Michael Payette

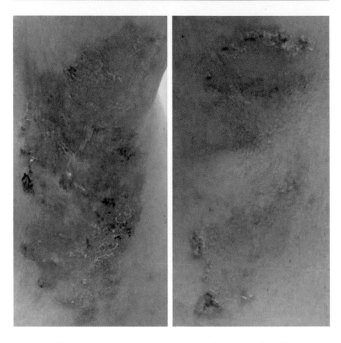

Hailey-Hailey affecting the axilla, pre and post treatment with CO_2 laser.

Hailey–Hailey disease (benign familial pemphigus) is a rare genodermatosis first described by two medical brothers in 1939. It is characterized by recurrent flares of vesicles, painful erosions, and weeping plaques, particularly involving the flexural areas. Symptoms usually begin in the second to fourth decades. The disease is generally localized, although widespread and severe involvement can occur. The most commonly affected sites are intertriginous areas like the axillae, groin, neck, and inframammary folds. The disease can exhibit an isomorphic response and affect areas of trauma or sites of inflammation from other diseases.

Hailey–Hailey disease is a dominantly inherited condition with variable expressivity. The defective gene, ATPase secretory pathway Ca2+ transporting 1 (ATP2C1), encodes the protein Secretory-pathway Ca2+-ATPases (SCPA1), which is an ATP-dependent calcium and manganese channel pump on the Golgi membrane in which downstream manifestations disrupt desmosome function between keratinocytes. The clinical and histopathologic picture can be similar to Darier disease and Grover disease (see relevant chapters).

MANAGEMENT STRATEGY

The management of Hailey–Hailey disease is accomplished through a combination of lifestyle modifications and medical and/or surgical therapy. Because the lesions of Hailey–Hailey disease are frequently precipitated by friction and aggravated by heat and moisture, lifestyle changes to minimize these can help reduce the frequency and severity of disease.

Polymicrobial infections with bacteria, yeasts, and viruses also appear to be exacerbating factors, and secondary infection with these organisms can significantly worsen the disease and cause a pungent odor. Thus simple antiinfective agents, topical or systemic, reduce the severity of exacerbations and remain the mainstay of treatment. Topical *clindamycin, fusidic acid,* and *imidazoles* have all been recommended. *Tetracyclines* and *semisynthetic penicillins* are the best systemic agents. If secondary infection with herpes simplex is suspected, *appropriate oral antiviral therapy* should be instituted.

Combining antiinfective therapy with *topical corticosteroids* seems to be particularly helpful, but corticosteroids alone may reduce the severity of lesions. Generally, moderate to potent agents are required, though some patients gain benefit from milder preparations. Caution should be exercised with long-term use because intertriginous skin is particularly prone to atrophy. Topical calcineurin inhibitors, like *tacrolimus* and *pimecrolimus,* may be effective as monotherapy or in combination with topical corticosteroids, although some authors dispute this. Some success has also been recorded with *calcitriol.* If there is not an expected response to topical therapy, clinicians should consider patch testing, as these patients commonly develop allergic contact dermatitis.

Patients with major exacerbations may benefit from a short course of systemic corticosteroids; however, there may be a rebound of the disease on withdrawal. Systemic alternatives that have been tried include *dapsone, ciclosporin, methotrexate,* and *retinoids,* but there is little evidence for their effectiveness beyond anecdotal case reports. *Electron beam therapy* has been reported for recalcitrant disease. There are few reports of treatment with biologic agents with limited benefit.

Surgical modalities like *cryotherapy, excision with grafting, dermabrasion,* and *CO_2 and other lasers* may also be beneficial in some patients, specifically for localized disease. Injections of *botulinum toxin* appear to be efficacious in reducing the sweating in axillary Hailey–Hailey disease.

Specific Investigations

- Biopsy
- Microbiologic cultures for bacteria, yeast, and herpesvirus
- Consider patch testing to topical preparations

First-Line Therapies

• Topical antimicrobials and systemic antibiotics	C
• Topical corticosteroids	C

Hailey–Hailey disease: the clinical features, response to treatment and prognosis. Burge SM. Br J Dermatol 1992; 126: 275–82.

In this series 86% of patients found combinations of topical corticosteroids and antimicrobial agents helpful at the first sign of a flare.

Familial benign chronic pemphigus and doxycycline: a review of 6 cases. Le Saché-de Peufeilhoux L, Raynaud E, Bouchardeau A, Fraitag S, Bodemer C. J Eur Acad Dermatol Venereol 2014; 28: 370–3.

This is a review of six patients who received oral doxycycline 50 to 100 mg/day. Two patients had complete remission, and two patients had significant improvement with mild flares during 4 years of follow-up.

The first article remains a key review of clinical and therapeutic aspects of this disease. We recommend patients failing topical therapies be started on doxycycline as first-line systemic therapy.

Evidence Levels: **A** Double-blind study **B** Clinical trial ≥ 20 subjects **C** Clinical trial < 20 subjects **D** Series ≥ 5 subjects **E** Anecdotal case reports

Second-Line Therapies

• Topical calcineurin inhibitors	E
• Calcitriol	E
• Systemic corticosteroids	E
• Dapsone	E
• Ciclosporin	E
• Botulinum toxin	E
• Carbon dioxide laser	E

Topical tacrolimus ointment is an effective therapy for Hailey–Hailey disease. Sand C, Thomsen HK. Arch Dermatol 2003; 139: 1401–2.

A 67-year-old man was cleared with once-daily tacrolimus 0.1% within 1 month and was maintained with as-needed use.

Familial benign chronic pemphigus (Hailey–Hailey disease): use of topical immunomodulators as a modern treatment option. Tchernev G, Cardoso JC. Rev Med Chil 2011; 139: 633–7.

This is a report of a 51-year-old male responding well to pimecrolimus 1% cream twice daily.

Treatment of Hailey–Hailey disease with topical calcitriol. Bianchi L, Chimenti M, Giunta A. J Am Acad Dermatol 2004; 51: 475–6.

This report showed complete clearance of lesions for 3 months after completing 1 month of twice-daily calcitriol 3 mcg/g ointment.

Generalized Hailey–Hailey disease. Marsch WC, Stüttgen G. Br J Dermatol 1978; 99: 553.

The use of systemic corticosteroids was successful in controlling extensive disease, but cessation of therapy resulted in significant rebound.

Benign familial chronic pemphigus treated with dapsone. Sire DJ, Johnson BL. Arch Dermatol 1971; 103: 262.

Three 21- to 64-year-old patients were cleared with 100 to 200 mg of dapsone daily and one was maintained on 50 mg every other day.

Benign familial pemphigus (Hailey-Hailey disease) responsive to low dose ciclosporin. Nanda A, Khawaja F, Harbi R, Nanda M, Dvorak R, Alsaleh QA. Indian J Dermatol Venereol Leprol 2010; 76: 422–4.

The reported patient was treated with 2.5 mg/kg/day and achieved a lasting remission with topical tacrolimus for maintenance.

Remission of refractory benign familial chronic pemphigus (Hailey-Hailey disease) with the addition of systemic ciclosporin. Varada S, Ramirez-FORT MK, Argobi Y, Simkin AD. J Cutan Med Surg 2015; 19: 163–6.

This patient had improvement on 2.8 mg/kg/day but nearly cleared on 3.8 mg/kg/day and had significant improvement in pain and pruritus.

Botulinum toxin type A as an adjuvant treatment modality for extensive Hailey–Hailey disease. Koeyers WJ, Van Der Geer S, Krekels G. J Dermatolog Treat 2008; 19: 251–4.

Diminution of the hyperhidrosis that exacerbates Hailey–Hailey disease may also be accomplished by utilizing oral glycopyrrolate.

Carbon dioxide laser treatment for Hailey-Hailey disease: a retrospective chart review with patient-reported outcomes. Hochwalt PC, Christensen KN, Cantwell SR, Hocker TL, Otley CC, Brewer JD. Int J Dermatol 2015; 54: 1309–14.

Thirteen patients with refractory disease were treated with CO_2 laser, and all patients had no recurrence in the treated areas. Seventy percent had new disease outside of treated sites that responded to additional treatments.

Tacrolimus, pimecrolimus, and calcitriol are at least safe and a good option for steroid-sparing maintenance therapy. Dapsone is generally safe and may work in certain patients. Ciclosporin can be used safely if doses do not exceed 5 mg/kg and patients are properly monitored. There are now a number of reports suggesting that botulinum toxin and CO_2 laser may be less invasive and efficacious options for refractory local disease.

Third-Line Therapies

• Surgical excision (with healing by secondary intention or by grafting)	E
• Dermabrasion	E
• Laser therapy (excluding CO_2 laser – see earlier)	E
• Superficial irradiation (Grenz rays or electron beam)	E
• Methotrexate	E
• Oral retinoids	E
• Topical 5-fluorouracil	E
• Biologics	E
• Photodynamic therapy	E
• Narrowband ultraviolet B therapy	E

Surgical treatment of familial benign chronic pemphigus. Crotty CP, Scheen SR, Masson JK, Winkelmann RK. Arch Dermatol 1981; 117: 540–2.

This is a report of five patients who had excision followed by split-thickness skin grafting. Three patients had no recurrence in treated areas, and one patient had mild recurrence after 8 years.

Refractory Hailey–Hailey disease successfully treated with sandpaper dermabrasion. LeBlanc KG Jr, Wharton JB, Sheehan DJ. Skinmed 2011; 9: 263–4.

A 53-year-old female had a lasting improvement on the neck and popliteal fossae after fine sandpaper dermabrasion down to the superficial dermis; however, she did have recurrence in the axillae.

Successful treatment of refractory Hailey-Hailey disease with a 595-nm pulsed dye laser: a series of 7 cases. Hunt KM, Jensen JD, Walsh SB, Helms ME, Soong VY, Jacobson ES. J Am Acad Dermatol 2015; 72: 735–7.

This report showed varying amounts of improvement of clinical lesions in six of seven patients treated with 595-nm pulsed-dye laser.

Effective treatment of Hailey-Hailey disease with a long-pulsed (5 ms) alexandrite laser. Awadalla F, Rosenbach A. J Cosmet Laser Ther 2011; 13: 191–2.

A 35-year-old male had complete clearance after 13 treatments with long pulsed alexandrite laser for 1 year with occasional short courses of topical hydrocortisone. The fluences ranged from 12 to 20 J/cm² with 10- to 15-mm spot sizes.

Persistent improvement of previously recalcitrant Hailey–Hailey disease with electron beam therapy. Narbutt J, Chrusciel A, Rychter A, Fijuth J, Lesiak A, Sysa-Jedrzejowska A. Acta Derm Venereol 2010; 90: 179–82.

Three patients had improvement of lesions after 20 Gy in 10 fractions to 90% isodose to each axilla without recurrence in 38 months of follow-up.

Methotrexate for refractory Hailey–Hailey disease. Vilarinho C, Ventura F, Brito C. J Eur Acad Dermatol Venereol 2010; 24: 106.

A 42-year-old woman showed near clearance after 3 months of oral methotrexate 15 mg weekly and had no recurrence in 2 years of follow-up.

Vesiculobullous Hailey–Hailey disease: successful treatment with oral retinoids. Hunt MJ, Salisbury EL, Painter DM, Lee S. Australas J Dermatol 1996; 37: 196–8.

A 56-year-old male had significant improvement after 6 weeks of 25 mg of daily etretinate. The patient was recurrence free 2 months after completing a 6-month course.

Successful treatment of Hailey–Hailey disease with acitretin. Berger EM, Galadari HI, Gottlieb AB. J Drugs Dermatol 2007; 6: 734–6.

A 64-year-old male had significant improvement after 6 months of 25 mg of daily acitretin.

Successful treatment of Hailey–Hailey disease with topical 5-fluorouracil. Dammak A, Camus M, Anyfantakis V, Guillet G. Br J Dermatol 2009; 161: 967–8.

A 43-year-old male was treated with 5-fluorouracil 5% cream three times weekly for 3 months, followed by weekly applications for 3 months, and showed near clearance for 6 months after completion of therapy.

Case reports of etanercept in inflammatory dermatoses. Norman R, Greenberg RG, Jackson JM. J Am Acad Dermatol 2006; 54 (Suppl 2): S139–42.

A 47-year-old woman was treated with subcutaneous etanercept 25 mg weekly for 1 month, then increased to 50 mg for 6 months, and then to 75 mg weekly to improve response. She showed dramatic improvement in 10 months and continued to improve.

Experience with photodynamic therapy in Hailey–Hailey disease. Fernandez Guarino M, Ryan AM, Perez-Garcia B, Arrazola JM, Jaen P. J Dermatol Treat 2008; 19: 288.

Three patients were treated with methyl aminolevulinic acid for 3 hours and then exposed to 7.5 min of 630 nm red light. The patients had a lot of pain and did not have significant improvement.

Successful therapeutic use of targeted narrow-band ultraviolet B therapy for refractory Hailey-Hailey disease. Hamada T, Umemura H, Aoyama Y, Iwatsuki K. Acta Derm Venereol 2013; 93: 110–1.

This report showed efficacy of narrow band ultraviolet B (NbUVB) therapy conflicting with previous reports of exacerbation with ultraviolet (UV) light.

Surgery can be definitive and should be considered for refractory localized disease. Many authors report some recurrences, either around the edges of the treated areas or on further friction or trauma. Treatment is invasive, and the trauma of dressings may exacerbate the disease, so proper patient selection is important. The rest of the modalities in this section have few reports demonstrating their efficacy. They should be reserved for very recalcitrant disease in appropriate patients.

Evidence Levels: **A** Double-blind study **B** Clinical trial ≥ 20 subjects **C** Clinical trial < 20 subjects **D** Series ≥ 5 subjects **E** Anecdotal case reports

99

Hand and foot eczema (endogenous, dyshidrotic eczema, pompholyx)

Ivan D. Camacho, Anne E. Burdick

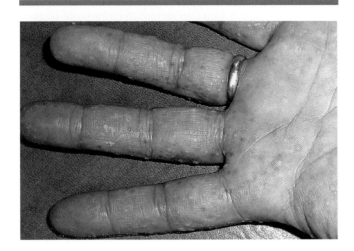

Endogenous hand and foot dermatitis occurs in two fairly distinct clinical patterns: pompholyx and hyperkeratotic dermatitis. There is considerable overlap, and both may occur in the same individual.

Pompholyx is usually episodic. Acute episodes of intense itching or burning are followed after a few hours by an eruption of vesicles, which expand and may coalesce to form large bullae. The sites most affected are the palms, soles, and the sides of hands, fingers, and toes. As the bullae rupture the dermatitis becomes highly exudative and very sore. The eruption tends to dry out after 2 weeks leading to painful fissuring of the skin in the subacute and chronic phase. The clinical course is highly variable, but in some cases recurrent attacks occur at 3- to 4-weekly intervals for months or years.

The hyperkeratotic pattern presents with pruritic, erythematous, scaly, fissured, hyperkeratotic patches on the palms and palmar surfaces of fingers and on the soles. The hyperkeratosis is variable but can cause distressing pain associated with deep fissures when pronounced.

Secondary infection of hand and foot dermatitis is common and may result in pustulation or lymphangitis.

Hand and foot dermatitis often occurs as a manifestation of atopy.

MANAGEMENT STRATEGY

Diagnosis of endogenous eczema requires exclusion of exogenous (irritant or allergic) dermatitis, hyperhidrosis, dermatophytosis, and other inflammatory skin diseases, notably psoriasis, which may be clinically indistinguishable. Although the pathogenesis is not completely understood, it is thought that overexpression of aquaporin 3 and aquaporin 10 proteins in the mid and upper epidermis with concomitant water exposure lead to skin dehydration and increased transepidermal water loss. Dyshidrotic eczema has also been reported to be induced by intravenous immunoglobulin (IVIG) therapy and during the immune reconstitution inflammatory syndrome.

Although endogenous eczema may resolve spontaneously, treatment is usually required to control pruritus, formation of vesicular lesions, and painful cracking and fissuring.

Topical corticosteroids are the mainstay of treatment. For mild localized disease, *mid- to-high-potency corticosteroid* creams or ointments are recommended. *Oral antihistamines* are useful for control of symptoms or as mild sedatives. *Emollients* are beneficial. The chronic, hyperkeratotic forms are dry, requiring occlusive emollients and keratolytic agents. A course of *oral antibiotics (cephalosporins or doxycycline)* is recommended for secondary impetiginization.

Topical tacrolimus or *pimecrolimus* is useful, alone or in combination with a corticosteroid, which may be delivered under occlusion for increased penetration. For severe disease, *systemic corticosteroids* are indicated: daily *prednisone* 0.5 to 1.0 mg/kg/day tapered over 2 weeks, or intramuscular *triamcinolone acetonide* (40–60 mg). Hand and foot narrowband phototherapy and *UVA*, alone or with *oral or topical psoralen*, are also effective. Paradoxically, sunlight has been reported to induce pompholyx, with positive provocation on phototesting.

Refractory hand and foot eczema may respond to systemic retinoids such as *alitretinoin*; immunosuppressive agents including *azathioprine, methotrexate, ciclosporin, mycophenolate mofetil*, or *etanercept*; and *radiotherapy*.

Intradermal botulinum toxin A and *oxybutynin* may be helpful as adjuvant therapy in dyshidrotic cases. *Low-nickel and low-cobalt diets* are recommended in nickel-sensitive patients who demonstrate a positive provocation test.

Specific Investigations
• Potassium hydroxide preparation
• Bacterial culture
• Patch testing

Pompholyx eczema as a manifestation of HIV infection, response to antiretroviral therapy. MacConnachie AA, Smith CC. Acta Derm Venereol 2007; 87: 378–9.

Pompholyx may present as both a manifestation of symptomatic HIV infection and as part of the immune reconstitution inflammatory syndrome. Conventional treatment for pompholyx may fail, but improvement may be observed with highly active antiretroviral therapy.

Pompholyx and eczematous reactions associated with intravenous immunoglobulin therapy. Gerstenblith MR, Antony AK, Junkins-Hopkins JM, Abuav R. J Am Acad Dermatol 2012; 66: 312–6.

A 3-year causative study of pompholyx in 120 patients. Guillet MH, Wierzbicka E, Guillet S, Dagregorio G, Guillet G. Arch Dermatol 2007; 143: 1504–8.

A prospective survey reported allergic contact pompholyx in 67.5% of cases (31.7% to cosmetic and hygiene products and 16.7% to metals), 15% idiopathic, 10% secondary to dermatophytes, and 6.7% due to ingestion of drugs, food, or nickel.

Role of contact allergens in pompholyx. Jain V, Passi S, Gupta S. J Dermatol 2004; 31: 188–93.

Patch testing with the Indian Standard Patch Test Battery was performed on 50 subjects, and 40% reacted to one or more allergens. Nickel sulfate was the most common allergen, followed by potassium dichromate, phenylenediamine, nitrofurazone, fragrance mix, and cobalt.

Low-cobalt diet for dyshidrotic eczema patients. Stuckert J, Nedorost S. Contact Derm 2008; 59: 361–5.

Restriction of dietary cobalt and nickel reduces flares of dyshidrotic eczema, regardless of patch test results.

Photoaggravated pompholyx. Nalluri R, Rhodes LE. Photodermatol Photoimmunol Photomed 2016; 32: 168–70.

Photoaggravated pompholyx must be considered if pompholyx worsens in summer.

First-Line Therapies	
• Topical corticosteroids	A
• Topical calcineurin inhibitors	C
• Oral antibiotics	D
• Oral antihistamines	D
• Oral corticosteroids	D
• Emollients	D
• Keratolytics	D

Pompholyx: a review of clinical features, differential diagnosis, and management. Wollina U. Am J Clin Dermatol 2010; 11: 305–14.

Acute and recurrent vesicular hand dermatitis. Veien NK. Dermatol Clin 2009; 27: 337–53.

Comprehensive review on chronic hand dermatitis.

Topical tacrolimus (FK 506) and mometasone furoate in treatment of dyshidrotic palmar eczema: a randomized, observer-blinded trial. Schnopp C, Remling R, Mohrenschlager M, Weigl L, Ring J, Abeck D. J Am Acad Dermatol 2002; 46: 73–7.

Topical tacrolimus 0.1% ointment was as effective as 0.1% mometasone furoate ointment after 4 weeks of twice-daily application, reducing the Dyshidrotic Area and Severity Index (DASI) to approximately 50% in 16 patients.

Efficacy and safety of pimecrolimus cream 1% in mild-to-moderate chronic hand dermatitis: a randomized, double-blind trial. Hordinsky M, Fleischer A, Rivers JK, Poulin Y, Belsito D, Hultsch T. Dermatology 2010; 221: 71–7.

Pimecrolimus 1% cream twice daily with overnight occlusion for 6 weeks improved pruritus and skin lesions in up to 30% of 652 treated patients.

Second-Line Therapies	
• Alitretinoin (9-*cis*-retinoic acid)	A
• UVA, PUVA, and narrowband UVB	B
• Intradermal botulinum A toxin	C
• Oxybutynin	C

Oral alitretinoin in chronic refractory hand eczema: a "real life" case-series of 12 patients. Kubica E, Ezzedine K, Lalanne N, Dartial Y, Taieb A, Milpied B. Eur J Dermatol 2011; 21: 454–6.

Twelve patients were treated with alitretinoin 30 mg daily for 3 to 6 months. Seven out of 10 patients responded within 1 to 3 months. Three stayed in remission for 6 months, and four relapsed within 10 days to 3 months after stopping the medication.

Successful retreatment with alitretinoin in patients with relapsed chronic hand eczema. Bissonnette R, Worm M, Gerlach B, Guenther L, Cambazard F, Ruzicka T, et al. Br J Dermatol 2010; 162: 420–6.

Alitretinoin 30 mg daily for 12 to 24 weeks showed 80% efficacy in 117 patients who were responders but relapsed within 24 weeks after a previous 24-week course of alitretinoin 30 mg daily.

Efficacy and safety of oral alitretinoin (9-*cis* retinoic acid) in patients with severe chronic hand eczema refractory to topical corticosteroids: results of a randomized, double-blind, placebo-controlled, multicentre trial. Ruzicka T, Lynde CW, Jemec GB, Diepgen T, Berth-Jones J, Coenraads PJ, et al. Br J Dermatol 2008; 158: 808–17.

Alitretinoin 30 mg daily monotherapy for 12 to 24 weeks improved symptoms and skin lesions in 48% of 409 patients with chronic hand eczema, regardless of clinical presentation.

Acitretin may also be of value in selected cases.

Local narrowband UVB phototherapy vs. local PUVA in the treatment of chronic hand eczema. Sezer E, Etikan I. Photodermatol Photoimmunol Photomed 2007; 23: 10–4.

Compared with PUVA, narrowband UVB was as effective in 12 patients treated three times a week, over a 9-week period. The initial dose of 150 mJ/cm² was increased by 20% until a final dose of 2000 mJ/cm² was reached.

Comparison of localized high-dose UVA1 irradiation versus topical cream psoralen–UVA for treatment of chronic vesicular dyshidrotic eczema. Petering H, Breuer C, Herbst R, Kapp A, Werfel T. J Am Acad Dermatol 2004; 50: 68–72.

Twenty-four of 27 patients treated with UVA1 irradiation to one hand and cream psoralen–UVA (PUVA) to the other showed a similar 50% improvement after a 3-week period of UV irradiation. One patient relapsed within the 3-week follow-up period.

Oral vs. bath PUVA using 8-methoxypsoralen for chronic palmoplantar eczema. Tzaneva S, Kittler H, Thallinger C, Hönigsmann H, Tanew A. Photodermatol Photoimmunol Photomed 2009; 25: 101–5.

Oral PUVA was as effective as bath PUVA in 29 patients with dyshidrotic eczema, who received treatment three times weekly for up to 20 weeks and were followed up for up to 40 months.

Regression of relapsing dyshidrotic eczema after treatment of concomitant hyperhidrosis with botulinum toxin-A. Kontochristopoulos G, Gregoriou S, Agiasofitou E, Nikolakis G, Rigopoulos D, Katsambas A. Dermatol Surg 2007; 33: 1289–90.

Two patients treated with 100 units of botulinum toxin A to each hand showed significant improvement of their dyshidrosis 1 week later, with no relapse after 8 weeks.

Pompholyx: what's new? Wollina U. Expert Opin Investig Drugs 2008; 17: 897–904.

Hyperhidrosis is an aggravating factor in approximately 40% of pompholyx patients. Botulinum toxin A, 100 units administered

Evidence Levels: A Double-blind study B Clinical trial ≥ 20 subjects C Clinical trial < 20 subjects D Series ≥ 5 subjects E Anecdotal case reports

intradermally to each hand, resulted in improvement of pruritus, lesions, and the starch iodine test for hyperhidrosis. The major disadvantages are the cost and the need for recurrent injections.

Remarkable improvement of relapsing dyshidrotic eczema after treatment of coexistent hyperhidrosis with oxybutynin. Markantoni V, Kouris A, Armyra K, Vavouli C, Kontochristopoulos G. Dermatol Ther 2014; 27: 365–8.

Improvement was reported with oxybutynin 5 mg twice a day for the first month and once a day for the second month. Patients experienced dry mouth, constipation, headache, and mild urine retention.

Third-Line Therapies	
• Ciclosporin	B
• Methotrexate	D
• Azathioprine	C
• Mycophenolate mofetil	D
• Etanercept	D
• Radiotherapy	D

Long-term follow-up of eczema patients treated with cyclosporine. Granlund H, Erkko P, Reitamo S. Acta Derm Venereol 1998; 78: 40–3.

Twenty-seven patients with chronic hand eczema treated with ciclosporin 3 mg/kg/day for 6 weeks had reduced disease activity of 54% and sustained improvement for 1 year, without topical treatment.

Low-dose oral methotrexate treatment for recalcitrant palmoplantar pompholyx. Egan CA, Rallis TM, Meadows KP, Krueger GG. J Am Acad Dermatol 1999; 40: 612–4.

In five patients with severe pompholyx 12.5 to 22.5 mg of methotrexate weekly resulted in a reduced dose or discontinuation of prednisone. Superpotent corticosteroids were continued topically.

Azathioprine in dermatological practice. An overview with special emphasis of its use in non-bullous inflammatory dermatoses. Scerri L. Adv Exp Med Biol 1999; 455: 343–8.

Six patients with severe dyshidrotic eczema received azathioprine monotherapy 100 to 150 mg daily with a mean duration of treatment of 34 months; three had excellent, one had good, and two had fair responses.

Dyshidrotic eczema treated with mycophenolate mofetil. Pickenacker A, Luger TA, Schwarz T. Arch Dermatol 1998; 134: 378–9.

One patient with recurrent dyshidrotic eczema refractory to topical and systemic corticosteroids and UVA1 had complete resolution after 4 weeks of mycophenolate mofetil at a dose of 1.5 g twice daily and 12 months of 1 g daily.

Recalcitrant hand pompholyx: variable response to etanercept. Ogden S, Clayton TH, Goodfield MJ. Clin Exp Dermatol 2006; 31: 145–6.

One patient responded significantly to etanercept 25 mg twice weekly for 6 weeks. The remission lasted 4 months. A subsequent flare was unresponsive to etanercept 50 mg twice weekly.

Long-term results of radiotherapy in patients with chronic palmo-plantar eczema or psoriasis. Sumila M, Notter M, Itin P, Bodis S, Gruber G. Strahlenther Onkol 2008; 184: 218–23.

Twenty-eight patients irradiated with a single dose of either 1 Gy or 0.5 Gy twice weekly, up to a total dose of 4 to 5 Gy, demonstrated significant improvement that was maintained during the 20-month follow-up period.

Hemangiomas

Daniel A. Grabell, Adam V. Nguyen, Adelaide A. Hebert

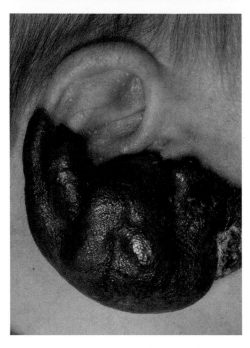

Hemangiomas are a neoplastic proliferation of endothelial cells that are generally benign but have been associated with local tissue damage, functional impact, and ulceration. The true incidence of the disease is unknown but is reported as 5% in Caucasian infants. Hemangiomas occur more frequently in Caucasian female infants with a predilection for premature infants, especially of low birth weight or multiple gestations. Most hemangiomas arise spontaneously during infancy, but an autosomal-dominant pattern of inheritance has rarely been reported as well.

MANAGEMENT STRATEGY

Cutaneous hemangiomas appear in the first few weeks of life and reach 80% of size by 3 months, with spontaneous involution in most cases by age 10. Early evaluation and treatment, if necessary, are critical to limit the patient's functional impairment and disfigurement. About half of the children with hemangiomas will have normal skin after involution, but the rest may have residual changes, including telangiectasias, atrophy, fibrofatty residuum, and scarring.

Differentiating benign common hemangiomas from other vascular anomalies is essential, as the pathophysiology, treatment modalities, and prognoses are significantly different. Vascular malformations and tumors, such as the kaposiform hemangioendothelioma (KE) and tufted angioma (TA), differ from hemangioma in both clinical and histologic appearance as well as growth rate and involutional tendencies. In particular, KE and TA are associated with the Kasabach–Merritt syndrome and its accompanying coagulopathy, whereas common hemangiomas are not. The majority of common hemangiomas occur as solitary lesions

but can be a sign of multisystem involvement such as diffuse neonatal hemangiomatosis, LUMBAR syndrome (lower body congenital infantile hemangiomas and other skin defects, urogenital anomalies and ulceration, myelopathy, bony deformities, anorectal malformations and arterial anomalies, and rectal anomalies), and PHACES syndrome (posterior fossa malformation, hemangiomas, cardiac anomalies, eye abnormalities, and sternal cleft/supraumbilical raphe).

Although the natural course of hemangiomas is self-limited and is often treated with active nonintervention, pharmaceutical intervention is indicated for hemangiomas that ulcerate, grow rapidly, compress, obstruct, or distort vital structures, such as the larynx, eyes, ears, and nose. In addition, hemangiomas associated with systemic involvement and large disfiguring facial hemangiomas should be treated. Medical management is generally centered on the administration of topical and systemic beta-blockers or corticosteroids. Surgical excision is a less frequently used management option.

Topical and systemic beta-blockers have become the preferred first-line therapy in hemangiomas that warrant treatment. The first case report of a hemangioma being successfully treated with propranolol was published in 2008. Oral propranolol hydrochloride solution was approved by the FDA for use in infants with an escalating starting dose of 1.2 mg/kg/day to a target dose of 3.4 mg/kg/day divided into two daily doses. Adverse events include the masking of hypoglycemia, hypotension, and bradycardia, which can be minimized by administering the medication after feeding and monitoring the heart rate and blood pressure after dose increases. Timolol, available as a solution or a gel, has been shown in small randomized clinical trials to be safe and effective for superficial infantile hemangiomas with twice-daily topical application.

Systemic corticosteroids may be used in patients who have contraindications to or do not respond to beta-blockers. Steroids are usually indicated during the growth phase. Prednisone or prednisolone can be given at doses from 2 to 4 mg/kg daily for 2 to 6 months and then gradually tapered over several months. Stopping treatment before adequate therapeutic response may result in rebound growth. Approximately one third of the patients will show an accelerated rate of involution, but another one third may have no response to this treatment modality. Reported risks include hypothalamopituitary–adrenal axis suppression, growth delays, pseudotumor cerebri, infections, and avascular bone necrosis. Surgical excision, either alone or in combination with corticosteroids, may also be employed in certain cases.

For the exceptional recalcitrant hemangioma, other treatments include cyclophosphamide, vincristine, bleomycin, and embolization.

Specific Investigations

- Ultrasound with Doppler
- Magnetic resonance imaging (MRI)
- Biopsy with immunohistochemistry

The diagnosis of a hemangioma is usually made clinically, and the previous investigations may only be needed in atypical cases to confirm the diagnosis, monitor the progress of treatment, establish the extent of the vascular lesion, or screen for other complications.

Soft-tissue vascular anomalies: utility of US for diagnosis. Paltiel HJ, Burrows PE, Kozakewich HPW, Zurakowski D, Mulliken JB. Radiology 2000; 214: 747–54.

Doppler ultrasonography is a low-cost, noninvasive method to confirm the diagnosis of a vascular anomaly, monitor

Evidence Levels: **A** Double-blind study   **B** Clinical trial ≥ 20 subjects   **C** Clinical trial < 20 subjects   **D** Series ≥ 5 subjects   **E** Anecdotal case reports

therapeutic response, or preclude the involvement of visceral organs. Hemangiomas can be differentiated from vascular malformations on ultrasonography by distinguishing features such as the presence of a solid tissue mass.

Although not specifically mentioned in this article, infants less than 3 months of age with a midline back or perineal hemangioma should be imaged with ultrasound of the spine to rule out LUMBAR syndrome and a tethered cord. A referral to a pediatric neurosurgeon and possible MRI may be needed as follow-up.

Hemangioma from head to toe: MR imaging with pathologic correlation. Vilanova JC, Barcelo J, Smirniotopoulos JG, Pérez-Andrés R, Villalón M, Miró J, et al. Radiographics 2004; 24: 367–85.

MRI is a useful noninvasive imaging technique to diagnose, characterize, and determine the extent of vascular lesions. On T_2-weighted images, hemangiomas have the characteristic appearance of multiple lobules, similar to a bunch of grapes.

Although not specifically mentioned in this article, infants with large, segmental, plaque-like facial hemangiomas should have an MRI of the head for possible posterior fossa brain abnormalities as a component of PHACES syndrome.

GLUT 1: a newly discovered immunohistochemical marker for juvenile hemangiomas. North PE, Waner M, Mizeracki A, Mihm MC Jr. Hum Pathol 2001; 31: 11–22.

Immunohistochemical staining can serve as a useful adjunct to distinguish between infantile hemangiomas and other common vascular malformations or vascular neoplasms that present during infancy. GLUT-1 (glucose transporter 1) stain is shown to be highly specific and uniformly positive in the endothelial vasculature of infantile hemangiomas.

Staining for placenta-associated vascular antigens Fc gamma RII, Lewis Y antigen (LeY), and merosin in infantile hemangiomas has shown a high specificity and holds promise for the development of an infantile hemangioma-specific immunohistochemical panel.

First-Line Therapies	
• Systemic beta-blockers	A
• Topical beta-blockers	B
• Topical corticosteroids	D
• Intralesional corticosteroids	B
• Systemic corticosteroids	B

Oral propranolol is the mainstay of therapy for life-threatening or endangering hemangiomas with active nonintervention or topical timolol reserved for relatively uncomplicated cases.

A randomized, controlled trial of oral propranolol in infantile hemangioma. Leaute-Labreze C, Hoeger P, Mazereeuw-Hautier J, Guibaud L, Baselga E, Posiunas G, et al. N Engl J Med 2015; 372: 735–46.

A randomized, double-blind, multicenter, two-stage adaptive trial of 460 infants to assess the efficacy of oral propranolol in treating infantile hemangiomas. In the first stage, the infants were randomized to receive either a placebo or one of four propranolol regimens of either 1 mg/kg/day or 3 mg/kg/day of propranolol for a duration of 3 or 6 months. After an interim analysis, new infants were treated with either a placebo or 3 mg/kg/day of propranolol for 6 months. Sixty percent of all infants receiving this regimen had complete or nearly complete resolution of the target hemangioma. Common adverse events include diarrhea, sleep disorder, and bronchitis.

Initiation and use of propranolol for infantile hemangioma: report of a consensus conference. Drolet BA, Frommelt PC, Chamlin SL, Haggstrom A, Bauman NM, Chiu YE, et al. Pediatrics 2013; 131: 128–40.

A multidisciplinary consensus conference reviewed the existing research on the use of oral propranolol for the treatment of infantile hemangiomas, with a primary goal of formulating a standardized set of guidelines that dermatologists could follow. Data compiled from 85 articles, including 1175 total patients, were reviewed. Based on the evidence, a starting dose of 1 mg/kg/day divided three times daily with a titration to a target dose of 2 mg/kg/day was recommended. Escalations should occur every 3 to 7 days as tolerated.

Propranolol treatment of infantile hemangiomas does not negatively affect psychomotor development. Movakine AV, Hermans DJ, Fuiikschot J, van der Vleuten CJ. J Am Acad Dermatol 2015; 73: 341–2.

A total of 103 patients previously started on oral propranolol between September 2008 and May 2013 were retrospectively assessed for possible psychomotor developmental delay caused by the medication. Data were collected from the Dutch Well Child Preventive Health Care Clinics and interpreted using the Van Wiechen scheme. Overall study results detected no evidence of psychomotor developmental delay in infants treated with propranolol for infantile hemangiomas.

Topical timolol maleate treatment of infantile hemangiomas. Puttgen K, Lucky A, Adams D, Pope E, McCuaig C, Powell J, et al. Pediatrics 2016; 138.

This multicenter retrospective cohort study of 731 patients evaluated the efficacy of topical timolol by scoring digital photographs of the infantile hemangioma utilizing a visual analog scale for color, size, extent, and volume. At 6 to 9 months of treatment 92.3% of patients had improved color and 76.6% had improvement in size, extent, and volume. The best response to therapy occurred in superficial hemangiomas <1 mm thick.

Timolol maleate 0.5% or 0.1% gel-forming solution for infantile hemangiomas: a retrospective, multicenter, cohort study. Chakkittakandiyil A, Phillips R, Frieden IJ, Siegfried E, Lara-Corrales I, Lam J, et al. Pediatr Dermatol 2011; 29: 28–31.

This retrospective cohort study reviewed 73 patients with infantile hemangioma. The mean age at initiation of therapy was 8 months, with 85% of patients dosed at 0.5% strength and the remainder being treated with 0.1%. All patients were treated twice daily and without occlusion. Mean treatment period was 3.4 months, and photos were evaluated by investigators to correspond to a 0 to 100 visual analog scale. Mean visual analog scale improvement was 45 units at the last visit. Longer treatment period was associated with greater improvement. The incidence of adverse events was extremely low—only one patient. No skin-related adverse events were noted in any subjects. No rebound growth was observed after discontinuation at 3 to 6 months.

Ultrapotent topical corticosteroid treatment of hemangiomas of infancy. Garzon MC, Lucky AW, Hawrot A, Frieden IJ. J Am Acad Dermatol 2005; 52: 281–6.

A retrospective review of 34 patients with hemangiomas treated with class I topical steroids showed good response in 35%, partial response in 38%, and no response in 27%. Treatment protocols varied between patients.

Intralesional corticosteroid therapy in proliferating head and neck hemangiomas: a review of 155 cases. Chen MT, Yeong EK, Horng SY. J Pediatr Surg 2000; 35: 420–3.

In this retrospective study, 155 hemangiomas of the head and neck region treated with intralesional corticosteroid injections (three to six injections of triamcinolone acetonide 10 mg/mL at monthly intervals, with an average of four injections per lesion) were analyzed. At the 1-month visit, 85% of hemangiomas showed greater than 50% reduction, with superficial hemangiomas showing the most improvement. Perioral hemangiomas appeared the most recalcitrant to intralesional corticosteroid treatment.

Oral corticosteroid use is effective for cutaneous hemangiomas. Bennett ML, Fleischer AB, Chamlin SL, Frieden IJ. Arch Dermatol 2001; 137: 1208–13.

This meta-analysis of 10 case series with 184 patients analyzed the efficacy of systemic corticosteroids in the treatment of cutaneous hemangiomas. The mean age of infants at the initiation of therapy was 4.5 months with an average prednisone dose equivalent to 2.9 mg/kg. The mean response rate was 84%, and the mean rate of rebound growth after treatment cessation was 36%. Treatment with higher doses of corticosteroids resulted in a higher response rate but greater adverse events. The average incidence of side effects was 35% (behavior changes, irritability, cushingoid appearance, and transient growth delay).

Second-Line Therapies	
• Surgical excision	D
• Becaplermin gel for ulcerated lesions	D

Surgical treatment of facial infantile hemangiomas: an analysis based on tumor characteristics and outcomes. Goldenberg DC, Hiraki PY, Marques TM, Koga A, Gemperli R. Plast Reconstr Surg 2016; 137: 1221–31.

A retrospective case review of 74 patients treated surgically was analyzed to evaluate outcomes based on tumor-related clinical features. The best candidates for emergency surgery were nonresponders to pharmacologic therapy with segmental periorbital hemangiomas, whereas those undergoing elective surgery were patients with localized lip, nasal, or eyelid hemangiomas in the proliferative phase.

Although most patients with infantile hemangiomas should be managed with pharmacotherapy, surgery remains an important option. The exact algorithm of when to operate remains controversial.

Response of ulcerated perineal hemangiomas of infancy to becaplermin gel, a recombinant human platelet-derived growth factor. Metz BJ, Rubenstein MC, Levy ML, Metry DW. Arch Dermatol 2004; 140: 867–70.

Eight infants were treated with becaplermin gel 0.01% for ulcerated perineal hemangiomas of infancy. Rapid ulcer healing occurred in all patients within 3 to 21 days (average, 10.25 days).

The rapid healing achieved with 0.01% becaplermin gel allows a reduction in the risk of secondary infection, pain, and the need for hospitalization, as well as in the costs that often accumulate from multiple follow-up visits and long-term therapy.

Third-Line Therapies	
• Vincristine	E
• Imiquimod	C
• Bleomycin	B

Vincristine as a treatment for a large haemangioma threatening vital functions. Fawcett SL, Grant I, Hall PN, Kelsall AW, Nicholson JC. Br J Plast Surg 2004; 57: 168–71.

A 21-month-old infant with a large, deep hemangioma in the beard distribution, necessitating multiple hospital admissions for respiratory and feeding difficulties, was treated with vincristine after failing to respond to systemic corticosteroid therapy. Vincristine (1.5 mg), administered weekly for 1 month, improved the patient's feeding and speech, as well as the external appearance of the lesion with no adverse events.

Although there are literature reports of success achieved with vincristine, the data are anecdotal at best.

Topical imiquimod in the treatment of infantile hemangiomas: a retrospective study. Ho NTC, Lansang P, Pope E. J Am Acad Dermatol 2007; 56: 63–8.

Eighteen children (median age of 18 weeks) treated with imiquimod 5% cream three or five times weekly for a mean of 17 weeks showed improvement in superficial hemangiomas and accelerated ulcer healing; no change was seen in deep hemangiomas. A 31% clearance rate was reported. Adverse events included crusting and inflammation.

Unfortunately, this study lacked a control arm, and the results may represent the natural course of untreated infantile hemangiomas.

Role of intralesional bleomycin in the treatment of complicated hemangiomas: prospective clinical study. Omidvari S, Nezakatgoo N, Ahmadloo N, Mohammadianpanah M, Mosalaei A. Dermatol Surg 2005; 31: 499–501.

Thirty-two patients with complicated hemangiomas (median age of 45 months) were treated with intralesional bleomycin (1–2 mg/cm^2 every 2 weeks for four to six courses). After the initial swelling and erythema, 56% of patients had 70% to 100% regression, whereas 21.9% had 50% to 70% regression. No severe adverse events were reported.

eudated androgens are unsuitable

101

Hereditary angioedema

Tabi A. Leslie, Malcolm W. Greaves

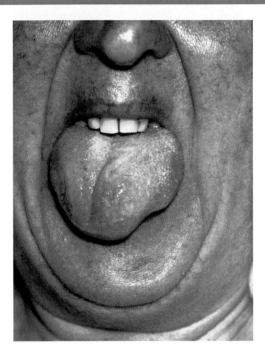

There are three types of hereditary angioedemas (HAEs). Types I and II HAEs—the most common forms—are autosomal dominantly inherited with a prevalence of 1:50,000 due to mutations in the C1-esterase inhibitor (C1INH) gene on chromosome 11q12-q13.1. However, de novo mutations of the gene controlling C1INH *(SERPING1)* can occur, accounting for approximately 25% of C1INII-HAE cases. Type I (85%) is characterized by a quantitative abnormality of the C1INH, and type II (15%) is due to a functional defect of the inhibitor of the first component of complement C1INH. These HAEs are mediated by the protease kallikrein and the nonapeptide bradykinin, acting on B$_2$ receptors, and are manifested by painless, nonpruritic swellings of subcutaneous (SC) and submucosal tissues, including abdominal organs and the upper airway. The third type of HAE, previously known as *HAE type III* (or the estrogen-dependent type), is now referred to as *HAE with normal C1INH*. This type is associated with a positive family history, occurring predominantly in women, with no detectable abnormality of C1INH or other complement components. A mutation in the gene encoding for factor 12 *(F12)*, which encodes for the Hageman factor (HAE–FX11), has been identified in some of these families. Acute abdominal pain simulating an "acute abdomen" is an important presentation in any type of HAE, and fatalities are possible (due to laryngeal obstruction). Associations with autoimmune disorders, mainly lupus erythematosus, occur in type I HAE but are rare in type II.

MANAGEMENT STRATEGY

Therapy for HAE is dependent on three considerations:

- Relief of acute angioedema (AAE), especially preservation of the airway

- Long-term prophylaxis
- Prevention of relapse due to dental and surgical interventions (short-term prophylaxis)

ACUTE ANGIOEDEMA

Acute presentations of HAE are treated optimally with intravenous (IV) *plasma-derived C1INH concentrate* at 20 units/kg body weight. This treatment is safe, and no proven cases of viral transmission have been reported. Reduction in swelling is usually significant within minutes and substantial within 2 to 3 hours. A recombinant C1INH preparation is now available. Patients can be taught to self-administer for a more rapid resolution of symptoms and to prevent further progression of the attack(s). *Fresh frozen plasma (FFP)*, which contains C1INH, can be used in an emergency if concentrate is unavailable. However, FFP carries a higher risk of inadvertent viral transmission (HIV, hepatitis) and theoretically could exacerbate angioedema due to the presence of C1 esterase substrate. The kallikrein–bradykinin mediator pathway is the target of current approaches to treatment of acute HAE. The swellings of HAE are mediated by bradykinin, a product of the action of kallikrein on its substrate kininogen. Bradykinin acts on B2 receptors, and its specific antagonist *icatibant* 30 mg subcutaneously has been proven effective in acute attacks of HAE. Icatibant may be the preferred therapy because it is given subcutaneously and can be administered in a domiciliary setting by health care professionals or even by self-administration after appropriate training. *Ecallantide*, a kallikrein inhibitor given subcutaneously in a dose of 30 mg, has been proven to be safe and effective for acute attacks. Laryngeal edema may require *tracheostomy, intubation*, and/or other life-support measures. Patients are routinely admitted for 24 hours after acute episodes, as life-threatening relapses are common.

Long-Term Prophylaxis

Long-term prophylaxis is appropriate in those patients with at least one or more attacks of angioedema per month and in those with severe symptoms. However, patients could have infrequent attacks and still present with laryngeal edema. Even first-episode angioedema can be fatal. Prophylactic treatment with plasma-derived C1INH is now the first-line therapy if available. IV infusions of 1000 units administered twice weekly can lead to less severe symptoms and even attack prevention. Other treatments include the 17α-alkylated ("attenuated") androgens *danazol* (100–200 mg daily) or *stanozolol* (up to 5.0 mg once or twice daily), which are used as second-line prophylactic medications that may be effective in preventing angioedema in some patients with type I or II HAE. The lowest effective dose of androgen should be used to obtain clinical remission. Side effects include hirsutism, deepening of voice, and menorrhagia. These attenuated androgens are unsuitable for long-term treatment of HAE in children, pregnant women, or the treatment of acute attacks. However, they are safe and effective in adults, provided they are closely supervised with clinical biochemical and radiologic assessments. In some patients, less frequent dosage of danazol (100 mg) on weekdays only or stanozolol (2 mg) on alternate days can be effective. Hepatocellular adenoma and hepatocellular carcinoma have been reported in patients on long-term danazol. Liver function tests and lipid levels should be monitored, with liver ultrasound scans performed every 2 years, although hepatic adenoma/carcinoma can occur in patients receiving attenuated androgens in the absence of any disturbance of liver function tests. Other less effective prophylactic therapies include *antifibrinolytics, tranexamic acid (TA)* (2.0–4.5 g daily), or *epsilon-aminocaproic acid (EACA)* (12–18 g daily) but should be avoided in patients with a history of thrombotic diseases. They are useful for short-term prophylaxis, especially for those where C1INH is not available or other therapies are contraindicated. In patients with mild infrequent attacks *avoidance of provoking factors,* including estrogens and angiotensin-converting enzyme (ACE) inhibitors, may be sufficient. For long-term management in selected cases, patients' caretakers can be trained to administer IV C1INH for occasional acute attacks if no medical facilities are at hand, thereby obviating the necessity for regular prophylaxis. Although not yet licensed for domiciliary administration, there is mounting evidence that C1INH concentrate can be safely and effectively self-administered by the SC route.

Prevention of Relapse Due to Dental and Surgical Interventions

In all patients, before elective surgical, dental, or other invasive procedures, *higher dose androgens can be used for 5 to 10 days.* Antifibrinolytics can be used 48 hours before and up to 2 to 5 days after the procedure. If an emergency procedure is necessary, C1INH concentrate or FFP can be administered. Patients with HAE should all wear a *MedicAlert disk* stating the diagnosis and emergency treatment.

Specific Investigations

- Complement levels (C4, C2, C1q)
- C1INH immunoreactive level
- Functional assay for C1INH

Angioedema. Kaplan AP, Greaves MW. J Am Acad Dermatol 2005; 53: 373–88.

Type I HAE is characterized by low antigenic and functional plasma levels of normal C1INH. Type II HAE is characterized by normal or elevated antigenic levels of a dysfunctional mutant C1INH together with functional C1INH. In those patients with a low C4 but normal C1INH levels, a functional assay should be obtained to identify type II disease. A depressed C1q level in addition to low C4 and C1INH levels is characteristic of acquired C1INH-deficient angioedema. Causes include B-cell lymphoma, cryoglobulinemia, and the presence of autoantibodies against C1INH itself.

Immunoregulatory disorders associated with hereditary angioedema. 1. Clinical manifestations of autoimmune disease. Brickman CN, Tsokos GC, James E. J Allergy Clin Immunol 1986; 77: 749–57.

One hundred fifty-seven HAE patients were systematically evaluated for manifestations of autoimmunity. Clinical immunoregulatory diseases were present in 19 of these (12%). Autoimmune diseases with a known human histocompatibility antigen association had developed in eight HAE patients, and all of these developed an associated disease. Four patients developed sicca syndrome or Sjögren's syndrome, and a further nine manifested part of the sicca complex. There were also HAE patients found with features (e.g., Raynaud disease, idiopathic pancreatitis) that suggested an immune-based abnormality.

An evaluation of tests used for the diagnosis and monitoring of C1 inhibitor deficiency: normal serum C4 does not exclude hereditary angioedema. Tarzi MD, Hickey A, Förster T, Mohammadi M, Longhurst HJ. Clin Exp Immunol 2007; 149: 513–6.

Although C4 is the single best screening test, it is not a definitive test. False-negative results may occur in patients, because normal C4 may occasionally present in HAE. Therefore assay of C1 inhibitor antigen and function should be performed, regardless of serum C4 levels, when clinical suspicion of HAE is high.

Genetic test indications and interpretations in patients with hereditary angioedema. Weiler CR, van Dellen RG. Mayo Clin Proc 2006; 81: 958–72.

Differentiating between HAE and AAE caused by C1INH deficiency can be aided by C1q testing. Genetic testing would be especially helpful in patients with borderline C1q levels and no family history of angioedema. Many patients with acquired C1INH deficiency have autoantibodies against C1INH. Measuring these autoantibodies would be helpful; however, the test is only available in research laboratories.

ACUTE ANGIOEDEMA

First-Line Therapy

- C1INH concentrate

Prospective study of rapid relief provided by C1 esterase inhibitor in emergency treatment of acute laryngeal attacks in hereditary angioedema. Craig TJ, Wasserman RL, Levy RJ, Bewtra AK, Schneider L, Packer F, et al. J Clin Immunol 2010; 30: 823–9.

Thirty-nine acute laryngeal attacks occurring in a prospective open-label study of 16 patients were treated with C1INH concentrate (Berinert). A single dose of 20 U/kg body weight was successful in treating all attacks with a median time to onset of relief of 15 minutes and a median time to complete resolution of all symptoms of 8.25 hours.

Nanofiltered C1 inhibitor concentrate for treatment of hereditary angioedema. Zuraw BL, Busse PJ, White M, Jacobs J, Lumry W, Baker J, et al. N Engl J Med 2010; 363: 513–22.

A placebo-controlled study of IV administration of nanofiltered pasteurized C1 inhibitor concentrate in 65 patients with HAE demonstrated that treatment shortened the acute attack from over 4 hours to 2 hours.

Pharmacokinetics of plasma-derived C1-esterase inhibitor after subcutaneous versus intravenous administration in subjects with mild or moderate hereditary angioedema: the PASSION study. Martinez-Saguer I, Cicardi M, Suffritti C, Rusicke E, Aygören-Pürsün E, Stoll H, et al. Transfusion 2014; 54: 1552–61.

Twenty-four subjects with mild or moderate HAE were randomly assigned to groups receiving 1000 units of C1INH concentrate by IV or SC administration. After SC administration, the mean relative bioavailability of functional C1INH was 39.7%, with maximum C1INH activity occurring within 48 hours and persisting for longer than IV administration. The mean half-life of functional C1INH was 120 hours after SC administration, compared with 62 hours after IV administration. The SC administration was well tolerated, with a higher incidence of mild injection site reactions than IV administration, as expected.

Evidence Levels: **A** Double-blind study **B** Clinical trial ≥ 20 subjects **C** Clinical trial < 20 subjects **D** Series ≥ 5 subjects **E** Anecdotal case reports

Subcutaneous self-injection of C1 inhibitor – an effective and safe treatment in a patient with hereditary angioedema. Weller K, Kruger R, Maurer M, Magerl M. Clin Exper Dermatol 2016; 41: 91–3.

A 25-year-old female patient diagnosed with HAE due to C1 inhibitor deficiency used an SC infusion kit to administer SC injections of C1 inhibitor 1000 U in 10 mL twice weekly. In the subsequent 2 years she has remained completely free of symptoms.

C1INH concentrate has also been effective as short-term prophylaxis in labor induction, tonsillectomy, and maxillofacial surgery. Long-term prophylaxis has not generally been advocated due to lack of availability, cost, and the potential for infectious transmission. However, this may be considered in children, pregnant women, and patients who do not respond to or tolerate androgens or antifibrinolytics, or if these drugs are contraindicated.

Suppliers of C1INH products include Berinert, Cinryze (human C1INH), and Ruconest (recombinant C1INH).

Second-Line Therapies

- FFP
- Icatibant
- Ecallantide

The safety of fresh frozen plasma for the treatment of hereditary angioedema. Prematta M, Thomas D, Scarupa M, Li C, Mende C, Rhoads C. J Allergy Clin Immunol 2008; 121: S99.

FFP was found to be effective in 76 of 82 acute attacks of HAE, and no patients developed significant adverse reactions.

FFP is effective and can be used if C1INH concentrate is unavailable. It is not virally inactivated and, being larger in volume, requires a longer infusion time. Apart from the risk of virus infection, using FFP carries the theoretical potential for exacerbation of attacks due to its content of complement substrates.

Treatment of acute edema attacks in hereditary angioedema with a bradykinin receptor-2 antagonist (icatibant). Bork K, Frank J, Grundt B, Schlattmann P, Nussberger J, Kreuz W. J Allergy Clin Immunol 2007; 119: 1497–503.

Fifteen patients with 20 attacks were treated with icatibant, with significant improvement relative to previous episodes as assessed using visual analog scales. Symptom intensity decreased within 4 hours after administration.

Icatibant, a new bradykinin receptor antagonist in hereditary angioedema. Cicardi M, Banerji F, Bracho F, Malbrán A, Rosenkranz B, Riedl M, et al. N Engl J Med 2010; 363: 532–41.

In two randomized double-blind trials relief of symptoms occurred in 2.5 hours versus 4.6 hours with placebo and 2.0 hours versus 12.0 hours with TA.

Ecallantide for the treatment of acute attacks in hereditary angioedema. Cicardi M, Levy RJ, McNeil DL, Li HH, Sheffer AL, Campion M. N Engl J Med 2010; 363: 523–31.

In a randomized double-blind trial in 71 patients ecallantide caused relief of symptoms in 165 minutes compared with over 240 minutes with placebo

Icatibant, a synthetic decapeptide, is a bradykinin B2 receptor antagonist recently licensed in the European Union for treatment of acute episodes of HAE. The recommended dose is one subcutaneous injection of 30 mg, preferably in the abdominal area. Mild reactions at the injection site are common. Ecallantide, a kallikrein inhibitor recently licensed in the United States (but not Europe) for the same indication, is also administered subcutaneously in a dosage of 30 mg.

LONG-TERM PROPHYLAXIS OF HEREDITARY ANGIOEDEMA

First-Line Therapies

- Danazol
- Stanozolol

How do we treat patients with hereditary angioedema? Cicardi M, Zingale L. Transfus Apheresis Sci 2003; 29: 221–7.

In a study of 141 patients, danazol and stanozolol proved equally effective; <10% of patients failed to obtain significant remission. Normalization of C1INH is not required. These authors start with a run-in period of 400 to 600 mg daily of danazol for 1 month, slowly tapering to 100 to 200 mg daily to determine the minimum dose that will maintain remission (C1INH level around 50% of normal; C4 within normal range; complete remission of angioedema).

Benefits and risks of danazol in hereditary angioedema: a long-term survey of 118 patients. Bork K, Bygum A, Hardt J. Ann Allergy Asthma Immunol 2008; 100: 153–61.

Data generated from patients who were treated with danazol for 2 months to 30 years showed that it was highly beneficial, with 111 out of 118 patients responding. Fifty-four (45.8%) patients had <1 attack per year or became symptom free. In the other patients during danazol treatment, the frequency of acute attacks decreased and became milder. Laryngeal edema decreased to 4.8%. Risk of adverse effects was high, with 93 patients suffering effects, including weight gain, menstrual irregularity, virilization, depression, headache, and liver adenomas, and 30 patients discontinuing the therapy.

Long-term prophylaxis of hereditary angioedema with androgen derivates: a critical appraisal and potential alternatives. Maurer M, Magerl M. J Dtsch Dermatol Ges 2011; 9: 99–107.

The IV substitution of C1INH and SC administration of icatibant are both well tolerated and reliable in controlling swelling attacks of HAE. Therefore long-term prophylactic treatment of HAE patients with androgen derivatives such as danazol may be reconsidered. Patients might benefit from either the withdrawal or dose reduction of androgen prophylaxis and rely on demand-oriented acute treatment of attacks using C1INH or icatibant.

Side effects in female patients may be troublesome, including menstrual disturbance, deepening of the voice, and hirsutism. In males, prostate changes should be monitored. All patients should have regular liver function tests. Attenuated androgens are contraindicated in pregnancy.

Second-Line Therapies

- TA
- Epsilon aminocaproic acid

Hereditary and acquired C1-inhibitor deficiency: biological and clinical characteristics in 235 patients. Agostoni A, Cicardi M. Medicine (Baltimore) 1992; 71: OK206–15.

Twelve of 15 patients had initially effective prophylaxis with TA, but this agent was only effective long term in 28% of patients, whereas danazol was effective long term in 97% of patients.

Tranexamic acid therapy in hereditary angioneurotic edema. Sheffer AL, Austen KF, Rosen FS. N Engl J Med 1972; 287: 452–4.

A randomized, placebo-controlled, double-blind crossover trial over a 4- to 13-month period. Seven of 12 patients receiving TA 1 g three times daily achieved a complete or near-complete cessation of attacks. Four additional patients experienced a moderate response.

TA is more potent than EACA and has been reported to cause fewer side effects.

Epsilon aminocaproic acid therapy of hereditary angioneurotic edema: a double blind study. Frank MM, Sergent JS, Kane MA, Alling DW. N Engl J Med 1972; 286: 808–12.

EACA (16 g daily) in a double-blind crossover trial prevented attacks of angioedema in four of five patients over a 2-year period. Common side effects consisted of weakness and increased fatigability. A follow-up open trial led to control of symptoms on 7 to 10 g of EACA daily.

Higher dose therapy (24–30 g) has led to elevation of creatine phosphokinase and aldolase levels and muscle necrosis. EACA therapy can also be used as short-term prophylaxis for minor procedures, but because of its potential thrombotic effects it should be discontinued before major surgery.

Third-Line Therapy

- C1INH concentrate

Cinryze (C1-inhibitor) for the treatment of hereditary angioedema. Gompels MM, Lock RJ. Expert Rev Clin Immunol 2011; 7: 569–73.

In a double-blind, placebo-controlled crossover trial, a plasma-derived concentrate of C1INH (pdC1INH) was used to treat HAE patients as a prophylaxis, with the frequency of attacks reducing by half to 6.26 per 12 weeks (compared with 12.73 per 12 weeks in the placebo group). Attacks were milder and of shorter duration. Patients with acute attacks receiving pdC1INH, 1000 units, reported time to onset of relief was 2 hours, compared with >4 hours in the placebo group.

PREVENTION OF RELAPSE DUE TO DENTAL AND SURGICAL INTERVENTIONS

First-Line Therapies

- FFP
- Danazol
- C1INH concentrate

Short-term prophylaxis in hereditary angioedema due to deficiency of the C1-inhibitor – a long-term survey. Farkas H, Zotter Z, Csuka D, Szabó E, Nébenfűhrer Z, Temesszentandrási G, et al. Allergy 2012; 67: 1586–93.

Retrospective analysis of 137 patients with HAE evaluated the efficacy of drugs administered for short-term prophylaxis. C1INH concentrate was found to be safe and effective in reducing edematous episodes after surgical procedures. Danazol may be used as an alternative to C1INH concentrate for prophylaxis before medical interventions.

WAO guideline for the management of hereditary angioedema. Craig T, Aygören-Pürsün E, Bork K, Bowen T, Boysen H, Farkas H, et. al. World Allergy Organ J 2012; 5: 182–99.

Androgens (danazol at 2.5–10 mg/kg/day, maximum 600 mg; stanozolol at 4–6 mg/d) may be used for 5 days before and 2 to 5 days postevent for preprocedural/short-term prophylaxis.

TA has been used in the past for preprocedural/short-term prophylaxis although with low efficacy in suppressing breakthrough attacks. The recommended oral dose is 25 mg/kg two to three times daily, maximum 3 to 6 g daily (not fully established).

Other preoperative options include 500 to 1000 units of C1INH concentrate or antifibrinolytic agents.

TREATMENT IN CHILDREN

Pediatric hereditary angioedema due to C1-inhibitor deficiency. Farkas H. Allergy Asthma Clin Immunol 2010; 6:18.

C1INH replacement therapy, antifibrinolytics, and attenuated androgens are currently favored medicinal products for the treatment of HAE in children, with regular monitoring and follow-up being vital. C1INH replacement therapy is effective and a safe agent for use in children. Antifibrinolytics have a favorable long-term safety profile and are therefore recommended but may lack efficacy. Attenuated androgens are another option in children, to be administered in the lowest effective dose.

HEREDITARY ANGIOEDEMA WITH NORMAL C1INH

Hereditary angioedema type 3, angioedema associated with angiotensin II receptor antagonists and female sex. Bork K. Am J Med 2004; 116: 644.

Two unrelated female patients with normal C1INH and C4 levels experienced severe exacerbations of HAE after the administration of losartan and valsartan, respectively.

Acute attacks of HAE with normal C1INH do not respond to C1INH concentrate, and antihistamines or corticosteroids are ineffective. The value of antifibrinolytics is unproven. For prevention danazol is worth trying in nonpregnant patients, but substantiation of its value is awaited. All patients should avoid angiotensin-2-receptor antagonists (sartans) and estrogens because these are known to provoke attacks in affected women. Bradykinin antagonists, such as icatibant, or kallikrein inhibitors, such as ecallantide, may offer benefit to these patients, although their benefit is unproven.

Evidence Levels: **A** Double-blind study **B** Clinical trial ≥ 20 subjects **C** Clinical trial < 20 subjects **D** Series ≥ 5 subjects **E** Anecdotal case reports

102

Hereditary hemorrhagic telangiectasia

Mitchell S. Cappell, Oscar Lebwohl

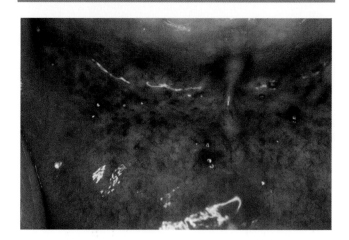

Hereditary hemorrhagic telangiectasia (HHT, or Osler–Weber–Rendu syndrome), an autosomal-dominant disease, produces a syndrome of multiple orocutaneous telangiectasias, especially on the face, lips, tongue, oral mucosa, and fingertips, together with multiple internal telangiectasias, especially on the mucosa of the nose and gastrointestinal (GI) tract. Individual telangiectasias typically are 3 to 10 mm wide, macular, bright red, non-pulsatile, and spidery or punctate in shape with a fine reticular internal structure. They tend to blanch under pressure (with diascopy) and refill immediately after releasing the pressure. They generally slowly increase in size and number with age. The basic lesion in HHT is a defect in the wall of small vessels that leads to direct arteriovenous communications without intervening capillaries. The prevalence of HHT is estimated at 1 per 6000 individuals. HHT is reliably diagnosed when three or more criteria are satisfied among a clinical tetrad (Curaçao criteria), listed later. HHT is possible or suspected when two criteria are satisfied. HHT is highly unlikely in adult patients satisfying only one or none of these criteria. About 85% of cases of HHT are due to underlying genetic mutations either in the gene encoding endoglin (ENG) that produces HHT1 or in the gene encoding activin receptor-like kinase (ACVRL1, previously called *ALK-1*) that produces HHT2. The remaining cases are caused by six other known families of mutations. Genetic mutations located on chromosome 5 cause HHT3, mutations located on chromosome 7 cause HHT4, and mutations located in the *MADH4* gene cause HHT associated with juvenile polyposis. The diagnosis can be confirmed by genetic tests for the individual mutations, but such tests are generally not necessary for diagnosis or clinical management.

Patients with rosacea or lupus erythematosus may have telangiectasias solely on the face but lack other manifestations of HHT. Patients with sporadic GI angiodysplasia are differentiated from patients with HHT by clinical presentation in old age, paucity of lesions, negative family history, and exclusive GI involvement without epistaxis or intranasal telangiectasia.

Clinical (Curaçao) criteria for diagnosis of hereditary hemorrhagic telangiectasia

Organ or other parameter	Characteristic finding
Nose	Recurrent, spontaneous epistaxis
Mucocutaneous	Telangiectasias on lips, oral cavity, nasal mucosa, or fingers
Gastrointestinal	Mucosal telangiectasias (or visceral arteriovenous malformations)
Family history	One or more first-degree relatives with HHT

HHT, hereditary hemorrhagic telangiectasia.

MANAGEMENT STRATEGY

The two major clinical complications of HHT are significant epistaxis and GI bleeding from nasal and GI telangiectasias. The bleeding may be chronic because these telangiectasias have thin and fragile vessel walls. Chronic blood loss may cause iron-deficiency anemia, whereas acute blood loss may cause hypovolemia and systemic hypotension. Internal shunts created by direct arteriovenous communications in HHT uncommonly cause clinical manifestations, including hypoxia from pulmonary arteriovenous shunts; cerebral ischemia, hemorrhage, or abscesses from intracerebral shunts; and portal hypertension, biliary tract disease, or high-output cardiac failure from intrahepatic shunts. Dermatologic telangiectasias are usually only a minor, cosmetic problem.

Specific Investigations

For epistaxis or gastrointestinal bleeding
- Serial hematocrit determinations — to assess severity of bleeding
- Serum iron, total iron binding capacity (TIBC), and ferritin levels – to diagnose iron-deficiency anemia

For epistaxis
- Nasal examination using fine-caliber, rigid, nasal endoscope
- Flexible nasal endoscopy – alternative technique of examination

For gastrointestinal bleeding
- Esophagogastroduodenoscopy (EGD) – for suspected upper GI bleeding
- Colonoscopy – for suspected lower GI bleeding
- Capsule endoscopy or double-balloon enteroscopy – for GI bleeding after a nondiagnostic EGD and colonoscopy
- Angiography – for ongoing bleeding after nondiagnostic endoscopic examinations

For epistaxis, bleeding severity is determined by inspection, vital signs, and laboratory tests. The bleeding site is precisely localized by nasal examination with a fine-caliber rigid tube (endoscope), using spot suction, and bright, shadow-free illumination, with a headlight, head mirror, or cold fiber-optic illumination. Flexible nasal endoscopy is a recent alternative examination technique. For GI bleeding, the bleeding severity is indicated by patient history, vital signs, physical findings, rectal examination, nasogastric aspiration, and transfusion requirements. The bleeding site and source are conclusively diagnosed by GI endoscopy.

Serial hematocrit determinations are important, particularly for acute bleeding, to determine need for transfusions of packed erythrocytes. Serum levels of iron, TIBC, and ferritin are important, particularly for chronic bleeding, to determine the need for iron replacement therapy.

Upper GI bleeding, usually manifested by hematemesis or melena, should be investigated by esophagogastroduodenoscopy (EGD). Lower GI bleeding, usually manifested by hematochezia or fecal occult blood, and occasionally by melena, should be investigated by colonoscopy. Small intestinal bleeding, usually manifested by hematochezia, melena, or fecal occult blood, can be investigated by capsule endoscopy after exclusion of upper and lower GI bleeding by EGD and colonoscopy, respectively. Double-balloon enteroscopy is often used at tertiary medical centers instead of capsule endoscopy to investigate small intestinal bleeding because of its greater diagnostic sensitivity and therapeutic capabilities despite its greater costs.

At endoscopy, telangiectasias appear as intensely red maculae due to the high oxygen content in erythrocytes within vessels supplied by arteries without intervening capillaries. The GI lesions resemble the cutaneous telangiectasias in size and shape. Telangiectasias are distinguished from lesions due to endoscopic trauma by identification during endoscopic intubation, as opposed to identification during endoscopic extubation with trauma; by a finely reticular (fernlike) internal structure due to a vascular tuft; by an irregular (fernlike) border as opposed to a round border with trauma; by an abrupt lesion margin as opposed to an indistinct margin with trauma; and by lesions lying flush (coplanar) with mucosa. Additionally, colonic lesions from endoscopic trauma usually occur at sharp colonic turns, during endoscopic looping, or after endoscopic suctioning.

Angiography is indicated for active GI bleeding if EGD and colonoscopy fails to diagnose the source of bleeding. The angiographic hallmarks of telangiectasias are a vascular tuft or tangle resulting from the local aggregation of irregular vessels; an early and intensely filling vein resulting from direct arteriovenous connection without intervening capillaries; and persistent opacification beyond the normal venous phase (slowly emptying vein), attributed to vascular tortuosity. Telangiectasias bleed only intermittently, and extravasation of contrast material from telangiectasias is infrequently detected at angiography.

Hereditary hemorrhagic telangiectasia: from molecular biology to patient care. Dupuis-Girod S, Bailly S, Plauchu H. J Thromb Haemostasis 2010; 8:1447–56.

Clinically oriented review of the genetics, pathophysiology, clinical presentation, diagnosis, and therapy of HHT.

Liver disease in patients with hereditary hemorrhagic telangiectasia. Garcia-Tsao G, Korzenik JR, Young L, Henderson KJ, Jain D, Byrd B, et al. N Engl J Med 2000; 343: 931–6.

Review of clinical findings caused by intrahepatic shunts with HHT, including eight patients with high-output cardiac failure, six patients with portal hypertension, and five patients with biliary tract disease.

Evidence of small-bowel involvement in hereditary hemorrhagic telangiectasia: a capsule-endoscopic study. Ingrosso M, Sabba C, Pisani A, Principi M, Gallitelli M, Cirulli A, et al. Endoscopy 2004; 36: 1074–9.

Study demonstrates a high frequency of small intestinal telangiectasias in elderly patients with HHT as detected by capsule endoscopy. Chronic blood loss from these intestinal telangiectasias may contribute to iron-deficiency anemia from HHT.

Evaluation of patients with hereditary hemorrhagic telangiectasia with video capsule endoscopy: a single-center prospective study. Chamberlain SM, Patel J, Carter Balart J, Gossage JR Jr, Sridhar S. Endoscopy 2007; 39: 516–20.

Prospective study of 80 patients evaluated by capsule endoscopy for small intestinal bleeding. The 32 patients with known HHT had significantly more GI telangiectasias than did 48 control patients without HHT (75% vs. 8.3% of patients had five or more telangiectasias). This study demonstrates the high sensitivity of capsule endoscopy in diagnosing small intestinal telangiectasias in patients who have HHT.

First-Line Therapies

For epistaxis or gastrointestinal bleeding

• Transfuse packed erythrocytes for significant, acute bleeding	A
• Oral iron therapy for iron-deficiency anemia from chronic blood loss	A
• Nonspecific therapy: avoid aspirin, other antiplatelet drugs, and anticoagulation	A
• Reverse severe coagulopathy if patient is actively bleeding (e.g., transfuse platelets for severe thrombocytopenia and transfuse fresh frozen plasma for elevated INR (international normalized ratio)	A
• Oral estrogen with progesterone	B

For epistaxis

• Nonspecific therapy: room humidification and nasal moisteners	A
• Nasal packing	A
• Septal dermoplasty	A
• Bevacizumab	B

For gastrointestinal bleeding

• Endoscopic therapy: argon plasma coagulation, thermocoagulation, electrocoagulation, or photocoagulation	B
• Angiographic embolization for bleeding refractory to endoscopic therapy	B
• Segmental bowel resection – for refractory bleeding	A

For cutaneous lesions

• Cosmetic therapy: laser or other focal ablation techniques for cutaneous lesions	A

The choice of therapy depends on bleeding site, severity, and chronicity as well as individual physician expertise. Severe bleeding requires hospitalization and insertion of two large-bore IV lines. Significant acute blood loss is treated with intravenous fluid resuscitation and transfusion of packed erythrocytes as needed. Chronic blood loss is treated with iron supplementation as needed.

Nonspecific therapy for bleeding from HHT includes *avoidance of aspirin, nonsteroidal antiinflammatory drugs (NSAIDs), other antiplatelet drugs, and anticoagulants* and administration of iron for patients with significant iron-deficiency anemia.

Nasal moisteners and room humidification promote mucosal integrity and reduce nasal mucosal injury and epistaxis. Epistaxis is initially treated by nonspecific local therapy such as *nasal packing*

Evidence Levels: **A** Double-blind study **B** Clinical trial ≥ 20 subjects **C** Clinical trial < 20 subjects **D** Series ≥ 5 subjects **E** Anecdotal case reports

to tamponade the bleeding. *Estrogen with progesterone* is used to prevent or arrest chronic epistaxis by promoting vascular integrity. Mutations in the different forms of HHT result in highly elevated levels of vascular endothelial growth factor (VEGF) that can cause an abnormal, immature vasculature with resultant telangiectasias. *Bevacizumab*, a recombinant humanized monoclonal antibody to VEGF, may reverse the telangiectasias occurring in HHT by inhibiting VEGF (antiangiogenesis). Preliminary clinical data, including one prospective open-label trial (described later), have shown IV bevacizumab may significantly reduce epistaxis in patients with HHT. Risks of IV bevacizumab include hypertension, bleeding in other organs, and bowel perforation. Submucosal or topical intranasal administration of bevacizumab may avoid much of the systemic toxicity of IV therapy with similar efficacy.

Several studies have reported a markedly reduced incidence of chronic epistaxis from telangiectasias after instituting estrogen therapy, either alone or with progesterone, due to the promotion of endothelial integrity. *Estrogen therapy* can be combined with other therapies, such as local endoscopic therapy, to increase efficacy. Despite controversy concerning efficacy, estrogen therapy should be considered before performing nasal surgery for chronic epistaxis because of its low risk and the risk of recurrent bleeding after surgery. Estrogen therapy is less desirable in males than in females because it can cause feminization.

Significant, refractory, chronic epistaxis is definitively treated by *septal dermoplasty*. Septal dermoplasty is indicated for severe, recurrent epistaxis, especially from anterior nasal mucosa. In this procedure, skin removed from the upper thigh is grafted on to the anterior nasal septum and floor to cover and protect the fragile mucosal telangiectasias from local trauma. The procedure is well tolerated using only local anesthesia, and complications, other than recurrent epistaxis, are rare. Septal dermoplasty is effective in >75% of cases. Failure results from inadequate graft coverage with bleeding from telangiectasias at or beyond the border of the grafted area. Focal laser therapy can be used to ablate discrete bleeding intranasal lesions.

Chronically bleeding GI telangiectasias may also be treated with estrogen and progesterone. Multiple individual case reports have described cessation of GI bleeding from telangiectasia in HHT. At endoscopy, actively bleeding, individual GI telangiectasias are treated with endoscopic *argon plasma coagulation* (APC), *thermocoagulation, electrocoagulation, or photocoagulation*. Endoscopists increasingly prefer APC because of its easy application and its potentially greater safety due to more superficial tissue ablation. Nonetheless, all these endoscopic therapies are relatively safe and highly successful at achieving hemostasis when performed by an experienced endoscopist. Nonbleeding lesions are generally not treated at endoscopy unless the lesions are particularly large and thus likely to bleed. However, patients with HHT often rebleed from other, untreated GI telangiectasias after an initial session of endoscopic therapy and therefore require multiple sessions of endoscopic therapy to treat these other lesions.

Segmental bowel resection is reserved for severe active bleeding, localized to a single region and refractory to medical and endoscopic therapy. Where available, *angiographic embolization* can obviate the need for GI surgery. Surgery or angiographic embolization often provides only intermediate-term relief due to formation of telangiectasias at other GI sites.

Treatment of bleeding gastrointestinal vascular malformations with oestrogen-progesterone. van Custen E, Rutgeerts P, Vantrappen G. Lancet 1990; 335: 953–5.

In a double-blind, placebo-controlled crossover trial of 10 patients with frequent and severe GI bleeding from HHT, the number of transfusions decreased significantly from a mean of 10.9 units of packed erythrocytes in controls receiving placebo

to a mean of 1.1 units in patients treated with estrogen-progesterone during a 6-month period.

Use of estrogen in treatment of familial hemorrhagic telangiectasia. Harrison DFN. Laryngoscope 1982; 92: 314–20.

Report of successful control of epistaxis with estrogen therapy in 67 patients with HHT, with few complications.

Treatment of hereditary hemorrhagic telangiectasia with submucosal and topical bevacizumab therapy. Karnezis TT, Davidson TM. Laryngoscope 2012; 122: 495–7.

In a prospective trial of 19 patients, the epistaxis severity score significantly decreased to 2.00 2 months after intranasal, submucosal injection of bevacizumab compared with the baseline, pretreatment severity score of 8.12 ($p < 0.0001$). Bevacizumab therapy statistically significantly protected against epistaxis for all 12 months of the clinical trial.

Bevacizumab in patients with hereditary hemorrhagic telangiectasia and severe hepatic vascular malformations and high cardiac output. Dupuis-Girod S, Ginon I, Saurin JC, Marion D, Guillot E, Decullier E, et al. JAMA 2012; 307: 948–55.

In a prospective, open-label study, 25 adult patients with severe HHT received bevacizumab intravenously for 2.5 months. The mean duration of epistaxis decreased from 221 min/mo at baseline to 43 min/mo at 6 mo ($p = 0.008$), and the mean number of episodes decreased from 26 episodes/mo at baseline to 11 episodes/mo at 6 mo. This study suggests that IV bevacizumab may decrease the frequency and duration of epistaxis in patients with HHT.

Outcome of septal dermoplasty in patients with hereditary hemorrhagic telangiectasia. Fiorella ML, Ross D, Henderson KJ, White RI Jr. Laryngoscope 2005; 115: 301–5.

Retrospective study reporting outcome of 32 consecutive patients undergoing septal dermoplasty in whom accurate records of transfusion requirements were available. Mean blood transfusion requirements declined significantly from a mean of 21 units of packed erythrocytes in the year before surgery to a mean of 1 unit in the year after surgery ($p < 0.001$). This study illustrates the fairly extensive literature supporting the efficacy of septal dermoplasty for treating recurrent, relatively severe epistaxis from HHT.

Diagnosis and management of gastrointestinal bleeding in patients with hereditary hemorrhagic telangiectasia. Longacre AV, Gross CP, Gallitelli M, Henderson KJ, White RI Jr, Proctor DD. Am J Gastroenterol 2003; 98: 59–65.

In a nonrandomized, long-term, observational study, the mean hemoglobin level increased and the chronic transfusion requirements decreased in about three quarters of 17 patients after instituting chronic estrogen hormonal therapy, either alone or with other therapies, for GI bleeding from HHT.

Argon plasma coagulation is an effective treatment for hereditary hemorrhagic telangiectasia patients with severe nosebleeds. Pagella F, Matti E, Chu F, Pusateri A, Tinelli C, Olivieri C, et al. Acta Otolaryngol 2013; 133: 174–80.

In this retrospective study, 26 patients with HHT were followed by telephone calls one or more years after undergoing APC treatment of nasal mucosa for severe epistaxis requiring blood transfusions. The epistaxis severity score decreased significantly from 8.5 before APC therapy to 4.3 after therapy ($p < 0.005$), as did the number of patients requiring blood transfusions ($p < 0.02$). The frequency, intensity, and duration of epistaxis also decreased significantly after APC therapy compared with baseline ($p < 0.0001$). The beneficial effects of therapy lasted 22.9 months. This work demonstrates that APC is an effective therapy for severe epistaxis from HHT.

Long-term outcome of argon plasma ablation therapy for bleeding in 100 consecutive patients with colonic angiodysplasia. Olmos JA, Marcolongo M, Pogorelsky V, Herrera L, Tobal F, Davalos JR. Dis Colon Rectum 2006; 49: 1507–16.

In this prospective trial, 85 of 100 patients with moderate to severe bleeding from colonic angiodysplasia treated at colonoscopy with APC (mean 3.9 angiodysplasias treated per patient) had no further overt bleeding and had a stable hemoglobin level without further blood transfusions or iron therapy during a mean follow-up of 20 months. Only two minor procedure complications occurred. Although not specifically addressing APC for telangiectasias in HHT, this large prospective study demonstrated high efficacy of this therapy for preventing rebleeding from the similar lesions of sporadic colonic angiodysplasia.

Second-Line or Temporizing Therapies

For epistaxis

• Arterial ligation	B
• Topical vasoconstrictors	B
• Cryosurgery/electrical cautery/argon plasma coagulation	B
• Unilateral or bilateral surgical closure of nostrils	B
• Arterial embolization	B
• Tamoxifen	B
• Submucosal resection	C
• Topical aminocaproic acid	D

For gastrointestinal bleeding

• Bevacizumab	C
• Oral aminocaproic acid therapy	D
• α-Interferon	D

Some recent data support use of *tamoxifen*, an estrogen antagonist, to prevent bleeding from telangiectasia in HHT. A few patients have responded to therapy with α-interferon, which has known antiangiogenic properties, but this therapy is currently experimental because of insufficient data.

Local nonspecific therapy of *arterial ligation, cryosurgery, electrical cautery, APC, or submucosal resection* provides temporary relief of epistaxis from HHT. However, these treatments can cause mucosal scarring, which diminishes the efficacy of subsequent septal dermoplasty. Topical intranasal therapy with vasoconstrictors or aminocaproic acid rarely produces scarring. Nonspecific therapies are indicated only for temporary relief of acute bleeding. Life-threatening epistaxis refractory to septal dermoplasty is treated by surgical closure of one or both nostrils, depending on the bleeding source.

Bevacizumab is considered a second-line therapy for GI bleeding from telangiectasias because of limited data on efficacy for this indication. *Aminocaproic acid* promotes thrombosis and retards bleeding by inhibiting fibrinolysis. Oral aminocaproic acid therapy has had mixed success with HHT. This therapy rarely causes hypotension or rhabdomyolysis. Aminocaproic acid is a temporary, second-line therapy.

Antiestrogen therapy for hereditary hemorrhagic telangiectasia: a double-blind placebo-controlled clinical trial. Yaniv E, Preis M, Hadar T, Shvero J, Haddad M. Laryngoscope 2009; 119: 284–8.

In a randomized, placebo-controlled trial of 21 patients with HHT, 9 of 10 patients (90%) treated with orally administered tamoxifen, an estrogen antagonist, had cessation of clinically significant epistaxis versus 3 of 11 patients receiving placebo ($p = 0.01$). This small, placebo-controlled trial suggests that tamoxifen may be effective in preventing epistaxis in HHT.

Evidence Levels: A Double-blind study B Clinical trial ≥ 20 subjects C Clinical trial < 20 subjects D Series ≥ 5 subjects E Anecdotal case reports

103

Herpes genitalis

Ramya Vangipuram, Laura Karas, Kevin Sharghi, Jarad Peranteau, Stephen K. Tyring

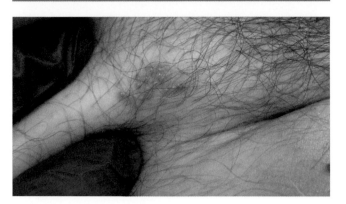

Herpes genitalis, or genital herpes, is a recurrent vesicular eruption of the skin and mucosa in the region between the navel and the buttocks, usually preceded by prodromal symptoms including itching, burning, and tingling. It is a common sexually transmitted disease caused predominantly by herpes simplex virus type 2 (HSV-2) but can also be caused by HSV-1. First-episode genital herpes due to HSV-1 has become increasingly common in certain populations—namely, heterosexual women and men who have sex with men (MSM). Primary infection may have associated influenza-like systemic signs and symptoms, including fever, headache, malaise, and myalgias, which occur 2 to 20 days after exposure. Lesions of the initial genital herpes infection typically last 2 to 3 weeks, during which time the lesions demonstrate a progression from grouped papules on an erythematous base, to vesicles, to ulcers with eventual crusting. Recurrences generally lack systemic symptoms and are less severe than the primary outbreak. Recurrent lesions occur in the same area but are fewer in number and heal more quickly, typically lasting 5 to 10 days. Genital herpes infection due to HSV-1 results in fewer symptomatic recurrences than infection caused by HSV-2. Residual hypopigmentation, hyperpigmentation, an scarring may occur with healing.

MANAGEMENT STRATEGY

Because no cure exists for herpes genitalis, treatment is aimed at reducing the number of recurrences using suppressive therapy and at promoting rapid healing when a recurrence is present. In addition, treatment aims to reduce infectivity by reducing viral shedding and to reduce complications such as urinary retention and aseptic meningitis. In the past, *acyclovir*, both topical and oral, was used as a first-line treatment for recurrences. Given acyclovir's low bioavailability, it requires frequent dosing. The standard dosing of oral acyclovir for a recurrence is 200 mg five times daily for 5 days. Alternative regimens have also been shown to be effective, including 400 mg three times daily for 5 days, 800 mg three times daily for 2 days, and 800 mg twice daily for 5 days. The frequent dosing of acyclovir led to the development of *valacyclovir* and *famciclovir* (the prodrugs of acyclovir and penciclovir, respectively) as

alternative therapies with improved bioavailability. The use of topical acyclovir should be discouraged, as it is less effective than oral acyclovir. Valacyclovir has been shown to be effective when dosed 500 mg twice daily for 3 days or 1000 mg once daily for 5 days. A dosing regimen of oral valacyclovir, given 2000 mg twice daily for 1 day, has been studied and shown to be more convenient; however, further comparative studies are needed. Famciclovir is effective when prescribed as 1000 mg twice daily for 1 day. It may also be taken as 125 mg twice daily for 5 days. Acyclovir, valacyclovir, and famciclovir may all be used for suppressive therapy.

Immunocompromised individuals have more frequent recurrences and can develop more severe lesions, thus requiring longer treatment periods with higher doses than those used in the immunocompetent. Severe cases may require intravenous therapy. Suppressive dosage regimens have been used in this population. Long-term therapy may lead to the selection of resistant strains of virus. In acyclovir-resistant cases, intravenous therapy with foscarnet may be required.

Addressing psychosocial issues is another important aspect of genital herpes management. The recurrent nature of genital HSV infection can have severe emotional and psychological impact on patients. Counseling serves to help them cope with the infection and to prevent sexual and perinatal transmission.

Specific Investigations

- Type-specific serologic testing
- Polymerase chain reaction (PCR)
- Viral culture
- Skin biopsy of atypical lesion

Type-specific laboratory testing should be performed to distinguish HSV-2 infections from HSV-1 infections, as this has implications for disease course and patient counseling. Patients with confirmed genital herpes should be offered testing for HIV and other sexually transmitted diseases. Severe or refractory cases may be due to underlying immunosuppression, which should be investigated further.

Precision of the Kalon herpes simplex virus type 2 IgG ELISA: an international interlaboratory assessment. Patel EU, Manucci J, Kahle EM, Lingappa JR, Morrow RA, Piwowar-Manning E, et al. BMC Infect Dis 2015; 15: 398.

Performance of the Focus HerpeSelect-2 EIA for the detection of herpes simplex virus type 2 antibodies in seven African countries. Mujugira A, Morrow RA, Celum C, Lingappa J, Delany-Moretlwe S, Fife KH, et al. Sex Transm Infect 2011; 87: 238–41.

Effect of sexually transmitted disease (STD) coinfections on performance of three commercially available immunosorbent assays used for detection of herpes simplex virus type 2-specific antibody in men attending Baltimore, Maryland, STD clinics. Summerton J, Riedesel M, Laeyendecker O, Gaydos C, Maldeis NE, Hardick A, et al. Clin Vaccine Immunol 2007; 14: 1545–9.

Using the evidence base on genital herpes: optimizing the use of diagnostic tests and information provision. Scoular A. Sex Transm Infect 2002; 78: 160–5.

Polymerase chain reaction for detection of herpes simplex virus (HSV) DNA on mucosal surfaces: comparison with HSV isolation in cell culture. Wald A, Huang M-L, Carrell D, Selke S, Corey L. J Infect Dis 2003; 188: 1345–51.

First-Line Therapies	
• Valacyclovir (Valtrex)	A
• Acyclovir (Zovirax)	A
• Famciclovir (Famvir)	A

Primary Genital Infection

Antiviral treatment should be initiated promptly, ideally within 72 hours of the appearance of lesions, and should be continued for 7 to 10 days. Treatment duration may be extended if adequate healing has not occurred. The following regimens may be used: acyclovir 400 mg three times daily or 200 mg five times daily; valacyclovir 1000 mg twice daily; or famciclovir 250 mg three times daily. Acyclovir, valacyclovir, and famciclovir demonstrate similar efficacy. Therefore the initial drug choice may be influenced by factors such as provider preference, cost, and availability. Valacyclovir may be preferable due to the convenience of twice-daily dosing.

Genital herpes. Gnann JW Jr, Whitley RJ. N Engl J Med 2016; 375: 666–74.

Genital herpes. Gupta R, Warren T, Wald A. Lancet 2007; 370: 2127–37.

Acute Reactivation Episodes

Standard-dose and high-dose daily antiviral therapy for short episodes of genital HSV-2 reactivation: three randomised, open-label, crossover trials. Johnston C, Saracino M, Kuntz S, Magaret A, Selke S, Huang ML, et al. Lancet 2012; 379: 641–7. Erratum in: Lancet 2012; 379: 616.

Three separate complementary open-label crossover studies compared no medication with acyclovir 400 mg twice daily (standard dose), valacyclovir 500 mg daily (standard dose) with acyclovir 800 mg three times daily (high dose), and standard-dose valacyclovir with valacyclovir 1 g three times daily (high dose). High-dose acyclovir was associated with less viral shedding than standard-dose valacyclovir, but there was no significant difference in time to lesion healing between the groups. High-dose valacyclovir had less viral shedding and shorter lesion healing time compared with its standard dose. Viral shedding persisted even in high-dose regimens.

Single-day therapy for recurrent genital herpes. Tyring S, Berger T, Yen-Moore A, Tharp M, Hamed K. Am J Clin Dermatol 2006; 7: 209–11.

A multicenter, randomized, double-blind, placebo-controlled clinical trial found that famciclovir 1000 mg twice daily for 1 day, taken within 6 hours of prodrome onset, resulted in a significant reduction in lesion healing time and reduced the time of all symptom resolution compared with placebo. A greater proportion of subjects who took famciclovir did not progress to a full genital herpes outbreak compared with those taking placebo (23.3% vs. 12.7%, respectively).

Sexually transmitted diseases treatment guidelines 2015. Centers for Disease Control and Prevention. MMWR Recomm Rep 2015; 64: 27–32.

Antiviral therapy should be initiated during the prodrome or within 24 hours of the appearance of lesions. Therefore it is important that patients have a supply of drug on hand in order to initiate treatment promptly.

Single-day patient initiated famciclovir therapy for recurrent genital herpes: a randomized, double-blind, placebo-controlled trial. Aoki FY, Tyring S, Diaz-Mitoma F, Gross G, Gao J, Hamed K. Clin Infect Dis 2006; 42: 8–13.

This study proved that in addition to being convenient (potentially a boon for increased patient compliance), single-day therapy is safe and effective for the treatment of recurrent genital herpes. Subjects receiving 1000 mg famciclovir orally twice daily for 1 day healed approximately 2 days faster than those on placebo.

A randomized, placebo-controlled comparison of oral valacyclovir and acyclovir in immunocompetent patients with recurrent genital herpes infections. Tyring SK, Douglas JM, Corey LC, Spruance SL, Esmann J. Arch Dermatol 1998; 134: 185–91.

This multicenter, double-blind, placebo-controlled, randomized, parallel-design study showed that oral valacyclovir 1000 mg twice daily for 5 days was as effective and well tolerated as acyclovir five times daily for 5 days for the treatment of recurrent genital herpes.

Prophylactic Treatment

Prophylactic treatment for frequent reactivation, recurrent severe attacks, at bone marrow transplantation, or before delivery.

Effect of valacyclovir on viral shedding in immunocompetent patients with recurrent herpes simplex virus 2 genital herpes: a US-based randomized, double-blind, placebo-controlled clinical trial. Fife KH, Warren TJ, Ferrera RD, Young DG, Justus SE, Heitman CK, et al. Mayo Clin Proc 2006; 81: 1321–7.

Over a 60-day period 1 g of valacyclovir daily was well tolerated and effectively reduced clinical and subclinical HSV-2 shedding compared with placebo.

Once-daily valacyclovir to reduce the risk of transmission of genital herpes. Corey L, Wald A, Patel R, Sacks SL, Tyring SK, Warren T, et al. N Engl J Med 2004; 350: 11–20.

Among heterosexual HSV-2 discordant couples, once-daily valacyclovir (500 mg) significantly reduced the risk of transmission of genital herpes. Clinically symptomatic HSV-2 infection was reduced by 75%, and acquisition of HSV-2 was reduced by 48% in the valacyclovir group versus placebo.

Valacyclovir therapy to reduce recurrent genital herpes in pregnant women. Andrews WW, Kimberlin DF, Whitley R, Cliver S, Ramsey PS, Deeter R. Am J Obstet Gynecol 2006; 194: 774–81.

This double-blind, placebo-controlled, randomized trial showed that daily valacyclovir, initiated at 36 weeks' gestation in HSV-positive pregnant women with a history of recurrences, significantly reduced the number of women with subsequent clinical HSV recurrences. However, this suppressive regimen did not reduce shedding of HSV within 7 days of delivery compared with placebo. The number of women with clinical HSV lesions at delivery was similar for both the placebo and the treatment group.

Effect of serologic status and cesarean delivery on transmission rates of herpes simplex virus from mother to infant. Brown ZA, Wald A, Morrow RA, Selke S, Zeh J, Corey L. JAMA 2003; 289: 203–9.

Evidence Levels: **A** Double-blind study **B** Clinical trial ≥ 20 subjects **C** Clinical trial < 20 subjects **D** Series ≥ 5 subjects **E** Anecdotal case reports

Among women with HSV in genital secretions at the time of labor, the risk of neonatal HSV was significantly reduced in those who had a cesarean delivery.

Sexually transmitted diseases treatment guidelines 2015. Centers for Disease Control and Prevention. MMWR Recomm Rep 2015; 64: 27–32.

Severe HSV infection, or complications requiring hospitalization, such as disseminated infection, pneumonitis, hepatitis, meningitis, or encephalitis, requires intravenous antiviral therapy. A regimen of acyclovir 5 to 10 mg/kg intravenously every 8 hours for a minimum of 2 days until clinical improvement occurs is recommended. Transition to oral antiviral therapy is recommended to complete a 10-day course.

Frequent reactivation of herpes simplex virus among HIV-1-infected patients treated with highly active antiretroviral therapy. Posavad CM, Wald A, Kuntz S, Huang ML, Selke S, Krantz E, et al. J Infect Dis 2004; 190: 693–6.

In HIV-infected individuals, antiretroviral therapy reduced the frequency and severity of symptomatic genital herpes. However, frequent asymptomatic viral shedding occurred.

Sexually transmitted diseases treatment guidelines 2015. Centers for Disease Control and Prevention. MMWR Recomm Rep 2015; 64: 27–32.

Acyclovir, valacyclovir, and famciclovir are safe to use in immunocompromised patients. Treatment duration is generally for 5 to 10 days of the following: acyclovir 400 mg three times daily, famciclovir 500 mg twice daily, or valacyclovir 1 g twice daily. Intravenous therapy may be required in severe cases.

Valacyclovir prophylaxis for the prevention of herpes simplex virus reactivation in recipients of progenitor cell transplantation. Dignani MC, Mykietiuk A, Michelet M, Intile D, Mammana L, Desmery P, et al. Bone Marrow Transplant 2002; 29: 263–7.

In over 100 patients after bone marrow transplantation, equal efficacy between intravenous acyclovir and oral valacyclovir was seen compared with no prophylaxis.

Second-Line Therapies

• Foscarnet	B
• Cidofovir	A

A multicenter phase I/II dose escalation study of single-dose cidofovir gel for treatment of recurrent genital herpes. Sacks SL, Shafran SD, Diaz-Mitoma F, Trottier S, Sibbald RG, Hughes A, et al. Antimicrob Agents Chemother 1998; 42: 2996–9.

A randomized, double-blind, clinic-initiated, sequential dose-escalation pilot study compared the safety and efficacy of single applications of 1%, 3%, and 5% cidofovir gel with placebo in the treatment of early lesional recurrent genital herpes. At all strengths, cidofovir significantly reduced the median time to negative virus culture in a dose-dependent fashion. Single-dose application of cidofovir gel confers a significant antiviral effect on lesions of recurrent genital herpes.

Clinical potential of the acyclic nucleoside phosphonates cidofovir, adefovir, and tenofovir in treatment of DNA virus and retrovirus infections. De Clercq E. Clin Microbiol Rev 2003; 16: 569–96.

The acyclic nucleoside phosphonate HPMPC (cidofovir) was proven effective in vitro and in vivo against a wide variety of DNA virus and retrovirus infections, including HSV types 1 and 2.

Foscarnet treatment of acyclovir-resistant herpes simplex virus infection in patients with acquired immunodeficiency syndrome: preliminary results of a controlled, randomized, regimen-controlled trial. Hardy WD. Am J Med 1992; 92: 30s–5s.

Twenty-five patients with AIDS and acyclovir-resistant HSV infection were treated with foscarnet infusions for 2 weeks, followed by 8 more weeks either with 40 mg/kg daily or without further treatment. Lesions healed most quickly in those treated for a total of 10 weeks.

Third-Line Therapies

• Aspirin	B
• Resiquimod	A
• Topical imiquimod	E

Aspirin in the management of recurrent herpes simplex virus infection. Karadi I, Karpati S, Romics L. Ann Intern Med 1998; 128: 696–7.

This study showed that patients treated with aspirin 125 mg daily had significantly fewer days of active HSV infection than controls who took no antiviral or antiinflammatory drugs. Of the 21 subjects, only 2 had recurrent genital HSV; the remainder had recurrent oral HSV.

Topical resiquimod 0.01% gel decreases herpes simplex virus type 2 genital shedding: a randomized, controlled trial. Mark KE, Corey L, Meng TC, Magaret AS, Huang ML, Selke S, et al. J Infect Dis 2007; 195: 1324–31.

A randomized, double-blind, vehicle-controlled trial assessed the efficacy of resiquimod 0.01% gel for reducing human anogenital HSV-2 mucosal reactivation. Adults with genital HSV-2 applied topical resiquimod or vehicle to anogenital lesions twice weekly for 3 weeks. The median lesion and shedding rates were lower for the treatment group than in the vehicle group for both sampling periods. The length of recurrence was not influenced by resiquimod treatment.

Treatment of recalcitrant herpes simplex virus with topical imiquimod. Hirokawa D, Woldow A, Lee SN, Samie F. Cutis 2011; 88: 276–7.

In this case report, an HIV-positive man with valacyclovir-resistant genital HSV-2 was successfully treated with topical imiquimod 5% cream three times weekly for 8 weeks.

NOVEL AND OTHER THERAPIES

- Helicase-primase inhibitors
- Psychosocial counseling
- Hygiene techniques

Effect of pritelivir compared with valacyclovir on genital HSV-2 shedding in patients with frequent recurrence: a randomized clinical trial. Wald A, Timmler B, Magaret A, Warren T, Tyring S, Johnston C, et al. JAMA 2016; 316: 2495–2503.

This phase II, randomized, double-blind, crossover trial compared oral pritelivir, a novel HSV helicase-primase inhibitor, dosed at 100 mg once daily, to oral valacyclovir 500 mg once daily. The study demonstrated a significantly lower rate of genital HSV shedding and lesions in the pritelivir arm versus the valacyclovir arm. Pritelivir thus appears to be significantly more effective than valacyclovir, though further investigation into long-term safety and efficacy is needed.

Sexually transmitted diseases treatment guidelines 2015. Centers for Disease Control and Prevention. MMWR Recomm Rep 2015; 64: 27–32.

Counseling of infected individuals serves to prevent sexual and perinatal infection and to help individuals cope with infection. Education for infected individuals seems to be of benefit both at the time of diagnosis and after resolution of the acute infection to further their understanding of the chronic nature of the disease.

Genital herpes: a review. Beauman JG, Maj MC. Am Fam Phys 2005; 72: 1527–34, 1541–2.

Prevention of secondary infection and spread of the infection can be achieved by keeping the affected area clean and dry, wearing loose-fitting clothing and cotton underwear, avoiding contact with the lesions, and washing hands immediately should contact with any sores occur.

PREVENTION

- Condoms
- Vaccine
- Disclosure to sexual partners

A pooled analysis of the effect of condoms in preventing HSV-2 acquisition. Martin ET, Krantz E, Gottlieb SL, Magaret AS, Langenberg A, Stanberry L, et al. Arch Intern Med 2009; 169: 1233–40.

This pooled analysis of over 5000 HSV-2–negative individuals at baseline showed that consistent use of condoms was associated with a 30% reduction in risk of acquiring HSV-2 compared with those with no condom use (HR of 0.70, 95% confidence interval (CI), 0.40–0.94, $p = 0.01$).

Knowledge of partners' genital herpes protects against herpes simplex virus type 2 acquisition. Wald A, Krantz E, Selke S, Lairson E, Morrow RA, Zeh J. J Infect Dis 2006; 194: 42–52.

This study utilized a time-to-event design to demonstrate that disclosure of genital herpes to an individual's partner increased the mean time to HSV-2 acquisition (270 days vs. 60 days, $p = 0.03$) compared with those who did not disclose their condition. Disclosure of HSV-2 infection to sexual partners has the potential to serve as a protective factor against HSV-2 transmission.

Effect of condoms on reducing the transmission of herpes simplex virus type 2 from men to women. Wald A, Langenberg AG, Link K, Izu AE, Ashley R, Warren T, et al. JAMA 2001; 285: 3100–6.

In heterosexual discordant couples in which the male is infected with HSV-2, the use of condoms confers protection against transmission in susceptible women. A concurrent reduction in sexual activity when the source partner had lesions also occurred as a result of counseling on sexual behavior.

Therapeutic vaccine for genital herpes simplex virus-2 infection: findings from a randomized trial. Bernstein D, Wald A, Warren T, Fife K, Tyring S, Lee P, et al. J Infect Dis 2017; 215: 856–64.

This double-blind, placebo-controlled, dose-escalation study evaluated a purified protein subunit vaccine currently in development for HSV-2. The vaccine was shown to have an acceptable safety profile. It demonstrated immunogenicity and reduced recurrent episodes of viral shedding and days with lesions. Further investigation is needed to determine the optimal dose and the duration of the protective effects.

Efficacy results of a trial of a herpes simplex vaccine. Belshe RB, Leone PA, Bernstein DI, Wald A, Levin MJ, Stapleton JT, et al. N Engl J Med 2012; 366: 34–43.

In this randomized, double-blind trial, 8323 women seronegative for HSV-1 and HSV-2 received the investigational vaccine (20 µg of glycoprotein D from HSV-2 with alum and 3-O-deacylated monophosphoryl lipid A as an adjuvant) at months 0, 1, and 6. The vaccine was found to be effective in preventing HSV-1, but not HSV-2, disease and infection.

Evidence Levels: **A** Double-blind study **B** Clinical trial ≥ 20 subjects **C** Clinical trial < 20 subjects **D** Series ≥ 5 subjects **E** Anecdotal case reports

Herpes labialis

Jane C. Sterling

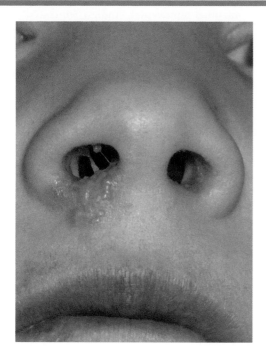

Herpes simplex virus (HSV) infects skin and mucous membranes, damaging keratinocytes and causing intense inflammation, seen as small blisters with erythema. Infections around the mouth or elsewhere on the skin are usually due to HSV-1, whereas genital infection is most commonly caused by HSV-2. The primary infection may be obvious or subclinical; once latency is established in sensory ganglia, reactivation can occur at variable intervals. In immunosuppression, disease can be chronic, and antiviral resistance can develop.

MANAGEMENT STRATEGY

Both primary and reactivation episodes are usually self-limiting and may require no treatment. Antiseptic creams, alcohol-based tinctures, or surface dressings can be soothing self-help remedies. Antiviral therapy, such as *aciclovir* and related drugs, is available for topical and systemic use and is an effective form of treatment. Although anogenital herpes responds well, *topical aciclovir*, applied five times daily for 5 days, in cutaneous herpes results in marginal benefit. The effect in trials, when compliance is usually good, is reported to be a reduction in pain and healing time of approximately 12 hours. Application of aciclovir with an adhesive patch inside the mouth, resulting in continuous local therapy, reduces time to healing by 1 day compared with placebo. Aciclovir 5% in combination with 1% hydrocortisone cream applied 5 times per day is safe and appears to reduce the risk of ulceration. *Oral aciclovir*, 200 mg five times daily for 5 days, will usually reduce the time to healing and duration of virus shedding more effectively than topical treatment. Shorter treatment courses with higher dose aciclovir produce similar effects. Topical or systemic treatment for an acute episode should be started early in the episode to have most benefit. In addition, pain relief may be necessary. Occlusion with gel or an adhesive patch can reduce pain and discomfort.

A failure of response to aciclovir may be due to the poor absorption and rapid clearance after ingestion or to the emergence of aciclovir resistance. *Valaciclovir*, a prodrug of aciclovir, and *famciclovir*, a prodrug of penciclovir, have improved bioavailability, and dosing is once or twice daily. A short course (single day) treatment with oral *famciclovir* can hasten healing if taken at the start of a reactivation episode. Efficacy of oral valaciclovir can be as good as intravenous aciclovir.

In frequently recurrent disease, or in immunosuppressed individuals when episodes may be severe, prophylactic antiviral treatment can be considered together with avoidance of any precipitating factors. *UV protection* may help to reduce viral reactivation in herpes labialis. To reduce frequency and severity of attacks, antiviral treatment needs to be continuous for several weeks or months. Aciclovir 400 mg twice daily is likely to produce a decrease in the frequency of reactivation episodes; valaciclovir or famciclovir may be prescribed as alternatives. There is a potential risk of selection of resistant strains of virus with long-term therapy, but this is rare even in immunosuppressed patients. Oral antivirals may be taken as a relatively short-term course to reduce the risk of a reactivation episode before and during intense sun exposure or before dental or cosmetic procedures.

Low-intensity light from a diode laser has been shown to increase the recurrence-free interval.

In immunosuppressed individuals with spreading or persistent infection, intravenous therapy with aciclovir, or the more toxic *foscarnet* or *cidofovir*, may be necessary. Topical preparations of cidofovir have been shown to have effect but are not commercially available. *Vidarabine, interferons,* and *interleukin-2* and other agents have also been used but without reliable effect. Herpes simplex is a common precipitating cause of episodes of recurrent erythema multiforme (see page NPI), which can be reduced in frequency by prophylactic antiviral therapy.

Other treatments reported to have some effect in acute attacks include the antivirals *idoxuridine, trifluorothymidine* (*TFT*), *inosine pranobex,* and *docosanol,* used topically, and low-level light therapy.

Specific Investigations

- Polymerase chain reaction (PCR) of blister fluid or biopsy
- Viral culture from swab of lesion
- Immunocytology of blister floor cells
- Electron microscopy of blister fluid
- Skin biopsy of atypical lesion
- Herpes simplex serology
- Assessment of immune function

The diagnosis is usually obvious clinically. In atypical disease, laboratory confirmation is essential. In unexplained persistent or severe disease, immunodeficiency should be excluded.

First-Line Therapies

Topical aciclovir	A
Topical aciclovir with hydrocortisone	A
Oral aciclovir	A
Occlusion with gel or patch	B

Primary cutaneous infection

Treatment of herpes simplex gingivostomatitis with aciclovir in children: a randomized double blind placebo controlled study. Amir J, Harel L, Smetana Z, Varsano I. BMJ 1997; 314: 1800–3.

A total of 61 children with herpetic gingivostomatitis were treated with aciclovir suspension 15 mg/kg or placebo five times daily for 7 days. Aciclovir reduced the duration of lesions from 10 to 4 days and reduced the period of viral shedding.

Acute reactivation episodes

Aciclovir cream for treatment of herpes simplex labialis: results of 2 randomized, double-blind, vehicle-controlled multicenter clinical trials. Spruance SL, Nett R, Marbury T, Wolff R, Johnson J, Spaulding T. Antimicrob Agents Chemother 2002; 46: 2238–43.

In two studies of a total of 1385 patients with recurrent herpes labialis, aciclovir 5% cream applied five times a day for 4 days reduced time to healing to an average of 4.4 days compared with 5.0 days when placebo was used.

Efficacy and safety of aciclovir mucoadhesive buccal tablet in immunocompetent patients with labial herpes (LIP Trial): a double-blind, placebo-controlled, self-initiated trial. Bieber T, Chosidow O, Bodsworth N, Tyring S, Hercogova J, Bloch M, et al. J Drugs Dermatol 2014; 13: 791–8.

A large double-blind, placebo-controlled study of adherent buccal patch containing either aciclovir or placebo showed a reduction in time to healing of 1 day and fewer reactivation episodes in the 9 months after a single treatment.

Effectiveness of topical corticosteroids in addition to antiviral therapy in the management of recurrent herpes labialis: a systematic review and meta-analysis. Arain N, Paravastu SC, Arain MA. BMC Infect Dis 2015; 15: 82.

In-depth review of four studies concluding that the combination of topical aciclovir and corticosteroid reduced ulceration but did not decrease the healing rate compared with aciclovir alone.

Treatment of recurrent herpes simplex labialis with oral aciclovir. Spruance SL, Stewart JCB, Rowe NH, McKeough MB, Wenerstrom G, Freeman DJ. J Infect Dis 1990; 161: 185–90.

Herpes labialis was less painful and quicker to heal in 114 patients treated early with 400 mg aciclovir, five times daily for 5 days, compared with 60 given placebo treatment. The blister development and lesion size were not affected by treatment.

Evaluation of the efficacy and safety of a CS20 protective barrier gel containing OGT compared with topical aciclovir and placebo on functional and objective symptoms of labial herpes recurrences: a randomized clinical trial. Khemis A, Duteil L, Coudert AC, Tillet Y, Dereure O, Ortonne JP. J Eur Acad Dermatol Venereol 2012; 26: 1240–6.

Application five times a day of either aciclovir cream or the glycerol-containing gel gave similar time to healing, but those using the gel had less pain.

Second-Line Therapies	
• Topical penciclovir	B
• Oral valaciclovir	A
• Oral famciclovir	A
• Low-level infrared, light	B

Recurrent herpes labialis: efficacy of topical therapy with penciclovir compared with aciclovir. Femiano F, Gombos F, Scully C. Oral Dis 2001; 7: 31–3.

Aciclovir 5% cream or penciclovir 1% cream was applied every 2 hours during waking hours for 4 days. Penciclovir treatment reduced the duration of symptoms by 1 day.

High-dose, short-duration, early valaciclovir therapy for episodic treatment of cold sores: results of two randomized, placebo-controlled multicenter studies. Spruance S, Jones T, Blatter MM, Vargas-Cortez M, Barber J, Hill J, et al. Antimicrob Agents Chemother 2003; 47: 1072–80.

Immediate treatment with either 2 g twice daily for 1 day or 2 g twice daily for 1 day plus 1 g twice daily for 1 day reduced the duration of the episode (5–5.5 days with placebo) by 0.5 to 1 day. The chance of an aborted episode was increased.

Single-dose, patient-initiated famciclovir: a randomized, double-blind, placebo-controlled trial for episodic treatment of herpes labialis. Spruance SL, Bodsworth N, Resnick H, Conant M, Oeuvray C, Gao J, et al. J Am Acad Dermatol 2006; 55: 47–53.

Famciclovir 750 mg twice daily for 1 day or famciclovir 1500 mg as a single dose were compared with placebo with 375 patients completing the study. Lesions healed in approximately 4 days in both groups taking famciclovir compared with 6 days for the placebo group.

Evaluation of the efficacy of low-level light therapy using 1072 nm infrared light for the treatment of herpes simplex labialis. Dougal G, Lee SY. Clin Exp Dermatol 2013; 38: 713–8.

In a randomized, placebo-controlled study, the light treatment, given in 3-minute irradiations six times over 2 days, reduced healing time to 5 days compared with 7 days for placebo.

Third-Line Therapies	
• Intravenous aciclovir	A
• Intravenous vidarabine	C
• Intravenous foscarnet	C
• Intravenous cidofovir	C
• Topical cidofovir	C

Multicenter collaborative trial of intravenous aciclovir for treatment of mucocutaneous herpes simplex virus infection in the immunocompromised host. Meyers JD, Wade JC, Mitchell CD, Saral R, Lietman PS, Durack DT, et al. Am J Med 1982; 73: 229–35.

Aciclovir given intravenously (250 mg/m^2, three times per day for 7 days) to immunocompromised patients with active HSV infection (85% oral disease) was superior to placebo in reduction of pain and healing time, plus reduction in duration of virus shedding.

Foscarnet treatment of aciclovir-resistant herpes simplex virus infection in patients with acquired immunodeficiency syndrome: preliminary results of a controlled, randomized, regimen-controlled trial. Hardy WD. Am J Med 1992; 92 (Suppl 2A): 30s–5s.

Twenty-five patients with acquired immune deficiency syndrome (AIDS) and aciclovir-resistant HSV infection were treated with foscarnet infusions for 2 weeks and then either for a further 8 weeks with 40 mg/kg daily or without further maintenance therapy. Healing of lesions was quickest in those treated for 10 weeks.

Evidence Levels: **A** Double-blind study **B** Clinical trial ≥ 20 subjects **C** Clinical trial < 20 subjects **D** Series ≥ 5 subjects **E** Anecdotal case reports

A controlled trial comparing foscarnet with vidarabine for aciclovir-resistant mucocutaneous herpes simplex in the acquired immunodeficiency syndrome. Safrin S, Crumpacker C, Chatis P, Davis R, Hafner R, Rush J, et al. N Engl J Med 1991; 325: 551–5.

Foscarnet 40 mg/kg every 8 hours produced healing of aciclovir-resistant herpetic lesions within 4 weeks in eight patients with AIDS, whereas no improvement occurred in six similar patients treated with vidarabine 15 mg/kg daily.

Treatment with intravenous (S)-1-[hydroxy-2-(phosphonylmethoxy)propyl]-cytosine of aciclovir-resistant mucocutaneous infection with herpes simplex virus in a patient with AIDS. Lalezari JP, Drew WL, Glutzer E, Miner D, Safrin S, Owen WF, et al. J Infect Dis 1994; 170: 570–2.

Treatment with four intravenous infusions of 5 mg/kg/week of HPMPC (cidofovir) produced 95% healing in a patient with severe resistant herpetic lesions.

A randomized, double-blind, placebo-controlled trial of cidofovir gel for the treatment of aciclovir-unresponsive mucocutaneous herpes simplex virus infection in patients with AIDS. Lalezari J, Schacker T, Feinberg J, Gathe J, Lee S, Cheung T, et al. J Infect Dis 1997; 176: 892–8.

Twenty patients with AIDS applied 0.3% or 1% cidofovir gel once daily for 5 days; 50% healed or improved compared with 0% of the 10 placebo-treated patients. Cidofovir produced local inflammation in a quarter of patients.

Prophylactic Treatment	
• Sunscreen	A
• Oral aciclovir	A
• Oral valaciclovir	A
• Oral famciclovir	B
• Low-intensity diode laser	B

Prevention of ultraviolet-light-induced herpes labialis by sunscreen. Rooney JF, Bryson Y, Mannix ML, Dillon M, Wohlenberg CR, Banks S, et al. Lancet 1991; 338: 1419–22.

Using an experimental UV exposure to induce reactivation of herpes, lesions developed in 71% of 38 patients using a placebo but none in 35 patients using sunscreen.

Oral aciclovir to suppress frequently recurrent herpes labialis: a double-blind, placebo-controlled trial. Rooney JF, Straus SE, Mannix ML, Wohlenberg CR, Alling DW, Dumois JA, et al. Ann Int Med 1993; 118: 268–72.

Twenty patients completed a randomized 4-month crossover study receiving aciclovir 400 mg twice a day or placebo. During active treatment, there were an average of 0.85 reactivation episodes compared with 1.8 during placebo treatment.

Valaciclovir prophylaxis for the prevention of herpes simplex virus reactivation in recipients of progenitor cell transplantation. Dignani MC, Mykietiuk A, Michelet M, Intile D, Mammana L, Desmery P, et al. Bone Marrow Transplant 2002; 29: 263–7.

Comparison of intravenous aciclovir, oral valaciclovir, or no prophylaxis after bone marrow transplantation in over 100 patients showed equal efficacy of the two antivirals.

Famciclovir prophylaxis of herpes zoster virus reactivation after laser skin resurfacing. Alster TS, Nanni CA. Dermatolog Surg 1999; 25: 242–6.

The expected rate of HSV reactivation after facial cosmetic laser or chemical peel procedures is approximately 10%. With oral famciclovir, 250 or 500 mg twice daily for 10 days, the reactivation rate was similar for both doses.

The efficacy of valaciclovir in preventing recurrent herpes simplex virus infections associated with dental procedures. Miller CS, Cunningham LL, Lindroth JE, Avdiushko SA. J Am Dent Assoc 2004; 135: 1311–8.

In a placebo-controlled trial of 125 adults with recurrent herpes labialis, valaciclovir (2 g twice a day on the day of dental treatment, with 1 g twice a day the following day) reduced the incidence of reactivation episodes from 20% (placebo) to 11% with antiviral treatment.

Low-intensity laser therapy is an effective treatment for recurrent herpes simplex infection. Results from a randomized double-blind placebo-controlled study. Schindl A, Neumann R. J Invest Dermatol 1999; 113: 221–3.

Forty-eight patients with monthly reactivation were irradiated daily for 2 weeks with either placebo or 690 nm light from a diode laser during quiescence. During the 1-year follow-up period, median recurrence-free interval was 3 weeks in the placebo group and 37.5 weeks in the treatment group.

OTHER THERAPIES

Multicenter randomized study of inosine pranobex versus aciclovir in the treatment of recurrent herpes labialis and recurrent herpes genitalis in Chinese patients. You Y, Wang L, Li Y, Wang Q, Cao S, Tu Y, et al. J Dermatol 2015; 42: 596–601.

One hundred forty-four patients received either oral inosine pranobex 1 g four times per day plus placebo aciclovir or aciclovir 200 mg five times per day plus placebo inosine pranobex. The two groups were comparable in symptoms and time to healing.

Clinical efficacy of topical docosanol 10% cream for herpes simplex labialis: a multicenter, randomized, placebo-controlled trial. Sacks SL, Thisted RA, Jones TM, Barbarash RA, Mikolich DJ, Ruoff GE, et al. J Am Acad Dermatol 2001; 45: 222–30.

Docosanol 10% cream applied five times a day until healing reduced symptoms and healing by approximately 1 day.

105

Herpes zoster

Zeena Nawas, Michael M. Hatch, Stephen K. Tyring

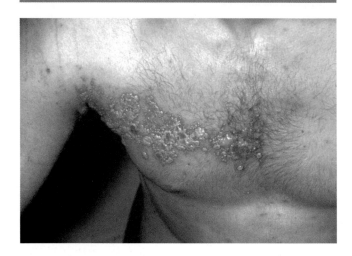

Reactivation of latent varicella zoster virus (VZV) produces the clinical syndrome herpes zoster (shingles), which manifests as a unilateral eruption along a single dermatome and is usually preceded by prodromal pain and paresthesia. The eruption lasts around 7 to 10 days and progresses from erythematous macules and papules to vesicles, then pustules, and finally crusts over. One of the most common complications of herpes zoster is postherpetic neuralgia (PHN), which is dermatomal pain persisting longer than 3 months.

MANAGEMENT STRATEGY

Early treatment—within the first 72 hours of vesicle formation—is important for antiviral efficacy, time to lesion healing, and minimizing zoster-associated pain (although initiating treatment after 72 hours may still be effective). *Aciclovir, valaciclovir,* and *famciclovir* are guanosine analogs that are phosphorylated by thymidine kinase to a triphosphate form that inhibits viral deoxyribonucleic acid (DNA) polymerase. The oral bioavailability of the antivirals determines the number of daily administrations. Patient compliance tends to decrease as the number of daily administrations increases. The most common side effects seen are nausea, headache, and gastrointestinal upset, but these drugs are otherwise safe and well tolerated. Patients with renal insufficiency will need an adjusted dose, as these medications are excreted by the kidneys.

Aciclovir-resistant VZV infections have been reported in immunocompromised patients (i.e., acquired immune deficiency syndrome (AIDS), transplant patients), and in these cases *foscarnet* (given intravenously 40 mg/kg three times daily) can be used as an alternative.

Acutely, *corticosteroids* may reduce zoster-associated pain, but they are associated with a risk of serious adverse events and have shown no benefit in reducing time to complete cessation of pain or prevention of PHN.

Pain management is especially difficult with conventional analgesics in zoster patients who develop PHN. Calcium channel α2-δ ligands (gabapentin and pregabalin), tricyclic antidepressants, opioids, topical lidocaine (Table 105.1), selective serotonin and norepinephrine reuptake inhibitors (duloxetine and venlafaxine), and topical capsaicin have been shown to reduce the pain associated with PHN. Of these medications, only gabapentin, pregabalin, 5% lidocaine patch, and 8% capsaicin patch have been approved by the Food and Drug Administration (FDA) specifically for the treatment of PHN. Adding gabapentin to an antiviral in patients with acute herpes zoster appears to significantly reduce the incidence of PHN. In January 2011, the FDA approved Gralise as a once-daily medication for the treatment of postherpetic neuralgia. Gralise is an extended-release form of gabapentin that not only has been shown to significantly decrease PHN pain scores but may also be associated with fewer side effects than its immediate-release counterpart. In 2012 the FDA approved Horizant, gabapentin enacarbil, for the once-daily therapy of PHN.

Vaccination of patients aged 50 years and over is the most promising option for the prevention of herpes zoster and therefore PHN. As of April 2016, the only FDA-approved zoster vaccine for adults is Zostavax. In a clinical trial involving more than 38,000 adults 60 years of age or older, the vaccine was shown to reduce the incidence of herpes zoster by 51% and the incidence of PHN by 67%. In 2006 the Advisory Committee on Immunization Practices recommended a single dose of zoster vaccine for adults 60 years of age or older, whether or not they have had a previous episode of herpes zoster. A subsequent clinical trial that studied Zostavax in patients aged 50 to 59 years showed that the vaccine efficacy for preventing herpes zoster was 69.8% in this age group. In 2011 the FDA approved Zostavax for patients 50 to 59 years of age. An adjuvanted herpes zoster subunit vaccine (HZ/su), which is currently being studied but is not yet approved, was shown to significantly reduce the risk of herpes zoster among adults who were 50 years of age or older. However, unlike Zostavax, the HZ/su vaccine efficacy was well preserved among participants who were 70 years of age or older.

Specific Investigations

No investigation is usually required
- Tzanck smear
- Virology (culture, serology [acute plus chronic], electron microscopy, polymerase chain reaction)

First-Line Therapies

Aciclovir 800 mg five times daily for 7 days	A
Famciclovir 500 mg three times daily for 7 days	A
Valaciclovir 1 g three times daily for 7 days	A

Valaciclovir compared with aciclovir for improved therapy for herpes zoster in immunocompetent adults. Beutner KR, Friedman DJ, Forszpaniak C, Andersen PL, Wood MJ. Antimicrob Agents Chemother 1995; 39: 1546–53.

Valaciclovir is comparable to aciclovir in the resolution of zoster eruption, but it accelerates the resolution of pain compared with aciclovir and is more convenient.

Factors influencing pain outcome in herpes zoster: an observational study with valaciclovir. Decroix J, Partsch H, Gonzalez R, Mobacken H, Goh CL, Walsh L, et al. Valaciclovir Zoster Assessment Group (VIZA). J Eur Acad Dermatol Venereol 2000; 14: 23–33.

Table 105.1 Treatment options for postherpetic neuralgia

Drug class	Examples	Initial daily dose (mg)	Titration to maximum dose
Calcium channel α2-δ ligands	Gabapentin	100–300	Start once at night and increase to three times daily dosing; increase by 100–300 mg every 3 days to total dose of 1800–2400 mg/day
	Gabapentin enacarbil		600 mg once daily in the morning for 3 days, then increase to 600 mg twice daily
	Pregabalin	150	Titrate up to 300 or 600 mg/day
Opioids	Hydrocodone	5–10	No titration
	Oxycodone (extended release)	20	Titrate up to 60 mg daily
Tricyclic antidepressants	Nortriptyline	10–25	Increase by 10–25 mg weekly, with a target dose of 75–150 mg daily; single dose or two divided doses
	Amitriptyline	10–25	Titrate up to 100 mg daily; single dose
	Desipramine	10–25	Increase every 3 days as needed up to 150 mg daily; single dose

An open-label study using a 7-day course of valaciclovir to treat 1897 immunocompetent patients. Valaciclovir was safe, effective (even when initiated more than 72 hours after the first vesicle), and associated with very few adverse events.

Famciclovir for the treatment of acute herpes zoster: effects on acute disease and postherpetic neuralgia. A randomized, double-blind, placebo controlled trial. Tyring S, Barbarash RA, Nahlik JE, Cunningham A, Marley J, Heng M, et al. Ann Intern Med 1995; 123: 89–96.

Famciclovir recipients had faster resolution of pain after an acute episode than those receiving placebo.

Double-blind, randomized, aciclovir-controlled, parallel-group trial comparing the safety and efficacy of famciclovir and aciclovir in patients with uncomplicated herpes zoster. Shen MC, Lin HH, Lee SS, Chen YS, Chiang PC, Liu YC. J Microbiol Immunol Infect 2004; 37: 75–81.

Famciclovir is comparable to aciclovir in the resolution of zoster cutaneous eruption but is more convenient and had a more favorable adverse event profile.

A comparative study to evaluate the efficacy and safety of aciclovir and famciclovir in the management of herpes zoster. Gopal MG, Shannoma, Kumar S, Ramesh M, Nandini AS, Manjunath NC. Clin Diagn Res 2013; 7: 2904–7.

Oral famciclovir given at 250 mg three times daily for 7 days is as effective as aciclovir 800 mg five times daily.

Oral aciclovir therapy accelerates pain resolution in patients with herpes zoster: a meta-analysis of placebo-controlled trials. Wood MJ, Kay R, Dworkin RH, Soong SJ, Whitley RJ. Clin Infect Dis 1996; 22: 341–7.

In four placebo-controlled studies aciclovir was clearly shown to accelerate pain resolution.

Antiviral treatment for preventing postherpetic neuralgia. Chen N, Li Q, Yang J, Zhou M, Zhou D, He L. Cochrane Database Syst Rev 2014; 2: CD006866.

Oral aciclovir does not significantly reduce the incidence of PHN.

Second-Line Therapies

Agents to reduce postherpetic neuralgia
- Calcium channel α2-δ ligands (gabapentin, pregabalin)   A
- Tricyclic antidepressants   A
- Lidocaine patch   A
- Oxycodone   A

Pregabalin for the treatment of postherpetic neuralgia: a randomized, placebo-controlled trial. Dworkin RH, Corbin AE, Young JP, Sharma U, LaMoreaux L, Bockbrader H, et al. Neurology 2003; 60: 1274–83.

Pregabalin is effective in the treatment of pain and sleep interference associated with PHN.

Efficacy and safety of gabapentin 1800 mg treatment for postherpetic neuralgia: a meta-analysis of randomized controlled trials. Fan H, Yu W, Zhang Q, Cao H, Li J, Wang J, et al. J Clin Pharm Ther 2014; 39: 334–42.

A meta-analysis of randomized controlled trials found gabapentin 1800 mg to significantly reduce postherpetic neuralgia up to 14 weeks. Treatment at this dose was safe up to 24 weeks. Comparison between once-daily and divided-dose gabapentin for the treatment of PHN showed no significant difference in efficacy.

Incidence of postherpetic neuralgia after combination treatment with gabapentin and valaciclovir in patients with acute herpes zoster: open-label study. Lapolla W, Digiorgio C, Haitz K, Magel G, Mendoza N, Grady J, et al. Arch Dermatol 2011; 147: 901–7.

The addition of gabapentin to valaciclovir produced a significant reduction in PHN. Therefore it is recommended that gabapentin be initiated in addition to antivirals for the treatment of acute zoster with moderate to severe pain at presentation.

Gabapentin versus nortriptyline in postherpetic neuralgia patients: a randomized, double blind clinical trial: the

GONIP Trial. Chandra K, Shafiq N, Pandhi P, Gupta S, Malhotra S. Int J Clin Pharmacol Ther 2006; 44: 358–63.

Gabapentin and nortriptyline are equally efficacious, but gabapentin is better tolerated.

Nortriptyline versus amitriptyline in postherpetic neuralgia: a randomized trial. Watson CP, Vernich L, Chipman M, Reed K. Neurology 1998; 51: 1166–71.

Nortriptyline is equally as effective as amitriptyline but is better tolerated.

The effects of preemptive treatment of postherpetic neuralgia with amitriptyline: a randomized, double-blind, placebo-controlled trial. Bowsher D. J Pain Symptom Manage 1997; 13: 327–31.

Low-dose amitriptyline given at the time of the acute zoster rash may reduce the incidence of PHN.

Topical lidocaine for the treatment of postherpetic neuralgia. Khaliq W, Alam S, Puri N. Cochrane Database Syst Rev 2007; 2: CD004846.

A meta-analysis combining two studies found that lidocaine is more effective than placebo, but there is insufficient evidence to recommend it as a first-line therapy. The studies cited in the review used 5% lidocaine gel applied for 8 to 24 hours or 5% lidocaine patch applied up to three times daily.

Efficacy of oxycodone in neuropathic pain: a randomized trial in postherpetic neuralgia. Watson CPN, Babul N. Neurology 1998; 50: 1837–41.

Patients on slow-release oxycodone had significantly greater pain relief and reduction in allodynia and disability.

Third-Line Therapies	
• Vaccination of adults	A
• Contact with varicella or with children	C
• Topical capsaicin	A
• Topical nonsteroidal antiinflammatory cream	C
• Tramadol	A
• Sympathetic nerve block	B
• Transcutaneous electrical stimulation	B
• Methylcobalamin injection	B

A vaccine to prevent herpes zoster and postherpetic neuralgia in older adults. Oxman MN, Levin MJ, Johnson GR, Schmader KE, Straus SE, Gelb LD, et al. N Engl J Med 2005; 352: 2271.

A randomized, double-blind, placebo-controlled trial of live attenuated Oka/Merck VZV vaccine enrolled 38,546 immunocompetent adults aged 60 years or over. The vaccine significantly reduced morbidity from herpes zoster and PHN. It was safe and well tolerated.

Efficacy, safety, and tolerability of herpes zoster vaccine in persons aged 50 to 59 years. Schmader KE, Levin MJ, Gnann Jr, JW, McNeil SA, Vesikari T, Betts RF, et al. Clin Infect Dis 2012; 54: 922–8.

The Merck Zostavax vaccine was shown to reduce the incidence of herpes zoster by 69.8% in patients aged 50 to 59 years and was well tolerated.

Family history and herpes zoster risk in the era of shingles vaccination. Hernandez PO, Javed S, Mendoza N, Lapolla W, Hicks LD, Tyring SK. J Clin Virol 2011; 52: 344–8.

The most important risk factor for development of zoster, after age and immune status, is a family history of shingles. Therefore patients over age 50 with a family history of shingles should be particularly encouraged to receive the zoster vaccine.

Contacts with varicella or with children and protection against herpes zoster in adults: a case controlled study. Thomas SL, Wheeler JG, Hall AJ. Lancet 2002; 360: 678–82.

Social contact with many children outside the household, or occupational contacts with children ill with chickenpox, results in a graded protection against zoster.

A randomized vehicle-controlled trial of topical capsaicin in the treatment of postherpetic neuralgia. Watson CP, Tyler KL, Bickers DR, Millikan LE, Smith S, Coleman E. Clin Ther 1993; 15: 510–26.

Capsaicin 0.075% cream applied three to four times per day was effective. The only side effect was burning or stinging at sites of application.

Benzydamine cream for the treatment of postherpetic neuralgia: minimum duration of treatment periods in a cross-over trial. McQuay HJ, Carroll D, Moxon A, Glynn CJ, Moore RA. Pain 1990; 40: 131–5.

Some patients benefit from 3% benzydamine hydrochloride cream applied six times daily.

Tramadol in postherpetic neuralgia: a randomized, double-blind, placebo-controlled trial. Boureau F, Legallicier P, Kabir-Ahmadi M. Pain 2003; 104: 323–31.

A double-blind study with 127 patients found tramadol to be effective in reducing pain intensity and increasing the percentage of pain relief compared with placebo. All patients were treated for 6 weeks with doses ranging from 100 to 400 mg based on therapeutic response. Patients over 75 years of age received divided doses (morning and night); others received a single-dose regimen.

Neuraxial and sympathetic blocks in herpes zoster and postherpetic neuralgia: an appraisal of current evidence. Kumar V, Krone K, Mathieu A. Regional Anesth Pain Med 2004; 29: 454–61.

Sympathetic blocks for herpes zoster and PHN appear to be useful but require randomized, controlled trials for validation.

Modified Jaipur block for the treatment of post-herpetic neuralgia. Puri N. Int J Dermatol 2011; 50: 1417–20.

Subcutaneous injections of 2% Xylocaine and 0.5% bupivacaine in 4 mg/mL methylprednisolone can provide significant pain relief in persistent PHN. Approximately 90% of patients in a recent study experienced complete pain relief after three rounds of subcutaneous injections administered at 6-week intervals.

Transcutaneous electrical nerve stimulation for chronic postherpetic neuralgia. Ing MR, Hellreich PD, Johnson DW, Chen JJ. Int J Dermatol. 2015; 54: 476–80.

A randomized study of patients with PHN refractory to other medical treatments found that transcutaneous electrical nerve stimulation produced a statistically significant reduction in pain scores.

Cryoanalgesia for postherpetic neuralgia: a new treatment. Calandria L. Int J Dermatol 2011; 50: 746–50.

Liquid nitrogen applied in a nonfreezing manner can safely reduce PHN pain. In a recent study, 75% of patients reported a >70% reduction in pain after a total of five weekly sessions.

Evidence Levels: **A** Double-blind study **B** Clinical trial ≥ 20 subjects **C** Clinical trial < 20 subjects **D** Series ≥ 5 subjects **E** Anecdotal case reports

A single-center randomized controlled trial of local methylcobalamin injection for subacute herpetic neuralgia. Xu G, Lv ZW, Feng Y, Tang WZ, Xu GX. Pain Med 2013; 14: 884–94.

Local methylcobalamin injection was effective in relieving pain and discomfort caused by subacute herpetic neuralgia and was well tolerated.

Corticosteroids for preventing postherpetic neuralgia. Han Y, Zhang J, Chen N, He L, Zhou M, Zhu C. Cochrane Database Syst Rev 2013; 3: CD005582.

A systematic review and meta-analysis of randomized controlled trials found moderate-quality evidence that corticosteroids given acutely during herpes zoster infection are ineffective in preventing postherpetic neuralgia.

Hidradenitis suppurativa

Noah Scheinfield, Gregor Jemec

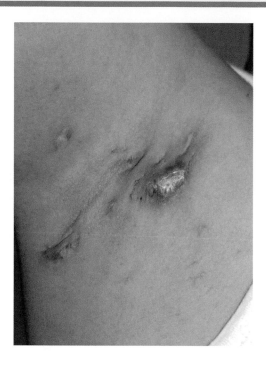

Hidradenitis suppurativa (HS) is a common, chronically relapsing skin disease characterized by recurring inflamed painful nodules, abscess and sinus formation, and scarring most likely due to aberrant cellular immunity stimulated by commensal bacteria (most commonly coagulase-negative *Staphylococcus* [CONS]). The disease can occur on any area where hair follicles are located. It is a follicular disease, distinct from acne vulgaris and staphylococcosis or other simple primary infections. Pain and suppuration cause considerable morbidity and significantly reduce quality of life in patients. The disease is associated with important comorbidities and an increased all-cause mortality compared with healthy controls and an increased cardiovascular mortality compared with psoriasis patients. Diseases associated with HS may include depression, obesity, smoking, polycystic ovarian disease, ulcerative colitis, Crohn disease, pyoderma gangrenosum, hormonal abnormalities, spondyloarthropathy, arthritis, metabolic syndrome, dyslipidemia, psychiatric disorders, drug dependence, hypertension, diabetes, thyroid disease, alcohol dependence, and lymphoma.

MANAGEMENT STRATEGY

HS is a clinical diagnosis, based on the identification of morphology, location, and the chronic/recurrent nature of lesions. The morphology may include noninflamed or inflamed nodules, abscesses, nondraining or draining sinus tracts (tunnels), and scars. The locations are bilateral and must involve one or more of these areas: axillae, inframammary area, and groin (including

genitals). Chronicity may be defined as at least two flares in 6 months. No pathognomonic test exists. Preclinical follicular changes can be identified with ultrasound or histologic investigation. Age of onset is usually in the third decade of life and is rare before puberty. An underlying endocrine disorder must be considered in prepubertal cases.

Hurley stage I lesions are often "blind" boils (i.e., deep and rounded nodules). These may be transient and flare to become abscesses that subside. Gradually scarring and sinus formation occur in separate areas of the affected regions (stage II), and ultimately scarring and sinuses coalesce to form stage III lesions. Early lesions can remit without treatment. Sinus tracts and scars limit nonsurgical treatment options. Clinically HS can often be distinguished from furunculosis (often large randomly occurring boils and not limited to inverse areas) or epidermal cysts (usually solitary, clinically stable lesions), pyogenic granulomas, and scarring folliculitis. HS is fundamentally a sterile disease, and cultures are usually negative because CONS is usually sifted on bacterial culture. Microbiology is most useful when presentations are atypical and in later stages of disease when superinfection may occur. If suspicion exists that a mimic of HS is present, for example, mycobacterial infection, squamous cell carcinoma, or Crohn disease, skin biopsies and/or additional relevant tests should be performed.

Current medical practice is mainly empiric. International guidelines have been suggested for the management of HS. A three-pronged approach gives structure to patient management: The first prong consists of adjuvant therapy, which includes pain management, treatment of established superinfections, weight loss, and tobacco cessation. Treatment of superinfections is defined by bacterial culture sensitivities. Patients should be provided access to appropriate bandaging of suppurating lesions.

The second prong involves medical therapy, which may be topical in mild cases. *Topical clindamycin* has been shown to have an effect on early lesions. *Topical gentamycin* may also be useful. Intralesional corticosteroids (single dose) or *resorcinol 15%* BID can be used as first-line treatment for HS. Systemic tetracycline (500 mg BID) or doxycycline may be used as an alternative for more disseminated disease. Cohort studies support coadministering *oral clindamycin 300 mg BID*, and *rifampicin 300 mg BID* may induce a remission of limited HS. Adalimumab has been shown effective in moderate to severe HS when administered in routine inflammatory bowel disease doses (week 0: 160 mg, week 2: 80 mg, and from week 4: 40 mg every week). Onset of effect has been shown to be at week 2 of treatment. A post hoc analysis of a smaller randomized controlled trial (RCT) indicated that infliximab 5 mg/kg may also be effective. Anakinra (100 mg daily) has also been found effective in a small trial. Although intravenous antibiotic therapy involving an imipenem-class drug has been reported, more research needs to be done before this can be recognized as part of the therapeutic ladder for HS.

Palliative medication includes systemic antiinflammatory drugs such as *oral corticosteroid*, *dapsone*, and *ciclosporine*. Patients may also benefit from *acitretin* 25 mg BID/TID, although this treatment is often limited by side effects and teratogenicity. Hormonal therapy with *cyproterone acetate* may be helpful in some females but requires high and continued use, which raises safety concerns. A study found that spironolactone at doses ranging from 25 mg BID to 100 mg BID might be useful in the treatment of HS.

An initial antiinflammatory response may be followed by relapse; continued and sustained immune responses can cause the HS to worsen, increasing morbidity, clinical manifestation of HS, and complication. HS shows little sign of improvement with isotretinoin.

The third prong of treatment is surgery. In milder cases this involves *minor surgery*—that is, localized excisions or exteriorization of sinus tracts. Only fluctuating obvious abscesses should undergo lancing. Lancing of inflamed nodules is painful to the patient and causes scarring. Nonfluctuating symptomatic lesions are better treated using intralesional corticosteroids. A CO_2 laser can be used to evaporate lesions. More advanced cases require major surgery, which should involve excision of the affected tissue or careful exteriorization (deroofing) of all sinus tracts (tunnels). The recurrence rate is inversely proportional to the extent of surgery, and wide excisions therefore offer a better chance of remission. Similarly, it is suggested that secondary intentional healing is superior to primary closure of postexcisional wounds. Secondary healing requires longer periods of wound management but generally does not preclude resumption of work after 3 to 4 weeks of treatment.

SPECIFIC INVESTIGATION

The diagnosis is clinical based on morphology, location, and chronicity/recurrence. Specific investigation may be necessary to rule out differential diagnosis depending on clinical findings.

First-Line Therapies	
• Antibiotics – topical clindamycin or oral tetracycline	B
• Oral clindamycin and rifampin for 10 weeks	B
• Surgery	B
• Intralesional Kenalog	D

Topical treatment of hidradenitis suppurativa with clindamycin. Clemmensen OJ. Int J Dermatol 1983; 22: 325–8.

Topical clindamycin for 3 months was significantly more effective than placebo in early lesions.

A randomised trial of topical clindamycin vs. systemic tetracycline in hidradenitis suppurativa with special reference to disease assessment. Jemec GBE, Wendelboe P. J Am Acad Dermatol 1998; 39: 971–4.

Clinical equivalence of efficacy between topical clindamycin and oral tetracycline in 46 patients.

Combination therapy with clindamycin and rifampicin for hidradenitis suppurativa: a series of 116 consecutive patients. Gener G, Canoui-Poitrine F, Revuz JE, Faye O, Poli F, Gabison G, et al. Dermatology 2009; 219: 148–54.

Disease severity assessed by Sartorius score reduced by 50% after 10 weeks.

De-roofing: a tissue-saving surgical technique for the treatment of mild to moderate hidradenitis suppurativa lesions. van der Zee HH, Prens EP, Boer J. J Am Acad Dermatol 2010; 63: 475–80.

Deroofing appears to be a useful form of limited surgery of sinus tracts (tunnels).

Recurrence of hidradenitis suppurativa after surgical management: a systematic review and meta-analysis. Mehdizadeh A, Hazen PG, Bechara FG, Zwingerman N, Moazenzadeh M, Bashash M, et al. J Am Acad Dermatol 2015; 73 (Suppl 1): S70–7.

Drainage alone carries a recurrence rate of up to 100%; radical excision has a recurrence rate of 25% at a median interval of 20 months. Success of surgery is affected by such variables as location, extent, and duration of disease.

Intralesional corticosteroid injections as a treatment option for acute lesions in patients diagnosed with hidradenitis suppurativa. Maini P, Posso-De Los Rios C, Gooderham M. J Amer Acad Derm 2015; 72 (Suppl 1): AB51.

A total of 33 (29%) patients received intralesional triamcinolone acetonide injections at concentrations of 2.5 mg/mL (14.3%), 3.33 mg/mL (34.7%), 5.0 mg/mL (38.8%), or 10 mg/mL (12.2%) as treatment to control acute lesions. Only 6/25 (25%) female subjects treated with intralesional injections required concomitant systemic antibiotics during flare-ups. The mean follow-up duration was 10.1 months for females and 23.2 months for males. An 8-year experience involving intralesional triamcinolone injections effectively treated inflammatory HS and reduced the use of systemic antibiotics.

Second-Line Therapies	
• Metformin	C
• Acitretin	C
• Quinolone with rifampin and metronidazole	C
• Spironolactone	C
• 1064 nm (for prevention rather than treatment of lesions) surgery	B
• CO_2 laser	B

Metformin for the treatment of hidradenitis suppurativa: a little help along the way. Verdolini R, Clayton N, Smith A, Alwash N, Mannello B. J Eur Acad Dermatol Venereol 2013; 27: 1101–8.

Open case series describing benefits of monotherapy using metformin.

Acitretin treatment for hidradenitis suppurativa: a prospective series of 17 patients. Matusiak L, Bieniek A, Szepietowski JC. Br J Dermatol 2014; 171: 170–4.

Eight of 17 patients (47%) experienced benefit; relapses occurred 2 to 8 months after stopping therapy.

A study on the management of hidradenitis suppurativa with retinoids and surgical excision. Puri N, Talwar A. Indian J Dermatol 2011; 56: 650–1.

The relapse rate after surgery was reduced from 40% to 20% by subsequent treatment with acitretin.

Efficacy of rifampin-moxifloxacin-metronidazole combination therapy in hidradenitis suppurativa. Join-Lambert O, Coignard H, Jais JP, Guet-Revillet H, Poirée S, Fraitag S, et al. Dermatology 2011; 222: 49–58.

Twenty-eight consecutive HS patients, including 6, 10, and 12 Hurley stage I, II, and III patients, respectively. Complete remission, defined as a clearance of all inflammatory lesions, including hypertrophic scars, was obtained in 16 patients, including 6/6, 8/10, and 2/12 patients with Hurley stage I, II, and III, after up to 12 months of treatment.

A case series of 20 women with hidradenitis suppurativa treated with spironolactone. Lee A, Fischer G. Australas J Dermatol 2015; 56: 192–6.

A total of 17 out of 20 (85%) responded to spironolactone who had failed other therapies at a 3-month follow-up from initial presentation.

Prospective controlled clinical and histopathologic study of hidradenitis suppurativa treated with the long-pulsed neodymium:yttrium-aluminium-garnet laser. Mahmoud BH, Tierney E, Hexsel CL, Pui J, Ozog DM, Hamzavi IH. J Am Acad Dermatol 2010; 62: 637–45.

In patients with milder disease treated with topical benzoyl peroxide and clindamycin, weekly treatment with long-pulsed neodymium:yttrium-aluminum-garnet laser for 4 months was significantly more effective than the aforementioned topical treatment alone.

Surgical treatment of chronic hidradenitis suppurativa: CO$_2$ laser stripping-secondary intention technique. Lapins J, Marcusson JA, Emtestam L. Br J Dermatol 1994; 131: 551–6.

CO$_2$ evaporation of diseased tissue under visual control, followed by secondary healing.

Third-Line Therapies	
• TNF-alpha monoclonal antibodies	A
• Immunosuppressants	D

Adalimumab for the treatment of moderate to severe hidradenitis suppurativa: a parallel randomized trial. Kimball AB, Kerdel F, Adams D, Mrowietz U, Gelfand JM, Gniadecki R, et al. Ann Intern Med 2012; 157: 846–55.

Significant effect of adalimumab 40 mg every week was noted during 12 weeks of treatment.

Efficacy and safety of adalimumab in patients with moderate to severe hidradenitis suppurativa: results from PIONEER II, a phase 3, randomized, placebo-controlled trial. Jemec G, Gottlieb A, Forman S, et al. J American Acad Dermatol 2015; 72 (Suppl 1): AB45.

The FDA approved dose adalimumab dosage in HS dosed at week 0: 160 mg, week 2: 80 mg, and from week 4: 40 mg every week, there after for 12 weeks effectively treated hidradenitis..

Two Phase 3 Trials of Adalimumab for Hidradenitis Suppurativa. Kimball AB, Okun MM, Williams DA, Gottlieb AB, Papp KA, Zouboulis CC, et al. N Engl J Med 2016; 375: 422–34.

In 2 phase 3 studies entitled PIONEER, 307 patients were enrolled in PIONEER I and 326 were enrolled in PIONEER II. Clinical response rates at week 12 were significantly higher for the groups receiving adalimumab 40 mg weekly than for the placebo groups: 41.8% versus 26.0% in PIONEER I (p=0.003) and 58.95 versus 27.6% in PIONEER II (P<0.001). Patients receiving adalimumab had significantly greater improvement than the placebo groups in rank-ordered secondary outcomes (lesions, pain, and the modified Sartorius score for disease severity) at week 12 in PIONEER II only. In PIONEER I, patients receiving oral antibiotic agents for hidradenitis suppurativa were required to stop treatment for at least 28 days before baseline; in PIONEER II, patients were allowed to continue treatment with antibiotics (tetracycline class) in stable doses.

Infliximab therapy for patients with moderate to severe hidradenitis suppurativa: a randomized, double-blind, placebo-controlled crossover trial. Grant A, Gonzalez T, Montgomery MO, Cardenas V, Kerdel FA. J Am Acad Dermatol 2010; 62: 205–17.

A randomized controlled trial indicating the effect of infliximab in post hoc analysis.

Safety and efficacy of anakinra in severe hidradenitis suppurativa: a randomized clinical trial. Tzanetakou V, Kanni T, Giatrakou S, Katoulis A, Papadavid E, Netea MG, et al. JAMA Dermatol 2016; 152: 52–9.

Seven out of nine (78%) achieved clinical response in the actively treated group (100 mg daily).

Dapsone therapy for hidradenitis suppurativa: a series of 24 patients. Yazdanyar S, Boer J, Ingvarsson G, Szepietowski JC, Jemec GB. Dermatology 2011; 222: 342–6.

Nine of 24 patients (38%) experienced benefits from therapy with dapsone.

Ciclosporin treatment of severe hidradenitis suppurativa – a case series. Anderson MD, Zauli S, Bettoli V, Boer J, Jemec GB. J Dermatolog Treat 2016; 27: 247–50.

Nine of 18 previously extensively treated patients (50%) experienced benefits from therapy with ciclosporin.

Evidence Levels: **A** Double-blind study **B** Clinical trial ≥ 20 subjects **C** Clinical trial < 20 subjects **D** Series ≥ 5 subjects **E** Anecdotal case reports

107

Histoplasmosis

Mahreen Ameen, Wanda Sonia Robles

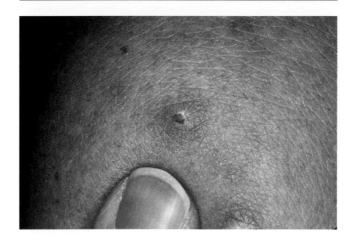

Histoplasmosis is an endemic mycosis caused by a dimorphic fungus, *Histoplasma capsulatum*, of which there are two varieties that are pathogenic to humans. The most common variety worldwide is *H. capsulatum var. capsulatum*, which is highly endemic in the United States, particularly in the Mississippi and Ohio valleys. *H. capsulatum var. duboisii* is endemic only in Central and West Africa (where it coexists with *H. capsulatum var. capsulatum*), and it is therefore sometimes referred to as *African histoplasmosis*. The infection is usually contracted through inhalation of spores in dry soil or bird or bat droppings. Disease progression and severity depend on the intensity of exposure to *H. capsulatum* and host immunity. There is a wide clinical spectrum of disease. Acute pulmonary disease is the most common presentation, and most cases are either asymptomatic or mild and self-limiting. Chronic pulmonary histoplasmosis, usually occurring in patients with underlying lung disease, produces cavities and later progression to pulmonary fibrosis. Hematogenous dissemination occurs within the first few weeks but resolves with the development of cell-mediated immunity to *H. capsulatum*. Progressive disseminated histoplasmosis occurs in the immunocompromised. Patient groups at risk include those with AIDS or hematologic malignancies, those on immunosuppressive therapy (including corticosteroids and tumor necrosis factor [TNF] antagonists), transplant recipients, and infants. Disseminated histoplasmosis is an AIDS-defining illness. It is usually a reactivation of prior infection and a sign of advanced immunosuppression, generally occurring in those with CD4 counts <150 cells/mm³.

Disseminated histoplasmosis can involve every organ system, most commonly presenting with hepatosplenomegaly and mucocutaneous lesions. Molluscum-like papules, nodules, or ulcerative lesions affect the skin and are usually localized to the face, upper chest, and arms. Oropharyngeal ulcers affect the buccal mucosa, tongue, gingiva, lips, pharynx, and larynx. Histoplasmosis may also present to the dermatologist as a cause of erythema multiforme or erythema nodosum, which are thought to be a hypersensitivity response to the *H. capsulatum* antigen. Rarely, primary cutaneous lesions may arise from direct inoculation.

MANAGEMENT STRATEGY

Pulmonary forms of histoplasmosis in the acute phase usually resolve spontaneously and only require treatment if symptoms persist for more than 1 month. Oral itraconazole is the treatment of choice for mild to moderate histoplasmosis. Severe pulmonary infection, disseminated histoplasmosis, and infection in the immunocompromised, particularly in association with AIDS, should be treated with amphotericin B (AmB) formulations (AmB deoxycholate, liposomal AmB, or AmB lipid complex). The lipid formulations carry a lower risk of nephrotoxicity but are more expensive. Treatment is commenced with AmB until there is clinical improvement and then stepped down to oral itraconazole. Fluconazole and ketoconazole are second-line alternatives to itraconazole. Ketoconazole carries higher risks of adverse effects than do the other azoles. The new triazoles, voriconazole and posaconazole, demonstrate in vitro activity against *H. capsulatum* and have been successfully used in individual cases for different forms of histoplasmosis infection.

Patients with AIDS-related histoplasmosis who undergo antiretroviral treatment have better outcomes than do those who are not treated with antiretrovirals. Some clinicians defer commencement of antiretroviral therapy until there is a reduction in fungal burden to avoid precipitating immune reconstitution inflammatory syndrome (IRIS). However, IRIS is a rare complication of histoplasmosis and is not usually severe. Therefore others advocate early antiretroviral therapy to improve cellular immunity, a key defense against *H. capsulatum*.

Specific Investigations

- Culture
- Histology
- Serology
- Serology for HIV (where relevant)
- Imaging studies to detect disseminated disease (chest x-ray/computed tomography/magnetic resonance imaging)

The gold-standard method for diagnosing histoplasmosis is the isolation of *H. capsulatum* from culture. The use of several specimens (sputum, bronchoalveolar lavage, skin lesions, blood, bone marrow, or liver) for culture will increase the yield. Culture is highly specific but is limited by slow growth, and plates must be kept for as long as 12 weeks. Blood culture using the lysis-centrifugation system is more rapid and increases sensitivity. Histopathology is also more rapid, but its sensitivity is <50% in patients with disseminated disease and even lower in pulmonary histoplasmosis. Biopsy specimens may demonstrate the distinctive 2- to 4-μm oval, narrow-based budding yeasts of *H. capsulatum*. Serologic tests are rapid but may be falsely negative in immunosuppressed patients and during the first 2 months after exposure while antibodies are still developing. In addition, elevated antibody titers persist for several years after initial infection. Antigen detection is a rapid means of diagnosis and can be useful in individuals who are immunocompromised when antibody production may be impaired. Sensitivity is greater with urine and plasma compared with other body fluids. Antigen quantitation enables treatment response to be monitored.

In disseminated disease, general laboratory tests will reveal a pancytopenia, hyperbilirubinemia, elevated liver enzyme, and serum lactate dehydrogenase levels.

Histoplasmosis: up-to-date evidence-based approach to diagnosis and management. Hage CA, Azar MM, Bahr N, Loyd J, Wheat LJ. Semin Respir Crit Care Med 2015; 36(5): 729–45.

This is a comprehensive and up-to-date review. Liposomal amphotericin B is recommended for more severe cases and itraconazole for milder cases and "step-down" therapy after response to amphotericin B.

Histoplasmosis complicating tumor necrosis factor-α blocker therapy: a retrospective analysis of 98 cases. Vergidis P, Avery RK, Wheat LJ, Dotson JL, Assi MA, Antoun SA, et al. Clin Infect Dis 2015; 61(3): 409–17.

Disseminated histoplasmosis is a potential complication of anti-TNF-α therapy. This is a multicenter retrospective review of 98 patients diagnosed with histoplasmosis between 2000 and 2011. The most commonly used biologic agent was infliximab (67.3%). Based on these data the authors recommend that antifungal therapy be administered for at least 12 months. Thereafter resumption of TNF-α blocker therapy appears safe. They also conclude that disease outcomes were generally favorable.

Histoplasmosis in HIV-infected patients: a review of new developments and remaining gaps. Adenis AA, Aznar C, Couppié P. Curr Trop Med Rep 2014; 1: 119–28.

This review outlines the impact of HIV on the prevalence and clinical manifestations of histoplasmosis. It assesses the data on clinical trials of drug therapy for histoplasmosis in HIV-infected individuals and discusses the relative merits of amphotericin and itraconazole and their limitations in terms of drug interactions in HIV-infected individuals.

First Line Therapies	
• Amphotericin B	**B**
• Itraconazole	**B**

Disseminated histoplasmosis in patients with AIDS in Panama: a review of 104 cases. Gutierrez ME, Canton A, Sosa N, Puga E, Talavera L. Clin Infect Dis 2005; 40(8): 1199–202.

In this study from Panama, the authors report that before the spread of AIDS, disseminated histoplasmosis was rarely seen. Now it is often the first manifestation of AIDS in this region and must be suspected in anyone with fever, respiratory symptoms, weight loss, diarrhea, and a CD4 cell count <100 cells/μL. One hundred of 104 (96%) patients with AIDS-related disseminated histoplasmosis received amphotericin B deoxycholate induction therapy, most receiving 1 g in total before being switched over to oral itraconazole. Forty patients had therapy-related adverse effects with hypokalemia reported in 50% and an increased creatinine level in 43%.

Itraconazole therapy for blastomycosis and histoplasmosis. NIAID Mycoses Study Group. Dismukes WE, Bradsher RW Jr, Cloud GC, Kauffman CA, Chapman SW, George RB, et al. Am J Med 1992; 93(5): 489–97.

This was a prospective, nonrandomized, multicenter open trial where 37 patients with histoplasmosis received itraconazole 200 to 400 mg daily. Eighty-one percent (n = 30) were cured after a median treatment period of 9 months. Treatment failure occurred only in those patients with chronic cavitary pulmonary disease. Twenty-nine percent (n = 25) experienced minor adverse effects, requiring therapy withdrawal in only one patient.

Itraconazole treatment of disseminated histoplasmosis in patients with the acquired immunodeficiency syndrome. AIDS Clinical Trial Group. Wheat J, Hafner R, Korzun AH, Limjoco MT, Spencer P, Larsen RA, et al. Am J Med 1995; 98: 336–42.

A multicenter, nonrandomized prospective trial. Itraconazole 300 mg twice daily for 3 days followed by 200 mg twice daily was given for 12 weeks. Evaluation of 59 patients showed that 50 (85%) responded well to therapy. Five withdrew from the study because of progressive infection. One died within the first week of therapy, and two withdrew because of itraconazole-related adverse effects. Resolution of systemic symptoms occurred after a median of 3 weeks in the less severely affected, and 6 weeks in the moderately severe cases. Fungemia cleared after a median period of 1 week.

Itraconazole demonstrates efficacy in the treatment of mild disseminated histoplasmosis in patients with AIDS. For patients with moderately severe or severe histoplasmosis, amphotericin B is the drug of first choice, which can be switched to itraconazole after clinical improvement.

Safety and efficacy of liposomal amphotericin B compared with conventional amphotericin B for induction therapy of histoplasmosis in patients with AIDS. Johnson PC, Wheat LJ, Cloud GA, Goldman M, Lancaster D, Bamberger DM, et al. US National Institute of Allergy and Infectious Diseases Mycoses Study Group. Ann Intern Med 2002; 137: 105–9.

A multicenter, randomized, controlled trial compared amphotericin B deoxycholate with liposomal amphotericin B for induction therapy of moderate to severe disseminated histoplasmosis in patients with AIDS. The trial demonstrated a higher response rate (88% vs. 64%) and lower mortality rate (2% vs. 13%) in patients who were treated with liposomal amphotericin (n = 51) than in those treated with amphotericin B deoxycholate (n = 22). Infusion-related side effects were greater with amphotericin B deoxycholate (63%) than with liposomal amphotericin B (25%) ($p = 0.002$). Nephrotoxicity was also higher with amphotericin B deoxycholate (37%) than with liposomal amphotericin B (9%) ($p = 0.003$).

This study demonstrated that liposomal amphotericin is associated with higher efficacy, lower mortality, and better tolerance during induction treatment of disseminated histoplasmosis.

Safety of discontinuation of maintenance therapy for disseminated histoplasmosis after immunologic response to antiretroviral therapy. Goldman M, Zackin R, Fichtenbaum CJ, Skiest DJ, Koletar SL, Hafner R, et al. AIDS Clinical Trials Group A5038 Study Group. Clin Infect Dis 2004; 38: 1485–89.

Traditionally, lifelong maintenance therapy with itraconazole had been the standard of care in order to reduce the risk of relapse of histoplasmosis infection. This was a prospective observational study to assess the safety of stopping maintenance therapy for disseminated histoplasmosis in patients with HIV infection after treatment with antiretroviral therapy. The study concluded that discontinuation of antifungal therapy after 12 months appears to be safe in patients with previously treated disseminated histoplasmosis that have sustained immunologic improvement with antiretroviral therapy.

Disseminated histoplasmosis: a comparative study between patients with acquired immunodeficiency syndrome and non-human immunodeficiency virus-infected individuals. Tobon AM, Agudelo CA, Rosero DS, Ochoa JE, De Bedout C, Zuluaga A, et al. Am J Trop Med Hyg 2005; 73(3): 576–82.

In this study of 52 patients with disseminated histoplasmosis, 30 patients had AIDS. Skin lesions were significantly higher in patients with AIDS, occurring in 53% of them ($p = 0.001$).

348

H. capsulatum was isolated more often in AIDS patients (*p* < 0.05), but antibodies to *H. capsulatum* were detected more frequently in non-HIV patients (*p* < 0.05). Itraconazole treatment was less effective in AIDS patients (*p* = 0.012), but in this group, too, highly active antiretroviral therapy (HAART) improved the response to antifungals compared with individuals who were not given HAART (*p* = 0.003), who exhibited higher mortality rates (*p* = 0.025). These results indicate the need to promote restoration of the immune system in patients with AIDS and histoplasmosis.

The authors highlight that the skin constitutes a more important target organ for H. capsulatum *in HIV-infected Latin American patients than in HIV-infected North American patients.*

Literature review and case histories of *Histoplasma capsulatum var. duboisii* infections in HIV-infected patients. Loulergue P, Bastides F, Baudouin V, Chandenier J, Mariani-Kurkdjian P, Dupont B, et al. Emerg Infect Dis 2007; 13(11): 1647–52.

African histoplasmosis caused by *H. capsulatum var. duboisii* is much rarer than histoplasmosis caused by variety *capsulatum*, and its association with HIV infection is rarely reported. This article reports three such cases and reviews the literature on similar cases. All cases were successfully treated initially with amphotericin B, which was subsequently switched to itraconazole. No clinical trials or efficacy studies have been performed for African histoplasmosis, and therefore its treatment is usually extrapolated from the guidelines of the Infectious Diseases Society of America established for histoplasmosis due to variety *capsulatum*.

Disseminated primary cutaneous histoplasmosis successfully treated with itraconazole. Singhi MK, Gupta L, Kacchawa D, Gupta D. Indian J Dermatol Venereol Leprol 2003; 69(6): 405–7.

Primary cutaneous histoplasmosis is rare. This is a report of a case of disseminated primary cutaneous histoplasmosis caused by *H. capsulatum* in an immunocompetent patient. The patient presented with a 2-year history of progressive erythematous nodules and plaques distributed mainly over the trunk. There was no evidence of systemic involvement. There was an excellent response to itraconazole 100 mg BID. Lesions began improving within 4 weeks and cleared within 16 weeks, and the total treatment period was 24 weeks. There was no recurrence 6 months after cessation of treatment.

Second-Line Therapies	
• Ketoconazole	B
• Fluconazole	B
• Posaconazole	D
• Voriconazole	D

Treatment of blastomycosis and histoplasmosis with ketoconazole. Results of a prospective randomized clinical trial. Dismukes WE, Cloud G, Bowles C, National Institute of Allergy and Infectious Diseases Mycoses Study Group. Ann Intern Med 1985; 103(6 Pt 1): 861–72.

This was a multicenter, prospective, randomized trial evaluating the efficacy and toxicity of low-dose (400 mg/d) and high-dose (800 mg/d) oral ketoconazole in the treatment of histoplasmosis. Among 19 patients with chronic cavitary histoplasmosis treated for 6 months or more, both regimens were equally effective (overall success rate, 84%). In 20 patients with localized or disseminated histoplasmosis treated for 6 months or more, low-dose

treatment was more effective (100% vs. 57% success rate, *p* = 0.03). The success rate for all patients with histoplasmosis treated for 6 months or more was 85%. Adverse effects occurred in 60% of patients and were more common with the high-dose regimen. Ketoconazole is effective for non–life-threatening histoplasmosis in immunocompetent patients. Because of the higher frequency of side effects associated with the high dose, the authors suggested that ketoconazole therapy should be initiated at the lower dose.

With the availability of better-tolerated and new-generation azoles, there are no recent studies evaluating ketoconazole therapy for histoplasmosis. However, it is still a drug that is commonly used in endemic settings because of its availability and low cost.

Fluconazole therapy for histoplasmosis. The National Institute of Allergy and Infectious Diseases Mycoses Study Group. McKinsey DS, Kauffman CA, Pappas PG, Cloud GA, Girard WM, Sharkey PK, et al. Clin Infect Dis 1996; 23(5): 996–1001.

Twenty-seven patients were enrolled in this trial. Two had acute pulmonary histoplasmosis, 11 had chronic pulmonary histoplasmosis, and 14 had disseminated histoplasmosis. Twenty patients received fluconazole 400 to 800 mg/day, and seven patients received fluconazole 200 mg daily. Successful treatment was reported in 17 patients (63%). There were no significant adverse effects. The authors concluded that fluconazole was only moderately effective and should be reserved for patients intolerant to itraconazole.

Treatment of histoplasmosis with fluconazole in patients with acquired immunodeficiency syndrome. National Institute of Allergy and Infectious Diseases, Acquired Immunodeficiency Syndrome Clinical Trials Group and Mycoses Study Group. Wheat J, MaWhinney S, Hafner R, McKinsey D, Chen D, Korzun A, et al. Am J Med 1997; 103: 223–32.

This was a multicenter, open-label, nonrandomized, prospective trial. The aim of the study was to assess the efficacy and safety of fluconazole in patients with AIDS and mild to moderate disseminated histoplasmosis. The initial protocol of fluconazole 1200 mg on day 1 followed by 600 mg daily for 8 weeks demonstrated a high failure rate of 50%. The therapy schedule was revised to 1600 mg on day 1 followed by 800 mg daily for 12 weeks, and then maintenance therapy with 400 mg daily for at least 1 year. Seven patients failed to respond to induction therapy, with progression of histoplasmosis leading to death in one patient. Two withdrew due to liver toxicity. Seventy-three percent (36/49 patients) responded, but 30.5% (11/36) subsequently relapsed, and one died. On the basis of historical comparison, maintenance therapy to prevent relapse with fluconazole 400 mg daily was less effective than itraconazole 200 to 400 mg daily or amphotericin B 50 mg weekly.

Fluconazole may have a role in the treatment of non–AIDS-related histoplasmosis. However, this study of AIDS-related infection demonstrated a comparatively poor efficacy rate with even high-dose fluconazole induction therapy and an unacceptably high relapse rate with maintenance therapy.

Salvage treatment of histoplasmosis with posaconazole. Restrepo A, Tobón A, Clark B, Graham DR, Corcoran G, Bradsher RW, et al. J Infect 2007; 54(4): 319–27.

Six patients with severe histoplasmosis infection were successfully treated with oral posaconazole (800 mg/day in divided doses) having previously failed on amphotericin B, itraconazole, fluconazole, or voriconazole. One patient had pulmonary disease and the rest had disseminated infection. Treatment duration ranged from 6 to 34 weeks. Significant clinical improvement was noted within the first month of treatment.

Although the patient numbers are small, this study suggests that posaconazole may be a useful treatment option for disseminated histoplasmosis refractory to other drug therapies.

Voriconazole use for endemic fungal infections. Freifeld A, Proia L, Andes D, Baddour LM, Blair J, Spellberg B, et al. Antimicrob Agents Chemother 2009; 53(4): 1648–51.

Nine patients with mostly disseminated histoplasmosis who had either failed or were intolerant of amphotericin B and itraconazole were treated with voriconazole. All of them improved or remained clinically stable after treatment, and responses were apparent within the first 2 months of voriconazole initiation. However, two of the patients whose response was "stable" had to discontinue treatment because of high costs. The others received treatment from 31 to 640 days.

Clinical practice guidelines for the management of patients with histoplasmosis: 2007 update by the Infectious Diseases Society of America. Wheat LJ, Freifeld AG, Kleiman MB, Baddley JW, McKinsey DS, Loyd JE, et al; Infectious Diseases Society of America. Clin Infect Dis 2007; 45(7): 807–25.

Evidence-based guidelines for the management of patients with histoplasmosis.

Mild Acute Pulmonary Histoplasmosis

Treatment is usually unnecessary unless symptoms persist for more than 1 month, when itraconazole is given at a loading dose (200 mg three times daily for 3 days) followed by 200 mg once or twice daily for 6 to 12 weeks.

Severe Acute Pulmonary Histoplasmosis

Parenteral amphotericin B (deoxycholate formulation, 0.7–10 mg/kg daily, or lipid formulation, 3–5 mg/kg daily) for 1 to 2 weeks followed by "step-down" itraconazole therapy, with an initial loading dose and then 200 mg twice daily for a total of 12 weeks.

Chronic Cavitary Pulmonary Histoplasmosis

Itraconazole, initial loading dose, and then 200 mg once or twice daily for at least 12 months.

Mild Disseminated Histoplasmosis

Itraconazole, initial loading dose, and then 200 mg twice daily for at least 12 months.

Severe Disseminated Histoplasmosis

Amphotericin B (doses as earlier for severe pulmonary infection) for 1 to 2 weeks followed by oral itraconazole, initial loading dose, and then 200 mg twice daily for at least 12 months.

Central Nervous System Histoplasmosis

Liposomal amphotericin B (5 mg/kg daily for a total of 175 mg/kg given over 4–6 weeks) followed by itraconazole 200 mg two or three times daily for at least 1 year and until resolution of cerebrospinal fluid (CSF) abnormalities, including *Histoplasma* antigen levels.

Treatment of Histoplasmosis in Pregnancy

Azoles are teratogenic, and therefore amphotericin B is recommended.

Immunosuppressed patients may require lifelong suppressive therapy with itraconazole (200 mg daily) if immunosuppression cannot be reversed. For those on long-term itraconazole therapy, blood itraconazole levels need to be measured 2 weeks after initiation of treatment. Women of childbearing age who are being treated with azoles need to use effective contraception during treatment and for 2 months after the drug is stopped.

An official American Thoracic Society statement: treatment of fungal infections in adult pulmonary and critical care patients. Limper AH, Knox KS, Sarosi GA, Ampel NM, Bennett JE, Catanzaro A, et al. American Thoracic Society Fungal Working Group. Am J Respir Crit Care Med 2011; 183(1): 96–128.

The American Thoracic Society convened a working group of experts in fungal infections to develop a concise clinical statement of current therapeutic options. The document discusses drug therapy for the different manifestations of histoplasmosis, including asymptomatic as well as symptomatic lung disease in immunocompetent hosts and disease in immunocompromised hosts.

Evidence Levels: **A** Double-blind study   **B** Clinical trial ≥ 20 subjects   **C** Clinical trial < 20 subjects   **D** Series ≥ 5 subjects   **E** Anecdotal case reports

108

Hydroa vacciniforme

Herbert Hönigsmann

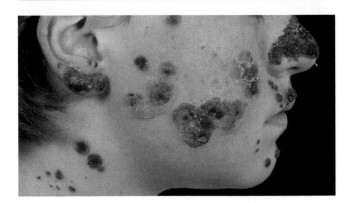

Hydroa vacciniforme (HV) is a very rare, idiopathic photodermatosis that mainly starts in childhood, frequently resolving by adolescence or young adulthood. Its prevalence is 0.1 to 0.5 cases per 100,000 per year. It is characterized by recurrent crops of papulovesicles or vesicles, most commonly on the face and the dorsa of the hands, but other sun-exposed areas of the skin, such as the lower lips, may also be involved. The vesicles resolve with pock-like scarring. The disease was first described by Bazin in 1862, and it is possible that before the clear definition of erythropoietic protoporphyria by Magnus et al. in 1961, some cases may have been protoporphyria rather than hydroa because of the similarity of symptoms. There are now many reports of an association with Epstein–Barr virus (EBV) infection originally from Japan and China, but not all these cases are typical: they are associated with natural killer (NK)/T-cell lymphoproliferative disorders with a frequently fatal outcome. More recently such cases were also reported from other areas in the world. These lesions are now classified as hydroa vacciniforme–like lymphomas.

MANAGEMENT STRATEGY

HV usually presents in childhood, sometimes with spontaneous improvement during adolescence. Parents generally seek specialist advice because their children are unable to tolerate sunshine (play outdoors or travel abroad) and because the eruption can result in considerable scarring, both of which cause significant morbidity.

HV is almost always refractory to any treatment, but *restriction of sun exposure, appropriate clothing, and regular use of broad-spectrum sunscreens with an effective UVA filter* can help in mild to moderate disease. Windows in the car and home can be covered with films that filter UV wavelengths less than 380 nm.

In patients with more severe disease, however, courses of *narrow-band UVB phototherapy* or *psoralen with UVA (PUVA)* administered as for polymorphic light eruption may help occasionally. Both phototherapy regimens usually consist of thrice-weekly treatments for an average of 3 to 4 weeks. It is important to administer these therapies carefully to avoid provoking disease exacerbations.

Antimicrobial therapy has also been tried, as have antimalarials and systemic immunosuppressive therapy, including intermittent oral corticosteroids, but although occasionally helpful, none of these appear to be reliably effective. β-Carotene, used in several studies, has mostly been ineffective.

For severe and refractory HV unresponsive to other therapies, immunosuppressive agents including *azathioprine* and *cyclosporine* may be effective, but *thalidomide* only exceptionally is. However, the use of immunosuppressive drugs for an admittedly unpleasant, but otherwise benign, disease should be carefully considered.

In four reports, *dietary fish oil* rich in omega-3 polyunsaturated fatty acids was associated with clinical improvement in three of four patients. The mechanism may be through inhibition of prostanoid production and by their proposed buffering effect against free radical–induced damage.

The rare nature of this condition means that there are no large or randomized trials. Evidence for treatment is based on case series or single reports.

Specific Investigations

- Erythrocyte and plasma protoporphyrin levels, red cell photohemolysis, and stool analysis
- Photoprovocation testing with UVA
- Serology for antinuclear antibody and extractable nuclear antigens
- Screening for EBV infection and detection of EBV-infected cells by T-cell receptor-γ gene rearrangement with polymerase chain reaction
- A porphyrin screen will exclude erythropoietic protoporphyria

Photoprovocation testing induces typical blisters. Light tests are abnormal in the UVA range. Photographs to the right of the figure show the result of photoprovocation with UVA (three times 30 J/cm^2 on 3 consecutive days): (A) after 24 hours; (B) after 48 hours; and (C) after 2 weeks.

Serology for antinuclear antibody and extractable nuclear antigens (anti-Ro, La, and Sm) will exclude bullous lupus erythematosus, which quite commonly can be ruled out by its clinical symptoms.

Rare cases have been associated with metabolic disorders, such as Hartnup disease, and so aminoaciduria should be ruled out.

Screening for EBV should be done in view of the increasing number of reports of the possible association.

Hydroa vacciniforme – aktionsspektrum. Jaschke E, Hönigsmann H. Hautarzt 1981; 32: 350–3.

Successful photoprovocation with UVA in one case.

Hydroa vacciniforme: a review of ten cases. Sonnex TS, Hawk JLM. Br J Dermatol 1988; 118: 101–8.

Successful photoprovocation with UVA in several cases.

Hydroa vacciniforme: a clinical and follow-up study of 17 cases. Gupta G, Man I, Kemmett D. J Am Acad Dermatol 2000; 42: 208–13.

Eight of 14 patients were sensitive in the UVA spectrum. UVA provocation tests showed a papulovesicular response in 6 of 14 patients.

There is now strong evidence that UVA radiation is the causal factor. In addition to reduced UVA minimal erythema dose values, repetitive broad-spectrum UVA has been shown to reproduce lesions that are clinically and histologically identical to those produced by natural sunlight and that heal with scarring. All cases seen so far by this author (H.H.) had their action spectrum in the UVA range.

Pathogenic link between hydroa vacciniforme and Epstein–Barr virus-associated hematologic disorders. Iwatsuki K, Satoh M, Yamamoto T, Oono T, Morizane S, Ohtsuka M, et al. Arch Dermatol 2006; 142: 587–95.

T cells positive for EBV-encoded small nuclear RNA (EBER) were detected to various degrees in cutaneous infiltrates in 28 (97%) of 29 patients, including all 6 patients with definite HV having a positive phototest reaction.

Hydroa vacciniforme is associated with increased numbers of Epstein-Barr virus-infected γδT cells. Hirai Y, Yamamoto T, Kimura H, Ito Y, Tsuji K, Miyake T, et al. J Invest Dermatol 2012; 132: 1401–8.

The observations indicate that cutaneous lesions of both typical and severe HV are induced by EBER+ T cells, associated with a larger number of EBER–cytotoxic T lymphocytes, without apparent involvement of NK cell infiltration.

Epstein-Barr virus involvement in the pathogenesis of hydroa vacciniforme: an assessment of seven adult patients with long-term follow-up. Verneuil L, Gouarin S, Comoz F, Agbalika F, Creveuil C, Varna M, et al. Br J Dermatol 2010; 163: 174–82.

EBV was involved in HV pathogenesis and persisted in adult patients with HV. A positive EBV DNA load, specific to HV in the spectrum of photosensitive disorders, might be a useful biomarker in HV.

Hydroa vacciniforme: a rare photodermatosis. Haddad JM, Monroe HR, Hardin J, Diwan AH, Hsu S. Dermatol Online J 2014: 20: pii: 13030/qt7961b22b.

The case of a 9-year-old girl with EBV-associated HV is presented. The discussion offers a good summary of the current diagnosis and management of HV.

First-Line Therapy

• High-factor broad-spectrum sunscreens and behavioral sunlight avoidance	C

Hydroa vacciniforme: a clinical and follow-up study of 17 cases. Gupta G, Man I, Kemmett D. J Am Acad Dermatol 2000; 42: 208–13.

Disease in 9 of 15 patients was controlled satisfactorily with high-factor broad-spectrum sunscreens and sunlight avoidance.

Hydroa vacciniforme: a review of ten cases. Sonnex TS, Hawk JLM. Br J Dermatol 1988; 118: 101–8.

Disease severity was reduced in 8 of 10 patients using either Coppertone Supershade 15 or RoC factor 10.

These sunscreens do not meet the standards as required nowadays. Modern sunscreens now must offer broad-spectrum protection against both UVB and UVA.

Borrowing from museums and industry: two photo-protective devices. Dawe R, Russell S, Ferguson J. Br J Dermatol 1996; 135: 1016–7.

The Museum 200 Film (manufactured by Sun Guard, Florida, USA) prevents transmission of all wavelengths less than 380 nm.

This is a clear, lightweight film that can be stuck on to any glass surface without causing visual impairment. It may be a useful adjunct in the treatment of most photodermatoses, but in some patients with HV, particularly those who are sensitive in the 380- to 400-nm wavelengths, it may not be beneficial.

Second-Line Therapies

• Narrowband UVB phototherapy (TL-01)	C
• PUVA	D
• Acyclovir/valacyclovir	D

Narrow-band UVB (TL-01) phototherapy: an effective preventative treatment for the photodermatoses. Collins P, Ferguson J. Br J Dermatol 1995; 132: 956–63.

This was an open clinical trial in which four patients were treated on average 10 times on a daily basis. Two of these patients reported an increase in tolerance to sunshine from 1 hour to 3 to 6 hours.

Hydroa vacciniforme: a clinical and follow-up study of 17 cases. Gupta G, Man I, Kemmett D. J Am Acad Dermatol 2000; 42: 208–13.

Five of 15 patients who had not responded to conservative measures were treated with narrowband UVB phototherapy. In three patients there was good or moderate disease control. In the other two, narrowband UVB phototherapy was not helpful.

Narrowband ultraviolet B (UVB) phototherapy in children. Jury CS, McHenry P, Burden AD, Lever R, Bilsland D. Clin Exp Dermatol 2006; 31: 196–9.

Narrowband UVB phototherapy is a useful and well-tolerated treatment for children with severe or intractable inflammatory skin disease.

Hydroa vacciniforme: a review of ten cases. Sonnex TS, Hawk JLM. Br J Dermatol 1988; 118: 101–8.

Two of 10 patients were treated with UVB and had improvement of their disease. There was a flare of the one patient treated with PUVA.

It is likely that broadband UVB was used in this report, but the methodology is unclear.

Hydroa vacciniforme – aktionsspektrum. Jaschke E, Hönigsmann H. Hautarzt 1981; 32: 350–3.

One patient received PUVA therapy and had good control of his disease.

Photosensitivity disorders: cause, effect and management. Millard TP, Hawk JL. Am J Clin Dermatol 2002; 3: 239–46.

A review of the management of various photodermatoses, with reference to the use of UVB and PUVA.

Antiviral therapy in children with hydroa vacciniforme. Lysell J, Wiegleb Edström D, Linde A, Carlsson G, Malmros-Svennilson J, Westermark A, et al. Acta Derm Venereol 2009; 89: 393–7.

Successful treatment in four children. Acyclovir/valacyclovir therapy is a safe treatment and should be tried. However, further studies are required to confirm these results.

Antiviral treatment of a boy with EBV-associated hydroa vacciniforme. Pahlow Mose A, Eisker N, Clemmensen O, Bygum A. BMJ Case Rep 2014; 2014: pii: bcr2014206488.

Marked improvement of EBV-associated HV in a young boy treated initially with acyclovir, followed by valacyclovir. The authors raise the intriguing question if antiviral therapy in patients

Evidence Levels: **A** Double-blind study   **B** Clinical trial ≥ 20 subjects   **C** Clinical trial < 20 subjects   **D** Series ≥ 5 subjects   **E** Anecdotal case reports

with EBV-associated HV could decrease the risk of lymphoproliferative disease in these patients.

Third-Line Therapies	
• Antimalarials	D
• β-Carotene	E
• Azathioprine	E
• Cyclosporine	E
• Dietary fish oil	E
• Thalidomide	E

Hydroa vacciniforme: a review of ten cases. Sonnex TS, Hawk JLM. Br J Dermatol 1988; 118: 101–8.

Four of 10 patients were treated with either hydroxychloroquine (2 patients) or chloroquine (2 patients). Hydroxychloroquine 100 mg daily was ineffective, but the two patients on chloroquine (100–125 mg daily) had a reduction in the severity of their disease.

Hydroa vacciniforme: an unusual clinical manifestation. Leenutaphong V. J Am Acad Dermatol 1991; 25: 892–5.

One patient treated with chloroquine phosphate 500 mg daily did not find it beneficial.

Hydroa vacciniforme. Ketterer R, Morier P, Frenk E. Dermatology 1994; 189: 428–9.

One patient treated with chloroquine 100 mg daily and broad-spectrum sunscreens showed good disease control.

It is unclear whether the response was due to chloroquine or the sunscreen.

Hydroa vacciniforme. Bickers DR, Demar LK, DeLeo V, Poh-Fitzpatrick MB, Aronberg JM, Harber LC. Arch Dermatol 1978; 114: 1193–6.

Two patients reported an improvement of their disease with β-carotene 180 mg daily.

Hydroa vacciniforme: induction of lesions with ultraviolet A. Halasz CLG, Leach EE, Walther RR, Poh-Fitzpatrick MB. J Am Acad Dermatol 1983; 8: 171–6.

The one patient treated with β-carotene 180 mg daily reported some subjective improvement.

Hydroa vacciniforme: diagnosis and therapy. Goldgeier MH, Nordlund JJ, Lucky AW, Sibrack LA, McCarthy MJ, McGuire J. Arch Dermatol 1982: 118: 588–91.

β-Carotene 120 mg daily for 2 months in the one patient was ineffective.

Hydroa vacciniforme presenting in an adult successfully treated with cyclosporin A. Blackwell V, McGregor JM, Hawk JLM. Clin Exp Dermatol 1998; 23: 73–6.

There was good control of disease with cyclosporine 3 mg/kg daily over a 2-month period.

The report does not provide details of follow-up.

Efficacy of ω-3 polyunsaturated fatty acids for the treatment of refractory hydroa vacciniforme. Durbec F, Reguiaï Z, Léonard F, Pluot M, Bernard P. Pediatr Dermatol. 2012; 29: 118–9.

One patient was successfully treated with dietary fish oil after unsuccessful treatment with other measures.

Dietary fish oil as a photoprotective agent in hydroa vacciniforme. Rhodes LE, White SI. Br J Dermatol 1998; 138: 173–8.

Three patients were treated with dietary fish oil, five capsules daily, for 3 months. A mild to good improvement was noted in two patients, but no improvement in the third. The latter patient responded to azathioprine.

Hydroa vacciniforme: major and minor forms. Cruces MJ, de la Torre C. Photodermatology 1986; 3: 109–10.

In the one patient treated with thalidomide there was initial improvement.

Thalidomide for the treatment of hydroa vacciniforme-like lymphoma: report of four pediatric cases from Peru. Beltrán BE, Maza I, Moisés-Alfaro CB, Vasquez L, Quiñones P, Morales D, et al. Am J Hematol 2014; 89: 1160–1.

Two out of four children responded.

Hydroa vacciniforme presenting in an adult successfully treated with cyclosporin A. Blackwell V, McGregor JM, Hawk JLM. Clin Exp Dermatol 1998; 23: 73–6.

In the one patient, thalidomide 100 mg daily was ineffective. Cyclosporine proved helpful at 3 mg/kg/day. Azathioprine 2.5 to 3.5 mg/kg daily was ineffective in the one patient studied.

Hyperhidrosis

James A.A. Langtry

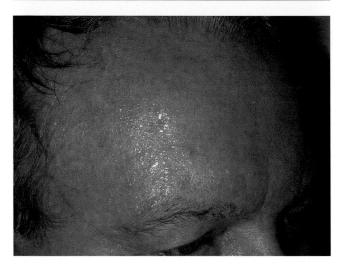

Hyperhidrosis is the result of increased secretion of eccrine sweat. This can be annoying, disabling (at work or socially), or indicative of an underlying systemic disease. The eccrine gland is unusual in that the sympathetic sudomotor fibers are cholinergic rather than adrenergic.

Hyperhidrosis can be classified as *idiopathic or pathologic. Idiopathic* hyperhidrosis is defined as excessive sweating that is symmetric; localized to the palms, soles, or axillae (singly or in combination); and independent of thermoregulation. Craniofacial hyperhidrosis is a similar but rarer condition. The other characteristics include its episodic nature, occurrence in response to stimuli, and onset at or after puberty; there is commonly a family history. There is an absence of bromhidrosis and little or no seasonal variation.

Pathologic hyperhidrosis may be localized or generalized. Localized hyperhidrosis may result from injury to the central or peripheral nervous systems, syringomyelia, neuritis, myelitis, tabes dorsalis, or localized vascular diseases, including cold injury, arteriovenous malformation, and erythrocyanosis. Localized hyperhidrosis can occur as a functional nevus in which a normal number of eccrine glands are oversensitive to acetylcholine. Localized areas of hyperhidrosis can develop as a compensatory phenomenon when extensive anhidrosis develops in Ross syndrome (bilateral Holmes Adie pupils, tendon areflexia, generalized anhidrosis). Hyperhidrosis may occur in hereditary conditions, including blue rubber bleb nevus syndrome. The causes of generalized hyperhidrosis include febrile illnesses; metabolic and endocrine diseases (diabetes, hyperthyroidism, gout, acromegaly, pregnancy, porphyria, pheochromocytoma, carcinoid syndrome, alcohol intoxication); congestive cardiac failure and shock; internal malignancy; central nervous system (CNS) diseases (tumors and injury); and hereditary syndromes (Chediak–Higashi syndrome and phenylketonuria).

MANAGEMENT STRATEGY

The treatments discussed here apply primarily to the symptomatic management of idiopathic hyperhidrosis.

Local treatments, including medical, electrical, or surgical modalities, aim to stop or reduce sweating sufficiently to control symptoms. Treatments with the lowest risk should be considered first, as dictated by the severity of the condition and a discussion with the patient to assess the balance of risk and benefit.

Topical aluminum chloride hexahydrate (ACH) 20% to 25% solution in ethanol is the first-line treatment. The mechanism of action may result from occlusion of the intraepidermal eccrine duct below the level of the stratum corneum. Correct application technique is critical to compliance: in the axillae, the solution should be applied nightly to the unshaven skin, with or without occlusion, and washed off the next morning before daytime sweating is established. The presence of moisture results in the formation of hydrochloric acid and resultant skin irritation. Mild-potency topical corticosteroids may be used to reduce the common problem of skin irritation, which is the usual reason for treatment failure. ACH solution should not be applied again in the morning. An oral anticholinergic (e.g., 1 mg of sodium glycopyrrolate) 45 minutes before the application of ACH may increase its efficacy by reducing sweating at the time of application, allowing the ACH to be retained on the skin and exert its effect on the sweat pores. The oral anticholinergic may be discontinued after several treatments have initiated a reduction in sweating. Hyperhidrosis may take 2 to 3 weeks to be controlled with topical ACH, at which time application can be reduced to once a week or at an interval that maintains control.

Other topical therapies include *formaldehyde*, which is a common contact sensitizer, and *glutaraldehyde*, which stains the skin. *Methenamine gel* releases formaldehyde but does not appear to produce contact allergy frequently. The anticholinergic *glycopyrrolate* in 1.5% to 2% concentrations topically in an aqueous cream base or as glycopyrrolate pads may be effective.

Iontophoresis is the process of introducing salt ions in solution through the skin into the tissues and may be effective in treating palmoplantar and axillary hyperhidrosis. Several iontophoretic devices are commercially available. Current is transmitted to electrodes in two trays filled with tap water, and the hands or feet are placed flat in the bottom of the trays. The current is increased until the patient experiences slight discomfort (average 15 mA on the palms and 20 mA on the soles). A special electrode for axillary use is available for some iontophoretic devices. The mechanism of reduction of sweating is not known. Current densities below the threshold of damage to the acrosyringium are employed, and mechanical obstruction does not occur. Iontophoresis is contraindicated in pregnancy and in patients with cardiac pacemakers and metal implants. Twenty-minute sessions three times a week are continued until sweating is sufficiently reduced; thereafter once- or twice-monthly maintenance therapies are instituted. Anticholinergic drugs such as glycopyrronium bromide may also be introduced by iontopheresis. A recent report suggests that botulinum toxin delivered by iontophoresis to the palms may be effective in the treatment of palmar hyperhidrosis.

Oral anticholinergic drugs and *minor tranquilizers* produce a dose-related inhibition of sweating and are therefore limited by side effects. Anticholinergic effects, including dry mouth, pupillary dilatation and photophobia, glaucoma, urinary retention, constipation, vomiting, and tachycardia, may, however, occur at doses that produce satisfactory sweat inhibition, thereby limiting their use. The oral anticholinergics most commonly used are *glycopyrronium bromide* (Robinul), up to 2 mg three times daily; *propantheline* 15 mg three times daily; or *oxybutynin* up to 5 mg twice daily. Oral glycopyrronium bromide is not licensed for use in hyperhidrosis in the UK.

Other systemic drugs that have been used include the calcium channel blocker *diltiazem*, the CNS inhibitor *clonidine*, and *tricyclic*

Evidence Levels: **A** Double-blind study **B** Clinical trial ≥ 20 subjects **C** Clinical trial < 20 subjects **D** Series ≥ 5 subjects **E** Anecdotal case reports

antidepressants, although these are the subject of few anecdotal reports.

More aggressive treatments may be sought as a result of treatment failure, inconvenience of the treatments, or side effects.

Botulinum toxin injected intradermally produces sustained anhidrosis and is shown to be effective in treating axillary, palmar, craniofacial, postamputation stump hyperhidrosis, compensatory sweating, and Frey syndrome. There are eight known serotypes of botulinum toxin, type A exotoxin (BTX-A). The commercially available BTX-A products differ in their potency and are not equivalent unit for unit. Botulinum toxin type B has been shown to be effective in the treatment of axillary hyperhidrosis and may be used as an alternative to BTX-A products, especially where antibody formation has resulted in a loss of clinical benefit to BTX-A. It is recommended that experience be gained with one of the products. BTX-A produces its effect by irreversibly blocking the release of acetylcholine from cholinergic junctions. Treatment of the axilla is simple and well tolerated. Multiple injections, 2 cm apart, are performed in the axillary vault corresponding to the area of maximum sweating (an area of approximately 200 cm^2). Palmar skin is painful to inject (may require a regional nerve block); injection is less well tolerated, and there is a potential for producing weakness of the intrinsic hand musculature. Administration of BTX-A to the palms by needle-free injector may be effective and less painful. It is not a practical treatment for plantar hyperhidrosis. Inactivation of affected cholinergic junctions is permanent, but new cholinergic junctions are produced through the natural process of tissue turnover and repair, so the effect is temporary. Onset of anhidrosis after injection occurs at 24 to 72 hours and lasts 3 to 6 months. A number of reports describe the increase in duration of efficacy of repeated BTX-A treatments over time for axillary hyperhidrosis. There are reports of efficacy of BTX-A utilizing iontophoresis and Dermojet as delivery systems to affected areas.

Surgical and physical techniques that have been employed in the management of axillary hyperhidrosis include:

- Cryotherapy (very painful and poorly tolerated).
- Thermal injury of localized sweat glands using a microwave-based device or Nd:YAG laser.
- Methods that remove subcutaneous tissue alone. A number of skin flaps/incisions are described to gain access to the subcutaneous axillary tissues, and the deep dermis and adjacent subcutis are trimmed away. Subcutaneous curettage and axillary liposuction are other methods described for achieving this objective.
- Methods that excise skin and subcutaneous tissue.
- Methods that combine cutaneous excision and resection of subcutaneous tissue.

Selective ablation of the sympathetic innervation of the palms, axillae, and soles reduces sweating effectively. A number of side effects are associated with sympathectomy, including compensatory hyperhidrosis, Horner syndrome, pneumothorax, and intraoperative cardiac arrest. Satisfactory long-term results are generally achieved, although recurrence of sweating usually occurs. It is best reserved for severe palmar hyperhidrosis (upper thoracic sympathectomy T2/T3 ganglia), avoiding denervation of the axillary sweat glands and thereby minimizing side effects. This is performed as an open surgical technique or endoscopically (by a transthoracic route) using electrocautery or laser. Percutaneous chemical sympathectomy with ethanol has also been used, a technique that may be employed in lumbar sympathectomy to treat plantar hyperhidrosis. However, this is not generally recommended given the significant risk of sequelae, including ejaculatory failure, impotence, and anorgasmia.

Specific Investigations

- Starch iodine to define areas of maximum sweating
- Gravimetric tests can be used for quantification

Tests are not necessary for diagnosis of idiopathic hyperhidrosis. Investigation appropriate to the clinical history and physical signs is necessary when hyperhidrosis is not idiopathic.

First-Line Therapy

• Topical ACH solution in ethanol	**B**

Aluminium chloride hexahydrate versus palmar hyperhidrosis. Evaporimeter study. Goh CL. Int J Dermatol 1990; 29: 368–70.

A single-blind study of unilateral palmar treatment with 20% ACH daily for 4 weeks in 12 patients. Efficacy was reported for all patients; however, four experienced skin irritancy, three patients clearing after 1 week of stopping treatment, and one patient withdrew from the study.

Axillary hyperhidrosis. Local treatment with aluminium-chloride hexahydrate 25% in absolute ethanol with and without supplementary treatment with triethanolamine. Glent-Madsen L, Dahl JC. Acta Dermatol Venereol 1988; 68: 87–9.

A randomized, double-blind, half-sided experiment in 30 volunteers. Triethanolamine in 50% ethanol was applied after treatment to one axilla to neutralize the pH and reduce skin irritation. The combined treatment was found to be less irritating, but also less effective in reducing sweating, although the reduction in efficacy was not noted by the volunteers.

Second-Line Therapies

• Topical anticholinergics	**B**
• Oral anticholinergics	**D**
• Iontophoresis	**B**
• Botulinum A neurotoxin	**A**
• Botulinum A neurotoxin delivered by Dermojet	**C**
• Botulinum A neurotoxin delivered by iontophoresis	**D**
• Botulinum B neurotoxin	**C**
• Liposuction and surgical excision (axillae only)	**C**
• Sympathectomy	**B**

Topical glycopyrrolate for patients with facial hyperhidrosis. Kim WO, Kil HK, Yoon KB, Yoon DM. Br J Dermatol 2008; 158: 1094–7.

Twenty-five patients were treated with 2% topical glycopyrrolate pads to one half of the forehead; the other side was treated with a placebo. Gravimetric testing showed a reduction in sweating on the treated side in the majority of patients.

Topical glycopyrrolate reduces axillary hyperhidrosis. Baker DM. J Eur Acad Dermatol Venereol 2016; 30: 2131–6.

A nonrandomized consecutive patient treatment comparison of 1% and 2% glycopyrrolate spray and subcutaneous botulinum toxin type A injections reporting effectiveness of 2% glycopyrrolate spray.

Propantheline bromide in the management of hyperhidrosis associated with spinal cord injury. Canaday BR, Stanford RH. Ann Pharmacother 1995; 29: 489–92.

Generalized hyperhidrosis after spinal injury was suppressed with careful titration of propantheline, starting at 15 mg daily and increasing to 15 mg three times daily.

Use of oral glycopyrronium bromide in hyperhidrosis. Baja V, Langtry JAA. Br J Dermatol 2007; 157: 118–21.

In this retrospective analysis of 19 patients with idiopathic hyperhidrosis of varying distribution, 79% reported response to treatment at a dose of 2 mg twice daily, increasing to 2 mg three times daily. In one third of patients treatment was limited by side effects.

Systemic therapy for primary hyperhidrosis: a retrospective study of 59 patients treated with glycopyrrolate or clonidine. Walling HW. J Am Acad Dermatol 2012; 66: 387–92.

Results of systemic anticholinergic treatment in 71 patients of whom 59 (mean age 29 years, 37 females, mean follow-up 19.5 months) had at least 2 months' follow-up data. Forty-two had palmoplantar or axillary, nine had generalized, and eight had craniofacial hyperhidrosis. Thirty out of 45 responded to glycopyrrolate at 1 to 2 mg twice daily. In the 15 treatment failures, 6 were nonresponders and 9 had adverse effects. Six out of 13 responded to clonidine 0.1 mg twice a day. In the seven treatment failures, three were nonresponders and four had adverse effects relating to hypotension. One patient responded to treatment with oxybutynin 5 mg twice a day.

A randomized placebo-controlled trial of oxybutynin for the initial treatment of palmar and axillary hyperhidrosis. Wolosker N, de Campos JRM, Kauffamn P, Puech-Leaon P. J Vasc Surg 2012; 55: 1696–700.

A study on 50 patients with palmar or axillary hyperhidrosis treated with either placebo or oxybutynin 5 mg twice a day for 6 weeks and assessed by clinical questionnaire and for quality of life. Improvement was noted in the oxybutynin-treated group in 70% with palmar and axillary hyperhidrosis, and in 90% with plantar hyperhidrosis; 65% showed improvement in quality of life, although 48% experienced dry mouth.

Iontophoresis with alternating current and direct current offset (AC/DC iontophoresis): a new approach for the treatment of hyperhidrosis. Reinauer S, Neusser A, Schauf G, Holzle E. Br J Dermatol 1993; 129: 166–9.

Palmar hyperhidrosis was controlled after an average of 11 treatments, with both the conventional DC and the AC/DC iontophoresis units studied. The AC/DC method, however, eliminated skin irritation and discomfort.

The effectiveness of tap water iontophoresis for palmoplantar hyperhidrosis using a Monday, Wednesday, Friday treatment regime. Siah TW, Hampton PJ. Dermatol Online J 2013; 19: 14.

A retrospective study of 23 patients reported effective treatment with this regimen.

Treatment of hyperhidrosis. Heymann WR. J Am Acad Dermatol 2005; 52: 509–10.

A review of the treatments available for hyperhidrosis, focusing on botulinum toxin.

Botulinum toxin A for axillary hyperhidrosis (excessive sweating). Heckmann M, Ceballos-Baumann AO, Plewig G. N Engl J Med 2001; 344: 488–93.

A multicenter trial in 145 patients with axillary hyperhidrosis comparing 200 U and 100 U of BTX-A (Dysport) per axilla. Changes in the rates of sweat production were measured gravimetrically. Two weeks after injection, sweat production was slightly less in the axilla injected with 200 U, and sweat reduction in both was significantly more than with placebo. After 24 weeks, sweat rates after 100 and 200 U were almost identical and less than half the baseline rate. Ninety-eight percent of the patients said they would recommend this therapy to others.

Botulinum toxin therapy for palmar hyperhidrosis. Shelley WB, Talanin NY, Shelley ED. J Am Acad Dermatol 1998; 38: 227–9.

Four patients with severe palmar hyperhidrosis were treated under regional nerve blocks of the median and ulnar nerve. Anhidrosis lasted for 12, 7, 7, and 4 months, respectively, and one patient experienced mild weakness of a thumb lasting 3 weeks.

A double-blind, randomized, comparative study of Dysport™ vs. Botox™ in primary palmar hyperhidrosis. Simonetta Moreau M, Cauhepe C, Magues JP, Senard JM. Br J Dermatol 2003; 149: 1041–5.

Eight patients were treated with intradermal injections of Botox in one palm and Dysport in the other (using a conversion factor of 1:4) after regional nerve blocks. Similar efficacy was reported for the two BTX-A products.

Effective treatment of frontal hyperhidrosis with botulinum toxin A. Kinkelin I, Hund M, Naumann M, Hamm H. Br J Dermatol 2000; 143: 824–7.

Ten men with focal frontal hyperhidrosis are reported to have had a good response to treatment with BTX-A injections.

Treatment of palmar hyperhidrosis with needle injection versus low-pressure needle-free jet injection of onabotulinum toxin A: an open label study. Vadeboncoeur S, Richer V, Nantel-Battista M, Benohanain A. Dermatol Surg 2017; 43: 264–9.

A prospective open-label study showing efficacy of onabotulinum toxin A treatment with needle-free injector.

BOTOX™ delivery by iontophoresis. Kavanagh GM, Oh C, Shams K. Br J Dermatol 2004; 151: 1093–5.

Two patients with palmar hyperhidrosis had treatment with BTX-A (Botox) delivered by iontophoresis. Control of approximately 70% was achieved for 3 months, without side effects.

Botulinum toxin type B: a new therapy for axillary hyperhidrosis. Nelson L, Bachoo P, Holmes J. Br J Plast Surg 2005; 58: 228–32.

The efficacy of BTX-B (NeuroBloc) was demonstrated in the treatment of 13 patients with axillary hyperhidrosis.

Liposuction for the treatment of axillary hyperhidrosis. Lillis PJ, Coleman WP. Dermatol Clin 1990; 8: 479–82.

The authors suggest that this technique shows promise as the surgical treatment of choice for axillary hyperhidrosis resistant to other modalities.

Surgical treatment of axillary hyperhidrosis in 123 patients. Bretteville-Jensen G, Mossing N, Albrechsten R. Acta Derm Venereol 1975; 55: 73–8.

Excision of the axillary vault and reconstruction with a modified Z-plasty is described. Of 123 patients, 57% achieved a 75% to 100% reduction of axillary sweating and 36% achieved a 50%

to 75% reduction. Complications included hematomas in 6 patients, limited flap necrosis in 5, and minor complications in 10 patients. There were no cases of keloid formation or restricted arm movement from wound contracture.

Transthoracic endoscopic sympathectomy for palmar hyperhidrosis in children and adolescents: analysis of 350 cases. Lin TS. J Laparoendosc Adv Surg Tech A 1999; 9: 331–4.

A total of 699 sympathectomies were performed in 350 patients aged 5 to 17 years (mean 12.9 years). There were no surgical deaths. The mean follow-up was 25 months (range 5–44 months), with highly satisfactory results reported in 95% of patients, although compensatory hyperhidrosis (86%) affected the axillae (12%), back (86%), abdomen (48%), or lower limbs (78%). The recurrence rates of palmar hyperhidrosis were 0.6% in the first year, 1.1% in the second, and 1.7% in the third.

Thoracoscopic sympathectomy for disabling palmar hyperhidrosis: a prospective randomized comparison between two levels. Baumgartner FJ, Reyes M, Sarkisayan GG, Iglesias A. Ann Thorac Surg 2011; 92: 2015–9.

Bilateral sympathectomy for severe palmar hyperhidrosis at the second costal head (R2 in 61 patients) versus the third costal head (R3 in 60 patients). R2 failed in 5 of 122 extremities and R3 in 5 of 120 extremities. R2 patients showed a trend toward higher levels of compensatory hyperhidrosis compared with R3 patients. R2 and R3 were found to be effective for disabling palmar hyperhidrosis with a low incidence of severe compensatory hyperhidrosis.

Severe plantar hyperhidrosis: an effective solution. Reisfeld R, Pasternack GA, Danials PD, Basseri E, Nish GK, Berliner KI. Ann Surg 2013; 79: 845–53.

Endoscopic lumbar sympathectomy using the clamping method was reported in 154 patients. Anhidrosis was achieved in 97% with two complications and six conversions to an open surgical procedure.

Third-Line Therapies

• Microwave-based devices	B
• Lasers and photodynamic therapy	D
• Biofeedback and behavioral modification	D
• Diltiazem	E
• Clonazepam	E
• Clonidine	E

Radiofrequency thermotherapy for treating axillary hyperhidrosis. Schick CH, Grallath T, Schick KS, Hashmonai M. Dermatol Surg 2016; 42: 624–30.

Thirty-three patients treated with radiofrequency thermotherapy with noninsulated microneedle three times at intervals of 6 weeks with average reduction of sweating reported to be 72%.

New treatment techniques for axillary hyperhidrosis. Mordon SR, Trelles MA, Leclere FM, Betrouni N. J Cosmet Laser Ther 2014; 16: 230–5.

The use of Nd:YAG laser, diode laser, and photodynamic therapy is described as potential new treatments for axillary hyperhidrosis.

Clinical evaluation of a microwave based device for treating axillary hyperhidrosis. Hong HC, Lupin M, O'Shaughnessy KF. Dermatol Surg 2012; 38: 728–35.

The aim is to selectively heat the interface between the skin and fat and thereby inhibit sweat gland excretion. Thirty-one patients with primary axillary hyperhidrosis had one to three treatments to both axillae over 6 months. At 12 months 90% had a 50% reduction in axillary sweating from baseline and 85% had a reduction of at least 5 points on the DLQI.

Use of biofeedback in treating chronic hyperhidrosis. Duller P, Gentry WD. Br J Dermatol 1980; 103: 143–8.

Biofeedback and behavioral modification can be tried, but is helpful in only a small number of patients.

Emotional eccrine sweating. A heritable disorder. James WD, Schoomaker EB, Rodman OG. Arch Dermatol 1987; 123: 925–9.

Two members of a family with palmar hyperhidrosis showed reduced palmar sweat secretion during administration of diltiazem.

Unilateral localized hyperhidrosis responding to treatment with clonazepam. Takase Y, Tsushimi K, Yamamoto K, Fukusako T, Morimatsu M. Br J Dermatol 1992; 126: 416.

A case of unilateral hyperhidrosis responding to this benzodiazepine antiepileptic agent.

Clonidine treatment in paroxysmal localized hyperhidrosis. Kuritzky A, Hering R, Goldhammer G, Bechar M. Arch Neurol 1984; 41: 1210–1.

Improvement of paroxysmal localized hyperhidrosis is described in two patients with oral clonidine hydrochloride 0.25 mg three times a day. Control of sweating was maintained with continuous treatment at 12-month follow-up.

Hypertrichosis and hirsutism

Shannon Harrison, Najwa Somani, Wilma F. Bergfeld

INTRODUCTION

Hirsutism is the excessive growth of terminal hairs in women in male androgen–dependent areas (face, breasts, upper thighs, abdomen, and back). It adversely affects quality of life. Although defined by a modified Ferriman–Gallwey (F-G) score of ≥8, race and ethnicity affect this criterion.

Hirsutism can result from endogenous androgens (ovarian or adrenal), exogenous androgens, or from increased hair follicle sensitivity to normal androgen levels. Common causes are polycystic ovarian syndrome (PCOS) and idiopathic hirsutism. Rarer causes are endocrinopathies, non-classical congenital adrenal hyperplasia and androgen-secreting tumors.

Hypertrichosis, by contrast, results from increased vellus hair growth in an androgen-independent, nonsexual distribution. Causes are familial or secondary to medications or an underlying systemic disorder.

Main Causes of Hirsutism

Ovarian

- **Polycystic ovary (PCOS) syndrome** (menstrual irregularities, infertility, and metabolic syndrome*)
- **HAIR-AN syndrome** (hyperandrogenism, severe metabolic syndrome*, acanthosis nigricans)
- **Hyperthecosis** (menstrual irregularities and metabolic syndrome*)
- **Ovarian tumors and hyperplasia** (irregular menses, virilization symptoms)

Adrenal

- **Congenital adrenal hyperplasia** – classical and nonclassical types (irregular menses, primary amenorrhea)
- **Cushing syndrome** (striae, fat redistribution, fragile skin, proximal muscle weakness, mood disturbance, insulin resistance)
- **Adrenal tumors** (virilization symptoms)

Pituitary**

- **Cushing disease** (striae, fat redistribution, fragile skin, proximal muscle weakness, mood disturbance, insulin resistance)
- **Acromegaly** (coarse facies and enlarged hands)
- **Hyperprolactinemia** (galactorrhea)

Idiopathic

- Occult functional hyperandrogenism
- Abnormalities in peripheral 5α-reductase or androgen receptor

Exogenous (androgenic medications)

- Testosterone, adrenocorticotropic hormone (ACTH), valproic acid, anabolic steroids, androgenic progestins

*Metabolic syndrome: obesity, insulin resistance/diabetes mellitus type 2, lipid abnormalities, cardiovascular disease.
**Pituitary tumors can also present with visual field disturbances.

MANAGEMENT STRATEGY

A thorough history and physical examination should identify any underlying cause of hypertrichosis and hirsutism. Offending drugs should be discontinued.

Most hirsute women have raised circulating androgen levels. In idiopathic hirsutism, circulating androgen levels appear normal, and menstrual cycles are regular. Polycystic ovarian syndrome (PCOS) and the rarer HAIR-AN syndrome and ovarian hypethecosis present with signs of hyperandrogenism and metabolic syndrome. In obese women, weight loss improves markers of metabolic syndrome and reduces cardiovascular risk. Body mass index (BMI) is the most important risk factor for hirsutism severity in PCOS.

Acute onset or rapid progression of hirsutism or presence of virilization indicate possible adrenal or ovarian tumor. In non-classical congenital adrenal hyperplasia, glucocorticoid therapy assists with ovulation induction, but hirsutism often requires systemic antiandrogen therapy. For classical congenital adrenal hyperplasia, glucocorticoids address both ovulation induction and hirsutism.

Physical hair removal methods

Mechanical hair removal is the first-line treatment choice for hirsutism and hypertrichosis. *Bleaching* with hydrogen peroxide preparations disguises dark facial hair but can irritate. Painless depilatory methods remove hair shafts at the skin surface. *Chemical depilatory creams* are quick to use but can irritate, and skin folds should be avoided. *Shaving* is inexpensive but is time consuming and not acceptable to most women except for the axillae and legs. Shaving does not affect the diameter or rate of growth of hair.

Epilatory hair removal methods remove the entire hair, including the root, and are painful. *Tweezing or plucking* is used in areas with fewer hairs. *Waxing* is used where hair density is higher. Epilation with *electrolysis* can achieve permanent reduction in hair growth but is time consuming, requires multiple treatments, and is operator dependent. It can be used on any skin or hair color. A fine needle is inserted into the hair follicle, which delivers direct current (galvanic electrolysis), high-frequency alternating current (thermolysis), or a blend of the two currents to damage the hair follicle. Side effects of all mechanical hair removal methods include erythema, folliculitis, pseudofolliculitis, infection, scarring, and dyspigmentation.

Photoepilation lasers include ruby (694 nm), alexandrite (755 nm), diode (800–810 nm), Nd:YAG (neodymium:yttrium-aluminum-garnet) laser (1064 nm) and IPL (intense pulsed light) noncoherent sources of 590 to 1200 nm. Lasers and IPL give partial short-term hair reduction up to 6 months, and efficacy improves with repeat treatments. No laser can achieve complete or persistent hair removal. Ideal candidates have fair skin and dark hair. Side effects include erythema, scarring, burns, dyspigmentation, and rarely with IPL, a paradoxical increase in hair growth.

Twice-daily *eflornithine hydrochloride* cream is approved by the Food and Drug Administration (FDA) for facial hirsutism and slows the rate of hair growth by irreversibly inhibiting ornithine decarboxylase. Benefits reverse after 8 weeks of discontinuation. Side effects include acne, pseudofolliculitis barbae, and irritant and allergic contact dermatitis. Adjuvant use with laser hair removal improves efficacy.

Systemic therapies for hirsutism

Although several meta-analyses and treatment guidelines are published, evidence supporting hirsutism treatments are limited due to small sample sizes and limited methodology of studies.

Combined oral contraceptive pills (estrogen and progestin OCP) are a first-line treatment for hirsutism. They reduce hyperandrogenism predominantly by suppressing ovarian androgen synthesis, increasing sex hormone–binding globulin levels, and suppressing free plasma testosterone levels. OCPs with low androgenic progestins (desogestrel or norgestimate) and progestins with antiandrogenic properties (cyproterone acetate, drospirenone) are preferred. However, potential risks (e.g., deep venous thrombosis) and benefits should be weighed, especially when choosing a second- or third-generation OCP. Clinical response requires 6 to 12 months of treatment. Combination treatment with another antiandrogen (e.g., spironolactone) is considered if response to monotherapy is limited.

Hirsutism can result from endogenous androgens (ovarian or adrenal), exogenous androgens, or from increased hair follicle sensitivity to normal androgen levels. Common causes are polycystic ovarian syndrome (PCOS) and idiopathic hirsutism. Rarer causes are endocrinopathies, non-classical congenital adrenal hyperplasia and androgen-secreting tumors.

Spironolactone is an antiandrogen that inhibits androgen biosynthesis and blocks the androgen receptor. The usual dose for hirsutism is 100 to 200 mg daily. Side effects include hyperkalemia, hypotension, and irregular menses. Tumorigenicity has been shown in animals, but relevance in humans is questionable. All antiandrogens, including spironolactone, have feminizing teratogenic potential and should be used with a reliable form of contraception. Hence, all pharmacologic therapy for hirsutism should not be commenced in women planning pregnancy.

Cyproterone acetate inhibits the androgen receptor. It can be used either in a sequential way for the first 10 days of the menstrual cycle (25–100 mg) with an OCP or a low dose (2 mg) in a combined OCP (Diane-35). Side effects are similar to OCPs. It is not available in the United States.

Finasteride is a type II 5-alpha-reductase inhibitor. It is pregnancy category X. Benefit is shown with oral therapy but not when used topically in a compounded formulation. No reports exist for dutasteride, a type I and II 5-alpha-reductase inhibitor for the treatment of hirsutism.

Flutamide and *insulin-lowering drugs* are not recommended for the treatment of hirsutism. Flutamide has specific indications but comes with significant risk of hepatotoxicity.

GnRH analogs are not recommended in the treatment of hirsutism unless oral contraceptives and antiandrogen treatments fail and hyperandrogenism is severe. Gonadotropin-releasing hormone (GnRH) treatment reduces estrogen to menopausal levels, causing hot flushes and osteoporosis risk.

Specific Investigations

Screening test
- Testosterone level (free and total)
- Consider βhCG level

If testosterone level raised or underlying endocrinopathy or tumor suspected
- Sex hormone–binding globulin level
- Dehydroepiandrosterone sulfate level

Androstenedione level
- Follicle-stimulating hormone level (FSH)

Luteinizing hormone level (LH)
- Serum prolactin
- 17-hydroxyprogesterone level (morning, follicular phase)

24-hour urinary free cortisol
- Somatomedin C level (IGF-1)
- Thyrotropin level

Special tests
- Transvaginal ovarian ultrasound
- Dexamethasone suppression test
- Computed tomography/magnetic resonance imaging (CT/MRI) abdomen or pelvis
- Cranial MRI

Investigations can identify underlying pathology. Moderate to severe hirsutism, hirsutism with signs of hyperandrogenism (e.g., clitoromegaly, central obesity, acanthosis nigricans, infertility, or irregular menstrual cycles), and acute-onset or rapidly progressing hirsutism should be investigated. Although controversy exists on obtaining androgen levels in mild isolated hirsutism (F-G score 8–15), we suggest testosterone screening on all patients.

An LH:FSH ratio >2 suggests, but does not confirm, PCOS. Transvaginal ultrasound detects polycystic ovaries, the presence or absence of which alone neither confirms nor refutes the diagnosis. Metabolic screening is essential. Early-morning serum 17-hydroxyprogesterone level detects nonclassical congenital adrenal hyperplasia. Twenty-four-hour urine cortisol and dexamethasone suppression tests evaluate for Cushing disease. Prolactin level and somatomedin-C (IGF-1) level screen for hyperprolactinemia and acromegaly, respectively. Suspicion of a pituitary tumor requires MRI scanning of the brain. Transvaginal ultrasound or abdominal CT or MRI scan can exclude an ovarian or adrenal tumor. Rarely, pregnancy and hypothyroidism can cause hirsutism and should be excluded.

The hirsute woman: challenges in evaluation and management. Paparodis R, Dunaif A. Endocrine Practice 2011; 17: 807–18.

A review of the etiology and diagnostic approach to hirsutism.

Epidemiology, diagnosis and management of hirsutism: a consensus statement by the Androgen Excess and Polycystic

Ovary Syndrome Society. Escobar-Morreale HF, Carmina E, Dewailly D, Gambineri A, Kelestimur F, et al. Hum Reprod Update 2012; 18: 146–70.

A review of the diagnosis and management of hirsutism.

The evaluation and treatment of androgen excess. Practice Committee of the American Society for Reproductive Medicine. Fertil Steril 2006; 86: S241–7.

This article reviews clinical diagnosis and laboratory testing for hirsutism.

The clinical evaluation of hirsutism. Somani N, Harrison S, Bergfeld WF. Dermatol Ther 2008; 21: 376–91.

The article has tables on history, examination templates, and diagnostic algorithms for evaluation of hirsutism.

First-Line Therapies

• Treat specific underlying pathology	
• Temporary hair removal/camouflage	B
• Weight loss if obese with PCOS	B
• Electrolysis	D
• Laser therapy and IPL	B
• Eflornithine	B
• Eflornithine with laser/IPL	C

American Association of Clinical Endocrinologists, American College of Endocrinology, and Androgen Excess and PCOS Society Disease State Clinical Review: guide to the best practices in the evaluation and treatment of polycystic ovarian syndrome – part 1. Goodman NF, Cobin RH, Futterweit W, Glueck JS, Legro RS, Carmina E. Endocrine Practice 2015; 21: 1291–300.

A thorough review of clinical features, investigations, and treatment for PCOS.

Lifestyle changes in women with polycystic ovary syndrome. Moran LJ, Hutchison SK, Norman RJ, Teede HJ. Cochrane Database Syst Rev 2011; 7: CD007506.

Limited studies show a small benefit from counseling on lifestyle modification in conjunction with other treatments for hirsutism, especially in PCOS. Smoking cessation, particularly in the case of OCPs use, is prudent.

Hirsutism. Mofid A, Alinaghi SA, Zansieh S, Yazdani T. Int J Clin Pract 2008; 62: 433–43.

A review of diagnostic strategies with user-friendly tables on hair removal methods and pharmacotherapies.

A comparative study of axillary hair removal in women: plucking versus the blend method. Urushibata O, Kasa K. J Dermatol 1995; 22: 738–42.

There are no randomized controlled trials on electrolysis. This small comparative study showed electrolysis was more effective than plucking for reduction of axillary hair.

Electrolysis: observations from 13 years and 140,000 hours of experience. Richards RN, Meharg GE. J Am Acad Dermatol 1995; 33: 662–6.

Side effects and efficacy are operator dependent.

Laser and photoepilation for unwanted hair growth Haedersdal M, Gøtzsche PC. Cochrane Database Syst Rev 2006; 4: CD004684.

Diode and alexandrite lasers conferred short-term 50% hair reduction lasting up to 6 months after treatment. IPL, neodymium:YAG, or ruby lasers have limited evidence of benefit.

Evidence based review of hair removal using lasers and light sources. Haedersdal M, Wulf HC. J Eur Acad Dermatol Venerol 2006; 20: 9–20.

Meta-analysis showing laser and IPL hair reduction as more effective short term than shaving, waxing, electrolysis, and epilation. The relative efficacy of different hair removal lasers and IPL has been compared in several studies, but small sample sizes can introduce type 2 errors.

Meta-analysis of hair removal laser trials. Sadoghha A, Mohaghegh Zahed G. Lasers Med Sci 2009; 24: 21–5.

Hair reductions 6 months posttreatment were 57.5%, 42.3%, 54.7%, and 52.8% after three treatments for diode, Nd:YAG, alexandrite, and ruby lasers, respectively.

Photoepilation with a diode laser vs. intense pulsed light: a randomized, intrapatient left-to-right trial. Klein A, Steinert S, Baeumler W, Landthaler M, Babilas P. Br J Dermatol 2013; 168: 1287–93.

Diode laser more effectively decreased axillary hair counts in 30 patients compared with IPL. Mean reductions from baseline at 3 and 12 months after six treatment sessions were 59.7% and 69.2% for diode laser and 42.4% and 52.7% for IPL (P < 0.01), respectively. Diode treatment was more painful than IPL.

Randomized, double blind clinical evaluation of the efficacy and safety of topical eflornithine HCl 13.9% cream in the treatment of women with facial hair. Wolf JE Jr, Shander D, Huber F, Jackson J, Lin C-S, Mathes BM, et al. Eflornithine Study Group. Int J Dermatol 2007; 46: 94–8.

Using a physician's global rating, at week 24, 58% of eflornithine-treated patients were improved compared with 34% of vehicle-treated patients.

A randomized bilateral vehicle controlled study of eflornithine cream combined with laser treatment versus laser treatment alone for facial hirsutism in women. Hamzavi I, Tan E, Shapiro J, Lui H. J Am Acad Dermatol 2007; 57: 54–9.

Eflornithine cream combined with six sessions of long-pulse alexandrite laser resulted in statistically significant differences in hair count analysis (P < 0.01) and blinded patient grading (P < 0.029) compared with laser alone for upper lip hirsutism in 31 patients.

Second-Line Therapies

• Oral contraceptives	B
• Spironolactone	B
• Cyproterone acetate	B

Hirsutism: an evidence-based treatment update. Somani N, Turvy D. Am J Clin Dermatol 2014; 15: 247–66.

A detailed clinical update and literature review of treatments for hirsutism with informative treatment tables.

Evidence-based approach to cutaneous hyperandrogenism in women. Schmidt TH, Shinkai K. J Am Acad Dermatol 2015: 73: 672–690.

A detailed analysis of management and treatments for cutaneous hyperandrogenism, including hirsutism.

Evidence Levels: A Double-blind study **B** Clinical trial ≥ 20 subjects **C** Clinical trial < 20 subjects **D** Series ≥ 5 subjects **E** Anecdotal case reports

Interventions for hirsutism (excluding laser and photoepilation therapy alone): review. Van Zuuren EJ, Fedorowicz Z, Carter B, Pandis N. Cochrane Database Syst Rev 2015; 4: CD010334.

Overall, published evidence on hirsutism treatment is limited, with small sample sizes and lack of blinding. Pooled data for OCP with ethinyl estradiol (EE) and cyproterone acetate vs. an OCP with EE and desogestrel demonstrated that both were effective in reducing F-G scores without significant difference between the two (mean difference [MD]: -1.84, 95% confidence interval [CI]: -3.86 to -0.18). Spironolactone 100 mg daily was more effective than placebo in reducing F-G scores (MD: -7.69, 95% CI: -10.12 to -5.26). Flutamide and finasteride had similar efficacies. Finasteride 5 mg and GnRH analogs showed inconsistent results in several studies. GnRH has significant side effects. Metformin showed no benefit over placebo.

Cyproterone acetate for hirsutism. Van der Spuy ZM, Le Roux PA. Cochrane Database Syst Rev 2003; 4: CD001125.

There are no studies comparing cyproterone acetate alone with placebo. One small placebo-controlled trial exists with cyproterone acetate 2 mg with EE OCP showing that it was more effective than placebo in reducing hirsutism scores.

Spironolactone versus placebo or in combination with steroids for hirsutism and/or acne (review). Brown J, Farquher C, Lee O, Toomath R, Jepson RG. Cochrane Database Syst Rev 2009; 2: CD000194.

Subjective improvement in hair growth was noted with spironolactone compared with placebo.

Third-Line Therapies	
• Oral finasteride	B
• Topical finasteride	D
• Flutamide	B
• Insulin-lowering monotherapy	B
• GnRH agonist analogs	B

Antiandrogens for the treatment of hirsutism: a systematic review and meta-analyses of randomized controlled trials. Swiglo BA, Cosma M, Flynn DN, Kurtz DM, LaBella ML, Mullan RJ, et al. J Clin Endocrinol Metab 2008; 93: 1153–60.

Two trials showed spironolactone (100 mg/d) was superior to placebo in improving hirsutism. Meta-analysis showed both finasteride and flutamide to be superior to placebo in reducing F-G scores. Antiandrogens were superior to metformin, and when spironolactone or finasteride are combined with OCPs, or when flutamide is combined with metformin, these regimens are superior to monotherapy with OCPs and metformin, respectively.

A randomized double blind, vehicle controlled bilateral comparison study of the efficacy and safety of finasteride 0.5% solution in combination with IPL in the treatment of facial hirsutism. Farshi S, Mansouri P, Rafie F. J Cosmet Laser 2012; 14: 193–9.

Addition of 0.5% finasteride solution in a spilt-face, vehicle-controlled trial of 75 women with chin hirsutism who were treated with three sessions of IPL showed minimal additional clinical improvement.

Evaluation and treatment of hirsutism in premenopausal women: an Endocrine Society clinical practice guideline. Martin KA, Chang J, Ehrmann DA, Ibanez L, Lobo RA, Rosenfield RL, et al. J Clin Endocrinol Metab 2008; 93: 1105–20.

Combined analysis of studies showed that OCPs are associated with a reduction in hirsutism scores. Meta-analysis concluded that no therapeutic advantages exist for GnRH treatment compared with other antiandrogens and OCPs.

Insulin sensitizers for the treatment of hirsutism: a systematic review and metaanalyses of randomized controlled trials. Cosma M, Swiglo BA, Flynn DN, Kurtz DM, LaBella ML, Mullan RJ, et al. J Clin Endocrinol Metab 2008; 93: 1135–42.

Metformin and the thiazolidinediones provided little or no important benefit.

Hypopigmented disorders

Seemal Desai, Sneha Ghunawat

Hypomelanotic disorders are skin conditions presenting with light-colored areas due to reduced melanin content in the lesional skin. Depigmented lesions, on the other hand, present clinically as milky white patches secondary to total destruction of melanocytes in the lesion. The disorders can be classified according to age of onset, extent of lesion, and underlying cause. This chapter briefly reviews the common hypopigmented dermatosis along with a brief overview of treatment options available.

Postinflammatary Hypomelanosis

Many dermatoses such as psoriasis, atopic dermatitis, seborrheic dermatitis, lupus erythematosus, sarcoidosis, lichen striatus, etc., lead to hypopigmented patches on resolving. Cutaneous injuries, burn, and cosmetic procedure (dermabrasion, chemical peels, and cryosurgery) can also lead to pigment loss. This loss of pigment is proposed to be secondary to alternation in the melanogenic pathway, destruction of melanocytes, or decrease in melanosome transfer. The severity of the pigment loss is proportionate to the degree of initial inflammation. The distribution also coincides with the distribution of the original lesions. It is seen in all skin types but is more frequently reported among dark-skinned individuals due to marked color contrast with the normal skin. The tendency of an individual to develop hypopigmentation/hyperpigmentation after initial inflammation is determined by the "chromatic tendency" of the patient. It is genetically determined and has an autosomal-dominant inheritance. Light microscopy from the lesions reveals loss of melanin content with a variable degree of lymphohistiocytic infiltrate in the upper dermis with occasional melanophages. The lesions may repigment spontaneously, such as after the procedure or may remain depigmented permanently, such as after lesions of lupus erythematosus.

Pityriasis Alba

It is an eczematous disorder seen commonly among children with a personal or family history of atopy, such as atopic dermatitis, conjunctivitis, rhinitis, asthma, etc. Lesions present with hypopigmented macules 0.5 to 3 cm in diameter located commonly on the face, neck, shoulders, and upper extremities. The lesions are covered with fine white scales. Erythema and pruritus are other common findings. The lesions are self-limiting. The generalized form of pityriasis alba is seen in adolescents and young adults with no personal or family history of atopy. The lesions are numerous, persistent, and involve the trunk and extremities.

Pityriasis Versicolor

This condition, which is also known as *tinea versicolor,* is a superficial infection of the keratin layer of the epidermis. The etiologic agent is a lipophilic yeast, *Pityrosporum orbiculare,* that is part of the normal flora of the skin. The organism is found more commonly in the budding form. The disease is seen when the form changes to hyphae. Potassium hydroxide mount of the lesion demonstrates "spaghetti and meatball" appearance. The sites involved include those that possess a high density of sebaceous glands such as the shoulders and upper back. The lesions clinically present with well-defined hypopigmented macules, which often coalesce into small patches with overlying fine scaling. The hypopigmentation is attributed to the formation of dicarboxylic acid by the organism. One such product, azelaic acid, inhibits tyrosinase in the melanogenesis pathway. Rarely the lesions can also be hyperpigmented to erythematous in color.

Leprosy (Hansen Disease)

It is an infectious disorder caused by *Mycobacterium leprae.* The bacteria affect the skin and peripheral nerves. The cutaneous lesions present clinically as well- to ill-defined hypopigmented macules with variable degrees of scaling and induration. The lesions classically are hypoesthetic, and examination reveals enlarged peripheral nerves.

Hypopigmented Variants of Common Dermatosis

Many common skin dermatoses such as mycosis fungoides, sarcoidosis, morphea, and scleroderma present with hypopigmented variants.

The hypopigmented variant of mycosis fungoides presents with ill-defined, light-colored macules and patches distributed primarily on sun-protected sites such as the back and buttocks. Histopathology reveals the presence of atypical lymphocytes in the epidermis (epidermotropism).

Lichen sclerosus is a chronic inflammatory disorder presenting clinically with hypopigmented to depigmented porcelain white plaques. The disease affects women in the fifth to sixth decades of life. The mechanism of depigmentation includes a decrease in melanin content and lack of transfer to melanosomes. Common sites of involvement are anogenital areas.

Morphea and systemic sclerosis also commonly present with hypopigmentation. The lesions are classically indurated. The typical presentation of the lesions includes a "salt and pepper" appearance. This refers to the perifollicular hyperpigmentation seen in hypopigmented patches. Differentiation from repigmenting patches of vitiligo can be difficult.

Evidence Levels: **A** Double-blind study **B** Clinical trial ≥ 20 subjects **C** Clinical trial < 20 subjects **D** Series ≥ 5 subjects **E** Anecdotal case reports

Hypopigmented variants of sarcoidosis are a less common presentation of the disease. It is more common among darker-colored individuals. The lesions favor the extremities. Clinical clues to the diagnosis include induration and yellowish tinge on diascopy.

Idiopathic Guttate Hypomelanosis

Idiopathic guttate hypomelanosis, also called *senile depigmented spots* and *symmetric progressive leukopathy of extremities*, is a common cause of acquired leukoderma seen in older patients and occasionally in young adults. It presents clinically with porcelain-white, guttate, oval-to-round lesions 2 to 5 mm in diameter present over the sun-exposed area of extremities. The number of lesions tends to increase with age. Although the lesions are asymptomatic, it is a cause of cosmetic concern for the patient. Etiology of this disorder is largely unknown. Multiple factors have been implicated such as HLA DQ 3, trauma, chronic sun exposure, and autoimmunity. Light microscopy reveals hyperkeratotic stratum corneum, atrophic epidermis, and flattened rete ridges. Decrease in the number of melanocytes and melanin content is noted in the lesions. The dermis shows changes of actinic damage such as elastorrhexis, collagen homogenization, and basophilia.

Progressive Macular Hypomelanosis

It is an acquired cause of hypomelanosis presenting commonly in individuals of mixed genetic background with skin type IV to VI. Common synonyms of this condition include *idiopathic multiple large macule hypomelanosis, nummular and confluent hypomelanosis of the trunk, cutis trunci variata*, and *creole dyschromia*. The etiology of this disorder is largely unknown. The presence of hormonal influences and *Propionibacterium* spp. has been implicated, although the exact pathogenic factors still need to be identified. It presents clinically with round, pale, coalescent macules over the back and less frequently on the abdomen. The lesions tend to be confluent in the midline. Microscopy reveals disruption in the maturation and distribution of melanosomes in the lesional skin. The clinical course of this disorder is unpredictable; spontaneous cure is reported over decades to years.

Chemical Leukoderma

The lesions present as depigmented macules initially developing at the sites of contact with industrial chemicals such as phenols, catechol, and hydroquinone. The lesions later spread to distant sites. The lesions are depigmented and clinically resemble vitiligo. Careful history is thus important in establishing the diagnosis. History of exposure to offending chemicals, along with similar history in other people at the workplace, is crucial in establishing the diagnosis.

Vitiligo is the subject of a separate chapter.

MANAGEMENT STRATEGY

The importance of a good history and thorough clinical examination cannot be underestimated when dealing with hypopigmented dermatosis. Detailed history regarding the age of onset, history of preceding lesions, associated symptoms, exposure to chemicals, family history, etc., is indispensable for reaching a correct diagnosis. Detailed note of the nature of pigmentary loss (hypo/depigmentation); site and distribution of lesions; and presence of associated findings such as induration, scaling, and sensory loss is to be made to reach a correct diagnosis.

Wood lamp examination helps to differentiate between hypopigmented and depigmented lesions. Progressive macular hypomelanosis displays punctate red fluorescence, whereas pityriasis versicolor displays a coppery-orange hue. Confocal laser scanning microscopy helps to access the melanin content and distribution patterns. Histopathology aids in identifying the primary disease process.

Sun exposure helps in repigmentation of lesions when there are residual functional melanocytes. Ultraviolet light stimulates melanocytes and melanin synthesis. However, overexposure may also carry a risk of increased color contrast due to skin tanning.

First-Line Therapies

- Photochemotherapy — D
- Topical corticosteroids — D
- Topical calcineurin inhibitors — D

Laser resurfacing induced hypopigmentation: histologic alterations and repigmentation with topical photochemotherapy. Grimes PE, Bhawan J, Kim J, Chiu M, Lask G. Dermatol Surg 2001; 27: 515–20.

Ten patients of post–laser resurfacing hypopigmentation were included in the study. Baseline biopsies were performed and accessed for epidermal melanin content, melanophages in dermis, perivascular inflammation, and dermal fibrosis. Patients underwent treatment with topical 0.001% 8 methoxypsoralen twice a week. The hydrophilic ointment was applied on the lesions for 30 minutes followed by ultraviolet A exposure at an initial dose of 0.2 to 0.5 J/cm^2 and increased by 0.2 to 0.5 J/cm^2 weekly. Topical photochemotherapy-induced moderate to excellent repigmentation was seen in 71% of patients. Adverse effects reported were minimal.

Topical 0.05% clobetasol propionate versus 1% pimecrolimus ointment in vitiligo. Coskun B, Saral Y, Turgut D. Eur J Dermatol 2005; 15: 88–91.

Ten vitiligo patients with bilaterally symmetric lesions were included in the study. Clobetasol propionate 0.05% was applied twice daily on the right side, whereas 1% pimecrolimus ointment was applied twice daily on the left side. Both sides showed comparable repigmentation at the end of the study.

Pilot trial of 1% pimecrolimus cream in the treatment of seborrheic dermatitis in African American adults with associated hypopigmentation. High WA, Pandya AG. J Am Acad Dermatol 2006; 54: 1083–8.

Five African Americans suffering from seborrheic dermatitis with hypopigmentation were in the pilot trial. Pimecrolimus was applied on the affected areas twice daily for 16 weeks. Hypopigmentation was assessed using a Mexameter. Marked improvement was noted 2 weeks onward.

Second-Line Therapies

- Laser — D
- Cosmetic camouflage — B
- Melanocyte grafting — C

The safety and efficacy of the 308-nm excimer laser for pigment correction of hypopigmented scars and striae alba. Alexiades-Armenakas MR, Bernstein LJ, Friedman PM, Geronemus RG. Arch Dermatol 2004; 140: 955–60.

Total of 31 adults with hypopigmented scars (22) and striae alba (9) were enrolled. Lesions were treated with xenon chloride excimer laser (308 nm, 3.2 cm², 30 ns). Initially treatment was started at 50 mJ/cm² minus the minimal erythema dose of the patient. Treatment was done biweekly until 50% to 75% pigment reaction was obtained, followed by two weekly sessions until a maximum of 10 treatment sessions, 75% calorimetric measurement, and 100% visual pigment correction. If no improvement was noted, the dose was increased by 50 mJ/cm² per treatment; otherwise, the same dose was maintained. Posttreatment evaluation was done in 1, 2, and 4 months. Statistically significant improvement was noted using colorimetric analysis after the first treatment. Sixty percent to 70% visual improvement was noted compared with control sites.

Melanocyte autologous grafting for treatment of leukoderma. Suvanprakorn P, Dee-Ananlap S, Pongsomboon C, Klaus SN. J Am Acad Dermatol 1985; 13: 968–74.

Patients with vitiligo, idiopathic guttate hypomelanosis, and postinflammatory hypomelanosis were included in the study. Blisters were created by suction/liquid nitrogen at the affected and healthy site. The roof of the bullae from the donor site was transferred to the affected area. Repigmentation was noted 7 to 14 days later.

Cosmetic camouflage. Antoniou C, Stefanaki C. J Cosmet Dermatol 2006; 5: 297–301.

A good cosmetic camouflage has been shown to be helpful for patients not relieved by conventional treatment, especially when a lesion is located over a cosmetically important site such as the face. The products may be oil or water based, depending on the skin type.

Evidence Levels: **A** Double-blind study **B** Clinical trial ≥ 20 subjects **C** Clinical trial < 20 subjects **D** Series ≥ 5 subjects **E** Anecdotal case reports

112

Ichthyoses

Rajani Nalluri, Georgina Devlin, Timothy H. Clayton

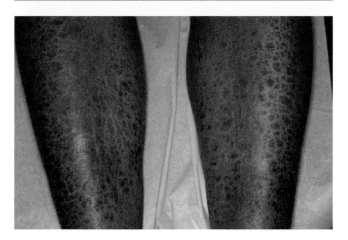

The ichthyoses represent a group of disorders of keratinization characterized by scaly skin. They may be inherited or acquired. Severity and extent vary widely from mild ichthyosis vulgaris (IV) to life-threatening harlequin ichthyosis. Inherited ichthyosis is classified broadly into syndromic and nonsyndromic ichthyosis, keratinopathic ichthyosis, and autosomal-recessive congenital ichthyosis. Whole genome sequencing is a comprehensive approach to diagnosing inherited ichthyoses at an early stage; a gene therapy approach and topical targeted therapy are future treatments with the potential to alleviate and even prevent disease in susceptible individuals.

MANAGEMENT STRATEGY

The key to management, where possible, is to establish an exact diagnosis. This provides a platform to plan therapy, discuss prognosis, and consider genetic counseling. It is important to identify the age of onset; the presence or absence of collodion membrane; blistering or erythroderma in the neonatal period; and the type, color, and distribution of scale. Family members should be examined. The Ichthyosis Support Group (ISG) provides a support network for families with resources and information sheets (www.ichthyosis.org.uk). In the United States families should contact the Foundation for Ichthyosis and Related Skin Types (FIRST) (www.firstskinfoundation.org).

Causative genes for a number of the inherited ichthyoses have recently been identified. IV is the most common disorder of cornification, with an incidence of 1:250. It is not usually present at birth. Clinical features include dry skin with associated fine white powdery scale on extensor surfaces, palmar hyperlinearity, and keratosis pilaris. Mutations in the *filament aggregating protein (filaggrin) gene (FLG)* have recently been identified as the cause of IV. Loss-of-function mutations in FLG have also been strongly associated with atopic dermatitis. Patients with ichthyosis have reduced epidermal barrier function, increased transepidermal water loss, and reduced pliability of the stratum corneum and hyperkeratosis. Topical treatment involves hydration, lubrication, and keratolysis. Emollients are widely used as a first-line

treatment. The effect of moisturizers in atopic dermatitis and related disorders has been documented in a large number of clinical trials of varying design and quality, but data are lacking on comparisons among different emollients. In mild to moderate cases urea-containing emollients alone are often sufficient, as they may have a humectant and keratolytic effect. Increasing the environmental humidity has also been shown to be beneficial. *Emollient baths* aid in softening the stratum corneum and facilitate mechanical debridement of thickened hyperkeratosis.

Keratolytics such as salicylic acid, urea, lactic acid, and propylene glycol reduce the adhesion of keratinocytes. However, because of the impaired barrier function, care should be taken to prevent salicylate toxicity. We do not advocate the use of topical salicylic acid in children due to the increased surface area–to–volume ratio. Cutaneous infection occurs as a result of impaired barrier function, and consideration should be given to prophylactic measures, such as antiseptic soaps or baths. Skin infection may require topical and systemic *antibacterials*, particularly *in epidermolytic ichthyosis (EI) (formerly referred to as epidermolytic hyperkeratosis, EHK)*, which often requires long-term antibiotic therapy.

Topical retinoids (e.g., tretinoin, adapalene, tazarotene) may be beneficial. *N*-acetylcysteine is a new addition to the topical treatments. They reduce the cohesiveness of epithelial cells, stimulate mitosis and turnover, and suppress keratin synthesis.

The severe ichthyoses usually respond to *systemic retinoid therapy. Acitretin* (1 mg/kg/day) and *isotretinoin* (1–2 mg/kg/day) have been shown to reduce scaling and discomfort and improve heat tolerance and sweating. However, recurrence of ichthyotic skin occurs on discontinuing treatment, thereby necessitating long-term use. Long-term treatment involves a higher risk of chronic skeletal toxicity, such as calcification of tendons and ligaments, hyperostoses, and osteoporosis, which requires regular monitoring. *Alitretinoin* may provide a safer alternative to a*citretin*, and further studies are necessary to assess its efficacy.

Retinoic acid metabolism-blocking agents have been shown to inhibit the cytochrome P450-dependent 4-hydroxylation of retinoic acid, resulting in increased tissue levels of retinoic acid and a reduction in epidermal proliferation and scaling. *Liarozole* showed clinical improvement and tolerability in a recent phase II/III trial.

Acquired ichthyoses are associated with a number of systemic disorders, including HIV, malignancy, sarcoidosis, leprosy, thyroid disease, hyperparathyroidism, nutritional disorders, chronic renal failure, and autoimmune diseases. They will often improve with treatment of the underlying condition. There have been few publications in recent years relating to acquired ichthyosis.

Specific Investigations

- Follow algorithm (see the figure later)
- Genetic screening: refer to www.genetests.org
- Fatty alcohol: NAD + oxidoreductase activity (Sjögren–Larsson)
- Steroid sulfatase activity
- Vitamin D status

Acquired ichthyosis

- Malignancy screening
- Infection screen, including HIV
- Metabolic screening
- Skin biopsy

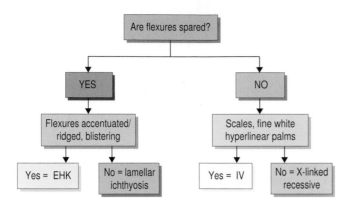

Are flexures spared?

YES → Flexures accentuated/ridged, blistering → Yes = EHK / No = lamellar ichthyosis

NO → Scales, fine white hyperlinear palms → Yes = IV / No = X-linked recessive

Revised nomenclature and classification of inherited ichthyoses: results of the First Ichthyosis Consensus Conference in Soréze 2009. Oji V, Tadini G, Akiyama M, Bardon CB, Bodemer C, Bourrat E, et al. J Am Acad Dermatol 2010; 69: 607–41.

A useful reference for all clinicians and an aid for future research.

Impact of next generation sequencing on diagnostics in a genetic skin disease clinic. Takeichi T, Nanda A, Liu L, Salam A, Campbell P, Fong K, et al. Exp Dermatol 2013; 22: 825–31.

The role of whole-exome sequencing as a comprehensive approach to diagnosing inherited skin diseases at an early stage is discussed.

Update on autosomal recessive congenital ichthyosis: mRNA analysis using hair samples is a powerful tool for genetic diagnosis. Sugiura K, Akiyama M. J Dermatol Sci 2015; 79: 4–9.

Autosomal recessive congenital ichthyosis (ARCI) includes harlequin ichthyosis, lamellar ichthyosis, and congenital ichthyosiform erythroderma. To date nine genes are causally associated with ARCI. This is an update on the molecular mechanisms, causative genes, clinical phenotypes, and possible effective therapies. It also discusses mRNA analysis of hair samples and next-generation sequencing as a genetic diagnosis method.

Expanding the keratin mutation database: novel and recurrent mutations and genotype–phenotype correlation in 28 patients with epidermolytic ichthyosis. Arin MJ, Oji V, Emmert S, Housser I, Traupe H, Krieg T, et al. Br J Dermatol 2011; 164: 442–7.

This paper discusses the identification of novel mutations and genotype–phenotype correlations in EHK, which allows improved understanding of disease pathogenesis and improved patient management.

Clinical expression and new SPINK5 splicing defects in Netherton syndrome: unmasking a frequent founder synonymous mutation and unconventional intronic mutations. Lacroix M, Lacaze-Buzy L, Furio L, Tron E, Valari M, Van der Weir G, et al. J Invest Dermatol 2012; 132: 575–82.

Netherton syndrome (NS) results from loss-of-function mutations in SPINK5 (serine protease inhibitor Kazal type 5), which encodes the serine protease inhibitor LEKTI (lymphoepithelial Kazal-type related inhibitor). A description of new SPINK5 defects in 12 patients, widening the clinical and molecular spectrum of NS.

The multifunctional role of filaggrin in allergic skin disease. McAleer MA, Irvine AD. J Allergy Clin Immunol 2013; 131: 280–91.

The role of mutations in the human filaggrin gene (FLG), which confer risk not only for atopic dermatitis but also for the associated allergic diseases of food allergy, asthma, and allergic rhinitis, is described.

Comprehensive analysis of the gene encoding filaggrin uncovers prevalent and rare mutations in ichthyosis vulgaris and atopic eczema. Sandilands A, Terron-Kwiatkowski A, Hull PR, O'Regan GM, Clayton TH, Watson RM, et al. Nature Genet 2007; 39: 650–4.

Common FLG null mutations cause ichthyosis vulgaris and predispose to eczema and secondary allergic diseases. This paper illustrates that the common European mutations are ancestral variants carried on conserved haplotypes.

Vitamin D deficiency and rickets in children and adolescents with ichthyosiform erythroderma in type IV and V skin. Chouhan K, Sethuraman G, Gupta N, Sharma VK, Kabra M, Khaitan BK, et al. Br J Dermatol 2012; 166: 608–15.

A controlled study examining the prevalence of vitamin D deficiency in adolescents with ichthyosiform erythroderma due to keratinizing disorders. All patients in the disease group had clinical, biochemical, or radiologic evidence of rickets.

The potential for vitamin D deficiency should be considered in patients with an ichthyotic disorder.

Acquired ichthyosis. Patel N, Spencer LA, English JC, Zirwas MJ. J Am Acad Dermatol 2006; 55: 647–56.

This review provides a useful algorithm for the evaluation of patients presenting with acquired ichthyosis.

First-Line Therapies	
• Humidification of environment	E
• Bathing/soaking	E
• Emollients	A

Association of glycerol and paraffin in the treatment of ichthyosis in children: an international, multicentric, randomized, controlled, double-blind study. Blanchet-Bardon C, Tadini G, Machado Matos M, Delarue A. J Eur Acad Dermatol Venereol. 2012; 26:1014-9.

This large study assessed the efficacy of a 15% glycerol and 10% paraffin (plus vehicle) emollient (Dexeryl) compared with placebo in a heterogeneous group of children with various ichthyotic disorders. Significant improvement was observed, and treatment was well tolerated.

Clinical effectiveness of moisturizers in atopic dermatitis and related disorders: a systematic review. Lindh JD, Bradley M. Am J Clin Dermatol 2015; 16: 341–59.

The majority of studies have shown that moisturizers have beneficial effects on clinical symptoms, and it is well documented for urea- and glycerin-based emollients.

Evidence Levels: **A** Double-blind study **B** Clinical trial ≥ 20 subjects **C** Clinical trial < 20 subjects **D** Series ≥ 5 subjects **E** Anecdotal case reports

Second-Line Therapies

- Keratolytics (salicylic acid [avoid in children], urea, α-hydroxy acids [e.g., lactic acid], propylene glycol)   A
- Topical retinoids (tretinoin, tazarotene)   C
- Topical liarozole   C
- Topical calcipotriol   C
- Topical N-acetylcysteine   D
- Topical pimecrolimus 1%   E
- Narrowband Ultraviolet B (UVB) phototherapy (Netherton syndrome)   E

Efficacy of urea therapy in children with ichthyosis. A multicenter randomized, placebo-controlled, double-blind, semilateral study. Kuster W, Bohnsack K, Rippke F, Upmeyer HJ, Groll S, Traupe H. Dermatology 1998; 196: 217–22.

Sixty children were treated for 8 weeks with 10% urea lotion on one side and lotion base on the other. Improvement was 78% after 8 weeks for 10% urea lotion and 72% for urea-free lotion base.

Improved topical treatment of lamellar ichthyosis: a double-blind study of four different cream formulations. Gånemo A, Virtanen M, Vahlquist A. Br J Dermatol 1999; 141: 1027–32.

Combination preparation of 5% lactic acid and 20% propylene glycol reduced scaling and dryness significantly and was preferred in most patients compared with 5% urea.

Treatment of ichthyosiform diseases with topically applied tazarotene: risk of systemic absorption. Nguyen V, Cunningham BB, Eichenfield LF, Alió AB, Buka RL. J Am Acad Dermatol 2007; 57: 123–5.

This open-label pilot study of nine patients showed that little systemic absorption was observed when tazarotene 0.05% or 0.1% cream or gel was used daily for 1 month on 20% to 90% body surface area (BSA). Treatment may be safe for longer, as the majority of patients were using it for over 12 months.

Successful topical adapalene treatment for the facial lesions of an adolescent case of epidermolytic ichthyosis. Ogawa M, Akiyama M. J Am Acad Dermatol 2014; 71: e103–5.

An adolescent with epidermolytic ichthyosis showed significant improvement of hyperkeratosis after 6 months of topical 0.1% adapalene gel.

Topical liarozole in ichthyosis: a double-blind, left–right comparative study followed by a long-term open maintenance study. Lucker GPH, Verfaille CJ, Heremans AMC, Vanhoutte FP, Boegheim JPJ, Steijlen PPM. Br J Dermatol 2005; 152: 566–9.

Liarozole 5% cream improved a range of ichthyoses in this study on 12 adults.

Successful treatment with topical N-acetylcysteine in urea in five children with congenital lamellar ichthyosis. Bassotti A, Moreno S, Criado E. Pediatr Dermatol 2011; 28: 451–5.

Topical 10% N-acetylcysteine emulsion prepared in urea 5% applied twice daily showed marked improvement in five children after 4 months.

The safety and efficacy of pimecrolimus 1%, cream for the treatment of Netherton syndrome. Yan AC, Honig PJ, Ming ME, Weber J, Shah KN. Arch Dermatol 2010; 146: 57–62.

A single-arm, open-label study of three children treated for a period of 18 months with 1% pimecrolimus. Treatment was well tolerated, with improvement in quality of life and severity scores. Serum levels of pimecrolimus were much lower than expected despite application to up to 50% BSA.

Narrowband UVB phototherapy as a novel treatment for Netherton syndrome. Kaminska EC, Ortel B, Sharma V, Stein SL. Photodermatol Photoimmunol Photomed 2012; 28: 162–4.

A case report of a 16-year-old patient with a clinical diagnosis of Netherton syndrome responsive to narrowband ultraviolet B (NB-UVB). Oral prednisolone (20 mg once daily) was started in a tapering dose at NB-UVB initiation. UVB was continued over a 4-year period.

The authors suggest NB-UVB may be useful for the atopic component of Netherton syndrome. Further studies are required.

Third-Line Therapies

- Acitretin/etretinate   B
- Isotretinoin   B
- Alitretinoin   E
- Liarozole   B

Oral retinoid therapy for disorders of keratinization: single-center retrospective 25 years' experience on 23 patients. Katugampola RP, Finlay AY. Br J Dermatol 2006; 154: 267–76.

This study provides the longest follow-up safety data on children and adults with disorders of keratinization on oral retinoid therapy. One patient developed diffuse idiopathic skeletal hyperostosis after 21 years of retinoid therapy. Abnormalities of the fasting lipid profile and liver function were seen in a small percentage.

Oral alitretinoin in congenital ichthyosis: a pilot study shows variable effects and risk of central hypothyroidism. Gånemo A, Sommerlund M, Vahlquist A. Acta Derm Venereol 2012; 92: 256–7.

An uncontrolled study of four patients with ichthyosis treated with alitretinoin 10 to 30 mg once daily. If no improvement was observed after 1 month, the dose was increased to 40 to 60 mg daily. Higher doses were needed in patients with lamellar ichthyosis. Thyroid disturbance was observed in two of the cases.

Alitretinoin may be an alternative to acitretin in those contemplating pregnancy and has a quicker washout period. Further trial data are required.

Oral liarozole in the treatment of patients with moderate/severe lamellar ichthyosis: results of a randomized, double-blind, multinational, placebo-controlled phase II/III trial. Vahlquist A, Blockhuys S, Steijlen P, van Rossem K, Didona B, Blanco D, et al. Br J Dermatol 2014; 170: 173–81.

Once-daily oral liarozole, 75 and 150 mg, improved scaling and Dermatology Life Quality Index (DLQI) and was well tolerated in patients with moderate/severe lamellar ichthyosis, although the primary efficacy variable was not statistically significant in this study involving 64 patients.

Oral liarozole versus acitretin in the treatment of ichthyosis: a phase II/III multicenter, double-blind, randomized, active-controlled study. Verfaille CJ, Vanhoutte FP, Blanchet-Bardon C, van Steensel MA, Steijlen PM. Br J Dermatol 2007; 156: 965–73.

Thirty-two patients were randomized to either liarozole 75 mg twice daily or acitretin 10 mg in the morning and 2 5mg at night for 12 weeks. Improvement was seen in both groups. Retinoid side effects were observed less frequently in the liarozole group.

Sjögren–Larsson syndrome: a study of clinical symptoms and dermatologic treatment in 34 Swedish patients. Gänemo A, Jagell Vahlquist A. Acta Derm Venereol 2009; 89: 68–73.

An observational study of all patients with Sjögren-Larsson syndrome (SLS) in Sweden. Fifty-six percent of patients were on oral acitretin (10 mg/week–25 mg once daily). The majority improved on introduction of acitretin, and ichthyosis severity scores were lower than in those not on oral retinoids.

This study is a useful reference regarding clinical variation, treatment, and long-term follow-up of a large cohort of patients with SLS.

High survival rate of harlequin ichthyosis in Japan. Shibata A, Ogawa Y, Sugiura K, Muro Y, Abe R, Suzuki T, et al. J Am Acad Dermatol 2014; 70: 387–8.

In this study, 91.7% of patients who were administered systemic retinoids survived, whereas only 50% who did not receive oral retinoids survived. Of these 62.5% received intensive care in a neonatal intensive care unit (NICU).

Improving outcomes for harlequin ichthyosis. Milstone LM, Choate KA. J Am Acad Dermatol 2013; 69: 808–9.

The article describes respiratory failure as a major contributing factor in 50% of neonatal deaths and suggests a lower threshold for considering intubation and intensive neonatal care.

Harlequin ichthyosis: a review of clinical and molecular findings in 45 cases. Rajpopat S, Moss C, Mellerio J, Vahlquist A, Gånemo A, Hellstrom-Pigg M, et al. Arch Dermatol 2011; 147: 681–6.

A review of 45 cases of harlequin ichthyosis. Overall survival rate was 56%. Ages of survivors ranged between 10 months and 25 years at the time of the study. Early introduction of oral retinoids may improve survival. All deaths were associated with homozygous mutations.

Evidence Levels: **A** Double-blind study **B** Clinical trial ≥ 20 subjects **C** Clinical trial < 20 subjects **D** Series ≥ 5 subjects **E** Anecdotal case reports

113

Impetigo

Michael Sladden, Robert M. Burd

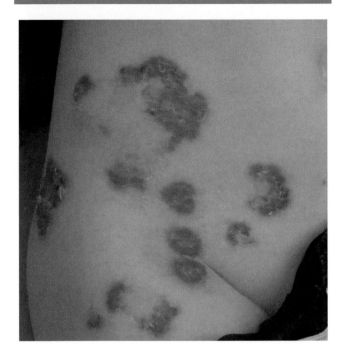

Impetigo is a common superficial bacterial infection of the skin, caused by *Staphylococcus aureus* or *Streptococcus pyogenes*. The infection is highly contagious and can easily spread to other body sites or close contacts. Impetigo usually affects children but can occur in people of any age. The worldwide population of children suffering from impetigo at any one time is estimated at 162 million, making impetigo a global major public health problem.

Impetigo can be primary, with direct bacterial invasion of previously normal skin, or secondary, where infection develops when the skin barrier is disrupted by underlying disease, such as scabies.

Impetigo is classified as nonbullous or bullous. In the more common nonbullous form, thin-walled vesicles rupture to form superficial erosions with yellowish-brown crusts, which eventually heal without scarring. Bullous impetigo is characterized by larger bullae or blisters, which may continue to develop for several days.

Most cases of nonbullous impetigo are caused by *S. aureus* but *S. pyogenes, alone or in combination with S. aureus,* may also be implicated. In cooler climates, staphylococcal impetigo predominates, whereas in warmer and more humid climates, streptococcal impetigo is more common. Bullous impetigo is almost always caused by exfoliative toxin-producing strains of *S. aureus*. Secondary impetigo is usually caused by *S. aureus*.

MANAGEMENT STRATEGY

The main aim of treatment is to eradicate the infecting bacteria to allow rapid skin healing and control the spread of infection. The ideal treatment should be effective, inexpensive, easily accessible, have limited adverse effects, and not promote bacterial resistance.

This requires the use of an appropriate antimicrobial delivered in an effective manner. Antibiotics may be administered either orally or topically. The choice between topical or oral therapy depends on:

- The experience of the practitioner
- The preference of the patient
- The extent and severity of the disease
- The local bacterial resistance patterns
- The cost and availability of local resources

Topical or oral antibiotics with proven efficacy against *S. aureus* are the first choice of therapy. It is reasonable to use short courses of topical antibiotics for mild, limited impetigo, while reserving oral antibiotics for recalcitrant, extensive disease. Globally, the majority of isolates of *S. aureus* are resistant to penicillin, and erythromycin resistance is also becoming more common. It is important to consider local patterns of antibiotic resistance when choosing appropriate therapy.

In developing countries, where *Streptococcus* is often the predominant pathogen, topical agents are expensive and may be unavailable. Treatment strategies have to be sufficiently flexible to meet local needs.

Historically, topical treatment of impetigo was difficult due to bacterial resistance and contact sensitivity to topical agents. More recently introduced topical antibiotics appear as effective as traditional oral antibiotics. When used in courses of less than 2 weeks, bacterial resistance does not seem to be a major problem. Recent studies of topical retapamulin indicate that it is effective and safe in the treatment of primary impetigo.

Strains of bacteria causing impetigo are often extremely virulent. Patients therefore need to be educated on personal hygiene methods to avoid the spread of infection. Evidence regarding the value of disinfecting measures is limited. However, common sense would indicate that cleaning lesional skin with soap and water or a mild, nonirritant antiseptic will aid the application of topical antibiotics and reduce the spread of infection.

Nasal carriage of *S. aureus* occurs in a high proportion of both patients and asymptomatic family members. Therefore in recurrent cases or multiple familial cases, *treatment of nasal and pharyngeal carriage* may be necessary.

Increasingly, methicillin-resistant *Staphylococcus aureus* (MRSA) has become an important cause of impetigo. MRSA poses a challenge because of its enhanced virulence and resistance to standard antibiotic therapy. Antibiotic treatment should be guided by knowledge of the likely causative agent and local resistance patterns, as well as bacterial susceptibility testing.

Specific Investigations

- Skin swabs for microbiologic assessment (Gram stain), culture, and sensitivity
- Nasal swabs from patients and immediate relatives in recalcitrant cases

A Gram stain of a swab from the lesion or exudate will reveal gram-positive cocci, confirming the clinical diagnosis. Bacterial culture and sensitivity from a pretreatment swab are useful to assess suitable alternative antibiotics in cases that do not respond to conventional treatment.

Interventions for impetigo (Cochrane Review). Koning S, van der Sande R, Verhagen AP, van Suijlekom-Smit LW, Morris AD, Butler CC, et al. Cochrane Database Syst Rev 2012; 1: CD003261.

Reviews the epidemiology and treatment of impetigo. Worldwide, bacteria causing impetigo show increasing rates of resistance for commonly used antibiotics. No resistance has yet been reported for retapamulin.

The global epidemiology of impetigo: a systematic review of the population prevalence of impetigo and pyoderma. Bowen AC, Mahé A, Hay RJ, Andrews RM, Steer AC, Tong SY, et al. PLoS One 2015; 28; 10: e0136789.

The global prevalence of childhood impetigo is estimated to be in excess of 162 million.

Contemporary causes of skin and soft tissue infections in North America, Latin America, and Europe: report from the SENTRY Antimicrobial Surveillance Program (1998–2004). Moet GJ, Jones RN, Biedenbach DJ, Stilwell MG, Fritsche TR. Diagn Microbiol Infect Dis 2007; 57:7–13.

Antimicrobial surveillance confirms that *S. aureus* is the predominant pathogen causing skin and soft tissue infections in all studied geographic areas.

Impetigo in epidemic and nonepidemic phases: an incidence study over 4½ years in a general population. Rortveit S, Rortveit G. Br J Dermatol 2007; 157: 100–5.

S. aureus was the causal bacterium in 89% (117/132) and 68% (84/123) of impetigo cases during epidemic and nonepidemic periods, respectively (*p* < 0.01). *S. aureus* was resistant to fusidic acid in 84% (98/117) and 64% (54/84) of cases in epidemic and nonepidemic periods, respectively (*p* < 0.01).

DNA heterogeneity of *Staphylococcus aureus* strains evaluated by Sma1 and SgrA1 pulsed field gel electrophoresis in patients with impetigo. Capoluongo E, Giglio A, Leonetti F, Belardi M, Giannetti A, Caprilli F, et al. Res Microbiol 2000; 151: 53–61.

Samples from lesional skin, nose, and pharynx were taken from 26 patients and their families, and the strain of *S. aureus* was typed; 54% of the patients had the same strain in both the nose and the lesion. In over half the families at least one other family member was found to be carrying the same strain as the patient's lesion.

NVC-422 topical gel for the treatment of impetigo. Iovino SM, Krantz KD, Blanco DM, Fernández JA, Ocampo N, Najafi A, et al. Int J Clin Exp Pathol 2011; 4: 587–95.

In 129 patients with clinically diagnosed impetigo, the majority of the infections were caused by *S. aureus* alone (106/125, 85%), of which 10% were MRSA.

First-Line Therapies	
• Topical mupirocin, fusidic acid, or retapamulin	A
• Oral flucloxacillin, cloxacillin, dicloxacillin, cephalexin, or erythromycin	A

Interventions for impetigo (Cochrane Review). Koning S, van der Sande R, Verhagen AP, van Suijlekom-Smit LW, Morris AD, Butler CC, et al. Cochrane Database Syst Rev 2012; 1: CD003261.

A systematic review of 68 trials, including 5578 participants, reporting on 50 different treatments, including placebo. There is good evidence that topical mupirocin and topical fusidic acid are equal to, or possibly more effective than, oral antibiotics for people with limited impetigo. Fusidic acid, mupirocin, and retapamulin are probably equally effective. Due to lack of studies in patients with extensive impetigo, it is unclear whether oral antibiotics are superior to topical antibiotics in this group.

No clear preference can be given for B-lactamase–resistant narrow-spectrum penicillins such as flucloxacillin, cloxacillin, or dicloxacillin or for broad-spectrum penicillins such as amoxicillin with clavulanic acid, cephalosporins, or macrolides. Penicillin was not as effective as most other antibiotics.

Impetigo: diagnosis and treatment. Hartman-Adams H, Banvard C, Juckett G. Am Fam Physician 2014; 15; 90: 229–35.

This review tabulates treatment regimens for impetigo.

Treatment of impetigo: oral antibiotics most commonly prescribed. Bolaji RS, Dabade TS, Gustafson CJ, Davis SA, Krowchuk DP, Feldman SR. J Drugs Dermatol 2012; 11: 489–94.

Oral antibiotics are the most common class of medications used to treat impetigo. There is an opportunity for physicians to take advantage of the equally efficacious topical antibiotics for treating impetigo. A shift toward topical antibiotics would likely decrease adverse effects associated with use of oral agents.

Common skin infections in children. Sladden MJ, Johnston GA. Br Med J 2004; 329: 95–9.

The authors suggest using topical mupirocin TID (three times per day) or fusidic acid TID for 7 days in mild impetigo. Oral antibiotics should be reserved for recalcitrant or extensive disease.

Topical retapamulin ointment, 1%, versus sodium fusidate ointment, 2%, for impetigo: a randomized, observer-blinded, noninferiority study. Oranje AP, Chosidow O, Sacchidanand S, Todd G, Singh K, Scangarella N, et al. Dermatology 2007; 215: 331–40.

Retapamulin 1% ointment BID (twice daily) for 5 days and sodium fusidate ointment 2% TID for 7 days had comparable clinical efficacies (94.8% and 90.1%). Success rates in the small numbers of sodium fusidate-, methicillin, and mupirocin-resistant *S. aureus* were good for retapamulin (9/9, 8/8, and 6/6, respectively). Both drugs were well tolerated. Retapamulin is a highly effective and convenient new treatment option for impetigo, with efficacy against isolates resistant to existing therapies.

Topical retapamulin ointment (1% wt/wt) twice daily for 5 days versus oral cephalexin twice daily for 10 days in the treatment of secondarily infected dermatitis: results of a randomized controlled trial. Parish LC, Jorizzo JL, Breton JJ, Hirman JW, Scangarella NE, Shawar RM, et al. J Am Acad Dermatol 2006; 55: 1003–13.

Retapamulin was as effective as cephalexin 500 mg BID (clinical success rates: 85.9% and 89.7%, respectively) in the treatment of patients with secondarily infected dermatitis. Microbiologic success rates were 87.2% for retapamulin and 91.8% for cephalexin. Retapamulin was well tolerated, and the topical formulation was preferred over the oral drug.

Topical mupirocin treatment of impetigo is equal to oral erythromycin therapy. Mertz PM, Marshall DA, Eaglstein WH, Piovanetti Y, Montalvo J. Arch Dermatol 1989; 125: 1069–73.

Seventy-five patients were treated in an investigator-blinded study comparing topical mupirocin applied three times daily with oral erythromycin 30 to 50 mg/kg daily. The mupirocin-treated patients experienced similar clinical results to those

370

treated with oral erythromycin, although mupirocin was superior in the microbiological eradication of *S. aureus*.

The emergence of resistance to penicillin and erythromycin is so common in isolates of S. aureus *that alternative antibiotics should be considered.*

Second-Line Therapies

- Intravenous antibiotics   **C**
- Other oral antibiotics, depending on sensitivity, including rifampicin and fusidic acid   **B**
- Topical antiseptics   **B**

Fusidic acid tablets in patients with skin and soft-tissue infection: a dose-finding study. Carr WD, Wall AR, Georgala-Zervogiani S, Stratigos J, Gouriotou K. Eur J Clin Res 1994; 5: 87–95.

Fusidic acid tablets, 250 mg twice daily, 500 mg twice daily, and 500 mg thrice daily, were compared in a randomized, double-blind study in 617 patients with skin and soft tissue infections. Each treatment was given for 5 to 10 days. Cure rates after 5 days of treatment were 34.7%, 37.8%, and 37.2%, respectively. End of treatment cure rates were 75.5%, 81.1%, and 74.0%, respectively.

Addition of rifampin to cephalexin therapy for recalcitrant staphylococcal skin infections – an observation. Feder Jr HM, Pond KE. Clin Pediatr 1996; 35: 205–8.

Two children with staphylococcal infections failing to respond to standard antibiotics responded when rifampin was added.

Hydrogen peroxide cream: an alternative to topical antibiotics in the treatment of impetigo contagiosa. Christensen OB, Anehus S. Acta Dermatol Venereol 1994; 74: 460–2.

A prospective comparison of hydrogen peroxide 1% cream with fusidic acid 2% cream (both applied two to three times daily) in 256 patients with impetigo. Over a 3-week treatment period, 92 patients of 128 (72%) in the hydrogen peroxide group were classified as healed, compared with 105 of 128 (82%) in the fusidic acid group. This difference was not statistically significant.

Effect of handwashing on child health: a randomised controlled trial. Luby SP, Agboatwalla M, Feikin DR, Painter J, Billhimer W, Altaf A, et al. Lancet 2005; 366: 225–33.

In squatter settlements in Karachi, children younger than 15 years in households that received plain soap and handwashing promotion had a 34% lower incidence of impetigo than controls (95% CI, –52% to –16%).

Third-Line Therapy

- Systemic antibiotic, topical antibiotic plus a formal antistaphylococcal regimen to reduce nasal and pharyngeal carriage to prevent cross infection   **E**

Use of 0.3% triclosan (Bacti-Stat) to eradicate an outbreak of methicillin-resistant *Staphylococcus aureus* in a neonatal nursery. Zafar AB, Butler RC, Reese DJ, Gaydos LA, Mennonna PA. Am J Infect Control 1995; 23: 200–8.

A nosocomial outbreak of infection with MRSA in a neonatal nursery proved difficult to control even with aggressive conventional measures. Additional use of a handwashing and bathing soap containing 0.3% triclosan immediately ended the outbreak.

Prevention and control of nosocomial infection caused by methicillin-resistant *Staphylococcus aureus* in a premature infant ward: preventive effect of a povidone-iodine wipe of neonatal skin. Aihara M, Sakai M, Iwasaki M, Shimakawa K, Kozaki S, Kubo M, et al. Postgrad Med J 1993; 69: S117–21.

An outbreak of MRSA causing impetigo was halted by wiping the body surface of the infants once daily with a diluted Isodine solution (10% povidone–iodine; 1:100 dilution).

Treatment of bullous impetigo and the staphylococcal scalded skin syndrome in infants. Johnston GA. Expert Rev Anti Infect Ther 2004; 2: 439–46.

It is important to swab the skin for bacteriologic confirmation and antibiotic sensitivities. Nasal swabs from the patient and immediate relatives should be performed to identify asymptomatic nasal carriers of *Staphylococcus aureus*. In the case of outbreaks on wards and in nurseries, health care professionals should also be swabbed.

Failure of first-line therapy suggests the presence of bacterial resistance or poor patient compliance. The choice of antibiotic should be based on the sensitivities of organisms cultured from the pretreatment swab. In recurrent cases, consider the possibility of nasal or pharyngeal colonization with pathogenic S. aureus *in either the patient or a close family member. This may require eradication by the use of a systemic antibiotic in conjunction with the nasal application of a topical antibiotic and an antiseptic skin cleanser. Topical antiseptics have also proved useful in nosocomial outbreaks.*

An example of a 5-day Staphylococcus *decolonization procedure used by one of the authors (MS) consists of daily hair and body washing with 4% chlorhexidine solution and thrice-daily application of nasal mupirocin ointment. Personal clothing and underwear, towels, washcloths, and bed linens are washed daily for 5 days. For resistant cases, oral antibiotics are also used (rifampicin 300 mg BID and fusidic acid 500 mg BID).*

114

Inducible urticarias, aquagenic pruritus, and cholinergic pruritus

Clive E.H. Grattan, Frances Lawlor

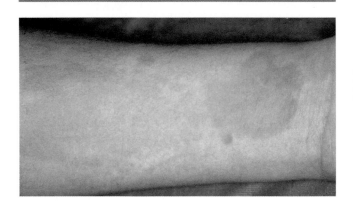

INDUCIBLE URTICARIAS

About 25% of patients with chronic urticaria have a definable and reproducible inducing trigger that distinguishes them from those with spontaneous urticaria and urticarial vasculitis. Inducible urticarias are defined by the predominant inducing stimulus (Table 114.1). More than one inducing stimulus elicits urticaria in some patients, and inducible urticarias can overlap with spontaneous urticaria. Physical urticarias caused by a physical stimulus (symptomatic dermographism, delayed pressure, heat and cold contact and solar urticarias, and vibratory angioedema) are now included within the inducible urticarias.

MANAGEMENT STRATEGY

Pharmacologic

The presentation of inducible urticarias may vary in morphology and severity. Milder forms may require little more than

avoidance of triggers and a preemptive dose of H_1 *antihistamine* before anticipated exposure, whereas a very severe attack involving anaphylaxis could potentially require emergency treatment with *intramuscular epinephrine (adrenaline)*. Acute presentations of severe inducible urticaria may require short courses of *oral corticosteroids* (e.g., prednisolone 0.5 mg/kg body weight daily for 5 days) in addition to regular nonsedating H_1 antihistamines. Drug management should be guided by the degree of disability or impairment in quality of life.

Nonpharmacologic

The triggering stimulus should be avoided where possible. Cold tolerance induction in cold urticaria and exercise tolerance induction in cholinergic urticaria has been described but is difficult to achieve and sustain. There is no evidence that exclusion diets are effective.

Specific Investigations

- Challenge (provocation) tests
- Blood tests (cryoproteins, specific IgE)

With the exceptions of testing for cryoglobulins in cold urticaria and specific IgE in food- and exercise-induced anaphylaxis, laboratory investigations are unnecessary and should not be undertaken except to monitor treatment or screen for eligibility (e.g., glucose-6-phosphatase dehydrogenase in patients being considered for dapsone or sulfasalazine).

The EAACI/GA(2) LEN/EDF/WAO Guideline for the definition, classification, diagnosis, and management of urticaria: the 2013 revision and update. Zuberbier T, Aberer W, Asero R, Bindslev-Jensen C, Brzoza Z, Canonica GW, et al. Allergy 2014; 69: 868–87.

The latest and most quoted European guideline on urticaria.

The definition, diagnostic testing and management of chronic inducible urticarias—update and revision of the EAACI/GA(2) LEN/EDF/UNEV 2009 consensus panel recommendations. Magerl M, Altrichter S, Borzova E, Giménez-Arnau A, Grattan CE, Lawlor F. Allergy 2016; 71: 780–802.

A comprehensive updated summary of provocation testing protocols.

Table 114.1 Classification of inducible urticarias by the eliciting stimulus (in approximate reducing frequency of occurrence)

Symptomatic dermographism	Stroking or rubbing the skin
Cholinergic urticaria (pale, papular wheals with red flares)	Rise in core temperature and other causes of sweating (exercise, hot baths, spicy food, and stress)
Cold urticaria	Rewarming of skin after cooling (localized or systemic)
Delayed pressure urticaria	Sustained perpendicular pressure
Solar urticaria	Ultraviolet or visible solar radiation
Localized heat urticaria	Local heat contact
Aquagenic urticaria	Local water contact at any temperature
Exercise-induced anaphylaxis	Exercise, but not hot baths
Food- and exercise-induced anaphylaxis	Exercise after a heavy food load or eating specific foods
Vibratory angioedema	Vibration

Evidence Levels: **A** Double-blind study   **B** Clinical trial ≥ 20 subjects   **C** Clinical trial < 20 subjects   **D** Series ≥ 5 subjects   **E** Anecdotal case reports

Cold urticaria syndromes: historical background, diagnostic classification, clinical and laboratory characteristics, pathogenesis and management. Wanderer AA. J Allergy Clin Immunol 1990; 85: 965–81.

A review of cold urticaria and its investigation.

Food-dependent exercise-induced anaphylaxis. Kidd JM, Cohen SH, Sosman AJ, Fink JN. J Allergy Clin Immunol 1983; 71: 407–11.

Anaphylaxis may rarely result from exercise after a heavy food load or eating certain foods (e.g., wheat, prawns, beef) for which specific IgE can be demonstrated by skin prick or ImmunoCAP testing.

First-Line Therapy

- Nonsedating ("second generation") antihistamines   **A**

Nonsedating antihistamines (Table 114.2) should always be prescribed in preference to classical antihistamines, which are often sedating and can impair psychomotor performance. Up-dosing of second-generation H_1 antihistamines is now widely practiced, although sedation at higher-than-licensed doses is a potential risk.

Therapeutic effects of cetirizine in delayed pressure urticaria: clinicopathological findings. Kontou-Fili K, Maniatakou G, Demaka P, Gonianakis M, Palaiologos G, Aroni K. J Am Acad Dermatol 1991; 24: 1090–3.

A double-blind, placebo-controlled study in 11 patients, showing a reduction in weight-induced wheal area and lesional eosinophil numbers on cetirizine 10 mg three times daily.

High-dose desloratadine decreases wheal volume and improves cold provocation thresholds compared with standard-dose treatment in patients with acquired cold urticaria: a randomized, placebo-controlled, cross-over study. Siebenhaar F, Degener F, Zuberbier T, Martus P, Maurer M. J Allergy Clin Immunol 2009; 123: 672–9.

Fourfold up-dosing a second-generation antihistamine has additional inhibitory effects on wheal formation in cold urticaria.

Rupatadine and its effects on symptom control, stimulation time, and temperature thresholds in patients with acquired cold urticaria. Metz M, Scholz E, Ferrán M, Izquierdo I, Giménez-Arnau A, Maurer M. Ann Allergy Asthma Immunol 2010; 104: 86–92.

A crossover, randomized, double-blind, placebo-controlled study of double-dose rupatadine, a second-generation H_1 antihistamine. Fifty-two percent of patients showed a complete response.

Table 114.2 Examples of nonsedating and mildly sedating H_1 antihistamines

Acrivastine	Nonsedating, three-times-daily dosing
Bilastine	Nonsedating, once-daily dosing
Cetirizine	Mildly sedating, once-daily dosing
Levocetirizine	The active enantiomer of cetirizine
Fexofenadine	Nonsedating, once-daily dosing
Loratadine	Nonsedating, once-daily dosing
Desloratadine	The active metabolite of loratadine
Mizolastine	Nonsedating, once-daily dosing
Rupatadine	Nonsedating, once-daily dosing

There was also a significant improvement in critical cold stimulation time and critical temperature threshold.

Second-Line Therapies

Symptomatic dermographism

• Narrowband UVB phototherapy	C
• Omalizumab	D
• H_2 antihistamines	B

Cholinergic urticaria

• Danazol	B
• Omalizumab	D
• Anticholinergics	E

Cold urticaria

• Omalizumab	D
• Leukotriene receptor antagonists	E
• Antibiotics "curative therapy"	E
• Cold tolerance (desensitization)	E

Heat urticaria

• Omalizumab	D

Delayed pressure urticaria

• Omalizumab	D
• Leukotriene receptor antagonists	B
• Sulfasalazine	C
• Dapsone	C

Solar urticaria

• Induction of tolerance (phototherapy and photochemotherapy)	D
• Omalizumab	D

Narrow-band ultraviolet B phototherapy is beneficial in antihistamine-resistant symptomatic dermographism: a pilot study. Borzova E, Rutherford A, Konstantinou G, Leslie K, Grattan CEH. J Am Acad Dermatol 2008; 59: 752–7.

A small open study of H_1 antihistamine–unresponsive symptomatic dermographism showing subjective and objective improvement in itch and whealing after 6 weeks' treatment, but relapse 6 to 12 weeks after stopping.

Anti-immunoglobulin E treatment of patients with recalcitrant physical urticaria. Metz M, Altricher S, Ardelean E, Kessler B, Krause K, Magerl M, et al. Int Arch Allergy Immnuol 2011; 154; 177–80.

One of two patients with symptomatic dermographism cleared completely within days of their first injection of omalizumab and remained clear on continuing treatment in this report, although other patients did not respond.

Retreatment with omalizumab results in rapid remission in chronic spontaneous and inducible urticaria. Metz M, Ohanyan T, Church MK, Maurer M. JAMA Dermatol 2014; 150: 288–90.

In dermographic urticaria H_2 receptor antagonists have a small but therapeutically irrelevant additional effect compared with H_1 antagonists alone. Sharpe GR, Shuster S. Br J Dermatol 1993; 129: 575–9.

In this double-blind, crossover study, 19 patients were randomized to treatment with cetirizine 10 mg at night plus either ranitidine 150 mg twice daily or placebo. There was an increase in whealing threshold with additional H_2 blockade, but no subjective benefit on itch.

Addition of an H_2 to an H_1 antihistamine may provide better control of some inducible urticarias despite the lack of trial evidence.

Beneficial effects of danazol on symptoms and laboratory changes in cholinergic urticaria. Wong E, Eftekhari N, Greaves MW, Milford Ward A. Br J Dermatol 1987; 116: 553–6.

Seventeen male patients treated with danazol 200 mg three times daily in a double-blind crossover study had sustained improvement in the number of exercise-induced wheals over 12 weeks.

Anabolic steroids should only be considered for severe cholinergic urticaria not responding adequately to up-dosed H_1 antihistamines, because of their potential for virilization and hepatotoxicity. Danazol should be reserved for severe cases and avoided during pregnancy. Androgenic adverse effects may be dose-limiting in women.

Successful treatment of cholinergic urticaria with anti-immunoglobulin E therapy. Metz M, Bergmann P, Zuberbier T, Maurer M. Allergy 2008; 63: 247–8.

One patient with highly symptomatic cholinergic urticaria who had not responded to several antihistamines, montelukast, and propranolol made a complete and sustained response to omalizumab 300 mg every 2 weeks.

Failure of omalizumab in cholinergic urticaria. Sabroe R. Clin Exp Dermatol 2009; 35:e217–9.

A patient with disabling cholinergic urticaria was completely unresponsive to omalizumab subcutaneously at 300 mg every 2 weeks for 4 months.

Clinical experience with omalizumab for cholinergic urticaria indicates that it can be highly effective but not every patient will respond. Cholinergic urticaria is an unlicensed indication.

Severe cholinergic urticaria successfully treated with scopolamine butylbromide in addition to antihistamines. Ujiie H, Shimizu T, Natsuga K, Arita K, Tomizawa K, Shimizu H. Clin Exp Dermatol 2006; 31: 978–81.

Although this case report suggests that anticholinergics may be successful for cholinergic urticaria, the general experience with this class of drugs is disappointing, and unwanted effects often outweigh any benefits.

Successful treatment of cold-induced urticaria/anaphylaxis with anti-IgE. Boyce JA. J Allergy Clin Immunol 2006; 117: 1414–8.

A trial of omalizumab in a 12-year-old atopic girl with increasingly severe cold-contact urticaria led to complete resolution of her symptoms over 5 months, but her symptoms recurred when she missed two doses of omalizumab.

An increasing number of reports illustrate the good response that some patients with cold urticaria have with omalizumab given off-license.

Improvement of cold urticaria by treatment with the leukotriene receptor antagonist montelukast. Hani N, Hartmann K, Casper C, Peters T, Schneider LA, Hunzelmann N, et al. Acta Derm Venereol 2000; 80: 229.

A case report of a patient with acquired cold-contact urticaria responding subjectively and objectively to montelukast 10 mg daily after only 4 days.

It is not clear whether montelukast was given as monotherapy or in combination with an antihistamine.

Treatment of acquired cold urticaria with cetirizine and zafirlukast in combination. Bonadonna P, Lombardi C, Senna G, Canonica GW, Passalacqua G. J Am Acad Dermatol 2003; 49: 714–6.

Two patients with severe cold-contact urticaria improved subjectively and objectively on a combination of cetirizine 10 mg once daily and zafirlukast 20 mg twice daily. Combination therapy was better than either drug alone.

Further studies are required to clarify what place (if any) leukotriene receptor antagonists have in the management of antihistamine-unresponsive cold urticaria.

Acquired cold urticaria: clinical picture and update on diagnosis and treatment. Siebenhaar F, Weller K, Mlynek A, Magerl M, Altrichter S, Vieira Dos Santos R, et al. Clin Exp Dermatol 2007; 32: 241–5.

Examples of antibiotic regimens used for "curative therapy" are given as phenoxymethylpenicillin 1 MU/day for 2 to 4 weeks, intramuscular benzylpenicillin 1 MU/day for 20 days, or doxycycline 200 mg/day for 3 weeks.

The authors claim that occasional patients respond to high-dose antibiotics even if no underlying infection can be detected, but personal experience suggests little or no benefit.

Cold urticaria: a clinico-therapeutic study in 30 patients, with special emphasis on cold desensitization. Henquet JM, Martens BPM, van Volten WA. Eur J Dermatol 1992; 2: 75–7.

Cold desensitization in four patients with severely disabling cold urticaria resulted in symptom-free follow-up ranging from 4 to 14 years. Induction of cold tolerance took 1 to 2 weeks.

Patients had to take cold showers (around 15 °C) for 5 minutes twice a day to maintain the tolerance, so this approach is not for the faint-hearted. Cold tolerance is now outdated.

Cold urticaria: tolerance induction with cold baths. Von Mackensen YA, Sticherling M. Br J Dermatol 2007; 157: 799–846.

Nine of 23 patients desensitized with cold water immersions 15 years earlier responded to a questionnaire survey. Only one of them was able to continue the cold baths for 6 months, two for 3 months, and the others stopped almost immediately.

This report introduces a little realism concerning the likelihood of cold desensitization being an effective and well-tolerated long-term therapy for cold-contact urticaria.

Heat urticaria: a revision of published cases with an update on classification and management. Pezzolo E, Peroni A, Gisondi P, Girolomoni G. Br J Dermatol 2016; 175: 473–8.

A comprehensive review of this rare subtype of inducible urticaria.

Rapid response to omalizumab in 3 cases of delayed pressure urticaria. Quintero OP, Arrondo AP, Veleiro B. J Allergy Clin Immunol Pract 2017; 5: 179–80.

Effective treatment of different phenotypes of chronic urticaria with omalizumab: case reports and review of literature. Kasperska-Zajac A, Jarząb J, Żerdzińska A, Bąk K, Grzanka A. Int J Immunopathol Pharmacol 2016; 29: 320–8.

Omalizumab is increasingly being reported as a successful treatment of delayed pressure urticaria. It is also effective for patients with chronic spontaneous urticaria and delayed pressure urticaria.

Efficacy of montelukast, in combination with loratadine, in the treatment of delayed pressure urticaria. Nettis E, Pannafino A, Cavallo E, Ferrannini A, Tursi A. J Allergy Clin Immunol 2003; 112: 212–3.

In a small randomized study, objective pressure rechallenge after 15 days showed that montelukast 10 mg once daily with loratadine 10 mg once daily was more effective than either drug alone.

Evidence Levels: **A** Double-blind study **B** Clinical trial ≥ 20 subjects **C** Clinical trial < 20 subjects **D** Series ≥ 5 subjects **E** Anecdotal case reports

Desloratadine in combination with montelukast suppresses the dermographometer challenge test papule, and is effective in the treatment of delayed pressure urticaria: a randomized, double-blind, placebo-controlled study. Nettis E, Colanardi MC, Soccio AL, Ferrannini A, Vacca A. Br J Dermatol 2006; 155: 1279–82.

Although this study suggests that pressure urticaria can be controlled without steroids, clinical experience with montelukast in delayed pressure urticaria is usually disappointing.

Delayed pressure urticaria: response to treatment with sulfasalazine in a case series of seventeen patients. Swerlick RA, Puar N. Dermatol Ther 2015; 28: 318–22.

This open study supports the use of sulfasalazine in delayed pressure urticaria.

Potential side effects include bone marrow depression and hypersensitivity reactions, so patients need careful monitoring. Sulfasalazine should only be considered in patients who are not sensitive to aspirin and other nonsteroidal drugs.

Delayed pressure urticaria—dapsone heading for first-line therapy. Grundmann SA, Kiefer S, Luger TA, Brehler R. J Dstch Dermatol Ges 2011; 9: 908–12.

Seventy-four percent of 31 patients with pressure urticaria treated with dapsone over a 6-year period surveyed retrospectively showed a good or very good response.

Dapsone can also be a useful and inexpensive treatment of delayed pressure urticaria.

Narrowband ultraviolet B phototherapy is a suitable treatment option for solar urticaria. Calzavara-Pinton P, Zane C, Rossi M, Sala R, Venturini M. J Am Acad Dermatol 2012; 67: e5–9.

Patients without an urticarial response to phototesting with NB-UVB were given an alternate-day exposure for 4 weeks. Those with an urticarial response to phototesting with NB-UVB were treated three times a day for 5 days in the first week and then subsequently the same as the first group for 3 weeks. Thirty-nine patients completed the study and reported good tolerance to the sun afterward.

Solar urticaria: long-term rush hardening by inhibition spectrum narrow-band UVB 311 nm. Wolf R, Herzinger T, Grahovac M, Prinz JC. Clin Exp Dermatol. 2013; 38: 446–7.

UVA rush hardening for the treatment of solar urticaria. Beissert S, Ständer H, Schwarz T. J Am Acad Dermatol 2000; 42: 1030–2.

Protection was achieved within 3 days of exposing three patients to multiple incremental UVA irradiations at 1-hour intervals. Rush hardening with UVA did not cause sunburn reactions and provided protection against visible light and UVB-induced urticaria in two of the three patients.

UV-induced tolerance should be considered for patients who need more than antihistamines.

Successful and long-lasting treatment of solar urticaria with UVA rush hardening therapy. Masuoka E, Fukunga A, Kishigami K, Jimbo H, Nishioka M, Uchimura Y, et al. Br J Dermatol 2012, 167: 198–201.

Two patients with solar urticaria who reacted to intradermal injection of their own serum that had been preirradiated with visible light were treated with multiple UVA incremental exposures at 1-hour intervals for 2 to 3 days and became symptom free, and their postirradiation skin tests became negative. Maintenance UVA exposures were performed every 1 or 2 weeks for 4 months in one patient and 5 months in the other. The first patient remained clear off treatment for 6 months.

Successful treatment with UVA rush hardening in a case of solar urticaria. Mori N, Makino T, Matsui K, Takegami Y, Murayama S, Shimizu T. Eur J Dermatol 2014; 24: 117–9.

A direct comparison between NB-UVB, PUVA, and UVA hardening for solar urticaria has not been performed to date.

Omalizumab in patients with severe and refractory solar urticaria: a phase II multicentric study. Aubin F, Avenel-Audran M, Jeanmougin M, Adamski H, Peyron JL, Marguery MC, et al. J Am Acad Dermatol 2016; 74: 574–5.

Failure of omalizumab in the treatment of solar urticaria. Müller S, Schempp CM, Jakob T. J Eur Acad Dermatol Venereol 2016; 30: 524–5.

As in all types of urticaria, omalizumab does not work for every patient.

Third-Line Therapies	
• Intravenous immunoglobulins	D
• Ciclosporin	E
• Plasmapheresis	E
• Etanercept	E

Effect of high-dose intravenous immunoglobulin in delayed pressure urticaria. Dawn G, Urcelay M, Ah-Weng A, O'Neill SM, Douglas WS. Br J Dermatol 2003; 149: 836–40.

Three of eight patients went into remission after one or more infusions of intravenous immunoglobulin (IVIG) at 2 g/kg and two improved, but confirmation of pressure-induced wheals by objective testing was not done, and all patients had spontaneous chronic urticaria. It was not clear whether the benefit of treatment was mainly on the pressure urticaria or the spontaneous urticaria.

Cold urticaria responding to systemic cyclosporine. Marsland AM, Beck MH. Br J Dermatol 2003; 149: 214.

One patient with acquired cold-contact urticaria of over 1 year's duration and unresponsive to antihistamines improved within a week of starting ciclosporin at 3 mg/kg daily, and the improvement was maintained at 1.7 mg/kg/day. It was not stated what happened on stopping treatment.

There is currently no good evidence that acquired cold-contact urticaria is an autoimmune disease, so the use of immunomodulating drugs should be regarded as speculative and of unproven benefit. The benefit seen in some patients probably relates to partial inhibition of histamine release. H_1 antihistamines should be given concurrently.

Cyclosporin A therapy for severe solar urticaria. Edström DW, Ros AM. Photodermatol Photoimmunol Photomed 1997; 13: 61–3.

A clinically useful reduction in sensitivity to visible or UV light occurred while taking ciclosporin at 4.5 mg/kg daily, but the symptoms recurred within 1 to 2 weeks of stopping treatment. The authors suggest that this treatment might be appropriate for severe disease when other treatments have failed, especially in countries where treatment is necessary only for a few months during summer.

Solar urticaria—effective treatment by plasmapheresis. Duschet P, Leyen P, Schwarz T, Höcker P, Greiter J, Gschnait F. Clin Exp Dermatol 1987; 12: 185–8.

A refractory period of at least 12 months followed a single treatment with 3 L plasmapheresis.

Successful treatment of delayed pressure urticaria with anti-TNF-α. Magerl M, Philipp S, Manasterski M, Friedrich M, Maurer M. J Allergy Clin Immunol 2007; 119: 752–4.

Single case report of a complete response of pressure urticaria symptoms within a week of starting etanercept for concurrent psoriasis.

Successful treatment of systemic cold contact urticaria with etanercept in a patient with psoriasis. Gualdi G, Monari P, Rossi MT, Crotti S, Calzavara-Pinton PG. Br J Dermatol 2012; 166: 1373–4.

A patient with long-standing cold-contact urticaria and psoriasis treated with etanercept underwent resolution of both conditions within weeks of starting treatment, relapse on withdrawal, and improvement on reintroduction.

AQUAGENIC PRURITUS

Aquagenic pruritus is diagnosed when itching, prickling, burning, buzzing, or other skin discomfort, which may be intense, is provoked by contact with water. There are no visible skin changes. The sensation is associated with feelings of anger, irritability, or depression in approximately half of patients. The symptoms are provoked at any water temperature and degree of salinity. They occur within minutes rather than hours and start either during a bath or shower or soon afterward. The discomfort may be present for between 10 minutes and 2 hours. Any part of the body may be affected. Patients may also itch when the ambient temperature changes. Spontaneous remission is rare. The pathogenesis of the condition is not clear.

MANAGEMENT STRATEGY

Other chronic skin diseases must be ruled out by taking a full history and by clinical examination (particularly aquagenic pruritus of the elderly manifesting as xerosis and other inducible urticarias). Direct questioning is necessary regarding cold-induced symptoms and whealing; water-induced whealing or syncope; exercise-, heat-, or emotion-induced symptoms and whealing; and friction-induced itching and whealing. The well-recognized "bath itch" that occurs in approximately 40% of patients with polycythemia rubra vera must be ruled out before aquagenic pruritus is diagnosed. Rarely, other hematologic abnormalities have also been associated. Occasionally, antimalarial drugs have induced an aquagenic pruritus–like picture in patients with lupus erythematosus. When the diagnosis is reached, it is important to explain that aquagenic pruritus is a recognized skin condition, which, although very unpleasant and difficult to manage, has no immediate implications with regard to the patient's general health. Therapy is usually based on the use of *antihistamines, adding sodium bicarbonate to the water,* and *phototherapy.*

Specific Investigations

- Complete blood count (repeated yearly)
- Water induction

First-Line Therapies

• Explanation	E
• Minimally sedating antihistamine	C
• Sodium bicarbonate added to bath water	D

Antihistamines are used by these authors in the management of aquagenic pruritus. There is no consensus regarding the first-line treatment, as the response of each patient is individual and no single treatment is effective in all cases; however, it would seem reasonable to start by advising a minimally sedating antihistamine 2 hours before the bath or shower on a regular basis. Patients may have a good response to antihistamines. Not all patients respond to antihistamine treatment, however, and, of those who do, the response may consist of a diminution rather than an abolition of symptoms.

Aquagenic pruritus. Greaves MW, Black AK, Eady RAJ, Coutts A. Lancet 1981; 282: 2008–11.

Aquagenic pruritus. Steinman HK, Greaves MW. J Am Acad Dermatol 1985; 13: 91–6.

Aquagenic pruritus: pharmacological findings and treatment. Greaves MW, Handfield-Jones SE. Eur J Dermatol 1992; 2: 482–4.

Aquagenic pruritus may respond to the addition of sodium bicarbonate to the bath water. Advice about the amount of sodium bicarbonate to be added varies. In those who have responded, 200 g, 100 g, and 25 g have been added. The most practical approach might be to start with approximately 200 g per bath, and if there is a satisfactory response, to reduce gradually to a level that continues to suppress the itching. In a series of 25 patients, 25% improved with this treatment; however, in some cases the response may be temporary. Large quantities of sodium bicarbonate may be purchased economically at bakers' wholesalers.

Baking soda baths for aquagenic pruritus. Bayoumi AHM, Highet AS. Lancet 1986; 11: 464.

Aquagenic pruritus treatment with sodium bicarbonate and evidence for a seasonal form. Bircher AJ. J Am Acad Dermatol 1989; 21: 817.

Second-Line Therapies

• UVB	C
• Narrowband UVB	E
• Combined UVA/narrowband UVB therapy	E

Due to the necessity for hospital attendance, UVB should be considered a second-line treatment for aquagenic pruritus. A response usually occurs between 2 and 4 weeks of treatment, but relapse normally occurs within months of stopping treatment, which may then be repeated as necessary or maintenance therapy instituted as the condition is ongoing.

A good response to NB-UVB is described in two patients to whom it was administered three times per week. The improvement occurred at about 2 months of treatment and was maintained on weekly treatment in the ensuing months. In one of the patients desloratadine was added during the maintenance period. NB-UVB may prove to be an effective form of phototherapy.

Combined UVA and UVB treatment was used to treat one patient with good response.

Ultraviolet phototherapy for pruritus. Rivard J, Lim HW. Dermatol Ther 2005; 18: 344–54.

Narrow band ultraviolet B in aquagenic pruritus. Xifra A, Carrascosa JM, Ferrandiz C. Br J Dermatol 2005; 158: 1233.

Evidence Levels: **A** Double-blind study **B** Clinical trial ≥ 20 subjects **C** Clinical trial < 20 subjects **D** Series ≥ 5 subjects **E** Anecdotal case reports

Aquagenic pruritus responding to combined ultraviolet A/narrowband UVB therapy. Jean M, Koh A, Chong WS. Photodermatol Photoimmunol Photomedicine 2009; 25: 169.

Third-Line Therapies	
• Bath oil	E
• Emulsifying ointment in the bath water	E
• PUVA	E
• Propranolol	E, C
• Transdermal nitroglycerin	E
• Naltrexone	E

PUVA treatment has been effective in the bath itch of polycythemia vera and has been used successfully both in a series of five patients and in individual patients, although either maintenance or repeated courses of therapy are necessary to maintain control of the condition. PUVA with oral psoralens may be regarded as a third-line treatment for practical reasons.

Aquagenic pruritus responding to intermittent photochemotherapy. Holme SA, Anstey AV. Clin Exp Dermatol 2001; 26: 40–1.

Repeated PUVA treatment of aquagenic pruritus. Goodkin R, Bernhard JD. Clin Exp Dermatol 2002; 27: 164–5.

Aquagenic pruritus responds to propranolol. Thomsen K. J Am Acad Dermatol 1990; 22: 697.

Treatment with propranolol of six patients with idiopathic aquagenic pruritus. Nosbaum A, Pecquet C, Bayrow O, Amsler E, Nicholas JF, Berard F, et al. J Allergy Clin Immunol 2011; 28: 113.

After a report of successful treatment of two patients with propranolol, six patients were treated with propranolol 10 to 40 mg/day for 3 months depending on their tolerance of the drug. Either relief or elimination of symptoms occurred in five after 7 days. Relapse took place after stopping, and one patient needed retreatment, which was effective.

Aquagenic pruritus response to the exogenous nitric oxide donor, transdermal nitroglycerin. Goihan Yahr M. Int J Dermatol 1994; 33: 752.

Transdermal nitroglycerin has been used effectively in one patient.

Efficacy and safety of naltrexone, an oral opiate receptor antagonist, in the treatment of pruritus and dermatological diseases. Metze D, Reinmann S, Beissert S, Luger T. J Am Acad Dermatol 1999; 41: 533–9.

Successful treatment of refractory aquagenic pruritus with naltrexone. Ingber S, Cohen PD. J Cutan Med Surg 2005; 9: 215–6.

Naltrexone at a dose of 50 mg daily controlled the condition in two patients with aquagenic pruritus to whom it was given.

CHOLINERGIC PRURITUS

Cholinergic pruritus occurs when patients itch, sting, or prickle after a rise in body temperature. The provoking stimuli are exercise (walking, running, dancing, going to the gym), including housework (ironing, vacuuming), heat (hot room, hot food, hot bath, sunny day), and emotion (excitement, stress, embarrassment) or fever. A combination of factors may cause a more pronounced itch (e.g., walking on a sunny day). The intensity, extent, and duration of the itching seem to be directly proportional to the strength of the eliciting stimulus. By definition, no whealing occurs on the skin during an attack. Although the prevalence of this condition is not known, it is the authors' impression that many people itch when they become warm, although this itching is frequently insufficiently severe or incapacitating to present at a dermatology clinic. Cholinergic pruritus can be regarded as a variant of cholinergic urticaria. There is one case report that describes a patient presenting initially with cholinergic pruritus who progressed to cholinergic urticaria. Because there are no visible skin lesions, it is important to be aware of the condition and to differentiate it from aquagenic pruritus in those who describe itching after a bath or shower.

MANAGEMENT STRATEGY

Explaining the provoking factors and stressing that the condition is not an allergy, related to diet, or related to any underlying disease is helpful. If possible, *minimizing situations in which the itching occurs* can be helpful, and cooling the skin as quickly as possible may lessen the duration of the itching. It is not possible to tell the patient how long the condition will be present before remission takes place. Therapeutic agents typically utilized are *antihistamines*, although *danazol* has been reported to be beneficial.

Specific Investigations
• Exercise induction
• Warm bath induction (40°–41°C)

First-Line Therapies	
• Explanation	E
• Second generation H$_1$ antihistamines	E

An explanation is the most important part of treatment. The patient needs to understand the relationship between the itching and heat and the importance of keeping cool. Treatment with minimally sedating antihistamines generally produces an improvement, although they are unlikely to suppress the condition completely. Antihistamines should be taken regularly every morning or 2 hours before an expected stimulus in order to assess any response. If the antihistamine proves helpful, the same dose could be repeated 9 to 12 hours later if necessary.

Second-Line Therapy	
• Danazol	C

Cholinergic pruritus, erythema, and urticaria: a disease spectrum responding to danazol. Berth-Jones J, Graham Brown RAC. Br J Dermatol 1989; 121: 235–37.

Danazol, which has been used in cholinergic urticaria, may rarely be effective in very severely affected individuals. The recommended dose is 200 mg three times daily. This dose could be continued for approximately 1 month and reduced to the minimum that controls the condition.

115

Irritant contact dermatitis

Nathaniel K. Wilkin

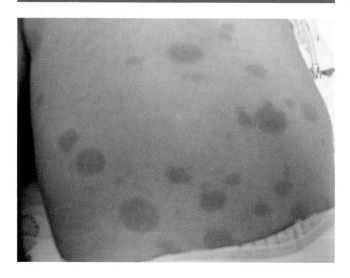

Irritant contact dermatitis (ICD) is the most common form of contact dermatitis and is defined as the reaction to an exogenous substance—the irritant—that damages the epidermis through physical or chemical mechanisms, triggering an innate immunologic response only. Clinical manifestations of ICD vary in presentation and severity according to multiple factors: preexisting status of the skin (atopy, barrier disruption, etc.), the nature and number of irritants (corrosives or caustic), the duration and frequency of contact, and the conditions of exposure (moisture, occlusion, temperature). Acute ICD is usually attributable to a single irritant. Chronic ICD usually results from exposure to multiple irritants, often in association with endogenous factors such as atopy or stress. Chronic cumulative ICD usually involves the hands.

ICD is common, often has a poor prognosis, has a significant economic impact on society, and seriously degrades the quality of life of affected individuals beyond the ability to work.

MANAGEMENT STRATEGY

The first step in any management strategy is *prevention*. Patients should be educated about proper skin care and protection, including handwashing, the use of moisturizers and barrier creams, avoidance of common irritants, and the use of protective clothing such as gloves and aprons when handling potentially irritating substances.

Dermatologists can encourage primary prevention by counseling patients at higher risk because of endogenous factors (e.g., atopy) or exogenous factors (e.g., frequent occupational exposures, such as in hairdressing). Secondary prevention includes measures that enable patients to remain employed without interfering with the resolution of the ICD. Chronic hand dermatitis is a common presentation of ICD, and patient education can be facilitated with a handout on lifestyle management principles directed at handwashing and moisturizing, occlusive moisturizing therapy at night, special protective modalities (such as type of glove to exclude specific irritants), and specific agents to avoid.

Azathioprine, ciclosporin, oral retinoids, psoralen and UVA (PUVA), Grenz ray therapy, and *superficial radiotherapy* may be justified for short-term control in patients who are compliant with moisturizing, use of protective modalities (gloves), and application of topical corticosteroids and still have a severe disruption of their quality of life due to active ICD. Because the goal of these second- and third-line therapies is to reduce the severity such that first-line therapies may become sufficient, patient selection is critical.

Specific Investigations

- Patch testing to environmentally relevant allergens
- Detailed case history of patient's work, habits, and hobbies

Irritant contact dermatitis: a review. Slodownik D, Lee A, Nixon R. Australas J Dermatol 2008; 49: 1–11.

Treatment of ICD is based on determining all contributing factors to the patient's dermatitis and prevention of contact with the causative agents where possible.

Clues to an accurate diagnosis of contact dermatitis. Rietschel RL. Dermatol Ther 2004; 17: 224–30.

Patch testing with known environmentally relevant allergens that is negative and sufficiently comprehensive would point to ICD, especially in patients without atopy, dyshidrosis, or psoriasis. A careful history and documentation of specific morphologic changes on physical examination are essential when pursuing the presumptive diagnosis of ICD after negative patch testing.

Patch testing, a detailed history, and assessment of specific morphologic changes provide for an accurate diagnosis and can identify specific environmental factors the patient should avoid. Such documentation is also useful should medicolegal questions arise regarding impairment and job placement.

Allergic and irritant contact dermatitis. Nosbaum A, Vocanson M, Hennino A, Nicholas JF. Eur J Dermatol 2009; 19: 325–32.

ICD and allergic contact dermatitis can have similar presentations. In such cases where differentiation is difficult, immunologic assay techniques can be used to make the diagnosis.

First-Line Therapies

Physical skin protection	C
Emollients	C
Barrier creams	C
Topical corticosteroids	C
Topical calcineurin inhibitors	C

Current concepts of irritant contact dermatitis. English JS. Occup Environ Med 2004; 61: 722–6.

Avoiding exposure to irritants, relying on the use of personal protective equipment, and using moisturizing creams constitute the basis of treatment of ICD.

Evidence Levels: **A** Double-blind study **B** Clinical trial ≥ 20 subjects **C** Clinical trial < 20 subjects **D** Series ≥ 5 subjects **E** Anecdotal case reports

A review of the management of ICD cases from an occupational medicine perspective, which includes an excellent guide to various gloves that provide protection for specific types of hazards.

Therapeutic options for chronic hand dermatitis. Warshaw EM. Dermatol Ther 2004; 17: 240–50.

A review of the therapeutic alternatives for patients with recalcitrant hand dermatitis.

Effect of glove-occlusion on human skin (II). Ramsing DW, Agner T. Contact Dermatitis 1996; 34: 258–62.

Occlusive gloves worn for prolonged periods may impair skin barrier function. Wearing cotton gloves under the occlusive gloves can prevent this negative effect.

High-fat petrolatum-based moisturizers and prevention of work-related skin problems in wet-work occupations. Mygind K, Sell L, Flyvholm MA, Jepsen KF. Contact Dermatitis 2006; 54: 35–41.

Detailed analyses revealed that protective gloves are the overall most effective protection and did not indicate that a high-fat moisturizer could successfully replace gloves.

Protective gloves should be used for as short a time as possible and with cotton gloves under the occlusive gloves. Gloves provide better protection than, and should not be replaced by, moisturizers or barrier creams.

A randomized comparison of an emollient containing skin-related lipids with a petrolatum-based emollient as adjunct in the treatment of chronic hand dermatitis. Kucharekova M, Van de Kerkhof PCM, Van der Valk PGM. Contact Dermatitis 2003; 48: 293–9.

The frequent use of emollients is associated with significant improvement in hand dermatitis. No significant difference in the improvement was demonstrated for the emollient containing skin-related lipids.

The frequent use of emollients is an essential component of therapy. Traditional petrolatum-based emollients are accessible, inexpensive, and just as effective as an emollient containing skin-related lipids.

Double-blind, randomized trial of scheduled use of a novel barrier cream and an oil-containing lotion for protecting the hands of health care workers. McCormick RD, Buchman TL, Maki DG. Am J Infect Control 2000; 28: 302–10.

The scheduled use of petrolatum oil–containing lotion or a barrier cream was associated with a marked improvement (69% and 52%, respectively) in chronic hand irritant dermatitis.

It is debatable whether the distinction between "skin care" and "skin protection" is real. Side effects with emollients and barrier creams are irritation and sensitization to their ingredients. A useful procedure is to include patch tests of those emollients and barrier creams anticipated to be used by the patient in the initial comprehensive patch-testing evaluation of the chronic contact dermatitis.

Clinical efficacy evaluation of a novel barrier protective cream. Slade HB, Fowler J, Draeolos ZD, Reece BT, Cargill DI. Cutis 2008; 82: 21–8.

Cor806.805 (Tetrix cream) was associated with beneficial results regarding the establishment of a barrier against common irritants lasting at least 6 hours.

Breakdown of the skin's barrier function occurs early in the ICD disease process. Reestablishing the skin's protective barrier is a critical step in the healing process.

Do topical corticosteroids modulate skin irritation in human beings? Assessment by transepidermal water loss and visual scoring. Van der Valk PGM, Maibach HI. J Am Acad Dermatol 1989; 21: 519–22.

Neither the corticosteroid products nor the vehicle significantly influenced barrier function during repeated application of an irritant, sodium lauryl sulfate, in low concentration.

The first step must be the elimination, to the fullest extent possible, of exposure to irritants. Until proven otherwise, no therapy should be considered sufficiently potent as to overcome the effects of continuing exposure to irritants.

Short-term glucocorticoid treatment compromises both permeability barrier homeostasis and stratum corneum integrity: inhibition of epidermal lipid synthesis accounts for functional abnormalities. Kao JS, Fluhr JW, Man MQ, Fowler AJ, Hachem JP, Crimrine D, et al. J Invest Dermatol 2003; 120: 456–64.

ICD can be treated with glucocorticoids; however, there may be a secondary compromise in barrier function, which might be correctable with topical application of lipids.

An open-label pilot study to evaluate the safety and efficacy of topically applied tacrolimus ointment for the treatment of hand and/or foot eczema. Thelmo MC, Lang W, Brooke E, Osborne BE, McCarty MA, Jorizzo JL, et al. J Dermatol Treat 2003; 14: 136–40.

Pimecrolimus cream 1%: a potential new treatment for chronic hand dermatitis. Belsito DV, Fowler JF, Marks JG, Pariser DM, Hanifin J, Duarte IA, et al. Cutis 2004; 73: 31–8.

The topical calcineurin inhibitor led to improvements over baseline in the open-label study, and there was a trend toward greater clearance than with vehicle in the pimecrolimus study.

Topical calcineurin inhibitors may have a role as an alternative to low-potency topical corticosteroids in chronic irritant dermatitis in patients with mild inflammatory changes who do not experience a burning sensation when the product is applied.

Second-Line Therapies	
• Ciclosporin	C
• UVB therapy	C
• PUVA therapy	C
• Bexarotene gel	C

Novel treatment of chronic severe hand dermatitis with bexarotene gel. Hanifin JM, Stevens V, Sheth P, Breneman D. Br J Dermatol 2004; 150: 545–53.

A phase I to II open-label, randomized clinical study of bexarotene gel, alone and in combination with a low- and a midpotency steroid, was conducted in 55 patients with chronic severe hand dermatitis at two academic clinics. Patients using bexarotene gel monotherapy reached a 79% response rate for at least 50% clinical improvement and a 39% response rate for at least 90% clearance of hand dermatitis. Adverse events possibly related to treatment in all patients were stinging or burning (15%), flare of dermatitis (16%), and irritation (29%). Bexarotene gel appears to be safe and tolerated by most patients, with useful therapeutic activity in chronic severe hand dermatitis.

Comparison of cyclosporine and topical betamethasone 17,21-dipropionate in the treatment of severe chronic hand eczema. Granlund H, Erkko P, Eriksson E, Reitamo S. Acta Derm Venereol 1996; 76: 371–6.

Low-dose oral ciclosporin at 3 mg/kg daily was compared with topical 0.05% betamethasone dipropionate in a randomized, double-blind study of 41 patients with chronic hand dermatitis and an inadequate response to treatment with topical halogenated corticosteroids for at least 3 to 4 weeks and/or PUVA and avoidance of relevant contact allergens. Both treatment groups had similar improvement and similar relapse rates after successful treatment. Adverse events were slightly more common in patients treated with ciclosporin.

Low-dose cyclosporine may be a useful alternative treatment, although very high-potency topical corticosteroids can be effective in patients who do not have an adequate response to other mid- to high-potency topical corticosteroids.

PUVA-gel vs. PUVA-bath therapy for severe recalcitrant palmoplantar dermatoses. A randomized, single-blinded prospective study. Schiener R, Gottlöber P, Müller B, Williams S, Pillekamp H, Peter RU, et al. Photodermatol Photoimmunol Photomed 2005; 21: 62–7.

PUVA-gel therapy can be an effective therapeutic alternative to conventional PUVA-bath therapy in treating localized dermatoses of the palms and soles. The advantages of PUVA-gel therapy are simplicity of use and low cost.

Local narrowband UVB phototherapy vs. local PUVA in the treatment of chronic hand eczema. Sezer E, Etikan I. Photodermatol Photoimmunol Photomed 2007; 23: 10–4.

There was a statistically significant improvement with both treatment modalities; however, the difference in clinical response between the two was not statistically significant. Local narrowband UVB phototherapy regimen is as effective as paint-PUVA therapy in patients with chronic hand eczema of both dry and dyshidrotic types.

Given the similar improvement in chronic hand dermatitis and the increased side effects with paint-PUVA therapy, it would be prudent to begin treatment with local narrowband UVB therapy and only use paint-PUVA therapy if the response is inadequate.

Third-Line Therapies	
• Superficial radiotherapy	A
• Oral alitretinoin	A

Oral alitretinoin (9-*cis*-retinoic acid) therapy for chronic hand dermatitis in patients refractory to standard therapy: results of a randomized, double-blind, placebo-controlled, multicenter trial. Ruzicka T, Larsen FG, Galewicz D, Horváth A, Coenraads PJ, Thestrup-Pedersen K, et al. Arch Dermatol 2004; 140: 1453–9.

Alitretinoin given at well-tolerated doses induced substantial clearing of chronic hand dermatitis in patients refractory to conventional therapy.

Alitretinoin: its use in intractable hand eczema and other potential indications. Petersen B, Jemec GB. Drug Des Dev Ther 2009; 3: 51–7.

Alitretinoin has significant therapeutic potential for the treatment of chronic recalcitrant hand eczema.

Alitretinoin is not currently approved for use in the United States. Although teratogenicity might occur at any clinically relevant dose, most other side effects are dose dependent. This drug should be reserved for patients whose chronic hand dermatitis is refractory to conventional therapies and prescribed for only as long as it takes to achieve control, which can be maintained with safer therapies.

Efficacy and patient perception of Grenz ray therapy in the treatment of dermatoses refractory to other medical therapy. Schalock PC, Zug KA, Carter JC, Dhar D, MacKenzie T. Dermatitis 2008; 19: 90–4.

Many patients treated with Grenz ray therapy (GRT) for recalcitrant dermatitis reported that this was an effective therapy in reducing the discomfort and severity of their skin condition. Overall, slightly more than half of treated patients believed GRT was a worthwhile therapy that they would use again.

Grenz ray therapy in the new millennium: still a valid treatment option? Warner JA, Cruz Jr PD. Dermatitis 2008; 19: 73–80.

Grenz ray or superficial radiotherapy is not an obvious "go to" treatment when one second-line treatment does not provide a sufficient response, but it may be tried for some additional advantage as an adjunct to intensive first-line treatment with or without low-dose ciclosporin.

Evidence Levels: **A** Double-blind study **B** Clinical trial ≥ 20 subjects **C** Clinical trial < 20 subjects **D** Series ≥ 5 subjects **E** Anecdotal case reports

Jellyfish stings

Christopher Sladden, Jamie Seymour, Michael Sladden

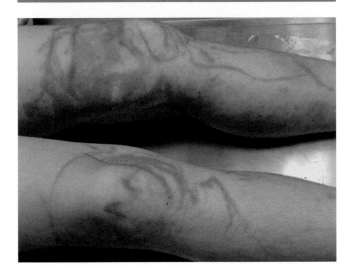

Jellyfish are members of the phylum Cnidaria, which consists of five classes: Cubozoa (box jellyfish), Hydrozoa (Portuguese man-of-war), Schyphozoa (true jellyfish), Staurozoa (staromedusans), and Anthozoans (corals). They are found in every ocean and some fresh water, from the surface to the depths of the seas. They often consist of a bell-shaped body, ranging from 1 millimeter to over 2 meters in diameter, with tentacles up to 30 meters long.

Jellyfish envenomings can occur during recreational and commercial pursuits, both in the water and when encountering living or dead animals on the shore. Jellyfish sting their prey using nematocysts, stinging structures located in specialized cells called *cnidocytes*. The nematocyst is a highly coiled, hollow, harpoonlike microtubule responsible for venom injection. Contact with a jellyfish tentacle can trigger millions of nematocysts to pierce the skin and inject venom. Those providing care to sting victims should avoid being stung by adherent tentacles on the victim.

Severity of jellyfish stings depends on many factors. These include the species and age of the jellyfish involved, the geographic location, the location of the nematocysts involved (bell or tentacle), patient age and general health, the amount of skin involved, and the number of nematocysts triggered.

Most jellyfish stings are self-limiting causing localized pain and skin lesions. However, symptoms can range from local discomfort, to severe pain, through to cardiovascular collapse and death. Immediate management of jellyfish stings occurs at the beach with first aid and resuscitation, and then if needed in a hospital. Immediate cutaneous reactions include wheals, blisters, and angioedema. Dermatologists are most likely to become involved later to manage the delayed sequelae of jellyfish stings.

In this chapter we discuss the most important type of jellyfish stings, the different symptoms and management of these stings, as well as strategies for prevention of jellyfish stings.

CLINICAL FEATURES

Major box jellyfish *(Chironex fleckeri)*

Chironex fleckeri is only found in northern Australian waters and is widely considered the most venomous animal in the world. However, several other species of chiropdropids (or multitentacled box jellyfish) found throughout non-Australian tropical realms are also capable of inflicting life-threatening envenomings. The toxin is dermonecrotic, cardiotoxic, and neurotoxic. Stings cause immediate and excruciating pain. Skin manifestations include large welts and whiplike purple-red plaques. Severe envenomation is rare but can cause cardiovascular collapse and death. Victims can drown before reaching shore. Many deaths occur within minutes of envenomation, at a time when the antivenom often is unavailable.

Irukandji jellyfish *(Carukia barnesi)*

Irukandji syndrome is a poorly defined set of symptoms occurring after envenoming by certain species of box jellyfish, usually *Carukia barnesi*. The initial sting is often barely noticed with minimal skin symptoms. The symptoms of Irukandji syndrome develop after 20 to 30 minutes with victims showing three patterns of symptoms: pain, catecholamine-like effects, and cardiopulmonary decompensation. Symptoms range from headaches, through severe pain, nausea, vomiting, and pulmonary edema, to hypertension and cardiac dysfunction, sometimes resulting in death. Although the syndrome is well documented in coastal northern Australia, it appears that Irukandji syndrome is an increasing marine problem worldwide.

Bluebottles or Portuguese man-of-war (*Physalia* species)

Bluebottle stings cause immediate intense pain and a linear red eruption at the sting site but rarely systemic effects. However, the Portuguese man-of-war (*Physalia physalis*), found in the Atlantic, Pacific, and Indian oceans, deserves special attention because it is potentially lethal.

True jellyfish (Schyphozoans)

The majority of jellyfish envenomings throughout the world occur from the Schyphozoans. Symptoms may range from mild irritation through to significant welts on the envenomed victim, which may result in skin necrosis in some instances. Life-threatening complications from these envenomings are rare.

Corals and sea anemones (Anthozoans)

Sea anemone stings range from mild erythema and tingling to painful urticarial and vesiculobullous lesions. Stings from corals are usually mild. "Coral cuts" from the hard coral exoskeleton are more serious and may introduce debris, bacteria, and other infection into the wound.

Seabather's eruption

This is an acute dermatitis caused by larvae of thimble jellyfish (*Linuche unguiculate*) and sea anemone (*Edwardsiella lineata*). It has been reported in Florida, the Bahamas, Bermuda, southeast Asia,

Brazil, and New York. The rash, usually confined to underneath the bathing suit, is a highly pruritic and erythematous papular eruption. Symptoms usually begin hours to 15 days after exposure.

CUTANEOUS MANIFESTATIONS OF JELLYFISH STINGS

Immediate cutaneous reactions include wheals and blisters at the site of the sting. In more severe stings, partial- or full-thickness skin necrosis can occur. Delayed, persistent, or recurrent eruptions have been reported at the initial envenomation site, consisting of erythema, urticarial lesions, papules, and plaques. Delayed hypersensitivity reactions occur infrequently. Other sequelae include dermatitis, secondary infections, postinflammatory hyperpigmentation and scarring, and erythema nodosum.

MANAGEMENT STRATEGY

First-Line Therapies

Prevention of jellyfish stings

- Stinger suits worn next to the skin reduce contact with jellyfish tentacles — E
- Beach/ocean stinger nets to provide physical barrier between jellyfish and swimmers (NB: These are only effective on jellyfish that are larger than the net mesh size) — E
- Proprietary Safe Sea cream (NB: This treatment may cause the discharge of more nematocysts in some species) — A
- Removing (and washing) bathing suits and showering to reduce/prevent seabather's eruption — E

Immediate management of stings

- Sting victims should be removed from the water — E
- Those providing care to sting victims must avoid being stung by the jellyfish — E
- Immediately remove any tentacles (dermis on fingers is usually thick enough to prevent significant envenoming to the first-aider) — E
- Wash sting site with sea water (not fresh water) — E
- Identify type of jellyfish involved — E
- Cardiopulmonary resuscitation if needed (usually only necessary for box jellyfish) — E

Topical agents to provide analgesia

- Lignocaine — C
- Ice — C
- Hot water — A

Major box jellyfish (*Chironex fleckeri*) stings

- Apply liberal amounts of vinegar to sting site to inactivate any undischarged nematocysts — C
- Cardiac monitoring, supportive care, and cardiopulmonary resuscitation if required — D

All but very minor box jellyfish stings require transport to hospital for:
- Oral and parenteral analgesia — C
- Administration of intravenous antivenom — D
- Administration of intravenous magnesium — D

Irukandji jellyfish stings

- Apply liberal amounts of vinegar to sting — C

The majority of stings require hospital admission for:
- Oral and parenteral analgesia — C
- Cardiac monitoring, supportive care, and cardiopulmonary resuscitation if required — D

Bluebottle and Portuguese man-of-war stings

- Application of hot water (45°C) gives rapid and significant relief — A

Interventions for the symptoms and signs resulting from jellyfish stings. Li L, McGee RG, Isbister GK, Webster AC. Cochrane Database Sys Rev 2013; 12: CD009688.

This review located seven trials that assessed a variety of different interventions applied in different ways and in different settings. Although heat appears to be an effective treatment for *Physalia* (bluebottle) stings, this evidence is based on a single trial of low-quality evidence.

Evidence-based treatment of jellyfish stings in North America and Hawaii. Ward NT, Darracq MA, Tomaszewski C, Clark RF. Ann Emerg Med 2012; 60: 399–414.

Systematic review of the evidence supporting various treatments for envenomation by jellyfish (cnidarian) and related organisms in North America and Hawaii. Hot water and topical lidocaine seem beneficial in improving pain symptoms. If not available, remove nematocysts and wash the area with salt water. Vinegar causes pain exacerbation or nematocyst discharge in the majority of species (but is useful in box jellyfish stings).

Efficacy of a jellyfish sting inhibitor in preventing jellyfish stings in normal volunteers. Kimball AB, Arambula KZ, Stauffer AR, Levy V, Davis VW, Liu M, et al. Wilderness Environ Med 2004; 15: 102–8.

This randomized controlled trial (RCT) showed that the topical barrier cream Safe Sea reduced incidence and severity of certain jellyfish stings.

A randomised controlled trial of hot water (45 degrees C) immersion versus ice packs for pain relief in bluebottle stings. Loten C, Stokes B, Worsley D, Seymour JE, Jiang S, Isbister GK. Med J Aust 2006; 184: 329–33.

Hot water immersion was more effective than cold packs at reducing pain in nematocyst-confirmed stings. Immersion in water at 45°C for 20 minutes provides effective and practical analgesia from bluebottle stings.

Evaluation of the effects of various chemicals on discharge of and pain caused by jellyfish nematocysts. Birsa LM, Verity PG, Lee RF. Comp Biochem Physiol C Toxicol Pharmacol 2010; 151: 426–30.

Immediate relief was reported when lidocaine was sprayed on the skin of testers in contact with jellyfish tentacles. Acetic acid, ammonia, meat tenderizer, baking soda, and urea may stimulate nematocyst discharge in *Chrysaora quinquecirrha* (sea nettle), *Chiropsalmus quadrumanus* (sea wasp), and *Physalia physalis* (Portuguese man-of-war) stings.

First aid treatment of jellyfish stings in Australia. Response to a newly differentiated species. Fenner PJ, Williamson JA, Burnett JW, Rifkin J. Med J Aust 1993; 158: 498–501.

Evidence Levels: A Double-blind study B Clinical trial ≥ 20 subjects C Clinical trial < 20 subjects D Series ≥ 5 subjects E Anecdotal case reports

Vinegar inhibits nematocyst discharge in box jellyfish stings and is accepted first aid treatment. However, it should not be used in *Physalia* (bluebottles) because it causes discharge of nematocysts.

First aid for jellyfish stings: do we really know what we are doing? Little M. Emerg Med Australas 2008; 20: 78–80.

First aid guidelines in Australia still suggest the use of ice, but little evidence exists to support this. There is more evidence for the use of hot water.

Is there a role for the use of pressure immobilization bandages in the treatment of jellyfish envenomation in Australia? Little M. Emerg Med (Fremantle) 2002; 14: 171–4.

A review of the literature indicates no benefit from applying compression bandages in jellyfish stings as recommended in some other envenomations.

Antivenom efficacy or effectiveness: the Australian experience. Isbister GK. Toxicology 2010; 268: 148–54.

A number of recent studies in Australia bring into question the effectiveness of some antivenoms, including box jellyfish antivenoms. The author notes this does not prove ineffectiveness, but suggests the need for more studies.

Australian venomous jellyfish, envenomation syndromes, toxins and therapy. Tibballs J. Toxicon 2006; 48: 830–59.

Case studies suggest antivenom for the major box jellyfish may be moderately efficacious.

Second-Line Therapies

Seabather's eruption

• Topical and oral antihistamines	E
• Topical and oral corticosteroids	E

Treatment of dermatitis and hyperpigmentation due to jellyfish stings

• Oral antihistamines	E
• Topical corticosteroids	E
• The immune modulators tacrolimus and pimecrolimus	E
• Hydroquinone	E

Secondary infections and long-term treatment

Dermonecrosis is a frequent outcome of *jellyfish* stings; however, many resolve spontaneously. Treating dermonecrosis from these envenomings as a burn, with specific attention to avoiding secondary bacterial infection, significantly decreases the risk of permanent scarring.

Seabather's eruption – a case of Caribbean itch. MacSween RM, Williams HC. BMJ 1996; 312: 957–8.

Reports one case of seabather's eruption successfully treated with topical 0.05% clobetasol propionate. In addition, the second case required 2 weeks of oral steroids, which relieved the symptoms, but the rash took 4 weeks to fade and left behind some faint atrophic scars at 8 weeks, follow-up.

Clinical perspectives on seabather's eruption, also known as "sea lice." Tomchik RS, Russell MT, Szmant AM, Black NA. JAMA 1993; 269: 1669–72.

Seabather's eruption is usually a benign clinical syndrome that resolves spontaneously. Treatment is symptomatic and involves the use of antihistamines and steroids.

Recurrent dermatitis after solitary envenomation by jelly fish partially responded to tacrolimus ointment 0.1%. Rallis E, Limas C. J Eur Acad Dermatol Venereol 2007; 21: 1287–8.

Topical tacrolimus produced improvement in symptoms in jellyfish-induced dermatitis.

Successful management of a delayed and persistent cutaneous reaction to jellyfish with pimecrolimus. Di Costanzo L, Balato N, Zagaria O, Balato A. J Dermatolog Treat 2009; 20: 179–80.

Topical pimecrolimus produced improvement in dermatitis.

Delayed cutaneous reaction to jellyfish. Veraldi S, Carrera C. Int J Dermatol 2000; 39: 28–9.

Oral hydroxyzine and topical hydrocortisone butyrate provided relief and reduced duration of a delayed dermatitis secondary to contact with an unknown jellyfish.

Granulomatous jellyfish dermatitis. Ulrich H, Landthaler M, Vogt T. J Dtsch Dermatol Ges 2007; 5: 493–5.

Topical therapy with tacrolimus 0.1% for two 2-week treatment periods led to healing of the skin changes with a slight scar in a patient with a granulomatous dermatitis.

Treatment of a pigmented lesion induced by a *Pelagia noctiluca* sting. Kokelj F, Burnett JW. Cutis 1990; 46: 62–4.

Hyperpigmentation, present 4 years after a jellyfish sting, was successfully treated within 4 days of using 1.8% hydroquinone.

Jessner lymphocytic infiltrate

Joanna E. Gach

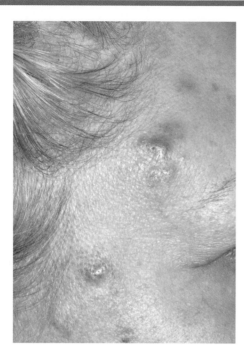

Jessner lymphocytic infiltrate (JLI) is a chronic inflammatory condition presenting with erythematous or reddish-brown papules or annular or arciform plaques, which can expand peripherally and sometimes develop central healing. The lesions are usually seen in adults and affect the face, neck, or upper trunk. Although they are frequently asymptomatic, some patients report itch or burning. A case report noted ectropion as a complication. The lesions can persist from weeks to years and disappear without sequelae but may recur. Additionally, JLI has been reported as a manifestation of borreliosis and an angiotensin-converting enzyme (ACE) inhibitor–induced drug eruption.

MANAGEMENT STRATEGY

JLI runs a waxing and waning course marked by intermittent improvement and subsequent exacerbations, which makes the evaluations of therapeutic effectiveness difficult. Patients demand treatment because they find the lesions disfiguring or itchy.

Potent topical steroids applied once or twice daily for 4 weeks are the first-line treatment for many dermatologists. Unfortunately, the results of treatment are variable and, most important, only short lasting. If the response is inadequate, injection of *intralesional corticosteroids* into localized lesions or the use of *potent topical steroids under occlusive dressing* may be beneficial but is associated with a greater risk of skin atrophy. *Topical tacrolimus* may be a safer alternative.

In cases where ultraviolet exposure has been reported to induce or exacerbate lesions, additional therapy with sunscreen may be needed. This group of patients may respond to *antimalarials*, in particular, hydroxychloroquine.

A variety of other therapies have been reported to be effective in the management of JLI. *Thalidomide, oral gold,* and *retinoids* proved to be helpful in some cases, but their use may be limited by the adverse effects, which may be difficult for the patient and physician to accept, especially as JLI is harmless.

Many other treatments, including nicotinamide, vitamin E, penicillin, chlortetracycline, minocycline, dapsone, quinacrine (mepacrine), and radiotherapy, have been tried unsuccessfully.

Specific Investigations

- Skin biopsy
- Lesional skin for direct immunofluorescence
- Antinuclear antibodies/extractable nuclear antigen

The diagnosis can be made on clinical grounds. The investigations are helpful in differentiating the condition from discoid lupus erythematosus, lupus erythematosus tumidus, and cutaneous lymphoma.

The heterogeneity of Jessner's lymphocytic infiltration of the skin. Immunohistochemical studies suggesting one form of perivascular lymphocytoma. Cerio R, Oliver GF, Jones EW, Winkelmann RK. J Am Acad Dermatol 1990; 23: 63–7.

Skin biopsy of the lesion shows normal epidermis and a moderate, dense, sleevelike perivascular and periadnexal infiltrate in the middle dermis. This consists of normal-looking lymphocytes with the B cells grouped in close proximity to the superficial vessels and T cells at the periphery, and occasionally, plasma cells.

Could Jessner's lymphocytic infiltrate of the skin be a dermal variant of lupus erythematosus? An analysis of 210 cases. Lipsker D, Mitschler A, Grosshans E, Cribier B. Dermatology 2006; 213: 15–22.

Immunofluorescence studies of lesional skin showed a lupus band with IgG, IgM ± C3 in 9.5% of cases of JLI. Antinuclear antibodies were present in 45% of cases.

Plasmacytoid dendritic cells: an overview of their presence and distribution in different inflammatory diseases, with special emphasis on Jessner's lymphocytic infiltrate of the skin and cutaneous lupus erythematosus. Tomasini D, Mentzel T, Hantschke M, Cerri A, Paredes B, Rütten A, et al. J Cutan Pathol 2010; 37: 1132–9.

Distribution of distinct perivascular and periadnexal clusters of plasmacytoid dendritic cells in JLI and tumid lupus erythematosus is identical.

First-Line Therapies

Potent topical/intralesional corticosteroids	C
Topical immunomodulators	E

Jessner's lymphocytic infiltration of the skin. A clinical study of 100 patients. Toonstra J, Wildschut A, Boer J, Smeenk G, Willemze R, van der Putte SC, et al. Arch Dermatol 1989; 125: 1525–30.

A series of 100 patients with JLI assessing clinical manifestations, duration, clinical course, and treatments. Forty-three of 91

Evidence Levels: A Double-blind study B Clinical trial ≥ 20 subjects C Clinical trial < 20 subjects D Series ≥ 5 subjects E Anecdotal case reports

patients treated with topical steroids had an excellent (*n* = 13) or good (*n* = 30) response, with temporary regression of the lesions. Many patients had no response.

Childhood Jessner's lymphocytic infiltrate of the skin. Higgins CR, Wakeel RA, Cerio R. Br J Dermatol 1994; 131: 99–101.

A case report of an 11-year-old boy with JLI responding to intralesional corticosteroids.

Effective treatment of chronic inflammatory skin diseases. Once a week occlusion therapy with clobetasol propionate and DuoDERM. Volden G. Tidsskr Nor Laegeforen 1992; 112: 1272–4.

JLI was among other chronic skin diseases that were treated once a week with clobetasol propionate lotion left under the completely occlusive hydrocolloid dressing DuoDERM. The lesions cleared within a few weeks.

Topical calcineurin inhibitors in treating Jessner's lymphocytic infiltration of the skin: report of a case. Tzung TY, Wu JC. Br J Dermatol 2005; 152: 383–4.

Tacrolimus 0.1% ointment twice daily produced an improvement after 2 weeks but had to be withdrawn because of diffuse erythema and desquamation that occurred 2 weeks later. The same effect occurred on rechallenge and settled with a single 5-mg dose of dexamethasone administered by intramuscular injection. Subsequently, pimecrolimus 1% cream cleared the rash within 6 weeks, with no relapse 2 months later.

Second-Line Therapies	
• Systemic corticosteroids	E
• Antimalarials	D
• Retinoids	E
• Photodynamic therapy	E
• Methotrexate	E
• Laser therapy	E
• Proquazone	C

Jessner's lymphocytic infiltrate treated with auranofin. Farrell AM, McGregor JM, Staughton RC, Bunker CB. Clin Exp Dermatol 1999; 24: 500.

Intramuscular injection of 40 mg Kenalog led to temporary improvement in this patient before oral gold was used successfully.

Jessner's lymphocytic infiltration of the skin. A clinical study of 100 patients. Toonstra J, Wildschut A, Boer J, Smeenk G, Willemze R, van der Putte SC, et al. Arch Dermatol 1989; 125: 1525–30.

Antimalarial drugs (chloroquine sulfate and hydroxychloroquine sulfate) were used in 15 patients, with a good response in 6. There were no details given regarding doses or treatment regimens.

Hydroxychloroquine 200 mg once or twice a day or chloroquine 200 mg daily was used in other case reports.

Satisfactory resolution of Jessner's lymphocytic infiltration of the skin following treatment with etretinate. Morgan J, Adams J. Br J Dermatol 1990; 122: 570.

One case of JLI was treated with etretinate 50 mg daily for 3 months and 25 mg daily for another 3 months. The rash subsided within 4 weeks of treatment and did not recur for 9 months after stopping treatment.

Isotretinoin 20 mg daily was used in other case reports but was not helpful.

Photodynamic therapy: new treatment for refractory lymphocytic infiltration of the skin. Park KY, Kim HK, Li K, Kim BJ, Seo SJ, Kim MN, et al. Clin Exp Dermatol 2012; 3: 235–7.

Remission was observed after two sessions of methyl 5-aminolevulinic acid cream photodynamic therapy with Aktilite 1 lamp, 630 nm.

Successful treatment of Jessner's lymphocytic infiltration of the skin with methotrexate. Laurinaviciene R, Clemmensen O, Bygum A. Acta Derm Venereol 2009; 89: 542–3.

Oral methotrexate 15 mg weekly for 6 months produced clearance. No recurrence 2 years after withdrawal of the drug.

Pulsed-dye laser treatment of Jessner lymphocytic infiltration of the skin. Borges da Costa J, Boixeda P, Moreno C. J Eur Acad Dermatol Venereol 2009; 23: 595–6.

Single treatment with 595-nm pulsed-dye laser cleared all lesions. New lesions were treated 2 months later.

Proquazone: a treatment for lymphocytic infiltration of the skin. Comparative study with 2 other nonsteroid antiinflammatory drugs. Johansson EA. Dermatologica 1987; 174: 117–21.

Eight of the 15 patients treated with proquazone (1-isopropyl-4-phenyl-7-methyl-2[IH]) 600 mg daily healed completely after 1 to 2 months of treatment. Recurrence of the rash in two cases responded to 600 mg daily for 3 to 4 days, on alternate months. Two further patients from among the initial responders showed a partial remission. Indomethacin (50–75 mg daily) and ibuprofen (1200 mg daily) were tried, without effect.

Third-Line Therapies	
• Auranofin	E
• Thalidomide	A

Jessner's lymphocytic infiltrate treated with auranofin. Farrell AM, McGregor JM, Staughton RC, Bunker CB. Clin Exp Dermatol 1999; 24: 500.

A marked improvement within 3 weeks of starting auranofin 3 mg orally twice daily. This case was unresponsive to chloroquine, hydroxychloroquine, minocycline, dapsone, and isotretinoin. Monitoring of the therapy includes monthly full blood count for thrombocytopenia and urinalysis to detect nephritis.

Crossover study of thalidomide vs. placebo in Jessner's lymphocytic infiltration of the skin. Guillaume JC, Moulin G, Dieng MT, Poli F, Morel P, Souteyrand P, et al. Arch Dermatol 1995; 131: 1032–5.

Twenty of 27 patients achieved complete remission after 2 months of therapy with thalidomide 100 mg daily. Sixteen (59%) patients were in complete remission 1 month after stopping therapy. Side effects included sleepiness, constipation, dry mouth, and sensorimotor neuropathy in two patients.

Juvenile plantar dermatosis

Stephen K. Jones

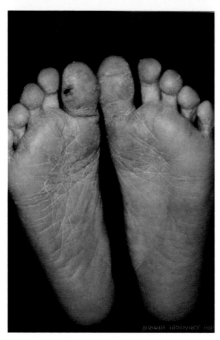

Courtesy of Joseph Bikowski, MD.

Juvenile plantar dermatosis (JPD) is a specific condition comprising symmetric erythema (with a polished "billiard ball" appearance), scaling, and fissuring, primarily of the pressure areas of the foot. Vesiculation is never found. The most common sites involved are the plantar aspects of the great toe, forefoot, heel, and rarely the fingertips and palms. The instep and interdigital skin are rarely affected. The condition occurs almost exclusively in children and clears around puberty.

MANAGEMENT STRATEGY

JPD usually presents between 4 and 7 years of age. Most series suggest that it is a "disease of school years," with clearing in most by puberty. It is uncommon in adults. Spontaneous resolution occurs in the majority of patients.

The main etiologic factor is thought to be the occlusive effect of "trainer" sports shoes and manmade fibers in hosiery, resulting in hyperhidrosis. This, some suggest, washes away surface lipids, which are already reduced because of the relative lack of sebaceous glands on the plantar surface of the foot. This hyperhidrosis is, therefore, followed by rapid dehydration of the skin on removal of footwear. It is proposed that this maceration/dehydration renders the skin susceptible to trauma (e.g., from sport). Avoidance of vigorous exercise may therefore be helpful in these patients.

The role of atopy is debated. Some series have found an increased incidence of atopy in patients and families, and, indeed, this condition was first referred to as "atopic winter feet." It has been argued that the atopic diathesis predisposes the skin of the foot to the traumatic effects of sport and vigorous activity and the effects of alternating hyperhidrosis and dehydration. Other series, however, have found no increased incidence of atopy.

Investigations are unlikely to be helpful, but positive patch tests have been found in between 10% and 29% of cases. Even when these are to footwear-related allergens, however, there is debate as to whether allergen avoidance affects clinical outcome. Increased numbers of bacteria have been suggested to cause inflammation of the sweat ducts and thereby inhibit sweat secretion, but this has not been a consistent finding.

Changing to nonocclusive footwear along with cotton socks or open footwear has been proposed as a therapeutic maneuver. *Emollients*, both to reduce fissuring and to reduce the dehydration occurring on removing occlusive footwear, are reported to be helpful. *Topical corticosteroids* may be beneficial if there is an inflammatory component. *Occlusive bandages* containing zinc ointment, ichthammol, or tar may help if hyperkeratosis and fissuring are a prominent feature. All these often only help temporarily, and regular rotation of emollients may be required.

It is the impression of most dermatologists that this condition has become less common in recent years, possibly related to changes in teenage fashion and footwear materials.

Specific Investigation

- Patch tests

Juvenile plantar dermatosis: a new entity. Mackie RM, Hussain SL. Clin Exp Dermatol 1976; 1: 253–60.

Thirteen of 102 patients showed a positive patch test. Eight were reactions to footwear constituents, but subsequent changes in footwear did not affect the clinical outcome.

Common pediatric foot dermatoses. Guenst BJ. J Pediatr Health Care 1999; 13: 68–71.

A practical review differentiating the various forms of tinea pedis and shoe dermatitis from JPD.

Sole dermatitis in children: patch testing revisited. Darling MI, Horn HM, McCormack SK, Schofield OM. Pediatr Dermatol 2011; 29: 254–7.

Of 14 children with JPD, 29% had clinically relevant reactions.

First-Line Therapy

• Await spontaneous resolution	C

Juvenile plantar dermatosis – an 8 year follow-up of 102 patients. Jones SK, English JSC, Forsyth A, Mackie RM. Clin Exp Dermatol 1987; 12: 5–7.

Of 50 patients traced, the condition had resolved in 38. The mean age of remission was 14 years.

Second-Line Therapies

• Change to nonocclusive footwear	C
• Sport avoidance	C
• Emollients	C
• Topical corticosteroids	C
• Rotation of topical agents	C
• Topical tacrolimus	C

Evidence Levels: A Double-blind study B Clinical trial ≥ 20 subjects C Clinical trial < 20 subjects D Series ≥ 5 subjects E Anecdotal case reports

Juvenile plantar dermatosis. Can sweat cause foot rash and peeling?. Gibbs NF. Postgrad Med 2004; 115: 73–5.

A review of the disease, its etiology, and its treatment.

Juvenile plantar dermatosis. Graham RM, Verbov JL, Vickers CFH. Br J Dermatol 1987; 12: 468–70.

Although there was no association with any particular sport, intensive exercise causing skin cracking, soreness, and bleeding was a common complaint; 75% of parents said that a change in footwear had not been helpful.

In contrast to Jones et al. earlier, only 30% of cases in this series had resolved (mean age 11.8 years), though the ages of the remaining 70% were not stated.

Juvenile plantar dermatosis responding to topical tacrolimus. Shipley DR, Kennedy CTC. Clin Exp Dermatol 2005; 31: 453–4.

Topical 0.1% tacrolimus twice daily in conjunction with a regular emollient produced improvement within 4 weeks, with the feet appearing almost normal after 2 months. Intermittent tacrolimus was useful for relapses.

Third-Line Therapies	
• Zinc oxide/impregnated bandages	C
• Bed rest/footwear avoidance	E

Juvenile plantar dermatosis. Graham RM, Verbov JL, Vickers CFH. Br J Dermatol 1987; 12: 468–70.

Occlusion with zinc paste or ichthammol-impregnated bandages was among the most beneficial of treatments.

The etiology of juvenile plantar dermatosis. Shrank AB. Br J Dermatol 1979; 100: 641–8.

Bed rest or avoidance of shoes/hosiery for 3 weeks resulted in disease clearance (thought to be related to the time taken for the sweat duct apparatus in the foot to regrow).

Juvenile xanthogranuloma

Megan Mowbray, Lynsey Taylor

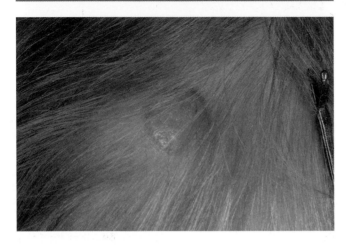

Juvenile xanthogranuloma (JXG) is a benign disorder characterized by solitary or multiple yellow-red nodules in the skin and, occasionally, in other organs. Lesions usually regress spontaneously by age 6 months to 3 years. JXG is most common in infancy and early childhood, but adults may be affected. Treatment is only recommended for systemic lesions if their location interferes with organ function.

MANAGEMENT STRATEGY

The diagnosis of JXG is usually made clinically, but a biopsy is required for atypical clinical variants (giant, plaquelike, paired, clustered, infiltrative, lichenoid, linear, subcutaneous, and intramuscular) and if multiple lesions are present. JXG is classified as a "non-Langerhans cell histiocytosis" and characterized histologically by an accumulation of foamy histiocytes lacking Birbeck granules (non-Langerhans cells) and multinucleated Touton-type giant cells. Immunohistochemical staining of lesions shows expression of factor XIIIa, cluster of differentiation (CD68), CD163, fascin, Human leukocyte antigen-antigen D related (HLA-DR), and CD14 but not S100 or CD1a. This pattern of expression suggests that the cell of origin of JXG is the dermal dendrocyte. The histogenesis of this group of conditions is unclear, but the relationship to Langerhans cell histiocytosis (LCH) is thought to be divergent differentiation from a common precursor CD34+ myeloid cell. Cases of the two conditions reported in the same individual suggest that this divergent maturation is not irreversible. B-Raf proto-oncogene (BRAF) Valine (V) substituted by glutamic acid (E) at codon 600 (V600E) mutations have been found in high frequency in LCH and Erdheim–Chester disease (ECD), suggesting a common origin of these diseases, but not, however, in any of the other histiocytoses.

The JXG family can be divided into three groups:

- Cutaneous – JXG, benign cephalic histiocytosis, generalized eruptive histiocytosis, adult xanthogranuloma, progressive nodular histiocytosis

- Cutaneous with a major systemic component – xanthoma disseminatum
- Systemic – ECD, rarely seen in children

In the most common solitary type of JXG (60%–89% of all cases), there is a male-to-female preponderance of 1.5:1. The usual affected sites are the head, neck, and upper trunk. In young infants with multiple lesions the male:female ratio increases to 12:1. In the majority of cases no further investigation is required, with lesions regressing spontaneously within months or years without the need for follow-up. Because involvement of other organs can occasionally occur in the cutaneous group, a review of systems and general examination is recommended to exclude extracutaneous involvement and to examine for café au lait macules (see later).

Eye involvement

The eye is the most commonly affected extracutaneous site of JXG. Uveal lesions are the most frequently reported, but lesions affecting the eyelid, orbit, conjunctiva, cornea, and optic nerve have also been described. Ocular symptoms and signs include unilateral redness and tearing, hyphema (hemorrhage into the anterior chamber), retinal detachment, and/or visible lesions of the corneal limbus, eyelids, optic nerve, or papilla. Iris lesions may lead to hyphema and glaucoma. The incidence of eye involvement in cutaneous JXG is only 0.2% to 0.4%, but ocular JXG can occur without cutaneous disease and can be locally aggressive.

Systemic JXG

Systemic JXG is classically defined as involvement of two or more visceral organs in addition to multiple cutaneous and subcutaneous lesions. However, there are many reports of extracutaneous involvement occurring both with and without cutaneous lesions. After the eye, the subcutis, central nervous system (CNS), lung, liver, and spleen are the most common sites, but there are reports of every organ system in the body being affected (testes, spine, tongue, and heart, among others). *Given the differential diagnosis is usually neoplasia, it is imperative to determine an accurate diagnosis.* As with the skin, extracutaneous lesions regress spontaneously, and treatment is therefore *only indicated in cases where organ function is compromised.*

Triple association of JXG, NF-1, and JMML

It is likely that there is an association of JXG with NF-1 (neurofibromatosis-1). Children with NF-1 have a 200- to 500-fold greater risk of developing juvenile myelomonocytic leukemia (JMML), and the triple association of JXG, NF-1, and JMML has also been reported. JMML is an aggressive myeloproliferative disorder of childhood that has an annual incidence of 1.2 per million, and although the absolute incidence is not known, it is possible that in a population of children with NF-1, the incidence of JMML could be between 1/2000 and 1/5000. An awareness of the increased risk of JMML in NF-1 and in cases with both JXG and NF-1 is important to ensure early diagnosis. Furthermore, the high frequency of JXG in NF-1 has been found useful diagnostically in children under 2 years with NF-1, as the seven clinical criteria required for diagnosis are of limited value before the age of 2 years. As well as JXG, naevus anemicus (NA) is found in high frequency in patients with NF-1, especially in children under 2 years with fewer than two diagnostic criteria.

Association of JXG and hematologic malignancy in adults

In adults there have been sporadic reports of xanthogranulomas preceding or arising concurrently with hematologic malignancies.

Specific Investigations

- In most cases, no specific investigations are required
- Ophthalmologic assessment in children under the age of 2 years with multiple lesions
- Full blood count and/or pediatric referral in children with JXG and café au lait macules, NF-1, or a family history of NF
- Biopsy in cases of unusual clinical variants
- Biopsy in cases with systemic manifestations to avoid unnecessary invasive diagnostic procedures

---

High prevalence of BRAF V600E mutations in Erdheim-Chester disease but not in other non-Langerhans cell histiocytoses. Haroche J, Charlotte F, Arnaud L, von Deimling A, Hélias-Rodzewicz Z, Hervier B. Blood 2012; 120: 2700–3.

BRAF status obtained in 93 cases. BRAF mutations were detected in 54% ECD, 38% LCH, and none of the other histiocytoses.

Radiological and clinicopathological features of orbital xanthogranuloma. Miszkiel KA, Sohaib SAS, Rose GE, Cree IA, Moseley IF. Br J Ophthalmol 2000; 84: 251–8.

Of 150 cases of intraocular JXG, none was identified on routine screening of individuals with cutaneous JXG. Of those children with eye involvement, 92% were under the age of 2 years, and if present, cutaneous lesions tended to be multiple.

Juvenile xanthogranuloma. Hernandez-Martin A, Baselga E, Drolet BA, Esterley NB. J Am Acad Dermatol 1997; 36: 355–67.

Recommendations are made in this review article following assessment of previously reported cutaneous and extracutaneous cases. In general, an awareness of the possibility of extracutaneous involvement is important.

The risk of intraocular juvenile xanthogranuloma: survey of current practices and assessment of risk. Wu Chang M, Frieden IJ, Good W. J Am Acad Dermatol 1996; 34: 445–9.

A postal survey of pediatric dermatologists (27% response rate) and ophthalmologists (44% response rate) revealed the difference in incidence of ocular xanthogranuloma presenting to both groups. Children under the age of 2 years with multiple skin lesions have the highest risk of intraocular involvement and should be screened by an ophthalmologist.

Juvenile xanthogranuloma associated with neurofibromatosis-1: 14 patients without evidence of hematologic malignancies. Cambhiangi SD, Restano L, Caputo R. Pediatr Dermatol 2004; 21: 97–101.

A retrospective review of 14 individuals affected by JXG and NF-1. The onset of JXG was within the first 2 years of life in 13 patients. Mean follow-up was for 4.3 years (range 1–10 years) in

11 patients, and none of these children developed hematologic malignancy during this period.

JXG, NF-1 and JMML: alphabet soup or a clinical issue?. Burgdorf WH, Zelger B. Pediatr Dermatol 2004; 21: 174–6.

An editorial comment and review on this triple association, which concludes that there is no evidence to support an increased risk of JMML in children with the combination of JXG and NF-1 compared with those children with NF-1 alone.

Juvenile xanthogranuloma in a child with previously unsuspected NF1 and JMML. Raygada M, Arthur DC, Wayne AS, Rennert OM, Toretsky JA, Stratakis CA. Pediatr Blood Cancer 2010; 54: 173–5.

Case report of a 9-month-old male with the triple association of JXG, NF-1, and JMML.

NF-1 diagnosed in a child based on multiple JXG and JMML. Jans SR, Schomerus E, Bygum A. Paediatr Dermatol 2015; 31: e29–31.

Case report of a 9-month-old male with multiple JXGs and NF-1 who developed JMML at 20 months of age.

Juvenile xanthogranuloma and naevus anemicus in the diagnosis of neurofibromatosis type 1. Ferrari F, Masurel A, Olivier-Faivre L, Vabres P. JAMA Dermatol 2014; 150: 142–6.

Among 72 patients with NF-1, 23 had JXG or NA. Both lesions were more frequent in those younger than 2 years. None of those with JXG developed chronic myelomonocytic leukemia.

First-Line Therapies

• None	E
• Surgical resection for symptomatic cutaneous and extracutaneous lesions	D

Juvenile xanthogranuloma: forms of systemic disease and their clinical implications. Freyer DR, Kennedy R, Bostrom BC, Kohut G, Dehner LP. J Pediatr 1996; 129: 227–37.

Surgery can be an effective cure for symptomatic extracutaneous lesions of JXG.

Update on juvenile xanthogranuloma: unusual cutaneous and systemic variants. Wu Chang M. Semin Cutan Med Surg 1999; 18: 195–205.

In adults, lesions tend not to resolve spontaneously and can last up to 7 years; excision may therefore be considered appropriate.

Second-Line Therapies

• Topical and intralesional corticosteroids for ocular lesions	D
• Oral corticosteroids	E
• Ocular surgery	E
• CO_2 laser for cutaneous lesions	E

Early treatment of juvenile xanthogranuloma of the iris with subconjunctival steroids. Casteels I, Olver J, Malone M, Taylor D. Br J Ophthalmol 1993; 77: 57–60.

Ocular lesions have been successfully treated with topical and intralesional corticosteroids.

Severe congenital systemic juvenile xanthogranuloma in monozygotic twins. Chantorn Wisuthsarewong W, Aanpreung P, Sanpakit K, Manonukul J. Pediatr Dermatol 2008; 25: 470–3.

Monozygotic twins with multiple cutaneous JXG, hepatosplenomegaly, liver failure, and bone marrow involvement. Treatment with systemic prednisolone 1 mg/kg/day with regression of lesions.

Infiltrative subcutaneous juvenile xanthogranuloma of the eyelid in a neonate. Kuruvula R, Escaravage GK Jr, Finn AJ, Dutton JJ. Ophthal Plast Reconstr Surg 2009; 25: 330–2.

Successful treatment with a combination of intralesional and oral corticosteroids.

Juvenile xanthogranuloma of the corneoscleral limbus. Lim-I-Linn Z, Li L. Cornea 2005; 24: 745–7.

Case report of successful surgical excision and grafting of a limbal juvenile xanthogranuloma in a child without cutaneous lesions.

Multiple juvenile xanthogranulomas successfully treated with CO_2 laser. Klemcke CD, Held B, Dippel E, Goerdt S. J Deutsch Dermatol Ges 2007; 144: 481–2.

Case report describing successful treatment of cutaneous JXG with CO_2 laser, with no recurrence at 5-year follow-up.

Third-Line Therapies	
• Chemotherapy, including oral corticosteroids	D
• Radiotherapy	D
• Oral methotrexate	E
• Pulsed methylprednisolone	E
• Vemurafenib	E

Use of radiation in treatment of CNS JXG. Vijapura CA, Fulbright JM. Paediatr Hematol Oncol 2012; 29: 440–5. Case report of a 13-year-old successfully treated with adjuvant radiotherapy for intracranial and leptomeningeal JXG. Literature review to identify all previous CNS JXG cases utilizing radiation, with six of eight patients demonstrating temporary or long-term improvement of neurologic disease.

Treatment of JXG. Stover DG, Alapati S, Regueira O, Turner C, Whitlock JA. Pediatr Blood Cancer 2008; 51: 130–3.

Two case reports of multisystem JXG. Treatment with LCH-based chemotherapy regimens resulted in prompt resolution of symptoms. This paper includes a literature review of all reported multisystem JXG cases treated with chemotherapy. Ten prior studies describe 15 cases (29 chemotherapeutic regimens of multisystem JXG). Twelve of the 15 patients received some form of corticosteroid; 9 of the 12 receiving corticosteroid had stable disease (SD), partial response (PR), or complete resolution (CR). Regimens that included corticosteroids and a vinca alkaloid had the highest and those without corticosteroids the lowest rates of CR, PR, or SD, respectively.

Pediatric lymphomas and histiocytic disorders of childhood. Allen CE, Kelly KM, Bollard CM. Pediatr Clin North Am 2015; 62: 139–65.

A comprehensive review of the current science and treatment strategies for all pediatric patients with lymphoma and histiocytic disorders. Cladribine and clofarabine have been reported as effective in patients with refractory or recurrent JXG. Therapies for ECD have included interferon (IFN-α) and recently vemurafenib.

Cladribine is highly effective in the treatment of Langerhans cell histiocytosis and rare histiocytic disorders of the juvenile xanthogranuloma group. Adam Z, Szturz P, Pour L, Krejčí M, Zahradová L, Tomíška M, et al. Vnitr Lek 2012; 58: 455–65.

This paper presents a survey of published experience with cladribine (2-CdA) in patients with LCH and JXG. Seven publications describe therapy response in certain JXG variants (ECD, disseminated JXG, and localized form of plain xanthoma type) to cladribine.

Juvenile xanthogranulomatosis with bilateral and multifocal ocular lesions of the iris, cornealscleral limbus, and choroid. Longmuir S, Dumitrescu A, Kwon Y, Boldt HC, Hong S. JAAPOS 2011; 15: 598–600.

Case report of 14-month-old boy with JXG skin lesions presenting with increased intraocular pressure, hyphema, anterior uveitis, iris mass, and subconjunctival limbal mass of the right eye with subsequent development of subretinal mass in the left eye. Ophthalmic disease responded to periocular injections of triamcinolone, topical prednisolone, oral prednisolone, and methotrexate. First published case using methotrexate as adjunctive treatment of JXG in a child.

Evidence Levels: **A** Double-blind study **B** Clinical trial ≥ 20 subjects **C** Clinical trial < 20 subjects **D** Series ≥ 5 subjects **E** Anecdotal case reports

Kaposi sarcoma

Niraj Butala, Sandra Pena, Steven M. Manders

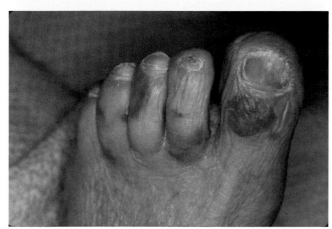

Kaposi sarcoma (KS) is a distinct, often multifocal, endothelial neoplasm etiologically linked to Kaposi sarcoma herpesvirus (KSHV) or human herpesvirus 8 (HHV8), predominantly transmitted via saliva but also by solid organ transplantation. In the United States, epidemic or acquired immunodeficiency syndrome (AIDS)-associated KS is the most common presentation; however, transplant or iatrogenic immunosuppression-related KS is on the increase. In clinical practice, classic and endemic KSs are also encountered. Therapy is similar for each type.

MANAGEMENT STRATEGY

Generally, the goals of therapy target cosmetic improvement, palliation, or cessation of progression. For treatment purposes, patients can be divided into several groups. Dermatologists most often encounter limited cutaneous KS, defined as fewer than 10 skin lesions, a lack of oral or visceral involvement, and the absence of tumor-associated lymphedema. Treatment options include *cryotherapy, intralesional vinblastine, radiotherapy,* and *alitretinoin gel.* Because treatment is essentially for cosmesis, side effects such as pigmentary changes and pain become important in therapeutic decisions.

For patients with resistant limited disease, extensive cutaneous involvement, systemic KS, or tumor-associated lymphedema, treatment modalities include liposomal anthracyclines (pegylated liposomal doxorubicin or liposomal daunorubicin), taxanes (paclitaxel), and interferon-α. For epidemic KS, effective antiretroviral therapy (ART) can by itself be sufficient to halt disease progression and has been found to have a synergistic effect with the *liposomal anthracyclines, paclitaxel,* and *interferon-α.* However, several cases of worsening of KS with the initiation of ART have been reported as part of an immune reconstitution syndrome. Iatrogenic immunosuppression–associated KS can respond to a reduction in treatment doses or a change in the immunosuppressive regimen to *sirolimus.* *Radiotherapy* remains an alternative treatment option for this group of patients.

Treatment of oral lesions is problematic because of inaccessibility to cryotherapy and radiation-induced mucositis. Options include *intralesional vinblastine,* sclerosing agents such as *sodium tetradecyl sulfate,* or systemic treatments.

An increasing number of investigational therapeutics have been explored for the treatment and prevention of KS, including antiangiogenic agents, antiviral agents, orally active matrix metalloproteinase inhibitors, tyrosine kinase inhibitors, and agents targeting interleukin (IL)-12.

Specific Investigations

- Serology for human immunodeficiency virus (HIV), CD4+ T-lymphocyte counts, viral load (if HIV positive)
- Complete blood count, renal and hepatic function
- Chest radiograph
- Stool for occult blood

Management of AIDS-related Kaposi's sarcoma. Di Lorenzo G, Konstantinopoulos PA, Pantanowitz L, Di Trolio R, De Placido S, Dezube BJ. Lancet Oncol 2007; 8: 167–76.

Review of current treatment strategies and ongoing investigations.

Update on KSHV epidemiology, Kaposi sarcoma pathogenesis, and treatment of Kaposi sarcoma. Uldrick TS, Whitby D. Cancer Lett 2001; 30: 150–62.

Comprehensive review of KS, including etiology and treatment options.

First-Line Therapies

Pegylated liposomal doxorubicin	A
Paclitaxel	A
Antiretroviral therapy	B
Cryotherapy	B
Radiotherapy	B
Alitretinoin gel	A

PEGylated liposomal doxorubicin plus highly active antiretroviral therapy versus highly active antiretroviral therapy alone in HIV patients with Kaposi's sarcoma. Martin-Carbonero L, Barrios A, Saballs P, Sirera G, Santos J, Palacios R, et al; Caelyx/KS Spanish Group. AIDS 2004; 18: 1737–40.

Randomized study comparing pegylated liposomal doxorubicin (20 mg/m² every 3 weeks) plus ART versus ART alone showed a greater response rate (76% vs. 20%, respectively, in the intent-to-treat analysis) in the former group.

Liposomal doxorubicin is currently the chemotherapeutic agent of choice.

A randomized controlled trial of highly active antiretroviral therapy versus highly active antiretroviral therapy and chemotherapy in therapy-naive patients with HIV-associated Kaposi sarcoma in South Africa. Mosam A, Shaik F, Uldrick TS, Esterhuizen T, Friedland GH, Scadden DT, et al. JAIDS 2012; 60: 150–7.

Fifty-nine treatment-naïve patients were randomized to ART (stavudine, lamivudine, and nevirapine) and 53 to ART and chemotherapy (triomune plus bleomycin, doxorubicin, and vincristine). Overall KS response was 39% in the ART arm and 66% in the combination therapy arm. There was no survival difference.

Multicenter trial of low-dose paclitaxel in patients with advanced AIDS-related Kaposi sarcoma. Tulpule A, Groopman J, Saville MW, Harrington Jr W, Friedman-Kien A, Espina BM, et al. Cancer 2002; 95: 147–54.

Phase II trial of 107 patients showed a complete or partial response, with or without concomitant protease inhibitor of 59% and 54%, respectively.

Randomized trial of paclitaxel versus pegylated liposomal doxorubicin for advanced human immunodeficiency virus-associated Kaposi sarcoma. Cianfrocca M, Lee S, Von Roenn J, Tulpule A, Dezube BJ, Aboulafia DM, et al. Cancer 2010; 116: 3969–77.

Seventy-three patients with advanced HIV–associated KS were randomized to paclitaxel versus pegylated liposomal doxorubicin, both of which resulted in significant improvement of pain and swelling. Overall incidence of toxicity was greater in those treated with paclitaxel.

Highly active antiretroviral therapy in AIDS-associated Kaposi's sarcoma: implications for the design of therapeutic trials in patients with advanced, symptomatic Kaposi's sarcoma. Krown SE. J Clin Oncol 2004; 22: 399–402.

This article reviews the evidence regarding the use of monotherapy in KS. In patients with early disease (stage T_0), 80% of patients who had not previously received ART showed regression with ART alone.

Cryotherapy for cutaneous Kaposi's sarcoma (KS) associated with acquired immune deficiency syndrome (AIDS): a phase II trial. Tappero JW, Berger TG, Kaplan LD, Volberding PA, Kahn JO. JAIDS 1991; 4: 839–46.

Subjects received an average of three treatments per lesion resulting in a 70% cosmetic response rate.

Radiotherapy of classic and human immunodeficiency virus-related Kaposi's sarcoma: results in 1482 lesions. Caccialanza M, Marca S, Piccinno R, Eulisse G. J Eur Acad Dermatol Venereol 2008; 22: 297–302.

A 98% clearance rate was reported in classic lesions, and a 91% clearance rate in HIV-associated lesions, with good overall tolerability.

Phase III vehicle-controlled, multicentered study of topical alitretinoin gel 0.1% in cutaneous AIDS-related Kaposi's sarcoma. Bodsworth NJ, Bloch M, Bower M, Donnell D, Yocum R, International Panretin Gel KS Study Group. Am J Clin Dermatol 2001; 2: 77–87.

Response rate was 37% (compared with 7% treated with vehicle).

Marginal response rate and exorbitant cost make the usefulness of this modality questionable. Tretinoin gel may be a reasonable alternative topical retinoid option (Topical treatment of epidemic Kaposi's sarcoma with all-transretinoic acid. Bonhomme L, Fredj G, Averous S, Szekely AM, Ecstein E, Trumbic B, et al. Ann Oncol 1991; 2: 234–5).

Second-Line Therapies

• Intralesional interferon	C
• Interferon-α_{2b}	C
• Intralesional vinblastine	C

Intralesional interferon-alpha and zidovudine in epidemic Kaposi's sarcoma. Dupuy J, Prize M, Lynch G, Bruce S, Schwartz M. J Am Acad Dermatol 1993; 28: 966–72.

Intralesional interferon-α (1 million units three times weekly for 6 weeks) showed a response rate of 85%, but this was not statistically significant.

Interferon-alpha2b with protease inhibitor-based antiretroviral therapy in patients with AIDS-associated Kaposi sarcoma: an AIDS malignancy consortium phase I trial. Krown SE, Lee JY, Lin L, Fischl MA, Ambinder R, Von Roenn JH. AIDS 2006; 41: 149–53.

The authors observed that the administration of interferon-α_{2b} led to limited improvement in KS lesions. The maximum tolerated dose was 5 million IU/day.

Intralesional vinblastine for cutaneous Kaposi's sarcoma associated with acquired immunodeficiency syndrome. Boudreaux AA, Smith LL, Cosby CD, Bason MM, Tappero JW, Berger TG. J Am Acad Dermatol 1993; 28: 61–5.

Responses were achieved in 88% of treated lesions, but pain and hyperpigmentation are common. Pain was minimized by the addition of bicarbonate-buffered lidocaine to the diluent.

Third-Line Therapies

• Bevacizumab	C
• Sorafenib	E
• Gemcitabine	E
• Lenalidomide	E
• Thalidomide	B
• Liposomal all-trans retinoic acid, intravenous	B
• Photodynamic therapy	B
• 9-*cis*-retinoic acid	B
• Etoposide	B
• Mechanistic target of rapamycin (mTOR) inhibitors (sirolimus/rapamycin)	C
• IL-12	C
• Matrix metalloproteinase inhibitor Col-3	C
• Halofuginone	C
• Imiquimod 5% cream	C
• Sodium tetradecyl sulfate 3%	C
• Surgical excision	E
• Antiviral agents (ganciclovir, valganciclovir, foscarnet)	B
• Intramuscular immunoglobulin	E

Phase II study of bevacizumab in patients with HIV-associated Kaposi's sarcoma receiving antiretroviral therapy. Uldrick TS, Wyvill KM, Kumar P, O'Mahony D, Bernstein W, Aleman K, et al. J Clin Oncol 2012; 30: 1476–83.

Seventeen patients with HIV-associated KS were treated with bevacizumab, an anti-vascular endothelial growth factor A (VEGFA) monoclonal antibody. Overall response rate (complete response plus partial response) was 31%.

A Kaposi's sarcoma complete clinical response after sorafenib administration. Ardavanis A, Doufexis D, Kountourakis P, Rigatos G. Ann Oncol 2008; 19: 1658–9.

This is a report of a clinical response of KS to sorafenib (400 mg by mouth twice daily) when administered as treatment for renal cell carcinoma.

Gemcitabine for the treatment of classic Kaposi's sarcoma: a case series. Zustovich F, Ferro A, Toso S. Anticancer Research 2013; 33: 5531–4.

Four patients with classic KS successfully responded to gemcitabine as monotherapy.

Lenalidomide in treating AIDS-related Kaposi's sarcoma. Martinez V, Tateo M, Castilla MA, Melica G, Kirstetter M, Boué F. AIDS 2011; 25: 878–80.

Three cases are described of HIV-associated KS successfully treated by lenalidomide, an analog to thalidomide.

A retrospective analysis of thalidomide therapy in non-HIV-related Kaposi's sarcoma. Ben M'barek L, Fardet L, Mebazaa A, Thervet E, Biet I, Kérob D, et al. Dermatology 2007; 215: 202–5.

Only 3 of 11 patients achieved remission, with sensory neuropathy and vertigo limiting therapy in 27%.

A multicenter phase II study of the intravenous administration of liposomal tretinoin in patients with acquired immunodeficiency syndrome-associated Kaposi's sarcoma. Bernstein ZP, Chanan-Khan A, Miller KC, Northfelt DW, Lopez-Berestein G, Gill PS. Cancer 2002; 95: 2555–61.

A thrice-weekly dosing schedule (60 mg/m^2 escalating to 90 mg/m^2 and then to 120 mg/m^2 if tolerated) was more effective than once a week, without any significant difference in toxicity.

New photodynamic therapy protocol to treat AIDS-related Kaposi's sarcoma. Tardivo JP, Del Giglio A, Paschoal LH, Baptista MS. Photomed Laser Surg 2006; 24: 528–31.

Case report describing successful treatment of a solitary patient with epidemic KS.

9-cis-retinoic acid capsules in the treatment of AIDS-related Kaposi sarcoma: results of a phase 2 multicenter clinical trial. Aboulafia DM, Norris D, Henry D, Grossman RJ, Thommes J, Bundow D, et al. Arch Dermatol 2003; 139: 178–86.

Overall response was 19%. Moderate efficacy and substantial toxicity at higher doses limit use.

Phase II evaluation of low-dose oral etoposide for the treatment of relapsed or progressive AIDS-related Kaposi's sarcoma: an AIDS Clinical Trials Group clinical study. Evans SR, Krown SE, Testa MA, Cooley TP, Von Roenn JH. J Clin Oncol 2002; 20: 3236–41.

Overall response rate was 36.1%; neutropenia and opportunistic infections were the most common side effects.

Sirolimus for Kaposi's sarcoma in renal-transplant recipients. Stallone G, Schena A, Infante B, Di Paolo S, Di Paolo S, Loverre A, et al. N Engl J Med 2005; 352: 1317–23.

All of 15 transplant patients achieved total remission when switched from ciclosporin to sirolimus for immunosuppression.

Classic Kaposi's sarcoma treated with topical rapamycin. Diaz-Ley B, Grillo E, Rios-Buceta L, Paoli J, Moreno C, Vano-Galvan S, et al. Dermatol Ther 2015; 28: 40–3.

An immunocompetent patient improved after 16 weeks of treatment with topical rapamycin.

Phase 2 study of pegylated liposomal doxorubicin in combination with interleukin-12 for AIDS-related Kaposi sarcoma. Little RF, Aleman K, Kumar P, Wyvill KM, Pluda JM, Read-Connole E, et al. Blood 2007; 110: 4165–71.

Thirty of 36 patients had a good response to liposomal doxorubicin with IL-12 for six 3-week cycles followed by twice-weekly IL-12 for maintenance for 3 years. No control group was included, and patients received highly active antiretroviral therapy (HAART) in addition to the experimental regimen.

Activity of subcutaneous interleukin-12 in AIDS-related Kaposi sarcoma. Little RF, Pluda JM, Wyvill KM, Rodriguez-Chavez IR, Tosato G, Catanzaro AT, et al. Blood 2006; 107: 4650–7.

IL-12 was administered twice weekly at varying doses. Significant results were observed at doses >100 ng/mg; side effects limited dosing above 500 ng/kg.

Randomized phase II trial of matrix metalloproteinase inhibitor COL-3 in AIDS-related Kaposi's sarcoma: an AIDS Malignancy Consortium Study. Dezube BJ, Krown SE, Lee JY, Bauer KS, Aboulafia DM. J Clin Oncol 2006; 24: 1389–94.

A response rate of 41% was observed at a dose of 50 mg/day. The medication was well tolerated overall.

Phase II AIDS malignancy consortium trial of topical halofuginone in AIDS-related Kaposi's sarcoma. Koon HB, Fingleton B, Lee JY, Geyer JT, Cesarman E, Parise RA, et al. JAIDS 2011; 56: 64–8.

Twenty-six patients with HIV and KS limited to the skin were treated with halofuginone (angiogenesis inhibitor) with response rate of 35%.

Imiquimod 5% cream for treatment of HIV-negative Kaposi's sarcoma skin lesions: a phase I to II, open-label trial in 17 patients. Célestin Schartz NE, Chevret S, Paz C, Kerob D, Verola O, Morel P, et al. J Am Acad Dermatol 2008; 585–91.

Imiquimod was applied under occlusion three times a week for 24 weeks. Eight of 17 patients showed some response, with 6 of 17 demonstrating tumor progression.

Intralesional vinblastine vs. 3% sodium tetradecyl sulfate for the treatment of oral Kaposi's sarcoma. A double blind, randomized clinical trial. Ramírez-Amador V, Esquivel-Pedraza L, Lozada-Nur F, De la Rosa-García E, Volkow-Fernández P, Súchil-Bernal L, et al. Oral Oncol 2002; 38: 460–7.

Sixteen patients were randomized to each arm. Results were equivocal but suggested a possibly greater tolerability of sodium tetradecyl sulfate.

Local therapy for mucocutaneous Kaposi's sarcoma in patients with acquired immunodeficiency syndrome. Webster GF. Dermatol Surg 1995; 21: 205–8.

Surgery can occasionally be helpful for isolated lesions, but recurrence is frequent; therefore this modality is of limited value.

Oral ganciclovir for patients with cytomegalovirus retinitis treated with a ganciclovir implant. Martin DF, Kupperman BD, Wolitz RA, Palestine AG, Li H, Robinson CA. N Engl J Med 1999; 340: 1063–70.

In this randomized controlled trial, intravenous and oral ganciclovir resulted in a decrease in the development of KS.

Effect of antiviral drugs used to treat cytomegalovirus end organ disease on subsequent course of previously diagnosed

Kaposi's sarcoma in patients with AIDS. Robles R, Lugo D, Gee L, Jacobson MA. J AIDS Hum Retrovirol 1999; 20: 34–8.

In patients being treated for cytomegalovirus with foscarnet, progression of KS was markedly delayed.

Valganciclovir for suppression of human herpesvirus 8 replication: a randomized, double-blind, placebo-controlled, crossover trial. Casper C, Krantz EM, Corey L, Kuntz SR. J Inject Dis 2008; 198: 23–30.

Valganciclovir was noted to reduce the shedding frequency and quantity of HHV-8.

Successful treatment of classical Kaposi sarcoma with low-dose intramuscular immunoglobulins. Thoms KM, Hellriegel S, Krone B, Beckmann I, Ritter K, Schon MP, et al. Br J Dermatol 2011; 164: 1107–9.

Improvement was noted in a patient with intramuscular globulins.

Evidence Levels: **A** Double-blind study **B** Clinical trial ≥ 20 subjects **C** Clinical trial < 20 subjects **D** Series ≥ 5 subjects **E** Anecdotal case reports

121

Kawasaki disease

Michael Pan, Lauren Geller, Ranon Mann, Adam Friedman, Adam Wulkan

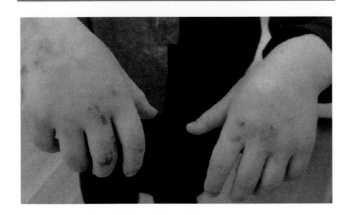

Kawasaki disease (KD), seen primarily in infants and children, is an acute febrile multiorgan vasculitic process known for its mucocutaneous and nodal involvement. Although KD was described in Japan several decades ago, its pathogenesis has yet to be clarified. Increasing evidence supports an infectious etiology.

MANAGEMENT STRATEGIES

The primary goal when treating a patient with KD is the prevention of cardiac complications, including coronary artery disease, aneurysm formation, myocardial infarction, and sudden death. Historically, the mainstay of therapy has been the use of high-dose *salicylates* (e.g., aspirin) and *intravenous γ-globulin* (IVIG) in order to manage the acute inflammatory characteristics of this condition and to prevent the aforementioned cardiovascular sequelae.

In the acute inflammatory phase, aspirin, a potent inhibitor of prostaglandin synthesis, is initially dosed at 80 to 100 mg/kg/day orally, divided four times per day, for 2 weeks. After the patient is afebrile for 48 hours, the dose is reduced to 3 to 5 mg/kg orally daily and continued for 6 to 8 weeks until the erythrocyte sedimentation rate (ESR) and platelet count normalize. Multiple trials have failed to elucidate the benefit of high-dose aspirin therapy with regard to outcomes; therefore current evidence is insufficient to support the use of salicylates as an integral component of first-line therapy in KD.

IVIG is a known first-line therapy in the treatment of KD. IVIG, which can lead to rapid defervescence, is able to neutralize circulating myelin antibodies and to downregulate proinflammatory cytokines, including interferon-γ (INF-γ). The pediatric dosing, which is equivalent to the adult dosing, is 400 mg/kg/day intravenously over 2 hours as a single daily infusion for 4 consecutive days; alternatively, a single dose of 2 g/kg can be intravenously infused over 12 hours. Failure of IVIG therapy has been linked to a gene polymorphism in the plasma platelet–activating factor acetylhydrolase. No specific regimen has been assigned for these nonresponding cases.

Specific Investigations
• ESR, complete blood count + platelet count, lactate dehydrogenase
• Multidetector computed tomography (CT)
• Echocardiography

Kawasaki disease: an overview. Pinna GS, Kafetzis D, Tselkas O, Skevaki CL. Curr Opin Infect Dis 2008; 21: 263–70.

Echocardiography, stress imaging, angiography, magnetic resonance imaging (MRI), and ultrafast CT scans have been useful in the diagnosis of coronary aneurysms, occlusions, and stenosis. Echocardiography is recommended both at the time of diagnosis and after 2 to 6 weeks. It has recently been demonstrated that multidetector CT is preferable to transthoracic echocardiography or MRI. CT can detect calcification and estimate soft plaques and offers rapid data collection and simple interpretation of images, all of which serve as an advantage over other diagnostic modalities. Conversely, MRI cannot offer rapid capture of images, thus prolonging the time under anesthesia and its associated risks. Transthoracic echocardiography can only image the proximal arteries and therefore cannot reliably detect stenosis.

The diagnosis and treatment of Kawasaki disease. Royle J, Burgner D, Curtis NJ. Pediatr Child Health 2005; 41: 87–93.

These guidelines highlight the difficulties in the diagnosis of KD. A meta-analysis of recent data offers insight that may assist in the early recognition of this important pediatric disease. The clinical features are common to many other childhood illnesses, so the diagnostic criteria are not highly sensitive. Blood serologies and chemistries may be helpful, but none is diagnostic and most have a low specificity. The echocardiogram should not be used as a diagnostic test. A normal echo does not exclude KD, as coronary lesions generally occur in the convalescent phase and may develop as late as 6 to 8 weeks after the onset of fever. Because there is no specific diagnostic test for KD, increased awareness of the epidemiology and the spectrum of clinical presentation is essential for early recognition and optimal management.

First-Line Therapies	
• Immunoglobulin	A
• Aspirin	B

Kawasaki disease: an update on diagnosis and treatment. Kuo HC, Yang KD, Chang WC, Ger LP, Hsieh KS. Pediatr Neonatol 2012; 53: 4–11.

An update on treatment modalities, including methylprednisolone, TNF-α antagonists, statins, plasma exchange, and cytotoxic agents. It concludes that high-dose aspirin does not appear to decrease the incidence of coronary artery lesions (CALs), although further studies are required.

Treating KD refractory to IVIG is a therapeutic challenge. Recent studies have shown associations of age, platelet count, ESR, hemoglobin, C-reactive protein (CRP), eosinophil count, lactate dehydrogenase (LDH), albumin, and alanine aminotransferase (ALT) with failure of primary treatment with IVIG. Because IVIG failure has an increased risk of CALs, it is essential to treat such patients with a second dose of IVIG, intravenous methylprednisolone, or a TNF-α inhibitor.

Resistance to intravenous immunoglobulin in children with Kawasaki disease. Tremoulet AH, Best BM, Song S, Wang S, Corinaldesi E, Eichenfield JR, et al. J Pediatr 2008; 153: 117–21.

IVIG treatment for the acute stage of KD has been shown to be effective and safe. However, it is known that 10% to 20% of patients are resistant to initial therapy (2 g/kg IV). These patients are at increased risk for the development of coronary artery abnormalities. Using demographic and laboratory information on IVIG-resistant cases, this retrospective study attempted to develop a scoring system to help identify future resistant cases among patients in San Diego County. This would perhaps indicate the need for secondary therapies early in the treatment of these patients. Unfortunately, the diversity of the patient population did not allow for the development of an accurate and clinically useful scoring system.

Analysis of potential risk factors associated with nonresponse to initial intravenous immunoglobulin treatment among Kawasaki disease patients in Japan. Uehara R, Belay ED, Maddox RA, Holman RC, Nakamura Y, Yashiro M, et al. Pediatr Infect Dis J 2008; 27: 155–60.

Some KD patients do not respond to initial treatment with IVIG. The purpose of this study was to determine potential risk factors associated with IVIG nonresponse among KD patients in Japan. The results emphasize that physicians should consider IVIG nonresponse in patients with recurrent KD, as well as in KD patients diagnosed and treated before the fifth day of illness who continue to have laboratory values associated with nonresponse, such as low platelet count and elevated ALT and CRP. These patients may benefit from the administration of a second-line treatment early during the illness in addition to the initial IVIG treatment.

Treatment of acute Kawasaki disease: aspirin's role in the febrile stage revisited. Hsieh KS, Weng KP, Lin CC, Huang TC, Lee CL, Huang SM. Pediatrics 2004; 114: 689–93.

In North America, high-dose aspirin (80–100 mg/kg/day orally) is widely used during the acute phase of KD. However, the necessity of this therapy has yet to be elucidated. This study indicated that treatment in the acute stage of KD without aspirin had no effect on the response rate of IVIG therapy, duration of fever, or incidence of coronary abnormalities. This response was seen when children were treated with high-dose (2 g/kg) IVIG as a single infusion, regardless of whether treatment was commenced before or after day 5 of illness. Therefore the available data show no appreciable benefit of aspirin in preventing IVIG nonresponse, aneurysm formation, or shortening of fever duration.

High-dose aspirin is associated with anemia and does not confer benefit to disease outcomes in Kawasaki disease. Kuo HC, Lo MH, Hsieh KS, Guo MM, Huang YH. PLoS One 2015; 10: e0144603.

This retrospective study analyzed 851 KD patients who had received single-dose IVIG along with either (1) high-dose aspirin until defervescence followed by low-dose aspirin (*n* = 305) or (2) low-dose aspirin only (*n* = 546). There were no significant differences in IVIG resistance rate, CALs, or duration of hospital stay. Furthermore, this study found that after IVIG, the group that received high-dose aspirin had lower hemoglobin levels and higher serum CRP and hepcidin levels with delay in normalization. The authors concluded that high-dose aspirin does not confer any benefit and is unnecessary in the acute phase of KD.

Second-Line Therapies

• Corticosteroids	A
• Retreatment with immunoglobulin	D

Efficacy of immunoglobulin plus prednisolone for prevention of coronary artery abnormalities in severe Kawasaki disease (RAISE study): a randomised, open-label, blinded-endpoints trial. Kobayashi T, Saji T, Otani T, Takeuchi K, Nakamura T, Arakawa H. Lancet 2012; 379: 1613–20.

This multicenter, prospective, randomized trial took place at 74 hospitals in Japan. Individuals with severe KD were randomized to receive either current standard of care IVIG (2 g/kg/day given over 24 hours) and aspirin (30 mg/kg/day) or IVIG and aspirin (same dose as control) plus prednisolone (2 mg/kg/day with 15-day taper after normalization of CRP). There were 125 assigned to the intervention group and 123 received only IVIG. The incidence of CALs was significantly decreased in the intervention arm with intravenous prednisolone (4 patients) versus the control arm (28 patients). Larger studies involving individuals from various ethnic backgrounds are needed.

Effects of steroid pulse therapy on immunoglobulin-resistant Kawasaki disease. Furukawa T, Kishiro M, Akimoto K, Nagata S, Shimizu T, Yamashiro Y. Arch Dis Child 2008; 93: 142–46.

In this nonrandomized study, the effectiveness of intravenous methylprednisone (IVMP) was compared with that of additional IVIG (2 g/kg 12–24 hours) and aspirin (30 mg/kg/day) as second-line therapy for KD. Fever was rapidly alleviated after IVMP administration (30 mg/kg/day for 3 consecutive days with heparin infusion 10–20 U/kg/h) in all IVIG-resistant patients in the study; 77% recovered without recurrence of KD and did not develop coronary artery aneurysms. The findings suggested that early IVMP treatment in IVIG-resistant patients is as effective as treatment with additional IVIG as second-line therapy.

Risk factors associated with the need for additional intravenous gamma-globulin therapy for Kawasaki disease. Muta H, Ishii M, Furui J, Nakamura Y, Matsuishi T. Acta Paediatr 2006; 95: 189.

The goal of this study, using data from a nationwide survey in Japan, was to identify the characteristics of patients who needed retreatment with IVIG. Elevated ESR, anemia, and high LDH are known predictive values for necessitating IVIG retreatment. In this study, male gender, incomplete and recurrent cases of KD, and treatment with IVIG at a dose of 1 g/kg or less within 4 days of illness onset were identified as independent risk factors associated with the need for retreatment. Identification of these risk factors would be beneficial to predict which patients might need IVIG retreatment. This could help physicians initially create a strategy to prevent cardiovascular complications in these patients.

Third-Line Therapies

• Ciclosporin	B
• Ticlopidine	E
• Pentoxifylline	B
• Ulinastatin	B
• Infliximab	A
• Plasma exchange	B
• Rituximab	E
• Dipyridamole	E
• Cardiac transplantation	E
• Coronary artery bypass grafting	B

Evidence Levels: **A** Double-blind study **B** Clinical trial ≥ 20 subjects **C** Clinical trial < 20 subjects **D** Series ≥ 5 subjects **E** Anecdotal case reports

Cyclosporin A treatment for Kawasaki disease refractory to initial and additional intravenous immunoglobulin. Suzuki H, Terai M, Hamada H, Honda T, Suenaga T, Takeuchi T, Hooshyar H, et al. Pediatr Infect Dis J 2011; 30: 610–5.

In this trial involving 28 individuals who failed IVIG therapy, ciclosporin 4 to 8 mg/kg/day oral administration was shown to be a safe, well tolerated, and efficacious option. Of the 28, 18 were afebrile within 3 days of therapy, 4 were afebrile within 4 to 5 days, and the remaining 6 failed to respond to treatment.

Response of refractory Kawasaki disease to pulse steroid and cyclosporin A therapy. Raman V, Kim J, Sharkey A. Pediatr Infect Dis J 2001; 20: 635–37.

A case of aggressive and protracted KD with coronary aneurysms, myocarditis, pericarditis, and valvular insufficiency, despite repeated administration of IVIG, responded to combination therapy with pulse and high-dose corticosteroids and ciclosporin 3 mg/kg/day.

Ulinastatin, a urinary trypsin inhibitor, for the initial treatment of patients with Kawasaki disease: a retrospective study. Kanai T, Ishiwata T, Kobayashi K, Sato H, Takizawa M, Kawamura Y, et al. Circulation 2011; 124: 2822–28.

This is a retrospective study comparing 369 patients with KD who were treated with a combination of ulinastatin (UTI) at 15,000 U/kg/day divided into three doses, aspirin (30 mg/kg/day), and IVIG (1–2 g/kg) versus 1178 patients treated with IVIG and aspirin. Those treated in the UTI group experienced fewer CALs (3%) than those in the control group (7%). Thus treatment with UTI was associated with fewer rescue treatments and CALs.

Infliximab for intravenous immunoglobulin resistance in Kawasaki disease: a retrospective study. Son MB, Gauvreau K, Burns JC, Corinaldesi E, Tremoulet AH, Watson VE, et al. J Pediatr 2011; 158: 644–49.

This study, performed between 2000 and 2008, assessed fever duration and coronary artery dimensions in patients refractory to IVIG therapy who subsequently received either infliximab (5 mg/kg) or additional IVIG (2 g/kg). Individuals treated with infliximab experienced decreased fever duration and shorter hospitalization, yet similar coronary artery dimensions, compared with the control group.

Infliximab for intensification of primary therapy for Kawasaki disease: a phase 3 randomised, double-blind, placebo-controlled trial. Tremoulet AH, Jain S, Jaggi P, Jimenez-Fernandez S, Pancheri JM, Sun X, et al. Lancet 2014; 383(9930): 1731–38.

In this study, 196 patients were enrolled to receive either infliximab (single dose 5 mg/kg, $n = 98$) or placebo ($n = 98$) in addition to IVIG standard therapy. There was no significant difference in the rate of treatment resistance. However, there was a significant reduction in left anterior descending coronary artery Z-score, days of fever, and inflammatory markers in the group that received infliximab. No serious adverse events could be attributed to infliximab.

Resistant Kawasaki disease treated with anti-CD20. Sauvaget E, Bonello B, David M, Chabrol B, Dubus JC, Bosdure E. J Pediatr 2012; 160: 875–76.

A 6-year-old boy with KD refractory to IVIG and systemic steroids was successfully treated with rituximab (15 mg/kg/day), an anti-CD20 monoclonal antibody, initiated on day 20 of disease onset. Within 2 days of rituximab therapy, the child's fever had dissipated, and the echocardiography revealed improvement of the CALs.

Long-term efficacy of plasma exchange treatment for refractory Kawasaki disease. Hokosaki T, Mori M, Nishizawa T, Nakamura T, Imagawa T, Iwamoto M, et al. Pediatr Int 2012; 54: 99–103.

A retrospective study involving 125 patients with KD refractory to IVIG therapy treated with plasma exchange (PE) therapy. The success of PE therapy was dependent on both the presence of CALs before PE and on what day of disease onset the PE therapy was initiated. CALs remained in 2.8% of individuals treated with PE when PE was initiated before day 9 of the onset of KD. For those with CALs in whom PE was started after day 9 of KD onset, sequelae remained 15% of the time. For the 105 patients in whom the coronary arteries were normal before PE initiation, none of them went on to develop CALs. Thus PE therapy is optimal for refractory KD when used before the development of CALs.

Prevention of thrombosis of coronary aneurysms in patients with a history of Kawasaki disease. Suda K, Kudo Y, Sugawara Y. Nippon Rinsho 2008; 66: 355–59.

To prevent coronary thrombosis in KD, long-term antithrombotic therapy using antiplatelet drugs such as aspirin, dipyridamole, ticlopidine, clopidogrel, and abciximab, with or without warfarin, is recommended by official guidelines.

Optimal time of surgical treatment for Kawasaki coronary artery disease. Yamauchi H, Ochi M, Fujii M, Hinokiyama K, Ohmori H, Sasaki T, et al. J Nippon Med Sch 2004; 71: 279–86.

The authors studied 21 patients with KD and coronary complications who underwent coronary artery bypass grafting (CABG) over a 12-year period. They conclude that CABG is successful when completed shortly after the acute onset of disease.

Keloids

Brian Berman, Ran Huo, Martha Viera,
Andrea Maderal

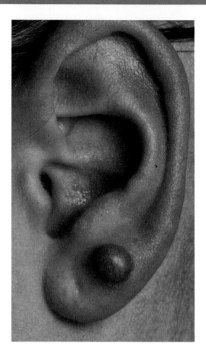

Keloids are dermal hyperproliferative growths with excessive accumulation of dense fibrous tissue that may appear in areas of trauma. By definition, keloids are scars that extend beyond the borders of the original wound and do not regress spontaneously. In addition to the cosmetic disfigurement and negative psychological impact that keloids may cause the patient, these scars can often present with intense pain and pruritus.

MANAGEMENT STRATEGY

The therapeutic options for keloids are numerous; however, there is no one modality that is considered to be universally safe and effective. Prevention of recurrence should be the main determinant in treatment selection. The initial rule of treatment involves *prevention* and *patient education*. It is of the utmost importance to close wounds with minimal tension and inflammation. Nonessential cosmetic surgery should be avoided in patients predisposed to developing keloids. These scars commonly develop in high-tension areas of the body. Incision sites in the skin of the midchest and skin overlying joints should be avoided, and surgical wounds should parallel skin creases.

Common therapeutic modalities include occlusive dressings, compression therapy, intralesional corticosteroid injections, intralesional interferon injections, intralesional 5-fluorouracil injections, cryosurgery, surgical excision, radiation therapy, and laser therapy. Because no single therapy is vastly superior or universally efficacious, combination therapies have led to the best success rates.

Intralesional corticosteroids have been the mainstay of treatment for keloids. The most commonly used is triamcinolone acetonide in concentrations of 10 to 40 mg/mL administered intralesionally

with a 25- to 27-gauge needle at 4- to 6-week intervals. *Topical corticosteroids and topically applied corticosteroid-impregnated tape* are also used frequently; the basis for the latter involves recent data demonstrating that occlusion enhances percutaneous penetration of steroid by the formation of a drug reservoir within the stratum corneum. *Silicone gel sheets and silicone occlusive dressings* have antikeloidal effects, which appear to be a result of hydration.

Pressure devices are thought to induce local tissue hypoxia and have been shown to have a thinning effect on keloids. A novel idea in the treatment of keloids and hypertrophic scars is the use *of intralesional interferon-α_{2b},* which has been used successfully to reduce scar height and postoperative recurrences, via a mechanism of collagen synthesis inhibition. *Interferon-γ* has also been evaluated in the treatment of keloids, with modest results.

Cryotherapy can be used as monotherapy or in conjunction with other treatment modalities, most commonly triamcinolone, with reported efficacy. Its mechanism of action involves the induction of vascular damage and tissue anoxia that ultimately leads to necrosis. However, some reported side effects have included hypopigmentation and postoperative pain. A specialized intralesional needle cryoprobe method has been recently reported to result in better efficacy and fewer side effects.

Radiation therapy has been used as monotherapy or as an adjuvant to surgical excision. The carcinogenesis risks of radiotherapy are extremely small; however, the concept of using potentially harmful radiation to treat benign lesions is a persistent and important issue.

Surgical excision alone yields widely varying results with high (55%–100%) recurrence rates. The *combination of surgical excision with other modalities, such as intralesional corticosteroids or with pressure dressing, x-ray therapy, interstitial radiation, and brachytherapy,* reduces recurrence rates to a range of 10% to 50%.

CO_2 and argon lasers have been used in the past in the treatment of keloids but have recently been replaced by the *Nd:YAG and 585-nm pulsed-dye laser* because of their better efficacy and fewer adverse effects. *Intralesional injection of 5-fluorouracil* has been beneficial for hypertrophic scars and for keloids. *Bleomycin, retinoic acid, intralesional verapamil, and mitomycin C* have all been reported to have good efficacy in small clinical trials, but more clinical experience with these agents is needed.

Specific Investigation
• Skin biopsy

Dermatofibrosarcoma protuberans is a unique fibrohistiocytic tumor expressing CD34. Aiba S, Tabata N, Ishii H, Ootani H, Tagami H. Br J Dermatol 1992; 127: 79–84.

Dermatofibrosarcoma protuberans can be easily misdiagnosed as a keloid. Histopathology may help differentiate the two, but expression of CD34 by tumor cells occurs only in dermatofibrosarcoma protuberans.

First-Line Therapies	
• Intralesional corticosteroids	B
• Compression	B
• Occlusive dressing	B
• Intralesional 5-fluorouracil	B

Evidence Levels: A Double-blind study B Clinical trial ≥ 20 subjects C Clinical trial < 20 subjects D Series ≥ 5 subjects E Anecdotal case reports

A new uniform protocol of combined corticosteroid injections and ointment application reduces recurrence rates after surgical keloid/hypertrophic scar excision. Hayashi T, Furukawa H, Oyama A, Funayama E, Saito A, Murao N, et al. Dermatol Surg 2012; 38: 893–7.

Twenty-one keloids were treated with surgical excision, then corticosteroid injections after removal of the sutures and every 2 weeks (for five more times) thereafter. In addition, all postsurgical wounds received self-administered steroid ointment application twice daily for 6 months after suture removal. Recurrence occurred in 3 of the 21 keloid cases (14.3%) and one of the six hypertrophic scar cases (16.7%).

Keloids treated with topical injections of triamcinolone acetonide. Immediate and long term results. Kiil J, Scand J Plast Reconstruct Surg 1977; 11: 169–72.

In a prospective clinical trial of 52 patients, intralesional injections of triamcinolone acetonide alone resulted in significant flattening and reduction of pruritus in 93% of the keloids. One third had partial recurrence at 1 year, and at 5 years more than 50% had recurred. All recurrences were successfully treated with further triamcinolone acetonide injections.

Outcomes of surgical excision with pressure therapy using magnets and identification of risk factors for recurrent keloids. Park TH, Seo SW, Kim JK, Chang CH. Plast Reconstr Surg 2011; 128: 431–9.

In this study, 1436 ear keloids in 883 patients were treated with surgical excision followed by pressure therapy using magnets. The overall recurrence-free rate was 89.4% after a follow-up period of 18 months. Keloid recurrence was significantly associated with the presence of prior treatment history, keloid low growth rate, and high patient body mass index.

A surgical approach for earlobe keloid: keloid fillet flap. Kim DY. Plast Reconstr Surg 2004; 113: 1668–74.

Surgical revision of keloids on earlobes followed by intradermal scaffold/linear surgical incision was performed in 19 subjects (26 earlobe keloids). At 12 months, the recurrence rate was 19.2%. There were no device-related adverse events.

Comparison of a silicone gel-filled cushion and silicone gel sheeting for the treatment of hypertrophic or keloid scars. Berman B, Flores F. Dermatol Surg 1999; 25: 484–6.

In this study of 32 keloid patients, 53% treated with silicone gel cushion and 36.3% treated with silicone gel sheeting had a reduction in keloid volume.

Clinical evaluation of a new self-drying silicone gel in the treatment of scars: a preliminary report. Signorini M, Clementoni MT. Aesthet Plast Surg 2007; 31: 183–7.

A prospective trial involving 160 patients that compared postoperative treatment with a self-drying transparent silicone gel with no treatment. Sixty-seven percent of patients in the treatment group had a significant improvement in scar quality.

Combination of different techniques for the treatment of earlobe keloids. Akoz T, Gideroglu K, Akan M. Aesthet Plast Surg 2002; 26: 184.

Nine patients were treated with surgical excision of their earlobe keloids, followed by triamcinolone acetonide injection and silicone gel sheets. No recurrences occurred in eight of the nine patients.

Intralesional 5-fluorouracil in keloid treatment: a systemic review. Bijlard E, Steltenpool S, Niessen FB. Acta Derm Venereol 2015; 95: 778–82.

Systematic review of 18 publications with 482 patients. 5-fluorouracil treatment was effective in 45% to 96% of patients, but only triamcinolone with 5-fluorouracil performed better than triamcinolone alone.

Comparison of the efficacy of intralesional triamcinolone acetonide and 5-fluorouracil tattooing for the treatment of keloids. Sadeghinia A, Sadeghinia S. Dermatol Surg 2012; 38: 104–9.

Forty patients were randomized to treatment with either intralesional triamcinolone acetonide injection or 5-fluorouracil tattooing every 4 weeks for 12 weeks. At 44-week follow-up, superior improvement was observed in the 5-fluorouracil group for lesion erythema, pruritus, height, surface, and induration. No side effect was detected in either of the groups.

Second-Line Therapies	
• Intralesional interferon-α_{2b}	B
• Cryosurgery	A
• Radiation	B

Recurrence rates of excised keloids treated with postoperative triamcinolone acetonide injections or interferon alfa-2b injections. Berman B, Flores F. J Am Acad Dermatol 1997; 37: 755–7.

There was a statistically significant reduction in the recurrence of 124 excised keloids with postexcision interferon-α_{2b} (18.7% recurrence) versus excision alone (51.1%) and versus treatment with postoperative intralesional triamcinolone (58.4%).

Effects of interferon-α2b on keloid treatment with triamcinolone acetonide intralesional injection. Lee JH, Kim SE, Lee A-Y. Int J Dermatol 2008; 47: 183–6.

Forty keloid lesions from 19 patients were treated either with triamcinolone acetonide intralesional (TAIL) combined with interferon-α_{2b} or with TAIL alone. Superior results were obtained with combination therapy, with more than 80% improvement in lesion depth and volume in most patients.

Cryotherapy in the treatment of keloids. Rusciani L, Paradisi A, Alfano C, Chiummariello S, Rusciani A. J Drugs Dermatol 2006; 5: 591–5.

Of 135 patients with 166 keloids treated with cryotherapy between 1990 and 2004, 79.5% responded very well with a volume reduction of 80% or more after three treatments. Median follow-up time was 4 years. The most common adverse effects included atrophic depressed scars and, in 75% of cases, residual hypopigmentation.

A comparison of the combined effect of cryotherapy and corticosteroid injections versus corticosteroids and cryotherapy alone on keloids: a controlled study. Yosipovitch G, Widijanti Sugeng M, Goon A, Chan YH, Goh CL. J Dermatol Treat 2001; 12: 87–90.

Ten patients with 28 keloids were treated with cryotherapy alone, steroid injection alone, or cryotherapy and steroid injection. At 8 months' follow-up the combination therapy was significantly better at reducing keloid thickness and pruritus than either treatment alone. None of the keloids treated with combination therapy recurred. No significant side effects were noted.

Hypofractionated electron-beam radiation therapy for keloids: retrospective study of 568 cases with 834 lesions. Shen J, Lian X, Sun Y, Wang X, Hu K, Hou X, et al. J Radiat Res 2015; 56: 811–7.

Retrospective study of 568 patients with 834 keloids treated with radiotherapy. Relapse rate was 9.59% and time to relapse 6 to 28 months. No radiation-induced cancers were observed.

Keloids can be forced into remission with surgical excision and radiation, followed by adjuvant therapy. Yamawaki S, Naitoh M, Ishiko T, Muneuchi G, Suzuki S. Ann Plast Surg 2011; 67: 402–6.

The authors treated 91 keloids in total, with 51 keloids (56.0%) resolved completely, by a combination of surgical excision and postoperative irradiation. Eighty-one keloids (89.0%) showed good results with additional treatment of intralesional steroid injections.

Treatment of keloids by surgical excision and immediate postoperative single-fraction radiotherapy. Ragoowansi R, Cornes PG, Moss AL, Glees JP. Plast Reconstruct Surg 2003; 111: 1853–9.

In a retrospective study of 80 patients treated with postoperative single-fraction radiotherapy, 9% of keloids relapsed after 1 year and 16% relapsed after 5 years.

Retrospective analysis of treatment of unresectable keloids with primary radiation over 25 years. Malaker K, Vijayraghavan K, Hodson I, Al Yafi T. Clin Oncol J Roy Coll Radiol 2004; 16: 290–8.

In this retrospective study involving 86 keloids in 64 patients, 97% of keloids showed significant regression after completing radiotherapy with either kilovoltage x-rays or electron beams, without significant side effects. The patients were treated with a total of 3750 cGy administered in five once-weekly fractions.

Postoperative high-dose-rate brachytherapy in the prevention of keloids. Veen RE, Kal HB. Int J Radiat Oncol Biol Phys 2007; 69: 1205–8.

Postoperative ^{192}Ir brachytherapy showed better cosmetic results at higher dosages, with only one keloid recurrence out of 38 observed after a once-administered 6-Gy and twice-administered 4-Gy regimen.

Postkeloidectomy irradiation using high-dose-rate superficial brachytherapy. Kuribayashi S, Miyashita T, Ozawa Y, Iwano M, Ogawa R, Akaishi S, et al. J Radiat Res 2011; 52: 365–8.

A total of 36 keloids were treated with high-dose-rate superficial brachytherapy after keloidectomy. The median follow-up period was 18 months (range 9–29 months). Only three keloids (9.7%) showed local recurrence.

Surgical excision with adjuvant irradiation for treatment of keloid scars: a systemic review. van Leeuwen MC, Stokmans SC, Bulstra AE, Meijer OW, Heymans MW, Ket JC, et al. Plast Reconstr Surg Glob Open 2015; 3: e440.

Systematic review of 33 articles that contained 3130 patients with 3470 keloid scars treated with excision followed by low-dose or high-dose brachytherapy. High-dose brachytherapy showed lower recurrence rates compared with low-dose brachytherapy and external radiation, and a short time (<7 hours) interval postexcision was associated with lower recurrence rate compared with long time interval (>24 hours).

Third-Line Therapies	
• Laser surgery	C
• Imiquimod	A
• Mitomycin C	B
• Intralesional interferon-γ	C
• Topical retinoic acid	B
• Intralesional bleomycin	B
• Verapamil	B
• Surgery	B

Management of ear lobule keloids using 980-nm diode laser. Kassab AN, El Kharbotly A. Eur Arch Otorhinolaryngol 2012; 269: 419–23.

Twelve patients with a total of 16 lobule keloids were treated with 980-nm diode laser and subsequent intralesional triamcinolone acetonide injection. Between two and five treatment sessions led to 75% of patients with more than 75% reduction of keloid size, with no recurrence in the past 12 months.

Effect of pulse width of a 595-nm flashlamp-pumped pulsed dye laser on the treatment response of keloidal and hypertrophic sternotomy scars. Manuskiatti W, Wanitphakdeedecha R, Fitzpatrick RE. Dermatol Surg 2007; 33: 152–61.

In 19 patients with keloidal or hypertrophic median sternotomy scars, pulsed dye laser with pulse width of 0.45 ms was significantly effective in reducing scar volume and improving elasticity. However, the reported reduction in scar volume was only 24.4% after three treatments.

The effect of carbon dioxide laser surgery on the recurrence of keloids. Norris JEC. Plast Reconstruct Surg 1991; 87: 44–9.

In this retrospective study, 23 patients had adequate follow-up. One had no recurrence, 9 required corticosteroids to suppress recurrence, and 13 were considered to be treatment failures.

Pilot study of the effect of postoperative imiquimod 5% cream on the recurrence rate of excised keloids. Berman B, Kaufman J. J Am Acad Dermatol 2002; 47: S209–11.

Thirteen keloids were treated with excision and imiquimod 5% cream every night for 8 weeks. Ten patients with 11 keloids completed the 6-month study, and there were no recurrences.

Role of mitomycin C in reducing keloid recurrence: patient series and literature review. Gupta M, Narang T. J Laryngol Otol 2011; 125: 297–300.

Twenty patients with 26 earlobe keloids were treated with surgical shave excision and topical mitomycin C. No recurrences were noted after 24 months.

Intralesional interferon gamma treatment for keloids and hypertrophic scars. Larrabee WF, East CA, Jaffe HS, Stephenson C, Peterson KE. Arch Otolaryngol Head Neck Surg 1990; 116: 1159–62.

Five of the 10 study patients had a reduction in their scar size by at least 50% in linear dimensions. The treatment protocol was one treatment per week for 10 weeks. Up to 0.05 mg of interferon-γ was injected weekly.

Evidence Levels: **A** Double-blind study **B** Clinical trial ≥ 20 subjects **C** Clinical trial < 20 subjects **D** Series ≥ 5 subjects **E** Anecdotal case reports

The local treatment of hypertrophic scars and keloids with topical retinoic acid. Janssen de Limpens AMP. Br J Dermatol 1980; 103: 319–23.

There was a reduction in keloid size and symptoms in 77% of 28 intractable keloids treated with topical retinoic acid.

Treatment of keloids and hypertrophic scars using bleomycin. Aggarwal H, Saxena A, Lubana PS, Mathur RK, Jain DK. J Cosmet Dermatol 2008; 7: 43–9.

Over 3 months, four courses of bleomycin were administered through a multiple superficial puncture technique in 50 patients with keloids and hypertrophic scars. Forty-four percent of patients experienced complete flattening of lesions, and 22% showed more than 75% lesion regression.

Comparison of intralesional verapamil with intralesional triamcinolone in the treatment of hypertrophic scars and keloids. Margaret Shanthi FX, Ernest K, Dhanraj P. Indian J Dermatol Venereol Leprol 2008; 74: 343–8.

In this randomized, single-blind, parallel group study in which 54 patients were allocated to receive either verapamil (2.5 mg) or triamcinolone (40 mg) every 3 weeks up to 6 months, there was a reduction in vascularity, pliability, height, and width of the scar with both the drugs after 3 weeks of treatment. Triamcinolone had a faster reduction rate, but verapamil had a lower rate of hypopigmentation.

123

Keratoacanthoma

M. Laurin Council, George J. Hruza

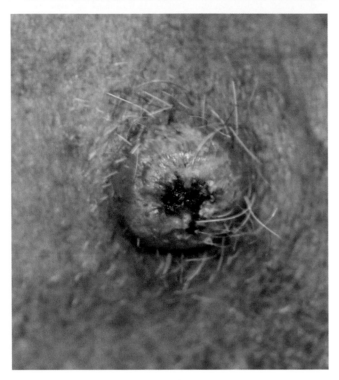

The Keratoacanthoma (KA) is a unique tumor of the skin with characteristics of both benign and malignant neoplasia. Typically, the lesion presents as a rapidly growing (weeks to months) crateriform nodule on sun-exposed skin of the middle aged or elderly Caucasian. During the proliferative phase, lesions grow quickly and can reach an impressive size. Once mature, KA stops growing before involuting. If observed, resolution of a KA classically occurs within several months. Clinically and histologically, a KA shares several characteristics with well-differentiated cutaneous squamous cell carcinoma (SCC). Histologically, for example, lesions appear as a symmetric exoendophytic proliferation of glassy keratinocytes with a central keratin-filled crater. Because a KA can be impossible to discern from a well-differentiated SCC, some dermatopathologists refer to the lesions as *SCC, KA-type.* Unlike SCC, the lesions are often clinically self-limited and spontaneously regress. Before regression, a KA can cause significant local destruction and morbidity. Because of these features, many consider KA a form of aborted SCC or low-grade malignancy. Although KAs appear most commonly as solitary lesions, multiple lesions may occur in the setting of a genodermatosis (e.g., Ferguson–Smith, Witten and Zak, Grzybowski, or Muir–Torre syndrome); during koebnerization (after surgery, phototherapy, laser, or placement of a tattoo); or as eruptive lesions in response to certain systemic medications, such as ciclosporin, BRAF inhibitors, and vismodegib.

MANAGEMENT STRATEGY

Because an accurate distinction between a clinically low-grade KA and a more aggressive SCC is challenging histologically, lesions should be removed in their entirety whenever possible. Although several features have been described to distinguish a self-involuting KA from its more aggressive counterpart (such as fewer mitoses, less pleomorphism, and good demarcation), these histologic criteria can be noted in both lesions. Complete removal aids in diagnosis and prevents further growth and proliferation, with associated local destruction, and decreases the likelihood of metastasis in the event of histologic misclassification of a SCC as KA.

Once a diagnosis has been established, management aims to stimulate resolution, prevent local destruction, minimize the risk of recurrence, and achieve a favorable cosmetic outcome. Management of a KA is therefore dependent on the size and location of the lesion(s), the rate of growth, and the causative factors (if known).

Small, solitary lesions are best treated with *excision,* with complete margin analysis (Mohs micrographic surgery) where appropriate. Low-risk lesions in select candidates may be treated with destructive methods such as *cryotherapy or electrodesiccation and curettage.* If confidence in a diagnosis can be ascertained, observation can be entertained, but with great caution. *Large lesions may be treated with topical (imiquimod or 5-fluorouracil) or intralesional (5-fluorouracil, methotrexate, or bleomycin) chemotherapy or x-ray therapy.* Eruptive KAs are best treated by removal of the cause, when known and practical, by systemic therapy, or by field treatment with photodynamic therapy (PDT) or other topical mechanisms, such as 5-fluorouracil, with or without occlusion.

The level of evidence in the literature for the treatment of KAs is poor—typically anecdotal evidence of single case reports. Nevertheless, larger studies encompassing SCC can be pertinent to management of these unique lesions.

Specific Investigation

- Biopsy

Solitary keratoacanthoma

First-Line Therapies

Mohs micrographic surgery	C
Excision	C

AAD/ACMS/ASDSA/ASMS 2012 appropriate use criteria for Mohs micrographic surgery: a report of the American Academy of Dermatology, American College of Mohs Surgery, American Society for Dermatologic Surgery Association, and the American Society for Mohs Surgery. Ad Hoc Task Force, Connolly SM, Baker DR, Coldiron BM, Fazio MJ, Storrs PA, et al. J Am Acad Dermatol 2012; 67: 531–50.

Expert consensus panel recommends Mohs micrographic surgery as appropriate treatment for primary keratoacathomas of any size on the head, neck, hands, feet, pretibial shin and genitalia; for lesions >1 cm on the trunk and extremities; for recurrent KAs of any size or location; and for keratocanthomas >0.5 cm on the trunk and extremities in immunocompromised patients.

Prognostic factors for local recurrence, metastasis, and survival rates in squamous cell carcinoma of the skin, ear, and lip. Rowe DE, Carroll RJ, Day Jr. CL. J Am Acad Dermatol 1992; 26: 976–90.

Authors evaluated the medical literature over a 50-year period to determine which treatment modality offers the best cure rate for SCC of the skin and lip. For primary tumors of the skin, Mohs micrographic surgery reportedly had a 3.1% recurrence rate at 5 years compared with 8.1% for surgical excision. For locally recurrent lesions, Mohs micrographic surgery reduced the rate of recurrence from 23.3% to 10%, compared with simple excision.

Keratoacanthomas treated with Mohs' micrographic surgery (chemosurgery). A review of forty-three cases. Larson PO. J Am Acad Dermatol 1987; 16: 1040–4.

During a 6- to 24-month follow-up period, one patient recurred (2.4%).

Second-Line Therapies	
• Destruction	C
• Observation	C
• Intralesional chemotherapy	C
• Topical therapy	D
• Photodynamic therapy	D
• Radiation	C

Cryosurgery for skin cancer: 30-year experience and cure rates. Kuflik EG. Dermatol Surg 2004; 30: 297–300.

The author reports his experience using cryosurgery to a temperature of –50° to –60°C for 4406 new and recurrent skin cancers in 2932 patients. Of the 132 treated SCCs, no lesions recurred at 5-year follow-up.

Evaluation of curettage and electrodesiccation in the treatment of keratoacanthoma. Nedwich JA. Australas J Dermatol 1991; 32: 137–41.

A retrospective series of 111 KAs in 106 patients treated with curettage and electrodesiccation. A recurrence rate of 3.6% is noted after 3 to 26 months.

Natural course of keratoacanthoma and related lesions after partial biopsy: clinical analysis of sixty-six tumors. Takai T, Misago N, Murato Y. J Dermatol 2015; 42: 353–62.

Regression rate of KA was 98.1%, and that of KA-like SCC was 33.3%. No regression was noted in lesions classified histologically as crateriform or infundibular SCC.

Intralesional methotrexate treatment for keratoacanthoma tumors: a retrospective case series. Aubut N, Alain J, Claveau J. J Cutan Med Surg 2012; 16: 212–7.

Complete response of 74% was noted in 46 cases; no significant adverse events. An average of 1.8 injection sessions was necessary, for a mean total dose of 10 mg.

Successful treatment of keratoacanthoma with intralesional fluorouracil. Goette DK, Odom RB. J Am Acad Dermatol 1980; 2: 212–6.

Case series of forty-one KAs in 30 patients were treated with weekly injections of 5-fluorouracil. Forty lesions cleared after an average of three injections.

Treatment of keratoacanthoma with intralesional bleomycin. Sayama S, Tagami H. Br J Dermatol 1983; 109: 449–52.

Six patients with biopsy-proved KA were treated with one or two injections of varying volumes of 0.5% bleomycin. All lesions regressed within 2 to 6 weeks of therapy.

Intralesional interferon alfa-2b treatment of keratoacanthomas. Oh CK, Son HS, Lee JB, Jang HS, Kwon KS. J Am Acad Dermatol 2004; 51: S177–80.

Four patients with histologically confirmed KA of the head or neck were treated with weekly interferon alfa-2b injections. All lesions resolved completely in 5 to 7 weeks.

Treatment of keratoacanthomas with 5% imiquimod cream and review of the previous report. Jeon HC, Choi M, Paik SH, Ahn CH, Park HS, Cho KH. Ann Dermatol 2011; 23: 357–61.

Complete regression was seen after 9 to 11 weeks in four patients with KA treated with imiquimod cream 5% three to four times weekly. In addition, the authors summarize seven other prior reports of imiquimod use in 14 total patients with KA of the face or hand. Complete remission was noted in all reported cases within 4 to 11 weeks; application frequencies ranged from twice daily to three times weekly.

Clinical efficacy of short contact topical 5-fluorouracil in the treatment of keratoacanthomas. Thompson BJ, Ravits M, Silvers DN. J Clin Aesthet Dermatol 2014; 7: 35–7.

Nine patients with biopsy-proven KA were treated with twice-daily 5-fluorouracil until complete resolution of the lesion (4–6 weeks). Two patients experienced temporary erythema, and all reported satisfaction with the treatment.

Efficacy of topical photodynamic therapy for keratoacanthomas: a case-series of four patients. Farias MM, Hasson A, Navarrete C, Nicklas C, Garcia-Huidobro I, Gonzalez S. Indian J Dermatol Venereol Leprol 2012; 78: 172–4.

Four solitary lesions cleared after three sessions of PDT with methyl aminolevulinic acid cream. No evidence of recurrence was noted, and excellent cosmetic outcomes were reported at 3 years of follow-up.

Radiation therapy of giant aggressive keratoacanthomas. Goldschmidt H, Sherwin WK. Arch Dermatol 1993; 129: 1162–5.

A retrospective review of 16 aggressive KAs, 14 of which had recurred after surgery, responded to a fractionated course of superficial radiation therapy with complete resolution and satisfactory cosmesis.

Multiple keratoacanthomas

First-Line Therapies	
• Oral acitretin	E
• Oral isotretinoin	E
• Oral erlotinib	E
• Combination	D
• Radiation	C

Acitretin induces remission in generalized eruptive keratoacanthoma of Grzybowski. Sami N, Bussian A. Int J Dermatol 2015; 54: e67–9.

A 66-year-old woman presented with generalized eruptive KAs. After 6 months of acitretin 25 mg/d, all initial lesions resolved and no new lesions developed. The patient remained in remission at the time of reporting, 6 months after the discontinuation of the drug.

Generalized eruptive keratoacanthomas of Grzybowski treated with isotretinoin. Vandergriff T, Nakamura K, High WA. J Drugs Dermatol 2008; 7: 1069–71.

A 68-year-old man with generalized eruptive KAs of Grzybowski was started on 20 mg isotretinoin daily for 1 month. The dosage was increased to 40 mg daily an additional 3 months. Regression of lesions was noted, and no new lesions appeared. Two years after discontinuation of the medication, the patient remained in complete remission.

Treatment of multiple keratoacanthomas with erlotinib. Reid DC, Guitart J, Agulnik M, Lacouture ME. Int J Clin Oncol 2010; 15: 413–5.

An 82-year-old man with multiple KAs was started on 150 mg/day of the epidermal growth factor receptor inhibitor, erlotinib, which resulted in rapid clinical improvement.

Successful treatment of multiple keratoacanthoma with topical imiquimod and low-dose acitretin. Barysch MJ, Kamarashev J, Lockwood LL, Dummer R. J Dermatol 2011; 38: 380–2.

An 86-year-old woman with multiple KA of the lower extremity, recurrent after excision and radiation, was started on imiquimod 5%. Improvement, but not clearance, was noted until addition of acitretin 25 mg daily. Lesions resolved within 2 months of combination therapy and recurred abruptly upon discontinuation of therapy. Resumption of the topical and systemic treatments resulted in a sustained remission for 1.5 years while on treatment.

Superficial radiotherapy for multiple keratoacanthomas. Bruscino N, Corradini D, Campolmi P, Massi D, Palleschi GM. Dermatol Ther 2014; 27: 163–7.

A 76-year-old woman with multiple KAs was successfully treated with superficial radiotherapy. At 1 year's follow-up, resolution of the lesions was noted.

Keratoacanthomas related to predisposing factors

First-Line Therapies	
• Cessation or completion of therapy	C
• Photodynamic therapy	E

Eruptive keratoacanthoma-type squamous cell carcinomas in patients taking sorafenib for the treatment of solid tumors. Smith KJ, Haley H, Hamza S, Skelton HG. Dermatol Surg 2009; 35: 1766–70.

Fifteen patients taking the multikinase inhibitor sorafenib for solid tumors developed multiple KAs during therapy. Lesions resolved upon completion of sorafenib.

Eruptive keratoacanthomas associated with leflunomide. Tidwell WJ, Malone J, Callen JP. JAMA Dermatol 2016; 152: 105–6.

Case report of eruptive KAs associated with leflunomide for arthritis, which resolved upon cessation of leflunomide and initiation of oral isotretinoin.

Photodynamic therapy for multiple eruptive keratoacanthomas associated with vemurafenib treatment for metastatic melanoma. Alloo A, Garibyan L, LeBoeuf N, Lin G, Wechniak A, Hodi FS, et al. Arch Dermatol 2012; 148: 363–6.

Case report of multiple KAs in the setting of vemurafenib therapy treated with multiple cycles of photodynamic therapy. Treated areas experienced significant clinical regression.

Evidence Levels: **A** Double-blind study **B** Clinical trial ≥ 20 subjects **C** Clinical trial < 20 subjects **D** Series ≥ 5 subjects **E** Anecdotal case reports

124

Keratosis pilaris and variants

Christina M. Correnti, Anna L. Grossberg

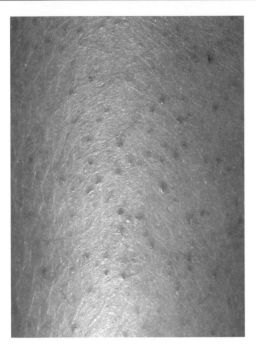

Keratosis pilaris (KP) is a common inherited disorder of unknown etiology characterized by tenacious keratin plugging of follicular orifices affecting characteristic body sites. It typically presents in childhood on the extensor aspects of the upper arms, anterior surfaces of the thighs, and lateral aspects of the cheeks. In more extensive cases, it may extend onto the distal extremities, shoulders, back, and buttocks. Perifollicular erythema is common, and a background of erythema on the cheeks may also be seen in keratosis pilaris rubra (KPR). Other variants of KP include erythromelanosis follicularis faciei et colli (EFFC) and keratosis pilaris atrophicans (KPA), which includes keratosis pilaris atrophicans faciei (ulerythema ophryogenes), keratosis follicularis spinulosa decalvans (KFSD), folliculitis spinulosa decalvans (FSD), and atrophoderma vermiculatum; these subtypes are also addressed in this chapter.

KP may be seen in conjunction with other skin disorders, such as atopic dermatitis; it may also arise or become exacerbated in association with various medical conditions or states, including pregnancy, and may be a feature of infants presenting with cutaneous stigmata of malnutrition. Extensive or persistent disease has also been observed in patients with Down syndrome and cardiofaciocutaneous syndrome, among others. KP has also developed in the setting of certain medications, notably Raf inhibitors.

MANAGEMENT STRATEGY

KP is very commonly asymptomatic and often does not require treatment. Those with extensive or symptomatic involvement often desire treatment, and even mild KP may cause patients cosmetic distress to the point of seeking therapy. It often becomes less prominent with increasing age, even without directed therapy.

Initial treatment aims to decrease excessive skin roughness and follicular accentuation. *Keratolytic agents* such as glycolic acid, ammonium lactate, salicylic acid, and urea-containing humectants are the mainstays of treatment. Use of a compound of salicylic acid 2% in 20% urea cream or salicylic acid 6% in propylene glycol combines the properties of an emollient with a keratolytic agent. Twice-daily application of one of these agents for at least a 3-week trial is recommended. The addition of gentle massage with a polyester sponge during a shower or bath may provide additional benefit. Vigorous scrubbing can lead to irritation and should be avoided. Once adequate relief of symptoms has been achieved, maintenance therapy of weekly or twice-weekly application of a topical keratolytic agent is recommended.

Topical retinoids may be utilized in some cases but must be gradually uptitrated in strength to avoid irritation. Tazarotene 0.05% cream has been shown to decrease the pruritus, erythema, and roughness of KP in a recent placebo-controlled trial. *Oral isotretinoin* has been helpful in some patients with ulerythema ophryogenes and atrophoderma vermiculatum.

If a significant inflammatory component is present, the inflammation can be treated for defined short time periods with a *medium-potency topical corticosteroid* in an emollient base. Once inflammation has abated, corticosteroids should be discontinued, and treatment should transition to keratolytics.

Cutaneous laser and light therapies have been utilized for several variants of KP (Table 124.1).

Specific Investigations

- Consider serum testosterone levels in obese females
- Ophthalmologic examination in cases of keratosis pilaris atrophicans

The prevalence of cutaneous manifestations in young patients with type 1 diabetes. Pavlović MD, Milenković T, Dinić M, Misović M, Daković D, Todorović S, et al. Diabetes Care 2007; 30: 1964–7.

The presence and frequency of skin manifestations were examined and compared in 212 unselected type 1 diabetic patients and 196 healthy sex- and age-matched control subjects. KP affected 12% of the diabetic patients compared with 1.5% of control subjects.

Other conditions associated with KP include high body mass index, ichthyosis, atopic conditions, pregnancy, cardiofaciocutaneous syndrome, and hyperandrogenism in obese females. KP-like lesions have been observed in patients treated with vemurafenib for metastatic melanoma.

Keratosis pilaris atrophicans. One heterogeneous disease or a symptom in different clinical entities? Oranje AP, van Osch LD, Oosterwijk JC. Arch Dermatol 1994; 130: 500–2.

Patients with keratosis pilaris atrophicans are reported to have increased incidence of ocular abnormalities, including photophobia, corneal deposits, juvenile cataracts, and corneal dystrophy.

This review also clarifies the confusing nosology of KP variants (ulerythema ophryogenes or KP atrophicans faciei, atrophoderma vermiculatum, keratosis follicularis spinulosa, FSD).

Table 124.1 Cutaneous laser and light therapies in the treatment of keratosis pilaris (KP) and variants

Variant	Modality	Details
Keratosis pilaris spinulosa decalvans	Non-Q-switched, high-energy, pulsed ruby laser	One case of KPSD of the scalp was complicated by recurrent secondary infection with limited response to multiple oral antibiotics and topical corticosteroids. Five treatments with a normal mode, non-Q-switched, high-energy, pulsed ruby laser at fluences of 19–21 J/cm^2 at 6-week intervals led to a significant reduction of inflammation in treated areas, at the expense of a persistent diminution of hair growth at 8-month follow-up.[a]
KP atrophicans (KPA)	585-nm pulsed-dye laser (PDL)	Twelve patients received two to eight treatments with energies ranging from 6.0–7.5 J/cm^2 resulting in erythema improvement but not textural improvement.[b]
Keratosis rubra pilaris (KRP)	532-nm potassium titanyl phosphate laser	A fluence of 12–14 J/cm^2 and pulse width of 510 ms was used for an initial seven treatments at 6- to 8-week intervals, then two treatments at 4-month intervals, resulting in cosmetic clearance of keratotic papules and reduction in facial erythema.[c]
KRP	595-nm PDL	Seven treatments spaced 6 weeks apart with spot size of 7 mm, a density energy up to 12 J/cm^2, and a pulse duration of 3 ms maintained marked improvement in erythema and follicular hyperkeratosis for 9 months.[d]
KPA	Intense pulsed light (IPL)	Four women were treated with five to nine sessions with an IPL system with a cut filter of 570 nm, power density between 40 and 47 J/cm^2 divided into two pulses of 3 ms, with a delay between both of 20 ms, resulting in over 75% reduction in erythema, observed reduced roughness, and no recurrence after 10 months.[e]
KRP or KPA	PDL	Ten patients with either condition were treated with two to seven sessions using PDL of 595 nm, spot size of 7 or 10 mm, pulse duration of 0.5 or 1.5 ms, and a fluence from 5–9 J/cm^2, resulting in over 75% to total resolution of erythema, with one case of postinflammatory hyperpigmentation.[f]
KP	Q-switched 1064-nm Nd:YAG laser	Twelve patients with KP were treated with 10 sessions every 2 weeks at 4.0–5.0 J/cm^2, 4-mm spot size, for three passes, resulting in more than grade 2 improvements in skin texture and dyspigmentation.[g]
KP	Long-pulsed 1064-nm Nd:YAG laser	Eighteen patients with untreated KP were treated three times at 4-week intervals using a 30-msec pulse width and fluence of 34 J/cm^2, with the contralateral arm serving as a control, resulting in significant improvements in erythema and the number of keratotic papules.[h]
KP	Combination of 595-nm PDL, long-pulsed 755-nm alexandrite laser, and microdermabrasion	Twenty-nine sites in 26 patients with KP were treated using a combination therapy, including 595-nm PDL with nonpurpuragenic fluences, a long-pulsed 755-nm alexandrite laser, and microdermabrasion. Pretreatment and posttreatment photographs and patient satisfaction rates were compared 3 months after treatment: 41.4% of sites demonstrated grade 3 clinical improvement, 34.5% had grade 2 improvement, 13.8% had grade 1 improvement, and 10.3% had grade 4 improvement. Improvements were noted in erythema, skin texture, and brown discoloration. Prolonged scaling was a potential adverse event.[i]
KP	810-nm diode laser	Of 18 Fitzpatrick type I–III patients completing this randomized, split-body, placebo-controlled trial, 3 were lost to follow-up and 2 withdrew due to laser-induced postinflammatory hyperpigmentation. After three treatments spaced 4–5 weeks apart, two blinded dermatologists rated the sites at 12 weeks. Skin texture improved significantly, but baseline erythema was not improved.[j]

[a] Chui CT, Berger TG, Price VH, Zachary CB. Recalcitrant scarring follicular disorders treated by laser-assisted hair removal: a preliminary report. Dermatol Surg 1999; 25: 34–7.

[b] Clark SM, Mills CM, Lanigan SW. Treatment of keratosis pilaris atrophicans with the pulsed tunable dye laser. J Cutan Laser Ther 2000; 2: 151–6.

[c] Dawn G, Urcelay M, Patel M, Strong AMM. Keratosis rubra pilaris responding to potassium titanyl phosphate laser. Br J Dermatol 2002; 147: 822–4.

[d] Kaune KM, Haas E, Emmet S, Schvan MP, Zutt M. Successful treatment of severe keratosis pilaris rubra with a 595-nm pulsed dye laser. Dermatol Surg 2009; 35: 1592–5.

[e] Rodríguez-Lojo R, Pozo JD, Barja JM, Piñeyro F, Pérez-Varela L. Keratosis pilaris atrophicans: treatment with intense pulsed light in four patients. J Cosmet Laser Ther 2010; 12: 188–90.

[f] Alcántara González J, Boixeda P, Truchuelo Díez MT, Fleta Asín B. Keratosis pilaris rubra and keratosis pilaris atrophicans faciei treated with pulsed dye laser: report of 10 cases. J Eur Acad Dermatol Venereol 2011; 25: 710–4.

[g] Park J, Kim BJ, Kim MN, Lee CK. A pilot study of Q-switched 1064-nm Nd:YAG laser treatment in the keratosis pilaris. Ann Dermatol 2011; 23: 293–8.

[h] Saelim P, Pongprutthipan M, Pootongkam S, Jariyasethavong V, Asawanonda P. Long-pulsed 1064-nm Nd:YAG laser significantly improves keratosis pilaris: a randomized, evaluator-blind study. J Dermatolog Treat 2013; 24: 318–22.

[i] Lee SJ, Choi MJ, Zheng Z, Chung WS, Kim YK, Cho SB. Combination of 595-nm pulsed dye laser, long-pulsed 755-nm alexandrite laser, and microdermabrasion treatment for keratosis pilaris: retrospective analysis of 26 Korean patients. J Cosmet Laser Ther 2013; 15: 150–4.

[j] Ibrahim O, Khan M, Bolotin D, Dubina M, Nodzenski M, Disphanurat W, et al. Treatment of keratosis pilaris with 810-nm diode laser: a randomized clinical trial. JAMA Dermatol 2015; 151: 187–91.

Evidence Levels: **A** Double-blind study **B** Clinical trial ≥ 20 subjects **C** Clinical trial < 20 subjects **D** Series ≥ 5 subjects **E** Anecdotal case reports

Red face revisited: disorders of hair growth and the pilosebaceous unit. Ramos-e-Silva M, Pirmez R. Clin Dermatol 2014; 32: 784–99.

This comprehensive review of diseases of the hair and pilosebaceous unit that may cause a red face includes epidemiology, clinical presentation, pathogenesis, and therapy of inflammatory follicular keratotic syndromes, ulerythema ophryogenes, atrophoderma vermiculatum, KFSD, and FSD.

First-Line Therapies

• 10% lactic acid cream	B
• 5% salicylic acid cream	B
• Sodium lactate and urea cream	B
• Polyester sponge	D
• Salicylic acid in urea	D
• Topical corticosteroids	D

Epidermal permeability barrier in the treatment of keratosis pilaris. Kootiratrakarn T, Kampirapap K, Chunhasewee C. Dermatol Res Pract 2015; 2015: 205012.

A blinded, prospective, randomized, split-side trial of 50 KP patients compared twice-daily 10% lactic acid (LA) and 5% salicylic acid (SA) for 3 months of therapy and 4 weeks after completion. The mean reduction of the lesions from baseline was statistically significant for both 10% LA (66%) and 5% SA (52%), with LA being statistically more effective ($p > 0.05$).

The authors suggest LA be tried first, given faster improvement and greater efficacy, despite its potential side effect of mild localized skin irritation.

Evaluation of a sodium lactate and urea créme to ameliorate keratosis pilaris. Weber TM, Kowcz A, Rizer R. J Am Acad Dermatol 2004; 50 (Suppl 1): 47.

A formulation containing sodium lactate and urea was tested on 32 subjects with mild to severe KP. The authors reported progressive, statistically significant improvements in overall condition, skin roughness, and skin tone at 3, 6, and 12 weeks of use.

Practical management of widespread, atypical keratosis pilaris. Novick NL. J Am Acad Dermatol 1984; 11: 305–6.

Thirty patients with widespread atypical or psychologically troubling KP were treated for prevention of excessive skin drying with application of salicylic acid 2% to 3% in 20% urea cream using a polyester sponge and use of emollient-based topical corticosteroids if a prominent inflammatory component was present. All patients reported satisfaction with cosmetic results. Clearing of lesions was noted in 75% to 100% of cases, with elimination of most lesions achieved within 2 to 3 weeks of daily therapy.

Keratosis pilaris decalvans nonatrophicans. Drago F, Maietta G, Parodi A, Rebora A. Clin Exp Dermatol 1993; 18: 45–6.

This is the first case report of a patient with an eruption of keratosis pilaris decalvans nonatrophicans with follicular keratotic papules on the limbs and trunk and body hair loss without scarring. The patient was treated with emollients and multivitamins, and the eruption spontaneously cleared with hair regrowth after 3 months.

Traditional methods of treated KP seem to be effective in treating cases of keratosis pilaris decalvans.

Second-Line Therapies

• Topical tazarotene	A
• Topical tretinoin	D
• Isotretinoin	E
• Topical tacrolimus	A
• Aquaphor	A
• Dermabrasion (for atrophoderma vermiculatum)	E

A comparative trial comparing the efficacy of tacrolimus 0.1% ointment with Aquaphor ointment for the treatment of keratosis pilaris. Breithaupt AD, Alio A, Friedlander SF. Pediatr Dermatol 2011; 28: 459–60.

This was a bilateral, paired comparison, double-blind study that showed improvement but no difference between Aquaphor and tacrolimus 0.1% ointment in 27 patients.

Topical tacrolimus was more likely to lead to >75% improvement (six tacrolimus sites vs. one Aquaphor site), though this failed to reach statistical significance, likely due to small sample size.

Tazarotene 0.05% cream for the treatment of keratosis pilaris. Bogle MA, Ali A, Bartel H. J Am Acad Dermatol 2004; 50 (Suppl 1): 39.

A randomized, placebo-controlled, double-blind prospective study of tazarotene 0.05% cream for the treatment of KP on the posterior arms of 33 patients resulted in statistically significant improvement in pruritus, erythema, and roughness of KP lesions.

Natural history of keratosis pilaris. Poskitt L, Wilkinson JD. Br J Dermatol 1994; 130: 711–3.

This retrospective questionnaire study of 49 patients with KP yielded 14 patients who had benefited from a variety of treatments. Of these patients, 8 reported therapy with topical tretinoin cream to be helpful.

Two reported dramatic improvement with oral tetracyclines; however, the questionnaire did not permit exclusion of possible coincident acne.

Clinical findings, cutaneous pathology, and response to therapy in 21 patients with keratosis pilaris atrophicans. Baden HP, Byers HR. Arch Dermatol 1994; 130: 469–75.

Twenty-one patients with keratosis pilaris atrophicans were treated with various agents, including keratolytics, antibiotics, topical corticosteroids, and oral retinoids, all with very limited response. Treatment of four patients with isotretinoin 1 mg/kg resulted in little or no improvement in three patients and exacerbation of the condition in one patient.

A case of atrophoderma vermiculatum responding to isotretinoin. Weightman W. Clin Exp Dermatol 1998; 23: 89–91.

Atrophoderma vermiculatum is a rare variant of KP that results in reticular or honeycomb scarring of the face. In this case report, two 6-month therapeutic courses of 0.50 mg/kg/day of isotretinoin, 2 weeks apart, halted progression of further atrophy, and the patient remained free of new lesions after 1 year.

In severe cases of atrophoderma vermiculatum with significant scarring, a trial of isotretinoin therapy may be worthwhile to halt progression of the disease.

Atrophoderma vermiculatum. Case reports and review. Frosch PJ, Brumage MR, Schuster-Pavlovic C, Bersch A. J Am Acad Dermatol 1988; 18: 538–42.

Dermabrasion may be used to reduce eventual scarring.

A case of ulerythema ophryogenes responding to isotretinoin. Layton AM, Cunliffe WJ. Br J Dermatol 1993; 129: 645–6.

Ulerythema ophryogenes, a variant of KP, begins in the eyebrows as small, discrete, horny, pinhead-sized, follicular-based papules that spread to the forehead and scalp. Atrophy and alopecia of the eyebrows and scalp may result. There is a variable response to isotretinoin.

Third-Line Therapies

• Tetracyclines: oxytetracycline, minocycline	E
• Long-pulse, non-Q-switched, ruby laser (KP spinulosa decalvans)	E
• Dapsone (keratosis folliculitis decalvans)	E
• Pulsed tunable dye laser (KP atrophicans)	C
• Intense pulsed light (KP atrophicans)	E
• Potassium titanyl phosphate laser (keratosis rubra pilaris)	E
• Pulsed dye laser (keratosis rubra pilaris)	E
• Pulsed dye laser (KP or KP atrophicans faciei)	C
• Q-switched 1064-nm neodymium-doped yttrium aluminium garnet laser	C
• Long-pulsed 1064-nm neodymium-doped yttrium aluminium garnet laser	C
• 810-nm diode laser	C

Keratosis pilaris rubra: a common but underrecognized condition. Marqueling AL, Gilliam AE, Prendiville J, Zvulunov A, Antaya RJ, Sugarman J, et al. Arch Dermatol 2006; 142: 1611–6.

This series of 27 cases distinguishes the clinical presentation of KPR compared with EFFC and other overlapping variants of KP. EFFC is very similar to KPR, with follicular papules of the face and/or neck, except it tends to develop later in life, most frequently in the second decade, more commonly in males, and possesses the differentiating features of a lack of torso involvement and the presence of hyperpigmentation. Treatments given for KPR in these patients included emollients; urea, LA, SA, topical corticosteroids, or a combination of these ingredients; topical agents containing cholecalciferol; and topical or systemic retinoid agents. In most patients, there was no substantial improvement with these treatments. One patient had excellent response with pulsed dye laser (PDL).

Some authors consider KPR and EFFC to be forms of the same condition, whereas others have considered EFFC as a part of the KPA group.

Folliculitis spinulosa decalvans: successful therapy with dapsone. Kunte C, Loeser C, Wolff H. J Am Acad Dermatol 1998; 39: 891–3.

In this case report, a patient presented with FSD with keratotic follicular papules on the trunk and extremities; lateral eyebrow alopecia; and erythema, scaling, and follicular hyperkeratoses on the scalp. Isotretinoin and topical corticosteroids were ineffective. Dapsone (100 mg/day) led to the resolution of inflammation and pustulation on the scalp within 1 month. The scarring alopecia did not expand after dapsone therapy.

Complete eradication of chronic long standing eczema and keratosis pilaris following treatment with dextroamphetamine sulfate. Check JH, Chan S. Clin Exp Obstet Gynecol 2014; 41: 202–4.

Dextroamphetamine sulfate treatment for sympathetic nervous system hypofunction markedly improved chronic eczema in two patients as well as KP in one of the patients.

Eczema and KP are two more chronic dermatologic conditions, aside from chronic urticaria and prurigo nodularis, that may improve with dextroamphetamine sulfate treatment.

Photopneumatic therapy for the treatment of keratosis pilaris. Ciliberto H, Farshidi A, Berk D, Bayliss S. J Drugs Dermatol 2013; 12: 804–6.

In this small unblinded study of 10 patients, photopneumatic therapy improved both the erythema and redness associated with KP for at least 1 month after one treatment.

Dermatologic toxicities to targeted cancer therapy: shared clinical and histologic adverse skin reactions. Curry JL, Torres-Cabala CA, Kim KB, Tetzlaff MT, Duvic M, Tsai KY, et al. Int J Dermatol 2014; 53: 376–84.

In this review of published reports of dermatologic toxicities with multiple targeted cancer therapies, RAF inhibitors (vemurafenib and sorafenib) were associated with multiple cutaneous epithelial proliferations, including KP, seborrheic keratosis, verruca vulgaris, actinic keratosis, keratoacanthoma, and squamous cell carcinoma.

Evidence Levels: **A** Double-blind study **B** Clinical trial ≥ 20 subjects **C** Clinical trial < 20 subjects **D** Series ≥ 5 subjects **E** Anecdotal case reports

125

Langerhans cell histiocytosis

Catherine Borysiewicz, Anthony C. Chu

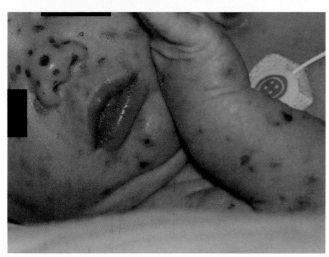

Langerhans cell histiocytosis (LCH) is a reactive condition defined by the accumulation/proliferation of a clonal population of epidermal Langerhans cells. Recent studies showing mutation in cell proliferation/regulatory pathways, however, suggest that it should be considered a neoplasm of myeloid origin. Patients can have either single or multiple organ involvement. Children tend to have more aggressive disease than adults.

LCH encompasses the diseases previously known as *histiocytosis X, eosinophilic granuloma, Hand–Schuller–Christian disease, Letter Siwe disease, congenital self-healing reticulohistiocytosis (Hashimoto–Pritzker), Langerhans cell granulomatosis,* and *nonlipid reticuloendotheliosis.*

MANAGEMENT STRATEGY

Before institution of therapy, a full investigation must be completed. A definitive diagnosis can be made histologically by identification of Langerhans cells that express CD1a by immunohistochemistry and the finding of Birbeck granules by electron microscopy.

Treatment depends on the organ(s) involved and the severity of the disease and thus should be tailored to the individual patient. Most published data are based on case reports and small case series in children, and this evidence may not always be directly applicable to adults. Patients are staged as single system disease (with bone involvement, this is further stratified into monoostotic and polyostotic bone disease), multisystem disease, and multisystem disease with evidence of organ dysfunction. Although some patients with LCH may undergo spontaneous remission, the disease is unpredictable, and many patients progress from single system disease to multisystem disease. Organs most commonly involved include the bone, skin, lymph nodes, pituitary, liver, lungs, central nervous system, gastrointestinal tract, spleen, bone marrow, and endocrine system.

Single system bone or skin disease has a good prognosis and may not require treatment. *Curettage* or *intralesional steroid*

injections can also be used in single system bone disease. Single system skin disease may respond to local measures with *topical steroids, topical nitrogen mustard, topical tacrolimus,* or *phototherapy.* Single system lung disease may respond to *prednisolone* at 2 mg/kg/day. In single system disease that does not respond to these measures, single system lymph node disease, and multisystem disease without organ dysfunction, systemic treatment with *azathioprine* (2 mg/kg/day), with or without low-dose, weekly *methotrexate* (5–10 mg/week), may lead to resolution.

In recalcitrant disease or in multisystem disease with evidence of organ dysfunction, treatment will depend on the age of the patient. Organ dysfunction of key organs—liver, lungs, spleen, and bone marrow—carries the worst prognosis. Trials have demonstrated that in pediatric patients, *prednisolone with vinblastine* is the treatment of choice. This combination is less effective in adults, who are also more sensitive to their side effects. In adult patients, first-line treatment is *etoposide*. In pediatric studies the use of maintenance therapy has been shown to reduce the overall morbidity of the disease. Adults often have a more chronic and relapsing course to their disease, and maintenance therapy with *azathioprine* for 1 year should be considered in all patients with multisystem disease. In both children and adults with multisystem disease with organ dysfunction, there remains a small group who do not respond to conventional therapy. In these patients, *2-chlorodeoxyadenosine* has proved useful and, in severe disease, *bone marrow transplantation* has been successful. A number of drugs have been used in various stages of the disease, but most are anecdotal case reports.

There has been great interest in the last 4 years in the finding of BRAF V600E and MAP2K1 mutations in LCH, and this has led to treatment in a few patients with recalcitrant disease with vemurafenib.

Long-term morbidity can be correlated to organ involvement or occur as a direct consequence of treatment and includes skeletal deformities, risk of secondary malignancies (particularly with the use of alkylating agents and radiotherapy), endocrine dysfunction, and infertility.

Specific Investigations

Routine investigations

- Biopsy of organ involved for staining for S100 and CD1a or electron microscopy for Birbeck granules. The presence of Birbeck granules may also be demonstrated by immunohistochemical staining of langerin (CD207)
- Full blood count with differential
- Coagulation tests (prothrombin time [PT], activated partial thromboplastin time [APTT])
- ESR
- Liver function tests
- C-reactive protein
- Chest x-ray
- Whole body position emission tomography (PET) computed tomography (CT) is the most effective way to identify both skeletal and nonskeletal disease

Indicated investigations

- Lung function tests in patients with lung disease
- High-resolution CT chest for all adult smokers or children with chest signs or symptoms
- Bronchoalveolar lavage for CD1a + cells or open lung biopsy if evidence of lung involvement
- CT brain and pituitary fossa if signs of diabetes insipidus
- Plasma and urine osmolality if signs of diabetes insipidus (plus a water deprivation test, if required)

- Full hormone screen if diabetes insipidus confirmed
- Magnetic resonance imaging (MRI) brain if lytic skull lesions, diabetes insipidus, or symptoms suggestive of central nervous system (CNS) involvement
- Panorthogram if gum involvement
- Bone marrow biopsy if hematologic abnormalities
- Abdominal ultrasound and liver biopsy if abnormal liver function
- Multiple bowel biopsies if evidence of malabsorption or failure to thrive in an infant

Histiocytosis syndromes in children: approach to the clinical and laboratory evaluation of children with Langerhans cell histiocytosis. Broadbent V, Gadner H, Komp DM, Ladisch S. Med Pediatr Oncol 1989; 17: 492–5.

Multiple organ systems may be affected in patients with LCH. Therefore the following studies are recommended for all patients at diagnosis: a complete blood count with white blood cell differential, liver function tests, coagulation times (PT and PTT), chest radiograph, and radiographic skeletal survey (more sensitive than a radionuclide bone scan for detecting bone lesions). A measurement of urine osmolality after overnight water deprivation should also be obtained. Further evaluations should be tailored to patients based on specific presenting signs and symptoms.

BRAF V600E mutation correlates with suppressive tumour immune microenvironment and reduces disease free survival in Langerhans cell histiocytosis. Zeng K, Wang Z, Ohshima K, Liu Y, Zhang W, Wang L, et al. Oncoimmunology 2016; 5: e1185582.

Study in 97 patients with LCH showed BRAF V600E mutation in 37.1% of patients, and this was significantly correlated with increased program cell death 1 ligand 1 (PDL1) expression and that BRAF V600E mutation and PDL1 were independent prognostic factors for disease survival in this disease.

BRAF V600E and MAP2K1 mutations in Langerhans cell histiocytosis occur predominantly in children. Zeng K, Ohshima K, Liu Y, Zhang W, Wang L, Fan L, et al. Hematol Oncol 2016; 10.1002/hon.2344 [Epub ahead of print].

Study in 97 patients with LCH showed BRAF V600E and MAP2K1 mutations in 32% and 17.5%, respectively. These mutations were significantly more common in children than in adults ($p = 0.001$).

First-Line Therapies

Skin disease

• Topical nitrogen mustard	C
• Phototherapy (PUVA, narrowband UVB)	E
• Topical tacrolimus	E

Multisystem disease

• Vinblastine	B
• Etoposide (VP16)	B

Topical nitrogen mustard: an effective treatment for cutaneous Langerhans cell histiocytosis. Sheehan MP, Atherton DJ, Broadbent V, Pritchard J. J Pediatr 1991; 119: 317–21.

Sixteen children with multisystem LCH with severe skin involvement were treated with topical nitrogen mustard with rapid clinical improvement. One child developed a contact allergy after use.

Long term follow up of topical mustine treatment for cutaneous Langerhans cell histiocytosis. Hoeger PH, Nanduri VR, Harper JI, Atherton DA, Pritchard J. Arch Dis Child 2000; 82: 483–7.

Topical nitrogen mustard (0.02% mechlorethamine hydrochloride mustard) was found to be safe in cutaneous disease. Follow-up in this study was an average of 8.3 years.

Topical nitrogen mustard ointment with occlusion for Langerhans' cell histiocytosis of the scalp. Treat JR, Suchin KR, James WD. J Dermatolog Treat 2003; 14: 46–7.

Topical nitrogen mustard ointment 0.01% under occlusion cleared a patient with scalp LCH in 3 weeks without irritation.

Topical nitrogen mustard in patients with Langerhans cell histiocytosis. Lindahl LM, Fenger-Gron M, Iversen L. Br J Dermatol 2012; 166: 642–5.

Ten children and four adults with skin involvement with LCH treated with nitrogen mustard and studied retrospectively. In five patients the skin improved, but in four patients systemic disease progressed; six patients developed contact dermatitis.

Topical nitrogen mustard is the best studied and most effective topical therapy. Contact allergy and risk of cutaneous carcinogenicity limit its use. It is not recommended for disease involving large areas of skin.

Satisfactory remission achieved by PUVA therapy in Langerhans cell histiocytosis in an elderly patient. Sakai H, Ibe M, Takaahashi H, Matsuo S, Okamoto K, Makino I, et al. J Dermatol 1996; 23: 42–6.

Case report of a 74-year-old man with cutaneous LCH and diabetes insipidus. Five weeks of PUVA therapy led to complete clearance of skin lesions. The endocrinopathy persisted.

Cutaneous Langerhans cell histiocytosis in an elderly man successfully treated with narrowband ultraviolet B. Imafuku S, Shibata S, Tashiro A, Furue M. Br J Dermatol 2007; 157: 1277–9.

Doses of 0.4 J/cm^2 to 1.0 J/cm^2 were given incrementally (total irradiation of 9.3 J/cm^2). Eleven sessions led to almost complete resolution in a Japanese man, which persisted at least 12 months after therapy was discontinued.

Etoposide in recurrent childhood Langerhans cell histiocytosis: an Italian cooperative study. Ceci A, De Terlizzi M, Colella R, Balducci D, Toma MG, Zurlo MG, et al. Cancer 1988; 62: 2528–31.

Twelve of 18 patients with recurrent LCH had a complete response and 3 a partial response after treatment with etoposide (200 mg/m^2/day given 3 days every 3 weeks).

Langerhans cell histiocytosis in childhood: results from the Italian Cooperative AIEOP-CNR-H.X. '83 study. Ceci A, de Terlizzi M, Colella R, Loiacono G, Balducci D, Surico G, et al. Med Pediatr Oncol 1993; 21: 259–64.

Ninety patients were divided into those with and without organ dysfunction. Monotherapy with either vinblastine or etoposide was an effective treatment in patients without organ dysfunction.

A randomised trial of treatment for multisystem Langerhans' cell histiocytosis. Gadner H, Grois N, Arico M, Broadbent V, Ceci A, Jakobson A, et al. J Pediatr 2001; 138: 728–34.

This controlled trial of 24 weeks of vinblastine (6 mg/m^2, IV weekly) or etoposide (150 mg/m^2/day for 3 days every 3 weeks)

Evidence Levels: **A** Double-blind study **B** Clinical trial ≥ 20 subjects **C** Clinical trial < 20 subjects **D** Series ≥ 5 subjects **E** Anecdotal case reports

and an initial dose of methylprednisolone (30 mg/kg/day for 3 days) recruited 143 untreated children with multisystem LCH. The two treatments were found to be equally effective with response rates of 58% for vinblastine and 69% for etoposide. Vinblastine is considered safer for use in children.

Etoposide has been consistently shown to be effective in multifocal LCH. However, the small risk of secondary leukemia after treatment in children with etoposide limits its use to the most high-risk pediatric patients.

Second-Line Therapies	
• Prednisolone	B
• 6-Mercaptopurine	B
• Thalidomide	C
• Methotrexate	C
• Cytosine arabinoside (Ara-C)	C
• 2-Chlorodeoxyadenosine (2-CdA)	C

Improved outcome in multisystem Langerhans cell histiocytosis is associated with therapy intensification. Gadner H, Grois N, Pötschger U, Minkov M, Aricò M, Braier J, et al. Histiocyte Society. Blood 2008; 111: 2556–62.

This randomized controlled trial had 193 patients with multisystem disease. Arm A consisted of 4 weeks of prednisone 40 mg/m^2 once daily tapering over 2 weeks, vinblastine 6 mg/m^2 IV weekly for 6 weeks followed by 18 weeks of 6-mercaptopurine 50 mg/m^2 daily with vinblastine (6 mg/m^2), and prednisolone (40 mg/m^2 for 5 days) pulses every 3 weeks; etoposide 150 mg/m^2 weekly for the first 6 weeks followed by pulsed therapy every 3 weeks was added in arm B. Both regimens had similar response rates (63% vs. 71%), 5-year survival probability (74% vs. 79%), and relapse rate (46% vs. 46%). *The more intense chemotherapy regimen with etoposide was better in patients with liver, lung, spleen, and hematopoietic system involvement.*

Treatment strategy for disseminated Langerhans cell histiocytosis. Gadner H, Heitger A, Grois N, Gatterer-Menz I, Ladisch S. Med Pediatr Oncol 1994; 23: 72–80.

A study of 106 patients divided into three groups: group A (multifocal bone disease), group B (soft tissue disease without organ dysfunction), and group C (patients with organ dysfunction). All patients received 6 weeks of etoposide, vinblastine, and prednisone, followed by continuation therapy with 1 year of 6-mercaptopurine, vinblastine, and prednisone. Patients in group B also received etoposide during continuation therapy, and group C received both etoposide and methotrexate. A complete response was seen in 89% of group A, 91% of group B, and 67% of group C patients.

This study treated patients with 1 year of "maintenance" chemotherapy, which has not been shown to be superior to the use of intermittent treatment for disease exacerbations.

A case of adult Langerhans cell histiocytosis showing successfully regenerated osseous tissue of the skull after chemotherapy. Suzuki T, Izutsu K, Kako S, Ohta S, Hangaishi A, Kanda Y, et al. Int J Hematol 2008; 87: 284–8.

A case report of an adult with large osteolytic lesions in the skull that successfully responded to 6 weeks of prednisolone and vinblastine, followed by the addition of 6-mercaptopurine for a further 12 months. After treatment x-ray examination confirmed bone regeneration.

Successful treatment of cutaneous Langerhans cell histiocytosis with thalidomide. Sander CS, Kaatz M, Elsner P. Dermatology 2004; 208: 149–52.

Thalidomide 200 mg once daily was given to a 38-year-old male with recurrent mucocutaneous LCH. He had significant improvement within 4 weeks and complete healing after 3 months. Treatment was continued at 100 mg once daily without relapse.

Langerhans cell histiocytosis with vulvar involvement and responding to thalidomide therapy—case report. Fernandes LB, Guerra JG, Costa MB, Paiva IG, Duran FP, Jaco DN. An Bras Dermatol 2011; 86: S78–81.

A 57-year-old woman with extensive skin involvement, including the scalp, face, trunk, axillae, and vulva. Systemic steroids and thalidomide at 100 mg/day led to complete resolution after 4 months. Disease relapsed on stopping treatment but was brought under control with thalidomide at 50 mg/day as maintenance therapy.

A phase II trial using thalidomide for Langerhans cell histiocytosis. McClain KL, Kozinetz CA. Pediatr Blood Cancer 2007; 48: 44–9.

Sixteen patients with LCH who had relapsed once or twice despite treatment were included in the trial. Six patients were considered high risk. The rest consisted of patients with skin and/or bone and/or brain involvement. Adults were commenced at 100 mg (children 50 mg) daily, which was increased by 50 mg per month until efficacy or toxicity was achieved. No high-risk patient responded to treatment. Four low-risk patients had complete responses, three had partial responses, and two did not respond.

Oral methotrexate and alternate-day prednisone for low-risk Langerhans cell histiocytosis. Womer RB, Anunciato KR, Chehrenama M. Med Pediatr Oncol 1995; 25: 70–3.

Thirteen low-risk children were treated successfully with prednisone 40 mg/m^2/day on alternate days and weekly methotrexate 20 mg/m^2 for a minimum of 3 months. Toxicity was minimal, and recurrences were treated with the same regimen.

Cytosine-arabinoside, vincristine, and prednisolone in the treatment of children with disseminated Langerhans cell histiocytosis with organ dysfunction: experience at a single institution. Egeler RM, de Kraker J, Voûte PA. Med Pediatr Oncol 1993; 21: 265–70.

Eighteen patients with multiorgan involvement (8 with organ dysfunction and 10 without organ dysfunction) received chemotherapy containing cytosine–arabinoside, vincristine, and prednisolone. Sixty-three percent of patients with organ dysfunction and 80% without the organ dysfunction had sustained remission.

This regimen is well tolerated and avoids the risk of secondary malignancies associated with etoposide. Results compare satisfactorily with other chemotherapeutic regimens.

Successful treatment of Langerhans cell histiocytosis with 2-chlorodeoxyadenosine. Goh NS, McDonald CE, MacGregor DP, Pretto JJ, Brodie GN. Respirology 2003; 8: 91–4.

A young man with LCH involving lungs and bone who had previously failed to respond to two chemotherapy regimens. Complete symptomatic remission was achieved after five cycles of 2-CdA (0.1 mg/kg/day for 7 days per cycle) with no evidence of recurrence at 5 years.

Efficacy of continuous infusion 2-CdA (cladribine) in pediatric patients with Langerhans cell histiocytosis. Stine KC, Saylors RL, Saccente S, McClaine KL, Becton DL. Pediatr Blood Cancer 2004; 43: 81–4.

Ten children with reactivated LCH or high-risk disease were treated with 2-CdA (initially 5 mg/m²/day for 3 days increasing to 6.5 mg/m²/day for 3 days). All 10 had clinical responses. Seven patients remained disease free for a median of 50 months. Three patients needed further drug therapy but were clinically in remission.

Cladribine (2-chlorodeoxyadenosine) in frontline chemotherapy for adult Langerhans cell histiocytosis: a single centre study of seven cases. Adam Z, Szturz P, Vanicek J, Moulis M, Pour L, Krejci M, et al. Acta Oncol 2013; 52: 994–1001.

Retrospective study of six males with multisystem disease and one male with multifocal bone disease treated with cladribine at 5 mg/m² subcutaneously in five cases or intravenously in two. Treatment was enhanced with cyclophosphamide and corticosteroids in two patients. Durable complete remissions were achieved in six patients with a median follow-up of 37 months. One patient had an early relapse.

This confirms the efficacy of 2-CdA in LCH, particularly in patients who have failed on other forms of treatment.

Third-Line Therapies	
Radiotherapy	B
Ciclosporin	B
Bone marrow transplantation	C
Trimethoprim–sulfamethoxazole	C
Vemurafenib	C
Interferon-α	D
2-Deoxycoformycin	E
Interleukin-2	E
Isotretinoin	E
Acitretin	E
Lenalidomide	E
Photodynamic therapy	E
Clofarabine	E
Mistletoe	E

Results of treatment of 127 patients with systemic histiocytosis (Letterer-Siwe syndrome, Schüller-Christian syndrome, and multifocal eosinophilic granuloma). Greenberger JS, Crocker AC, Vawter G, Jaffe N, Cassady JR. Medicine 1981; 60: 311–38.

Many patients discussed in this retrospective study achieved remission from local radiation therapy for bone and soft tissue lesions.

Chemotherapy is now generally preferred due to the slight risk of secondary malignancy, but also the fact that LCH is often a generalized disease and local treatment is thus limited.

Cyclosporin A therapy for multisystem Langerhans cell histiocytosis. Minkov M, Grois N, Broadbent V, Ceci A, Jakobson A, Ladisch S. Med Pediatr Oncol 1999; 33: 482–5.

Twenty-six patients with refractory LCH were treated with ciclosporin alone or in combination with prednisolone, vinblastine or etoposide, and/or antithymocyte globulin. The median dose was 6 mg/kg/day (range 2–12 mg/kg/day) for a median duration of 4.5 months. One patient had a complete response, and three had a partial response.

Ciclosporin has been effective in only a small number of patients with LCH, and remissions tend to be short.

Hematopoietic stem cell transplantation in patients with severe Langerhans cell histiocytosis and hematological dysfunction: experience of the French Langerhans Cell Study Group. Akkari V, Donadieu J, Piguet C, Bordigoni P, Michel G, Blanche S, et al. Bone Marrow Transpl 2003; 31: 1097–103.

Eight patients with LCH and hematologic dysfunction received a hematopoietic stem cell transplant (three autologous and five allogeneic). All had responded poorly to initial chemotherapy. Autologous transplant failed in all patients. Three patients had a complete response, and two died from toxicity after the allogeneic transplant. Ultimately only two patients had no recurrences after 21 months and 7 years of follow-up.

Improved outcome of treatment resistant high risk Langerhans cell histiocytosis after allogeneic stem cell transplantation with reduced-intensity conditioning. Steiner M, Matthes Martin S, Attarbaschi A, Minkov M, Grois N, Unqer E, et al. Bone Marrow Transpl 2005; 36: 215–25.

Treatment-related mortality after hematopoietic stem cell transplant for multisystem refractory LCH is unacceptably high (50%). Therefore a novel approach is to use a reduced intensity conditioning (RIC) protocol. Nine patients with multisystem-risk, organ-positive LCH who had active disease despite numerous therapies underwent RIC allogeneic stem cell transplant; 78% (seven of nine) were alive without evidence of disease after 1 year. Two patients died.

Stem cell transplant for refractory LCH can be highly toxic but can achieve sustained disease control. Several other case reports have documented long-term remissions after bone marrow transplantation. This approach is generally reserved for patients with fulminant disease not responding to chemotherapy.

Effect of trimethoprim-sulphamethoxazole in Langerhans cell histiocytosis: preliminary observations. Tzortzatou-Stathopoulou F, Xaidara A, Mikraki V, Moschovi M, Arvantis D, Ageloyianni P, et al. Med Pediatr Oncol 1995; 25: 74–8.

Twenty-three children with both single and multisystem disease were treated for a 4-week to 3-month duration. Patients with single system disease responded well, whereas those with multisystem disease had a more limited response.

Dramatic efficacy of vemurafenib in both multisystemic and refractory Erdheim Chester disease and Langerhans cell histiocytosis harboring the BRAF V600E mutation. Haroche J, Cohen-Aubart F, Emile JF, Arnaud L, Maksud P, Charlotte F, et al. Blood 2013; 121: 1495–500.

Two patients with skin or lymph node LCH showing BRAF V600E mutation were treated with vemurafenib for 4 months. Patients responded, but persistent active disease was still observed.

Widespread skin-limited Langerhans cell histiocytosis: complete remission with interferon alpha. Kwong YL, Chan ACL, Chan TK. J Am Acad Dermatol 1997; 36: 628–9.

Subcutaneous interferon-α at 6 MU daily for 9 months followed by 3 MU for 9 months led to resolution of a patient with extensive single system cutaneous disease.

Intralesional interferon-α has been used for localized cutaneous disease also.

Successful treatment of two children with Langerhans' cell histiocytosis with 2'-deoxycoformycin. McCowage GB, Frush DP, Kurtzberg J. J Pediatr Hematol Oncol 1996; 18: 154–8.

Evidence Levels: A Double-blind study B Clinical trial ≥ 20 subjects C Clinical trial < 20 subjects D Series ≥ 5 subjects E Anecdotal case reports

Two patients (aged 3 and 5) who were refractory to multiple chemotherapeutic agents were treated with 2'-deoxycoformycin 4 mg/m^2 intravenously weekly for 8 weeks, then every 2 weeks for at least 16 months. Both patients achieved sustained remission with continued treatment. Toxicity was limited to asymptomatic grade III to IV lymphopenia and abnormalities of lymphocyte mitogen responses.

Interleukin-2 therapy of Langerhans cell histiocytosis.
Hirose M, Saito S, Yoshimoto T, Kuroda Y. Acta Pediatr 1995; 84: 1204–6.

A 20-month-old girl with disseminated LCH who had failed chemotherapy achieved a transient remission with intravenous IL-2.

Langerhans cell histiocytosis: complete remission after oral isotretinoin therapy.
Tsambaos D, Georgiou S, Kapranos N, Monastirli A, Stratigos A, Berger H. Acta Derm Venereol 1995; 75: 62–4.

A patient with single system cutaneous disease achieved a complete response to oral isotretinoin at 1.5 mg/kg/day for 9 months with no relapse at 5 years.

Langerhans cell histiocytosis in an adult: good response of cutaneous lesions to acitretin.
Cardoso JC, Cravo M, Cardosos R, Brites MM, Reis JP, Tellechea O, et al. Clin Exp Dermatol 2010; 35: 627–30.

Erosive LCH in the groin was treated with acitretin 25 mg/day and topical steroids. After 1 year the patient was free of skin lesions and treatment was stopped. No follow-up was documented.

Lenalidomide induced therapeutic response in a patient with aggressive multi-system Langerhans cell histiocytosis resistant to 2-chlorodeoxyadenosine and early relapse after high dose BEAM chemotherapy with autologous peripheral stem cell transplant.
Adam Z, Rehak Z, Koukalova R, Szturz P, Krejci M, Pour L, et al. Vnitr Lek 2012; 58: 62–71.

An adult patient with multisystem LCH had relapsed after treatment with a combination of etoposide and cyclophosphamide, then cladribine, and then BEAM chemotherapy (carmustine, etoposide, cytarabine, melphalan) with autologous stem cell transplant. Treatment was started with lenalidomide 25 mg/day for 21 days in 28-day cycles. After four cycles, 50% reduction in size of lymph nodes was noted on imaging. With further cycles, etoposide 100 mg on days 22, 23, and 24 was added. After five cycles, complete remission was achieved, and the patient underwent allogeneic bone marrow transplant 4 months later.

Photodynamic therapy for multi-resistant cutaneous Langerhans cell histiocytosis.
Failla V, Wauters O, Caucanas M, Nikkels-Tassoudji N, Nikkels AF. Rare Tumours 2010; 2: e34.

An 18-month-old boy with severe skin involvement failed to respond to topical steroids and topical nitrogen mustard. Systemic corticosteroids and vinblastine improved the trunk, but not the scalp. Methyl aminolevulinate–based photodynamic therapy resulted in significant regression of the scalp lesions. Follow-up for 6 months showed no recurrence.

Clofarabine in refractory Langerhans cell histiocytosis.
Rodriguez-Galindo C, Jeng M, Khuu P, McCarville MB, Jeha S. Pediatr Blood Cancer 2008; 51: 703–6.

Two children with LCH refractory to treatment (including 2-CdA) were treated with five or six cycles of clofarabine (optimized to 25 mg/m^2/day for 5 days), which induced remission in both patients.

Response to subcutaneous therapy with mistletoe in recurrent multisystem Langerhans cell histiocytosis.
Seifert G, Laengler A, Tautz C, Seeger K, Henze G. Pediatr Blood Cancer 2007; 48: 591–2.

A patient with multisystem disease, recurrent relapses, and persistent cutaneous lesions, despite chemotherapy, was treated with an aqueous extract of mistletoe (Helixor) subcutaneously three times a week, alternating doses weekly between 1 mg, 2.5 mg, and 5 mg. Cutaneous lesions cleared after 4 weeks of treatment, and the patient remained in remission after 5 years on continuous treatment.

Leg ulcers

David J. Margolis

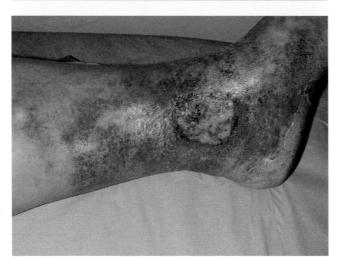

Chronic leg wounds are likely related to the fact that legs are on the most distal aspects of the circulatory, lymphatic, and nervous system supply, in addition to the fact that the legs are the bearers of weight and gravity. Arterial and venous problems, infection, trauma, and systemic problems such as diabetes add to impaired healing. Leg ulcers secondary to other causes such as infection, keratinocyte cancers, or pyoderma gangrenosum are discussed elsewhere. Management of leg ulcers is at least partially based on the etiology of the wound.

MANAGEMENT STRATEGY

Wound care

Many chronic wounds are contaminated by microorganisms, but most are likely not infected. It is generally believed that *debridement* is the first step toward treating wound contamination. The presence of microorganisms and necrotic tissue causes local tissue inflammation resulting in high levels of proinflammatory cytokines and tissue proteases. Debridement and aggressive cleaning can be done mechanically with curettage, scissors, or scalpel. It can also be accomplished with pressurized liquids, ultrasound, biomechanically (i.e., maggots), and enzymatically.

Dressing

Wound dressings should be chosen to address exudate control, wound protection, and pain relief. The goal is to provide a moist wound environment to promote granulation tissue formation and epithelialization. Using *hydrocolloids, hydrogels, alginates, transparent films*, and other bandages provides coverage and may promote the function of these enzymes. However, excessive exudate can saturate the wound bed, diminishing these beneficial properties, and macerate surrounding tissue, making it more prone to injury. Finally, choosing a dressing that does not adhere to the wound bed can be important to assure that it does not disrupt reepithelialization when it is removed.

Accurately identifying the key cause of wounds is essential in the management of leg ulcers though many wounds are complex and may be of more than one etiology. The following are specific approaches to different leg ulcers.

Venous leg ulcers

Venous insufficiency caused by venous reflux and/or deep venous thrombosis (DVT) is a cause of ambulatory venous hypertension, which leads to venous leg ulcers. The diagnosis of superficial or deep venous abnormality can be with a duplex ultrasound but may also be apparent on clinical examination.

Calf muscle pump function is critical for venous outflow; thus venous ulcer management hinges on good lower limb compression. The use of *compression bandages* for venous leg ulcers has been carefully studied and is the standard care. For prevention, it is recommended that patients wear graduated *compression stockings. Leg elevation and weight reduction* reduce swelling severity.

Arterial ulcers

Ulcers can be caused by chronic limb ischemia, usually the result of peripheral vessel disease. Those with diabetes tend to have involvement of smaller arterioles. Lower limb ischemia causes pain and limb pallor. Arterial circulation can be evaluated non-invasively with ankle brachial index (ABI) and pulse volume recordings (PVR). The PVR may be nondiagnostic in patients with advanced calcification such as those with diabetes. In this setting a duplex ultrasound or computed tomography (CT) angiography is necessary. Treatment including proximal obstructive lesions causing ischemia may require invasive interventions such as *angioplasty* or *arterial bypass grafting*. Patients with poor arterial circulation can develop deep soft tissue infection, osteomyelitis, or gangrene, leading to amputation.

Diabetic neuropathy

Unperceived trauma and/or pressures can lead to wounding and ulcer formation in diabetic neuropathy. A 5.07 Semmes–Weinstein monofilament can be used to test for protective sensation.

Pressure ulcers

Pressure ulcers most often occur in patients with limited mobility, such as bed-ridden elderly patients or those with spine or brain injury, and are most commonly seen in areas bearing weight from sitting or lying over a bony prominence close to the surface of the skin, such as the sacrum or trochanter. Efforts should be aimed at off-loading the affected area.

First-Line Therapies

- Depending on wound etiology (e.g., surgical revascularization, compression therapy, and/or off-loading)
- Debridement of devitalized tissue and antibiotics (often not necessary)
- Wound dressings to maximize the wound environment depending on the wound setting

Evidence Levels: A Double-blind study **B** Clinical trial ≥ 20 subjects **C** Clinical trial < 20 subjects **D** Series ≥ 5 subjects **E** Anecdotal case reports

Chronic venous ulcers: a comparative effectiveness review of treatment modalities. Zenilman J, Valle MF, Malas MB, Maruthur N, Qazi U, Suh Y, et al. Comparative Effectiveness Review No. 127. AHRQ Publication No. 13-EHC121-EF. Rockville, MD: Agency for Healthcare Research and Quality. December 2013.

General evidence-based review on the therapy for venous leg ulcers.

Compression for venous leg ulcers. O'Meara S, Cullum NA, Nelson EA. Cochrane Database Syst Rev 2012; 11: CD000265.

Compression increases ulcer healing rates compared with no compression.

Antibiotics and antiseptics for venous leg ulcers. O'Meara S, Al-Kurdi D, Ologun Y, Ovington LG. Cochrane Database Syst Rev 2010; 1: CD003557.

No evidence supports routine use of systemic antibiotics. However, lack of evidence does not mean that it is ill advised. Recommendations are that antibacterial preparations should only be used in clinical infections.

Compression for preventing recurrence of venous ulcers. Nelson EA, Bell-Syer SEM. Cochrane Database Syst Rev 2015; 9: CD002303.

Evidence from one trial exists that compression hosiery reduces the rate of reulceration among those with venous leg ulcers.

Diabetes, lower extremity amputation and death. Hoffstad O, Mitra N, Walsh J, Margolis DJ. Diabetes Care 2015; 38: 1852–7.

Individuals with diabetes and a lower extremity amputation are nearly three times more likely to die at any given point in time than those with diabetes who do not have an amputation. The cause of death is only partially explained by known complications of diabetes.

Second-Line Therapies

- Ablation of incompetent superficial and perforator veins for venous leg ulcers
- Cell-based therapy (e.g., living or nonviable allographs)
- Device-based therapy (e.g., hyperbaric oxygen, negative pressure therapy, etc.)
- Systemic therapy (e.g., pentoxifylline, etc.)

The impact of ablation of incompetent superficial and perforator veins on ulcer healing rates. Harlander-Locke M, Lawrence PF, Alktaifi A, Jimenez JC, Rigberg D, DeRubertis B. J Vasc Surg 2012; 55: 458–64.

Significant reduction in ulcer size and ultimate healing after ablation of incompetent superficial and perforator veins in patients who have failed conventional compression therapy.

A factorial, randomized trial of pentoxifylline or placebo, four-layer or single-layer compression, and knitted viscose or hydrocolloid dressings for venous ulcers. Nelson EA, Prescott RJ, Harper DR, Gibson B, Brown D, Ruckley CV. J Vasc Surg 2007; 45: 134–41.

Pentoxifylline increased the proportion of healing compared with placebo.

Hyperbaric oxygen therapy for chronic wounds. Kranke P, Bennett MH, Martyn-St James M, Schnabel A, Debus SE. Cochrane Database Syst Rev 2015; 6: CD004123.

Hyperbaric oxygen therapy may improve the healing of diabetic foot ulcers in the short term but not the long term.

Hyperbaric oxygen therapy does not reduce indications for amputation in patients with diabetes with nonhealing ulcers of the lower limb: a prospective, double blinded, randomized controlled clinical trial. Fedorko L, Bowen JM, Jones W, Oreopoulos G, Goeree R, Hopkins RB, et al. Diabetes Care 2016; 39: 392–9.

A randomized clinical trial that did not demonstrate an advantage of hyperbaric oxygen therapy when added to comprehensive wound care for the treatment of a chronic diabetic foot ulcer.

Skin grafting and tissue replacement for treating foot ulcers in people with diabetes. Santema TB, Poyck PPC, Ubbink DT. Cochrane Database Syst Rev 2016; 2: CD011255.

Diabetic foot ulcers may benefit from the use of skin grafts and tissue replacements.

Advanced wound care therapies for nonhealing diabetic, venous and arterial ulcers. Greer N, Foman NA, MacDonald R, Dorrian J, Fitzgerald P, Rutks I, et al. Ann Intern Med 2013; 159: 532–42.

Advanced therapies can improve the likelihood that an individual with a nonhealing wound will heal.

Stem cells in wound healing: the future of regenerative medicine? A minireview. Duscher D, Wond VW, Maan ZN, Whittam AJ, Januszyk M, Gurtner GC. Gerontology 2016; 62: 216–25.

Review describing evidence to date on the use of stem cells for the treatment of chronic wounds and the challenges of conducting studies to show the clinical usefulness of this therapy.

Comparative effectiveness of a bioengineered living cellular construct vs. a dehydrated human amniotic membrane allograft for the treatment of diabetic foot ulcers in a real world setting. Kirsner RS, Sabolinski ML, Parsons NB, Skornicki M, Marston WA. Wound Repair Regen 2015; 23: 737–44.

An electronic medical records database cohort study comparing two advanced therapies. Both therapies appeared to be effective, although the living cellular construct was superior.

The use of human amnion/chorion membrane in the clinical setting of lower extremity repair: a review. Zelen CM, Snyder RJ, Serena TE, Li WW. Clin Podiatr Med Surg 2015; 32: 135–46.

A summary of several studies on the use of amniotic-based products to improve wound outcomes.

Leiomyoma

Nick Collier, Ian Coulson

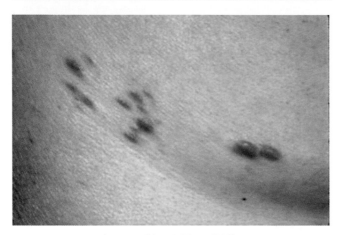

Courtesy of Joseph Bikowski, MD.

Cutaneous leiomyomas are rare benign neoplasms originating from smooth muscle. Three types exist: (1) piloleiomyoma, the most common type, arising from the arrectores pilorum muscle; (2) dartoic myoma, or genital leiomyoma, arising from scrotal/labial dartos muscle or smooth muscle of the nipple; and (3) angioleiomyoma, arising from vascular wall muscle. Piloleiomyomas frequently occur as multiple lesions (80%). Multiple leiomyomas can be inherited in an autosomal dominant fashion in association with uterine leiomyoma (Reed syndrome, *m*ultiple *c*utaneous and *u*terine *l*eiomyomata [MCUL1; OMIM 150800]). Familial multiple leiomyomata can rarely be associated with renal cell cancer (*h*ereditary *l*eiomyomatosis and *r*enal *c*ell *c*ancer [HLRCC; OMIM 605839]). Both familial forms are caused by mutations in the fumarate hydratase gene (coding for an enzyme in the tricarboxylic acid cycle) on 1q42.1, which is hypothesized to act as a tumor suppressor gene through an unknown mechanism. Clinically, cutaneous leiomyomas present as flesh-colored or brownish-red dermal papules or nodules up to 2 cm in diameter, typically distributed on the trunk and extensor surfaces of extremities. They often appear from the second to fourth decade and gradually increase in number and size. Paroxysmal pain, described as stabbing, burning, or pinching, may be triggered by cold or mechanical stimulation and is possibly due to muscle contraction or compression of entrapped nerves. Angioleiomyomas are less frequently symptomatic, whereas genital leiomyomas are asymptomatic.

MANAGEMENT STRATEGY

Symptomatic solitary lesions are best *excised*. Symptomatic multiple leiomyomas are therapeutically challenging because they involve a large area and recur after excision in 50% of cases. Selective excision of larger painful lesions may be considered, provided patients are warned of the relatively high chance of recurrence. *CO₂ laser* ablation of symptomatic lesions may be successful. Other therapeutic methods aim to inhibit smooth muscle contraction, and thus pain, by interfering with local tissue mediators (e.g., norepinephrine, epinephrine, and acetylcholine). There are reports of success with oral *doxazosin* (a selective α_1-blocker)

1 to 4 mg daily, oral *nifedipine* (calcium channel blocker) 10 mg three times daily, *amlodipine* (calcium channel blocker) 5 mg twice daily, *phenoxybenzamine* (nonselective α-blocker) 10 mg twice daily, topical 9% *hyoscine hydrobromide* (anticholinergic), and oral *glyceryl trinitrate* (nitroglycerin) 0.8 to 1.6 mg as needed. Analgesics that target neuropathic pain, for example, oral *gabapentin* 300 mg three times daily and *duloxetine,* have been beneficial. Potential triggers should be avoided. Intralesional injection of *botulinum toxin A* (5 units per cm²) has shown some benefit.

Women, particularly those with a family history, should undergo gynecologic review to exclude possible uterine involvement ("fibroids"). Menorrhagia may necessitate hysterectomy, and leiomyosarcoma, although rare, should be excluded. Potential familial forms require referral to a clinical geneticist with informed consent for mutational analysis of the fumarate hydratase gene. Individuals considered to have HLRCC will require renal ultrasound surveillance to detect the development of renal tumors.

Specific Investigations

- Biopsy
- Biochemical assay of fumarate hydratase – for low/absent activity
- Genetic analysis – for fumarate hydratase gene mutations

Cutaneous smooth muscle neoplasms: clinical features, histologic findings and treatment options. Holst VA, Junkins-Hopkins JM, Elenitas R. J Am Acad Dermatol 2002; 46: 477–90.

A well-referenced review covering leiomyoma and angioleiomyoma. On histologic examination, leiomyomas stained with special stains such as Masson trichrome reveal brick-red smooth muscle fibers. Immunohistochemical techniques demonstrating desmin, smooth muscle actin, or muscle-specific actin confirm tumor origin.

Germline mutations in FH predispose to dominantly inherited uterine fibroids, skin leiomyomata and papillary renal cell cancer. Tomlinson IP, Alam NA, Rowan AJ, Barclay E, Jaeger EE, Kelsell D, et al. Multiple Leiomyoma Consortium. Nature Genet 2002; 30: 406–10.

The authors demonstrate that the gene predisposing to uterine fibroids, cutaneous leiomyoma, and renal cell carcinoma encodes fumarate hydratase. This enzyme acts as a tumor suppressor in familial leiomyomas, and its measured activity in the tumor is very low or absent. Mutations of the fumarate hydratase gene are found in individuals with dominantly inherited susceptibilities to multiple cutaneous and uterine leiomyomatosis and renal cancer.

Evidence for a new fumarate hydratase gene mutation in a unilateral type 2 segmental leiomyomatosis. Parmentier L, Tomlinson I, Happle R, Borradori L. Dermatology 2010; 221: 149–53.

A novel mutation, c.695delG, leading to a truncated protein, p.Gly232AspfsX24, was found.

First-Line Therapy

- Surgical excision   **D**

Evidence Levels: **A** Double-blind study   **B** Clinical trial ≥ 20 subjects   **C** Clinical trial < 20 subjects   **D** Series ≥ 5 subjects   **E** Anecdotal case reports

Leiomyomas of the skin. Fisher WC, Helwig EB. Arch Dermatol 1963; 88: 510–20.

The clinical findings and natural course of 54 cutaneous leiomyomas from 38 patients are described. Surgically excised leiomyomas were found to have a high recurrence rate of 50%.

Second-Line Therapies	
• Doxazosin	E
• Phenoxybenzamine	E
• Topical hyoscine hydrobromide	E
• Nifedipine	E
• Amlodipine	E
• Oral glyceryl trinitrate	E
• Cryotherapy	E
• Simple analgesics	E
• Gabapentin	E
• Duloxetine	E
• Botulinum toxin A	E
• CO_2 laser	E

The rarity of the condition means that most publications on therapy are case reports. The therapeutic agents are not consistently effective.

Successful treatment of pain in two patients with cutaneous leiomyomata with the oral alpha-1 adrenoceptor antagonist, doxazosin. Batchelor RJ, Lyon CC, Highet AS. Br J Dermatol 2004; 150: 775–6.

Two women with symptomatic cutaneous leiomyoma were treated with oral doxazosin 1 to 4 mg daily, a reversible α_1-blocker that, unlike phenoxybenzamine, is selective. Doxazosin was well tolerated, and patients experienced "dramatic improvement"/complete relief of symptoms that was sustained for 6 months in one patient.

Pharmacologic modulation of cold-induced pain in cutaneous leiomyomata. Archer CB, Whittaker S, Greaves MW. Br J Dermatol 1988; 118: 255–60.

Two cases of cutaneous leiomyoma. One patient responded only to phenoxybenzamine 10 mg twice daily, and the other responded to hyoscine hydrobromide (the response lasted only 6 hours). The latter patient also improved with cryotherapy.

Therapy for painful cutaneous leiomyomas. Thompson JA. J Am Acad Dermatol 1985; 13: 865–7.

A 24-year-old man with multiple painful leiomyomas treated successfully with nifedipine 10 mg three times daily for 8 months. The dosage was increased to 10 mg four times daily after the onset of cool weather and increased pain.

Leiomyomatosis cutis et uteri. Engelke H, Christophers E. Acta Derm Venereol 1979; 59: 51–4.

A woman with cutaneous leiomyoma who responded to oral glyceryl trinitrate 0.8 to 1.6 mg for acute attacks, with maintenance nifedipine 20 mg and phenoxybenzamine 60 mg administered during 2 years of follow-up.

Disseminated cutaneous leiomyomatosis treated with oral amlodipine. Aggarwal S, De D, Kanwar AJ, Saikia UN, Khullar G, Mahajan R. Indian J Dermatol Venereol Leprol 2013; 79: 136.

A 32-year-old male with multiple painful cutaneous leiomyomas, who was intolerant of nifedipine due to headaches, experienced significant pain reduction and reduced side effects using amlodipine.

Gabapentin treatment of multiple piloleiomyoma-related pain. Alam M, Rabinowitz AD, Engler DE. J Am Acad Dermatol 2002; 46: S27–9.

A 54-year-old woman with numerous cutaneous leiomyomas who experienced near-complete pain relief with gabapentin 300 mg three times daily introduced gradually.

Successful pain relief of cutaneous leiomyomata due to Reed syndrome with the combination treatment of pregabalin and duloxetine. Kostopanagiotou G, Arvaniti C, Kitsiou MC, Apostolaki S, Chatzimichael K, Matsota P. J Pain Symptom Manage 2009; 38: e3–5.

A combination of pregabalin 600 mg daily and duloxetine 60 mg daily was used successfully to treat a 34-year-old woman with multiple leiomyomas. This produced complete pain relief that was maintained over a 12-month follow-up period.

Efficacy of intralesional botulinum toxin A for treatment of painful cutaneous leiomyomas: a randomized clinical trial. Naik HB, Steinberg SM, Middelton LA, Hewitt SM, Zuo RC, Linehan WM, et al. JAMA Dermatol 2015; 151: 1096–102.

Eighteen participants received either placebo or 5 units per cm^2 of botulinum toxin A. There was a 4-point fall in the skin-related Dermatology Life Quality Index (DLQI). There was a reduction in resting leiomyoma-related pain but not after ice provocation.

Treatment of multiple cutaneous leiomyomas with CO_2 laser ablation. Christenson LJ, Smith K, Arpey CJ. Dermatol Surg 2000; 26: 319–22.

A 73-year-old woman not eligible for pharmacologic therapy who had multiple cutaneous leiomyomas. CO_2 laser ablation of six symptomatic cutaneous leiomyomas induced complete pain relief that was sustained during 9 months of follow-up.

Successful treatment of multiple cutaneous leiomyomas with carbon dioxide laser ablation. Michajłowski I, Błażewicz I, Karpinsky G, Sobjanek M, Nowicki R. Postepy Dermatol Alergol 2015; 32: 480–11.

Leiomyomas over the deltoid were treated with CO_2 laser ablation, with each lesion being treated on four occasions at monthly intervals. The cosmetic result was suboptimal, but pain was greatly diminished.

Leishmaniasis

Suhail M. Hadi, Ali S. Hadi

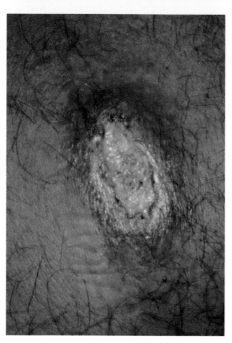

Courtesy of Joseph Bikowski, MD.

Leishmaniasis is a flagellate protozoan disease caused by many species of the genus *Leishmania*. It can be classified into three clinical forms: visceral (kala azar), which is the most severe form; mucocutaneous, which may lead to extensive destruction of the mucous membranes; and cutaneous (Old and New World), which affects mainly exposed parts of the body, causing ulcers and eventually scarring.

Generalized and mucosal leishmaniasis may be seen in patients with human immunodeficiency virus (HIV) infection and acquired immune deficiency syndrome (AIDS). Subclinical forms of the disease do exist. Leishmaniasis is transmitted mainly by the bite of the infected female phlebotomine sandfly. However, other possible routes of transmission exist, including transfusion, needle sharing, congenital, sexual, and person-to-person contact. Only the management of cutaneous leishmaniasis (CL) will be addressed here.

Many faces of cutaneous leishmaniasis. Bari AU, Rahman SB. Indian J Dermatol Venereol Leprol 2008; 74: 23–7.

A total of 718 patients with CL were analyzed; 5.7% had unusual presentations. The most common of these presentations was lupoid leishmaniasis.

Cutaneous leishmaniasis mimicking inflammatory and neoplastic processes: a clinical, histopathological and molecular study of 57 cases. Saab J, Fedda F, Khattab R, Yahya L, Loya A, Satti M, et al. J Cutan Pathol 2012; 39: 251–62.

Skin biopsies from 145 patients were studied; 125 were confirmed as CL by polymerase chain reaction (PCR). Eighteen cases presented with a prebiopsy clinical diagnosis that ranged from dermatitis to neoplasm. Of the 125 cases, 57 showed a histopathologic pattern other than CL.

MANAGEMENT STRATEGY

CL presents with a typical lesion and a history of exposure. A skin scraping for microscopic analysis is the simplest test. Cultures from an exudate or scraping show good results. PCR offers a rapid, highly sensitive, and specific modality of diagnosis. Serologic tests can be used and include the indirect immunofluorescent antibody test, direct agglutination test, fast agglutination screening test, and enzyme-linked immunosorbent assay (ELISA).

A new vaccine has been recently studied for its protection against CL. Results showed durable protective immunity. It has the advantages of being inexpensive and administered by a non-invasive nasal route.

Pentavalent antimonials are the first-line therapy. *Meglumine antimoniate* is the drug of choice. It can be given intralesionally with local anesthetic (particularly in children, because of pain) or systemically 10 mg/kg daily for 2 weeks. *Leishmania recidivans* requires higher doses for longer periods. *Sodium stibogluconate* can be infiltrated into individual lesions 1 to 2 mL/week. In widespread severe cases it can be given intramuscularly or intravenously in a dose of 10 mg/kg/day for 2 weeks.

Pentavalent antimoniate use is complicated by a high rate of side effects, including arthralgia; fatigue; gastrointestinal (GI) upset; elevation of amylase, lipase, and liver enzyme levels; leukopenia; anemia; and electrocardiogram (ECG) abnormalities. Side effects appear to be dose related and are more common in patients with renal and liver impairment and those with cardiac arrhythmias. *Amphotericin B* has been used in antimony-resistant cases.

Pentamidine isethionate (aromatic diamidine) is effective for diffuse CL. Side effects of pentamidine include hypoglycemia, diabetes mellitus, hypotension (if administered too rapidly), GI upset, and headache.

Allopurinol has antileishmanial activity, and other oral drugs such as miltefosine, zinc sulfate, rifampin, doxycycline, and azoles are also beneficial. γ-Interferon was shown to be effective as monotherapy treatment. Topical preparations such as *paromomycin* ointment and 5% *imiquimod* show considerable therapeutic potential.

Good cure rates have been achieved with both thermotherapy and cryotherapy. Lasers have been used, but further studies are needed to support their benefit. Additional treatment modalities are presented next.

Specific Investigations

- Skin biopsy
- Fine needle aspiration
- Slit-skin smear, press imprint smear
- Culture
- Leishmanin (Montenegro) skin test
- Serology
- Polymerase chain reaction (PCR) for leishmanial deoxyribonucleic acid (DNA)

The margin of the lesion contains amastigotes, whereas the center has dead skin and debris. Accordingly, the margin is preferred when performing a slit-skin smear. The aspirate can then be sent for culture or histology, which shows Leishman–Donovan bodies inside macrophages using Giemsa stain.

The gold-standard medium for culture is Novy–MacNeal–Nicolle, with positive results in 1 to 3 weeks, or Schneider *Drosophila* medium, which gives positive results in 1 week.

Evidence Levels: **A** Double-blind study **B** Clinical trial ≥ 20 subjects **C** Clinical trial < 20 subjects **D** Series ≥ 5 subjects **E** Anecdotal case reports

Microculture is a new culture medium that has higher carbon dioxide concentrations and lower oxygen and pH, which encourages more rapid amastigote to promastigote differentiation. Culture is not a reliable method in older lesions, as the organisms become scarce and difficult to isolate.

Serologic tests aim to detect the presence of antibodies against *Leishmania*. They are particularly valuable in visceral and mucocutaneous leishmaniasis.

PCR is a sensitive and powerful method of diagnosis of CL. Recently it was found that important genes involved in the innate immune response to *Leishmania* are downregulated in natural killer (NK) cells from patients with diffuse CL, particularly toll-like receptors (TLRs) and janus kinase/signal transducer and activator of transcription (JAK/STAT) signaling pathways.

Comparison of molecular, microscopic, and culture methods for diagnosis of cutaneous leishmaniasis. Rasti S, Ghorbanzadeh B, Kheirandish F, Mousavi SG, Pirozmand A, Hooshyar H, et al. J Clin Lab Anal 2016; 30: 610–5.

One hundred thirty patients were tested, and 66.9%, 56.2%, 75.4%, 73.8%, and 76.2% were positive for microscopic culture, PCR, nested PCR, and combined PCR and microscopy (proposed method), respectively. Sensitivity, specificity, and positive and negative predictive values of PCR were 99%, 100%, 100%, and 96.9%, respectively, for microscopy; 87.9%, 100%, 100%, and 72.1%, for culture; 72.7%, 100%, 100%, and 53.4%; and 97%, 100%, 100%, and 91.2% for nested PCR. kDNA-PCR was the most sensitive method for diagnosis of CL.

Molecular detection of *Leishmania* spp. isolated from cutaneous lesions of patients referred to Herat Regional Hospital, Afghanistan. Mosawi SH, Dalimi A. East Mediterr Health J 2016; 21: 878–84.

Light microscopy examination was positive in 58%, whereas PCR was positive in 78% of cases.

Press imprint smear: a rapid, simple, and cheap method for the diagnosis of cutaneous leishmaniasis caused by *Leishmania (Viannia) braziliensis*. Sousa AQ, Pompeu MM, Frutuoso MS, Lima JW, Tinel JM, Pearson RD. Am J Trop Med Hyg 2014; 91: 905–7.

Amastigotes were seen in 92% of 75 patients. The press imprint smear was positive in 85.3%, and histopathology was positive in 44%. It is a rapid and relatively sensitive method for the diagnosis of CL.

Performance of an ELISA and indirect immunofluorescence assay in serologic diagnosis of zoonotic cutaneous leishmaniasis in Iran. Sarkari B, Ashrafmansori M, Hatam G, Habibi P, Abdolahi Khabisi S. Interdiscip Perspect Infect Dis 2014; 505: 134.

Sixty-one sera from parasitologically confirmed CL patients and 50 sera from healthy controls, along with 50 sera from non-CL patients, were studied. Indirect fluorescent antibody (IFA) was used to detect anti-*Leishmania* IgG, ELISA was used to detect anti-*Leishmania* IgM, total IgG, or IgG 1 and IgG4. Sensitivity and specificity of IFA were 91.6% and 81%, respectively. ELISA showed reasonable sensitivity and specificity. Serologic tests can be used for proper diagnosis of CL.

Down-regulation of TLR and JAK/STAT pathway genes is associated with diffuse cutaneous leishmaniasis: a gene expression analysis in NK cells from patients infected with *Leishmania mexicana*. Fernández-Figueroa EA, Imaz-Rosshandler I, Castillo-Fernández JE, Miranda- Ortíz H, Fernández- López JC, Becker I, et al. PLoS Negl Trop Dis March 31, 2016; 10: e0004570.

First-Line Therapies

Pentavalent antimonials

• Meglumine antimoniate	B
• Sodium stibogluconate antimony	B

Clinical features, epidemiology, and efficacy and safety of intralesional antimony treatment of cutaneous leishmaniasis: recent experience in Turkey. Uzun S, Durdu M, Culha G, Allahverdiyev AM, Memisoglu HR. J Parasitol 2004; 90: 853–9.

Intralesional meglumine antimoniate was given as first-line therapy for 890 patients with CL. A weekly dose of 0.2 to 1 mL was given for up to 20 weeks or until complete cure. It was found to have an efficacy of 97.2%, with a low relapse rate (3.9%) and no serious side effects.

Clinical efficacy of intramuscular meglumine antimoniate alone and in combination with intralesional meglumine antimoniate in the treatment of Old World cutaneous leishmaniasis. Munir A, Janjua SA, Hussain I. Acta Dermatovenerol Croat 2008; 16: 60–4.

Sixty patients were studied. A combination of intramuscular meglumine antimoniate 20 mg/kg/day plus intralesional meglumine antimoniate 0.5 mL daily for 21 days was superior to intralesional treatment alone, with 75% complete cure for the former.

Intralesional antimony for single lesions of Bolivian cutaneous leishmaniasis. Soto J, Rojas E, Guzman M, Verduguez A, Nena W, Maldonado M, et al. Clin Infect Dis 2013; 56: 1255–60.

A randomized, open-label trial of 80 patients in Bolivia divided patients into three groups, one receiving either intralesional antimony, cryotherapy, or placebo. At 6 months the cure rate was 70% for the antimony, 20% for cryotherapy group, and 17% for placebo.

Second-Line Therapies

• Pentamidine isethionate	B
• Rifampin	A
• Azoles	B, A
• Cryotherapy	A, B
• Thermotherapy	B
• Hypertonic sodium chloride	A

Recurrent American cutaneous leishmaniasis. Gangneux JP, Sauzet S, Donnard S, Meyer N, Cornillet A, Pratlong F, et al. Emerg Infect Dis 2007; 13: 1436–8.

Twenty-one patients with recurrent CL were enrolled. Intravenous or intramuscular pentamidine isethionate (4 mg/kg) on alternate days cured the lesions within 1 to 3 months.

The role of rifampicin in the management of cutaneous leishmaniasis. Kochar DK, Aseri S, Sharma BV, Bumb RA, Mehta RD, Purohit SK. Q J Med 2000; 93: 733–7.

Sixty-four patients were enrolled: 32 received rifampin 600 mg twice daily for 4 weeks, and 32 received placebo. Of the rifampin group, 73.9% had complete healing of their lesions, compared with 4.3% of the placebo group. Rifampin is suitable for multiple lesions and is well tolerated.

Fluconazole for the treatment of cutaneous leishmaniasis caused by Leishmania major. Alrajhi AA, Ibrahim EA, De Vol EB, Khairat M, Faris RM, Maguire JH. N Engl J Med 2002; 346: 891–5.

Patients (n = 106) received fluconazole 200 mg daily, and 103 received placebo for 6 weeks. Healing was complete in 79% of the fluconazole group and 34% of the placebo group at 3 months, follow-up.

Comparison of oral itraconazole and intramuscular meglumine antimoniate in the treatment of cutaneous leishmaniasis. Saleem K, Rahman A. J Coll Phys Surg Pak 2007; 17: 713–6.

Two hundred patients with wet and dry CL were studied. Itraconazole (100 mg twice daily for 6–8 weeks) was superior to meglumine antimoniate in achieving complete clinical and parasitologic cure (75% compared with 65%), with fewer side effects.

Intralesional sodium stibogluconate alone or its combination with either intramuscular sodium stibogluconate or oral ketoconazole in the treatment of localized cutaneous leishmaniasis: a comparative study. El-Sayed M, Anwar AE. J Eur Acad Dermatol Venereol 2010; 24: 335–40.

Ten patients were treated with intralesional sodium stibogluconate (SSG) alone (group 1). Ten patients were treated with the combination of intralesional SSG + intramuscular SSG (group 2). Ten patients were treated with the combination of intralesional SSG and oral ketoconazole (group 3). Treatment period was 12 weeks. Cure rate was 58.3% in group 1, 93.3% in group 2, and 92.3% in group 3. Combination of oral ketoconazole with intralesional SSG is more effective than intralesional SSG alone.

Efficacy of a weekly cryotherapy regimen to treat Leishmania major cutaneous leishmaniasis. Mosleh IM, Geith E, Natsheh L, Schönian G, Abotteen N, Kharabsheh S. J Am Acad Dermatol 2008; 58: 617–24.

Patients (n = 120) were treated with cryotherapy once weekly over one to seven sessions; 84% of lesions were cured after one to four sessions. The side effects were minimal.

Evaluation of thermotherapy for the treatment of cutaneous leishmaniasis in Kabul, Afghanistan: a randomized controlled trial. Case AJ, Safi N, Davis GD, Nadir M, Hamid H, Robert LL Jr. Mil Med 2012; 177: 345–51.

Patients (n = 382) with CL were randomly assigned to two treatment groups and followed for 6 months. The cure rate for the thermotherapy group was 82.5%, compared with 74% in the glucantime group. A single localized treatment with thermotherapy was more effective than 5 days of intralesional glucantime. Also, thermotherapy was cost effective, with fewer side effects, and better patient compliance than intralesional glucantime.

Thermotherapy effective and safer than miltefosine in the treatment of cutaneous leishmaniasis in Colombia. López L, Cruz C, Godoy G, Robledo SM, Vélez ID. Rev Inst Med Trop Sao Paulo 2013; 55: 197–204.

In an open-label trial, one group received oral miltefosine 50 mg daily for 28 days, and the other group received thermotherapy of 50°C on the lesion and perilesional area. There was no statistically significant difference in efficacy between the two groups, but the miltefosine group experienced GI discomfort.

Randomized, double-blind, controlled, comparative study on intralesional 10% and 15% hypertonic saline versus intralesional sodium stibogluconate in Leishmania donovani cutaneous leishmaniasis. Ranawaka RR, Weerakoon HS, de Silva SH. Int J Dermatol 2015; 54: 555–63.

This was a randomized, double-blind, controlled study of 10% and 15% hypertonic saline injections compared with that of sodium stibogluconate. Four hundred forty-four patients were studied and followed for 18 months. All three groups had cure rates above 90%. The 15% hypertonic saline group showed cutaneous necrosis in 30.6% of lesions, compared with 3.1% of lesions in the 10% hypertonic group. Ten percent hypertonic saline can be considered an alternative to SSG.

Third-Line Therapies	
Miltefosine (hexadecylphosphocholine)	A, B
Imiquimod 5%	D
Paromomycin ointment	B
Photodynamic therapy	B
Direct current electrotherapy	D
CO_2 laser	B
Intralesional zinc sulfate	A
Pentoxifylline	B
Amphotericin	C
Trichloroacetic acid	B
Radiofrequency heat therapy	B
Immunization	A

Miltefosine in the treatment of cutaneous leishmaniasis caused by Leishmania braziliensis in Brazil: a randomized and controlled trial. Machado PR, Ampuero J, Guimarães LH, Villasboas L, Rocha AT, Schriefer A, et al. PLoS Negl Trop Dis 2010; 21: e912.

Ninety patients were enrolled; 60 received miltefosine orally and 30 received pentavalent antimony. Six months later, the cure rate was 53.3% in the pentavalent antimony group and 75% in the miltefosine group. Apoptosis-like death of Leishmania donovani may be a possible explanation of the mode of action of miltefosine.

Role of imiquimod and parenteral meglumine antimoniate in the initial treatment of cutaneous leishmaniasis. Arevalo I, Tulliano G, Quispe A, Spaeth G, Matlashewski G, Llanos-Cuentas A, et al. Clin Infect Dis 2007; 44: 1549–54.

Combination treatment with imiquimod and meglumine antimoniate gave superior results, with rapid healing and better cosmetic outcome. Imiquimod kills the intracellular Leishmania amastigotes in vitro by activating macrophages to release nitric oxide.

Topical paromomycin with or without gentamicin for cutaneous leishmaniasis. Ben Salah A, Ben Messaoud N, Guedri E, Zaatour A, Ben Alaya N, Bettaieb J, et al. N Engl J Med 2013; 368: 524–32.

A randomized, controlled study of 375 patients using topical paromomycin with and without gentamicin for ulcerative CL. Three groups received 15% topical paromomycin and 0.5% gentamicin, paromomycin alone, or control. Treatment continued for 20 days; cure rates were 81%, 82%, and 58% for the paromomycin–gentamicin, paromomycin, and control groups, respectively.

Comparison between the efficacy of photodynamic therapy and topical paromomycin in the treatment of Old World cutaneous leishmaniasis: a placebo-controlled, randomized clinical trial. Asilian A, Davami M. Clin Exp Dermatol 2006; 31: 634–7.

Evidence Levels: **A** Double-blind study **B** Clinical trial ≥ 20 subjects **C** Clinical trial < 20 subjects **D** Series ≥ 5 subjects **E** Anecdotal case reports

This study compared the parasitologic and clinical efficacy of photodynamic therapy (PDT) and topical paromomycin in 60 patients. Topical PDT was given weekly for 4 weeks. Complete improvement was seen in 93.5% of patients treated with topical PDT versus 41.2% in the topical paromomycin group.

The parasiticidal effect of electricity on *Leishmania major*, both in vitro and in vivo. Hejazi H, Eslami G, Dalimi A. Ann Trop Med Parasitol 2004; 98: 37–42.

Exposure to direct current of 3, 6, 9, and 12 V (at 0.2–10.7 mA) killed all promastigotes (in culture) within 10 to 15 minutes. Three weeks of electrotherapy at 3 V for 10 minutes twice weekly appeared to cure all the lesions in mice.

Efficacy of CO_2 laser for treatment of anthroponotic cutaneous leishmaniasis, compared with combination of cryotherapy and intralesional meglumine antimoniate. Shamsi Meymandi S, Zandi S, Aghaie H, Heshmatkhah A. J Eur Acad Dermatol Venereol 2011; 25: 587–91.

Single treatment session of CO_2 laser was more effective in treating dry-type CL than combined cryotherapy and intralesional glucantime with a shorter healing time (6 weeks vs. 12 weeks).

Comparison of intralesionally injected zinc sulfate with meglumine antimoniate in the treatment of acute cutaneous leishmaniasis. Iraji F, Vali A, Asilian A, Shahtalebi MA, Momeni AZ. Dermatology 2004; 209: 46–9.

A total of 104 patients with acute cutaneous leishmaniasis (ACL) were studied. The duration of treatment was 6 weeks. Thirty-five patients received meglumine antimoniate, and 31 received intralesional zinc sulfate. Cure rates were 60% for meglumine antimoniate and 83.8% for zinc sulfate. Intralesional injection of 2% zinc sulfate is a good alternative for the treatment of ACL.

Clinical and immunologic outcome in cutaneous leishmaniasis patients treated with pentoxifylline. Brito G, Dourado M, Polari L, Celestino D, Carvalho LP, Queiroz A, et al. Am J Trop Med Hyg 2014; 90: 617–20.

Thirty-six patients with CL were studied. One group received intralesional antimony along with pentoxifylline, and the other received antimony with placebo. The pentoxifylline group showed a decrease in tumor necrosis factor-alpha (TNF-α) and interferon-gamma levels compared with the placebo group. Cure rate was higher in the pentoxifylline group, but not statistically significant. Pentoxifylline has an antiinflammatory effect.

Liposomal amphotericin B treatment of cutaneous leishmaniasis due to *Leishmania tropica*. Solomon M, Pavlotsky F, Leshem E, Ephros M, Trau H, Schwartz E. J Eur Acad Dermatol Venereol 2011; 25: 973–7.

Thirteen patients received liposomal amphotericin B (5 consecutive days of 3 mg/kg, followed by a sixth dose on day 10); 85% had facial lesions. Eleven of 13 patients (84%) achieved complete clinical cure within 2 months. There were no reported relapses after 11 months, and the side effects were mild.

The efficacy of 5% trichloroacetic acid cream in the treatment of cutaneous leishmaniasis lesions. Ali NM, Fariba J, Elaheh H, Ali N. J Dermatolog Treat 2012; 23: 136–9.

Sixteen patients with CL were treated with 5% trichloroacetic acid cream twice daily for 8 weeks. Mean area of the lesions was $38.81 + 81.9$ mm^2. After 6 months, it was $3.6 + 9.1$ mm^2. All patients were cured by week 8. No side effects.

Long-term efficacy of single-dose radiofrequency-induced heat therapy vs. intralesional antimonials for cutaneous leishmaniasis in India: RFHT for cutaneous leishmaniasis. Bumb RA, Prasad N, Khandelwal K, Aara N, Mehta RD, Ghiya BC, et al. Br J Dermatol 2013; 168: 1114–9.

One hundred patients with CL were studied. Fifty patients received one treatment of radiofrequency-induced heat therapy (RFHT); the other 50 received intralesional SSG injections. Follow-up was for 18 months. After 6 months, the cure rate was 98% in the RFHT group and 95% in the SSG group. No relapse in any patient.

Cluster randomised trial to evaluate the effectiveness of a vaccine against cutaneous leishmaniasis in the Caratinga microregion, south-east Brazil. Mayrink W, Mendonca-Mendes A, de Paula JC, Siqueira LM, Marrocos Sde R, Dias ES, et al. Trans R Soc Trop Med Hyg 2013; 107: 212–9.

A randomized trial of 8734 patients in a Brazilian area with a high frequency of CL were given a killed vaccine from 2002 to 2011. They showed a significantly lower number of individuals infected with CL in the vaccine group compared with the placebo group.

Lentigo maligna

Aaron S. Farberg, Darrell S. Rigel

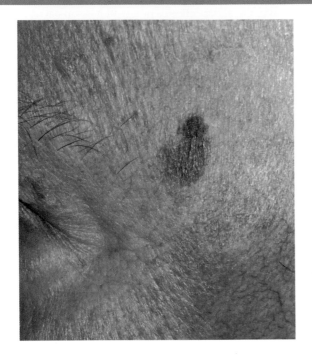

Lentigo maligna (LM) is a subtype of preinvasive intraepidermal melanoma that classically presents as widespread pigmented patches of atypical melanocytes in the background of long-standing sun damage. The lifetime risk of LM progressing to invasive lentigo malignant melanoma (LMM) varies from 2.2% to 4.7%, depending on patient age at diagnosis. LMM represents 4% to 15% of all melanomas, and its incidence is increasing at a greater rate than any other melanoma subtype. The widespread atypical melanocytes often originate on the head or neck and spread slowly. LM has traditionally been challenging to diagnose because it is difficult to distinguish nonmalignant atypical melanocytic hyperplasia from melanoma in situ (MIS) in chronically sun-damaged skin. Treatment of LM remains complex, with recurrence rates that remain high (2%–50%) due to subclinical extension and difficulty of determining tumor margins.

MANAGEMENT STRATEGY

Successful management of LM depends on early diagnosis and definitive removal. The differential diagnosis includes solar lentigo, macular seborrheic keratosis, pigmented actinic keratosis, pigmented squamous cell carcinoma in situ, and pigmented superficial basal cell carcinoma. Confirmatory biopsy is necessary before definitive treatment. The use of a Wood lamp may help to determine the perimeter of the lesion. Dermoscopy may also be helpful. Excisional biopsy of the entire lesion is ideal in order to ascertain its maximum depth. However, the lesion tends to be large (>1 cm) due to its propensity for extensive radial growth before vertical growth into the dermis. Therefore biopsy of part of the lesion is often performed. Treatment is primarily surgical, although eradication by other methods may be considered.

Patients with a history of LM should have periodic full-body skin examinations by a dermatologist to allow for early detection of recurrence, progression, or a second primary skin cancer. Patients with LM also require a consultation about sun protection behaviors.

Specific Investigation

- Skin biopsy and patient evaluation

Diagnosis and treatment of early melanoma. NIH Consensus Statement. 1992; 10: 1–26.

Biopsy of sufficient depth is critical for diagnosis and management of pigmented lesions. Punch, saucerization, excision, or incisional biopsy may be acceptable. On microscopic examination LM is characterized by increased numbers of atypical melanocytes at the epidermal-dermal junction, which may be solitary or arranged in nests but do not invade the dermis. Evaluation should include a personal and family history, complete skin examination, and palpation of regional lymph nodes. Blood tests or imaging studies are not indicated.

First-Line Therapies

• Excision	A
• Mohs micrographic surgery	D
• Modified Mohs surgery	D
• Staged excision	D

Diagnosis and treatment of early melanoma. NIH Consensus Statement. 1992; 10: 1–26.

Current recommendations are based on the National Institutes of Health (NIH) consensus for MIS, which suggests excision of the lesion or biopsy site with a margin of 0.5 cm of clinically normal skin and layer of subcutaneous tissue. In general, margins of 0.5 to 1.0 cm are suggested for LM where feasible. Difficulties may arise in determination of clinical margins due to diffuse background sun damage. A Wood lamp may be useful in defining subclinical extension. Reflectance confocal microscopy (RCM) may also improve diagnostic accuracy of LM by identifying optimal biopsy sites. RCM may assist in presurgical mapping, intraoperative margin assessment, assessing response to nonsurgical therapies, and monitoring for recurrence. Accurate determination of margins is key because LM is likely to recur after inadequate excision.

Usefulness of the staged excision for lentigo maligna and lentigo maligna melanoma: the "square" procedure. Johnson TM, Headington JT, Baker SR, Lowe L. J Am Acad Dermatol 1997; 37: 758–64.

With this technique, a margin of 0.5 to 1.0 cm is outlined with angled corners to facilitate processing. A peripheral strip of tissue 2 to 4 cm wide is excised and processed for evaluation of permanent sections. Residual tumor is subsequently excised in a directed fashion based on mapping. There were no recurrences in 35 patients at 2 years.

Mohs micrographic surgery is accurate 95.1% of the time for melanoma in situ: a prospective study of 167 cases. Bene NI, Healy C, Coldiron BM. Dermatol Surg 2008; 34: 660–4.

Evidence Levels:　**A** Double-blind study　**B** Clinical trial ≥ 20 subjects　**C** Clinical trial < 20 subjects　**D** Series ≥ 5 subjects　**E** Anecdotal case reports

Patients (*n* = 116) with MIS in sun-exposed skin of LMM type were treated by Mohs micrographic surgery (MMS) with subsequent evaluation of the final margin with paraffin-embedded sections that were cut en face over a period of 12 years (mean follow-up, 50 months; median 48 months; 594.5 patient-years). The clearance rate by MMS technique using frozen sections was 94.1% for the MIS LM type. The cure rate was 99.0% for the MIS LM type.

MMS is a viable option for treatment of MIS that may increase cure rate and reduce the size of the defect, especially in cosmetically and functionally sensitive areas.

Conventional surgery compared with slow Mohs micrographic surgery in the treatment of lentigo maligna: a retrospective study of 62 cases. Hilari H, Llorca D, Traves V, Villanueva A, Serra-Guillén C, Requena C, et al. Actas Dermosifiliogr 2012; 103: 614–23.

A review of the clinical records of patients with LM of the head treated definitively with conventional surgical excision or slow MMS at the dermatology department of Instituto Valenciano de Oncología between January 1993 and April 2011 was reported. Surgical margins larger than 0.5 cm were required in 69.2% of recurrent LM and 26.5% of primary LM. Factors associated with the need for wider margins were prior treatment that might have interfered with the clinical delineation of the border, lesions in the center of the face, and skin phototypes III to V. Surgical margins of 0.5 cm are inadequate for the treatment of a considerable number of LM lesions located on the head, particularly if these are recurrent. Slow MMS using paraffin-embedded sections appears to be the treatment of choice in such cases, particularly for recurrent lesions or lesions with poorly defined borders or possible subclinical extension.

A potential disadvantage of relying on "slow Mohs" is the amount of time added to each procedure. In addition, the technique depends on off-site tissue processing and interpretation, thereby magnifying the possibility of error.

Recurrence rate of lentigo maligna after micrographically controlled staged surgical excision. De Vries K, Greveling K, Prens LM, Munte K, Koljenovic, van Doorn MBA, et al. Br J Dermatol 2016; 174: 588–93.

This is a retrospective review of records of all patients at an academic medical center in the Netherlands diagnosed with LM treated with staged surgical excision between 2002 and 2011. Recurrences were identified through the nationwide network registry with a 5-year mean follow-up. Of 100 patients identified, 4 had a recurrence. Staged surgical excision may provide a high clearance and low recurrence rate.

Five-year outcomes of wide excision and Mohs micrographic surgery for primary lentigo maligna in an academic practice cohort. Hou JL, Reed KB, Knudson RM, Mirzoyev SA, Lohse CM, Frohm ML, et al. Dermatol Surg 2015; 41: 211–8.

This retrospective study evaluated the outcomes of MMS versus wide excision with 5-mm margins in a cohort from a single academic practice. Four hundred twenty-three LM lesions were treated with either wide excision (269) or Mohs (154). Recurrence rates were 1.9% for the Mohs-treated group and 5.9% for the wide excision group. The study concluded Mohs surgery may offer increased cure rates and avoid the need for repeat surgery and thus may be the preferred treatment for LM.

Geometric staged excision for the treatment of lentigo maligna and lentigo maligna melanoma: a long-term experience with literature review. Abdelmalek M, Loosemore MP, Hurt MA, Hruza G. Arch Dermatol 2012; 148: 599–604.

All patients with a diagnosis of LM and LMM were treated by staged excision from 1999 to 2007. The rate of recurrence after geometric staged excision was 1.7% (4 of 239), with a mean of 32.3 months of follow-up. The mean margin to clearance after excision was 6.6 mm for LM and 8.2 mm for LMM. A total of 11.7% of LMM was initially diagnosed as LM on biopsy, with the invasive component discovered during the excision.

Staged excision for lentigo maligna and lentigo maligna melanoma: a retrospective analysis of 117 cases. Hazan C, Dusza SW, Delgado R, Busam KJ, Halpern AC, Nehal KS. J Am Acad Dermatol 2008; 58: 142–8.

The authors conducted a retrospective study of 117 LM and LMM cases treated with a staged margin-controlled excision technique with rush paraffin-embedded sections. The mean total surgical margin required for excision of LM was 0.71 cm and was 1.03 cm for LMM. The study concluded that the standard excision margins for LM and LMM are often inadequate, and occult invasive melanoma occurs in LM.

Intraoperative real-time reflectance confocal microscopy for guiding surgical margins of lentigo maligna melanoma. Hibler BP, Cordova M, Wong RJ, Rossi AM. Dermatol Surg 2015; 41: 980–3.

This case study demonstrates the utility of RCM in augmenting the management of LM. It may be used to guide surgical management to verify surgical margins to decrease patient morbidity. Initial cost and the associated learning curve are limitations to widespread use of the technology.

Videodermatoscopy-assisted Mohs micrographic surgery vs. other treatments for lentigo maligna in 54 patients with a long-term follow-up. Dika E, Fanti PA, Christman H, Piraccini BM, Misciali C, Vaccari S, et al. J Eur Acad Dermatol Venereol 2016; 30: 1440–1.

This retrospective single-center study included patients with LM on the head and neck referred for surgical excision with at least 5 years of follow-up. Videodermatoscopy-assisted MMS was used to evaluate all margins, and additional excision was performed where positive for frozen sections. Patients were divided into three groups: standard excision, MMS, and videodermatoscopy-assisted MMS. Videodermatoscopy-assisted MMS reduced the number of steps and overall timing of the surgical procedure. Recurrence was 24% for standard excision, 5% of MMS, and 0% in the videodermatoscopy-assisted MMS group.

AAD/ACMS/ASDSA/ASMS 2012 appropriate use criteria for Mohs micrographic surgery: a report of the American Academy of Dermatology, American College of Mohs Surgery, American Society for Dermatologic Surgery Association, and the American Society for Mohs Surgery. Connolly SM , Baker DR, Coldiron BM, Fazio MJ, Storrs PA, Vidimos AT, et al. J Am Acad Dermatol 2012; 67: 531–50.

Of all the clinical scenarios for LM as determined by this consortium, five were deemed appropriate for Mohs surgery, one uncertain, and zero inappropriate with consensus reached for all scenarios. MMS was deemed appropriate for primary LM in areas H and M (face, genitalia, hands, feet, nails, pretibial surface, ankles, areolae) for healthy and immunocompromised patients. Locally recurrent LM was rated appropriate for MMS in all body locations for both healthy and immunocompromised patients. The use of MMS for primary LM in healthy or immunocompromised patients was determined to be uncertain when located on area L (trunk and extremities excluding pretibial, hands, feet, nails, ankles).

Radiotherapy for lentigo maligna: a literature review and recommendations for treatment. Fogarty GB, Scolyer RA, Lin E, Haydu L, Guitera P, Thompson J. Br J Dermatol 2013; 170: 52–8.

Nine studies described 537 patients with LM treated with definitive primary radiotherapy. There was a 5% recurrence rate of 349 assessable patients. Salvage was successful in most recurrent cases. Progression to LMM occurred in 5 patients. Marginal and in-field recurrence rates were 4% and 5%, respectively. Median study follow-up was 3 years.

Grenz ray treatment of lentigo maligna and early lentigo maligna melanoma. Hedblad MA, Mallbris L. J Am Acad Dermatol 2012; 67: 60–8.

Patients ($n = 593$) were treated with Grenz rays (GR) (primary therapy, $n = 350$; partial excision followed by GR, $n = 71$; radical excision followed by GR as recurrence-prophylactic treatment, $n = 172$) at the Department of Dermatology, Karolinska University Hospital, Stockholm, Sweden, between 1990 and 2009. The treatment was given twice a week over 3 consecutive weeks in total doses of 100 to 160 Gy. Dosage depended on the stage of LM and the depth of periadnexal atypical melanocytic extension in histologically examined materials before treatment. Four hundred twenty-five patients have been followed up for at least 2 years and, of these, 241 for 5 years. Overall, 520 of 593 patients (88%) showed complete clearance after one fractionated treatment. Residual lesions were seen in 15 patients, and 58 relapsed, 53 of whom (72%) within 2 years.

One of the advantages of this soft x-ray or Miescher technique is exclusion of underlying bone and minimization of risk of bony necrosis. The potential disadvantage is inadequate depth of penetration.

Cryosurgery for lentigo maligna. Kuflik E, Gage A. J Am Acad Dermatol 1994; 31: 75–8.

Thirty white patients were treated with cryosurgery. The lesions ranged from 1.3 to 4.5 cm in diameter. Treatment consisted of freezing with liquid nitrogen delivered by open spray. Lesions recurred in two patients, yielding a recurrence rate of 6.6% during the average follow-up period of 3 years. The two recurrent lesions were successfully retreated with cryosurgery. Eleven patients observed for more than 5 years showed no recurrence.

Q-switched neodymium:yttrium-aluminum-garnet laser treatment of lentigo maligna. Orten SS, Waner M, Dinehart SM, Bardales RH, Flock ST. Otolaryngol Head Neck Surg 1999; 120: 296–302.

Eight patients with LM were treated with the neodymium-doped yttrium aluminium garnet laser. Three patients were treated with both 532 and 1064 nm. Two of these had complete eradication without recurrence at 3.5 years. The other showed a partial response but died of unrelated causes before completion of therapy.

The Nd:YAG laser emits energy at 532 nm and 1064 nm, which may be especially suited to LM. Melanin has greater absorption at 532 nm, whereas the longer wavelength, 1064 nm, may provide deeper penetration.

Carbon dioxide laser treatment for lentigo maligna: a retrospective review comparing 3 different treatment modalities. Lee H, Sowerby LJ, Temple CL, Yu E, Moore CC. Arch Facial Plast Surg 2011; 13: 398–403.

Seventy-three patients aged 39 to 93 years (mean age, 64.8 years) were included in the study. Twenty-seven patients were treated with surgical excision, 31 patients with radiation therapy, and 15 patients with CO$_2$ laser ablation. The median follow-up times were 16.6 months for surgical excision, 46.3 months for radiation therapy, and 77.8 months for CO$_2$ laser ablation ($p < 0.001$). Recurrence rates by treatment modality were 4.2% (1 of 27) for surgical excision, 29.0% (9 of 31) for radiation therapy, and 6.7% (1 of 15) for CO$_2$ laser ablation. A trend toward lower recurrence rates with surgical excision and CO$_2$ laser ablation was identified, but the results were not statistically significant.

CO$_2$ laser ablation may have a role as an alternative treatment for lentigo maligna among patients in whom standard treatments, such as surgical excision and radiation therapy, are declined or carry significant morbidity.

Intralesional interferon treatment of lentigo maligna. Cornejo P, Vanaclocha F, Polimon I, Del Rio R. Arch Dermatol 2000; 136: 428–30.

Interferon-α is a biological response modifier indicated for adjunctive treatment of high-risk melanoma. The mechanism involves both immunomodulation and direct antiproliferative effects. Successful treatment of 11 LM lesions in 10 patients at doses of 3×10^6 to 6×10^6 IU administered three times weekly is reported, with clearance in all patients after between 12 and 29 doses.

Topical 5% imiquimod in the treatment of lentigo maligna. Wong JG, Toole JW, Demers AA, Musto G, Wiseman MC. J Cutan Med Surg 2012; 16: 245–9.

Twenty-seven patients were reviewed. There were 20 responders (74.1%) and 7 failures. The mean tumor size (area of an ellipse) was 6.69 cm^2, and the mean treatment duration was 17.7 weeks. Neither the size of the tumor ($p = 0.86$) nor treatment duration ($p = 0.18$) was related to resolution of the lesion. Imiquimod is an effective treatment for LM that provides patients with a cosmetically favorable outcome when standard surgery is not an option.

A quantitative systematic review of the efficacy of imiquimod monotherapy for lentigo maligna and an analysis of factors that affect tumor clearance. Mora AN, Karia PS, Nguyen BM. J Am Acad Dermatol 2015; 73: 205–12.

This systematic review based on 347 tumors from 45 studies revealed histologic and clinical clearance rates to be 76.2% and 78.3%, respectively. The incidence of clinical recurrence was 2.3% with a mean follow-up of 34 months. Treatment with more than 60 total applications or more than 5 applications per week was associated with a higher likelihood of clearance.

Evidence Levels: **A** Double-blind study **B** Clinical trial ≥ 20 subjects **C** Clinical trial < 20 subjects **D** Series ≥ 5 subjects **E** Anecdotal case reports

Imiquimod 5% cream as primary or adjuvant therapy for melanoma in situ, lentigo maligna type. Swetter SM, Chen FW, Kim DD, Egbert BM. J Am Acad Dermatol 2015; 72: 1047–53.

Fifty-eight cases analyzed for local recurrence after topical imiquimod 5% treatment for either primary therapy or adjuvant after narrow-margin excision. In this study 86.2% demonstrated clinical clearance at mean follow-up of 42.1 months; 72.7% primary and 94.4% adjuvant. Imiquimod cream appears to be a viable option for primary or adjuvant treatment of LM in patients who are poor surgical candidates.

Treatment of lentigo maligna with imiquimod cream: a long-term follow-up study of 10 patients. Van Meurs T, Van Doorn R, Kirtschig G. Dermatol Surg 2010; 36: 853–8.

Ten patients with LM were treated with imiquimod 5% cream between 2004 and 2007 with a median follow-up of 31 months (range 11–56 months). Histologic clearance was assessed in all patients using posttreatment biopsies. Complete clinical clearance was achieved in 9 of 10 patients after treatment with imiquimod. During follow-up, three clinical and histologic recurrences were observed at 9, 10, and 27 months after treatment cessation. In a fourth patient, histologic recurrence without clinical signs was demonstrated 17 months after treatment. Five of 10 patients were in sustained clinical remission.

Treatment of lentigo maligna with tazarotene 0.1% gel. Chimenti S, Carrozzo AM, Citarella L, De Felice C, Peris K. J Am Acad Dermatol 2004; 50: 101–3.

In this series, two elderly patients with facial LM were treated with daily application of tazarotene gel 0.1% for 6 to 8 months. No recurrence in either patient was observed after follow-up periods of 18 and 30 months, respectively. These results should be interpreted with caution, considering the relatively short follow-up.

The use of photodynamic therapy in the treatment of lentigo maligna. Karam A, Simon M, Lemasson G, Misery L. Pigment Cell Melanoma Res 2013; 26: 275–7.

This study included 15 cases from a retrospective single-center review of patients with LM on the face. Patients underwent aminolevulinate treatment before red light therapy (40–90 J/cm^2) from three to nine sessions at 3-week intervals. Initial clinical evaluation occurred after three sessions, and three immediate failures were observed. Clinical and histologic healing was observed in the other patients with a 10- to 29-month follow-up.

A randomized trial of the off-label use of imiquimod 5% cream with vs. without tazarotene 0.1% gel for the treatment of lentigo maligna, followed by conservative staged excisions. Hyde MA, Hadley ML, Tristani-Firouzi P, Goldgar D, Bowen GM. Arch Dermatol 2012; 148: 592–6.

Ninety patients with 91 LMs were randomized into two groups. One group received imiquimod 5% cream 5 days a week for 3 months, whereas the other group also received tazarotene 0.1% gel 2 days a week for 3 months. After topical therapy, all patients underwent staged excisions and frozen section analysis with melan-A immunostaining to confirm negative margins. Forty-six patients with 47 LMs were randomized to receive monotherapy: 42 of 47 LMs reached the intended treatment duration, with 27 complete responses (64%). Forty-four patients with 44 LMs were randomized to receive combined therapy. Thirty-seven of 44 LMs reached the intended treatment duration, with 29 complete responses (78%). This difference did not reach statistical significance ($p = 0.17$). There have been no recurrences to date, with a mean follow-up period of 42 months.

Pretreating LM with imiquimod 5% cream may decrease surgical defect sizes; however, total reliance on topical imiquimod as an alternative to surgery may put the patient at increased risk of a local recurrence.

A two-staged treatment of lentigo maligna using ablative laser therapy followed by imiquimod: excellent cosmesis, but frequent recurrences on the nose. Greveling K, de Vries K, van Doorn MB, Prens EP. Br J Dermatol 2016; 174: 1134–6.

Retrospective study of ablative laser therapy followed by 6 weeks of topical imiquimod 5% cream (5 days/week). Thirty-five patients were treated with median follow-up of 42 and 14 months for different cohorts. A strong inflammatory response was found in 100% of the subjects in contrast to imiquimod monotherapy where there were nonresponders. After 2 and 3 years of follow-up, cumulative incidence of recurrence was 23.5%, with five of six being on the nose. Patient self-rated cosmetic outcome was 8.5/10.

Leprosy (including reactions)

Anne E. Burdick, Ivan D. Camacho

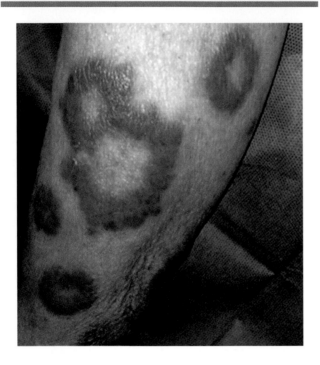

Leprosy, or Hansen disease, is an infection caused by *Mycobacterium leprae (M. leprae)*, affecting the skin, respiratory mucosa, peripheral nerves, and other organs. The cardinal features are anesthetic skin lesions, enlarged peripheral nerves, and peripheral neuropathy with acid-fast bacilli (AFB) in tissue biopsies or skin slit smears. A patient's cell-mediated immunity against *M. leprae* determines his or her presentation of leprosy in the Ridley–Jopling spectrum: tuberculoid (TT), borderline tuberculoid (BT), midborderline (BB), borderline lepromatous (BL), and lepromatous (LL). A patient with TT leprosy has high cell-mediated immunity to *M. leprae* and few well-demarcated lesions located on cooler parts of the body. A patient with LL leprosy has low cell-mediated immunity to *M. leprae* and numerous disseminated infiltrated erythematous papules, plaques, and nodules, often presenting with peripheral neuropathy. BB leprosy patients have multiple annular "dimorphous" plaques (see figure). On biopsy, TT lesions reveal rare and sometimes absence of AFB; polymerase chain reaction (PCR) may be positive. LL lesions have innumerable AFB. Indeterminate (I) leprosy presents as a single or a few hypopigmented patches that tend to resolve spontaneously but may progress to leprosy anywhere on the spectrum. Pure neural leprosy is limited to peripheral nerve involvement without skin lesions.

Leprosy reactions occur in 25% to 50% of patients before, during, or after treatment. BT, BB, and BL patients may develop a delayed hypersensitivity reaction, a type 1 "reversal" reaction, with the reappearance of red edematous lesions and an acute peripheral neuritis. Patients on etanercept, infliximab, and adalimumab may manifest leprosy and a type 1 reversal reaction

if they have concomitant subclinical leprosy. HIV patients may develop BT lesions and a type 1 reversal reaction as an immune reconstitution inflammatory syndrome within 6 months of starting highly active antiretroviral therapy if they also have a subclinical leprosy infection.

Erythema nodosum leprosum, a type 2 reaction, is an immune complex reaction that develops in BL and LL cases. In a type 2 reaction, crops of new red, indurated, tender papules, plaques, or nodules develop, usually with fever and occasionally with iritis or orchitis. Lucio phenomenon, a rare vasculitic reaction, presents as tender purpuric and necrotic lesions in BL and LL cases.

MANAGEMENT STRATEGY

Leprosy treatment consists of multidrug therapy with *rifampicin and dapsone, with or without clofazimine.* For treatment purposes, the World Health Organization (WHO) classifies I, TT, and BT cases as paucibacillary and recommends monthly rifampicin 600 mg and daily dapsone 100 mg for 6 months. WHO classifies BB, BL, and LL cases as multibacillary and recommends monthly rifampicin 600 mg, daily dapsone 100 mg, and clofazimine 300 mg monthly and 50 mg daily for 12 months.

The U.S. National Hansen's Disease Program guidelines are different. For paucibacillary cases, daily rifampicin 600 mg and daily dapsone 100 mg are recommended for 12 months. For multibacillary cases, daily rifampicin 600 mg, daily dapsone 100 mg, and daily clofazimine 50 mg are recommended for 24 months. In the United States, clofazimine is available only through the National Hansen's Disease Program as an investigational drug.

If clofazimine is not available or declined due to skin hyperpigmentation, or if a patient cannot take rifampicin or dapsone, alternative antibiotics are *minocycline* 100 mg, *ofloxacin* 400 mg, *Levaquin* 500 mg, *clarithromycin* 500 mg, or *moxifloxacin* 400 mg. Rifampicin is often prescribed monthly for patients on prednisone, warfarin, oral contraceptives, and other drugs with metabolism affected by rifampicin. If multidrug therapy is interrupted for any reason, it should be resumed when possible for the remaining months required to complete the recommended duration of multidrug therapy.

Multidrug therapy should be continued during reactions. Mild type 1 reversal reactions and type 2 reactions are treated with *nonsteroidal antiinflammatory drugs.* For a severe type 1 reversal reaction with acute neuritis, particularly involving the face, aggressive therapy with systemic steroids is started to prevent potentially irreversible nerve damage. *Prednisone* 0.5 to 1 mg/kg daily should be started and tapered slowly, 5 to 10 mg every 2 to 4 weeks, for 3 to 6 months or longer depending on the patient's response. Because high doses of steroids are often required to control a type 1 reversal reaction, the addition of a steroid-sparing drug should be considered. *Methotrexate* and *ciclosporin* are effective for a type 1 reversal reaction, permitting a decreased dose or discontinuation of prednisone.

A severe type 2 reaction also responds to prednisone 0.5 to 1 mg/kg daily and often requires a slower taper of 6 months or longer. *Thalidomide,* a known teratogen, is the drug of choice for men and for women who are postmenopausal, surgically sterile, or are using appropriate contraceptives. The initial thalidomide dose ranges from 100 to 300 mg nightly depending on the type 2 reaction severity. The dose is decreased slowly over several months to a maintenance dose of 50 to 100 mg nightly to prevent recurrences. Other drugs for type 2 reaction include *methotrexate, azathioprine, infliximab,* and *etanercept.* Lucio phenomenon is treated with prednisone, *low-dose aspirin,* and wound care.

Evidence Levels: **A** Double-blind study **B** Clinical trial ≥ 20 subjects **C** Clinical trial < 20 subjects **D** Series ≥ 5 subjects **E** Anecdotal case reports

After completion of multidrug therapy, the National Hansen's Disease Program advises paucibacillary patients to be screened annually for 5 years and multibacillary patients for 8 years. Household contacts who lived with a leprosy patient during the 3 years before multidrug therapy was started should have one screening examination according to WHO. The National Hansen's Disease Program also recommends one screening for paucibacillary leprosy contacts and advises an annual screening for 5 years for multibacillary leprosy contacts.

For leprosy neuropathy and neuritis, *gabapentin*, *pregabalin*, or *amitriptyline* alleviates the pain.

Specific Investigations

- Skin biopsy from periphery of lesion for diagnosis and annually
- PCR for diagnosis if a paucibacillary lesion biopsy does not show
- Slit skin smears
- Neurosensory testing
- Chemistry panel, complete blood count
- Glucose-6-phosphate dehydrogenase level before dapsone
- Urinalysis (type 2 reaction)
- Purified protein derivative (PPD) or QuantiFERON Gold before immunosuppression
- Hepatitis screening
- HLA-B13 in Asians with increased risk of dapsone hypersensitivity reaction

First-Line Therapies

Rifampicin and dapsone (paucibacillary and multibacillary)	B
Clofazimine (in addition to rifampicin and dapsone, for multibacillary and, in high doses, for type 2 reaction)	B
Nonsteroidal antiinflammatory drugs (type 1 reversal reaction and type 2 reaction)	D
Prednisone (type 1 reversal reaction and type 2 reaction)	D
Thalidomide (type 2 reaction)	D

Leprosy. Britton WJ, Lockwood DN. Lancet 2004; 363: 1209–19.
Review of clinical features, diagnostic criteria, and treatment of leprosy and reactions.

Treatment of leprosy/Hansen's disease in the early 21st century. Worobec SM. Dermatol Ther 2009; 22: 518–37.
Review of leprosy and reactions.

Leprosy: forgotten, but not gone (yet). Dinubile MJ, Keystone JS. Int J Dermatol 2011; 50: 1024–6.
Comparison of type 1 reversal reaction and type 2 reaction features.

Human immunodeficiency virus and leprosy: an update. Lockwood DN, Lambert SM. Dermatol Clin 2011; 29: 125–8.

Leprosy and HIV co-infection: a critical approach. Massone C, Talhari C, Ribeiro-Rodrigues R, Sindeaux RH, Mira MT, Talhari S, et al. Expert Rev Anti Infect Ther 2011; 9: 701–10.

The role of thalidomide in the management of erythema nodosum leprosum. Walker SL, Waters MF, Lockwood DN. Lepr Rev 2007; 78: 197–215.

Secondary leprosy infection in a patient with psoriasis during treatment with infliximab. Teixeira FM, Vasconcelos LM, Rola Cde A, Prata de Almeida TL, Valença JT Jr, Nagao-Dias AT. J Clin Rheumatol 2011; 17: 269–71.
A psoriatic man on infliximab for 2 years developed BL lesions and neuropathy.

Leprosy reaction manifesting after discontinuation of adalimumab therapy. Camacho ID, Valencia I, Rivas MP, Burdick AE. Arch Dermatol 2009; 145: 349–51.
An undiagnosed BT patient presented with a type 1 reversal reaction after discontinuing adalimumab 5 weeks prior for presumed seronegative arthritis.

Second-Line Therapies

Minocycline, Levaquin, ofloxacin, clarithromycin, moxifloxacin,	B
Methotrexate (type 1 reversal reaction and type 2 reaction)	B
Ciclosporin (type 1 reversal reaction)	D
Azathioprine (type 2 reaction)	D
Infliximab (type 2 reaction)	D
Etanercept (type 2 reaction)	D
Gabapentin or pregabalin (neuropathy and neuritis)	D
Amitriptyline (neuropathy and neuritis)	D

Response to cyclosporine treatment in Ethiopian and Nepali patients with severe leprosy type 1 reactions. Marlowe SN, Leekassa R, Bizuneh E, Knuutilla J, Ale P, Bhattarai B, et al. Trans R Soc Trop Med Hyg 2007; 101: 1004–12.
Forty-one patients with type 1 reversal reaction treated with ciclosporin 5 to 7.5 mg/kg/day for 12 weeks had 67% to 100% improvement after 24 weeks. Neuritis recurred when discontinued.

Cyclosporin A treatment of leprosy patients with chronic neuritis is associated with pain control and reduction in antibodies against nerve growth factor. Sena CB, Salgado CG, Tavares CM, Da Cruz CA, Xavier MG, Do Nascimento JL. Lepr Rev 2006; 77: 121–9.
Twenty patients with neuritis unresponsive to 40 mg/day prednisone had improved sensation, strength, and pain after ciclosporin 5 mg/kg/day with a 12-month taper.

Using methotrexate to treat patients with ENL unresponsive to steroids and clofazimine: a report on 9 patients. Hossain D. Lepr Rev 2013; 82: 105–12.
Nine patients with type 2 erythema nodosum leprosum resistant to prednisone and clofazimine responded well to prednisolone (30–40 mg/day for 3–6 months, then dose was halved and tapered slowly over 2.5–3 years) with methotrexate (7.5 mg weekly for 24–36 months). Patients remained relapse free for 2.5 years.

Methotrexate treatment for type 1 (reversal) leprosy reactions. Biosca G, Casallo S, López-Vélez R. Clin Infect Dis 2007; 45: e7–9.
A BL patient with type 1 reversal reaction and poor tolerance to corticosteroids responded to methotrexate 7.5 mg weekly. Prednisone was stopped in 2 months, and lesions resolved in 6 months.

Methotrexate in resistant ENL. Kar BR, Babu R. Int J Lepr Other Mycobact Dis 2004; 72: 480–2.

A patient with a type 2 reaction unresponsive to prednisolone 50 mg daily improved with methotrexate 15 mg weekly for 2 weeks. Prednisolone was tapered to 20 mg daily with continued improvement on methotrexate 7.5 mg weekly.

Azathioprine as a steroid sparing agent in leprosy type 2 reactions: report of nine cases. Duraes SM, Salles SA, Leite VR, Gazzeta MO. Lepr Rev 2011; 82: 304–9.

Review of nine reports of type 2 reaction cases refractory to prednisone and clofazimine responding to azathioprine 2 to 3 mg/kg/day. The prednisone dose was decreased in 4 weeks and halved after 12 weeks with fewer type 2 reactions.

Clinical outcomes in a randomized controlled study comparing azathioprine and prednisolone versus prednisolone alone in the treatment of severe leprosy type 1 reactions in Nepal. Marlowe SN, Hawksworth RA, Butlin CR, Nicholls PG, Lockwood DN. Trans R Soc Trop Med Hyg 2004; 98: 602–9.

Forty patients with type 2 reversal reaction randomized to prednisolone 40 mg daily vs. prednisolone 40 mg daily with azathioprine 3 mg/kg daily for 12 weeks had no difference in outcome.

Severe refractory erythema nodosum leprosum successfully treated with the tumor necrosis factor inhibitor etanercept. Ramien ML, Wong A, Keystone JS. Clin Infect Dis 2011; 52: e133–5.

An LL patient who had type 2 reactions for 6 years despite daily thalidomide 100 mg and multiple courses of 40 to 60 mg/day of prednisone improved on etanercept 50 mg subcutaneously weekly for 6 weeks. Prednisone and thalidomide were stopped in 6 months.

Treatment of recurrent erythema nodosum leprosum with infliximab. Faber WR, Jensema AJ, Goldschmidt WF. N Eng J Med 2006; 355: 739.

A BL patient with type 2 reaction multidrug therapy refractory to daily prednisolone 40 mg and thalidomide 300 mg responded promptly to three doses of infliximab 5 mg/kg every other week with no recurrence for 1 year after the last dose.

131

Leukocytoclastic vasculitis

Nicole Fett, Jeffrey P. Callen

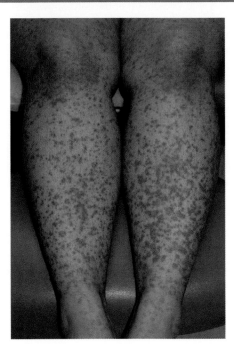

Vasculitis is best classified based on the size of the vessels involved. Large vessel vasculitides, giant cell arteritis and Takayasu arteritis, involve large arteries and rarely have associated cutaneous findings. Pure medium vessel vasculitides such as polyarteritis nodosa and cutaneous polyarteritis nodosa affect vessels with muscular walls. Cutaneous features of medium vessel vasculitides include livedo reticularis, retiform purpura, nodules, ulcers, and infarcts. Vasculitides that involve both medium and small vessels include granulomatosis with polyangiitis (GPA, previously Wegener granulomatosis), eosinophilic granulomatous angiitis (EGPA, previously Churg–Strauss syndrome), and microscopic polyangiitis. Overlap medium and small vessel vasculitides may present with features of medium vessel involvement and features classic for small vessel involvement (urticaria, palpable purpura). Cryoglobulinemia can be associated with either a small vessel vasculitis or an occlusive vasculopathy and frequently is associated with hepatitis C viral infection. This condition is manifest with purpuric skin lesions usually. Lastly, pure small vessel vasculitides include IgA vasculitis (previously Henoch–Schönlein purpura [HSP]), erythema elevatum diutinum, urticarial vasculitis (UV), and cutaneous small vessel vasculitis (CSVV, previously leukocytoclastic vasculitis [LCV]). LCV is a histopathologic term that describes the pattern seen on skin biopsy and should not be used as a clinical diagnosis. The majority of patients labeled with LCV have CSVV; however, the most common cutaneous manifestations of antineutrophil cytoplasmic antibody (ANCA)–associated vasculitis is LCV, and therefore careful evaluation for systemic involvement is necessary in patients whose skin biopsies reveal LCV. CSVV is frequently secondary to exposure to medications or associated with infections. Most, perhaps roughly 60% of the time, CSSV is self-limiting.

MANAGEMENT STRATEGY

Management of small vessel vasculitis requires evaluation for systemic involvement, removal of potential causative agents or treatment directed at associated diseases, management of symptoms in those patients with self-limiting disease, and targeted or empiric therapy for patients with recurrent or recalcitrant disease. Patients with systemic vasculitis, particularly when involving the kidneys, lungs, or central nervous system, require immediate referral to rheumatology, nephrology, or other specialists and frequently require *hospitalization* for treatment with *systemic corticosteroids and immunosuppressive/immunomodulatory agents.*

Patients with CSVV in whom there is an identifiable cause, such as a drug, are treated symptomatically in addition to removing the presumed causative agent. Symptomatic measures include *rest, elevation, gradient support stockings*, and *antihistamines.*

The challenge is to treat the patient who has chronic CSVV without a defined etiology and without systemic involvement. In patients with asymptomatic disease who are not bothered by the appearance of their vasculitic lesions, no treatment may be needed. For those patients who develop pain, ulcerations, or psychological distress, the risks and benefits of therapy should be discussed. Treatment recommendations for CSVV are largely based on case reports, case series, and expert opinion. If systemic therapy is considered for disease "confined to the skin," *colchicine* and *dapsone* are first-line agents, given their relative safety. *Immunosuppressive/immunomodulatory agents including methotrexate* and *azathioprine* have been used in patients who are refractory to colchicine and dapsone. *Systemic corticosteroids* should be avoided due to the narrow window between therapeutic effect and toxicity.

Specific Investigations

For all patients

- Careful history for drugs, preceding illness, and signs of systemic involvement
- Serologic tests for infectious diseases (hepatitis C, hepatitis B, human immunodeficiency virus)
- Complete blood count
- Comprehensive blood biochemistry
- Urinalysis
- Chest radiograph

For patients with chronic or recurrent disease

- Skin biopsy of *new* lesions
- ANCAs
- Antinuclear antibody (ANA), rheumatoid factor, anti-Ro/SS-A, etc.
- Complement levels

For selected patients

- Urine toxicology screen for cocaine/levamisole
- Echocardiography
- Visceral angiography
- Malignancy screening tests

The purpose of evaluating the patient with cutaneous vasculitis is to identify a cause of the process and assess for the presence of systemic involvement. The evaluation begins with a careful history and physical examination, followed by selected testing based on the acuteness of the process and the findings from the history and physical examination. Direct immunofluorescence (DIF) is required to differentiate IgA vasculitis, which might be associated with a higher risk of renal involvement, from other causes of CSVV.

Cutaneous vasculitis in children and adults: associated diseases and etiologic factors in 303 patients. Blanco R, Martinez-Taboada VM, Rodriguez-Valverde V, Garcia-Fuentes M. Medicine 1998; 77: 403–18.

Diagnoses and associated diseases of 172 adults and 131 children who presented to a medical center over a 19-year period. Of the 131 children, only 1 had a secondary vasculitis. In contrast, approximately 30% of the adults had systemic involvement or secondary vasculitis. The authors therefore recommend less intensive investigations in children than in adults.

A practical approach to the diagnosis, evaluation, and management of cutaneous small-vessel vasculitis. Goeser MR, Laniosz V, Wetter DA. Am J Clin Dermatol 2014; 15: 299–306.

An approach to the patient with small vessel vasculitis and a very useful algorithm for evaluation and treatment.

Drug-associated cutaneous vasculitis: study of 239 patients from a single referral center. Ortiz-Sanjuán F, Blanco R, Hernández JL, Pina T, González-Vela MC, Fernández-Llaca H, et al. J Rheumatol 2014; 41: 2201–7.

This retrospective review spanning 36 years assessed 773 patients with a diagnosis of cutaneous vasculitis. Of these, 30.9% met the 2012 Chapel Hill Consensus Conference (CHCC) definition for drug-induced cutaneous vasculitis. Antibiotics were implicated as the causative agent in 62.3% of cases. 45.2% required systemic immunosuppression, and 18.4% of them relapsed over 5 months. A large percentage of patients had systemic manifestations (joint 51%, gastrointestinal 38.1%, nephropathy 34.7%) and laboratory abnormalities (cryoglobulins 26%, ANAs 21.1%, anemia 18.8%, leukocytosis 24.7%, positive rheumatoid factor 17.5%), which suggests misclassification and would explain the high proportion of patients who required systemic immunosuppression and who relapsed.

Single-organ cutaneous small-vessel vasculitis according to the 2012 revised International Chapel Hill Consensus Conference Nomenclature of Vasculitides: a study of 60 patients from a series of 766 cutaneous vasculitis cases. Loricera J, Blanco R, Ortiz-Sanjuán F, Hernández JL, Pina T, González-Vela MC, et al. Rheumatology 2015; 54: 77–82.

This retrospective review spanning 35 years assessed 766 patients with a diagnosis of cutaneous vasculitis. Of these patients, 60 (7.8%) met the 2012 CHCC definition of single-organ cutaneous small vessel vasculitis (SoCSVV). The etiology of the SoCSVV was medication related in 52% and infection related in 34%. Approximately a quarter of patients with SoCSVV were treated with systemic corticosteroids or nonsteroidal antiinflammatory drugs (NSAIDs). Complete recovery was noted in all patients within 4 months; however, 8% of them developed recurrence.

First-Line Therapies

• Observation	D
• Removal or withdrawal of the causative agent (e.g., drug)	D
• Colchicine	C
• Dapsone	C
• Nonsteroidal antiinflammatory drugs	C

Colchicine in the treatment of cutaneous leukocytoclastic vasculitis: results of a prospective, randomized controlled trial. Sais G, Vidaller A, Jucgla A, Gallardo F, Peyri J. Arch Dermatol 1995; 131: 1399–402.

Forty subjects with CSVV were randomized to receive colchicine or topical emollients. The study was powered to detect a 40% difference between groups. The study failed to detect a statistically significant difference between groups; however, the colchicine-treated group included all patients who had failed to respond to dapsone and a disproportionate amount of subjects who had failed other therapies. Thus the colchicine arm included patients with more recalcitrant disease, and this may have contributed to the negative result. It was also noted that the subjects' disease flared with withdrawal of the colchicine.

Colchicine is effective in controlling chronic cutaneous leukocytoclastic vasculitis. Callen JP. J Am Acad Dermatol 1985; 13: 193–200.

This open-label study involved 13 patients. This is the largest case series of colchicine use in CSVV.

Colchicine use in CSVV is supported by four case series. An inadvertently imbalanced randomized controlled trial (RCT) of colchicine in CSVV failed to show statistically significant improvement.

Sulfone therapy in the treatment of leukocytoclastic vasculitis. Report of three cases. Fredenberg MF, Malkinson FD. J Am Acad Dermatol 1987; 16: 772–8.

Three patients with CSVV were successfully treated with moderate doses of dapsone (100–150 mg daily).

Dapsone therapy for Henoch-Schönlein purpura: a case series. Iqbal H, Evans A. Arch Dis Child 2005; 90: 985–6.

Eight children with HSP were treated with dapsone. Cutaneous vasculitis improved within 1 week of therapy. Six relapsed when treatment was stopped and subsequently cleared with reinstitution of dapsone.

Dapsone in Henoch-Schönlein purpura. Sarma PS. Postgrad Med J 1994; 70: 464–5.

Case series of six adults with HSP treated with dapsone 100 mg daily. Four of 6 had clearance of arthritis and purpura within 1 week.

There are several single cases reporting efficacy of dapsone in CSVV and four small case series supporting its use.

The therapeutic response of urticarial vasculitis to indomethacin. Millns JL, Randle HW, Solley GO, Dicken CH. J Am Acad Dermatol 1980; 3: 349–55.

Open-label trial of 10 patients with UV treated with indometacin 25 mg three times daily to 50 mg four times daily. Six cleared within 17 days. Three had partial improvement.

Two case series report success with indometacin use.

Second-Line Therapies

• Systemic corticosteroids	A
• Azathioprine	C
• Methotrexate	C
• Ciclosporin	C
• Mycophenolate mofetil	C
• Rituximab (for cryoglobulinemic and ANCA-associated vasculitis)	A

Early prednisone therapy in Henoch-Schönlein purpura: a randomized, double-blind, placebo-controlled trial. Ronkainene J, Koskimies O, Ala-Houhala M, Antikainen M, Merenmies J, Rajantie J, et al. J Pediatr 2006; 149: 241–7.

Evidence Levels: **A** Double-blind study **B** Clinical trial ≥ 20 subjects **C** Clinical trial < 20 subjects **D** Series ≥ 5 subjects **E** Anecdotal case reports

One hundred seventy-one children with HSP were randomized to receive 1 mg/kg/day of prednisone for 2 weeks and 2 additional weeks of tapered prednisone versus placebo. The prednisone group had a statistically significant decrease in abdominal and joint pain and renal dysfunction. Prednisone did not prevent the development of renal symptoms. The authors conclude that prednisone may be used in children with HSP to treat abdominal pain, arthritis, and renal involvement.

The clinical and histopathologic spectrums of urticarial vasculitis: study of forty cases. Sanchez NP, Winkelmann RK, Schroeter AL, Dicken CH. J Am Acad Dermatol 1982; 7: 599–605.

Case series of 40 patients with UV. Thirteen of 17 patients treated with prednisone 40 mg daily or greater had complete remission or decreased severity in clinical urticaria.

Chronic urticaria-like lesions in systemic lupus erythematosus. A review of 12 cases. O'Loughlin S, Schroeter AL, Jordon RE. Arch Dermatol 1978; 114: 879–83.

Twelve patients with systemic lupus erythematosus (SLE) and UV. Ten of 12 treated with prednisone and improved. Doses ranged from 50 mg to 10 mg daily.

A randomized placebo-controlled study supports the use of prednisone in HSP. Three case series report vasculitis clearance with prednisone in urticarial vasculitis.

The clinical spectrum and therapeutic management of hypocomplementemic urticarial vasculitis: data from a French nationwide study of fifty-seven patients. Jachiet M, Flageul B, Deroux A, Le Quellec A, Maurier F, Cordoliani F, et al. Arthritis Rheumatol 2015; 67: 527–34.

Patients were treated with many different agents, and the study is limited by the lack of untreated controls. Approximate complete response rates were 25% hydroxychloroquine, 18% colchicine, 18% dapsone, 20% corticosteroids, 45% azathioprine, 0% methotrexate, 55% mycophenolate mofetil, 80% ciclosporin, and 70% rituximab.

Azathioprine. An effective, corticosteroid-sparing therapy for patients with recalcitrant cutaneous lupus erythematosus or with recalcitrant cutaneous leukocytoclastic vasculitis. Callen JP, Spencer LV, Burruss JB, Holtman J. Arch Dermatol 1991; 127: 515–22.

An open-label trial involving six patients who had failed to respond to "less toxic" therapies.

Azathioprine therapy for steroid-resistant Henoch-Schönlein purpura: a report of 6 cases. Fotis L, Tuttle PV 4th, Baszis KW, Pepmueller PH, Moore TL, White AJ. Pediatr Rheumatol Online J. 2016 Jun 23;14(1):37. doi: 10.1186/s12969-016-0100-x.

Six children with relapsing HSP without significant renal involvement were treated with azathioprine. All patients had relapsing symptoms despite corticosteroid use. They were successfully treated with azathioprine and were tapered off of corticosteroids. The duration of azathioprine therapy ranged from 7–21 months and no adverse events were reported.

Prednisone plus azathioprine treatment in patients with rheumatoid arthritis complicated by vasculitis. Heurkens AH, Westedt ML, Breedveld FC. Arch Intern Med 1991; 151: 2249–54.

Twenty-eight patients with rheumatoid arthritis–associated vasculitis were studied. Nine patients with severe systemic vasculitis improved with 60 mg of prednisone and 2 mg/kg/body weight of azathioprine daily. The remaining 19 patients with cutaneous vasculitis were randomized to prednisone plus azathioprine treatment versus continuation of a previous regimen. Although measures of both vasculitis and arthritis activity improved to a greater degree in the patients treated with prednisone plus azathioprine in the first 3 months of therapy, and this therapy was associated with a low incidence of relapse of vasculitis, there was not a statistically significant difference between the two treatment protocols at the end of the follow-up period.

Case reports and series, totaling 21 patients, have been published supporting the use of azathioprine. A randomized alternative-therapy–controlled trial of 19 patients with rheumatoid vasculitis failed to detect a statistically significant difference in number of vasculitic lesions.

Methotrexate in patients with moderate systemic lupus erythematosus (exclusion of renal and central nervous system disease). Gansauge S, Breitbart A, Rinaldi N , Schwarz-Eywill M. Ann Rheum Dis 1997; 56: 382–5.

Open-label trial of methotrexate involving 22 patients with SLE. Nine of the 22 patients had vasculitis. Six of 9 had resolution of their vasculitis with methotrexate.

Methotrexate use has been reported in 13 patients with CSVV in case reports and series.

Cyclosporin A in the treatment of cutaneous vasculitis. Clinical and cellular effects. Tosca A, Ioannidou DJ, Katsantonis JC, Kyriakis KP. JEADV 1996; 6: 135–41.

Twelve patients received 5 mg/kg/day for 2 months and then 2 months of prednisone ranging from 10 to 40 mg/day. Five had complete clearance and no relapses over a follow-up time of 4 to 12 months. Six responded but then relapsed during a follow-up range of 4 to 20 months.

Treatment of complicated Henoch-Schönlein purpura with mycophenolate mofetil: a retrospective case series report. Nikibakhsh AA, Mahmoodzadeh H, Karamyyar M, Hejazi S, Noroozi M, Macooie AA, et al. Int J Rheumatol 2010; 2010: 5. Article ID: 254316.

Six children with steroid-resistant HSP were treated with mycophenolate mofetil 30 mg/kg/day. Five had improvement in their cutaneous symptoms or were reported to have "all manifestations resolved."

Mycophenolate mofetil is effective for maintenance therapy of hypocomplementaemic urticarial vasculitis. Worm M, Sterry W, Kolde G. Br J Dermatol 2000; 143: 1324.

Two women were initially treated with cyclophosphamide–dexamethasone and then transitioned to mycophenolate mofetil, 2 gm daily. No vasculitis flares occurred during 15 months of maintenance therapy.

Efficacy of mycophenolate is supported by one open-label trial, case reports, and series.

A randomized controlled trial of rituximab following failure of antiviral therapy for hepatitis C-associated cryoglobulinemic vasculitis. Sneller M, Hu Z, Langford CA. Arthritis Rheum 2012; 64: 835–42.

Twenty-four patients who failed to improve with antiviral therapy were randomized to rituximab versus standard immunosuppression. Ten patients in the rituximab group (83%) were in remission at study month 6, compared with 1 patient in the control group (8%) (*p* < 0.001).

A randomized, controlled trial of rituximab for treatment of severe cryoglobulinemic vasculitis. De Vita S, Quartuccio L, Isola M, Mazzaro C, Scaini P, Lenzi M, et al. Arthritis Rheum 2012; 64: 843–53.

Fifty-nine patients with CV and related skin ulcers, active glomerulonephritis, or refractory peripheral neuropathy who failed or were not candidates for antiviral therapy were randomized to receive rituximab or conventional treatment (glucocorticoids, cyclophosphamide or azathioprine, and plasma exchange). Rituximab showed statistically significant improvement over conventional treatment in all outcomes.

Retreatment regimen of rituximab monotherapy given at the relapse of severe HCV-related cryoglobulinemic vasculitis: long-term follow up data of a randomized controlled multicenter study. Quartuccio L, Zuliani F, Corazza L, Scaini P, Zani R, Lenzi M, et al. J Autoimmun 2015; 63: 88–93.

Retrospective evaluation of the 30 patients randomized to receive rituximab in the 2012 trial. Patients received this as monotherapy for vasculitis flares. After their initial treatment 43.3% were in complete remission and did not require additional rituximab, 56.7% required at least one retreatment with rituximab. Of those who were retreated, 66% responded to retreatment.

Efficacy of low-dose rituximab for the treatment of mixed cryoglobulinemia vasculitis: phase II clinical trial and systematic review. Visentini M, Tinelli C, Colantuono S, Monti M, Ludovisi S, Gragnani L, et al. Autoimmun Rev 2015; 14: 889–96.

Fifty-two patients with hepatitis C virus (HCV)-associated mixed cryoglobulinemic vasculitis were treated with low-dose rituximab (250 mg/m^2 twice). Response, time to relapse, and adverse events were compared with published historical controls who were treated with standard doses of rituximab (375 mg/m^2 given four times). No differences were found in treatment response, time to relapse, and adverse events. The use of historical controls is a significant limitation of this study.

Management of noninfectious mixed cryoglobulinemia vasculitis: data from 242 cases included in the CryoVas survey. Terrier B, Krastinova E, Marie I, Launay D, Lacraz A, Belenotti P, et al. Blood 2012; 119: 5996–6004.

Retrospective analysis of patients who did not have hepatitis C. Thirty percent had a connective tissue disease, 22% had B-cell lymphoma, and 48% were essential (idiopathic). These authors compared outcomes of patients treated with rituximab plus corticosteroids, those with corticosteroids alone, and those with corticosteroids and immunosuppressive therapies. They found that those treated with rituximab were more likely to achieve complete clinical, serologic, and renal responses and were more likely to be on doses of prednisone below 10 mg/d than those treated with other regimens. However, rituximab-treated patients had more infectious complications (perhaps related to combination with high-dose corticosteroids). The mortality in the groups was identical.

Successful use of rituximab for cutaneous vasculitis. Chung L, Funke AA, Chakravarty EF, Callen JP, Fiorentino DF. Arch Dermatol 2006; 142: 1407–10.

Two women with recalcitrant CSVV, one of whom with a history of non-Hodgkin lymphoma, responded to infusions of rituximab.

Successful treatment of rheumatoid vasculitis-associated cutaneous ulcers using rituximab in two patients with rheumatoid arthritis. Hellmann M, Jung N, Owczarczyk K, Hallek M, Rubbert A. Rheumatology 2008; 47: 929–30.

These two reports document improvement with rituximab in a total of four patients, two with rheumatoid arthritis and two with a history of lymphoma.

Rituximab has become standard of care for cryoglobulinemic vasculitis refractory to antiviral therapy based on RCTs. However, with the

approval of new antiviral therapies that cure hepatitis C infection in 96% to 98% of patients, additional therapies for hepatitis C–associated vasculitides may not be needed in the future. Rituximab use in CSVV is supported by case series.

Third-Line Therapies	
• Antihistamines	E
• Pentoxifylline	E
• Plasma exchange	D
• Intravenous immunoglobulin (IVIG)	E
• Infliximab	E
• Tacrolimus	E

Synergistic effects of pentoxifylline and dapsone in leucocytoclastic vasculitis. Nurnberg W, Grabbe J, Czarnetzki BM. Lancet 1994; 343: 491.

Three cases of CSVV that resolved with pentoxifylline (1200 mg per day) and dapsone (100 mg per day).

Chronic leukocytoclastic vasculitis associated with polycythemia vera: effective control with pentoxifylline. Wahba-Yahav AV. J Am Acad Dermatol 1992; 26: 1006–7.

A single case improved with pentoxifylline 400 mg three times daily.

Plasma exchange in refractory cutaneous vasculitis. Turner AN, Whittaker S, Banks I, Jones RR, Pusey CD. Br J Dermatol 1990; 122: 411–5.

Eight patients with intractable CSVV were treated with plasma-exchange therapy. Seven improved.

Case report: steroid sparing effect of intravenous gamma globulin in a child with necrotizing vasculitis. Gedalia A, Correa H, Kaiser M, Sorensen R. Am J Med Sci 1995; 309: 226–8.

A 2½-year-old boy with fever, arthritis, and necrotizing CSVV was able to taper off of prednisone after intravenous γ-globulin administration.

Successful treatment of chronic leucocytoclastic vasculitis and persistent ulceration with intravenous immunoglobulin. Ong CS, Benson EM. Br J Dermatol 2000; 143: 447–9.

A 24-year-old woman with chronic ulcerating CSVV refractory to multiple immunosuppressants cleared with IVIG.

Therapy for severe necrotizing vasculitis with infliximab. Mang R, Ruzicka T, Stege H. J Am Acad Dermatol 2004; 51: 321–2.

A 62-year-old female with chronic ulcerating CSVV refractory to prednisone, IVIG, and topical tacrolimus healed with two infusions of infliximab. Unfortunately, recurrent infections limited further use. It must also be noted that tumor necrosis factor alpha therapies have also been reported to cause CSVV.

Response of deep cutaneous vasculitis to infliximab. Uthman IW, Touma Z, Sayyad J, Salman S. J Am Acad Dermatol 2005; 53: 353–4.

A 15-year-old female cleared with infliximab.

Treatment of severe and difficult cases of systemic lupus erythematosus with tacrolimus. A report of three cases. Duddridge M, Powell RJ. Ann Rheum Dis 1997; 56: 690–2.

Two of the three had clearing of CSVV.

Evidence Levels: **A** Double-blind study **B** Clinical trial ≥ 20 subjects **C** Clinical trial < 20 subjects **D** Series ≥ 5 subjects **E** Anecdotal case reports

132

Lichen myxedematosus

Jessica A. Kaffenberger, Joslyn S. Kirby

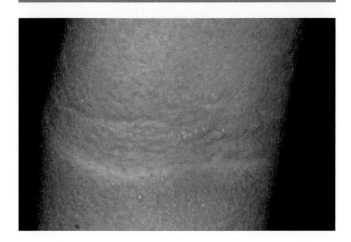

Lichen myxedematosus (LM) is a rare, chronic disease characterized by infiltration of the skin with mucin-producing fibroblasts. Typical examination findings include shiny, skin-colored to erythematous papules, nodules, and plaques on the face and/or extremities. Extensive disease can cause widespread firm, thickened skin, including leonine facies. The systemic form, scleromyxedema, can be associated with a monoclonal IgG lambda gammopathy, esophageal dysmotility, myopathy, and dermatoneuro syndrome. Localized forms do not have these associations and include acral persistent papular mucinosis, self-healing papular mucinosis, discrete LM, nodular LM, and cutaneous mucinosis of infancy.

MANAGEMENT STRATEGY

The treatment of LM remains a challenge. The absence of controlled studies makes comparison of different drugs or drug regimens difficult.

Localized forms may be observed or treated with topical medications *(steroids or calcineurin inhibitors)* or destructive therapies such as *cryotherapy, dermabrasion,* or *hyaluronidase.*

The systemic form, scleromyxedema, is treated more aggressively, and patients may require treatment with multiple medications. Given the association between scleromyxedema and monoclonal gammopathy, some therapies for systemic LM parallel the treatment of multiple myeloma. *Melphalan* has shown beneficial results when used alone or in combination with other therapies, including *plasmapheresis, oral prednisone,* or *autologous stem cell transplant.* However, melphalan use is severely limited by adverse effects, including malignancy, sepsis, and death. Other immunosuppressive agents, including *bortezomib, 2-chlorodeoxyadenosine (cladribine), cyclophosphamide, ciclosporin, methotrexate, thalidomide,* or a combination of *dexamethasone, octreotide, and sirolimus* have demonstrated some efficacy.

Alternatives to immunosuppressive agents include *intravenous immunoglobulin (IVIG), isotretinoin, interferon-α_{2b}, intralesional triamcinolone acetonide, psoralen with UVA (PUVA),* and *extracorporeal photochemotherapy.*

Specific Investigations

* Serum protein electrophoresis
* Tests for HIV infection
* Thyroid function testing
* Tests for hepatitis C infection

Scleromyxedema. Hummers LK. Curr Opin Rheumatol 2014; 26: 658–62.

An abnormal paraprotein, most commonly a monoclonal IgG lambda, is found in most patients (>80%) with scleromyxedema. Esophageal dysmotility can affect about 50% and myopathy about 10% to 50%. Associations with HIV and hepatitis C virus infections are rare. The cause of the disease is unknown, and it must be distinguished from thyroid-related mucinoses.

Scleromyxedema secondary to hepatitis C virus and successfully treated with antiviral therapy. Smith JA, Kalimullah FA, Erickson CP, Peng LS. Dermatol Online J 2015; 21: 9.

Small studies have associated scleromyxedema with hepatitis C infection. This appears more common in Japanese patients. A handful of cases outside Japan have been reported, including this patient who improved with ribavirin and interferon-α_{2b}.

First-Line Therapies

• Intravenous immunoglobulin	C
• Melphalan	C
• Systemic corticosteroids	D
• Plasmapheresis	D

Scleromyxedema: a case series highlighting long-term outcomes of treatment with intravenous immunoglobulin (IVIG). Blum M, Wigley FM, Hummers LK. Medicine 2008; 87: 10–20.

Eight patients had dramatic improvement of their cutaneous and visceral disease and were subsequently maintained with IVIG. Numerous other case reports and series, including several reports of patients with dermatoneuro syndrome, also demonstrated skin and systemic symptom improvement with IVIG (0.5–2 g/kg). IVIG has also been shown to be beneficial in combination with several therapies, including plasmapheresis, prednisone, melphalan, and thalidomide,

Scleromyxedema. Dinneen AM, Dicken CH. J Am Acad Dermatol 1995; 33: 37–43.

A review of 17 patients treated with melphalan. Twelve of the patients revealed improvement in their cutaneous symptoms; however, eight of the patients had only temporary improvement. Ten of the treated patients died from complications of the disease or treatment.

Scleromyxedema: an experience using treatment with systemic corticosteroid and review of the published work. Lin YC, Wang HC, Shen JL. J Dermatol 2006; 33: 207–10.

A case report of successful treatment with prednisolone 0.3 mg/kg/day divided four times daily for 1 week then tapered for 3 more weeks. Other studies have successfully used prednisone 60 mg four times daily for 4 to 6 weeks with gradual taper or pulse dexamethasone. However, other reports demonstrate a mixed success rate with steroids alone. Several case reports show a benefit of combining dexamethasone with bortezomib and/or thalidomide.

Scleromyxedema with monoclonal gammopathy and neurological involvement: recovery from coma after plasmapheresis. do Prado AD, Schmoeller D, Bisi MC, Piovesan DM, Dias FS, Staub HL. Int J Dermatol 2012; 51: 1013–5.

A man with severe cutaneous and central nervous system disease (dermatoneuro syndrome) underwent three consecutive courses of plasmapheresis with remarkable neurologic improvement. There is mixed success in other case reports.

Second-Line Therapies	
• Autologous stem cell transplantation	D
• Bortezomib	D
• Isotretinoin/etretinate	D
• Topical or intralesional corticosteroids	E
• Topical calcineurin inhibitors	E

Scleromyxedema: role of high-dose melphalan with autologous stem cell transplantation. Donato ML, Feasel AM, Weber DM, Prieto VG, Giralt SA, Champlin RE, et al. Blood 2006; 107: 463–6.

All seven patients survived, five had a complete remission of the skin, and visceral disease greatly improved. However, there is a report of a patient with scleromyxedema who developed dermatoneuro syndrome after autologous stem cell transplantation.

Response to bortezomib of a patient with scleromyxedema refractory to other therapies. Migkou M, Gkotzamanidou M, Terpos E, Dimopoulos MA, Kastritis E. Leuk Res 2011; 35: e209–11.

A case report of a patient with a history of numerous unsuccessful treatments treated with 21-day cycles of bortezomib 1.3 mg/m^2 on days 1, 4, 8, and 11 and dexamethasone 40 mg on days 1 to 4. The patient experienced sensory peripheral neuropathy after the second cycle, so the bortezomib dose was reduced to 1 mg/m^2. Eight cycles of bortezomib with dexamethasone were completed with near resolution at 24 months.

Treatment of recalcitrant scleromyxedema with thalidomide in 3 patients. Sansbury J, Cocuroccia B, Jorizzo J, Gubinelli E, Gisondi P, Girolomoni G. J Am Acad Dermatol 2004; 51: 126–31.

Three patients had marked improvement of cutaneous lesions, joint mobility, and reduction of paraprotein levels. Several successful cases of thalidomide (50–400 mg/day) were reported, including in combination with other therapies such as IVIG, dexamethasone, and chemotherapeutic agents.

Generalized papular and sclerodermoid eruption: scleromyxedema. Serdar ZA, Altunay IK, Yasar SP, Erfan GT, Gunes P. Indian J Dermatol Venereol Leprol 2010; 76: 592.

A report of scleromyxedema improving with isotretinoin 60 mg daily for 6 months. Previous case reports of scleromyxedema treated with isotretinoin demonstrate mixed results.

Nodular-type lichen myxedematosus: a case report. Ogita A, Higashi N, Hosone M, Kawana S. Case Rep Dermatol 2010; 2: 195–200.

A case report of a complete response to intralesional triamcinolone acetonide for nodular-type lichen myxedematosus. Other case reports showed mixed results with topical or intralesional steroids.

Treatment of localized lichen myxedematosus of discrete type with tacrolimus ointment. Rongioletti F, Zaccaria E, Cozzani E, Parodi A. J Am Acad Dermatol 2008; 58: 530–52.

Two patients with near-complete resolution of lichen myxedematosus with twice-daily application for 8 weeks. One patient did not respond to topical steroids.

Third-Line Therapies	
• Allogeneic stem cell transplantation	E
• Cyclophosphamide	E
• Ciclosporin	E
• Dexamethasone + octreotide + sirolimus	D
• Methotrexate	E
• Extracorporeal photopheresis	E
• PUVA	E
• Radiation	E
• Vincristine	E

Allogenic stem cell transplantation for the treatment of refractory scleromyxedema. Shayegi N, Alakel N, Middeke JM, Schetelig J, Mantovani-Loffler L, Bornhauser M. Transl Res 2015; 165: 321–4.

A patient with scleromyxedema associated with severe neurologic involvement continued to relapse despite numerous therapies, including autologous stem cell transplant. A rapid clinical remission occurred after allogeneic hematopoietic stem cell transplant from a sibling.

Scleromyxedema with subclinical myositis. Prasad PV, Joseph JM, Kaviarasan PK, Viswanathan P. Indian J Dermatol Venereol Leprol 2004; 70: 36–8.

A case report of a patient with scleromyxedema and myositis treated with cyclophosphamide 50 mg twice a day and prednisolone 40 mg/day. The patient had a 75% improvement at 1 month.

Successful treatment of intractable scleromyxedema with cyclosporin A. Saigoh S, Tashiro A, Fujita S, Matsui M, Shibata S, Takeshita H, et al. Dermatol 2003; 207: 410–1.

After failing PUVA, oral prednisone, and plasmapheresis, a patient's condition improved with ciclosporin at doses of 50 to 100 mg/day. There was a 50% improvement at 4 months and near resolution at 18 months.

Scleromyxedema: a novel therapeutic approach. El-Darouti MA, Hegazy RA, Fawzy MM, Mahmoud SB, Dorgham DA. J Am Acad Dermatol 2013; 69: 1062–6.

Five cases of scleromyxedema were successfully treated with 6 months of combination therapy of dexamethasone 120 mg intramuscularly over 2 consecutive days per week, octreotide 200 µg subcutaneous every other day, and oral sirolimus 1 g BID. Sirolimus was continued for an additional 6 months.

Arndt Gottron scleromyxedema: successful response to treatment with steroid minipulse and methotrexate. Mehta V, Balachandran C, Rao R. Indian J Dermatol 2009; 54: 193–5.

A single report of a patient who had over 75% improvement in cutaneous induration after treatment with minipulses of betamethasone 3 mg twice weekly and methotrexate 10 mg weekly.

Cutaneo-systemic papulosclerotic mucinosis (scleromyxedema): remission after extracorporeal photochemotherapy and corticoid bolus. D'Incan M, Franck F, Kanold J, Bacin F, Achin R, Beyvin AJ, et al. Ann Dermatol Venereol 2001; 128: 38–41.

A complete cutaneous therapeutic response was obtained in one patient after 12 extracorporeal photopheresis courses and four pulse treatments of prednisolone.

Evidence Levels: **A** Double-blind study **B** Clinical trial ≥ 20 subjects **C** Clinical trial < 20 subjects **D** Series ≥ 5 subjects **E** Anecdotal case reports

Scleromyxedema: treatment of widespread cutaneous involvement by total skin electron-beam therapy. Rampino M, Garibaldi E, Ragona R, Ricardi U. Int J Dermatol 2007; 46: 864–7.

The report of one patient successfully treated with radiation therapy and a review of previous reports.

Vincristine, idarubicin, dexamethasone and thalidomide in scleromyxoedema. Laimer M, Namberger K, Massone C, Koller J, Emberger M, Pleyer L, et al. Acta Derm Venereol 2009; 89: 631–5.

A case report of a patient treated with the chemotherapeutic regimen of vincristine, idarubicin, and dexamethasone (VID regimen) in addition to daily oral thalidomide that led to clinical and laboratory remission in 12 weeks.

Lichen nitidus

133

Andrew L. Wright

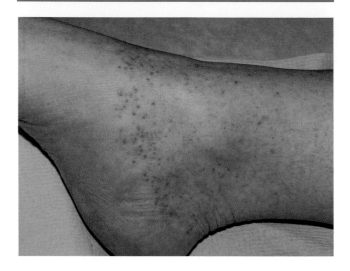

Lichen nitidus is an uncommon idiopathic condition presenting with 1- to 2-mm-diameter flat-topped or domed papules. They usually remain discrete but may be grouped. They can occur on any part of the body but mainly affect the forearms, penis, abdomen, chest, and buttocks. Palmar lesions may be hemorrhagic.

MANAGEMENT STRATEGY

Lichen nitidus persists for long periods but is generally asymptomatic, and *treatment may not be necessary*. No large controlled clinical trials have been reported; most treatments are based on anecdotal reports.

In patients with localized disease, *potent topical corticosteroids and topical tacrolimus* can be successful in clearing lesions. For more extensive disease *phototherapy* (psoralen plus UVA [PUVA] and UVB) has been reported to be successful. *Antihistamines*, including *astemizole* and *cetirizine*, are reported to have cleared lesions. Generalized lesions have cleared with *PUVA, UVB,* and *acitretin.*

Specific Investigation

- Biopsy

First-Line Therapies

• Topical corticosteroids	E
• UVB	D

Successful treatment of lichen nitidus. Wright S. Arch Dermatol 1984; 120: 155–6.

A 24-year-old woman with a 12-year history of extensive lesions cleared with 1 month's treatment using 0.05% fluocinonide cream twice daily. No recurrence was noted at 12-month follow-up.

Treatment of generalized lichen nitidus with narrow band ultraviolet light. Park JH, Choi YL, Kim WS, Lee DY, Yang JM, Lee ES, et al. J Am Acad Dermatol 2006; 54: 545–6.

A 33-year-old man with a 3-year history of generalized disease was reported as almost clear after 28 treatments and remained clear 11 months after cessation of therapy. A 10-year-old with generalized disease was reported as completely clear after 41 treatments and was clear at the 6-month follow-up.

Two cases of generalized lichen nitidus treated successfully with narrow band UVB phototherapy. Kim YC, Shim SD. Int J Dermatol 2006; 45: 615–7.

A 7-year-old girl and a 10-year-old boy, both with generalized lichen nitidus, were treated with narrowband UVB phototherapy, receiving between 17 and 30 treatments with maximum 9.5 J/cm². Both were reported as almost clear at the end of treatment and remained clear for at least 11 months.

A case of generalized lichen nitidus successfully treated with narrow-band ultraviolet B treatment. Bilgili SG, Karadag AS, Calka O, Ozdemir S, Kosem M. Photodermatol Photoimmunol Photomed 2013; 29: 215–7.

A 15-year-old girl with generalized lichen nitidus was treated with 25 sessions of UVB over a 2-month period with complete clearance.

Second-Line Therapies

• Topical tacrolimus	E
• Antihistamines	D
• PUVA	E
• Oral retinoids	E
• Ciclosporin	E
• Topical pimecrolimus	E

Lichen nitidus treated with topical tacrolimus. Dobbs CR, Murphy SJ. J Drugs Dermatol 2004; 3: 683–4.

A 32-year-old man with lichen nitidus confined to the penis was treated with twice-daily tacrolimus 0.1%. The lesion was reported to be clear after 4 weeks' treatment and had not relapsed after 4 months.

Generalised lichen nitidus: a report of two cases treated with astemizole. Ocampo J, Torne R. Int J Dermatol 1989; 28: 49–51.

Two patients treated with astemizole, a 65-year-old man with a 3-month history and a 48-year-old woman with a 4-month history, were either cleared or dramatically improved with 6 to 12 days of astemizole 10 mg daily.

Lichen nitidus treated with astemizole. Thio HB. Br J Dermatol 1993; 129: 342.

A 20-year-old woman with widespread disease responded to astemizole 10 mg daily after relapsing after a successful course of PUVA. There was no recurrence of lesions at 2-year follow-up.

It should be noted that astemizole has been discontinued because of cardiotoxicity noted with certain drug interactions. It is presumed that safer antihistamines might also be valuable.

Evidence Levels: **A** Double-blind study **B** Clinical trial ≥ 20 subjects **C** Clinical trial < 20 subjects **D** Series ≥ 5 subjects **E** Anecdotal case reports

Treatment of generalized lichen nitidus with PUVA. Randle HW, Sander HM. Int J Dermatol 1986; 25: 330–1.

A 29-year-old woman with an 8-month history of a generalized eruption was treated with PUVA three times weekly. Lesions cleared after 46 treatments (290 J) and remained clear 5 years later.

Association of lichen planus and lichen nitidus – treatment with etretinate. Aram H. Int J Dermatol 1988; 27: 117.

A 35-year-old woman with a 4-month history cleared with 8 weeks of etretinate 25 mg/50 mg on alternate days. Treatment was stopped 1 month later. There was no recurrence 5 months after completing the treatment.

Treatment of palmoplantar lichen nitidus with acitretin. Lucker GPH, Koopman RJJ, Steijlen PM, Van der Valk PG. Br J Dermatol 1994; 130: 791–3.

A 23-year-old man had a 14-month history of hand and foot involvement that failed to clear with acitretin 50 mg daily but was reported to have improved significantly on 75 mg daily.

A case of generalized lichen nitidus treated with low dose cyclosporine. Lee YK, Choi KW, Lee CW, Kim KH. Korean J Dermatol 2007; 45: 1311–4.

A 16-year-old girl with generalized lichen nitidus was significantly improved with 8 weeks of ciclosporin 2 mg/kg/day.

Generalized lichen nitidus successfully treated with pimecrolimus 1% cream. Farshi S, Mansouri P. Dermatol Online J 2011; 17: 11.

Lesions were reduced and flattened after treatment twice daily for 8 weeks.

Generalized lichen nitidus: successful treatment with systemic isotretinoin. Topal IO, Gokdemir G, Sahin IM. Indian J Dermatol Venereol Leprol 2013; 79: 554.

A 15-year-old female patient cleared completely with 4 months of isotretinoin 40 mg daily.

Treatment of lichen planus and lichen nitidus with itraconazole: reports of six cases. Libow LF, Coots NV. Cutis 1998; 62: 247–8.

A report of two cases showing partial clearance of lichen nitidus after 2 weeks of itraconazole 200 mg twice daily.

Improvement of lichen nitidus after topical dinitrochlorobenzene application. Kano Y, Otake Y, Shiohara T. J Am Acad Dermatol 1998; 39: 305–8.

This paper reports a patient treated with 0.1% dinitrochlorobenzene (DNCB) applied at 2-weekly intervals after sensitization with 1% DNCB. The lesions were said to have cleared after 7 months of treatment, compared with a control area. Six months after cessation of treatment, lesions were said to be recurring in the treated area.

Generalised lichen nitidus in a child: response to cetirizine dihydrochloride/levamisole. Sehgal VN, Jain S, Kumar S, Bhattacharya SN, Singh N. Australas J Dermatol 1998; 39: 60.

A 6-year-old boy with a 6-month history of generalized involvement showed complete regression/healing of lesions over a 4-week period of treatment with cetirizine dihydrochloride 5 mg daily and levamisole 50 mg on alternate days for 4 weeks.

Generalised lichen nitidus is successfully treated with an antituberculous agent. Kubota Y, Kirya H, Nakayama J. Br J Dermatol 2002; 146: 1081–3.

A 10-year-old Japanese girl with a 2-year history of lichen nitidus showed almost complete clearance after a 6-month course of oral isoniazid.

Facial actinic lichen nitidus successfully treated with hydroxychloroquine: a case report. Bouras M, Benchikhi H, Ouakkadi A, Zamiati S. Dermatol Online J 2013; 19: 20406.

Treatment with a combination of topical steroids and hydroxychloroquine produced complete clearance in 4 weeks in a 23-year-old female with facial lichen nitidus.

Third-Line Therapies

• Itraconazole	E
• Dinitrochlorobenzene	E
• Cetirizine dihydrochloride and levamisole	E
• Isoniazid	E

Lichen planopilaris

Anwar Al Hammadi, Eric Berkowitz

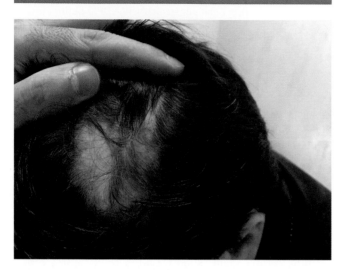

Lichen planopilaris (LPP), also known as *follicular lichen planus*, is a clinical syndrome consisting of lichen planus (LP) associated with cicatricial scalp alopecia. The condition is more common in women and presents with perifollicular erythema and keratotic plugs at the margins of the expanding alopecia. The follicular involvement is limited to the infundibulum and the isthmus, both demonstrating lichenoid inflammation. The main complications of follicular LP are atrophy and scarring, with permanent hair loss. Three forms of LPP are recognized: classic LPP; Graham–Little syndrome, characterized by the triad of multifocal scalp cicatricial alopecia, nonscarring alopecia of the axilla and/or groin, and keratotic follicular papules; and frontal fibrosing alopecia that affects mainly postmenopausal women and appears as cicatricial alopecia of the frontoparietal hairline and is associated with nonscarring alopecia of the eyebrows.

MANAGEMENT STRATEGY

Therapeutic management for LPP is challenging. However, if the associated inflammation can be controlled in its early stages, follicular units may be preserved and hair regrowth may be possible. A good therapeutic response would include a reduction in associated symptoms along with stabilization of the disease and some regrowth of hair in the active perimeter of the alopecic patch. For the most part, therapeutic reports are anecdotal. *Oral antihistamines* may be used to control pruritus, and *high-potency topical corticosteroids* are used to control the inflammation in early lesions. *Intralesional injections of 3 to 5 mg/mL of triamcinolone acetonide* are effective in well-developed lesions. *Hydroxychloroquine* may be efficacious. *Retinoids* have demonstrated some effect in the treatment of LP and therefore provide a possible alternative to corticosteroid treatment. Other agents that have been reported to be of use are *cyclosporine* and *mycophenolate mofetil*. There is some rationale for trying biologic agents such as tumor necrosis factor (TNF)–blocking agents for this condition.

- Skin biopsy
- Immunofluorescence studies
- Dermoscopy

A histologic review of 27 patients with lichen planopilaris. Tandon YK, Somani N, Bergfeld WF. J Am Acad Dermatol 2008; 59: 91–8.

Characteristic features of LPP include the absence of arrector pili muscles and sebaceous glands, a perivascular and perifollicular lymphocytic infiltrate, mucinous perifollicular fibroplasia with absence of interfollicular mucin, and superficial perifollicular wedge-shaped scarring.

Immunofluorescence abnormalities in lichen planopilaris. Ioannides D, Bystryn JC. Arch Dermatol 1992; 128: 214–6.

Direct immunofluorescence studies were performed on biopsied lesions of patients with LPP and LP. All of the LPP studies demonstrated abnormal linear deposits of immunoglobulin, consisting of IgG or IgA restricted to the basement membrane. The biopsies from those with LP demonstrated fibrillar deposits.

These different appearances suggest different disease processes for LPP and LP.

Dermatoscopy: alternative uses in daily clinical practice. Micali G, Lacarrubba F, Massimino D, Schwartz R. J Am Acad Dermatol 2011; 64: 1135–46.

Video dermatoscopy is performed with a video camera equipped with lenses providing magnification ranging from ×10 to ×1000 and shows the reduction to total absence of orifices, hyperkeratotic perifollicular scales, and erythema. In addition, perifollicular arborizing vessels, pigmented networks, and white pale or blue-gray dots in dark-skinned individuals, corresponding to focal decrease in melanin content, can also be observed.

The use of anti-keratin 903 antibodies to visualize colloid bodies and diagnose lichen planopilaris. Lanoue J, Yanofsky VR, Mercer SE, Phelps RG. Am J Dermatopathol 2016; 38: 353–8.

CK-903 is a useful adjunctive tool that will allow for a quicker, less costly, and more accurate diagnosis of LPP given its ability to identify colloid bodies even in the setting of significant inflammation and fibrosis and its advantages over direct immunofluorescence of low cost, short preparation time, and lack of need for a specialized fluorescent microscope.

• High-potency corticosteroids	**D**
• Intralesional corticosteroids	**C**

Lichen planopilaris: report of 30 cases and review of the literature. Chieregato C, Zini A, Barba A, Magannini M, Rosina P. Int J Dermatol 2003; 42: 342–5.

This clinical trial reports good therapeutic benefit from early treatment with high-potency topical steroids. Only four patients did not respond to the therapy and needed other treatments.

Scarring alopecia. Newton RC, Hebert AA, Freese TW, Solomon AR. Dermatol Clin 1987; 5: 603–18.

High-potency topical corticosteroids may be used to control inflammation in early scalp lesions. Intralesional injections with triamcinolone acetonide at concentrations of 3 to 5 mg/mL are more effective in well-developed lesions. Additionally, oral corticosteroids have been used in short tapering dosages to control severe disease.

Second-Line Therapies	
• Oral corticosteroids	C
• Retinoids	C
• Antimalarials	C
• Tetracycline	D

Postmenopausal frontal fibrosing alopecia: a frontal variant of lichen planopilaris. Kossard S, Lee MS, Wilkinson B. J Am Acad Dermatol 1997; 36: 59–66.

Oral corticosteroids and antimalarials were found to slow the course of LPP.

Lichen planopilaris: clinical and pathologic study of forty-five patients. Mehregan DA, Van Hale HM, Muller SA. J Am Acad Dermatol 1992; 27: 935–42.

This large study of 45 patients involved multiple different therapeutic modalities. High-potency topical steroids and oral steroids (30–40 mg daily) for 3 months demonstrated the highest success rates.

Oral treatment of keratinizing disorders of skin and mucous membranes with etretinate. Comparative study of 113 patients. Mahrle G, Meyer-Hamme S, Ippen H. Arch Dermatol 1982; 118: 97–100.

This paper reports the comparative results of the effects of the aromatic retinoid etretinate on various skin disorders.

Retinoids have been found to have a significant impact in cases of LP and have therefore been tried with some success in cases of LPP. Isotretinoin may be preferred over acitretin, as the latter agent has been associated with hair loss, but long-term therapy with low-dose acitretin has been studied in psoriasis and is well tolerated.

A case-series of 29 patients with lichen planopilaris. The Cleveland Clinic Foundation experience on evaluation, diagnosis, and treatment. Cevasco NC, Bergfeld WF, Remzi BK, de Knott HR. J Am Acad Dermatol 2007; 57: 47–53.

In this retrospective study of 29 patients, researchers found that the most commonly prescribed treatments for the reduction of primary symptoms associated with LPP were ketoconazole shampoo (86%), topical steroids (83%), multivitamins with minerals (76%), intralesional steroids (69%), topical minoxidil (41%), and tetracycline (38%). The most common treatment combination was topical steroid, ketoconazole shampoo, tetracycline, and multivitamins with minerals (14%).

Although patient response to any of these therapies was minimal, tetracycline (1 g/day) was the only treatment associated with a significant number of positive responses (6 of 11 patients).

Hydroxychloroquine and lichen planopilaris: efficacy and introduction of Lichen Planopilaris Activity Index scoring system. Chiang C, Sah D, Cho BK, Ochoa BE, Price VH. J Am Acad Dermatol 2010; 62: 387–92.

This retrospective study of 40 adult patients showed significant efficacy of hydroxychloroquine in the treatment of LPP. After 6 months, 69% of patients (26 of 38) were full or partial responders. After 12 months, 83% of patients (33 of 40) were full or

partial responders. Of the nine responders at 12 months, six were able to discontinue hydroxychloroquine and had a sustained remission with no systemic medication for at least 1 year.

Third-Line Therapies	
• Mycophenolate mofetil	D
• Cyclosporine	D
• Tacrolimus	E
• Thalidomide	E
• TNF-blocking drugs	E
• Low-dose excimer 308-nm laser	D
• Pioglitazone	D

Efficacy and safety of mycophenolate mofetil for lichen planopilaris. Cho BK, Sah D, Chwalek J, Roseborough I, Ochoa B, Chiang C, et al. J Am Acad Dermatol 2010; 62: 393–7.

In this retrospective study of 16 adult patients mycophenolate mofetil was effective at reducing the signs and symptoms of active LPP in 83% of patients (10 of 12 completers) who had failed multiple prior treatments after at least 6 months of treatment. Five of 12 patients were complete responders, 5 of 12 patients were partial responders, and 2 of 12 patients were treatment failures. Four patients withdrew from the trial because of adverse events.

Short course of oral cyclosporine in lichen planopilaris. Mirmirani P, Willey A, Price V. J Am Acad Dermatol 2003; 49: 667–71.

The authors present three patients with recalcitrant LPP unresponsive to hydroxychloroquine, high-potency topical steroids, and intralesional steroids who were treated with cyclosporine. The duration of treatment ranged from 3 to 5 months, with resolution of symptoms, no progression of hair loss, and no evidence of disease activity. One of the patients had a mild recurrence, which resolved with topical 0.1% tacrolimus in Cetaphil lotion.

Thalidomide-induced remission of lichen planopilaris. Boyd AS, King LE Jr. J Am Acad Dermatol 2002; 47: 967–8.

The authors describe the case of a patient who was diagnosed with LPP and treated with hydroxychloroquine, azathioprine, isotretinoin, cyclophosphamide, dapsone, cyclosporine, levamisole, chloroquine, acitretin, methotrexate, clofazimine, and enoxaparin, all without any benefit. The patient was then started on thalidomide 50 mg orally twice a day, with resolution of the symptoms. Side effects limited the ability to continue the medication. Initially, the patient only complained of fatigue and constipation; however, at 4 months, mild numbness and tingling of the fingers and toes developed, and the patient experienced significant depression, necessitating discontinuation of the medication.

Thalidomide's mechanism of action in this disorder may involve TNF inhibition, suggesting that medications such as adalimumab, etanercept, or infliximab may be beneficial. There has, however, been a case report of LPP developing in a patient treated with etanercept.

Low-dose excimer 308-nm laser for treatment of lichen planopilaris. Navarini AA, Kolios AG, Prinz-Vavricka BM, Haug S, Trüeb RM. Arch Dermatol 2011; 147: 1325–6.

In this small study of 13 patients with biopsy-proven active classic LPP or variants, pruritus and pain improved in all patients who had these complaints before the treatment. Erythema reduced in five patients and decreased inflammatory lesions in seven patients. An increased growth of hair after 4 to 8 weeks was observed in three patients, with stable remission in two patients.

Lichen planopilaris treated with a peroxisome proliferator-activated receptor γ-agonist. Mirmirani P, Karnik P. Arch Dermatol 2009; 145: 1363–6.

A 47-year-old man with LPP recalcitrant to therapy responded to pioglitazone at a dose of 15 mg/day.

Because of the theoretical basis for the use of peroxisome proliferator-activated receptor (PPAR) agonists in LPP, further studies are warranted to determine whether this treatment is genuinely efficacious for the disorder.

The use of oral pioglitazone in the treatment of lichen planopilaris. Mesinkoyska NA, Tellez A, Dawes D, Piliang M, Bergfeld W. J Am Acad Dermatol 2015; 72: 355–6.

Retrospective case analysis of the 22 patients who were prescribed pioglitazone hydrochloride for at least 1 month, and clinical follow-up longer than 3 months showed that pioglitazone was effective in controlling the symptoms, inflammation, and disease progression in 16 patients (72.7% of the patients). Moreover, new hair regrowth was noted in six patients (27.3%). From the responders, only two patients (9%) experienced relapse after discontinuation of pioglitazone.

Evidence Levels: **A** Double-blind study **B** Clinical trial ≥ 20 subjects **C** Clinical trial < 20 subjects **D** Series ≥ 5 subjects **E** Anecdotal case reports

135

Lichen planus

Roselyn Kellen, Mark G. Lebwohl

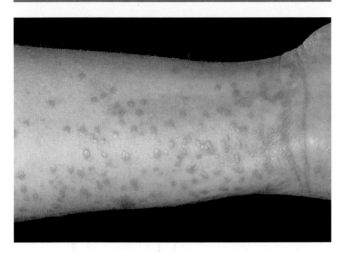

Lichen planus is a pruritic papulosquamous disease with characteristic histopathologic and clinical features. Classically, lesions are described with the 6 "P's": purple, pruritic, planar, polygonal, papule, and plaque. In some patients, fine white lines are visible across the surface of the lesions, known as *Wickham striae*. Oral erosive lichen planus, a painful erosive condition affecting mucous membranes, is addressed in a separate chapter.

MANAGEMENT STRATEGY

Although lichen planus can resolve spontaneously, treatment is often required because pruritus can be severe and interfere with sleep and quality of life. An association with underlying diseases such as hepatitis C is still controversial. Physicians should obtain a detailed medical history, as there are numerous reports of lichen planus or lichenoid eruptions occurring after vaccinations, particularly hepatitis B, and after the use of certain medications.

In patients with localized disease, *superpotent corticosteroids* should be applied twice daily for 2 to 4 weeks. If the response is inadequate, *intralesional injection of corticosteroids* into localized lesions may be beneficial. Topical antipruritic agents containing *menthol, phenol, camphor, lidocaine, pramoxine,* or *doxepin hydrochloride* can be useful. *Oral antihistamines* may offer limited benefit in severely pruritic patients. Sedating antihistamines can be helpful at bedtime.

Traditionally, patients with extensive lichen planus have been treated with systemic corticosteroids. *Oral prednisone* 30 to 60 mg daily for 2 to 6 weeks, or its equivalent, tapered over the ensuing 2 to 6 weeks, is often effective. Unfortunately, even in patients who clear with systemic corticosteroids, relapses are frequent. If patients require more than two courses of high-dose systemic corticosteroids over the span of a few months, alternative treatments should be sought. Fortunately, there is evidence in the literature for steroid-sparing treatments, including several agents that have been studied in clinical trials.

Oral metronidazole has emerged as a safe and effective alternative to systemic corticosteroids: 500 mg twice daily for 20 to 60 days has proved beneficial in many patients. *Sulfasalazine* has

been studied in a randomized, double-blind trial. Patients are started on 500 mg twice daily, and the dosage is increased by 500 mg every 3 days until a dose of 2.5 g daily is reached, for a total of 3 to 6 weeks. The use of *narrowband ultraviolet B* three times a week for 6 weeks has helped patients achieve partial and complete remission. *PUVA (Psoralen + UltraViolet A)* has been particularly beneficial in the lichen planus–like eruption associated with graft-versus-host disease. However, in one retrospective study, the recurrence rate was higher in patients who received PUVA compared with narrowband UVB. *Isotretinoin* in doses of 10 mg orally twice daily for 2 months has been reported to clear lichen planus in several patients, and *acitretin* 30 mg daily has also resulted in marked improvement or remission.

More recent studies have supported the evidence for certain therapies or evaluated the use of new agents. Oral *methotrexate* (15 mg/week for adults and 0.25 mg/kg/week for children) has helped patients achieve complete remission after 24 weeks, with most side effects reported as mild. The use of subcutaneous *enoxaparin* (5 mg weekly for 8 weeks) enabled more patients to achieve complete remission compared with the use of oral prednisone (0.5 mg/kg). *Apremilast* (20 mg twice daily for 12 weeks) has helped some patients improve their Physician Global Assessment score and maintain this improvement for 4 weeks after treatment.

For *severe and refractory lichen planus* unresponsive to other therapies, *antimicrobials* (antibiotics, antifungals), immunosuppressive agents (*mycophenolate mofetil, azathioprine, ciclosporin, antimalarials*), *tumor necrosis factor (TNF) blockers (adalimumab), thalidomide, topical calcineurin inhibitors, vitamin D analogs,* and *alitretinoin* have been used with success in some patients.

Palmoplantar lichen planus has been successfully treated with *acitretin* 35 mg/day (0.5 mg/kg) for 2 months, *UVA-1 laser therapy* three times a week for 4 weeks (100 J/cm²), and *ciclosporin* 3.5 mg/kg daily.

For *nail lichen planus,* there are case reports detailing the use of 30 mg *alitretinoin* daily, *ciclosporin* 3 mg/kg daily, and *etanercept* (25 mg subcutaneous twice a week for 6 months and then 50 mg weekly).

Specific Investigations

- Detailed medication history
- Liver function tests
- Serology for hepatitis B and C

Hepatitis C virus infection and lichen planus: a systematic review with meta-analysis. Lodi G, Pellicano R, Carrozzo M. Oral Dis 2010; 16: 601–12.

This meta-analysis included 33 studies that compared the prevalence of hepatitis C in patients with lichen planus and 6 studies that reported on the prevalence of lichen planus in patients with hepatitis C. Among patients with lichen planus, the odds ratio of being seropositive for hepatitis C was 4.85. Among patients with hepatitis C, the odds ratio of having lichen planus was 4.47.

There is conflicting data regarding the association between lichen planus and hepatitis C. This may be partially explained by geographic location and rates of hepatitis infection, genetic factors, the age of patients included in studies, and the size of previous studies.

Drug-induced lichen planus. Thompson DF, Skaehill PA. Pharmacotherapy 1994; 14: 561–71.

β-Blockers, methyldopa, penicillamine, quinidine, quinine, and nonsteroidal antiinflammatory agents play a role in the development of lichen planus. There is insufficient evidence to implicate angiotensin-converting enzyme inhibitors, sulfonylurea agents, carbamazepine, gold, lithium, and other drugs.

Many drugs and chemicals have been associated with lichenoid drug eruptions, which can be difficult to distinguish from true lichen planus. In addition to those mentioned here, hepatitis B and influenza vaccinations, allopurinol, tetracyclines, furosemide, hydrochlorothiazide, isoniazid, phenytoin, and etanercept are reported to cause lichenoid eruptions.

First-Line Therapies

• Topical corticosteroids	C
• Intralesional corticosteroids	D
• Antihistamines	C

Betamethasone-17,21-dipropionate ointment: an effective topical preparation in lichen rubra planus. Bjornberg A, Hellgren L. Curr Med Res Opin 1976; 4: 212–7.

Patients with lichen planus that had become resistant to betamethasone valerate ointment were treated with betamethasone dipropionate ointment once or twice daily for 2 to 3 weeks. Fourteen of 19 patients achieved better improvement with betamethasone dipropionate ointment.

Although topical and intralesional corticosteroids are first-line treatments for lichen planus, their use has been based on anecdotal reports rather than on controlled clinical trials. This is one of very few comparative trials of topical therapies for lichen planus.

Treatment of generalized cutaneous lichen planus with dipropionate and betamethasone disodium phosphate: an open study of 73 cases. Pitche P, Saka B, Kombate K, Tchangai-Walla K. Ann Dermatol Venereol 2007; 134: 237–40.

Injections of systemic corticosteroids performed at 2-week intervals resulted in complete remission in 61 of 73 (83.6%) patients with lichen planus; 8.2% of patients experienced partial remission, and another 8.2% failed this therapy. At 3 months, the relapse rate of initial responders was 23.3% and at 6 months 31.5% had relapsed.

Second-Line Therapies

• Metronidazole	B
• Sulfasalazine	A
• Systemic corticosteroids	B
• Isotretinoin, acitretin	A
• Narrowband or broadband UVB	B
• PUVA	C
• Methotrexate	B

Efficacy of oral metronidazole in treatment of cutaneous and mucosal lichen planus. Rasi A, Behzadi AH, Davoudi S, Rafizadeh P, Honarbakhsh Y, Mehran M, et al. J Drugs Dermatol 2010; 9: 1186–90.

Forty-nine patients participated in this open trial of oral metronidazole 250 mg every 8 hours for 12 weeks. Twenty patients (40.82%) had a complete response and 16 (32.65%) a partial response. Thirteen (26.53%) did not improve.

Metronidazole has also been studied in a dose of 500 mg twice daily for 20 to 60 days. The safety of oral metronidazole has led many dermatologists to use this treatment as first-line therapy for lichen planus.

Efficacy of sulfasalazine in the treatment of generalized lichen planus: randomized double-blinded clinical trial on 52 patients. Omidian M, Ayoobi A, Mapar MA, Feily A, Cheraghian B. J Eur Acad Dermatol Venereol 2010; 24: 1051–4.

Forty-four patients completed a double-blind study of sulfasalazine or placebo taken for 3 to 6 weeks. Sulfasalazine doses were started at 1 g per day and increased by 0.5 g every 3 days until a dosage of 2.5 g daily was achieved. Study medications were continued for 3 to 6 weeks. After 6 weeks of treatment, 19 patients (82.6%) in the sulfasalazine group achieved improvement compared with 2 patients (9.6%) in the placebo group. Pruritus improved in 14.3% of placebo patients and 91.3% in sulfasalazine-treated patients. Mild response (<50% of lesions cleared) occurred in 21.7% of patients in the sulfasalazine group, moderate response (>50% of lesions cleared) in 52.2%, and excellent clearing of lesions (>80%) in 8.7%. Gastrointestinal upset and headache were the most common side effects and occurred in 30.7% of patients, leading three patients to leave the study. Mild skin rash also occurred in one patient.

Although complete clearing occurred in a minority of patients, the authors did not continue this study beyond 6 weeks. Perhaps longer therapy would result in greater rates of clearing.

Treatment of lichen planus with acitretin. A double-blind, placebo-controlled study in 65 patients. Laurberg G, Geiger JM, Hjorth N, Holm P, Hou-Jensen K, Jacobsen KU, et al. J Am Acad Dermatol 1991; 24: 434–7.

Acitretin resulted in marked improvement or remission in 64% of patients compared with 13% of placebo-treated patients in a double-blind trial in 65 subjects. Acitretin doses of 30 mg daily were used, leading to mucocutaneous side effects (dryness of the mouth, lips, nose, and skin and hair loss) and hyperlipidemia.

Isotretinoin in doses of 10 mg orally twice daily has been effective in the treatment of oral lichen planus, and anecdotal use suggests efficacy in generalized lichen planus as well. A recent case report described a patient with palmoplantar lichen planus that cleared after 2 months of acitretin 35mg/kg/day (0.5 mg/kg). The latter isotretinoin regimen has fewer mucocutaneous side effects than higher doses of acitretin. Restrictions on the use of isotretinoin in the United States may make this less practical.

Comparison of the narrow band UVB versus systemic corticosteroids in the treatment of lichen planus: a randomized clinical trial. Iraji F, Faghihi G, Asilian A, Siadat AH, Larijani FT, Akbari M. J Res Med Sci 2011; 162: 1578–82.

In this randomized clinical trial, 46 patients were administered either prednisolone 0.3 mg/kg for 6 weeks ($n = 23$) or narrowband UVB (nbUVB) three times a week for 6 weeks ($n = 23$) with a maximum dose of 9 J/cm^2. More patients in the nbUVB group achieved complete response (12/23) compared with those in the steroid group (3/23) ($p < 0.05$). No side effects were reported.

Several other retrospective studies highlight the efficacy of UVB, especially nbUVB, for the treatment of generalized cutaneous lichen planus.

Psoralen plus UVA vs. UVB-311 nm for the treatment of lichen planus. Wackernagel A, Legat FJ, Hofer A, Quehenberger F, Kerl H, Wolf P. Photodermatol Photoimmunol Photomed 2007; 23: 15–9.

This retrospective chart review compared 15 patients treated with PUVA to 13 patients treated with nbUVB. Sixty-seven percent of the PUVA-treated patients achieved complete remission, and 33% achieved a partial clinical response. Thirty-one percent

442

of patients treated with nbUVB achieved complete remission and 46% a partial response. The mean duration of therapy was 10.5 weeks for PUVA and 8.2 weeks for nbUVB, and the mean number of treatments was 25.9 PUVA treatments compared with 22.5 nbUVB treatments. Lichen planus recurred in 47% of PUVA-treated patients but only in 30% of nbUVB-treated patients.

Long-term efficacy of PUVA treatment in lichen planus: comparison of oral and external methoxsalen regimens. Helander I, Jansen CT, Meurman L. Photodermatology 1987; 4: 265–8.

Good or excellent clearing occurred in 10 of 13 patients after 8 to 46 bath-PUVA treatments, compared with 5 of 10 patients after 8 to 30 oral PUVA treatments. However, examination of patients months after PUVA suggested that treatment might prolong the duration of lichen planus.

Methotrexate for treatment of lichen planus: old drug, new indication. Kanwar AJ, De D. J Eur Acad Dermatol Venereol 2013; 27: e410–3.

Twenty-four patients with generalized lichen planus were treated with oral methotrexate (15 mg/week in adults or 0.25 mg/kg/week for children). After 2 weeks, 7 patients (30%) had at least 50% improvement in disease severity. By the end of 24 weeks, 14 patients (58%) had complete remission. Fifty percent of patients reported side effects; most were mild and only 1 patient had to discontinue therapy due to abnormal liver function tests. There were no relapses during the 3 months' follow-up.

Third-Line Therapies

• Trimethoprim–sulfamethoxazole	E
• Griseofulvin	E
• Itraconazole	C
• Terbinafine	E
• Antimalarials	E
• Tetracycline or doxycycline	C
• Ciclosporin, FK 506	E
• Mycophenolate mofetil	E
• Azathioprine	E
• Etanercept	E
• Adalimumab	E
• Interferon	E
• 0.1% tacrolimus ointment	E
• Pimecrolimus cream	E
• Alitretinoin	E
• Thalidomide	D
• UVA1	D
• Low-molecular-weight heparin	B
• Apremilast	C

Antimicrobials

Treatment of lichen planus with Bactrim. Abdel-Aal H, Abdel-Aal MA. J Egypt Med Assoc 1976; 59: 547–9.

Oral trimethoprim–sulfamethoxazole, two tablets twice daily for 5 days, cleared lichen planus within 2 weeks only to have the skin lesions relapse 2 months later. The trimethoprim–sulfamethoxazole was again effective when readministered to patients who experienced relapse.

Histopathological evaluation of griseofulvin therapy in lichen planus: a double-blind controlled study. Sehgal VN, Bikhchandani R, Koranne RV, Nayar M, Saxena HM. Dermatologica 1980; 161: 22–7.

Griseofulvin 500 mg/day for 2 months was effective in 18 of 22 patients.

Pulsed itraconazole therapy in eruptive lichen planus. Khandpur S, Sugandhan S, Sharma VK. J Eur Acad Dermatol Venereol 2009; 23: 98–101.

Sixteen patients with eruptive lichen planus were treated with itraconazole 200 mg twice daily pulsed for 1 week each month for 3 months. By the end of the first month, 9 of 16 patients (56.25%) stopped developing new lesions. Only 9 of the patients were followed for 3 months, and 7 of the 9 (77.7%) stopped developing new lesions. All of the 9 patients reported improvement of pruritus, and 5 of the 9 had complete relief of pruritus. By the end of 3 months, partial flattening was present in 6 of 9 patients (66.66%) and complete flattening in 3 (33.33%).

Given the partial response seen at 3 months, longer therapy may be warranted.

The use of oral terbinafine or topical ciclopirox for lichen planus. Click JW, Wilson BB. Cutis 2009; 84: 42.

A patient with topical corticosteroid–refractory lichen planus was treated with terbinafine 250 mg daily for 3 weeks and the lichen planus cleared. Upon recurrence of the lichen planus, the terbinafine was again given for 3 weeks. The patient's lichen planus began to resolve within 3 days of restarting the oral terbinafine. A second patient with lichen planus was treated with ciclopiroxolamine cream for tinea pedis, and her lichen planus also resolved.

It is unclear why antifungal therapy is effective in the treatment of lichen planus, but there are numerous reports of various antifungal agents working for this condition.

Systemic immunosuppressive agents

Childhood actinic lichen planus: successful treatment with antimalarials. Ramírez P, Feito M, Sendagorta E, González-Beato M, De Lucas R. Australas J Dermatol 2012; 53: e10–3.

Lichen planus actinicus is a photosensitive variant that presents in sun-exposed areas of the body, including the face, V of the neck, and arms. This report documents an excellent response to hydroxychloroquine and photoprotection in an 8-year-old girl.

Successful treatment of resistant hypertrophic and bullous lichen planus with mycophenolate mofetil. Nousari HC, Goyal S, Anhalt GJ. Arch Dermatol 1999; 135: 1420–1.

Mycophenolate mofetil was reported to successfully treat resistant hypertrophic and bullous lichen planus.

Generalized severe lichen planus treated with azathioprine. Verma KK, Sirka CS, Khaitan BK. Acta Derm Venereol 1999; 79: 493.

Generalized severe lichen planus has been successfully treated with azathioprine.

Palmoplantar lichen planus with umbilicated papules: an atypical case with rapid therapeutic response to ciclosporin. Karakatsanis G, Patsatsi A, Kastoridou C, Sotiriadis D. J Eur Acad Dermatol Venereol 2007; 21: 1006–7.

A 63-year-old woman with lichen planus of the palms, forearms, soles, and feet was treated with ciclosporin 3.5 mg/kg daily. Pruritus improved within 2 weeks, and clinical improvement occurred within 4 weeks, at which point ciclosporin was tapered over the next 4 weeks.

In a different case report, a patient with 20 dystrophic fingernails noted improvement within 2 months of starting ciclosporin 3 mg/kg daily, but she required the addition of valsartan for hypertension.

Successful treatment of lichen planus with adalimumab. Holló P, Szakonyi J, Kiss D, Jokai H, Horváth A, Kárpáti S. Acta Derm Venereol 2012; 92: 385–6.

A 39-year-old woman with extensive lichen planus refractory to systemic corticosteroids, acitretin, and PUVA was treated with adalimumab 80 mg followed by 40 mg every other week. Pruritus decreased after 2 weeks, and skin lesions resolved within 2 months, leaving only hyperpigmentation.

Nail lichen planus: successful treatment with etanercept. Irla N, Schneiter T, Haneke E, Yawalkar N. Case Rep Dermatol 2010; 2: 173–6.

There are a number of case reports of lichen planus of the nails responding to treatment with TNF-α blockers. Unless the nail involvement is treated early, it is difficult to imagine that any therapy would reverse the pterygium that develops in late disease. There are also a number of reports of lichen planus induced by TNF-α blockers.

Other

Lichen planus and chronic hepatitis C: exacerbation of the lichen under interferon therapy. Areias J, Velho GC, Cerqueira R, Barbédo C, Amaral B, Sanches M, et al. Eur J Gastroenterol Hepatol 1996; 8: 825–8.

Given the association between lichen planus and hepatitis C, one might expect interferon to benefit both diseases. There are reports of interferon benefiting patients with lichen planus and exacerbating the condition in others.

Treatment of cutaneous lichen planus with thalidomide. Moura AK, Moure ER, Romiti R. Clin Exp Dermatol 2009; 34: 101–3.

Eight patients with cutaneous lichen planus were treated with thalidomide 100 mg daily at bedtime. Three patients withdrew because of transient neuropathy of the legs and transient weakness that began shortly after the treatment started. Five patients noted improvement of pruritus within a few days after starting thalidomide. Skin lesions regressed in a mean of 4 weeks, and complete remission was achieved in a mean of 3 months.

Ultraviolet A1 in the treatment of generalized lichen planus: a report of 4 cases. Polderman MC, Wintzen M, van Leeuwen RL, de Winter S, Pavel S. J Am Acad Dermatol 2004; 50: 646–7.

Four patients with refractory generalized lichen planus were treated with UVA1 45 J/cm² 5 days per week for two 4-week treatment periods with a 3-week rest in between. All four improved, with one patient achieving 98% clearance.

There is also a case report detailing the treatment of palmoplantar lichen planus with UVA-1 laser therapy three times a week for 4 weeks (100 J/cm²); the patient was still symptom free 1 year later.

Topical tacrolimus in the treatment of lichen planus in a child. Fortina AB, Giulioni E, Tonin E. Pediatr Dermatol 2008; 25: 570–1.

A child with lichen planus did not respond to topical corticosteroids, but her condition resolved upon treatment with tacrolimus 0.03% ointment.

Tacrolimus 0.1% has also been used successfully to treat lichen planus in adults. In addition, case reports describe the successful use of topical pimecrolimus for cutaneous lichen planus.

Comparison of therapeutic effect of low-dose low-molecular-weight heparin (enoxaparin) vs. oral prednisone in treatment of patients with lichen planus: a clinical trial. Iraji F, Asilian A, Saeidi A, Siadat AH, Saeidi AR, Hassanzadeh A. Adv Biomed Res 2013; 2: 76.

Patients were given subcutaneous enoxaparin 5 mg weekly ($n = 25$) or 0.5 mg/kg prednisone daily ($n = 23$) until complete remission or a maximum of 8 weeks. The average time until improvement was 25.2 ±13 days in the enoxaparin group compared with 9.7 ± 6 days in the oral prednisone group. In the enoxaparin group, 8 patients (32%) achieved complete remission, and 10 (40%) experienced partial improvement. In the oral prednisone group, 16 patients (69.6%) had complete remission, and 6 patients (26.1%) had partial improvement ($p < 0.05$). The mean lesion size after treatment was lower in the prednisone group ($p < 0.05$). The relapse rate was not significantly different between the enoxaparin and prednisone groups (33% vs. 40.9%, respectively). No serious complications were found in the enoxaparin group, whereas 22% of the patients on prednisone experienced side effects, with the most common being dyspepsia.

Response of recalcitrant lichen planus to alitretinoin in 3 patients. Brehmer F, Haenssle HA, Schön MP, Emmert S. J Am Acad Dermatol 2011; 65: e58–60.

One patient with a 15-year history of cutaneous lichen planus and severe pruritus, a second patient with oral lichen planus, and a third patient with cutaneous and mucocutaneous lichen planus were treated with alitretinoin. The first patient was treated with 30 mg daily, and the other two patients were treated with 10 mg daily. All three patients responded dramatically to the alitretinoin within 4 weeks.

Alitretinoin is a retinoid that was developed for the treatment of hand eczema. There are several case reports of efficacy in the treatment of lichen planus, including two patients with nail lichen planus. As with other retinoids, elevation of serum lipids can occur.

An open-label pilot study of apremilast for the treatment of moderate to severe lichen planus: a case series. Paul J, Foss CE, Hirano SA, Cunningham TD, Pariser DM. J Am Acad Dermatol 2013; 68: 255-61.

Ten patients were treated with 20 mg apremilast twice daily for 12 weeks. After 12 weeks, 3 patients (30%) had at least a two-grade improvement in Physician Global Assessment, but all 10 patients had improvements in secondary end points such as lesion count. There was no loss of benefit when patients were assessed 28 days after the end of treatment. There were no serious adverse events.

Evidence Levels: **A** Double-blind study **B** Clinical trial ≥ 20 subjects **C** Clinical trial < 20 subjects **D** Series ≥ 5 subjects **E** Anecdotal case reports

136

Lichen sclerosus

Fiona M. Lewis

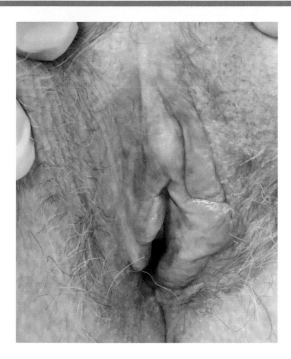

Lichen sclerosus (LS) is a chronic scarring dermatosis that has a predilection for the anogenital skin. It occurs in both sexes but is more common in females and has two peaks of incidence—in girls before puberty and in women after menopause. It can also affect the extragenital skin. It appears to be lymphocyte mediated, and there is a strong association with other autoimmune disorders and the presence of circulating antibodies in females but not in males. It is postulated that an inflammatory response to chronic exposure to urine in occluded skin may be an important etiologic factor in male genital lichen sclerosus. A small number of patients with genital LS (<5%) will develop a squamous cell carcinoma (SCC).

MANAGEMENT STRATEGY

The aims of management are to alleviate symptoms, reduce scarring and hence maintain function, and, by careful follow-up, to detect any premalignant and malignant change.

The most common symptom of LS in females is pruritus, but soreness and pain can occur if the skin fissures. In children, constipation is often the presenting symptom. White atrophic plaques are the typical clinical feature, with ecchymosis being a frequent observation. Occasionally, the plaques may be thickened and hyperkeratotic. Perianal involvement occurs in a figure-of-eight pattern in females but is hardly ever seen in men. If untreated, scarring will lead to changes in the vulval architecture. The labia minora may be resorbed, and the clitoral hood can seal. Narrowing of the introitus can cause dyspareunia, and fusion of the labia minora may eventually lead to difficulties with micturition.

In males, tightening of the foreskin causes phimosis and subsequently problems with sexual function. Meatal stenosis leads to difficulties with micturition.

Secondary pain syndromes can develop in both sexes, and it is important to recognize these sensory disorders (vulvodynia, penile dysesthesia), as management must be directed to these rather than alter the treatment for LS. Any psychosexual issues must be recognized and addressed.

The first-line treatment for LS in adults and children of both sexes is an ultrapotent topical steroid. The general recommended regimen is clobetasol propionate 0.05% ointment once a day for a month, on alternate days for a month, and then twice weekly for a further month. After this 3-month period, the patient can apply treatment once daily if any symptoms occur. A 30-g tube should last at least 3 months in an adult and 6 months in a child, but the majority of patients use much less than this. With successful treatment, the ecchymosis, fissuring, and hyperkeratosis should resolve and scarring should not progress. The pallor will often remain and any scarring present before treatment starts will not reverse. There is no direct evidence that shows that treatment can reduce the risk of developing an SCC.

Soap substitutes (e.g., emulsifying ointment) are helpful symptomatically, and barrier preparations are recommended if there is urinary incontinence. Stool softeners can be helpful in children if constipation is an issue.

In women, surgery is only recommended for excision of any malignant lesion that develops or to release labial adhesions that are causing severe introital narrowing. However, in males circumcision may be a very helpful part of management.

Specific Investigations

- Biopsy
- Autoimmune screen if clinically indicated

A diagnosis of LS can often be made on the classic clinical appearances. Biopsy is mandatory if there are unusual or atypical features or in those who have failed to respond to first-line treatment.

Light microscopic criteria for the diagnosis of early vulvar lichen sclerosus: a comparison with lichen planus. Fung MA, LeBoit PE. Am J Surg Pathol 1998; 22: 473–8.

Nine out of 68 cases of LS reviewed were found to have sections that showed a transition from a lichenoid reaction to pathognomonic LS (dermal sclerosis or edema), thus demonstrating the early histopathologic signs of LS. A psoriasiform lichenoid pattern, basilar epidermotropism, loss of papillary dermal elastic fibers, basement membrane thickening, and epidermal atrophy were shown to be much more suggestive of LS than lichen planus.

Association of autoimmune diseases with lichen sclerosus in 532 male and female patients. Kreuter A, Kryvosheyeva Y, Terras S, Moritz R, Mollenhoff K, Altmeyer P, et al. Acta Derm Venereol 2013;93(2):238-41.

Concomitant autoimmune disease and circulating autoantibodies were found significantly more often in females than males with LS.

First-Line Therapies

Ultrapotent topical steroids	A
Emollients	E
Use of soap substitutes	E

Topical interventions of genital lichen sclerosus. Chi CC, Kitschig G, Baldo M, Brackenbury F, Lewis F, Wojnarowska F. Cochrane Database Syst Rev 2011; 7: CD008240.

A Cochrane review, including seven randomly controlled trials with a total of 249 patients and investigating six treatments. This concluded that topical clobetasol propionate 0.05% and mometasone furoate were effective in treating LS, compared with placebo. No significant benefit was found for topical testosterone, dihydrotestosterone, and progesterone.

A double-blind, randomized prospective study evaluating topical clobetasol propionate 0.05% versus topical tacrolimus 0.1% in patients with vulvar lichen sclerosus. Funaro D, Lovett A, Leroux N, Powell J. J Am Acad Dermatol 2014; 71: 84–91.

In this randomized, double-blind controlled trial, 28 patients were treated with tacrolimus 1% ointment and 27 with clobetasol propionate 0.05% ointment once daily for 3 months. Signs and symptoms improved in both groups. However, clobetasol propionate was significantly more effective than tacrolimus.

The response of balanitis xerotica obliterans to local steroid application compared with placebo in children. Kiss A, Csontai A, Pirot L, Nyirady P, Merksz M, Kiraly L. Urol 2001; 165: 219–20.

A double-blind, placebo-controlled, randomized study of 40 boys comparing 0.05% mometasone furoate against placebo. The application of a potent topical steroid produced clinical improvement in phimosis in histologic early and intermediate disease and slowed deterioration in the late stages.

Treatment of vulval lichen sclerosus with topical corticosteroids in children: a study of 72 children. Casey G, Cooper S, Powell JJ. Clin Exp Dermatol 2015; 40: 289–92.

Sixty-two girls were treated prospectively with clobetasol propionate 0.05% ointment for 3 months. Ten others responded to a moderately potent steroid. 72.6% had complete resolution of symptoms compared with 32.2% of 31 patients who had used a moderately potent steroid.

First randomized trial of clobetasol propionate and mometasone furoate in the treatment of vulvar lichen sclerosus: results of efficacy and tolerability. Virgili A, Minghetti S, Corazza M, Borghi A. Brit J Dermatol 2014; 171: 388–96.

Fifty-four patients were randomized to apply clobetasol propionate 0.05% or mometasone furoate 0.1% on a tapering regimen for 12 weeks. Both showed equal efficacy with a response rate of 89% and were well tolerated.

Continuous versus tapering application of the potent topical corticosteroid mometasone furoate in the treatment of vulvar lichen sclerosus: results from a randomized trial. Borghi A, Corazza M, Minghetti S, Giulia T, Virgili A. Brit J Dermatol 2015; 173: 1381–6.

Sixty-four patients applied mometasone furoate 0.1% ointment on a reducing regimen over 12 weeks or continuously for 5 days per week. The response rate as reported by objective and subjective scores showed similar efficacy in both regimens.
This confirms that a tapering regimen is equally effective as continuous treatment.

Does treatment of vulvar lichen sclerosus influence its prognosis? Cooper S, Gao X-H, Powell JJ, Wojnarowska F. Arch Dermatol 2004; 140: 702–6.

A study of 327 females (74 children and 253 adults) with response to treatment recorded in 255 patients at least 3 months after the start of topical application. Symptoms improved in 96% of those treated with an ultrapotent topical steroid. Clinical signs were recorded in 253 patients; 23% showed a complete response with return of normal texture and color, 68% had a partial response, and 7% a poor response.

Second-Line Therapies	
• Circumcision	B
• Topical tacrolimus	B
• Topical pimecrolimus	A

Lichen sclerosus of the male genitalia and urethra: surgical options and results in a multicenter international experience of 215 patients. Kulkarni S, Barbagli G, Kirpekar D, Mirri F, Lazzeri M. Eur Urol 2009; 55: 945–54.

A large retrospective observational study comparing circumcision and/or meatotomy, one- or two-stage penile oral mucosal graft urethroplasty, and definitive perineal urethrostomy. Circumcision alone or together with meatotomy was successful in 100% of cases, meatotomy alone in 80%, and various forms of urethroplasty in 73% to 91%.
It is not stated whether any of these patients who required surgery for persistent phimosis had received any topical treatment first.

Multicenter, phase II trial on the safety and efficacy of topical tacrolimus ointment for the treatment of lichen sclerosus. Hengge UR, Krause W, Hofmann H, Stadler R, Gross G, Meurer M, et al. Br J Dermatol 2006; 155: 1021–8.

A prospective study of 84 patients (49 women, 32 men, and 3 girls) treated with 0.1% topical tacrolimus ointment twice daily for up to 24 weeks. Thirty-six percent had a complete, and 29% a partial, clinical response.
Topical calcineurin inhibitors decrease immune surveillance and can reactivate infection. There are therefore major concerns about using them in a disease such as LS where malignancy can develop.

A double-blind, randomized controlled trial of clobetasol versus pimecrolimus in patients with vulvar lichen sclerosus. Goldstein AT, Creasey A, Pfau R, Phillips D, Burrows LJ. J Am Acad Dermatol 2011; 64: 99e–104e.

A group of 38 women were treated for 12 weeks. Clobetasol propionate 0.05% was superior in improving inflammation as seen in posttreatment biopsies. Both treatments showed improvement in symptoms and a decreased clinical evaluation score.

Third-Line Therapies	
• Acitretin	A
• CO_2 laser	B

Acitretin for severe lichen sclerosus of male genitalia: a randomized, placebo controlled study. Ioannides D, Lazaridou E, Apalla Z, Sotiriou E, Gregoriou S, Rigopoulos D. J Urol 2010; 183: 1395–9.

Men (n = 52) with severe long-standing LS were treated with acitretin 35 mg/day or placebo for 20 weeks. A complete response was achieved in 36.4% vs. 6.3% of controls.

Evidence Levels: **A** Double-blind study **B** Clinical trial ≥ 20 subjects **C** Clinical trial < 20 subjects **D** Series ≥ 5 subjects **E** Anecdotal case reports

The double-blind nature of this study is limited because of the expected side effects of oral acitretin as opposed to placebo.

Is carbon dioxide laser treatment of lichen sclerosus effective in the long run? Windahl T. Scand J Urol Nephrol 2006; 40: 208–11.

A retrospective review of 62 men who had failed to respond adequately to a topical steroid, although the potency is not specified. They were treated with CO_2 laser (15–20 W output with defocused beam) with vaporization of macroscopically abnormal areas on the glans penis. Of 50 patients who were contacted up to 14 years after treatment, 80% had no symptoms or visible lesion. Two men were found to have SCC at follow-up.

Other Therapies

• Photodynamic therapy with 5-aminolevulinic acid	B
• Topical calcipotriol	B
• Topical tretinoin	B
• Oxatomide gel	B
• Topical testosterone	B
• Oral stanozolol	B
• Low-dose ultraviolet A1 phototherapy	C
• Antibiotics	D
• Intralesional triamcinolone	D
• Surgery for clitoral phimosis	D
• Cryosurgery	D
• Ciclosporin	D
• Potassium *p*-aminobenzoate	D
• Adipose-derived mesenchymal cells and platelet-rich plasma	D
• Focused ultrasound therapy	D
• Hydroxycarbamide	E
• Hydroxyurea	E
• Methotrexate	E
• Oral calcitriol	E
• Extracorporeal photopheresis	E

Low-dose ultraviolet A1 phototherapy for extragenital lichen sclerosus: results of a preliminary study. Kreuter A, Gambichler T, Avermaete A, Happe M, Bacharach-Buhles M, Hoffmann K, et al. J Am Acad Dermatol 2002; 46: 251–5.

A series of 10 patients (8 female and 2 male) were treated with low-dose (ultraviolet A1) four times a week for 10 weeks with a cumulative UVA1 dose of 800 J/cm². A marked reduction in clinical score, decrease in skin thickness, and increase in dermal density was seen in all patients who also reported a subjective improvement.

UVA1 phototherapy for genital lichen sclerosus. Beattie PE, Dawe RS, Ferguson J, Ibbotson SH. Clin Exp Dermatol 2006; 31: 343–7.

Five out of seven patients had moderate (three patients) or minimal (two patients) improvement after at least 15 treatments with UVA1 three to five times weekly.

The extragenital lesions of LS appear to respond better to UVA1. There are also concerns about an increased potential for the development of SCC with phototherapy.

Open-label trial of ciclosporin for vulvar lichen sclerosus. Bulbul Baskan E, Turan H, Tunali S, Cikman Toker S, Saricaoglu H. J Am Acad Dermatol 2007; 57: 276–8.

A retrospective study of five women with recalcitrant LS unresponsive to several topical treatments treated with ciclosporin 3 to 4 mg/kg/day for 3 months. An improvement in symptoms was seen in all patients. There was no relapse on discontinuation of the drug, and in the 12-month follow-up any recurrent symptoms were controlled with clobetasol dipropionate cream.

Again, there is a potentially increased risk of SCC with the use of immunosuppressants in LS.

Efficacy of photodynamic therapy in vulvar lichen sclerosus treatment based on immunohistochemical analysis of CD34, CD44, myeline basic protein and Ki67 antibodies. Olejek A, Steplewska K, Gabriel A, Kozak-Darmas I, Jarek A, Kellas-Sleczka S, et al. Int J Gynecol Cancer 2010; 20: 879–87.

One hundred women were treated with photodynamic therapy with improvement in signs and symptoms.

Treatment of lichen sclerosus with antibiotics. Shelley WB, Shelley ED, Amurao CV. Int J Dermatol 2006; 45: 1104–6.

A retrospective review of 15 patients (9 females and 4 males) treated with oral or intramuscular penicillin or cephalosporin for 3 to 21 months. Four patients cleared completely, and the rest reported an improvement in symptoms.

The rationale for using antibiotic therapy was based on the debatable evidence for an infectious etiology for LS, in particular, the possibility of Borrelia burgdorferi as a causative agent.

Lichen simplex chronicus

Michael Renzi, Lacy L. Sommer, Donald J. Baker

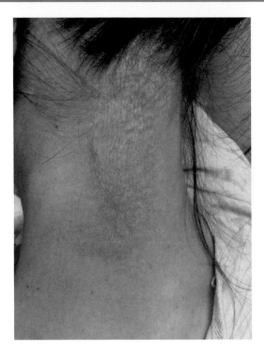

Lichen simplex chronicus (LSC, or neurodermatitis circumscripta) is characterized by pruritic, lichenified plaques that most often occur on the neck, anterior tibias, ankles, wrists, and anogenital region in response to chronic localized scratching or rubbing. Primary LSC evolves on apparently normal skin from pruritus of unclear etiology, whereas secondary LSC is superimposed upon preexisting dermatoses, especially atopic dermatitis, psoriasis, or dermatophytosis.

Psychogenic factors can play an important contributory role, and psychopathology, such as anxiety and obsessive-compulsive disorder, has been found at higher rates in LSC groups compared with control groups. Neurologic abnormalities may sometimes be a factor in the etiology of LSC, as an association between long-standing LSC on the limbs and chronic cervical or lumbar radiculopathy has been reported.

MANAGEMENT STRATEGY

The objective of treatment is to remove environmental triggers, break the itch–scratch cycle, and treat any underlying cutaneous or systemic disease. Patients' understanding of their role in the itch–scratch cycle is essential if their cooperation in avoiding scratching is to be enlisted, thereby facilitating a more complete and permanent recovery. Recurrences are frequent, and complete resolution often requires multiple approaches to therapy. Environmental triggers such as harsh skin care products or bathing regimens, friction, and excessive moisture or dryness should be minimized or eliminated. High-potency *topical corticosteroids*, such as clobetasol, diflorasone, and betamethasone, as creams

or ointments, are the initial treatments of choice. The potency and/or frequency of application of topical corticosteroids should be decreased as the lesion resolves to avoid atrophy with their long-term use. Adjunctive therapies such as *doxepin cream* may be introduced if topical corticosteroids are not easily tapered. Occlusion has been found to be a successful aid to therapy because it provides a physical barrier to prevent scratching and permits enhanced and prolonged application of topical medications. *Occlusive plastic film* or hydrocolloid dressings have been used alone or over mid-potency corticosteroids. *Flurandrenolide tape* is very effective as both an occlusive and antiinflammatory measure and is usually changed once daily, although a short occlusion-free period each day will help minimize the side effects of occlusion therapy. In chronic, difficult cases on the lower leg, an Unna boot (a gauze roll impregnated with zinc oxide) may be applied for up to 1 week, provided there is no concomitant infection of the occluded area. *Calcineurin inhibitors* such as *tacrolimus* and *pimecrolimus* also have been successfully used as monotherapy to treat LSC and offer a good alternative for treatment in steroid-sensitive areas such as the genitalia.

Intralesional injections of triamcinolone at monthly intervals can rapidly induce involution. Although highly effective, repeated injections may cause depigmentation or thinning of the epidermis; therefore other therapies should be used if several treatments with intralesional corticosteroids do not clear LSC. Infected areas should not be injected with corticosteroids because of the risk of abscess formation. Secondary infections should be treated with appropriate topical or systemic antibiotics. Intralesional *botulinum toxin* has been reported to offer lasting relief in patients with recalcitrant LSC.

A variety of other therapies have been reported to be effective in the management of LSC. *Doxepin cream, capsaicin cream,* and *aspirin/dichloromethane solution* are occasionally of value as monotherapy but are probably best used as adjunctive therapy when LSC does not quickly clear with topical or intralesional corticosteroids. *Oral antihistamines* may be useful for their sedative effect on patients who scratch during their sleep. *Surgical excision* has been used infrequently to treat nodular LSC. Noninvasive *transcutaneous electrical nerve stimulation (TENS)* has emerged as a possible effective treatment for pruritic dermatoses such as LSC. Pruritus and neuralgia of varying etiologies have responded to the anticonvulsant *gabapentin*, which may explain its usefulness in treating LSC. In more severe or recalcitrant conditions, *psychotherapy* and/or the use of *psychopharmacologic agents* may be needed for sustained improvement. *Benzodiazepines, amitriptyline, pimozide,* and *doxepin* have been used to treat neurotic excoriations and severe neurodermatitis. Neurodermatitis has improved with habit-reversal *behavioral therapy, biofeedback,* and *hypnotherapy* in certain individuals. *Acupuncture* and *electroacupuncture* are labor intensive but have been effective in treating some cases of LSC. *Alitretinoin* was used successfully in a single case of LSC on the hands. Adjuvant therapy with *narrowband ultraviolet B (UVB) phototherapy* and *silk fabrics* may prove useful for cases of vulvar LSC.

Specific Investigation

- Skin biopsy with periodic acid–Schiff stain

LSC that is atypical in appearance or poorly responsive to therapy should be biopsied and cultured to look for preexisting dermatoses and underlying cutaneous malignancy or infection. Squamous cell carcinoma, though rare, has been reported to develop within long-standing LSC. Lesions should be surveyed

Evidence Levels: A Double-blind study **B** Clinical trial ≥ 20 subjects **C** Clinical trial < 20 subjects **D** Series ≥ 5 subjects **E** Anecdotal case reports

carefully, and fixed plaques or proliferating nodules should raise suspicion for malignant transformation.

First-Line Therapies

• Topical corticosteroids	A
• Occlusion – flurandrenolide tape	C
• Intralesional corticosteroids	C

A double-blind, multicenter trial of 0.05% halobetasol propionate ointment and 0.05% clobetasol 17-propionate ointment in the treatment of patients with chronic, localized atopic dermatitis or lichen simplex chronicus. Datz B, Yawalkar S. J Am Acad Dermatol 1991; 25: 1157–60.

In 127 patients with chronic, localized atopic dermatitis or LSC, healing was reported in 65.1% of those treated with halobetasol propionate ointment (a superpotent group I topical corticosteroid) compared with 54.7% of those treated with clobetasol propionate (a weaker group I topical corticosteroid). Success rates, early onset of therapeutic effect, and adverse effects were similar in the two treatment groups.

Group I topical corticosteroids should not be used for more than 2 weeks. They are therefore best combined with adjuvant therapies such as topical doxepin or pimecrolimus cream.

Flurandrenolone tape in the treatment of lichen simplex chronicus. Bard JW. J Ky Med Assoc 1969; 67: 668–70.

Of the 18 patients in the study, 10 used flurandrenolone tape, and 8 used a topical corticosteroid preparation without occlusion. Lasting remissions were seen in 70% of those using the tape versus 25% of those using topical corticosteroids without occlusion. Duration of therapy is not mentioned.

The use of occlusion with topical corticosteroids is considered the treatment of choice for LSC despite the lack of adequate clinical trials.

Update on intralesional steroid: focus on dermatoses. Richards RN. J Cutan Med Surg 2010; 14: 19–23.

In the absence of any formal clinical studies since the 1960s, Richards compiled a review of peer-reviewed literature, six standard dermatology textbooks, and questionnaires from dermatologists to summarize the available information on the use of intralesional steroids in localized dermatoses. Pooled clinical experience is presented in this review, which suggests that triamcinolone acetonide 2.5 mg/mL administered in total doses of 7.5 to 20 mg intralesionally every 3 to 4 weeks has proven to be a safe, economical, and highly effective treatment for localized dermatoses such as LSC.

Corticosteroid injections are considered first-line therapy despite the lack of adequate controlled clinical trials.

Second-Line Therapies

• Doxepin cream	B
• Pimecrolimus cream	C
• Tacrolimus ointment	B
• Capsaicin cream	E

The antipruritic effect of 5% doxepin cream in patients with eczematous dermatitis. Doxepin Study Group. Drake LA, Millikan LE. Arch Dermatol 1995; 131: 1403–8.

A multicenter, double-blind trial conducted to evaluate the safety and antipruritic efficacy of 5% doxepin cream in patients with LSC ($n = 136$), nummular eczema ($n = 87$), or contact dermatitis ($n = 86$). Patients treated with doxepin versus vehicle had significantly greater pruritus relief. Of doxepin-treated patients, 60% experienced relief from pruritus within 24 hours with a response rate of 84% by the end of the study.

Pimecrolimus 1% cream for pruritus in postmenopausal diabetic women with vulvar lichen simplex chronicus: a prospective noncontrolled case series. Kelekci HK, Uncu HG, Yilmaz B, Ozdemir O, Sut N, Kelekci S. J Dermatolog Treat 2008; 19: 274–8.

Twelve postmenopausal diabetic women with vulvar LSC were treated with pimecrolimus 1% cream twice daily for 3 months. All patients experienced a statistically significant reduction in pruritus when evaluated at 4 weeks and 12 weeks. After 3 months of treatment, 10 women (83.3%) had a complete cure, and the pruritus was improved in the 2 remaining women.

Effective treatment of scrotal lichen simplex chronicus with 0.1% tacrolimus ointment: an observational study. Tan ES, Tan AS, Tey HL. J Eur Acad Dermatol Venereol 2015; 29: 1448–9.

In this prospective, observational study, 29 men presenting with scrotal LSC were treated with 0.1% tacrolimus ointment twice daily for 6 weeks. After treatment, there were statistically significant improvements ($p \leq 0.001$) in mean itch score, mean itch frequency, mean sleep score, degree of skin modification, and mean affected scrotal surface area. The mean onset of action was 3.5 days. Six patients experienced intolerable burning sensation and discontinued treatment.

Treatment of prurigo nodularis, chronic prurigo and neurodermatitis circumscripta with topical capsaicin. Tupker RA, Coenraads PJ, van der Meer JB. Acta Derm Venereol 1992; 72: 463.

In this small, open study, two patients with corticosteroid-unresponsive neurodermatitis circumscripta were treated with 0.25% capsaicin, applied five times daily, resulting in flatter lesions and marked relief of itching.

Third-Line Therapies

• Transcutaneous electrical stimulation	B
• Acupuncture and electroacupuncture	C
• Botulinum toxin	D
• Aspirin	A
• Gabapentin	D
• Psychotherapy	E
• Hypnosis	E
• Psychopharmacotherapy	E
• Surgical excision	E
• Alitretinoin	E
• Phototherapy	E
• Silk underwear	A

Use of transcutaneous electrical nerve stimulation for chronic pruritus. Mohammad Ali BM, Hegab DS, El Saadany HM. Dermatol Ther 2015: 28: 210–5.

Ten patients with atopic dermatitis (group I), 20 patients with LSC (group II), and 16 with chronic intractable pruritus from chronic liver disease (group III) had their most pruritic, distressing lesions treated with TENS. Treatment occurred during three 30-minute sessions each week and continued for a maximum of 12 sessions or until symptomatic resolution was obtained. The results showed statistically significant mean reductions in visual analog scale (VAS) scores at weeks 2 and 4 compared with baseline for all groups. At the 1-month follow-up mean reductions in visual analog itch scores from baseline remained statistically significant for groups I and II but were found to be statistically insignificant for group III.

Acupuncture treatment of 139 cases of neurodermatitis. Yang Q. J Tradit Chin Med 1997; 17: 57–8.

Acupuncture was used to treat 96 patients with localized neurodermatitis and 43 patients with generalized neurodermatitis. A course of treatment was 10 days, with 3- to 5-day rest periods between multiple courses of therapy. An 81% cure rate and 14% improvement rate were reported, but the number of courses of therapy and long-term follow-up were not specified.

Acupuncture and electroacupuncture (where acupuncture needles are stimulated with low-voltage, high-frequency stimulation) may be used to reduce the proinflammatory neuropeptide state in pruritic and inflamed skin and thereby promote a more normal state of neuropeptide homeostasis.

Botulinum toxin type A injection in the treatment of lichen simplex: an open pilot study. Heckmann M, Heyer G, Brunner B, Plewig G. J Am Acad Dermatol 2002; 46: 617–9.

Four patients received 20 units of botulinum toxin type A (100 U/mL) per 2 cm × 2 cm area of an LSC plaque. One week after injection, there was a noticeable reduction in pruritus. Three patients were free of itching, and the remaining patient had >50% reduction in itching. After 12 weeks, three patients remained asymptomatic.

The effect of topically applied aspirin on localized circumscribed neurodermatosis. Yosipovitch G, Sugeng M, Chan YH, Goon A, Ngim S, Goh CL. J Am Acad Dermatol 2001; 45: 910–3.

In this double-blind, crossover, placebo-controlled study, 29 patients with LSC were randomized to receive aspirin/dichloromethane solution treatment followed by placebo or vice versa. In the aspirin/dichloromethane treatment group 46% achieved a significant response, and 12% of the placebo group achieved a comparable improvement.

Therapeutic hotline: treatment of prurigo nodularis and lichen simplex chronicus with gabapentin. Gencoglan G, Inanir I, Gunduz K. Dermatol Ther 2010; 23: 194–8.

Five patients with LSC and four with prurigo nodularis refractory to antihistamines, corticosteroids, phototherapy, and antidepressants were treated with gabapentin. Gabapentin therapy was initiated at 300 mg/day and titrated up by 300 mg/day every 3 days to a final dose of 900 mg/day. Doses were subsequently decreased during a total treatment period ranging from 4 to 10 months. After 2 months, some reduction in pruritus was noted in all patients. Clinical improvement was maintained during the 3-month follow-up period after patients discontinued gabapentin. All patients had improvement in their pruritus, with residual itching responding to topical lubricants. Side effects were limited to tolerable sedation in some patients.

The behavioral treatment of neurodermatitis through habit-reversal. Rosenbaum MS, Ayllon T. Behav Res Ther 1981; 19: 313–8.

Four patients with neurodermatitis received a single treatment session in which they learned to substitute a competing response for their urges to scratch. There was a rapid reduction in scratching in all patients. At 6 months, scratching had been eliminated in one patient and markedly reduced in three patients.

Brief hypnotherapy of neurodermatitis: a case with 4-year followup. Lehman RE. Am J Clin Hypn 1978; 21: 48–51.

One patient with extensive neurodermatitis was treated with eight sessions of hypnotherapy. She was clear within 2 weeks after her last session and remained clear at 4-year follow-up.

Improvement of chronic neurotic excoriations with oral doxepin therapy. Harris BA, Sherertz EF, Flowers FP. Int J Dermatol 1987; 26: 541–3.

Two patients with chronic neurotic excoriations had improvement in symptoms and in clinical signs of their skin condition within several weeks of receiving oral doxepin (30–75 mg daily).

Nodular lichen simplex of the scrotum treated by surgical excision. Porter WM, Bewley A, Dinneen M, Walker CC, Fallowfield M, Francis N, et al. Br J Dermatol 2001; 144: 343–6.

Two patients with nodular LSC of the scrotum were treated by surgical excision of LSC plaques with remission lasting over 12 months.

Efficacy of treatment with oral alitretinoin in patient suffering from lichen simplex chronicus and severe atopic dermatitis of hands. D'Erme AM, Milanesi, N, Angoletii AF, Maio V, Massi D, Gola M. Dermatol Ther 2014; 27: 21–3.

One patient with LSC of the hands and underlying atopic dermatitis received alitretinoin 30 mg daily and topical emollients for 12 weeks. Substantial clinical improvement was achieved with no recurrence observed 4 months after the end of treatment.

Phototherapy for vulvar lichen simplex chronicus: an "off-label use" of comb light device. Virgili A, Minghetti S, Borghi A, Corazza M. Photodermatol Photoimmunol Photomed 2014; 30: 332–4.

One patient with vulvar LSC received narrowband UVB phototherapy with a 211-nm comblike instrument marketed for scalp dermatitis. Treatment was performed three times per week for 14 weeks with dose titration up to 980 mJ/cm^2. Clinical characteristics and symptoms began to improve after 4 weeks. Marked improvement was reported at 10 weeks with complete resolution at 14 weeks.

Effectiveness of silk fabric underwear as an adjuvant tool in the management of vulvar lichen simplex chronicus: results of a double-blind randomized controlled trial. Corazza M, Borghi A, Minghetti S, Toni G, Virgili A. Menopause 2015; 22:850-6.

In this double-blind study 20 women with vulvar LSC were entered into a 1-week, open-label, active treatment phase in which they applied 0.1% mometasone furoate (MMF) ointment once daily to the affected vulva. Participants entered a 4-week maintenance phase in which they were randomly assigned to wear either silk or cotton briefs. At the end of the maintenance phase, the silk group was shown to have fewer MMF applications, an increased mean symptom-free interval, and greater improvement in symptom severity compared with the cotton group.

138

Linear IgA bullous dermatosis

Neil J. Korman

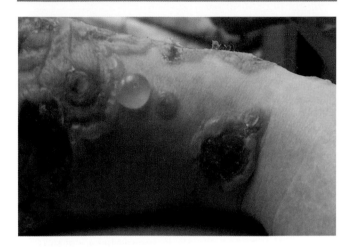

Linear IgA bullous dermatosis is an acquired autoimmune blistering disease of the skin and mucous membranes. The skin lesions consist of papulovesicles or blisters that may have an arcuate pattern, with a "cluster of jewels" grouping of blisters along with urticarial plaques. Involvement of the oral mucous membranes is common, and ocular involvement, with subsequent scarring of the conjunctiva, may uncommonly occur. Although originally believed to be a distinct entity, it is now clear that chronic bullous disease of childhood is the childhood counterpart of adult linear IgA bullous dermatosis. Direct immunofluorescence studies demonstrate that all patients have linear IgA deposits at the epidermal basement membrane zone, and the diagnosis of linear IgA bullous dermatosis is dependent on this finding. The target antigens involved are 97 kDa and, less commonly, 290 kDa. The 97-kDa antigen is an anchoring filament protein that is part of the 180-kDa bullous pemphigoid antigen-2, and antibodies directed against the 290-kDa protein represent an IgA response directed against type VII collagen. Several reports stress the association with ulcerative colitis. Drug-induced disease is a well-recognized entity, and vancomycin is the most commonly implicated agent.

MANAGEMENT STRATEGY

If drug-induced disease is considered, the suspect trigger drug must be withdrawn. Treatment of linear IgA bullous dermatosis is dictated by the severity of disease and the areas of involvement. All patients should be evaluated by an ophthalmologist to ensure the absence of ocular disease. Because linear IgA bullous dermatosis tends to be chronic, it is important to be aware of the potential not only for short-term, but also for long-term, toxicities in any treatment used. In addition, treatment of children with chronic bullous disease of childhood (the childhood counterpart of linear IgA bullous dermatosis of adults) requires special consideration to ensure that any medications used have no specific contraindications in children.

The majority of patients with disease limited to the skin will respond well to treatment with *dapsone*, and this is the first-line therapy for patients with linear IgA bullous dermatosis. Dapsone generally works quite rapidly, with responses often occurring in the first few days of starting the drug. It is most effective for the skin lesions of linear IgA bullous dermatosis, with the mucous membrane lesions being more resistant.

The dosage of dapsone for patients with linear IgA bullous disease should be individually titrated to determine the best dose that effectively controls the disease. Typically, initial dosages in adults range from 50 to 100 mg/day. If sufficient control is not achieved after 6 to 8 weeks, a higher dosage may be tried (as high as 150–200 mg/day), typically increasing the dose by 25 mg per month while monitoring laboratory studies. After disease control is attained, the dosage can then be slowly reduced to the minimum that maintains appropriate control.

Because of a dose-related oxidant stress on normal aging red blood cells, all patients treated with dapsone will experience some degree of hemolysis that is usually dose dependent. A reduction of approximately 2 to 3 g of hemoglobin is often observed. As long as this decrease is relatively gradual and patients have no history of cardiovascular disease or anemia, this is usually well tolerated. It is important to measure levels of glucose-6-phosphate dehydrogenase (G6PD) in patients to be treated with dapsone because those with a deficiency in this enzyme can develop severe hemolysis. Methemoglobinemia, which is also dosage dependent, occurs in most patients but is usually asymptomatic. More worrisome toxicities include bone marrow suppression and even agranulocytosis, which usually occurs early in the course of therapy, and a dapsone-induced neuropathy, which occurs more commonly in patients treated for several years with more than 200 mg of dapsone daily. Less commonly, hepatitis, nephritis, pneumonitis, erythema multiforme, and the dapsone hypersensitivity syndrome have all been reported.

For those patients who fail to achieve satisfactory control of their disease with dapsone as first-line therapy, it is often of value to add *systemic corticosteroids*. This combination is considered second-line therapy. The dosage of prednisone required is often in the 20-to 40-mg daily range. Often the addition of prednisone will not only cause significant clinical improvement, but it may also allow the dosage of dapsone to be reduced, thereby minimizing its potential toxicity.

Other viable second-line therapies include *colchicine, sulfapyridine*, and the combination of *doxycycline or minocycline* and *niacinamide plus sulfapyridine* at doses of approximately 1 to 3 g daily, and colchicine has been reported to be beneficial at doses of 1.0 to 1.5 mg daily. The combination of doxycycline or minocycline and niacinamide, usually at doses of 1.5 g of niacinamide and 200 mg of doxycycline or minocycline, has been used with success. Doxycycline and minocycline should not be used in children under 9 years of age because they can both permanently stain teeth.

Third-line therapies include sulfamethoxypyridazine, dicloxacillin, erythromycin, mycophenolate mofetil, azathioprine, ciclosporin, methotrexate, interferon-α, and intravenous immunoglobulin (IVIG). Toxicity profiles and financial considerations favor using erythromycin, dicloxacillin, or sulfamethoxypyridazine before treatment with the immunosuppressive agents or IVIG. Although there is a role for the use of rituximab in the treatment of most of the other autoimmune blistering diseases, there is a question as to whether rituximab is of value in the treatment of linear IgA bullous dermatosis.

Specific Investigations

- Skin biopsy of blister for histology
- Perilesional skin biopsy for direct immunofluorescence
- Indirect immunofluorescence
- Consider G6PD level before dapsone use
- Consider thiopurine methyl transferase estimation before azathioprine use
- Ophthalmology consult

Linear IgA disease in adults. Leonard JN, Haffenden GP, Ring NP, McMinn RM, Sidgwick A, Mowbray JF, et al. Br J Dermatol 1982; 107: 301–16.

A clinicopathological study of mucosal involvement in linear IgA disease. Kelly SE, Frith PA, Millard PR, Wojnarowska F, Black MM. Br J Dermatol 1988; 119: 161–70.

Cicatrizing conjunctivitis as predominant manifestation of linear IgA bullous dermatosis. Webster GF, Raber I, Penne R, Jacoby RA, Beutner EH. J Am Acad Dermatol 1994; 30: 355–7.

Chronic bullous disease of childhood, childhood cicatricial pemphigoid, and linear IgA disease of adults. A comparative study demonstrating clinical and immunopathologic overlap. Wojnarowska F, Marsden RA, Bhogal B, Black MM. J Am Acad Dermatol 1988; 19: 792–805.

Linear immunoglobulin A bullous dermatosis. Fortuna G, Marinkovich MP. Clin Dermatol 2012; 30: 38–50.

These are excellent reviews of the clinical and immunologic features of linear IgA bullous dermatosis.

Vancomycin-induced linear IgA bullous dermatosis. Baden LA, Apovian C, Imber MJ, Dover JS. Arch Dermatol 1988; 124: 1186–8.

Litt's Drug Eruption Reference Manual, 10th ed. (Taylor & Francis, New York, 2004) implicates acetaminophen, aldesleukin, amiodarone, ampicillin, atorvastatin, candesartan, captopril, carbamazepine, cefamandole, ceftriaxone, cotrimoxazole, ciclosporin, diclofenac, furosemide, glyburide, granulocyte–macrophage colony-stimulating factor, ibuprofen, interferon-α, lithium, metronidazole, naproxen, penicillins, phenytoin, piroxicam, rifampin, sulfamethoxazole, and vancomycin as drug triggers for linear IgA disease. The extent of disease may sometimes simulate toxic epidermal necrolysis.

The diagnosis of linear IgA bullous dermatosis requires routine histologic studies as well as direct and indirect immunofluorescence studies. Once the diagnosis is confirmed, laboratory studies to be obtained will depend on the specific treatment anticipated.

First-Line Therapy

• Dapsone	C

Linear IgA dapsone responsive bullous dermatosis. Wojnarowska F. J Roy Soc Med 1980; 73: 371–3.

One of the first reports of this condition and response to dapsone. Since then, most series have demonstrated dapsone to be the most effective first-line monotherapy.

Second-Line Therapies

• Dapsone and prednisone	D
• Sulfapyridine	C
• Colchicine	D
• Tetracycline and niacinamide	E

Colchicine as a novel therapeutic agent in chronic bullous dermatosis of childhood. Banodkar DD, Al-Suwaid AR. Int J Dermatol 1997; 36: 213–6.

Eight patients were given colchicine, five of whom showed complete remission within 4 to 6 weeks. The remaining three also responded but required concurrent steroids to maintain remission.

Treatment of pemphigus and linear IgA dermatosis with nicotinamide and tetracycline. Chaffins ML, Collison D, Fivenson DP. J Am Acad Dermatol 1993; 28: 998–1001.

Sublamina densa-type linear IgA bullous dermatosis successfully treated with oral tetracycline and niacinamide. Yomoda M, Komani A, Hashimoto T. Br J Dermatol 1999; 141: 608–9.

There are four reports of successful use of 2 g of tetracycline and 1.5 g of nicotinamide daily in adults only.

Third-Line Therapies

• Sulfamethoxypyridazine	E
• Dicloxacillin	E
• Flucloxacillin	E
• Erythromycin	E
• Trimethoprim–sulfamethoxazole	E
• Methotrexate	E
• Interferon-α	E
• Mycophenolate mofetil	E
• Azathioprine	E
• Ciclosporin	E
• IVIG	E
• Thalidomide	E
• Immunoabsorption	E

Sulphamethoxypridazine for dermatitis herpetiformis, linear IgA disease, and cicatricial pemphigoid. McFadden JP, Leonard JN, Powles AV, Rutman AJ, Fry L. Br J Dermatol 1989; 121: 759–62.

Reports of sulfamethoxypyridazine (0.25–1.5 g daily) use as monotherapy in four patients with linear IgA disease who were intolerant of dapsone.

Treatment of chronic bullous dermatosis of childhood with oral dicloxacillin. Skinner RB, Totondo CK, Schneider MA, Raby L, Rosenberg EW. Pediatr Dermatol 1995; 12: 65–6.

Chronic bullous disease of childhood: successful treatment with dicloxacillin. Siegfried EC, Sirawan S. J Am Acad Dermatol 1998; 39: 797–800.

Mixed immunobullous disease of childhood: a good response to antimicrobials. Powell J, Kirtschig G, Allen J, Dean D, Wojnarowska F. Br J Dermatol 2001; 144: 769–74.

Linear IgA bullous dermatosis responsive to trimethoprim-sulfamethoxazole. Peterson JD, Chan LS. Clin Exp Dermatol 2007; 32: 756–8.

Linear IgA disease: successful treatment with erythromycin. Cooper SM, Powell J, Wojnarowska F. Clin Exp Dermatol 2002; 27: 677–9.

Treatment of linear IgA bullous dermatosis of childhood with flucloxacillin. Alajlan A, Al-Khawajah M, Al-Sheikh O, Al-Saif F, Al-Rasheed S, Al-Hoqail I, et al. J Am Acad Dermatol 2006; 54: 652–6.

Antibiotics have been used largely in childhood disease and are a reasonable option because of their low toxicity.

Treatment of linear IgA bullous dermatosis of childhood with mycophenolate mofetil. Farley-Li J, Mancini AJ. Arch Dermatol 2003; 139: 1121–4.

Successful treatment of oral linear IgA disease using mycophenolate. Lewis MA, Yaqoob NA, Emanuel C, Potts AJ. Oral Surg Oral Med Oral Pathol Oral Radiol Endod 2007; 103: 483–6.

The adult dose is usually 35 to 45 mg/kg, which is about 1.5 g twice daily for a 75-kg adult.

Methotrexate and cyclosporine are of value in the treatment of adult linear IgA disease. Burrows NP, Jones RR. J Dermatol Treat 1992; 3: 31–3.

Linear IgA disease: successful treatment with cyclosporine. Young HS, Coulson IH. Br J Dermatol 2000; 143: 204–5.

Therapy-resistant blistering responding to ciclosporin 4 mg/kg daily.

Interferon alpha for linear IgA bullous dermatosis. Chan LS, Cooper KD. Lancet 1992; 340: 425.

High-dose intravenous immune globulin is also effective in linear IgA disease. Kroiss MM, Vogtt T, Landthaler M, Stolz W. Br J Dermatol 2000; 142: 582–4.

Successful treatment of linear IgA disease with salazosulphapyridine and intravenous immunoglobulins. Goebeler M, Seitz C, Rose C, Sitaru C, Jeschke R, Marx A, et al. Br J Dermatol 2003; 149: 912–4.

Upper aerodigestive tract complications in a neonate with linear IgA bullous dermatosis. Gluth MB, Witman PM, Thompson DM. Int J Pediatr Otorhinolaryngol 2004; 68: 965–70.

A newborn with skin involvement had life-threatening respiratory compromise from disease affecting the larynx, subglottis, trachea, and esophagus. Management with both tracheostomy and gastrostomy tube placement was necessary. Treatment included systemic corticosteroids, dapsone, and IVIG.

High-dose intravenous immunoglobulins for the treatment of autoimmune mucocutaneous blistering diseases: evaluation of its use in 19 cases. Segura S, Iranzo P, Martínez-de Pablo I, Mascaró JM Jr, Alsina M, Herrero J, et al. J Am Acad Dermatol 2007; 56: 960–7.

As the use of IVIG therapy for autoimmune blistering diseases has evolved, it has become clear that to obtain optimal results, patients should receive treatment with high-dose IVIG, defined as 2 g/kg per cycle, typically given at 4-week intervals.

Linear IgA bullous dermatosis of childhood: response to thalidomide. Madnani NA, Khan KJ. Indian J Dermatol Venereol Leprol 2010; 76: 427–9.

An 8-year-old boy demonstrated a dramatic response with thalidomide with total clearance in 1 month, and while on treatment he was disease free for 1 year. The authors postulate that thalidomide works by inhibition of interleukin-12, which is a potent proinflammatory cytokine. Development of neuropathy is a concern with long-term use.

Linear IgA disease: successful application of immunoadsorption and review of the literature. Kasperkiewicz M, Meier M, Zillikens D, Schmidt E. Dermatology 2010; 220: 259–63.

Immunoadsorption has been previously successfully applied in severe and/or otherwise treatment-resistant IgG-mediated immunobullous disorders.

139

Lipodermatosclerosis

Cecilia A. Larocca, Tania J. Phillips

Specific Investigations

- Biopsy
- Duplex ultrasound
- Laser Doppler scanning
- Ultrasound indentometry
- Capillary microscopy
- Magnetic resonance imaging

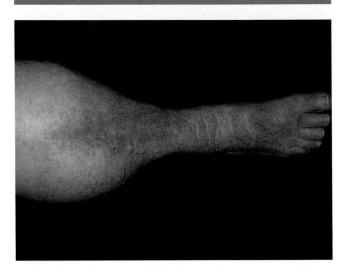

Lipodermatosclerosis (LDS) is the result of a progressive fibrotic process of the skin and subcutaneous fat induced by chronic venous insufficiency. It usually presents as a sclerotic region, often surrounding venous ulcers, above the medial malleolus on the lower leg. The diagnosis is based on clinical findings. LDS more often affects middle-aged to elderly obese women with venous abnormalities. Pain is the most consistent presenting symptom. Two stages of LDS have been described: acute and chronic. The acute form presents with painful, tender, and slightly indurated plaques. Often, clinicians mistake the acute form for cellulitis, phlebitis, erythema nodosum, inflammatory morphea, or panniculitis. The chronic variant, which is strongly associated with venous insufficiency, is densely indurated and less painful than the acute form. It may be associated with hyperpigmentation. In its late stages, chronic LDS alters the shape of the leg, making it look like an inverted bottle, with extreme fibrosis and sclerosis in the dermis and subcutaneous tissue. Acute or chronic presentations may also occur.

MANAGEMENT STRATEGY

The current treatment of choice is the *combination of stanozolol and compression therapy*. However, patients with acute LDS often find compression therapy painful. In this case stanozolol is used alone. Stanozolol is contraindicated in patients with uncontrolled hypertension and heart failure. Of note, although stanozolol is no longer commercially available in the United States, danazol has been used as an alternative. However, stanozolol is still available in Europe, and its purchase is unregulated online. *Pentoxifylline* is an alternative that stimulates fibrinolysis but may cause gastrointestinal upset. *Niacin* has some fibrinolytic properties and has also been used. Other treatments, such as *antibiotics, antiinflammatory agents, antimetabolites, and long-term cimetidine*, have also been proposed. Intralesional triamcinolone, platelet-rich plasma, and topical capsaicin may be helpful. *Surgical approaches* include *subfascial perforator endoscopic surgery (SEPS), perforator vein sclerotherapy, ultrasound therapy,* and *complete excision of LDS followed by split-thickness skin graft repair.*

The clinical spectrum of lipodermatosclerosis. Kirsner RS, Pardes JB, Eaglstein WH, Falanga V. J Am Acad Dermatol 1993; 28: 623–7.

The diagnosis of LDS is based on clinical findings. In most cases, biopsy is not advised because 50% of biopsy sites do not heal.

Acute lipodermatosclerosis is associated with venous insufficiency. Greenberg A, Hasan A, Montalvo BM, Falabella A, Falanga A. J Am Acad Dermatol 1996: 35: 566–8.

One third to one fifth of patients with acute LDS lack evidence of venous disease with routine venous evaluation. Chronic LDS may present after or independently of acute LDS.

Lipodermatosclerosis: the histologic spectrum with clinical correlation to the acute and chronic forms. Hurwitz D, Kirsner RS, Falanga V, Elgard GW. J Clin Pathol 1996; 23: 78.

Biopsy specimens of acute LDS showed little epidermal change or capillary proliferation. In the subcutis, there was lobular and septal panniculitis with eosinophils, fibrin thrombi, and purpura. Biopsies of chronic LDS showed dermal changes associated with venous insufficiency, including capillary proliferation, hemosiderin deposition, and fibrosis. Epidermal hypertrophy was also found.

Lipodermatosclerosis: a clinicopathological study of 25 cases. Walsh SN, Santa Cruz DJ. J Am Acad Dermatol 2010; 62: 1005–12.

Biopsies may distinguish LDS from other fibrosing entities. Most cases show pseudoxanthoma elasticum–like elastic fiber calcification within the septae.

Skin iron deposition characterises lipodermatosclerosis and leg ulcer. Caggiati A, Rosi C, Casini A, Cirenza M, Petrozza V, Acconcia MC, et al. Eur J Vasc Endovasc Surg 2010; 40: 777–82.

Lipodermatosclerosis is always accompanied by hemosiderin deposition.

Duplex venous imaging: role for a comprehensive lower extremity examination. Badgett DK, Comerota MC, Khan MN, Eid IG, Kerr RP, Comerota AJ. Ann Vasc Surg 2000; 14: 73–6.

Results of duplex scanning of 205 lower extremities with varices: 106 not previously operated and 99 previously operated for varicose veins. Egeblad K, Baekgaard N. Ugeskr Laeger 2003; 3016–8.

Color duplex ultrasound can accurately detect the specific location of lower extremity venous insufficiency that often leads to LDS.

Quantifying fibrosis in venous disease: mechanical properties of lipodermatosclerosis and healthy tissue. Geyer MJ, Brienza DM, Chib V, Wang J. Adv Skin Wound Care 2004; 17: 131–42.

Evidence Levels: **A** Double-blind study **B** Clinical trial ≥ 20 subjects **C** Clinical trial < 20 subjects **D** Series ≥ 5 subjects **E** Anecdotal case reports

Ultrasound indentometry was used to quantify fibrotic tissue in LDS.

Excision of lipodermatosclerotic tissue: an effective treatment for non-healing venous ulcer. Ahnlide I, Bjellerup M, Akesson H. Acta Derm Venereol 2000; 80: 28–30.

In seven cases, laser Doppler scanning showed an increase in blood flow in lipodermatosclerotic skin, which decreased after surgical removal of the affected area.

Microangiopathy in chronic venous insufficiency: quantitative assessment by capillary microscopy. Howlader MH, Smith PD. Eur J Vasc Endovasc Surg 2003; 26: 325–31.

Advanced venous disease (LDS and healed ulcer) was associated with a reduced number of capillaries and increased capillary convolution.

Magnetic resonance imaging as a diagnostic tool for extensive lipodermatosclerosis. Chan CC, Yang CY, Chu CY. J Am Acad Dermatol 2008; 58: 525–7.

In a single case, magnetic resonance imaging (MRI) was in agreement with histopathologic findings. Additional studies are necessary to validate this technique.

First-Line Therapies

• Compression therapy	A
• Stanozolol	B
• Compression therapy plus stanozolol	B
• HR (O-[beta-hydroxymethyl]-rutosides)	B

The clinical spectrum of lipodermatosclerosis. Kirsner RS, Pardes J, Eaglstein WH, Falanga VJ. Am Acad Dermatol 1993; 28: 623–7.

Traditionally LDS has been treated with compression using graded stockings or elastic bandages. The authors suggest open-toe and below-the-knee graded stockings, with 30- to 40-mm Hg pressure. Stockings with a zipper in the back are easier for elderly patients to use. Patients with acute LDS often have too much pain to use compression stockings; in these patients, stanozolol 2 mg twice daily dramatically reduced pain and tenderness.

Graduated compression stockings reduce lipodermatosclerosis and ulcer recurrence. Vandongen YK, Stacey MC. Phlebology 2000; 25: 33–7.

A randomized controlled trial of 150 patients showed that elastic stockings alone can improve the skin changes of LDS and lower risk of recurrence.

Removal of dermal edema with class I and II compression stockings in patients with lipodermatosclerosis. Gniadecka M, Karlsmark T, Bertram A. J Am Acad Dermatol 1998; 39: 966–70.

In this study, ultrasonography demonstrated that low levels of compression, class I (18–26 mm Hg), in lipodermatosclerosis are as effective as class II (26–36 mm Hg) in the removal of dermal edema.

Venous lipodermatosclerosis: treatment by fibrinolytic enhancement and elastic compression. Burnand K, Clemenson G, Morland M, Jarrett PE, Browse NL. Br Med J 1980; 280: 7–11.

Stanozolol 5 mg twice daily with compression was shown to reduce extravascular fibrin and area of LDS but not leg dimensions. Patients reported improvement in LDS but could not distinguish response during placebo from stanozolol treatment.

Patients taking stanozolol should be carefully monitored for excessive fluid retention, hirsutism, acne, liver function, and plasma fibrinogen concentration. Stanozolol is contraindicated in patients with uncontrolled hypertension or congestive heart failure.

Acute lipodermatosclerosis: an open clinical trial of stanozolol in patients unable to sustain compression. Vesikovic J, Medenica LJ, Pavlovic MD. Dermatol Online J 2008; 14: 1.

In an open trial of 17 patients, stanozolol 2 mg twice daily, without compression, decreased pain and dermal thickness.

HR (Paroven, Venoruton; O-(beta-hydroxyethyl)-rutosides) in venous hypertensive microangiopathy. Incandela L, Belacaro G, Renton S, DeSanctis MT, Cesarone MR, Bavera P, et al. J Cardiovasc Pharmacol Ther 2002; 7: S7–10.

HR reduced signs and symptoms of chronic venous insufficiency and LDS.

Second-Line Therapies

• Superficial venous surgery	B
• Subfascial perforator endoscopic surgery (SEPS)	C
• Pentoxifylline	C

Long term results of compression therapy alone versus compression plus surgery in chronic venous ulceration (ESCHAR): randomised controlled trial. Gohel MS, Barwell JR, Taylor M, Chant T, Foy C, Earnshaw JJ, et al. BMJ 2007; 335: 83.

Surgical correction of superficial venous reflux (saphenous vein ablation) with compression reduced ulcer recurrence at 4 years compared with treatment with compression alone.

The effects on LDS were not specifically mentioned in this study.

Midterm results of endoscopic perforator vein interruption for chronic venous insufficiency: lessons learned from the North American Subfascial Endoscopic Perforatory Surgery registry. Gloviczki P, Bergan JJ, Rhodes JM, Canton LG, Harmsen MS, Ilstrup DM. J Vasc Surg 1999; 29: 489–502.

In this prospective registry of 148 patients who underwent SEPS ablations for LDS, patients reported improved overall LDS symptoms, including less pain, edema, and hyperpigmentation, as well as more rapid ulcer healing. Seventy-one percent of patients had a concomitant venous procedure (e.g., saphenous vein ablation).

Pentoxifylline for treating venous leg ulcer. Jull AB, Waters J, Arroll B. Cochrane Database Syst Rev 2002; 1: CD001733.

Pentoxifylline is a dimethylxanthine derivative that increases red blood cell flexibility, alters fibroblast physiology, and stimulates fibrinolysis. The dose of 400 mg three times daily may be increased to 800 mg three times daily if no improvement occurs.

Pentoxifylline is a good alternative in those intolerant to stanozolol. Side effects include nausea, dizziness, heartburn, and, occasionally, vomiting.

Third-Line Therapies

• Ultrasound	D
• Excision of lipodermatosclerotic tissue	D
• Intralesional triamcinolone injections	D
• Hydroxychloroquine	D
• Danazol	E
• Oxandrolone	E
• Niacin	E
• Sclerotherapy	E
• Antibiotics	E
• Intralesional platelet-rich plasma	E
• Topical capsaicin	E

Ultrasound therapy for lipodermatosclerosis. Damian DL, Yiasemides E, Gupta S, Armour K. Arch Dermatol 2009; 145: 330–2.

Eight patients treated with 3-MHz continuous ultrasound three times weekly for 4 to 8 weeks showed decreased skin hardness and erythema. Patients also wore grade II compression stockings.

Excision of lipodermatosclerotic tissue: an effective treatment for nonhealing venous ulcer. Ahnlide I, Bjellerup M, Akesson H. Acta Derm Venereol 2000; 80: 28–30.

In this combined retrospective and prospective study, six of seven patients' nonhealing venous ulcers healed after excision of lipodermatosclerotic tissue and split-skin graft.

Surgical removal of ulcer and lipodermatosclerosis followed by split-skin grafting (shave therapy) yields good long-term results in "non-healing" venous leg ulcers. Schmeller W, Gaber Y. Acta Derm Venereol 2000; 80: 267–71.

In 41 patients with LDS and recalcitrant leg ulcers, despite prior treatment with compression and surgical venous ablation, shave excision with meshed split-thickness skin grafts demonstrated 67% ulcer healing at an average follow-up of 2.4 years.

Intralesional triamcinolone in the management of lipodermatosclerosis. Campbell LB, Miller OF 3rd. J Am Acad Dermatol 2006; 55: 166–8.

A retrospective chart review of 28 patients showed improvement in pain, erythema, edema, and induration after one to three intralesional injections of 5 to 10 mg/mL triamcinolone.

Adjunct therapies were used in the majority of the patients.

Lipodermatosclerosis: improvement noted with hydroxychloroquine and pentoxifylline. Choonhakarn C, Chaowattanapanit S. J Am Acad Dermatol 2012; 66: 1013–4.

A retrospective chart review of 32 patients showed improvement in pain, erythema, edema, and induration after treatment with hydroxychloroquine (maximum <6.5 mg/kg/d) and pentoxifylline (1200 mg/d) within 2 weeks to 6 months.

An acute case of lipodermatosclerosis successfully treated with danazol. Hammerman S, Mamakos L, Falanga V. J Am Acad Dermatol 2012; 66 (Suppl 1): AB42.

One patient with LDS resistant to leg elevation, aspirin, and niacin was treated with oral danazol, with improvement of pain and disease extension. With 100 mg twice daily, erythema and induration also improved. After 4 months, the patient transitioned to compression only without recurrence of LDS.

Danazol is an anabolic androgen, with fibrinolytic activity similar to stanozolol.

Lipodermatosclerosis: successful treatment with danazol. Hafner C, Wimmershoff M, Lanthaler M, Vogt T. Acta Derm Venereol 2005; 85: 365–6.

Pain and induration from LDS improved after administration of 400 mg oral danazol daily.

Treatment of lipodermatosclerosis with oxandrolone in a patient with stanozolol-induced hepatotoxicity. Segal S, Cooper J, Bolognia J. J Am Acad Dermatol 2000; 43: 558–9.

Oxandrolone is another anabolic androgen similar to stanozolol with known fibrinolytic activity but with a lower incidence of hepatotoxicity. A single patient with LDS initially improved within 2 weeks with stanozolol (2 mg daily) but developed hepatotoxicity. Oxandrolone 10 mg twice daily reduced pain and induration of the legs with 3 months of treatment.

Lipid lowering and enhancement of fibrinolysis with niacin. Holvoet P, Collen D. Circulation 1995; 92: 698–9.

Niacin, at 100 to 150 mg three to five times a day, improved the hyperlipidemia often associated with LDS. In large doses it causes vasodilation and stimulates fibrinolysis.

Niacin is another alternative for patients who cannot tolerate stanozolol.

The effect of ultrasound-guided sclerotherapy (UGS) of incompetent perforator veins on venous clinical severity and disability scores. Masuda EM, Kessler DM, Lurie F, Puggioni A, Kistner RL, Eklof B. J Vasc Surg 2006; 43: 551–6.

In this 68-patient series, ultrasound-guided sclerotherapy (UGS) was an effective modality in the treatment of incompetent perforator veins and associated venous hypertension.

Severe chronic venous insufficiency treated by foamed sclerosant. Pascarella L, Bergan JJ, Mekenas LV. Ann Vasc Surg 2006; 20: 83–91.

In this prospective study, sclerotherapy with 1% to 3% polidocanol foam with compression is superior to compression alone for venous ulcer healing.

Lipodermatosclerosis is not specifically addressed.

Hypodermatitis sclerodermiformis and unusual acid-fast bacteria. Cantwell A, Kelso D, Rowe L. Arch Dermatol 1979; 115: 449–52.

There is little evidence to support the use of antibiotics, antiinflammatory agents, or antimetabolites.

Refractory lipodermatosclerosis treated with intralesional platelet-rich plasma. Jeong K, Shin M, Kim N. J Am Acad Dermatol 2011; 65: e157–8.

This is a single case report of LDS and recalcitrant venous leg ulcer treated intralesionally with the patient's own platelet-rich plasma. Ulcer healing occurred with improvement in LDS and no ulcer recurrence over 6 months.

Topical capsaicin for the treatment of acute lipodermatosclerosis and lobular panniculitis. Yosipovitch G, Mengesha Y, Facliaru D, David M. J Dermatolog Treat 2005; 16: 178–80.

Two cases of acute LDS resolved with topical capsaicin 0.075% applied five times daily to an area pretreated with topical anesthetic EMLA (eutectic mixture of lidocaine 2.5% and prilocaine 2.5%). Mechanism of action is unclear.

Evidence Levels: **A** Double-blind study **B** Clinical trial ≥ 20 subjects **C** Clinical trial < 20 subjects **D** Series ≥ 5 subjects **E** Anecdotal case reports

140

Livedo reticularis

Ruwani P. Katugampola, Andrew Y. Finlay

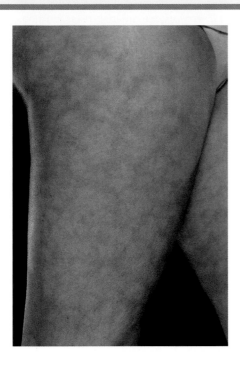

Livedo reticularis (LR) is the netlike, mottled, violaceous discoloration of the skin secondary to dilatation and stagnation of blood within dermal capillaries. The unaffected normal-colored islands of skin are the areas where blood supply is sufficient; in the network areas the supply is insufficient. This commonly occurs on the legs, arms, and trunk, but can be diffuse, and is more pronounced after exposure to cold. LR can be physiologic (cutis marmorata), can occur as a primary phenomenon (idiopathic LR), or secondary to a number of diseases that cause dermal vessel wall thickening and/or lumen occlusion. Secondary causes of LR include systemic lupus erythematosus, polyarteritis nodosa, antiphospholipid syndrome cryoglobulinemia, oxalosis, cholesterol emboli, hypercalcemia (secondary to malignancy, hyperparathyroidism, renal failure), underlying malignancy (as a paraneoplastic phenomenon), and medications. Idiopathic LR may be congenital (cutis marmorata telangiectatica congenita) or associated with painful ulcers (livedoid vasculitis) or with cerebrovascular involvement (Sneddon syndrome). LR has been reported as a paraneoplastic phenomenon associated with metastatic breast cancer, renal cell carcinoma, and multiple myeloma. LR has also been reported as a complication of accidental intraarterial filler injections, such as hyaluronic acid fillers and use of silicone implants for soft tissue augmentation.

MANAGEMENT STRATEGY

The etiology of physiologic and primary LR is unknown, and no definitive treatment is available. The management of primary LR depends on the presence of associated ulcers (anomalies [congenital form]) and systemic involvement (Sneddon syndrome). In secondary LR, the underlying cause needs to be identified and treated.

Physiologic LR, which occurs in healthy children and adults in response to cold weather, is diffuse, mild, temporary, and usually asymptomatic. No specific treatment is required for this condition except *avoidance of cold exposure*, protection from cold exposure with *warm clothing*, and *rewarming* the affected area.

Cutis marmorata telangiectatica congenita is rare and presents at birth or soon after birth. A small proportion of affected children have associated congenital anomalies such as hemangiomas, glaucoma, limb atrophy, cardiac malformation, or psychomotor retardation that need to be identified and referred for appropriate specialist care. The LR in these children usually spontaneously disappears or markedly improves with age.

Patients with Sneddon syndrome are at risk of cerebrovascular disease and may benefit from *antithrombotic treatment*. The timing of such treatment is debated, as LR may precede the neurologic events by up to 10 or more years. Advice regarding other risk factors predisposing to cerebrovascular events such as smoking, obesity, hypertension, and oral contraceptives is important.

Although a number of agents, including antiplatelet therapy, danazol, pentoxifylline, and systemic steroids, have been used to treat ulcers associated with LR, no single agent has been shown to completely resolve the LR itself.

Several medications, including those used in dermatology, have been associated with LR. The decision to withdraw the suspected medication should be based on the clinical judgment, alternative treatments, and other side effects rather than the appearance of LR per se.

Specific Investigations

- Skin biopsies for microscopy and direct immunofluorescence (adults)
- Full blood count and renal function
- Rheumatologic serologic tests
- Cryoglobulin level
- Anticardiolipin antibodies
- Coagulation screen
- Serum lipid profile
- Serum calcium

A detailed clinical history followed by physical examination is essential, especially in diagnosing Sneddon syndrome, identifying congenital anomalies in infants, and in excluding secondary causes of LR. The histology of LR is noninflammatory thickening of dermal vessel walls with eventual occlusion of the lumen.

Livedo reticularis and related disorders. Dean SM. Curr Treat Options Cardiovasc Med 2011; 13: 179–91.

Livedo reticularis: a review of the literature. Sajjan VV, Lunge S, Swamy MB, Pandit AM. Indian Dermatol Online J 2015; 6: 315–21.

Both of these reviews of LR include an extensive list of its systemic associations. The authors conclude that management of secondary LR should be directed toward the underlying cause and that all patients with either primary or secondary LR should be encouraged to avoid the use of tobacco and vasoconstricting medications.

Livedo reticularis: an update. Gibbs MM, English JC, Zirwas MJ. J Am Acad Dermatol 2005; 52: 1009–19.

The authors of this review conclude that several deep punch biopsies, at least one from the central normal skin and one from the peripheral violaceous skin, be obtained to identify causes of secondary LR. In addition to cold avoidance, limb elevation and compression stockings are suggested for symptomatic patients based on the authors' clinical experience.

The histopathological characteristics of livedo reticularis. In SI, Han JH, Kang HY, Lee ES, Kim YC. J Cutan Pathol 2009; 36: 1275–8.

A survey of 16 patients with LR concluded that multiple skin biopsies from both the peripheral erythematous and central whitish areas in LR increase diagnostic yield.

Diagnostic impact and sensitivity of skin biopsies in Sneddon's syndrome. A report of 15 cases. Wohlrab J, Fisher M, Wolter M, Marsch WC. Br J Dermatol 2001; 145: 285–8.

Deep 4-mm punch biopsies from the central white part of the LR demonstrated a sensitivity of 27% with one biopsy, 53% with two biopsies, and 80% with three biopsies of diagnosing Sneddon syndrome in clinically suspected cases. The authors concluded that the positive histology was important for commencing prophylaxis of cerebrovascular events in patients initially presenting with LR.

Livedo reticularis: an underutilized diagnostic clue in cholesterol embolization syndrome. Chaudhary K, Wall BM, Rasberry RD. Am J Med Sci 2001; 321: 348–51.

Six out of 8 patients with unexplained acute renal failure due to suspected cholesterol emboli syndrome (CES) demonstrated cholesterol emboli in skin biopsies of LR. Deep skin biopsies of LR are proposed as a safe diagnostic procedure to confirm CES, thus avoiding increased morbidity associated with biopsy of visceral organs.

The spectrum of livedo reticularis and anticardiolipin antibodies. Asherson RA, Mayou SC, Merry P, Black MM, Hughes GRV. Br J Dermatol 1989; 120: 215–21.

In this retrospective study of 65 patients with LR (idiopathic and secondary), there was a statistically significant increase in the incidence of strokes, transient ischemic attacks, venous thrombosis, fetal loss, and valvular heart disease in 28 anticardiolipin-positive patients compared with 37 anticardiolipin-negative patients.

First-Line Therapy	
• Aspirin	**D** (Sneddon syndrome)

Sneddon's syndrome: generalized livedo reticularis and cerebrovascular disease – importance of hemostatic screening. Devos J, Bulcke J, Degreef H, Michielsen B. Dermatology 1992; 185: 296–9.

Two cases of Sneddon syndrome are described, one of whom was shown to have twice the normal level of tissue plasminogen activator antigen, fourfold the normal level of plasminogen activator inhibitor, abnormal thrombin time, and elevated levels of factor XII during a neurologic event. Aspirin was commenced at 300 mg daily with normalization of the hemostatic parameters after 4 months of treatment and freedom from neurologic symptoms at 10 months.

There was no change to the patient's LR with aspirin treatment.

Second-Line Therapies	
• Corticosteroids	**D**
• Psoralen plus ultraviolet A phototherapy (PUVA)	**D**
• Pentoxifylline + methylprednisolone	**E**

Cholesterol emboli syndrome in type 2 diabetes: the disease history of a case evaluated with renal scintigraphy. Piccoli GB, Sargiotto A, Burdese M, Colla L, Bilucaglia D, Magnano A, et al. Rev Diabetic Stud 2005; 2: 92–6.

A 75-year-old obese, diabetic, hypertensive man with moderate dyslipidemia who developed CES after endovascular intervention manifesting as acute renal failure and LR of both feet. Methylprednisolone 300 mg intravenously for 3 days followed by oral prednisolone 25 mg daily and tapered over 2 months, commenced in view of deteriorating renal function, resulted in improvement in serum creatinine and disappearance of LR within 2 days of starting treatment.

Livedo reticularis and livedoid vasculitis responding to PUVA therapy. Choi HJ, Hann SK. J Am Acad Dermatol 1999; 40: 204–7.

Two patients with ulcers due to livedoid vasculitis of the lower legs resistant to treatment with other systemic treatment, including aspirin, prednisolone, and pentoxifylline, were treated with systemic PUVA using methoxsalen. Only the lower legs were exposed to UVA initially with 4 J/cm^2 three times a week and subsequent 1 J/cm^2 increments. No significant ulcers had recurred at 3 and 6 months, follow-up of the two patients after the last treatment. Improvement in the discoloration of the skin affected by LR was noted in one of the patients at completion of PUVA treatment.

Widespread livedoid vasculopathy. Marzano AV, Vanotti M, Alessi E. Acta Derm Venereol 2003; 83: 457–60.

A 37-year-old woman with widespread LR and recurrent painful ulcers on all limbs, trunk, and scalp was treated with intravenous methylprednisolone 80 mg/day for 5 days, followed by intramuscular and subsequent tapering oral dose to 32 mg/day and with pentoxifylline 400 mg twice daily for 2 months. There was a marked clinical improvement within 2 weeks of treatment, and the intensity of the LR faded but did not completely resolve.

Third-Line Therapies	
• Chemical lumbar sympathectomy	**C**
• Withdrawal of causative medications (minocycline, interferon α2b, or amantadine)	**D**
• Simvastatin	**E**

Chemical lumbar sympathectomy in the treatment of idiopathic livedo reticularis. Wang WH, Zhang L, Li X, Zhao J, Zhuang JM, Dong GX. J Vasc Surg 2015; 62: 1018–22.

Ten women with idiopathic LR were treated with L3–4 chemical lumbar sympathectomy (CLS) using 5% phenol, 2 mL in each injection site. Seven patients were "clear or almost clear" of LR after CLS; LR recurred in two of these patients ≤1 year during follow-up, but achieved "clear or almost clear" skin after repeat CLS.

The women recruited for this study were bothered by the social inhibition caused by LR and "showed a very strong desire for treatment by seeking medical treatment at least twice and waiting for at least 1 week to make a decision" [to have the procedure].

Minocycline induced arthritis associated with fever, livedo reticularis and pANCA. Elkayam O, Yaron M, Caspi D. Ann Rheum Dis 1996; 55: 769–71.

Three women treated with long courses of oral minocycline for acne developed LR of the lower legs associated with fever and arthritis/arthralgia associated with elevated titers of perinuclear neutrophil antibodies (pANCA) during treatment. Symptoms resolved after discontinuation of treatment but recurred after

Evidence Levels: A Double-blind study B Clinical trial ≥ 20 subjects C Clinical trial < 20 subjects D Series ≥ 5 subjects E Anecdotal case reports

rechallenge. The specific outcome of LR after discontinuation of treatment is not clearly stated.

Livedo reticularis associated with interferon α therapy in two melanoma patients. Ruiz-Genao DP, García-F-Villalta MJ, Hernández-Núñez A, Ríos-Buceta L, Fernández-Herrera J, García-Díez A. J Eur Acad Dermatol Venereol 2005; 19: 252–4.

Two patients treated with subcutaneous interferon α2b as adjuvant therapy for malignant melanoma (American Joint Committee on Cancer stage IIA and IIB, respectively) developed LR on legs and trunk 2 weeks after commencing treatment. LR cleared completely with no further recurrence after treatment was discontinued for other reasons.

Amantadine-induced livedo reticularis – case report. Quaresma MV, Gomes AC, Serruya A, Vendramini DL, Braga L, Buçard AM. An Bras Dermatol 2015; 90: 745–7.

A 79-year-old man with Parkinson disease treated with amantadine, carbidopa, and levodopa developed LR. This resolved with the discontinuation of amantadine. Amantadine is one of the more common drugs to cause LR.

Livedo reticularis caused by cholesterol embolization may improve with simvastatin. Finch TM, Ryatt KS. Br J Dermatol 2000; 143: 1319–20.

A 69-year-old man with LR without ulceration of the legs extending to the lower abdomen due to cholesterol embolization failed to respond to low-dose aspirin and low-fat diet. Fasting serum cholesterol was 6.9 mmol/L^{-1} and serum triglyceride was normal. Three months after initiation of simvastatin 10 mg daily the serum cholesterol decreased to 4.9 mmol/L^{-1} with associated reduction in extent and prominence of the LR.

141

Livedoid vasculopathy

Sultan A. Mirza, Bethany R. Hairston,
Mark D.P. Davis

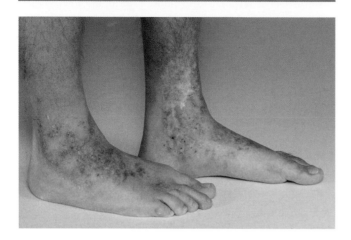

Livedoid vasculopathy, or livedoid vasculitis, is a painful ulcerative condition of the lower extremities with characteristic clinical and histopathologic features. Pain is a prominent feature, associated with infarctive, tiny, shallow ulcerations most often involving the legs around the feet and ankles. This condition is difficult to treat and often recalcitrant to therapy. Healed ulcers have the nonspecific appearance of atrophie blanche, characterized by smooth, porcelain-white lesions surrounded by punctate telangiectasia and hyperpigmentation; this appearance also may be seen in the context of healed ulcers due to venous insufficiency.

MANAGEMENT STRATEGY

Clinicopathologic correlation for a diagnosis of livedoid vasculopathy is necessary before treatment options can be considered. Histologic identification of the characteristic segmental hyalinized appearance of the dermal blood vessels is important to exclude other causes of lower extremity ulcerative disease. Increasing numbers of reports suggest that the disease has a procoagulant predisposition, with both hereditary and acquired hypercoagulable states; therefore a comprehensive coagulation screen is recommended.

Typically shallow and numerous, the ulcers in livedoid vasculopathy are painful and slow healing. *Wound care* is an important facet of treatment. *Excellent dressings* and *topical products* are available to treat chronic ulcerative diseases, and selection depends on the moisture content of the wound and the possibility of superinfection. *Pain management* is also essential.

Because of the potential procoagulant mechanisms involved in disease etiology, medical therapy involves prevention and treatment of dermal vessel thrombosis and improvement of vascular perfusion. Medical management has included *aspirin (acetylsalicylic acid)*, *niacin (nicotinic acid)*, *pentoxifylline*, *dipyridamole*, *warfarin*, and *danazol*. Systemic corticosteroids are not considered a primary therapy; however, some patients' conditions have improved with immunosuppressants in combination therapy. *Psoralen with ultraviolet A (PUVA)* has also been used. Patients with livedoid vasculitis recalcitrant to traditional management have been treated with *minidose heparin, subcutaneous low-molecular-weight heparin injections, rivaroxaban, certain prostanoids, intravenous immunoglobulin (IVIG)*, and a *tissue-type plasminogen activator (tPA)*.

Specific Investigations

- Skin biopsy, including routine histology and direct immunofluorescence
- Wound and tissue cultures
- Hemogram
- Serum homocysteine
- Cryoglobulin
- Thrombophilia investigations: anticardiolipin antibody, anti-β_2-glycoprotein I antibodies, factor V Leiden R506Q and prothrombin G20210A mutations, biologic activity and antigen levels of protein C and S, functional and immunologic levels of antithrombin III protein, detection of lupus anticoagulant, lipoprotein(a), and fibrinopeptide A levels
- Noninvasive venous and arterial function testing: continuous-wave Doppler, venous duplex imaging, plethysmography, and transcutaneous oximetry

Livedoid vasculopathy: an intriguing cutaneous disease. Criado PR, Rivitti EA, Sotto MN, Valente NYS, Aoki V, de Carvalho JF, et al. An Bras Dermatol 2011; 86: 961–77.

Livedoid vasculopathy was originally described as a clinical expression of vasculitis; however, current understanding of the main pathogenetic mechanism suggests a vasoocclusive phenomenon due to intraluminal thrombosis of dermal vessels. The authors review etiologic associations, publications on livedoid vasculopathy associated with hypercoagulable conditions, and options for treatment.

Livedoid vasculopathy: an in-depth analysis using a modified Delphi approach. Alavi A, Hafner J, Dutz JP, Mayer D, Sibbald RG, Criado PR, et al. J Am Acad Dermatol 2013; 69: 1033–42.

This article reviews nomenclature changes with this condition. An illustrative approach to diagnosis and review of treatments are well presented.

Association between peripheral vascular endothelial dysfunction and livedoid vasculopathy. Yang CH, Shen SC, Hui RC, Huang YH, Chu PH, Ho WJ. J Am Acad Dermatol 2012; 67: 107–12.

Sixteen patients diagnosed with livedoid vasculopathy were compared with 16 matched control subjects in this prospective study using flow-mediated vasodilation of the brachial artery, an indicator of vascular endothelial function, using high-resolution, two-dimensional ultrasonic imaging. Peripheral vascular endothelial dysfunction was demonstrated in patients, providing some evidence of endothelial dysfunction in the development of the disease. Decreased nitric oxide bioavailability may be the main reason for this dysfunction; however, the authors noted that more studies are needed to clarify the mechanism.

Livedoid vasculopathy: further evidence for procoagulant pathogenesis. Hairston BR, Davis MD, Pittelkow MR, Ahmed I. Arch Dermatol 2006; 142: 1413–8.

This retrospective study of 45 patients with biopsy-proven livedoid vasculopathy analyzed the presence of coagulation abnormalities. The laboratory results revealed numerous heterogeneous

Evidence Levels: A Double-blind study B Clinical trial ≥ 20 subjects C Clinical trial < 20 subjects D Series ≥ 5 subjects E Anecdotal case reports

coagulation abnormalities, including factor V Leiden mutations, protein C or S abnormalities, prothrombin G20210A gene mutations, lupus anticoagulant, anticardiolipin antibodies, and elevated homocysteine, thus providing further evidence of procoagulant mechanisms for this disease.

Livedoid vasculopathy: the role of hyperhomocysteinemia and its simple therapeutic consequences. Meiss F, Marsch WC, Fischer M. Eur J Dermatol 2006; 16: 159–62.

Hypercoagulability due to hyperhomocysteinemia was recognized as a potentially contributing factor to livedoid vasculopathy in a 49-year-old woman.

Livedoid vasculopathy and its association with factor V Leiden mutation. Yong AA, Tan AW, Giam YC, Tang MB. Singapore Med J 2012; 53: 258–60.

Two cases of livedo vasculopathy with factor V Leiden mutations are described.

Livedoid vasculopathy associated with heterozygous protein C deficiency. Boyvat A, Kundakci N, Babikir MO, Gurgey E. Br J Dermatol 2000; 143: 840–2.

Livedoid vasculitis in association with protein C deficiency is described in one patient.

Livedoid vasculitis: a manifestation of the antiphospholipid syndrome. Acland KM, Darvay A, Wakelin SH, Russell-Jones R. Br J Dermatol 1999; 140: 131–5.

Four patients with ulcerative livedoid vasculitis are described, all of whom had associated elevated anticardiolipin antibody levels but no other evidence of systemic disease.

Atrophie blanche: a disorder associated with defective release of tissue plasminogen activator. Pizzo SV, Murray JC, Gonias SL. Arch Pathol Lab Med 1986; 110: 517–9.

Plasma from eight patients with atrophie blanche was analyzed for release of vascular tPA before and after venous occlusion. The average plasma level of releasable tPA was only 0.03 IU/mL compared with 0.70 IU/mL for 118 healthy controls.

First-Line Therapies

• Wound care (including bed rest and leg elevation)	C
• Aspirin	C
• Dipyridamole	C
• Pentoxifylline	D

Atrophie blanche: a clinicopathological study of 27 patients. Yang LJ, Chan HL, Chen SY, Kuan YZ, Chen MJ, Wang CN, et al. Changgeng Yi Xue Za Zhi 1991; 14: 237–45.

Twenty-seven patients were reviewed with respect to mean age at onset, disease duration, natural course, and clinical morphology. Thirteen patients responded to local wound care, bed rest, and low-dose aspirin plus dipyridamole as treatment for the first attack or recurrent episodes.

Livedoid vasculopathy associated with sickle cell trait: significant improvement on aspirin treatment. El Khoury J, Taher A, Kurban M, Kibbi AG, Abbas O. Int Wound J 2012; 9: 344–7.

The authors describe a patient with sickle cell trait diagnosed with livedoid vasculopathy; treatment with aspirin led to significant improvement in the cutaneous ulcers.

Livedo vasculitis: therapy with pentoxifylline. Sams WM Jr. Arch Dermatol 1988; 124: 684–7.

Eight patients with disease unresponsive to a variety of medications were treated with pentoxifylline. Three experienced complete healing and four were much improved, whereas only one was unchanged after treatment.

Second-Line Therapies

• Low-molecular-weight heparin	C
• Warfarin	D
• Hyperbaric oxygen	D
• Danazol	D

Frequency of thrombophilia determinant factors in patients with livedoid vasculopathy and treatment with anticoagulant drugs – a prospective study. Di Giacomo TB, Hussein TP, Souza DG, Criado PR. J Eur Acad Dermatol Venereol 2010; 24: 1340–6.

Thirty-four patients diagnosed with livedoid vasculopathy were tested for prothrombin time, activated partial thromboplastin time, antithrombin activity, protein C and S activity, anticardiolipin antibodies, lupus anticoagulant, prothrombin gene mutation, factor V Leiden mutation, methylenetetrahydrofolate reductase mutation, plasma homocysteine, and fibrinogen; 18 (52%) presented laboratory abnormalities of procoagulant conditions. Thirteen of the 34 patients were treated with anticoagulant drugs (either warfarin or heparin), with clinical improvement in 11 patients.

Livedoid vasculopathy in a pediatric patient with elevated lipoprotein(a) levels: prompt response to continuous low-molecular-weight heparin. Goerge T, Weishaupt C, Metze D, Nowak-Göttl U, Sunderkötter C, Steinhoff M, et al. Arch Dermatol 2010; 146: 927–8.

The authors describe a pediatric patient with livedoid vasculopathy who had elevated levels of lipoprotein(a). Treatment with low-molecular-weight heparin (enoxaparin) showed remission of the ulcers and pain.

Treatment of livedoid vasculopathy with low-molecular-weight heparin: report of 2 cases. Hairston BR, Davis MD, Gibson LE, Drage LA. Arch Dermatol 2003; 139: 987–90.

Two patients with livedoid vasculitis recalcitrant to conventional first- and second-line therapies had a beneficial response to subcutaneous injections of low-molecular-weight heparin.

Difficult management of livedoid vasculopathy. Frances C, Barete S. Arch Dermatol 2004; 140: 1011.

Fourteen of 16 patients treated with either low-molecular-weight heparin or a vitamin K antagonist (fluindione) had more effective results than with antiplatelet drugs. One patient responded partially to aspirin and dipyridamole; the remaining patient responded to no treatments.

The authors recommend that the benefit-to-risk ratio, cost, and quality of life be considered when prescribing either low-molecular-weight heparin or vitamin K antagonists.

Ulcerations caused by livedoid vasculopathy associated with a prothrombotic state: response to warfarin. Davis MD, Wysokinski WE. J Am Acad Dermatol 2008; 58: 512–5.

Warfarin therapy healed ulcerations in a 50-year-old woman who had a lifelong history of painful ulcerations; the patient was a heterozygous carrier of factor V Leiden and prothrombin gene mutations.

A case of livedoid vasculopathy associated with factor V Leiden mutation: successful treatment with oral warfarin. Kavala M, Kocaturk E, Zindanci I, Turkoglu Z, Altintas S. J Dermatol Treat 2008; 19: 121–3.

A 19-year-old man with a 4-year history of recurrent leg ulcerations had rapid improvement with oral warfarin therapy after laboratory diagnosis of protein C and factor V Leiden mutations.

Warfarin therapy for livedoid vasculopathy associated with cryofibrinogenemia and hyperhomocysteinemia. Browning CE, Callen JP. Arch Dermatol 2006; 142: 75–8.

A 50-year-old man with abnormal cryofibrinogen and homocysteine levels had a dramatic response to oral warfarin therapy after being refractory to treatment with multiple other medications.

Livedoid vasculopathy: long-term follow-up results following hyperbaric oxygen therapy. Juan WH, Chan YS, Lee JC, Yang LC, Hong HS, Yang CH. Br J Dermatol 2006; 154: 251–5.

Eight patients completed a prospective study evaluating the efficacy of hyperbaric oxygen on healing the ulcers of livedoid vasculopathy. Leg ulcers in all eight patients healed completely at a mean of 3.4 weeks; however, six patients had relapses of ulceration but responded to additional hyperbaric oxygen therapy.

Livedoid vasculopathy and high levels of lipoprotein(a): response to danazol. Criado PR, de Souza Espinell DP, Valentef NS, Alavi A, Kirsner RS. Dermatol Ther 2015; 28: 248–53.

The authors present four patients with livedoid vasculopathy who were successfully treated with low-dose danazol (200 mg daily orally); clinical characteristics and laboratory workup, including the level of lipoprotein(a), are also presented.

Low-dose danazol in the treatment of livedoid vasculitis. Hsiao GH, Chiu HC. Dermatology 1997; 194: 251–5.

Six of seven patients treated with low-dose danazol (200 mg daily orally) had rapid cessation of new lesion formation, prompt reduction in pain, and healing of active ulceration.

Third-Line Therapies

• Tissue plasminogen activator	C
• Intravenous immunoglobulin	C
• PUVA	C
• Sulfapyridine	D
• Rivaroxaban	E
• Cilostazol	E
• Prostanoids (PGE-1, prostacyclin)	E

Tissue plasminogen activator for treatment of livedoid vasculitis. Klein KL, Pittelkow MR. Mayo Clin Proc 1992; 67: 923–33.

In a prospective study, six patients who had nonhealing ulcers caused by livedoid vasculitis and in whom numerous conventional therapies had failed were treated with low-dose tPA. In five of the six patients, dramatic improvement with almost complete healing of the ulcers occurred during hospitalization. Several were maintained with warfarin therapy after their inpatient treatment.

Successful long-term use of intravenous immunoglobulin to treat livedoid vasculopathy associated with plasminogen activator inhibitor-1 promoter homozygosity. Tuchinda P, Tammaro A, Gaspari AA. Arch Dermatol 2011; 127: 1224–5.

A 33-year-old patient diagnosed with livedoid vasculopathy associated with plasminogen activator inhibitor-1 promoter homozygosity was treated with IVIG after failing antiinflammatory, antiplatelet, and tPA therapies. She was successfully treated for over 4 years without complications with IVIG, 0.5 g/kg every 2 weeks, given intravenously by an implanted Port-A-Cath. The authors also describe several preventative regimens that may help to decrease the risk of thromboembolic events related to IVIG infusion.

Efficacy of intravenous immunoglobulins in livedoid vasculopathy: long-term follow-up of 11 patients. Monshi B, Posch C, Vujic I, Sesti A, Sobotka S, Rappersberger K. J Am Acad Dermatol 2014; 71: 738–44.

In this retrospective study, the authors analyzed IVIG therapy in 11 patients. Most patients received IVIG added to an existing regimen, primarily aspirin, oral anticoagulants, or low-molecular-weight heparin, alone or in combination. Reduction of disease activity and improved quality of life were achieved after 6 rounds of IVIG.

Refractory livedoid vasculitis responding to PUVA: a report of four cases. Tuchinda C, Leenutaphong V, Sudtim S, Lim HW. Photodermatol Photoimmunol Photomed 2005; 21:154–6.

Four patients with refractory livedoid vasculopathy responded to PUVA therapy; however, two of the four patients had recurrent lesions within a few months after cessation of therapy.

Livedoid vasculitis responding to PUVA therapy. Lee JH, Choi HJ, Kim SM, Hann SK, Park YK. Int J Dermatol 2001; 40: 153–7.

Eight patients treated with systemic PUVA had rapid cessation of new lesion formation, notable symptom relief, and complete healing of primary lesions without unacceptable adverse effects.

Clinical studies of livedoid vasculitis (segmental hyalinizing vasculitis). Winkelmann RK, Schroeter AL, Kierland RR, Ryan TM. Mayo Clin Proc 1974; 49: 746–50.

Clinical, laboratory, and histologic studies of 37 patients with livedoid vasculitis were presented. Treatment options included niacin (nicotinic acid), which was effective because of the inhibiting effect of nicotinate on contraction of vascular smooth muscle of the skin. Nine of 12 patients had sustained remission of their livedoid vasculopathy. Rest and wet-dressing therapy produced short remissions. Six of 11 patients responded to sulfapyridine, and 3 of 8 responded to guanethidine. Corticosteroids, sympathectomy, and other forms of chemotherapy were not successful.

Rivaroxaban prevents painful cutaneous infarctions in livedoid vasculopathy. Kerk N, Drabik A, Luger TA, Schneider SW, Goerge T. Br J Dermatol 2013; 168: 898–9.

Three patients were treated with rivaroxaban (10 mg daily) for livedoid vasculopathy. Pain levels and the frequency of new ulcers were noted to improve significantly within 1 month and 3 months, respectively.

Response of livedoid vasculopathy to rivaroxaban. Winchester DS, Drage LA, Davis MD. Br J Dermatol 2015; 172: 1148–50.

Two patients treated with rivaroxaban (10–20 mg daily) noted relief of pain and complete healing in ulcers within 2 months.

Cilostazol: a novel agent in recalcitrant livedoid vasculopathy. Mendiratta V, Malik M, Yadav P, Nangia A. Indian J Dermatol Venereol Leprol 2016; 82: 222–4.

A 25-year-old woman with recalcitrant livedoid vasculopathy was initially treated with oral cilostazol (50 mg daily), with reduction in pain and burning and improvement of the ulcers, then twice

Evidence Levels: **A** Double-blind study   **B** Clinical trial ≥ 20 subjects   **C** Clinical trial < 20 subjects   **D** Series ≥ 5 subjects   **E** Anecdotal case reports

daily for a short time during a flare. Within a few months, medication was tapered off, and no relapse was noted within a year.

Treatment of livedoid vasculopathy with alprostadil (PGE-1): case report and review of published literature. Mofarrah R, Aberer W, Aberer E. J Eur Acad Dermatol Venereol 2013; 27: 252–4.

This article discusses the diagnosis and treatment of livedoid vasculopathy in patients. It examines a 47-year-old patient with livid reticular discoloration and ulceration on both legs. It informs of a vasodilatory effect of prostaglandins and that prostaglandin E1 (PGE-1) is a promising drug used for the treatment of livedoid vasculopathies.

Lyme borreliosis

Matthew Grant, David Banach

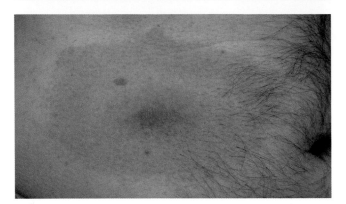

Courtesy of Yale Dermatology Residents Slide Collection.

Lyme disease is a multisystem illness caused by spirochetes of the genus *Borrelia*. In North America, the causative agent is *Borrelia burgdorferi*, whereas in Europe, disease is caused primarily by *B. afzelii* and *B. garinii*. Clinical manifestations of Lyme disease depend on the stage of illness and may be limited to the skin or involve the nervous system, joints, or heart. Lyme disease is the most common vectorborne disease in the United States. It is endemic in the Northeast, the mid-Atlantic, and parts of Wisconsin and Minnesota. The most common vector for Lyme disease in the United States is the *Ixodes scapularis* tick. *I. pacificus* has been linked to transmission of *B. burgdorferi* in the northwestern United States.

Mice and deer are the major reservoirs of *B. burgdorferi*. After hatching in the spring, tick larvae acquire *B. burgdorferi* while feeding on white-footed mice. The following spring, the larvae develop into nymphs and are then capable of transmitting infection. Nymph or adult female forms slowly deposit spirochetes into human skin during feeding. Ticks must remain attached and feed for over 48 hours to transmit a sufficient inoculum of spirochetes for illness to occur.

MANAGEMENT STRATEGY

Routine antimicrobial prophylaxis or serologic testing after a tick bite is not recommended. It is reasonable to offer single-dose prophylaxis to patients residing in endemic areas who remove engorged *I. scapularis* ticks attached for >36 hours. This recommendation is based on the result of a randomized trial of single-dose doxycycline (200 mg), which prevented 87% of Lyme infections if administered within 72 hours of tick removal. Regardless of whether prophylaxis is taken, patients who remove a tick attached for more than a day should be monitored for up to 30 days for the occurrence of local skin lesions or fever.

The best mode of preventing Lyme disease is avoidance of tick-infested areas. If tick exposure is unavoidable, then one should ideally wear permethrin-treated clothes with long sleeves and long pants tucked into socks. Exposed skin should be treated with a DEET-based repellent, which has activity against ticks in addition to mosquitoes and most biting insects.

Skin self-inspection within 36 hours of tick exposure and bathing within 2 hours of exposure have both been associated with decreased risk of developing Lyme borelliosis. Daily inspection of the entire body, including the scalp, is recommended because attached ticks removed within 24 to 36 hours are unlikely to transmit *B. burgdorferi*. *Ixodes* ticks are small: larvae are less than 1 mm in size, and adult females are 2 to 3 mm in size. Attached ticks should be removed with tweezers by carefully pulling on the mouth apparatus close to the skin, taking care not to retain mouth parts of the embedded tick.

Lyme disease generally occurs in stages, with different signs and symptoms at each stage. Therapeutic recommendations vary depending on the stage of disease and the presence of extracutaneous manifestations.

Early localized Lyme disease

The most common clinical manifestation of early Lyme disease is erythema migrans (EM). This characteristic skin lesion occurs at the site of the bite a median of 10 days after inoculation, beginning as an erythematous papule and evolving into an expanding annular patch with a distinct edge. Although central clearing of erythema leading to a bull's-eye or targetoid appearance is characteristic, many lesions do not demonstrate this finding, and absence of central clearing should not exclude an EM diagnosis. The lesion may be accompanied by nonspecific symptoms, including fever, regional lymphadenopathy, arthralgia, fatigue, and headache. About 75% of patients with Lyme disease in the United States are diagnosed during the early localized stage with a single primary lesion. Untreated lesions usually fade within 3 to 4 weeks.

Administration of doxycycline 100 mg twice daily, amoxicillin 500 mg three times daily, or cefuroxime axetil 500 mg twice daily for at least 14 days is recommended for early localized or early disseminated Lyme disease associated with EM. Doxycycline has the advantage of also treating human granulocytic anaplasmosis caused by *Anaplasma phagocytophilum*, which can be cotransmitted by *I. scapularis* bites. Doxycycline can cause photosensitivity and is contraindicated during pregnancy or breastfeeding and for children less than 8 years old.

A rare skin manifestation of early Lyme infection described predominantly in Europe is borrelial lymphocytoma (BL). This solitary bluish-red nodule occurs at the site of a tick bite typically preceding or concomitantly with EM. Commonly involved sites are the ear lobes in children and near or on the nipple in adults. BL may develop within weeks to months after a tick bite and if untreated can persist for months to years. Treatment regimens used to treat EM can be used to treat BL.

Early disseminated Lyme disease

Early dissemination of the spirochete occurs via blood or lymphatics over several weeks in untreated infection. Multiple annular skin lesions resembling primary EM can arise when spirochetes are deposited at skin sites remote from the initial bite—notably these lesions are generally smaller. Other common symptoms include fever, lethargy, myalgia, headache, and neck stiffness. Patients may present with atrioventricular (AV) conduction disturbances, iritis or uveitis, aseptic meningitis (lymphocytic pleocytosis in cerebrospinal fluid [CSF] with normal glucose), cranial nerve palsies (notably facial nerve palsies), or peripheral radiculopathy. In adults, intravenous ceftriaxone 2 g daily for 14 to 28 days is recommended for early Lyme disease presenting with neurologic or advanced cardiac conduction abnormalities. Parenteral

Evidence Levels: **A** Double-blind study **B** Clinical trial ≥ 20 subjects **C** Clinical trial < 20 subjects **D** Series ≥ 5 subjects **E** Anecdotal case reports

penicillin or cefotaxime are second-line agents. Temporary pacing may be required for patients with high-degree AV block (PR interval ≥0.30 seconds). Insertion of a permanent pacemaker is not necessary, as conduction defects usually resolve with medical treatment alone. Isolated facial nerve palsy and first-degree AV block can be treated with oral doxycycline.

Late Lyme disease

Late Lyme disease can occur months to years after previously untreated or inadequately treated initial infection. Lyme arthritis is the most common manifestation of late Lyme disease, although its incidence is decreasing due to improved recognition of early disease. Lyme arthritis is oligoarticular and presents as recurrent swelling of large joints, primarily the knees. Persistent swelling is atypical. Positive serologic testing is required to confirm the diagnosis, and positive polymerase chain reaction (PCR) results from synovial fluid strengthen the diagnosis.

Late neuroborreliosis is rare and can manifest as peripheral neuropathy, encephalomyelitis, or a subacute encephalopathy characterized by memory disturbances, mood alterations, and somnolence.

A rare dermatologic finding associated with late Lyme disease is acrodermatitis chronica atrophicans (ACA). ACA has been predominantly described in elderly female patients and has rarely been seen in the United States but is more common in European patients with *B. afzelii*. ACA presents months to years after initial infection with a poorly demarcated area of violaceous discoloration and swelling of involved skin. These lesions usually involve the extensor surfaces of the extremities, including the dorsum of the hands. Over time the lesions become atrophic, with a characteristic hyperpigmented, hairless, and translucent appearance. Involvement of peripheral nerves can also result in sensory neuropathy.

Lyme arthritis without neurologic symptoms can be treated with a 28-day oral regimen of either doxycycline 100 mg twice daily or amoxicillin 500 mg three times daily. Adults with evidence of concurrent neurologic involvement should receive intravenous ceftriaxone. Recurrent or persistent joint swelling after an oral regimen can be retreated with another 28-day course of oral antimicrobials or with a 2- to 4-week parenteral regimen. Adults with late neurologic disease should be treated with a parenteral regimen for 2 to 4 weeks. Repeated or prolonged therapy is not recommended.

Posttreatment symptoms

Persistent arthritic complaints appear to be immunologically mediated and are most common in individuals with the HLA-DR4 haplotype. Research studies have not consistently demonstrated microbiologic persistence of *Borrelia* in patients with symptoms after completion of treatment for Lyme. Moreover, prolonged or multiple courses of antimicrobials are unhelpful and may be harmful. Symptomatic treatment with nonsteroidal agents, intraarticular corticosteroids, disease-modifying antirheumatic drugs, or in severe nonremitting cases, arthroscopic synovectomy may provide relief.

Reinfection and vaccination

Patients treated for early Lyme disease, specifically EM, do not develop protective immunity and if reexposed may become reinfected. The clinical presentation associated with reinfection is similar to primary infection. At this time there is no vaccine available to protect against Lyme disease.

SPECIFIC INVESTIGATIONS

Testing

Prospective study of serologic tests for Lyme disease. Steere A, McHugh G, Damle N, Sikand V. Clin Inf Dis 2008; 47: 188–95.

Early Lyme disease is a clinical diagnosis with 80% of patients in endemic areas presenting with EM. Only one third of patients presenting with EM and early Lyme disease have positive serology, but sensitivity increases during the convalescent phase. Two-step testing with enzyme-linked immunosorbent assay (ELISA) and Western immunoblot remains the gold standard for diagnosing later stages of Lyme disease. In this study, over 90% of patients with disseminated disease and 100% of patients with late Lyme disease had positive two-step test results. The authors were also able to demonstrate increased sensitivity using a single-step IgG C6 peptide ELISA. This test warrants further investigation in a broader patient population.

Prevention

Peridomestic Lyme disease prevention. Results of a population based case-control study. Connally NP, Durante AJ, Yousey-Hindes M, Meek JI, Nelson RS, Heimer R. Am J Prev Med 2009; 37: 201–6.

This was a 32-month case-control study comparing 364 patients with Lyme disease to neighborhood-matched controls to evaluate the impact of prevention measures on risk. In multivariate analysis, checking for ticks within 36 hours after spending time in the yard, bathing within 2 hours after exposure, and fencing around the yard were associated with decreased risk of EM.

Prophylaxis

Prophylaxis with single-dose doxycycline for the prevention of Lyme disease after an *Ixodes scapularis* tick bite. Nadelman RB, Nowakowski J, Fish D, Falco RC, Freeman K, McKenna D, et al; Tick Bite Study Group. N Engl J Med 2001; 345: 79–84.

In this investigation, 482 patients were randomized to receive 200 mg doxycycline or placebo within 72 hours of removal of an *I. scapularis* tick. One of 235 subjects (0.4%) who received doxycycline, compared with 8 of 247 (3.2%) who received placebo, developed EM. No asymptomatic seroconversions occurred and no subject developed extracutaneous Lyme disease. Prophylaxis was effective at decreasing the development of Lyme disease. More gastrointestinal symptoms occurred with doxycycline.

Treatment

The clinical assessment, treatment, and prevention of Lyme disease, human granulocytic anaplasmosis, and babesiosis: clinical practice guidelines by the Infectious Diseases Society of America. Wormser GP, Dattwyler RJ, Shapiro ED, Halperin JJ, Steere AC, Klempner MS, et al. Clin Infect Dis 2006; 43: 1089–134.

First-Line Therapies

Early localized disease (erythema migrans)*

- Doxycycline[†] 100 mg twice daily for 14 days · · · · · A
- Amoxicillin 500 mg three times daily for 14 days · · · · · A
- Cefuroxime axetil 500 mg twice daily for 14 days · · · · · A

Early neurologic (meningitis or radiculopathy)

- Ceftriaxone 2 g IV daily for 14 days · · · · · B
- Penicillin G 18–24 million units IV daily
  (divided and dosed every 4 hours) for 14 days · · · · · B

Cardiac disease including atrioventricular block

- Can be treated with oral or parenteral
  regimens recommended for early localized or
  early neurologic disease for 14 days[‡] · · · · · C

Lyme arthritis without neurologic involvement

- Doxycycline[†] 100 mg twice daily for 28 days
  or amoxicillin 500 mg three times daily for
  28 days · · · · · B

Lyme arthritis with neurologic involvement

- Ceftriaxone 2 g IV daily for 14–28 days · · · · · B
- Penicillin G 18–24 million units IV daily (divided
  and dosed every 4 hours) for 14–28 days · · · · · B

Recurrent arthritis

- Retreatment with a 28-day course of oral
  antibiotics · · · · · D

Late neuroborreliosis

- Ceftriaxone 2 g IV daily for 14–28 days · · · · · B
- Penicillin G 18–24 million units IV daily (divided
  and dosed every 4 hours) for 14–28 days · · · · · B

Acrodermatitis chronic atrophicans

- Doxycycline 100 mg twice daily for 21 days · · · · · C
- Amoxicillin 500 mg three times daily for 21 days · · · · · C
- Cefuroxime axetil 500 mg twice daily for 21 days · · · · · D

*Level B recommendation for borrelial lymphocytoma and early Lyme disease
with isolated cranial nerve palsy.
[†]Doxycycline is contraindicated in pregnancy and in children <8 years old.
[‡]Initial treatment with parenteral regimen recommended in hospitalized
patients.

Second-Line Therapies

Early localized disease

- Erythromycin 250 mg orally four times
  daily for 14 days · · · · · B
- Azithromycin 500 mg daily for 7 days · · · · · B

Neurologic involvement or advanced cardiac conduction block

- Doxycycline 100 mg twice a day for
  10–28 days · · · · · B

Second-line therapies are to be used in the setting of contraindication to first-line treatments (e.g., severe allergy).

Amoxicillin plus probenecid versus doxycycline for treatment of erythema migrans borreliosis. Dattwyler RJ, Volkman DJ, Conaty SM, Platkin SP, Luft BJ. Lancet 1990; 336: 1404–6.

Seventy-two adults with early Lyme disease were randomized to either amoxicillin 500 mg three times daily or doxycycline 100 mg twice daily for 3 weeks. Both groups had 100% cure rates of their EM and were asymptomatic after a 6-month follow-up period.

Comparison of cefuroxime axetil and doxycycline in the treatment of early Lyme disease. Nadelman RB, Luger SW, Frank E, Wisniewski M, Collins JJ, Wormser GP. Ann Intern Med 1992; 117: 273–80.

A randomized, multicenter, investigator-blinded trial treated 123 patients with EM for 20 days with either cefuroxime axetil 500 mg twice daily ($n = 63$) or doxycycline 100 mg twice daily ($n = 60$). Cure or improvement was achieved in 51 of 55 (93%) evaluable patients treated with cefuroxime axetil and in 45 of 51 (88%) patients treated with doxycycline. At 1-year post treatment, the percentage of patients who achieved a satisfactory outcome was comparable between the two groups. Cefuroxime was associated with more diarrhea than was doxycycline and is more expensive than doxycycline or amoxicillin.

Two controlled trials of antibiotic treatment in patients with persistent symptoms and a history of Lyme disease. Klempner MS, Hu LT, Evans J, Schmid CH, Johnson GM, Trevino RP, et al. N Engl J Med 2001; 345: 85–92.

Patients with persistent symptoms after previously treated Lyme disease were randomized to receive either intravenous ceftriaxone 2 g daily for 30 days followed by oral doxycycline 200 mg daily for 60 days or matching placebos. This study was halted after planned interim analysis of the first 107 subjects indicated that the study would be unlikely to reveal a significant difference in outcomes.

Azithromycin compared with amoxicillin in the treatment of erythema migrans. A double-blind, randomized, controlled trial. Luft BJ, Dattwyler RJ, Johnson RC, Luger SW, Bosler EM, Rahn DW, et al. Ann Intern Med 1996; 124: 785–91.

In this report, 246 adults with EM were randomized to either amoxicillin 500 mg three times daily for 20 days or azithromycin 500 mg once daily for 7 days. Those treated with amoxicillin were more likely to achieve complete resolution of disease at day 20 (88% for amoxicillin compared with 76% for azithromycin; $p = 0.024$). More azithromycin recipients (16%) than amoxicillin recipients (4%) had relapses.

Treatment of Erythema Migrans With Doxycycline for 10 Days Versus 15 Days. Stupica D, Lusa L, Ruzić-Sabljić E, Cerar T, Strle F. Clin Infect Dis 2012; 55: 343–50.

In this study 117 patients with EM received doxycycline 100 mg twice daily for 10 or 15 days. Resolution of EM was similar in both groups, and at 12 months 93% of the 15-day group and 92% of patients in the 10-day group showed complete response, and most had complete response within 2 months. There was a higher rate of photosensitivity in the 15-day group.

Antibiotic treatment duration and long-term outcomes of patients with early Lyme disease from a Lyme disease hyperendemic area. Kowalski TJ, Tata S, Berth W, Mathiason MA, Agger WA. Clin Infect Dis 2010; 50: 512–20.

This retrospective cohort study provides follow-up data of 617 patients diagnosed with early localized or disseminated Lyme disease. The 2-year treatment failure-free survival rates of patients treated with ≤10, 11 to 15, and ≥16 days of antibiotics were 99.0%, 98.9%, and 99.2%, respectively.

Evidence Levels: **A** Double-blind study **B** Clinical trial ≥ 20 subjects **C** Clinical trial < 20 subjects **D** Series ≥ 5 subjects **E** Anecdotal case reports

Lymphangioma circumscriptum

Patrick O.M. Emanuel, Kevin McKerrow

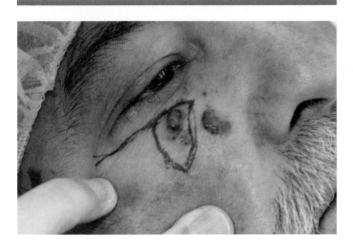

Lymphangioma circumscriptum is an uncommon lymphatic malformation. It presents on the skin surface as grapelike groups of thin-walled, translucent, lymph-filled vesicles, often compared with frog spawn. Hemorrhage within the lesions can create a deep red or black appearance.

More commonly congenital, they are typically noted at birth or appear during childhood. They are most commonly found around the shoulder girdle and proximal limbs. There is a morphologically identical acquired variant related to lymphatic obstruction as a consequence of surgery, radiation, or malignancy.

MANAGEMENT STRATEGIES

Although observation is an appropriate option for many cases, cosmetic concern is the typical indication for treatment. Other indications may include persistent leakage of lymphatic fluid or blood and recurrent infection. The risk of developing angiosarcoma and squamous cell carcinoma is trivial and should not be used to rationalize full surgical excision.

Treatment is challenging and often thwarted by local recurrences due to the persistence of deep lymphatic cisterns, which may delve deep into the subcuticular adipose tissue, skeletal muscle, and nerves. Every treatment option has associated recurrence rates/complication profiles. Consequently, there is disagreement in the literature as to which treatment option is the most effective. Although *complete surgical excision* has the lowest recurrence rates, it has the highest rate of complications; more extensive lesions may be deemed inoperable.

Sclerotherapy using a variety of sclerosants has been advocated as a less invasive and effective treatment modality, which is either a first-line alternative or an adjunct to surgery.

Other authorities suggest that after definitive diagnosis and radiologic mapping, surgical excision and postoperative histologic assessment of excision margins provide the most effective treatment options.

Resurfacing of the lesions can be attempted and achieved even if proper surgical excision is not possible and/or sclerotherapy fails, but recurrence rates are usually higher than with other therapies. The high-energy, short-pulse CO_2 laser has been found to yield functionally and cosmetically acceptable results. This seals communicating channels to the deeper cisterns by vaporizing the superficial lymphatics and is said to have fewer complications than more aggressive treatment alternatives. Other laser methods, particularly the pulsed dye laser, have also been shown to be effective in selected superficial cases.

Specific Investigations

- Biopsy
- Imaging studies
- Magnetic resonance imaging (MRI)
- Lymphangiography
- Ultrasound

In the majority of cases the clinical diagnosis is straightforward. In some, the differential diagnosis may be broad: genital lesions are often associated with verrucous changes, which give them a warty appearance and are often confused with viral warts or squamous cell carcinoma; discoloration of the vesicles can lead to confusion with hemangiomas and even malignant melanoma; herpetic infection and dermatitis herpetiformis are less frequent differential diagnoses. Biopsy is diagnostic for clinically unusual cases and exhibits numerous thin-walled, dilated lymphatic channels encroaching onto the epidermis (which may become hyperkeratotic), expanding the papillary dermis and extending deep into the dermis and subcutis. Immunostaining with VEGFR3 and D2-40 decorates the vessels and confirms their lymphatic origin.

MRI can define the entire anatomy of a lesion and, when used preoperatively, can help prevent unnecessarily extensive or incomplete surgical resection. Computed tomography (CT), ultrasound, and lymphoscintigraphy have also been useful in determining the extent of a lesion.

Secondary lesions may be investigated for an underlying cause if the cause is not clinically obvious. Lymphangiomas may be associated with rare disorders such as Proteus, Cobb, and Klippel–Trenaunay syndromes, and so appropriate investigations and consultations should be sought if these conditions are suspected.

First-Line Therapies

• Conservative/observation	A
• Antibiotics	D
• Sclerotherapy	A
• OK-432	A
• Hyperosmolar saline	D
• Sodium tetradecyl sulfate	E
• Surgery	A

Intralesional sclerotherapy with group A *Streptococcus pyogenes* of human origin (OK-432) has emerged as an effective sclerosing agent.

OK-432 therapy in 64 patients with lymphangioma. Ogita S, Tsuto T, Nakamura K, Deguchi E, Iwai N. J Pediatr Surg 1994; 29: 784–5.

A case of unresectable lymphangioma circumscriptum of the vulva successfully treated with OK-432 in childhood. Ahn SJ, Chang SE, Choi JH, Moon KC, Koh JK, Kim DY. J Am Acad Dermatol 2006; 55: S106–7.

Treatment of lymphangioma in children: our experience of 128 cases. Okazaki T, Iwatani S, Yanai T, Kobayashi H, Kato Y, Marusasa T, et al. J Pediatr Surg 2007; 42: 386–9.

The main advantage of OK-432 over other sclerosing agents is the absence of perilesional fibrosis. OK-432 is an effective agent for cases of a single or limited numbers of vesicles. In larger lesions the technique is useful as a pretreatment adjunct to surgical excision.

Treatment of lymphangioma circumscriptum with sclerotherapy: an ignored effective remedy. Al Ghamdi KM, Mubki TF. J Cosmet Dermatol 2011; 10: 156–8.

Lymphangioma circumscriptum: treatment with hypertonic saline sclerotherapy. Bikowski JB, Dumont AM. J Am Acad Dermatol 2005; 53: 442–4.

Hypertonic saline has been reported to be effective for the management of lymphangioma circumscriptum to the shoulder, although wider use of this agent in comparison with other treatments for lymphangioma circumscriptum has not been reported.

Percutaneous sclerotherapy of lymphangioma. Molitch HI, Unger EC, Witte CL, van Sonnenberg E. Radiology 1995; 194: 343–7.

Five patients with unresectable lymphangiomas of the pelvis ($n = 2$), neck ($n = 1$), abdomen ($n = 1$), or leg ($n = 1$) were treated at two medical centers with sclerotherapy, using doxycycline as the sclerosant.

Treatment of unusual vascular lesions: usefulness of sclerotherapy in lymphangioma circumscriptum and acquired digital arteriovenous malformation. Park CO, Lee MJ, Chung KY. Dermatol Surg 2005; 31: 1451–3.

Two cases of lymphangioma circumscriptum were treated with a sclerosant, sodium tetradecyl sulfate, and were almost cleared with several treatments of sclerotherapy.

Surgery

Treatment of lymphangioma in children: our experience of 128 cases. Okazaki T, Iwatani S, Yanai T, Kobayashi H, Kato Y, Marusasa T, et al. J Pediatr Surg 2007; 42: 386–9.

Primary surgical excision was significantly more successful than sclerotherapy, but the results are often unsatisfactory because of complications, including damage to surrounding structures, particularly nerves and blood vessels, scarring, and recurrence due to incomplete excision. Ultrasound and MRI demonstrate deep cisterns, thereby ensuring deeper excision of these structures and less risk of recurrence.

Surgical management of "lymphangioma circumscriptum." Browse NL, Whimster I, Stewart G, Helm CW, Wood JJ. Br J Surg 1986; 73: 585–9.

Confirmation of the completeness of excision can be obtained using frozen section analysis of the lateral and deep margins.

Lymphangioma circumscriptum of the vulva mimicking genital wart: a case report and review of literature. Sah SP, Yadav R, Rani S. J Obstet Gynaecol Res 2001; 27: 293–6.

A case report of vulval lymphangioma circumscriptum, clinically diagnosed as a genital wart. After biopsy, the patient required extensive vulval surgery, and there was no recurrence after 16 months.

Surgical management of penoscrotal lymphangioma circumscriptum. Latifoglu O, Yavuzer R, Demir Y, Ayhan S, Yenidünya S, Atabay K. Plast Reconstruct Surg 1999; 103: 175–8.

An extensive lymphangioma circumscriptum of the penis and scrotum that was treated by wide excision in single-stage surgery. At the fourteenth postoperative month the patient was free of recurrence.

Lymphangioma circumscriptum: pitfalls and problems in definitive management. Bond J, Basheer MH, Gordon D. Dermatol Surg 2008; 34: 271–5.

Two cases of surgical excision with no recurrence at 1 and 2 years. Imaging of deep communicating structures and histologic assessment of excision margins provide the greatest chance of nonrecurrence.

Second-Line Therapies	
• CO_2 laser	D
• Pulsed dye laser	D
• Radiotherapy	E
• Cryotherapy	D
• Argon laser	D
• Suction-assisted lipectomy	D
• Topical imiquimod	D

Carbon dioxide laser vaporization of lymphangioma circumscriptum. Bailin PL, Kantor GR, Wheeland RG. J Am Acad Dermatol 1986; 14: 257–62.

CO_2 laser in a vaporization mode successfully ablated superficial cutaneous lesions in seven patients with lymphangioma circumscriptum.

Lymphangioma circumscriptum: review and evaluation of carbon dioxide laser vaporization. Eliezri YD, Sklar JA. J Dermatol Surg Oncol 1988; 14: 357–64.

Three patients were treated with CO_2 laser vaporization, with good to excellent cosmetic results and complete resolution of their symptoms.

CO_2 laser therapy of vulval lymphangiectasia and lymphangioma circumscriptum. Huilgol SC, Neill S, Barlow RJ. Dermatol Surg 2002; 28: 575–7.

Focal recurrence and an area of localized persistence were noted in both patients with lymphangioma circumscriptum treated with CO_2 laser therapy.

CO_2 laser therapy of vulval lymphangiectasia and lymphangioma circumscriptum. Haas AF, Narurkar VA. Dermatol Surg 1998; 24: 893–5.

A difficult case of lymphangioma circumscriptum was treated successfully with a high-energy, short-pulse CO_2 laser after two failed surgical excisions.

CO_2 laser ablation of lymphangioma circumscriptum of the scrotum. Treharne LJ, Murison MS. Lymphat Res Biol 2006; 4: 101–3.

Widespread disease of the scrotum had excellent symptomatic relief after treatment with the CO_2 laser.

Evidence Levels: **A** Double-blind study **B** Clinical trial ≥ 20 subjects **C** Clinical trial < 20 subjects **D** Series ≥ 5 subjects **E** Anecdotal case reports

Treatment of lymphangioma circumscriptum with the intense pulsed light system. Thissen CA, Sommer A. Int J Dermatol 2007; 46: 16–8.

An intense pulsed light source led to good cosmetic results.

Treatment of lymphangioma circumscriptum with combined radiofrequency current and 900 nm diode laser. Lapidoth M, Ackerman L, Amitai DB, Raveh E, Kalish E, David M. Dermatol Surg 2006; 32: 790–4.

Treatment was rated as "excellent" in four patients and "good" in two. Swelling, erythema, and pain were present in all patients and ulcers and scarring in two.

Lymphangioma circumscriptum treated with pulsed dye laser. Lai CH, Hanson SG, Mallory SB. Pediatr Dermatol 2001; 18: 509–10.

A child with a symptomatic lymphangioma circumscriptum was treated with pulsed dye laser, with good results.

Radiotherapy in congenital vulvar lymphangioma circumscriptum. Yildiz F, Atahan IL, Ozhar E, Karcaaltincaba M, Cengiz M, Ozyigit G, et al. Int J Gynecol Cancer 2008; 18: 556–9.

A patient was treated successfully with a course of external radiotherapy after failed attempts with sclerosing agents and surgery.

Radiotherapy is a useful treatment for lymphangioma circumscriptum: a report of two patients. Denton AS, Baker-Hines R, Spittle MF. Clin Oncol (R Coll Radiol) 1996; 8: 400–1.

Localized radiotherapy has been successfully used.

Treatment of lymphangioma circumscriptum with topical imiquimod 5% cream. Wang JY, Liu LF, Mao XH. Dermatol Surg 2012; 38: 1566–9.

Lymphedema

*Peter C. Lambert, Giuseppe Micali,
Robert A. Schwartz*

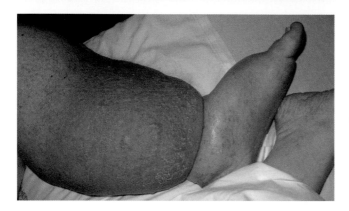

Lymphedema is a chronic, progressive, and sometimes debilitating condition. It is due to abnormal accumulation of protein-rich lymphatic fluid in interstitial spaces. Lymphedema is classified into primary and secondary types.

Primary lymphedema is caused by a developmental malformation of the lymphatic system. It may be classified by age of onset into congenital lymphedema, lymphedema praecox, and lymphedema tarda. Primary congenital lymphedema, or Milroy disease, occurs at age less than 2 years and is an uncommon autosomal dominant disorder due, in some families, to one of several known missense mutations that interfere with vascular endothelial growth factor-3 (VEGF-3) signaling, resulting in abnormal vascular lymphatic function. Lymphedema praecox, also known as *Meige disease*, has its onset between age 2 and 35 years, with a marked tendency to arise during puberty or during pregnancy. Finally, lymphedema tarda has an age of onset later than 35 years.

Secondary lymphedema is due to obstruction of or damage to an otherwise normal lymphatic system. Common causes are malignancy, surgery, radiation therapy, and, globally, filariasis.

Once lymphedema has become established, biophysical influences, such as the law of La Place (which causes dilated structures to expand, regardless of what caused them to begin with) and pathophysiologic responses, such as fibrosis, make it progressive and difficult to treat. Chronic lymphedema may lead to striking verrucous proliferative changes in the overlying skin known as *elephantiasis nostra*. Lymphedema may also predispose the affected tissue to recurrent infection and to a usually aggressive form of *angiosarcoma*, in a condition known as *Stewart–Treves syndrome*.

MANAGEMENT STRATEGIES

Lymphedema must be distinguished from cutaneous and soft tissue lymphedema due to other causes, particularly of cardiac, hepatic, or renal etiology. Not infrequently, there may be more than one cause acting simultaneously or in sequence. Chronic lymphedema is characterized clinically by brawny, nonpitting edema, unlike lymphedema due to cardiac, hepatic, or renal causes, which tend to produce pitting edema. *Lymphoscintigraphy* (lymphography using an isotope; LSG) is a first-line imaging modality useful to evaluate and diagnose disorders of lymphatic vasculature.

The goal of therapy for lymphedema is to reduce stasis of protein-rich lymph in the interstitium and to improve outflow of the lymphatic circulation.

The primary treatment step should be a *conservative approach with medical and physical therapy.*

Complex decongestive therapy (CDT) is an effective first-line treatment option. CDT is a four-component plan composed of *multilayer compression bandaging, manual lymphatic drainage, skin care,* and *exercise.* Therapeutic efficacy is highly dependent on patient compliance. Because of this, strict adherence to the treatment protocol should be encouraged. *Pneumatic compression therapy* has been widely used to control lymphedema as a second-line alternative approach. Because of its poor outcomes as a monotherapy, however, its use has become limited. Recent advances in these modalities have produced beneficial results. In contrast, medications, such as *diuretics,* have been ineffective, showing limited or no benefit. *Meticulous skin care and hygiene* may reduce the incidence of secondary bacterial and fungal infections. If infection does occur, *topical or systemic antibiotics* should be initiated at the first sign of the infection, as infections may lead to further lymphatic injury.

Surgery is reserved for patients refractory to conservative management. *Microsurgical lymphatic-venous anastomoses* have yielded promising results, particularly in repairing traumatic injury. *Excisional surgical therapy* has been performed to reduce limb size and to improve mobility in advanced cases of chronic lymphedema. A notable more recent innovation has been *vascularized lymph node transfer* from one region of the body to another. Reports using this technique are extremely promising.

The scheme proposed here, outlining a two-step conservative therapy and a third-step surgical approach, is for a hypothetical average patient. However, no such individual exists. Preferred therapy varies widely and should be shaped to meet the specific needs of each patient.

Specific Investigations

- Lymphoscintigraphy
- Magnetic resonance imaging (MRI)
- Computed tomography (CT)
- Indocyanine green lymphography

Advances in imaging of lymph flow disorders. Witte CL, Witte MH, Unger EC, Williams WH, Bernas MJ, McNeill GC, et al. Radiographics 2000; 20: 1697–719.

A review illustrating cases in which lymphoscintigraphy, MRI, and CT were used in evaluating and diagnosing primary or secondary lymphedema.

Indocyanine green (ICG) lymphography is superior to lymphoscintigraphy for diagnostic imaging of early lymphedema of the upper limbs. Mihara M, Hara H, Araki J, Kikuchi K, Narushima M, Yamamoto T, et al. PLoS One 2012; 7: e38182.

Indocyanine green combined with MRI had a higher sensitivity in diagnosing early upper limb lymphedema in comparison to other imaging modalities.

First-Line Therapy

- Complex (or complete) decongestive therapy   **C**

Prospective trial of intensive decongestive physiotherapy for upper extremity lymphedema. Karadibak D, Yavuzsen T, Saydam S. J Surg Oncol 2008; 97: 572–7.

This study of 62 women with breast cancer–related lymphedema of an upper extremity demonstrated the effectiveness of CDT by decreasing limb volume and proscribing activity.

Synergic effect of compression therapy and controlled active exercises using a facilitating device in the treatment of arm lymphedema. Godoy Mde F, Pereira MR, Oliani AH, de Godoy JM. Int J Med Sci 2012; 9: 280–4.

A randomized controlled trial of 20 women resulted in the reduction of lymphedematous arms from breast cancer treatment by combining compression therapy with controlled exercises using a facilitating device.

Primary lymphedema: clinical features and management in 138 pediatric patients. Schook CC, Mulliken JB, Fishman SJ, Grant FD, Zurakowski D, Greene AK. Plast Reconstr Surg 2011; 127: 2419–31.

Successful management with compression garments without the need for surgical intervention.

Can manual treatment of lymphedema promote metastasis? Godette K, Mondry TE, Johnstone PA. J Soc Integr Oncol 2006; 4: 8–12.

Contraindications to CDT include hypertension, paralysis, diabetes mellitus, bronchial asthma, acute infections, and congestive heart failure. Malignant disease is also widely considered a contraindication; however, this opinion is not unequivocally supported by current cancer research.

Second-Line Therapy

- Pneumatic compression therapy   **B**

Direct evidence of lymphatic function improvement after advanced pneumatic compression device treatment of lymphedema. Adams KE, Rasmussen JC, Darne C, Tan IC, Aldrich MB, Marshall MV, et al. Biomed Opt Express 2010; 1: 114–25.

This study supports the effectiveness of pneumatic compression device treatment by showing lymphatic function improvement in both controlled subjects and breast cancer–related lymphedema patients.

Third-Line Therapies

- Surgery   **B**
- Low-level laser therapy   **A**

Microsurgery for lymphedema: clinical research and long term results. Campisi C, Bellini C, Campisi C, Accogli S, Bonioli E, Boccardo F. Microsurgery 2010; 30: 256–60.

A retrospective study of 1800 subjects undergoing microsurgery for the treatment of peripheral lymphedema resulting in marked improvement in 83% of patients.

Overview of surgical treatments for breast cancer-related lymphedema. Suami H, Chang DW. Plast Reconstr Surg 2010; 126; 1853–63.

A review of surgical procedures for the treatment of breast cancer–related lymphedema and current issues in the management of lymphedema with surgical treatment.

Treatment of postmastectomy lymphedema with laser therapy: double blind placebo control randomized study. Ahmed Omar MT, Abd-El-Gayed Ebid A, El Morsy AM. J Surg Res 2011; 165: 82–90.

Fifty patients were studied, 25 receiving laser and 25 placebo. Low-level laser therapy reduced limb volume and increased shoulder mobility and hand grip strength in 93% of 50 women with breast cancer–related lymphedema.

Indocyanine green lymphographic evidence of surgical efficacy following microsurgical and supermicrosurgical lymphedema reconstructions. Chen WF, Zhao H, Yamamoto T, Hara H, Ding J. J Reconstr Microsurg 2016; 32: 688–98.

Twenty-one patients were noted to have experienced significant improvement with microsurgical reconstruction of lymphedema using newer techniques despite persistence of limb enlargement.

Vascularized lymph node transfer from the thoracodorsal axis for congenital and post filarial lymphedema of the lower limb. Venkatramani H, Kumaran S, Chethan S, Sapapathy SR. J Surg Oncol 2017; 115: 78–83.

Success with an exciting new technique using lymph node transplants from one part of the body to another to correct intractable lymphedema is reported.

A number of similar reports have now been published.

Lymphocytoma cutis

Fiona J. Child

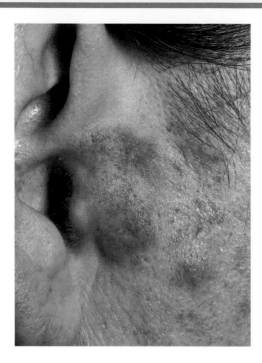

Lymphocytoma cutis (cutaneous lymphoid hyperplasia, cutaneous B-cell pseudolymphoma, Spiegler–Fendt sarcoid) is an entity encompassing a spectrum of benign B-cell lymphoproliferative diseases that share clinical and histopathologic features. Various antigenic stimuli can induce lymphocytoma cutis, but in most cases the cause is not known. It is more common in females, with a female-to-male ratio of approximately 2:1. Most cases are characterized by localized erythematous, plum-colored nodules and plaques that may be difficult to distinguish from cutaneous B-cell lymphoma. Less frequently the generalized form may present with multiple miliary papules that measure a few millimeters in diameter. Lymphocytoma cutis secondary to *Borrelia* infection is most frequently seen at sites where skin temperature is low, such as the earlobes, nipples, nose, and scrotum.

MANAGEMENT STRATEGY

A skin biopsy for histopathology and immunohistochemistry is required to confirm the diagnosis, but the distinction between lymphocytoma cutis and cutaneous B-cell lymphoma may be difficult on both clinical and histopathologic evaluation. There are no agreed histologic criteria; however, features that suggest lymphocytoma cutis include an unaffected epidermis, separated by a Grenz zone, below which are well-formed, nonexpanded, reactive germinal centers. The majority of the infiltrate consists of small, round lymphocytes with a B:T cell ratio of <3:1, without cellular atypia, and polytypic expression of kappa and lambda light chains. A further feature is the presence of numerous tangible-body macrophages within the lymphoid follicles. Molecular analysis of the immunoglobulin heavy chain gene has shown that a significant proportion harbor B-cell clones, which suggests that many cases previously thought to

be lymphocytoma cutis represent indolent low-grade primary cutaneous B-cell lymphomas (PCBCL). Therefore in cases with a detectable B-cell clone, a careful evaluation to exclude systemic disease (a thorough clinical examination, thoracoabdominopelvic computed tomography [CT] scan, and bone marrow biopsy) is required, with adequate long-term follow-up.

A history of possible stimuli known to cause lymphocytoma cutis should be sought; these include *Borrelia burgdorferi* infection, *Leishmania* infection, trauma, vaccinations, allergy hyposensitization injections, ingestion of drugs, arthropod bites, acupuncture, gold pierced earrings, tattoos, treatment with leeches *(Hirudo medicinalis)*, and post–herpes zoster scars, but in most cases the etiology is unknown.

The course of the disease varies but tends to be chronic and indolent, and some lesions may resolve spontaneously without treatment. There is no therapy of proven value for lymphocytoma cutis, with only anecdotal case reports and small series reported and no clinical trials in the literature.

If a cause can be identified, the causative agent should be removed. If infection with *B. burgdorferi* is suspected, treatment with appropriate *antibiotics* (*amoxicillin* 500–1000 mg three times per day, or *doxycycline* 100 mg two to three times per day for 14–21 days) should be initiated.

Localized disease can be treated by simple *excision* and may respond to *intralesional injection of corticosteroids, local irradiation,* or *intralesional interferon-α.* More widespread (generalized) disease is traditionally treated with *oral antimalarials,* most commonly *hydroxychloroquine* (maximum dose 6.5 mg/kg/day); however, lesions may fail to respond to treatment or may recur after cessation of therapy. Other treatment modalities include *subcutaneous interferon-α and oral thalidomide.* Effective responses to destructive therapies, including *cryotherapy* and the *argon laser,* have been reported. A subtype of generalized lymphocytoma cutis may be exacerbated by light, and therefore *sun avoidance* and the use of *sun block* are important.

Specific Investigations

- Serology for *B. burgdorferi* (antibodies identified in 50% of patients with borrelial lymphocytoma)
- Skin biopsy for histology, immunophenotype, and immunoglobulin gene analysis
- Patch testing (if a possible contact allergen is suspected)

The spirochetal etiology of lymphadenosis benigna cutis solitaria. Hovmark A, Asbrink E, Olsson I. Acta Derm Venereol 1986; 66: 479–84.

Of 10 patients investigated, four reported a previous tick bite. Positive *Borrelia* serology was found in six of nine patients, and spirochetes were cultured from one of two skin biopsies.

***Borrelia burgdorferi*-associated lymphocytoma cutis: clinicopathologic, immunophenotypic, and molecular study of 106 cases.** Colli C, Leinweber B, Müllegger R, Chott A, Kerl H, Cerroni L. J Cutan Pathol 2004; 31: 232–40.

A total of 106 cases of *B. burgdorferi*–associated lymphocytoma cutis in a region endemic for *Borrelia* infection were studied retrospectively. The most common sites affected were the earlobe, genital area, and nipple (these locations may be due to the predilection of *B. burgdorferi* spirochetes for cooler body sites). In some cases the histopathologic, immunophenotypic, and molecular features were misleading, and it was concluded that integration of all data is necessary to obtain the correct diagnosis.

Evidence Levels: **A** Double-blind study **B** Clinical trial ≥ 20 subjects **C** Clinical trial < 20 subjects **D** Series ≥ 5 subjects **E** Anecdotal case reports

Borrelial lymphocytoma in adult patients. Maraspin V, Nahtigal Klevišar M, Ruzic-Sabljic E, Lusa L, Strle F. Clin Infect Dis 2016; 63: 914–21.

Cases of borrelial lymphocytoma diagnosed in 144 adults from a single institution were followed for 1 year. Breast and earlobe were the most common sites of involvement, and 72% had concomitant erythema migrans. Ninety percent of patients responded to a course of antibiotics. Those with features of disseminated Lyme borreliosis were most likely to fail treatment, but all responded to retreatment.

Cutaneous lymphoid hyperplasia and cutaneous marginal zone lymphoma: comparison of morphologic and immunophenotypic features. Baldassano MF, Bailey EM, Ferry JA, Harris NL, Duncan LM. Am J Surg Pathol 1999; 23: 88–96.

The histologic and immunophenotypic features of 14 cases of lymphocytoma cutis and 16 cases of cutaneous marginal zone lymphoma were compared.

Differential diagnosis of cutaneous infiltrates of B lymphocytes with follicular growth pattern. Leinweber B, Colli C, Chott A, Kerl H, Cerroni L. Am J Dermatopathol 2004; 26: 4–13.

The histopathologic, immunophenotypic, and molecular features of *B. burgdorferi*–associated lymphocytoma cutis, primary cutaneous follicle center cell lymphoma, and primary cutaneous marginal zone lymphoma were compared. Features that favored lymphocytoma cutis were the presence of tingible-body macrophages, strong proliferation rate of follicular cells, BCL-2-negative follicular cells, and the absence of monoclonality.

Immunophenotypic and genotypic analysis in cutaneous lymphoid hyperplasias. Hammer E, Sangueza O, Suwanjindar P, White CR, Braziel R. J Am Acad Dermatol 1993; 28: 426–33.

Of 11 patients with histologic and immunophenotypic features of lymphocytoma cutis, clonal rearrangements were detected in two, both of whom subsequently developed B-cell lymphoma.

Polymerase chain reaction analysis of immunoglobulin gene rearrangement analysis in cutaneous lymphoid hyperplasias. Bouloc A, Delfau-Larue M-H, Lenormand B, Meunier F, Wechsler J, Thomine E, et al. Arch Dermatol 1999; 135: 168–72.

Twenty-four patients with a diagnosis of lymphocytoma cutis according to clinical, histopathologic, and immunophenotypic criteria underwent polymerase chain reaction (PCR) analysis of the immunoglobulin heavy chain gene using DNA from lesional skin. In one patient, a B-cell clone was detected. In the other 23 a polyclonal result was obtained.

Cutaneous B-cell lymphomas are known to have a relatively high false-negative rate using PCR due to somatic hypermutation, which affects the variable region of the immunoglobulin heavy chain gene and may prevent primer binding. The number of false-negative results may be significantly reduced by using multiple primer sets for different parts of the variable region and for the kappa light chain gene. This paper only used one set of primers, and therefore the detection of only one B-cell clone may be a significant underestimate.

A review of 55 cases of cutaneous lymphoid hyperplasia: reassessment of the histopathologic findings leading to reclassification of 4 lesions as cutaneous marginal zone lymphoma and 19 as pseudolymphomatous folliculitis. Arai E, Shimizu M, Hirose T. Hum Pathol 2005; 36: 505–11.

The histopathologic features of 55 cases of cutaneous lymphoid hyperplasia were reassessed. Of these, nine were reclassified as marginal zone lymphoma, distinguished by patchy or diffuse centrocyte-like cells, with plasma cells at the periphery of the infiltrate, monotypic light chain restriction, and a clonal immunoglobulin heavy chain gene rearrangement.

Clonality assessment of cutaneous B-cell lymphoid proliferations: a comparison of flow cytometry immunophenotyping, molecular studies, and immunohistochemistry/in situ hybridization and review of the literature. Schafernak KT, Variakojis D, Goolsby CL, Tucker RM, Martínez-Escala ME, Smith FA, et al. Am J Dermatopathol 2014; 36: 781–95.

Flow cytometry immunophenotyping, which is not routinely applied to the skin, was performed on 73 cutaneous lymphoid infiltrates; B-cell clones were detected in 68% of infiltrates diagnosed as B-cell lymphoma, in contrast to none of the 14 cases of cutaneous lymphoid hyperplasia.

Lymphomatoid contact reaction to gold earrings. Fleming C, Burden D, Fallowfield M, Lever R. Contact Derm 1997; 37: 298–9.

A rare entity characterized by nodules at sites of piercing with gold jewelry and the histologic features of lymphocytoma cutis. Patch tests to gold sodium thiosulfate are positive.

Vaccination-induced cutaneous pseudolymphoma. Maubec E, Pinquier L, Viguier M, Caux F, Amsler E, Aractingi S, et al. J Am Acad Dermatol 2005; 52: 623–9.

Nine patients developed cutaneous lymphoid hyperplasia at the site of hepatitis vaccinations. Aluminum deposits were identified in all nine biopsy specimens, and the authors suggest that cutaneous lymphoid hyperplasia is a possible adverse effect of vaccinations that include aluminum oxide as an adjuvant.

Diffuse cutaneous pseudolymphoma due to therapy with medicinal leeches. Altamura D, Calonje E, Liau JL, Rogers M, Verdolini R. JAMA Dermatol 2014; 150: 783–4.

Scattered papules and plaques on her back, confirmed histologically as cutaneous lymphoid hyperplasia, developed in a female after application of medicinal leeches for fibromyalgia. The lesions resolved with the application of a topical steroid.

First-Line Therapies

Localized

• Excision	E
• Topical corticosteroids	E
• Intralesional corticosteroids	E
• Oral antibiotics (if positive *Borrelia* serology)	E
• CO_2 or Nd:YAG laser (if occurring within a tattoo)	E

Generalized

• Antimalarials	E
• Sun avoidance/sun block (light exacerbated)	E

Treatment of cutaneous pseudolymphoma with hydroxychloroquine. Stoll DM. J Am Acad Dermatol 1983; 8: 696–9.

A case report of a 40-year-old woman with generalized lymphocytoma cutis that cleared with 400 mg hydroxychloroquine daily.

Cutaneous lymphoid hyperplasia (pseudolymphoma) in tattoos: a case series of 7 patients. Kluger N, Vermeulen C, Moguelet P, Cotton H, Koeb MH, Balme B, et al. J Eur Acad Dermatol Venereol 2010; 24: 208–13.

Two of seven patients with cutaneous lymphoid hyperplasia occurring within their tattoos were treated with CO_2 or Nd:YAG laser with improvement.

Second-Line Therapies

Localized

• Superficial radiotherapy	E
• Intralesional interferon-α	E
• Argon laser	E
• Cryotherapy	D
• Topical 0.1% tacrolimus ointment	E
• Intralesional rituximab	E
• Topical photodynamic therapy	E

Generalized

• Subcutaneous interferon-α$_{2b}$	E
• Thalidomide	E

Cutaneous lymphoid hyperplasia: results of radiation therapy. Olson LE, Wilson JF, Cox JD. Radiology 1985; 155: 507–9.

Four cases of lymphocytoma cutis were treated with radiation therapy. Over a follow-up period of 8 months to 7 years there were no recurrences.

Local orthovolt radiotherapy in primary cutaneous B-cell lymphoma. Pimpinelli N, Vallecchi C. Skin Cancer 1999; 14: 219–24.

Data from 115 patients with PCBCL produced a 98.2% complete remission rate and a median disease-free period of 55 months; recurrences were mostly limited to the skin. In view of the difficulties in distinguishing between PCBCL and lymphocytoma cutis, many groups have used superficial radiotherapy in cases of lymphocytoma cutis, although evidence remains anecdotal.

In our experience these cases are relatively radioresistant compared with PCBCL.

Treatment of cutaneous pseudolymphoma with interferon alfa-2b. Tomar S, Stoll HL, Grassi MA, Cheney R. J Am Acad Dermatol 2009; 60: 172–4.

One patient with multiple nodules and plaques was treated with intralesional interferon-α$_{2b}$ (1 MU in 1 mL saline) every 2 weeks for a total of 5 weeks with complete resolution of all lesions except for one that was subsequently excised.

Role of the argon laser in treatment of lymphocytoma cutis. Wheeland RG, Kantor GR, Bailin PL, Bergfeld WF. J Am Acad Dermatol 1986; 14: 267–72.

The argon laser improved cosmetic appearance and alleviated symptoms of lymphocytoma cutis, but failed to provide complete histologic clearing in a young man who had failed to respond adequately to initial therapy with hydroxychloroquine.

Lymphocytoma cutis: a series of five patients successfully treated with cryosurgery. Kuflik AS, Schwartz RA. J Am Acad Dermatol 1992; 26: 449–52.

Five patients with lymphocytoma cutis underwent therapy with liquid nitrogen to individual lesions using a single cycle of 15 to 20 seconds per lesion, with complete clinical resolution of all lesions treated within 3 to 6 weeks.

Spiegler–Fendt type lymphocytoma cutis: a case report of two patients successfully treated with interferon alpha-2b. Hervonen K, Lehtinen T, Vaalasti A. Acta Derm Venereol 1999; 79: 241–2.

Two men who had generalized lymphocytoma cutis and had failed to respond to other therapies were treated with subcutaneous interferon-α$_{2b}$ 2.5 MU three times per week, with complete resolution of all lesions by 3 months. However, lesions recurred in both men between 6 and 23 months after the completion of treatment.

Treatment of cutaneous lymphoid hyperplasia with thalidomide: report of two cases. Benchikhi H, Bodemer C, Fraitag S, Wechsler J, Delfau-Larue M-H, Gounod N, et al. J Am Acad Dermatol 1999; 40: 1005–7.

Two cases of lymphocytoma cutis involving the nose that showed complete regression after treatment with thalidomide for 3 months at a dose of 100 mg once daily for 2 months and 50 mg once daily for the third month. There was no recurrence at 36 and 31 months follow-up, respectively.

Disseminated cutaneous lymphoid hyperplasia of 12 years' duration triggered by vaccination. Pham-Ledard A, Vergier B, Doutre MS, Beylot-Barry M. Dermatology 2010; 220: 176–9.

A 17-year old-girl with long-standing hepatitis B vaccination–induced cutaneous lymphoid hyperplasia was treated with oral thalidomide with a complete clinical response.

Lymphocytoma cutis treated with topical tacrolimus. El-Dars LD, Statham BN, Blackford S, Williams N. Clin Exp Dermatol 2005; 30: 305–7.

Two cases of lymphocytoma cutis affecting the face were treated with topical tacrolimus 0.1% twice daily. In both cases the lesions completely resolved after 8 months, application.

Treatment of cutaneous lymphoid hyperplasia with the monoclonal anti-CD20 antibody rituximab. Martin SJ, Duvic M. Clin Lymphoma Myeloma Leuk 2011; 11: 286–8.

One case of lymphocytoma cutis was treated with intralesional rituximab with notable clinical improvement. Persistent and recurrent erythematous areas were subsequently treated with topical tacrolimus with further improvement.

Successful treatment of lymphadenosis benigna cutis with topical photodynamic therapy with delta-aminolevulinic acid. Takeda H, Kaneko T, Harada K, Matsuzaki Y, Nakano H, Hanada K. Dermatology 2005; 211: 264–6.

Two females were treated with five treatments of topical δ-aminolevulinic acid photodynamic therapy (ALA-PDT) with dramatic clinical and histopathologic improvement

Evidence Levels: **A** Double-blind study **B** Clinical trial ≥ 20 subjects **C** Clinical trial < 20 subjects **D** Series ≥ 5 subjects **E** Anecdotal case reports

146

Lymphogranuloma venereum

Frederick A. Pereira

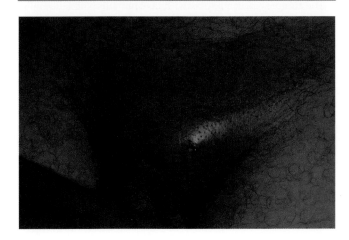

Classic lymphogranuloma venereum (LGV) is an uncommon, sexually transmitted infection (STI) occurring in the tropics. It is characterized by three stages of disease: (1) transient genital ulceration; (2) painful, suppurative inguinal lymphadenopathy; and (3) fibrosis, lymphatic obstruction, and genital elephantiasis. A new LGV syndrome has emerged in the industrialized world among men who have sex with men (MSM). The clinical picture consists of proctitis with associated tenesmus, mucopurulent discharge, abdominal pain, and perianal ulceration. Lymphadenopathy is not a prominent feature of the proctitis syndrome. Asymptomatic infection can occur in all forms of LGV. LGV is a systemic disease of lymphoid tissue caused by serovars L1, L2, and L3 of *Chlamydia trachomatis*. It can be associated with extragenital manifestations such as erythema nodosum, myalgia, reactive arthritis, fever, fatigue, and weight loss.

MANAGEMENT STRATEGY

The long-term sequelae of untreated LGV are horrific, and treatment should be started immediately on the basis of clinical suspicion, epidemiologic information, and exclusion of other diagnoses. Treatment should *not* be delayed pending positive laboratory confirmation. Nucleic acid amplification testing (NAAT) is the method of choice to detect *C. trachomatis*. Material can be obtained from an ulcer base, rectal mucosa, or bubo aspirate. That material is then tested with a screening NAAT to detect chlamydia. If *C. trachomatis* is detected, a second NAAT is used to identify the specific serovar. If NAAT testing is not available, a single complement fixation test in titer greater than 1:64 or a fourfold rise in titer over a few weeks is strongly suggestive of LGV.

The treatment of choice is *doxycycline* 100 mg twice daily for 3 weeks. *Fluoroquinolones* and *tetracyclines* are contraindicated in pregnant and lactating women. These women should be treated with *erythromycin* 500 mg four times daily for 3 weeks. Children

with LGV should be treated with erythromycin. *Azithromycin* 1 g once a week for 3 weeks has been used successfully as an alternative to erythromycin. Moxifloxacin has antichlamydial activity, but there are only anecdotal reports of its use in LGV. HIV-positive patients are treated with the same regimens; however, these patients may require prolonged treatment, and they must be closely monitored for treatment failure and relapse. Fluctuant buboes should be drained by needle aspiration through normal skin at the superior pole. Buboes should not be incised because of danger of sinus formation.

All patients with LGV should be tested for other STIs and bloodborne diseases, particularly HIV and hepatitis B and C. Intensive and repeated safe-sex counseling is necessary because most patients continue to engage in high-risk behaviors. Sex partners should be evaluated, tested for infection, and then presumptively treated with azithromycin 1 g orally or doxycycline 100 mg twice a day for 7 days.

Specific Investigations
• NAAT
• Chlamydial serology

Lymphogranuloma venereum 2015: clinical presentation, diagnosis, and treatment. Stoner BP, Cohen SE. Clin Infect Dis 2015; 61(Suppl 8): S865–73.

Proctitis and proctocolitis are now the most common clinical manifestations of LGV. The classic inguinal presentation with buboes is becoming increasingly uncommon.

Lymphogranuloma venereum among men who have sex with men. An epidemiologic and clinical review. De Vrieze NH, de Vreis HJ. Expert Rev Anti Infect Ther 2014; 12: 697–704.

Approximately 25% of infections are asymptomatic. MSM who have had receptive anal intercourse in the past 6 months should be screened. Asymptomatic carriers are a reservoir of infection, and these persons should be treated.

2013 European guideline on the management of lymphogranuloma venereum. De Vries HJ, Zingoni A, Kreuter A, Moi H, White JA. J Eur Acad Dermatol Venereol 2015; 29: 1–6.

After resolution of signs and symptoms after a full 21 days of treatment, a microbiological "test of cure" is not considered necessary. Patients should be tested for other STIs and hepatitis B and C. In addition, they should be warned of the risks of unprotected sex and mucosally traumatic sexual practices such as enemas and use of sexual toys.

Lymphogranuloma venereum presenting as perianal ulceration: an emerging clinical presentation? Singhrao T, Higham E, French P. Sex Transm Infect 2011; 87: 123–4.

LGV, along with herpes simplex, chancroid, and syphilis, must be included in the differential diagnosis of anal ulcers, particularly in MSM. Herpes simplex remains the most common cause.

Lymphogranuloma venereum. Herring A, Richens J. Sex Transm Infect 2006; 82: 23–5.

The laboratory diagnosis of LGV consists of detection of *C. trachomatis*-specific DNA followed by genotyping to identify serovars L1, L2, or L3. Culture of chlamydiae is technically difficult, and few laboratories have the facilities to do this. Complement fixation studies can be useful for diagnosis. High or rising titers in a symptomatic patient are suggestive of LGV.

The association between lymphogranuloma venereum and HIV among men who have sex with men: systematic review and meta-analysis. Rönn MM, Ward H. BMC Infect Dis 2011; 11: 70.

In 13 studies the prevalence of HIV among MSM with LGV ranged from 67% to 100%. HIV + MSM are disproportionately affected by LGV.

Persistent high-risk sexual behavior in men who have sex with men after symptomatic lymphogranuloma venereum proctitis. Van den Bos RR, van der Meijden WI. Int J STD AIDS 2007; 18: 715–6.

After treatment of LGV proctitis, 17 of 26 patients (65%) were subsequently treated for another STI within 3 years. Health education and counseling efforts must be intensified because patients continue to engage in high-risk sexual activities.

First-Line Therapy

- Doxycycline 100 mg orally twice daily for 21 days **B**

Centers for Disease Control and Prevention. Sexually transmitted disease treatment guidelines, 2015. Workowski KA, Bolan GA. MMWR Recomm Rep 2015; 64: 1–137.

Second-Line Therapies

- Erythromycin base 500 mg orally four times daily for 21 days **B**
- Azithromycin 1.0 g orally once weekly for 3 weeks **C**
- Moxifloxacin 400 mg daily for 10 days **E**
- Aspiration of buboes **B**

Treatment of lymphogranuloma venereum. McLean CA, Stoner BP, Workowski KA. Clin Infect Dis 2007; 44: 147–52.

Doxycycline 100 mg twice daily for 3 weeks is recommended as first-line treatment for LGV. Azithromycin 1.0 g orally once weekly for 3 weeks appears to be effective against LGV. Erythromycin base 500 mg four times a day orally is the preferred treatment for pregnant women with LGV.

Doxycycline failure in lymphogranuloma venereum. Méchaï F, de Barbayrac B, Aoun O, Mérens A, Umbert P, Rapp C. Sex Transm Infect 2010; 86: 278–9.

The authors report a patient with LGV proctitis who failed a full 3-week course of doxycycline. The patient achieved rapid clinical cure with a 10-day course of moxifloxacin 400 mg daily. Failure of doxycycline is unusual.

An audit on the management of lymphogranuloma venereum in a sexual health clinic in London, UK. Hill SC, Hodson L, Smith A. Int J STD AIDS 2010; 21: 772–6.

Fifty-five patients were treated with doxycycline, and seven patients were treated with azithromycin 1 g per week for 3 weeks. All patients treated with azithromycin achieved clinical cure, and microbiological cure was proven in six. Half of the treated patients returned for follow-up within 3 months; a notable proportion tested positive for newly acquired STIs. Patients continue to engage in high-risk behaviors after treatment, and safe-sex counseling efforts need to be intensified.

Lymphogranuloma venereum. Becker LE. Int J Dermatol 1976; 15: 26–33.

Incision and drainage of buboes is not recommended. Fluctuant buboes should be aspirated at the superior pole through normal skin with a large-bore needle.

Evidence Levels: **A** Double-blind study **B** Clinical trial ≥ 20 subjects **C** Clinical trial < 20 subjects **D** Series ≥ 5 subjects **E** Anecdotal case reports

147

Lymphomatoid papulosis

Rachel S. Klein, Elisha Singer, Jacqueline M. Junkins-Hopkins, Carmela C. Vittorio, Alain H. Rook, Ellen J. Kim

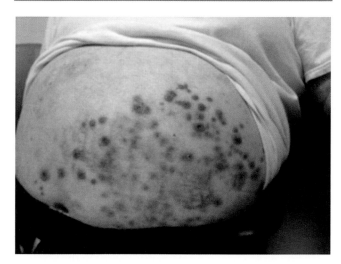

Lymphomatoid papulosis (LyP) is a distinct subset of CD30+ lymphoproliferative disorders in the World Health Organization/ European Organization for the Research and Treatment of Cancer (WHO/EORTC) classification of cutaneous lymphomas, defined histologically by a variable infiltrate of CD30+ lymphocytes, in conjunction with the clinical presentation of crops of recurrent, self-healing papulonodules. Patients may present with very few or with multiple lesions, which may evolve into a crusted or necrotic stage, which often heal with a scar. Less common presentations include regional, isolated acral, and oral disease. Itching can occur. LyP affects adults and children as young as 11 months of age and may persist for years to decades. Approximately 5% to 25% of patients with LyP may present with or develop a lymphoproliferative malignancy, such as mycosis fungoides (MF – cutaneous T-cell lymphoma, CTCL), anaplastic large cell lymphoma (ALCL), and Hodgkin or non-Hodgkin lymphomas. There may also be a slight risk of developing a nonhematologic neoplasm. The same clone has been documented in some patients with LyP and the associated lymphoma (including MF and ALCL), supporting the concept that LyP lies within the spectrum of CTCL. Clinical and histologic overlap may also be seen with LyP and arthropod bites, pityriasis lichenoides, and folliculitis.

MANAGEMENT STRATEGY

Most important, the management of LyP begins with understanding the natural history of the disease. LyP is defined as a recurrent, self-healing (remission of every individual lesion), papulonodular eruption, with histology suggesting CTCL. There are six histologic variants, including type A (wedge-shaped infiltrate containing eosinophils and histiocytes), type B (epidermotropism, resembles MF), type C (cohesive sheets of CD30+ cells, resembles ALCL), type D (CD8/CD30+, resembles primary cutaneous aggressive epidermotropic CD8+ cytotoxic T-cell lymphoma), type E (CD30+ with angioinvasion), and type F (CD30+, follicular). Long-term survival does not appear to vary among the histologic subtypes, but associated lymphomas may be seen more commonly with subtypes B and C. A minor subset of LyP patients may have chromosomal rearrangements involving the DUSP22-IRF4 (dual specificity protein phosphatase 22/interferon regulatory factor 4) locus on 6p25.3, which has been observed in some cutaneous ALCL patients.

Clinical evaluation should include a complete history assessing for atypical features, including previous lymphoid neoplasms, constitutional symptoms, lymphadenopathy, or laboratory abnormalities on complete blood counts, blood chemistry, and lactate dehydrogenase. Patients with abnormal findings should undergo computed tomography (CT) or positron emission tomography (PET)/CT scanning to exclude a systemic lymphoma. Distinguishing LyP from primary cutaneous ALCL is important, although this may be difficult because of clinical and histologic overlap, including spontaneous regression.

Persistent lesions greater than 2 to 3 cm in diameter favor primary cutaneous ALCL; however, some patients do not fit well into either category. Such "borderline" cases have similar biological behavior to LyP and can be managed as such.

Treatment of LyP should be tailored to the disease burden, because treatment has not been proven to alter the natural course of LyP, nor does treatment prevent the development of associated lymphomas. Treatment should be reserved for symptomatic or cosmetically bothersome cases. First-line therapies include *topical corticosteroids*, *low-dose methotrexate*, and *phototherapy*. A response may be seen within the first few weeks of treatment, including the development of fewer lesions, faster resolution of individual lesions, and occasionally induction of remission. Large or borderline lesions can be treated with *local radiotherapy* or *excision*. Therapies that are beneficial in MF may also be used, including topicals such as *carmustine* (BCNU), *mechlorethamine* (nitrogen mustard), *bexarotene*, and *imiquimod* cream 5%. Systemic biologic agents such as *interferon-α* and the retinoid X receptor agonist *bexarotene* are also effective for suppression of lesions. In severe cases, the anti-CD30 antibody, *brentuximab vedotin*, is effective; however, this must be balanced by the risks of peripheral neuropathy, neutropenia, and rarely, progressive multifocal leukoencephalopathy (PML). Multiagent chemotherapy is not indicated, despite histologic features that may suggest ALCL. LyP can recur for decades, requiring careful consideration of treatment side effects and continued monitoring for the development of lymphoma.

Specific Investigations

- Biopsy and histologic review to confirm the diagnosis
- Exclusion of constitutional ("B") symptoms, clinical hepatosplenomegaly/lymphadenopathy, or laboratory abnormalities
- Ongoing surveillance for a lymphoproliferative neoplasm

EORTC, ISCL, and USCLC consensus recommendations for the treatment of primary cutaneous CD30-positive lymphoproliferative disorders: lymphomatoid papulosis and primary cutaneous anaplastic large-cell lymphoma. Kempf W, Pfaltz K, Vermeer M, Cozzio A, Ortiz-Romero P, Bagot M, et al. Blood 2011; 118: 4024–35.

These consensus guidelines give recommendations for the management of the spectrum of CD30+ cutaneous lymphoproliferative disease. Typical LyP does not require staging procedures if there is a normal physical examination and review of systems. Long-term follow-up is required for all subtypes.

Lymphomatoid papulosis. Reappraisal of clinicopathologic presentation and classification into subtypes A, B, and C. El Shabrawi-Caelen L, Kerl H, Cerroni L. Arch Dermatol 2004; 140: 441–7.

A retrospective review of 85 patients with LyP documented histologic overlap between subtypes A, B, and C and between type B and MF. Eight percent of patients had more than one histologic subtype of LyP. The authors also stress the tight overlap with LyP and CD30 lymphoma. A variety of clinicohistopathologic presentations of LyP, including those with histology showing follicular mucinosis, syringotropism, vesicle formation, MF-like bandlike infiltrates, and associated keratoacanthoma, are discussed.

A variant of lymphomatoid papulosis simulating primary cutaneous aggressive epidermotropic CD8+ cytotoxic T-cell lymphoma. Description of 9 cases. Saggini A, Gulia A, Argenyi Z, Fink-Puches R, Lissia A, Magaña M, et al. Am J Surg Pathol 2010; 34: 1168–75.

A variant of LyP, termed *LyP type D*, is described in nine patients with clinical aspects of LyP but with histopathologic features resembling primary cutaneous aggressive epidermotropic CD8+ cytotoxic lymphoma. The histology of LyP type D is of medium sized CD8+ CD30+ pleomorphic cells with prominent, pagetoid reticulosis–like epidermotropism. None of the patients developed a lymphoproliferative malignancy during a mean follow-up of 84 months.

Accurate clinicopathologic correlation is necessary to avoid misdiagnosing LyP type D patients.

Angioinvasive lymphomatoid papulosis: a new variant simulating aggressive lymphomas. Kempf W, Kazakov DV, Schärer L, Rütten A, Mentzel T, Paredes BE, et al. Am J Surg Pathol 2013; 37: 1–13.

Another variant of LyP is retrospectively described in 16 patients with oligolesional papules that ulcerated, with histology showing CD30+, often CD8+ angioinvasive T cells, termed *type E LyP*. Such histology can overlap with cytotoxic cutaneous lymphomas, but none of the patients developed extracutaneous disease.

Follicular lymphomatoid papulosis revisited: a study of 11 cases, with new histopathological findings. Kempf W, Kazakov DV, Baumgartner HP, Kutzner H. J Am Acad Dermatol 2013; 68: 809–16.

Follicular LyP is a variant of LyP with involvement of hair follicles, mostly in the form of perifollicular infiltrate with variable degrees of folliculotropism. Other changes, including hyperplasia of the follicular epithelium, rupture of hair follicle, and follicular mucinosis, are less common. Rarely, intrafollicular pustules can be seen in the follicular epithelium; such lesions manifest clinically as pustules.

Some propose that follicular LyP should be termed LyP type F; others propose it is a subtype of types A and C.

Primary and secondary cutaneous CD30+ lymphoproliferative disorders: a report from the Dutch Cutaneous Lymphoma Group on the long-term follow-up data of 219 patients and guidelines for diagnosis and treatment. Bekkenk MW, Geelen FAMJ, van Voorst Vader PC, Heule F, Geerts ML, van Vloten WA, et al. Blood 2000; 95: 3653–61.

Guidelines are proposed for the diagnosis and treatment of patients with CD30+ lymphoproliferative disorders based on long-term follow-up of 219 patients, 118 of whom had LyP (4% had tumors). Fifty-two of 118 patients received no treatment or topical corticosteroids. The remainder received a variety of standard treatments, none of which was associated with complete, sustained remission. Staging of patients with type C LyP failed to reveal extracutaneous disease. Nineteen percent developed an associated lymphoma. Induction of remission of the secondary lymphoma had no effect on the natural course of LyP. The calculated risk for extracutaneous disease was 4% at 10 years.

Lymphomatoid papulosis: treatment response and associated lymphomas in a study of 180 patients. Wieser I, Oh CW, Talpur R, Duvic M. J Am Acad Dermatol 2016; 74: 59–67.

In this retrospective chart review of 180 patients diagnosed with LyP between 1995 and 2015 at a specialty clinic, 47.2% of patients had histologic subtype A, 17.2% type B, 22.8% type C, 7.8% type D, 0.6% type E, and 4.4% mixed subtype. One hundred fourteen other lymphomas were observed in 93 patients (51.6% of cohort), with the most common being MF (61.4%) and ALCL (26.3%). Risk factors for development of lymphoma included male sex and histologic subtypes B and C. Number of lesions and symptom severity were not associated with lymphoma development. Patients with type D were less likely to have lymphomas. The presence of T-cell clonality was not associated with increased lymphoma risk. Treatment provided symptomatic relief but did not prevent progression to lymphoma.

The overall higher association (40%) with lymphoma compared with other studies may represent a referral bias.

CD30+ cutaneous lymphoproliferative disorders: the Stanford experience in lymphomatoid papulosis and primary cutaneous anaplastic large cell lymphoma. Liu HL, Hoppe RT, Kohler S, Harvell JD, Reddy S, Kim YH. J Am Acad Dermatol 2003; 49: 1049–58.

In 19 of 31 cases with LyP, a higher than previously reported associated coexisting hematolymphoid malignancy (61% with one or more) was noted. Most had MF, which occurred before, during, or after the diagnosis of LyP. Some had two hematolymphoid malignancies. Three progressed to ALCL, with an interval ranging from 77 to 152 months. The overall 5- and 10-year survival of patients with LyP was 100% and 92%, respectively, and none died of LyP. Those with ALCL had a favorable course. LyP subtype did not predict the risk of associated malignancy.

The higher association with malignancy may represent selection bias.

Lymphomatoid papulosis in children: a series of 25 cases. Miquel J, Fraitag S, Hamel-Taillac D, Molina T, Brousse N, de Prost Y, et al. Br J Dermatol 2014; 171: 1138–46.

This is a retrospective analysis of lymphomatoid papulosis in 25 children up to 15 years of age (15 male, 10 female; median age 7.5 years) diagnosed with LyP (82% were type A, remainder type C). Marked eosinophilic infiltrate was common (44%). No associated lymphomas were observed during median follow-up of 10 years. Pityriasis lichenoides chronica (PLC) was observed in 36% of patients and atopic dermatitis in 28%.

In children, PLC may be a predisposing factor for LyP.

Lymphomatoid papulosis in children: a retrospective cohort study of 35 cases. Nijsten T, Curiel-Lewandrowski C, Kadin ME. Arch Dermatol 2004; 140: 306–12.

In a retrospective cohort analysis of 35 patients diagnosed with LyP during childhood (less than 18 years old) followed over a mean

Evidence Levels: A Double-blind study   B Clinical trial ≥ 20 subjects   C Clinical trial < 20 subjects   D Series ≥ 5 subjects   E Anecdotal case reports

duration of 9 years, 3 patients (9%) developed a malignant non-Hodgkin lymphoma. No clinical risk factors were identified. Patients with childhood LyP were also significantly more likely to have atopy.

Children with LyP have an approximate 10% risk of developing a hematologic malignancy during their lives and thus require careful life-long monitoring.

Single cell analysis of CD30+ cells in lymphomatoid papulosis demonstrates a common clonal T-cell origin. Steinhoff M, Hummel M, Anagnostopoulos I, Kaudewitz P, Seitz V, Assaf C, et al. Blood 2002; 100: 578–84.

The large CD30+ cells in LyP type A represent a single clone within each individual case, whereas the majority of CD30– cells are polyclonal. The identical T-cell clone can be identified in separate skin lesions and at different time points, demonstrating the persistence of the T-cell clone in LyP.

Assessment for clonality will not help differentiate borderline cases of LyP from ALCL or MF.

Lymphomatoid papulosis associated with mycosis fungoides: a study of 21 patients including analyses for clonality. Zackheim H, Jones C, LeBoit PE, Kashani-Sabet M, McCalmont TH, Zehnder J. J Am Acad Dermatol 2003; 49: 620–3.

Of 54 patients with LyP, 39% had MF. LyP preceded (67%), followed (19%), or was concurrent with (14%) a diagnosis of MF, and 95% had type A LyP. Of those checked (7 patients) 100% had an identical clone in MF and LyP lesions.

Large cell transformation mimicking regional lymphomatoid papulosis in a patient with mycosis fungoides. Nakahigashi K, Ishida Y, Matsumura Y, Kore-eda S, Ohmori K, Fujimoto M, et al. J Dermatol 2008; 35: 283–8.

The authors report a 57-year-old man with stage III MF who developed a regional eruption of either transformed MF or type C LyP on his chest. Spontaneous resolution supported the diagnosis of LyP.

The importance of differentiating LyP from large cell transformation of MF is stressed. In contrast to LyP, which is associated with a better prognosis, in patients with MF, those with large cell transformation have a worse prognosis.

First-Line Therapies

• Therapy not required	**B**
• PUVA (Psoralen ultraviolet A) phototherapy	**B**
• Low-dose methotrexate	**B**
• Topical corticosteroids	**E**

Practical management of CD30+ lymphoproliferative disorders. Hughey LC. Dermatol Clin 2015; 33: 819–33.

This recent review discusses current therapies for symptomatic LyP. Given the excellent long-term prognosis, it may be reasonable to simply monitor off therapy. The remaining specific treatment options are discussed in further detail.

PUVA-treatment in lymphomatoid papulosis. Wantzin GL, Thompsen K. Br J Dermatol 1982; 107: 687–90.

Five patients with LyP, including one patient with tumors, were treated with PUVA (51–124 J/cm² for classic LyP and 481 J/cm² for tumors). There was a reduction in the number of lesions and shortening of the life cycle of each individual lesion to 1 week from 3 to 6 weeks. Remission was achieved in one patient.

Methotrexate is effective therapy for lymphomatoid papulosis and other primary cutaneous CD30+ lymphoproliferative disorders. Vonderheid EC, Sajjadian A, Kadin ME. J Am Acad Dermatol 1996; 34: 470–81.

A 20-year experience of methotrexate therapy in 45 patients with LyP, CD30+ lymphoma, and borderline cases is reviewed. Patients responded within 4 weeks (15–20 mg weekly). Maintenance doses were given at 10- to 14-day intervals (range 7–28 days); 29% had concomitant MF, requiring other therapies (mechlorethamine hydrochloride, carmustine, standard UV (ultraviolet) therapy, and PUVA), which offered some additional benefit, but the relative effectiveness was less than with methotrexate. LyP and CD30+ lymphoma responded similarly. Three patients had diminished responsiveness, suggesting resistance to methotrexate. Severe exacerbations occurred upon abrupt drug discontinuation.

This is considered first-line therapy for symptomatic disease, with disease control typical but remission off drug uncommon.

Lymphomatoid papulosis: successful weekly pulse superpotent topical corticosteroid therapy in three pediatric patients. Paul MA, Krowchuk DP, Hitchcock MG, Jorizzo JL. Pediatr Dermatol 1996; 13: 501–6.

Three children with LyP were treated with halobetasol or clobetasol propionate twice daily for 2 to 3 weeks, followed by weekly pulsed application, resulting in complete resolution of nearly all cutaneous lesions. Adjuvant intralesional triamcinolone was used for three ulcerated lesions.

Although this modality is unlikely to alter the disease course, it is a reasonable treatment approach because it has a relatively low complication profile.

Second-Line Therapies

• Topical mechlorethamine (nitrogen mustard)	**B**
• Topical carmustine	**C**
• Topical bexarotene	**C**

Long-term efficacy, curative potential, and carcinogenicity of topical mechlorethamine chemotherapy in cutaneous T cell lymphoma. Vonderheid EC, Tan ET, Kantor AF, Shrager L, Micaily B, Van Scott EJ. J Am Acad Dermatol 1989; 20: 416–28.

Seven patients with LyP and 17 with concomitant LyP and MF were treated with 10 to 20 mg of mechlorethamine dissolved in 40 to 60 mL water and applied once daily to the entire skin surface except for the genitalia, until at least 2 weeks after complete clearance of lesions. Four of the seven with LyP achieved a complete response, with one lasting for more than 8 years of follow-up. A slightly increased risk of squamous and basal cell carcinomas, Hodgkin disease, and colon cancer was noted.

A common side effect of mechlorethamine therapy is an allergic hypersensitivity reaction, which may occur less frequently when mechlorethamine is prepared in an ointment base.

Topical carmustine therapy for lymphomatoid papulosis. Zacheim HS, Epstein EH, Crain WR. Arch Dermatol 1985; 121: 1410–4.

Seven patients with LyP were treated with once-daily total skin applications of topical carmustine. Total doses ranged from 280 to 1180 mg. Local treatment of individual lesions after the total skin course included twice-daily application of 2 mg/mL or 4 mg/mL 95% ethanol. All patients had a rapid reduction in the number and size of lesions. Lesions cleared faster and did not scar with maintenance therapy, but remission was not seen. Rare persistent telangiectases were noted.

Third-Line Therapies

• Oral bexarotene	C
• Recombinant interferon	C
• Excimer laser	E
• Radiotherapy	E
• Topical methotrexate	E
• Imiquimod cream	E
• Brentuximab vedotin	B

Bexarotene is a new treatment option for lymphomatoid papulosis. Krathen RA, Ward S, Duvic M. Dermatology 2003; 206: 142–7.

Oral bexarotene, started at 300 mg daily, was associated with more rapid disappearance, less necrosis, and a reduction in new lesions. One of three patients had a complete response. Topical bexarotene used in patients with less than 10% body surface area involved had a similar benefit.

Oral bexarotene is often used in conjunction with levothyroxine and lipid-lowering agents because of frequently seen central hypothyroidism and hyperlipidemia.

Therapeutic use of interferon-alpha for lymphomatoid papulosis. Schmuth M, Topar G, Illersperger B, Kowald E, Fritsch PO, Sepp NT. Cancer 2000; 89: 1603–10.

Five patients were treated with subcutaneous interferon-α, 3 to 15 million IU (international units) three times per week. Three were treated for 12 to 13 months, and each achieved a complete response that was durable for at least 1 year after discontinuation of therapy. Two were treated for 5 to 7 months: one had a partial response and one had complete response; however, neither was durable after discontinuation of therapy. Only one of six controls achieved spontaneous remission.

308-nm excimer laser for the treatment of lymphomatoid papulosis and stage IA mycosis fungoides. Kontos AP, Kerr HA, Malick F, Fivenson DP, Lim HW, Wong HK. Photodermatol Photoimmunol Photomed 2006; 22: 168–71.

A patient with LyP who had a failed response to PUVA and methotrexate was treated with the 308-nm excimer pulse laser, 13 treatments three times per week, with a maximum fluence of 500 mJ/cm². This resulted in 75% clearance, with minimal recurrence and postinflammatory hyperpigmentation.

This handheld device allows delivery of higher fluences, with a diminished risk of carcinogenesis.

Persistent agmination of lymphomatoid papulosis: an equivalent of limited plaque mycosis fungoides type of cutaneous T-cell lymphoma. Heald P, Subtil A, Breneman D, Wilson LD. J Am Acad Dermatol 2007; 57: 1005–11.

Seven cases of regional LyP were treated as if they were localized MF, with local radiotherapy, resulting in long-standing remissions. The radiation doses ranged from 30 to 46 Gy in fractionated doses. One patient also had topical bexarotene and localized electron beam therapy. At follow-up (2–6 years), six of the seven had no recurrences. One patient with recurrence subsequently achieved complete remission with interferon-α and PUVA.

Treatment of regional LyP with localized radiation therapy as if it were MF may offer prolonged remission of LyP, but, as demonstrated, these patients may still develop an associated lymphoma. Long-term follow-up is critical.

Treatment of lymphomatoid papulosis with imiquimod 5% cream. Hughes PH. J Am Acad Dermatol 2006; 54: 546–7.

A 13-year-old boy with LyP was reported to have a complete response within 2 weeks with lesional application of imiquimod 5% cream three times per week.

Patients' responses to imiquimod are variable, and patients should be warned of possible inflammation. The usefulness of imiquimod is limited by its cost.

Results of a phase II trial of brentuximab vedotin for CD30+ cutaneous T-cell lymphoma and lymphomatoid papulosis. Duvic M, Tetzlaff MT, Gangar P, Clos AL, Sui D, Talpur R. J Clin Oncol 2015; 33: 3759–65.

Brentuximab vedotin is a monoclonal antibody to CD30 that is conjugated to the tubulin toxin monomethyl auristatin E, that was initially approved by the Food and Drug Administration (FDA) for refractory Hodgkin lymphoma and systemic ALCL. This single-center, open-label phase II study demonstrated efficacy in CD30 expressing CTCLs (primary cutaneous ALCL, LyP, or transformed MF/Sézary syndrome). At a dose of 1.8 mg/kg given intravenously every 3 weeks, overall response rate in 48 patients was 73% (35% achieved complete response). All patients with LyP (n = 9) and primary cutaneous ALCL (n = 2) responded; time to response was 3 weeks (range, 3–9 weeks), and median duration of response was 26 weeks (range, 6–44 weeks). The most common adverse event was peripheral neuropathy (65% of patients, grade 1 or 2), which can persist.

Brentuximab vedotin has considerable efficacy in a variety of CD30-expressing CTCLs with reasonable side effect profile. However, peripheral neuropathy is common, and though not seen in this study, the FDA issued a black box warning on brentuximab vedotin due to the development of PML (in five patients reported thus far) treated with it. Of note, these patients were heavily pretreated with immunosuppressive medications, which is generally not the case in LyP patients. Given the overall favorable prognosis of LyP, brentuximab vedotin should be reserved for only severe refractory LyP cases.

Evidence Levels: **A** Double-blind study **B** Clinical trial ≥ 20 subjects **C** Clinical trial < 20 subjects **D** Series ≥ 5 subjects **E** Anecdotal case reports

148

Malignant atrophic papulosis

Noah Scheinfeld

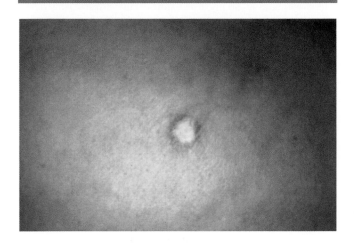

Malignant atrophic papulosis (MAP), also known as *Degos disease (DD)*, is a disorder characterized by occlusive vasculopathy; it possesses purely cutaneous and systemic variants. They are starkly divided by their prognosis, with purely cutaneous DD being wholly benign in course, and systemic DD usually being fatal within a few years of onset. Cutaneous DD can precede the development of systemic DD, and no factor has yet been defined that will predict those with cutaneous DD who will go on to develop systemic DD. The cause of death in systemic DD is related to perforation of blood vessels, bleeding, and intestinal perforation. Systemic MAP can involve the nervous, ophthalmologic, gastrointestinal (GI), cardiothoracic, and hepatorenal systems

MANAGEMENT STRATEGY

It is likely that the purely cutaneous type of DD is underdiagnosed as it is banal and benign. The disease is more commonly reported in men and young adults, but this may simply be sampling error.

Cutaneous and systemic DD have similar cutaneous eruptions. In the skin, DD occurs as erythematous, pink or red papules (2–15 mm), which evolve into scars with central, porcelain-white atrophic centers. The papules of MAP usually have a peripheral telangiectatic rim and can be domed or atrophic. The papules can have central crusts. Urticaria, ulceropustular, and/or gummalike nodules can manifest. All areas of the body, with the exception of the face, can be involved.

Viruslike inclusions, observable with an electron microscope, are frequently present in the endothelial cells and fibroblasts of patients with DD. C3 deposits are sometimes noted. There can be intracytoplasmic cylinders in the histiocytes.

Pathologically, the tissue affected by DD reveals an occlusive arteriopathy involving small-caliber vessels resulting in tissue infarction. The bland appearance of MAP vasculopathy (or an endovasculitis) on histologic examination does not equate with the serious nature of systemic DD.

No specific laboratory test can be used to diagnose DD. Cases of DD can manifest antiphospholipid antibodies and antinuclear antibodies, but these seem to be correlative rather than causative antibodies. Some reports note increased plasma fibrinogen levels, increased platelet aggregations, and a decrease of local and systemic fibrinolytic activity. There are cases of systemic lupus erythematosus and other collagen vascular diseases that display DD-like atrophic porcelain-white papules; however, these cases likely do not represent cases of DD.

Histopathology shows a wedge-shaped degeneration of collagen with a prominent interface reaction with squamatization of the dermoepidermal junction, melanin incontinence, and epidermal atrophy.

The role of imaging and laboratory investigations is to establish if systemic MAP is present so that treatment with newer agents can be considered. A patient with purely cutaneous DD should be given regular stool guaiac tests to test for internal bleeding. Tissue specimens can help strengthen the diagnosis of DD, but many clinical and histologic features of DD can rarely be found in patients with lupus; therefore a patient's clinical, histologic, and laboratory data must be integrated to definitively support the diagnosis of DD.

Older treatments for MAP and cutaneous DD include anticoagulation with either *coumarins* or *heparin*, platelet inhibitors such as *aspirin* and *dipyridamole*, and agents with fibrinolytic activity, including *phenformin*, and immunosuppression with either *ciclosporin* or *azathioprine*. Intravenous *immunoglobulin* has been used but with limited success. Topical *nicotine patches* have been used with success.

MAP is no longer an incurable disease. Reports have noted that initiation and continuing treatment with *eculizumab*, a monoclonal antibody directed against the complement protein C5, can put patients with systemic MAP into remission. Although the sample size of the use of eculizumab is small and most of the cases are unpublished, it seems that eculizumab is the treatment of choice for systemic MAP. The dosing for this treatment is still not clear, but is likely at the high end of published doses (900 mg intravenously or perhaps higher given continuously for treatment of MAP). The success of eculizumab suggests that MAP is a vascular rather than an immune disease. As eculizumab is a very expensive complex treatment, its use is not recommended for purely cutaneous DD. *Treprostinil*, a synthetic analog of prostacyclin (PGI2), has shown some promise when combined with eculizumab.

Specific Investigations

- Physical examination
- Tissue biopsy (skin primarily, but also tissue from the intestines and other internal organs)
- Complete blood count
- Stool guaiac
- Antinuclear antibody titer
- Protein C, protein S, and factor V Leiden; antithrombin III; and homocysteine levels
- Anticardiolipin antibody titer
- Antiphospholipid antibody titer
- Endoscopy of the GI tract (i.e., stomach, esophagus, duodenum, colon, rectum)
- Laparoscopy of the intestine
- Clinical integration of the aforementioned data

First-Line Therapies

• Eculizumab	D
• Treprostinil	D

A 32-year-old man with a rash, myalgia, and weakness. Burgin S, Stone JH, Shenoy-Bhangle AS, McGuone D. N Engl J Med 2014; 370: 2327–37.

A man with a rash, myalgia, and weakness. Shapiro L, Whelan P, Magro C. N Engl J Med 2014; 371: 1361.

The effects of eculizumab on the pathology of malignant atrophic papulosis. Magro CM, Wang X, Garrett-Bakelman F, Laurence J, Shapiro LS, DeSancho MT. Orphanet J Rare Dis 2013; 8: 185.

Effective treatment of malignant atrophic papulosis (Köhlmeier-Degos disease) with treprostinil — early experience. Shapiro LS, Toledo-Garcia AE, Farrell JF. Orphanet J Rare Dis 2013. 8: 52.

Degos disease: a C5b-9/interferon-α-mediated endotheliopathy syndrome. Magro CM, Poe JC, Kim C, Shapiro L, Nuovo G, Crow MK, et al. Am J Clin Pathol 2011; 135: 599–610.

Commentary on Degos disease: a C5b-9/interferon-α-mediated endotheliopathy syndrome by Magro et al: a reconsideration of Degos disease as hematologic or endothelial genetic disease. Scheinfelt N. Dermatol Online J 2011; 17: 6.

The initial enthusiasm for eculizumab as monotherapy may have faded. Burgin et al note that eculizumab (900 mg/d) failed as treatment for advanced systemic atrophic papulosis with GI involvement, with death as the outcome. Shapiro et al. note that only two patients initially given eculizumab as monotherapy are still alive; they instead use a combination of subcutaneous treprostinil and eculizumab. Eculizumab, if given early enough, may help abate malignant atrophic papulosis, but as monotherapy it is not instrumental in controlling it. With four patients treated, there have been no deaths. The first two are now 6-year survivors. Each of them had been critically ill in ICU settings before therapy. This information is important because malignant atrophic papulosis without treatment or hope of treatment is lethal, and patients should be directed toward those experienced with treatment, as eculizumab alone may not work.

Other reports have supported the use of eculizumab for systemic Degos disease, but informal communication to the author noted that despite treatment with eculizumab, some patients with systemic Degos disease have died. One report noted two patients with Degos disease in whom eculizumab failed. One had overlapping lupus, and the other had pulmonary hypertension. The pulmonary hypertension patient was treated with treprostinil, and cutaneous MAP lesions resolved but disabling digital pain remained. In the patient with Degos disease and lupus, treprostinil temporarily resulted in clearing of hematuria and central nervous system (CNS) symptoms, and magnetic resonance imaging (MRI) finding improvements.

Malignant atrophic papulosis. Degos R. Br J Dermatol 1979; 100: 21–35.

Numerous clinical manifestations have been reported and can affect the skin, mucosa, GI tract, viscera, and CNS and may require surgical intervention or fibrinolytic therapy. Anticoagulants have shown the most favorable responses.

Malignant atrophic papulosis: treatment with aspirin and dipyridamole. Stahl D, Thomsen K, Hou-Jensen K. Arch Dermatol 1978; 114: 1687–9.

A case report of a patient treated with aspirin 0.5 g twice daily and dipyridamole 50 mg three times daily arrested the development of both cutaneous lesions and systemic symptoms. Discontinuation of therapy resulted in no relapses 4 months posttherapy.

Malignant atrophic papulosis in an infant. Torrelo A, Sevilla J, Mediero I, Candelas D, Zambrano A. Br J Dermatol 2002; 146: 916–8.

A 7-month-old female with cutaneous lesions, vomiting, and poor weight gain was treated successfully with aspirin 12 mg/kg daily and dipyridamole 4 mg/kg daily in three divided doses.

Effect of fibrinolytic treatment in malignant atrophic papulosis. Delaney TJ, Black MM. Br Med J 1975; 3: 415.

The further development of cutaneous disease was halted in a 42-year-old female patient placed on phenformin 50 mg twice daily and ethylestrenol 2 mg four times daily. Withdrawal of therapy resulted in relapse that responded to reinstitution of therapy.

Penile ulceration in fatal malignant atrophic papulosis (Degos disease). Thompson KF, Highet AS. Br J Dermatol 2000; 143: 1320–2.

A fatal outcome in a patient who initially presented with penile ulceration and was treated with aspirin and dipyridamole but could not tolerate the therapy. Ciclosporin resulted in clinical improvement. Neurologic and GI symptoms developed, and lansoprazole resulted in healing of gastric ulceration. Atrial fibrillation and pleuritic pain were treated with heparin with clinical improvement. Continued symptoms prompted trials of tacrolimus, prednisolone, azathioprine, and cyclophosphamide, without success.

A case of malignant atrophic papulosis successfully treated with nicotine patches. Kanekura T, Uchino Y, Kanzaki T. Br J Dermatol 2003; 149: 660–2.

Nicotine patches that released 5 mg every 24 hours were applied daily and resulted in clearing of skin lesions. Three weeks after withdrawal of the patches, lesions recurred and again responded to therapy. The patient had no systemic involvement.

Second-Line Therapies	
• Coumadin (warfarin)	E
• Heparin	E
• Aspirin	E
• Dipyridamole	E
• Phenformin	E
• Ethylestrenol	E
• Nicotine patches	E
• Lansoprazole (for GI ulceration)	E
• Ciclosporin	E

Third-Line Therapies	
• Azathioprine	E
• Cyclophosphamide	E
• Tacrolimus	E
• Intravenous immunoglobulin	E
• Ultraviolet B therapy	E

Inefficacy of intravenous immunoglobulins and infliximab in Degos' disease. De Breucker S, Vandergheynst F, Decaux G. Acta Clin Belg 2008; 63: 99–102.

Evidence Levels: **A** Double-blind study **B** Clinical trial ≥ 20 subjects **C** Clinical trial < 20 subjects **D** Series ≥ 5 subjects **E** Anecdotal case reports

A 60-year-old man who presented with systemic Degos disease died despite anticoagulants, prednisone, intravenous immunoglobulins, and infliximab (Remicade).

The use of intravenous immunoglobulin in cutaneous and recurrent perforating intestinal Degos disease (malignant atrophic papulosis). Zhu KJ, Zhou Q, Lin AH, Lu ZM, Cheng H. Br J Dermatol 2007; 157: 206–7.

A 38-year-old Chinese woman with Degos disease unresponsive to a variety of therapies was treated with one course of high-dose IVIG therapy (0.4 g/kg) daily for 5 days. A week later a dramatic improvement of the lesions and general condition was noticed. During the next 11 months of follow-up, the patient had no new skin lesions or GI complaints.

A fatal case of malignant atrophic papulosis (Degos' disease) in a man with factor V Leiden mutation and lupus anticoagulant. Hohwy T, Jensen MG, Tøttrup A, Steiniche T, Fogh K. Acta Derm Venereol 2006; 86: 245–7.

A 33-year-old man presented with a widespread skin eruption consistent with malignant atrophic papulosis and died 2.5 years after onset of the disease. The patient was treated with narrow-band ultraviolet (UV) B, prednisolone, and, later, aspirin, pentoxifylline, and warfarin without effect.

A case of systemic malignant atrophic papulosis (Köhlmeier-Degos' disease). Fernández-Pérez ER, Grabscheid E, Scheinfeld NS. J Natl Med Assoc 2005; 97: 421–5.

Despite use of ciclosporin, prednisone, cidofovir, IVIG, and anticoagulant therapy a young male patient died. The therapy had no effect on the course of the patient's disease.

Malignant atrophic papulosis of Degos. Report of a patient who failed to respond to fibrinolytic therapy. Howsden SM, Hodge SJ, Herndon JH, Freeman RJ. Arch Dermatol 1976; 112: 1582–8.

A 21-year-old female died of complications from MAP after therapy with phenformin, ethylestrenol, aspirin, niacin, and low-molecular-weight dextran.

Benign familial Degos disease worsening during immunosuppression. Powell J, Bordea C, Wojnarowska J, Farrell AM, Morris PJ. Br J Dermatol 1999; 141: 524–7.

A 61-year-old woman with Degos disease underwent a cadaveric kidney transplant. Her condition worsened with the use of prednisolone, azathioprine, and ciclosporin.

[An autopsy case of Degos disease with ascending thoracic myelopathy]. Sugai F, Sumi H, Hara Y, Kajiyama K, Morino H, Fujimura H. Rinsho Shinkeigaku 1998; 38: 1049–53. [In Japanese].

Aggressive therapies, including pulsed-dose methylprednisolone and cyclophosphamide, were not successful in this 44-year-old man with Degos disease complicated by thoracic transverse myelopathy, with the patient ultimately succumbing to respiratory failure.

149

Malignant melanoma

Sarah Utz, Philip Friedlander, Orit Markowitz

Table 149.1 Current melanoma excisional margin guidelines

Tumor thickness	Recommended clinical margins
In situ	0.5 cm
≤1.0 mm	1.0 cm
1.01–2 mm	1–2 cm
2.01–4 mm	2.0 cm
>4 mm	2.0 cm

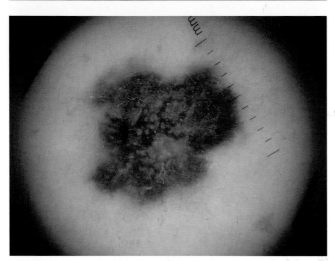

Melanoma is the leading cause of death among all cutaneous diseases in the United States. In 2015 it was estimated that 73,870 new cases of melanoma were diagnosed in the United States, and nearly 9940 patients died from this cancer.

MANAGEMENT STRATEGY

Early detection of melanoma is paramount in its management. Physicians and patients must become familiar with the *ABCDE signs of melanoma:* Asymmetry, Border, Color, Diameter, and Evolution. A specificity of 88% and sensitivity of 73% have been reported if two out of three of the following characteristics are noted on physical examination: irregular outline, diameter >6 mm, and color variegation. Even expert clinicians misdiagnose melanoma in up to one third of cases, and only *biopsy and histologic examination* can provide a definitive diagnosis.

Important in the management of melanoma is *primary prevention* (risk reduction) and *secondary prevention* (early detection). The National Institutes of Health (NIH) stresses the importance of screening programs and regular skin examinations by health professionals. The American Academy of Dermatology Task Force recommends follow-up one to four times a year for 2 years after a diagnosis of melanoma, depending on the thickness of the lesion and other risk factors, such as a family history of melanoma, and then once or twice a year thereafter. Other modalities such as *dermoscopy* and the recently Food and Drug Administration (FDA)-approved *MelaFind* are noninvasive tools aiding in identification of high-risk pigmented lesions.

The first step in the diagnosis of suspected melanoma is to obtain a biopsy. If total excision is not practical, a full-thickness incisional biopsy is acceptable.

The goal of surgical management of primary cutaneous melanoma is to achieve negative histologic margins with wide local excision to prevent recurrence and metastases. The current surgical margin guidelines from the National Comprehensive Cancer Network (NCCN) are based on Breslow depth (Table 149.1).

The standard treatment for stage IA melanoma is *wide local excision.* Total excision of primary melanoma with wide margins offers the best chance for cure. However, melanoma cells may extend noncontiguously for several millimeters beyond the visible lesion. The current recommendation for melanoma in situ may need to be extended to 9-mm margins.

The NCCN suggests that *sentinel lymph node (SLN) biopsy* be discussed and offered to patients in those with melanomas greater than 1 mm thick or 0.76 to 1 mm with ulceration or additional adverse features such as increased mitotic rate or lymphovascular invasion. The presence of melanoma in the SLN is the most significant factor in the prognosis of a patient with localized cutaneous melanoma. If the SLN is positive, a *completion lymphadenectomy* of all involved nodal basins is considered. The overall effect of completion lymphadenectomy after a positive SLN has yet to show survival benefit. An *elective lymphadenectomy* may also be performed, but it can result in significant morbidity and remains controversial.

For patients with clinically positive lymph nodes, a diagnostic nodal biopsy (e.g., fine-needle biopsy) is recommended, and, if positive, a *therapeutic lymphadenectomy* is performed. Adjuvant therapy approved by the FDA for the management of stage III or deep stage II melanomas includes high-dose *interferon (IFN)-α_{2b}*, which most consistently confers a disease-free survival benefit. More recently, *ipilimumab*, an immune checkpoint modulator that blocks cytotoxic T-lymphocyte–associated antigen 4 (CTLA-4), was approved for the adjuvant management of patients with melanoma involving regional lymph nodes >1 mm who have undergone complete lymph node dissection. The approval was based on recurrence-free survival benefit in patients treated with ipilimumab relative to placebo. Patients with satellitosis or in-transit metastases on an extremity are candidates for regional treatment with *isolated limb hyperthermic perfusion/infusion* with chemotherapeutic agents such as melphalan. *Talimogene laherparepvec*, an oncolytic herpesvirus engineered to secrete granulocyte-macrophage colony-stimulating factor (GM-CSF), was approved for intratumoral injection as treatment of unresectable subcutaneous, cutaneous, and nodal lesions.

Stage IV melanoma has a very poor prognosis, with patients demonstrating a 5-year survival below 5%. The presence of BRAF mutations has transformed the systemic management of stage IV melanoma. Until 2011, only two treatments, *dacarbazine and high-dose interleukin-2* (HD-IL-2), were FDA approved for the treatment of stage IV melanoma. HD-IL-2 requires administration as an inpatient and can carry significant toxicity risks, including capillary leak syndrome, renal failure, and neurologic toxicity. Given its toxicity profile, only a very limited number of patients are appropriate candidates for this treatment.

It has become increasingly evident that melanoma is a molecularly heterogeneous disease. Recently sequencing of components of the MAPK pathway in a panel of cancer cell lines identified activating mutations in the downstream BRAF protein in 50% to 60% of melanomas. Over 90% of the mutations in BRAF occur at position 600, with the most common being a V600E mutation.

Vemurafenib and *dabrafenib* are potent inhibitors of V600E-mutated BRAF. Randomized phase III studies using V600E inhibitors as first-line systemic therapy in patients with stage IV melanoma demonstrated statistically significant survival benefit after treatment with a BRAF inhibitor compared with dacarbazine treatment. However, median progression-free survival is limited to approximately 6 months. As such, elucidating resistance mechanisms is extremely important. Inhibition of the MAPK pathway downstream of BRAF by using the MEK inhibitor *trametinib* also confers a significant overall survival benefit relative to treatment with chemotherapy in patients with V600-mutated melanoma. Concurrent inhibition of BRAF and MEK confers higher response rates and improved progression-free duration than single-agent treatment. Two combination regimens, vemurafenib plus cobimetinib and dabrafenib plus trametinib, are FDA approved as treatment in V600 BRAF–mutated melanoma. Treatment with the combination of dabrafenib plus trametinib has demonstrated overall survival benefit relative to single-agent vemurafenib treatment.

A subset of melanomas contains a mutation in the KIT gene as opposed to BRAF; these tumors have shown response to oral inhibitors of KIT but also with limited durability.

Immunotherapies offer the potential for longer lasting benefit than BRAF inhibition as demonstrated by the small subset of patients who develop durable responses to HD-IL-2. CTLA-4 is an immunomodulatory protein that downregulates T-cell activity. Inhibition of CTLA-4 using the monoclonal antibody ipilimumab has shown significant antitumor activity in melanoma. Treatment of stage IV melanoma patients with ipilimumab has an overall survival benefit compared with treatment with a peptide vaccine. An overall survival benefit is also seen after treatment with the combination of ipilimumab and dacarbazine compared with treatment with single-agent dacarbazine.

Over the past few years, it has become increasingly clear that antibody-mediated inhibition of immunomodulatory proteins other than CTLA-4 are also efficacious. Targeting either the programmed death 1 protein (PD-1) or its ligand PD-L1 produced durable responses in a subset of patients with melanoma. PD-1 is an inhibitory receptor on T cells whose immunosuppressive ligand, PD-L1, is expressed on many melanomas. Two PD-1 inhibitors, *pembrolizumab* and *nivolumab*, are FDA approved as single agents for systemic treatment of stage IV melanoma. A randomized phase III trial demonstrated an overall survival benefit after treatment with nivolumab relative to dacarbazine. The rate of high-grade autoimmune toxicity also was lower in patients who received treatment with the PD-1 inhibitor. The Checkmate 067 phase III study compared treatment with ipilimumab alone, nivolumab alone, or combined ipilimumab plus nivolumab treatment in 945 patients with stage IV melanoma who have not received prior systemic therapy for advanced disease. Although median progression-free survival was 2.9 months, 6.9 months, and 11.5 months, respectively, the combination therapy led to higher rates of high-grade toxicity, with 55% of patients developing a grade 3 or higher adverse event. Overall survival data are not yet presented. At present, the optimal sequencing of targeted and immune therapies is still unclear.

Specific Investigations

- Dermoscopy
- Biopsy of primary site
- Sentinel lymph node biopsy
- Laboratory and imaging studies: chest radiograph, computed tomography (CT), magnetic resonance imaging (MRI), positron emission tomography (PET) scans
- MelaFind

Final version of 2009 American Joint Committee on Cancer (AJCC) melanoma staging and classification. Balch CM, Gershenwald JE, Soong SJ, Thompson JF, Atkins MB, Byrd DR, et al. J Clin Oncol 2009; 27: 6199–206.

This paper describes the updated staging system for cutaneous melanoma based on a multivariate analysis of 30,946 patients with stages I, II, and III and 7972 patients with stage IV. Specifically, in patients with localized melanoma, tumor thickness, mitotic rate, and ulceration were the most important prognostic factors. Mitotic rate replaced tumor invasion when defining T1b melanomas. In patients with regional metastases, the N category was determined by number of metastatic nodes, tumor burden, and ulceration of the primary lesion. All patients with microscopic nodal metastases are classified as stage III regardless of tumor burden. Elevated lactose dehydrogenase (LDH) was also included as an independent predictor of poor outcomes in patients with stage IV melanoma.

National Comprehensive Cancer Network. Clinical practice guidelines in oncology. V 1.2013. Coit DG, Andtbacka R, Anker CJ, Bichakjian CK, Carson WE 3rd, Daud A, et al. Available online: http://www.nccn.org/professionals/physician_gls/pdf/melanoma.pdf.

Mitotic rate was added to the initial stratification of stage I and II melanoma. The extent of initial workup is controversial. Most agree that chest radiography and blood work are not necessary for stage IA melanoma. For stage IB and stage IIA melanomas, a baseline chest radiograph is optional because it is not sensitive or specific. Other imaging studies, such as CT, MRI, and/or PET scans, should be performed only to evaluate specific signs or symptoms or for stages III and IV. Fine-needle aspiration is indicated for stage III with macrometastases or in-transit metastases and stage IV. LDH is only indicated for stage IV. These guidelines also discuss frequency of follow-up visits and appropriate follow-up tests, both of which depend on the stage of the melanoma as well as other risk factors.

Incisional biopsy and melanoma prognosis. Bong JL, Herd RM, Hunter JA. J Am Acad Dermatol 2002; 46: 690–4.

A large retrospective case analysis using matched controls to investigate the influence of incisional biopsy on melanoma prognosis. A total of 5727 biopsied melanoma patients were examined, with 5.6% having undergone incisional biopsies. The authors conclude that melanoma prognosis is not influenced by an incisional procedure before definitive excision of the tumor. Because of the histologic limitations of this procedure, however, the authors recommend that incisional biopsies be reserved for lesions that cannot be excised primarily or when clinical suspicion for melanoma is low.

The role of sentinel lymph node biopsy for melanoma: evidence assessment. Johnson TM, Sondak VK, Bichakjian CK, Sabel MS. J Am Acad Dermatol 2006; 54: 19–27.

In reviewing 1198 articles regarding melanoma sentinel node biopsy this paper discusses the evidence base behind the sentinel node hypothesis. The authors state that the available evidence overwhelmingly supports SLN status as the most powerful independent factor predicting survival, with highest sensitivity and specificity of any nodal staging test. They also discuss that SLN biopsy results in improved regional disease control. The article claims that, based on available evidence, there is a potential subset survival benefit for subclinical detection of nodal disease followed by immediate complete lymph node dissection (CLND). The article reviews the Multicenter Selective Lymphadenectomy Trial I (MSLT-1) interim results and discusses the morbidities of SLN biopsy. The authors conclude that current evidence supports the use of SLN biopsy in the management of melanoma.

Atlas of Dermoscopy. Marghoob AA, Braun R, Kopf AW, eds. London: Parthenon Publishing, 2005.

Dermoscopy increases the diagnostic sensitivity of melanoma in appropriately trained clinicians. In high-risk patients, the availability of baseline images for comparison permits the detection of melanomas that are growing or changing. Three-month-interval digital dermoscopy mole monitoring has demonstrated 93% sensitivity for lentigo maligna and in situ melanoma, and 96% sensitivity for invasive melanoma diagnosis. This clinician-oriented atlas is an up-to-date multiauthored text reviewing virtually every aspect of dermoscopy.

The performance of MelaFind: a prospective multicenter study. Monheit G1, Cognetta AB, Ferris L, Rabinovitz H, Gross K, Martini M, et al. Arch Dermatol 2011; 147: 188–94.

MelaFind is a fully automatic, noninvasive, computerized diagnostic system approved by the FDA in 2011. MelaFind identifies high-risk pigmented lesions that should be considered for biopsy to rule out melanoma, with a high sensitivity of 98.4% for thin pigmented melanomas over 2 mm in diameter.

First-Line Therapies	
• Surgical excision	B
• Selective lymphadenectomy	C
• Elective lymphadenectomy	C

Surgical margins for melanoma in situ. Kunishige JH, Brodland DG, Zitelli JA. J Am Acad Dermatol 2012; 66: 438–44.

The previously accepted 5-mm margin to surgically excise melanoma in situ was shown to be inadequate in several studies. This prospective series of 1072 patients with 1120 melanomas in situ investigated the minimal surgical margins required to remove 97% of all tumors. This group determined that 86% of all melanomas in situ were completely excised with 6-mm margins, and the minimum surgical margin required to successfully remove 98.9% of all melanomas in situ was 9 mm. The 9-mm margin was found to be statistically superior to the 6-mm margin.

Excision margins in high-risk malignant melanoma. Thomas JM, Newton-Bishop J, A'Hern R, Coombes G, Timmons M, Evans J, et al. N Engl J Med 2004; 350: 757–66.

This is a randomized clinical trial with 900 subjects comparing 1-cm and 3-cm margins in high-risk tumors. The median follow-up was 60 months. A 1-cm margin was associated with a significantly increased risk of locoregional recurrence. There were 128 deaths attributable to melanoma in the group with 1-cm margins, compared with 105 in the group with 3-cm margins, but overall survival was similar in the two groups.

Overview and update of the phase III Multicenter Selective Lymphadenectomy Trials (MSLT-I and MSLT-II) in melanoma. Morton DL. Clin Exp Metastasis 2012; 29: 699–706.

The Multicenter Selective Lymphadenectomy Trial II (MSLT-II) was designed to investigate if SLN biopsy may be therapeutic as well as diagnostic and if complete lymph node dissection could therefore be avoided in most patients with SLN metastases. Its primary outcome is melanoma-specific survival. MSLT-II is a randomized phase III trial of SLN biopsy plus complete lymph node dissection versus SLN biopsy plus high-definition ultrasound observation of lymph nodes in patients with SLN metastases confirmed by histopathology or reverse transcription polymerase chain reaction (RT-PCR). High-definition ultrasound can detect metastases as small as 4 mm.

Sentinel lymph node biopsy for melanoma: American Society of Clinical Oncology and Society of Surgical Oncology joint clinical practice guideline. Wong SL, Balch CM, Hurley P, Agarwala SS, Akhurst TJ, Cochran A, et al. Ann Surg Oncol 2012; 19: 3313–24.

This practice guideline was developed by the American Society of Clinical Oncology and Society of Surgical Oncology in an effort to provide an evidence-based guideline for the use of SLN biopsy in staging patients with newly diagnosed melanoma. A systematic review of 73 studies concluded that SLN biopsy is recommended for patients with intermediate-thickness melanomas of any anatomic site. Additionally, SLN biopsy may be recommended for staging purposes and to facilitate regional disease control. Complete lymph node dissection is recommended for all patients with a positive SLN biopsy and achieves good regional disease control.

Elective lymph node dissection in patients with melanoma: systematic review and meta-analysis of randomized controlled trials. Lens MB, Dawes M, Goodacre T, Newton-Bishop JA. Arch Surg 2002; 137: 458–61.

This is a large systematic review and meta-analysis of randomized controlled trials comparing elective lymph node dissection with surgery delayed until the time of clinical recurrence. Elective lymphadenectomy shows no significant overall survival benefit for patients undergoing elective lymph node dissection.

Second-Line Therapies	
• Pegylated IFN-α_{2b}	A
• Paclitaxel and carboplatin	D
• Imiquimod	E
• Interleukin-2	B
• Isolated limb perfusion	E
• Bcl-2 antisense and dacarbazine	A
• Dacarbazine	A
• Vemurafenib	A
• Trametinib	B
• Imatinib	B
• Ipilimumab	A
• Pembrolizumab	A
• Vemurafenib and cobimetinib	A
• Nivolumab and ipilimumab	A
• Ipilimumab plus dacarbazine	A

The Society for Immunotherapy of Cancer consensus statement on tumor immunotherapy for the treatment of cutaneous melanoma. Kaufman HL, Kirkwood JM, Hodi FS, Agarwala S, Amatruda T, Bines SD, et al. Nat Rev Clin Oncol 2013;10: 588-98.

This comprehensive review provides recommendations for the immunotherapy use in patients with high-risk and advanced-stage melanoma in the United States. The recommendations were made by a panel of clinicians, nurses, and patient advocates that used a literature review of high-quality, peer-reviewed studies from 1992–2012. The panel identified roles for IFN-α_{2b}, pegylated-IFN-α_{2b}, interleukin-2 (IL-2), and ipilimumab.

Adjuvant therapy with pegylated interferon alfa-2b versus observation alone in resected stage III melanoma: final results of EORTC 18991, a randomised phase III trial. Eggermont AM, Suciu S, Santinami M, Testori A, Kruit WH, Marsden J, et al. Lancet 2008; 372: 117-26.

This study assessed whether long-term (5 years) adjuvant pegylated IFN-α_{2b} therapy could be well tolerated while maintaining recurrence-free survival. A total of 1256 patients with

Evidence Levels: **A** Double-blind study   **B** Clinical trial ≥ 20 subjects   **C** Clinical trial < 20 subjects   **D** Series ≥ 5 subjects   **E** Anecdotal case reports

resected stage III melanoma were randomly assigned to an observation group (n = 629) or pegylated IFN-α_{2b} group (n = 627) for 5 years. Relapse-free survival was significantly better in the IFN treatment group compared with the observation group (45.6% vs. 38.9%), but there was no significant benefit to overall survival. Subsequently, pegylated IFN-α_{2b} was approved by the FDA in 2011 as adjuvant therapy for patients with stage III melanoma.

Adjuvant ipilimumab versus placebo after complete resection of high-risk stage III melanoma (EORTC 18071): a randomised, double-blind, phase 3 trial. Eggermont AM, Chiarion-Sileni V, Grob JJ, Dummer R, Wolchok JD, Schmidt H, et al. Lancet Oncol 2015; 16: 522.

This study aimed to address whether ipilimumab could have a role as adjuvant therapy for patients with completely resected stage III melanoma at high risk of recurrence. In a double-blind phase III trial looking at 951 patients, ipilimumab was found to significantly improve recurrence-free survival for patients with completely resected, high-risk, stage III melanoma.

Improved survival with ipilimumab in patients with metastatic melanoma. Hodi FS, O'Day SJ, McDermott DF, Weber RW, Sosman JA, Haanen JB, et al. N Engl J Med 2010; 363: 711–23.

The FDA approved ipilimumab, a monoclonal antibody against the immune checkpoint receptor CTLA-4, based on this randomized phase III trial. A total of 676 patients with unresectable stage III or IV melanoma were assigned to three groups: ipilimumab plus glycoprotein 100 peptide vaccine (gp100) (n = 403), ipilimumab alone (n = 137), or gp100 alone (n = 136). Ipilimumab, with or without gp100 vaccine, compared with gp100 alone, significantly improved overall survival in patients with previously treated metastatic melanoma (10.1 months for ipilimumab alone, 10.0 months for combination therapy, vs. 6.4 months for gp100 alone).

Pembrolizumab versus ipilimumab in advanced melanoma. Robert C, Schachter J, Long GV, Arance A, Grob JJ, Mortier L, et al. N Engl J Med 2015; 372: 2521–32.

This study was a phase III randomization of 834 patients with stage IV melanoma, who were not previously treated with an inhibitor of CTLA-4 or PD-1, to treatment with ipilimumab or pembrolizumab. A statistically significant improvement in response rate, 6-month progression-free survival, and 12-month overall survival favoring PD-1 inhibitor treatment was observed. The rate of high-grade autoimmune toxicity was also lower in patients who received treatment with the PD-1 inhibitor.

Combined vemurafenib and cobimetinib in BRAF-mutated melanoma. Larkin al J, Ascierto PA, Dréno B, Atkinson V, Liszkay G, Maio M, et al. N Engl J Med 2014; 371: 1867–74.

This study randomly assigned 495 patients with previously untreated, unresectable, locally advanced or metastatic BRAF V600 mutation–positive melanoma to either vemurafenib and cobimetinib combination or vemurafenib and placebo. Median progression-free survival showed a statistically significant difference of 9.9 months in the combination group and 6.2 months in the control.

Nivolumab in previously untreated melanoma without BRAF mutation. Robert C, Long GV, Brady B, Dutriaux C, Maio M, Mortier L, et al. N Engl J Med 2015; 372: 320–30.

This study randomly assigned 418 previously untreated patients with metastatic melanoma without a BRAF mutation to either nivolumab or dacarbazine. At 1 year, there was statistically significant increase in overall survival, with 72.9% in the nivolumab group compared with 42.1% in the dacarbazine group. Median

progression-free survival was 5.1 months in the nivolumab group versus 2.2 months in the dacarbazine group.

Combined nivolumab and ipilimumab or monotherapy in untreated melanoma. Larkin J, Hodi FS, Wolchok JD. N Engl J Med 2015; 373: 23–34.

The Checkmate 067 phase III study compared treatment with ipilimumab alone, nivolumab alone, or combined ipilimumab plus nivolumab treatment in 945 patients with stage IV melanoma who have not received prior systemic therapy for advanced disease. Although median progression-free survival was 2.9 months, 6.9 months, and 11.5 months, respectively, the combination therapy led to higher rates of high-grade toxicity, with 55% of patients developing a grade 3 or higher adverse event. Overall survival data are not yet presented.

Combination of paclitaxel and carboplatin as second-line therapy for patients with metastatic melanoma. Rao RD, Holtan SG, Ingle JN, Croghan GA, Kottschade LA, Creagan ET, et al. Cancer 2006; 106: 375–82.

This was a retrospective review article including 31 patients who received combination treatment after other treatment failures, most of which were post-temozolomide (post-TMZ) or post-dacarbazine (post-DTIC). The authors concluded that the clinical benefit rates appear to be at least as good as for most other therapies considered standard for metastatic melanoma (albeit in the prebiologic era), and the data provide justification for further testing of this drug combination in the first-line setting.

Locoregional cutaneous metastases of malignant melanoma and their management. Wolf IH, Richtig E, Kopera D, Kerl H. Dermatol Surg 2004; 30: 244–7.

This article discussed the palliative benefits seen with application of topical imiquimod 5% cream three times weekly to cutaneous metastases with a 1-cm margin. In a five-patient sample, complete clinical and histopathologic remission of locoregional cutaneous metastases of malignant melanoma occurred in two and partial remission occurred in one, with no regression in the remaining two patients.

High-dose recombinant interleukin 2 therapy for patients with metastatic melanoma: analysis of 270 patients treated between 1985 and 1993. Atkins MB, Lotze MT, Dutcher JP, Fisher RI, Weiss G, Margolin K, et al. J Clin Oncol 1999; 17: 2105–16.

In this intention-to-treat analysis, 270 patients with metastatic melanoma were entered into eight clinical trials conducted between 1985 and 1993. These patients received at least one dose of high-dose recombinant IL-2 by IV infusion every 8 hours for up to 14 consecutive doses over 5 days as clinically tolerated, with a second cycle performed after 6 to 9 days of rest. Additional courses were repeated every 6 to 12 weeks as tolerated in stable or responding patients. The overall response rate was 16%, with 6% of patients achieving complete responses. The median response duration in partial responders was 5.9 months. Severe toxicities reversed rapidly after therapy was completed.

Durable complete responses with high-dose bolus interleukin-2 in patients with metastatic melanoma who have experienced progression after biochemotherapy. Tarhini AA, Kirkwood JM, Gooding WE, Cai C, Agarwala SS. J Clin Oncol 2007; 25: 3802–7.

In this intention-to-treat clinical trial, 26 patients with metastatic melanoma with disease progression on or after biochemotherapy

(BCT) (cisplatin, vinblastine, dacarbazine, IL-2, and IFN-α_{2b}) received high-dose bolus IL-2. All patients except three received at least two cycles. Four patients (all with stage M1a disease) experienced complete responses.

Management of in-transit melanoma of the extremity with isolated limb perfusion. Fraker DL. Curr Treat Options Oncol 2004; 5: 173–84.

The primary use of ILP (isolated limb perfusion) is in the treatment of satellitosis and in-transit metastasis. ILP involves very high doses of chemotherapeutic agents, usually melphalan, administered through femoral, iliac, or axillary vessels to isolated anatomic regions. Reports have shown that the addition of tumor necrosis factor to melphalan may improve response rates, but no clear benefit has been demonstrated.

Bcl-2 antisense (oblimersen sodium) plus dacarbazine in patients with advanced melanoma: the Oblimersen Melanoma Study Group. Bedikian AY, Millward M, Pehamberger H, Conry R, Gore M, Trefzer U, et al. J Clin Oncol 2006; 24: 4738–45.

In one of the largest randomized controlled studies in advanced melanoma, 771 patients were randomly assigned to treatment with oblimersen–dacarbazine (386 patients) or dacarbazine (385 patients). The use of oblimersen with dacarbazine safely improves outcomes in patients with advanced melanoma, particularly those with normal baseline LDH. Because the patients in this study had advanced stage III and IV melanoma, the authors suggest examination of patients with less advanced disease in whom Bcl-2 expression has been confirmed.

Inhibition of mutated, activated BRAF in metastatic melanoma. Flaherty KT, Puzanov I, Kim KB, Ribas A, McArthur GA, Sosman JA, et al. N Engl J Med 2010; 363: 809–19.

This landmark multicenter, phase I, dose-escalation trial of PLX4032, an oral inhibitor of V600E-mutated BRAF, demonstrated complete or partial tumor regression in the majority of patients with metastatic melanoma. Fifty-five patients (49 had melanoma) were enrolled in the dose-escalation phase, with an additional 32 patients with V600E-mutated BRAF melanomas enrolled in the extension phase, allowing the maximum dose that could be administered without adverse effects. In the dose-escalation cohort, among 16 patients with V600E-mutated BRAF melanoma, 10 patients demonstrated partial response and 1 had a complete response. In the extension cohort, 24 patients had a partial response and 2 had a complete response. Median progression-free survival for all patients was over 7 months. Interestingly, responses to PLX4032 were seen as early as 14 days after initiating treatment, as seen on fludeoxyglucose (FDG)-labeled PET imaging.

Improved survival with vemurafenib in melanoma with BRAF V600E mutation. Chapman PB, Hauschild A, Robert C, Haanen JB, Ascierto P, Larkin J, et al. N Engl J Med 2011; 364: 2507–16.

Vemurafenib, a specific inhibitor of the V600E mutation, was FDA approved in 2011 based on this phase III randomized controlled trial comparing vemurafenib with dacarbazine in 675 patients with previously untreated melanoma with the V600E BRAF mutation. At 6 months, the overall survival in the vemurafenib group was 84% compared with 64% in the dacarbazine group. At interim analysis of this trial, crossover from dacarbazine to vemurafenib was recommended due to the significantly improved rates of overall and progression-free survival in the vemurafenib group.

Improved survival with MEK inhibition in BRAF-mutated melanoma. Flaherty KT, Robert C, Hersey P, Nathan P, Garbe C, Milhem, et al. N Engl J Med 2012; 367: 107–14.

In previous trials, MEK inhibition by trametinib showed promise. In this phase III open-label trial, trametinib, compared with chemotherapy, significantly improved rates of progression-free and overall survival among patients with metastatic melanoma containing the V600E or V600K BRAF mutation. A total of 322 patients were randomly assigned to receive either oral trametinib daily or chemotherapy in a 2:1 ratio (intravenous dacarbazine or paclitaxel) every 3 weeks. Patients in the chemotherapy cohort who demonstrated disease progression were permitted to cross over to receive trametinib. Median progression-free survival was 4.8 months in the trametinib group and 1.5 months in the chemotherapy group. At 6 months, the overall rate of survival was 81% in the trametinib group and 67% in the chemotherapy group despite crossover.

KIT as a therapeutic target in metastatic melanoma. Carvajal RD, Antonescu CR, Wolchok JD, Chapman PB, Roman RA, Teitcher J, et al. J Am Med Assoc 2011; 305: 2327–34.

In this single-group, open-label, phase II trial, treatment with the KIT inhibitor imatinib showed significant clinical responses in patients with advanced melanoma harboring KIT mutations. Patients ($n = 205$) with metastatic melanoma were screened for the presence of KIT mutations. Fifty-one patients were identified with this mutation, and 28 patients from this group were treated. These 28 patients had advanced unresectable melanoma arising from acral, mucosal, and chronically sun-damaged areas. Imatinib was administered orally twice daily. The overall durable response rate was 16% with a median time to progression of 12 weeks and median overall survival of 46.3 weeks.

Third-Line Therapies	
• Radiation therapy	B
• Mohs micrographic surgery	B

The benefits of adjuvant radiation therapy after therapeutic lymphadenectomy for clinically advanced, high-risk, lymph node-metastatic melanoma. Agrawal S, Kane JM 3rd, Guadagnolo BA, Kraybill WG, Ballo MT. Cancer 2009; 115: 5836–44.

This large retrospective review evaluated the role of adjuvant radiation therapy on regional recurrence and survival after therapeutic lymphadenectomy for clinically advanced lymph node metastatic melanoma. A total of 615 patients were chosen based on criteria for high risk of regional nodal relapse. At a follow-up period of 5 years, regional recurrence was found in 10.2% of patients in the adjuvant radiation therapy group compared with 40.6% in the observation group.

Mohs micrographic surgery for the treatment of melanoma. Hui AM, Jacobson M, Markowitz O, Brooks NA, Siegel DM. Dermatol Clinics 2012; 30: 503–15.

The article discusses the current literature on the utility of Mohs micrographic surgery for the treatment of melanoma in situ, with an extensive review of Mohs technique, the latest advances in immunohistochemical staining, and outcomes.

Mastocytoses

Nicholas A. Soter

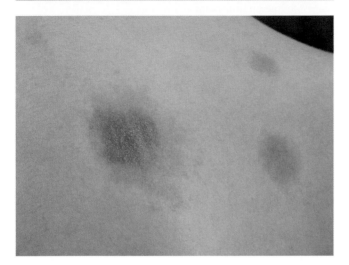

The mastocytoses are a group of disorders of mast cell proliferation that may exhibit both cutaneous and systemic features. Clinical manifestations result from mast cell activation and from infiltration of various organs. The World Health Organization has classified mastocytosis into disease categories: cutaneous mastocytosis, indolent systemic mastocytosis, systemic mastocytosis with a nonmast-cell clonal hematologic disorder, aggressive systemic mastocytosis, mast cell leukemia, mast cell sarcoma, and extracutaneous mastocytoma. The most frequent site of organ involvement in individuals with mastocytosis is the skin. Cutaneous forms include urticaria pigmentosa (shown here), mastocytoma, diffuse and erythrodermic cutaneous mastocytosis, and telangiectasia macularis eruptiva perstans. An international task force has proposed a revised classification of cutaneous mastocytosis into maculopapular cutaneous mastocytosis with monomorphic and polymorphic variants, diffuse cutaneous mastocytosis, and cutaneous mastocytoma, with the elimination of telangiectasia macularis eruptiva perstans. The cutaneous forms of mastocytosis may be present with or without systemic manifestations. In pediatric patients, the cutaneous lesions usually are not associated with systemic involvement and often have spontaneous resolution around puberty. In adult patients, the cutaneous lesions usually are chronic and are associated with systemic mastocytosis. Adult patients should be classified because the type and stage of systemic mastocytosis has therapeutic and prognostic implications. Only the treatment of the cutaneous features will be discussed.

MANAGEMENT STRATEGY

An important aspect of therapy of the cutaneous lesions of mastocytosis is avoidance of triggering factors, which may include temperature changes, friction, physical exertion, ingestion of alcohol, the use of nonsteroidal antiinflammatory agents or opiate analgesics, and emotional stress. Of concern is the possibility of anaphylaxis after stings by *Hymenoptera* spp., which may occur even in patients receiving venom immunotherapy.

A history seeking systemic features should be undertaken, as well as a physical examination to determine the types of skin lesions and to assess for lymphadenopathy and hepatosplenomegaly. The presence of specific systemic manifestations will determine the type of specialty physician to whom a referral should be made for further evaluation.

Patients with systemic mastocytosis require long-term follow-up because associated nonmast-cell clonal hematologic disorders, such as myelodysplastic or myeloproliferative syndromes and lymphoproliferative disorders, may develop.

A skin biopsy should be obtained in all individuals with cutaneous lesions. A complete blood count with differential analysis, a blood chemistry profile that includes liver function tests, and a blood tryptase level should be obtained in all patients with cutaneous lesions, except those with mastocytomas.

In many cases cutaneous mastocytomas may involute spontaneously; they rarely are described in adults. Childhood urticaria pigmentosa regresses spontaneously in approximately 50% of cases and urticaria pigmentosa in adults in 10%. Diffuse and erythrodermic cutaneous mastocytosis usually resolves spontaneously during childhood. Telangiectasia macularis eruptiva perstans tends to be a chronic condition.

Most of the therapeutic reports have been in patients with urticaria pigmentosa and, to a lesser extent, in diffuse and erythrodermic cutaneous mastocytosis. The major therapeutic measure is the administration of *oral H₁ antihistamines* to alleviate pruritus and whealing. *Oral disodium cromoglycate* has been efficacious in some individuals. The role and efficacy of topical high-potency glucocorticoid preparations with plastic-film occlusion, of narrowband ultraviolet B (NB-UVB) phototherapy, of psoralens and ultraviolet A (PUVA) photochemotherapy, and UVA1 phototherapy have not been subjected to controlled clinical trials or remain anecdotal. Cytoreductive therapy to reduce mast cell proliferation is not recommended in patients with only cutaneous manifestations. There is no therapy that will eradicate the mast cells in the cutaneous lesions.

Specific Investigation

- Skin biopsy

Cutaneous manifestations in patients with mastocytosis: consensus report of the European Competence Network on Mastocytosis; the American Academy of Allergy, Asthma & Immunology; and the European Academy of Allergology and Clinical Immunology. Hartmann K, Escribano L, Grattan C, Brackow K, Carter MC, Alvarez-Twose I, et al. J Allergy Clin Immunol 2016; 37: 35–45.

The major criterion for cutaneous involvement in patients with mastocytosis is typical skin lesions that are associated with Darier sign. Minor criteria include increased numbers of mast cells in biopsy specimens of lesional skin and an activating KIT mutation in lesional skin tissue. In lesional skin biopsy specimens, the number of mast cells is increased four to eightfold, which is about 40 mast cells/mm². The use of an antibody against tryptase should be the standard histochemical marker to detect and quantitate mast cells. No specific, aberrantly expressed marker of clonal cutaneous mast cells has been identified.

First-Line Therapies

• H₁ antihistamines	A
• H₂ antihistamines	D
• Disodium cromoglycate	A

Comparison of azelastine and chlorpheniramine in the treatment of mastocytosis. Friedman BS, Santiago ML, Berkebile C, Metcalfe DD. J Allergy Clin Immunol 1993; 92: 520–6.

In a double-blind, randomized, crossover trial in 13 subjects with urticaria pigmentosa and systemic mastocytosis, the administration of both azelastine and chlorpheniramine for 4 weeks was associated with a reduction in pruritus.

Rupatadine improves quality of life in mastocytosis: a randomized, double-blind, placebo-controlled trial. Siebenhaar F, Főrtch A, Krause K, Weller K, Metz M, Magerl M, et al. Allergy 2013; 68: 949–52.

In a double-blind, randomized, placebo-controlled, crossover trial in 7 patients with cutaneous mastocytosis and in 23 with indolent systemic mastocytosis, the administration of rupatadine for 28 days was associated with a 16.1% reduction ($p = 0.004$) in the mean ItchyQoL total score and 30.3% reduction ($p = 0.001$) in pruritus.

Comparison of the therapeutic efficacy of cromolyn sodium with that of combined chlorpheniramine and cimetidine in systemic mastocytosis: results of a double-blind clinical trial. Frieri M, Alling DW, Metcalfe DD. Am J Med 1985; 78: 9–14.

Five of six patients with systemic mastocytosis had less pruritus and four of six had less urticaria while receiving chlorpheniramine and cimetidine. There was no beneficial effect in those receiving disodium cromoglycate.

Oral disodium cromoglycate in the treatment of systemic mastocytosis. Soter NA, Austen KF, Wasserman SI. N Engl J Med 1979; 301: 465–9.

In a double-blind, crossover study in five patients with systemic mastocytosis and urticaria pigmentosa, in 15 of 18 trials oral disodium cromoglycate ameliorated pruritus and whealing.

Urticaria pigmentosa: clinical picture and response to oral disodium cromoglycate. Czarnetzki BM, Behrendt H. Br J Dermatol 1981; 105: 563–7.

In a blind, crossover trial, 3 children and 10 adults with urticarial pigmentosa were treated with oral disodium cromoglycate or placebo for 1 month, respectively. Relief of pruritus was observed in 67.7% of children and in 70% of adults.

Oral and topical sodium cromoglycate in the treatment of diffuse cutaneous mastocytosis in an infant. Edwards AM, Čapková Š. BMJ Case Reports 2011; 2011: http://dx.doi.org/10.1136/bar.02.2011.3910.

In a single infant with diffuse cutaneous mastocytosis, there was improvement in pruritus, whealing, and flushing after the administration of oral disodium cromoglycate and topical 4% sodium cromoglycate emulsion.

Second-Line Therapies

• Topical glucocorticoid with plastic-film occlusion	C
• NB-UVB phototherapy	D
• Oral PUVA photochemotherapy	D
• Psoralen baths plus UVA photochemotherapy	D
• UVA1 phototherapy	D

Urticaria pigmentosa: systemic evaluation and successful treatment with topical steroids. Guzzo C, Lavker R, Roberts LJ II, Fox K, Schechter N, Lazarus G. Arch Dermatol 1991; 127: 191–6.

In seven of nine adult patients with urticaria pigmentosa, the topical application of betamethasone dipropionate ointment 0.05% under occlusion overnight to one half of the body for 6 weeks was associated with resolution of the lesions, with a maximum response within 3 to 12 weeks after the cessation of treatment. Lesions began to recur between 6 and 9 months after completing therapy. Retreatment for 6 months followed by once-weekly application of betamethasone dipropionate ointment under occlusion kept the patients clear of lesions, with the longest follow-up time being 2.5 years.

The appropriate method for using topical glucocorticoids in patients with urticaria pigmentosa needs to be determined in controlled trials.

Topical corticosteroids versus "wait and see" in the management of solitary mastocytoma in pediatric patients: a long-term follow-up. Patrizi A, Tabanelli M, Neri I, Virdi A. Dermatol Ther 2015; 28: 57–61.

In 130 patients with mastocytomas, 62 were treated with clobetasol cream, and 68 were untreated. A retrospective analysis showed no statistical differences between the two groups in the number of resolved or partially improved subjects. Complete remission occurred in an average of 16.4 months with treatment and 37.5 months without treatment. Average follow-up time was 56.3 months, with a range of 4 to 142 months.

Although the resolution of mastocytomas may occur with or without treatment, the time to resolution is faster with treatment using topical glucocorticoids, which are effective and safe considering the long time for resolution.

Cutaneous mastocytosis: successful treatment with narrowband ultraviolet B phototherapy. Prignano F, Troiano M, Lotti T. Clin Exp Dermatol 2010; 35: 914–5.

In seven adult patients with urticaria pigmentosa, the pruritus was reduced after three cycles of 12 treatments with narrowband UVB phototherapy.

Indolent systemic mastocytosis treated with narrow-band UVB phototherapy: study of five cases. Brazzelli V, Grasso V, Marina G, Barbaccia V, Merante S, Bouer E, et al. J Eur Acad Dermatol Venereol 2012; 26: 465–9.

In five adult patients with indolent systemic mastocytosis, the pruritus was controlled and urticaria pigmentosa resolved after a median of 3.5 months of therapy. At a 6-month follow-up evaluation, there was no relapse of the pruritus or urticaria pigmentosa.

Due to its excellent side effect profile, NB-UVB phototherapy is preferred to PUVA photochemotherapy or UVA1 phototherapy.

Short- and long-term effectiveness of oral and bath PUVA therapy in urticaria pigmentosa and systemic mastocytosis. Godt O, Proksch E, Streit V, Christophers E. Dermatology 1997; 195: 35–9.

In 20 patients with urticaria pigmentosa treated with PUVA photochemotherapy, improvement in pruritus was seen in 8 of 15 patients. Darier sign was suppressed in 7 and reduced in 8 patients. There was follow-up for 18 years; 25% showed improvement for more than 5 years. Bath PUVA photochemotherapy with 8-methoxypsoralen was without effect. The success of PUVA photochemotherapy lasted from only a few weeks to more than 10 years.

Photochemotherapy of dominant, diffuse, cutaneous mastocytosis. Smith ML, Orton PW, Chu H, Weston WL. Pediatr Dermatol 1990; 7: 251–5.

In three infants and one child with diffuse cutaneous mastocytosis treated with oral PUVA photochemotherapy twice weekly for 3 to 5 months, there was reduced pruritus, reduced blister formation, and a less thick skin, with persistence of dermographism.

Evidence Levels: **A** Double-blind study **B** Clinical trial ≥ 20 subjects **C** Clinical trial < 20 subjects **D** Series ≥ 5 subjects **E** Anecdotal case reports

Medium- versus high-dose ultraviolet A1 therapy for urticaria pigmentosa: a pilot study. Gobello T, Mazzanti C, Sordi D, Annessi G, Abeni D, Chinni LM, et al. J Am Acad Dermatol 2003; 49: 679–84.

In 12 patients with urticaria pigmentosa, treatment with both medium-dose UVA1 (60 J/cm^2) for 15 days and high-dose UVA1 (130 J/cm^2) for 10 days was associated with less pruritus, with a decrease in the number of mast cells and a change in the number of lesions over a 6-month period.

The appropriate method and schedules for the use of oral PUVA photochemotherapy, UVA1 phototherapy, and even narrowband UVB phototherapy need to be determined by controlled trials.

Third-Line Therapies

• Interferon-α	D
• Topical calcineurin inhibitors	E
• Leukotriene receptor inhibitors	E
• Thalidomide	E
• Surgical excision	E
• Flashlamp-pumped pulsed dye and Nd:YAG lasers	E
• Electron beam radiation	E
• Tyrosine kinase inhibitors	B
• Cladribine	B
• Omalizumab	E

Treatment of urticaria pigmentosa using interferon alpha. Kolde G, Sunderkötter C, Luger TA. Br J Dermatol 1995; 133: 91–4.

Six adult patients with urticaria pigmentosa, were treated with subcutaneous interferon-alpha started at a daily dose of 0.5×10^6 U, increasing to 5×10^6 U within 10 days. This dose was given five times a week for 6 to 20 weeks then, reduced to three injections a week for 6 to 38 weeks. There was marked improvement of pruritus and whealing and Darier sign became negative. There was no reduction in the number or appearance of the macular and papular skin lesions or in the number or structural organization of the lesional mast cells in light or electron microscopic studies.

Cutaneous mastocytosis: two pediatric patients treated with topical pimecrolimus. Correia O, Duarte AF, Quirino P, Azevedo R, Delgado L. Dermatol Online J 2010; 16: 8.

In two children, 14 to 26 months, with a mastocytoma and in four children, 7 to 16 months, with urticaria pigmentosa, pimecrolimus cream was applied twice daily, and substantial improvement was noted within 3 months.

Leukotriene-receptor inhibition for the treatment of systemic mastocytosis. Tolar J, Tope WD, Neglia JP. N Engl J Med 2004; 350: 735–6.

In a 2-month-old boy with systemic mastocytosis and skin lesions, wheezing, and hepatomegaly, when montelukast 0.25 mg/kg twice daily was not given, wheezing and cutaneous vesicles reappeared and subsided when the drug was readministered.

The leukotriene-receptor inhibitors should be evaluated in mastocytosis in a controlled trial.

Thalidomide in systemic mastocytosis: results from an open-label, multicenter, phase II study. Gruson B, Lortholary O, Canioni D, Chandesris O, Lanterner F, Bruneru J, et al. Br J Hematol 2013; 161: 434–42.

In a prospective, open-label, multicenter study on 19 patients with systemic mastocytosis, 14 of whom had urticaria pigmentosa and 1 of whom had diffuse cutaneous mastocytosis, thalidomide was used for 6 months. Of the patients with skin lesions or symptoms, the overall response rate was 61%, with improvement or disappearance of pruritus in 64%.

Solitary mastocytoma in an adult: treatment by excision. Ashinoff R, Soter NA, Freedberg IM. J Dermatol Surg Oncol 1993; 19: 487–8.

In a 33-year-old woman, a solitary mastocytoma was excised.

Treatment of an unusual solitary mast cell lesion with the pulsed dye laser resulting in cosmetic improvement and reduction in the degree of urticarial reaction. Rose RF, Daly BM, Sheehan-Dave R. Dermatol Surg 2007; 31: 851–3.

In a 12-year-old girl with a solitary mast cell lesion with features of solitary mastocytoma and telangiectasia macularis eruptiva perstans treated with a 585-nm pulsed dye laser, there were cosmetic improvement and reduction in the severity of wheals after six treatments.

The treatment of urticaria pigmentosa with the frequency-doubled Q-switch ND-YAG laser. Bedlow AJ, Gharrie S, Harland CC. J Cutan Laser Ther 2000; 2: 45–7.

In a 30-year-old woman with urticaria pigmentosa treated with a frequency-doubled Q-switched Nd:YAG laser, there was initial improvement in the clinical appearance, but the lesions recurred after 9 months.

The cosmetic treatment of urticaria pigmentosa with Nd-YAG laser at 532 nanometers. Resh B, Jones E, Glaser DA. Cosmet Dermatol 2005; 4: 78–82.

In a 19-year-old man with urticaria pigmentosa treated with a 532-nm diode-pumped Nd:YAG laser there was a reduction in the number of lesions.

The efficacy of lasers in the treatment of various forms of cutaneous skin lesions of mastocytosis remains unknown.

Complete response after imatinib mesylate therapy in a patient with well-differentiated systemic mastocytosis. Alvarez-Twose J, González P, Morgado JM, Jara-Acevedo M, Sánchez-Muñoz L, Matito A, et al. J Clin Oncol 2012; 30: e126–9.

In a 65-year-old man with well-differentiated systemic mastocytosis and urticaria pigmentosa, imatinib mesylate, a tyrosine kinase inhibitor, was administered and improvement of the skin lesions was noted at 8 months, with total remission at 18 months when imatinib mesylate was discontinued. Eight months after discontinuing the treatment, the skin lesions remained in remission.

Imatinib mesylate in the treatment of diffuse cutaneous mastocytosis. Morren M-A, Hoppé A, Renard M, Rychter MD, Uyttebroeck A, Dubreuil P, et al. J Pediatr 2013; 162: 205–7.

In a 3-month-old girl and in an 11-month-old girl with diffuse cutaneous mastocytosis and an activating KIT mutation in exon 8 (p. Asp 419 del) in the skin lesions, with the administration of imatinib mesylate for 9 months and 1 year, respectively, there were no relapses with a 2-year and 6-month follow-up, respectively.

Masitinib for the treatment of systemic and cutaneous mastocytosis with handicap: a phase 2a study. Paul C, Sans B, Suarez F, Casassus P, Barete S, Lanternier F, et al. Am J Hematol 2010; 85: 921–5.

In a multicenter, open-label trial in 7 patients with cutaneous mastocytosis and in 18 patients with systemic mastocytosis, the administration of masitinib mesylate, a tyrosine kinase inhibitor, resulted in a reduction of mast cells in skin biopsy specimens in 7 of 14 patients and a decrease in pruritus and flushing in 10 of 25 patients.

Cladribine therapy for systemic mastocytosis. Kluin-Nelemans HC, Oldhoff JM, van Doormaal JJ, van't Wout JW, Verhoef G, Gerrits WBJ, et al. Blood 2003; 102: 4270–6.

In each of seven patients with systemic mastocytosis and urticaria pigmentosa treated with cladribine, which is a synthetic purine analog cytoreductive agent, there was a reduction in the number of skin lesions to near disappearance and a reduction in mast cells in skin biopsy specimens.

Long-term efficacy and safety of cladribine (2-CdA) in adult patients with mastocytosis. Barete S, Lortholary O, Damaj G, Hirsh I, Chandesris MO, Elle C, et al. Blood 2015; 20: 1009–16.

In a nationwide retrospective study in France over one decade in 68 adult patients with various types of systemic mastocytosis who were treated with cladribine, those with urticaria pigmentosa showed improvement in the skin with a decrease in the number of mast cells in skin biopsy specimens.

Successful treatment of cutaneous mastocytosis and Ménière disease with anti-IgE therapy. Siebenhaar F, Kühn W, Zuberbier T, Maurer M. J Allergy Clin Immunol 2007; 120: 213–5.

In a 56-year-old woman with cutaneous mastocytosis, described as red-brown macules and papules with an increase in mast cells in a skin biopsy specimen, treatment with omalizumab controlled wheal formation and pruritus, although the skin lesions persisted.

Cutaneous and gastrointestinal symptoms in two patients with systemic mastocytosis successfully treated with omalizumab. Lieberoth S, Thomsen SF. Case Rep Med 2015; 2015: 903541.

In a 48-year-old woman and in a 57-year-old man with systemic mastocytosis and severe pruritus, the administration of omalizumab was associated with a reduction in pruritus.

Tyrosine kinase inhibitors, cytoreductive agents, and omalizumab have been used in patients with systemic mastocytosis, with improvement of the skin symptoms in some patients. The use of these therapeutic agents in extensive cutaneous mastocytosis without systemic disease warrants further investigation.

Evidence Levels: **A** Double-blind study **B** Clinical trial ≥ 20 subjects **C** Clinical trial < 20 subjects **D** Series ≥ 5 subjects **E** Anecdotal case reports

151

Melasma

Stephanie Ogden, Christopher E.M. Griffiths

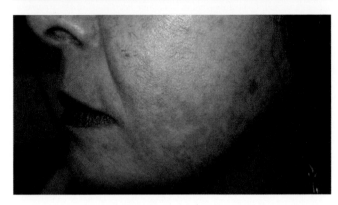

Melasma is an acquired hypermelanosis that most commonly affects females of childbearing age, although males may also be affected. The condition can be classified according to the pattern of facial involvement, which includes centrofacial (forehead, cheeks, chin, and upper lip), malar, and mandibular. Less frequently the neck, arms, and chest may be affected. Melasma is more prevalent in individuals with Fitzpatrick skin types III and above and can have a significant psychosocial impact.

Three histologic subtypes of melasma exist—epidermal, dermal, and mixed—which may be differentiated by the use of a Wood lamp, where epidermal melasma shows enhanced contrast and dermal melasma less contrast. More recently, in vivo reflectance confocal microscopy has been studied as a noninvasive method of evaluating melasma. Histologic features of melasma include increased epidermal and dermal melanin, solar elastosis, damage to the basement membrane, increased vascularity, and increased numbers of dermal mast cells and CD4+ T cells. Epidermal melasma is the most responsive to treatment.

The pathogenesis of melasma is not fully understood; however, hormonal factors, in particular pregnancy and the use of oral contraceptives, are the most common precipitants. Exposure to ultraviolet (UV) radiation both precipitates and exacerbates. Other etiologic factors include phototoxic medications, genetic predisposition, and thyroid disease.

MANAGEMENT STRATEGY

Melasma is often difficult to treat due to the recalcitrant and recurrent nature of the condition and the risk of postinflammatory hyperpigmentation associated with some treatments, particularly in individuals with darker skin. Pregnancy-induced melasma may resolve spontaneously postpartum, and females taking the oral contraceptive pill may be advised to change to *an alternative form of contraception.*

Sun exposure increases melanin production and may exacerbate melasma; therefore all patients should receive sun protection advice and use a *high-factor broad-spectrum sunscreen with good protection against UVA.* Recent evidence suggests that *sunscreen with protection against visible light* may provide additional benefit. Patients may also wish to use *camouflage makeup.*

Current treatment options include *topical depigmenting agents, chemical peels, laser therapies,* and *tranexamic acid.* The response to monotherapy is often limited, and therefore a combination of treatments may optimize outcome. Commonly used treatments include 2% to 5% hydroquinone, tretinoin, triple combination creams (containing hydroquinone, tretinoin, and fluocinolone), and azelaic acid. Glycolic acid is the most commonly reported peeling agent and may be used as an adjunct to topical depigmenting agents. The results of laser therapies are mixed, and treatment carries a significant risk of relapse and postinflammatory hyperpigmentation depending on the type of laser used.

Specific Investigation

- Thyroid function tests

Evaluation of autoimmune thyroid disease in melasma. Rostami Mogaddam M, Iranparvar Alamdari M, Maleki N, Safavi Ardabili N, Abedkouhi S. J Cosmet Dermatol 2015; 14: 167–71.

The prevalence of thyroid abnormalities in 70 nonpregnant females with melasma compared with 70 age-matched controls was 18.5% (15.7% positive anti-thyroid peroxidase antibodies) versus 4.3% (5.7% positive anti-thyroid peroxidase antibodies).

First-Line Therapies

• Triple combination cream	A
• Hydroquinone	A
• Tretinoin	A
• Sunscreen	A

Systematic review of randomized controlled trials on interventions for melasma: an abridged Cochrane Review. Jutley GS, Rajaratnam R, Halpern J, Salim A, Emmett C. J Am Acad Dermatol 2014; 70: 369–73.

This review included 20 studies and concluded that triple combination cream was more effective than hydroquinone or any agent in dual combination. Azelaic acid (20%) was superior to 2% hydroquinone in lightening melasma, and tretinoin led to greater objective improvement in melasma than placebo.

Efficacy and safety of a new triple-combination agent for the treatment of facial melasma. Taylor SC, Torok H, Jones T. Cutis 2003; 72: 67–72.

Two multicenter, randomized studies compared a formulation containing tretinoin 0.05%, hydroquinone 4%, and fluocinolone acetonide 0.01% with the three possible dual combinations of the three agents in 641 patients with melasma (Fitzpatrick skin types I–IV). The triple combination formulation was significantly more effective than any of the dual combinations. At week 8 a 75% reduction in melasma/pigmentation was observed in more than 70% of patients treated, compared with 30% in patients using dual therapy.

Commonly reported adverse effects with triple combination cream include mild erythema, burning, and peeling.

A histologic examination for skin atrophy after 6 months of treatment with fluocinolone acetonide 0.01%, hydroquinone 4%, and tretinoin 0.05% cream. Bhawan J, Grimes P, Pandya AG, Keady M, Byers HR, Guevara I, et al. Am J Dermatopathol 2009; 31: 794–8.

This study found no evidence of clinical or histologic atrophy in 30 melasma patients after daily use of triple combination cream for 24 weeks.

Topical tretinoin (retinoic acid) improves melasma. A vehicle-controlled, clinical trial. Griffiths CEM, Finkel LJ, Ditre CM, Hamilton TA, Ellis CN, Voorhees JJ. Br J Dermatol 1993; 129: 415–21.

A study of 0.1% tretinoin once daily in 38 Caucasian women for 40 weeks found that 68% of tretinoin-treated patients were improved or much improved, compared with only 5% in the vehicle-treated group. Erythema and desquamation were more common in the tretinoin group.

The efficacy of a broad spectrum sunscreen in the treatment of melasma. Vasquez M, Sanchez JL. Cutis 1983; 92: 95–6.

Broad-spectrum sunscreen compared with vehicle used alongside hydroquinone led to improvement in 96% of subjects compared with 81% of those using vehicle.

Near-visible light and UV photoprotection in the treatment of melasma: a double-blind randomized trial. Castanedo-Cazares JP, Hernandez-Blanco D, Carlos-Ortega B, Fuentes-Ahumada C, Torres-Alvarez B. Photodermatol Photoimmunol Photomed 2014; 30: 35–42.

A randomized study of 68 patients with melasma treated with 4% hydroquinone and sunscreen with either broad-spectrum UV protection alone or with iron oxide as a visible light–absorbing pigment. Patients using sunscreen with additional protection against visible light experienced significantly greater improvement in melasma.

The vast majority of recent clinical trials for melasma treatments include regular use of a high-factor sunscreen as part of the regimen.

Second-Line Therapies	
• Azelaic acid	A
• Glycolic acid peels	A
• Adapalene	A

The treatment of melasma: 20% azelaic acid versus 4% hydroquinone cream. Balina LM, Graupe K. Int J Dermatol 1991; 30: 893–5.

A double-blind, randomized study of over 300 women. After the 24-week treatment period, 65% of azelaic acid–treated patients had good or excellent results. No significant treatment differences were observed between azelaic acid– and hydroquinone-treated patients.

Glycolic acid peels/azelaic acid 20% cream combination and low potency triple combination lead to similar reduction in melasma severity in ethnic skin: results of a randomized controlled study. Mahajan R, Kanwar AJ, Parsad D, Kumaran MS, Sharma R. Indian J Dermatol 2015; 60: 147–52.

A 12-week randomized study of 40 patients treated with either low-potency triple combination cream (hydroquinone 2%, tretinoin 0.05%, fluocinolone 0.01%) or glycolic acid peels (starting at 20% and gradually increasing to 70% repeated at 2-week intervals) in combination with 20% azelaic acid cream at night (apart from 2 days before and after peels).

Efficacy and safety of serial glycolic acid peels and a topical regimen in the treatment of recalcitrant melasma. Erbil H, Sezer E, Tastan B, Arca E, Kurumlu Z. J Dermatol 2007; 34: 25–30.

Twenty-eight patients were randomized to receive eight peels, starting at 20% glycolic acid and increasing gradually to 70% on alternate weeks combined with azelaic acid 20% cream and adapalene 0.1% applied at night, or the topical agents alone, over a 20-week treatment period. A significant improvement in the melasma area and severity index (MASI) was seen in both groups at 20 weeks, although there was greater improvement in the chemical peel group.

Use of superficial peels may speed and enhance the response to topical agents. Other peeling agents that have been used in the treatment of melasma include salicylic acid, tretinoin 1%, Jessner solution, and trichloroacetic acid.

Adapalene in the treatment of melasma: a preliminary report. Dogra S, Kanwar AJ, Parasad D. J Dermatol 2002; 29: 539–40.

A randomized split-face study of 30 women comparing adapalene 0.1% and tretinoin 0.05% for 14 weeks. Both retinoids produced a similar significant improvement in melasma. Adapalene was better tolerated.

Third-Line Therapies	
• Niacinamide	A
• Kojic acid	A
• Lignin peroxidase	A
• Rucinol	A
• Topical tranexamic acid	A
• Laser and intense pulsed light (IPL)	B
• Oral tranexamic acid	B

A double-blind, randomized clinical trial of niacinamide 4% versus hydroquinone 4% in the treatment of melasma. Navarrete-Solis J, Castanedo-Cazares J, Torres-Alvarez B, Oros-Ovalle C, Fuentes-Ahumada C, Gonzalez FJ, et al. Dermatol Res Pract 2011; 2011: 379173.

Twenty-seven patients with Fitzpatrick skin types IV or V were enrolled in this 8-week study. The MASI scores improved from 4 to 1.2 in the hydroquinone-treated skin and from 3.7 to 1.4 in the niacinamide-treated skin.

Kojic acid vis-à-vis its combinations with hydroquinone and betamethasone valerate in melasma: a randomized, single blind, comparative study of efficacy and safety. Deo KS, Dash KN, Sharma YK, Virmani NC, Oberai C. Indian J Dermatol 2013; 58: 281–5.

A single-blind, randomized study of 80 patients treated with either kojic acid 1% cream; kojic acid 1% and hydroquinone 2% cream; kojic acid 1% and betamethasone valerate 0.1% cream; or kojic acid 1%, hydroquinone 2%, and betamethasone valerate 0.1% cream. All groups demonstrated improvement in MASI score; however, the greatest response was seen with kojic acid used in combination with hydroquinone.

Kojic acid is derived from fungi and is considered to have high sensitizing potential.

A split-face evaluation of a novel pigment-lightening agent compared with no treatment and hydroquinone. Draelos ZD. J Am Acad Dermatol 2015; 72: 105–7.

In this investigator-blind 12-week study of 60 women with Fitzpatrick skin types I–IV, twice-daily topical therapy with lignin peroxidase was compared with either no treatment or 4%

Evidence Levels: **A** Double-blind study **B** Clinical trial ≥ 20 subjects **C** Clinical trial < 20 subjects **D** Series ≥ 5 subjects **E** Anecdotal case reports

hydroquinone. Significant improvement in MASI scores was noted with lignin peroxidase, with comparable results to that seen with hydroquinone.

Lignin peroxidase is an enzyme derived from a tree fungus that breaks down melanin. Further work to evaluate this treatment is warranted.

Evaluation of efficacy and safety of rucinol serum in patients with melasma: a randomized controlled trial. Khemis A, Kaiafa A, Queille-Roussel C, Duteil L, Ortonne JP. Br J Dermatol 2007; 156: 997–1004.

A double-blind, randomized, split-face study of rucinol 0.3% (4-n-butylresorcinol) serum or vehicle for 12 weeks in 28 women, which revealed a significant improvement in clinical pigmentation score in rucinol-treated compared with vehicle-treated skin. The treatment was well tolerated.

Efficacy and safety of liposome-encapsulated 4-n-butyl resorcinol 0.1% cream for the treatment of melasma: a randomized controlled split-face trial. Huh SY, Shin J, Na J, Huh C, Youn S, Park K. J Dermatol 2010; 37: 311–5.

This study of 23 Korean women with melasma found a significantly greater improvement in the melanin index in patients receiving the active treatment, although the reduction was modest.

Rucinol is a resorcinol derivative that inhibits tyrosinase and tyrosinase-related protein-1 activity in vitro.

Topical tranexamic acid as a promising treatment for melasma. Ebrahimi B, Naeini FF. J Res Med Sci 2014; 19: 753–7.

A randomized, double-blind, split-face study of 3% tranexamic acid solution compared with 3% hydroquinone and 0.01% dexamethasone, both applied twice daily for 12 weeks. Thirty-nine patients with epidermal melasma completed the study with comparable significant improvements in MASI scores.

Tranexamic acid is thought to reduce melanin synthesis through inhibition of the plasminogen/plasmin pathway. One split-face, vehicle-controlled study of a liposome gel formulation of tranexamic acid reported no significant difference compared with vehicle in terms of change in MASI. More studies to determine the long-term effects, optimum formulation, and effects of combination of topical tranexamic acid with established treatments are required.

Nonablative 1550-nm fractional laser therapy versus triple topical therapy for the treatment of melasma: a randomized controlled pilot study. Kroon MW, Wind BS, Beek JF, van der Veen JP, Nieuweboer-Krobotov L, Bos J, et al. J Am Acad Dermatol 2011; 64: 516–23.

This observer-blinded study of 20 women with melasma compared triple combination cream with four sessions of nonablative 1550-nm fractional laser therapy over an 8-week period. Both treatments resulted in a significant improvement in melasma, although there was evidence of recurrence in half the patients in each group at 6-month follow-up.

The results of open-label studies of fractional photothermolysis for melasma are variable. A number of uncontrolled studies have reported

a significant incidence of postinflammatory hyperpigmentation. The treatment has little or no "downtime." One study found no additional benefit of fractional photothermolysis plus Q-switched neodymium doped yttrium-aluminum-garnet (Nd:YAG) laser treatment versus Nd:YAG alone.

A comparison of low-fluence 1064-nm Q-switched Nd:YAG laser with topical 20% azelaic acid cream and their combination in melasma in Indian patients. Bansal C, Naik H, Kar HK, Chauhan A. J Cutan Aesthet Surg 2012; 5: 266–72.

Sixty patients (Fitzpatrick skin type III–V) were randomized to receive treatment with Nd:YAG laser ($0.5-1 \text{ J/cm}^2$) alone or in combination with 20% azelaic acid twice daily. Combination therapy was more effective in improving MASI score at 12 weeks.

Higher energy settings have been associated with an increased risk of postinflammatory hyperpigmentation. There are reports of mottled hypopigmentation after use of this laser, which can be long lasting; furthermore recurrence of melasma or rebound hyperpigmentation after treatment is common. Laser therapy may be more effective when combined with other topical treatments such as triple combination cream.

Single-session intense pulsed light combined with stable fixed-dose triple combination topical therapy for the treatment of refractory melasma. Figueiredo Souza L, Trancoso Souza S. Dermatol Ther 2012; 25: 477–80.

A randomized study of 62 patients (Fitzpatrick skin types II–V) who received either a single session of IPL followed by triple combination cream or triple combination cream alone. Assessment at 6 months demonstrated a significantly greater improvement in melasma in the IPL-treated group. Three patients developed postinflammatory hyperpigmentation in the IPL group.

Melasma-like hyperpigmentation has been reported in patients treated with IPL. Further controlled trials with longer follow-up are required to determine the safety of IPL for melasma, as well as the risk of recurrence.

Oral tranexamic acid with fluocinolone-based triple combination cream versus fluocinolone-based triple combination cream alone in melasma: an open labeled randomized comparative trial. Padhi T, Pradhan S. Indian J Dermatol; 2015; 60: 520.

Forty patients were included in this randomized, open-label study, which compared oral tranexamic acid 250 mg twice daily and triple combination cream daily with the cream alone. There was a greater improvement in MASI scores at 8 weeks in the tranexamic acid–treated group. No recurrences were noted at 6-month follow-up.

Tranexamic acid is contraindicated in individuals with a history of thromboembolic disease. Further controlled studies are required to determine safety, efficacy, and optimal dosing regimens.

Cysteamine 5% cream and topical undecylenoyl phenylalanine 2% have been reported to be effective in treating melasma in single short-term, placebo-controlled studies; further longer-term studies comparing these treatments with established treatments such as hydroquinone/triple combination cream are warranted.

Merkel cell carcinoma

Maryam Liaqat, Warren R. Heymann

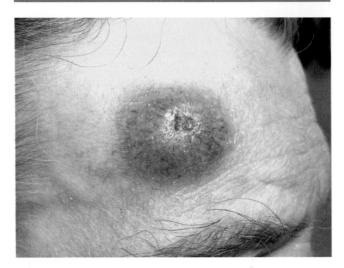

Merkel cell carcinoma (MCC) is a rare, cutaneous, neuroendocrine carcinoma with aggressive clinical behavior initially described by Toker in 1972. Classically presenting as a firm, dome-shaped, red to purple nodule, MCC typically affects older individuals, with the median patient age being 69 years. Immunosuppressive conditions such as chronic lymphocytic leukemia, human immunodeficiency virus, and solid organ transplantation have been linked to an increased risk of developing MCC. In terms of the pathogenesis of MCC, evidence exists for both infectious and environmental factors. Support for viral-promoted oncogenesis came with the discovery in 2008 of the Merkel cell polyomavirus. Ultraviolet (UV) radiation has also been described as a risk factor for the development of MCC, as most of these tumors develop at sites of sun damage with UV-associated cutaneous malignancies. The most common location is the head and neck region followed by the trunk. There is a high mortality rate associated with MCC, reported to range from 33% to 46%. Rarely, MCC may display spontaneous regression.

MANAGEMENT STRATEGY

Given the rarity of this malignancy, randomized controlled trials for therapies are lacking. As such, much of the data regarding the success of treatment modalities such as surgery, radiation, and chemotherapy stem from case series or retrospective analyses of patient data. An algorithmic approach to treatment has been put forth by the National Comprehensive Cancer Network (NCCN).

Imaging is employed for the initial workup and staging (as clinically indicated) to detect regional or distant metastases. This may be performed with either computed tomography (CT), magnetic resonance imaging (MRI), or FDG/somatostatin receptor positron emission tomography–CT (PET-CT), although studies have not shown a convincing advantage for functional imaging modalities.

Surgical removal of the primary tumor is an important component of any treatment strategy, either with standard wide local excision or Mohs micrographic surgery. In addition to excision of the primary tumor, sentinel lymph node biopsy (SLNB) is often recommended, if feasible, given the tendency of the tumor to metastasize. Evidence of clinically positive lymphadenopathy at the time of presentation will often prompt lymphadenectomy.

There are no approved therapies for advanced disease. Radiation may be used adjunctively for disease control to the primary site as well as the draining lymph node basin. Not all studies have shown a statistically significant benefit with radiation therapy. Moreover, recurrences may respond less well to radiation therapy. Chemotherapy is sometimes employed, though less evidence supports its use. Isolated limb perfusion or infusion has been used successfully for in-transit metastases. Finally, recent use of checkpoint inhibitors against programmed death-ligand 1 in advanced disease has shown positive results.

Specific Investigations

- Diagnostic imaging
- Prognostic serology
- Sentinel lymph node biopsy

Complete spontaneous regression of Merkel cell carcinoma (1986–2016): a 30 year perspective. Walsh NM. J Cutan Pathol 2016; 43: 1150–4.

A review of spontaneous regression of MCC, which usually results in a cure. The author speculates on the role of the MCC polyomavirus in the process.

Somatostatin receptor positron emission tomography/computed tomography imaging in Merkel cell carcinoma. Sollini M, Taralli S, Millela M, Erba PA, Rubagotti S, Fraternali A, et al. J Eur Acad Dermatol Venereol 2016; 30: 1507–11.

A retrospective study of 23 consecutive MCC patients who underwent a somatostatin receptor PET-CT imaging. PET-CT was used to detect primary tumor site (4/23) or to stage (8/23) or restage (11/23) patients. Sensitivity, specificity, and diagnostic accuracy of PET-CT were 92%, 73%, and 83%, respectively.

Somatostatin PET-CT has high diagnostic performance, resulting in changing the management of 7/23 patients. However, it failed to identify the site of unknown primary MCC similarly to conventional imaging.

Interest of (18)F-FDG PET-CT scanning for staging and management of Merkel cell carcinoma: a retrospective study of 15 patients. Maury G, Dereure O, Du-Thanh A, Mariano-Goulart D, Guillot B. J Eur Acad Dermatol Venereol 2011; 25: 1420–7.

This retrospective study of 15 patients compared clinical staging with (18)FDG PET-CT as well as conventional CT. Investigators found that FDG PET-CT imaging did not change disease staging and/or management based on a combination of clinical examination, SLNB, and conventional CT. Conventional CT and FDG PET-CT demonstrated identical sensitivity and specificity in this small patient cohort.

These results support data of other studies that have shown similar sensitivities when comparing functional and anatomic imaging modalities.

Prognostic value of antibodies to Merkel cell polyomavirus T antigens and VP1 protein in patients with Merkel cell carcinoma. Samimi M, Molet L, Fleury M, Laude H, Carlotti A, Gardair C, et al. Br J Dermatol 2016; 174: 715–6.

Evidence Levels: **A** Double-blind study **B** Clinical trial ≥ 20 subjects **C** Clinical trial < 20 subjects **D** Series ≥ 5 subjects **E** Anecdotal case reports

A retrospective and prospective trial at 11 French hospitals where 143 samples were included in the study. Antibodies against T antigens were associated with disease burden and therefore thought to be a useful marker of disease recurrence or progression when detected >12 months after diagnosis. In contrast, antibodies to major capsid VP1 protein have a favorable prognostic value when detected at high levels at baseline.

Absolute lymphocyte count: a potential prognostic factor for Merkel cell carcinoma. Johnson ME, Zhu F, Li T, Wu H, Galloway TJ, Farma JM, et al. J Am Acad Dermatol 2014; 70: 1028–35.

At a single institution, a retrospective study of 64 patients with MCC complete blood count was obtained in the month before definitive surgery, chemotherapy, or radiation. An absolute lymphocyte count (ALC) of 1.1 k/mm^3 was noted to be associated with overall, but not disease-free, survival. The authors concluded that ALC, a simple test, may provide additional prognostic information.

Sentinel lymph node biopsy in Merkel cell carcinoma: a 15-year institutional experience and statistical analysis of 721 reported cases. Gunaratne DA, Howle JR, Veness MR. Br J Dermatol 2016; 174: 273–81.

A comprehensive literature review of MCC patients undergoing SLNB. SLNBs were taken from 736 regional sites with 29.6% recorded as positive. Distant relapse was noted more commonly with positive SLNB.

Merkel cell carcinoma: value of sentinel lymph-node status and adjuvant radiation therapy. Servy A, Maubec E, Sugier PE, Grange F, Mansard S, Lesimple T, et al. Ann Oncol 2016; 27: 914–9.

SLNB positivity was noted in 21 of 87 patients with MCC. Patients with SLNB negativity were noted to have a longer disease-free survival and overall survival in stage I and II disease.

Recurrence and survival in patients undergoing sentinel lymph node biopsy for Merkel cell carcinoma: analysis of 153 patients from a single institution. Fields RC, Busam KJ, Chou JF, Panageas KS, Pulitzer MP, Kraus DH, et al. Ann Surg Oncol 2011; 18: 2529–37.

SLNB was positive in 29% of patients with clinically negative nodes in this retrospective review of 153 patients. Primary tumor size and the presence of lymphovascular invasion were associated with sentinel lymph node positivity. The status of the sentinel lymph node was not associated with disease-specific survival or disease recurrence.

Sentinel lymph node biopsy for evaluation and treatment of patients with Merkel cell carcinoma: the Dana-Farber experience and meta-analysis of the literature. Gupta SG, Wang LC, Peñas PF, Gellenthin M, Lee SJ, Nghiem P. Arch Dermatol 2006; 142: 685–90.

This study presented a combination of a single-institution retrospective review (30 patients) and literature-based meta-analysis (92 patients) for a total of 122 patients, and it found that SLNBs can detect clinically and radiographically occult disease. CT scans of lymph node basins have a low sensitivity (20%) for detecting both regional and distant metastases. Patients with positive SLNBs were more likely to receive adjuvant therapy and benefit from such therapy (improved relapse-free survival). The median follow-up period of this study of 12 to 15 months did not allow investigators to report disease-specific survival. Instead, only relapse-free survival data were reported.

First-Line Therapies

• Wide surgical excision	C
• Mohs micrographic surgery	C/E

Mohs micrographic surgery for the treatment of Merkel cell carcinoma. Kline L, Coldiron B. Dermatol Surg 2016; 42: 945–51.

This study was a retrospective chart review of 22 patients treated with Mohs surgery at a single institution. The recurrence rate was noted to be 5%. Regional lymph node metastasis was 14%, and no distant metastases were reported.

Merkel cell carcinoma. Comparison of Mohs micrographic surgery and wide excision in eighty-six patients. O'Connor WJ, Roenigk RK, Brodland DG. Dermatol Surg 1997; 23: 929–33.

Examining 86 patients with MCC in their retrospective review, standard wide local excision was noted to be associated with a high rate of local persistence and regional metastasis (32% and 49%, respectively) compared with Mohs micrographic surgical excision (8.3% for local persistence and 33.3% for regional metastasis). The mean follow-up for patients treated with standard surgical excision was 60 months, whereas the follow-up for those treated with Mohs excision was 36 months. Adjuvant radiation therapy reduces local persistence of tumor and regional metastases in Mohs-treated patients.

This review only included 13 patients who received Mohs excision. In addition, the extended follow-up period for patients treated with standard surgical excision compared with Mohs excision selects for more recurrences and metastases in the former group.

Second-Line Therapies

• Radiation	C
• Chemotherapy and isolated limb perfusion/infusion	C
• Check point inhibitors	E/B

Radiation therapy is associated with improved outcomes in Merkel cell carcinoma. Strom T, Carr M, Zager J, Naghavi A, Smith FO, Cruse CW, et al. Ann Surg Oncol 2016; 23: 3572–8.

This study included 171 patients with nonmetastatic MCC and pathologic nodal evaluation in whom the majority underwent wide local excision. The study demonstrated a higher rate of local control, local regional control, and survival with the use of radiation therapy. Additionally, radiation therapy was beneficial regardless of tumor margin status.

Adjuvant radiation therapy is associated with improved survival in Merkel cell carcinoma of the skin. Mojica P, Smith D, Ellenhorn JD. J Clin Oncol 2007; 25: 1043–7.

This was a retrospective study of 1487 patients who received some form of cancer-directed surgery as part of their treatment. Those who also received adjuvant radiation therapy showed improved median survival compared with those who did not undergo radiation.

Although this study included a large number of patients, the methods and regimens of radiation therapy delivered varied, with some patients receiving external beam radiation therapy and others receiving radioisotopes, implants, or some combination of these.

Adjuvant radiation therapy and chemotherapy in Merkel cell carcinoma: survival analyses of 6908 cases from the National Cancer Database. Bhatia S, Storer BE, Iyer JG, Moshiri A, Parvathaneni U, Byrd D, et al. J Natl Cancer Inst 2016; 108: djw042.

In the largest cohort of MCC patients to date, the authors evaluated the role of adjuvant radiation therapy and chemotherapy in survival. As previously reported, adjuvant radiation therapy was found to improve overall survival in MCC stage I and II disease. However, neither chemotherapy nor radiation therapy resulted in overall survival for stage III MCC.

Although 6908 MCC patients represents a very large cohort, this is a retrospective, nonrandomized analysis. Additionally, details regarding chemotherapy were lacking in the review.

In-transit Merkel cell carcinoma treated with isolated limb perfusion or isolated limb infusion: a case series of 12 patients. Zeitouni NC, Giordano CN, Kane JM. Dermatol Surg 2011; 37: 357–64.

In this series of 12 patients (two from the authors' institution and 10 from the literature), isolated limb infusion was found to be less invasive than isolated limb perfusion. Two patients from the authors' institution were treated with isolated limb infusion, whereas those reported from review of the literature had been treated with isolated limb perfusion. All patients were able to avoid limb amputation. Complete response was seen in 11/12 patients. One patient had a partial response. Mean duration of response was 21.8 months. The mean follow-up period was 25.3 months.

Although both techniques appear to be reasonable options for the treatment of in-transit disease, the inclusion of only two cases of isolated limb infusion compared with 10 cases of isolated limb perfusion makes comparison of their respective efficacies difficult. Both isolated limb infusion and isolated limb perfusion allow for the regional treatment of in-transit or advanced local disease with high-dose chemotherapy while minimizing systemic effects; however, isolated limb infusion is less invasive (percutaneous catheter placement) than isolated limb perfusion. In addition, isolated limb infusion may be performed in areas of prior lymphadenectomy with scarred vessels permitting repeat treatments as needed. Moreover, isolated limb infusion utilizes a low-flow, hypoxic system with subsequently shorter treatment times.

Avelumab in patients with chemotherapy-refractory metastatic Merkel cell carcinoma: a multicentre, single-group, open-label, phase 2 trial. Kaufman H, Russell J, Hamid O, Bhatia S, Terheyden P, D'Angelo SP, et al. Lancet Oncol 2016; 17: 1374–85.

An open-label, single-group, international, phase II trial of an anti PD-L1 monoclonal antibody for patients with chemotherapy-refractory stage IV MCC. Eighty-eight patients were enrolled and received one dose of avelumab. Nine percent of patients had a complete response, whereas 23% had a partial response. The medication was tolerated well, with only five grade 3 treatment-related adverse effects, and there were no grade 4 events or deaths.

PD-L1 expression is noted to be high in the majority of MCCs; therefore use of PD-L1 inhibitors to regulate the immune system interactions appears intuitive. The results of the study are promising, and similar outcomes have been noted with other checkpoint inhibitors. This study included patients previously treated with chemotherapy, suggesting that avelumab has higher efficacy.

PD-1 blockade with pembrolizumab in advanced Merkel-cell carcinoma. Nghiem PT, Bhatia S, Lipson EJ, Kudchadkar RR, Miller N, Annamalai L, et al. N Engl J Med 2016; 374: 2542–52.

A multicenter, phase II, noncontrolled study in patients with advanced MCC with no previous systemic therapy who were treated with pembrolizumab at dose levels approved for melanoma. A total of 26 patients received at least one dose. Pembrolizumab was noted to have an objective response rate of 56%: four patients with a complete response and ten patients with a partial response. Grade 3 or 4 treatment-related adverse events were observed in four of the 26 patients.

Similar to other checkpoint inhibitors, responses to pembrolizumab were observed irrespective of Merkel cell polyomavirus status. Note there were grade 4 treatment-related adverse reactions in this study, one of which was noted to be myocarditis. However, this improved on discontinuation of therapy and initiation of glucocorticoid treatment. Overall, checkpoint blockade may be the best option to treat patients with advanced MCC.

Evidence Levels: **A** Double-blind study **B** Clinical trial ≥ 20 subjects **C** Clinical trial < 20 subjects **D** Series ≥ 5 subjects **E** Anecdotal case reports

Methicillin-resistant *Staphylococcus aureus* and Panton–Valentine leukocidin *Staphylococcus aureus* infections

Dirk M. Elston

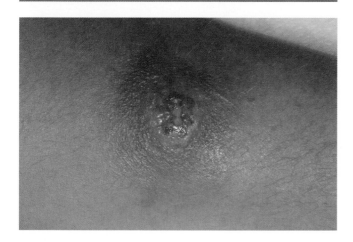

Methicillin- resistant *Staphylococcus aureus* (MRSA) bacteria have developed resistance to beta-lactam antibiotics such as methicillin, dicloxacillin, nafcillin, and oxacillin and the cephalosporins through horizontal gene transfer and natural selection. Although not necessarily more virulent than sensitive strains, infection caused by them is more difficult to treat due to their resistance to standard antibiotics. Although originally described in health care settings (hospitals and care homes), it is now endemic in community as well as livestock settings.

Panton–Valentine leukocidin (PVL) is a toxin that destroys leukocytes and is a virulence factor in some strains of *S. aureus* (SA). Strains of PVL-SA producing a new pattern of disease have emerged in the UK and worldwide. In the UK the genes encoding for PVL are carried by <2% of clinical isolates of *S. aureus* submitted to the National Reference Laboratory, whether methicillin-sensitive *S. aureus* (MSSA) or MRSA. Like other *S. aureus* strains, PVL-SA predominantly causes skin and soft tissue infections (SSTI) but can also cause invasive infections (myositis, osteomyelitis). The most serious of these is a necrotizing hemorrhagic pneumonia with a high mortality, which often follows a "flulike" illness and may affect otherwise healthy young people in the community. PVL skin infections may be remarkably severe, painful, and recurrent, producing folliculitis, furunculosis cellulitis, and skin necrosis. Transmission has been associated with family groups, contact sports, gymnasium use, and military camps.

MANAGEMENT STRATEGY (MRSA)

Health care–type strains of MRSA are associated with sepsis and are common colonists of chronic wounds, where debridement is typically the best strategy. Community-type MRSA infections typically present as an abscess or furunculosis. The most important intervention for an abscess remains surgical drainage. Purulent material can reform rapidly, so a punch or cruciate incision is advised, as it tends to remain open longer to allow adequate drainage. A curette is used to probe the wound and ensure that all pockets of purulent material have been adequately drained. Irrigation can be helpful, but packing is discouraged, as purulent material often reforms behind the packing material. Evidence suggests that antibiotics are often unnecessary if an abscess is adequately drained. There are obvious reasons to avoid antibiotics when they are not needed, including the risk of Stevens–Johnson syndrome, antibiotic-associated diarrhea, and selection of resistant strains.

Patients with significant surrounding cellulitis, refractory infection, or systemic manifestations may require antibiotic therapy. Most community-associated (CA) MRSA strains are sensitive to trimethoprim–sulfamethoxazole. Most strains are also sensitive to doxycycline and minocycline, but doxycycline does not penetrate well into the nares. Clindamycin resistance is emerging in many communities. For serious infections, therapy should be guided by culture and sensitivity. Vancomycin, linezolid, dalbavancin, telavancin, and daptomycin are often effective. Rifampin improves the intracellular killing of bacteria by vancomycin. Quinupristin–dalfopristin and tigecycline may also be effective, but quinupristin–dalfopristin, like daptomycin, may not penetrate reliably into pulmonary tissue, and tigecycline has a significant incidence of nausea. Ceftobiprole and oritavancin appear promising.

Spread occurs through skin-to-skin contact and via fomites. Decolonization may be indicated for prevention of recurrence or prevention of serious invasive disease in close contacts. The most effective decolonization regimens address the nares, intertriginous, and anogenital sites, as well as eczematous skin. In some patients, gut colonization may also be an issue.

SPECIFIC INVESTIGATIONS

Cultures should be obtained from the contents of purulent infections and resistant infections. New molecular diagnostic tests are being developed to screen for MRSA and identify genes associated with resistance.

Screening for mupirocin resistance in *Staphylococcus*. Sanju AJ, Kopula SS, Palraj KK. J Clin Diagn Res 2015; 9: DC09–10.

In a study of 100 stains of *Staphylococcus*, higher levels of resistance were noted by the minimum inhibitory concentration (MIC) method than by the disc diffusion method.

When screening for mupirocin resistance, the disk diffusion method may fail to identify low-level mupirocin resistance.

High vancomycin minimum inhibitory concentration is a predictor of mortality in methicillin-resistant *Staphylococcus aureus* bacteremia. Wi YM, Kim JM, Joo EJ, Ha YE, Kang CI, Ko KS, et al. Int J Antimicrob Agents 2012; 40: 108–13.

A retrospective cohort study of 137 patients with MRSA bacteremia demonstrated a 30-day cumulative survival of 53.8% for patients infected with isolates having an MIC ≥1 µg/mL and

79.8% for patients infected with isolates having an MIC <1 µg/mL (log-rank test, $p = 0.026$).

Although data has been mixed, this study suggests early consideration of an alternative agent in seriously ill patients with MRSA bacteremia whose isolate demonstrates high vancomycin MICs.

Epidemiology

Genome-wide association study reveals a locus for nasal carriage of *Staphylococcus aureus* in Danish crossbred pigs. Skallerup P, Espinosa-Gongora C, Jørgensen CB, Guardabassi L, Fredholm M. BMC Vet Res 2015; 11: 290.

Pigs have been identified as a major reservoir of MRSA, and the use of antibiotics in livestock has been associated with transmission of resistant organisms to humans. A single nucleotide polymorphism on chromosome 12 was found to be associated with nasal carriage of *S. aureus* in pigs, suggesting it may be possible to select pigs genetically resistant to *S. aureus* colonization.

The emerging ST8 methicillin-resistant *Staphylococcus aureus* clone in the community in Japan: associated infections, genetic diversity, and comparative genomics. Iwao Y, Ishii R, Tomita Y, Shibuya Y, Takano T, Hung WC, et al. Kansenshogaku Zasshi 2015; Suppl 13: 15–27.

Japanese ST8 CA-MRSA, a new strain with SCCmecIV1, has emerged in Japan. It is associated with SSTIs, colitis, and invasive infections (sepsis, epidural abscesses, and necrotizing pneumonia). It lacks the Panton–Valentine leukocidin phage and arginine catabolic mobile element present in our typical USA300 strain.

This new strain has already spread to Hong Kong and can be expected to appear elsewhere.

Prognosis

Treatment failure outcomes for emergency department patients with skin and soft tissue infections. May LS, Zocchi M, Zatorski C, Jordan JA, Rothman RE, Ware CE, et al. West J Emerg Med 2015; 16: 642–52.

In this study of 272 patients, 198 (72.8%) completed 1-week follow-up, and 10.2% of patients reported 1-week treatment failure. The use of packing was associated with a higher risk of treatment failure, and the odds of treatment failure were 66% lower for patients who received antibiotics after incision and drainage.

Data is emerging that the use of packing is associated with treatment failure after drainage of an abscess. Some data suggests that the addition of an antibiotic may be associated with improved outcomes.

Pathogenesis

Skin commensal staphylococci may act as reservoir for fusidic acid resistance genes. Hung WC, Chen HJ, Lin YT, Tsai JC, Chen CW, Lu HH, et al. PLoS One 2015; 10: e0143106.

In a study of 59 healthy volunteers, a total of 34 fusidic acid–resistant staphylococcal strains were isolated from 22 individuals. All were coagulase negative, and resistance genes fusB or fusC were present in *Staphylococcus epidermidis*, *Staphylococcus capitis* subsp. *urealyticus*, *Staphylococcus hominis* subsp. *hominis*, *Staphylococcus warneri*, and *Staphylococcus haemolyticus*.

These findings suggest that the skin commensal staphylococci may act as reservoirs for fusidic acid resistance genes.

First-Line Therapy	
Treatment of MRSA abscesses	
• Surgical drainage alone	B
• Surgical drainage plus trimethoprim–sulfamethoxazole	B
• Minocycline	B
• Doxycycline	B
• Clindamycin	B
Eradication of colonization: nares	
• Mupirocin	B
• Tea tree oil	B
Eradication of colonization: skin	
• Bleach baths	D
• Chlorhexidine	B
• Triclosan	B
• Tea tree oil soap	B
• Undecylenamidopropyltrimonium methosulfate/phenoxyethanol	C
• Octenidine dihydrochloride	C

Microbiology and initial antibiotic therapy for injection drug users and noninjection drug users with cutaneous abscesses in the era of community-associated methicillin-resistant *Staphylococcus aureus*. Jenkins TC, Knepper BC, Jason Moore S, Saveli CC, Pawlowski SW, Perlman DM, et al. Acad Emerg Med 2015; 22: 993–7.

Injection drug use is a risk factor for abscesses and MRSA infection. In a study of seven academic and community hospitals in Colorado, antibiotic regimens started in the emergency department were compared between injection drug users and noninjection drug users.

Among the 323 patients with cutaneous abscesses, 104 (32%) occurred in injection drug users. Surprisingly, among the 235 cases where at least one microorganism was identified by culture, *S. aureus* was identified less commonly among injection drug users compared with noninjection drug users (55% vs. 75%, $p = 0.003$), with similar patterns observed for MRSA (33% vs. 47%, $p = 0.054$) and MSSA (17% vs. 26%, $p = 0.11$).

Compared with noninjection drug users, cutaneous abscesses in injection drug users were less likely to involve *S. aureus*, including MRSA, and more likely to involve streptococci and anaerobes. Although clindamycin provides coverage against all of these pathogens, trimethoprim–sulfamethoxazole provides inadequate coverage for streptococci and anaerobes. This suggests that the choice of antibiotic should take factors like IV drug abuse into account.

Epidemiology, microbiology, and antibiotic susceptibility patterns of skin and soft tissue infections, Joint Base San Antonio-Lackland, Texas, 2012 to 2014. Fisher A, Webber BJ, Pawlak MT, Johnston L, Tchandja JB, Yun H. MSMR 2015; 22: 2–6.

An outbreak of MRSA infection was reported among military families in San Antonio in 2014. Of the 772 total cases studied, 254 were cultured and 196 resulted in growth of one or more pathogens. MRSA was the most common pathogen ($n = 110$). MSSA ($n = 68$), other gram-positive cocci ($n = 5$), and gram-negative rods ($n = 18$) were also isolated. In vitro activity of commonly

Evidence Levels: **A** Double-blind study **B** Clinical trial ≥ 20 subjects **C** Clinical trial < 20 subjects **D** Series ≥ 5 subjects **E** Anecdotal case reports

used antibiotics against *S. aureus* isolates dropped from the previous surveillance period.

Outbreaks of MRSA infection with decreased antimicrobial susceptibility warrant enhanced local preventive efforts and close adherence to evidence-based treatment algorithms.

Trimethoprim-sulfamethoxazole therapy reduces failure and recurrence in methicillin-resistant *Staphylococcus aureus* skin abscesses after surgical drainage. Holmes L, Ma C, Qiao H, Drabik C, Hurley C, Jones D, et al. J Pediatr 2016; 169: 128–34.

Patients age 3 months to 17 years of age with uncomplicated skin abscess that required surgical drainage were randomized to receive either 3 or 10 days of oral trimethoprim–sulfamethoxazole therapy. Among those with MRSA infection, those treated for only 3 days were more likely to experience treatment failure (*P* = 0.03, rate difference 10.1%, 95% confidence interval [CI], 2.1%–18.2%) and recurrent infection within 1 month (*P* = 0.046, rate difference 10.3%, 95% CI, 0.8%–19.9%).

Although the primary treatment for a MRSA abscess remains thorough drainage, this study and others suggest that antibiotics may reduce the risk of treatment failure and recurrence. A full 10 days of treatment is superior to an abbreviated 3-day course.

Recurrent skin and soft tissue infections in HIV-infected patients during a 5-year period: incidence and risk factors in a retrospective cohort study. Hemmige V, McNulty M, Silverman E, David MZ. BMC Infect Dis 2015; 15: 455.

Risk factors for recurrent infection in a multivariable Cox regression model were nonhepatitis liver disease, the presence of an intravenous catheter, and a history of intravenous drug use.

Highly active antiretroviral therapy (HAART), CD4+ count, trimethoprim–sulfamethoxazole or azithromycin use, and diabetes mellitus were not associated with recurrence.

Randomized controlled trial of cephalexin versus clindamycin for uncomplicated pediatric skin infections. Chen AE, Carroll KC, Diener-West M, Ross T, Ordun J, Goldstein MA, et al. Pediatrics 2011; 127: e573–80.

This was a comparison of clindamycin and cephalexin for the treatment of uncomplicated SSTIs caused predominantly by CA-MRSA. Of the 200 enrolled patients, 69% demonstrated MRSA on wound cultures. Spontaneous drainage or a drainage procedure occurred in 97% of subjects. There is no significant difference between cephalexin and clindamycin in this study.

The data presented here is similar to previous data. The treatment for an uncomplicated abscess remains drainage, and the use of an antibiotic has little effect on outcome.

Comparative effectiveness of antibiotic treatment strategies for pediatric skin and soft-tissue infections. Williams DJ, Cooper WO, Kaltenbach LA, Dudley JA, Kirschke DL, Jones TF, et al. Pediatrics 2011; 128: e479–87.

In a study of 6407 children who underwent drainage for MRSA infections, there were 568 treatment failures (8.9%). The rate of recurrence was high (22.8%). The adjusted odds ratios for treatment failure were 1.92 (95% CI, 1.49–2.47) for trimethoprim–sulfamethoxazole and 2.23 (95% CI, 1.71–2.90) for β-lactams. Among the 41,094 children without a drainage procedure, there were 2435 treatment failures (5.9%), but the rate of recurrence was similar to the rate in those who required drainage (18.2%). The adjusted odds ratios for treatment failure were 1.67 (95% CI,

1.44–1.95) for trimethoprim–sulfamethoxazole and 1.22 (95% CI, 1.06–1.41) for β-lactams. The authors concluded that, compared with data for clindamycin, use of either trimethoprim–sulfamethoxazole or β-lactams was associated with an increased risk of treatment failure.

MRSA abscesses typically respond to drainage alone, and it is the adequacy of the drainage procedure rather than the choice of antibiotic that is the prime determinant of outcome. It would also be important to know the local prevalence of inducible clindamycin resistance before recommending clindamycin over trimethoprim–sulfamethoxazole when an antibiotic is needed.

Prevention of recurrent staphylococcal skin infections. Creech CB, Al-Zubeidi DN, Fritz SA. Infect Dis Clin North Am 2015; 29: 429–64.

Staphylococcal infections often cluster within households, and asymptomatic carriers serve as reservoirs for transmission. A household approach to decolonization and fomite control is more effective than measures performed by individuals alone.

Staphylococcus aureus colonization and strain type at various body sites among patients with a closed abscess and uninfected controls at U.S. emergency departments. Albrecht VS, Limbago BM, Moran GJ, Krishnadasan A, Gorwitz RJ, McDougal LK, et al. J Clin Microbiol 2015; 53: 3478–84.

Staphylococcal-infected subjects were usually colonized with the infecting strain. Among MRSA-infected subjects, the most common site was the groin.

Moist areas of skin are commonly colonized with MRSA. Interventions that only address nasal carriage are inferior to those that also address skin carriage, especially in the groin, axillae, and umbilicus.

The impact of hospital-acquired methicillin-resistant *Staphylococcus aureus* in a burn population after implementation of universal decolonization protocol. Johnson AT, Nygaard RM, Cohen EM, Fey RM, Wagner AL. J Burn Care Res 2016; 37: e525–30.

Universal decolonization of all patients with daily chlorhexidine baths and a 5-day course of nasal mupirocin was effective in reducing mortality in an adult and pediatric burn unit.

Effectiveness of simple control measures on methicillin-resistant *Staphylococcus aureus* infection status and characteristics with susceptibility patterns in a teaching hospital in Peshawar. Rafiq MS, Rafiq MI, Khan T, Rafiq M, Khan MM. J Pak Med Assoc 2015; 65: 915–20.

Barrier precautions remain a key intervention to prevent the spread of MRSA infection.

Prospective investigation of nasal mupirocin, hexachlorophene body wash, and systemic antibiotics for prevention of recurrent community-associated methicillin-resistant *Staphylococcus aureus* infections. Miller LG, Tan J, Eells SJ, Benitez E, Radner AB. Antimicrob Agents Chemother 2012; 56: 1084–6.

In a prospective study of 31 patients with recurrent CA-MRSA skin infections who received nasal mupirocin, topical hexachlorophene body wash, and an oral anti-MRSA antibiotic, the mean number of infections after the intervention decreased significantly (0.03 vs. 0.84 infections/month, *p* ≤ 0.0001).

Among patients with recurrent infection, some data suggest that decolonization can reduce the rate of future recurrences.

Targeted intranasal mupirocin to prevent colonization and infection by community-associated methicillin-resistant *Staphylococcus aureus* strains in soldiers: a cluster randomized controlled trial. Ellis MW, Griffith ME, Dooley DP, McLean JC, Jorgensen JH, Patterson JE, et al. Antimicrob Agents Chemother 2007; 51: 3591–8.

Second-Line Therapy	
• Vancomycin ± rifampin	B
• Linezolid and newer oxazolidinones	A
• Dalbavancin	B
• Telavancin	B
• Daptomycin	B
Eradication of colonization: nares	
• Retapamulin	D
• Triple antibiotic ointment	D
• Silver sulfadiazine cream	D
Eradication of colonization: skin	
• Benzoyl peroxide soap	E
• Zinc pyrithione soap	E

Weight-based antibiotic dosing in a real-world European study of complicated skin and soft-tissue infections due to methicillin-resistant *Staphylococcus aureus*. Lawson W, Nathwani D, Eckmann C, Corman S, Stephens J, Solem C, et al. Microbiol Infect 2015; 21 (Suppl 2): S40–6.

Real-world dosing of weight-based intravenous (IV) antibiotic therapy in patients hospitalized for complicated MRSA SSTIs were assessed by means of data from 12 European countries. Patients had been treated with IV vancomycin, teicoplanin, or daptomycin. Low, standard (labeled), and high dosing groups were assessed in 1502 patients. The majority of patients receiving first-line teicoplanin and daptomycin (96% and 80%, respectively) received higher than labeled complicated SSTI doses. In contrast, vancomycin doses were lower than labeled doses in >40% of patients.

This real-world data reveals significant deviations from labeled antibiotic dosing and suggests that fear of vancomycin toxicity may affect management.

Randomized controlled noninferiority trial comparing daptomycin to vancomycin for the treatment of complicated skin and skin structure infections in an observation unit. Shaw GJ, Meunier JM, Korfhagen J, Wayne B, Hart K, Lindsell CJ, et al. J Emerg Med 2015; 49: 928–36.

In a study of 100 patients, daptomycin was not inferior to vancomycin in the treatment of complicated SSTIs.

An open-label, pragmatic, randomized controlled clinical trial to evaluate the comparative effectiveness of daptomycin versus vancomycin for the treatment of complicated skin and skin structure infection. Kauf TL, McKinnon P, Corey GR, Bedolla J, Riska PF, Sims M, et al. BMC Infect Dis 2015; 15:503.

The primary end point of this study was infection-related length of stay. Secondary end points included health care resource utilization, cost, clinical response, and patient-reported outcomes. There were no significant differences between the two, although vancomycin was associated with a lower likelihood of day 2 clinical success (odds ratio [OR] = 0.498, 95 % CI, 0.249–0.997; $P < 0.05$).

Other factors, including cost, may be more important than efficacy in driving the decision of which therapy to use.

Dalbavancin: a novel lipoglycopeptide antibiotic with extended activity against gram-positive infections. Smith JR, Roberts KD, Rybak MJ. Infect Dis Ther 2015; 4: 245–58.

Lipoglycopeptides have extended half-lives and are effective against MRSA.

In vitro activity of ceftaroline against bacterial pathogens isolated from skin and soft tissue infections in Europe, Russia and Turkey in 2012: results from the Assessing Worldwide Antimicrobial Resistance Evaluation (AWARE) surveillance programme. Karlowsky JA, Biedenbach DJ, Bouchillon SK, Iaconis JP, Reiszner E, Sahm DF. J Antimicrob Chemother 2016; 71: 162–9.

Most ceftaroline-nonsusceptible isolates were from Russia, Turkey, Italy, and Hungary. Ceftaroline susceptibility was 99% for *S. aureus* isolates submitted by 7 of 17 countries.

In most areas, ceftaroline continues to demonstrate potent in vitro activity against contemporary strains of bacteria, including MRSA.

In vitro activities of tedizolid and linezolid against gram-positive cocci associated with acute bacterial skin and skin structure infections and pneumonia. Chen KH, Huang YT, Liao CH, Sheng WH, Hsueh PR. Antimicrob Agents Chemother 2015; 59: 6262–5.

Tedizolid is a novel, expanded-spectrum oxazolidinone with potent activity against a wide range of gram-positive pathogens. This study of 425 isolates of gram-positive bacteria from patients with acute bacterial skin and skin structure infections or pneumonia included 100 MRSA isolates. Tedizolid exhibited better in vitro activities than linezolid against MRSA (MIC90s, 0.5 vs. 2 µg/mL) as well as MSSA (MIC90s, 0.5 vs. 2 µg/mL), *S. pyogenes* (MIC90s, 0.5 vs. 2 µg/mL), *S. agalactiae* (MIC90s, 0.5 vs. 2 µg/mL), *Streptococcus anginosus* group (MIC90s, 0.5 vs. 2 µg/mL), *Enterococcus faecalis* (MIC90s, 0.5 vs. 2 µg/mL), and vancomycin-resistant enterococci (VRE) (MIC90s, 0.5 vs. 2 µg/mL).

Tedizolid exhibited two- to fourfold better in vitro activities against a variety of gram-positive cocci compared with linezolid.

Third-Line Therapies	
• Tigecycline	B
• Ceftobiprole, ceftaroline	C
• Oritavancin	C
• Honey and bee venom	D
• Topical simvastatin	E
• Topical celecoxib	E
• Nanoparticles	E
• Confectioner's sugar	E
• Sugar and povidone iodine	E
• Botanical extracts	D

Dalbavancin and oritavancin: an innovative approach to the treatment of gram-positive infections. Roberts KD, Sulaiman RM, Rybak MJ. Pharmacotherapy 2015; 35: 935–48.

In 2014, the U.S. Food and Drug Administration approved two new lipoglycopeptides, oritavancin and dalbavancin, for the treatment of acute bacterial skin and skin structure infections. They demonstrate increased potency against MRSA compared with vancomycin.

Currently, there is more data concerning dalbavancin than oritavancin, but both are promising additions to our armamentarium.

Evidence Levels: A Double-blind study B Clinical trial ≥ 20 subjects C Clinical trial < 20 subjects D Series ≥ 5 subjects E Anecdotal case reports

Exploration of alginate hydrogel/nano zinc oxide composite bandages for infected wounds. Mohandas A, Kumar PTS, Raja B, Lakshmanan VK, Jayakumar R. Int J Nanomedicine 2015; 10 (Suppl 1): 53–66.

The prepared composite bandages exhibited excellent antimicrobial activity against MRSA.

These bandages have a nontoxic nature at lower concentrations of nano zinc oxide.

Melittin, a honeybee venom-derived antimicrobial peptide, may target methicillin-resistant *Staphylococcus aureus*. Choi JH, Jang AY, Lin S, Lim S, Kim D, Park K, et al. Mol Med Rep 2015; 12: 6483–90.

Both honey and melittin demonstrate activity against MRSA.

Exploring simvastatin, an antihyperlipidemic drug, as a potential topical antibacterial agent. Thangamani S, Mohammad H, Abushahba MF, Hamed MI, Sobreira TJ, Hedrick VE, et al. Sci Rep 2015; 5: 16407.

Simvastatin, used systemically as a lipid-lowering agent, demonstrated broad-spectrum antibacterial activity against gram-positive organisms, including MRSA, when used topically. It also demonstrated the ability to suppress production of the key MRSA toxins α-hemolysin and Panton–Valentine leukocidin.

The most intriguing finding of this study was that simvastatin exhibits excellent antibiofilm activity against established staphylococcal biofilms.

Repurposing celecoxib as a topical antimicrobial agent. Thangamani S, Younis W, Seleem MN. Front Microbiol 2015 28; 6: 750.

Celecoxib, a marketed inhibitor of cyclooxygenase-2, exhibits broad-spectrum antimicrobial activity against gram-positive pathogens, including MRSA. The primary antimicrobial mechanism of action is dose-dependent inhibition of ribonucleic acid (RNA), deoxyribonucleic acid (DNA), and protein synthesis.

Topical application of celecoxib significantly reduced the mean bacterial count in a mouse model of MRSA skin infection.

Nordihydroguaiaretic acid enhances the activities of aminoglycosides against methicillin-sensitive and resistant *Staphylococcus aureus* in vitro and in vivo. Cunningham-Oakes E, Soren O, Moussa C, Rathor G, Liu Y, Coates A, et al. Front Microbiol 2015; 6: 1195.

Nordihydroguaiaretic acid (NDGA) is an antioxidant compound extracted from the plant *Larrea tridentata*. Antimicrobial activity targets the bacterial cell membrane.

In this study of 200 clinical isolates of MRSA and MSSA, NDGA demonstrated synergy with aminoglycosides in a murine skin infection model.

Effect of medical honey on wounds colonised or infected with MRSA. Blaser G, Santos K, Bode U, Vetter H, Simon A. J Wound Care 2007; 16: 325–8.

In seven patients with nonhealing wounds infected or colonized with MRSA who had failed other antiseptics and antibiotics, honey resulted in complete healing.

My grandmother, Anny Elston, MD, reported that as a World War I medic she used confectioner's sugar to treat infected ulcers in returning prisoners of war. All ulcers healed. The treatment is inexpensive, and resistance to the desiccating effects of sugar is unlikely.

PVL-SA MANAGEMENT STRATEGY

Microbiologic swabs should be taken and PVL polymerase chain reaction (PCR) testing requested, as this may not be routinely undertaken. Small abscesses require drainage only. Lesions should be covered, and towels and other possible fomites should not be shared. Lesions over 5 cm in diameter or when there is also cellulitis require antibiotics (flucloxacillin or clindamycin), usually orally for 5 to 7 days. Where MRSA PVL infection is suspected, rifampicin plus either doxycycline, fusidic acid or trimethoprim, or clindamycin as monotherapy. For severe and invasive infections, such as pyomyositis or toxic shock, parenteral vancomycin, teicoplanin, daptomycin, or linezolid have been used in combination with high-dose intravenous immunoglobulin (IVIG) (2 day) in addition to drainage and debridement.

Decolonization is recommended to prevent transmission to close contacts with 4% chlorhexidine soap or 2% triclosan for 5 days and mupirocin nasal cream daily for 5 days to the nares.

Specific Investigations
• Swabs for culture and PVL PCR
• If PVL infection is suspected, it is important to specifically request PVL PCR, as it is not routinely performed

First-Line Therapy	
• Drainage of small abscesses	C
• Drainage and antibiotics for larger abscesses (over 5 cm) and if cellulitis evident	
• Flucloxacillin 500 mg four times a day for 5 days	C
• Clindamycin 450 mg four times a day for 5 days	C
• Decolonization	C
If PVL MRSA is suspected or confirmed	
• Rifampicin 300 mg twice daily plus doxycycline100 mg twice daily	C
• Rifampicin 300 mg twice daily plus fusidic acid 500 mg three times a day	C
• Rifampicin 300 mg twice a day plus trimethoprim 200 mg twice a day	C
• Clindamycin 450 mg four times a day	C

Guidance on the diagnosis and management of PVL-associated *Staphylococcus aureus* Health Protection Agency UK 2008. Available online at www.hpa.org.uk.

This document gives detailed advice regarding PVL infection, including patient information leaflets and practical advice about decolonization.

Decolonization is performed with either chlorhexidine body wash or shampoo or 2% triclosan. The product is applied to wetted skin directly without dilution daily for 5 days –it should be washed off after 1 minute. Individual towels are needed and, if possible, changed daily. Mupirocin nasal cream (about a matchstick head–sized amount) should be applied to the inner surface of each nostril on a cotton bud and massaged inside the nostrils thrice daily for 5 days.

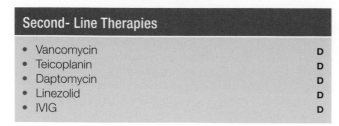

Second-Line Therapies

- Vancomycin   D
- Teicoplanin   D
- Daptomycin   D
- Linezolid   D
- IVIG   D

Guidance on the diagnosis and management of PVL-associated *Staphylococcus aureus*. Health Protection Agency UK 2008. Serious life-threatening infection will need advice from microbiologists and infectious disease specialists.

Evidence Levels: **A** Double-blind study   **B** Clinical trial ≥ 20 subjects   **C** Clinical trial < 20 subjects   **D** Series ≥ 5 subjects   **E** Anecdotal case reports

Miliaria

Kelly R. Kane, Sandra Pena, Warren R. Heymann

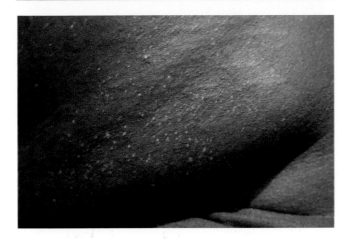

Miliaria is a benign, transient disorder caused by occlusion and resultant injury in the eccrine duct. It is subdivided into miliaria crystallina, miliaria rubra, and miliaria profunda, based on the level of obliteration. Miliaria crystallina, the most superficial form (sudamina), occurs with occlusion of the sweat duct in the stratum corneum. It is self-limiting and typically appears as clear vesicles without significant erythema. Miliaria rubra ("prickly heat") is the most common, presenting as numerous pruritic nonfollicular papules or vesicles with surrounding erythema. The obstruction occurs within the eccrine duct in the stratum malpighii. Typically it occurs on the trunk, neck, or back but can affect other areas and has been reported to occur under splints or braces and military uniforms because of the warm occlusive environment. Miliaria profunda is uncommon, classically occurring at the dermoepidermal junction or dermis; however, advances in imaging have begun to cause physicians to question this understanding. Miliaria profunda is typically seen after repeated cases of miliaria rubra in tropical settings. These patients can also have associated systemic symptoms related to overheating.

MANAGEMENT STRATEGY

Miliaria most typically occurs as a result of excessive sweating in hot, humid conditions, prolonged perspiration, or after extended febrile illness. There are other less common reports of congenital miliaria, miliaria occurring after medication administration in the intensive care setting, and in association with congenital illnesses such as pseudohypoaldosteronism (PHA) and with hypernatremia. Miliaria is often exacerbated by tight clothing and high humidity. Management begins with *removal of the inciting factors.* There is no strong evidence for the various treatment options.

Adults often develop miliaria during travel in the tropics, military service, or with heavy exercise. *Gradual exposure* helps to acclimatize to a hot and humid environment, but this may take a few months. *Loose-fitting clothing, fans,* and *cool showers* may minimize the symptoms. With the use of any topical lotion or cream, care must be taken to ensure that the product applied does not occlude the skin, further exacerbating the condition. In the case of

severe itching, *antihistamines, cold packs,* and *topical corticosteroids* may be used. *Oatmeal baths* have been anecdotally reported to provide relief. However, all these measures will prove ineffective if the sweating is not reduced. All cases will respond to *air conditioning, exposure of the involved skin,* and the use of *antipyretics* in appropriate circumstances. Miliaria profunda has been reported to respond to oral retinoids and anhydrous lanolin.

Miliaria may be complicated by superinfection; it should be treated with *systemic antibiotics* aimed at Staphylococci as the likely pathogen. Clinicians should make patients aware that anhidrosis in the area of the eruption may occur and persist up to 3 weeks (or sometimes even longer) after the onset of lesions, and increased heat retention may occur if a large surface area was initially affected. Thus patients at risk of heat exhaustion or heat stroke should take precautions to remain in air-conditioned environments during hot weather. A biopsy may be helpful in atypical cases of miliaria.

Specific Investigations

- None usually required

In atypical cases

- Microbiology—swab for bacteria and yeasts
- Histology
- Advanced imaging—high-definition optical coherence tomography (HD-OCT)

Nonneoplastic disorders of the eccrine glands. Wenzel FG, Horn TD. J Am Acad Dermatol 1998; 38: 1–7.

The histology and pathophysiology of eccrine sweat ducts are reviewed. The erythematous macule or papule of miliaria rubra occurs with an obstruction of the sweat duct at the stratum malpighii. In the case of miliaria crystallina, the disruption is in the stratum corneum and, with miliaria profunda, at or beneath the dermoepidermal junction. The pathogenesis of miliaria is reviewed, describing the role of resident bacteria and periodic acid–Schiff (PAS)-positive extracellular polysaccharide substance blocking eccrine ducts.

Duct disruption, a new explanation of miliaria. Shuster S. Acta Derm Venereol 1997; 77: 1–3.

A hypothesis is presented that ascribes miliaria crystallina to mechanical disruption of the eccrine duct, rather than the commonly accepted pathogenesis of duct plugging. This disruption is attributed to ultraviolet irradiation causing a split between upper epidermal cells and the stratum corneum.

The role of extracellular polysaccharide substance produced by *Staphylococcus epidermidis* in miliaria. Mowad CM, McGinley KJ, Foglia A, Leyden JJ. J Am Acad Dermatol 1995; 33: 729–33.

The ability of various strains of coagulase-negative staphylococci to induce miliaria under an occlusive dressing was evaluated. *Staphylococcus epidermidis* was the only strain that induced miliaria. The authors conclude that PAS-positive extracellular polysaccharide substance produced by *S. epidermidis* plays a central role in the pathogenesis of miliaria by obstructing sweat delivery.

A novel finding in atopic dermatitis: film-producing *Staphylococcus epidermidis* as an etiology. Allen HB, Meuller JL. Int J Dermatol 2011; 50: 992–3.

S. epidermidis biofilm was cultured in a patient with atopic dermatitis. The authors proposed subclinical miliaria contributes to pruritus in atopic patients.

The pathogenesis of miliaria rubra: role of the resident microflora. Holzle E, Kligman AM. Br J Dermatol 1978; 99: 117–37.

The degree of miliaria rubra and anhidrosis induced in 55 subjects was directly correlated with the density of resident flora present on occluded areas of skin, as measured by detergent scrub and culture. A historical overview of research into the pathogenesis of miliaria rubra is included.

Miliaria crystallina in an intensive care setting. Haas N, Martens F, Henz BM. Clin Exp Dermatol 2004; 29: 32–4.

Two cases of miliaria crystallina occurring in an intensive care setting are presented. The authors hypothesize that the mechanism is secondary to transient poral closure due to the drugs used in the intensive care setting that may have stimulated sweating.

Pruritus, papules and perspiration. LaShell M, Tankersley M, Guerra A. Ann Allergy Asthma Immunol 2007; 98: 299–302.

This article reviews common exercise-induced eruptions, with miliaria rubra being discussed as the cause of the patient's recurring, self-limited eruption occurring with indoor exercise or hot tub exposure. Exercise challenge re-created the clinical picture and confirmed the diagnosis.

Miliaria-rash after neutropenic fever and induction chemotherapy for acute myelogenous leukemia. Nguyen TA, Stevens MP. An Bras Dermatol 2011; 86: 104–6.

A 40-year-old female developed miliaria crystallina after developing neutropenic fevers while on treatment with idarubicin and cytarabine. Treatment of the underlying fever led to resolution of cutaneous lesions. A review of miliaria and excessive perspiration associated with medications, including doxorubicin, bethanechol, salbutamol, and clonidine, is discussed.

Newborn with pseudohypoaldosteronism and miliaria rubra. Akcakus M, Koklu E, Poyrazoglu H, Kurtoglu S. Int J Dermatol 2006; 45: 1432–4.

Autosomal-recessive type I PHA as a cause of miliaria is discussed in a patient who developed miliaria rubra specifically during salt depletion crises. The rash cleared after stabilization of electrolytes and reappeared upon hyponatremia. The miliaria rubra seen in this patient was felt to be due to high concentrations of sodium chloride in the sweat directly damaging eccrine ducts.

Miliaria rubra and thrombocytosis in pseudohypoaldosteronism: case report. Onal H, Erdal A, Ersenb A, Onal Z, Keskindemircia G. Platelets 2012; 23: 645–7.

The authors report a case of miliaria rubra and thrombocytosis in a 6-month-old girl with PHA. They hypothesize that sympathetic activation provides vascular tonus during sodium excretion in sweat, and salt depletion crisis may play a role in the development of skin lesions and thrombocytosis in patients with PHA.

Widespread miliaria crystallina in a newborn with hypernatremic dehydration. Engür D, Türkmen MK, Savk E. Pediatr Dermatol 2013; 30: e234–5.

The authors present a case of extensive, widespread miliaria crystallina that developed in a newborn with severe hypernatremic dehydration. They propose the destruction of sweat ducts with excretion of sweat with high levels of sodium as a possible mechanism.

In vivo imaging of miliaria profunda using high-definition optical coherence tomography: diagnosis, pathogenesis, and treatment. Tey HL, Tay EY, Cao T. JAMA Dermatol 2015; 151: 346–8.

Two cases of miliaria profunda were evaluated using HD-OCT. In the epidermis, the authors identified dilated spiraling acrosyringium and an adjacent hyperrefractile substance, which they believed to be keratin. As a result of their finding, the authors challenge our prior understanding of the location of the obstruction.

First-Line Therapies	
• Prevention	D
• Frequent showering	D E
• Air conditioning	B
• Oatmeal baths	E
• Topical antiseptics	E
• Antipyretics	E

Miliaria rubra of the lower limbs in underground miners. Donoghue AM, Sinclair MJ. Occup Med (Lond) 2000; 50: 430–3.

Case series of 25 miners working in a hot and humid environment who developed miliaria. Symptoms resolved after 4 weeks of sedentary duties in the air-conditioned areas. This report also analyzed coexisting dermatologic conditions in these patients.

Diseases of the eccrine and apocrine sweat glands. Miller JL. In: Bolognia JL, Jorizzo JL, Rapini RP, eds. Dermatology. Philadelphia: Mosby, 2012; 34–11.

Preventative measures, such as a cool environment, for days to weeks is the primary goal to prevent excessive sweating and maceration of the stratum corneum.

Goosefleshlike lesions and hypohidrosis. Dimon NS, Fullen DR, Helfrich YR. Arch Dermatol 2007; 43: 1323–8.

Numerous treatments for miliaria are described, including anhydrous lanolin, oral isotretinoin, regular bathing to remove salt and bacteria, and antibiotics.

Congenital miliaria crystallina in a term neonate born to a mother with chorioamnionitis. Babu TA, Sharmila V. Pediatr Dermatol 2012; 29: 306–7.

A case report of a full-term infant, whose birth was complicated by chorioamnionitis, presented at delivery with miliaria crystallina that self-resolved in 3 days. The authors proposed that prolonged rupture of membranes, maternal fever, and warm amniotic fluid may have contributed to fetal sweating and development of miliaria. Conservative and preventative measures are emphasized.

Second-Line Therapies	
• Topical corticosteroids	E
• Systemic antibiotics	E

Miliaria rubra. Siddiqi A. In: Domino FJ, ed. 5-Minute Clinical Consult (online). Philadelphia: Lippincott Williams & Wilkins, 2012; 1–4.

For relief of pruritus, 0.1% betamethasone twice daily for 3 days may be applied over the affected area. In the event of superimposed infection, an antistaphylococcal agent such as dicloxacillin (flucloxacillin) 250 mg four times daily for 10 days may be used.

Evidence Levels: **A** Double-blind study **B** Clinical trial ≥ 20 subjects **C** Clinical trial < 20 subjects **D** Series ≥ 5 subjects **E** Anecdotal case reports

Heat illness: prickly heat. Platt M, Vicario S. In: Marx JA, ed. Rosen's Emergency Medicine: Concepts and Clinical Practice, 7th edn. Vol 2. Philadelphia: Mosby, 2009; 1887.

If a case of miliaria rubra becomes diffuse or pustular, oral erythromycin has been shown to be helpful. During the most acute phase of miliaria rubra, chlorhexidine lotion or cream can be used as an antibacterial agent, with salicylic acid 1% three times daily over small areas to aid in desquamation (not to be used in children).

Third-Line Therapies	
• Anhydrous lanolin/isotretinoin	E
• Ascorbic acid	B
• Intramuscular steroids	E

Miliaria profunda. Kirk JF, Wilson BB, Chun W, Cooper PH. J Am Acad Dermatol 1996; 35: 854–6.

This case report describes a 23-year-old man with miliaria profunda successfully treated with both anhydrous lanolin and isotretinoin after a poor response to topical corticosteroids. The impact of either as an individual treatment is therefore difficult to assess.

The effects of administration of ascorbic acid in experimentally induced miliaria and hypohidrosis in volunteers. Hindson TC, Worsley DE. Br J Dermatol 1969; 81: 226–7.

Miliaria and hypohidrosis were induced in 36 subjects, half of whom were given 1 g daily of ascorbic acid and half a placebo, beginning on the day of wrapping the skin with polythene occlusion. Compared with the placebo group, the ascorbic acid group developed less severe miliaria and hypohidrosis, had quicker healing of visible lesions, and had notable improvement in hypohidrosis at 1 week.

Patients presenting with miliaria while wearing flame resistant clothing in high ambient temperatures: a case series. Carter R, Garcia AM, Souhan BE. J Med Case Reports 2011; 5: 474.

Two cases of miliaria rubra are reported in military personnel wearing flame-resistant army combat uniforms (FRACU) in arid environments. Both patients received 250 mg intramuscular methylprednisolone, and one was continued on triamcinolone acetonide 0.1% cream twice daily for 1 week. Resolution was achieved; however, relapse with repeated FRACU use occurred.

Molluscum contagiosum

Ian H. Coulson, Tashmeeta Ahad

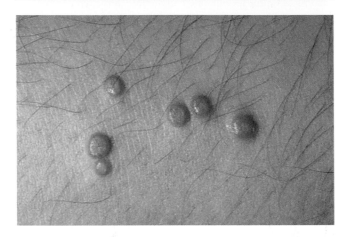

Molluscum contagiosum (MC) is a common, self-limiting pox-virus infection of the skin and occasionally mucous membranes. Lesions occur in children, usually on the trunk and body folds, and in young adults, if sexually transmitted, in the genital region. They typically present as multiple 1- to 10-mm-diameter, discrete, pearly white or flesh-colored, umbilicated papules. They may be surrounded by an eczematous reaction, which can be managed with topical steroids if symptomatic. Mollusca may be very extensive and recalcitrant to treatment in all forms of cell-mediated immunosuppression, especially in patients with AIDS.

MANAGEMENT STRATEGY

There is no specific antiviral therapy for MC. Physical and chemical destructive methods of treatment, as well as topical and systemic immunostimulatory therapies, have been tried, but no single intervention has been convincingly shown to be effective. Only a few have been subjected to the rigors of placebo-controlled studies, important for a condition that has a high spontaneous resolution rate. A Cochrane systematic review performed in 2009 reviewing randomized trials investigating the efficacy of treatments for MC found insufficient evidence to conclude that any treatment was definitively effective.

The choice of therapy will depend on the age and immune status of the patient, as well as the number and location of the lesions. In immunocompetent patients with few lesions, it is reasonable to *await spontaneous resolution*, which will usually occur within a few months. Secondarily infected MC may need *topical antiseptic or antibiotic* treatment to minimize the risk of atrophic scarring. Active intervention may be justified for cosmetic reasons, in immunodeficient states, or to hasten resolution, in order to prevent autoinoculation or transmission of the virus to close contacts. Avoidance of communal bathing and restriction of the sharing of towels should also help prevent the spread of infection to others.

A commonly used and inexpensive treatment is the *manual extrusion* of individual lesions using gloved fingers or fine forceps. This has proved more effective than *cryotherapy single treatment for 5 to 10 seconds, applied every 2 to 3 weeks. Curettage and electrodesiccation* of larger lesions may result in scarring and also requires pain alleviation, especially in children, by the prior application of a eutectic mixture of local anesthetics (lidocaine and prilocaine cream). Topically applied caustic agents have been used with variable results. Good success rates are reported with topical application of *0.5% podophyllotoxin applied twice daily for three consecutive days per week up to 4 weeks.* Other topical applications include *40% silver nitrate paste one to three applications (after 2% lidocaine gel), 10% povidone–iodine with 50% salicylic acid applied daily, 5% acidified nitrite, applied nightly with 5% salicylic acid under occlusion,* and *topical salicylic acid 12% gel.* Significant scarring has been documented with both *potassium hydroxide (5% or 10% KOH frequency ranging from three times a week to twice daily)* and *phenol,* and the latter is no longer recommended. *Cantharidin,* a clinician-applied topical blistering agent washed off 2 to 6 hours later, has proved to be an effective treatment but is not readily available. There has been some controversy about the use of *imiquimod 5% cream* for MC, as two unpublished large randomized control trials have shown lack of efficacy. In patients with AIDS, both *1% imiquimod* and *topical cidofovir 3%,* a competitive inhibitor of DNA polymerase, have proved successful for treating MC. Recovery of immune function with *highly active antiretroviral therapy (HAART)* may also result in the resolution of MC in these patients.

Specific Investigation

- Methylene blue staining of a smear to look for molluscum bodies or histopathology of a curetted specimen
  This is only required when the diagnosis is in doubt.

First-Line Therapies

- Await spontaneous resolution   **B**
- Manual extrusion with gloved fingers or fine forceps   **B**

Time to resolution and effect on quality of life of molluscum in children in the UK: a prospective community cohort study. Olsen JR, Gallacher J, Finlay AY, Piguet V, Francis NA. Lancet Infect Dis 2015; 15: 190–5.

In 306 children, aged between 4 and 15, mean time to resolution of molluscum was 13·3 months. Eighty (30%) of 269 cases had not resolved by 18 months, and 36 (13%) had not resolved by 24 months. MC had a small effect on quality of life for most participants, although 33 (11%) of 301 participants had a very severe effect on quality of life (Children's Dermatology Life Quality Index score >13).

Scarring in molluscum contagiosum: comparison of physical expression and phenol ablation. Weller R, O'Callaghan CJ, MacSween RM, White MI. Br Med J 1999; 319: 1540.

There was no difference in overall efficacy of the two methods, but phenol resulted in significantly more scarring.

For manual extrusion, wear gloves and squeeze or use fine forceps and discard extruded curdlike material. Lesions may take 1 to 2 weeks to improve.

Evidence Levels: **A** Double-blind study   **B** Clinical trial ≥ 20 subjects   **C** Clinical trial < 20 subjects   **D** Series ≥ 5 subjects   **E** Anecdotal case reports

Second-Line Therapies

• Cryotherapy	C
• Topical 0.5% podophyllotoxin	A
• Topical 5% acidified nitrite coapplied with 5% salicylic acid	A
• Topical salicylic acid gel 12%	A
• Topical 10% povidone–iodine and 50% salicylic acid	B
• Topical 40% silver nitrate paste	B

Molluscum contagiosum in children: evidence-based treatment. White MI, Weller R, Diack P. Clin Exp Dermatol 1997; 22: 51.

This study compared the efficacy and the potential for scarring of manual extrusion, cryotherapy, and topical phenol. Manual extrusion was more effective than cryotherapy. Phenol was associated with significant scarring and is not recommended for the treatment of MC.

Despite the lack of large placebo-controlled trials exploring cryotherapy, treatment is usually rapid, and therefore its use is supported. Cryotherapy should be applied once, for 5 to 10 seconds, directly on the lesion. This can be repeated every 2 to 3 weeks until the lesion has gone. A topical anesthetic (such as lidocaine/prilocaine cream) 1 hour before treatment, can be used, especially if a cluster of lesions is being treated. Potential adverse effects include scarring or hypopigmentation.

Topical 0.3% and 0.5% podophyllotoxin cream for self-treatment of molluscum contagiosum in males. A placebo-controlled, double-blind study. Syed TA, Lundin S, Ahmad M. Dermatology 1994; 189: 65–8.

In this randomized trial of 150 males aged 10 to 26 with lesions mostly located on the thighs or genitalia, 0.5% podophyllotoxin cream, 0.3% podophyllotoxin cream, or placebo cream was applied twice daily for three consecutive days per week for a duration of up to 4 weeks. Cure rates were 92%, 52%, and 16%, respectively.

Podophyllotoxin is an antimitotic agent, the safety and efficacy of which have not yet been definitively established in young children. Potential adverse effects include pruritus, burning, and inflammation.

Molluscum contagiosum effectively treated with a topical acidified nitrite, nitric oxide liberating cream. Ormerod AD, White MI, Shah SAA, Benjamin N. Br J Dermatol 1999; 141: 1051–3.

A double-blind study in 30 children of sodium nitrite 5% coapplied nightly with 5% salicylic acid under occlusion resulted in a cure rate of 75%, compared with 21% with salicylic acid alone. Mean duration to cure was 1.83 months. Adverse effects included staining of the skin and irritation.

Topical therapy with salicylic gel as a treatment for molluscum contagiosum in children. Leslie KS, Dootson G, Sterling JC. J Dermatol Treat 2005; 16: 336–40.

One hundred fourteen children with MC were treated with monthly 70% alcohol vehicle, monthly phenol 10%, or salicylic acid gel 12% applied once or twice weekly. Salicylic acid was well tolerated and significantly better (87%) than the vehicle alone (59%) or phenol (56%) at clearing MC. There was no difference in efficacy when analyzed on an "intention to treat" basis.

Molluscum contagiosum treated with iodine solution and salicylic acid plaster. Ohkuma M. Int J Dermatol 1990; 29: 443–5.

Povidone–iodine solution 10% and 50% salicylic acid plaster applied daily to MC in 20 patients was significantly more effective than either agent used alone, with a mean duration to clearance of 26 days and with no adverse effects.

Treatment of molluscum contagiosum with silver nitrate paste. Niizeki K, Hashimoto K. Pediatr Dermatol 1999; 16: 395–7.

In 389 patients, topical 40% silver nitrate paste was applied after 2% lidocaine gel; 70% cleared after one application, 97.7% after three applications. Treatment was well tolerated, and no scarring was reported. It was easier to apply than a 40% aqueous solution of silver nitrate.

Third-Line Therapies

Physical destruction

• Curettage with topical local anaesthesia cream	C
• Pulsed dye laser	C
• Photodynamic therapy	D

Topical therapy

• Application of duct tape	E
• Cantharidin	B
• 10% potassium hydroxide solution	A
• Topical 1%–5% imiquimod	A
• Diphencyprone	C
• Australian lemon myrtle	C
• Topical cidofovir	E
• Tretinoin	E
• Adapalene	E
• *Melaleuca alternifolia* and iodine	C
• Ingenol mebutate 0.015%	E
• Sinecatechins 10% ointment	E

Systemic therapy

• *Candida* antigen – intralesional	C
• Cimetidine	D
• Interferon-α – subcutaneous	E

Treatment of molluscum contagiosum using a lidocaine/prilocaine cream (EMLA) for analgesia. de Waard-van der Speck FB, Oranje AP, Lillieborg S, Hop WC, Stolz E. J Am Acad Dermatol 1990; 23: 685–8.

A double-blind study in 83 children showed efficacy of EMLA cream applied for less than 60 minutes in reducing the pain of curettage, though no comment was made on clearance rates.

Curettage treatment for molluscum contagiosum: a follow-up survey study. Simonart T, De Maertelaer V. Br J Dermatol 2008; 159: 1144.

In this 2-month prospective study of 73 patients treated with curettage, 66% of patients were not cured after a single session, and 45% of patients failed to clear after two sessions. Risk factors for treatment failure included higher number of lesions and atopic dermatitis.

A prospective randomized trial comparing the efficacy and adverse effects of four recognized treatments of molluscum contagiosum in children. Hanna D, Hatami A, Powell J,

Marcoux D, Maari C, Savard P, et al. Pediatr Dermatol 2006; 23: 574–9.

A prospective randomized study comparing four common treatments for MC in 124 children (curettage with topical anesthesia, cantharidin 0.7% (applied for 2–4 hours), salicylic acid 16.7% plus lactic acid 16.7% (Duofilm) three times per week, and imiquimod 5% three times per week). Curettage was the most effective, with 80% cure rate and the fewest side effects. Cantharidin and salicylic acid produced irritation. Imiquimod was promising, but the optimum dosing regimen is still to be determined.

Treatment of molluscum contagiosum with the pulsed dye laser over a 28-month period. Hancox JG, Jackson J, McCagh S. Cutis 2003; 71: 414–6.

All treated lesions in 43 patients resolved, and in 15 of them no further lesions developed after two treatments.

Photodynamic therapy for molluscum contagiosum infection in HIV-coinfected patients: review of 6 cases. Moiin A. J Drugs Dermatol 2003; 6: 637–9.

Treatment of six patients with 5-aminolevulinic acid (ALA) and photodynamic therapy (PDT) resulted in a reduction in lesion count and severity.

Use of duct tape occlusion in the treatment of recurrent molluscum contagiosum. Lindau MS, Munar MY. Pediatr Dermatol 2004; 21: 609.

Case report of well-tolerated and successful home therapy of multiple MC used over 2 months.

Childhood molluscum contagiosum: experience with cantharidin therapy in 300 patients. Silverberg NB, Sidbury R, Mancini AJ. J Am Acad Dermatol 2000; 43: 503–7.

A retrospective study of topical cantharidin applied to nonfacial MC for 4 to 6 hours was complicated by the use of other concurrent therapies. Of 300 children, over 90% cleared after a mean of 2.1 treatments; 90% experienced blistering at the treated site, but none developed bacterial infections.

Cantharidin is a topical blistering agent that should be applied by a clinician. Application is directly onto lesions with a blunt wooden end of a cotton swab and occluded to prevent spread. This is then washed off 2 to 6 hours later or at the first sign of blistering. Treatment can be repeated every 2 to 4 weeks until fully resolved. Adverse effects include burning, erythema, pruritus, and dyspigmentation.

Double randomized, placebo-controlled study of the use of topical 10% potassium hydroxide solution in the treatment of molluscum contagiosum. Short KA, Fuller LC, Higgins EM. Pediatr Dermatol 2006; 23: 279–81.

A double-randomized, placebo-controlled study in 20 children with 10% potassium hydroxide or normal saline applied twice daily until signs of inflammation: 70% (7/10) of the active group compared with 20% (2/10) of the placebo group achieved complete resolution. This difference was not statistically significant. Dosing studies are required to minimize irritancy.

Five percent or 10% concentrations of potassium hydroxide can be used with frequencies ranging from three times per week to twice daily.

Dermatologists, imiquimod, and treatment of molluscum contagiosum in children: righting wrongs. Katz KA. JAMA Dermatol 2015; 151: 125–6.

The use of imiquimod 5% cream for MC has been controversial, as two large unpublished randomized trials of children treated with imiquimod 5% cream or vehicle three times weekly for up to 16 weeks did not show efficacy. The first study showed 24% (52/217) complete clearance rate in the imiquimod group versus 26% (28/106) complete clearance rate in the placebo group. The second study showed a 24% (60/253) versus a 28% (35/126) complete clearance rate in the imiquimod 5% group and placebo group, respectively. This contradicts favorable responses seen in uncontrolled studies and case series, which suggests spontaneous resolution may account for efficacy seen in these studies.

Treatment of molluscum contagiosum in males with an analog of imiquimod 1% cream: a placebo controlled, double-blind study. Syed TA, Goswami J, Ahmadpour OA, Ahmad SA. J Dermatol 1998; 25: 309–13.

One hundred male patients applied either the analog cream or placebo to their mollusca three times daily for 5 days each week for 1 month; 82% cleared with active treatment, compared with 16% of those using placebo. The treatment was well tolerated.

Treatment of molluscum contagiosum with topical diphencyprone therapy. Kang SH, Lee D, Park JH, Cho SH, Lee SS, Park SW. Acta Derm Venereol 2005; 85: 529–30.

Weekly application of 0.0001% diphencyprone in 22 sensitized children over 8 weeks. There was 63.6% complete clearance over a mean treatment period of 5.1 weeks.

Essential oil of Australian lemon myrtle (*Backhousia citriodora*) in the treatment of molluscum contagiosum. Burke BE, Baillie JE, Olson RD. Biomed Pharmacother 2004; 58: 245–7.

Once-daily application of a 10% solution of *Backhousia citriodora* gave over 90% reduction in lesions in 9 of 16 children, compared with none of 16 in the control group (vehicle alone).

Topical cidofovir. A novel treatment for recalcitrant molluscum contagiosum in children infected with human immunodeficiency virus 1. Toro JR, Wood LV, Patel NK, Turner ML. Arch Dermatol 2000; 136: 983–5.

Topical 3% cidofovir applied daily for 5 days per week for 8 weeks cleared previously recalcitrant lesions in two children.

Comparative study of 5% potassium hydroxide solution versus 0.05% tretinoin cream for molluscum contagiosum in children. Rajouria EA, Amatya A, Karn D. Kathmandu Univ Med J 2011; 9: 291–4.

Fifty children were treated with either 5% KOH solution or 0.05% tretinoin cream at bedtime (25 in each group). Both treatments were effective in reducing the lesion count, but response to KOH was quicker. Side effects were less noticeable with tretinoin cream.

Topical retinoids such as tretinoin and adapalene have been tried for MC in small case reports. Frequency can range from every alternate day and titrated up to twice daily as tolerated. Adverse effects include erythema, dryness, and irritation.

Treatment of molluscum contagiosum: a brief review and discussion of a case successfully treated with adapalene. Scheinfeld N. Dermatol Online J 2007; 13: 15.

A single case report of successful topical adapalene therapy.

Combination of essential oil of *Melaleuca alternifolia* and iodine in the treatment of molluscum contagiosum in children. Markum E, Baillie J. J Drugs Dermatol 2012; 11: 349–54.

Fifty-three children were treated with twice-daily essential oil of *Malaleuca alternifolia* (the tea tree) alone (TTO), a combination of *Malaleuca alternifolia* and iodine (TTO-I), or iodine alone. After 30 days 48 children were followed up. There was

510

a 90% reduction in lesions in the TTO-I group—significantly higher than in the other groups.

Treatment of molluscum contagiosum with ingenol mebutate. Javed S, Tyring SK. J Am Acad Dermatol 2014; 70: e105.

Single case report of a 4-year-old girl treated with two repeated 3-day applications of ingenol mebutate 0.015% leading to resolution of lesions.

Recalcitrant molluscum contagiosum successfully treated with sinecatechins. Padilla España L, Mota-Burgos A, Martinez-Amo JL, Benavente-Ortiz F, Rodríguez-Bujaldón A, Hernández-Montoya C. Dermatol Ther 2016; 29: 217–8.

Case of a 5-year-old girl with a 2-year history of more than 50 MC lesions, already treated with potassium hydroxide 10% for 1 month. Sinecatechins 10% ointment (derived from green tea) applied twice daily for 4 weeks led to resolution of all lesions with no recurrence at 3-month follow-up.

One-year experience with *Candida* antigen immunotherapy for warts and molluscum. Marron M, Salm C, Lyon V, Galbraith S. Pediatr Dermatol 2008; 25: 189–92.

One-year follow-up in 25 of 47 patients with molluscum treated with intralesional *Candida* antigen therapy. There was complete resolution in 56%, partial clearing in 28%, and no improvement in 16%.

Treatment of molluscum contagiosum with oral cimetidine: clinical experience in 13 patients. Dohil M, Prenderville JS. Pediatr Dermatol 1996; 13: 310–2.

Thirteen children were treated with a 2-month course of oral cimetidine 40 mg/kg/day. All but three children who completed treatment experienced clearance of all lesions.

Interferon alpha treatment of molluscum contagiosum in immunodeficiency. Hourihane J, Hodges E, Smith J, Keefe M, Jones A, Connett G. Arch Dis Child 1999; 80: 77–9.

MC in two children with combined immunodeficiency cleared with subcutaneous interferon-α.

Interferon-alpha treatment of molluscum contagiosum in a patient with hyperimmunoglobulin E syndrome. Kilic SS, Kilicbay F. Paediatrics 2006; 117: e1253–5.

Successful treatment with 6 months of subcutaneous interferon-α of MC resistant to multiple therapies in an immunodeficient child.

Resolution of disseminated molluscum contagiosum with highly active antiretroviral therapy (HAART) in patients with AIDS. Calista D, Boschini A, Landi G. Eur J Dermatol 1999; 9: 211–3.

Three patients with recalcitrant MC cleared 6 months after commencing HAART.

Morphea

Jack C. O'Brien, Heidi T. Jacobe

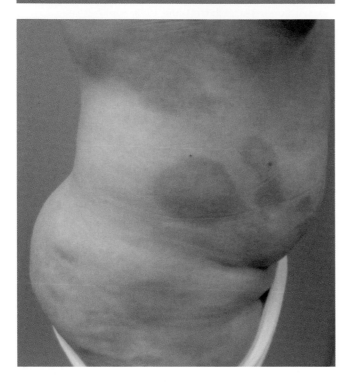

Morphea, also known as *localized scleroderma* (a term that should be discouraged because of unnecessary confusion with systemic sclerosis), is an autoimmune disorder characterized by inflammation and sclerosis of the dermis and in some cases the underlying subcutis, fascia, and muscle. Although previously considered self-limited, a growing body of evidence suggests a remitting relapsing course may be common. Further, untreated lesions may leave behind permanent cosmetic and functional disfigurement, warranting treatment to prevent these sequelae. Morphea has a spectrum of manifestations, ranging from skin only to internal involvement, with musculoskeletal complaints (e.g., synovitis) being the most common extracutaneous manifestation.

Morphea is classified into subtypes, including circumscribed, linear, or generalized. Any subtype may have involvement of the subcutis. Onset is bimodal and can occur in childhood, where linear morphea is most common, or in adults, where circumscribed and generalized predominate.

Notably, morphea is distinct from systemic sclerosis, and there is no progression to systemic sclerosis or involvement of heart, lungs, gastrointestinal tract, or kidneys in morphea. Further, scleroderma hallmark autoantibodies (anticentromere antibody, antitopoisomerase antibody, anti-RNA polymerase III) are absent in morphea, as is Raynaud phenomenon.

MANAGEMENT STRATEGY

The management of morphea centers first on determining the extent of disease activity and then assessing disease severity, including functional or cosmetic impairment. Active disease is defined as new or expanding lesions with peripheral induration and erythema. An important feature is the depth of involvement. Morphea may be limited to the dermis or involve the subcutis. Recent evidence suggests deeper involvement may have more serious sequelae. Patients with active morphea with involvement of deeper tissues should generally be treated with methotrexate and steroids and not topical therapies, particularly when lesions are extensive or involve cosmetically or functionally sensitive sites. The overarching goal for management of active lesions is to shut down activity to prevent damage.

Patients with en coup de sabre, or hemifacial atrophy, should be assessed for ophthalmologic complaints and referred for an ophthalmologic evaluation of possible subclinical eye involvement. In addition, assess neurologic or dental complaints and refer to a neurologist or dentist if symptoms or abnormalities are noticed. Patients with widespread superficial plaques (particularly in postmenopausal women) require assessment for genital involvement.

Patients with inactive morphea lesions also merit close attention, as studies show inactive disease can have a significant impact on life quality. In this case, multidisciplinary supportive care rather than treatment aimed at eradicating disease activity is warranted.

Once the evaluation is complete, treatment decisions should be based on activity and damage, depth of involvement (dermal vs. deeper tissues), area of involvement, and disease progression. The goal of therapy is to shut down inflammation in active or expanding lesions to avoid long-term sequelae of unchecked active disease.

In general, limited dermal inflammatory lesions that are not rapidly progressing or cosmetically or functionally threatening may be treated with topical therapies *(calcipotriene, calcitriol, tacrolimus, or topical steroids)* or *intralesional triamcinolone.* These patients should be closely followed, and, if their lesions multiply or spread, suppressive therapy is indicated *(phototherapy or methotrexate ± steroids)* to prevent continued development of new lesions. In general, patients with extensive active lesions involving the deep dermis, subcutis, or below, or those with cosmetically or functionally threatening lesions such as en coup de sabre or hemifacial atrophy, should receive methotrexate and systemic steroids. Widespread active morphea limited to the dermis may be treated with *phototherapy, preferably UVA1,* or, if unavailable, *UVA without psoralen or narrowband UVB.* Serial photography and skin scores are invaluable to determine response to treatment. The goal of therapy is to prevent progression of existing lesions and abrogate inflammation. Complete resolution of lesions does not occur (unless lesions are very early) and should not be considered a therapeutic end point.

In addition to treating active disease, it is imperative to assess for features of disease damage, as these have been shown to have significant impairment in quality of life for patients with morphea. Patients with limitation in range of motion, contracture, or weakness in an affected limb should be referred to occupational or physical therapy. In cases where limb length discrepancy is suspected, refer to prosthetics and orthotics for shoe inserts. For deep lesions in cosmetically sensitive areas (e.g., en coup de sabre), referral to plastic surgery can be offered as long as disease is stable and inactive.

The evidence currently does not support the use of topical steroids, oral or topical calcipotriol, D-penicillamine, interferon-γ, or antimalarials. Therefore the use of these treatments is discouraged in severe cases of morphea where function or cosmesis is threatened. Penicillamine also has a significant side effect profile, including nephrotoxicity, and should be avoided.

Evidence Levels: **A** Double-blind study   **B** Clinical trial ≥ 20 subjects   **C** Clinical trial < 20 subjects   **D** Series ≥ 5 subjects   **E** Anecdotal case reports

Specific Investigations

- Localized Scleroderma Cutaneous Assessment Tool (LoSCAT)
- Serial digital photography
- Histopathology
- Ultrasound and Doppler ultrasound
- Magnetic resonance imaging (MRI)

Development of consensus treatment plans for juvenile localized scleroderma. Li SC, Torok KS, Pope E, Dedeoglu F, Hong S, Jacobe HT, et al. Arthritis Care Res (Hoboken) 2012; 64: 1175–85.

This paper outlines the consensus evaluation and treatment plans for juvenile moderate to severe morphea as determined by a focus group with expertise in morphea and the current literature.

The Localized Scleroderma Cutaneous Assessment Tool: responsiveness to change in a pediatric clinical population. Kelsey CE, Torok KS. J Am Acad Dermatol 2013; 69: 214–20.

This is a validation study for the LoSCAT demonstrating that the mLoSSI, the activity measure of the LoSCAT, is a valid and responsive measure of disease activity of morphea in children.

The use of Doppler ultrasound to evaluation lesions of localized scleroderma. Li SC, Liebling MS. Curr Rheumatol Rep 2009; 11: 205–11.

Disease-related structural changes, such as tissue thickening, atrophy, and architectural alterations, can be readily detected using ultrasound. High spatial resolution enables monitoring of changes in tissue thickness over the course of disease and treatment, offering another method to document therapeutic efficacy in the hands of an experienced ultrasonographer.

MRI findings in deep and generalized morphea (localized scleroderma). Horger M, Fierlbeck G, Kuemmerle-Deschner J, Tzaribachev N, Wehrmann M, Claussen C, et al. Am J Roentgenol 2008; 190: 32–9.

This paper describes MRI findings in morphea. MRI allows for establishment of the depth of involvement and degree of activity based on signal intensity. This article also provides images of MRI findings in morphea.

First-Line Therapies

Extensive dermal lesions

• Phototherapy: BB-UVA, NB-UVB, UVA1	**A**

Moderate to severe morphea/deep involvement

• Methotrexate + IV corticosteroids	**C**
• Methotrexate + oral steroids	**A**

Limited dermal lesions

• Topical tacrolimus under occlusion	**C**
• Intralesional steroids	**C**

One limited deep lesion

• Intralesional steroids	**C**

A systematic review of morphea treatments and therapeutic algorithm. Zwischenberger BA, Jacobe HT. J Am Acad Dermatol 2011; 65: 925–41.

An evaluation and treatment algorithm is proposed for all types of morphea based on current literature and expert opinion.

Update on morphea part II. Outcome measures and treatment. Fett N, Werth VP. J Am Acad Dermatol 2011; 64: 231–42.

The authors discuss outcome measures and treatment options and provide algorithms for treatment of generalized, linear, and limited plaque morphea.

A randomized controlled study of low-dose UVA1, medium-dose UVA1, and narrowband UVB phototherapy in the treatment of localized scleroderma. Kreuter A, Hyun J, Stucker M, Sommer A, Altmeyer P, Gambichler T. J Am Acad Dermatol 2006; 54: 440–7.

Low- and medium-dose UVA1 (20 and 50 J/cm^2) was compared with narrowband (NB) UVB in a randomized trial. All patients showed a significant decrease in skin scores. Medium-dose UVA1 had a significantly greater decrease compared with NB-UVB; there were no differences between low-dose UVA1 and NB-UVB.

Medium-dose is more effective than low-dose ultraviolet A1 phototherapy for localized scleroderma as shown by 20-MHz ultrasound assessment. Sator PG, Radakovic S, Schulmeister K, Hönigsmann H, Tanew A. J Am Acad Dermatol 2009; 60: 786–91.

Ultrasound-measured dermal thickness was the primary outcome measure in this randomized controlled trial (RCT) comparing low (20 J/cm^2) and high dose (70 J/cm^2). High doses resulted in significant decrease in dermal thickness measured by ultrasound but no significant differences in clinical score.

Different low doses of broad-band UVA in treatment of morphea and systemic sclerosis. El-Mofty M, Mostafa W, El-Darouty M, Bosseila M, Nada H, Yousef R, et al. Photodermatol Photoimmunol Photomed 2004; 20: 148–56.

Sixty-three patients with both progressive systemic sclerosis and morphea were treated with various doses of UVA without psoralen. Results were similar between 5, 10, and 20 J/cm^2. This offers a more widely available alternative to UVA1.

Methotrexate treatment in juvenile localized scleroderma: a randomized, double-blinded, placebo-controlled trial. Zulian F, Martini G, Vallongo C, Cittadello F, Falcini F, Patrizi A, et al. Arthritis Rheum 2011; 63: 1998–2006.

Seventy patients were randomized to receive oral methotrexate (15 mg/m^2, maximum 20 mg) or placebo once weekly for 12 months. Both groups received oral prednisone (1 mg/kg/day, maximum 50 mg) for the first 3 months. Using a composite outcome measure, the methotrexate treatment group had a higher rate of remission and less recurrence. This is the first randomized placebo-controlled trial to demonstrate efficacy in the treatment of morphea.

Pulsed high-dose corticosteroids combined with low-dose methotrexate in severe localized scleroderma. Kreuter A, Gambichler T, Breuckmann F, Rotterdam S, Freitag M, Stuecker M, et al. Arch Dermatol 2005; 141: 847–52.

Methotrexate 15 mg/week plus intravenous methylprednisolone 100 mg/day for 3 days per month was administered to 15 adults. Fourteen of 15 improved, and no correlation was found between duration of disease and response to treatment.

Localized scleroderma: response to occlusive treatment with tacrolimus ointment. Mancoso G, Berdondini RM. Br J Dermatol 2005; 152: 180–2.

Tacrolimus 0.1% ointment applied twice daily to a target plaque and occluded was compared with petrolatum in seven adults. Early inflammatory lesions resolved and late sclerotic lesions softened, without improvement in atrophy and scarring.

Efficacy of topical tacrolimus 0.1% in active plaque morphea: randomized, double-blind, emollient-controlled pilot study. Kroft EB, Groeneveld TJ, Seyger MM, de Jong EM. Am J Clin Dermatol 2009; 10: 181–7.

In this randomized, double-blind, emollient-controlled study of 10 patients with active plaque morphea, the authors concluded that topical tacrolimus applied twice a day for 12 weeks effectively decreases skin thickness, dyspigmentation, erythema, telangiectasia, and atrophy.

Second-Line Therapies	
Extensive dermal lesions	
• PUVA (bath or cream)	B
Moderate to severe morphea	
• Mycophenolate mofetil	C
• Abatacept	D
Limited dermal lesions	
• Imiquimod	C
• Calcipotriene under occlusion	
• Calcipotriol–betamethasone	C
• Pirfenidone 8% gel	D

UVA/UVA1 phototherapy and PUVA photochemotherapy in connective tissue disease and related disorders: a research based review. Breuckmann F, Gambichler T, Altmeyer P, Kreuter A. BMC Dermatol 2004; 4: 11.

These authors systematically review the literature on UVA/UVA1 and PUVA therapy in various skin conditions, including morphea, and conclude that significant softening of the skin occurs with all modalities used.

Successful treatment of severe or methotrexate-resistant juvenile localized scleroderma with mycophenolate mofetil. Martini G, Ramanan AV, Falcini F, Girschick H, Goldsmith DP, Zulian F. Rheumatology (Oxford) 2009; 48: 1410–3.

Ten children with morphea already taking methotrexate and systemic steroids with limited improvement had mycophenolate mofetil added to their treatment. Nine of the 10 patients reported improvement.

First case series on the use of calcipotriol-betamethasone dipropionate for morphoea. Dytoc MT, Kossintseva I, Ting PT. Br J Dermatol 2007; 157: 615–8.

Calcipotriol in combination with betamethasone dipropionate was reported to have efficacy in the treatment of morphea in a prospective study of six patients with plaque morphea.

Topical calcipotriene for morphea/linear scleroderma. Cunningham BB, Landells ID, Langman C, Sailer DE, Paller AS. J Am Acad Dermatol 1998; 39: 211–5.

Uncontrolled trial evaluated topical calcipotriene 0.005% ointment applied under occlusion to active target lesions twice daily. All 12 patients showed significant decrease in subjective/clinical sclerosis scales.

First case series on the use of imiquimod for morphoea. Dytoc M, Ting PT, Man J, Sawyer D, Fiorillo L. Br J Dermatol 2005; 153: 815–20.

The authors used 5% imiquimod cream, an inducer of interferon-γ known to inhibit TGF-β, to treat 12 patients. Dyspigmentation, induration, and erythema improved. The histology of the skin showed a reduction of dermal thickness.

Pirfenidone gel in patients with localized scleroderma: a phase II study. Rodriguez-Castellano M, Tlacuilo-Parra A, Sanchez-Enriquez S, Velez-Gomez E, Guevara-Gutierrez E. Arthritis Res Ther 2014; 16: 510.

This was an open-label trial of pirfenidone 8% gel applied three times a day for 6 months in adults with morphea. The authors report the mLoSSI score was improved at 3 and at 6 months from baseline and there was histologic improvement.

Third-Line Therapies	
• Ciclosporin	E
• Infliximab	E

Combining UVA therapy with systemic immunosuppressives to treat progressive diffuse morphoea. Rose RF, Goodfield MJ. Clin Exp Dermatol 2005; 30: 226–8.

The authors discuss the various treatments used in morphea and comment that combination therapies may hold promise. Of note, ciclosporin and mycophenolate should not be used in combination with PUVA due to risk of photocarcinogenesis.

Good response to linear scleroderma in a child to ciclosporin. Strauss RM, Bhushan M, Goodfield MJ. Br J Dermatol 2004; 150: 790–2.

A 12-year-old child with rapidly expanding linear morphea was first treated with clobetasol twice a day. Because there was little improvement in her condition, ciclosporin 3 mg/kg daily was added to the regimen with rapid improvement and softening of the lesion on her thigh.

A case report of successful treatment of recalcitrant childhood localized scleroderma with infliximab and leflunomide. Ferguson ID, Weiser P, Torok KS. Open Rheumatol J 2015; 9: 30–5.

A 14-year-old female with severe progressive morphea was treated with infliximab and then leflunomide after not tolerating methotrexate with steroids and mycophenolate mofetil. She had improvement in mLoSSI, joint function, and global assessment. The authors felt the improvement was largely due to infliximab.

157

Mucoceles

Noah Scheinfeld

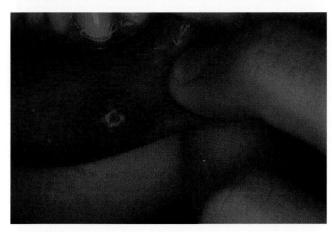

Labial mucoceles fall into two categories: the mucous extravasation cyst and the mucous retention cyst. The mucous extravasation cyst describes a false cyst because the mucous extravasation cyst lacks an epithelial lining arising from the partially or totally severed salivary gland duct, resulting in the accumulation of saliva in the adjacent soft tissue. At this point the mucocele is cut off by a fibrous connective tissue pseudocapsule. Ductal epithelium lines the mucous retention cyst. The mucous retention cyst develops from partial obstruction of a duct in the presence of the salivary gland's continued mucus secretion. The extravasation mucocele manifests most commonly and on the young person's lower lip. The retention mucocele is more apt to occur on the buccal cheek or soft palate of an older patient.

To expand this further, mucous extravasation cysts arise from trauma to salivary gland ducts. This trauma leads to rupture of ducts and leakage of mucin from the minor salivary glands. The mucin subsequently forms pseudocystic aggregations, most commonly on the lower lip. These aggregations are referred to as *mucoceles*. Mucoceles manifest with a variety of tones and color that range from flesh color to red to translucent blue. The shape of mucoceles is round or oval, and their surface is smooth. They usually possess a soft, fluctuant, or gel-like consistency. Single or multiple mucoceles can manifest and can range from 0.1 to 2 cm in diameter. A variant of a mucocele termed *superficial mucocele* can manifest on the palate, retromolar pad, and posterior buccal mucosa as single or multiple vesicles, which can break down into an ulcer. Despite healing after a few days, superficial mucoceles recur often in the same location. A mucocele is termed a *ranula* when on the floor of the mouth, and an *epulis* when on the gums.

MANAGEMENT STRATEGY

The natural history of mucoceles can involve their expansion and periodic rupture and sometimes spontaneous resolution. There is some morbidity associated with mucoceles that ranges from discomfort to suboptimal cosmetic appearance of a nodule with a hardened consistency due to scarring and tissue consolidation.

A clinical diagnosis can be supported, when necessary, by histology and ultrasound imaging. In addition to conservative treatment, a range of surgical and other techniques can be employed.

Specific Investigations

- Biopsy
- Doppler ultrasonography
- Color Doppler imaging

First-Line Therapies

• Cryotherapy	C
• Intralesional corticosteroids	D
• Do nothing	D

A simple cryosurgical method for treatment of oral mucous cysts. Toida M, Ishimaru JI, Hobo N. Int J Oral Maxillofac Surg 1993; 22: 353–5.

Twelve female and six male patients with mucous cysts on the lower lip and the tip of the tongue were treated by direct application of liquid nitrogen with a cotton swab. Each lesion was exposed to four or five cycles composed of freezings of 10 to 30 s and thawings of double the freezing times. No anesthesia was required. All lesions had disappeared completely 2 to 4 weeks after one or two treatment courses of cryosurgery. In all cases, neither scarring nor recurrence was noted during the 6 months to 5 years of follow-up.

Histopathology of mucoceles infiltrated with steroids. Merida FMT. Med Cutan Ibero Lat Am 1976; 4; 15–8.

Eight cases of lip mucocele with intralesional infiltration of triamcinolone acetonide (Kenacort). In three cases there was complete regression of the lesion after a variable period between the first and the fourth infiltration. In five cases the results were negative. The patients who reacted positively to treatment were followed up for a year afterward.

A review of common pediatric lip lesions: herpes simplex/ recurrent herpes labialis, impetigo, mucoceles, and hemangiomas. Bentley JM, Barankin B, Guenther LC. Clin Pediatr 2003; 42: 475–82.

After a diagnosis is made, treatment is often not needed as smaller and more superficial mucoceles are likely to rupture and spontaneously heal. The patient's future as it relates to mucoceles is good whether or not surgery is involved.

Clinical characteristics, treatment, and evolution of 89 mucoceles in children. Mínguez-Martinez I, Bonet-Coloma C, Ata-Ali-Mahmud J, Carrillo-García C, Peñarrocha-Diago M, Peñarrocha-Diago M. J Oral Maxillofac Surg 2010; 68: 2468–71.

In a series of 89 cases, mucoceles were more commonly located on the lower lip; 43.8% resolved spontaneously, and 8% of the surgically removed mucoceles reappeared.

Second-Line Therapy

• Punch biopsy	E

Two simple treatments for lower lip mucocoeles. Gill D. Australas J Dermatol 996; 37: 220.

Punch is a useful technique for treating mucocele and has the added benefit of providing a histologically certain diagnosis.

Third-Line Therapies

- CO_2 laser — **B**
- Surgical excision — **B**
- Marsupialization — **D**
- Micromarsupialization — **D**
- Nonablative lasers — **E**

Treatment of mucocele of the lower lip with carbon dioxide laser. Huang IY, Chen CM, Kao YH, Worthington P. J Oral Maxillofac Surg 2007; 65: 855–8.

Eighty-two patients with biopsy-confirmed mucocele of the lower lip were treated with CO_2 laser vaporization with no bleeding and minimal scar formation. There were two recurrences. Researchers noted mild discomfort and rare complications. At the operative site, one patient felt temporary numbness. Due to the fact that the operative time is shorter than for excision, carbon dioxide laser appears useful for children and for less cooperative patients.

Clinicostatistical study of lower lip mucoceles. Yamasoba T, Tayama N, Syoji M, Fukuta M. Head Neck 1990; 12: 316–20.

Researchers reported 70 patients with lower lip mucoceles for patient characteristics, clinical features, and histopathologic findings. Patients were divided almost equally between males and females, with ages ranging from 2 to 63 years, with the highest incidence of lesions occurring in the second decade. Mucocele life span ranged a few days to 3 years. Size did not affect outcome. The upper lateral incisor was the most commonly involved area. Of 70 biopsies, 68 were mucous extravasation cysts and 2 were mucous retention cysts. Surgical excision was the treatment of choice, with recurrence of the lesion in only two cases.

Conventional surgical treatment of oral mucocele: a series of 23 cases. Bahadure RN, Fulzele P, Thosar N, Badole G, Baliga S. Eur J Paediatr Dent 2012; 13: 143–6.

Conventional surgical procedure with excision of minor salivary glands was effective in 23 patients and was considered with 3-year follow-up to have a low recurrence rate.

Clinical and histopathologic study of salivary mucoceles. Kang SK, Kim KS. Taehan Chikkwa Uisa Hyophoe Chi 1989; 27: 1059–71.

In a series of 112 patients, surgeons treated 107 mucoceles (95%) by excision and only 5 by marsupialization. Eighteen of 112 cases (16%) recurred. Only 3 of the 112 cases revealed an epithelial lining. This incidence indicates that the mucus extravasation by damage of excretory duct rather than the ductal dilatation by mucus retention may play a critical role in the production of these lesions. In 81 cases (72.3%) minor salivary glands were included in the excision biopsy specimen.

Treatment of mucus retention phenomena in children by the micromarsupialization technique: case reports. Delbem AC, Cunha RF, Vieira AE, Ribeiro LL. Pediatr Dent 2000; 22: 155–8.

Micromarsupialization requires neither injections nor surgery and was studied in 14 patients. Micromarsupialization basically involves placing a topical anesthetic gel on the mucocele for 3 minutes, passing a 4 to 0 silk suture through the body of the mucocele, and tying a surgeon's knot. The suture material is removed 7 days later, at which time the mucocele is resolved. The advantages of this technique include simplicity and relative lack of pain. Micromarsupialization is not indicated for fibrotic lesions, lesions of the palate, or lesions inside of the cheek. Of the original 14 patients treated by the micromarsupialization technique, 12 presented full regression 1 week after treatment. Two cases recurred.

Excision of oral mucocele by different wavelength lasers. Romeo U, Palaia G, Tenore G, Del Vecchio A, Nammour S. Indian J Dent Res 2013; 24: 211–5.

In three cases excision was performed using two different techniques (circumferential incision technique and mucosal preservation technique) and three different laser wavelengths (Er, Cr:YSGG 2780 nm, diode 808 nm, and KTP 532 nm). All the tested lasers, regardless of wavelength, showed many advantages (bloodless surgical field, no postoperative pain, relative speed, and easy execution). The most useful surgical technique depends on clinical features of the lesion.

Mucocele of the minor salivary glands in an infant: treatment with diode laser. Paglia M, Crippa R, Ferrante F, Angiero F. Eur J Paediatr Dent 2015; 16: 139–42.

A report of one case of mucocele in a 3-month-old infant in the right labial commissure noted excision by diode laser of different wavelengths (635–980 nm), with an average power of 1.8 W, in continuous wave mode, using 300- to 320-micron optical fibers. The healing occurred in 10 days. There were no adverse effects, and the patient was carefully followed up until complete healing.

Evidence Levels: **A** Double-blind study **B** Clinical trial ≥ 20 subjects **C** Clinical trial < 20 subjects **D** Series ≥ 5 subjects **E** Anecdotal case reports

158

Mucous membrane pemphigoid

Caroline Allen, Vanessa Venning

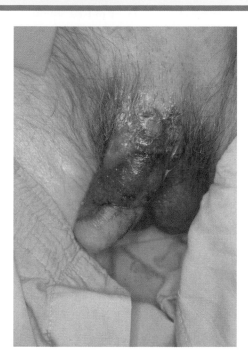

Mucous membrane pemphigoid (MMP) formerly known as *cicatricial pemphigoid,* is a heterogeneous group of chronic acquired autoimmune subepidermal blistering diseases. It is characterized by blistering and erosions of one or more mucous membranes (eyes, oral mucosa, esophagus, genitals) and to a lesser extent the skin. This may lead to permanent scarring of the affected area, particularly the conjunctiva.

MANAGEMENT STRATEGY

MMP is a chronic disease and does not generally remit spontaneously; disease activity will fluctuate without treatment, and treatments are disease modifying rather than curative.

Optimal treatment for MMP is unclear as there is little evidence in the form of randomized control trials; international consensus guides treatment strategy, based on the site, severity, extent, and rate of progression of disease. Patient comorbidities must also be considered, and a multidisciplinary approach is vital.

World Workshop on Oral Medicine VI: a systematic review of the treatment of mucous membrane pemphigoid. Taylor J, McMillan R, Shephard M, Setterfield J, Ahmed R, Carrozzo M; et al. Oral Surg Oral Med Oral Pathol Oral Radiol 2015; 120: 161–71.e20.

Interventions for mucous membrane pemphigoid and epidermolysis bullosa aquisitia. Kirtshig G, Murrell D, Wojnarowska F, Khumalo N. Cochrane Database Syst Rev 2003; CD004056.

The first international consensus on mucous membrane pemphigoid: definition, diagnostic criteria, pathogenic factors, medical treatment and prognostic indicators. Chan LS, Ahmed AR, Anhalt GJ, Bernauer W, Cooper KD, Elder MJ, et al. Arch Dermatol 2002; 138: 370–9.

Specific Investigations

For diagnosis

- Direct immunofluorescence
- Indirect immunofluorescence on salt split skin

For treatment

- Complete blood count (CBC), liver function tests (LFTs), renal function
- Glucose 6 phosphate dehydrogenase (G6PD) activity
- Thiopurine methyltransferase (TPMT)

First-Line Therapies

Topical corticosteroids	C
Dapsone	C
Antiinflammatory antibiotics	D
Systemic corticosteroids	C
Cyclophosphamide	C

Mild disease

The management of oral mucous membrane pemphigoid with dapsone and topical corticosteroid. Arash A, Shirin L. J Oral Pathol Med 2008; 37: 341–4.

Five patients with mild MMP had a good response to triamcinolone in orobase.

Treatment of severe erosive gingival lesions by topical application of clobetasol propionate in custom trays. Gonzales-Moles MA, Ruiz Avila I, Rodriguez-Archilla A, Morales-Garcia P, Mesa-Aguado F, Bascones-Martinez A, et al. Oral Surg Oral Med Oral Pathol Oral Radiol Endodont 2003; 95: 688–92.

Improvement in all 22 patients with oral MMP treated with topical clobetasol propionate with nystatin applied via a gingival tray.

Treatment-resistant or severe disease

Dapsone efficacy and adverse events in the management of mucous membrane pemphigoid. Hegarty AM, Ormond M, Sweeney M, Hodgson T. Eur J Dermatol 2010; 20: 223–4.

Eight out of 20 patients improved with dapsone. One failed to respond, and 11 developed side effects necessitating cessation.

The management of oral mucous membrane pemphigoid with dapsone and topical corticosteroid. Arash A, Shirin L. J Oral Pathol Med 2008; 37: 341–4.

All 15 patients had a significant response to topical corticosteroids and dapsone 25 to 100 mg daily. Ten had complete resolution.

Dapsone therapy of cicatricial pemphigoid. Rogers RS III, Mehregan DA. Semin Dermatol 1988; 7: 201–5.

Seventy-seven patients with oral, ocular or generalized MMP benefited from either 150 mg dapsone per day or 1500 to 3000 mg sulfapyridine per day for at least 12 weeks.

Sulphamethoxypyridazine for dermatitis herpetiformis, linear IgA disease and cicatricial pemphigoid. McFadden JP, Leonard JN, Powles AV, Rutman AJ, Fry L. et al. Br J Dermatol 1989; 121: 759–62.

Sulfamethoxypyridazine 500 to 1500 mg was partially effective in 10 of 15 patients with oral and generalized MMP.

Treatment with dapsone 50 to 200 mg/daily and sulfonamides 500 to 1500 mg sulfapyridine or sulfamethoxypyridazine is effective in some patients.

Antiepiligrin cicatricial pemphigoid of the larynx successfully treated with a combination of tetracycline and niacinamide. Sakamoto K, Mori K, Hashimoto T, Yancey KB, Nakashima T. Arch Otolaryngol Head Neck Surg 2002; 128: 1420–3.

Successful therapy with tetracycline and nicotinamide in cicatricial pemphigoid. Kreyden OP, Borradori L, Trueb RM, Burg G, Nestle FO. Hautarzt 2001; 52: 247–50.

Single case reports of effective treatment with tetracycline 1500 mg/day and nicotinamide (500–3000 mg/day).

Systemic minocycline as a therapeutic option in predominantly oral mucous membrane pemphigoid: a cautionary report. Carrozzo M, Arduino P, Bertolusso G, Cozzani E, Parodi A. Int J Oral Maxillofac Surg 2009; 38: 1071–6.

Seven of nine patients with oral disease responded to minocycline 200 mg/day; however, side effects limited treatment in five.

Combination therapy with nicotinamide and tetracyclines for cicatricial pemphigoid: further support for its efficacy. Reiche L, Wojnarowska F, Mallon E. Clin Exp Dermatol 1998; 23: 254–7.

Minocycline 50 to 100 mg/day combined with 2.5 to 3 g nicotinamide per day was beneficial in five of eight patients.

Antiinflammatory antibiotics can be of benefit. Side effects may limit treatment. Nicotinamide may confer additional protection.

Mucous membrane pemphigoid. Treatment experience at two institutions. Lamey PJ, Rees TD, Binnie WH, Rankin KV. Oral Surg Oral Med Oral Pathol 1992; 74: 50–3.

Fourteen patients with oral MMP were treated with a combination of systemic and topical steroids: eight became asymptomatic, five improved, and one was unchanged.

Cicatricial pemphigoid: a re-evaluation of therapy. Nayar M, Wojnarowska F. J Dermatol Treat 1993; 4: 89–93.

Five of 15 patients with generalized MMP benefited from prednisolone 40 to 60 mg/day, but it was ineffective in oral disease.

Treatment with systemic corticosteroids seems helpful at doses of prednisolone 0.5 to 2 mg/kg/day. Most studies used a combination of systemic steroids and a steroid-sparing drug; a small randomized trial supported combination treatment in ocular MMP (see later).

Cyclophosphamide for ocular inflammatory diseases. Pujari SS, Kempen JH, Newcomb CW, Gangaputra S, Daniel E, Suhler EB, et al. Ophthalmology 2010; 117: 356–65.

Retrospective cohort study of 98 patients with MMP treated with cyclophosphamide (75–150 mg/daily) and oral prednisolone.

Forty-two patients achieved complete remission within 6 months, increasing to 67 at 1 year.

Management of ocular mucous membrane pemphigoid with immunosuppressive therapy. Thorne JE, Woreta FA, Jabs JA, Anhalt GJ. Ophthalmology 2008; 115: 2146–52.

Retrospective cohort study. Forty out of 44 patients treated with cyclophosphamide (2 mg/kg/day) and prednisolone (initially 1 mg/kg/day tapering over 1–2 months) achieved remission within 2 years; 5 subsequently relapsed.

Analysis of a novel protocol of pulsed intravenous cyclophosphamide for recalcitrant or severe ocular inflammatory disease. Suelves AM, Arcinue CA, González-Martín JM, Kruh JN, Foster CS. Ophthalmology 2013; 120: 1201–9.

Retrospective case series of 65 patients (110 eyes) of patients with ocular disease treated with pulsed intravenous cyclophosphamide (starting dose 1 g/m^2 body surface area [BSA] in 1000 mL saline over 1 hour; subsequent doses calculated based on hemogram by absolute numbers) in combination with methylprednisolone (1000 mg in 1000 mL normal saline over 1 hour). Complete remission was achieved in 54 patients (84%).

Oral cyclophosphamide without corticosteroids to treat mucous membrane pemphigoid. Munyangango EM, Le Roux-Villet C, Doan S, Pascal F, Soued I, Alexandre M, et al. Br J Dermatol 2013; 168: 381–90.

Retrospective case series of 13 patients with severe refractory MMP. Oral cyclophosphamide (2 mg/kg/day) without corticosteroids was commenced on a background of previous treatments (dapsone, sulfasalazine, or topicals) in the absence of corticosteroids. Nine out of 13 patients responded to treatment, with 7/13 achieving complete remission, 4 of whom maintained this at 6 months after the study. Ten out of 13 patients suffered lymphopenia, leading to withdrawal of cyclophosphamide in 6/13.

In patients with severe ocular disease combination treatment with cyclophosphamide (oral or intravenous) and prednisolone is first line; oral and intravenous treatments seem equally effective. Cyclophosphamide has been shown to be effective in the absence of corticosteroids. In mild to moderate MMP, dapsone in combination with corticosteroids may be used first line.

Second-Line Therapies	
• Topical mitomycin	C
• Mycophenolate mofetil	C
• Azathioprine	D
• Methotrexate	D
• Ciclosporin	D

Intraoperative mitomycin C in the treatment of cicatricial obliterations of conjunctival fornices. Secchi AG, Tognon MS. Am J Ophthalmol 1996; 122: 728–30.

Intraoperative topical mitomycin was useful in 4/4 patients.

Subconjunctival mitomycin C for the treatment of ocular cicatricial pemphigoid. Donnenfeld ED, Perry HD, Wallerstein A, Caronia RM, Kanellopoulos AJ, Sforza PD, et al. Ophthalmology 1999; 106: 72–9.

No disease progression occurred in 8/9 eyes treated with subconjunctival mitomycin C.

Ocular cicatricial pemphigoid review. Foster CS, Sainz De La Maza M. Curr Opin Allergy Clin Immunol 2004; 4: 435–9.

Evidence Levels: **A** Double-blind study **B** Clinical trial ≥ 20 subjects **C** Clinical trial < 20 subjects **D** Series ≥ 5 subjects **E** Anecdotal case reports

Subconjunctival mitomycin did not prevent progression of scarring.

The benefit of mitomycin is uncertain.

Mycophenolate mofetil for ocular inflammation. Daniel E, Thorne JE, Newcomb CW, Pujari SS, Kaçmaz RO, Levy-Clarke GA, et al. Am J Ophthalmol. 2010; 149: 423–32.

Retrospective cohort study of 18 patients with ocular MMP treated with mycophenolate mofetil in combination with prednisolone. Forty-one percent achieved complete control at 6 months, increasing to 71% at 1 year; most relapsed on discontinuation of prednisolone, but the authors report a steroid-sparing effect. Doses were not specified.

Long-term results of therapy with mycophenolate mofetil in ocular mucous membrane pemphigoid. Doycheva D, Deuter C, Blumenstock G, Stuebiger N, Zierhut M. Ocul Immunol Inflamm 2011; 19: 431–8.

Retrospective study of 10 patients (19 eyes) with ocular MMP treated with mycophenolate mofetil (1 g/day) with prednisolone (initially 1 mg/kg/day, tapered to 5 mg/day). Control of inflammation achieved in 58% (11/19 eyes). Progression was prevented in 47% (9/19 eyes).

Treatment of mucous membrane pemphigoid with mycophenolate mofetil. Nottage JM, Hammersmith KM, Murchison AP, Felipe AF, Penne R, Raber I. Cornea 2013; 32: 810–5.

Retrospective case series of 23 consecutive patients with ocular disease. Sixteen patients achieved control with mycophenolate as monotherapy, a further 3 in combination with other treatments. Treatment was stopped in 5 patients; in 4 this was due to failure to obtain inflammatory control, and the fifth suffered an adverse reaction.

Treatment of mucous membrane pemphigoid with the combination of mycophenolate mofetil, dapsone, and prednisolone: a case series. Staines K, Hampton PJ. Oral Surg Oral Med Oral Pathol Oral Radiol 2012; 114: e49–56.

Six patients with skin and oral disease treated with mycophenolate mofetil (1–1.5 g/day) with dapsone 50 mg and prednisolone 0.5 mg/kg/day. At 18 months all had complete resolution of skin, oral, and pharyngeal disease.

Cicatricial pemphigoid: treatment with mycophenolate mofetil. Ingen-Housz-Oro S, Prost-Squarcioni C, Pascal F, Doan S, Brette MD, Bachelez H, et al. Ann Dermatol Venereol 2005; 132: 13–6.

Mycophenolate mofetil (1.5 g/day or 2 g/day) helped to control the disease in 10 of 14 patients; most also received cyclophosphamide or dapsone.

Immunosuppressive therapy for ocular mucous membrane pemphigoid strategies and outcomes. Saw VP, Dart JK, Rauz S, Ramsay A, Bunce C, Xing W, et al. Ophthalmology 2008; 115: 253–61.e1.

In a retrospective noncomparative study of 115 patients, azathioprine 1 to 2.5 mg/kg daily was effective in 47%. Side effects limited treatment in 40%. Combination of sulfur/steroid/myelosuppresive may be superior to single therapy. Control of inflammation does not necessarily prevent progression.

Azathioprine for ocular inflammatory diseases. Pasadhika S, Kempen JH, Newcomb CW, Liesegang TL, Pujari SS, Rosenbaum JT, et al. Am J Ophthalmol 2009; 148: 500–9.

Retrospective cohort of 33 patients with ocular disease treated with azathioprine and oral prednisolone. Forty-four percent achieved control by 6 months, with 12% off prednisolone treatment. This increased to 67% controlled by 1 year, with 17% off prednisolone. Doses were not specified.

Methotrexate for ocular inflammatory diseases. Gangaputra S, Newcomb CW, Liesegang TL, Kaçmaz RO, Jabs DA, Levy-Clarke GA, et al; Systemic Immunosuppressive Therapy for Eye Diseases Cohort Study. Ophthalmology 2009; 116: 2188–98.

Retrospective cohort study of 58 patients with ocular MMP. A reported 39.5% achieved complete control of inflammation at 6 months, increasing to 65.0% at 1 year with 26.8% off prednisolone at 1 year. Doses of methotrexate were not specified.

Methotrexate therapy for ocular cicatricial pemphigoid. McCluskey P, Chang JH, Singh R, Wakefield D. Ophthalmology 2004; 111: 796–801.

In 12 of 17 patients with mainly ocular MMP oral methotrexate (and topical treatment) prevented progression of scarring. Methotrexate was given orally as a single weekly dose at a starting dose of 5 to 15 mg determined empirically and approximately based on body weight.

Cyclosporine for ocular inflammatory diseases. Kaçmaz RO, Kempen JH, Newcomb C, Daniel E, Gangaputra S, Nussenblatt RB, et al. Ophthalmology 2010; 117: 576–84.

Ciclosporin was minimally effective even at doses in excess of 3.5 mg/kg/day. All patients remained on corticosteroids.

Ocular autoimmune pemphigoid and cyclosporine. Alonso A, Bignone ML, Brunzini M, Brunzini R. Allergol Immunopathol (Madr) 2006; 34: 113–5.

Treatment-resistant ocular pemphigoid in 82 patients was treated with ciclosporin 100 mg/day, with an attendant reduction in the dose of steroids.

There is evidence that the immunosuppressive agents are effective. Mycophenolate mofetil 0.5 to 1 g twice daily and azathioprine 1 to 3 mg/kg/day are used most frequently. Methotrexate 5 to 25 mg/week and ciclosporin 2 to 4 mg/kg/day are less widely used.

Third-Line Therapies	
• Intravenous immunoglobulins	C
• Plasmapheresis	E
• Rituximab	D
• Etanercept	E
• Infliximab	E
• Topical tacrolimus	E
• Pentoxifylline	C
• Colchicine	E
• Low-level laser	E

Consensus statement on the use of intravenous immunoglobulin therapy in the treatment of autoimmune mucocutaneous blistering diseases. Ahmed AR, Dahl MV. Arch Dermatol 2003; 139: 1051–9.

Good review on uses and regimens.

Treatment of epidermolysis bullosa acquisita with intravenous immunoglobulin in patients non-responsive to conventional therapy: clinical outcome and post-treatment long-term follow-up. Ahmed AR, Gürcan HM. J Eur Acad Dermatol Venereol 2012; 26: 1074–83.

Retrospective case series of 10 patients with epidermolysis bullosa acquisita (EBA), 7 of whom had mucosal disease. Intravenous immunoglobulin (IVIG) was used as monotherapy with 2 g/kg/cycle given over 3 days initially monthly, then tapering. Complete clinical response occurred in all with prolonged remission.

Intravenous immunoglobulins and mucous membrane pemphigoid. Mignogna MD, Leuci S, Piscopo R, Bonovolontà G. Ophthalmology 2008; 115: 752.

IVIG treatment was beneficial in six patients with generalized MMP also affecting the eyes.

IVIG at doses 0.5 to 2 g/day (over 3–5 days) initially once monthly is justified in rapidly progressive or recalcitrant disease, either in combination with other treatments or as monotherapy.

Combination of rituximab and intravenous immunoglobulin for recalcitrant ocular cicatricial pemphigoid: a preliminary report. Foster CS, Chang PY, Ahmed AR. Ophthalmology 2010; 117: 861–9.

Six patients were treated with a combination of IVIG and rituximab. Disease progression was arrested in all six.

A dose of 375 mg/m^2 of rituximab was given once weekly for 8 consecutive weeks. Thereafter, for the subsequent 4 months, it was given once monthly

The dose of IVIG was 2 g/kg per cycle. The total dose was divided into three equal parts on 3 consecutive days. The frequency of the IVIG was monthly until the B-cell level returned to normal. Thereafter, IVIG was continued, and the intervals between infusions were increased to 6, 8, 10, 12, 14, and 16 weeks. The last cycle was given at the 16-week interval.

Rituximab for treatment-refractory pemphigus and pemphigoid: a case series of 17 patients. Kasperkiewicz M, Shimanovich I, Ludwig RJ, Rose C, Zillikens D, Schmidt E. J Am Acad Dermatol 2011; 65: 552–8.

Five patients with refractory MMP were treated with rituximab. Complete remission occurred in three patients, partial remission in the other two. No serious side effects were noted.

Rituximab for patients with refractory mucous membrane pemphigoid. Le Roux-Villet C, Prost-Squarcioni C, Alexandre M, Caux F, Pascal F, Doan S, et al. Arch Dermatol 2011; 147: 843–9.

Twenty-five patients with severe refractory MMP received one or two cycles of rituximab; complete response occurred in 22 patients and partial response in 1. Two patients died from infectious complications; these patients also received high-dose immunosuppression for laryngeal and tracheal edema.

One or two cycles of rituximab (375 mg/m^2 weekly for 4 weeks).

Twenty-one of the patients were receiving concomitant therapy with dapsone and/or sulfasalazine therapy, which was maintained during rituximab cycles.

Bullous and mucous membrane pemphigoid show a mixed response to rituximab: experience in seven patients. Lourari S, Doffoel-Hantz V, Meyer N, Bulai-Livideanu C, Viraben R, et al. J Eur Acad Dermatol Venereol 2011; 25: 1238–40.

Two patients with MMP were treated with rituximab, leading to complete remission in one and partial remission in the other. Four infusions of rituximab were given at weekly intervals at a dose of 375 mg/m^2.

Rituximab preserves vision in ocular mucous membrane pemphigoid. Rübsam A, Stefaniak R, Worm M, Pleyer U. Expert Opin Biol Ther 2015; 15: 927–33.

Retrospective case series of six patients treated with rituximab at high doses either as monotherapy (3/6) or with concomitant immunosuppression (3/6). Five patients had ocular disease, and one had extensive disease. After one cycle all achieved short-term complete remission. After a second cycle, 2/6 achieved complete remission and 3/6 partial remission. Mean follow-up was 22 months. Two patients experienced infusion reactions.

Rituximab combined with conventional therapy versus conventional therapy alone for the treatment of mucous membrane pemphigoid (MMP). Maley A, Warren M, Haberman I, Swerlick R, Kharod-Dholakia B, Feldman R. J Am Acad Dermatol 2016; 74: 835–40.

Retrospective review of 49 patients comparing outcomes of 24 who received rituximab and 25 who received conventional immunosuppression. All patients in the rituximab group achieved disease control with a mean time to disease control of 10.2 months, compared with 10 (40%) of the patients in the conventional immunosuppression group, with a mean time to disease control of 37.7 months. Adverse events were seen in 33% of the rituximab group compared with 48% of the conventional group. The two groups were not matched, nor were they randomized; rituximab dosing was not uniform.

Ten patients were initially treated with the lymphoma protocol for rituximab (four weekly infusions of 375 mg/m^2), and 14 patients were initially treated with the rheumatoid arthritis protocol (two infusions of 1000 mg given 15 days apart). Eleven patients were treated with a single course of rituximab, whereas 13 required additional therapy. The mean total infusions of rituximab were 5.25 (range 2–16, SD 3.98).

Data from two larger and several small retrospective case series suggest benefit of rituximab; further evidence is needed.

Therapeutic effect of etanercept in anti-laminin 5 (laminin 332) mucous membrane pemphigoid. Schulz S, Deuster D, Schmidt E, Bonsmann G, Beissert S. Int J Dermatol 2011; 50: 1129–31.

Recalcitrant cicatricial pemphigoid treated with the anti-TNF-alpha agent etanercept. Kennedy JS, Devillez RL, Henning JS. J Drugs Dermatol 2010; 9: 68–70.

Treatment of ocular cicatricial pemphigoid with the tumour necrosis factor alpha antagonist etanercept. Prey S, Robert PY, Drouet M, Sparsa A, Roux C, Bonnetblanc JM, et al. Acta Dermatol Venereol 2007; 87: 74–5.

Successful treatment of mucous membrane pemphigoid with etanercept in 3 patients. Canizares MJ, Smith DI, Conners MS, Maverick KJ, Heffernan MP. Arch Dermatol 2006; 142: 1457–61.

Cicatricial pemphigoid and therapy with the TNF inhibitor etanercept. Labrecque PG, Null M. J Am Acad Dermatol 2004; 50: 48.

Treatment of recalcitrant cicatricial pemphigoid with the tumor necrosis factor alpha antagonist etanercept. Sacher C, Rubbert A, König C, Scharffetter-Kochanek K, Krieg T, Hunzelmann N. J Am Acad Dermatol 2002; 46: 113–5.

These case reports describe eight patients who responded to etanercept 50 mg/week subcutaneously, including five with ocular disease. Two patients maintained remission after cessation of the drug, and another relapsed.

Evidence Levels: **A** Double-blind study **B** Clinical trial ≥ 20 subjects **C** Clinical trial < 20 subjects **D** Series ≥ 5 subjects **E** Anecdotal case reports

Successful treatment of mucous membrane pemphigoid with infliximab. Heffernan MP, Bentley DD. Arch Dermatol 2006; 142: 1268–70.

Treatment comprised 5 mg/kg week 0, 2, and every 8 weeks IV.

Mucous membrane pemphigoid in a series of 7 children and a review of the literature with particular reference to prognostic features and treatment. Veysey EC, McHenry P, Powell J, Crone M, Harper JI, Allen J, et al. Eur J Pediatr Dermatol 2007; 17: 218–26.

Two cases with MMP benefited from infliximab; disease was ocular and oral in both and esophageal in one.

The biologics, particularly the anti-TNF agent etanercept, may have a role, but evidence is limited.

Pentoxifylline (anti-tumor necrosis factor drug): effective adjunctive therapy in the control of ocular cicatricial pemphigoid. El Darouti MA, Fakhry Khattab MA, Hegazy RA, Hafez DA, Gawdat HI. Eur J Ophthalmol 2011; 21: 529–37.

Randomized blinded study of 30 patients with ocular MMP treated with IV methylprednisolone and cyclophosphamide, either with or without adjuvant pentoxifylline (IV then oral).

Patients in both groups received pulsed steroid therapy (500 mg IV methylprednisolone daily for 5 days) with cyclophosphamide (500 mg in 2 L saline given on day 1 of the pulse steroid therapy). Adjuvant IV pentoxifylline was given at a dose of 400 mg tds for the first 3 days to the treatment group. Both cycles were repeated weekly until cessation of progression. Then the cycles were spaced to be given with pulsed oral steroid (60 mg prednisolone for 2 consecutive days) administered between cycles for both groups, with the addition of daily oral pentoxifylline (400 mg) in the treatment group. This was repeated until the end of the study, for a total duration 6 months.

Inflammation and progression of scarring were reduced in patients receiving pentoxifylline.

Adjuvant pentoxifylline appears beneficial in control of ocular disease; further evidence is needed.

Oral mucous membrane pemphigoid: complete response to topical tacrolimus. Lee HY, Blazek C, Beltraminelli H, Borradori L. Acta Derm Venereol 2011; 91: 604–5.

Single case of a complete response to oral suspension of tacrolimus 0.03% in aqueous solution, twice daily as an oral rinse.

Successful treatment of mucous membrane pemphigoid with tacrolimus. Suresh L, Martinex Caixto LE, Radfar L. Spec Care Dentist 2006; 26: 66–70.

Case report: patient treated with tacrolimus ointment. 0.1% tds for 6 weeks.

Single case reports suggest topical tacrolimus may be of benefit.

Low-level laser therapy for oral mucous membrane pemphigoid. Cafaro A, Broccoletti R, Arduino PG. Lasers Med Sci 2012; 27: 1247–50.

Laser light may improve the symptoms of oral lesions of cicatricial pemphigoid: a case report. Oliveira PC, Reis Junior JA, Lacerda JA, Silveira NT, Santos JM, Vitale MC, et al. Photomed Laser Surg 2009; 27: 825–8.

Laser phototherapy (GaAlAs diode laser, 660-nm wavelength, 30 mW, continuous wave, diameter approx. 3 mm, 60 J/cm^2 per session) was used in association with oral prednisolone (40 mg).

Low-level laser therapy in the treatment of mucous membrane pemphigoid: a promising procedure. Yilmaz HG, Kusakci-Seker B, Bayindir H, Tözüm TF. J Periodontol 2010; 81: 1226–30.

Single case report of patient treated with 810-nm diode laser. The lesions were treated by low-light laser therapy over a period of 7 days using a continuous waveform for 40 seconds and an energy density of 5 J/cm^2.

Five patients with oral disease have received treatment with low-level laser, either as an adjunct or alone, with benefit reported.

Mycetoma: eumycetoma and actinomycetoma

Mahreen Ameen, Wanda Sonia Robles

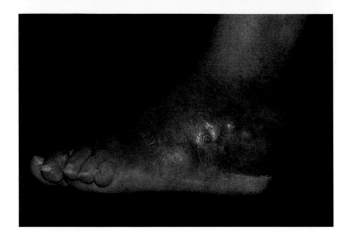

Mycetomas (Madura foot) are endemic in the tropics and subtropics. They are chronic, granulomatous, subcutaneous infections caused by either actinomycetes bacteria or eumycetes fungi, giving rising to actinomycetomas and eumycetomas, respectively. The infectious agents are saprophytes existing in soil or plants, and infection usually results from traumatic inoculation into the skin. Consequently, the disease most commonly affects agriculturalists and those who are barefoot. The disease is characterized by abscesses, draining sinuses, and discharging grains, and it slowly progresses with risk of bone and visceral involvement. The discharging grains represent aggregates of fungal hyphae or bacterial filaments. Actinomycetomas are produced by agents of the genera *Nocardia*, *Actinomadura*, *Streptomyces*, and *Nocardiopsis*. *Nocardia* is the most common agent, particularly in the Americas, but *Streptomyces somaliensis* is more common in Sudan and the Middle East. Eumycetomas are caused by a large number of fungi: *Madurella mycetomatis* is of particular significance as it is the most prevalent causative agent in regions of India and Africa.

MANAGEMENT STRATEGY

Treatment of mycetomas is generally difficult, and management varies from a very conservative approach to chemotherapy and surgery. Effective chemotherapy is available for actinomycetomas; however, eumycetomas are more refractory to drug therapy.

Eumycetomas may sometimes be managed conservatively as they are usually indolent and seldom life threatening. Treatment is then symptomatic with relief of pain and applications of dressings to affected areas, particularly the sinuses. Any secondary bacterial infection requires treatment. More active management consists of long courses of antifungals, 18 to 24 months or even longer, together with aggressive surgical excision and debulking. Antifungal therapy is initiated before surgery and continued afterward to reduce the risk of recurrence. Small lesions have a more favorable prognosis as they are more easily excised completely. Advanced disease with bony involvement characteristically shows

poor therapy response and often requires surgical amputation. Of all the antifungal drugs, azoles have been most commonly used. Fluconazole has been found to be ineffective but ketoconazole and itraconazole have both demonstrated efficacy, particularly at high doses (200–400 mg daily for ketoconazole and 300–400 mg daily for itraconazole). Itraconazole is preferred as it is better tolerated for longer periods and is thought to demonstrate greater efficacy than ketoconazole, although there are no published studies comparing their efficacy. There are reports of the high tolerability and efficacy of the newer broad-spectrum triazoles, such as voriconazole and posaconazole, against *Madurella* species and *Scedosporium apiospermum* infection. This is supported by in vitro susceptibility testing. However, their high costs are prohibitive for use in most endemic regions. Griseofulvin appears to be ineffective. Amphotericin has shown variable responses in the few cases in which it has been used. High-dose terbinafine (500 mg twice daily) has demonstrated limited clinical efficacy, which correlates with in vitro susceptibility testing, which has shown only moderate efficacy of terbinafine against some black-grain mycetomas. In vitro studies have not demonstrated any efficacy of echinocandins against *Madurella mycetomatis*.

Actinomycetomas are usually amenable to antibiotic therapy, but cure rates vary widely from 60% to 90%. Combined drug therapy is preferred in order to prevent the development of drug resistance, as well as to eradicate any residual infection. The duration of drug therapy depends on clinical response. Cure is defined by a lack of clinical activity, absence of grains, and negative cultures. Treatment with sulfonamides and sulfonamide combinations such as trimethoprim–sulfamethoxazole (cotrimoxazole) are usually first line. Aminoglycosides, tetracyclines, rifampicin, ciprofloxacin, and amoxicillin–clavulanate have also been successfully used. Parenteral amikacin and oral cotrimoxazole combination therapy is especially advocated for cases at risk of bone or visceral involvement. Actinomycetomas seldom require surgical management.

Specific Investigations

- Direct microscopy
- Culture
- Histopathology

It is imperative to differentiate between eumycetomas, which respond poorly to chemotherapy, and actinomycetomas, which generally respond well. Furthermore, species identification is important as it has treatment and prognostic implications—some species having demonstrated higher efficacy to some chemotherapy regimens than others.

The clinical diagnosis can be confirmed by the demonstration and identification of grains, which can be obtained by direct extraction, fine needle aspiration, or deep tissue biopsy. Direct microscopy of a crushed grain in 20% potassium hydroxide gives an indication of the size and shape of the grain, which provides an initial clue to the causative agent, whether bacterial or fungal. Histopathology of a deep surgical biopsy demonstrates a granulomatous, inflammatory reaction with abscesses containing grains. Culture of grains using Sabouraud or blood agar media permits species identification. However, fungal culture can be particularly difficult, as morphologic differentiation of fungi may be poor or delayed. Molecular tests have therefore been developed for species identification of several black-grained eumycetoma, including species-specific polymerase chain reaction (PCR) analysis. Serologic tests such as enzyme-linked immunosorbent assay (ELISA) are employed by some centers to support diagnosis as well as to assess therapy response. Radiology and ultrasound enable assessment of disease extent and bony involvement. Helical computed tomography can provide detailed assessments of soft tissue and visceral involvement.

Hand mycetoma: The Mycetoma Research Centre experience and literature. Omer RF, Seif El Din N, Abdel Rahim FA, Fahal AH. PLoS Negl Trop Dis 2016; 10: e0004886.

Data is discussed on 533 patients with hand mycetoma managed over a period of 24 years at the Mycetoma Research Centre, Khartoum, Sudan. A reported 83.3% had eumycetoma, which were treated with ketoconazole (400–800 mg daily) or itraconazole (200–400 mg daily). Actinomycetomas were treated with streptomycin sulfate (1 gram daily), dapsone (100 mg daily), or streptomycin and trimethoprim–sulfamethoxazole (8/40 mg/kg/day), which was sometimes combined with amikacin (15 mg/kg/day) and given in cycles.

The surgical treatment of mycetoma. Suleiman SH, Wadaella el S, Fahal AH. PLoS Negl Trop Dis 2016; 10: e0004690.

The Mycetoma Research Centre, Khartoum, Sudan, has extensive experience in the surgical management of mycetomas and discusses different surgical options, including wide local excision, repetitive debridement, and amputation.

Mycetoma: a unique neglected tropical disease. Zijlstra EE, van de Sande WW, Welsh O, Mahgoub el S, Goodfellow M, Fahal AH. Lancet Infect Dis 2016; 16: 100–12.

A comprehensive up-to-date review discussing current therapeutics and future challenges.

Mycetoma in the Sudan: an update from the Mycetoma Research Centre, University of Khartoum, Sudan. Fahal A, Mahgoub el S, El Hassan AM, Abdel-Rahman ME. PLoS Negl Trop Dis 2015; 9: e0003679.

This world-renowned center, which has seen the greatest number of mycetoma cases, describes their experience of 6792 patients seen during the period 1991 to 2014. *Madurella mycetomatis* eumycetoma was the most common type found in 70%.

Eumycetoma and actinomycetoma—an update on causative agents, epidemiology, pathogenesis, diagnostics and therapy. Nenoff P, van de Sande WW, Fahal AH, Reinel D, Schöfer H. J Eur Acad Dermatol Venereol 2015; 29: 1873–83.

This article covers both fungal and bacterial mycetomas and presents data on their treatment.

Mycetoma: experience of 482 cases in a single center in Mexico. Bonifaz A, Tirado-Sánchez A, Calderón L, Saúl A, Araiza J, Hernández M, et al. PLoS Negl Trop Dis 2014; 8: e3102.

This is a retrospective study reporting epidemiologic, clinical, and microbiologic data on all cases of mycetoma seen over a 33-year period (1980–2013) in Mexico City. Ninety-two percent of cases were actinomycetomas, and 78% of these were due to *Nocardia brasiliensis*.

Mycetoma medical therapy. Welsh O, Al-Abdely HM, Salinas-Carmona MC, Fahal AH. PLoS Negl Trop Dis 2014; 8: e3218.

Drug therapies for both actinomycetomas and eumycetomas are comprehensively covered.

First-Line Therapies

• Sulfonamides	B
• Aminoglycosides	B
• Itraconazole	C

Actinomycetomas in Senegal. Study of 90 cases. Dieng MT, Niang SO, Diop B, Ndiaye B. Bull Soc Pathol Exot Filiales 2005; 98: 18–20.

Ninety patients with actinomycetomas (*A. pelletieri*, n = 60; *A. madurae*, n = 25; *S. somaliensis*, n = 5) in Senegal were treated with sulfamethoxazole monotherapy. Despite bone involvement in 55% of cases, cure was achieved after 1 year of treatment in 83% of patients. Fifty percent of these cases were localized to the foot. Despite treatment two patients died of visceral involvement.

Mycetoma in children: experience with 15 cases. Bonifaz A, Ibarra G, Saul A, Paredes-Solis V, Carrasco-Gerard E, Fierro-Arias L. Pediatr Inf Dis J 2007; 26: 50–2.

Mycetomas are very rare in children, but the clinical presentation and course are similar to that in adults. There were 13 cases of *Nocardia* actinomycetoma and 2 cases of *M. mycetomatis* eumycetoma. Sulfonamide combinations were advocated as first-line therapy for actinomycetomas and amoxicillin–clavulanate as second-line therapy. Itraconazole and ketoconazole were used in the management of eumycetomas.

A modified two-step treatment for actinomycetoma. Ramam M, Bhat R, Garg T, Sharma VK, Ray R, Singh MK et al. Indian J Dermatol Venereol Leprol 2007; 73: 235–9.

The authors emphasize that although parenteral therapy regimens demonstrate high efficacy, they are costly in terms of inpatient stays. They describe a reduced parenteral regimen (intravenous gentamicin 80 mg twice daily together with oral cotrimoxazole 320–1600 mg twice daily for 1 month), followed by a longer phase of oral medication (doxycycline 100 mg twice daily together with cotrimoxazole at the same dose). All 21 patients demonstrated significant clinical response at the end of the parenteral phase of treatment. The oral phase needed to be continued for 3.5 to 16 months (mean 9.1 months) until cure, and in the majority of these patients this included a treatment period of 5 to 6 months after complete healing of the lesions to prevent any relapse.

Clinical and mycologic findings and therapeutic outcome of 27 mycetoma patients from São Paulo, Brazil. Castro LG, Piquero-Casals J. Int J Dermatol 2008; 47: 160–3.

This article describes the treatment of 13 cases of eumycetoma (with itraconazole) and 14 cases of actinomycetoma (with cotrimoxazole). Combination drug therapy was used in more than half of the cases. There was higher efficacy in three patients with actinomycetoma treated with cotrimoxazole in combination with amikacin. However, two of these patients developed hearing loss after treatment. The authors emphasize the problems of diagnostic testing, even in secondary and tertiary health centers, and were only able to identify the etiologic agent in fewer than half of their cases.

Improvement of eumycetoma with itraconazole. Smith EL, Kutbi S. J Am Acad Dermatol 1997; 34: 279–80.

This study from Saudi Arabia treated 25 patients with a follow-up period of 12 years. The authors recommend a combination itraconazole drug therapy together with surgical excision or debulking. Drainage of sinuses with removal of grains that can cause inflammation reduced pain and swelling.

Mycetoma in children. Fahal AH, Sabaa AH. Trans R Soc Trop Med Hyg 2010; 104: 117–21.

A large retrospective study of 722 children (age range 4–17 years) with confirmed mycetoma seen at the Mycetoma Research Centre, Sudan, during a 20-year period until 2009. Diagnosis was established by cytologic and ultrasound examinations of the lesions and histologic examination of the surgical biopsies. Most of the patients had eumycetomas. Combined medical treatment and surgical excision was the standard treatment. Disease recurrence after surgical excision was reported in 17.9% of patients.

The safety and efficacy of itraconazole for the treatment of patients with eumycetoma due to *Madurella mycetomatis*. Fahal AH, Rahman IA, El-Hassan AM, Rahman ME, Zijlstra EE. Trans R Soc Trop Med Hyg 2011; 105: 127–32.

This prospective study of 13 patients demonstrated that preoperative treatment with a 1-year course of itraconazole enhances lesion encapsulation, which facilitates wide local excision, avoiding unnecessary mutilating surgery. Itraconazole was given at 400 mg daily for 3 months followed by a reduced dose of 200 mg daily for 9 months. All patients showed a good clinical response to the 400-mg daily dose but a slower response to the 200-mg daily dose. Posttreatment surgical exploration demonstrated that all lesions were well localized and encapsulated and easily removed. There was only a single recurrence after a follow-up period of 18 to 36 months.

Second-Line Therapies	
• Amoxicillin–clavulanate	B
• Terbinafine	B
• Ketoconazole	C
• Posaconazole	D
• Imipenem	D
• Voriconazole	D
• Oxazolidinones	E

Last generation triazoles for imported eumycetoma in eleven consecutive adults. Crabol Y, Poiree S, Bougnoux ME, Maunoury C, Barete S, Zeller V et al. PLoS Negl Trop Dis 2014; 8: e3232.

Data is presented on 11 cases of eumycetoma (*Fusarium solani* complex *n* = 3; *Madurella mycetomatis n* = 3; *Exophiala jeanselmei n* = 1) that were treated by either voriconazole or posaconazole for a mean duration of 25.9 ± 18 months. There was complete response (major clinical and magnetic resonance imaging [MRI] improvement) in 5/11, partial response in 5/11, and failure in 1/11. Optimal outcome was associated with fungal species and initiation of drug therapy <65 months since first symptoms.

Treatment of actinomycetoma due to *Nocardia* spp. with amoxicillin-clavulanate. Bonifaz A, Flores P, Saul A, Carrasco-Gerard E, Ponce RM. Br J Dermatol 2007; 156: 308–11.

This study advocates amoxicillin–clavulanate as rescue therapy in patients with *Nocardia* spp. refractory to other therapy regimens. Twenty-one patients who had previously failed on other therapy regimens were treated with oral amoxicillin–clavulanate 875/125 mg twice daily. There was clinical and microbiologic cure in 15 (71%) patients after a mean treatment period of 10 months. Patients with bone and visceral involvement required longer treatment periods.

Clinical efficacy and safety of oral terbinafine in fungal mycetoma. N'Diaye B, Dieng MT, Perez A, Stockmeyer M, Bakshi R. Int J Dermatol 2006; 45: 154–7.

High-dose terbinafine, 500 mg twice daily, was given to 23 patients with eumycetomas in Senegal. After 24 to 48 weeks of treatment mycologic cure was seen in 25% patients, and a further 55% of patients demonstrated clinical improvement. Treatment was well tolerated.

This is the only study of terbinafine monotherapy for the treatment of eumycetomas, perhaps because the drug is prohibitively expensive in countries endemic for the infection.

Ketoconazole in the treatment of eumycetoma due to *Madurella mycetomii*. Mahgoub ES, Gumaa SA. Trans R Soc Trop Med Hyg 1984; 78: 376–9.

This trial consisted of 13 patients treated in the Sudan and Saudi Arabia. Ketoconazole was given at doses of 200 to 400 mg daily for 3 to 36 months (median 13 months). Treatment was well tolerated. Five patients were cured, and a further 4 improved. Response appeared to be dose dependent. The authors recommend a 400-mg daily dose of ketoconazole and a minimum treatment period of 12 months where there is bony involvement irrespective of clinical improvement.

Given the availability of newer antifungals, there are a few recent trials evaluating the use of ketoconazole for eumycetomas. However, it is a less expensive drug than itraconazole and therefore is more commonly used in endemic regions.

Posaconazole treatment of refractory eumycetoma and chromoblastomycosis. Negroni R, Tobon A, Bustamante B, Shikanai-Yasuda MA, Patino H, Restrepo A. Rev Inst Med Trop Sao Paulo 2005; 47: 339–46.

In this study from Argentina, posaconazole (800 mg daily in divided doses) was given to six patients with eumycetoma (*M. grisea, n* = 3; *M. mycetomatis, n* = 2; *S. apiospermum, n* = 1) resistant to standard therapy. There was partial and complete clinical response in five of the six patients. Treatment was well tolerated, even after long-term administration of more than 2 years.

Efficacy of imipenem therapy for *Nocardia* actinomycetomas refractory to sulphonamides. Ameen M, Arenas R, Vásquez del Mercado, Torres E, Zacarias R. J Am Acad Dermatol 2010; 62: 239–46.

Eight patients with severe and protracted infection (two with visceral and a further two with bone involvement) refractory to previous sulfonamide monotherapy received a 3-week course of parenteral imipenem (1.5 g daily, *n* = 3) given as either monotherapy or in combination with amikacin (1 g daily, *n* = 5). Treatment cycles were repeated at 6-month intervals. Oral cotrimoxazole was also given and continued between cycles. Treatment was well tolerated, and four patients achieved clinical and microbiologic cure after one to two cycles of treatment, with the others demonstrating greater than 75% clinical improvement and negative culture results.

This study also demonstrated that sulfonamides are effective for limited disease of relatively short duration. Their partial efficacy in severe cases was the reason for continuing treatment with sulfonamides in combination with imipenem.

***Madurella mycetomatis* mycetoma treated successfully with oral voriconazole.** Lacroix C, De Kerviller E, Morel P, Derouin F, Feuilhade de Chavin M. Br J Dermatol 2005; 152: 1067–8.

Voriconazole has been reported to be effective in the management of disseminated fungal infections with *Scedosporium* and *Fusarium* spp. This is the first report of successful treatment of a eumycetoma with oral voriconazole monotherapy given for 16 months at a dose of 300 mg twice daily. The treatment was well tolerated, and the patient remained disease free 4 years after the end of treatment.

Scedosporium apiospermum mycetoma with bone involvement successfully treated with voriconazole. Porte L, Khatibi S, Hajj LE, Cassaing S, Berry A, Massip P, et al. Trans R Soc Trop Med Hyg 2006; 100: 891–4.

Scedosporium apiospermum mycetoma usually requires limb amputation. This case with bone involvement that had previously failed with itraconazole, fluconazole, and cotrimoxazole was given voriconazole 400 mg daily for 18 months. There was a good clinical response, and MRI demonstrated impressive regression of bony lesions. Treatment, however, was discontinued because of hepatic impairment.

This report suggests voriconazole as a promising treatment option for S. apiospermum *mycetomas.*

Clinical experience with linezolid for the treatment of *Nocardia* infection. Moylett EH, Pacheco SE, Brown-Elliott BA, Perry TR, Buescher ES, Birmingham MC. Clin Infect Dis 2003; 36: 313–8.

Oral linezolid belongs to the new broad-spectrum oxazolidinones. This report describes its successful use in *Nocardia* infection. There was only a single case of cutaneous infection with *N. brasilienesis.* Linezolid produced clinical cure after only 2 months of treatment at a dose of 600 mg twice daily.

Third-Line Therapies	
• Rifampicin	C
• Amphotericin B	D

Modified Welsh regimen: a promising therapy for actinomycetoma. Damle DK, Mahajan PM, Pradhan SN, Belgaumkar VA, Gosavi AP, Tolat SN, et al. J Drugs Dermatol 2008; 7: 853–6.

Eighteen patients with poor responses to previous therapies were treated with the standard "Welsh regimen" consisting of amikacin and cotrimoxazole in combination with rifampicin. Sixteen patients who completed treatment were cured and remained in remission during a follow-up period of up to 18 months.

This study has demonstrated efficacy and tolerability of these three drugs in combination. There are also reported cases of rifampicin being added to sulfonamides to improve efficacy.

Scedosporium infection in immunocompromised patients: successful use of liposomal amphotericin B and itraconazole. Barbaric D, Shaw PJ. Med Pediatr Oncol 2001; 37: 122–5.

A report of five cases of *Scedosporium* infection in immunosuppressed patients. Three of these patients died despite treatment with various combinations of amphotericin B and itraconazole. Two patients were successfully treated with liposomal amphotericin B and itraconazole.

Mycobacterial (atypical) skin infections

Ure Eke, John Berth-Jones

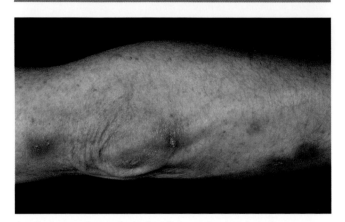

Atypical, or "nontuberculous" mycobacterial infections are being increasingly recognized and reported. Over 150 species in this genus are now recognized and are broadly divided into slow-growing and rapidly growing mycobacteria. Most outbreaks of infection arise from various sources of contaminated water, in a diverse range of domestic, occupational, clinical, and environmental settings. Cutaneous infection is often opportunistic, after preexisting trauma or inflammation of the skin, and nosocomial infections have been associated with a range of cosmetic and surgical procedures. Mycobacteria exhibit high levels of resistance to disinfectants and antiseptics, and have often been isolated from sources that may be considered "clean," such as chlorinated tap water.

Specific Investigations

- Histology
- Tissue culture
- Polymerase chain reaction (PCR)

Although some classical presentations are diagnosed clinically, mycobacterial infection is often unexpected, so a high level of awareness of these infections may be required. Histology is often helpful, and culture enables antimicrobial sensitivity to be investigated. Definitive diagnosis is achieved by PCR and related methodologies, and precise identification of the species involved will often assist with treatment.

FISH TANK (SWIMMING POOL) GRANULOMA

Fish tank granuloma is an infection of the skin caused by *Mycobacterium marinum*, presenting with plaques and nodules, commonly on the upper extremities, which may spread in a sporotrichoid fashion after an incubation period of 2 to 6 weeks. The most common sources of infection are tropical fish aquariums and swimming pools. The infection is commonly limited to the

skin, but tenosynovitis, osteomyelitis, and arthritis have been reported with deeper infections. Rarely, disseminated infection may occur, especially in the immunocompromised. There are reports of the development of cutaneous *M. marinum* infection during treatment with infliximab and adalimumab, although paradoxically, infliximab has been found to be a useful adjunctive therapy in the management of *M. marinum* infection.

MANAGEMENT STRATEGY

Diagnosis is often suspected from the history and clinical features. Histology shows noncaseating granulomas, but a complete absence of epithelioid cells and multinucleate giant cells is not unusual in acute lesions. Suppurative, tuberculoid, and palisading patterns of granulomas have been described. Dermal small vessel proliferation with mixed inflammation may be a good indicator of cutaneous atypical mycobacterial infections. Ziehl–Nielsen staining is positive for acid-fast bacilli in 30% of biopsies. Culture of the biopsy specimen at 30 to 33°C yields pigmented colonies of *M. marinum*. In vitro sensitivity studies have not been uniformly predictive of clinical response to the antibiotics. They do not have a routine role in directing initial treatment but may be useful in resistant cases. PCR is rapid and sensitive and can be performed on formalin-fixed, paraffin-embedded specimens.

Spontaneous resolution may occur within 3 years, but treatment is recommended for rapid recovery and prevention of dissemination. Although controlled trials are lacking, successful treatment is reported with various *antibiotics* given singly or in combination. The mean duration of treatment in various reports ranges from 6 to 20 weeks. No statistical difference in efficacy between treatments has been demonstrated. Lesions can often be effectively treated by *simple excision*, but occasionally this seems to result in a prolonged infection. The second-line treatments described later have been so designated as there is less published experience with them. The third-line treatments (e.g., *heat treatment*) are probably best regarded as adjunctive.

First-Line Therapies

• Minocycline 100–200 mg once daily for 6–12 weeks	C
• Doxycycline 100 mg twice daily for 3–4 months	C
• Clarithromycin 500 mg once or twice daily for 3–4 months	C
• Rifampicin 600 mg and ethambutol 1.2 g daily for 3–6 months	D
• Co-trimoxazole 2–3 tablets twice daily for 6 weeks	D
• Clarithromycin 250 mg twice daily and ethambutol 800 mg once daily for 2–6 months	D

Epidemiologic, clinical, and therapeutic pattern of *Mycobacterium marinum* infection: a retrospective series of 35 cases from southern France. Eberst E, Dereure O, Guillot B, Trento C, Terru D, van de Perre P, et al. J Am Acad Dermatol 2012; 66: e15–6.

Thirty-four of 35 (97%) had complete clearance of skin lesions with one course of oral antimicrobial therapy given over a period of 4 to 24 weeks (median 12.4 weeks). Single antibiotic therapy was successful in 25 patients. Fourteen of these received minocycline 200 mg daily, 5 patients received doxycycline 200 mg daily, and 6 clarithromycin 500 mg daily. Nine patients had dual antibiotic therapy using a combination of clarithromycin with doxycycline, minocycline, rifampicin, or ofloxacin.

Sixty-three cases of *Mycobacterium marinum* infection. Clinical features, treatment and antibiotic susceptibility of causative isolates. Aubry A, Chosidow O, Caumes E, Robert J, Cambau E. Arch Intern Med 2002; 162: 1746–5.

All patients were treated with antibiotics and 48% underwent surgery. Clarithromycin, doxycycline, and rifampicin were the most commonly prescribed antibiotics. Forty patients had drug combinations, commonly clarithromycin and rifampicin or tetracyclines, tetracyclines and rifampicin or ethambutol.

Soft tissue infections caused by marine bacterial pathogens: epidemiology, diagnosis, and management. Finkelstein R, Oren I. Curr Infect Dis Rep 2011; 13: 470–7.

The authors support the use of dual antibiotic therapy to reduce the risk of resistance while advocating monotherapy for limited superficial infection. Suggested recommended treatment regimens include rifampicin with ethambutol, clarithromycin with ethambutol, clarithromycin with minocycline, and clarithromycin or minocycline monotherapy. They suggest that antibiotics should be given for 3 or 4 months and treatment should be continued for 1 to 2 months after resolution of lesions to reduce the chance of relapse.

Atypical mycobacterial cutaneous infections in Hong Kong: 10 year retrospective study. Ho MH, Ho CK, Chong LY. Hong Kong Med J 2006; 12: 21–6.

Seventeen cases of *M. marinum* were identified over a 10-year period. Thirteen responded to treatment with oral tetracycline alone (9 minocycline and 4 doxycycline). Two patients had antituberculous drugs initially but were subsequently switched to minocycline. One patient had a combination of isoniazid, rifampicin, ethambutol, and minocycline. The average duration of treatment was 20 weeks. The authors recommend minocycline 100 mg twice daily as the treatment of choice.

Cutaneous non-tuberculous mycobacterial infections: a clinical and histopathological study of 17 cases from Lebanon. Abbas O, Marrouch N, Kattar MM, Zeynoun S, Kibbi AG, Rached RA, et al. J Eur Acad Dermatol Venereol 2011; 25: 33–42.

Ten out of 11 patients were successfully treated with either minocycline 100 mg twice a day (6 patients) or clarithromycin 500 mg twice a day monotherapy (4 patients). Patients were treated for an average of 4.8 months (range 3–8 months).

Second-Line Therapies

- Ciprofloxacin 500 mg + clarithromycin 250 mg twice daily for 4 months   E
- Rifabutin 600 mg + clarithromycin 500 mg twice daily + ciprofloxacin 500 mg twice daily for 4 months   E
- Azithromycin 500 mg three times a week for 2 months   E
- Lymecycline 150 mg daily for 55 days   E
- Rifampicin 450 mg daily, clarithromycin 500 mg twice daily, amikacin 400 mg intravenously once daily for 6 months   E

Successful treatment of refractory cutaneous infection caused by *Mycobacterium marinum* with a combined regimen containing amikacin. Huang Y, Xu X, Liu Y, Wu K, Zhang W, Liu P, et al. Clin Interv Aging 2012; 7: 533–8.

A rapidly progressive infection failing to respond to rifampicin, clarithromycin, and moxifloxacin settled promptly when the listed regimen containing amikacin.

Third-Line Therapies

- Simple excision   E
- Curettage and electrodesiccation   E   E
- Incision and drainage   E
- Heat therapy by gloves, hot water, or heated armlet   E
- Photodynamic therapy   E   E
- Cryotherapy   E
- Adjunctive anti-TNF-α inhibitors   E

Treatment of *Mycobacterium marinum* cutaneous infections. Rallis E, Koumantaki-Mathioudaki E. Expert Opin Pharmacother 2007; 8: 2965–78.

Review article. Surgical treatment may not be necessary or may even be contraindicated in some patients and should be reserved for cases with isolated superficial lesions that are nonresponsive to systemic therapy. Cryotherapy, electrodessication, photodynamic therapy, and local hyperthermic therapy have also been reported with some success.

Efficacy of oral minocycline and hyperthermic treatment in a case of atypical mycobacterial skin infection by *Mycobacterium marinum*. Hisamichi K, Hiruma M, Yamazaki M, Matsushita A, Ogawa H. J Dermatol 2002; 29: 810–1.

Minocycline 200 mg daily and local hyperthermic treatment (a disposable chemical pocket warmer) was used every evening for 5 to 6 hours over 2.5 months. Although there have been four cases in Japan where patients have been treated with hyperthermic treatment alone, the authors advocate it to be used in conjunction with minocycline.

Mycobacterium marinum infection cured by photodynamic therapy. Wiegell SR, Kongshoj B, Wulf HC. Arch Dermatol 2006; 142: 1241–2.

A patient intolerant of antibiotics was cured by treatment with methyl aminolevulinate applied for 3 hours, followed by illumination with 37 J/cm^2 of red light, undertaken once weekly for 3 weeks.

Possible role of anti-TNF monoclonal antibodies in the treatment of *Mycobacterium marinum* infection. Garzoni C, Adler S, Boller C, Furrer H, Villiger PM. Rheumatology 2010; 49: 1991–3.

A patient with PCR-confirmed *M. marinum* synovial infection of the foot was given triple combination therapy of ethambutol, clarithromycin, and rifampicin for 4 months. Clinical improvement was noted with the subsequent addition of infliximab 5 mg/kg/month.

Mycobacterium marinum infection of the hand and wrist. Cheung JP, Fung B, Wong SS, Ip WY. J Orthop Surg 2010; 18: 98–103.

In this review article the authors support the use of combination therapy with rifampicin, ethambutol, and clarithromycin for

M. marinum infection of the hand and wrist, which may be complicated by tenosynovitis leading to joint immobilization and contractures. They advocate surgical debridement for deep-seated infections.

MYCOBACTERIUM ULCERANS

Mycobacterium ulcerans (Buruli ulcer) is the third most common mycobacterial infection, after leprosy and tuberculosis, in immunocompetent hosts. It occurs most commonly in wetlands of tropical and subtropical countries (Africa and Australia). Children under 15 years of age are most commonly affected. After inoculation into the skin, *M. ulcerans* proliferates and produces a toxin, mycolactone, which enters the cells and causes necrosis of the dermis, panniculus, and deep fascia. Initially firm, painless nodules, papules, or plaques are seen. As the necrosis spreads, overlying ulceration develops over 1 or 2 months. The ulcers have a characteristic undermined edge and necrotic base. Although indolent in the majority, the ulcers can grow rapidly to more than 15 cm, with resultant extensive scarring and deformity. Up to 13% of patients may develop systemic involvement.

MANAGEMENT STRATEGY

There are anecdotal reports of spontaneous resolution of cutaneous *M. ulcerans* infection, but early treatment is recommended to limit disease progression and prevent contractures. The World Health Organization recommends *combination chemotherapy* with oral rifampicin and intramuscular streptomycin as first-line treatment. Adjunctive *surgical excision* may be required for necrotic or unhealed skin tissue. Antimicrobial therapy may reduce the extent of surgical excision. Recent combined therapy options contain oral preparations, which are easier to administer and show similar efficacy. There can be paradoxical clinical deterioration peaking around week 8 of antimicrobial therapy before subsequent improvement. This response does not indicate treatment failure and may be the result of temporary immunostimulation from antimicrobial treatment. Adequate wound care and the use of bed nets offer protection against *M. ulcerans* infections in endemic areas. Independent risk factors for relapse after surgery alone include incomplete excision, age under 16 years, leg edema, and plaque-like lesions before ulceration.

Smears from the necrotic base of ulcers often reveal clumps of acid-fast bacilli on Ziehl–Nielsen staining. Appropriately selected biopsy specimens that include the necrotic base and the undermined edge of lesions with subcutaneous tissue are nearly always diagnostic. Histology reveals necrosis of the deep dermis and panniculitis. Inflammatory cells are few, presumably due to the immunosuppressive activity of the toxin. With healing, there is a granulomatous response, and the ulcerated area is eventually replaced by a depressed scar, which may result in functional disability. *M. ulcerans* can be cultured from exudates or tissue fragments, but visible growth often requires 6 to 8 weeks, incubation at 33°C. PCR is quicker and has the highest sensitivity compared with microscopy, culture, and histopathology. For PCR, a 3-mm punch biopsy is the best sample for nonulcerative lesions, whereas a swab is best for ulcerative lesions.

Screening of all cases for coinfection with HIV is recommended in locations where the latter is endemic.

First-Line Therapies

- Oral rifampicin daily at 10 mg/kg and streptomycin intramuscularly at 15 mg/kg daily for 8 weeks **B**
- Rifampicin 10 mg/kg daily and clarithromycin 7.5 mg/kg twice daily for 8 weeks **B**
- Rifampicin 10 mg/kg/day and moxifloxacin 400 mg once daily for 8 weeks (for adults) **C**
- Adjunctive surgery with antibiotics **B**
- Wide surgical excision alone **B**
- Local heat (40°C) **C**

Treatment of *Mycobacterium ulcerans* disease (Buruli ulcer); guidance for health workers. World Health Organization, Switzerland, Geneva 2012. http://onlinelibrary.wiley.com/doi/10.1111/tmi.12342/full#tmi12342-bib-0040.

A nice review including advice on treatment. Rifampicin and streptomycin is recommended as standard treatment using the regimen noted earlier (although contraindicated in pregnancy). In Australia and French Guiana rifampicin is used with clarithromycin or moxifloxacin previously mentioned.

Antimicrobial treatment for early, limited *Mycobacterium ulcerans* infection: a randomised controlled trial. Nienhuis WA, Stienstra Y, Thompson WA, Awuah PC, Abass KM, Tuah W, et al. Lancet 2010; 375: 664–72.

In this open-label, randomized, multicenter trial, early lesions of *M. ulcerans* were treated with oral rifampicin 10 mg/kg/day and intramuscular streptomycin 15 mg/kg/day alone for 8 weeks or rifampicin and streptomycin for 4 weeks followed by oral rifampicin and clarithromycin 7.5 mg/kg/day for 4 weeks. Seventy-three patients (96%) in the former group and 68 (91%) in the latter had complete healing at 1 year with no recurrences. The authors recommend switching to oral clarithromycin at week 4 to limit the number of injections with streptomycin.

Clinical efficacy of combination of rifampin and streptomycin for treatment of *Mycobacterium ulcerans* disease. Sarfo FS, Phillips R, Asiedu K, Ampadu E, Bobi N, Adentwe E, et al. Antimicrob Agents Chemother 2010; 54: 3678–85.

A study of 160 patients with confirmed *M. ulcerans* infection treated with oral rifampicin 10 mg/kg/day and intramuscular streptomycin 15 mg/kg daily for 8 weeks. Ninety-five percent (152 patients) with early and late forms of disease responded to therapy without surgery. In eight cases, surgical excision followed by split-skin graft repair was carried out at week 8 due to progressive lesions or nonhealing lesions. Complete healing was achieved between 2 and 48 weeks. There were no recurrences in 158 (98%) of cases. Treatment was generally well tolerated. Two patients changed from streptomycin to oral moxifloxacin 400 mg daily due to nausea, vomiting, and dizziness.

Successful outcomes with oral fluoroquinolones combined with rifampicin in the treatment of *Mycobacterium ulcerans*: an observational cohort study. O'Brien DP, McDonald A, Callan P, Robson M, Friedman ND, Hughes A, et al. PLoS Negl Trop Dis 2012; 6: e1473.

A prospective study of 147 cases: 47 had surgery alone with 30% treatment failure, 90 had combined surgical and medical treatment with no treatment failure. In the latter group, rifampicin and ciprofloxacin were used in 61% of patients and rifampicin and clarithromycin in 23% of cases. There was no evident difference in clinical efficacy between antibiotic regimens. Paradoxical reactions were seen in eight (9%) of the antibiotic-treated cases.

Effect of a control project on clinical profiles and outcomes in Buruli ulcer: a before/after study in Bas-Congo, Democratic Republic of Congo. Phanzu DM, Suykerbuyk P, Imposo DB, Lukanu PN, Minuku JB, Lehman LF, et al. PLoS Negl Trop Dis 2011; 5: e1402.

A prospective observational study in Congo comparing clinical outcomes of patients admitted with *M. ulcerans* ulcers. Between 2004 and 2007, 64 patients were treated with surgery alone resulting in healing in 48 patients; 15 patients were left with disability; 12 patients died due to sepsis. Between 2005 and 2007, 107/190 patients were treated with rifampicin and streptomycin. The majority of these patients were also treated with surgery. In this group, healing occurred in 176 of 190 patients, 37 were left with functional disability, and death occurred in 6 patients. Sepsis, malnutrition and anemia, and postsurgical shock were reported causes of fatality.

Histopathological changes and clinical responses of Buruli ulcer plaque lesions during chemotherapy: a role for surgical removal of necrotic tissue? Ruf MT, Sopoh GE, Brun LV, Dossou AD, Barogui YT, Johnson RC, et al. PLoS Negl Trop Dis 2011; 5: e1334.

Of the 12 patients in the study, 9 were treated with limited surgical excision of necrotic tissues followed by skin grafting between 7 and 39 days after antimicrobial therapy. Surgical excision was not required in 3 of the 12 patients.

Pretreatment with antibiotics limits the extent of surgical excision required and thereby reduces post-treatment morbidity.

Phase change material for thermotherapy of Buruli ulcer: a prospective observational single center proof-of-principle trial. Junghanss T, Um Boock A, Vogel M, Schuette D, Weinlaeder H, Pluschke G. PLoS Negl Trop Dis 2009; 3: e380.

In this series, six patients with confirmed ulcerative Buruli lesions received thermotherapy for 28 to 31 days in lesions less than 2 cm (three patients) and 50 to 55 days in lesions equal to or larger than 2 cm (three patients). All had good outcomes with no recurrences 18 months after therapy.

MYCOBACTERIUM KANSASII

This organism most commonly causes pulmonary disease; skin lesions are rare. Most reported cases have occurred in immunocompromised subjects. The gross morphology of such lesions varies greatly and can be verrucous, nodular, pustular, ulcerated, or sporotrichoid. Cutaneous lesions may progress slowly or run an acute course.

MANAGEMENT STRATEGY

Although conventional combination chemotherapy with *antituberculous drugs* is effective, the choice of treatment should be determined by in vitro sensitivity. Resolution of *M. kansasii* infection has been reported after antiretroviral medication for HIV.

Lesions caused by *M. kansasii* may yield a variety of histopathologic features. They may be granulomatous in the chronic

form or show necrosis with an intense inflammatory infiltrate composed of polymorphonuclear cells in the more acute form. The organisms grow best on Lowenstein–Jensen culture medium at 37°C.

First-Line Therapies	
• Combination of antituberculous drugs for 6–18 months	D
• Antituberculous drugs with intramuscular kanamycin 500 mg three times a week for 3 months	E
• Minocycline 100–200 mg daily for 16 weeks	E
• Erythromycin 2 g daily for 6 months	E

Current treatment of nontuberculous mycobacteriosis: an update. Esteban J, García-Pedrazuela M, Muñoz-Egea MC, Alcaide F. Expert Opin Pharmacother 2012; 13: 967–86.

In this review the authors recommend isoniazid, rifampicin, and ethambutol for 18 months with at least 12 months of negative cultures. They conclude that there is a 6.9% risk of relapse with a 12-month multidrug regimen. In cases of resistance or adverse reactions, they recommend a 3-month course of streptomycin or amikacin followed by intermittent therapy with one of these drugs. Alternative treatments include clarithromycin, levofloxacin and moxifloxacin, and linezolid.

***Mycobacterium kansasii* infection presenting as cellulitis in a patient with systemic lupus erythematosus.** Hsu PY, Yang YH, Hsiao CH, Lee PI, Chiang BL. Formos Med Assoc 2002; 101: 581–4.

In this case report the authors describe successful treatment of *M. kansasii* infection with rifampicin 600 mg daily, clarithromycin 500 mg twice a day, isoniazid 300 mg daily, and ethambutol 1200 g daily for total of 1 year in a patient with known systemic lupus erythematosus (SLE).

Primary cutaneous *Mycobacterium kansasii* infection in a child. Chaves A, Torrelo A, Mediero IG, Menéndez-Rivas M, Ortega Calderón A, Zambrano A. J Pediatr Dermatol 2001; 18: 131–4.

A case of *M. kansasii* infection in the elbow of an immunocompetent 6-year-old girl treated successfully with surgical excision and a 5-month course of erythromycin 50 mg/kg/day.

RAPIDLY GROWING MYCOBACTERIA

Mycobacterium fortuitum, Mycobacterium chelonae, and *Mycobacterium abscessus* are environmental pathogens also known as *rapidly growing mycobacteria (RGM)*, so termed because colonies are visible to the naked eye within 7 days of culture. Cutaneous lesions due to these pathogens usually occur after surgery, percutaneous catheter insertion, or accidental inoculation. Dark red nodules develop, with abscess formation and clear fluid drainage. Disseminated disease occurs most commonly in immunosuppressed hosts.

MANAGEMENT STRATEGY

RGM should be individually identified and in vitro sensitivity tests performed before treatment. *M. fortuitum* and *M. chelonae* are resistant to most antituberculous drugs except kanamycin and amikacin. *M. fortuitum* may also be susceptible to cefoxitin, ciprofloxacin, and imipenem. *M. abscessus* is usually sensitive to amikacin, cefoxitin, and clarithromycin. Tobramycin and clarithromycin are more effective than amikacin in the treatment of *M. chelonae*. The wide variability in antibiotic sensitivity means that each case must be considered individually. For persistent nonhealing cutaneous lesions, wide excisional surgery with delayed closure or skin grafting can be undertaken. The duration of therapy can vary from 6 weeks to 7 months and is dictated by clinical and microbiological response.

Histology reveals polymorphonuclear microabscess and granuloma formation with foreign body–type giant cells. Acid-fast bacilli may be demonstrated in the microabscesses. Diagnosis is usually confirmed by culture. PCR systems can also be used for diagnosis and species identification in selected cases.

First-Line Therapies

Mycobacterium chelonae

- Clarithromycin 500 mg twice a day for 3–8 months ± surgery — **C**
- Azithromycin 250 mg daily for at least 6 months — **E**
- Clarithromycin as part of dual or triple therapy with ciprofloxacin, tobramycin, and tigecycline — **E**

Systematic review of tattoo-associated skin infection with rapidly growing mycobacteria and public health investigation of a cluster in Scotland 2010. Conaglen PD, Laurenson IF, Sergeant A, Thorn SN, Rayner A, Stevenson J. Euro Surveill 2013; 18: 20553.

This article summarizes 25 previous reports (142 cases), from 11 countries, published between 2003 and 2012, of RGM infection associated with tattoos. Causative agents included *M. chelonae* (most frequently), *M. abscessus*, and *M. fortuitum*, among others. Spontaneous resolution was documented in several cases; others generally responded to a diverse range of antibiotics, including macrolides and tetracyclines, used alone or in combination, with surgery being required for nine cases in one report.

Clinical management of rapidly growing mycobacterial cutaneous infections in patients after mesotherapy. Regnier S, Cambau E, Meningaud JP, Guihot A, Deforges L, Carbonne A, et al. Clin Infect Dis 2009; 49: 1358–64.

Sixteen patients were diagnosed with cutaneous infection due to RGM after an outbreak after mesotherapy in France. *M. chelonae* was identified in 11 patients and *M. frederiksbergense* in 2 patients. Patients were treated with drug regimens containing clarithromycin. Six received triple therapy initially, and 8 received dual therapy. Fourteen received clarithromycin 1 to 2 g/day, 6 received intravenous tobramycin 3 mg/kg/day, 14 received ciprofloxacin 500 mg twice a day, and 6 received intravenous tigecycline initially at 100 mg followed by 50 mg/day. Patients were treated for a mean duration of 14 weeks (range 1–24 weeks), with time to healing estimated at 6.2 months (range 1–15 months). Success was noted in all but one patient.

First-Line Therapies

Mycobacterium fortuitum

- Clarithromycin 500 mg twice a day and levofloxacin 500 mg twice a day for 3–6 months — **B**
- Clarithromycin 250–500 mg twice a day ± intramuscular amikacin 250 mg three times a week for 3–6 months — **C**
- Ciprofloxacin 500 mg twice a day for 3–6 months — **C**
- Ciprofloxacin 500 mg twice a day, clarithromycin 500 mg twice a day, and amoxicillin–clavulanic acid 500 mg twice a day for 6 weeks — **E**
- Co-trimoxazole 800/160 mg twice a day, clarithromycin 500 mg twice a day, and amoxicillin–clavulanic acid 500 mg twice a day for 6 weeks — **E**
- Levofloxacin 300 mg daily — **E**
- Trimethoprim — **D**

An outbreak of *Mycobacterium fortuitum* cutaneous infection associated with mesotherapy. Quiñones C, Ramalle-Gómara E, Perucha M, Lezaun ME, Fernández-Vilariño E, García-Morrás P, et al. J Eur Acad Dermatol Venereol 2010; 24: 604–6.

Thirty-nine patients were suspected of having cutaneous *M. fortuitum* infection after mesotherapy in a beauty clinic. Twelve had culture-confirmed *M. fortuitum*. All were successfully treated with clarithromycin 500 mg twice a day and levofloxacin 500 mg daily for 3 to 6 months. Two underwent excision of localized lesions.

Cutaneous infection with *Mycobacterium fortuitum* after localized microinjections (mesotherapy) treated successfully with a triple drug regimen. Nagore E, Ramos P, Botella-Estrada R, Ramos-Níguez JA, Sanmartín O, Castejón P. Acta Derm Venereol 2001; 81: 291–3.

One case received a combination of ciprofloxacin 500 mg twice a day, clarithromycin 500 mg twice a day, and amoxicillin–clavulanic acid 500 mg twice a day for 6 weeks. One received treatment with clarithromycin, cotrimoxazole 800/160 mg twice a day, and amoxicillin–clavulanic acid. The third was given ciprofloxacin 500 mg twice a day, clarithromycin 500 mg twice a day, and co-trimoxazole 800/160 mg twice a day for 3 weeks followed by clarithromycin 500 mg twice a day. All lesions healed within 2 to 6 weeks.

Successful treatment of a widespread cutaneous *Mycobacterium fortuitum* infection with levofloxacin. Nakagawa K, Tsuruta D, Ishii M. Int J Dermatol 2006; 45: 1098–9.

An immunocompromised patient treated successfully with levofloxacin 300 mg daily. Duration not specified.

First-Line Therapies

Mycobacterium abscessus

- Clarithromycin 1 g/day for adults and 0.5 g/day for children for 3–6 months + adjunctive surgery — **B**
- Clarithromycin 250 mg twice a day + moxifloxacin 400 mg daily for 4–5 months — **B**
- Clarithromycin 250–500 mg twice a day ± intramuscular amikacin 250 mg three times a week for 3–6 months — **B**
- Multiple antibiotic therapy + adjunctive interferon-γ for refractory lesions — **E**

Evidence Levels: **A** Double-blind study **B** Clinical trial ≥ 20 subjects **C** Clinical trial < 20 subjects **D** Series ≥ 5 subjects **E** Anecdotal case reports

Report on an outbreak of postinjection abscesses due to *Mycobacterium abscessus*, **including management with surgery and clarithromycin therapy and comparison of strains by random amplified polymorphic DNA polymerase chain reaction.** Villanueva A, Calderon RV, Vargas BA, Ruiz F, Aguero S, Zhang Y, et al. Clin Infect Dis 1997; 24: 1147–53.

A cohort of 350 patients was clinically diagnosed with *M. abscessus* infections after an outbreak in a physician's office in Columbia (205 cases culture confirmed). Patients received either surgery alone or clarithromycin alone or combination of drugs and surgery. Of 35 patients treated with clarithromycin alone, 8 patients were cured (23%). Of 22 patients treated with surgical resection alone, 7 were cured (32%). Of 148 patients treated with combined surgery and clarithromycin, 140 were cured (95%). Clarithromycin was given at a dose of 1 g/day in adults and 0.5 g/day in children for 3 to 6 months.

Clarithromycin and amikacin vs. clarithromycin and moxifloxacin for the treatment of postacupuncture cutaneous infections due to *Mycobacterium abscessus*: **a prospective observational study.** Choi WS, Kim MJ, Park DW, Son SW, Yoon YK, Song T, et al. Clin Microbiol Infect 2011; 17: 1084–90.

A series of 52 patients with *M. abscessus* infection after acupuncture. Thirty-three were treated with oral clarithromycin 250 mg twice a day plus intramuscular amikacin 250 mg three times a week, and 19 were treated with oral clarithromycin 250 mg twice a day plus oral moxifloxacin 400 mg daily. The median time to resolution of lesions in the clarithromycin plus moxifloxacin-treated group was significantly shorter (17 vs. 20 weeks, respectively, $p = 0.017$).

Treatment of refractory disseminated *Mycobacterium abscessus* **infection with interferon gamma therapy.** Colsky AS, Hanly A, Elgart Kerdel FA. Arch Dermatol 1999; 135: 125–7.

Successful treatment of *M. abscessus* infection not responding to combination antibiotic therapy with kanamycin, cefotaxime, and clarithromycin given for 3 months, after adjunctive interferon-γ 50 μg/m² subcutaneously three times a week for 7 months.

Mycosis fungoides and Sézary syndrome

Pierluigi Porcu, Henry K. Wong

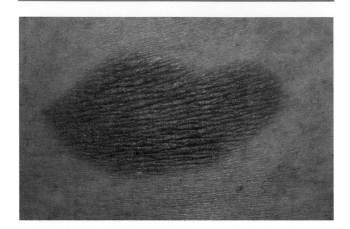

Mycosis fungoides (MF) and Sézary syndrome (SS) are the most common subtypes of cutaneous T-cell lymphoma (CTCL), a heterogeneous group of extranodal non-Hodgkin lymphomas (NHLs) of the skin that includes the CD30-positive lymphoproliferative disorders. The identity of the T-cell subset and the specific immune compartment (blood, skin, or lymph nodes) initially targeted by the transforming event in CTCL are not known. The tumor cell in MF is a mature, CD45RO+, CD4+, CLA+, skin-homing, effector memory T-cell lacking CCR7. In Sézary syndrome, the phenotype is a mature CD4+ T cell with the CCR7 central memory variant. Functional studies of T cells from patient samples have provided valuable insight into the pathogenesis and clinical aspects of MF. Decreased production of cytokines such as interferon (IFN) and IL-12, upregulation of inhibitory molecules such as CTLA-4 and PD1, and a diminished T-cell immune repertoire contribute to an increased risk of infections and of secondary malignancies. Highly selective skin trafficking, mediated by the chemokine receptors CCR4 and CCR10, target the skin across all stages of MF, even though tumor cells can be detected with highly sensitive methods in the blood and the lymph nodes. Finally, in the advanced stage of MF and SS, the presence of extensive gene mutations, complex chromosomal abnormalities, aberrant gene expression, unresponsiveness to growth-inhibitory signals, and defective apoptosis can drive the transformation into a highly aggressive and lethal malignancy.

MF accounts for 65% to 75% of all CTCL cases. It usually presents in the fifth to sixth decade, but can affect all ages, and is more common in males. The course tends to be more aggressive in African Americans. The current best estimate for the number of new MF cases in the United States is about 3000/year. Prevalence is much higher, due to the long survival.

MANAGEMENT STRATEGY

An effective treatment strategy depends on making an accurate and prompt diagnosis, which in early-stage MF can be challenging. The key histologic finding is epidermal invasion by atypical lymphoid cells with a convoluted "cerebriform" nucleus on histopathology in the proper clinical context. The International Society of Cutaneous Lymphomas (ISCL) has developed consensus standards for diagnosis based on a four-point scale, which is grounded on clinical, pathologic, and immunophenotypic criteria. Although imperfect, these consensus criteria should increase concordance in clinical practice and treatment recommendations. Often, multiple visits and skin biopsies are needed during the evolution of MF before the distinctive histologic features appear and the consensus ISCL standards for a diagnosis of MF are reached.

Once diagnosis is confirmed, determining the clinical stage is important in the decision process for treatment. Staging aims at defining the specific sites of involvement and the overall disease burden for each patient, drives the management strategy, and predicts outcomes. The current staging system for MF and SS is the product of a joint effort of the ISCL and the European Organisation for Research and Treatment of Cancer (EORTC). This system, built on the original TNM classification developed by the U.S. National Cancer Institute in 1979, includes assessment of the peripheral blood compartment—hence TNMB—and allows optimal definition of SS and stratification of patients for clinical trials. This staging requires the integration of clinical findings and laboratory assays, such as flow cytometry and T-cell receptor (TCR) gene clonality analysis, that may not always be available and whose interpretation can be affected by confounding factors. Based on this classification, for clinical purposes, for decisions on treatment and discussion of survival, patients can be divided into "early stage" (IA–IIA) or "advanced stage" (IIB–IVB), with very different progression and survival rates.

MF typically demonstrates slow and predictable clinical progression, which can very often be inferred by the behavior and evolution of the lesions in the skin. Although many cases can be treated conservatively using skin-directed therapies, without resorting to systemic therapy, and enjoy a normal lifespan, a subset experience incomplete clearance and progress to more advanced stages with significant morbidity and mortality. Because MF is an indolent malignancy for most patients, long-term outcome studies based on large patient populations are required to estimate true rates of disease relapse, progression, transformation, and survival. Recent publications have addressed this need and offer a better assessment of the natural history of MF and SS.

Patients with MF should ideally be managed by a multidisciplinary team, including a dermatologist, a medical oncologist, a dermatopathologist familiar with skin lymphoma, and a radiation oncologist. The availability of nursing staff with expertise in dealing with skin care and skin malignancies is also desirable. This approach minimizes management errors and increases patient satisfaction. An initial consultation at a cancer center with an experienced cutaneous lymphoma team should be strongly considered. Finally, optimal patient support and education are paramount for an effective treatment strategy, and new patients should be encouraged to contact patient advocacy organizations that provide those resources.

Treatment objectives depend on the stage at diagnosis. For patients presenting with early-stage MF (IA–IIA), the goals are to control symptoms, clearing all visible disease in the skin; to slow or prevent progression; and to minimize distress, costs, and side effects. Avoidance of immunosuppressive therapies is a key objective. In a few patients, this can be achieved with minimal topical therapy (steroids). In most patients, however, this will require a coordinated effort and a sequence of skin-directed treatments to induce, and then maintain, a clinical response. Finally, in some patients, this objective will only be achieved with combinations of skin-directed and systemic therapies. Early studies have demonstrated that traditional cytotoxic chemotherapy, such

Evidence Levels: A Double-blind study   B Clinical trial ≥ 20 subjects   C Clinical trial < 20 subjects   D Series ≥ 5 subjects   E Anecdotal case reports

as CHOP, does not improve survival compared with conservative skin-directed treatment regardless of stage of disease.

With many modalities available for skin-directed and systemic therapy, there are often several options for disease management, and the strategy for each patient may depend on the availability and accessibility of specific treatments. The goal is to initiate a treatment plan that the patient can adhere to reliably, to induce clinical response. Whether a cure is achievable in early-stage MF remains debatable. Nevertheless there are occasional patients who do not have recurrence of the disease after 5 to 10 years or longer. In most cases the disease recurs at some later point, with lesions often reappearing in the skin as patches or plaques, which often respond again to skin-directed treatments. Reinstitution of treatments that were previously effective is a wise and effective approach to patients with early-stage MF and is currently recommended in the NCCN guidelines.

In stage I MF, response may occasionally be achieved with *emollients*, but often *potent topical corticosteroids* are necessary. Other skin-directed therapies may be effective as monotherapy. These include *topical chemotherapy, retinoids, or phototherapy*. Phototherapy (UVB, UVA) or *photochemotherapy (PUVA)* is effective and can clear involved areas. In poorly responsive disease, combination treatment with topical and phototherapy may yield greater response. As disease stage advances, treatment strategy should adapt to reflect the disease velocity and burden. Applying more potent therapy can produce a complete response, but the chance of a complete response is reduced.

In stage II MF, achieving a clinical response is a higher priority based on reduced survival of patients in this group; thus combining a systemic therapy with skin-directed therapy leads to a higher likelihood of response. Many patients will respond to combinations of topical treatment as before with *NBUVB* or *PUVA*. Also the addition of a systemic agent is beneficial in regimens such as *PUVA plus retinoids* or *PUVA plus interferon-α_{2a}*. Local radiotherapy is very effective at controlling persistent plaques or tumors, and *total skin electron beam (TSEB)* therapy is a good option when skin involvement is widespread and refractory to other approaches. *Topical chemotherapy (nitrogen mustard)* may still be effective.

For patients with advanced-stage MF (IIB–IVB) the goal of therapy is to induce remission, avoid any further reduction of immune competence, and prevent infections. Inability to realize these goals is likely to result in further disease progression, severe morbidity, and death. In these patients, treatment decisions are complex, and highly effective options for therapy remain limited.

Due to the natural history of MF, with multiple relapses and gradual progression over many years from limited (IA) to extensive (IB) patch/plaque disease, by the time patients have developed advanced-stage (IIB–IVB) disease they are likely to have been exposed to combined skin-directed and systemic therapy, most frequently *interferons* and *bexarotene*. Thus very few patients with advanced-stage MF are systemic therapy naïve, and the concept of "first-line" versus "second-line" choice may not easily apply. The best examples of chemo-naïve CTCL patients are those with tumor stage d'emblée and patients with SS. In all other cases, progression is subtle and does not occur en bloc. Patients have a gradation of skin lesions, exhibiting differential response to the ongoing therapy. The initial management of advanced-stage MF often focuses on strategies aimed at buttressing the existing treatment plan, rather than drastically changing direction. Skin-directed therapy is generally continued because most patients have areas of persistent patch/plaque disease that need to be optimally controlled. Likewise, some of the systemic drugs in use at the time of progression may be continued if there is evidence of residual, if inadequate, activity and they are well tolerated.

Older front-line drugs (*bexarotene, interferons*), shown to be effective in advanced-stage MF, are now being used in the treatment of earlier stages, in combination with skin-directed therapies, and newer drugs (*vorinostat, romidepsin*) are increasingly being introduced as primary choices in patients who progress from early to advanced-stage resistant disease. The drug *denileukin diftitox* is no longer available from the manufacturer in the United States, although a substitute drug may become available in the future.

Patients with SS may be stage III to IVB. These patients present a particularly challenging problem due to drug resistance; severe, often intractable, pruritus; greater risk of infections; and difficulty with venous access, which may be required for infusional therapy, photopheresis, and disease monitoring. For patients with low tumor burden, *extracorporeal photopheresis (ECP)* can be effective, although durable complete responses are not common and its effect on survival is unclear. More frequently, patients with SS require combined modality therapy with *bexarotene, interferons*, and *ECP* (see article by Raphael et al.). Chemotherapy should rarely be used in the management of SS.

In stage IV MF outcomes are generally poor, regardless of the treatment. Incomplete response and quick relapses after treatment are the rule. *CHOP* and similar combination chemotherapy regimens can be used for patients who may need rapid debulking, followed by more effective long-term strategies, such as *allogeneic hematopoietic stem cell transplant. Local radiotherapy* is useful for bulky nodal disease and symptomatic skin lesions. Effective palliation requires consideration of symptoms such as nausea, constipation, pain, anorexia, infections, pruritus, and depression.

Specific Investigations

- Adequate skin biopsy reviewed by a pathologist with expertise in cutaneous lymphoma. Immunophenotype and TCR gene analysis are recommended, but not essential
- Complete physical examination, with assessment of % body surface area (BSA) and degree of pruritus
- Comprehensive metabolic panel, LDH, hematology, differential white blood cell count, Sézary cell count (if available), or peripheral blood flow cytometry (preferred) and TCR gene analysis if flow is abnormal or SS is suspected
- Imaging with CT or PET-CT scans is recommended in patients with tumor lesions and palpable lymph nodes
- Lymph node biopsy with histology, immunophenotype, and TCR gene analysis, if enlarged
- HTLV-1 serology in populations at risk

The diagnostic studies and initial clinical assessment in patients with MF can be complex. In the United States, the NCCN publishes guidelines for the diagnosis and therapy of MF and SS. Similar guidelines are produced by the European Society of Medical Oncology (ESMO) and other national societies in Europe. The NCCN guidelines are updated annually and represent the consensus view of a panel that includes dermatologists, medical oncologists, radiation oncologists, and pathologists. The NCCN guidelines suggest a combination of essential and nonessential investigations, which the treating physician can select as clinically indicated in individual patients.

Many of the clinical assessment tools and laboratory investigations have been recently reviewed and integrated into new clinical end points and response criteria for MF, through a collaborative effort of the ISCL, EORTC, and the United States Cutaneous Lymphoma Consortium (USCLC).

Defining early mycosis fungoides. Pimpinelli N, Olsen EA, Santucci M, Vonderheid E, Haeffner AC, Stevens S, et al. J Am Acad Dermatol 2005; 53: 1053–63.

Revisions to the staging and classification of mycosis fungoides and Sézary syndrome: a proposal of the International Society for Cutaneous Lymphomas (ISCL) and the cutaneous lymphoma task force of the European Organisation of Research and Treatment of Cancer (EORTC). Olsen E, Vonderheid E, Pimpinelli N, Willemze R, Kim Y, Knobler R, et al. Blood 2007; 110: 1713–22.

These papers describe a consensus approach to the diagnosis and clinical staging of MF/SS. These focus on MF/SS and exclude other types of CTCL and the cutaneous B-cell lymphomas (CBCL), which are staged differently. Several retrospective studies of the applicability of the ISCL criteria have been published, and they support their validity across different patient populations. The two largest studies by Agar et al. and Talpur et al. are discussed later.

Clinical end points and response criteria in mycosis fungoides and Sézary syndrome: a consensus statement of the International Society for Cutaneous Lymphomas (ISCL), the United States Cutaneous Lymphoma Consortium (USCLC), and the Cutaneous Lymphoma Task Force of the European Organisation for Research and Treatment of Cancer (EORTC). Olsen EA, Whittaker S, Kim YH, Duvic M, Prince HM, Lessin SR, et al. J Clin Oncol 2011; 29: 2598–607.

This paper, together with the earlier one (2007) by Olsen et al., provides a complete set of guidelines and rules not only to diagnose and stage disease in MF/SS, but also to assess responses to treatment. Standardized response criteria are absolutely essential for clinical trials and to facilitate communication among physicians from different institutions.

Survival outcomes and prognostic factors in mycosis fungoides/Sézary syndrome: validation of the revised International Society for Cutaneous Lymphomas/European Organisation for Research and Treatment of Cancer staging proposal. Agar NS, Wedgeworth E, Crichton S, Mitchell TJ, Cox M, Ferreira S, et al. J Clin Oncol 2010; 28: 4730–9.

A multicenter cohort of 1502 British CTCL patients observed over 1980 to 2009 and classified according to the current ISCL/ EORTC criteria. The large size and the long-term follow-up allowed a better estimate of rates of progression (34%) and disease-specific mortality (26%). These rates suggest that long-term morbidity and mortality may be greater than expected. The rate of progression in patients with stage IA and IB at 20 years may be higher than previously recognized (18% and 47%, respectively). Furthermore, a significant difference in survival and progression was noted for patients with early-stage disease having patches alone (T1a/T2a) compared with those having patches and plaques (T1b/T2b). Multivariate analysis also showed that advanced skin (T) stage, presence of the tumor clone in the peripheral blood without Sézary cells (B0b), increased LDH, and folliculotropic MF were independent predictors of survival and progression.

Long-term outcomes of 1,263 patients with mycosis fungoides and Sézary syndrome from 1982 to 2009. Talpur R, Singh L, Daulat S, Liu P, Seyfer S, Trynosky T, et al. Clin Cancer Res 2012; 18: 5051–60.

A cohort of patients at the MD Anderson Cancer Center between 1982 and 2009, mean age at diagnosis ~55 years, ~71% with early stage. Disease progression for early-stage patients (12%) and disease-specific mortality for the entire cohort (8.1%)

were lower than those observed by Agar et al. Risk factors associated with progression or deaths were advanced age, plaque stage, LDH, and tumor area.

Second lymphomas and other malignant neoplasms in patients with mycosis fungoides and Sézary syndrome: evidence from population-based and clinical cohorts. Huang KP, Weinstock MA, Clarke CA, McMillan A, Hoppe RT, Kim YH. Arch Dermatol 2007; 143: 45–50.

This study analyzed Stanford (1973–2001) and SEER-9 registry data (1984–2001) for a cumulative population of >2200 patients and estimated relative risk for various malignancies, excluding nonmelanoma skin cancers, by using the standardized incidence ratio (SIR). In both cohorts there was a very significant increase in the risk of Hodgkin lymphoma. The risk of non-Hodgkin lymphoma was increased in the SEER-9 cohort. Cumulative incidence of second malignancies in the Stanford cohort was estimated to be 10% at 8.6 years. Therefore updated SEER (population based) and Stanford (clinic based) data confirm increased risk of lymphoma in patients with MF/SS.

A look at the National Comprehensive Cancer Network guidelines for cutaneous lymphomas. Porcu P. Clin Lymphoma Myeloma Leuk 2010; 10(Suppl. 2): S109–11.

This article highlights the importance of a multidisciplinary approach in the management of MF/SS and the general strategy of gradual escalation of systemic therapy, leaving cytotoxic drugs for later. In addition, the strategy of "looping back" is integral to the NCCN guidelines. This concept is based on the observation that disease relapse or progression in MF/SS does not necessarily imply advancement to a higher stage (i.e., from T1 to T2, or T3). Rather, patients who start with T1 disease and achieve remission may relapse back to T1 disease.

First-Line Therapies	
Early stage (IA–IIA)	
• Emollients	E
• Topical corticosteroids	B
• UVB or PUVA	B
• Excimer 308-nm laser	D
• Photodynamic therapy	D
• Imiquimod 5% cream	D
• Topical chemotherapy	B
• Local radiotherapy	B
• Topical bexarotene and other retinoids	B
Advanced stage (IIB–IVB)	
• Oral bexarotene and other retinoids	B
• Interferons	B
• Extracorporeal photopheresis (ECP)	B
• Low-dose methotrexate	B
• PUVA ± retinoids	C
• PUVA ± interferons	C
• Denileukin diftitox	A

Topical steroids for mycosis fungoides – experience in 79 patients. Zackheim HS, Kashani-Sabet M, Smita A. Arch Dermatol 1998; 134: 949–54.

Topical corticosteroids are a safe first-line treatment. However, if there is poor clinical response and worsening of the disease,

Evidence Levels: **A** Double-blind study **B** Clinical trial ≥ 20 subjects **C** Clinical trial < 20 subjects **D** Series ≥ 5 subjects **E** Anecdotal case reports

then additional treatment is valuable. Steroids are most often effective for the poikilodermatous variant of MF. Thicker lesions are often less responsive and benefit from additional skin-directed treatment.

Long-term follow-up of patients with early-stage cutaneous T-cell lymphoma who achieved complete remission with psoralen plus UV-A monotherapy. Querfeld C, Rosen ST, Kuzel TM, Kirby KA, Roenigk HH, Prinz BM, et al. Arch Dermatol 2005; 141: 305–11.

A single-center analysis of patients with early MF who achieved long-term remission with PUVA. Sixty-six of 104 patients with clinical stages IA to IIA MF achieved complete remission (CR) after PUVA monotherapy between 1979 and 1995. The long-term survival rates at 5, 10, and 15 years were 94%, 82%, and 82%, respectively, in patients with stage IA, and 80%, 69%, and 58% in patients with stage IB/IIA. The major complication from PUVA was that one third of the patients developed signs of chronic photodamage and secondary cutaneous malignancies.

PUVA is an effective treatment for MF capable of inducing long-term remissions and perhaps, in some cases, "cure."

Narrowband UVB and psoralen-UVA in the treatment of early-stage mycosis fungoides: a retrospective study. Diederen PV, van Weelden H, Sanders CJ, Toonstra J, van Vloten WA. J Am Acad Dermatol 2003; 48: 215–9.

A retrospective study comparing NBUVB and PUVA examining response to treatment, relapse-free interval, and irradiation dose in 56 patients with stage IA and IB MF. A total of 21 patients were treated with narrowband UVB (311 nm); 35 were treated with PUVA. Narrowband UVB led to complete remission in 17 (81%) and partial remission in 4 (19%), and none showed progressive disease. PUVA treatment led to complete remission in 25 (71%) and partial remission in 10 (29%), and none showed progressive disease. Thus NBUVB is effective for patients with early-stage MF.

Monochromatic excimer light (308 nm) in patch-stage IA mycosis fungoides. Mori M, Campolmi P, Mavilia L, Rossi R, Cappugi P, Pimpinelli N. J Am Acad Dermatol 2004; 50: 943–5.

This was effective in the treatment of patch stage IA MF. The authors treated seven patch lesions in four patients with unequivocal diagnosis of MF. All lesions achieved complete clinical and histologic remission. The total dose ranged from 5 to 9.3 J/cm^2 (mean 7.1 J/cm^2; median 7 J/cm^2), and remission was maintained with a follow-up of 3 to 28 months without significant side effects reported.

Photodynamic therapy with methyl-aminolaevulinic acid for mycosis fungoides. Kim ST, Kang DY, Kang JS, Baek JW, Jeon YS, Suh KS. Acta Derm Venereol 2012; 92: 264–8.

Ten patients received two sessions of PDT at 1-week intervals. Five showed complete response on biopsy, and two showed partial responses. During follow-up (8–31 months), six of the seven patients remained in stable remission. For patients with limited skin involvement, likely <5%, PDT may be an alternative option to consider.

Treatment of patch and plaque stage mycosis fungoides with imiquimod 5% cream. Deeths MJ, Chapman JT, Dellavalle RP, Zeng C, Aeling JL. J Am Acad Dermatol 2005; 52: 275–80.

This treatment showed safety and efficacy in patch and plaque stage MF in six patients, stage IA to IIB, using topical imiquimod 5% cream three times per week for 12 weeks in an open-label pilot study. After response with biopsies pretreatment and posttreatment, there was a 50% response with histologic clearance of

disease in index lesions. Irritation at the application site was seen in patients responding to treatment.

Long-term efficacy, curative potential, and carcinogenicity of topical mechlorethamine chemotherapy in cutaneous T cell lymphoma. Vonderheid EC, Tan ET, Kantor AF, Shrager L, Micaily B, Van-Scott EJ. J Am Acad Dermatol 1989; 20: 416–28.

A retrospective review of 331 patients, 195 with initial complete response with stage I to IVA. Of these patients, 65 had remission greater than 4 years, and 35 greater than 8 years. Complete responses lasting more than 8 years were also described in nine patients with stage II/III. Patients often continued maintenance therapy for an average of 3 years. Risks of nitrogen mustard include sensitization to the application, squamous and basal cell carcinoma, Hodgkin disease, and colon cancer.

Topical mechlorethamine (nitrogen mustard), 10 mg in 60 mL water, or as ointment, is effective in stage I and II MF. As with phototherapy, earlier-stage disease responds more quickly and for longer. Topical carmustine (BCNU) is also effective and causes less contact allergic dermatitis, but each treatment is limited to 3 to 4 weeks because of the risk of myelosuppression, which may be cumulative.

Phase 1 and 2 trial of bexarotene gel for skin-directed treatment of patients with cutaneous T-cell lymphoma. Breneman D, Duvic M, Kuzel T, Yocum R, Truglia J, Stevens VJ. Arch Dermatol 2002; 138: 325–32.

Sixty-seven patients with stage IA to IIA CTCL used this topical retinoid in incremental doses. There was a 21% complete response and 42% partial response. The median time to relapse was 23 months.

Topical 1% bexarotene gel has been approved by the Food and Drug Administration (FDA) for refractory or persistent stage IA to IIA MF. Local irritation can occur, particularly with increased frequency of application. Treatment is initially applied on alternate days, increasing gradually to a maximum of four times daily.

Comparison of pegylated interferon α-2b plus psoralen PUVA versus standard interferon α-2a plus PUVA in patients with cutaneous T-cell lymphoma. Hüsken AC, Tsianakas A, Hensen P, Nashan D, Loquai C, Beissert S, et al. J Eur Acad Dermatol Venereol 2012; 26: 71–8.

This 17-patient retrospective study compared the safety and efficacy of pegylated interferon-α2b (1.5 µg/kg weekly) versus standard IFN-α (9 MIU three times a week) in combination with PUVA. Myelosuppression and liver toxicity were more frequent with PEG-IFN-α2b, whereas fatigue and other adverse events leading to discontinuation were more frequent with standard IFN- α2a. The response rate in the PEG-IFN-α2b plus PUVA group seemed superior.

Predictors of response to extracorporeal photopheresis in advanced mycosis fungoides and Sézary syndrome. McGirt LY, Thoburn C, Hess A, Vonderheid EC. Photodermatol Photoimmunol Photomed 2010; 26: 182–91.

Sézary syndrome: immunopathogenesis, literature review of therapeutic options, and recommendations for therapy by the United States Cutaneous Lymphoma Consortium (USCLC). Olsen EA, Rook AH, Zic J, Kim Y, Porcu P, Querfeld C, et al. J Am Acad Dermatol 2011; 64: 352–404.

Olsen et al. summarize published treatment options for SS. Extracorporeal photopheresis (ECP), a procedure that treats pheresed blood with Oxsoralen, received FDA approval in 1988 as a medical device for the treatment of CTCL. ECP is well tolerated and should be considered for all patients with SS. Treatment is given every 2 to 4 weeks, with responses typically seen at 3 to 6 months. Oral bexarotene and interferons should be combined with ECP in all but those cases where the peripheral blood burden of Sézary cells is minimal.

High clinical response rate of Sézary syndrome to immunomodulatory therapies: prognostic markers of response. Raphael BA, Shin DB, Suchin KR, Morrissey KA, Vittorio CC, Kim EJ, et al. Arch Dermatol 2011; 147: 1410–5.

Outcomes in 98 patients with SS according to ISCL/EORTC criteria seen over a 25-year period at the University of Pennsylvania. Patients were treated with at least 3 months of ECP and one or more systemic agents. A total of 73 patients had significant improvement with multimodality therapy: 30% had complete response, with clearing of all disease. Lower CD4/CD8 ratio and median percentage of CD4+/CD26– and CD4+/CD7– cells at baseline predicted for complete response. Eosinophilia was shown in one study to predict a favorable response to ECP, but this remains to be confirmed.

Second-Line Therapies

Early stage (IA–IIA)

• Retinoids plus PUVA	B
• Interferons	B
• Total skin electron beam (TSEB) radiotherapy	B
• Oral bexarotene	B
• Low-dose methotrexate	B

Advanced stage (IIB–IVB)

• TSEB radiotherapy	B
• Vorinostat	B
• Depsipeptide	B
• Brentuximab vedotin	B
• Alemtuzumab	B
• Liposomal doxorubicin	B
• Gemcitabine	B
• Pralatrexate	B
• Purine analogs	B

Phase IIb multicenter trial of vorinostat in patients with persistent, progressive, or treatment refractory cutaneous T-cell lymphoma. Olsen EA, Kim YH, Kuzel TM, Pacheco TR, Foss FM, Parker S, et al. J Clin Oncol 2007; 25: 3109–15.

A pivotal, open-label, phase II trial that enrolled 74 patients with stage >IB CTCL who had failed two systemic therapies (one of which must have been bexarotene). Patients received vorinostat 400 mg daily, with planned dose reductions for toxicity. The objective response rate, assessed by the Severity-Weighted Assessment Tool (SWAT), was 30%, and the median response duration was ~6 months.

Final results from a multicenter, international, pivotal study of romidepsin in refractory cutaneous T-cell lymphoma. Whittaker SJ, Demierre MF, Kim EJ, Rook AH, Lerner A, Duvic M, et al. J Clin Oncol 2010; 28: 4485–91.

Romidepsin was administered as a 4-hour infusion (14 mg/m^2) on days 1, 8, and 15 of a 28-day cycle. The average number of cycles received by the patients was 4, and the median number of doses was 12. The objective response rate was 34%, the complete response rate was 6%, and the median duration of response was >12 months. In pruritus assessment, 43% of the patients experienced "clinically significant" improvement. As for vorinostat, the most common adverse effects were fatigue, nausea, vomiting, anorexia, and thrombocytopenia. Although electrocardiographic changes were common, no serious cardiac events were observed.

Romidepsin was approved by the FDA in 2009 for relapsed/refractory CTCL based on two phase II trials (Whittaker et al.) that enrolled a total of 167 patients with relapsed or refractory CTCL.

Vorinostat and romidepsin are FDA-approved histone deacetylase (HDAC) inhibitors (HDACi), a promising class of drugs with activity in CTCL. Vorinostat, an oral agent, was approved in 2006 for relapsed and refractory CTCL. Romidepsin, an intravenous agent, was approved in 2009 for CTCL and more recently in 2011 for the treatment of peripheral T-cell lymphoma (PTCL). These agents modulate chromatin condensation and potentially alter abnormal gene transcription and expression in cancer cells. They affect multiple functions in cancer cells, including proliferation, apoptosis, and angiogenesis. A subset of T-cell lymphomas, including MF and SS, may be sensitive to the antitumor effect of HDACi. Although not as myelosuppressive as conventional chemotherapy, HDACi may have some immune-suppressive effects, altered electrolytes, and association with thrombocytopenia.

Phase II investigator-initiated study of brentuximab vedotin in mycosis fungoides and Sézary syndrome with variable CD30 expression level: a multi-institution collaborative project. Kim YH, Tavallaee M, Sundram U, Salva KA, Wood GS, Li S, et al. J Clin Oncol 2015; 33: 3750–8.

Brentuximab vedotin (SGN-35) is an anti-CD30 monoclonal antibody conjugated to monomethyl auristin E, which releases the cytotoxic moiety intracellularly. The antibody is given IV every 3 weeks at 1.8 mg/mg. The objective response was 70%. Limiting side effects include peripheral neuropathy. The response rate was not necessarily dependent on CD30 expression.

Alemtuzumab for relapsed and refractory erythrodermic cutaneous T-cell lymphoma: a single institution experience from the Robert H. Lurie Comprehensive Cancer Center. Querfeld C, Mehta N, Rosen ST, Guitart J, Rademaker A, Gerami P, et al. Leuk Lymphoma 2009; 50: 1969–76.

Low-dose intermittent alemtuzumab in the treatment of Sézary syndrome: clinical and immunologic findings in 14 patients. Bernengo MG, Quaglino P, Comessatti A, Ortoncelli M, Novelli M, Lisa F, et al. Haematologica 2007; 92: 784–94.

Alemtuzumab (campath-1H) is a humanized monoclonal antibody against CD52, a molecule expressed on almost all leukocytes, including malignant T cells and B cells. The drug is approved for refractory chronic lymphocytic leukemia (CLL), but has activity in T-cell lymphoma and leukemia. The phase II study by Querfeld et al. specifically investigated the activity of alemtuzumab in patients with erythrodermic CTCL (including SS). Ten patients received alemtuzumab intravenously using an escalating dose regimen with a final dose of 30 mg three times weekly for 4 weeks followed by subcutaneous administration for 8 weeks. Nine patients were treated with only the subcutaneous or IV dosing. The overall response rate was 84%, with nine (47%) complete and seven (37%) partial remissions. The median follow-up was 24 months (range, 6–62+ months). Median overall survival was 41 months, whereas median progression free survival was 6 months. Toxicities included myelosuppression and infections, but most were moderate and transient. Although the conventional dose of alemtuzumab is 30 mg thrice weekly, Bernengo et al. studied a lower-dose intermittent schedule with the goal of avoiding excessive toxicity. The drug, given subcutaneously, was held once circulating Sézary cells fell below a certain threshold and resumed when the Sézary cell count increased. This approach appears to be safer, but it needs to be compared with the conventional schedule for efficacy.

Evidence Levels: A Double-blind study B Clinical trial ≥ 20 subjects C Clinical trial < 20 subjects D Series ≥ 5 subjects E Anecdotal case reports

Third-Line Therapies

• Topical bexarotene gel and other retinoids	B
• Single-agent chemotherapy	B
• Combination chemotherapy	B
• Allogeneic bone marrow transplantation	D
• Liposomal doxorubicin	B
• Gemcitabine	B
• Pralatrexate	B
• Purine analogs	B

Total skin electron beam and non-myeloablative allogeneic hematopoietic stem-cell transplantation in advanced mycosis fungoides and Sézary syndrome. Duvic M, Donato M, Dabaja B, Richmond H, Singh L, Wei W, et al. J Clin Oncol 2010; 28: 2365–72.

Allogeneic hematopoietic stem cell transplantation (HSCT) leverages the antitumor immune effect of the allograft, known as *graft versus lymphoma (GVL) effect*. However, allogeneic HSCT has significant mortality (up to 30%). Selecting the best time window, remission-inducing therapy, and condition regimen for patients with refractory CTCL is important. Duvic et al. studied the use of TSEBR in the preparatory regimen for allogeneic HSCT. Nineteen patients with heavily pretreated advanced CTCL and median age 50 years received TSEBR followed by fludarabine and melphalan conditioning and allogeneic HSCT between 2001 and 2008. Eighteen patients experienced engraftment, and 15 achieved full donor chimerism. Twelve experienced graft-versus-host disease. Four patients died in remission from transplant complications, and two died from progressive disease. Five of eight patients who relapsed in the skin regained complete response with reduced immunosuppression or donor lymphocyte infusions. Eleven of 13 were in complete remission, with median follow-up of 19 months.

Myiasis

Chen "Mary" Chen, Robert G. Phelps

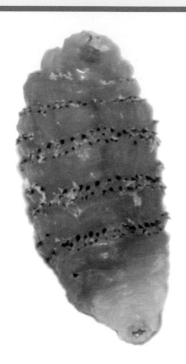

Myiasis is the infestation of human and animal tissue by the larval or pupal stages of two-winged true flies (Diptera), most commonly the *Dermatobia hominis* (botfly) and *Cordylobia anthropophaga* (tumbu fly). It is typically found in tropical and subtropical regions and is rare elsewhere. Its development is associated with poor hygiene, poor housing conditions, and overall debilitated state. Patients present with enlarging insect bites, ulceration, furuncle, or wound ulceration with sensation of irritation and lancinating pain. Larvae infest necrotic or viable skin but may also infest the eyes, ears, nose, and gastrointestinal (GI) or genitourinary (GU) sites.

MANAGEMENT STRATEGY

Myiasis was a major public health concern in the early twentieth century. Improvements in hygiene and wound care have significantly decreased its incidence. Nosocomial outbreaks, however, continue to occur sporadically. Manner of transmission differs depending on the species of flies. Furuncular myiasis is the most common and occurs through larvae burrowing into the skin.

Therapy objectives include complete larvae removal and prevention of secondary infestations and bacterial infections. Risk of exposure is linked to travel to Central and South America and parts of Africa. Visitors to rural regions should be *covered at all times with long-sleeved garments and hats*. Because many larvae vectors include bloodseeking arthropods, sleeping with a *mosquito net* at night is recommended. Liberal use of *insect repellents* is likewise useful. All clothing should be *hot ironed and thoroughly dried* to remove any residual eggs. To prevent barefoot transmission of fly eggs from the soil, *appropriate footwear* should be utilized. Wound myiasis can be prevented using *antiseptic techniques*. Wound cleaning, irrigation, and regular dressing changes are usually sufficient. As a precaution, patients with large wounds should sleep indoors only and with windows closed.

Once infestation has occurred, therapy consists of *surgical removal of all larvae* with minimal trauma to the organisms. Simple infiltration of the area with lidocaine and surgical removal is standard of care when few organisms are present. *Occlusive therapy* (using petroleum jelly or strips of bacon), inducing larvae to protrude their abdomen to reach air, may be helpful when many larvae are present. Careful technique must be used to extract the larvae whole; otherwise a considerable foreign body reaction may ensue. If there is secondary pyogenic infection, this should be treated with antibiotics. Supplemental treatments including *isopropyl alcohol*, *Dakin solution*, *iodine*, or *hydrogen peroxide* can be included in wound care. Anecdotal reports suggest use of *topical and systemic ivermectin* for complicated conditions (extensive or multiple lesions, substantial involvement of orbital or oral cavities, or failure of surgical extraction).

Specific Investigations

- Detailed travel history
- Morphologic and molecular identification of the parasite

A blow to the fly—*Lucilia cuprina* draft genome and transcriptome to support advances in biology and biotechnology. Anstead CA, Batterham P, Korhonen PK, Young ND, Hall RS, Bowles VM, et al. Biotechnol Adv 2016; 34: 605–20.

Draft genome and transcriptome of the blow fly gives new and global insights into its biology, interactions with the host animal, and aspects of insecticide resistance at the molecular level. The genetic resource will also aid the design of new and improved interventions for myiasis.

Molecular identification of two species of myiasis-causing *Cuterebra* by multiplex PCR and RFLP. Noel S, Tessier N, Angers B, Wood DM, Lapointe FJ. Med Vet Entomol 2004; 18: 161–6.

The fly larvae should be extracted whole and specific identification attempted. Each larva may molt and have several instars, each with a slightly different morphology, complicating identification. The adult fly should be identified, if possible. Consultation with an entomologist in difficult cases is helpful. Scanning electron microscopy and multiplex polymerase chain reaction (PCR) may aid identification.

Identification of subcutaneous myiasis using bedside emergency physician performed ultrasound. Schechter E, Lazar J, Nix ME, Mallon WK, Moore CL. J Emerg Med 2011; 40: e1–3.

Ultrasound diagnosis of patient with *C. anthropophaga* maggot infestation with hyperechoic areas.

Evidence Levels: **A** Double-blind study **B** Clinical trial ≥ 20 subjects **C** Clinical trial < 20 subjects **D** Series ≥ 5 subjects **E** Anecdotal case reports

First-Line Therapies	
Surgical therapy	
• Surgical removal with local anesthesia with or without adjuvant suffocation techniques	D
Asphyxiation therapy	
• Vaseline therapy	E
• Bacon therapy	E
• Pork fat therapy	E
• Hair gel therapy	E
• Occlusion with *chimo* (pastelike form of smokeless tobacco)	E
• Small wad of cotton soaked in the sap of the *Thevetia ahouai* (Apocynaceae) tree	E

Second-Line Therapies	
• Systemic ivermectin	E
• Topical ivermectin	E
• Chlorhexidine gluconate rinses	E
• Pyrantel pamoate	E
• Radiation therapy	E
• Chloroform/ether	E
• Mineral turpentine	E
• Ethanol spray	E
• Oil of betel leaf	E
• Mineral turpentine	E

Myiasis in travelers. Lachish T, Marhoom E, Kosta Y, Mumcuoglu KY, Tandlich M, Schwartz E. J Travel Med 2015; 22: 232–6.

This retrospective observational study identified 90 patients diagnosed with myiasis from posttravel clinics in Israel. Seventy-six percent of the cases were managed by manual extraction, which can be performed after covering the central pore of the lesion with a sealing ointment such as paraffin.

Myiasis: a traveler's dilemma. Mammino J, Lal K. J Clin Aesthet Dermatol 2013; 6: 47–9.

Scalp myiasis successfully extracted with excisional biopsy technique under local anesthesia. This assures that the larvae, along with the subcutaneous tissue surrounding the implanted larvae, is removed.

Cutaneous myiasis. Krajewski A, Allen B, Hoss D, Patel C, Chandawarkar RY. J Plast Reconstr Aesthet Surg 2009; 62: e383–6.

The favored treatment modality is complete surgical extraction of larvae from the lesion to prevent the risk of secondary infection associated with retained larvae.

One catches not only mice with bacon. An atraumatic treatment for cutaneous myiasis. Schulte C, Schunk M, Krebs B. Dtsch Med Wochenschr 2002; 127: 266–8.

A piece of raw bacon, serving as occlusion material, was fixated on the affected skin for 2 hours. The larvae emerged due to oxygen deficiency. After retraction of the bacon it was possible to grasp the emerged end of the larvae with tweezers and pull them out completely.

Alternatives to bacon therapy. Biggar RJ. JAMA 1994; 271: 901–2.

The authors use Vaseline over the wound to smother the larvae, and they emerge spontaneously.

Traditional methods encourage the larva to exit on its own, taking advantage of its need for oxygen, by using various occlusive dressings to suffocate it.

Dermal myiasis: the porcine lipid cure. Sauder DN, Hall RP, Wurster CF. Arch Dermatol 1981; 117: 681–2.

Pork fat was placed on the lesions and covered with an occlusive tape, and the emerging larvae were extracted with forceps.

Oral myiasis: a rare case report and literature review. Shikha S, Prasad Guru R, Ashutoshdutt P, Meenakshi S. J Dent (Tehran) 2015; 12: 456–9.

For extensive disease in the oral cavity, the treatment was given systemic ivermectin 6 mg once daily for three days and oral amoxicillin 250 mg three times daily for 7 days. Mouth rinse twice daily with 0.2% chlorhexidine gluconate for 15 days under supervision.

Use of ivermectin in the treatment of orbital myiasis caused by *Cochliomyia hominivorax*. De Tarso P, Pierre-Filho P, Minguuini N, Pierre LM, Pierre AM. Scand J Infect Dis 2004; 36: 503–5.

One dose of ivermectin (200 µg/kg) was used for infestation with *Hypoderma lineatum*, and led to spontaneous migration of the maggots.

Myiasis owing to *Dermatobia hominis* in a HIV-infected subject: treatment by topical ivermectin. Clyti E, Nacher M, Merrien L, El Guedj M, Roussel M, Sainte-Marie D, Couppié P. Int J Dermatol 2007; 46: 52–4.

Human immunodeficiency virus (HIV) infection did not modify the pathogenicity of myiasis but did contribute unusually extensive and voluminous inflammatory nodules. Use of topical ivermectin killed the larvae and facilitated their extraction.

Myiasis: successful treatment with topical ivermectin. Victoria J, Trujillo R, Barreto M. Int J Dermatol 1999; 38: 142–4.

Four patients presented with traumatic myiasis caused by *C. hominivorax* with 50–100 larvae each. One topical treatment with 1% ivermectin in a propylene glycol solution was applied to the affected area. The topical solution was left for 2 hours, followed by gentle washing with normal saline or sterile water. Within 1 hour, almost all larvae stopped moving, and within 24 hours, all died.

Nasal myiasis: a case report. White ZL, Chu MW, Hood RJ. Ear Nose Throat J 2015; 94: e24–5.

Two patients without necrosis or large masses were successfully treated with conservative therapy, consisting of a single dose of pyrantel pamoate, daily sinus irrigation with saline, and daily bedside endoscopic debridement.

Head and neck myiasis, cutaneous malignancy, and infection: a case series and review of the literature. Jennifer A, Villwock JA, Harris TM. J Emerg Med 2014; 47: e37–41.

One patient in the case series received radiation beam therapy for her concurrent squamous cell carcinoma, which serendipitously eradicated the larvae infection. Use of this modality for myiasis treatment has not been previously reported.

Dissanayake, larvicidal effects of mineral turpentine, low aromatic white spirits, aqueous extracts of *Cassia alata*, **and aqueous extracts, ethanolic extracts and essential oil of betel leaf (*Piper betle*) on *Chrysomya megacephala*.** Kumarasinghe SP, Karunaweera ND, Ihalamulla RL, Arambewela LS. Int J Dermatol 2002; 41: 877–80.

Evidence Levels: **A** Double-blind study **B** Clinical trial ≥ 20 subjects **C** Clinical trial < 20 subjects **D** Series ≥ 5 subjects **E** Anecdotal case reports

163

Myxoid cyst

David de Berker

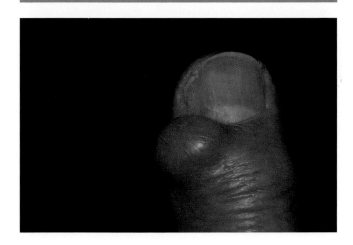

Myxoid cysts are also known as *digital mucus cysts* or *pseudocysts* and represent a ganglion of the distal interphalangeal joint. They arise in different forms in soft tissues, typically above or distal to the distal interphalangeal joint. The most common presentation is as a translucent nodule on the dorsum of the digit. Additional patterns of presentation include as a pseudofibroma emerging between the proximal nail fold and dorsal aspect of the nail plate, or as a tumor beneath the nail matrix causing a red lunula, increased transverse curvature of the nail, and sometimes its disintegration.

MANAGEMENT STRATEGY

Myxoid cysts contain gelatinous material that has escaped from the distal interphalangeal joint. Treatment can involve evacuation combined with measures to prevent further escape from the joint. *Simple drainage* through an incision can achieve the first, but normally there is recurrence within a few weeks. Measures to prevent the further accumulation of fluid are directed at reducing joint pathology or blocking the pathway of escape of fluid. The first category includes the use of *injected triamcinolone,* which might reduce synovial inflammation and the pressure of fluid within the joint, and *surgery* for osteophytes. Osteophytes appear to weaken the joint capsule and possibly contribute to joint pathology and synovial fluid production. Their removal is associated with resolution of the myxoid cyst but at risk of alteration of joint function.

Blockage of the path of fluid escape is achieved by a range of traumatic and scarring procedures. The challenge is to produce an effective scar over the joint without excess morbidity or a long-term nail dystrophy.

A practical compromise of morbidity, complexity of treatment, and efficacy is to employ *cryosurgery* in the first instance. This is best used with a distal block using lidocaine or bupivacaine. The cyst is then incised and drained. Two freezes of between 10 and 20 seconds with liquid nitrogen are given, with a complete thaw in between. Over the next 2 weeks the wound is dressed. This results in success in about 50% of cases involving fingers. Those that fail can be retreated in the same way or proceed to surgery. Morbidity

is least when there is *precise surgery* to the path of fluid escape. This can be identified by methylene blue injection into the joint and then raising a flap in a distal-to-proximal path, containing the cyst in the roof of the flap. The pathway is dyed and can be tied with absorbable ligature. The flap is sutured back in place, and success is reported as 94% in the fingers. In some instances patient preference or medical considerations may mean that surgery is the first-line therapy.

Specific Investigations

- Transillumination
- Pricking and expression of gelatinous material
- Ultrasound
- Magnetic resonance imaging (MRI)

Transillumination is a useful clinical aid. Where there is diagnostic doubt, simple incision can be helpful to demonstrate the gelatinous material. Alternatively, high-resolution ultrasound or MRI can be employed. The first can only help define whether the structure is cystic or not. The latter provides better anatomic definition and in over 80% of cases allows location of the pedicle communicating between the cyst and joint. Plain x-ray may reveal osteophytes of osteoarthritis, but this will not usually alter treatment.

Benign tumors and pseudotumors of the nail: a novel application of sonography. Wortsman X, Wortsman J, Soto R, Saavedra T, Honeyman J, Sazunic I, et al. J Ultrasound Med 2010; 29: 803–16.

MR imaging of digital mucoid cysts. Drapé JL, Idy Peretti I, Goettmann S. Radiology 1996; 200: 531–6.

First-Line Therapies

• Cryosurgery	**B**
• Puncture	**D**
• Laser therapy	**C**
• Sclerosant	**C**

Myxoid cysts of the finger: treatment by liquid nitrogen spray cryosurgery. Dawber RPR, Sonnex T, Leonard J, Ralphs I. Clin Exp Dermatol 1983; 8: 153–7.

Fourteen patients were treated with two 30-second freezes and no evacuation of the cyst. Follow-up was between 14 and 40 months, with an 86% cure rate. One patient had a significant nail dystrophy as a long-term complication.

Removal of the overlying cyst or evacuation of the contents might reduce the duration of cryosurgery needed. Longer freeze times increase morbidity and risk of scarring.

Specific indications for cryosurgery of the nail unit. Kuflik EG. J Dermatol Surg Oncol 1992; 18: 702–6.

Forty-nine patients were treated with a range of single cryosurgical doses, from 20 to 30 seconds using open spray, and 30 to 40 seconds using the cryoprobe. This was combined with curettage in 23 patients and simple deroofing in the remainder. There was resolution in 63% over the follow-up period of 1 to 60 months.

A simple technique for managing digital mucous cysts. Epstein E. Arch Dermatol 1979; 115: 1315–6.

Repeated puncture of myxoid cysts in 40 patients led to resolution in 72% after two to five treatments, but no follow-up period is given.

Blunt force may be an effective treatment for ganglion cysts. Trivedi NN, Schreiber JJ, Daluiski A. HSS J 2016; 12: 100–4.

Review of reports of aspiration treatment suggests overall success rate of 53%.

Blunt force alone may be sufficient as reported by Trivedi et al. based on online self-reporting. But details are not well documented, as it is usually done as self-care.

Treatment of digital myxoid cysts with carbon dioxide laser vaporization. Huerter CJ, Wheeland RG, Bailin PL, Ratz JL. J Dermatol Surg Oncol 1987; 13: 723–7.

Carbon dioxide laser cured 10 patients with follow-up of 35 months.

Treatment of digital mucous cysts with intralesional sodium tetradecyl sulfate injection. Park SE, Park EJ, Kim SS, Kim CW. Dermatol Surg 2014; 40: 1249–54.

The sclerosant sodium tetradecyl sulfate 1% (fingers) or 3% (toes) 0.2 to 0.5 mL was injected into a lesion after aspiration of the gel. It was then repeated every 4 weeks if the cyst persisted, up to 7 times (mean 2.3), with eventual resolution in 80% and subsequent relapse in a further 2 patients (10%) after a mean follow-up of 16 months (range 2–38 months).

Treatment of 63 subjects with digital mucous cysts with percutaneous sclerotherapy using polidocanol. Esson GA, Holme SA. Dermatol Surg. 2016; 42: 59–62.

Three percent polidocanol (0.02–0.5 mL) is a sclerosant that can be used in a similar way with similar results.

Some reports have described necrosis of the nail fold, but this is seldom extensive. The theoretical complication of sclerosant entering the joint does not appear to occur.

Second-Line Therapy

• Surgery	B

Marginal osteophyte excision in treatment of mucous cysts. Eaton RG, Dobranski AI, Littler JW. J Bone Joint Surg 1973; 55A: 570–4.

Forty-four patients with surgery entailing tracing of the communication between cyst and joint, excision of the cyst, and in some instances surgery to the osteophytes provided success in 43 of 44 patients, with follow-up of between 6 months and 10 years.

There is a theoretical possibility of operating on the osteophytes alone, leaving the cyst in place and allowing it to involute once the precipitating pathology has been removed.

Etiology and treatment of the so-called mucous cyst of the finger. Kleinert HE, Kutz JE, Fishman JH, McCraw LH. J Bone Joint Surg 1972; 54: 1455–8.

Similar surgery, but with less emphasis on osteophyte debridement, resulted in success for all of 36 patients followed for between 12 and 18 months postoperatively.

Use of Wolfe graft for the treatment of mucous cysts. Jamnadas-Khoda B, Agarwal R, Harper R, Page RE. J Hand Surg Eur 2009; 34: 519–21.

Forty-nine patients with 51 myxoid cysts underwent excision of the cyst on the dorsum of a finger with repair using a full-thickness graft taken from the flexor crease of the wrist. Recurrence rate rose from zero at 4 months to at least 4% longer term.

Proximal nail fold flap dissection for digital myxoid cysts – a 7 year experience. Eke U, Ahmed I, Ilchyshyn A. Dermatol Surg 2014; 40: 206–8.

Flap repair with a longer follow-up in 18 patients revealed 37% relapse rate over 5 to 84 months (median 29.7).

Ganglion of the distal interphalangeal joint (myxoid cyst): therapy by identification and repair of the leak of joint fluid. de Berker D, Lawrence C. Arch Dermatol 2001; 137: 607–10.

A study of 54 patients used methylene blue dye injected into the distal interphalangeal joint to identify the communication between the joint and the cyst. A skin flap was designed around the cyst. The communication was sutured and the flap replaced with no tissue excision. In 89% of patients the communication was identified. At 8 months, 48 patients remained cured with no visible scarring. Myxoid cysts of the toes had a higher relapse rate than those of the fingers.

Skin excision and osteophyte removal is not required in the surgical treatment of digital myxoid cysts. Lawrence C. Arch Dermatol 2005; 141: 1560–4.

The procedure in this study was limited to raising a flap overlying the distal interphalangeal joint, draining the mucoid content of the cyst, and cauterizing the underlying soft tissues on the joint. The flap was sutured back in place. Over 8 months, 24 of 26 (92%) of finger myxoid cysts remained cured. Cure rate for myxoid cysts of the toes was 33.3%.

Third-Line Therapy

• Flurandrenolide tape	D

The most likely course of action after failure of surgery is either to repeat the surgery or to modify the surgical approach to include osteophyte surgery if these were not treated in the first instance. If a CO_2 laser is available, this might also be chosen, given the good results reported in the small published series. Alternatively, sclerosant could be used, although again, multiple treatments could be anticipated.

Treatment of myxoid cyst with flurandrenolide tape. Ronchese F. R I Med J 1970; 57: 154–5.

After the failure of electrodesiccation, five patients were treated with corticosteroid tape for 2 to 3 months, and success was reported in all during a follow-up of 2 to 3 years. The rationale for this choice is where the joint appears inflamed with more marked osteoarthritis and managing the inflammation may diminish the production and efflux of synovial fluid.

Evidence Levels: **A** Double-blind study **B** Clinical trial ≥ 20 subjects **C** Clinical trial < 20 subjects **D** Series ≥ 5 subjects **E** Anecdotal case reports

164

Nail psoriasis

Waqas Shaikh, Joy Wan, Adam I. Rubin

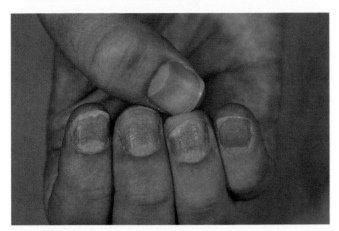

Clinical features of nail psoriasis can be divided by the site of origin within the nail unit. Signs of nail matrix psoriasis include pitting, red spots in the lunula, leukonychia, and nail plate crumbling. Signs of nail bed psoriasis include onycholysis, splinter hemorrhages, oil spots, and subungual hyperkeratosis. It is important to distinguish among these diverse manifestations of nail psoriasis, as they influence treatment selection and the response to therapy.

MANAGEMENT STRATEGY

Nail psoriasis can be challenging to diagnose and treat, but this is an important entity, causing significant emotional and physical impairments. Nails are easily visible. In professions where frequent interpersonal interactions are the norm, such as salespeople, nail psoriasis can have a detrimental impact on careers. In severe cases, the ability to manipulate small objects and accomplish routine daily tasks can be diminished significantly.

Considering the known link among nail psoriasis, enthesitis, and psoriatic arthritis, it is imperative to ask patients about current or prior history of joint pain, joint swelling, and morning stiffness lasting longer than 1 hour. A basic joint examination should also be performed. Positive findings should be further investigated with radiologic imaging and/or referral to a rheumatologist.

There are overlapping clinical features of nail psoriasis and onychomycosis, so it is important to evaluate patients for the latter possibility and remember that nail psoriasis and onychomycosis can coexist in the same patient. If present, onychomycosis should be treated first.

In cases where the diagnosis is equivocal, a nail unit biopsy may be considered for additional diagnostic information. Although nail clippings can show histologic features of psoriasis, the features seen in nail clippings alone are nonspecific. The most definitive diagnosis can be obtained from a combination of nail plate and soft tissue findings. The best anatomic area of the nail unit to biopsy corresponds to the origin of the physical signs noted. For example, if subungual hyperkeratosis is present, the nail bed would be the most appropriate location to biopsy, as the anatomic origin of this clinical sign is the nail bed.

Treatment should be tailored to the individual patient, taking into account the severity of nail disease, age, the types of clinical signs present, the extent of psoriasis on the skin, the presence or absence of concurrent psoriatic arthritis, the patient's occupation, and other comorbidities, as well as insurance coverage/regulations or lack thereof.

General nail care is of utmost importance to prevent worsening of the nail changes and to help treat existing lesions. The nail plate should be clipped back to the point of its attachment to the nail bed if possible. This prevents repetitive minor trauma. The Koebner phenomenon can affect the nails and may impede resolution, worsen existing lesions, or promote the development of new lesions on the nails. Additionally, when subungual hyperkeratosis is prominent, patients may use instruments to clean out this material from under the nail plate. However, this type of maneuver also causes trauma to the nail and has the same consequences as described earlier. Avoidance of excessive nail care such as filing can also diminish excess trauma. Use of gloves can be helpful during wet work, cleaning, or gardening to help protect the nails. Nail cosmetics, such as acrylic nails, may cause additional trauma in their application or removal and should be avoided.

For mild or moderate disease, topical therapies generally improve the nails. It is critical to select a therapy that will be beneficial based on the signs of nail psoriasis present. For example, with onycholysis, if the nail plate is clipped back to the point of attachment to the nail bed, topical medications can easily be applied to the specific site of psoriasis involvement (the nail bed in this case). In contrast, nail plate signs, such as nail plate crumbling and pitting, are caused by psoriatic inflammation affecting the nail matrix and will not be adequately treated by topical medications, which do not penetrate the proximal nail fold sufficiently to diffuse into the matrix. In these cases where nail matrix psoriasis is present, intralesional steroids can be effective.

Severe nail psoriasis or concomitant nail psoriasis and psoriatic arthritis would qualify for systemic therapy. If psoriatic arthritis is present, the choice of medication may be coordinated with the patient's rheumatologist and may depend on other comorbidities. Traditional systemic psoriasis medications such as acitretin and methotrexate have evidence supporting their effectiveness for nail psoriasis. However, the treatment of psoriasis has been revolutionized by the advent of biologic medications, which may have more favorable safety and efficacy profiles than the traditional systemic medications. The selection of any particular systemic medication for nail psoriasis entails a holistic view of the patient, including age, comorbidities, and insurance coverage, as well as the impact of severe nail psoriasis on quality of life.

Specific Investigations

- Record Nail Psoriasis Severity Index (NAPSI)
- Biopsy (in selected cases)

NAPSI is a commonly used tool to assess nail psoriasis severity. Each nail is divided into four quadrants. For each quadrant, signs of nail bed psoriasis (onycholysis, splinter hemorrhages, hyperkeratosis, and oil-drop dyschromia) are identified. For each nail, a score of 0 to 4 is given for nail bed signs based on the number of quadrants involved. Similarly, nail matrix psoriasis signs (pitting, leukonychia, crumbling, and red spots in lunula) are identified in each quadrant. For each nail, a score of 0 to 4 is given for nail matrix signs based on the number of quadrants involved. The scores are added to give a total score of 0 to 8 for each nail. The maximum NAPSI is 80 for all 10 fingernails. This method can be applied to the toenails as well but is not often done.

Several other severity scoring systems for nail psoriasis also exist, but none is uniformly applied.

Nail Psoriasis Severity Index: a useful tool for evaluation of nail psoriasis. Rich P, Scher RK. J Am Acad Dermatol 2003; 49: 206–12.

First-Line Therapies	
• Topical corticosteroids	A
• Topical vitamin D analogs	A
• Topical tazarotene	A
• Topical tacrolimus	B
• Intralesional triamcinolone acetonide	C

Comparison of nail lacquer clobetasol efficacy at 0.05%, 1% and 8% in nail psoriasis treatment: prospective, controlled and randomized pilot study. Nakamura RC, Abreu L, Duque-Estrada B, Tamler C, Leverone AP. An Bras Dermatol 2012; 87: 203–11.

A split-hand study of 15 patients was performed with application of 0.05%, 1%, or 8% clobetasol nail lacquer on the left hand and base coat nail lacquer on the right hand twice a week for 16 weeks. The treated left hand group showed 51% improvement in modified NAPSI compared with baseline. No significant difference was observed across the different concentrations of clobetasol nail lacquer. No adverse effects were observed.

Calcipotriol ointment in nail psoriasis: a controlled double-blind comparison with betamethasone dipropionate and salicylic acid. Tosti A, Piraccini BM, Cameli N, Kokely F, Plozzer C, Cannata GE, et al. Br J Dermatol 1998; 139: 655–9.

This study compared twice-daily application of calcipotriol ointment (50 µg/g) to betamethasone dipropionate (64 mg/g) plus salicylic acid (0.03 g/g) ointment to the nails of 58 patients for 3 to 5 months. There was 49.2% and 51.7% reduction in fingernail subungual hyperkeratosis and 20.1% and 22.9% reduction in toenail subungual hyperkeratosis in the calcipotriol and betamethasone dipropionate plus salicylic acid groups, respectively; however, the difference between the two treatment groups was not statistically significant. Adverse effects were mild and included erythema, periungual irritation, burning, and diffuse urticaria.

In our experience, calcipotriol is well tolerated by patients. It is available as a solution, which can be helpful to treat areas of the nail that may be difficult to access.

Tazarotene 0.1% gel in the treatment of fingernail psoriasis: a double-blind, randomized, vehicle-controlled study. Scher RK, Stiller M, Zhu YI. Cutis 2001; 68: 355–8.

A study of 31 patients randomized to tazarotene 0.1% gel or vehicle gel nightly to two fingernails (one finger under occlusion and one without occlusion) for up to 24 weeks. The tazarotene group showed a significant reduction in onycholysis. Compared with the nonoccluded nails, the occluded nails had a more rapid onset of improvement in onycholysis and showed significant improvement in nail pitting. Adverse effects in the tazarotene group included skin peeling and paronychia.

In our experience, tazarotene may be irritating, and reduction of the dosage schedule can provide therapeutic improvements while decreasing the intensity of the irritation.

Tacrolimus 0.1% ointment in nail psoriasis: a randomized controlled open-label study. De Simone C, Maiorino A, Tassone F, D'Agostino M, Caldarola G. J Eur Acad Dermatol Venereol 2013; 27: 1003–6.

A single-blind, split-hand study of 21 patients treated with tacrolimus 0.1% ointment nightly for 12 weeks showed a significant 13-point reduction in NAPSI in the treated hands and a 3-point reduction in the untreated hands compared with baseline. One patient developed acute paronychia in the tacrolimus-treated hand. No other adverse effects were observed.

In our experience, topical tacrolimus is well tolerated by patients with nail psoriasis.

Treatment of nail psoriasis with intralesional triamcinolone acetonide using a needle-free jet injector: a prospective trial. Nantel-Battista M, Richer V, Marcil I, Benohanian A. J Cutan Med Surg 2014; 18: 38–42.

A pre–post comparative trial of 17 patients treated with monthly intralesional triamcinolone acetonide for 4 months led to a 46.25% decrease in target nail NAPSI compared with baseline.

The site of injection is dependent on nail pathology. Injections that target the nail matrix (at the proximal nail fold) are recommended for nail pitting, surface ridging, and nail plate thickening. Nail bed injections (often at the lateral nail fold directed medially toward the nail bed) are recommended for oil spots, onycholysis, and subungual hyperkeratosis. Nail bed injections can be uncomfortable, and topical medications may be a better choice if the medication can access the zone of involvement in the nail bed. In general, 0.1 to 0.3 mL of 2.5 to 10 mg/mL triamcinolone acetonide is injected per site. Frequencies vary from weekly to monthly to every 2 months. Potential adverse effects include injection site pain, subungual hematomas, paresthesias, skin atrophy, and terminal phalanx atrophy ("disappearing digit"). In our clinic, we offer patients a topical anesthetic or a vibratory device to help minimize discomfort with the injections. Dilution of the steroid with lidocaine may also decrease discomfort with the procedure.

Second-Line Therapies	
• Acitretin	B
• Methotrexate	A
• Etanercept	B
• Adalimumab	A
• Infliximab	A
• Ustekinumab	A
• Secukinumab	A
• Apremilast	A
• Ixekizumab	A
• Golimumab	A
• Certolizumab	A

Evaluation of the efficacy of acitretin therapy for nail psoriasis. Tosti A, Ricotti C, Romanelli P, Cameli N, Piraccini BM. Arch Dermatol 2009; 145: 269–71.

Thirty-six patients with moderate to severe nail psoriasis were treated with low-dose acitretin (0.2–0.3 mg/kg/day) for 6 months in a pre–post comparative trial. There was a 41% reduction in NAPSI and 50% reduction in modified NAPSI of the target nail. Twenty-five percent showed almost complete clearance, 27% showed moderate improvement, 33% mild improvement, and 11% no improvement. Except for one patient developing severe periungual dryness and multiple pyogenic granulomas, there were no clinical or laboratory adverse effects.

Evidence Levels: **A** Double-blind study **B** Clinical trial ≥ 20 subjects **C** Clinical trial < 20 subjects **D** Series ≥ 5 subjects **E** Anecdotal case reports

Use of acitretin may be limited by patient comorbidities and in females of childbearing potential, considering its category X pregnancy designation.

A 52-week trial comparing briakinumab with methotrexate in patients with psoriasis. Reich K, Langley RG, Papp KA, Ortonne JP, Unnebrink K, Kaul M, et al. N Engl J Med 2011; 365: 1586–96.

A 52-week, double-blind, randomized trial in 317 patients with moderate to severe psoriasis comparing briakinumab and methotrexate 5 to 25 mg weekly showed a reduction in NAPSI from 4.8 to 1.2 (75% improvement) and 4.8 to 3 (38% improvement), respectively.

Briakinumab was previously under investigation for the treatment of psoriasis but is not currently available.

A 24-week randomized clinical trial investigating the efficacy and safety of two doses of etanercept in nail psoriasis. Ortonne JP, Paul C, Berardesca E, Marino V, Gallo G, Brault Y, et al. Br J Dermatol 2013; 168: 1080–7.

A 24-week, randomized, dose-comparison trial was performed in 72 patients with moderate to severe psoriasis treated with etanercept. Group 1 received etanercept 50 mg twice weekly for 12 weeks followed by once weekly for 12 weeks. Group 2 received etanercept 50 mg once weekly for 24 weeks. NAPSI score decreased from 6.0 to 1.7 (72% improvement) in group 1 and decreased from 5.8 to 1.4 (75% improvement) in group 2 at 24 weeks compared with baseline. Target fingernail NAPSI-50 was achieved by 82.3% and 80.7% of patients in group 1 and group 2, respectively. Common adverse events were nasopharyngitis and headache.

Adalimumab for treatment of moderate to severe chronic plaque psoriasis of the hands and feet: efficacy and safety results from REACH, a randomized, placebo-controlled, double-blind trial. Leonardi C, Langley RG, Papp K, Trying SK, Wasel N, Vender R, et al. Arch Dermatol 2011; 147: 429–36.

A double-blind, placebo-controlled, randomized trial evaluated adalimumab (80 mg week 0, 40 mg week 1, and 40 mg every other week thereafter) for 16 weeks in 72 patients with moderate to severe chronic plaque psoriasis of hands/feet. At 16 weeks, there was 50% improvement in NAPSI in the adalimumab group compared with 8% improvement in the placebo group. At 28 weeks, the adalimumab group had a 54% NAPSI improvement. The most frequently reported adverse events were nasopharyngitis, headache, diarrhea, and injection site reaction.

Baseline nail disease in patients with moderate to severe psoriasis and response to treatment with infliximab during 1 year. Rich P, Griffiths CE, Reich K, Nestle FO, Scher RK, Li S, et al. J Am Acad Dermatol 2008; 58: 224–31.

In a 50-week, double-blind, randomized, placebo-controlled, crossover trial of infliximab (5 mg/kg given at weeks 0, 2, 6, and every 8 weeks thereafter) in 305 patients with nail psoriasis showed 44.7% rate of nail disease clearance and 57.2% decrease in NAPSI in the infliximab group, in contrast to 5.1% rate of nail disease clearance and 4.1% increase in NAPSI in the placebo group.

A comparative study examining infliximab, adalimumab, and etanercept showed significant improvement in NAPSI scores (95.1%, 89.5%, and 92.8%, respectively) at 48 weeks with the most rapid improvement in the infliximab group.

Ustekinumab improves nail disease in patients with moderate-to-severe psoriasis: results from PHOENIX 1. Rich P,

Bourcier M, Sofen H, Fakharzadeh S, Wasfi Y, Wang Y, et al. Br J Dermatol 2014; 170: 398–407.

A double-blind, randomized, placebo-controlled, crossover trial in 545 patients with nail psoriasis treated with ustekinumab (45 mg or 90 mg at weeks 0 and 4 with a maintenance dose every 12 weeks) showed NAPSI improvement of 46.5% in the 45-mg group and 48.7% in the 90-mg group at 24 weeks.

Secukinumab improves hand, foot and nail lesions in moderate-to-severe plaque psoriasis: subanalysis of a randomized, double-blind, placebo-controlled, regimen-finding phase 2 trial. Paul C, Reich K, Gottlieb AB, Mrowietz U, Philipp S, Nakayama J, et al. J Eur Acad Dermatol Venereol 2014; 28: 1670–5.

Three hundred four patients with nail psoriasis from a randomized, double-blind, placebo-controlled trial were examined in this post hoc analysis. Induction regimens of secukinumab 150 mg were single dose (week 0), monthly (weeks 0, 4, and 8), or early (weeks 0, 1, 2, and 4). At 12 weeks, the composite fingernail scores improved with the early (–19.1%) and monthly (–10.6%) regimens, worsened with placebo (+14.4%), and remained stable with the single-dose regimen (–3.7%) compared with baseline.

Apremilast, an oral phosphodiesterase 4 inhibitor, in patients with difficult-to-treat nail and scalp psoriasis: results of 2 phase III randomized, controlled trials (ESTEEM 1 and ESTEEM 2). Rich P, Gooderham M, Bachelez H, Goncalves J, Day RM, Chen R, et al. J Am Acad Dermatol 2016; 74: 134–42.

In a trial with 1255 patients with moderate to severe plaque psoriasis, NAPSI changed by –22.5% to –29.0% in the apremilast 30 mg twice daily group and –7.1% to +6.5% in the placebo group, compared with baseline. Common adverse events included diarrhea, nausea/vomiting, abdominal pain, weight loss, nasopharyngitis, upper respiratory tract infections, and headache. Rare serious adverse effects included depression, suicidal thoughts, and suicidal behavior.

Improvement of scalp and nail lesions with ixekizumab in a phase 2 trial in patients with chronic plaque psoriasis. Langley RG, Rich P, Menter A, Krueger G, Goldblum O, Dutronc Y, et al. J Eur Acad Dermatol Venereol 2015; 29: 1763–70.

In a post hoc analysis of a double-blind, placebo-controlled, randomized trial and open-label extension trial of patients with moderate to severe psoriasis, 58 patients were found to have nail psoriasis. Patients with nail psoriasis in the placebo, ixekizumab 75 mg, and ixekizumab 150 mg groups received injections at weeks 0, 2, 4, 8, 12, and 16. The placebo, ixekizumab 75 mg, and ixekizumab 150 mg groups had NAPSI reductions of 1.7%, 63.8%, and 52.6% at 20 weeks, respectively, compared with baseline. By week 48 in the open-label extension (ixekizumab 120 mg every 4 weeks) involving 51 patients, 51% of nail psoriasis patients treated with ixekizumab 120 mg showed complete nail psoriasis clearance.

Golimumab, a new human tumor necrosis factor α antibody, administered every 4 weeks as a subcutaneous injection in psoriatic arthritis: twenty-four-week efficacy and safety results of a randomized, placebo-controlled study. Kavanaugh A, McInnes I, Mease P, Krueger GG, Gladman D, Gomez-Reino J, et al. Arthritis Rheum 2009; 60: 976–86.

A double-blind, randomized, placebo-controlled, dose-escalation trial in 319 patients with psoriasis and psoriatic arthritis compared golimumab 50 mg every 4 weeks to golimumab 100 mg every 4 weeks. Secondary end point analysis of 287 patients with nail psoriasis showed a median percentage improvement in NAPSI at 24 weeks of 0%, 33%, and 54% in the placebo, golimumab 50 mg, and golimumab 100 mg groups, respectively. Reported adverse effects were nasopharyngitis, upper respiratory tract infections, injection site reactions, and transaminitis.

Effect of certolizumab pegol on signs and symptoms in patients with psoriatic arthritis: 24-week results of a Phase 3 double-blind randomised placebo-controlled study (RAPID-PsA). Mease PJ, Fleischmann R, Deodhar AA, Wollenhaupt J, Khraishi M, Kielar D, et al. Ann Rheum Dis 2014; 73: 48–55.

A double-blind, placebo-controlled, randomized trial of certolizumab (200 mg every 2 weeks or 400 mg every 4 weeks after loading dose regimen [400 mg at week 0, 2, and 4]) was performed in 409 patients with psoriatic arthritis. Within the 79.3% of patients with baseline nail disease, there was a change in mean NAPSI of −1.1 (32% decrease), −1.6 (52% decrease), and −2.0 (59% decrease) in the placebo, certolizumab 200 mg, and certolizumab 400 mg groups after 24 weeks, respectively. Common adverse effects were injection site reactions, diarrhea, headache, nasopharyngitis, upper respiratory tract infections, and transaminitis.

Third-Line Therapies

• Topical 5-fluorouracil	A
• Topical Psoralen and ultraviolet A (PUVA)	D
• Pulsed dye laser (PDL)	A
• Excimer laser	B
• Photodynamic therapy (PDT)	B
• Lindioil	B
• Ciclosporin	B
• Anthralin	D
• Intense pulsed light (IPL)	D
• Leflunomide	D
• Tofacitinib	A

Dystrophic psoriatic fingernails treated with 1% 5-fluorouracil in a nail penetration-enhancing vehicle: a double-blind study. De Jong EM, Menke HE, van Praag MC, van De Kerkhof PC. Dermatology 1999; 199: 313–8.

In a split-hand study of 57 patients with psoriatic fingernails, 1% topical 5-fluorouracil in a urea and propylene glycol vehicle (Belanyx lotion) and Belanyx lotion alone both led to 30% to 40% improvement in the total nail area severity (NAS) scores of a target nail and to improved patient- and investigator-reported outcomes after 12 weeks. No significant difference was observed between the two treatments, however.

Topical 5-fluorouracil can worsen onycholysis and should thus be used with caution in nail psoriasis patients who have onycholysis as the most prominent sign.

Local PUVA treatment for nail psoriasis. Handfield-Jones SE, Boyle J, Harman RR. Br J Dermatol 1987; 116: 280–1.

In a case series of five patients, 1% 8-methoxypsoralen (Meladinine) solution was applied from the proximal nail fold up to the terminal phalanx of affected fingernails followed by 0.5 J/cm² increasing up to a max of 2 J/cm² of ultraviolet A (UVA) two to three times a week. Two patients achieved sustained clearance for 4 to 8 months, two patients improved significantly, and one patient did not have sustained improvement. Onycholysis appeared to respond better to topical PUVA than did nail pits.

The effect of different pulse durations in the treatment of nail psoriasis with 595-nm pulsed dye laser: a randomized, double-blind, intrapatient left-to-right study. Treewittayapoom C, Singvahanont P, Chanprapaph K, Haneke E. J Am Acad Dermatol 2012; 66: 807–12.

Twenty patients were treated monthly with 6-ms pulse duration and 9 J/cm² PDL settings on one hand and 0.45-ms pulse duration and 6 J/cm² PDL settings on the other for 6 months. NAPSI improved significantly in both groups (roughly 40% decrease) within the first 3 months, but there was no significant difference between the two pulse duration groups. Participants reported greater pain with the longer pulse duration, and transient petechiae and hyperpigmentation were observed in both groups.

Single blinded left-to-right comparison study of excimer laser versus pulsed dye laser for the treatment of nail psoriasis. Al-Mutairi N, Noor T, Al-Haddad A. Dermatol Ther 2014; 4: 197–205.

Forty-two patients with psoriatic nail disease were treated with twice-weekly excimer laser on the right hand and monthly PDL on the left hand for up to 12 weeks in this unblinded study. The mean NAPSI scores decreased significantly in both treatment groups, but improvement was significantly greater with PDL (NAPSI decreased from 29.5–3.2 [89% reduction]) than excimer laser (NAPSI decreased from 29.8–16.3 [45% reduction]). Subungual hyperkeratosis and onycholysis were most responsive to laser treatment, whereas nail pitting was least responsive.

Pulsed dye laser vs. photodynamic therapy in the treatment of refractory nail psoriasis: a comparative pilot study. Fernandez-Guarino M, Harto A, Sanchez-Ronco M, Garcia-Morales I, Jaen P. J Eur Acad Dermatol Venereol 2009; 23: 891–5.

In an unblinded, intrapatient, split-hand study, 14 patients received PDT (methyl-aminolevulinic acid [MAL] with PDL) on one hand and PDL alone on the other hand monthly for 6 months. Both treatments resulted in improvements in NAPSI, but there was no significant difference between PDT and PDL.

Although the results suggest a lack of benefit with topical MAL, we cannot make any definitive conclusions about the efficacy of PDT for nail psoriasis based on this lone study.

A Chinese herb, *Indigo naturalis*, extracted in oil (Lindioil) used topically to treat psoriatic nails: a randomized clinical trial. Lin YK, Chang YC, Hui RC, See LC, Chang CJ, Yang CH, et al. JAMA Dermatol 2015; 151: 672–4.

In an investigator-blinded, split-hand study of Lindioil versus topical calcipotriol solution in 33 patients, significantly greater improvements in the single-hand NAPSI scores were seen in Lindioil-treated nails (51.3% improvement) compared with calcipotriol-treated nails (27.1% improvement) after 24 weeks. Two patients experienced irritation from Lindioil.

Evaluation of the efficacy of methotrexate and cyclosporine therapies on psoriatic nails: a one-blind, randomized study. Gumusel M, Ozdemir M, Mevlitoglu I, Bodur S. J Eur Acad Dermatol Venereol 2011; 25: 1080–4.

In an investigator-blinded, randomized trial, 34 patients received subcutaneous methotrexate (15 mg weekly for first 3 months, then 10 mg weekly for the second 3 months) or ciclosporin (5 mg/kg/day for the first 3 months, then 2.5–3.5 mg/kg/day for the second 3 months), which led to a moderate reduction in NAPSI scores by 43% and 37%, respectively, after 6 months. There was no significant difference between the two treatment groups. Methotrexate was associated with statistically significant

Evidence Levels: **A** Double-blind study **B** Clinical trial ≥ 20 subjects **C** Clinical trial < 20 subjects **D** Series ≥ 5 subjects **E** Anecdotal case reports

improvements in nail matrix findings, whereas ciclosporin was associated with statistically significant improvements in nail bed findings.

Topical anthralin therapy for refractory nail psoriasis. Yamamoto T, Katayama I, Nishioka K. J Dermatol 1998; 25: 231–3.

In the comparative prepost study of 20 patients who applied 0.4% to 2.0% anthralin in petrolatum daily for 5 months, 12 (60%) patients had greater than 50% improvement of their nails, and 4 (20%) patients had no response. Anthralin worked most effectively for onycholysis and thickened nails and variably for pitting, whereas transverse or longitudinal lines did not respond. The main side effect was reversible pigmentation of the nail plate.

Novel treatment of nail psoriasis using the intense pulsed light: a one-year follow-up study. Tawfik AA. Dermatol Surg 2014; 40: 763–8.

In the comparative prepost study, 20 patients with fingernail and toenail psoriasis were treated with IPL every 2 weeks until no further improvement or for a maximum of 6 months. After a mean of 8.6 treatments, significant improvements were observed in NAPSI scores, with 32.2% of patients improving on the nail matrix NAPSI and 71.2% of patients improving on the nail bed NAPSI. Nail disease relapsed in three patients after 6 months after treatment.

Leflunomide in psoriatic arthritis: results from a large European prospective observational study. Behrens F, Finkenwirth C, Pavelka K, Stolfa J, Sipek-Dolnicar A, Thaci D, et al. Arthritis Care Res 2013; 65: 464–70.

A subgroup analysis of nail psoriasis was performed within a prospective, 24-week observational study of 511 patients receiving leflunomide for treatment of psoriatic arthritis. Approximately 32% of patients with psoriatic nail lesions at baseline had significant improvement in their nails. In the overall study, 12% of patients experienced adverse effects, most frequently diarrhea, alopecia, hypertension, and pruritus. Three instances of serious drug reactions (transaminitis and hypertensive crisis) were observed.

Tofacitinib, an oral Janus kinase inhibitor, for the treatment of chronic plaque psoriasis: results from two randomized, placebo-controlled, phase III trials. Papp KA, Menter MA, Abe M, Elewski B, Feldman SR, Gottlieb AB, et al. Br J Dermatol 2015; 173: 949–61.

In subgroup analyses significant dose-dependent improvements in NAPSI were observed at week 16. NAPSI improved by a mean of 14% to 22% among the 408 patients with nail psoriasis who received tofacitinib 5 mg twice daily and by 26% to 42% among the 404 patients who received tofacitinib 10 mg twice daily. Although overall rates of adverse events were similar across treatment groups, there were 12 cases of herpes zoster in the tofacitinib groups in contrast to none in the placebo groups.

Necrobiosis lipoidica

Nicole Yi Zhen Chiang, Ian Coulson

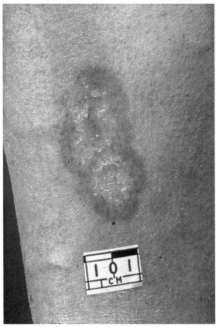

Necrobiosis lipoidica (NL) is a chronic cutaneous granulomatous condition with degenerative connective tissue changes. It is only seen in 1 in 300 diabetics but may be unassociated with glucose intolerance. NL may rarely be complicated by ulceration and squamous cell carcinoma.

MANAGEMENT STRATEGY

Smoking cessation and avoiding trauma to the affected shins are key factors to avoid transformation from an unsightly plaque into a painful, recalcitrant ulcer. The progression of new lesions may be halted by *intralesional or occluded potent topical corticosteroids* applied to the margins of the lesions. Once atrophy has developed, there is little that will reverse this, although *topical retinoids* may be tried. Telangiectasia is often marked and has been treated with *pulsed dye laser*. Extensive lesions may justify trials of *nicotinamide or prednisolone*. Antiplatelet therapy in the form of *aspirin or dipyridamole* has its enthusiasts, though responses are inconclusive. Phototherapy such as *topical psoralen and Ultraviolet VA (PUVA) and UVA-1*, as well as *photodynamic therapy*, have received recent interest and may arrest progression and improve the appearance. A variety of systemic antiinflammatory and immunosuppressive agents have been tried with some success, including *mycophenolate mofetil, fumaric acid esters, ciclosporin, antimalarials, thalidomide, and pentoxifylline*. *Infliximab and etanercept* have also been proposed.

The chronically ulcerated lesion is a challenge; antibiotics deal with secondary infection, appropriate dressings may be required, and growth factors such as *becaplermin and granulocyte–macrophage colony-stimulating factor (GM-CSF)* may accelerate healing. Because diabetics may have coexisting large vessel atherosclerosis that may contribute to ulceration, noninvasive arterial studies or angiography needs to be considered if clinically indicated.

Excision and grafting may transform the patient's quality of life and improve cosmesis. Work with the diabetologist to optimize diabetic control.

Specific Investigations

- Two-hour postprandial glucose
- Skin biopsy
- Consider angiography or venous circulation studies
- Consider a biopsy to exclude sarcoidosis, which may mimic NL, or if clinical features suggest, the rare development of squamous cell carcinoma
- Consider thyroid function tests

Squamous cell carcinoma arising in an area of long-standing necrobiosis lipoidica. Lim C, Tschuchnigg M, Lim J. J Cutan Pathol 2006; 33: 581–3.

Case report of a squamous cell carcinoma arising de novo in an area of NL.

Carcinoma cuniculatum arising in necrobiosis lipoidica. Porneuf M, Monpoint S, Barnéon G, Alirezai M, Guillot B, Guilhou JJ. Ann Dermatol Venereol 1991; 118: 461–4.

Although rare, squamous cell carcinomas may complicate any condition in which papillary dermal scarring is appreciable.

Unilateral necrobiosis lipoidica of the ischemic limb – a case report. Naschitz JE, Fields M, Isseroff H, Wolffson V, Yeshurun D. Angiology 2003; 54: 239–42.

A possible ischemic pathogenesis of NL emerges from a case of unilateral large vessel arteriosclerotic ischemia with ipsilateral NL.

The author has experience of a severely ulcerated area of NL that only started to heal after the disobliteration of severe femoropopliteal atheroma.

Updated results of 100 patients on clinical features and therapeutic options in necrobiosis lipoidica in a retrospective multicenter study. Erfurt-Berge C, Dissemond J, Schwede K, Seitz AT, Al Ghazal P, Wollina U, et al. Eur J Dermatol 2015 25:595–601.

This multicenter retrospective study included 100 patients with NL lesions on the lower leg. Thyroid disorders were found in 15% of all cases.

First-Line Therapies

- Stop smoking and optimize diabetic control   C
- Intralesional or topical corticosteroids under occlusion   D

Necrobiosis lipoidica diabeticorum: association with background retinopathy, smoking, and proteinuria. A case controlled study. Kelly WF, Nicholas J, Adams J, Mahmood R. Diabet Med 1993; 10: 725–8.

Stop smoking and control diabetes mellitus with vigilance. Fifteen diabetics with NL were each matched with five control subjects with diabetes mellitus. Background retinopathy, proteinuria, and smoking were all more common with NL. No differences were noted between those with NL and controls in the prevalence of vascular

Evidence Levels: **A** Double-blind study   **B** Clinical trial ≥ 20 subjects   **C** Clinical trial < 20 subjects   **D** Series ≥ 5 subjects   **E** Anecdotal case reports

disease and neuropathy. Glycosylated hemoglobin concentrations were higher in patients with NL.

Granuloma annulare and necrobiosis lipoidica treated by jet injector. Sparrow G, Abell E. Br J Dermatol 1975; 93: 85–9.

Three of five cases of NL underwent complete resolution, and one had partial improvement with 5 mg/mL triamcinolone injection to the edges of lesions. No serious complications of this type of treatment were observed.

Treatment of psoriasis and other dermatoses with a single application of a corticosteroid left under a hydrocolloid occlusive dressing for a week. Juhlin L. Acta Dermatol Venereol 1989; 69: 355–7.

A 0.1% betamethasone alcoholic lotion under a hydrocolloid dressing was an effective, well-tolerated treatment, and three applications only were required.

Second-Line Therapies

• Systemic corticosteroids	D
• Aspirin and dipyridamole	C
• Pentoxifylline	E
• Nicotinamide	D
• Clofazimine	D
• Topical PUVA	D
• Topical tacrolimus	E

Necrobiosis lipoidica: treatment with systemic corticosteroids. Petzelbauer P, Wolff K, Tappeiner G. Br J Dermatol 1992; 126: 542–5.

Oral methylprednisolone was given to six patients with nonulcerating NL for 5 weeks; in all there was cessation of disease activity during the 7-month follow-up period. Initial dosage was 1 mg/kg daily for 1 week, then 40 mg daily for 4 weeks, followed by tapering and termination in 2 weeks. All patients, including the diabetics, tolerated the treatment well. There was no improvement in atrophy. Benefit was maintained at the end of the 7-month follow-up period.

Careful monitoring of blood glucose is mandatory in all diabetic patients with NL treated with systemic corticosteroids.

Pentoxifylline: an effective therapy for necrobiosis lipoidica. Wee E, Kelly R. Australas J Dermatol 2015 Nov 12 [Epub ahead of print].

Three cases of biopsy-proven NL were treated with pentoxifylline 400 mg three times daily. Patient 1 and 2 had early-stage NL, presenting with indurated, red-brown plaques. Pentoxifylline reversed the inflammation and induration completely after 7 and 12 months, respectively. No recurrence in activity was seen in patient 1 after 12 months. In patient 3, pentoxifylline was effective in reversing ulceration completely after 10 months of treatment. Some areas of atrophy remained in all patients. None of the patients reported significant side effects.

Healing of necrobiotic ulcers with antiplatelet therapy. Correlation with plasma thromboxane levels. Heng MC, Song MK, Heng MK. Int J Dermatol 1989; 28: 195–7.

NL in diabetics has been considered a cutaneous manifestation of diabetic microangiopathy. Seven diabetic patients with necrobiotic ulcers of recent onset that healed after administration of 80 mg/day of acetylsalicylic acid and 75 mg three times daily of dipyridamole had elevated thromboxane levels. Healing was associated with depression of the elevated thromboxane levels in all seven patients.

Treatment of necrobiosis lipoidica with low-dose acetylsalicylic acid. A randomized double-blind trial. Beck HI, Bjerring P, Rasmussen I, Zachariae H, Stenbjerg S. Acta Dermatol Venereol 1985; 65: 230–4.

No response was seen with the use of 40 mg acetylsalicylic acid daily for 24 weeks, despite documented platelet aggregation inhibition.

Necrobiosis lipoidica: a case with histopathological findings revealed asteroid bodies and was successfully treated with dipyridamole plus intralesional triamcinolone. Jiquan S, Khalaf AT, Jinquan T, Xiaoming L. J Dermatolog Treat 2008; 19: 54–7.

A 48-year-old woman with more than 2 years' history of NL plaques on her right leg responded to 25 mg three times daily of dipyridamole plus intralesional triamcinolone. After 4 weeks of therapy, she developed mild dizziness, and the dose was reduced to twice daily. The NL lesions healed completely after 2 months.

High dose nicotinamide in the treatment of necrobiosis lipoidica. Handfield-Jones S, Jones S, Peachey R. Br J Dermatol 1988; 118: 693–6.

An open study of high-dose nicotinamide (1.5 grams a day) in the treatment of 15 patients with NL. Of 13 patients who remained on treatment for more than 1 month, 8 improved. A reduction in pain, soreness, and erythema, and the healing of ulcers if present, was noted. There were no significant side effects, particularly with respect to diabetic control. Lesions tended to relapse if treatment was stopped.

Clofazimine – therapeutic alternative in necrobiosis lipoidica and granuloma annulare. Mensing H. Int J Dermatol 1989; 28: 195–7.

Ten patients with NL were treated with clofazimine 200 mg orally daily. Six of 10 patients responded; 3 of the responders achieved complete remission of the dermatosis. All the patients treated had reddening of the skin, but this was reversible after the end of therapy, as were the other side effects (i.e., diarrhea and dryness of the skin).

Topical PUVA treatment for necrobiosis lipoidica. McKenna DB, Cooper EJ, Tidman MJ. Br J Dermatol 2000; 143: 71.

Four of eight patients with NL responded favorably to topical PUVA using a 0.15% methoxsalen emulsion, with weekly treatments, starting with 0.5 J/cm² with 20% incremental increases until erythema developed at the edge of the lesions. The mean number of treatments administered was 39.

Successful treatment of chronic ulcerated necrobiosis lipoidica with 0.1% topical tacrolimus ointment. Clayton T, Harrison P. Br J Dermatol 2005; 152: 581–2.

A case report of ulcerated NL that healed successfully with 0.1% tacrolimus ointment applied twice daily for 1 month.

Third-Line Therapies

• Topical retinoids	E
• Ciclosporin	E
• Heparin	E
• Antimalarials	E
• Mycophenolate mofetil	E

Necrobiosis lipoidica treated with topical tretinoin. Heymann WR. Cutis 1996; 58: 53–4.

A case is presented in which atrophy was diminished by the application of topical tretinoin.

Persistent ulcerated necrobiosis lipoidica responding to treatment with cyclosporin. Darvay A, Acland KM, Russell-Jones R. Br J Dermatol 1999; 141: 725–7.

In two patients with severely ulcerated NL the ulceration healed completely after 4 months of cyclosporin therapy, and both patients have remained free of ulceration since. Effective doses were between 3 and 5 mg/kg daily. Three other reports of the effective use of cyclosporin therapy in ulcerated NL now exist.

Minidose heparin therapy for vasculitis of atrophie blanche. Jetton RL, Lazarus GS. J Am Acad Dermatol 1983; 8: 23–6.

The authors speculate that subcutaneous heparin 5000 IU twice daily may help NL because it helped the vasculitis associated with atrophie blanche. A subsequent letter informs that perilesional low-dose heparin has been successfully used in NL by Russian dermatologists.

Necrobiosis lipoidica diabeticorum treated with chloroquine. Nguyen K, Washenik K, Shupack J. J Am Acad Dermatol 2002; 46(Suppl Case Reports): S34–6.

Single successful report using oral chloroquine.

Significant improvement in ulcerative necrobiosis lipoidica with hydroxychloroquine. Kavala M, Sudogan S, Zindanci I, Kocaturk E, Can B, Turkoglu Z, et al. Int J Dermatol 2010; 49: 467–9.

A 62-year-old woman with type 2 diabetes mellitus and ulcerative NL on both shins achieved almost complete clearance of ulcerations after taking oral hydroxychloroquine, 200 mg twice daily, for 10 weeks.

Ulcerative necrobiosis lipoidica responsive to colchicine. Schofield C, Sladden MJ. Australas J Dermatol 2012; 53: e54–7.

Single report of 10 years of bilateral ulcerative NL achieved complete resolution of ulcers after 2 months of colchicine 500 µg twice daily.

Successful treatment of ulcerated necrobiosis lipoidica with mycophenolate mofetil. Reinhard G, Lohmann F, Uerlich M, Bauer R, Bieber T. Acta Dermatol Venereol 2000; 80: 312–3.

A 61-year-old woman with NL for over 30 years was started on mycophenolate mofetil 0.5 g twice daily, and the lesions regressed

within 4 weeks. The dose was reduced to 0.5 g over the next 4 months and then stopped. Within 14 days of stopping mycophenolate mofetil the ulceration recurred.

Photodynamic therapy of necrobiosis lipoidica – a multicenter study of 18 patients. Berking C, Hegyi J, Arenberger P, Ruzicka T, Jemec GB. Dermatology 2009; 218: 136–9.

A retrospective study of 18 patients with NL who were treated with photodynamic therapy (PDT) using methyl aminolevulinate or 5-aminolevulinic acid as topically applied photosensitizers. Complete response was seen in 1/18 patients after 9 PDT cycles and partial response in 6/18 patients (2–14 PDT cycles), giving an overall response rate of 39% (7/18).

Photodynamic therapy for necrobiosis lipoidica is an unpredictable option: three cases with different results. Truchuelo T, Alcántara J, Fernandez-Guarino M, Pérez B, Jaén P. Int J Dermatol 2013; 52: 1567–1624.

Three patients were treated with methyl aminolevulinic (MAL) acid cream (Metvix) under occlusion for 3 hours, followed by irradiation with red light (630 nm, 37 J/cm², 7.5 min). The intervals between treatment ranged from 1 to 3 months (patient 1: two sessions, patient 2: one session, and patient 3: three sessions). Patient 1 and 2 were nonresponders. Patient 3 experienced great improvement after the second session. Pain during irradiation was the most common side effect.

Effectiveness of platelet-rich plasma in healing necrobiosis lipoidica diabeticorum ulcers. Motolese A, Vignati F, Antelmi A, Saturni V. Clin Exp Dermatol 2015; 40: 39–41.

Fifteen patients with recalcitrant NL on the legs were treated with homologous platelet-rich plasma. All patients responded with a mean reduction in wound size of 79% after 84 to 126 days without any adverse effects.

Successful treatment of ulcerative necrobiosis lipoidica diabeticorum with intravenous immunoglobulin in a patient with common variable immunodeficiency. Barouti N, Qian Cao A, Ferrara D, Prins C. JAMA Dermatol 2013; 149: 879–81.

A 63-year-old female with recurrent ear, nose, and throat infections and 7 years of ulcerating NL lesions was found to have common variable immunodeficiency (CVID). The patient was treated with intravenous immunoglobulin (0.4 g/kg/d) for 5 consecutive days. Three weeks after this single cycle, all ulcerations healed completely with no recurrence after 2 years.

Intralesional infliximab in noninfectious cutaneous granulomas: three cases of necrobiosis lipoidica. Barde C, Laffitte E, Campanelli A, Saurat JH, Thielen AM. Dermatology 2011; 222: 212–6.

Three patients with NL had three cycles of three weekly injections of intralesional infliximab with a 1-week treatment interruption between each cycle. Two patients experienced almost complete remission for up to 18 months. The third patient showed partial improvement. No serious side effects were noticed, apart from pain at injection sites.

Treatment of refractory ulcerative necrobiosis lipoidica diabeticorum with infliximab: report of a case. Hu SW, Bevona C, Winterfield L, Qureshi AA, Li VW. Arch Dermatol 2009; 145: 437–9.

An 84-year-old woman with a 3-year history of ulcerative NL on the right leg responded to five infusions of intravenous infliximab (5 mg/kg) at weeks 0, 2, 6, 12, and 21. Complete wound healing was achieved at week 6 of infliximab therapy, with excellent

Evidence Levels: **A** Double-blind study **B** Clinical trial ≥ 20 subjects **C** Clinical trial < 20 subjects **D** Series ≥ 5 subjects **E** Anecdotal case reports

cosmesis. The patient experienced no adverse effects from infliximab and no recurrence for more than 1 year.

Treatment of necrobiosis lipoidica with etanercept and adalimumab. Zhang KS, Quan LT, Hsu S. Dermatol Online J 2009; 15: 12.

A 29-year-old with noninsulin-dependent diabetes and more than 9 years. history of NL on her legs and trunk received subcutaneous etanercept 50-mg injections twice weekly for 3 months and then weekly after that. She achieved significant improvement and complete pain resolution by 4 months. Due to insurance reasons, the patient was switched to subcutaneous adalimumab (40 mg) injections for 3 months, which did not result in any improvement. Six months after switching back to etanercept, the patient reported progressive improvement in the NL lesions. No significant side effects were reported apart from tiredness.

Treatment of necrobiosis lipoidica with the tumor necrosis factor antagonist etanercept. Zeichner JA, Stern DW, Lebwohl M. J Am Acad Dermatol 2006; 54: S120–1.

A 35-year-old woman with type 1 diabetes and NL plaque on her right shin was started on weekly intralesional etanercept (25 mg) injections into the dermis at 1-cm intervals throughout the surface area of the lesion. Initial improvement was observed by the first month of treatment, and the lesion continued to resolve over the next 8 months. The patient experienced no side effects from etanercept.

Fumaric acid esters in necrobiosis lipoidica: results of a prospective noncontrolled study. Kreuter A, Knierim C, Stücker M, Pawlak F, Rotterdam S, Altmeyer P, et al. Br J Dermatol 2005; 153: 802–7.

Eighteen patients with NL were given the standard Fumaderm regimen as used in psoriasis for at least 6 months. Three discontinued therapy, but the rest gained significant clinical, ultrasonographic, and histologic improvement.

The management of hard-to-heal necrobiosis with Promogran. Omugha N, Jones AM. Br J Nurs 2003; 15: S14–20.

A single case study with nonhealing ulcerated NL of 3 years' duration. Treatment with a new protease-modulating matrix (freeze-dried matrix composed of collagen and oxidized regenerated cellulose) resulted in complete healing of the ulcer after 8 weeks, where other dressing regimens had failed to effect healing over a period of 2.5 years.

Healing of chronic leg ulcers in diabetic necrobiosis lipoidica with local granulocyte–macrophage colony-stimulating factor treatment. Remes K, Ronnemaa T. J Diabetes Complications 1999; 13: 115–8.

Topical recombinant human GM-CSF healed two patients with ulcerated NL within 10 weeks. A reduction in the size of the ulcers was already evident after the first topical applications. The ulcers have remained healed for more than 3 years.

Becaplermin and necrobiosis lipoidicum diabeticorum: results of a case control pilot study. Stephens E, Robinson JA, Gottlieb PA. J Diabetes Complications 2001; 15: 55–6.

Five patients with type 1 diabetes mellitus and NL were treated with topical becaplermin gel (recombinant platelet-derived growth factor). The index patient had ulcerated NL, and this healed. Three of the five patients with nonulcerated NL reported a subjective improvement in sensation and lightening of color of the lesions. However, serial photographs and measurements over the 5-month treatment period showed no significant change in the size of the treated areas.

The surgical treatment of necrobiosis lipoidica diabeticorum. Dubin BJ, Kaplan EN. Plast Reconstruct Surg 1977; 60: 421–8.

Seven cases treated by excision of the lesions down to the deep fascia, ligation of the associated perforating blood vessels, and the use of split-skin grafts to cover the defects. There were no recurrences.

Thalidomide for the treatment of refractory necrobiosis lipoidica. Kukreja T, Peterson J. Arch Dermatol 2006; 142: 20–2.

A 51-year-old woman was treated successfully with a dose of thalidomide 150 mg daily, tapering to 50 mg twice weekly. A response was seen after 4 months and maintained after 2 years.

Treatment of ulcerated necrobiosis lipoidica with intravenous immunoglobulin and methylprednisolone. Batchelor JM, Todd PM. J Drugs Dermatol 2012; 11: 256–9.

The authors report a case of a female patient with recalcitrant ulcerated NL that was resistant to several systemic agents but who initially responded to intravenous immunoglobulin. However, this became less effective over time, but a course of intravenous methylprednisolone led to regression.

UVA1 phototherapy for treatment of necrobiosis lipoidica. Beattie PE, Dawe RS, Ibbotson SH, Ferguson J. Clin Exp Dermatol 2006; 31: 235–8.

Six patients with NL were treated with UVA1 irradiation. The minimum erythema dose was determined at 24 h, and 50% of this dose was used as a starting dose. Treatment was given three to five times weekly with increments of 20% at each visit. NL resolved completely in one patient after 29 exposures. Two subjects obtained moderate improvement after 15 and 24 exposures, whereas two had only minimal improvement after 15 and 51 exposures. The remaining patient had no improvement after 16 treatments.

Necrolytic acral erythema

Courtney Rubin, Carrie Kavorik

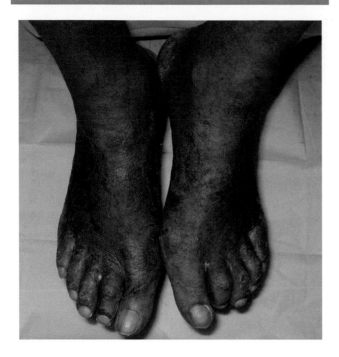

Necrolytic acral erythema (NAE) is characterized as sharply demarcated, erythematous to violaceous, hyperpigmented, hyperkeratotic plaques with variable scale and occasional erosions, surrounded by a rim of erythema. The lesions of NAE tend to affect the dorsal hands and feet (especially the great toe) but have also been reported to extend to the legs and trunk. The head, neck, palms, soles, nail plate, nail bed, and mucous membranes are typically spared, though exceptions have been noted. Less commonly, NAE may present with acute blistering lesions.

Hepatitis C virus (HCV) infection is one of the most common bloodborne infections globally, with approximately 3% of the world's population affected. Although HCV infection primarily affects the liver, it has also been associated with several mucocutaneous manifestations, including leukocytoclastic vasculitis, cryoglobulinemia, lichen planus, porphyria cutanea tarda, polyarteritis nodosa, and generalized pruritus. NAE is another distinct cutaneous manifestation of HCV infection that was first described in 1996 in Egypt in seven patients with chronic HCV infection.

MANAGEMENT STRATEGY

Some have categorized the evolution of NAE into three distinct stages. The initial stage consists of a small (2–3 mm) erythematous papule that grows in surface area and thickness to become covered in scale. The center of the papule may become dusky or develop an erosion. The fully developed stage consists of increasing surface area and confluence of the initial stage lesions, leading to sharply demarcated erythematous lichenified plaques with overlying scale. Thin crust, vesicles, pustules, and weeping may

also be seen in this stage. The late stage is characterized by thinning and hyperpigmentation of previously developed lesions, followed by spontaneous relapse and remission. The lesions of NAE are often locally pruritic, though in some cases the pruritus can be generalized. Other patients have complained that the lesions cause aching or burning pain.

Although the exact pathogenesis of NAE is not known, infection with hepatitis C seems to have an essential role in the development of it. The lack of NAE lesions in patients with other cirrhotic conditions such as alcoholic hepatitis or hepatitis B infection excludes chronic liver damage as the sole cause. Attempts to identify hepatitis C viral particles or RNA in NAE biopsies using electron microscopy and reverse transcription polymerase chain reaction (RT-PCR) have not been successful. Reduced amino acid levels, elevated glucagon levels, reduced fatty acid levels, reduced serum zinc, and reduced epidermal zinc have all been implicated in NAE and may be related to HCV-induced metabolic alterations. Zinc deficiency especially has been suggested as a pathogenic factor given the responsiveness of NAE to oral zinc sulfate. Although many patients with NAE who respond to oral zinc have normal zinc levels, some have postulated that cutaneous zinc levels may be low in these patients. The role of zinc in the pathogenesis of NAE remains unclear. Because zinc is believed to be antiapoptotic, some have postulated that its deficiency may lead to epidermal necrolysis. Zinc deficiency may also impair the transport of essential nutrients like vitamin A to the epidermis. Because not all patients with NAE are responsive to oral zinc supplementation, it is likely that the etiology of NAE is multifactorial.

In one study, 87% of patients diagnosed with NAE were unaware of their underlying HCV infection.

Early NAE may present with vesicular lesions on the dorsal hands or feet that may be confused with acute eczematous reactions, contact dermatitis, or stasis changes when it is limited to the feet and/or legs. Chronic NAE may mimic lichen simplex chronicus. The necrolytic erythemas include necrolytic migratory erythema, acrodermatitis enteropathica, pellagra, and NAE. Although these entities may all share some clinical and histologic features, they can be distinguished based on cutaneous distribution and underlying biochemical abnormalities. Necrolytic migratory erythema presents with elevated glucagon levels, whereas acrodermatitis enteropathica presents with depressed zinc levels, and pellagra is associated with niacin deficiency. NAE may also be distinguished based on its association with HCV and acral distribution.

On histology, NAE demonstrates psoriasiform hyperplasia, acanthosis, papillomatosis, and parakeratosis. Vascular ectasia can be seen within the dermal papillae, along with pigment incontinence. A superficial, patchy, dermal, perivascular lymphocytic and neutrophilic infiltrate with extension into the epidermis is often seen, along with necrotic keratinocytes in the superficial epidermis. In the absence of necrotic keratinocytes, NAE can be easily confused with psoriasis histologically. Because NAE lacks pathognomonic histology, a high index of suspicion and clinical-pathologic correlation is required for diagnosis.

Specific Investigations

- Liver function tests
- Serology for hepatitis C
- Skin biopsy

In patients who may have NAE, a hepatitis panel and liver function tests can help to clarify the diagnosis. Other tests that may

Evidence Levels: **A** Double-blind study **B** Clinical trial ≥ 20 subjects **C** Clinical trial < 20 subjects **D** Series ≥ 5 subjects **E** Anecdotal case reports

distinguish NAE from entities in the differential diagnosis include serum albumin, total protein, amino acids, zinc, biotin, and glucagon levels.

A cutaneous marker of viral hepatitis C. El Darouti M, Abu el Ela M. Int J Dermatol 1996; 35: 252–6.

A cutaneous sign of hepatitis C virus infection. Abdallah MA, Ghozzi MY, Monib HA, Hafez AM, Hiatt KM, Smoller BR, et al. J Am Acad Dermatol 2005; 53: 247–51.

Many patients diagnosed with NAE have historically been from Egypt, where the high burden of HCV infection has affected 15% to 20% of the population. The increased prevalence of NAE in Egypt may also be related to HCV genotype 4, which is endemic there, or a genetic predisposition in the population or environmental cofactor. In the United States the prevalence of NAE among patients with chronic HCV infection appears to be low, around 1.7%.

Low prevalence of necrolytic acral erythema in patients with chronic hepatitis C virus infection. Raphael B, Dorey-Stein ZL, Lott J, Amorosa V, Lo Re V, Kovarik C. J Am Acad Dermatol 2012; 67: 962–8.

Most patients in the United States with NAE are African American, and there does not appear to be a gender predilection. The vast majority of NAE has been observed in patients with HCV infection. However, several cases of seronegative NAE have been reported.

First-Line Treatments

- Zinc sulfate **C**
- Treatment of underlying hepatitis C **C**

Necrolytic acral erythema as a cutaneous marker of hepatitis C: report of two cases and review. Tabibian JH, Gerstenblith MR, Tedford RJ, Junkins-Hopkins JM, Abuav R. Dig Dis Sci 2010; 55: 2735–43.

Necrolytic acral erythema: a review of the literature. Geria AN, Holcomb KZ, Scheinfeld NS. Cutis 2009; 83: 309–14.

The cost, safety, and previous success of oral zinc supplementation in treating NAE make it first-line therapy. A response to oral zinc supplementation is usually observed within several weeks. The response to oral zinc seems to be dose dependent, with less improvement when a lower dose, such as 60 mg per day, is used. Although some patients successfully treated with oral zinc demonstrate low zinc levels, many are responsive to oral zinc supplementation despite normal zinc levels. Remission of lesions after a combination of oral zinc and intralesional injections of interferon alfa-2b has also been reported, suggesting that treatment with oral zinc may be enhanced by interferon.

Thus far, oral zinc supplementation with 220 mg oral zinc sulfate twice daily seems to be the most effective treatment for NAE with the fewest side effects. Many have reported improvement in and remission of NAE with long-term oral zinc supplementation. Successful treatment of NAE often leaves behind postinflammatory pigmentation with complete resolution of symptoms. The mechanism by which oral zinc treats NAE is not yet understood. It is possible that patients with HCV have metabolic derangements that lead to low zinc levels or that these patients have low cutaneous zinc levels even in the setting of normal plasma zinc. Zinc may also have an antiinflammatory, antiviral, and immune-stimulatory effect. Those patients being treated with long-term zinc supplementation should have serum copper levels monitored, as zinc therapy may alter copper bioavailability.

Second-Line Therapies

- Narrowband ultraviolet B (UVB) phototherapy **E**
- Topical tacrolimus **E**

Necrolytic acral erythema: successful treatment with topical tacrolimus ointment. Manzur A, Siddiqui AH. Int J Dermatol 2008; 47: 1073–5.

Patients have been reported to have modest improvement of NAE after narrowband UVB therapy, and one patient completely cleared and maintained remission after a liver transplant. Improvement in NAE has also been reported after treatment of the underlying HCV with interferon alpha, with or without ribavirin. However, NAE may relapse after the interferon treatment is discontinued. There is one report of complete resolution of NAE after application of 0.1% topical tacrolimus ointment for 4 weeks. NAE generally does not respond to topical corticosteroids or intralesional triamcinolone injections.

Necrolytic migratory erythema

Benedict C. Wu, Sandra A. Kopp, Analisa Vincent Halpern

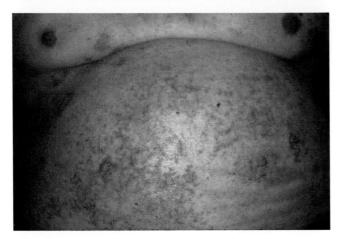

Necrolytic migratory erythema (NME) is a characteristic paraneoplastic cutaneous reaction classically associated with an underlying gastroenteropancreatic neuroendocrine tumor (NET), most commonly a pancreatic islet α-cell neoplasm. NME has also been associated with the pseudoglucagonoma syndrome (hyperglucagonemia in the absence of a glucagon-secreting tumor), metastatic NET, glucagon infusion–dependent states, hepatic disease, gluten-sensitive enteropathy, pancreatic insufficiency, glucagon cell adenomatosis, other malabsorption or malnutritional states, and cholangiocarcinoma. It may be associated with a polyfunctional endocrine tumor (MEN1).

NME is classically accompanied by weight loss, new-onset or worsening diabetes mellitus, normocytic anemia, and hyperglucagonemia.

The lesions begin as pruritic or painful erythematous patches with central bullae formation leading to the classic appearance of a centrally crusted, annular erosive plaque with a psoriasiform border.

NME can be widespread but has a predilection for areas subject to pressure and friction such as the buttocks, inferior abdomen, lower extremities, and intertriginous areas.

Parakeratosis and upper-level keratinocyte vacuolization are characteristic on histopathologic examination of early lesions. The pathogenesis of NME has not been fully elucidated, although several theories have emerged from observations of patient responses to various treatment strategies (e.g., tumor resection, parenteral nutrition with zinc, amino acids, essential fatty acids, etc.). One theory suggests that the catabolic effects of glucagon lead to a hypermetabolic state, resulting in the deficiency of zinc and essential fatty acids. Given the multitude of various diseases that have been associated with NME, a multifactorial model for the pathogenesis of the disease has been hypothesized: (1) hyperglucagonemia-induced hypoalbuminemia leads to deficiencies in zinc (Zn), essential fatty acids (EFA), and amino acids (AA) such as tryptophan (albumin binds and circulates Zn, AA, and EFA throughout the body); (2) Zn deficiency induces primary cutaneous inflammation, as Zn plays a major role in restoring

prostaglandin-mediated inflammatory response in the epidermis; and (3) subsequent tryptophan deficiency causes keratinocyte degradation without concomitant new cell formation. Tryptophan is essential for niacin biosynthesis; without adequate niacin, keratinocytes cannot regulate proper cellular turnover, capillary tone, and appropriate maturation of epidermis and mucosal epithelia. Theoretically, this constellation of elevated serum glucagon, hypoalbuminemia, zinc, EFA and AA deficiency, and potentially hepatic dysfunction ultimately leads to the increase in epidermal inflammation, breakdown, and necrolysis observed in NME.

Necrolytic acral erythema (NAE), often associated with hepatitis C virus (HCV) infection, is considered by some to be an acral variant of NME. Despite the predominantly acral lesions of classical NAE, there have been reports of NAE over the nails, trunk, and proximal extremities as well, and one should consider the diagnosis of atypical NAE in the differential diagnosis of NME.

MANAGEMENT STRATEGY

Addressing the underlying cause of NME is paramount for treatment. In the setting of glucagonoma, *surgical resection* of the tumor is ideal; however, metastasis is commonly present at the time of diagnosis, obfuscating complete cure. Glucagonomas grow slowly and tend to be encapsulated so if caught early and fully excised adjunctive therapy is usually unnecessary. Most traditional chemotherapies are not effective in treating glucagonomas; however, some combination chemotherapy with hormonal regimens can reduce tumor burden, resulting in symptomatic improvement of NME. The *somatostatin agonists*, octreotide and lanreotide, are considered the first-line treatment of choice in NME with or without associated glucagonoma. These agents reduce conversion of proglucagon to the active form of glucagon. The use of *combination chemotherapy* targeting selective islet cells can be considered for moderately and well-differentiated tumors. Additionally, a streptozotocin (STZ)–based combination therapy may be considered for moderately and well-differentiated NETs, particularly when the tumor is pancreatic in origin, intermediate or high grade based on mitotic index or Ki-67, or exhibiting rapid clinical or radiologic progression. It has been reported that STZ and doxorubicin (DOX) combination chemotherapy in pancreatic NETs resulted in a 38% response rate and 32 months' median overall survival. For poorly differentiated NETs a platinum-based chemotherapeutic regimen, such as STZ, 5-FU, and cisplatin (FCiSt), should be considered. *Peptide receptor radioligand* therapy with radiolabeled somatostatin agonists has been tried with moderate success. *Sunitinib*, an inhibitor of multiple receptor tyrosine kinases such as vascular endothelial growth factor (VEGF) and platelet-derived growth factor (PDGF), has demonstrated improved progression-free survival in patients with advanced pancreatic NETs. Adjunctive *deep vein thrombosis (DVT) prophylaxis* should also be advised due to the risk of thromboembolism with glucagonoma. It is clear that correcting any nutritional deficiencies in general (with correction of amino acids, essential fatty acids, or zinc specifically) should be undertaken immediately, as there is good evidence that supplementation has been associated with a marked improvement of the cutaneous lesions of NME.

A diagnosis of NME in the absence of glucagonoma should make one suspect possible underlying nutritional deficiencies or pseudoglucagonoma syndrome. These conditions can be encountered in hepatic disease and other causes of chronic malabsorption such as celiac disease, inflammatory bowel disease, chronic pancreatitis, or metastatic NET and cholangiocarcinoma. Glucagon cell adenomatosis, the diffuse enlargement of islets of Langerhans cells with resulting glucagon hypersecretion, should

Evidence Levels: **A** Double-blind study **B** Clinical trial ≥ 20 subjects **C** Clinical trial < 20 subjects **D** Series ≥ 5 subjects **E** Anecdotal case reports

be expected when there is no evidence of a detectable pancreatic mass on imaging. If MEN1 or a polyfunctional endocrine tumor is suspected, one should consider investigating levels of fasting *insulin, prolactin, parathyroid hormone, calcium, vasoactive intestinal peptide (VIP), gastrin,* and *adrenocorticotropic hormone (ACTH)* in the workup.

Specific Investigations

- Serum glucagon, chromogranin **A**
- Serum zinc, amino acids (tryptophan), total protein, albumin, essential fatty acid, riboflavin, niacin, pyridoxine (vitamin B_6), cyanocobalamin (vitamin B_{12}), biotin, folic acid, pantothenic acid, methylmalonic acid, and propionic acid levels
- Hemoglobin/hematocrit
- Serum fasting glucose
- Serum liver function tests and hepatitis B and C profile
- Abdominal computed tomography (CT) scan, endoscopic ultrasound, celiac angiography, and/or somatostatin receptor scintigraphy
- Multiple endocrine neoplasia type 1 (MEN1) gene
- Serum fasting insulin, prolactin, calcium, VIP, gastrin, parathyroid hormone, ACTH
- Skin biopsy (H&E)

Glucagonoma and glucagonoma syndrome: a case report with review of recent advances in management. Al-Faouri A, Ajarma K, Alghazawi S, Al-Rawabdeh S, Zayadeen A. Case Rep Surg 2016; 2016: Article ID: 1484089, 3 pp.

This case report emphasizes the importance of recognizing the rash of NME in patients with an underlying glucagonoma/glucagonoma syndrome. New advances in the management of metastatic pancreatic NETs include liver resection, liver transplantation, long-acting somatostatin analogs, targeted radiotherapy, radioembolization with selective internal radiation microspheres, and biologic therapy.

Guidelines for the management of gastroenteropancreatic neuroendocrine (including carcinoid) tumors (NETs). Ramage JK, Ahmed A, Ardill J, Bax N, Breen DJ, Caplin ME, et al. Gut 2012; 61: 6–32.

These guidelines have been revised by members of the UK and Ireland Neuroendocrine Tumor Society. The purpose of these guidelines is to identify and inform the key decisions to be made in the management of gastroenteropancreatic NETs. Chemotherapeutic agents included streptozotocin/doxorubicin and temozolomide/capecitabine. A streptozotocin-based combination should be considered for moderately and well-differentitated tumors, whereas a platinum-based regimen should be considered for poorly differentiated NETs.

Octreotide-responsive necrolytic migratory erythema in a patient with pseudoglucagonoma syndrome. Virani S, Prajapati V, Devani A, Mahmood M, Elliott J. J Am Acad Dermatol 2013; 68: e44–6.

A 56-year-old female with a history of ectopic Cushing syndrome with liver metastases was diagnosed with NME secondary to pseudoglucagonoma syndrome. The patient suffered from a 20-year history of recurrent painful cutaneous eruptions that failed to respond to a 2-week tapering course of prednisone. However, near resolution of lesions was observed after 4 weeks of subcutaneous administration of octreotide.

A rare but revealing sign: necrolytic migratory erythema. Compton N, Chien A. Am J Med 2013; 126: 387–9.

Patients with glucagonoma may present initially with NME. This case report highlights the importance of maintaining high clinical suspicion of underlying malignancy, such as glucagonoma, once a diagnosis of NME is made. In this case the patient's rash was completely resolved 6 days after resection of a pancreatic tumor.

Necrolytic migratory erythema-like presentation for cystic fibrosis. Koch LH, Lewis D, Williams JV. J Am Acad Dermatol 2008; 58: S29–30.

This case report supports the chronic malabsorption syndrome (CMS) theory as a cause of NME. Patients with CMS secondary to cystic fibrosis can present with psoriasiform lesions similar to NME. In this single case report, the patient's NME-like lesions resolved after beginning nutritional therapy with zinc and hydrolyzed protein formula.

Necrolytic migratory erythema without glucagonoma in patients with liver disease. Marinkovich MP, Botella R, Datloff J, Sangueza OP. J Am Acad Dermatol 1995; 32: 604–9.

In the absence of glucagonoma, hepatocellular dysfunction and hypoalbuminemia appear to be the most common factors associated with NME. NME may be a cutaneous marker for various liver diseases associated with malnutrition and low-protein states.

Glucagon cell adenomatosis: a new entity associated with necrolytic migratory erythema and glucagonoma syndrome. Otto AI, Marschalko M, Zalatnai A, Toth M, Kovacs J, Harsing J, et al. J Am Acad Dermatol 2001; 65: 458–9.

This report highlights a fatal case of NME in a newly recognized condition of the endocrine pancreas: glucagon cell adenomatosis.

First-Line Therapies

- Lanreotide **A**
- Radiolabeled somatostatin analog **B**
- Radioactive microspheres **B**
- Tumor resection **B**

Lanreotide in metastatic enteropancreatic neuroendocrine tumors. Caplin ME, Pavel M, Cwikla JB, Phan AT, Raderer M, Sedláčková E, et al. N Engl J Med 2014; 17: 224–33.

This randomized, double-blind, placebo-controlled, multinational study of the somatostatin analog lanreotide was shown to significantly prolong progression-free survival among patients with metastatic enteropancreatic NETs of grade 1 or 2.

Treatment with the radiolabeled somatostatin analog [177 Lu-DOTA 0,Tyr3] octreotate: toxicity, efficacy, and survival. Kwekkeboom DJ, de Herder WW, Kam BL, Van Eijck CH, Van Essen M, Kooji PP, et al. J Clin Oncol 2008; 26: 2124–30.

A total of 504 patients with gastropancreatic NETs were treated with a radiolabeled somatostatin analog with promising results for tumor-free survival, progression-free survival, and overall survival.

Radioembolization with selective internal radiation microspheres for neuroendocrine liver metastases. King J, Quinn R, Glenn DM, Janssen J, Tong D, Liaw W, et al. Cancer 2008; 1: 921–9.

This is a prospective study of 34 patients, all with nonresectable NETs with liver metastases treated with yttrium (^{90}Y) radioactive microspheres, who achieved long-term responses.

Surgical treatment of pancreatic neuroendocrine tumors: report of 112 cases. Gao C, Fu X, Pan Y, Li Q. Dig Surg 2010; 27: 197–204.

A retrospective review of 112 cases of pancreatic NETs. Pancreatic NETs can be safely resected with aggressive radical surgery to improve long-term survival. Patients' 5-year survival rate was significantly correlated with vascular invasion and resection margin.

Second-Line Therapy

• Nutritional supplementation with amino acids, zinc, or essential fatty acids	D

Glucagonoma syndrome: survival 21 years with concurrent liver metastases. Dourakis SP, Alexopoulou A, Georgousi KK, Delladetsima JK, Tolis G, Archimandritis AJ. Am J Med Sci 2007; 334: 225–7.

A report of unresectable glucagonoma treated symptomatically; the rash cleared with zinc supplementation.

Peripheral amino acid and fatty acid infusion for the treatment of necrolytic migratory erythema in the glucagonoma syndrome. Alexander EK, Robinson M, Staniec M, Dluhy RG. Clin Endocrinol (Oxf) 2002; 57: 827–31.

Long-term intermittent peripheral intravenous administration of amino acids and fatty acids led to significant improvement in NME symptoms.

Third-Line Therapies

• Streptozocin	B
• Doxorubicin	B
• Fluorouracil	B
• Everolimus	A
• Sunitinib	A
• Dacarbazine	D
• Liver transplantation	B

Fluorouracil, doxorubicin, and streptozocin in the treatment of patients with locally advanced and metastatic pancreatic endocrine carcinomas. Kouvaraki MA, Ajani JA, Hoff P, Wolff R, Evans DB, Lozano R, et al. J Clin Oncol 2004; 22: 4762–71.

This article is a retrospective look at 84 patients with locally or metastatic pancreatic endocrine carcinoma that had been treated with fluorouracil, doxorubicin, and streptozocin (FAS) to determine the role of systemic chemotherapy. The response rate to FAS was 39%, with a median response duration of 9.3 months. The 2-year progression-free survival rate was 41%, and the 2-year overall survival was 74%.

Therapeutic management of patients with gastroenteropancreatic neuroendocrine tumours. Khan MS, Caplin ME. Endocr Relat Cancer 2011; 18 Suppl 1: S53–74.

Review of therapies on the horizon for pancreatic NETs, such as peptide receptor radionuclide therapy, sunitinib, and everolimus.

Sunitinib malate for the treatment of pancreatic neuroendocrine tumors. Raymond E, Dahan L, Raoul J-L, Bang Y-J, Borbath I, Lombard-Bohas C, et al. N Engl J Med 2011; 364: 501–13.

A multinational, randomized, double-blind, placebo-controlled, phase III trial of sunitinib, a tyrosine kinase inhibitor, was done in patients with advanced, well-differentiated pancreatic NETs. Daily sunitinib improved progression-free survival, overall survival, and objective response rate compared with placebo.

Everolimus for advanced pancreatic neuroendocrine tumors. Yao JC, Shah MH, Ito T, Lombard-Bohas C, Wolin EW, Van Cutsem E, et al. N Engl J Med 2011; 364: 514–23.

In this multinational, randomized, double-blind trial, everolimus, an oral inhibitor of mammalian target of rapamycin (mTOR), was shown to significantly prolong progression-free survival among patients with progressive advanced pancreatic NETs.

Liver transplantation for the treatment of liver metastases from neuroendocrine tumors: an analysis of the UNOS database. Gedaly R, Daily MF, Davenport D, McHugh PP, Koch A, Angulo P, et al. Arch Surg 2011; 146: 953–8.

A retrospective analysis of 150 cases of treating liver metastases from neuroendocrine tumors with liver transplantation (LT). Longer wait times and disease stabilization before LT were associated with better outcome as well as longer progression-free survival.

Evidence Levels: **A** Double-blind study **B** Clinical trial ≥ 20 subjects **C** Clinical trial < 20 subjects **D** Series ≥ 5 subjects **E** Anecdotal case reports

168

Nephrogenic systemic fibrosis

Anjela Galan, Shawn E. Cowper

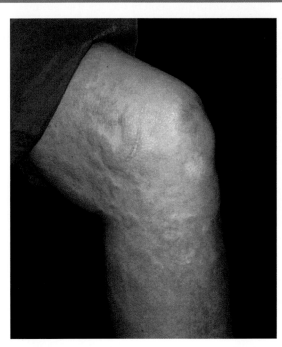

Brawny induration with a woodlike texture on the lower extremity of a patient with NSF. Reprinted from Cowper SE, Robin HS, Steinberg SM, Su LD, Leboit PE. Scleromyxedema-like cutaneous disease in renal dialysis patients. Lancet, 356(9234) 1000 to 1, 2000, with permission from Elsevier.

Nephrogenic systemic fibrosis (NSF) affects patients with renal impairment who have been exposed to gadolinium-containing contrast agents (GCCAs) for magnetic resonance imaging (MRI) studies. Onset is marked by cutaneous erythema, edema, hyperpigmentation, and woody induration. The clinical course commonly results in joint contractures and sometimes fibrosis of internal organs. Since the introduction of stricter use guidelines for GCCA in 2010, new cases of NSF have essentially vanished. Unfortunately, many patients exposed between 1997 and 2010 still suffer with its lingering effects. Because of the small number of affected patients and the absence of new cases, meaningful prospective human studies will likely never be possible. Animal models of NSF have been produced, however, and continue to serve as human surrogates in the development of newer and safer MRI contrast agents and in the search for future antifibrotic therapies.

MANAGEMENT STRATEGY

NSF is preventable but not curable. Three GCCAs (Magnevist, Omniscan, and Optimark) are contraindicated in patients with renal dysfunction (acute kidney injury or chronic kidney disease [estimated glomerular filtration rate (GFR) of <30 mL/min/1.73 m²]). Patients should be screened before the use of GCCAs to identify those at risk. Avoid GCCAs in patients with suspected or known impairment of drug elimination unless the need for the diagnostic information is essential and not available with alternative modalities. If exposure is unavoidable, optimal dosing and follow-up should involve the managing radiologist and nephrologist. Repeat administration of any GCCA during a single imaging session must be avoided, and sufficient time for its elimination must be allowed before reexposure. Although not proven to prevent NSF, immediate hemodialysis after exposure to a GCCA is recommended.

FDA Drug Safety Communication: new warnings for using gadolinium-based contrast agents in patients with kidney dysfunction. U.S. Food and Drug Administration; http://www.fda.gov/Drugs/DrugSafety/ucm223966.htm.

Specific Investigations

- Deep skin biopsy (incisional or substantial deep punch) followed by histologic and CD34 immunohistologic evaluation by an experienced dermatopathologist
- Renal function parameters (e.g., blood urea nitrogen and creatinine)
- Electrophoresis to exclude scleromyxedema-associated paraprotein
- Serologic autoantibody testing (e.g., ANA, Scl-70) to exclude systemic sclerosis and mixed connective tissue disease
- Hypercoagulability evaluation

There are no serologic tests for NSF. Diagnosis is based upon clinicopathologic correlation in a patient with renal disease. Gadolinium identification within skin samples is not sufficient to secure a diagnosis, and its absence does not exclude it. Consequently, testing for gadolinium is not fruitful.

Nephrogenic systemic fibrosis: clinicopathological definition and workup recommendations. Girardi M, Kay J, Elston DM, Leboit PE, Abu-Alfa A, Cowper SE. J Am Acad Dermatol 2011; 65: 1095–106.

First-Line Therapies

- Reestablishment of renal function
  - Transplantation **D**
  - Dialysis **D**
- Physical therapy **E**
- Pain management **E**

Transplantation, particularly if performed soon after NSF onset, is often the best therapeutic recourse. Although the benefit is limited (approximately 50%), complete resolution may be achieved. Significant clinical improvement may slowly accrue months or years after resumption of renal function. Treatment with dialysis has mixed results. In one study half of patients on dialysis had clinical improvement without complete resolution.

Rigorous physical therapy is mandatory to improve motion and maintain joint function.

Treatment of nephrogenic systemic fibrosis: limited options but hope for the future. Linfert DR, Schell JO, Fine DM. Semin Dial 2008; 21: 155–9.

The outcome of patients with nephrogenic systemic fibrosis after successful kidney transplantation. Leung N, Shaikh A, Cosio FG, Griffin MD, Textor SC, Gloor JM, et al. Am J Transplant 2010; 10: 558–62.

Clinical improvement of nephrogenic systemic fibrosis after kidney transplantation. Panesar M, Banerjee S, Barone GW. Clin Transplant 2008; 22: 803–8.

Renal transplantation for nephrogenic systemic fibrosis: a case report and review of literature. Cuffy MC, Singh M, Formica R, Simmons E, Abu Alfa AK, Carlson K, et al. Nephrol Dial Transplant 2011; 26: 1099–101.

Rehabilitation in nephrogenic systemic fibrosis. Ramaizel L, Sliwa JA. PMR 2009; 1: 684–6.

Second-Line Therapies	
• Extracorporeal photopheresis	E
• Pentoxifylline	E
• Imatinib mesylate	E

Extracorporeal photopheresis improves nephrogenic fibrosing dermopathy/nephrogenic systemic fibrosis: three case reports and review of literature. Mathur K, Morris S, Deighan C, Green R, Douglas KW. J Clin Apher 2008; 23: 144–50.

Extracorporeal photopheresis has been associated with symptomatic improvement in at least nine patients in the setting of ongoing renal failure. Another study suggests similar effects in three patients with end-stage renal disease with ongoing hemodialysis.

Nephrogenic systemic fibrosis: early recognition and treatment. Knopp EA, Cowper SE. Semin Dial 2008; 21: 123–8.

Pentoxifylline was associated with improvement in two patients.

Gadolinium – a specific trigger for the development of nephrogenic fibrosing dermopathy and nephrogenic systemic fibrosis? Grobner T. Nephrol Dial Transplant 2006; 21: 1104–8.

Imatinib mesylate treatment of nephrogenic systemic fibrosis. Kay J, High WA. Arthritis Rheum 2008; 58: 2543–8.

Antifibrotic effect after low dose imatinib mesylate treatment in patients with nephrogenic systemic fibrosis: an open-label nonrandomized, uncontrolled clinical trial. Elmholdt TR, Buus NH, Ramsing M, Olesen AB. J Eur Acad Dermatol Venereol 2013; 27: 779–84.

Evaluation of imatinib mesylate as a possible treatment of nephrogenic systemic fibrosis in a rat model. Hope TA, LeBoit PE, High WA, Fu Y, Brasch R. Magn Res Imag 2013; 32: 139–44.

Anecdotal experience in two patients treated with 400 mg of imatinib daily showed significant improvement in symptoms at 15 weeks. Clinical effects on skin, but not on joint mobility, have been reported in three patients treated with low-dose imatinib mesylate. Additional rare case reports with similar findings are found in the literature. Two additional patients showed improvement in joint mobility and tethering that reversed upon discontinuation of therapy. The optimal period of treatment has not been determined. Administration of imatinib in rats treated with gadolinium resulted in decreased lesion severity.

Third-Line Therapies	
• Sodium thiosulfate	E
• UVA1	E
• PUVA with retinoids	E
• Photodynamic therapy with methyl aminolevulinate	E
• Plasmapheresis	E
• Intravenous immunoglobulin (IVIG)	E
• Corticosteroids (topical, intralesional, and systemic)	E
• Methotrexate (systemic)	E
• Azathioprine	E
• Calcipotriene	E
• Alefacept	E
• Rapamycin	E

Nephrogenic systemic fibrosis: early recognition and treatment. Knopp EA, Cowper SE. Semin Dial 2008; 21: 123–8.

The treatments listed earlier are discussed in this review article. Most of these therapies lack large studies, reproducibility, or complete information upon which to evaluate efficacy.

The treatment of nephrogenic systemic fibrosis with therapeutic plasma exchange. Poisson JL, Low A, Park YA. J Clin Apher 2013; 28: 317–20.

Clinical symptom improvement, especially in pain levels, was reported in two patients with NSF after a series of therapeutic plasma exchange.

Evidence Levels: **A** Double-blind study **B** Clinical trial ≥ 20 subjects **C** Clinical trial < 20 subjects **D** Series ≥ 5 subjects **E** Anecdotal case reports

169

Neurofibromatosis, type 1

Elizabeth Ghazi, Rhonda E. Schnur

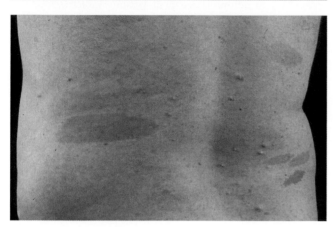

Type 1 neurofibromatosis (NF1), or von Recklinghausen disease, is an autosomal dominant multisystem disorder with highly variable expression. NF1 is caused by mutations of the neurofibromin gene on chromosome 17. The neurofibromin protein is a GTPase-activating protein that, in its normal role, negatively regulates RAS protein signal transduction. NF1 mutations lead to overly active RAS (RAS-GTP) and, subsequently, overactivation of the mTOR (mammalian target of rapamycin) cell-signaling pathway. Clinically, this results in excess cell growth and the potential for malignant transformation. The disorder has multisystem effects, including neurologic, cardiac, vascular, musculoskeletal, and endocrine manifestations, but cutaneous and ocular lesions (including Lisch nodules, optic gliomas, and orbital plexiform lesions) are the most characteristic. Cutaneous lesions include café au lait spots, neurofibromas, and plexiform neurofibromas. Neurofibromas may be small, benign, subcutaneous lesions or larger, plexiform tumors that follow nerves and/or extend into deeper bony and visceral structures. Malignant peripheral nerve sheath tumors (MPNSTs) may develop, particularly within larger plexiform lesions. Café au lait macules are typically the first lesions to appear in infancy and early childhood, and neurofibromas tend to proliferate during adolescence.

MANAGEMENT STRATEGY

The diagnosis of NF1 is established by well-defined clinical criteria. The sensitivity of mutation detection varies depending on the techniques used but has greatly improved. Mutation identification is useful in reproductive counseling, in confirming the diagnosis in uncertain cases, and in differentiating NF1 from other conditions with overlapping phenotypes such as the Legius and multiple lentigines syndromes. The nature of the mutation may also affect the prognosis; large deletions or null mutations are associated with more severe disease, including more severe intellectual disability and greater tumor burdens. Approximately 50% of NF1 cases represent de novo mutations.

There is currently no proven medical therapy to prevent or treat neurofibromas, but significant efforts are under way to develop targeted treatment approaches that exploit the molecular biology of the NF1 protein. Ketotifen has been used for pain, tenderness, and pruritus of neurofibromas, but there are no recent large studies using this drug. Otherwise, standard treatment for neurofibromas is currently limited to surgery. For benign neurofibromas, cosmetic concerns and discomfort are indications for removal. Most neurofibromas are small and can be removed by simple excision. Although there is little morbidity, surgery is not practical for large tumors.

A wire loop connected to a monopolar diathermy machine in the cutting mode has been used to treat hundreds of small lesions. Hemostasis is readily obtained, healing is by secondary intention, and cosmetic outcome is good. CO_2 laser vaporization has been used for small tumors with healing by secondary intention or for larger tumors in conjunction with primary closure. Hundreds of tumors can be removed in one outpatient session under local anesthesia. Unfortunately, surgery is not curative, and lesions may continue to progress, requiring repeated procedures.

Treatment of plexiform neurofibromas is particularly challenging because these tumors are often highly vascular and invasive. Symptomatic lesions should be evaluated by magnetic resonance imaging (MRI) or positron emission tomography (PET) scans because of the risk for evolution into MPNSTs. Unexplained pain or rapid growth within a plexiform neurofibroma and areas displaying necrosis or an unusual appearance on imaging studies merit biopsy to exclude malignant transformation. cDNA gene expression profiling may be used in the future to help distinguish benign from premalignant and malignant lesions. Nonsurgical treatments for plexiform neurofibromas and MPNSTs are under active investigation. Sirolimus, an allosteric inhibitor of mTOR, has been shown to slow the progression of plexiform neurofibromas. A new generation of therapeutic agents includes angiogenesis inhibitors and antiinflammatory agents that inhibit cell growth and induce apoptosis. Drugs that target RAS signal transduction or limit RAS posttranslational processing, such as farnesyl transferase inhibitors (tipifarnib), are also promising. In addition, agents that affect the microenvironment of NF1 tumors via limiting the induction of other signaling pathways and through interactions with other cell lines are being targeted. For example, the tyrosine kinase inhibitor, imatinib mesylate, targets PDGFRα, c-KIT, and c-ABL and is being studied in phase II clinical trials. Combinations of these agents with mTOR inhibitors are also being studied.

RAS-induced transformation requires isoprenylation (i.e., farnesylation or geranyl-geranylation), which can be blocked by farnesyl transferase inhibitors as well as by 3-hydroxy-3-methylglutaryl coenzyme A (HMG-CoA) reductase inhibitors. HMG-CoA reductase is the rate-limiting enzyme in the mevalonate pathway that leads to the synthesis of cholesterol and isoprenyl groups. Therefore statins are also being explored in the treatment of MPNSTs and NF1-related bone dysplasia and cognitive difficulties because of their known inhibition of p21Ras/mitogen-activated protein kinase (MAPK) activity. For tibial pseudoarthrosis, recombinant bone morphogenetic protein (an anabolic agent) and bisphosphonates (anticatabolic agents) have been used in combination to promote healing. Many of the aforementioned medications are undergoing phase II trials.

For mutations that alter gene splicing, antisense oligomers can restore splicing at the mRNA level in vitro. Tamoxifen, in vitro and in orthotopically xenografted mouse models, inhibits proliferation and survival of MPNST cells and may be a promising treatment modality.

Referral of a patient with aggressive MPNSTs to an oncologist for chemoradiotherapy may be warranted.

Information about ongoing clinical trials can be found at www.ctf.org./research/nf1 and www.ClinicalTrials.gov.

Specific Investigations

- Annual complete cutaneous examinations, particularly in those patients with large plexiform lesions
- Complete baseline ophthalmologic examination with slit lamp and dilated fundoscopy. Annual ocular examinations in children to screen for optic pathway gliomas should be continued through age 8 and every 2 years thereafter from ages 8 to 18
- Skin and eye examinations for first-degree relatives
- Regular developmental assessment in children: evaluation and management of learning disability and attention deficits, as needed
- Regular blood pressure checks to screen for renal artery stenosis or pheochromocytoma
- MRI of brain, optic nerves, and spinal cord, with and without contrast, should be performed if the patient is symptomatic and/or has focal neurologic signs
- MRI or PET scan, with and without contrast, to evaluate deep or changing plexiform neurofibromas
- Biopsy or excision of changing or suspicious lesions
- Radiographs if osseous involvement is suspected
- Genetic studies

Neurofibromatosis 1. Friedman JM. 1998 [Updated 2014]. In: Wallace SE, Amemiya A, Bean LJH. GeneReviews. Seattle: University of Washington. http://www.ncbi.nlm.nih.gov/books/NBK1109.

A frequently updated, comprehensive review.

First-Line Therapies

• Surgical excision	C
• Laser therapy	B

The role of surgery in children with neurofibromatosis. Neville HL, Seymour-Dempsey K, Slopis J, Gill BS, Moore BD, Lally KP, et al. J Pediatr Surg 2001; 36: 25–9.

A large study of 249 pediatric patients with NF1 and NF2: 50 (48 with NF1) had surgery; 14 of the 50 had malignancies, and 8 underwent multiple resections. Surgical and postoperative management are reviewed.

The megasession technique for excision of multiple neurofibromas. Onesti MG, Carella S, Spinelli G, Scuderi N. Dermatol Surg 2010; 36: 1488–90.

In 15 patients, electrosurgery under general anesthesia or deep sedation was used to treat multiple neurofibromas (average 330) in a single-stage procedure. The authors proposed this method because it caused minimal discomfort and had excellent esthetic results, with a short recovery time and relatively low cost.

Treatment of neurofibromas with a carbon dioxide laser: a retrospective cross-sectional study of 106 patients. Méni C, Sbidian E, Moreno JC, Lafaye S, Buffard V, Goldzal S, et al. Dermatology 2015; 230: 263–8.

CO_2 laser treatment was well tolerated with satisfactory outcomes in over 106 patients with both symptomatic and asymptomatic neurofibromas.

Management and prognosis of malignant peripheral nerve sheath tumors: the experience of the French Sarcoma Group (GSF-GETO). Valentin T, Le Cesne A, Ray-Coquard I, Italiano A, Decanter G, Bompas E, et al. Eur J Cancer 2016; 56: 77–84.

A total of 353 patients with MPNSTs, including 37% with NF1, were analyzed. Curative-intent surgery was undertaken in 294. Of these, 21% had neoadjuvant treatment (mainly chemotherapy), and 59% had adjuvant treatment (mainly radiotherapy). For operated patients, the median progression-free survival was 26.3 months. MPNST patients with NF1 who were treated with palliative chemotherapy showed worse survival than patients with sporadic forms of MPNSTs. This is the largest study of MPNST to date.

Second-Line Therapies

• Ketotifen	B
• Chemotherapy	D

Ketotifen suppression of NF1 neurofibroma growth over 30 years. Riccardi VM. Am J Med Genet A 2015; 167: 1570–7.

A single NF patient was observed to have arrested growth of neurofibromas.

Chemotherapy benefit for pediatric neurofibromatosis type I. Brower V. Lancet Oncol 2016; 17: e186.

Significantly better 5-year event-free survival (69%) was observed in 127 patients with NF1 and low-grade gliomas who were treated with carboplatin and vincristine, compared with 137 patients without NF1 who were similarly treated (39%).

Third-Line Therapies

• Imatinib	E
• mTOR inhibitor (sirolimus, rapamycin)	B, E
• VEGF/c-KIT inhibitor (bevacizumab, cediranib)	D, E
• Multikinase inhibitor (sorafenib)	E
• Tamoxifen	E
• Statins (simvastatin, lovastatin)	A, B
• Pirfenidone	B
• Radiofrequency	D
• BRAF inhibitors (vemurafenib)	E
• Interferon alpha	D
• Antisense morpholino oligomers	E

Imatinib mesylate for plexiform neurofibromas in patients with neurofibromatosis type 1: a phase 2 trial. Robertson KA, Nalepa G, Yang FC, Bowers DC, Ho CY, Hutchins GD, et al. Lancet Oncol 2012; 13: 1218–24.

Patients were treated with oral imatinib mesylate at 220 mg/m² twice daily for children and 400 mg twice daily for adults for 6 months. Of the 23 patients who received imatinib for at least 6 months, 6 (26%) had a 20% or more decrease in volume of one or more plexiform tumors. Adverse effects included reversible neutropenia and hyperglycemia.

Sirolimus for nonprogressive NF1–associated plexiform neurofibromas: an NF clinical trials consortium phase II

Evidence Levels: **A** Double-blind study **B** Clinical trial ≥ 20 subjects **C** Clinical trial < 20 subjects **D** Series ≥ 5 subjects **E** Anecdotal case reports

study. Weiss B, Widemann BC, Wolters P, Dombi E, Vinks AA, Cantor A, et al. Pediatr Blood Cancer 2014; 61: 982–6.

This trial studied 13 patients with nonprogressive plexiform neurofibromas using a starting dose of sirolimus of 0.8 mg/m^2 body surface area by mouth, given twice daily for a 28-day course. None of the patients had severe toxicity. However, sirolimus did not induce shrinkage of nonprogressive peripheral neurofibromas; therefore the authors suggested that sirolimus should not be considered as a treatment option for nonprogressive tumors. However, an unexpected significant improvement in the mean scores of the emotional and school domains in a quality of life questionnaire was reported in six individuals.

Sirolimus for progressive neurofibromatosis type 1-associated plexiform neurofibromas: a neurofibromatosis Clinical Trials Consortium phase II study. Weiss B, Widemann B, Wolters P, Dombi E, Vinks AA, Cantor A, et al. Neuro Oncol 2015; 17: 596–603.

This study was focused on patients with inoperable, NF1-associated, progressive plexiform neurofibromas. Twenty-nine patients were treated with sirolimus and 49 with placebo. Two subjects were removed from the trial for severe sirolimus toxicity (grade 2 pneumonitis; both cases reversed with cessation of therapy). Sirolimus prolonged the time to progression of plexiform neurofibromas by almost 4 months in these NF1 patients.

Prolonged survival in adult neurofibromatosis type I patients with recurrent high-grade gliomas treated with bevacizumab. Theeler BJ, Ellezam B, Yust-Katz S, Slopis JM, Loghin ME, de Groot JF. J Neurol 2014; 261: 1559–64.

Five patients with recurrent high-grade gliomas were treated with a median of 20 cycles of bevacizumab (ranging from 10–72 months). All five experienced prolonged postrecurrence survival. The median overall survival from the time of glioma diagnosis was 72.6 months. Three out of five patients developed vascular complications leading to discontinuation of the drug.

Tamoxifen inhibits malignant peripheral nerve sheath tumor growth in an estrogen-receptor independent manner. Byer S, Eckert JM, Brossier NM, Clodfelder-Miller BJ, Turk AN, Carroll AJ, et al. Neuro Oncol 2011; 13: 28–41.

A tamoxifen metabolite, 4-hydroxy-tamoxifen, inhibited proliferation and survival of MPNST cells in vitro and in an orthotopic xenograft mouse model.

A randomized placebo-controlled lovastatin trial for neurobehavioral function in neurofibromatosis I. Bearden CE, Hellemann GS, Rosser T, Montojo C, Jonas R, Enrique N, et al. Ann Clin Transl Neurol 2016; 3: 266–79.

Forty-four NF1 patients were randomly assigned to 14 weeks of lovastatin (maximum dose of 80 mg/day for adult participants and 40 mg/day for children) or placebo. Differential improvement favoring lovastatin treatment was observed for one primary outcome measure (working memory) and two secondary measures (verbal memory and adult self-reported internalizing problems).

Phase II trial of pirfenidone in children and young adults with neurofibromatosis type 1 and progressive plexiform neurofibromas. Widemann BC, Babovic-Vuksanovic D, Dombi E, Wolters PL, Goldman S, Martin S, et al. Pediatr Blood Cancer 2014; 61: 1598–602.

Thirty-six NF1 patients with progressive plexiform neurofibromas were treated with pirfenidone. The median time to progression for pirfenidone-treated patients was 13.2 months compared with 10.6 months for the placebo control group. No objective responses were observed. Pirfenidone was well tolerated but did not demonstrate sufficient beneficial activity to warrant its use.

Radiofrequency in the treatment of craniofacial plexiform neurofibromatosis: a pilot study. Baujat B, Krastinova-Lolov D, Blumen M, Baglin AC, Coquille F, Chabolle F. Plast Reconstruct Surg 2006; 117: 1261–8.

This five-patient pilot study demonstrated partial diminution or stabilization of plexiform neurofibromas using radiofrequency treatment. Treatment was well tolerated, with the best effects observed in the early stages of the disease.

Interferon-[alpha] for unresectable progressive and symptomatic plexiform neurofibromas. Kebudi R, Cakir FB, Gorgun O. J Pediatr Hematol Oncol 2013; 35: e115–7.

IFN-alpha 2a at a dose of 3,000,000 U/m^2/SC was given three times a week, every other day, to five patients. The dose was increased to 6,000,000 U/m^2 SC three times weekly and continued for 1 year. Four out of five patients had stable disease; one progressed to MPNST. Follow-up ranged from 2 to 10 years.

Chemotherapy for the treatment of malignant peripheral nerve sheath tumors in neurofibromatosis 1: a 10-year institutional review. Zehou O, Fabre E, Zelek L, Sbidian E, Ortonne N, Banu E, et al. Orphanet J Rare Dis 2013; 8: 127.

This retrospective review of 21 NF1 patients with MPNSTs who were treated with standard chemotherapy (anthracycline and/or ifosfamide) showed that conventional chemotherapy does not reduce mortality.

Nevoid basal cell carcinoma syndrome

Maral Kibarian Skelsey, Gary L. Peck

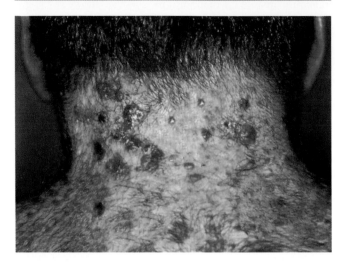

Nevoid basal cell carcinoma (Gorlin) syndrome (NBCCS) is an autosomal dominant syndrome characterized by basal cell carcinomas (BCCs) and multiple systemic manifestations. These may include palmar or plantar pits, odontogenic keratocysts of the jaw, ectopic intracranial calcification (falx cerebri), fused or bifid ribs, macrocephaly, cleft lip, coarse facies, hypertelorism, medulloblastomas, cardiac and ovarian fibromas, lymphomesenteric cysts, pectus deformity, and syndactyly of the digits.

For most patients NBCCS is caused by mutations in a tumor suppressor patched (PTCH)1 gene, mapped to the long arm of chromosome 9(q2231). The PTCH1 gene encodes a transmembrane protein that acts as a receptor to the hedgehog protein and affects the sonic hedgehog signaling pathway (SHH). The PTCH1 protein binds to the transmembrane protein, smoothened (SMO), and inhibits the SHH signal pathway. SMO promotes release of Gli proteins from suppressor of fused (SUFU), its inhibitor. Mutations in the PTCH1 gene result in an overexpression of the SHH pathway and formation of neoplasms and specific developmental anomalies. Patients without the PTCH gene mutation may have a mutation in SUFU, which results in overactivation of Gli transcription factors and cell proliferation. This subtype of NBCCS may exhibit medulloblastoma before age 5 and an absence of odontogenic keratocysts. Rarely, mutations in PTCH2 may also have an association with NBCCS.

MANAGEMENT STRATEGY

The management of NBCCS patients is focused on patient education, tumor prevention, and treatment of BCC while optimizing cosmesis and minimizing discomfort and cost.

Patient education should include information on *sunscreens, sun protective clothing and eyewear, UV films* for car windows, and the necessity of *avoiding radiation treatment*, as well as *genetic counseling*. Patients should be tested regularly for *vitamin D* deficiency, prescribed supplementation based on their laboratory values,

and be examined for clinical features of deficiency. Full-body skin examinations should be performed on an annual basis and at more frequent intervals after the development of the first skin cancer. The dermatologist has a role as an advocate and resource for these patients, who may need referrals to other specialists for diagnosis and treatment of the extracutaneous implications of NBCCS. In particular, annual ophthalmologic and dental examinations should be performed. Pediatric patients should be followed up and undergo developmental, vision, speech, and hearing screenings. A baseline echocardiogram can rule out a potentially dangerous cardiac fibroma. Pelvic ultrasound should be considered in girls who have reached puberty. As there is a need to limit radiation exposure, routine x-rays to establish syndrome criteria are unnecessary unless the diagnosis is uncertain. Digital imaging is preferable when possible. An annual magnetic resonance imaging (MRI) of the head is recommended until the age of 8 when medulloblastoma becomes rare.

Genetic testing can be limited to the following situations: (1) prenatal testing if the diagnosis is confirmed in a family member; (2) establishing the diagnosis in patients who do not meet sufficient criteria; and (3) screening an asymptomatic patient who is at risk because of an affected family member.

Patients with NBCSS need *emotional support* as they undergo multiple treatments that may result in scarring and deformity. They may benefit from regular screening for depression and referral to a support network where this is available (e.g., www.Gorlinsyndrome.org).

The size and numbers of tumors, especially in those with type I and II skin, the young age at presentation, and the distribution on the head and neck, pose challenges greater than those associated with sporadic BCC. Nonetheless, with the notable exception of radiotherapy, which should be avoided, treatment is based on the same modalities including *surgery; laser resurfacing; photodynamic therapy;* and topical, injectable, and systemic therapy, including *vismodegib*, an SHH pathway inhibitor that binds SMO, and *capecitabine*, a systemic fluorouracil prodrug.

The role of *chemoprevention* (prophylactic therapy to reduce the incidence of new BCCs) is still unclear. Evidence for efficacy in NBCCS is inconclusive, except for vismodegib, which is not well tolerated but may find a role here.

This chapter is focused largely on the literature specific to NBCCS, and the reader is referred to the chapter on BCC for a broader review of the management of this tumor.

Specific Investigations

- Radiologic studies
- Dermatoscopy
- Vitamin D level
- Genetic studies (in selected cases)

Consensus statement from the first international colloquium on basal cell nevus syndrome (BCNS). Bree AF, Shah MR. Am J Med Genet A 2011; 155: 2091–7.

This is a multidisciplinary consensus group's statement on the diagnostic criteria for NBCCS and protocols for evaluation and surveillance of pediatric and adult patients.

High prevalence of vitamin D deficiency in patients with basal cell nevus syndrome. Tang J, Wu A, Linos E, Parimi N, Lee W, Aszterbaum M, et al. Arch Dermatol 2010; 146: 1105–10.

Levels of 25-hydroxyvitamin D (25[OH]D) were measured in 41 ambulatory patients with NBCCS who were participating in a

2-year chemoprevention clinical trial. Population-based controls were selected and matched by age, sex, Fitzpatrick skin type, and season/geography. NBCCS patients were three times more likely to be vitamin D deficient (56% vs. 18%; $p < 0.001$).

First-Line Therapies

• Surgical management	B
• Mohs micrographic surgery	B
• Avoidance of ultraviolet light and radiotherapy	B

Consensus for nonmelanoma skin cancer treatment: basal cell carcinoma, including a cost analysis of treatment methods. Kauvar AN, Cronin T, Roenigk R, Hruza G, Bennett R. Dermatol Surg 2015; 41: 550–71.

Tumor factors associated with increased recurrence rates of BCC include location on the "mask" area of the midface, hands, feet, and genitalia; size over 20 cm on the torso or extremities and 10 mm or larger in the nonmask areas of the face; micronodular, infiltrative, sclerosing, morpheaform, or desmoplastic histologic subtypes; ill-defined margins; prior recurrence; and perineural invasion. Host factors linked to high-risk BCC include occurrence in a site of prior radiation or scar, immunosuppression, genetic syndrome, and age younger than 40.

The nevoid basal cell carcinoma syndrome: sensitivity to the ultraviolet and x-ray irradiation. Frentz G, MunchPetersen B, Wulf HC, Niebuhr E, da Cunha Bang F. J Am Acad Dermatol 1987; 17: 637–43.

Radiation therapy should be avoided in patients with NBCCS because these patients develop BCC as a consequence of radiotherapy within 6 months to 3 years, in contrast to the usual 20- to 30-year lag period for radiation-induced tumors seen in patients with sporadic BCC.

Sun exposure and basal cell carcinomas in the nevoid basal cell carcinoma syndrome. Goldstein AM, Bale SJ, Peck GL, DiGiovanna JJ. J Am Acad Dermatol 1993; 29: 34–41.

The distribution of tumors in NBCCS, favoring sun-exposed sites, would indicate that solar irradiation may be an exacerbating factor.

Second-Line Therapy

• Electrodesiccation and curettage	B

Basal cell and squamous cell skin cancers: clinical practice guidelines in oncology. Miller SJ, Alam M, Anderson J, Berg D, Bichakjian CK, Bowen G, et al. JNCCN 2010; 8: 836–64.

Surgery results in the highest cure rate and lowest recurrence for BCC. Electrodesiccation and curettage is effective for low-risk tumors in non–hair-bearing areas if fat is not reached. Pathology should be obtained to exclude high-risk tumor. Excisions with 4-mm clinical margins are usually adequate. High-risk tumors should be treated with Mohs surgery or excision with complete circumferential peripheral and deep margin assessment with frozen or permanent section.

Third-Line Therapies

• Photodynamic therapy (PDT)	A
• Imiquimod	A
• Cryosurgery	B
• 5-Fluorouracil (5FU)	B
• CO_2 laser	B
• Pulsed dye laser (PDL)	C
• Alexandrite laser	E
• Interferon	B
• Bleomycin	B
• Electrochemotherapy	E
• Retinoids	C
• Interleukin-2 (IL-2)	C
• Paclitaxel	E
• Capecitabine	E
• Chemical peel	E
• Dermabrasion	E
• Vismodegib (in locally advanced or metastatic BCC)	A
• Sonidegib	B
• Ingenol mebutate	D

Treatment of Gorlin syndrome (nevoid basal cell carcinoma syndrome) with methylaminolevulinate photodynamic therapy in seven patients, including two children: interest of tumescent anesthesia for pain control in children. Girard C, Debu A, Bessis D, Blatiére V, Dereure O, Guillot B. J Eur Acad Dermatol Venereol 2013; 27: e171–5.

Seven patients with 41 BCCs had prior superficial curettage for sBCCs or debulking for nBCCs, then had methyl aminolevulinic (MAL) acid applied topically to lesions 3 hours before illumination with 635 nm red light for 10 minutes. Overall clearance in patients was 60% after one session and 78% after three sessions. There were excellent cosmetic outcomes in all patients. Treatments were well tolerated in adults with moderate pain sensation during illumination, and a ropivacaine–lidocaine tumescent anesthesia was used on the youngest patient to ensure excellent pain tolerance.

Efficacy of photodynamic therapy as a treatment for Gorlin syndrome-related basal cell carcinomas. Loncaster J, Swindell R, Slevin F, Sheridan L, Allan D, Allan E. Clin Oncol 2009; 21: 502–8.

Thirty-three NBCCS patients (138 lesions) were treated with PDT, and lesion thicknesses were assessed using ultrasound, both before treatment and during follow-up. Topical PDT was used to treat superficial lesions (<2 mm thick) and a systemic photosensitizer + light delivered by interstitially placed optical fibers, which extended the remit of PDT, allowed for thicker lesions (>2 mm) to be treated. Local control rates of 56.3% at 12 months were achieved overall.

Consensus recommendations for the treatment of basal cell carcinomas in Gorlin syndrome with topical methylaminolevulinate-photodynamic therapy. Basset-Seguin N, Bissonnette R, Girard C, Haedersdal M, Lear JT, Paul C, et al. J Eur Acad Dermatol Venereol 2014; 28: 626–32.

Seven dermatologists developed consensus recommendations for the treatment of BCC with MAL-PDT in BCNS patients based on their extensive experience and review of the literature. They conclude that all superficial BCC (sBCC) and nodular BCC (nBCC) <2 mm in depth may be treated and that periorificial sBCC and nBCC may be considered for treatment. Multiple tumors may be treated simultaneously if pain management is adequate. Although MAL-PDT is not approved for pediatric use, the panel agreed, based on case studies and the experts' pediatric experience, that treatment of children may be considered.

Photodynamic therapy for patients with basal cell nevus syndrome. Gilchrest BA, Brightman LA, Thiele JJ, Wasserman DI. Dermatol Surg 2009; 35: 1576–81.

Seven cases were treated with aminolevulinic acid (ALA)-PDT intermittently at 15-month intervals over broad areas of the face and parts of the torso and extremities. A 20% ALA solution was applied for a 1-hour incubation and the area was exposed to blue light (417 nm) for 16 minutes, 40 seconds. Patients were followed for 7 years and experienced resolution of the majority of BCC and reduction in the number of new BCC, as well as improvement in their cosmetic appearance.

Photodynamic therapy versus topical imiquimod versus topical fluorouracil for treatment of superficial basal cell carcinoma: a single-blind, non-inferiority, randomized clinical trial. Arits AH, Mosterd K, Essers BA, Spoorenberg E, Sommer A, De Rooij MJ, et al. Lancet Oncol 2013; 14: 647–54.

In this trial, 601 patients with sBCC were randomized to receive two sessions of MAL-PDT (1-week interval), imiquimod cream once daily five times a week for 6 weeks, or fluorouracil 5% cream twice daily for 4 weeks. The percentage of tumor-free patients at both 3- and 12-month follow-up was 72.8% (95% confidence interval [CI], 66.8–79.4) for PDT, 83.4% (78.2–88.9) for imiquimod, and 80.1% (74.7–85.9) for fluorouracil.

Cryosurgery for cutaneous malignancy: an update. Kuflik EG. Dermatol Surg 1997; 23: 1081–7.

Cryosurgery is best suited for superficial noninfiltrating tumors with well-defined borders. Cryosurgery is not effective for morpheaform or infiltrating histologic subtypes, recurrent lesions, or deeply penetrating or very aggressive tumors.

Gorlin syndrome: the role of the carbon dioxide laser in patient management. Grobbelaar AO, Horlock N, Gault DT. Ann Plast Surg 1997; 39: 366–73.

Ultrapulse CO_2 used for the successful treatment of basal cell carcinomas found in patients with basal cell nevus syndrome. Nouri K, Chang A, Trent JT, Jiménez GP. Dermatol Surg 2002; 28: 287–90.

Three patients with multiple small BCCs were effectively treated with ultrapulse CO_2 laser, with complete histologic clearance and minimal scarring noted at follow-up.

Although sBCCs can be ablated to the mid-dermis or deeper with 100% clearance, large nBCCs with diameters greater than 10 mm cannot reliably be removed with this method.

Single treatment of nonmelanoma skin cancers using a pulsed-dye laser with stacked pulses. Tran HT, Lee RA, Oganesyan G, Jiang SB. Lasers Surg Med 2012; 44: 459–67.

Twenty patients with 23 biopsy-proven BCCs and squamous cell carcinoma (SCC) in situ were randomized to receive either no treatment or 595 nm PDL, either without or with double (stacked) pulses. The nonstacked treatment group had a clearance rate of 25% (similar to the nontreated group), whereas the double-stacked group had a clearance rate of 71%. The lesions with residual tumors were noted to be beyond the central treatment zone by histopathology and, if excluded, resulted in a clearance rate of 100%.

755 nm alexandrite laser for the reduction of tumor burden in basal cell nevus syndrome. Ibrahimi OA, Sakamoto FH, Tannous Z, Anderson RR. Lasers Surg Med 2011; 43: 68–71.

Targeting the vasculature has been recognized as a means of eradicating tumors; however, vascular lasers such as the PDL have limited efficacy in the treatment of BCC. The long-pulsed alexandrite can penetrate twice the depth of the PDL and can reach the vasculature of the dermis. A BCNS patient with a history of radiation therapy was treated on the upper extremities and anterior trunk with the 755 nm alexandrite laser with two passes at an energy of 100 J/cm^2, pulse length of 3 milliseconds, no dynamic cooling mode, and 8-mm spot size with 10% overlapping between pulses. Fifteen of 18 treated lesions showed complete clinical response and appeared at 7 months as a hypopigmented scar. Biopsy of a single lesion at 7 months showed no residual BCC.

Intralesional agents in the management of cutaneous malignancy: a review. Good LM, Miller MD, High WA. J Am Acad Derm 2011; 64: 413–22.

Intralesional treatment of skin cancer is a consideration when surgical intervention is not a viable option and for cases where cosmetic outcome may be compromised with surgery. Interferons alpha-2b (1.5 M IU, 3 times weekly for 3 weeks) and also beta-1a are used for BCC. There is little experience of this modality in NBCCS.

Successful treatment of multiple basaliomas with bleomycin-based electrochemotherapy: a case series of three patients with Gorlin-Goltz syndrome. Kis E, Baltas E, Kinyo A, Varga E, Nagy N, Gyulai R, et al. Acta Derm Venereol 2012; 92: 648–51.

In electrochemotherapy (ECT) tumors are destroyed when electric pulses are delivered at the same time as a chemotherapeutic agent is administered; this is thought to increase the local cytotoxicity of the anticancer drug. Three patients with BCNS and a total of 99 BCCs on the face, scalp, trunk, and extremities received intravenous bleomycin–based ECT at a dose of 15 mg/m^2 while under general sedation. Tumors ranged in size from 0.32 to 0.2 cm^3. Electrical pulses were delivered during the pharmacokinetic peak, 828 minutes after the intravenous administration of bleomycin. The types of electrodes used varied depending on the size and type of tumor. One patient underwent four treatment sessions spaced at 2-month intervals; the remainder were treated only once. Complete response (CR) of tumors occurred in 87%, with partial response in 12%. No recurrence was observed during a 10–28 month follow-up. Histology of two tumors confirmed CR. Side effects were limited to erythema and edema around treated lesions, necrosis of treated lesions for 2–3 weeks, and sore muscles at time of pulse delivery.

Electrochemotherapy: a valid treatment for Gorlin-Goltz syndrome. Curatolo P, Miraglia E, Rotunno R, Calvieri S, Giustini S. Acta Dermatovenerol Croat 2013; 21: 132–4.

A BCNS patient with a 5 × 10 cm BCC on the scalp was treated with bleomycin-based ECT at a dose of 15 mg/m^2. An initial necrotic eschar on the nodule reepithelialized at 4 weeks, at which time a second ECT was performed. After 4 weeks there was complete response of the tumor with no recurrence after 4 years.

Effect of perilesional injections of PEG-interleukin-2 on basal cell carcinoma. Kaplan B, Moy RL. Dermatol Surg 2001; 26:1037–40.

Evidence Levels: **A** Double-blind study **B** Clinical trial ≥ 20 subjects **C** Clinical trial < 20 subjects **D** Series ≥ 5 subjects **E** Anecdotal case reports

Twelve BCCs in eight patients were treated with intralesional pegylated IL2, with a 66% (8/12) clinical and histologic cure rate. Erythema, swelling, and pain occurred in 10/12 injection sites but resolved in a week's time, and only one patient experienced systemic flulike symptoms.

Successful treatment of an intractable case of hereditary basal cell carcinoma syndrome with paclitaxel. El Sobky RA, Kallab AM, Dainer PM, Jillella AP, Lesher JL Jr. Arch Dermatol 2001; 137: 827–8.

Novel approach to Gorlin syndrome: a patient treated with oral capecitabine. Beach DF, Somer R. J Clin Oncol 2011; 29: e397–401.

Capecitabine, a systemic prodrug of fluorouracil (FU), is metabolized in the liver and then converted to the active form of FU by cytidine deaminase, an enzyme found in tumor cells. A patient with NBCCS with only limited response to topical FU was treated with oral capecitabine 1500 mg orally every 12 hours for 14 days, every 3 weeks. After 6 months he had near-complete resolution of a 2 × 2.5 cm BCC on the scalp and near-complete resolution of a 2.5 × 1.5 cm BCC on the scapula. Multiple lesions completely cleared, and no new lesions developed during the 2 years the patient has been on the medication.

Efficacy and safety of vismodegib in advanced basal cell carcinoma. Sekulic A, Migden MR, Oro AE, Dirix L, Lewis KD, Hainsworth JD, et al. N Engl J Med 2012; 366: 217–9.

In a phase II pivotal study (ERIVANCE BCC), 104 patients with advanced BCC (71 locally advanced, 33 metastatic) received 150 mg of oral vismodegib (G DC0449) daily.

The response rate was 30% in patients with metastatic BCC and 43% in patients with locally advanced BCC, with complete responses in 21% of these patients. Adverse events occurring in more than 30% of patients were muscle spasms, alopecia, dysgeusia, weight loss, and fatigue. Serious adverse events were attributed to treatment with vismodegib in 4% of patients.

Surgical excision after neoadjuvant therapy with vismodegib for a locally advanced basal cell carcinoma and resistant basal cell carcinomas in Gorlin syndrome. Chang ALS, Atwood SX, Tartar DM, Oro AE. JAMA Dermatol 2013; 149: 639–41.

Treatment of an NBCCS patient with vismodegib 150 mg/day for 51 weeks resulted in regression of his advanced BCC, facilitating tumor extirpation. While on vismodegib, however, the patient acquired secondary resistance and developed new tumors.

Patient with Gorlin syndrome and metastatic basal cell carcinoma refractory to smoothened inhibitors. Zhu GA, Li AS, Chang AL. J Am Acad Dermatol 2014; 150: 877–9.

A patient with NBCCS and BCC metastatic to the lung was initially treated with a new SMO inhibitor saridegib at 130 mg/d. Because the tumor was unresponsive after 16 months, he was started on vismodegib and continued to experience growth of both preexisting and new nodules.

The use of vismodegib to shrink keratocystic odontogenic tumors in patients with basal cell nevus syndrome. Ally MS, Tang JU, Joseph T, Thompson B, Lindgren J, Raphael MA, et al. JAMA Dermatol 2014; 150: 542–5.

Vismodegib may be a nonsurgical treatment option for keratocystic odontogenic tumors (KCOTs) in NBCCS patients. In six patients with both BCNS and KCOT, tumor size was reduced by 50% after vismodegib 150 mg/d for a mean of 18 months. There was no new KCOT development during therapy. Long-term efficacy is unknown, and it is not clear why some patients did not respond.

An investigator-initiated open-label clinical trial of vismodegib as a neoadjuvant to surgery for high-risk basal cell carcinoma. Ally MS, Aasi S, Wysong A, Teng C, Anderson E, Bailey-Healy I, et al. J Am Acad Dermatol 2014; 71: 904–11.

Eleven patients with advanced BCC were treated with vismodegib 150 mg/day for a mean of 4 months, which reduced the surgical defect area by 27% (95% CI, 45.7%–7.9%; $p = 0.006$). Treatment was limited by severe side effects, and 29% of patients could not complete more than 3 months because of adverse events. No effect was seen with treatment less than 3 months.

Vismodegib exerts targeted efficacy against recurrent sonic hedgehog subgroup medulloblastoma: results from phase II pediatric brain tumor consortium studies PBTC025b and PBTC032. Robinson GW, Orr BA, Wu G, Gururangan S, Lin T, Qaddoumi I, et al. J Clin Oncol 2015; 33: 2646–54.

Phase II study of vismodegib in 31 pediatric and adult recurrent medulloblastoma (MB) patients showed that vismodegib retains activity against adult recurrent SHH-MB but not against non-SHH–MB. Data on pediatric patients were insufficient.

Topical treatment of basal cell carcinomas in nevoid basal cell carcinoma syndrome with a smoothened inhibitor. Skavara H, Kalthoff F, Meingassner JG, Wolff-Winiski B, Aschauer H, Kelleher JF, et al. J Invest Dermatol 2011; 131: 1735–44.

LDE225 (sonidegib) cream, a selective inhibitor of SMO, has shown inhibition of murine basaloid cells in organ cultures of PTCH1 heterozygotes. Eight BCNS patients participated in a double-blind, randomized, placebo-controlled study of 75% LDE225 cream or vehicle. After 4 weeks complete response was observed in 3 of 13 LDE225-treated BCC; 9 showed partial response. One had no clinical response. Treatment was well tolerated.

PEP005 (ingenol mebutate) gel for the topical treatment of superficial basal cell carcinoma: results of a randomized phase IIa trial. Siller G, Rosen R, Freeman M, Welburn P, Katsamas J, Ogbourne SM. Australas J Dermatol 2010; 51: 99–105.

Although developed for treatment of actinic keratoses, topical ingenol mebutate gel 0.05% showed histologic clearance of sBCC in 63% of patients ($n = 8$). Side effects included local skin reactions, application-site pain, and headache.

Chemoprevention	
• Retinoids	D
• Nonsteroidal antiinflammatory drugs (NSAIDs)	C
• Vismodegib	A

Chemoprevention of basal cell carcinoma with isotretinoin. Peck GL, Gross EG, Butkus D, DiGiovanna JJ. J Am Acad Dermatol 1982; 6(Suppl 2): 815–23.

Treatment and prevention of basal cell carcinoma with oral isotretinoin. Peck GL, DiGiovanna JJ, Sarnoff DS, Gross EG, Butkus D, Olsen TG, et al. J Am Acad Dermatol 1988; 19: 176–85.

Eight percent of 270 tumors due to NBCCS, arsenic exposure, or sunlight exposure in 12 patients treated with a mean dose of 3.1 mg/kg/day for 8 months underwent complete clinical and histologic regression. Lower doses given to 3 patients for 3 to 8 years were effective for chemoprevention of new BCCs.

Effectiveness of isotretinoin in preventing the appearance of basal cell carcinomas in basal cell nevus syndrome. Goldberg LH, Hsu SH, Alcalay J. J Am Acad Dermatol 1989; 21: 144–5.

Etretinate treatment of the nevoid basal cell carcinoma syndrome. Therapeutic and chemopreventive effect. Hodak E, Ginzburg A, David M, Sandbank M. Int J Dermatol 1987; 26: 606–9.

Efficacy of retinoids in preventing development of BCCs has been reported only in a few cases of NBCCS, and the sparsity of these reports renders them somewhat unconvincing.

Basal cell carcinoma chemoprevention with nonsteroidal anti-inflammatory drugs in genetically predisposed PTCH1$^{+/-}$ humans and mice. Tang JY, Aszterbaum M, Athar M, Barsanti F, Cappola C, Estevez N, et al. Cancer Prev Res 2010; 3: 253–4.

A 3-year, double-blind, randomized clinical trial in 60 PTCH1$^{+/-}$ patients with NBCCS assessed the effects of oral celecoxib on the development of BCCs. A trend for reducing BCC burden was detected ($p = 0.069$), and the effect appeared most pronounced in patients with less severe disease. The study was discontinued because of concern over enhanced cardiovascular risks.

Inhibiting the hedgehog pathway in patients with the basal cell nevus syndrome. Tang JY, Mackay-Wiggan JM, Aszterbaum M, Yauch RL, Lindgren J, Chang K, et al. N Engl J Med 2012; 366: 2180–8.

In a randomized, double-blind, placebo-controlled, 18-month study, vismodegib reduced the incidence of new, clinically significant BCC (2 vs. 29 cases per group per year, $p < 0.001$). Percent change in baseline size of BCC was found to be 65% versus –11%, $p = 0.003$. No tumors progressed while on vismodegib. Because of adverse events, 54% of patients discontinued vismodegib before the planned conclusion of the study.

Intermittent vismodegib therapy in basal cell nevus syndrome. Yang X, Dinehart SM. JAMA Dermatol 2016; 152: 223–4.

Two patients with NBCCS underwent intermittent therapy with vismodegib: one treated daily for 1 month with 2 months off and the other 2 months on and 2 months off. Side effects resolved within 1 month of the drug holiday, allowing the regimen to be well tolerated. Efficacy was comparable to other trials, with a mean of 1.4 new BCC per year, per patient.

Tazarotene: randomized, double-blind, vehicle-controlled, and open-label concurrent trials for basal cell carcinoma prevention and therapy in patients with basal cell nevus syndrome. Tang JY, Chiou AS, Mackay-Wiggan JM, Aszterbaum M, Chanana AM, Lee W, et al. Cancer Prev Res 2014; 7: 292–9.

In studies on 36 and 34 patients, respectively, topical tazarotene did not appear effective in curing or preventing BCCs in NBCCS.

Evidence Levels: **A** Double-blind study   **B** Clinical trial ≥ 20 subjects   **C** Clinical trial < 20 subjects   **D** Series ≥ 5 subjects   **E** Anecdotal case reports

171

Nevus sebaceus

Stuart R. Lessin, Clifford S. Perlis

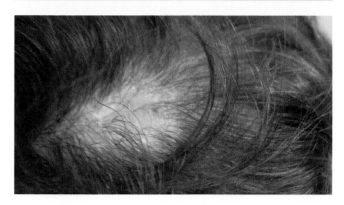

Nevus sebaceus, first described by Jadassohn in 1895, is a term for a congenital hamartoma of the epidermis and adnexal structures typically involving the scalp and face. It results from the mosaic expression of HRAS and KRAS gene mutations. It presents at birth or appears in early childhood as a pink, orange, or yellow waxy plaque with a granular pitted surface that is often hairless. The size and configuration can be variable. During puberty the lesion thickens and becomes verrucous as glands enlarge within the dermis. Development of cutaneous and adenexal neoplasms has been reported in 10% to 20% of lesions after puberty and in adulthood. These neoplasms are most commonly benign. Surgical treatment addresses cosmetic issues, as well as prophylaxis or treatment of neoplasms.

MANAGEMENT STRATEGY

For most lesions, clinical examination is sufficient to establish the diagnosis. A skin biopsy can confirm the clinical impression when indicated. Most neoplastic growths that arise in a nevus sebaceus do not develop until after the age of 16 years; the overwhelming majority is benign. These include syringocystadenoma papilliferum, trichoblastoma, tricholemmoma, sebaceoma, nevocellular nevus, and seborrheic keratosis. The most common malignancy that develops within a nevus sebaceus is a basal cell carcinoma, but the absolute incidence is very rare. Isolated case reports describe rare patients who have developed sebaceous carcinoma, squamous cell carcinoma, tricholemmal carcinoma, or microcystic adnexal carcinoma within nevus sebaceus.

In 2000 case series established that trichoblastoma was the most common neoplasm arising in nevus sebaceus. With this evidence of minimal risk of malignant neoplastic transformation, prophylactic surgery is not justified. Conservative management with clinical observation and biopsy of any lesions suspicious for malignancy appear to be most prudent.

Tumors arising in nevus sebaceus: a study of 596 cases. Cribier B, Scrivener Y, Grosshans E. J Am Acad Dermatol 2000; 42: 263–8.

Retrospective case series of 596 cases demonstrating a 1.7% occurrence of benign tumors in childhood. Most tumors arising in nevus sebaceus occurred in adults over 40; in these adults, 2.1% of the neoplasms were basal cell carcinomas. The authors conclude that prophylactic surgery in children is of uncertain benefit.

Trichoblastoma is the most common neoplasm developed in nevus sebaceus of Jadassohn: a clinicopathologic study of a series of 155 cases. Jaqueti G, Requena L, Sánchez Yus E. Am J Dermatopathol 2000; 22: 108–18.

Retrospective case series of 155 cases failed to reveal any cases of basal cell carcinoma. Trichoblastoma was the most common (7.7%) basaloid tumor. It appears that histologic misinterpretation of trichoblastomas as basal cell carcinomas has been responsible for the erroneous reporting of an increased risk of basal cell carcinoma development within nevus sebaceus. The authors concluded that early prophylactic surgery seems inappropriate.

Secondary neoplasms associated with nevus sebaceus of Jadassohn: a study of 707 cases. Idriss MH, Elston DM. J Am Acad Dermatol 2014; 70: 332–7.

Retrospective case series of 706 cases demonstrating that most secondary neoplasms arising in association with nevus sebaceus are benign. Trichoblastoma and syringocystadenoma papilliferum were the most frequent benign tumors, occurring in 7.4% and 5.2% of cases, respectively. Malignant tumors were present in 2.5% of the cases, with basal cell carcinoma being most common, and almost all were seen in adults. The authors conclude that it is reasonable to delay surgical management until adolescence.

Specific Intervention

- Skin biopsy

A skin biopsy may be performed to confirm a clinical diagnosis. Clinical changes suggestive of neoplastic transformation may be investigated by skin biopsy.

First-Line Therapies

Observation	D
Surgical excision	E

Based on recent case series and histologic analyses that demonstrate the incidence of basal carcinoma is rare, particularly in children, clinical observation should be considered as the first option for any intervention. Prophylactic surgical excision is not warranted based on current data. Elective surgical excision may be considered if lesions become symptomatic or affect appearance. In instances of biopsy-confirmed neoplastic transformation, management should be dictated by the histology of the specific tumor.

Nevus sebaceous revisited. Moody MN, Landau JM, Goldberg LH. Pediatr Dermatol 2012; 29: 15–23.

A comprehensive review of reported nevus sebaceus outcomes and recommendations for prophylactic excision are provided. It is recommended that all cases of nevus sebaceus be evaluated individually with a thorough medical history, physical examination, and review of therapeutic options in order to determine if prophylactic excision is warranted. Nevus sebaceus in cosmetically apparent regions in healthy children is recognized as a reasonable indication for consideration of prophylactic excision.

Second-Line Therapies

- Curettage and cautery   E
- Cryotherapy   E
- Laser resurfacing   E
- Photodynamic therapy   E

A variety of destructive methods have been described for treatment of nevus sebaceus and provide an alternative to surgical excision; however, they may not be as effective in removal of deeper structures.

Linear nevus sebaceus of Jadassohn treated with the carbon dioxide laser. Ashinoff R. Pediatr Dermatol 1993; 10: 189–91.

A case report of the use of a carbon dioxide laser to electively treat a nevus sebaceus of the nose in a 10-year-old boy. Carbon dioxide laser vaporization provided partial and superficial destruction with good palliative appearance-enhancing result. The treatment did not eliminate the need for continued clinical surveillance.

Topical photodynamic therapy for nevus sebaceous on the face. In S-I, Lee JY, Kim YC. Eur J Dermatol 2010; 20: 590–2.

A total of 12 patients were treated with topical 20% aminolevulinic acid (ALA) or methyl aminolevulinate (MAL) after CO_2 laser ablation. Lesions were irradiated with a light-emitting diode (LED) device. Treatment was repeated at 1- to 4-week intervals to each patient. All 12 patients responded with 3/12 (25%) mild (25%–50% improvement), 7/12 (58%) moderate (51%–75% improvement), and 2/12 (17%) marked (>75%) improvement. Two patients showed partial recurrences after completion of treatments. There were no significant side effects.

Evidence Levels: A Double-blind study   **B** Clinical trial ≥ 20 subjects   **C** Clinical trial < 20 subjects   **D** Series ≥ 5 subjects   **E** Anecdotal case reports

172

Notalgia paresthetica

Joanna Wallengren

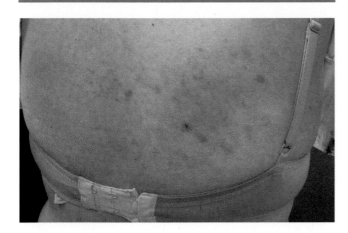

Notalgia paresthetica is a unilateral sensory neuropathy characterized by pruritus or burning pain at the medial inferior tip of the scapula. Accompanying pigmentation or mild lichenification is secondary to scratching. Occasionally the distribution may be bilateral, and a few hereditary cases have been described. Pruritus is believed to result from nerve impingement or chronic nerve trauma.

MANAGEMENT STRATEGY

Treatment aims to reduce the itch by altering peripheral or central nerve transmission. Topical corticosteroids are generally ineffective unless secondary inflammation is present.

Topical *capsaicin* 0.025% three times daily for 5 weeks depletes sensory nerve transmitters in the skin. In case of relapse, the treatment may be repeated for a few days or weeks until pruritus subsides. Capsaicin may be applied in higher concentrations such as 0.075% or 0.1%; with increasing concentrations there is more burning but the desensitization of the skin occurs sooner. High-dose (8%) capsaicin patch for 1 hour is associated with severe burning. It has shown considerable variability in efficacy, reducing notalgia paresthetica for 2 days to 3 months.

Local anesthesia with 5% lidocaine patch twice daily blocks peripheral nerve transmission, but there is a risk for contact allergy to the anesthetic.

Daily electrical stimulation using *cutaneous field stimulation (CFS)* or *transcutaneous electrical nerve stimulation (TENS)* for 2 to 5 weeks has been tried with good results, with the pruritus relapsing gradually.

Deep intramuscular *acupuncture* to the paravertebral muscles in the T2 to T6 dermatome once a week until the pruritus subsides, as well as spinal physiotherapy, has been reported in a few cases. Also, single treatments with *botulinum toxin* or an *anesthetic block* have been described in anecdotal case reports. The reduction of itch due to these treatments may last for months or years.

Oral therapy may be preferred in patients in whom repeated topical treatments may be difficult to perform. Anticonvulsants such as *gabapentin* or *oxcarbazepine* alter central nerve transmission. Gabapentin in doses of 900 mg a day is often required.

Most of these treatments offer only transient relief, and there is a considerable risk of relapse upon discontinuation of treatment.

Specific Investigations

- Skin biopsy
- Radiography of the thoracic spine
- Magnetic resonance imaging (MRI) of the thoracic spine

Notalgia paresthetica. Case reports and histologic appraisal. Weber PJ, Poulos EG. J Am Acad Dermatol 1988; 18: 25–30.

Skin biopsies from 14 patients revealed necrotic keratinocytes. Melanin and melanophages in the upper and mid-dermis were found in biopsies of patients with pigmented lesions.

Investigation of spinal pathology in notalgia paresthetica. Savk O, Savk E. J Am Acad Dermatol 2005; 52: 1085–7.

Forty-three patients with notalgia paresthetica underwent radiography of the spine. Thirty-seven skin lesions were accompanied by relevant spinal changes (60.7%).

Notalgia paresthetica associated with nerve root impingement. Eisenberg E, Barmeir E, Bergman R. J Am Acad Dermatol 1997; 37: 998–1000.

An impingement of the nerve root was confirmed by MRI in one patient.

Notalgia paresthetica is a clinical diagnosis, and none of the previously mentioned investigations are required in the clinical situation.

First-Line Therapies

• Capsaicin 0.025%	A
• Lidocaine 5% patch	E

Successful treatment of notalgia paresthetica with topical capsaicin: vehicle-controlled, double-blind, crossover study. Wallengren J, Klinker M. J Am Acad Dermatol 1995; 32: 287–9.

This double-blind crossover comparison between capsaicin 0.025% and vehicle cream was performed in 20 patients for 10 weeks, with the 4-week treatments being followed by 2 weeks of washout. The group treated with capsaicin first had a reduction of VAS (Visual Analog Scale) from 61% to 35% during the first period, whereas in the other group VAS was reduced from 52% to 27%. Most patients relapsed within a month.

Notalgia paraesthetica—report of three cases and their treatment. Layton AM, Cotterill JA. Clin Exp Dermatol 1991; 16: 197–8.

All three patients improved upon treatment with 2.5% lidocaine and 2.5% prilocaine; two patients relapsed, but pruritus was reduced.

Second-Line Therapies

• Cutaneous field stimulation	D
• TENS	D
• Gabapentin	E
• Oxcarbazepine	E

Cutaneous field stimulation (CFS) in treatment of severe localized itch. Wallengren J, Sundler F. Arch Dermatol 2001; 137: 1323–5.

Seventeen patients with different disorders of neuropathic pruritus completed the study. Four of five patients with notalgia paresthetica improved after daily use of CFS for 5 weeks, with VAS reduced from 65% to 40%. Itch gradually relapsed after the discontinuation of CFS.

Transcutaneous electrical nerve stimulation offers partial relief in notalgia paresthetica patients with a relevant spinal pathology. Savk E, Savk O, Sendur F. J Dermatol 2007; 34: 315–9.

Nine of 15 patients treated with TENS for 2 weeks improved substantially, with mean VAS being reduced from 100% to 45%.

Efficacy of gabapentin in the improvement of pruritus and quality of life of patients with notalgia paresthetica. Maciel AA, Cunha PR, Laraia IO, Trevisan F. An Bras Dermatol 2014; 89: 570–5.

A nonrandomized study of 20 patients, where 10 patients were treated with gabapentin 300 mg/day for 4 weeks. At the end of treatment, mean VAS for pruritus was decreased from 95% to 50%.

Open pilot study on oxcarbazepine for the treatment of notalgia paresthetica. Savk E, Bolukbasi O, Akyol A, Karaman G. J Am Acad Dermatol 2001; 45: 630–2.

Four patients were treated with oxcarbazepine for 6 months: two improved, with VAS reduced from 80% to 50% and from 90% to 40%, respectively.

Third-Line Therapies	
• Spinal physiotherapy with ultrasound and manipulation	D
• Botulinum toxin A	D
• Acupuncture (deep intramuscular stimulation) of the paravertebral muscles at T2–T6 once a week until pruritus subsides	E
• Anesthetic paravertebral block at dermatome T3–T6 with bupivacaine 0.75% and methylprednisolone on one occasion	E

Notalgia paresthetica: clinical, physiopathological and therapeutic aspects. A study of 12 cases. Raison-Peyron N, Meunier L, Acevedo M, Meynadier J. J Eur Acad Dermatol Venereol 1999; 12: 215–21.

Pruritus was reduced in four of six patients treated by spinal physiotherapy using ultrasound or manipulation. The improvement was sustained for 1 to 9 years.

Botulinum toxin type A for neuropathic itch. Wallengren J, Bartosik J. Br J Dermatol 2010; 163: 424–6.

Four patients with notalgia paresthetica received a total of 18 to 100 U of BTX-A (Botulinum toxin A) intradermally to the affected area. Mean VAS was reduced by 40% at 6-week follow-up. At follow-up after 18 months, pruritus relapsed.

Treatment of notalgia paresthetica with botulinum toxin A: a double-blind randomized controlled trial. Maari C, Marchessault P, Bissonnette R. J Am Acad Dermatol. 2014;70(6):1139–41.

In this double-blind, randomized, placebo-controlled study on 20 patients with notalgia paresthetica, a total dose of up to 200 U BTX-A or saline was administered intradermally. After an observation of 12 weeks after the treatment, the placebo group received BTX-A, and both groups were evaluated at week 24. There was no statistically significant difference between the patients treated with BTX-A and placebo.

Neurogenic pruritus: an unrecognised problem? A retrospective case series of treatment by acupuncture. Stellon A. Acupunct Med 2002; 20: 186–90.

Sixteen patients with different disorders of neuropathic pruritus completed the study. Four patients with notalgia paresthetica improved, with mean VAS reduced from 73% to 0%.

Successful treatment of notalgia paresthetica with a paravertebral local anesthetic block. Goulden V, Toomey PJ, Highet AS. J Am Acad Dermatol 1998; 8: 114–6.

Paravertebral block at dermatome T3 to T6 in one patient resulted in clearing of pruritus within a few days, lasting for 1 year of follow-up.

Evidence Levels: **A** Double-blind study **B** Clinical trial ≥ 20 subjects **C** Clinical trial < 20 subjects **D** Series ≥ 5 subjects **E** Anecdotal case reports

Onchocerciasis

Michele E. Murdoch

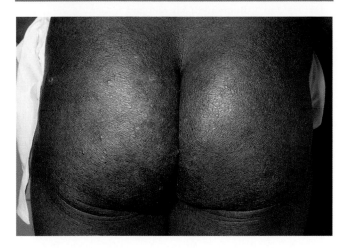

Onchocerciasis is a major tropical parasitic infection caused by the filarial worm *Onchocerca volvulus* and is transmitted by blood-sucking *Simulium* spp. blackflies, which breed near fast-flowing rivers. Global estimates suggest that 37 million people carry *O. volvulus*, most of whom live in Africa, and a total of 120 million people are considered at risk of infection because of where they live. The disease is endemic in 30 countries in sub-Saharan Africa, and small foci also exist in Yemen and Central and Southern America. Mass ivermectin treatment has now eliminated or interrupted transmission in 11 of the 13 foci in the Americas, and the World Health Organization has verified elimination of onchocerciasis in Colombia, Ecuador, Mexico and Guatemala. The first manifestation of infection is usually intense pruritus, and subsequently a wide variety of acute and chronic skin and eye changes develop. The socioeconomic consequences of onchocerciasis are most marked in hyperendemic areas in sub-Saharan Africa. Globally, approximately 270,000 people are blind and 500,000 have significant visual loss as a direct consequence of onchocerciasis. A multicountry study in Africa revealed that 42% of the adult population in endemic villages suffered from pruritus, and 28% of the population had onchocercal skin lesions.

MANAGEMENT STRATEGY

The mainstay of treatment is *ivermectin*. Ivermectin is a safe, effective microfilaricide (i.e., it kills the immature larval stages of filarial worms), but it does not kill the adult worms. After a few months of dosing, the numbers of microfilariae in the skin gradually increase back toward pretreatment levels, and treatment has to be repeated throughout the lifespan of the adult worm (10–14 years).

Wolbachia spp. symbiotic endobacteria have been identified as essential for the filarial worms' fertility and offer novel targets for treatment. Additional treatment with *doxycycline* to sterilize the worms significantly enhances ivermectin-induced suppression of microfilaridermia.

The approach to treatment of onchocerciasis varies for (1) treatment of individuals outside of endemic areas, (2) treatment of individuals within endemic areas, and (3) mass treatment programs.

Treatment of Individuals Outside of Endemic Areas

Treatment of individuals living outside of areas with ongoing transmission consists of a single dose of ivermectin (150 µg/kg), followed 1 week later by doxycycline (200 mg daily for 6 weeks). Alternative doxycycline regimens are doxycycline 200 mg daily for 4 weeks or 100 mg daily for 6 weeks.

If the patient is pregnant or less than 9 years of age, doxycycline is contraindicated.

Treatment of Individuals Within Endemic Areas

Treatment of individuals within areas of ongoing transmission consists of a single dose of ivermectin 150 µg/kg repeated every 3 to 6 months until the patient is asymptomatic. Treatment should be repeated if there is recurrence of pruritus, itchy papular rash, or eosinophilia. Treatment with ivermectin may be required for 10 years or more.

Mass Treatment Programs

Three regional programs have been established to coordinate global control. The Onchocerciasis Control Program (OCP, 1974–2002) successfully used *aerial larviciding* of rivers in West Africa to control the vector blackfly, and more recently it has distributed *ivermectin* to control any recrudescence. The Onchocerciasis Elimination Program in the Americas (OEPA), which started in 1991, uses 6-monthly mass ivermectin therapy and aims to eliminate onchocerciasis from the region. The largest program, the African Program for Onchocerciasis Control (APOC), commenced in 1995 and aims to eliminate onchocerciasis by 2025. It consists of large-scale, annual, community-directed treatment of ivermectin in 15 non-OCP countries and 4 ex-OCP countries. Its original aim was to reduce onchocerciasis until it was no longer a public health problem, but this was revised in 2010 to aim for elimination.

In forested areas of central Africa and Sudan, which are coendemic with loiasis, ivermectin cannot be used because it causes serious neurologic adverse reactions, including encephalopathy. Whereas lengthy doxycycline regimens are deemed impractical for main large-scale treatment of onchocerciasis, in areas coendemic with loiasis, doxycycline is a safe alternative as it is inactive against *Loa loa* because of the absence of *Wolbachia*.

Specific Investigations

- Skin snips
- Other parasitologic forms of diagnosis:
  - Detection of intraocular microfilariae using a slit lamp
  - Demonstration of adult worms by collagenase digestion of excised nodules
  - Full blood count (for eosinophilia)
  - Mazzotti test (only do if skin snips negative and hence patient likely to be lightly infected)
- Future investigative tools:
  - Diethylcarbamazine patch test
  - Serodiagnosis
  - Polymerase chain reaction
  - Antigen detection dipstick assay on urine

The effects of ivermectin on onchocercal skin disease and severe itching: results of a multicentre trial. Brieger WR, Awedoba AK, Eneanya CI, Hagan M, Ogbuagu KF, Okello DO et al. Trop Med Int Health 1998; 3: 951–61.

The effects of ivermectin were assessed in 3-monthly, 6-monthly, and annual doses in 4072 villagers in forest zones of Ghana, Nigeria, and Uganda who underwent interviews and clinical examinations at baseline and at five follow-up visits. Reactive skin lesions were categorized as acute papular onchodermatitis, chronic papular onchodermatitis, and lichenified onchodermatitis. From 6 months onwards there was a 40% to 50% reduction in the prevalence of severe itching after ivermectin treatment compared with the placebo group. Also, a greater reduction in prevalence and severity of reactive skin lesions over time was seen in those receiving ivermectin. The differences between the various ivermectin treatment regimens were not significant.

The African Programme for Onchocerciasis Control: impact on onchocercal skin disease. Ozoh GA, Murdoch ME, Bissek A-C, Hagan M, Ogbuagu K, Shamad M et al. Trop Med Int Health 2011; 16: 875–83.

Seven study sites in Cameroon, Sudan, Nigeria, and Uganda participated in two cross-sectional surveys of 5193 individuals at baseline and 5180 people after 5 or 6 years of annual ivermectin therapy. At follow-up, significant ($p < 0.001$) reductions were found in the risk of itching (odds ratio [OR] 0.32) and acute papular onchodermatitis (OR 0.28), chronic papular onchodermatitis (OR 0.34), depigmentation (OR 0.31), and nodules (OR 0.37). Reduction in the odds ratio of lichenified onchodermatitis was also significant (OR 0.54, $p < 0.03$).

A trial of a three-dose regimen of ivermectin for the treatment of patients with onchocerciasis in the UK. Churchill DR, Godfrey-Faussett P, Birley HDL, Malin A, Davidson RN, Bryceson ADM. Trans R Soc Trop Med Hyg 1994; 88: 242.

As ivermectin is also thought to suppress embryogenesis in adult worms, the efficacy of three doses of ivermectin given at monthly intervals was studied to determine whether such a regimen could lead to a greater suppression of microfilaridermia. Thirty-three patients (of whom 27 were European) with onchocerciasis were treated with a single dose of 150 to 200 µg/kg ivermectin and observed in hospital for 72 hours. Second and third doses were given as outpatient treatment, respectively, 1 and 2 months later. Patients were followed up at 3-, 6-, and 12-monthly intervals after the last dose of ivermectin. The patients with positive skin snips before treatment were compared with patients given a single dose of ivermectin in a previous study (Godfrey-Faussett P et al., 1991, see later). Relapses occurred slightly less frequently after three doses. In contrast to studies in West Africa, where reactions to ivermectin are rare, 17 patients (52%) had reactions. The authors therefore recommend that the first dose of ivermectin for lightly infected expatriates be given in hospital.

Ivermectin in the treatment of onchocerciasis in Britain. Godfrey-Faussett P, Dow C, Black ME, Bryceson ADM. Trop Med Parasitol 1991; 42: 82–84.

Thirty-one patients with early, light infection were treated with a single dose of 150 to 200 µg/kg ivermectin. Those who relapsed were retreated after an interval of not less than 5 months.

Approximately two thirds relapsed within 1 year. A similar pattern was seen after the second dose. A single dose of ivermectin, repeated every 3 to 6 months as necessary, was considered to be the treatment of choice for patients in nonendemic areas lightly infected with *O. volvulus*. One third of such patients may be cured with each treatment.

Effects of standard and high doses of ivermectin on adult worms of *Onchocerca volvulus*: a randomised controlled trial. Gardon J, Boussinesq M, Kamgno J, Gardon-Wendel N, Demanga-Ngangue, Duke BOL. Lancet 2002; 360: 203–10.

Ivermectin 150 µg/kg given at intervals of 0.5 to 3.0 months is known to cause slight but significant increased mortality of adult worms. In this randomized study of 657 Cameroonian patients with onchocerciasis, 3-monthly treatment with ivermectin killed more female adult worms than did annual treatment. There was no difference between standard (150 µg/kg) and high-dose schedules (800 µg/kg).

The feasibility of large-scale 3-monthly ivermectin treatment in endemic areas and its likely greater effect in reducing transmission have still to be determined.

An investigation of persistent microfilaridermias despite multiple treatments with ivermectin, in two onchocerciasis-endemic foci in Ghana. Awadzi K, Boakye DA, Edwards G, Opoku NO, Attah SK, Osei-Atweneboana MY et al. Ann Trop Med Parasitol 2004; 98: 231–49.

Some individuals in endemic areas have persistent microfilaridermia despite nine treatments with ivermectin. In this open, case-control study of 21 "suboptimal" responders, 7 amicrofilaridermic responders and 14 ivermectin-naive subjects, the results revealed that the persistent microfilaridermias are mainly due to nonresponsiveness of the adult female worms, raising the possibility that the worms have developed resistance to ivermectin.

Endosymbiotic bacteria in worms as targets for a novel chemotherapy in filariasis. Hoerauf A, Volkmann L, Hamelmann C, Adjei O, Autenrieth IB, Fleischer B et al. Lancet 2000; 355: 1242–43.

The activity of doxycycline against *Wolbachia* spp. and the fertility of adult female worms were assessed by examination of excised subcutaneous onchocercal nodules in 22 Ghanaian individuals treated with doxycycline 100 mg daily for 6 weeks and 14 untreated controls. Immunohistology with an antibody to bacterial heat shock protein-60 was used to assess the presence or absence of *Wolbachia* spp., and the morphology of female worms was examined. In addition, PCR reactions using, first, endobacterial primers, and, second, nematode primers, were performed. None of the treated worms had usual bacterial loads, and there was total suppression of normal embryonic worm development during early oocyte/morula stages, whereas nodules from untreated controls showed normal embryogenesis.

Depletion of *Wolbachia* endobacteria in *Onchocerca volvulus* by doxycycline and microfilaridermia after ivermectin treatment. Hoerauf A, Mand S, Adjei O, Fleischer B, Büttner DW. Lancet 2001; 357: 1415–16.

The Ghanaian participants in this study were not randomized because this was not acceptable to the village elders. Instead, the first 55 patients were allocated to ivermectin and doxycycline and the next 33 to ivermectin alone. Doxycycline 100 mg daily was given from the start of the study for 6 weeks. Subgroup A (31 doxycycline-treated and 24 controls) was given ivermectin 2.5 months after the start of the study, and subgroup B (24 doxycycline-treated

Evidence Levels: A Double-blind study **B** Clinical trial ≥ 20 subjects **C** Clinical trial < 20 subjects **D** Series ≥ 5 subjects **E** Anecdotal case reports

and 9 controls) 6 months after the onset of the study. The results suggested a complete block in worm embryogenesis for at least 18 months after treatment with ivermectin and doxycycline.

The principle of targeting Wolbachia *spp. with ivermectin in combination treatment offers the potential of interrupting transmission. Shorter anti-Wolbachia spp. regimens (either with other antibiotics or in combinations) are needed for mass treatment of endemic areas.*

Wolbachia endobacteria depletion by doxycycline as antifilarial therapy has macrofilaricidal activity in onchocerciasis: a randomized placebo-controlled study. Hoerauf A, Specht S, Büttner M, Pfarr K, Mand S, Fimmers R et al. Med Microbiol Immunol 2008; 197: 295–311.

In a randomized, placebo-controlled trial in Ghana, 67 onchocerciasis patients received 200 mg/day doxycycline for 4 or 6 weeks, followed by ivermectin after 6 months. After 6, 20, and 27 months, efficacy was evaluated by onchocercoma histology, PCR, and microfilariae determination. Administration of doxycycline resulted in endobacteria depletion and female worm sterilization. The 6-week treatment was macrofilaricidal, with >60% of the female worms found dead.

Macrofilaricidal activity after doxycycline only treatment of *Onchocerca volvulus* in an area of *Loa loa* co-endemicity: a randomized controlled trial. Turner JD, Tendongfor N, Esum M, Johnston KL, Langley RS, Ford L et al. PLoS Negl Trop Dis 2010; 4: e660.

Within a larger, double-blind, randomized trial, a group of 22 Cameroonian individuals coinfected with *O. volvulus* and low to moderate intensities of *L. loa* infection were treated with a course of 6 weeks of doxycycline 200 mg/day followed by ivermectin at 4 months. Doxycycline was well tolerated in patients coinfected with moderate intensities of *L. loa* microfilariae. A 6-week course of doxycycline yielded macrofilaricidal and worm-sterilizing effects, which were not dependent on coadministration of ivermectin.

Long term impact of large scale community-directed delivery of doxycycline for the treatment of onchocerciasis. Tamarozzi F, Tendongfor N, Enyong PA, Esum M, Faragher B, Wanji S et al. Parasites Vectors 2012; 5: 53.

In an area coendemic for *O. volvulus* and *L. loa*, 375 Cameroonian individuals who had been treated 4 years previously with doxycycline 100 mg daily for 6 weeks followed by one or two rounds of annual ivermectin mass drug treatment, plus 132 persons who had had one or two rounds of annual ivermectin alone, were evaluated. A statistically significant lower microfilarial prevalence and load were found in those who had received doxycycline followed by ivermectin compared with those who received ivermectin alone.

Second-Line Therapies

• Albendazole	A

Albendazole in the treatment of onchocerciasis: double-blind clinical trial in Venezuela. Cline BL, Hernandez JL, Mather FJ, Bartholomew R, De Maza SN, Rodulfo S et al. Am J Trop Med Hyg 1992; 47: 512–20.

Forty-nine individuals with onchocerciasis (26 treated and 23 controls) were treated with a 10-day course of albendazole (400 mg daily) or placebo. Patients in the albendazole-treated group with baseline microfilarial densities over 5 mf/mg skin showed a significant reduction in microfilarial densities at 12

months. Albendazole was well tolerated and is believed to interfere with embryogenesis in adult *O. volvulus* worms.

The co-administration of ivermectin and albendazole – safety, pharmacokinetics and efficacy against *Onchocerca volvulus*. Awadzi K, Edwards G, Duke BOL, Opoku NO, Attah SK, Addy ET et al. Ann Trop Med Parasitol 2003; 97: 165–78.

In a randomized, double-blind, placebo-controlled trial in 44 male patients with onchocerciasis in Ghana, the coadministration of ivermectin (200 µg/kg) with albendazole (400 mg) did not offer any advantage over ivermectin alone.

N.B. Onchocerciasis and lymphatic filariasis commonly coexist, and current integrated control programs use repeated annual mass treatment of endemic communities with ivermectin and albendazole.

OTHER THERAPIES

• Suramin	D
• Future therapies	
• Moxidectin	A
• New macrofilaricides	

Thirty-month follow-up of sub-optimal responders to multiple treatments with ivermectin, in two onchocerciasis-endemic foci in Ghana. Awadzi K, Attah SK, Addy ET, Opoku NO, Quartey BT, Lazdins-Helds JK et al. Ann Trop Med Parasitol 2004; 98: 359–70.

Suramin is both a macrofilaricide and a microfilaricide, but unfortunately a course of suramin requires weekly intravenous infusions and may have serious adverse effects, including nephrotoxicity.

In this paper, Awadzi et al. propose the use of suramin under hospital supervision in selected individuals with onchocerciasis who are resistant to multiple doses of ivermectin. The treatment regimen proposed was a total adult dose of 5.0 g (72.5–84.7 mg/kg) over 6 weeks.

Report of the 36th session of the Technical Consultative Committee (TCC), Ouagadougou, 11–15 March, 2013. World Health Organization/African Programme for Onchocerciasis Control (APOC). http://www.who.int/apoc/about/structure/tcc/TCC36_Final _Report_170513.pdf (accessed 23/3/16).

Moxidectin is a microfilaricidal drug that shows a higher potency than ivermectin in animal models. A phase III trial in humans in 1472 people aged 12 years and above in four study sites in Ghana, Liberia, and the Democratic Republic of Congo compared a single dose of 8 mg moxidectin with ivermectin (150 µg/kg). A reported 96.6% of moxidectin-treated and 97.2% of ivermectin-treated individuals completed 12 months follow-up. Preliminary results revealed that the average percent reduction in skin mf levels during 1-year posttreatment was significantly higher after moxidectin (95.0±1.9) than ivermectin (84.4±15.4). Moxidectin had a higher and more prolonged efficacy compared with ivermectin. Because moxidectin has the same mode of action as ivermectin, whether it could replace ivermectin in the event of resistance is unknown.

After an investment from the Global Health Investment Fund (GHIF) in 2015, Medicines Development for Global Health has commenced the registration process for moxidectin for human use.

In addition to being one of the sponsors for GHIF, the Bill & Melinda Gates Foundation is also supporting research to optimize other treatment regimens (Death of Onchocerciasis and Lymphatic Filariasis, DOLF; www.dolf.wustl.edu). Studies include attempts to reformulate flubendazole, a known effective macrofilaricide, in order to improve its bioavailability.

Oral lichen planus

Drore Eisen

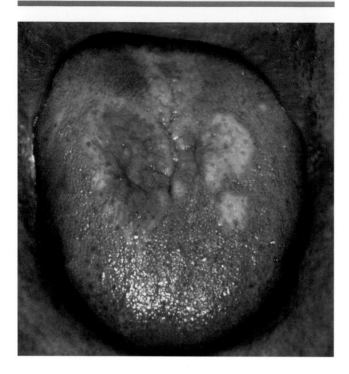

Oral lichen planus (OLP) is a common chronic inflammatory disorder affecting all areas of the oral mucosa that rarely undergoes complete remission, even with treatment.

MANAGEMENT STRATEGY

All treatment should be aimed at eliminating erythematous and ulcerative lesions, alleviating symptoms, and potentially reducing the risk of malignant transformation. Given the uncertainty of the premalignant nature of OLP, it is important to monitor all patients carefully and long term.

Although the etiology of OLP is unknown, the possibility of a hypersensitivity reaction (oral lichenoid reaction) should be considered when lesions are confined to mucosa in close proximity to a dental restoration. In such cases, identifying allergies to dental materials by patch testing and then removing the fillings with positive reactions or empirically removing the filling often results in resolution. Another uncommon cause of lichenoid reaction is drugs. A thorough medication history, with emphasis on nonsteroidal antiinflammatory drugs (NSAIDs) and angiotensin-converting enzyme (ACE) inhibitors is warranted, as drug-induced reactions are reversible when the implicated drug is withdrawn.

Exacerbating factors, including sharp dental restorations and poorly fitting dental appliances, should be eliminated. An optimal oral hygiene program that minimizes dental plaque and calculus can significantly improve gingival OLP.

All agents employed for the treatment of OLP are for off-label indications and lack adequate efficacy studies; thus optimal dose, duration of treatment, safety, and their true efficacy remain unknown.

The most useful agents for the treatment of OLP are *potent topical corticosteroids*. Asymptomatic reticular lesions do not require therapy. For intractable erosive lesions, *intralesional corticosteroids* repeated every 2 to 4 weeks are highly effective.

Unresponsive OLP may benefit from *topical immunomodulators* (i.e., tacrolimus, pimecrolimus, and ciclosporin), which may be used as alternatives to, or in conjunction with, topical corticosteroids. Relapses after cessation of therapy are to be expected. Their long-term safety for this chronic disease is unknown.

A number of *herbal preparations* have been reported to benefit OLP, including curcuminoids (6000 mg/d), lycopene (8 mg/day), and topical aloe vera (70% concentration).

A variety of *lasers, UV phototherapy,* and *photodynamic therapy* have also been shown to be beneficial in alleviating OLP symptoms.

For patients with severe oral disease or with extraoral manifestations, the addition of *systemic immunosuppressives* is indicated. The author has found that methotrexate (12.5–20 mg/week), azathioprine (100–150 mg/day), mycophenolate mofetil (1–2 g/day), acitretin (25–50 mg/day), and hydroxychloroquine (400 mg/day) are the most useful systemic agents. Ciclosporin, thalidomide, and Tumor necrosis factor-alpha (TNF-α) inhibitors may be used for refractory cases, but data are limited.

Systemic corticosteroids (30–80 mg of prednisone) should be reserved for acute flares and not as maintenance therapy. Secondary candidiasis frequently complicates all therapies and requires treatment with topical or systemic agents. All treatments for OLP are palliative and not curative, and patients should expect a chronic course with intermittent acute exacerbations.

Specific Investigations

- Biopsy for confirmation; direct immunofluorescence when indicated to exclude vesiculoerosive diseases
- Monitoring for malignant transformation
- Hepatitis serologies when risk factors are present
- Thyroid disease may constitute a comorbidity of OLP
- Consider contact and drug lichenoid reactions

Direct immunofluorescence in oral lichen planus. Buajeeb W, Okuma N, Thanakun S, Laothumthut T. JCDR 2015; 9: ZC34–7.

Biopsies of gingival OLP are often nondiagnostic. Immunofluorescence shows characteristic shaggy fibrinogen deposition at the basement membrane zone.

The malignant transformation of oral lichen planus and oral lichenoid lesions: a systematic review. Fitzpatrick SG, Hirsch SA, Gordon SC. J Am Dent Assoc 2014; 145: 45–56.

Although the malignant potential of OLP remains controversial, the overall rate of transformation approximates 1%, requiring continued regular observation of patients.

Course of oral lichen planus: a retrospective study of 808 northern Italian patients. Carbone M, Arduino PG, Carrozzo M, Gandolfo S, Argiolas MR, Bertolusso G, et al. Oral Dis 2009; 15: 235–43.

Routine hepatitis screening in northern European and American OLP patients without risk factors may not be warranted, but OLP is significantly associated with hepatitis C infections in southern Europe and Japan.

Association between oral lichenoid reactions and amalgam restorations. Pezelj-Ribaric S, Prpic J, Miletic I, Brumini G, Soskic MS, Anic I. J Eur Acad Dermatol Venereol 2008; 22: 1163–7.

Evidence Levels: A Double-blind study B Clinical trial ≥ 20 subjects C Clinical trial < 20 subjects D Series ≥ 5 subjects E Anecdotal case reports

When patch test reactions to mercury compounds were positive, partial or complete replacement of amalgam fillings led to a significant improvement in nearly all patients.

Thyroid disease and oral lichen planus as comorbidity: a prospective case-control study. Garcia-Pola MJ, Llorente-Pendas S, Seoane-Romero JM, Berasaluce MJ, Garcia-Martin JM. Dermatology 2016 [Epub ahead of print].

Diagnosis of thyroid disease was present in 15.3% of 215 OLP patients.

First-Line Therapies

- Topical corticosteroids   **B**
- Intralesional corticosteroids   **B**

Systemic and topical corticosteroid treatment of oral lichen planus: a comparative study with long-term follow-up. Carbone M, Goss E, Carrozzo M, Castellano S, Conrotto D, Broccoletti R, et al. J Oral Pathol Med 2003; 32: 323–9.

Patients treated with either topical clobetasol or prednisone and then clobetasol responded similarly, suggesting that prednisone should be reserved only for acute exacerbations.

High-potency preparations are more effective than midpotency ones. Once the disease becomes controlled, topical steroids may be used several times weekly to prevent flare-ups.

Efficacy of intralesional betamethasone for erosive oral lichen planus and evaluation of recurrence: a randomized, controlled trial. Liu C, Xie B, Yang Y, Lin D, Wang C, Lin M, et al. Oral Surg Oral Med Oral Pathol Oral Radiol 2013; 116: 584–90.

Intralesional triamcinolone and betamethasone are highly efficacious for erosive lesions.

Second-Line Therapies

Topical immunosuppressants
- Tacrolimus   **A**
- Pimecrolimus   **A**
- Ciclosporin   **A**

Systemic immunosuppressants
- Methotrexate   **E**
- Mycophenolate mofetil   **E**
- Azathioprine   **E**
- Hydroxychloroquine sulfate   **C**
- TNF-alpha inhibitors (adalimumab, etanercept)   **E**
- Levamisole   **C**

A comparative treatment study of topical tacrolimus and clobetasol in oral lichen planus. Radfar L, Wild RC, Suresh L. Oral Surg Oral Med Oral Pathol Oral Radiol Endod 2008; 105: 187–93.

In this 6-week, 30-patient study, tacrolimus was shown to be as useful as clobetasol.

Long-term efficacy and safety of topical tacrolimus in the management of ulcerative/erosive oral lichen planus. Hodgson TA, Sahni N, Kaliakatsou F, Buchanan JA, Porter SR. Eur J Dermatol 2003; 13: 466–70.

Of 50 patients who used tacrolimus for 2 to 39 months, 14% had complete resolution of ulcers, 80% had partial resolution, and 6% reported no benefit.

Randomized trial of pimecrolimus cream versus triamcinolone acetonide paste in the treatment of oral lichen planus. Gorouhi, F, Solhpour A, Beitollahi JM, Afshar S, Davari P, Hashemi P, et al. J Am Acad Dermatol 2007; 57: 806–13.

In a 20-patient, 2-month study, pimecrolimus was as effective as triamcinolone 0.1%.

Pimecrolimus 1% cream for oral erosive lichen planus: a 6-week randomized, double-blind, vehicle-controlled study with a 6-week open-label extension to assess efficacy and safety. McCaughey C, Machan M, Bennett R, Zone JJ, Hull CM. J Eur Acad Dermatol Venereol 2011; 25: 1061–7.

Highly effective when used twice daily for 6 weeks, but blood concentrations were detected in most patients. Relapses occurred in all patients after discontinuing therapy.

Clinical and serologic efficacy of topical calcineurin inhibitors in oral lichen planus: a prospective randomized controlled trial. Vohra S, Singal A, Sharma SB. Int J Dermatol 2016; 55: 101–5.

In an 8-week study involving 40 patients, pimecrolimus and tacrolimus were equally effective.

Tacrolimus and pimecrolimus are not always effective and, when discontinued, do not result in long-term benefits. Given the potential for systemic absorption, their safety for long-term use in the oral cavity remains unknown.

Ciclosporin vs. clobetasol in the topical management of atrophic and erosive oral lichen planus: a double-blind, randomized controlled trial. Conrotto D, Carbone M, Carrozzo M, Arduino P, Broccoletti R, Pentenero M, et al. Br J Dermatol 2006; 154: 139–45.

In this 2-month study, 40 patients (65%) improved with ciclosporin versus 95% with clobetasol. Two months after discontinuing treatment, one third of the clobetasol group remained clear, versus three quarters of the ciclosporin group.

Ciclosporin benefits are inconsistent. The high cost of swishing ciclosporin (500 mg/5 mL TID) limits its use, but swishing a smaller quantity or applying a finger rub dose (50 mg/day) has been shown to be beneficial and lowers the cost.

Oral lichen planus: a case series with emphasis on therapy. Torti DC, Jorizzo JL, McCarty MA. Arch Dermatol 2007; 143: 511–5.

About 50% treated with low doses of methotrexate (2.5–12.5 mg/week) responded to therapy.

Successful treatment of oral erosive lichen planus with mycophenolate mofetil. Dalmau J, Puig L, Roe E, Peramiquel L, Campos M, Alomar A. J Eur Acad Dermatol Venereol 2007; 21: 259–60.

A prospective study of findings and management in 214 patients with oral lichen planus. Silverman S Jr, Gorsky M, Lozada-Nur F, Giannotti K. Oral Surg Oral Med Oral Pathol Oral Radiol Endod 1991; 72: 665–70.

Azathioprine (50–150 mg/day) is effective but requires 3 to 6 months before maximal benefit is achieved.

Hydroxychloroquine sulfate (Plaquenil) improves oral lichen planus: an open trial. Eisen D. J Am Acad Dermatol 1993; 28: 609–12.

Nine out of 10 patients had an excellent response to hydroxychloroquine 200 to 400 mg/d for 6 months.

Adalimumab in the management of cutaneous and oral lichen planus. Chao TJ. Cutis 2009; 84: 325–8.

A single case report of "thick plaques" of lichen planus arising on the tongue and buccal mucosa responding to adalimumab.

Etanercept for the management of oral lichen planus. Yarom N. Am J Clin Dermatol 2007; 8: 121.

Levamisole monotherapy for oral lichen planus. Won TH, Park SY, Kim BS, Seo PS, Park SD. Ann Dermatol 2009; 21: 250–4.

In 11 patients taking levamisole 50 mg three times daily for three consecutive days per week, after 3 months, 5 patients reported complete improvement.

Although systemic agents offer significantly better results than topicals, none produces long-term remission when discontinued. Clinical benefits are achieved and maintained with long-term administration, and topicals should be administered concomitantly.

Third-Line Therapies	
• Topical and systemic retinoids	B
• Systemic ciclosporin	D
• Thalidomide	E
• Curcuminoids	C
• Lycopene	C
• Aloe vera gel	B
• Lasers, UV phototherapy, photodynamic therapy	B

Topical tretinoin therapy and oral lichen planus. Sloberg K, Hersle K, Mobacken H, Thilander H. Arch Dermatol 1979; 115: 716–8.

More than 70% of the 23 patients treated with 0.1% tretinoin improved.

Topical retinoids in oral lichen planus treatment: an overview. Petruzzi M, Lucchese A, Lajolo C, Campus G, Lauritano D, Serpico R. Dermatology 2013; 226: 61–7.

As a monotherapy, topical retinoids have limited value and should be used in combination with topical corticosteroids.

Treatment of lichen planus with acitretin: a double-blind, placebo-controlled study in 65 patients. Laurberg G, Geiger JM, Hjorth N, Holm P, Hou-Jensen K, Jacobsen KU, et al. J Am Acad Dermatol 1991; 24: 434–7.

In this 2-month study with 65 patients, some with OLP, acitretin (30 mg/day) resulted in remission or marked improvement in most cases. The majority of patients experienced adverse effects.

Efficacy and safety of oral alitretinoin in severe oral lichen planus – results of a prospective pilot study. Kunz M, Urosevic-Maiwald M, Goldinger SM, Frauchiger AL, Dreier J, Belloni B, et al. JEADV 2016; 30: 293–8.

In this study 30 mg oral alitretinoin for 24 weeks in 10 refractory patients resulted in improvement in 40% of patients.

Severe lichen planus clears with very low-dose cyclosporine. Levell NJ, Munro CS, Marks JM. Br J Dermatol 1992; 127: 66–7.

In this study ciclosporin 1 to 2.5 mg/kg/day was used in four patients with extensive disease until skin and oral disease clearance. Relapses could be then controlled with topical therapies on oral ciclosporin discontinuation.

Effective treatment of oral erosive lichen planus with thalidomide. Camisa C, Popovsky JL. Arch Dermatol 2000; 136: 1442–3.

A single report resolving with thalidomide (50–100 mg/d).

High-dose curcuminoids are efficacious in the reduction in symptoms and signs of oral lichen planus. Chainani-Wu N, Madden E, Lozada-Nur F, Silverman S, Jr. J Am Acad Dermatol 2012; 66: 752–60.

In 20 patients in this double-blind placebo study, curcuminoids (6000 mg/d) produced modest benefits.

Lycopene in the management of oral lichen planus: a placebo-controlled study. Saawarn N, Shashikanth MC, Saawarn S, Jirge V, Chaitanya NC, Pinakapani R. Indian J Dent Res 2011; 22: 639–43.

In 15 patients taking lycopene (8 mg/day) for 6 weeks 73% showed 70% to 100% benefit.

Efficacy of topical aloe vera in patients with oral lichen planus: a randomized double-blind study. Salazar-Sanchez N, Lopez-Jornet P, Camacho-Alonso F, Sanchez-Siles M. J Oral Pathol Med 2010; 39: 735–40.

In 32 patients taking a 70% concentration of aloe vera three times a day for 12 weeks most improved modestly.

A comparative pilot study of low intensity laser versus topical corticosteroids in the treatment of erosive-atrophic oral lichen planus. Jajarm HH, Falaki F, Mahdavi O. Photomed Laser Surg 2011; 29: 421–5.

A 630-nm diode laser versus dexamethasone wash was studied in 30 patients; both therapies were effective with equal response rates.

Phototherapy approaches in treatment of oral lichen planus. Pavlic V, Vujic-Aleksic V. Photodermatol Photoimmunol Photomed 2014; 30: 15–24.

This review showed no solid evidence for the effectiveness of UV phototherapy, lasers, or photodynamic therapy for OLP.

Evidence Levels: A Double-blind study B Clinical trial ≥ 20 subjects C Clinical trial < 20 subjects D Series ≥ 5 subjects E Anecdotal case reports

Orf

Jane C. Sterling

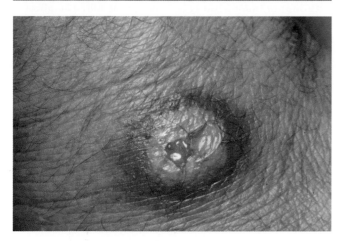

Orf (ecthyma contagiosum) is due to a parapoxvirus infection and is seen as an inflammatory papule that rapidly evolves to a necrotic blister. Orf usually presents as a single lesion, most commonly on the hands or occasionally the face, but lesions can be multiple or very large in immunosuppressed individuals. The infection is predominantly an occupational disease affecting livestock owners and veterinary workers because the orf virus is carried by sheep and occasionally goats or deer. It has also been reported as a result of animal contact with home husbandry or in association with religious observances, and there are rare cases of human-to-human transmission.

MANAGEMENT STRATEGY

Orf is a self-limiting infection, and *treatment is usually not necessary.* The immune response to the virus usually results in resolution of the disease within 2 to 7 weeks without any specific treatment. There is no available treatment that is specifically antiviral for the orf virus, and no human vaccine has been produced. Treatment is usually only indicated if there is secondary bacterial infection or immunosuppression. Erythema multiforme can be triggered by orf infection.

Preventive measures include vaccination of sheep before the lambing period to boost immune response and the wearing of gloves, if possible, when handling animals with any sign of the disease.

Various treatments have been reported anecdotally. *Idoxuridine, surgery,* and *cryotherapy* have been suggested to reduce the time to healing. For immunosuppressed individuals, infection with orf may result in a more persistent or progressive infection or giant orf. In such cases, interventional treatment is warranted, and often treatments can be combined. Surgery may be performed to remove the bulk of the infected tissue. Idoxuridine, cryotherapy, *cidofovir, interferon,* and topical *imiquimod* cream have been reported to show benefit.

Specific Investigations

- Electron microscopy of scrapings from lesion
- Biopsy
- Polymerase chain reaction (PCR)

Diagnosis is usually clinical but can be confirmed by the noted investigations if required. Electron microscopy is the diagnostic method used in the UK, whereas the Centers for Disease Control and Prevention (CDC) has adopted PCR.

The structure of the orf virus. Nagington J, Newton A, Horne RW. Virology 1964; 23: 4611–72.

The ultrastructural description of the orf virus.

Orf. Report of 19 human cases with clinical and pathological observations. Leavell UW, McNamara MJ, Muelling R, Talbert WM, Rucker RC, Dalton AJ. JAMA 1968; 204: 657–64.

Detailed description of clinical and histologic features of 19 cases of orf infection. Defines six stages of infection. Over half the lesions healed within 5 weeks.

Polymerase chain reaction for laboratory diagnosis of orf virus infections. Torfason EG, Gunadottir S. J Clin Virol 2002; 24: 79–84.

Method for molecular diagnosis of orf initially used as research tool but now used in the United States.

Ecthyma contagiosum (orf) – report of a human case from the United Arab Emirates and review of the literature. Al-Salam S, Nowotny N, Sohail MR, Kolodziejek J, Berger TG. J Cutan Pathol 2008; 35: 603–7.

More detailed method for molecular diagnosis of orf used in a clinical case.

First-Line Therapy

- No specific treatment usually necessary

Orf. Report of 19 human cases with clinical and pathological observations. Leavell UW, McNamara MJ, Muelling R, Talbert WM, Rucker RC, Dalton AJ. JAMA 1968; 204: 657–64.

Lymphangitis and lymphadenopathy occurred in 3 of 19 cases. *Awareness of the risk of secondary bacterial infection is important.*

Second-Line Therapies

• Surgery	D
• Cryotherapy	D
• Idoxuridine	E
• Cidofovir	E
• Interferon	E
• Imiquimod	D

Giant orf with prolonged recovery in a patient with psoriatic arthritis treated with etanercept. Rørdam OM, Grimstad Ø, Spigset O, Ryggen K. Acta Derm Venereol 2013; 93: 487–8.

During long-term treatment with etanercept, a sheep farmer developed giant orf. He was treated successfully with debulking surgery followed by repeated cryotherapy and imiquimod for a total of 17 weeks.

Orf infection: a clinical study at the Royal Medical Services Hospitals. Tawara MJ, Obaidat NA. J Roy Med Serv 2010; 17: 41–6.

A review of 64 cases observed and treated over 5 years in Jordan. Eleven were treated with cryotherapy and 13 with antibiotics. Most were treated symptomatically only.

A case of ecthyma contagiosum (human orf) treated with idoxuridine. Hunskaar S. Dermatologica 1984; 168: 207.

The orf lesion of a healthy female was treated with 40% idoxuridine in dimethyl sulfoxide three times daily for 6 days. The lesion healed in less than 4 weeks.

Parapoxvirus orf in kidney transplantation. Peeters P, Sennesael J. Nephrol Dial Transplant 1998; 13: 531.

A large lesion on the thumb recurred after excisional surgery. After 40% idoxuridine topically, further surgery, and repeated cryotherapy, the lesion resolved.

Giant orf in a patient with chronic lymphocytic leukaemia. Hunskaar S. Br J Dermatol 1986; 114: 631–4.

A large palmar orf lesion was excised and small local recurrences treated with 40% idoxuridine.

A case of human orf in an immunocompromised patient treated successfully with cidofovir cream. Geerinck K, Lukito G, Snoeck R, DeVos R, DeClercq E, Vanrenterghem Y, et al. J Med Virol 2001; 64: 543–9.

An immunosuppressed renal transplant patient developed a persistent giant orf lesion. Treatment with 1% cidofovir cream daily for five cycles of 5 days of treatment alternating with 5 rest days plus debridement as necessary led to full resolution of the lesion.

Recurrent orf in an immunocompromised host. Tan ST, Blake GB, Chambers S. Br J Plast Surg 1991; 44: 465–7.

A tumorlike orf lesion in an immunosuppressed patient was unresponsive to surgery and idoxuridine. Temporary improvement occurred after 2 weeks of daily intralesional interferon of 1 million IU per injection with clearance after repeat surgery with subcutaneous interferon (1 million IU daily).

Rapid improvement of human orf (ecthyma contagiosum) with topical imiquimod cream; report of four complicated cases. Erbağci Z, Erbağci I, Almila Tuncel A. J Dermatolog Treat 2005; 16: 353–6.

Treatment with imiquimod 5% applied twice daily for up to 10 days to orf lesions complicated by erythema multiforme, angioedema, or as giant orf possibly hastened clearance of the orf lesion and the secondary effects.

Progressive orf virus infection in a patient with lymphoma: successful treatment using imiquimod. Lederman ER, Green GM, DeGroot HE, Dahl P, Goldman E, Greer PW, et al. Clin Infect Dis 2007; 44: e100–3.

Giant and multifocal orf in a patient with non-Hodgkin lymphoma did not respond to debulking and topical cidofovir. Imiquimod 5% cream applied on alternate days led to improvement after a week and clearance within 2 months.

Evidence Levels: **A** Double-blind study **B** Clinical trial ≥ 20 subjects **C** Clinical trial < 20 subjects **D** Series ≥ 5 subjects **E** Anecdotal case reports

Palmoplantar keratoderma

Ravi Ratnavel

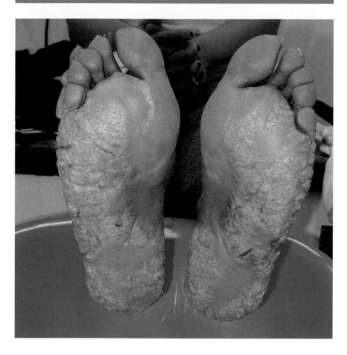

Palmoplantar keratodermas (PPKs) consist of a heterogeneous group of disorders characterized by thickening of the palms and soles. The condition may be subdivided into primary hereditary keratodermas, acquired forms, and conditions in which PPK is an associated secondary feature of a specific dermatosis.

MANAGEMENT STRATEGY

PPK may be localized to the hands and feet or develop as part of a more generalized skin disorder. It is important when making a diagnosis to establish its morphology and the presence of any associated ectodermal disease at sites other than the palms and soles. Biopsy may be necessary to distinguish between some hereditary forms of PPK. PPK can be associated with infections (dermatophytes, human papillomavirus, HIV, syphilis, and scabies), drugs (arsenic exposure), and internal malignancy (paraneoplastic phenomenon) or may be a cutaneous manifestation of systemic disease (myxedema, diabetes mellitus). Hyperkeratosis of the palms and soles can also be a feature of eczema, psoriasis, and cutaneous T-cell lymphoma.

Treatment of PPK is challenging. Most therapeutic options produce only short-term improvement and are frequently complicated by unwanted adverse effects. Treatment options range from simple measures such as *saltwater soaks* with physical paring of the skin and use of *topical keratolytics*, through to *systemic retinoids* and *reconstructive surgery* with total excision of the hyperkeratotic skin followed by grafting.

In patients with limited disease, *topical keratolytics* containing salicylic acid, lactic acid, or urea in a suitable emollient base may

be tried. Examples include 5% to 10% salicylic acid, 20% to 70% propylene glycol, or 10% lactic acid in aqueous cream or a combination therapy using 10% urea and 5% lactic acid in aqueous cream to be applied twice daily. These formulations can be made up on an individual basis or the closest proprietary product prescribed. The efficacy of these agents may be increased by occlusion at night. *Topical retinoids* such as tretinoin (0.01% gel and 0.1% cream) may also be tried; treatment is, however, often limited by skin irritation. *Potent topical corticosteroids*, such as clobetasol propionate 0.05%, with or without keratolytics, are occasionally of value in the management of inflammatory PPK. *5-Fluorouracil 5%* has produced dramatic results in spiny keratoderma, but its use in other keratodermas has not been evaluated.

The efficacy of the *oral retinoids* in keratoderma is well established. Good responses have been seen in mal de Meleda, Papillon–Lefèvre syndrome, and erythrokeratoderma variabilis. In some types of PPKs, particularly epidermolytic forms, hyperesthesia may limit the usefulness or practicality of treatment with retinoids. The potential risk of bone toxicity should also be assessed in patients on long-term therapy, although the risks are small. Periodic radiologic bone monitoring and, when possible, prescription of pulsed (intermittent) therapy are recommended. The optimal dosage of oral acitretin is 25 to 35 mg daily in adults or 0.6 mg/kg daily in children, which may be adjusted after 4 weeks of therapy. Oral isotretinoin 0.5 mg/kg is a less effective option. Oral alitretinoin 30 mg/day is a further option.

Psoralen plus UVA (PUVA) therapy or *re-PUVA* (a synergistic combination of oral retinoids and PUVA) may be effective in PPK secondary to psoriasis or eczema. In oculocutaneous tyrosinemia (an autosomal recessive condition characterized by focal palmoplantar keratosis, corneal ulceration, and mental retardation), *dietary restriction of phenylalanine and tyrosine* has led to resolution of PPK. *Oral administration of 1α,25-dihydroxyvitamin D_3* and *topical calcipotriol* ointment has been reported to be effective. Regular podiatry, careful selection of footwear, and treatment of secondary fungal infections are integral parts of management of all PPK. Regular intermittent use of terbinafine cream and other topical antifungals can reduce skin maceration and improve comfort. *Surgical or laser dermabrasion* is an option for some patients, with potential amelioration of symptoms and improved penetration of topical agents.

For severe refractory PPK *excision and skin grafting* may be considered. Excision should remove hyperkeratotic skin, including dermis, epidermis, and subcutis, to prevent any risk of recurrence.

Specific Investigations

- Scrapings for mycology
- Thyroid function tests

An epidemiologic investigation of dermatologic fungus infections in the northernmost county of Sweden (Norbotten) 1977–81. Gamborg Nielson P. Mykosen 1984; 27: 203–10.

In a 5-year survey of dermatophyte infections in Norbotten, Sweden, the frequency of dermatophytosis among patients with hereditary PPK was shown to be 35%, corresponding to a prevalence of 36.7%. The predominant feature of dermatophytosis in patients with hereditary PPK was scaling and fissuring. Treatment improved the clinical signs after 2 to 3 months.

Hereditary palmoplantar keratoderma and dermatophytosis in the northernmost county of Sweden (Norbotten).

Gamborg Nielson P. Acta Derm Venereol Suppl (Stockh) 1994; 188: 1–60.

In relatives of the original case, dermatophytosis was found in 65% of men, 22% of women, and 21% of children, resulting in a total frequency of 36.2%. Statistically, it was proved that *Trichophyton mentagrophytes* occurred more often in patients with hereditary PPK. Vesicular eruptions along the hyperkeratotic border occurred significantly more often in patients with dermatophytosis and were considered pathognomonic of secondary dermatophytosis.

Palmoplantar keratoderma in association with myxoedema. Hodak E, David M, Feuerman EJ. Acta Derm Venereol 1986; 66: 354–5.

A patient with myxedema and intractable PPK showed improvement after treatment with thyroid replacement therapy. The possibility of a causal relationship between hypothyroidism and PPK was questioned.

Severe palmar keratoderma with myxoedema. Tan OT, Sarkany I. Clin Exp Derm 1977; 2: 287–8.

A patient with myxedema and PPK showed rapid improvement in PPK after thyroxine treatment.

First-Line Therapies	
• Topical keratolytics	B
• Topical retinoids	B

Alleviation of the plantar discomfort caused by pachyonychia congenita with topical applications of aluminum chloride and salicylic acid ointments. Takayama M, Okuyama R, Sasaki Y, Ohura T, Tagami H, Aiba S. Dermatology 2005; 211: 302.

Aluminum chloride solution 10% once daily was used to reduce plantar sweating, which may exacerbate blistering and hyperkeratosis in this condition.

Vitamin A acid in the treatment of palmoplantar keratoderma. Gunther SH. Arch Dermatol 1972; 106: 854–7.

Nine patients with PPK were treated with once-daily retinoic acid 0.1% in petroleum jelly, and all improved within 4 months. Permanent remission ensued in two patients. Recurrence was observed in the majority of cases 8 weeks after the withdrawal of treatment. This was avoided by the topical application of vitamin A acid once or twice weekly.

Topical treatment of keratosis palmaris et plantaris with tretinoin. Touraine R, Revuz J. Acta Derm Venereol Suppl (Stockh) 1975; 74: 152–3.

Six patients were treated for 2 months with either tretinoin 0.1% lotion or 0.05% cream once daily. Improvement was seen in most patients. Better results were achieved with the use of occlusive dressings, mechanical paring before topical application, and when a higher concentration of topical tretinoin was used (0.3%).

Second-Line Therapy	
• Systemic retinoids	A

The treatment of keratosis palmaris et plantaris with isotretinoin. A multicenter study. Bergfeld WF, Derbes VJ, Elias PM, Frost P, Greer KE, Shupack JL. J Am Acad Dermatol 1982; 6: 727–31.

Five of six patients with PPK were safely and effectively treated with isotretinoin, with dramatic clearing of the keratoderma within the first 4 weeks of therapy. The mean dose was 1.95 mg/kg daily, and mean duration of therapy was 113 days.

Acitretin in the treatment of severe disorders of keratinisation. Results of an open study. Blanchet-Bardon C, Nazzaro VV, Rognin C, Geiger JM, Puissant A. J Am Acad Dermatol 1991; 24: 982–6.

An open noncomparative study to evaluate the clinical response to acitretin in patients with nonpsoriatic disorders of keratinization and to establish the optimal dosage for efficacy and tolerance. Thirty-three patients with ichthyoses, PPK, or Darier disease were treated for 4 months. Most showed a marked improvement. The optimal acitretin dosage providing the best efficacy with minimal side effects varied from patient to patient. The mean daily dose ($\pm$SD) was 27 $\pm$ 11 mg in adults and 0.7 $\pm$ 0.2 mg/kg in children.

A controlled study of comparative efficacy of oral retinoids and topical betamethasone/salicylic acid for chronic hyperkeratotic palmoplantar dermatitis. Capella GL, Fracchiolla C, Frigerio E, Altomare G. J Dermatolog Treat 2004; 15: 88–93.

A single-blind, matched-sample investigation was carried out in 42 patients with chronic hyperkeratotic palmoplantar dermatitis, who were administered acitretin 25 to 50 mg daily for 1 month controlled versus a conventional topical treatment (betamethasone/salicylic acid ointment). Acitretin was significantly better than the conventional treatment after 30 days (two-sided, p < 0.0001). The authors suggested that acitretin should be considered a first-choice treatment.

Acitretin in the treatment of mal de Meleda. Van de Kerkhof PC, Dooren-Greebe RJ, Steijlen PM. Br J Dermatol 1992; 127: 191–2.

Two patients with mal de Meleda treated with acitretin experienced a marked reduction of PPK. The optimal dosage was found to be 10 to 30 mg daily. Higher dosages resulted in hyperesthesia. Discontinuation of acitretin resulted in relapse within days.

Alitretinoin: a new treatment option for hereditary punctate palmoplantar keratoderma. Raone B, Raboni R, Patrizi P. J Am Acad Dermatol 2014; 71: e48–9.

A single patient case report demonstrating improvement of punctate keratoderma with alitretinoin 30 mg daily for 8 months.

Third-Line Therapies	
• Reconstructive surgery with total excision of hyperkeratotic skin followed by grafting	C
• Topical calcipotriol	E
• Oral vitamin D_3 analogs	E
• Topical corticosteroids with or without keratolytics	E
• PUVA or re-PUVA	D
• Dermabrasion	E
• CO_2 laser	B
• 5-Fluorouracil	E
• Tyrosine-restricted diet in oculocutaneous keratoderma	E

Evidence Levels: **A** Double-blind study **B** Clinical trial ≥ 20 subjects **C** Clinical trial < 20 subjects **D** Series ≥ 5 subjects **E** Anecdotal case reports

Plastic surgery in the management of palmoplantar kerato-derma (palmoplantar neoplasty). Farina R. Aesthet Plast Surg 1987; 11: 249–53.

Five cases of PPK were treated successfully by grafting skin taken from the calves and thighs.

Palmoplantar keratoderma and skin grafting: postsurgical long-term follow-up of two cases with Olmsted syndrome. Bédard MS, Powell J, Laberge L, Allard-Dansereau C, Bortoluzzi P, Marcoux D. Pediatr Dermatol 2008; 25: 223–9.

A 6- and 10-year follow-up of successful surgical correction of mutilating keratoderma.

Surgical correction of pseudoainhum in Vohwinkel syndrome. Pisoh T, Bhatia A, Oberlin C. J Hand Surg [Br] 1995; 20: 338–41.

Successful surgical correction of constricting rings in a patient with Vohwinkel syndrome.

Surgical correction of hyperkeratosis in the Papillon–Lefèvre syndrome. Peled IJ, Weinrauch L, Cohen HA, Wexler MK. J Dermatol Surg Oncol 1981; 7: 142–3.

A patient with Papillon–Lefèvre syndrome underwent successful surgical correction of hyperkeratosis of the palms.

Topical calcipotriol in the treatment of epidermolytic pal-moplantar keratoderma of Vorner. Lucker GP, Van de Kerkhof PC, Steijlen PM. Br J Dermatol 1994; 130: 543–5.

A patient with hereditary epidermolytic PPK of Vorner was successfully treated with topical calcipotriol.

Efficacy, tolerability, and safety of calcipotriol ointment in disorders of keratinisation. Results of a randomized, dou-ble blind vehicle-controlled, right/left comparative study. Kragballe K, Steijlen PM, Ibsen HH, van de Kerkhof PC, Esmann J, Sorensen LH, et al. Arch Dermatol 1995; 131: 556–60.

Twenty patients with PPK showed no therapeutic benefit with topical calcipotriol.

Improvement of palmoplantar keratoderma of nonheredi-tary type (eczema tyloticum) after oral administration of 1 alpha 25-dihydroxyvitamin D3. Katayama H, Yamane Y. Arch Dermatol 1989; 125: 1713.

A patient with acquired PPK was successfully treated with oral 1α,25-dihydroxyvitamin D, 0.5 µg daily for 3 months, with no side effects.

Oral psoralen photochemotherapy (PUVA) of hyperkera-totic dermatitis of the palms. Mobacken H, Rosen K, Swanbeck G. Br J Dermatol 1983; 109: 205–8.

PUVA was found to be effective in five patients with chronic hyperkeratotic dermatitis of the palms.

Dermabrasion of the hyperkeratotic foot. Daoud MS, Randle HW, Yarborough JM. Dermatol Surg 1995; 21: 243–4.

A patient with acquired PPK treated with dermabrasion and then 2% crude coal tar and 5% salicylic acid in petrolatum showed no evidence of recurrence after 6 months. The indications for dermabrasion include dry, fissured hyperkeratotic heels; psoriatic keratoderma before PUVA therapy; punctate keratoderma; and generalized keratoderma.

Methods and effectiveness of surgical treatment of lim-ited hyperkeratosis with CO_2 laser. Babaev OG, Bashilov VP, Zakharov AK. Khirurgiia (Mosk) 1993; 4: 74–9.

Five hundred two patients with limited hyperkeratosis were treated, with a favorable clinical effect. Recurrences were noted in only 4% of cases

Dietary management of oculocutaneous tyrosinemia in an 11-year-old child. Ney D, Bay C, Scheider JA, Kelts D, Nyhan WL. Am J Dis Child 1983; 137: 995–1000.

An 11-year-old girl with oculocutaneous tyrosinemia with plantar keratosis and keratitis demonstrated resolution of her keratitis and improvement of her plantar keratosis with dietary restriction of phenylalanine and tyrosine to less than 100 mg/kg.

Palmoplantar pustulosis

Sonja Molin, Thomas Ruzicka

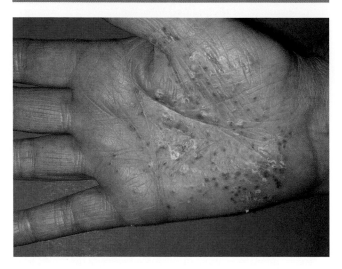

Palmoplantar pustulosis (PPP) is a skin disease characterized by chronic and relapsing pustular eruptions of palms and soles. Because its clinical and genetic characteristics differ from psoriasis vulgaris, PPP probably must be considered a separate entity.

MANAGEMENT STRATEGY

PPP is a common disease that is often refractory to treatment and shows a high recurrence rate. Unlike psoriasis, there are no reported associations with candidate genes within the PSORS1 locus, interleukin-36 receptor antagonist mutations, or tumor necrosis factor (TNF)-α promoter polymorphisms. Female predominance and high prevalence in smokers are characteristic. *Cessation of smoking* is essential for the treatment course of PPP. Consideration of comorbidities such as streptococcal or *Helicobacter pylori* infection, diabetes mellitus, thyroid disease, celiac disease, or osteoarthropathy is necessary. *Tonsillectomy* can be helpful if a streptococcal focus is found. A *gluten-free diet* is recommended if gluten intolerance is proved. At the beginning of therapy and in patients with milder symptoms of PPP, potent *topical corticosteroids* are the treatment of choice and are even more effective when used *under occlusion*. *Psoralen and ultraviolet A light (PUVA)* therapy is also effective. In more severe or recalcitrant courses of disease, systemic medication should be considered. The retinoid *acitretin* (starting dose 0.3–0.5 mg/kg body weight) is of proven value, but its practical use in women is limited due to teratogenicity. There is evidence that the combination of PUVA with systemic retinoids is superior to the individual treatments. Low-dose *ciclosporin* (1–4 mg/kg daily) and *methotrexate* (10–25 mg once weekly) can cause improvement of PPP but requires careful clinical and laboratory monitoring. *Fumaric acid esters* have also been reported to be effective.

A multitude of other therapeutic proposals for the treatment of PPP decorate the literature. A new approach might be the vitamin D analog *maxacalcitol* for topical treatment. First studies show benefit compared with placebo.

Reports on *TNF-α antagonist* therapy in PPP show conflicting results, with many reports highlighting even induction or

aggravation of the disease. Non-TNF-α–inhibiting biologic agents such as *ustekinumab* or *secukinumab*, as well as the new oral phosphodiesterase-4 inhibitor *apremilast*, might be promising new therapeutic options, especially in recalcitrant cases. Controlled clinical trials are needed to substantiate the evidence.

Specific Investigations

- Screen for infection with streptococci or *H. pylori*
- Gluten intolerance
- Thyroid disease
- Diabetes mellitus
- Osteoarthropathy
- Exclude SAPHO (synovitis, acne, pustulosis, hyperostosis, and osteitis)

Management of palmoplantar pustulosis: do we need to change? Mrowietz U, van de Kerkhof PC. Br J Dermatol 2011; 164: 942–6.

Overview on PPP, also discussing current data on tonsillectomy and a probable "tonsil-palmoplantar-skin axis."

Palmoplantar pustulosis associated with gastric *Helicobacter pylori* infection. Sáez-Rodríguez M, Noda-Cabrera A, García-Bustínduy M, Guimerá-Martín-Neda F, Dorta-Alom S, Escoda-García M, et al. Clin Exp Dermatol 2002; 27: 720.

Clearing of PPP in a patient with gastric *H. pylori* infection after eradication treatment with amoxicillin and clarithromycin in combination with omeprazole. No relapse of PPP during a 4-year follow-up.

Thyroid disease in pustulosis palmoplantaris. Agner T, Sindrup JH, Høier-Madsen M, Hegedüs L. Br J Dermatol 1989; 121: 487–91.

In 53% of 32 patients with PPP thyroid disease was detected compared with 16% in the control group.

Osteoarticular manifestations of pustulosis palmaris et plantaris and of psoriasis: two distinct entities. Mejjad O, Daragon A, Louvel JP, Da Silva LF, Thomine E, Lauret P, et al. Ann Rheum Dis 1996; 55: 177–80.

Comparison of 23 patients with PPP and 23 patients with psoriatic arthritis (PsoA). Clinical findings showed involvement of the anterior chest wall (e.g., sternoclavicular joints) in 19 out of 23 patients with PPP compared with 10 out of 23 with PsoA. Radiologic signs of arthropathy were demonstrated in 11 PPP patients and four PsoA patients.

SAPHO syndrome: a long-term follow-up study of 120 cases. Hayem G, Bouchaud-Chabot A, Benali K, Roux S, Palazzo E, Silbermann-Hoffman O, et al. Semin Arthritis Rheum 1999; 29: 159–71.

Significant association of PPP with axial osteitis in 120 reported cases with SAPHO syndrome.

Women with palmoplantar pustulosis have disturbed calcium homeostasis and a high prevalence of diabetes mellitus and psychiatric disorders: a case-control study. Hagforsen E, Michaëlsson K, Lundgren E, Olofsson H, Petersson A, Lagumdzija A, et al. Acta Derm Venereol 2005; 85: 225–32.

Disturbed calcium homeostasis was found frequently in 60 PPP patients compared with control group. Association with diabetes mellitus, psychiatric disorders, and gluten intolerance was also reported.

Evidence Levels: **A** Double-blind study **B** Clinical trial ≥ 20 subjects **C** Clinical trial < 20 subjects **D** Series ≥ 5 subjects **E** Anecdotal case reports

Palmoplantar pustulosis and gluten sensitivity: a study of serum antibodies against gliadin and tissue transglutaminase, the duodenal mucosa and effects of gluten-free diet. Michaëlsson G, Kristjánsson G, Pihl Lundin I, Hagforsen E. Br J Dermatol 2007; 156: 659–66.

Laboratory investigation of 123 patients with PPP showed IgA antibodies against gliadin in 18% and antibodies against tissue transglutaminase in 10% of cases. Celiac disease was found in 6% of patients. Gluten-free diet resulted in (nearly) total clearance of skin symptoms and decrease of antibody level.

First-Line Therapies

• Oral retinoids	A
• PUVA	B
• Topical corticosteroids	C

Interventions for chronic palmoplantar pustulosis. Marsland AM, Chalmers RJ, Hollis S, Leonardi-Bee J, Griffiths CE. Cochrane Database Syst Rev 2006; 1: CD001433.

An extensive review of literature concerning PPP treatment showed proven evidence of PUVA and systemic retinoids alone or in combination; effectiveness of topical corticosteroids under occlusion; and probable benefit of low-dose ciclosporin, tetracycline antibiotics, and Grenz ray therapy.

A detailed survey of evidence-based PPP treatment options, including the classical publications regarding PUVA and systemic retinoids.

A hydrocolloid occlusive dressing plus triamcinolone acetonide cream is superior to clobetasol cream in palmo-plantar pustulosis. Kragballe K, Larsen FG. Acta Derm Venereol 1991; 71: 540–2.

Complete clearance of PPP with use of medium-strength topical corticosteroid under hydrocolloid occlusion in 13 out of 19 patients in a left–right comparison with a highly potent topical corticosteroid alone (complete remission only in 3 out of 19 patients).

Second-Line Therapies

• Ciclosporin	A
• Methotrexate	B
• Fumaric acid esters	C
• Excimer light therapy (308 nm)	C

Double-blind placebo-controlled study of long-term low-dose ciclosporin in the treatment of palmoplantar pustulosis. Erkko P, Granlund H, Remitz A, Rosen K, Mobacken H, Lindelöf B, et al. Br J Dermatol 1998; 139: 997–1004.

Fifty-eight PPP patients treated with ciclosporin in a daily dose of 1 to 4 mg/kg body weight for 12 months. Low-dose treatment showed improvement in 13 of 27 patients compared with 6 of 31 in the placebo group. Benefit of long-term use only supposed.

Pustulosis palmaris et plantaris treated with methotrexate. Thomsen K. Acta Derm Venereol 1971; 51: 397–400.

Satisfactory response in 8 out of 25 patients receiving weekly oral doses of 25 mg methotrexate for 2 months.

Efficacy of fumaric acid ester monotherapy in psoriasis pustulosa palmoplantaris. Ständer H, Stadelmann A, Luger T, Traupe H. Br J Dermatol 2003; 149: 220–2.

Marked reduction of PPP Area and Severity Index (PPPASI) in 13 patients with PPP treated with fumaric acid esters for a period of 24 weeks.

Efficacy of excimer light therapy (308 nm) for palmoplantar pustulosis with the induction of circulating regulatory T cells. Furuhashi T, Torii K, Kato H, Nishida E, Saito C, Morita A. Exp Dermatol 2011; 20: 768–70.

Significant improvement of PPPASI score after 20 to 30 treatments with excimer light therapy in 17 patients.

Third-Line Therapies

• Liarozole	A
• Ustekinumab	B
• Apremilast	A
• Maxacalcitol	A

Dermatologic adverse reactions during anti-TNF treatments: focus on inflammatory bowel disease. Mocci G, Marzo M, Papa A, Armuzzi A, Guidi L. J Crohns Colitis 2013; 7: 769–79.

Review about the potential skin side effects of anti-TNF blockade, including psoriasiform lesions and PPP.

Benefit of TNF-α antagonist use in PPP is conflicting, with therapeutic efficacy, PPP initiation, or aggravation occurring.

Efficacy of ustekinumab in refractory palmoplantar pustular psoriasis. Morales-Múnera C, Vilarrasa E, Puig L. Br J Dermatol 2013; 168: 820–4.

Five PPP patients treated with ustekinumab responded.

Investigator-initiated, open-label trial of ustekinumab for the treatment of moderate-to-severe palmoplantar psoriasis. Au SC, Goldminz AM, Kim N, Dumont N, Michelon M, Volf E, et al. J Dermatolog Treat 2013; 24: 179–87.

Apremilast, an oral phosphodiesterase-4 inhibitor, in the treatment of palmoplantar psoriasis: results of a pooled analysis from phase II PSOR-005 and phase III Efficacy and Safety Trial Evaluating the Effects of Apremilast in Psoriasis (ESTEEM) clinical trials in patients with moderate to severe psoriasis. Bissonnette R, Pariser DM, Wasel NR, Goncalves J, Day RM, Chen R, et al. J Am Acad Dermatol 2016; 75: 99–105.

Compared with placebo, a significant improvement was achieved in patients with moderate to severe PPP during treatment with apremilast. However, the study did not evaluate the presence of pustules/palmoplantar pustular lesions separately.

Phase III clinical study of maxacalcitol ointment in patients with palmoplantar pustulosis: a randomized, double-blind, placebo-controlled trial. Umezawa Y, Nakagawa H, Tamaki K. J Dermatol 2016; 43: 288–93.

Significant improvement in PPP patients treated topically with the vitamin D analog 22-oxacalcitriol twice daily for 8 weeks compared with placebo.

178

Panniculitis

Carrie Ann R. Cusack, Christine M. Shaver

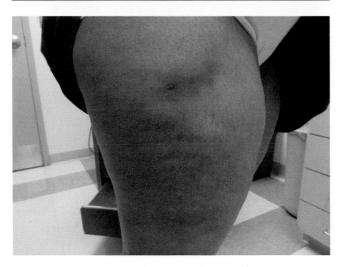

Panniculitis is a term used to describe the different inflammatory diseases of the subcutaneous fat. The subcutaneous fat is derived embryologically from mesenchymal cells, which differentiate into adipocytes, or fat cells. A collection of adipocytes is termed a *microlobule,* and groups of microlobules make up the individual lobules in the subcutaneous fat layer of the skin. Lobules are separated from each other by fibrous septae, and within these septae are the main arteries and veins that nourish fatty tissue. Knowledge of the basic subcutaneous architecture allows for classification of the different types of panniculitides, which relies on distinguishing whether inflammation is predominantly located in the lobules or in the fibrous septae. Based on this classification, we can better separate the individual disease processes.

The characteristic septal panniculitis is erythema nodosum, which is also the most common panniculitis. The majority of other panniculitides are predominantly lobular. However, some other rarer panniculitides have predominantly septal inflammation, such as subacute nodular migratory panniculitis, panniculitis of morphea/scleroderma, and α1-antitrypsin deficiency panniculitis. Within the lobular panniculitides, a further division can be made based on the presence of vasculitis.

The main lobular panniculitis with vasculitis is erythema induratum, or more aptly termed, *nodular vasculitis.* Rarer vasculitic panniculitides occur in the setting of leprosy with erythema nodosum leprosum and Lucio phenomenon.

The remaining lobular panniculitides are not associated with vasculitis but can be associated with systemic disease. Subtypes include lupus panniculitis, pancreatic panniculitis, cytophagic histiocytic panniculitis, panniculitis of dermatomyositis, infectious panniculitis, sclerosing panniculitis/lipodermatosclerosis, oxalosis, and those with needle-shaped clefts (sclerema neonatorum and subcutaneous fat necrosis of the newborn).

Previously the term *Weber–Christian disease (WCD)* has been described, which encompassed lobular panniculitides without vasculitis that also displayed nonspecific systemic features. It was largely a diagnosis of exclusion that has since fallen out of favor, as most cases previously classified as WCD have been able to be reclassified into newer and more specific diseases. A report by White and Winkelmann reviewed 30 cases of WCD and found that in all cases, a more specific diagnosis could be found. Therefore this terminology will not be used in our classification schema.

MANAGEMENT STRATEGY

Many studies can be performed in evaluating panniculitides; however, none is more important than the skin biopsy. Therefore it is extremely important that the biopsy includes a substantial portion of the subcutaneous fat. A punch biopsy alone is not enough. Although a double punch biopsy technique is better, the best way to get a sample of subcutaneous tissue is either through an excisional biopsy that extends through the subcutis or a narrow incisional biopsy that includes a significant amount of fatty tissue. If an infectious cause of the panniculitis is suspected, a small piece of this biopsy should be sent for Gram staining as well as culture for bacteria, mycobacteria, and fungi. If a mycobacterial infection is in consideration, the specimen should be grown at 24°, 30°, 37°, and 42°C.

Lupus panniculitis, also known as *lupus profundus,* makes up a small portion of cutaneous lupus erythematosus, comprising only 2% to 3%. In many instances, it is the first cutaneous sign of lupus erythematosus. It is associated mainly with discoid lupus erythematosus (DLE), occurring in more than one third of cases of DLE. Lesions of DLE often are present in the skin overlying the lesions of lupus profundus (Image 1). Lupus panniculitis occurs in approximately 10% to 15% of patients with systemic lupus erythematosus (SLE), which tends to have a chronic course with few systemic manifestations, usually arthralgias. The distribution of these lesions can be helpful in making the diagnosis, as they are typically located on the face, trunk, and proximal extremities, in contrast to erythema nodosum. Laboratory studies should include ANA, dsDNA, ssDNA, SSA, SSB, complement levels, CBC, and a chemistry panel. On biopsy, it shows a predominantly lobular inflammation of T lymphocytes and macrophages. A biopsy for direct immunofluorescence (DIF) should be performed to confirm the diagnosis in cases where the histopathology is not specific. In many cases, linear deposition of C3 and IgM is present along the dermoepidermal junction in the overlying skin. First-line therapy for lupus profundus consists of systemic *antimalarial agents* as well as sunscreen. The addition of a second antimalarial agent has proven helpful in patients who are resistant to one agent. In addition, *systemic corticosteroids* can be used first line; however, they are usually effective only in the early phases of disease.

Nodular vasculitis includes both tuberculous and nontuberculous causes. The tuberculous form is referred to as *erythema induratum (of Bazin).* Nontuberculous etiologies include other infectious agents, such as *Nocardia* or hepatitis C virus, and medications such as propylthiouracil. The nontuberculous form has sometimes been referred to as *erythema induratum of Whitfield.* Clinically, lesions appear on the posterior legs of middle-aged women and present as painful, erythematous nodules. In making the diagnosis, mycobacterial culture as well as polymerase chain reaction (PCR) of mycobacterial DNA should be ordered. Purified protein derivative as well as a Quantiferon-TB Gold test can be helpful in making the diagnosis caused by tuberculosis. On biopsy, it is typically a lobular panniculitis with a mixed inflammation of lymphocytes and neutrophils. The key is identifying vasculitis, as the majority of cases show inflammation of either arteries or veins. Treatment includes *multidrug antituberculous* agents in cases caused by tuberculosis, and other antibiotics

Evidence Levels: **A** Double-blind study **B** Clinical trial ≥ 20 subjects **C** Clinical trial < 20 subjects **D** Series ≥ 5 subjects **E** Anecdotal case reports

in cases of other infectious etiologies. Other effective therapies *include potassium iodide, colchicine, and corticosteroids.*

Pancreatic panniculitis can occur in many different pancreatic disorders that cause tissue necrosis. This includes acute or chronic pancreatitis, pancreatic carcinoma (most often the acinar cell type), pancreas divisum, and pancreatic pseudocysts. It occurs in about 2% to 3% of all cases of pancreatic diseases. The presence of panniculitis may precede the detection of pancreatic disease and warrants an investigation for potential etiologies. It may be a harbinger of metastasis in cases of pancreatic carcinoma. Lesions consist of subcutaneous nodules that usually occur on the legs (around the ankles and knees predominantly) but can occur in any location. The nodules may or may not be painful, but the majority of lesions ulcerate, discharging an oily brown substance. Histopathology shows fat necrosis, and formation of "ghost cells" is classic. Amylase and, more specifically, lipase are elevated in pancreatic panniculitis and should be ordered. A CBC should be ordered as well, as eosinophilia may be present in 60% of cases. Magnetic resonance imaging (MRI) can identify a pancreatic *malignancy. Treatment involves addressing the underlying pancreatic inflammation.* Octreotide has also been helpful.

Cytophagic histiocytic panniculitis is defined based on the presence of hemophagocytosis on histopathology. There are characteristic "bean-bag cells," which are macrophages that engulf lymphocytes, neutrophils, and erythrocytes. The vast majority of cases are caused by a lymphoma. The main types are Epstein–Barr virus–associated extranodal NK/T-cell lymphoma and primary cutaneous gamma/delta T-cell lymphoma. Clinically, painful subcutaneous nodules are present. Patients may have a prolonged clinical course with fever, hepatosplenomegaly, and pancytopenia secondary to hemophagocytosis of the bone marrow. Many cases of cytophagic histiocytic panniculitis are now being classified on a spectrum with subcutaneous panniculitis–like T-cell lymphoma (SPTCL) as the two diseases share many clinical and histopathologic characteristics. Treatment of cytophagic histiocytic panniculitis consists *of treating any underlying malignancy,* possibly with a bone marrow transplant. In cases where lymphoma has not been identified, cyclosporine has been effective.

α1-Antitrypsin deficiency panniculitis occurs in patients with a severe deficiency of this enzyme, a protease inhibitor. Many different alleles of the gene encode this protein, with the most common being the M allele. The most common phenotype for the protease inhibitor (Pi) is PiMM. Patients with the S or Z allele may exhibit a mild deficiency in the enzyme. Patients with the phenotype PiZZ have the most severe enzyme deficiency, and it is typically these patients who manifest the panniculitis. Inflammation in the subcutaneous fat occurs because lipase, elastase, and other enzymes are not neutralized. These patients have painful, often purpuric nodules that ulcerate and drain. On pathology, there is usually focal necrosis of the fat lobules with a predominantly neutrophilic inflammation. An elastin stain may be helpful to show the reduced elastic tissue, and gene phenotyping can reveal an enzyme mutation. The most effective treatment is *enzyme replacement* through intravenous injections. Other treatments include *dapsone, colchicine, and liver transplantation.*

Panniculitis can also occur in infants. The two main types are sclerema neonatorum and subcutaneous fat necrosis of the newborn. They both are characterized histologically by needle-shaped clefts within lipocytes. In sclerema neonatorum, an extremely rare condition, the skin becomes hardened on the buttocks or thighs and then rapidly spreads in the first few days of life, causing immobility. Death typically occurs in a few days. Treatment for this condition is disappointing. It *involves supportive care, treating any underlying condition, and exchange transfusions.* The prognosis for subcutaneous fat necrosis of the newborn, on the other hand, is good. This disease involves full-term infants in contrast to premature newborns in sclerema neonatorum. Clinically, this condition consists of localized, indurated plaques involving the trunk that form during the first few weeks of life. Most lesions resolve spontaneously, and treatment is supportive. It may be complicated by hypercalcemia and therefore serial monitoring of calcium levels for at least 4 months after disease resolution is suggested, and treatment of resultant hypercalcemia may be required.

Lipodermatosclerosis, or sclerosing panniculitis, is a condition that usually develops in patients with chronic venous insufficiency. It is classically located on the medial lower legs in middle-aged women. It has been described as looking like an "inverted champagne bottle." Histologically there are ischemia and necrosis of the central fat lobule, leading to characteristic lipomembranous changes. Treatment involves *correcting the venous insufficiency* with compression stockings and leg elevation. *Stanozolol* has also been helpful.

Panniculitis can also occur in the setting of other connective tissue diseases such as dermatomyositis and morphea/scleroderma. In morphea, usually there is a septal panniculitis with a plasma lymphocytic cell infiltrate. Indurated plaques appear on the trunk and extremities. In dermatomyositis, the panniculitis is more lobular, and the inflammation is primarily lymphocytic. Clinically, there are tender, indurated plaques that may ulcerate and heal with atrophy. Treatment of both conditions involves treating the underlying connective tissue disease.

The physical forms of panniculitis, such as those resulting from cold exposure, foreign body, or factitious causes, usually resolve by removal of the offending trigger or surgical removal of the foreign body. This is similar to panniculitis caused by silicone or paraffin that has been used for cosmetic purposes. There are also forms of panniculitis associated with chronic renal failure, with the main ones being calciphylaxis and oxalosis. Calciphylaxis can cause large areas of necrosis. Treatment involves *parathyroidectomy, sodium thiosulfate, binding agents, or renal transplantation.* Oxalosis is a crystalline deposit panniculitis. Calcium oxalate crystals typically are deposited on the palmar fingers, among other locations. Treatment for this is *renal transplantation.*

Finally, panniculitis may also be drug induced. Of note, vemurafenib, used in the treatment of unresectable or metastatic melanoma harboring the BRAF-V600E mutation, has led to 30 cases of associated panniculitis in the literature. The observed lesions are usually multiple, located on the lower limbs, and often of the lobular type. Withdrawal of the drug can result in resolution.

Specific Investigations

- Skin biopsy for routine microscopy (most important)
- Skin biopsy for culture and sensitivity (routine, mycobacterial, fungal)
- Skin biopsy for PCR
- Skin biopsy for immunoperoxidase and gene rearrangement studies
- ANA and other rheumatologic serologic tests
- Serum α1-antitrypsin levels
- Serum lipase and amylase
- Abdominal MRI
- Complete blood count with differential
- Chemistry panel

LUPUS PANNICULITIS

First-Line Therapies	
• Antimalarials	E
• Systemic corticosteroids	E

Connective tissue panniculitis: lupus panniculitis, derma-tomyositis, morphea/scleroderma. Hansen CB, Callen JP. Dermatol Ther 2010; 23: 341–9.

A review article that touts oral antimalarials and sunscreen as first-line treatment for lupus profundus. Hydroxychloroquine is recommended at 200 mg twice a day with a maximum dose of 6.5 mg/kg/day. The onset of action is around 4 to 8 weeks but can take up to 6 months for optimal benefit. Chloroquine is also recommended at 250 to 500 mg/day but has a higher risk of ophthalmologic toxicity.

Systemic lupus erythematosus presenting as panniculitis (lupus profundus). Diaz-Jouanen E, DeHoratius RJ, Alarcón-Segovia D, Messner RP. Ann Intern Med 1975; 82: 376–9.

A case study in which five or six patients improved after adding hydroxychloroquine to their systemic corticosteroid regimen.

Connective tissue panniculitis. Winkelmann RK, Padilha-Goncalves A. Arch Dermatol 1980; 116: 291–4.

Case report of a patient obtaining remission with hydroxychloroquine 200 mg twice daily and systemic corticosteroids. However, she developed SLE. A second patient on hydroxychloroquine was cleared of the condition after failing to respond to non-steroidal antiinflammatory drugs (NSAIDs), potassium iodide, and corticosteroids.

Lupus erythematosus panniculitis (profundus). Maciejewski W, Bandmann HJ. Acta Derm Venereol 1979; 59: 109–12.

Case report of a patient diagnosed with lupus profundus by direct immunofluorescence and treated with chloroquine.

Lupus erythematosus presenting as panniculitis. Verbov JL, Borrie PR. Proc R Soc Med 1971; 64: 28–9.

A case report of the condition clearing in one patient with hydroxychloroquine 200 mg twice daily.

Second-Line Therapies	
• Topical corticosteroids under occlusion	E
• Second antimalarial agent	E

Lupus erythematosus profundus treated with clobetasol propionate under a hydrocolloid dressing. Yell JA, Burge SM. Br J Dermatol 1993; 128: 103.

A single case of a cure with clobetasol under hydrocolloid dressing occlusion, changed weekly. The patient responded after 1 month.

Lupus panniculitis treated by a combination therapy of hydroxychloroquine and quinacrine. Chung HS, Hann SK. J Dermatol 1997; 24: 569–72.

In this case report, a 24-year-old male presented with non-tender, indurated plaques on the left facial and submandibular regions. Histopathologic and DIF studies confirmed the diagnosis of lupus profundus. The patient had marginal improvement with either hydroxychloroquine or systemic steroids alone. However,

combination of hydroxychloroquine and quinacrine together cleared the lesions.

Third-Line Therapies	
• Intravenous immunoglobulin (IVIG)	E
• Rituximab	E
• Gold	E
• Bismuth	E
• Thalidomide	E
• Cyclosporine	E
• Dapsone	E
• Mycophenolate mofetil	E

Intravenous immunoglobulin in lupus panniculitis. Santo JE, Gomes MF, Gomes MJ, Peixoto LC, Pereira S, Acabado A, et al. Clin Rev Allergy Immunol 2010; 38: 307–18.

The patient was a 51-year-old Caucasian female who initially developed nodular lesions on the abdomen and limbs. Pathology and DIF were consistent with lupus panniculitis. She was initially treated with hydroxychloroquine but developed transaminitis and had biopsy-proven hepatic inflammation. Systemic steroids and azathioprine yielded no response as well. On thalidomide 300 mg, the patient developed neuropathy and diarrhea. She was then started on dapsone but again developed transaminitis. After 15 years of failing different therapies, she was started on IVIG once monthly for 6 months and saw complete regression of the subcutaneous nodules. The doses were spread out to every 3 months, and the patient remained in remission.

Rituximab for the treatment of lupus erythematosus panniculitis. Moreno-Suarez F, Pulpillo-Ruiz A. Dermatol Ther 2013; 26: 415–8.

Two patients presented with lupus profundus refractory to several therapies and demonstrated brisk improvement after infusion of rituximab at a dosage of 375 mg/m²/week. Painful lesions resolved after the first infusion, and no further lesions appeared.

A case of "refractory" lupus erythematosus profundus responsive to rituximab [case report]. McArdle A, Baker JF. Clin Rheumatol 2009; 28: 745–6.

The patient was a 22-year-old African American female who presented with painful nodules on the buttocks, consistent with a diagnosis of lupus panniculitis. The patient was started on prednisolone 1 mg/kg and hydroxychloroquine but continued to worsen. Mycophenolate mofetil resulted in significant nausea and vomiting. Rituximab, an anti-CD20 monoclonal antibody, was then considered. The dosage was 1000 mg administered 2 weeks apart. Over a 1-month period, the patient had complete resolution of all signs of lupus profundus.

Lupus erythematosus profundus. Arnold HL Jr. Arch Dermatol 1956; 73: 14–26.

One patient had a partial response to IV gold followed by bismuth sodium thioglycolate.

Facets of lupus erythematosus: panniculitis responding to thalidomide. Wienart S, Gadola S, Hunziker T. J Deutschen Dermatologischen Gesellschaft 2008; 6: 214–6.

Lupus erythematosus profundus with partial C4 deficiency responding to thalidomide. Burrows NP, Walport MJ, Hammond AH, Davey N, Jones RR. Br J Dermatol 1991; 125: 62–7.

Evidence Levels: A Double-blind study   B Clinical trial ≥ 20 subjects   C Clinical trial < 20 subjects   D Series ≥ 5 subjects   E Anecdotal case reports

A female patient with disfiguring lupus erythematosus profundus from the age of 13 years was found to have an isolated partial C4 deficiency. Marked improvement in her cutaneous lesions occurred with thalidomide.

The dynamism of cutaneous lupus erythematosus: mild discoid lupus erythematosus evolving into SLE and SCLE and treatment-resistant lupus panniculitis. Wozniacka A, Salamon M, Lesiak A, McCauliffe DP, Sysa-Jedrzejowska A. Clin Rheumatol 2007; 26: 1176–9.

A 47-year-old woman with biopsy-proven lupus panniculitis responded to cyclosporine at a dose of 4 mg/kg/day in addition to methylprednisolone. After 10 days, there was improvement. The steroids were tapered and stopped after 3 months, and cyclosporine was gradually tapered to 2 mg/kg/day. The patient had previously failed antimalarials, systemic steroids, azathioprine, cyclophosphamide, methotrexate, and pulse doses of methylprednisolone.

Lupus erythematosus profundus successfully treated with dapsone: review of the literature. Ujiie H, Shimizu T, Ito M, Arita K, Shimizu H. Arch Dermatol 2006; 142: 399–401.

A 56-year-old woman with ulcerated, biopsy-proven lupus profundus responded to dapsone at a dose of 75 mg/day after 6 weeks.

NODULAR VASCULITIS

First-Line Therapies

• Potassium iodide	D
• Treat underlying tuberculosis	B

Potassium iodide in the treatment of erythema nodosum and nodular vasculitis. Horio T, Imamura S, Danno K, Ofuji S. Arch Dermatol 1981; 117: 29–31.

A case study in which 11 of 51 patients had nodular vasculitis. Seven of the 11 patients responded within 2 weeks to potassium iodide 300 mg three times daily.

Treatment of erythema nodosum and nodular vasculitis with potassium iodide. Schulz EJ, Whiting DA. Br J Dermatol 1976; 94: 75–8.

Sixteen of 17 patients responded to potassium iodide, usually with relief of symptoms within 2 days. The average duration of therapy was 3 weeks, and daily doses ranged from 360 to 900 mg.

Successful treatment of erythema induratum of Bazin following rapid detection of mycobacterial DNA by polymerase chain reaction. Degitz K, Messer G, Schirren H, Classen V, Meurer M. Arch Dermatol 1993; 129: 1619–20.

A single case of erythema induratum successfully treated with isoniazid, rifampin, and ethambutol.

Erythema induratum of Bazin. Cho KH, Lee DY, Kim CW. Int J Dermatol 1996; 35: 802–8.

A retrospective study of 32 patients with erythema induratum of Bazin. All improved with triple antituberculous therapy, but four relapsed and subsequently cleared.

Diagnosis and treatment of erythema induratum (of Bazin). Feiwel M, Munro DD. Br Med J 1965; 1: 1109–11.

Twelve patients were diagnosed with erythema induratum secondary to tuberculosis, and all responded well to two- to

three-drug therapy: streptomycin, p-aminosalicylic acid 12.5 mg daily, and isoniazid 200 to 260 mg daily for 9 months.

Second-Line Therapies

• NSAIDs	E
• Antimalarials	E
• Colchicine	E

Neutrophilic vascular reactions. Jorizzo JL, Solomon AR, Zanolli MD, Leshin B. J Am Acad Dermatol 1988; 19: 983–1005.

A review article in which nodular vasculitis is one of the causes of necrotizing vasculitis. NSAIDs may benefit serum sickness–like features but do not help cutaneous lesions.

Chloroquine-induced remission of nodular panniculitis present for 15 years. Shelley WB. J Am Acad Dermatol 1981; 5: 168–70.

One patient with nodular panniculitis responded within 1 month to chloroquine 250 mg/day after failing to respond to corticosteroids, NSAIDs, and tetracycline.

Cutaneous necrotizing vasculitis. Lotti T, Comacchi C, Ghersetich I. Int J Dermatol 1996; 35: 457–74.

By inhibiting neutrophil chemotaxis, oral colchicine in doses of 0.6 mg twice daily may be helpful in chronic forms of the disease.

Third-Line Therapies

• Gold	E
• Mycophenolate mofetil	E

Nodular vasculitis (erythema induratum): treatment with auranofin. Shaffer N, Kerdel FA. J Am Acad Dermatol 1991; 25: 426–9.

One patient with nodular vasculitis responded to oral gold 3 mg twice daily and improved after 3 weeks. She had previously failed to respond to prednisone, colchicine, D-penicillamine, sulindac, and bumetanide for suspected erythema nodosum.

Case reports: nodular vasculitis responsive to mycophenolate mofetil. Taverna JA, Radfar A, Pentland A, Poggioli G, Demierre MF. J Drugs Dermatol 2006; 5: 992–3.

A 70-year-old woman was treated with 1 g of mycophenolate mofetil twice daily. She slowly responded over a 1-year period.

PANCREATIC PANNICULITIS

First-Line Therapies

• Treat underlying pancreatic condition	E
• Resection of metastases of pancreatic cancer	E

Resolution of panniculitis after placement of pancreatic duct stent in chronic pancreatitis. Lambiase P. Am J Gastroenterol 1996; 91: 1835–7.

One patient with pancreatitis secondary to alcohol presented with chest pain and tender skin nodules on the shins. After a skin biopsy showed panniculitis, he was diagnosed with pancreatitis without abdominal pain but a high amylase. A stent was placed to correct a stricture in the pancreatic duct, leading to resolution of the symptoms and the skin lesions within 1 month.

Panniculitis caused by acinous pancreatic carcinoma. Heykarts B, Anseeuw M, Degreef H. Dermatology 1999; 198: 182–3.

One patient with skin nodules was found to have acinar pancreatic carcinoma upon surgical resection. She was initially unresponsive to high-dose corticosteroids and methotrexate, but the skin lesions resolved slowly after the resection. Subsequently, metastases were found in the right liver, and the patient failed to respond to fluorouracil.

Resolution of pancreatic panniculitis following metastasectomy. Banfill KE, Oliphant TJ, Prasad KR. Clin Exp Dermatol 2012; 37: 440–1.

A 69-year-old man presented with a 6-month history of painful skin lesions. Three months after developing the skin lesions, a computed tomography (CT) scan revealed a large necrotic mass in the liver consistent with a metastasis. The patient underwent resection of a solitary liver metastasis, which resulted in complete resolution of his panniculitis.

Second-Line Therapy	
• Octreotide	E

Liquefying panniculitis associated with acinous carcinoma of the pancreas responding to octreotide. Hudson-Peacock MJ, Regnard CF, Farr PM. J R Soc Med 1994; 87: 361–2.

One patient presented with increasing numbers of painful leg nodules secondary to poorly differentiated adenocarcinoma. She failed to respond to prednisolone, but octreotide 50 μg twice daily subcutaneously halted progression of the skin nodules. However, despite therapy, the patient died 3 weeks later.

CYTOPHAGIC HISTIOCYTIC PANNICULITIS

First-Line Therapies	
• Treat underlying T-cell lymphoma (chemotherapy)	E
• Prednisone	E E
• Cyclosporine	E

Cytophagic histiocytic panniculitis and subcutaneous panniculitis-like T-cell lymphoma: report of 7 cases. Marzano AV, Berti E, Paulli M, Caputo R. Arch Dermatol 2000; 136: 889–96.

A report of seven cases of cytophagic histiocytic panniculitis (CHP). Five patients had subcutaneous T-cell lymphoma and died after failing to respond to various chemotherapeutic agents. One patient has done well with prednisone for 13 months, and the other living patient has done well with systemic corticosteroids, cyclophosphamide, and dapsone for 36 years.

Successful treatment of cytophagic histiocytic panniculitis with modified CHOP-E: cyclophosphamide, adriamycin, vincristine, prednisone, and etoposide. Matsue K, Itoh M, Tsukuda K, Miyazaki K, Kokubo T. Am J Clin Oncol 1994; 17: 470–4.

One patient with CHP received eight courses of modified CHOP-E every 3 weeks and obtained a remission that has lasted 2 years.

Cytophagic histiocytic panniculitis. Case report with resolution after treatment. Alegre VA, Fortea JM, Camps C, Aliaga A. J Am Acad Dermatol 1989; 20: 875–8.

One patient with CHP for 2 months was treated with cyclophosphamide, vincristine, doxorubicin, and prednisone for nine cycles and achieved a cure. The authors recommend early, aggressive treatment.

Cytophagic histiocytic panniculitis – a syndrome associated with benign and malignant panniculitis: case comparison and review of the literature. Craig AJ, Cualing H, Thomas G, Lamerson C, Smith R. J Am Acad Dermatol 1998; 39: 721–36.

Case report of two patients with CHP. One patient responded to prednisone plus cyclosporine 15 mg/kg/day. The other patient died during treatment with chemotherapy for T-cell lymphoma.

Subcutaneous panniculitic T-cell lymphoma in children: response to combination therapy with cyclosporine and chemotherapy. Shani-Adir A, Lucky AW, Prendiville J, Murphy S, Passo M, Huang FS, et al. J Am Acad Dermatol 2004; 50: S18–22.

A case report of two adolescents with CHP. Both responded symptomatically to cyclosporine, and complete remission was obtained in one with chemotherapy.

Successful treatment of severe cytophagic histiocytic panniculitis with cyclosporine A. Ostrov BE, Athreys BH, Eichenfield AH, Goldsmith DP. Semin Arthritis Rheum 1996; 25: 404–13.

A 16-year-old patient with CHP who was on prednisone flared and cyclosporine was added. At a dose of 4 mg/kg/day, remission occurred.

Second-Line Therapies	
• Tacrolimus	E
• Bone marrow transplantation	E
• Potassium iodide	E
• Dapsone	E
• Cyclophosphamide	E
• Irradiation	E
• Anakinra	E

Successful treatment of cyclosporine-A-resistant cytophagic histiocytic panniculitis with tacrolimus. Miyabe Y, Murata Y, Baba Y, Ito E, Nagasaka K. Mod Rheumatol 2011; 21: 553–6.

A 34-year-old female with CHP initially failed treatment with high-dose prednisolone with cyclosporine. After changing cyclosporine to tacrolimus, the CHP responded.

Effective high-dose chemotherapy followed by autologous peripheral blood stem cell transplantation in a patient with the aggressive form of cytophagic histiocytic panniculitis. Koizumi K, Sawada K, Nishio M, Katagiri E, Fukae J, Fukada Y, et al. Bone Marrow Transplant 1997; 20: 171–3.

One patient with CHP was treated with CHOP-E and GM-CSF and achieved remission. He was subsequently treated with bone marrow transplant and remained disease free for 1 year.

Evidence Levels: **A** Double-blind study **B** Clinical trial ≥ 20 subjects **C** Clinical trial < 20 subjects **D** Series ≥ 5 subjects **E** Anecdotal case reports

Cytophagic histiocytic panniculitis is not always fatal. White JW Jr, Winkelmann RK. J Cutan Pathol 1989; 16: 137–44.

One patient with CHP was treated with potassium iodide and achieved remission for 15 years.

Successful treatment of a patient with subcutaneous panniculitis-like T-cell lymphoma with high-dose chemotherapy and total body irradiation. Mukai HY, Okoshi Y, Shimizu S, Katsura Y, Takei N, Hasegawa Y, et al. Eur J Haematol 2003; 70: 413–16.

One patient with CHP and T-cell lymphoma achieved remission after three courses of CHOP followed by total body irradiation and autologous stem cell transplant.

Interleukin 1 receptor antagonist to treat cytophagic histiocytic panniculitis with secondary hemophagocytic lymphohistiocytosis. Behrens EM, Kreiger PA, Cherian S, Cron RQ. J Rheumatol 2006; 33: 2081–4.

A 14-year-old girl with CHP who failed cyclosporine and etoposide responded to methylprednisolone and anakinra.

α₁-ANTITRYPSIN DEFICIENCY PANNICULITIS

First-Line Therapies	
• Doxycycline	E
• Dapsone	D
• α₁-Antitrypsin concentrate	E
• Liver transplant	E

Use of anticollagenase properties of doxycycline in treatment of alpha 1-antitrypsin deficiency panniculitis. Humbert P, Faivre B, Gibey R, Agache P. Acta Derm Venereol 1991; 71: 189–94.

Three patients with recurrent α₁-antitrypsin (A1AT) panniculitis were treated with doxycycline 200 mg daily for 3 months. All cleared within 8 weeks.

Clinical and pathologic correlations in 96 patients with panniculitis including 15 patients with deficient levels of alpha 1-antitrypsin. Smith KC, Su Pittelkow MR, Winkelmann RK. J Am Acad Dermatol 1989; 21: 1192–6.

Fifteen patients had A1AT panniculitis. Out of six treated with dapsone, five responded.

Unusual acute sequelae of alpha 1-antitrypsin deficiency: a myriad of symptoms with one common cure. Franciosi AN, McCarthy C, Carroll TP, McElvaney NG. Chest 2015; 148: 136–8.

A single case of biopsy-proven A1AT panniculitis that cleared after one dose of IV A1AT at a dose of 120 mg/kg.

Alpha 1-antitrypsin deficiency-associated panniculitis: resolution with intravenous alpha 1-antitrypsin administration and liver transplantation. O'Riordan K, Blei A, Rao MS, Abecassis M. Transplantation 1997; 63: 480–2.

Two patients with homozygous deficiency had panniculitis. One received cure with liver transplant, whereas the other received intravenous A1AT and was clear while on this medicine.

Treatment of alpha-1-antitrypsin deficiency, massive edema, and panniculitis with alpha-1 protease inhibitor. Furey NL, Golden RS, Potts SR. Ann Intern Med 1996; 125: 699.

A patient with red thigh nodules was found to have A1AT-deficiency panniculitis. The patient failed to respond to doxycycline and received α1-protease concentrate and improved within 24 hours.

Second-Line Therapies	
• Potassium iodide	E
• Plasmapheresis	E
• Cyclophosphamide	E
• Colchicine	E
• Prednisone	E

Atlantic Provinces Dermatology Association Society Meeting, May 3, 1986. Miller RAW, cited by Ross JB. J Can Dermatol Assoc 1986; 13–7.

One patient with A1AT-deficiency panniculitis failed to respond to prednisone and azathioprine but responded after switching to dapsone, potassium iodide, and plasmapheresis two to three times per week.

Cyclophosphamide therapy for Weber–Christian disease associated with alpha 1-antitrypsin deficiency. Strunk RW, Scheld WM. South Med J 1986; 79: 1425–7.

One patient with A1AT-deficiency panniculitis failed to respond to prednisone and heparin. Cyclophosphamide was added with good response.

Necrotic panniculitis with alpha-1 antitrypsin deficiency. Viraben R, Massip P, Dicostanzo B, Mathieu C. J Am Acad Dermatol 1986; 14: 684–7.

A patient with A1AT-deficiency panniculitis failed to respond to prednisolone, lincomycin, colchicine, and cyclophosphamide. Rapid improvement occurred after plasma exchange transfusions once daily for 8 weeks.

Familial occurrence of alpha 1-antitrypsin deficiency and Weber-Christian disease. Breit SN, Clark P, Robinson JP, Luckhurst E, Dawkins RL, Penny R. Arch Dermatol 1983; 119: 198–202.

A report of two cases of A1AT-deficiency panniculitis. One patient responded once cyclophosphamide was added to the initial treatment with dexamethasone. The other patient received colchicine and dicloxacillin and the panniculitis resolved.

Severe panniculitis caused by homozygous ZZ alpha 1-antitrypsin deficiency treated successfully with human purified enzyme (Prolastin). Chowdhury MM, Williams EJ, Morris JS, Ferguson BJ, McGregor AD, Hedges AR, et al. Br J Dermatol 2002; 147: 1258–61.

Life-threatening panniculitis and skin necrosis was cleared with Prolastin and prednisolone. She was put on a dose of 100 mg/kg every 6 days.

Papular urticaria

Hee J. Kim, Jacob O. Levitt

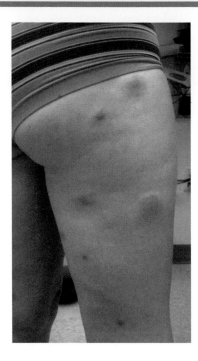

Papular urticaria is a common disease characterized by chronic or recurrent eruptions of 3- to 10-mm pruritic papules, wheals, vesicles, or bullae with central pallor caused by hypersensitivity to the bites of arthropods. Not all individuals who are bitten by an offending arthropod develop a reaction. However, when a bite results in a pruritic papular eruption more persistent than typical urticaria, such dermatologic manifestation is described as papular urticaria. These papules characteristically present as clusters on the extensor surfaces of arms and legs; however, location is largely dependent on the offending arthropod. Eruptions are less often found on the face, neck, trunk, buttocks, or thighs and typically spare the genital, perianal, and axillary regions. Individual lesions may last for 2 to 10 days and rarely longer. Intense pruritus associated with papular urticaria often leads to excoriations, lichenification, and secondary infection. Cases have been reported in infants as young as 2 weeks old but are generally seen in children 2 to 7 years old and in adult males. There is a predilection for the spring and summer months when insect populations peak.

MANAGEMENT STRATEGY

The exact cause of papular urticaria is often unidentified; hence, it is a diagnosis of exclusion. Initial evaluation should include complete blood count with differential, serum IgE, scratch test for dermographism, environmental evaluation, and even skin biopsy if considering systemic treatment.

Given the lack of evidence-based treatments for papular urticaria, we have suggested a therapeutic ladder that addresses (1) a presumed arthropod assault, (2) the pathophysiology of the allergic and inflammatory response, and (3) the severity of the inflammation at presentation.

The most effective treatment for papular urticaria is the *identification and removal of the offending arthropod*. This may require intense investigation by both physician and patient. *Empiric therapy for scabies* should be given because benefits outweigh the risks. This can be achieved with application of permethrin cream 5% or malathion lotion 0.5% once and re-application 3 to 7 days later. In the case of suspected bed bugs and fleas, *fumigation of the home* is required using professional services. Fumigation of the home should also be considered in recurrent cases of papular urticaria. Clothes and bedding should be laundered before and after treatment; specifically, they should be placed in a dryer at 60°C for 10 minutes to dehydrate and kill scabies and bed bugs. In persistent cases, application of diethyl-m-toluamide (DEET) before bed may help. If there are pets in the home, *aggressive flea control* and veterinary evaluation may be necessary. If the exposure is thought to be from the outdoors, prevention can be achieved through *protective clothing* and *insect repellents*.

While the cause of papular urticaria is being investigated and treated, symptomatic therapy should be implemented immediately for patient comfort. The goal of symptomatic therapy is to reduce and prevent inflammation. The degree of aggressiveness in therapy depends on the degree of inflammation at presentation. For milder cases, *topical steroids* should be prescribed, with choice of class depending on the severity of lesions. For individual refractory or severe lesion, *intralesional triamcinolone* is often helpful. If these are ineffective or if the inflammatory response is severe on initial presentation, proceed to systemic immunosuppression—for example, a 10-day *oral prednisone* taper starting at 1 mg/kg or 1 mg/kg of intramuscular triamcinolone. Systemic corticosteroids will often permanently blunt the inflammatory reaction, provided the antigenic stimulus has been removed. If papular urticaria becomes chronic in the context of two failed courses of systemic steroids and negative pest control investigations, other systemic immunosuppressants should be considered, such as *phototherapy, ciclosporin, or methotrexate*.

Pruritus control is often achieved with antihistamines. In milder cases, *nonsedating antihistamines* such as loratadine, desloratadine, fexofenadine, cetirizine, or levocetirizine can help alleviate symptoms. Doses above those given on the product labeling may be necessary. With more severe itching, *diphenhydramine and hydroxyzine* are favored. In chronic or recurrent cases, T-cell–mediated lesions, in contrast to the histamine-mediated lesions of early papular urticaria, may render antihistamines ineffective. In that case, topical agents, such as *camphor/menthol, calamine lotion, crotamiton, lidocaine, and pramoxine* can help.

Careful attention should be paid to any signs of infection secondary to scratching, and appropriate *topical or oral antibiotics* should be used.

Infrequently, cases of papular urticaria persist without the offending arthropod ultimately being identified. Although rare, hospitalizing the patient for a period of 3 to 7 days, while simultaneously treating for scabies on admission, results in resolution as reexposure to arthropod antigenic stimuli ceases in the hospital environment. In refractory cases, eruptions will continue until the patient is naturally hyposensitized over time. Hyposensitization can take years to develop, and the concept can be especially confusing to those who have no pets in the home or for those where only one family member is affected.

Specific Investigations

- Environmental evaluation
- Complete blood count with differential
- Serum IgE
- Scratch test for dermographism
- Skin biopsy (if systemic treatment is being given)

Bed bugs (*Cimex lectularius*) tend to live in wallpaper, mattress seams, couches, and headboards but can also be found in luggage, vehicles, and clothing. Importantly, they can live away from a host for up to 1 year after just one blood meal and can be spread via used furniture as well as travelers (clothing, baggage). They feed at night every 4 to 12 minutes and typically cause a painless bite of which the host is unaware. In vitro, bed bugs have been found to transmit hepatitis B, but there is no evidence for human transmission. Bed bugs are detected by human inspection, bed bug–sniffing dogs, and carbon dioxide–emitting monitoring systems.

Papular urticaria: a histopathologic study of 30 patients. Jordaan HF, Schneider JW. Am J Dermatopathol 1997; 19: 119–26.

More than half of cases reported mild acanthosis, mild spongiosis, exocytosis of lymphocytes, mild subepidermal edema, extravasation of erythrocytes, and a superficial and deep mixed inflammatory cell infiltrate of moderate intensity with interstitial eosinophils. Four subtypes are described: lymphocytic, eosinophilic, neutrophilic, and mixed. The authors conclude that type I hypersensitivity reaction is part of the pathogenesis of papular urticaria based on immunohistochemical evidence.

Differential Th1/Th2 balance in peripheral blood lymphocytes from patients suffering from flea bite-induced papular urticaria. Cuellar A, Rodriguez A, Rojas F, Halpert E, Gomez A, Garcia E. Allergol Immunopathol 2009; 37: 7–10.

Compared with age-matched healthy controls, 18 pediatric patients with papular urticaria had a lower frequency of Interferon-γ–producing CD4+ T cells and a higher frequency of IL-4–producing CD4+ T cells.

Specific pattern of flea antigen recognition by IgG subclass and IgE during the progression of papular urticaria caused by flea bite. Cuéllar A, Rodríguez A, Halpert E, Rojas F, Gómez A, Rojas A, et al. Allergol Immunopathol 2010; 38: 197–202.

Among children clinically diagnosed with papular urticaria caused by flea bites, those who had 2 to 5 years of symptoms responded to flea antigen with higher IgE bands than those who had a shorter or longer duration of symptoms. In addition, healthy controls responded to flea antigen with IgG1 and IgG3 rather than IgE.

Both immediate and delayed-type hypersensitivity reactions are thought to be involved.

First-Line Therapies

• Elimination of arthropod	D
• Antihistamines	A
• Topical steroids	D
• Topical antipruritics (e.g., camphor/menthol, calamine lotion, crotamiton, lidocaine, and pramoxine)	E

Papular urticaria in children. Howard R, Frieden IJ. Pediatr Dermatol 1996; 13: 246–9.

Definitive treatment is elimination of the arthropod source. Pets must be treated with insecticidal shampoos and be well groomed. Carpets, rugs, and cloth furniture should be thoroughly vacuumed and the vacuum bag should be disposed, as eggs could fall off the pet onto these surfaces. Fumigation of fleas should include outdoor areas that the pet frequents. Veterinarians and professional exterminators should be called upon when necessary.

Dermatologic infestations. Shmidt E, Levitt J. Int J Dermatol 2012; 51: 131–41.

Removal and avoidance of the offending arthropod is the best treatment. Preventive measures include use of insect repelents such as DEET and control of parasites infesting indoor pets. Empiric therapy with permethrin cream 5% or malathion lotion 0.5% is recommended. Anti-inflammatory therapy with topical steroids and control of pruritus with topical or oral antihistamines are discussed. A topical antibiotic such as mupirocin is recommended for impetiginized lesions.

Zoonoses of dermatologic interest. Parish LC, Scwartzman RM. Semin Dermatol 1993; 12: 57–64.

Animal fleas not only infest the pet but also live in the rugs and floors, visiting the pet for blood meals; therefore, the pet should be treated with insecticides, and the house should be fumigated.

Tropical rat mite dermatitis. Theis J, Lavoipierre MM, LaPerriere R, Kroese H. Arch Dermatol 1981; 117: 341–3.

Six cases of papular urticaria caused by the tropical rat mite (*Ornithonyssus bacoti*) are presented. Rodents were present in or around the home in most cases.

Effectiveness of bed bug monitors for detecting and trapping bed bugs in apartments. Wang C, Tsai WT, Cooper R, White J. J Econ Entomol 2011; 104: 274–8.

Authors compared the effectiveness of three bed bug–monitoring devices containing CO_2 as an attractant. A homemade dry ice trap was most effective, followed by the Cimex Detection Case (CDC3000) and then NightWatch; however, when NightWatch was used on consecutive nights, its efficacy increased. This study also confirmed the efficacy of Interceptor, an attractant-less monitoring system.

Evaluation of four bed bug traps for surveillance of the brown dog tick (*Acari ixodidae*). Carnohan LP, Kaufman PE, Allan SA, Gezan SA, Weeks EN. J Med Entomol 2015; 52: 260–8.

NightWatch and CO_2-baited ClimbUp traps were more effective than other trapping systems in capturing brown dog ticks.

Ability of bed bug-detecting canines to locate live bed bugs and viable bed bug eggs. Pfiester M, Koehler PG, Pereira RM. J Econ Entomol 2008; 101: 1389–96.

In a controlled experiment set-up in hotel rooms, the dogs were able to detect bed bugs with 98% accuracy.

Lethal effects of heat and use of localized heat treatment for control of bed bug infestations. Pereira RM, Koehler PG, Pfiester M, Walker W. J Econ Entomol 2009; 102: 1182–8.

Heat treatment of furniture for 2 to 7 hours at 49°C using equipment that costs less than $400 can successfully disinfect furniture.

Gaseous chlorine dioxide as an alternative for bedbug control. Gibbs SG, Lowe JJ, Smith PW, Hewlett AL. Infect Control Hosp Epidemiol 2012; 33: 495–9.

At all concentrations tested (362, 724, and 1086 ppm), chlorine dioxide resulted in 100% mortality of bedbugs 18 hours after the exposure. These concentrations can be safely achieved in a hospital room.

In conjunction with chemical treatment of the home, the following strategies can be used to prevent further infestation: a sealed, plastic cover for the mattress; moving the mattress away from the wall; keeping blankets off the floor; petrolatum applied to the legs of the bed; plastic cups with or without water under the legs of the beds; white sheets to make the bed bugs or blood more visible; removing lose wallpaper; and filling in cracks of floorboards, furniture, walls, and windowsills. To prevent infection while traveling, travelers should examine the bed and area around the bed, avoid using hotel drawers, keep suitcases zipped, and launder clothes with heated drying upon return.

Comparison of cetirizine, ebastine and loratadine in the treatment of immediate mosquito-bite allergy. Karppinen A, Kautiainen H, Petman L, Burri P, Reunala T. Allergy 2002; 57: 534–7.

A double-blind, placebo-controlled, crossover study compared prophylactic administration of daily cetirizine 10 mg, ebastine 10 mg, and loratadine 10 mg in 29 adults with mosquito bites. Cetirizine and ebastine significantly reduced the size of wheals and pruritus. Cetirizine was found to be most effective against pruritus but more sedative than ebastine and loratadine.

Levocetirizine for treatment of immediate and delayed mosquito bite reactions. Karppinen A, Brummer-Korvenkontio H, Petman L, Kautiainen H, Herve JP, Reunala T. Acta Derm Venereol 2006; 86: 329–31.

A double-blind, placebo-controlled, crossover study with levocetirizine 5 mg daily in 28 adults sensitive to mosquito bites. Patients were given the study drug for 4 days and exposed to mosquito bites on day 3. Levocetirizine reduced the size of wheals by 60% and pruritus by 62% compared to placebo.

Papular urticaria. Millikan LE. Semin Dermatol 1993; 12: 53–6.

Prevent papular urticaria by using repellents containing DEET if repeated exposure is suspected. Use antipruritics, including menthol, camphor, and pramoxine, for pruritus.

Second-Line Therapies	
• Intralesional steroids	E
• Oral steroids	E
• DEET	E

Insect bite-induced hypersensitivity and the SCRATCH principles: a new approach to papular urticaria. Hernandez RG, Cohen BA. Pediatrics 2006; 118: 189–96.

Authors advocate the use of intralesional steroids in older children and adults to suppress pruritus if more conservative measures fail.

The role of dexamethasone in papular urticaria. El-Nasr NS. J Egypt Med Assoc 1961; 44: 340–1.

Dexamethasone 0.25 mg PO twice or three times daily for 1 to 2 weeks was used with good results. Pruritus resolved within 48 hours.

Comparative activity of three repellents against bedbugs *Cimex hemipterus*. Kumar S, Prakash S, Rao KM. Indian J Med Res 1995; 102: 20–3.

DEET, diethyl phenyl-acetamide (DEPA), and dimethyl phthalate (DMP) were tested against bedbugs on the shaven skin of rabbits. DEET was superior to the other two repellents at all concentrations tested. At 75% concentration, DEET showed 85% repellency for up to 2 hours and 52% repellency 6 hours after treatment.

Insect repellents: an overview. Brown M, Hebert AA. J Am Acad Dermatol 1997; 36: 243–9.

DEET was highly effective at repelling mosquitoes, biting fleas, gnats, chiggers, and ticks. Permethrin works as both an insecticide and a repellent against lice, ticks, fleas, mites, mosquitoes, and black flies.

Third-Line Therapies	
• Phototherapy	E
• Ciclosporin	E
• Hospitalization	E

Papular dermatitis in adults: subacute prurigo, American style? Shertz EF. J Am Acad Dermatol 1991; 24: 697–702.

Twelve patients with pruritic papular eruptions were followed, and the majority were refractory to conservative symptomatic management but showed some control with oral steroids, ultraviolet B (UVB), or psoralen and ultraviolet A radiation (PUVA) treatment.

Papular urticaria and transfer of allergy following bone marrow transplantation. Smith SR, Macfarlane AW, Lewis-Jones MS. Clin Exp Dermatol 1988; 13: 260–2.

A 20-year-old male who underwent allogeneic bone marrow transplant developed papular urticaria as a result of transfer of allergy from the donor. Upon withdrawal of ciclosporin, the patient developed a papular eruption. This suggests a suppressive effect of ciclosporin on papular urticaria.

Papular urticaria. Rook A, Frain-Bell W. Arch Dis Child 1953; 28: 304–10.

Multiple cases of papular urticaria are reported where the eruption cleared when patients were hospitalized. Hospitalization removes the patient from the arthropod source of papular urticaria and allows for sufficient time to rid the home of the arthropods before the patient returns home.

Evidence Levels: **A** Double-blind study **B** Clinical trial ≥ 20 subjects **C** Clinical trial < 20 subjects **D** Series ≥ 5 subjects **E** Anecdotal case reports

180

Paracoccidioidomycosis (South American blastomycosis)

Wanda Sonia Robles, Mahreen Ameen

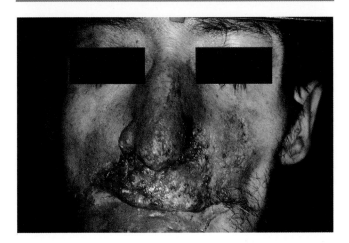

Paracoccidioidomycosis (PCM) is a chronic, progressive, granulomatous mycosis caused by the dimorphic fungus *Paracoccidioides brasiliensis*. It primarily affects the lungs and is believed to be acquired from inhalation of the fungus that resides in soil and plants of endemic regions. PCM is restricted to Latin America, where it is the most prevalent systemic endemic mycosis. It has been reported in nearly all countries from Mexico to Argentina, with the exception of the Caribbean islands and Chile. Eighty percent of cases occur in Brazil, with the highest incidence in the state of Sao Paulo. This is followed by Venezuela, Colombia, Ecuador, and Argentina. PCM characteristically affects those working in agriculture and in rural areas. Because of the long latency period, the disease may appear many years after a person has left an endemic region. Untreated PCM has one of the highest rates of mortality of all the systemic mycoses.

There are two main clinical forms: an acute or subacute form, and a unifocal or multifocal chronic form. The acute form affects young people of both sexes and involves mainly the reticuloendothelial system. This form of infection is often severe and carries a worse prognosis. The chronic form most commonly affects adult males and causes pulmonary and/or mucocutaneous disease. Most cases of pulmonary infection have an indolent course. Only 2% of those infected develop the disseminated form of disease. Dissemination occurs most commonly to the mucosae of the upper airways and upper gastrointestinal tract. Cutaneous and lymph node involvement is common, and other organ systems may be involved such as the adrenal glands (causing Addison syndrome), bones, and central nervous system. Oral lesions affect the gingivae, the hard palate, lips, and tongue. Nasal and pharyngeal ulcers can give rise to dysphagia and dysphonia. Ulcerative lesions can be painful and are characterized by a punctate vascular pattern over a granulomatous base. Cutaneous lesions are highly polymorphic, consisting of verrucous and ulcerative papules, plaques, and nodules. Centrofacial localization is typical and usually a result of dissemination of oral lesions. PCM is also characterized by massive and visible cervical and submandibular lymphadenopathy, which may progress to form abscesses with draining sinuses. Other lymph glands may also become enlarged. Primary mucocutaneous infection is rare, but can occur after direct inoculation of the skin or mucous membranes. It can arise from using twigs to clean the teeth, which is practiced in rural Brazil.

Disseminated infection is severe in the immunocompromised, including those coinfected with HIV. The mortality rate with HIV infection is high, ranging from 30% to 45%. However, the incidence of PCM in patients with AIDS in Latin America is low, and this has been attributed to the widespread use of trimethoprim–sulfamethoxazole as prophylaxis for *Pneumocystis carinii* pneumonia.

MANAGEMENT STRATEGY

P. brasiliensis is highly sensitive to antifungal drugs, and therefore a large therapeutic armamentarium exists to treat PCM. *Itraconazole* is the drug of choice for the treatment of mild to moderate acute and chronic clinical forms of PCM. It is given at a dose of 100 to 200 mg daily for a mean period of 6 months (range 3–12 months) depending on clinical response. It gives a cure rate of 90%, and recurrence rates of 0% to 15% have been reported after a median of 12 months, depending on comorbidities such as alcoholism, malnutrition, and AIDS. *Ketoconazole* (200–400 mg daily) is also highly effective, with 90% of patients responding after 6 to 12 months of treatment with only a 10% relapse rate. However, adverse effects are common especially with long-term treatment. With the availability of newer antifungals, its use has decreased. *Sulfonamides* (sulfadiazine, sulfamethoxypyridazine, sulfadimethoxine, trimethoprim–sulfamethoxazole) are an attractive option as they are inexpensive and well tolerated. However, therapy duration is characteristically long, usually 2 to 3 years. Compliance can therefore be a problem, which might explain their lower cure rate of only 70%. In addition, they have a significant relapse rate of 35%. They are still commonly used as first agents in endemic regions because of their ready availability and low cost. Parenteral *amphotericin B* (cumulative dose of 1–2 g based on clinical response) is the drug of choice for severe or refractory infection. The cure rate is only 60%, but consideration must be given to the fact that it is usually given to the most severely ill patients. The relapse rate with amphotericin B is generally higher than with *itraconazole*, occurring in 20% to 30% of cases. Long-term maintenance therapy with an azole or sulfonamide is therefore required. In cases of central nervous system (CNS) PCM, sulfadiazine appears to be equally effective as amphotericin B. Recently *voriconazole*, an extended-spectrum triazole, has demonstrated comparable efficacy and tolerability to itraconazole in the treatment of PCM. However, its high costs make it prohibitive for use in most endemic settings. There are few studies demonstrating the efficacy of *fluconazole* for PCM. It has been suggested that it may be useful in the management of CNS PCM given its excellent CNS penetration. Long-term follow-up after treatment of PCM is required, as relapse rates are unknown. More recently the use of amphotericin B lipid complex has been advocated.

Specific Investigations

- Direct microscopy
- Culture
- Histology
- Serologic tests
- Chest radiography
- Serology for HIV/AIDS infection (where relevant)

Rapid diagnosis may be achieved by direct microscopic examination of sputum or other exudates in potassium hydroxide. *P. brasiliensis* appears as large, round yeast cells with multiple budding. Culture of sputum, skin, lymph node, or bone marrow specimens on Sabouraud dextrose agar can recover the organism, but may require 20 to 30 days for growth. Biopsy specimens reveal granuloma formation, and Gomori methenamine silver stain reveals yeast cells. Several serologic tests detect antibodies against the fungus, and they can provide results earlier than culture or histopathology. The most common test is immunodiffusion, which has high specificity, but sensitivity varies depending on the type of antigen used. Therefore a negative serologic response does not exclude PCM, particularly in the immunocompromised.

Paracoccidioidomycosis and AIDS: an overview. Goldani L, Sugar AM. Clin Infect Dis 1995; 21: 1275–81.

This is the largest published review of paracoccidioidomycosis in association with AIDS. A wide spectrum of clinical manifestations was seen in the 27 patients described, ranging from indolent infection to rapidly progressive disease. There was multiorgan involvement in 70.4% of patients ($n = 19$), with disseminated disease being the most common form of paracoccidioidomycosis. The overall mortality among patients with AIDS is high (30%). The prognosis can be improved by earlier diagnosis and aggressive therapy with amphotericin B, followed by lifelong suppressive therapy with trimethoprim–sulfamethoxazole.

Paracoccidioidomycosis in patients with human immunodeficiency virus: review of 12 cases observed in an endemic region in Brazil. Paniago AM, de Freitas AC, Aguiar ES, Aguiar JI, da Cunha RV, Castro AR, et al. J Infect 2005; 51: 248–52.

This study demonstrated that the lymph nodes were the organ most commonly involved ($n = 10$, 83.3%), followed by the lung ($n = 7$, 58.3%). Papulonodular ulcerative skin lesions affected 50% ($n = 6$), and oral mucosal ulcerative lesions were present in 42% ($n = 5$). A single patient had pleural involvement with a secondary pathologic rib fracture. Seven patients had multiorgan involvement. All patients were treated with trimethoprim–sulfamethoxazole, and seven patients in addition received amphotericin B. However, eight patients (67%) died as a result of disease progression.

Pharmacologic management of paracoccidioidomycosis. Yasuda MA. Expert Opin Pharmacother 2005; 6: 385–97.

This article emphasizes the long duration of drug therapy required for both the treatment and maintenance of patients with severe infection. It explores the possibility of finding novel therapies among new classes of drugs, drug combinations, or agents capable of modulating the immune response, such as a peptide derived from the 43 kDa *P. brasiliensis* glycoprotein.

Drugs for treating paracoccidioidomycosis. Menezes VM, Soares BG, Fontes CJ. Cochrane Database Syst Rev 2006; 19: CD004967.

This was a critical evaluation of the current therapeutic armamentarium used for the treatment of paracoccidioidomycosis. On the basis of strict selection criteria, including randomized controlled trials, only a single study could be included for analysis (Shikanai-Yasuda MA et al., 2002) with a brief mention of other studies.

Treatment options for paracoccidioidomycosis and new strategies investigated. Travassos LR, Taborda CP, Colombo AL. Expert Rev Anti Infect Ther 2008; 6: 251–62.

This article highlights the significant and unresolved burden of relapses despite the use of long courses of drug therapies, which include sulfamethoxazole–trimethoprim, itraconazole, and amphotericin B. A peptide vaccine aimed at immunotherapy of paracoccidioidomycosis is being studied, and the authors suggest that it could be used as a vaccine to reduce the duration of chemotherapy and the risk of relapse.

Paracoccidioidomycosis. Ramos-E-Silva M, Saraiva Ldo E. Dermatol Clin 2008; 26: 257–69.

This review is written with dermatologists in mind, with a focus on the features of mucocutaneous presentation.

Central nervous system paracoccidioidomycosis: an overview. De Almeida SM. Braz J Infect Dis 2005; 9: 126–33.

CNS involvement with paracoccidioidomycosis has been found in 13% of patients with systemic disease. This review article covers the clinical presentation, diagnostic tests, and treatments for CNS infection. Sulfas are considered the drugs of choice, with sulfamethoxazole–trimethoprim (160/800 mg three times daily) being most commonly used. Amphotericin B is only used in cases of resistance or intolerance to sulfonamides. Of the azoles, itraconazole and particularly ketoconazole penetrate the blood–brain barrier poorly. Fluconazole, however, has excellent CNS penetration, making it a potentially suitable alternative to the other drug therapies.

Amphotericin B lipid complex in the treatment of severe paracoccidioidomycosis: a case series. Peçanha PM, de Souza S, Falqueto A, Grão-Veloso TR, Lírio LV, Ferreira CU Jr, et al. Int J Antimicrob Agents 2016; 48: 428–30.

First report of amphotericin B lipid complex (ABLC) used in the treatment of paracoccidioidomycosis with a cure rate of 100% in 28 patients.

First-Line Therapies	
• Itraconazole	**B**
• Sulfonamides	**B**
• Amphotericin B	**B**

Treatment of paracoccidioidomycosis with itraconazole. Naranjo MS, Trujillo M, Munera MI, Restrepo P, Gomez I, Restrepo A. J Med Vet Mycol 1990; 28: 67–76.

Forty-seven patients with mainly the chronic adult form of infection were treated with itraconazole 100 mg daily for a mean treatment period of 6 months (range 3–24 months). There was marked clinical improvement in 43 patients (89%) and complete resolution of disease in only 1 patient. The mycologic tests (direct examination and cultures) became negative during the first month of treatment in 87% of patients, and by the end of treatment there was a decline in specific antibody titers in 72% of patients. There was no clinical relapse in 15 patients during a 12-month follow-up period.

Randomized trial with itraconazole, ketoconazole and sulfadiazine in paracoccidioidomycosis. Shikanai-Yasuda MA, Benard G, Higaki Y, Del Negro GM, Hoo S, Vaccari EH, et al. Med Mycol 2002; 40: 411–7.

This study from Brazil included 42 patients with moderately severe paracoccidioidomycosis. They were randomized to receive itraconazole 50 to 100 mg daily ($n = 14$), ketoconazole 200 to 400 mg daily ($n = 14$), or sulfadiazine 150 mg/kg daily ($n = 14$) for an induction period of 4 to 6 months. This was followed by slow-release sulfa (sulfamethoxypyridazine) until negative serologic results were obtained. The majority of patients in all arms

Evidence Levels: **A** Double-blind study **B** Clinical trial ≥ 20 subjects **C** Clinical trial < 20 subjects **D** Series ≥ 5 subjects **E** Anecdotal case reports

were reported as cured after 6 months of treatment, and antibody levels reduced significantly by 10 months of treatment for all three drugs.

This study demonstrated that both sulfadiazine and the azoles were equally effective, and the cure rates for the individual drugs were similar to previous studies.

Paracoccidioidomycosis in children: clinical presentation, follow-up and outcome. Pereira RM, Bucaretchi F, Barison Ede M, Hessel G, Tresoldi AT. Rev Inst Med Trop Sao Paulo 2004; 46: 127–31.

This study from Brazil investigated 70 episodes of infection in 63 children under the age of 15 years (range 2–15 years). The juvenile and disseminated form of paracoccidioidomycosis was seen in 70% of episodes, most of them presenting with a febrile lymphoproliferative syndrome. The diagnosis was confirmed by lymph node biopsy (84%), bone biopsy (9%), and skin biopsy (7%). Treatment consisted of either sulfamethoxazole–trimethoprim monotherapy (*n* = 50), sulfamethoxazole–trimethoprim combined with amphotericin B (*n* = 9), or ketoconazole (*n* = 5). Follow-up revealed significant sequential improvement 1 and 6 months later. However, six patients died (9.3%) and four developed sequelae: portal hypertension in three and hypersplenism in one (6.3%). The authors attribute the deaths to the severity of disseminated infection in the context of profound immunosuppression caused by paracoccidioidomycosis as well as malnutrition. A long period of drug treatment, up to 2 years, is required in order to prevent any risk of relapse.

The authors suggest sulfamethoxazole–trimethoprim as first-line therapy in children because of its efficacy, low cost, and easy route of oral administration. It may also be infused intravenously for severe infection. They attributed therapy failure largely to noncompliance.

Paracoccidioidomycosis: a clinical and epidemiological study of 422 cases observed in Mato Gross do Sul. Paniago AM, Aguiar JI, Aguiar ES, da Cunha RV, Pereira GR, Londero A, et al. Rev Soc Bras Med Trop 2003; 36: 455–9.

In terms of treatment this paper illustrates how sulfamethoxazole–trimethoprim is commonly used in endemic areas for paracoccidioidomycosis; 90.3% of patients were treated with this drug, with the majority responding to treatment.

Clinical and serologic features of 47 patients with paracoccidioidomycosis treated by amphotericin B. De Campos EP, Sartori JC, Hetch ML, de Franco MF. Rev Inst Med Trop Sao Paulo 1984; 26: 212–7.

In this study of 47 patients with disseminated infection treated with amphotericin B (3 mg/kg, total dose of 2.0–3.0 g), clinical and serologic cure was obtained in 54% of patients.

Paracoccidioidomycosis: a comparative study of the evolutionary serologic, clinical and radiologic results for patients treated with ketoconazole or amphotericin B plus sulfonamides. Marques SA, Dillon NL, Franco MF, Habermann MC, Lastoria JC, Stolf HO, et al. Mycopathologia 1985; 89: 19–23.

This was a retrospective study comparing the use of ketoconazole (400 mg daily for 30 days followed by 200 mg daily for 18 months) in 22 patients against amphotericin B (1.5–1.75 mg/kg/day for 30–60 days) together with sulfonamide maintenance therapy for up to 18 months in 32 patients. Approximately one third of patients in each group had the acute form of the infection, and the rest had chronic disease. Patients treated with ketoconazole demonstrated better responses, but the results were not statistically significant. There was a sharper drop in antibody titers in patients treated with ketoconazole, but there was no difference in radiologic evolution between the treatments.

Failure of amphotericin B colloidal dispersion in the treatment of paracoccidioidomycosis. Dietze R, Flowler VG Jr, Steiner TS, Pecanha PM, Corey GR. Am J Trop Med Hyg 1999; 60: 837–9.

In this study four adults with the aggressive juvenile form of paracoccidioidomycosis were treated with amphotericin B colloidal dispersion. One patient was also coinfected with HIV. They all received a dose of 3 mg/kg/day for at least 28 days. Three patients, including the HIV-infected case, demonstrated a complete clinical response, but relapsed within 6 months. They were subsequently successfully treated with cotrimoxazole. The authors suggest possible reasons for failure might have been the dose, treatment duration, the drug formulation, inadequate drug delivery to sites of infection, and impaired host immunity. The authors also describe unpublished data on five further patients with chronic paracoccidioidomycosis treated with liposomal amphotericin 4 mg/kg/day. They also responded to treatment initially, but subsequently relapsed after treatment was stopped.

These results raise concerns about the use of short courses of lipid-based formulations to treat PCM. Further and larger studies are required to investigate their efficacy.

Paracoccidioidomycosis: epidemiological, clinical, diagnostic and treatment up-dating. Marques SA. An Bras Dermatol 2013; 88: 700–11.

A very good review article that outlines the treatment of paracoccidioidomycosis with itraconazole, sulfamethoxazole–trimethoprim, and amphotericin B as first-line interventions.

Paracoccidioidomycosis in Mexico: clinical and epidemiological data from 93 new cases (1972-2012). López-Martínez R, Hernández-Hernández F, Méndez-Tovar LJ, Manzano-Gayosso P, Bonifaz A, Arenas R, et al. 2014; 57: 525–30.

This very good review article reports itraconazole alone and the combination of itraconazole with sulfamethoxazole–trimethoprim as the most effective treatment.

Second-Line Therapies	
• Ketoconazole	B
• Fluconazole	B
• Voriconazole	B
• Terbinafine	E

Treatment of paracoccidioidomycosis with ketoconazole: a three-year experience. Restrepo A, Gómez I, Cano LE, Arango MD, Gutiérrez F, Sanín A, et al. Am J Med 1983; 74: 48–52.

Thirty-eight patients with active infection were treated with ketoconazole 200 mg daily for 6 months. Treatment was well tolerated. There was complete resolution of infection in 13 patients (34%) and significant improvement in the majority of the rest of the patients.

In a subsequent study, 24 of these patients were followed up for a 1- to 2-year period. Relapse was detected in only two patients. There are no recent studies evaluating ketoconazole for PCM, as its use has declined with the advent of newer antifungals.

A pan-American 5-year study of fluconazole therapy for deep mycoses in the immunocompetent host. Pan-American Study Group. Diaz M, Negroni R, Montero-Gei F, Castro LG, Sampaio SA, Borelli D, et al. Clin Infect Dis 1992; 14 (Suppl 1): S68–76.

Twenty-seven of 28 patients responded to treatment with fluconazole 200 to 400 mg daily given for at least 6 months.

Treatment was well tolerated. However, relapse was noted in one patient within the first year.

This is the only reported study of fluconazole therapy for PCM. A longer period of follow-up is required in order to evaluate drug efficacy.

An open-label comparative pilot study of oral voriconazole and itraconazole for long-term treatment of paracoccidioidomycosis. Queiroz-Telles F, Goldani LZ, Schlamm HT, Goodrich JM, Espinel-Ingroff A, Shikanai-Yasuda MA. Clin Infect Dis 2007; 45: 1462–9.

This multicenter study from Brazil investigated the efficacy, safety, and tolerability of voriconazole for the long-term treatment of acute or chronic paracoccidioidomycosis, with itraconazole as the control treatment. Patients were randomized (at a 2:1 ratio) to receive oral voriconazole (*n* = 35) or itraconazole (*n* = 18) for 6 to 12 months. Voriconazole was given at an initial loading dose of 800 mg in divided doses on day 1, followed by 200 mg twice daily. The dose of itraconazole was 100 mg twice daily. There was a satisfactory response rate in 88.6% of the voriconazole group and 94.4% of the itraconazole group. The response rate among treatment-evaluable patients was 100% for both treatment groups. No relapses were observed after 8 weeks of follow-up. Both drugs were well tolerated, although liver function test values were slightly higher in patients receiving voriconazole, necessitating the withdrawal of voriconazole from two patients.

This study has demonstrated equal efficacy and tolerability of oral voriconazole and itraconazole for the long-term treatment of paracoccidioidomycosis. This study also included a case of CNS paracoccidioidomycosis that responded to treatment. Voriconazole demonstrates good CNS penetration, having been successfully used in the treatment of other mycotic CNS infections. On the basis of these results the authors suggested that intravenous voriconazole should be evaluated as an alternative to amphotericin B for the initial treatment of severe paracoccidioidomycosis, given the high relapse rate and toxicity associated with amphotericin B therapy.

Chronic paracoccidioidomycosis in a female patient in Austria. Mayr A, Kirchmair M, Rainer J, Rossi R, Kreczy A, Tintelnot K, et al. Eur J Clin Microbiol Infect Dis 2004; 23: 916–9.

Case report of a Cuban female patient who was initially misdiagnosed with tuberculosis. She was successfully treated with amphotericin B (1 mg/kg/day) for 10 days followed by voriconazole 200 mg daily for 3 months.

Paracoccidioidomycosis (South American blastomycosis) successfully treated with terbinafine: first case report. Ollague JM, de Zurita AM, Calero G. Br J Dermatol 2000; 143: 188–91.

A case report of a 63-year-old male who presented with lesions of paracoccidioidomycosis in the perineal region. Initial treatment with trimethoprim–sulfamethoxazole failed. He was subsequently treated with terbinafine 250 mg twice daily for 6 months, which resulted in rapid resolution of all lesions without evidence of relapse for 2 years after treatment.

Terbinafine has demonstrated similar activity to itraconazole against P. brasiliensis in vitro.

Isavuconazole treatment of cryptococcosis and dimorphic mycoses. Thompson GR 3rd, Rendon A, Ribeiro Dos Santos R, Queiroz-Telles F, Ostrosky-Zeichner L, Azie N, et al. Clin Infect Dis 2016; 63: 356–62.

An open-label, nonrandomized, phase III trial to evaluate efficacy and safety of isavuconazole in the management of invasive fungal infections. Thirty-eight patients, of which 10 had paracoccidioidomycosis, received this treatment. The study reports that 63% of the total of patients had an overall successful response.

Evidence Levels: **A** Double-blind study **B** Clinical trial ≥ 20 subjects **C** Clinical trial < 20 subjects **D** Series ≥ 5 subjects **E** Anecdotal case reports

181

Parapsoriasis

James E. Miller, Graham A. Johnston

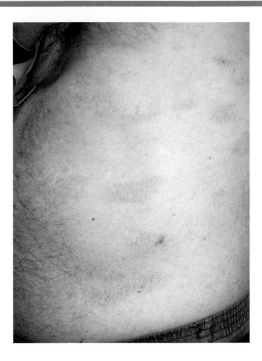

The use of the description parapsoriasis, even as an umbrella term, remains controversial, and debate remains whether the variants described in this chapter are in fact precursors of cutaneous T-cell lymphoma (CTCL). This chapter covers the entities small plaque parapsoriasis (SPP), which includes the synonyms chronic superficial scaly dermatitis, persistent superficial dermatitis, digitate dermatosis, and xanthoerythroderma perstans, and large plaque parapsoriasis (LPP), which includes the synonyms parakeratosis variegata, retiform parapsoriasis, atrophic parapsoriasis, and poikilodermatous parapsoriasis. Confusingly, the term *parapsoriasis en plaque* has been used for both SPP and LPP.

Parapsoriasis is often grouped with other cutaneous lymphoproliferative disorders, including pityriasis lichenoides et varioliformis acuta, pityriasis lichenoides chronica, lymphomatoid papulosis, and mycosis fungoides, all of which are the subjects of separate chapters.

MANAGEMENT STRATEGY

Although the diagnosis of parapsoriasis is initially considered on clinical grounds, histopathologic examination, with T-cell receptor gene rearrangement studies, is essential to exclude monoclonality and CTCL. However, monoclonality is not sensitive or specific for CTCL. Monoclonality has been identified in SPP, but it is reported more often in LPP. This does not appear to predict the risk of progression to CTCL. Regular repeat skin biopsies are recommended if a clinical or histologic progression to CTCL is suspected.

Although topical therapy is appropriate in mild or early cases, the potential for progression to cutaneous lymphoma in patients with parapsoriasis can justify the use of phototherapy in symptomatic or progressive cases.

Specific Investigations

- The diagnosis is initially suspected on clinical findings
- Histology is nonspecific but differs between small and large plaque types
- T-cell receptor (TCR) gene rearrangement studies can identify T-cell clones

---

Immunohistochemistry cannot differentiate between small and large plaque parapsoriasis.

Clonal T cell receptor gamma-chain gene rearrangement by PCR-based GeneScan analysis in the skin and blood of patients with parapsoriasis and early-stage mycosis fungoides. Klemke CD, Dippel E, Dembinski A, Pönitz N, Assaf C, Hummel M, et al. J Pathol 2002; 197: 348–54.

Although the authors of this paper concede that studies have shown T-cell clonality in both skin and peripheral blood, they argue that monoclonality is neither easily demonstrable nor ought to be a prerequisite for diagnosis.

The role of immunohistochemical analysis in the diagnosis of parapsoriasis. Bordignon M, Belloni-Fortina A, Pigozzi B, Saponeri A, Alaibac M. Acta Histochem 2011; 113: 92–5.

Given the lack of clinical and histologic markers of distinction between parapsoriasis and early CTCL, the use of immunohistochemical techniques has been explored to try to establish a more definitive diagnosis. However these techniques, including CD4/CD8 ratio, expression of T-cell antigens, and expression of proliferation markers, have been found unhelpful in distinguishing between parapsoriasis and early CTCL.

Defining early mycosis fungoides. Pimpinelli N, Olsen EA, Santucci M, Vonderheid E, Haeffner AC, Stevens S, et al. J Am Acad Dermatol 2005; 53: 1053.

To aid in the diagnosis of early CTCL an algorithm was devised by the International Society for Cutaneous Lymphomas (ISCL) encompassing clinical, histopathologic, immunohistochemistry, and T-cell gene arrangement characteristics. The study was proposed to validate the algorithm using a 4-point threshold. They found the algorithm to be statistically valid, but it was limited by a sensitivity of 87.5% and an even lower specificity at 60%. The authors felt that until sensitivity and specificity improved, existing clinicopathologic correlation will remain the gold standard.

SMALL PLAQUE PARAPSORIASIS

SPP consists of fixed, scaly erythematous plaques less than 5 cm in diameter. They are predominantly asymptomatic but can be mildly pruritic and occur mainly on the trunk and proximal extremities. The lesions sometimes appear to run in fingerlike lines parallel to the ribs (hence the synonym digitate dermatosis). Histology shows mild spongiosis with focal parakeratosis and small areas of perivascular lymphocytic infiltrate within the papillary dermis. SPP runs a chronic, indolent, and usually benign course.

First-Line Therapies

• Emollients, tar, topical corticosteroids	E
• Psoralen Ultraviolet A treatment	C
• Narrowband Ultraviolet B	C

Treatments with emollients, topical tar, and topical corticosteroid are widely used, but evidence is anecdotal and these treatments are therefore unreferenced.

Narrowband UVB phototherapy for small plaque parapsoriasis. Aydogan K, Karadogan SK, Tunali S, Adim SB, Ozcelik T. J Eur Acad Dermatol Venereol 2006; 20: 573–7.

Forty-five patients were treated with narrowband UVB therapy three to four times weekly. There was a complete response in 33 patients with a mean cumulative dose of 14.3 J/cm^2 after a mean number of 29 exposures. There was a partial response in 12 of the 45. Relapses occurred in 6 of the 45 patients within a mean of 7.5 months.

Treatment of small plaque parapsoriasis with narrow-band (311 nm) ultraviolet B: a retrospective study. Herzinger T, Degitz K, Plewig G, Rocken M. Clin Exp Dermatol 2005; 30: 379–81.

Sixteen patients had complete remission after a mean number of 33 exposures and a mean total dose of 35.4 J/cm^2. Relapse occurred after an average of 29 weeks showing similarity with the study by Aydogan et al.

Narrowband (311-nm) UV-B therapy for small plaque parapsoriasis and early-stage mycosis fungoides. Hofer A, Cerroni L, Kerl H, Wolf P. Arch Dermatol 1999; 35: 1377–80.

Fourteen patients with SPP were treated with narrowband UVB, three to four times weekly for 5 to 10 weeks. Complete response was achieved after an average of 20 exposures. All patients then relapsed after an average of 6 months. Topical corticosteroids were effective at producing a second clearance in an unspecified number of patients.

Retrospective study of 24 patients with large or small plaque parapsoriasis treated with ultraviolet B therapy. Arai R, Horiguchi Y. J Dermatol 2012; 39: 674–6.

A retrospective study of 24 patients given UVB for both small and large plaque parapsoriasis. Five patients resolved with treatment over a median duration of 3.5 years. Eighteen continued with active disease, although this cohort had a median duration of 2 years of treatment. The findings suggest longer treatment is required to cause remission, although the values were not significant. One patient progressed from LPP to CTCL. The study suggests long-term phototherapy is of clinical benefit.

Treatment of parapsoriasis and mycosis fungoides: the role of psoralen and long-wave ultraviolet light A (PUVA). Powell FC, Spiegel GT, Muller SA. Mayo Clin Proc 1984; 59: 538–46.

Seven patients with SPP had complete clearance with as few as 15 treatments (84 J/cm^2) of standard PUVA. Three patients reported recurrence at follow-up (mean of 13 months), and one of these was then successfully treated with topical corticosteroid.

Second-Line Therapy	
• Topical nitrogen mustard	C

Topical nitrogen mustard therapy in patients with mycosis fungoides or parapsoriasis. Lindahl LM, Fenger-Gron, M, Iversen L. J Eur Acad Dermatol Venereol 2013; 27: 163–8.

Seventy-one patients with parapsoriasis (no information on numbers of LPP and SPP) were treated with mechlorethamine hydrochloride between 1991 and 2009. A dose of 20 mg was dissolved in 40 mL water and applied daily to affected skin for a 14-day induction period. Maintenance therapy of two treatments every 4 to 8 weeks occurred until clear, insufficient response or side effects developed. The "overall" response was 90%, with a "complete" response of 41%. Relapse (no time given) was 62%. The main side effect was contact dermatitis resulting in withdrawal of treatment in 14% of patients.

LARGE PLAQUE PARAPSORIASIS

This is clinically similar to SPP but lesions are larger than 5 cm, irregularly shaped, and often atrophic or poikilodermatous. Lesions typically occur over the lower trunk and thighs.

Specific Investigations
• Skin biopsy
• TCR gene rearrangement studies

The diagnosis is suggested clinically. Histology demonstrates psoriasiform epidermal hyperplasia with areas of atrophy in poikilodermatous areas. There is vacuolization in the basal layer and a bandlike lymphocytic infiltrate in the papillary dermis. Pautrier microabscesses, a prominent feature of mycosis fungoides, are usually absent.

Progression of LPP to cutaneous T-cell lymphoma is reported, with one retrospective study demonstrating a figure of 35%. This same study also reported 10% of patients with SPP progressing to CTCL.

Large plaque parapsoriasis: clinical and genotypic correlations. Simon M, Flaig MJ, Kind P, Sander CA, Kaudewitz P. J Cutan Pathol 2000; 27: 57–60.

TCR gene rearrangement status was assessed in 12 patients. Six of 12 patients with LPP had a clonal T-cell population. One developed CTCL after a follow-up of 8 years. The other five patients did not progress after follow-up of 2 to 21 years.

The authors conclude that TCR gene rearrangement status has no prognostic significance and does not allow distinction between LPP and early CTCL.

A retrospective study of the probability of the evolution of parapsoriasis en plaques into mycosis fungoides. Väkevä L, Sarna S, Vaalasti A, Pukkala E, Kariniemi AL, Ranki A. Acta Derm Venereol 2005; 85: 318–23.

A 26-year retrospective analysis of 105 patients with SPP and LPP reported that 10% of patients with SPP and 35% of patients with LPP progressed to histologically confirmed CTCL over a median time of 10 and 6 years, respectively.

Subsequent cancers, mortality and causes of death in patients with mycosis fungoides and parapsoriasis: a Danish nationwide, population-based cohort study. Lindahl LM, Fenger-Gron M, Iversen L. J Am Acad Dermatol 2014; 71: 529.

Using the Danish nationwide population-based registry, 368 mycosis fungoides and 582 parapsoriasis patients were compared with the general population for subsequent cancers, mortality, and causes of death. Subsequent cancers were significantly increased in the parapsoriasis group, including non-Hodgkin lymphoma (NHL), hematologic cancers other than NHL, and nonhematologic cancers, with the highest incidence being in the gastrointestinal (GI) tract. Interestingly the incidence of these malignancies

Evidence Levels: **A** Double-blind study   **B** Clinical trial ≥ 20 subjects   **C** Clinical trial < 20 subjects   **D** Series ≥ 5 subjects   **E** Anecdotal case reports

was significantly higher within the first 5 years of diagnosis. In the mycosis fungoides group the only significantly increased cancer was NHL. Both groups had a significantly increased mortality compared with the general Danish population, with the mycosis fungoides group being more pronounced with the first 5 years of diagnosis.

First-Line Therapies

Topical steroids

* Ultraviolet A with 5-methoxypsoralen   C
* Ultraviolet A with 4,6,4′-trimethylangelicin   E

The use of topical steroids has not been evaluated in clinical trials, but its benefit has been observed in early-stage CTCL.

Photochemotherapy in cutaneous T cell lymphoma and parapsoriasis en plaque. Long-term follow-up in forty-three patients. Rosenbaum MM, Roenigk HH Jr, Caro WA, Esker A. J Am Acad Dermatol 1985; 13: 613–22.

Of the 43 patients included in the study 7 patients had LPP treated with oral psoralen and UVA (PUVA). A complete response was achieved in all 7, though the total dosages of PUVA are not stated. Average follow-up for all 43 patients was 38.4 months (range 4–67 months), and during that time relapse was observed in 5 out of the 7 patients with LPP.

The authors argue that because CTCL is in the differential diagnosis of LPP and PUVA is effective for both conditions, it may be useful in patients in whom it is difficult to distinguish between the two conditions.

Topical nitrogen mustard therapy in patients with mycosis or parapsoriasis. Lindahl LM, Fenger-Gron M, Iversen L. J Eur Acad Dermatol Venereol 2013; 27: 163–8.

Seventy-one patients with parapsoriasis (no information on numbers of LPP and SPP) were treated with mechlorethamine hydrochloride between 1991 and 2009. A dose of 20 mg was dissolved in 40 mL water and applied daily to affected skin for a 14-day induction period. Maintenance therapy of two treatments every 4 to 8 weeks occurred until clear, insufficient respone or side effects developed. The "overall" response was 90%, with a "complete" response of 41%. Relapse (no time given) was 62%. The main side effect was contact dermatitis resulting in withdrawal of treatment in 14% of patients.

Evaluation of a 1-hour exposure time to mechlorethamine (chlormethine) in patients undergoing topical treatment. Foulc P, Evrard V, Dalac S, Guillot B, Delaunay M, Verret JL, et al. Br J Dermatol 2002; 147: 926–30.

Three patients with LPP were included in this study. One patient stopped treatment because of the side effects, and two of the three resulted in complete remission. The mechlorethamine regimen, however, varied between the four centers included in the study and is not specified for the individual patient.

Paronychia

Richard B. Mallett, Cedric C. Banfield

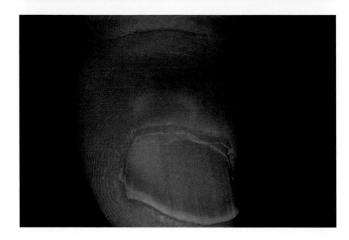

Paronychia is characterized by inflammation of the proximal and/or lateral nail folds, with the fingers being more commonly affected than the toes. Acute paronychia is a painful pyogenic infection that usually occurs after injury or minor trauma and is characteristically caused by *Staphylococcus aureus,* although other aerobic and anaerobic bacteria and herpetic viruses are also found.

Chronic paronychia, one of the most common inflammatory nail disorders, presents as tender erythema of the nail folds with thickening of the tissues, loss of the cuticle, and subsequent dystrophy of the nail plate. The causative factors are repetitive microtrauma and exposure to water, irritants, and allergens, causing a contact dermatitis with subsequent colonization by yeasts and bacteria. Other less common causes of chronic paronychia include retronychia, characterized by the disruption of the longitudinal growth of a nail due to acute traumatic injury or repetitive microtrauma, with resultant embedding of the old nail in the ventral surface of the proximal nail fold as the new nail regenerates. Also, cutaneous leishmaniasis may rarely present as an unusual chronic paronychia in endemic areas. Pemphigus vulgaris may present with either acute or chronic paronychia.

Drug-induced paronychia with pseudopyogenic granuloma is increasingly recognized and may occur with systemic retinoids, antiretroviral drugs such as indinavir, epidermal growth factor (EGF) receptor inhibitors, including gefitinib and cetuximab, and the novel anticancer mechanistic Target Of Rapamycin mTOR inhibitors such as everolimus.

Tumors, including Bowen's disease, keratoacanthomas, squamous cell carcinoma, enchondroma, and amelanotic melanoma, may masquerade as chronic paronychia. Dermoscopy has been used to diagnose periungual Bowen's disease mimicking chronic paronychia.

MANAGEMENT STRATEGY

Acute paronychia requires urgent effective treatment to prevent damage to the nail matrix. If the infection is superficial and pointing, then *incision and drainage* may be appropriate. Infection is often due to *S. aureus,* but β-hemolytic streptococci and anaerobic

organisms may also be found. A swab must be taken for bacterial culture and antibiotic sensitivity and a *broad-spectrum antibiotic* covering both aerobic and anaerobic organisms given. *Warm compresses with an astringent* (e.g., aluminum acetate lotion, if available) can help reduce edema and provide a hostile environment for bacteria. For deeper infections, if there has been no marked clinical improvement after 48 hours of antibiotic therapy, *surgical treatment* may be undertaken. Under local anesthesia, the proximal third of the nail plate is removed, and a gauze wick is laid under the proximal nail fold to allow drainage. Cases of antibiotic-resistant acute paronychia may be due to herpetic viruses, fungi, or noninfectious causes.

Chronic paronychia is usually due to dermatitis and often associated with wet work (e.g., in domestic workers, cooks, bartenders, fishmongers, etc.) and may be exacerbated by contact irritants or allergens. Immediate sensitivity to fresh foods can be a factor. In children, thumb sucking may initiate the condition. Eczema or psoriasis may predispose to chronic paronychia, as may poor peripheral circulation and rarely pemphigus vulgaris. Microtrauma, including overzealous manicuring of the cuticle, is also important. The middle and index fingers of the right hand and the middle finger of the left hand are most commonly affected, but any finger may be involved. Inflammation with bolstering of the nail fold and loss of the cuticle opens a space between the nail fold and the nail plate, which commonly becomes colonized with yeast, especially *Candida* species, and a wide range of other microorganisms. Acute exacerbations due to bacterial infection may occur.

Successful treatment relies on protection of the affected fingers from water, irritants, allergens, and trauma, together with antiinflammatory treatment using moderately potent or potent *topical corticosteroids. Tacrolimus* 0.1% ointment applied twice daily may also be effective. Swabs for yeast and bacteria should be taken, *anticandidal preparations* can be useful, and antibiotic preparations may also be needed. Treatment should be continued until the inflammation has subsided and the cuticle reformed and reattached to the nail plate (3 months or more). For repeated acute episodes, *intralesional or systemic corticosteroids plus systemic antibiotics* for a week may be useful. In cases where conservative management fails, surgery or *low-dose superficial radiotherapy* has been tried. For cases due to retronychia simple avulsion of the nail plate is normally curative, but conservative treatment using taping can be tried.

Drug-induced pseudopyogenic granulomatous paronychia responds to daily topical *2% mupirocin* with *clobetasol propionate* ointment. Additionally, for patients on EGF or mTOR inhibitors oral *doxycycline* 100 mg twice daily or dose reduction may be useful.

Specific Investigations

- Skin swabs
- Open patch tests against fresh foods

Anaerobic paronychia. Whitehead SM, Eykyn SJ, Phillips I. Br J Surg 1981; 68: 420–2.

Swabs were taken from 116 acute paronychias. Anaerobes or mixed aerobes and anaerobes were isolated in 30%. Of 81 paronychias with aerobic organisms only, *S. aureus* was isolated in 69%.

Clinical and cytologic features of antibiotic-resistant acute paronychia. Durdu M, Ruocco V. J Am Acad Dermatol 2014; 70: 120–6.

Evidence Levels: **A** Double-blind study **B** Clinical trial ≥ 20 subjects **C** Clinical trial < 20 subjects **D** Series ≥ 5 subjects **E** Anecdotal case reports

Antibiotic-resistant paronychia may be infectious or noninfectious. Cytologic examination may be useful diagnostically and may prevent unnecessary use of antibiotics and surgical drainage procedures.

Refractory purulent paronychia in a young girl. Pediatric dermatology photoquiz. Diagnosis paronychial cutaneous leishmaniasis. Topal I, Duman H, Baz V, Gungor S, Kocaturk E, Ozekinci S. Pediatr Dermatol 2016; 33: 93–4.

Case report and successful treatment with complete resolution using intralesional meglumine antimonite once a week for 5 weeks.

Chronic paronychia. Short review of 590 cases. Frain-Bell W. Trans St John's Hosp Dermatol Soc 1957; 38: 29–35.

On culture, *Candida albicans* was grown in 70% and bacteria, including *S. aureus*, in 10%.

An excellent overview.

Role of foods in the pathogenesis of chronic paronychia. Tosti A, Guerra L, Morelli R, Bardazzi F, Fanti PA. J Am Acad Dermatol 1992; 27: 706–10.

Nine of 20 food handlers with chronic paronychia had positive reactions to 20-minute open patch tests with suspected fresh foods, including wheat flour, egg, chicory, and tomatoes.

First-Line Therapies

Acute
- Amoxicillin with clavulanic acid — E
- Surgical drainage — E

Chronic
- Topical corticosteroid preparations — B
- Topical tacrolimus 0.1% ointment — B
- Topical clotrimazole drops — E
- Topical clindamycin solution — E

Due to retronychia
- Avulsion of nail plate — E

Drug-induced periungual granuloma
- Mupirocin and clobetasol propionate — E

EGF- or mTOR inhibitor–induced paronychia
- Doxycycline — E
- Dose reduction — E

Paronychia: a mixed infection, microbiology and management. Brook I. J Hand Surg [Br] 1993; 18: 358–9.

Culture from 61 patients with paronychia showed a mixture of both aerobic and anaerobic bacteria in 49%. The combination of amoxicillin with clavulanic acid is suggested as first-line treatment for acute bacterial paronychia, together with appropriate surgical drainage.

Nail surgery and traumatic abnormalities. Thomas L, Zook E, Rosio T, Dawber R, Haneke E, Baran R. In: Baran R, de Berker D, Holzberg M, Thomas L, eds. Baran and Dawber's Diseases of the Nails and Their Management, 4th edn. Wiley-Blackwell, 2012; 623–4.

For acute paronychia, under local anesthesia the proximal third of the nail plate is removed and a wick laid under the proximal nail fold.

Topical steroids versus systemic antifungals in the treatment of chronic paronychia: an open, randomized double-blind and double dummy study. Tosti A, Piraccini BM, Ghetti E. J Am Acad Dermatol 2002; 47: 73–6.

An open, randomized, double-blind trial of oral itraconazole, oral terbinafine, and topical methylprednisolone aceponate. Patients were treated for 3 weeks and observed for a further 6 weeks. Of 48 nails treated with methylprednisolone aceponate, 41 (85%) were improved or cured at the end of the study, compared with only 30 of 57 (53%) with itraconazole and 29 of 64 (45%) with terbinafine.

Efficacy and safety of tacrolimus ointment 0.1% vs. betamethasone 17-valerate 0.1% in the treatment of chronic paronychia: an unblinded randomized study. Rigopoulos D, Gregoriou S, Belyayeva E, Larios G, Kontochristopoulos G and Katsambas A. Br J Dermatol 2009; 160: 858–60.

This open study showed that both topical tacrolimus 0.1% and betamethasone 17-valerate 0.1% ointments applied twice daily to the affected perionychium gave statistically significantly better cure or improved rates compared with placebo. Also, in this study, tacrolimus 0.1% ointment appeared to be more effective than betamethasone 17-valerate 0.1% ointment.

The management of superficial candidiasis. Hay RJ. J Am Acad Dermatol 1999; 40: S35–42.

The central role of *Candida* in chronic paronychia is debatable, and other factors such as irritant or allergic dermatitis may play a role. Therefore, in addition to polyenes or imidazoles, concomitant use of a topical corticosteroid is a logical approach.

Diseases of the nails in infants and children: paronychia. Silverman RA. In: Callen JP, Dahl MV, Golitz LE, Schachner LA and Stegman SJ, eds. Advances in Dermatology. Vol. 5. Chicago: Mosby Year Book, 1990; 164–5.

Clotrimazole drops several times a day should inhibit fungal growth. Topical clindamycin solution applied to the fingers several times daily kills bacteria, has a bitter taste to discourage finger sucking, and has an alcohol–propylene glycol vehicle that dries out residual moisture. Side effects from oral absorption of these medications have not been reported.

Retronychia – clinical and pathophysiological aspects. Ventura F, Correia O, Duarte A, Barros A, Haneke E. JEADV 2016; 30: 16–9.

Review of 20 cases of retronychia. Avulsion of the nail confirms the diagnosis and is the curative treatment.

Paronychia associated with antiretroviral therapy. Tosti A, Piraccini BM, D'Antuono A, Marzaduri S. and Bettoli V. Br J Dermatol 1999; 140: 1165–8.

Six cases of periungual pseudopyogenic granuloma induced by indinavir, lamivudine, and zidovudine responded to daily applications of clobetasol propionate and mupirocin.

Doxycycline for the treatment of paronychia induced by the epidermal growth factor receptor inhibitor cetuximab. Suh K-Y, Kindler HL, Medenica M, and Lacouture M. Br J Dermatol 2006; 154: 191–2.

During treatment with cetuximab a patient developed painful paronychia, refractory to topical mupirocin and cephalexin but improved after treatment with doxycycline 100 mg twice daily.

Paronychia and pyogenic granuloma induced by new anti-cancer mTOR inhibitors. Sibaud V, Dalenc F, Mourey L and Chevereau C, et al. Acta Derm Venereol 2011; 91: 584–5.

Seven patients treated with mTOR inhibitors presenting with chronic paronychia were treated variously with topical steroids, silver nitrate, topical antibiotics, and oral doxycycline and pristinamycin; three patients required dose reduction.

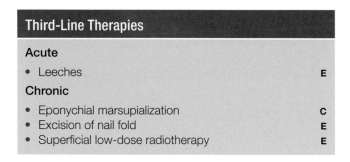

Second-Line Therapies

Chronic

- Nystatin ointment   E
- Intralesional or systemic corticosteroids and antibiotics   E

Treatment of chronic paronychia. Vickers HR. Br Med J 1979; 2: 1588.

A nystatin-containing ointment should be worked into the affected nail fold every time the patient is going to get the hands wet, for at least 6 weeks.

Fungal (onychomycosis) and other infections involving the nail apparatus. Hay RJ, Baran R. In: Baran R, deBerker D, Holzberg M, Thomas L, eds. Baran and Dawber's Diseases of the Nails and Their Management, 4th edn. Hoboken, NJ: Wiley-Blackwell, 2012; 239.

For frequent acute exacerbations of chronic paronychia, intralesional or systemic corticosteroids plus either erythromycin 1 g daily or tetracycline 1 g daily for a week is recommended.

Third-Line Therapies

Acute

- Leeches   E

Chronic

- Eponychial marsupialization   C
- Excision of nail fold   E
- Superficial low-dose radiotherapy   E

Thumb paronychia treated with leeches. Graham CE. Med J Aust 1992; 156: 512.

Acute paronychia successfully treated with leeches while trekking in Tasmania.

Eponychial marsupialization and nail removal for surgical treatment of chronic paronychia. Bednar MS, Lane LB. J Hand Surg [Am] 1991; 16: 314–7.

Twenty-eight fingers with chronic paronychia were treated with marsupialization of the dorsal roof of the proximal nail fold plus complete or partial removal of the nail in those patients with associated nail abnormality. Postoperative treatment was with hydrogen peroxide soaks and oral antibiotics for 5 to 14 days. Twenty-seven of 28 fingers were cured.

Surgical treatment of recalcitrant chronic paronychia of the fingers. Baran R, Bureau H. J Dermatol Surg Oncol 1981; 7: 106–7.

Description of the technique of simple excision of the affected nail fold without the need for marsupialization.

How we treat paronychia. Fliegelman MT, Lafayette GO. Postgrad Med 1970; 48: 267–8.

For recalcitrant cases of chronic paronychia, triamcinolone can be injected into the affected nail fold. For the most severe cases, a course of low-dose superficial radiotherapy may be given.

Periungual Bowen disease mimicking chronic paronychia and diagnosed by dermoscopy. Giacomel J, Lallas A, Zalaudek I, Argenziano G. J Am Acad Dermatol 2014; 71: e65–7.

183

Parvovirus infection

Andrea L. Zaenglein, Joanne E. Smucker

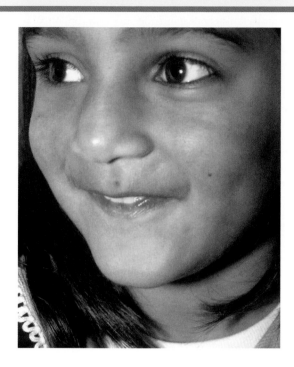

Infection with human parvovirus B19 (HPB19) causes a variety of well-described exanthems and can result in a spectrum of systemic illness. Erythema infectiosum, also known as *fifth disease* according to the original classification of childhood exanthems, is the classic and most common eruption associated with HPB19 infection. Outbreaks occur in the winter and spring and affect school-aged children between 5 and 15 years of age. The infection is transmitted via respiratory droplets. After a short variable prodrome of fever, malaise, diarrhea, and pharyngitis, the classic features of the exanthem appear. Bright pink macular erythema of the cheeks ("slapped cheek sign") together with nasal bridge and circumoral pallor precedes an evanescent macular, reticulated, or "lacelike" rash over the trunk and proximal limbs. The rash may last for up to 4 weeks and subsequently may recur after exposure to sun, warm temperature, and intense physical activity (see figure). Purpuric eruptions, most commonly the papular purpuric gloves-and-socks syndrome (PPGSS), are also reported in association with HBP19. Arthropathy is another common finding, particularly in older patients affected with HPB19. Other systemic manifestations of HBP19 infection include idiopathic thrombocytopenic purpura, hemophagocytic syndrome, lymphadenitis, meningitis and encephalitis, hepatitis, myocarditis, nephritis, and vasculitis. In patients with a predisposing hematologic condition, infection with HPB19 may cause a transient aplastic crisis. Chronic and secondary infections have been encountered in immunosuppressed patients and rarely in immunocompetent patients. Primary infection during pregnancy may place the fetus at risk for severe anemia, thrombocytopenia, hydrops fetalis, neurologic sequelae, and intrauterine fetal demise.

MANAGEMENT STRATEGY

Erythema infectiosum is typically a self-resolving exanthem. In the majority of cases, *supportive care and reassurance* are all that is required. The rash of erythema infectiosum is immune complex mediated so patients are assumed to be no longer infectious by the time that it appears. HPB19 IgG is detectable in the blood once the eruption occurs. Once a clinical diagnosis has been made, parents can be reassured and advised on simple supportive measures such as antipyretics, fluids, and simple emollients for the rash. The condition is self-resolving in the majority of immunocompetent patients.

The clinician should be aware of a variety of other less common cutaneous presentations of HPB19 infection, including both petechial and nonpetechial eruptions. The most common is the PPGSS. This consists of pruritic to painful edema, erythema, and petechiae of the hands and feet with a classic sharp demarcation at the wrist and ankles. This eruption may be seen together with the "slapped cheek" sign. An enanthem may occur with palatal, pharyngeal, labial, and lingual erythema, petechiae, and ulcerations. A diffuse papular exanthem, fever, and other nonspecific viral symptoms may accompany the eruption. PPGSS is seen more often in the spring and summer and typically occurs in adolescents and young adults. Unlike in erythema infectiosum, patients with PPGSS have been reported to be viremic while the rash is present and are thus contagious. The eruption typically resolves within 1 to 2 weeks with simple supportive measures. More generalized petechial eruptions have been reported either primarily or after classic erythema infectiosum. The acropetechial syndrome involves the perioral skin in addition to the hand and foot involvement classically seen in PPGSS. A petechial eruption in a bathing trunk distribution has also been described. Parvovirus should be suspected with all petechial rashes whose origin is undetermined. Asymmetric periflexural exanthema (unilateral lateral thoracic syndrome) and papular acrodermatitis of childhood (Gianotti–Crosti syndrome) have been described after HPB19 infection. HPB19 is also in the differential diagnosis of the "blueberry muffin" baby. Other possible associations with cutaneous manifestations include erythema nodosum, erythema multiforme, livedo reticularis, vasculitis, Sweet syndrome, and Behçet disease.

HPVB19 infection may cause a symmetric arthropathy in many adults, most commonly women, and up to 10% of children. It is similar to rheumatoid arthritis involving the wrists, ankles, knees, and metacarpophalangeal and proximal interphalangeal joints. Arthropathy may accompany the cutaneous eruption but frequently follows it. The arthritis is usually self-limited in both adults and children, requiring only *nonsteroidal antiinflammatory drugs (NSAIDs)* for symptomatic relief. Occasionally the arthritis may lead a more chronic course, and it has been suggested that infection with HPB19 may be a trigger for autoimmune arthritis and connective tissue disease.

HPB19 is extremely tropic for proerythroblasts, granulocytes, and platelets. It binds to globoside on the erythrocyte precursor cell membrane, where it is endocytosed, replicates, and causes cellular apoptosis. In predisposed individuals with either an underlying disorder of hemolysis, decreased erythrocyte production, or active bleeding, HPB19 infection can cause a transient aplastic crisis. This acute anemia may be self-limited and asymptomatic, but *transfusion* may be indicated if severe. In addition to anemia, there may be moderate neutropenia and thrombocytopenia. Potentially fatal marrow necrosis rarely occurs in very young children. Severe cases of transient aplastic crisis not responding to transfusion may require intravenous immunoglobulin (IVIG) and even *bone marrow transplantation*. Chronic HPB19 infection in immunosuppressed patients can result in pure red blood cell aplasia, a form of chronic anemia that results from the inability to create neutralizing antibodies to the virus. This is treated with IVIG, which is often curative. Of interest, parvovirus B19 can contaminate blood products, including bone marrow, and may have the ability to transmit infection through this means. Children who are already anemic due to other causes, such as malaria, malnutrition, or parasites, can become profoundly anemic with HPB19 infection.

Patients with AIDS and chronic anemia secondary to HPB19 infection, who are treated with highly active antiretroviral therapy *(HAART)*, with recovery of CD4 counts, have had resolution of their anemia with documented seroconversion from IgM to IgG antiparvovirus antibodies. Other AIDS patients started on HAART experienced an immune reconstitution syndrome. With the development of renewed immunity, AIDS patients can experience overwhelming systemic involvement of parvovirus, resulting in encephalitis, severe anemia, or other severe sequelae.

Fetal infection with parvovirus B19 may result in mild to severe anemia, thrombocytopenia, high-output congestive heart failure, nonimmune hydrops fetalis, and fetal death. Fetal stroke and other neurologic sequelae have been reported. Fetal infection occurs usually during the first 20 weeks of pregnancy, although third trimester hydrops-related and spontaneous nonhydrops-related fetal demise has been reported. One third or more of women of childbearing age do not have IgG antibodies to HPB19 and are susceptible to primary infection. Vertical transmission occurs in 33% of women, and fetal complications occur in 3% of infected women. Vertical transmission is higher during epidemics. Testing maternal serum for IgM and IgG titers and/or HPB19 DNA with polymerase chain reaction (PCR) analysis should be performed in pregnant women who develop symptoms of HBP19 infection or are in contact with children with a known parvovirus infection. If they have serologic evidence of primary infection, serial fetal ultrasonography should be performed to evaluate for signs of fetal anemia and hydrops fetalis. If hydrops fetalis is present, cordocentesis to confirm the presence of anemia and *intrauterine transfusion* should be strongly considered. Treatment with transfusion is lifesaving in appropriately selected patients and results in favorable long-term neurodevelopmental outcomes. If the pregnancy is near or at term, delivery should be considered. Pregnant women with normal immunity and IgG antibodies to HPB19, or those with a remote history of infection, can be reassured that exposure to HPB19 during pregnancy will not have adverse outcomes on their pregnancy.

Rarely additional systemic involvement, including renal, neurologic, hepatic, respiratory, ocular, and endocrine, has been reported during acute infection with HPB19. Viral myocarditis can also occur, resulting in significant morbidity and mortality, including ventricular dysfunction and heart failure. HPB19 infection can mimic various connective tissue disorders, in particular systemic lupus erythematosus, dermatomyositis, and vasculitis. Infection with HPB19 has also been shown to a play a role in the development of a multitude of chronic conditions, including, but not limited to, other connective tissue disease, hepatitis, nephritis, neurologic disease, and malignancy. However, a causal relationship has not been established.

Specific Investigations

- Hematology (complete blood count)
- Serology

Although most parvovirus infections are diagnosed clinically, there may be instances such as atypical presentations with systemic concerns or new-onset arthropathy of unknown cause where diagnostic testing may be warranted. Serologic testing includes analysis for IgM and IgG antibodies using enzyme-linked immunoassay (ELISA), radioimmunoassay, or immunofluorescence. IgM to HPB19 indicates recent infection. Sensitivity and specificity vary greatly based on the technical skill of the test performer. HPB19-specific IgG antibodies indicate past exposure and may be positive in over half the adult population.

A typical clinical appearance together with supportive serology is sufficient to establish the diagnosis in the majority of cases. In at-risk patients or those who have symptoms of anemia, a complete blood count will establish whether there is any significant level of anemia requiring transfusion.

It is possible to detect parvovirus DNA in both the blood and lesional skin. PCR techniques are considered extremely sensitive and may be useful in the following clinical scenarios: patients with an atypical presentation of HPB19 infection, where the clinical suspicion of infection is high and antibody studies are negative, and in immunocompromised patients who cannot mount an appropriate immunoglobulin response. In addition, a window period exists during the first 7 days after exposure when IgG and IgM are negative, and a second period exists where IgM has become undetectable. PCR may also be helpful during these periods.

Parvovirus B19. Young NS, Brown KE. N Engl J Med 2004; 350: 586–97.

A comprehensive review of HPB19 infection and its manifestations is detailed.

The cutaneous manifestations of human parvovirus B19 infection. Magro CM, Dawood MR, Crowson N. Hum Pathol 2000; 31: 488–97.

This is a description of the cutaneous manifestations in a series of 14 patients who were shown to have antecedent HPB19 infection with positive serology and/or B19 genome in skin samples.

Human parvovirus B19 specific IgG, IgA, and IgM antibodies and DNA in serum specimens from persons with erythema infectiosum. Erdman DD, Usher MJ, Tsou C, Caul EO, Gary GW, Kajigaya S, et al. J Med Virol 1991; 35: 110–5.

A study looking at the efficacy of testing for parvovirus infection with antigen-specific antibodies versus PCR.

First-Line Therapies

• Reassurance	E
• Antipyretics (e.g., acetaminophen [paracetamol], ibuprofen)	E

Human parvoviruses. Schneider E. In: Long S, Pickering L, Prober C, eds. Principles and Practices of Pediatric Infectious Diseases, 4th edn. Philadelphia: Elsevier, 2012; 1087–91.

Most children require no specific therapy. Simple supportive therapies may be used. No antiviral drug or vaccine is available. Viral vaccination is under development.

Second-Line Therapies

• NSAIDs	E
• Systemic corticosteroids	E
• Blood transfusion	C

Evidence Levels: **A** Double-blind study **B** Clinical trial ≥ 20 subjects **C** Clinical trial < 20 subjects **D** Series ≥ 5 subjects **E** Anecdotal case reports

Human parvovirus infection: rheumatic manifestations, angioedema, C1 esterase inhibitor deficiency, ANA positivity and possible onset of systemic lupus erythematosus. Fawaz-Estrup F. J Rheumatol 1996; 23: 1180–5.

A series of nine adult patients with serologic evidence of acute or recent HPB19 infection and polyarthralgia/polyarthritis. All patients responded to NSAIDs, although one patient also required pulsed intravenous methylprednisolone for a lupuslike illness.

In older children and adults the arthralgia/arthritis may be severe enough to warrant treatment with an NSAID. In the majority of cases the joint symptoms settle within a few days or weeks.

Parvoviruses and bone marrow failure. Brown KE, Young NS. Stem Cells 1996; 14: 151–63.

In patients with underlying hemolytic disorders, infection with HPB19 is the primary cause of a transient aplastic crisis, which may require transfusion. In immunocompromised patients, persistent infection may manifest as pure red cell aplasia and chronic anemia.

Third-Line Therapies

• Immunoglobulin infusion	C
• Bone marrow/stem cell transplantation	D
• Intrauterine transfusion	C
• HAART	E

Persistent B19 parvovirus infection in patients infected with human immunodeficiency virus type 1 (HIV-1): a treatable cause of anaemia in AIDS. Frickhofen N, Abkowitz J, Safford M, Berry JM, Antunez-de-Mayolo J, Astrow A, et al. Ann Intern Med 1990; 113: 926–33.

This is a series of seven patients who were HIV positive with persistent HPB19 infection and anemia. Six patients were treated with IVIG and showed rapid reduction in serum virus concentrations and subsequent resolution of their anemia. Two patients relapsed but again responded to further immunoglobulin.

Intravenous immunoglobulin therapy for pure red cell aplasia related to human parvovirus B19 infection: a retrospective study of 10 patients and review of the literature. Crabol Y, Terrier B, Rozenber F, Pestre V, Legendre C, Hermine O, et al. Clin Infect Dis 2013; 56: 968–77.

A review of efficacy of IVIG for therapy of pure red cell aplasia (PRCA) related to HPV-B19 infection. IVIG was found to be effective for short-term use in immunocompromised patients with HPV-B19 PRCA.

Intravenous immunoglobulin treatment of four patients with juvenile polyarticular arthritis associated with persistent parvovirus B19 infection and antiphospholipid antibodies. Lehmann HW, Plentz A, Von Landenberg P, Müller-Godeffroy E, Modrow S. Arthritis Res Ther 2004; 6: R1–6.

A small series of four children with oligoarthritis and polyarthritis and chronic HPB19 infection treated with IVIG (in addition to other therapies) with variable improvement in symptoms and quality-of-life measurements. Dosing for the IVIG was 0.4 g/kg/day for 5 successive days. Two cycles were given 1 month apart.

Mononeuropathy multiplex associated with acute parvovirus B19 infection: characteristics, treatment and outcome. Lenglet T, Haroche J, Schnuriger A, Maisonobe T, Viala K, Michel Y, et al. J Neurol 2011; 258: 1321–6.

The course of three patients with HPB19 virus–positive neuropathy is described. Treatment with IVIG resulted in good but incomplete improvement in symptoms.

Stem cell transplantation in 6 children with parvovirus B19-induced severe aplastic anaemia or myelodysplastic syndrome. Urban C, Lackner H, Müller E, Benesch M, Strenger V, Sovinz P, et al. Klin Padiatr 2011; 223: 332–4.

This is a small series of children infected with HPB19 with resultant refractory bone marrow failure treated with stem cell transplantation.

Parvovirus associated fulminant hepatic failure and aplastic anemia treated successfully with liver and bone marrow transplantation. Bathla L, Grant W, Mercer D, Vargas L, Gebhart C, Langnas A. Am J Transplant 2014; 14: 2645–50.

This is a report of two case reports of children with hepatic failure secondary to HPV-B19 complicated with aplastic anemia who underwent liver transplant and bone marrow transplantation with excellent outcomes.

Fetal morbidity and mortality after acute parvovirus B19 infection in pregnancy: prospective evaluation of 1018 cases. Enders M, Weidner A, Zoellner I, Searle K, Enders G. Prenat Diagn 2004; 24: 513–8.

Survival in fetuses with severe hydrops fetalis after intrauterine transfusion was 84.6% (11/13). All fetuses with severe hydrops who were not transfused died.

Parvovirus B19 in pregnancy: prenatal diagnosis and management of fetal complications. Dijkmans AC, de Jong EP, Dijkmans BA, Lopriore E, Vossen A, Walther FJ. Curr Opin Obstet Gynecol 2012; 24: 95–101.

This is a review of the current approach to women exposed to HPB19 in pregnancy.

Resolution of chronic parvovirus B19 induced anemia, by use of highly active antiretroviral therapy in a patient with acquired immunodeficiency syndrome. Ware M. Clin Infect Dis 2001; 32: E122–3.

A case of an AIDS patient with transfusion-dependent anemia caused by HPB19 that resolved with HAART therapy is reported.

Pediculosis

Hee J. Kim, Jacob O. Levitt

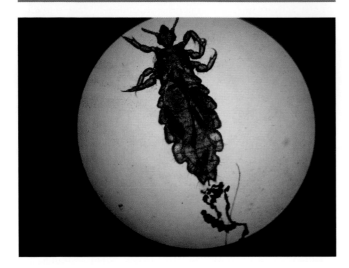

Lice are wingless, dorsoventrally flattened, blood-sucking insects that are obligate ectoparasites of birds and mammals. Pediculosis denotes an infestation by *Pediculus capitis* (head louse), *Pediculus humanus* (body or clothing louse), or *Phthirus pubis* (pubic or crab louse). The bites of lice are painless and can rarely be detected. The clinical signs and symptoms are the result of the host's reaction to the saliva, which has vasodilatory and anticoagulation properties. Saliva is injected into the dermis by the louse at the time of feeding. Depending on immune sensitivity and previous exposure, red macules or papules develop hours to days after feeding. Pruritus is the most common symptom of any type of pediculosis. If left untreated, superinfection of excoriations may lead to impetiginous crusts and regional lymphadenopathy.

PEDICULOSIS CAPITIS

MANAGEMENT STRATEGY

In the United States, an estimated 6 to 12 million people are infested with head lice every year. Children 3 to 12 years old and their parents are most commonly affected. Identification of live lice is the gold standard of diagnosis; however, finding nits alone in a patient who has not been treated warrants treatment. One study showed that around 20% of patients found to have nits alone eventually develop live lice. Nits are easier to spot, especially at the nape of the neck and behind the ears. Hatched nits are white; unhatched nits are brown. Detection combing of wet hair with a fine-toothed nit comb allows efficient recovery of lice and nits for diagnosis.

Management must take into consideration key elements of the head louse life cycle. It takes 4 days to develop a nervous system in the egg, 12 days at most to hatch, and 7 days after hatching for the nymph to lay eggs. Contrary to the direction of most non-ovicidal pediculicides, one retreatment in 7 days will not kill all viable nits. As such, therapies that do not kill

eggs require three weekly treatments. Pediculicides that are ovicidal require two treatments separated by 1 week. Agents that act on the louse nervous system will not affect ova that are less than 4 days old. Lice are sensitive to dehydration but can live off the host for up to 55 hours. Transmission is mainly by direct head-to-head contact. Indirect spread through fomites is also possible. Until definitive safety data are available, the occasional patient under 2 years old should be treated with *mechanical methods*.

Launderable items (worn clothing and used bedding, towels, scarves, and hats) should be *placed in a dryer at 60°C* (i.e., on high) for at least 10 minutes. Brushes, combs, and hair ornaments can be placed in hot (60°C or more) water for 10 minutes. Nonlaunderable items (i.e., certain stuffed animals) should be placed in a bag for 3 days (not 15 days, as eggs laid off a host are unlikely to hatch near a host to obtain their first blood meal). Clothes, furniture, and rugs should be vacuumed. Fumigation of the home is discouraged.

Contacts of index cases, including classmates and family members, *should be screened*. Empiric therapy for close household contacts, particularly if they share a bed, is justifiable. Those likely to have had head-to-head contact with the index case in the prior 4 to 6 weeks should be identified and screened. Children should not be excluded from school for head lice, as the infestation often has been ongoing for months before its detection. Hair grows 1 cm per month, and lice lay eggs close to the scalp where it is moist and warm. Nits detected 2 cm from the scalp represent a 2-month-old infestation. Requiring therapy within a week of the detected infestation is reasonable.

Considerations guiding therapy include safety and efficacy. The efficacy of chemical modalities depends on regional resistance patterns of lice. Because of widespread resistance to permethrin and lindane, *malathion* formulated in isopropyl alcohol with terpineol remains the most effective therapy due to its ovicidal and pediculicidal properties. *Topical ivermectin* lotion and *spinosad topical suspension* have proven to be effective alternatives. A less reliable topical option is *benzyl alcohol lotion*. Alternatives that do not act on the louse nervous system are *mechanical methods* such as louse occlusion, cuticle disruption, and physical removal. Barring shaving the head, these modalities are often unreliable and result in recurrent infestation between treatments and continued infectiveness.

Specific Investigations

- Examination for nits and lice via detection combing
- Dermoscopy

Plastic detection comb better than visual screening for diagnosis of head louse infestation. Balcioglu C, Burgess IF, Limoncu ME, Sahin MT, Ozbel Y, Bilac C, et al. Epidemiol Infect 2008; 136: 1425–31.

Detection combing is 3.84 times more effective than visual inspection for finding live head lice.

Dermoscopy for diagnosis and treatment monitoring of pediculosis capitis. Di Stefani A, Hofmann-Wellenhof R, Zalaudek I. J Am Acad Dermatol 2006; 54: 909–11.

A handheld noncontact dermatoscope can be used to differentiate eggs containing nymphs, empty cases of hatched lice, and

Evidence Levels: **A** Double-blind study **B** Clinical trial ≥ 20 subjects **C** Clinical trial < 20 subjects **D** Series ≥ 5 subjects **E** Anecdotal case reports

pseudo-nits. Treatment success can also be monitored using the dermatoscope.

Therapy for head lice based on life cycle, resistance, and safety considerations. Lebwohl M, Clark L, Levitt J. Pediatrics 2007; 119: 965–74.

This article highlights the importance of designing treatment schedules in accordance with the head lice life cycle. Malathion 0.5% in isopropyl alcohol 78% with terpineol 12% is a safe, resistance-breaking formulation approved by the Food and Drug Administration (FDA) as a first-line treatment for head lice. Two treatments 1 week apart correlate with the head lice life cycle. There is no evidence to suggest that the second application, 1 week later, is unsafe. A single treatment cures 70% to 80% of cases.

Knockdown resistance allele frequencies in North American head louse (Anoplura: Pediculidae) populations. Yoon KS, Previte DJ, Hodgdon HE, Poole BC, Kwon DH, El-Ghar GE, et al. J Med Entomol 2014; 51: 450–7.

A high frequency of kdr–type T917I mutation in head lice is reported: 84.4% in the United States from 1999 to 2009, increased to 99.6% from 2007 to 2009. This is responsible for complete insensitivity of the louse voltage-gated sodium channel to permethrin.

Effectiveness of Ovide against malathion-resistant head lice. Downs AM, Narayan S, Stafford KA, Coles GC. Arch Dermatol 2005; 141: 1318.

In this in vitro study, Ovide (containing malathion, terpineol, and isopropyl alcohol) killed 100% of British head lice resistant to malathion after a 60-minute exposure. Terpineol and malathion appear to be effective in overcoming resistance.

Efficacy of a reduced application time of Ovide lotion (0.5% malathion) compared with Nix crème rinse (1% permethrin) for the treatment of head lice. Meinking TL, Vicaria M, Eyerdam DH, Villar ME, Reyna S, Suarez G. Pediatr Dermatol 2004; 21: 670–4.

Reduced application time (20 minutes) of Ovide cured 98% (40 of 41) of subjects on day 15 compared to Nix (10 minutes), which cured 55% (12 of 22); 19.5% of Ovide patients and 40.9% of Nix patients required a second treatment on day 8. Reinfestation rates were 0% for Ovide and 23% for Nix.

Permethrin 1% obtained approval with well-done studies decades ago; however, resistance has caused permethrin cure rates to decline dramatically.

The clinical trials supporting benzyl alcohol lotion 5% (Ulesfia): a safe and effective topical treatment for head lice (pediculosis humanus capitis). Meinking TL, Villar ME, Vicaria M, Eyerdam DH, Paquet D, Mertz-Rivera K, et al. Pediatr Dermatol 2010; 27: 19–24.

Benzyl alcohol lotion 5% was studied in 695 subjects. Two multicenter, randomized, double-blind, placebo-controlled trials showed a cure rate of ~67% in 126 subjects.

Benzyl alcohol stuns breathing spiracles open, allowing the vehicle to asphyxiate the lice.

Assessment of topical versus oral ivermectin as a treatment for head lice. Ahmad HM, Abdel-Azim ES, Abdel-Aziz RT. Dermatol Ther 2014; 27: 307–10.

This study compared the efficacy of a single topical application of 1% ivermectin solution to a single dose of oral (200 µg/kg per dose) ivermectin. After 1 week, patients who received topical ivermectin had a significantly higher cure rate of 88%. No recurrence of infestation was observed after a 4-week end point.

Topical 0.5% ivermectin lotion for treatment of head lice. Pariser DM, Meinking TL, Bell M, Ryan WG. N Engl J Med 2012; 367: 1687–93.

Two placebo-controlled trials assessing the efficacy of a single 10-minute application of ivermectin lotion without nit combing were conducted in 765 individuals aged 6 months and older. Approximately 79% of subjects remained louse free for 15 days after a single treatment.

Efficacy and safety of spinosad and permethrin creme rinses for pediculosis capitis (head lice). Stough D, Shellabarger S, Quiring J, Gabrielsen AA Jr. Pediatrics 2009; 124: 389–95.

Two investigator-blinded studies compared 0.9% spinosad without nit combing to 1% permethrin with combing in 1038 subjects aged ≥6 months. The efficacy of spinosad (~86%) was statistically superior to permethrin (~44%). Spinosad did not require a combing step, and most patients required one rather than two applications.

Spinosad was more effective than permethrin, which is currently recommended first-line treatment by the American Academy of Pediatrics.

Single application of 4% dimeticone liquid gel versus two applications of 1% permethrin crème rinse for treatment of head louse infestation: a randomized controlled trial. Burgess IF, Brunton ER, Burgess NA. BMC Dermatol 2013; 13: 5.

In this single-center, parallel-group, randomized, controlled, open-label trial, one application of 4% dimeticone liquid gel for 15 minutes had a significantly higher success rate at 77.1% than that of 1% permethrin.

Dimeticone (also known as dimethicone) penetrates the respiratory spiracles of lice and interrupts oxygen supply, leading to organism death.

Randomised, controlled, parallel group clinical trials to evaluate the efficacy of isopropyl myristate/cyclomethicone solution against head lice. Burgess IF, Lee PN, Brown CM. Pharmaceut J 2008; 280: 371–5.

In this randomized, controlled, assessor-blind, parallel-group trial involving 168 subjects with head louse infestation, patients treated with 10-minute single application of isopropyl myristate/cyclomethicone (IPM/C) solution had a significantly higher cure rate of 82% on day 14 compared to those treated with permethrin 1%. IPM/C was easier to apply and less odorous.

A simple treatment for head lice: dry-on, suffocation-based pediculicide. Pearlman DL. Pediatrics 2004; 114: e275–9.

Cetaphil cleanser is applied to the hair and dried with a hair dryer, followed by nit combing. This is repeated three times at intervals of a week apart. A total of 133 patients were studied; 96% efficacy is claimed.

1,2-Octanediol, a novel surfactant, for treating head louse infestation: identification of activity, formulation, and randomised, controlled trials. Burgess IF, Lee PN, Kay K, Jones R, Brunton ER. PLoS One 2012; 7: e35419.

In this observer-blinded study of 520 subjects, the cure rate of an application of 1,2-octanediol 5% lotion was 70.9% for 2 to 2.5 hours and 87.9% for 8 hours/overnight, both more effective than 0.5% malathion liquid.

Octanediol eliminates lice by disrupting the insect's cuticular lipid and causing dehydration.

Tocopheryl acetate 20% spray for elimination of head louse infestation: a randomised controlled trial comparing with 1% permethrin creme rinse. Burgess IF, Burgess NA, Brunton ER. BMC Pharmacol Toxicol 2013; 14: 43.

Two treatments, 7 days apart, with tocopheryl acetate 20% spray (applied to dry hair for 20 minutes and then washed), had a cure rate of 73.9% (17/23) compared to 22.7% (5/22) with permethrin 1% crème rinse.

Tocopheryl acetate immobilizes lice and inhibits eggs from hatching via physical mechanism of action.

A single application of crotamiton lotion in the treatment of patients with pediculosis capitis. Karaci I, Yawalkar SJ. Int J Dermatol 1982; 21: 611–3.

Forty-seven of 49 subjects were cured with one application of crotamiton 10% lotion, and all were cured with a second application in 1 week.

The trial was open label and never independently validated.

A randomised, assessor blind, parallel group comparative efficacy trial of three products for the treatment of head lice in children—melaleuca oil and lavender oil, pyrethrins and piperonyl butoxide, and a "suffocation" product. Barker SC, Altman PM. BMC Dermatol 2010; 10: 6.

Cure rates were as follows: melaleuca (tea tree) oil and lavender oil (41/42; 98%); NeutraLice, a suffocation product (40/41; 98%); products containing pyrethrins and piperonyl butoxide (10/40; 25%).

Single blind, randomised, comparative study of the Bug Buster kit and over the counter pediculicide treatments against head lice in the United Kingdom. Hill N, Moor G, Cameron MM, Butlin A, Preston S, Williamson MS, et al. Br Med J 2005; 331: 384–7.

A cure rate of 57% (32/56) is reported for wet combing with conditioner in four sessions over 13 days.

Nit combing can be painful and time consuming but may be worthwhile for treatment of lice that are resistant to pharmacotherapy.

Third-Line Therapies	
• Oral ivermectin	A
• Oral trimethoprim–sulfamethoxazole	B
• Oral levamisole	B
• Albendazole 2% suspension	E
• Desiccation	B
• Head shaving	E

Lindane toxicity: a comprehensive review of the medical literature. Nolan K, Kamrath J, Levitt J. Pediatr Dermatol 2012; 29: 141–6.

Lindane has been associated with significant adverse reactions, including death, seizures, shortness of breath, and hematologic effects. Lindane has been banned in some U.S. states, including California and Michigan. It is no longer recommended for use in children younger than 10 years old, those weighing less than 50 kg, breastfeeding women, older adults, or people with compromised dermal barriers.

Given the significant toxicity associated with lindane and the availability of other safer treatments, lindane should be avoided.

Oral ivermectin versus malathion lotion for difficult-to-treat head lice. Chosidow O, Giraudeau B, Cottrell J, Izri A, Hofmann R, Mann SG, et al. N Engl J Med 2010; 362: 896–905.

This multicenter, cluster-randomized, double-blind, controlled trial conducted in 812 patients compared oral ivermectin (at a dose of 400 µg/kg body weight) with 0.5% malathion lotion, each given on days 1 and 8. Included were subjects who had live lice resistant to topical insecticide used 2 to 6 weeks prior to enrollment. In the intention-to-treat population, 95.2% of patients who received oral ivermectin were lice free on day 15, compared to 85.0% in those who used topical malathion. Oral ivermectin had superior efficacy without increase in side effects.

Safety studies of oral ivermectin in children are lacking.

Head lice infestation: single drug versus combination therapy with 1% permethrin and trimethoprim/sulfamethoxazole. Hipolito RB, Mallorca FG, Zuniga-Macaraig ZO, Apolinario PC, Wheeler-Sherman J. Pediatrics 2001; 107: E30.

Permethrin (1%) and trimethoprim (10 mg/kg/day divided BID)–sulfamethoxazole cured 38 of 40 (95%) of subjects by week 2. TMP–SMX monotherapy was 83% effective, and permethrin monotherapy was 79.5% effective.

Levamisole: a safe and economical weapon against pediculosis. Namazi MR. Int J Dermatol 2001; 40: 292–4.

Levamisole administered in a dose of 3.5 mg/kg for 10 days cured 67% (18/28) of children with head lice.

Treatment of pediculosis capitis with topical albendazole. Ayoub N, Maatouk I, Merhy M, Tomb R. J Dermatolog Treat 2012; 23: 78–80.

Four patients were successfully treated with topical albendazole 2% suspension.

Efficacy of the LouseBuster, a new medical device for treating head lice (Anoplura: Pediculidae). Bush SE, Rock AN, Jones SL, Malenke JR, Clayton DH. J Med Entomol 2011; 48: 67–72.

LouseBuster is a medical device designed to kill head lice in all life stages by delivering heated air (59 ± 1.5°C) at two to three times greater airflow than a regular blow dryer. After 30-min treatment, mortality of lice and eggs was ~94% for both experienced and novice operators.

PEDICULOSIS CORPORIS

MANAGEMENT STRATEGY

Because body lice live in the seams of clothing, treatment revolves around laundering of clothes and bedding in high heat (>60°C) for at least 10 minutes. Infested mattresses should be abandoned for 3 weeks. Given that resistance patterns in head lice follow those of body lice, topical malathion, carbaryl, and permethrin are good first choices. Oral ivermectin is another alternative. All household contacts should be treated. Patients should be monitored for symptoms of louseborne illnesses, specifically epidemic typhus (*Ricketssia prowazekii*), relapsing fever (*Borrelia recurrentis*), and trench fever (*Bartonella quintana*).

First-Line Therapies	
• Laundering of clothes and bedding	E
• Personal hygiene	E
• Malathion 0.5% lotion	E
• Permethrin 5% cream	E
• Oral ivermectin	B

Human lice and their management. Burgess IF. Adv Parasitol 1995; 36: 271–342.

A comprehensive review of human lice is provided. For body lice, laundering of clothing is stressed, and the use of pediculicides on the patient is questioned. In mass eradication, fomites can be dusted with malathion or permethrin.

Given the safety of topical therapy, two treatments applied for 8 to 12 hours 1 week apart outweigh the risk of stray lice on the host reestablishing infestation.

Oral ivermectin in the treatment of body lice. Foucault C, Ranque S, Badiaga S, Rovery C, Raoult D, Brouqui P. J Infect Dis 2006; 193: 474–6.

Administration of three doses of oral ivermectin 12 mg with a 7-day interval decreased the prevalence of subjects infested with body lice from 84.9% to 18.5% over a 14-day period. However, this effect was not sustained on day 45 after treatment. More studies need to be conducted to evaluate the efficacy of oral ivermectin.

PEDICULOSIS PUBIS

MANAGEMENT STRATEGY

Crab lice commonly affect pubic (mons and perianal), thigh, chest, and axillary hair, eyelashes, and rarely, scalp hair. Pediculicide should be applied to these areas to ensure eradication, and repeat application is recommended after 7 days. Eyelash infestation should be treated separately (see later). Household contacts and sexual partners of the prior month should be treated. Fomites should be laundered as for head lice. Screening for other sexually transmitted diseases is advised.

First-Line Therapies	
• Malathion 0.5% lotion	E
• Permethrin 1% crème rinse	B
• Permethrin 5% cream	E
• Pyrethrin 0.33% with piperonyl butoxide shampoo	E
• Oral ivermectin 200 µg/kilogram	E

Scabies and pediculosis pubis: an update of treatment regimens and general review. Leone PA. Clin Infect Dis 2007; 44 (Suppl 3): S153–9.

A comprehensive review of scabies and pediculosis pubis is provided. No significant treatment failure of pediculosis pubis has been reported since 1996. One study reported in vitro pubic lice resistance to pyrethrins; however, it was susceptible to permethrin 5% lotion. Lindane 1% shampoo is no longer recommended due to its toxicity.

PHTHIRIASIS PALPEBRARUM

MANAGEMENT STRATEGY

Phthiriasis palpebrarum is an infestation of the eyelashes by crab lice. In children, the infested mother is often the source of infestation. Patients should be treated with application of either permethrin 1% lotion for at least 10 minutes or an occlusive ointment such as petroleum jelly twice a day for 10 days. Alternatives include yellow mercuric oxide, physostigmine 1% eye ointment, and mechanical removal. Treatment of household and sexual contacts and fomites is warranted.

First-Line Therapies	
• Petroleum jelly	E
• Permethrin 1% lotion	E
• Yellow mercuric oxide 1% ointment	B
• Mechanical lice and nit removal	E
• Physostigmine 0.25% or 1% ointment	E

Yellow mercuric oxide: a treatment of choice for phthiriasis palpebrarum. Ashkenazi I, Desatnik HR, Abraham FA. Br J Ophthalmol 1991; 75: 356–8.

Yellow mercuric oxide 1% ointment was applied four times daily for 14 days in 35 patients with phthiriasis palpebrarum. Complete eradication of lice and eggs was reported.

Pediculosis ciliaris. Chin GN, Denslow GT. J Pediatr Ophthalmol Strabismus 1978; 15: 173–5.

Physostigmine 1% ointment applied to eyelid margins twice a day for 14 days is reported. Other suggestions for therapy include (1) thick application of petroleum jelly twice a day for 8 days; (2) mechanical removal of lice and nits with forceps and cotton-tipped swabs followed by application of yellow oxide of mercury 1% to 2% ointment twice a day for 1 week; or (3) cryotherapy.

Second-Line Therapies

- Argon laser   E
- Cryotherapy   E
- Gamma benzene hexachloride   E
- Oral ivermectin   E

Oral ivermectin therapy for phthiriasis palpebrum. Burkhart CN, Burkhart CG. Arch Ophthalmol 2000; 118: 134–5.

A single case of oral ivermectin use in lash pediculosis.

Evidence Levels: **A** Double-blind study   **B** Clinical trial ≥ 20 subjects   **C** Clinical trial < 20 subjects   **D** Series ≥ 5 subjects   **E** Anecdotal case reports

185

Pemphigus

Daniel Mimouni, Grant J. Anhalt

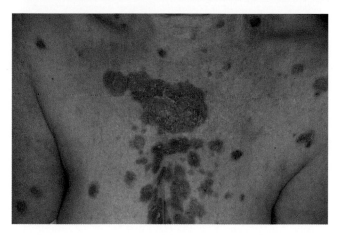

Pemphigus is an autoimmune blistering disease of the skin with an established immunologic basis but unknown etiology. Its histologic hallmark is the loss of cell-to-cell adhesion (acantholysis) mediated by autoantibodies to epidermal cell surface proteins. Pemphigus has three major variants: pemphigus vulgaris, pemphigus foliaceus, and paraneoplastic pemphigus, which are differentiated by the presence/absence of intraepithelial blisters and erosions of the skin and variable involvement of the mucous membranes. Their associated risks of morbidity and mortality vary greatly

Specific Investigations

- Skin biopsy for routine microscopy
- Skin biopsy for direct immunofluorescence
- Serum for indirect immunofluorescence
- Enzyme-linked immunoassay (ELISA) for antibodies to desmoglein 1 and/or desmoglein 3
- Malignancy screening tests in patients with paraneoplastic pemphigus

Making sense of antigens and antibodies in pemphigus. Anhalt GJ. J Am Acad Dermatol 1999; 40: 763–6.

Accuracy of indirect immunofluorescence testing in the diagnosis of paraneoplastic pemphigus. Helou J, Allbritton J, Anhalt GJ. J Am Acad Dermatol 1995; 32: 441–7.

The diagnosis of pemphigus is established by the fulfillment of three criteria; if one is missing, the diagnosis is uncertain:

- Appropriate clinical features
- Histologic changes showing acantholysis of affected epithelium
- Demonstration of IgG autoantibodies on the cell surface of affected epithelium or detection of antigen-specific autoantibodies in the blood

Pemphigus vulgaris is characterized by progressively evolving fragile blisters and erosions. Oral involvement essentially "always" occurs and is the major point to differentiate pemphigus

vulgaris from pemphigus foliaceus. Histologic changes include suprabasilar acantholysis and cell surface–bound IgG. Circulating autoantibodies are specific for desmoglein 3 alone when lesions are restricted to the mouth and for both desmoglein 3 and 1 when cutaneous lesions are present in addition to oral lesions. Definition of the specificity of desmoglein autoantibodies can be reliably gained by ELISA.

In pemphigus foliaceus, mucosal lesions "never" occur. This is the major clinical feature differentiating pemphigus foliaceus from pemphigus vulgaris. The cutaneous lesions are superficial scaling erosions. Immunopathologic studies reveal subcorneal acantholysis and tissue-bound and circulating antidesmoglein 1 antibodies.

Paraneoplastic pemphigus occurs in the context of several lymphoproliferative disorders: non-Hodgkin lymphoma, chronic lymphocytic leukemia, Castleman disease, thymoma, and retroperitoneal sarcoma. Intractable mucositis with lichenoid erosions is the most constant clinical finding. Polymorphous cutaneous involvement with lesions that resemble erythema multiforme, pemphigus, pemphigoid, or lichenoid eruptions is observed. Histologic study shows suprabasilar acantholysis or interface/lichenoid changes. The key diagnostic finding is the presence of antibodies against desmoglein 3 and 1 and additional autoantibodies against epithelial plakin proteins, such as desmoplakin, envoplakin, and periplakin, which may be identified by immunoblotting or immunoprecipitation techniques. They may also be inferred with immunofluorescent techniques showing their reactivity with murine bladder epithelium, although the lichenoid variant of paraneoplastic pemphigus has been occasionally reported with the complete absence of the characteristic autoantibodies.

MANAGEMENT STRATEGY

If pemphigus vulgaris is not treated definitively and promptly, the process "hardens," leading to epitope spreading, which makes the disease more difficult to control. Even if the initial presentation is limited, without systemic treatment, it will generalize. Animal studies have clearly shown that once enough autoantibody reaches the skin, blistering will occur, and this damage cannot be prevented by antiinflammatory agents or even pretreatment with high doses of *systemic corticosteroids*. Topical treatment of the mucous membranes or skin has no significant effect on the course of the disease, though *topical corticosteroids* or *intralesional injections of corticosteroids* may temporarily relieve pain and inflammation.

Other factors complicate management and include the following:

1. **Circulating autoantibodies have a degradative half-life of about 3 weeks. Lasting improvement can only occur with reduction of both existing and newly produced antibody, so improvement occurs very slowly unless the antibodies are physically removed by plasmapheresis, or their catabolism is increased by administration of high doses of exogenous normal human immunoglobulins (IVIG).**
2. **Pemphigus is notorious for its persistence. Spontaneous remissions typically do not occur, and remissions and relapses are common. Most people require some form of treatment for life.**
   Only a small repertoire of drugs is effective in reducing autoantibody synthesis, but these drugs are limited by high cost and potential toxicities.
3. **All forms of pemphigus are rare, precluding the performance of large controlled trials. The medical literature discussing**

therapeutic regimens is dominated by small series and case reports, which provide only a weak evidence base for the design of rational therapeutic regimens. However, there are excellent animal models of pemphigus, which have given clinicians a good understanding of the pathophysiology of the disease and are instrumental in the formulation of the treatment approach.

Thus the primary goal of treatment in all forms of pemphigus is to reduce the synthesis of autoantibodies by the immune system. It currently consists of three basic steps:

1. Administration of *rituximab* with systemic corticosteroids with the additional use of IVIG
2. Administration of *rituximab* with systemic corticosteroids plus an antimetabolite such as *azathioprine* or *mycophenolate mofetil (MMF)*
3. If rituximab is not applicable, corticosteroids plus cyclophosphamide with a possible addition of short-term plasmapheresis

The commitment to the use of cyclophosphamide is a serious one. This drug is extremely effective, but use of this alkylating agent is accompanied by short-term leucopenia and a long-term increased risk of leukemia, lymphoma, and bladder cancer, as well as the risk of sterility in younger patients. The increasing use of rituximab is being explored as a way to avert having to use cyclophosphamide.

All types of pemphigus are rare, making large controlled trials difficult to perform. The medical literature on therapeutic regimens is dominated by small series and case reports, which provide a weak evidence base for the design of rational treatment. Some studies have suggested other potential drugs, but they cannot yet be applied because the mechanism whereby they might effectively inhibit new antibody synthesis is unknown. This list includes tetracycline and niacin (nicotinamide), methotrexate, dapsone, and gold. A well-performed randomized trial showed no corticosteroid-sparing benefit of ciclosporin. It is therefore not recommended for the treatment of pemphigus vulgaris, although it may still play a role in the treatment of paraneoplastic pemphigus.

First-Line Therapies

Pemphigus vulgaris and foliaceus

• Systemic corticosteroids	B
• Rituximab	D

Pemphigus: a 20 year review of 107 patients treated with corticosteroids. Rosenberg FR, Sanders S, Nelson CT. Arch Dermatol 1976; 112: 962–70.

The first-line therapy for all forms of pemphigus is systemic corticosteroids. Corticosteroids work relatively quickly and are relatively safe when used in appropriate doses for limited periods. In the past, regimens of rapidly accelerating doses of corticosteroids were administered, but they were found to be associated with unacceptably high morbidity and mortality risks. Initial treatment should start at 1 mg/kg daily (lean body weight). A good clinical response, defined as a resolution of the majority of existing lesions and absence of newly developing lesions, should be evident within 2 to 3 months. The dose should then be reduced to 40 mg daily and subsequently tapered over 6 to 9 months, ideally to a maintenance dose of 5 mg

every other day. Tapering can be accomplished by reducing the prednisone by an average of 10 mg per month initially and 5 mg per month later. There are some advantages to beginning an alternate-dose regimen at 40 mg daily so that monthly reductions would ideally be 40/20 mg alternate days, 40/0 mg, 30/0 mg, 20/0 mg, 15/0 mg, and 10/0 mg and then 5/0 mg alternate days for maintenance.

In recent years there is more evidence that the addition of rituximab early in the course of the disease provides a safe and extremely effective treatment that allows an accelerated tapering of systemic corticosteroids, minimizing their devastating side effects.

The use of a second-line therapy is certainly indicated if significant corticosteroid side effects develop or are expected to develop during the ideal prednisone taper, if the disease does not improve sufficiently to allow continuous tapering, or the disease flares. With the introduction of better tolerated drugs such as MMF, it is reasonable to use a second agent from the start of therapy in all patients with moderate to severe disease from the start of therapy, in anticipation of steroid-sparing benefits.

Monthly pulse corticosteroids have been suggested as a less toxic alternative to daily oral therapy, but pemphigus is very persistent, and more consistent daily or alternate-day dosing is usually required to achieve suppression.

Patients must be monitored for corticosteroid-induced osteopenia by bone mineral density studies (DEXA scan) at the institution of therapy and annually thereafter. Patients without a history of renal calculi may be given prophylactic supplemental calcium 1500 mg daily and vitamin D 400 to 800 IU daily. In patients with osteopenia or osteoporosis, additional therapies may include hormonal replacement in women (estrogen/progesterone or raloxifene in those with a contraindication for estrogens, such as a history of breast carcinoma) or exogenous testosterone in men with low serum testosterone levels or a bisphosphonate such as alendronate or intranasal calcitonin.

In pemphigus vulgaris, therapy as outlined should commence in all patients once the diagnosis is confirmed. Even in cases with limited oral lesions, the disease will progress unless treated with systemic agents, and palliative therapy with topical agents or intralesional injections just delays definitive therapy. There is clinical evidence that early intervention with definitive treatment leads to a better long-term outcome. In pemphigus foliaceus, however, not every patient requires immediate treatment. Some patients have a very limited and smoldering disease and can therefore benefit from palliative treatment, such as topical corticosteroids. In cases of slowly progressive disease one can also consider the use of rituximab as monotherapy. Paraneoplastic pemphigus is usually relentlessly progressive, justifying the immediate institution of systemic corticosteroids and a second-line treatment. If a patient has an associated benign lymphoproliferative disorder, such as thymoma, hyaline vascular Castleman disease, or sarcoma, complete surgical removal should be attempted to prolong disease remission.

Successful treatment of pemphigus with biweekly one gram infusions of rituximab: a retrospective study of 47 patients. Leshem YA, Hodak E, David M, Anhalt GJ, Mimouni D. J Am Acad Dermatol 2013; 68: 404–11.

The aim of this study was to assess the clinical response of patients with pemphigus to a single cycle of rituximab at the dosage used in rheumatoid arthritis (RA) and to evaluate the response to repeated cycles of rituximab. Remission rates after the first treatment cycle reached 76%. Repeating the treatment further increased the remission rates to 91%. There was a 22% relapse rate at a median time of 8 months, but 75% of relapsing patients achieved remission again with additional cycles.

Evidence Levels: A Double-blind study B Clinical trial ≥ 20 subjects C Clinical trial < 20 subjects D Series ≥ 5 subjects E Anecdotal case reports

Treatment of refractory pemphigus vulgaris with rituximab (anti-CD20 monoclonal antibody). Dupuy A, Viguier M, Bedane C, Cordoliani F, Blaise S, Aucouturier F, et al. Arch Dermatol 2004; 140: 91–6.

A single cycle of rituximab for the treatment of severe pemphigus. Joly P, Mouquet H, Roujeau JC, D'Incan M, Gilbert D, Jacquot S, et al. N Engl J Med 2007; 357: 545–53.

Twenty-one patients with pemphigus that was refractory to corticosteroids (at least two relapses despite prednisone treatment with doses higher than 20 mg per day; corticosteroid-dependent disease) or who had severe contraindications to corticosteroids were treated with four weekly infusions of rituximab, 375 mg/m^2 body surface area. Eighteen showed complete remission at 3 months.

Efficacy of rituximab for pemphigus: a systematic review and meta-analysis of different regimens. Wang H, Wei Liu C, Li Y, Huang Y. Acta Derm Venereol 2015; 95: 928–32.

This meta-analysis examined the efficacy of different dosing regimens containing rituximab in treating pemphigus. The analysis included 578 patients with pemphigus from 30 studies. Seventy-six percent of patients achieved complete remission after one cycle of rituximab. No superiority of lymphoma protocol over RA or high-dose rituximab over low-dose rituximab was shown in outcome.

Durable remission of pemphigus with a fixed-dose rituximab protocol. Heelan K, Al-Mohammedi F, Smith MJ , Knowles S, Lansang P, Walsh S, et al. JAMA Dermatol 2014; 150: 703–8.

Ninety-two patients received rituximab. Complete remission rates with or without adjuvant treatment at final follow-up were 89%. No serious infectious adverse events occurred.

Subcutaneous veltuzumab, a humanized anti-CD20 antibody, in the treatment of refractory pemphigus vulgaris. Ellebrecht CT, Choi EJ, Allman DM, Tsai DE, Wegener WA, Goldenberg DM, et al. JAMA Dermatol 2014; 150: 1331–5.

Veltuzumab, a second-generation humanized anti-CD20 antibody, was administered as two 320-mg (188 mg/m^2) subcutaneous doses 2 weeks apart to a patient with refractory pemphigus vulgaris, resulting in complete remission of disease off therapy for 2 years. No serious adverse events occurred during 35 months of follow-up.

Depletion of CD20+ B cells by the use of anti-CD20 monoclonal antibody is emerging as a potentially powerful tool in many autoimmune diseases and is approved for use in RA. CD20 is not expressed on pre-B cells or plasma cells, so it is not profoundly immunosuppressive, and the effect only lasts 6 to 10 months, as the CD20+ cells are repopulated from stem cells. Currently approved dosing is 375 mg/m2 weekly × 4 for lymphoma or 1000 mg × 2, days 1 and 15, for RA. The original dosing regimen for lymphoma was designed to prevent tumor lysis syndrome in patients with bulky lymphomas. The authors have used the simpler, lower dose RA schedule in a small number of pemphigus vulgaris patients with equivalent efficacy. Toxicity of rituximab is minimal, but the addition of the drug to patients already exposed to corticosteroids and immunosuppressive drugs increases the risk of infection, including one reported fatal case of Pneumocystis jirovecii (formerly known as carinii) pneumonia (PJP) in a patient treated with rituximab and cyclophosphamide. PJP prophylaxis should be considered with the use of this drug. The drug can cause rapid reduction of autoantibody levels in even severely affected cases, with excellent results and often dramatic recoveries. It is possible that a second course of rituximab has an important consolidation role for durable remission. The addition of IVIG to rituximab is reasonable in explosive acute cases; however, according to the current studies its added value in less acute cases is questionable. Rituximab is used most commonly in paraneoplastic pemphigus, where it has a dual role of treating the underlying lymphoproliferative disease as well as the associated autoimmune disease.

Second-Line Therapies	
• MMF	B
• Azathioprine	C
• High-dose IVIG	C

Treatment of pemphigus vulgaris and foliaceus with mycophenolate mofetil. Mimouni D, Anhalt GJ, Cummins DL, Kouba DJ, Thorne JE, Nousari HC. Arch Dermatol 2003; 139: 739–42.

Forty-two patients were treated with MMF, 1.5 g twice daily, and standard prednisone therapy. Complete clinical remission was defined as achieving no new lesions with prednisone doses less than 10 mg daily. This was achieved in 70% of patients with pemphigus vulgaris and 55% of patients with pemphigus foliaceus. Therapy was discontinued in only two cases due to adverse effects—one secondary to febrile neutropenia and one for gastrointestinal intolerance.

For pemphigus vulgaris and foliaceus, two effective antimetabolite immunosuppressive drugs are azathioprine and MMF. Mycophenolate has an excellent safety profile, but it is very expensive. Azathioprine appears to be equally effective and is much cheaper, but has much more frequent toxicities. These drugs are added to the systemic corticosteroids, if the indications for their use are met. Once their beneficial effect is observed, the corticosteroids should be progressively tapered, while the second agent is used at full doses for up to 2 to 3 years to induce a durable remission. For both drugs, the doses required are greater than those needed to control other cutaneous diseases because only at high doses does one observe the required inhibition of the synthesis of autoantibodies by B cells.

MMF has approval for two dosing schedules: 1000 mg PO BID in renal transplantation, and 1500 mg PO BID in cardiac transplants. Both dosing regimens have been used in pemphigus, but there is insufficient evidence to recommend one over the other. Onset of action is slow, and remissions are observed in responders after 2 to 12 months of therapy. Monitoring of complete blood count and liver enzymes should be performed monthly, but cytopenias and hepatotoxicity are rarely observed. Some lymphopenia without neutropenia is common but has no adverse consequences and can correlate with a good clinical effect. Some nausea and diarrhea can occur but improve with dosage reduction. Avoidance of pregnancy is mandatory, as human fetal malformations have occurred with its use.

Azathioprine in the treatment of pemphigus vulgaris. A long term follow-up. Aberer W, Wolff-Schreiner EC, Stingl G, Wolff K. J Am Acad Dermatol 1987; 16: 527–33.

Azathioprine is given in a single daily dose of 3 to 4 mg/kg. At this dose, there is a risk of neutropenia, thrombocytopenia, hepatotoxicity, and severe or debilitating nausea. Monitoring should consist of complete blood count and liver enzymes, initially every 2 weeks. Patients with thiopurine methyltransferase deficiency (TPMT) cannot metabolize the drug effectively and can develop severe pancytopenia during the first 2 months of therapy. Late effects include elevation of liver enzymes and drug fever. The drug also requires 6 to 8 weeks of therapy before its effect on the disease can be judged. The drug is quite effective, but even if one screens patients for TPMT deficiency before starting treatment, the incidence of side effects is greater than with mycophenolate. It is still a useful second-line agent for those who cannot afford mycophenolate. There is also concern that exposure to this drug can increase one's lifetime risk of leukemia or lymphoma, but the risk is very much less than that associated with the use of alkylating agents.

A comparison of oral methylprednisolone plus azathioprine or mycophenolate mofetil for the treatment of pemphigus. Beissert S, Werfel T, Frieling U, Böhm M, Sticherling M, Stadler R, et al. Arch Dermatol 2006; 142: 1447–54.

A prospective, multicenter, randomized, nonblinded clinical trial to compare two parallel groups of patients with pemphigus treated with oral methylprednisolone plus azathioprine or oral methylprednisolone plus MMF. In 13 (72%) of 18 patients with pemphigus receiving oral methylprednisolone and azathioprine, complete remission was achieved after a mean 74 days compared with 20 (95%) of 21 patients receiving oral methylprednisolone and MMF in whom complete remission occurred after a mean 91 days. In 6 (33%) of 18 patients treated with azathioprine, severe adverse effects were documented in contrast to 4 (19%) of 21 patients who received MMF.

Randomized controlled open-label trial of four treatment regimens for pemphigus vulgaris. Chams-Davatchi C, Esmaili N, Daneshpazhooh M, Valikhani M, Balighi K, Hallaji Z, et al. J Am Acad Dermatol 2007; 57: 622–8.

The aim of this randomized study was to compare the efficacy and safety of four treatment regimens for new-onset pemphigus vulgaris (*n* = 121): prednisolone alone, prednisolone plus azathioprine, prednisolone plus mycophenolate mofetil, and prednisolone plus intravenous cyclophosphamide pulse therapy. Results after 1 year were better with adjuvant treatment than with corticosteroid treatment alone. The highest efficacy was noted for azathioprine, followed by cyclophosphamide (pulse therapy), and mycophenolate mofetil. Interestingly, there were no significant differences in side effects among the groups.

High-dose intravenous immune globulin for the treatment of autoimmune blistering diseases. Harman KE, Black MM. Br J Dermatol 1999; 140: 865–74.

Treatment of pemphigus with intravenous immunoglobulin. Bystryn JC, Jiao D, Natow S. J Am Acad Dermatol 2002: 358; 358–63.

Both studies used IVIG in addition to treatment with prednisone and immunosuppressive therapy. IVIG produced a rapid reduction of circulating autoantibody levels, which was accompanied by significant clinical improvement in some cases.

High-dose IVIG can be used for acute control of active pemphigus. This treatment seems to accelerate the catabolism of the autoantibody and reduce circulating levels as effectively as plasmapheresis. It is generally safe and well tolerated but has some risk. A small number of patients can develop thrombotic complications such as deep venous thrombosis or stroke. It is enormously expensive (as much as $12,000 per treatment for a 70-kg patient) and may lose its effectiveness after repeated treatment cycles. It can be given intravenously at a dose of 2 g/kg body weight, infused in divided doses over 2 to 5 days monthly.

IVIG is used frequently for acute control of severe cases. It can provide disease control for several months while slower acting drugs such as MMF are used and is safer than plasmapheresis. It can also be used effectively in combination with rituximab. The use of IVIG for extended periods to induce a remission is more controversial and requires better data.

Third-Line Therapies	
• Cyclophosphamide	B
• Cyclophosphamide plus plasmapheresis	E
• Chlorambucil	D

Dexamethasone-cyclophosphamide pulse therapy for pemphigus. Pasricha JS, Khaitan BK, Raman RS, Chandra M. Int J Dermatol 1995; 34: 875–82.

Alkylating agents such as cyclophosphamide have a profound effect on inhibition of autoantibody synthesis and are the most effective agents for inducing remission. They also have very significant potential toxicities, which restrict their use to third-line therapy. In countries where the high cost of rituximab limits its use, cyclophosphamide is still frequently used.

Cyclophosphamide is the preferred agent because any neutropenia associated with its use is predictable in onset, and withdrawal of the drug results in rapid recovery of neutrophils (within 1 week to 10 days). There are four ways to administer the drug:

1. **Daily orally at 2.5 mg/kg. A single morning dose is followed by aggressive fluid consumption throughout the day to rinse metabolites from the bladder and prevent hemorrhagic cystitis. Weekly complete blood counts and urinalysis are required. With this use, a durable remission can be obtained after 18 to 24 months of therapy in almost all cases. This exposure probably increases the patient's lifetime risk of leukemia, lymphoma, or bladder cancer by as much as 5% to 10% over the normal population. This risk is appreciated some 20 to 30 years after treatment. Such treatment can also cause sterility in young patients.**
2. **Monthly intravenous pulses at a dose of 750 mg/m² body surface area. Monthly intravenous administration reduces the risk of hemorrhagic cystitis, but this intermittent use is not as effective in suppressing the disease.**
3. **Monthly intravenous administration with lower dose oral daily maintenance. This can also be very effective in inducing a remission.**
4. **Single, very high-dose immunoablative therapy. This experimental treatment is effective in many autoimmune diseases. It employs a dose of intravenous cyclophosphamide of 200 mg/kg, given over 4 days, which induces profound marrow aplasia. Upon recovery, the patients often experience a complete remission. However, unlike the experience with disorders such as aplitic anemia, where remission may last many years, most patients with pemphigus relapse within 2 years of completion of therapy, limiting its usefulness.**

Synchronization of plasmapheresis and pulse cyclophosphamide therapy in pemphigus vulgaris. Euler HH, Loffler H, Christophers E. Arch Dermatol 1987; 123: 1205–10.

Plasmapheresis is the only method by which one can rapidly reduce autoantibody levels and is used in patients with very extensive and accelerated disease. Its use involves a total of six high-volume removals (3–3.5 L per removal, three times weekly for 2 consecutive weeks). This must be combined with the concomitant use of systemic corticosteroids and oral or pulse cyclophosphamide. If these drugs are not used, the reduction of autoantibodies removes feedback inhibition to the autoimmune B cells and causes a rebound flare of the disease. This can be blunted only by alkylating agents due to their preferential toxicity to rapidly proliferative B cells. This causes the induction of a durable remission, though cyclophosphamide must still be used at full doses for 18 to 24 months to harden that remission.

Evidence Levels: **A** Double-blind study **B** Clinical trial ≥ 20 subjects **C** Clinical trial < 20 subjects **D** Series ≥ 5 subjects **E** Anecdotal case reports

The use of chlorambucil with prednisone in the treatment of pemphigus. Shah N, Green AR, Elgart GW, Kerdel F. J Am Acad Dermatol 2000; 42: 85–8.

In patients who develop hemorrhagic cystitis from cyclophosphamide, chlorambucil can be substituted.

Chlorambucil is more difficult to use because the cytopenias induced by it are more unpredictable and when they occur may take months to resolve.

Ineffectiveness of ciclosporin as an adjuvant to corticosteroids in the treatment of pemphigus. Ioannides D, Chrysomallis F, Bystryn JC. Arch Dermatol 2000; 868: 505–6.

Thirty-three consecutive patients hospitalized with pemphigus vulgaris (*n* = 29) or foliaceus (*n* = 4) were randomized to receive either prednisolone or prednisolone plus ciclosporin, 5 mg/kg daily. The groups were similar in terms of disease severity and demographics. The addition of ciclosporin produced no change in the response to treatment or the total dose of corticosteroid administered. Complications were, however, more common in those patients who received ciclosporin.

Although there are anecdotal cases reporting benefit from the use of ciclosporin, this well-performed study with an impressive number of cases is good evidence that the drug should not be used in pemphigus vulgaris and foliaceus. There is still good anecdotal evidence that ciclosporin may have a role to play in the management of paraneoplastic pemphigus, a disease with a much more complex pathophysiology.

Perforating dermatoses

Roselyn Kellen, Mark G. Lebwohl

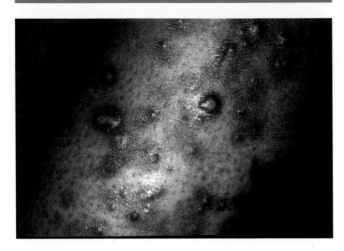

The perforating dermatoses are a varied group of conditions characterized by the transepidermal elimination of dermal material. Four primary conditions are included in the discussion of the perforating disorders:

- Reactive perforating collagenosis, which is characterized by the transepidermal elimination of collagen
- Elastosis perforans serpiginosa (EPS), characterized by transepidermal extrusion of elastic material
- Perforating folliculitis, in which epidermal perforation involves hair follicles
- Kyrle disease, in which dermal connective tissue perforates through the epidermis

MANAGEMENT STRATEGY

Definitive diagnosis of the perforating disorders depends on the demonstration of transepidermal elimination on skin biopsy. Differentiation between the different forms of perforating disorders can be accomplished by Masson trichrome stains for collagen (reactive perforating collagenosis), Verhoeff–van Gieson stains for elastic tissue (EPS), and step-sectioning to look for hair follicles (perforating folliculitis). Differentiation between these various disorders may be important, as EPS is associated with other diseases such as pseudoxanthoma elasticum, Down syndrome, osteogenesis imperfecta, Ehlers–Danlos syndrome, Rothmund–Thomson syndrome, Marfan syndrome, and penicillamine treatment. Reactive perforating collagenosis is commonly associated with diabetes and chronic kidney disease.

Acquired perforating dermatoses have been associated with several medications, including sorafenib, natalizumab, azathioprine, and telaprevir. In particular, acquired reactive perforating collagenosis has occurred in patients treated with indinavir, erlotinib, sorafenib, and sirolimus. Perforating folliculitis has been reported in patients treated with tumor necrosis factor-α blockers, nilotinib, lenalidomide, sorafenib; a patient with cystic fibrosis; and a patient who had previously suffered from varicella in the same distribution as the perforating folliculitis lesions.

Management of the perforating diseases involves determination of underlying etiologies. Most often, conditions such as diabetes mellitus and renal failure will be known to the patient who presents with perforating skin lesions. When the underlying cause is not apparent, serum chemistry for renal and liver function tests and oral glucose tolerance test or hemoglobin A_{1C} may be helpful.

Once the diagnosis of underlying diseases is ascertained, treatment is directed at associated symptoms. Pruritus can be managed initially with *topical or intralesional corticosteroids, topical anesthetics, and menthol,* as well as *oral antihistamines,* but the latter agents are usually not sufficiently effective. Minimizing pruritus is important because many of the perforating disorders typically exhibit a Koebner phenomenon, meaning that lesions develop in traumatized or scratched skin. Topical antipruritic agents such as menthol, phenol, or camphor and topical anesthetics such as lidocaine and pramocaine are useful. *Topical doxepin hydrochloride* or oral antihistamines may also be of some benefit. Trimming the fingernails to minimize trauma to the skin and avoidance of scratching are key elements of treatment. *Topical tretinoin* and *topical tazarotene* have been shown to be effective for some patients. For those patients whose condition is exacerbated by sun exposure, sunscreens may be helpful. Conversely, in patients with renal disease ultraviolet B (UVB) is dramatically effective for pruritus and has been reported to benefit perforating skin lesions as well. If UVB, narrowband UVB, and topical retinoids are ineffective, *oral retinoids, allopurinol,* or *antibiotics* can be tried. More recently, case reports have detailed improvement with *amitriptyline* (10–25 mg daily for several weeks) and topical vitamin D analogs, including *tacalcitol* and *maxacalcitol.*

Specific Investigations

- Skin biopsy with Masson trichrome stains and Verhoeff–van Gieson stains
- Serum blood urea nitrogen, creatinine, amino alanine transferase, aspartate amino transferase, alkaline phosphatase, bilirubin, uric acid
- Serum glucose, oral glucose tolerance test, or hemoglobin A_{1C}
- Hepatitis C virus antibodies
- Thyroid function tests

Clinicopathological features of 25 patients with acquired perforating dermatosis. Akoglu G, Emre S, Sungu N, Kurtoglu G, Metin A. Eur J Dermatol 2013; 23: 864–71.

Of the 25 patients with acquired perforating dermatosis, 17 (68%) had acquired reactive perforating collagenosis, 7 patients (28%) had perforating folliculitis, and 1 patient (4%) had Kyrle disease. The most commonly associated disease was diabetes mellitus (12 patients, 48%). Five patients (20%) had chronic kidney disease, 2 patients had thyroid disease, and 1 patient had hepatitis C.

First-Line Therapies

• Tretinoin 0.1%	D
• Tazarotene gel 0.1%	E
• UVB	E
• Narrowband UVB	D

Familial reactive perforating collagenosis: a clinical, histopathological study of 10 cases. Ramesh V, Sood N, Kubba A, Singh B, Makkar R. J Eur Acad Dermatol Venereol 2007; 21: 766–70.

Evidence Levels: A Double-blind study **B** Clinical trial ≥ 20 subjects **C** Clinical trial < 20 subjects **D** Series ≥ 5 subjects **E** Anecdotal case reports

Ten patients with familial reactive perforating collagenosis were studied. All the patients responded to topical retinoic acid. The authors suggested that sunscreens may benefit patients whose lesions develop in the summer.

Familial reactive perforating collagenosis may be a distinct entity that occurs in infancy or early childhood. It is of interest that sunlight might play a role in the development of this condition, as phototherapy is used therapeutically in adults with perforating disorders.

Tazarotene is an effective therapy for elastosis perforans serpiginosa. Outland JD, Brown TS, Callen JP. Arch Dermatol 2002; 138: 169–71.

A report of two patients with EPS who responded to daily treatment with 0.1% tazarotene gel. A 22-year-old woman had been treated unsuccessfully with liquid nitrogen cryotherapy, topical tretinoin, oral isotretinoin, and carbon dioxide (CO_2) laser surgery. A 56-year-old woman had failed to respond to cryotherapy, corticosteroids, tretinoin, and triamcinolone acetonide. Both patients were treated with tazarotene. The skin condition of the 22-year-old greatly improved, and that of the 56-year-old improved moderately.

Treatment of acquired perforating dermatosis with narrowband ultraviolet B. Ohe S, Danno K, Sasaki H, Isei T, Okamoto H, Horio TJ. J Am Acad Dermatol 2004; 50: 892–4.

Narrowband UVB resulted in complete clearing in all five patients treated with phototherapy two to three times per week. Narrowband UVB was started at 400 mJ/cm² and increased up to 1500 mJ/cm². Clearing occurred with 10 to 15 treatments. Disease recurred in three patients between 1 and 10 months after discontinuation of narrowband UVB. Two patients remained clear on narrowband UVB maintenance treatment until 7 and 8 months, respectively.

An 8-year-old boy with familial reactive perforating collagenosis affecting the face received narrowband UVB three times a week. After 25 exposures (total cumulative dose of 38,150 mJ/cm²) the lesions completely regressed and the patient was left with scars and pigmentation changes.

Broadband UVB is also a well-established modality for uremic pruritus. Because many patients with perforating diseases have associated renal failure, UVB phototherapy may dramatically benefit pruritus and reduce the number of skin lesions.

Second-Line Therapies	
• Allopurinol	D
• Isotretinoin	E
• PUVA	E
• Acitretin	E

Acquired reactive perforating collagenosis: four patients with a giant variant treated with allopurinol. Hoque SR, Ameen M, Holden CA. Br J Dermatol 2006; 154: 759–62.

All four patients failed topical and oral corticosteroids and antibiotics and were started on allopurinol 100 mg once daily despite normal serum uric acid levels. Three of the four experienced dramatic improvement at 2 to 4 months, with prevention of new lesions, a reduction in pruritus, and clearance of existing lesions. The fourth patient died before the follow-up examination.

In another case report, a patient treated with 100 mg allopurinol once daily experienced marked improvement within 4 weeks: the pruritus and the skin lesions resolved, and he was only left with postinflammatory hyperpigmentation. This response was maintained at follow-up 14 months later. Numerous anecdotal reports have documented improvement of perforating disorders with allopurinol treatment, regardless of whether uric acid levels are elevated or normal.

Reactive perforating collagenosis: a condition that may be underdiagnosed. Satchell AC, Crotty K, Lee S. Australas J Dermatol 2001; 42: 284–7.

Three patients with diabetes mellitus were treated for reactive perforating collagenosis. A 73-year-old woman was treated with 0.5% phenol with 10% glycerine in sorbolene cream. After 1 month of treatment the itch resolved and skin lesions diminished in number and size. A 75-year-old woman responded to treatment with narrowband UVB. The patient received phototherapy three times per week for 2 months, with resolution of her skin lesions. When the condition recurred 6 months later, it again cleared with 3 months of narrowband UVB. A 58-year-old woman who did not respond to corticosteroids, antihistamines, UVB, or PUVA was successfully treated with oral acitretin 25 mg daily, which resolved the itch and cleared the skin lesions.

Kyrle's disease. Effectively treated with isotretinoin. Saleh HA, Lloyd KM, Fatteh S. J Fla Med Assoc 1993; 80: 395–7.

A 63-year-old patient with Kyrle disease and chronic renal failure was treated with oral isotretinoin for 13 weeks. Cutaneous lesions cleared completely.

Reactive perforating collagenosis responsive to PUVA. Serrano G, Aliaga A, Lorente M. Int J Dermatol 1988; 27: 118–9.

A 21-year-old woman with a 10-year history of reactive perforating collagenosis was treated with PUVA four times per week. Improvement was noted in 2 weeks. Lesions stopped developing after completion of PUVA therapy (326 J/cm² total), and no new lesions were noted in over a year of posttreatment observations.

Third-Line Therapies	
• Doxycycline	E
• Oral metronidazole	E
• Oral clindamycin	E
• Oral hydroxychloroquine	E
• Imiquimod	E
• Surgical debridement	E
• Cryotherapy	E
• Cantharidin	E
• Ultrapulse laser	E
• CO_2 laser	E
• Photodynamic therapy	E
• Transcutaneous electrical nerve stimulation (TENS)	E
• Amitriptyline	E
• Tacalcitol, maxacalcitol	E

Successful treatment of acquired reactive perforating collagenosis with doxycycline. Brinkmeier T, Schaller J, Herbst RA, Frosch PJ. Acta Derm Venereol 2002; 82: 393–5.

An 87-year-old woman with acquired reactive perforating collagenosis responded to treatment with oral doxycycline 100 mg daily for 2 weeks. Within 5 days of initiation of treatment, new skin lesions ceased to form, and within 10 days of treatment most lesions had healed.

Regression of skin lesions of Kyrle's disease with metronidazole in a diabetic patient. Khalifa M, Slim I, Kaabia N, Bahri F, Trabelsi A, Letaief AO. J Infect 2007; 55: e139–40.

Metronidazole 500 mg twice daily for 1 month completely cleared lesions of Kyrle disease. Lesions did not recur during 12 months of follow-up.

Regression of skin lesions of Kyrle's disease with clindamycin: implications for an infectious component in the etiology of the disease. Kasiakou SK, Peppas G, Kapaskelis AM, Falagas ME. J Infect 2005; 50: 412–6.

A patient with old, uninflamed hyperkeratotic lesions of Kyrle disease and newer inflamed lesions was successfully treated with a combination of oral clindamycin and surgical removal of large lesions.

Sirolimus-induced inflammatory papules with acquired reactive perforating collagenosis. Lübbe J, Sorg O, Malé PJ, Saurat JH, Masouyé I. Dermatology 2008; 216: 239–42.

A patient with acquired reactive perforating collagenosis attributed to sirolimus after liver transplantation responded to oral hydroxychloroquine 200 mg daily even though the sirolimus was continued. Skin remained clear for 6 months, during which time the patient continued on hydroxychloroquine as well as sirolimus.

Imiquimod therapy for elastosis perforans serpiginosa. Kelly SC, Purcell SM. Arch Dermatol 2006; 142: 829–30.

A 14-year-old girl with elastosis perforans serpiginosa was treated with imiquimod cream applied every night for 6 weeks and then three times weekly for the next 4 weeks. After 10 weeks her skin cleared completely.

A new treatment for acquired reactive perforating collagenosis. Oziemski MA, Billson VR, Crosthwaite GL, Zajac J, Varigos GA. Australas J Dermatol 1991; 32: 71–4.

A single patient with reactive perforating collagenosis was successfully treated with surgical debridement and split-skin grafting of the affected areas.

Because skin lesions are often numerous, surgical removal and skin grafting may be impractical.

Elastosis perforans serpiginosa: treatment with liquid nitrogen cryotherapy and review of the literature. Humphrey S, Hemmati I, Randhawa R, Crawford RI, Hong CH. J Cutan Med Surg 2010; 14: 38–42.

A 13-year-old male with EPS of the face was successfully treated with liquid nitrogen cryotherapy.

Treatment of acquired perforating dermatosis with cantharidin. Wong J, Phelps R, Levitt J. Arch Dermatol 2012; 148: 160–2.

Cantharidin was used to successfully treat the acquired perforating dermatosis in a 65-year-old woman with diabetes and chronic renal failure.

Acquired perforating dermatosis successfully treated with photodynamic therapy. Sezer E, Erkek E. Photodermatol Photoimmunol Photomed 2012; 28: 50–2.

A 60-year-old woman with acquired perforating dermatosis and diabetes mellitus was successfully treated with photodynamic therapy.

Localized idiopathic elastosis perforans serpiginosa effectively treated by the coherent ultrapulse 5000C esthetic laser. Abdullah A, Colloby PS, Foulds IS, Whitcroft I. Int J Dermatol 2000; 39: 719–20.

Portions of lesions of EPS were treated by laser, with complete clearing of treated sites but no changes in untreated sites.

Response of elastosis perforans serpiginosa to pulsed CO_2, Er:YAG, and dye lasers. Saxena M, Tope WD. Dermatol Surg 2003; 29: 677–8.

A 17-year-old male presenting with EPS on the neck was treated with CO_2 laser on the right neck and erbium:yttrium aluminum garnet (Er:YAG) laser on the left neck. Only mild improvement of EPS was achieved, and subtle atrophic scarring occurred on the area treated with the CO_2 laser. The patient then received pulsed dye laser therapy on both sides of the neck, resulting in only minimal improvement of EPS.

Treatment of elastosis perforans serpiginosa with the pinhole method using a carbon dioxide laser. Yang JH, Han SS, Won CH, Chang SE, Lee MW, Choi JH, et al. Dermatol Surg 2011; 37: 524–6.

Conflicting reports concerning the usefulness of the CO_2 laser for EPS suggest that this modality may be useful as a last resort in some, but not all, patients with EPS.

Treatment of pruritus of reactive perforating collagenosis using transcutaneous electrical nerve stimulation. Chan LY, Tang WY, Lo KK. Eur J Dermatol 2000; 10: 59–61.

A 47-year-old woman and an 85-year-old woman, each of whom had failed to respond to treatment with topical steroids and antihistamines, received TENS therapy for 1 hour daily over the course of 3 weeks. Skin lesions cleared within 3 months of treatment in both patients.

Effective treatment of uremic pruritus and acquired perforating dermatosis with amitriptyline. Yong A, Chong WS, Tey HL. Australas J Dermatol 2014; 55: 54–7.

Two patients with a history of chronic kidney disease were diagnosed with acquired perforating dermatosis, both suffering from severe pruritus. The first patient, whose biopsy was consistent with Kyrle disease, received amitriptyline 25 mg daily. Within 1 week, his itch score markedly decreased and the nodules had flattened. The itch and lesions reappeared after discontinuing amitriptyline but responded to retreatment. The second patient received amitriptyline 10 mg daily and within 2 weeks, the itching resolved and the excoriated papules healed. His dose was later increased to 25 mg daily when the itch reappeared.

Tacalcitol in the treatment of acquired perforating collagenosis. Escribano-Stable JC, Domenech C, Matarredona J, Pascual JC, Jaen A, Vicente J. Case Rep Dermatol 2014; 6: 69–73.

A 65-year-old patient who had failed topical corticosteroids and antihistamines achieved complete remission after 2 months of topical tacalcitol once daily. The lesions returned 4 weeks after finishing treatment but responded to retreatment within 3 weeks.

In a different case report, pruritus and papules resolved after the use of 0.0025% maxacalcitol ointment twice daily (total of 60 g) for 2 months.

Acknowledgment

We would like to thank Sarah Markoff for her contributions to the previous edition of this chapter.

Evidence Levels: A Double-blind study **B** Clinical trial ≥ 20 subjects **C** Clinical trial < 20 subjects **D** Series ≥ 5 subjects **E** Anecdotal case reports

187

Perioral dermatitis

Antonios Kanelleas, John Berth-Jones

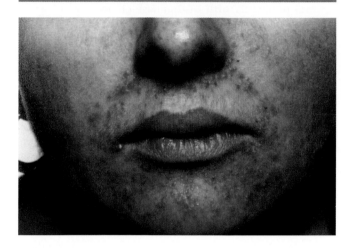

Perioral dermatitis is a persistent erythematous eruption of inflammatory papules (and sometimes pustules) on the chin, perioral areas, and nasolabial folds, characteristically sparing the skin immediately adjacent to the vermilion border. The main symptoms include pruritus, burning sensation, and soreness. It is usually seen in young women but also occurs in childhood.

The etiology is unknown; however, the development of perioral dermatitis is frequently preceded by intentional or inadvertent application of potent topical corticosteroids to the facial skin. The use of steroid inhalers may also induce perioral dermatitis. A similar eruption involving the eyelids and periorbital skin has been termed *periocular dermatitis*. The granulomatous subset of perioral dermatitis, which is seen in prepubertal children, presents with small flesh-colored or yellow-brown papules.

The suggested relationship of perioral dermatitis with infectious agents and infestations such as *Candida* spp., *Demodex folliculorum,* and fusiform bacteria has not been confirmed. However, a high prevalence of atopy has been found among patients with perioral dermatitis.

Although sometimes described as a variant of rosacea, perioral dermatitis is distinguished from this disease by its distribution, by the relatively monomorphic appearance of the lesions, by the absence of flushing and telangiectasia, and by its tendency to occur in younger patients. Differential diagnoses also include allergic and irritant contact dermatitis, which does not usually spare the lip margins; acne vulgaris; seborrhoeic dermatitis; and lupus miliaris disseminatus faciei.

MANAGEMENT STRATEGY

Many cases are associated with the use of *potent topical corticosteroids,* and *withdrawal* of this medication is the most important measure in this group. Patients must be warned that the condition may initially flare after this maneuver. Any cosmetic products applied on the area should also be discontinued. So discontinuation of all topical products is a perfectly acceptable initial approach. If the flare proves intolerable, temporary use of

a less potent topical corticosteroid can often be helpful. *Systemic tetracyclines* are also frequently employed, and a range of other modalities are used less frequently. In most cases there will be a permanent remission, but relapses may rarely occur. In case of treatment failure, the possibility of contact allergic dermatitis may need to be investigated by patch testing.

Specific Investigation

- No investigation is routinely required

First-Line Therapies

• Withdrawal of topical corticosterids	B
• Oral tetracyclines	B

Complications of topical hydrocortisone. Guin JD. J Am Acad Dermatol 1981; 4: 417–22.

Perioral dermatitis developed after the use of topical hydrocortisone.

Although usually associated with the use of potent topical corticosteroids, this case suggests that even hydrocortisone may induce perioral dermatitis.

Perioral dermatitis: aetiology and treatment with tetracycline. Macdonald A, Feiwel M. Br J Dermatol 1972; 87: 351–9.

Tetracycline 250 mg given three times daily for a week, then twice daily for 2 to 3 months, proved highly effective in this series of 29 cases.

Perioral dermatitis in renal transplant recipients maintained on corticosteroids and immunosuppressive therapy. Adams SJ, Davison AM, Cunliffe WJ, Giles GR. Br J Dermatol 1982; 106: 589–92.

A report of five cases where perioral dermatitis developed in patients on oral corticosteroids that could not be discontinued. A 2-month course of doxycycline was effective.

There are also a few recent reports that low-dose doxycycline (40 mg daily) has been useful in perioral dermatitis.

Second-Line Therapies

• Topical pimecrolimus	A
• Topical tetracycline	B
• Topical erythromycin	B
• Oral erythromycin	E
• Topical metronidazole	C
• Topical azelaic acid	D
• Oral isotretinoin	E
• Topical adapalene	E
• Photodynamic therapy	B
• Topical praziquantel	B
• Oral azithromycin	D
• Sodium sulfacetamide lotion	D

Pimecrolimus cream (1%) efficacy in perioral dermatitis: results of a randomized, double-blind, vehicle-controlled study in 40 patients. Oppel T, Pavicic T, Kamann S, Bräutigam M, Wollenberg A. J Eur Acad Dermatol Venereol 2007; 21: 1175–80.

Twenty patients were treated with topical pimecrolimus cream 1% twice a day for 4 weeks. The comparison group consisted of 20 patients treated with the vehicle compound. The Perioral Dermatitis Severity Index (PODSI) score was found to be significantly lower in the pimecrolimus group at the end of the treatment period, whereas no differences between the two groups were observed after a 4-week follow-up period.

A randomized, double-blind, vehicle-controlled study of 1% pimecrolimus cream in adult patients with perioral dermatitis. Schwarz T, Kreiselmaier I, Bieber T, Thaci D, Simon JC, Meurer M, et al. J Am Acad Dermatol 2008; 59: 34–40.

This multicenter, double-blind trial confirmed the findings of the earlier mentioned study. Patients treated with pimecrolimus also reported greater improvement in quality of life.

There are reports linking the use of topical calcineurin inhibitors with the induction of perioral dermatitis and rosacea-like eruptions after treatment for facial inflammatory dermatoses.

Topical tetracycline in the treatment of perioral dermatitis. Wilson RG. Arch Dermatol 1979; 115: 637.

Topical tetracycline, applied twice daily, proved highly effective in this series of 30 patients. Twenty-four cleared completely after 5 to 28 days.

A topical erythromycin preparation and oral tetracycline for the treatment of perioral dermatitis: a placebo-controlled trial. Weber K, Thurmayr R, Meisinger A. J Dermatol Treat 1993; 4: 57–9.

A comparison of the response to topical erythromycin (33 patients), oral tetracycline (35 patients), and placebo (31 patients). Oral tetracycline and topical erythromycin were comparable in efficacy, and both were superior to placebo.

Topical therapy for perioral dermatitis. Bikowski JB. Cutis 1983; 31: 678–82.

Six cases cleared with topical erythromycin.

Identical twins with perioral dermatitis. Weston WL, Morelli JG. Pediatr Dermatol 1998; 15: 144.

Two cases responded to oral erythromycin.

Topical metronidazole in the treatment of perioral dermatitis. Veien NK, Munkvad JM, Nielsen AO, Niordson AM, Stahl D, Thormann J. J Am Acad Dermatol 1991; 24: 258–69.

A prospective, randomized, double-blind trial with 109 patients. Both groups improved, but 1% metronidazole cream applied twice daily was less effective than oxytetracycline 250 mg twice daily over 8 weeks.

Topical metronidazole gel (0.75%) for the treatment of perioral dermatitis in children. Miller SR, Shalita AR. J Am Acad Dermatol 1994; 31: 847–8.

Three children with perioral or periocular eruptions were treated with topical metronidazole gel (0.75%) twice daily.

Significant improvement was observed after 2 months. Complete resolution occurred after 14 weeks.

Azelaic acid as a new treatment for perioral dermatitis: results from an open study. Jansen T. Br J Dermatol 2004; 151: 933–4.

Ten cases were treated with topical 20% azelaic acid cream applied twice daily. Complete clearing was reported in all cases after 2 to 6 weeks. The cream was well tolerated.

Perioral dermatitis with histopathologic features of granulomatous rosacea: successful treatment with isotretinoin. Smith KW. Cutis 1990; 46: 413–5.

Isotretinoin was used successfully in a resistant case.

Perioral dermatitis successfully treated with topical adapalene. Jansen T. J Eur Acad Dermatol Venereol 2002; 16: 175–7.

Successful treatment of one case of perioral dermatitis with topical adapalene gel once daily for 4 weeks. The patient had had no history of steroid use, and previous topical therapy with erythromycin had failed.

Photodynamic therapy for perioral dermatitis. Richey DF, Hopson B. J Drugs Dermatol 2006; 5: 12–6.

Twenty-one patients participated in this prospective split-face study. One half of the face was treated with 5-aminolevulinic acid (ALA)-PDT once weekly for approximately 4 weeks, and the other half was treated with topical clindamycin once daily. Out of 14 patients who completed the study, the sides treated with PDT had a mean clearance of 92.1%, compared with 80.9% for the clindamycin sides ($p = 0.0227$). The mean patient satisfaction level for PDT was also higher.

Topical praziquantel as a new treatment for perioral dermatitis: results of a randomized vehicle-controlled pilot study. Bribeche MR, Fedotov VP, Jillella A, Gladichev VV, Pukhalskaya DM. Clin Exp Dermatol 2014; 39: 448–53.

Praziquantel (an anthelmintic drug) 3% was applied as a 3% ointment twice daily for 4 weeks and was found to be superior to vehicle in this study with 46 adult subjects. Dermatology Life Quality Index (DLQI) also improved. No serious treatment-related side effects occurred in either group.

Pediatric periorificial dermatitis: clinical course and treatment outcomes in 222 patients. Goel NS, Burkhart CN, Morrell DS. Pediatr Dermatol 2015; 32: 333–6.

A retrospective review of 222 children treated for perioral and/or periocular dermatitis at a single center. A history of previous steroid use was reported in 58.1% before onset of the disease. Treatments employed included oral azithromycin, topical metronidazole, and sodium sulfacetamide lotion, often combining the systemic antibiotic with a topical modality. Ninety-four (72%) of 131 patients who returned for follow-up had complete resolution of symptoms. Adverse effects included pigmentary changes (1.8%), worsening of symptoms (1.8%), gastrointestinal upset (0.9%), irritant dermatitis (0.9%), and xerosis (0.5%).

Evidence Levels: **A** Double-blind study **B** Clinical trial ≥ 20 subjects **C** Clinical trial < 20 subjects **D** Series ≥ 5 subjects **E** Anecdotal case reports

188

Peutz–Jeghers syndrome

Chinmoy Bhate, Robert A. Schwartz

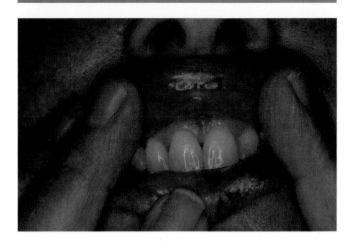

Peutz–Jeghers syndrome (PJS) is a rare hereditary disorder of polyposis. It is characterized by gastrointestinal polyps, mucocutaneous pigmentation, recurrent abdominal pain from intussusceptions, and an increased risk of intestinal and other malignancies.

The pigmented macules of PJS are typically found around the mouth, eyes, nostrils, and anus; they may also be seen on the hands and feet. These brown to black macules are often round or oval, 1 to 5 mm in diameter, and irregular in shape. They may occasionally manifest with a blue-gray hue. Clinically and histologically, these are simple lentigines.

Most patients with this autosomal dominant disorder have a germline mutation of the STK11/LKB1 (serine/threonine kinase 11) tumor suppressor gene, located at chromosome 19p13.3. A more recently identified second PJS disease locus exists at 19q13.4. The exact mechanism of cancer and hamartoma development remains unclear. Genetic testing may be useful in equivocal cases, as well as in counseling of at-risk families; however, it is not 100% sensitive.

MANAGEMENT STRATEGY

Management is predicated upon the potential for visceral complications and familial inheritance. This includes an evaluation for associated findings, including gastrointestinal polyps, which occur in nearly all PJS patients, recurrent intussusceptions, gastrointestinal bleeding, and a variety of other internal malignancies. Disease is most often discovered between the ages of 10 and 30 years. Any child seen with recurrent, unexplained abdominal pain should raise concern for intussusception, a medical emergency associated with PJS. Gastrointestinal polyps are most often found in the small bowel but may also be seen in the stomach, large bowel, and rectum; these polyps are at risk for malignant degeneration. Esophagogastroduodenoscopy, capsule endoscopy or balloon enteroscopy, and colonoscopy are important in the evaluation and treatment of gastrointestinal polyposis.

Cancers of the stomach, pancreas, esophagus, lung, uterus, and testes (Sertoli cell) all have an elevated relative risk in patients with PJS. Women with this disorder also carry an increased risk of bilateral breast cancer. Ovarian neoplasms, especially granulosa cell tumors, may be seen. Both in men and women, sex cord tumors with annular tubules and sex cord stromal tumors with sexual precocity may develop.

Genetic testing in suspected cases is critical in order to identify familial or de novo mutations. Genetic counseling of PJS patients and their relatives is indicated. Families should be reassured that the mucocutaneous macules are benign and may improve after puberty. Several therapies for these pigmented macules have been used with varying responses; removal may potentially mask the underlying disorder in patients with undiagnosed PJS.

The *Q-switched Nd:YAG laser* and *ruby laser (Q-switched and short pulsed)* have been used in the treatment of labial macules without sequelae or recurrences. Anesthesia is not usually required, and minimal wound care is necessary. The *CO_2, alexandrite, and argon lasers,* as well as *intense pulsed light,* have also been effective in the treatment of labial macules. Cryosurgery, surgical excision, electrodesiccation, and dermabrasion may lead to scarring and dyspigmentation, often without complete removal of the pigmented macules. Similarly, *trichloroacetic acid* may not produce total resolution.

> ### Specific Investigations
>
> - Gastrointestinal evaluation
> - Genetic testing (in some cases)
> - Histology of polyps and mucocutaneous macules (if diagnosis is in question)
> - Psychosocial evaluation

Rapid detection of germline mutations for hereditary gastrointestinal polyposis/cancers using HaloPlex target enrichment and high-throughput sequencing technologies. Kohda M, Kumamoto K, Eguchi H, Hirata T, Tada Y, Tanakaya K, et al. Fam Cancer 2016; 15: 553–62.

The authors discuss traditional means of molecular diagnostics as well as newer, high-throughput sequencing-based tests; they present methodology that may potentially promote more rapid screening with high efficiency and accuracy.

The STK11/LKB1 gene is one among many that are linked with hereditary gastrointestinal polyposis/cancer syndromes. Genetic testing is widely utilized in routine practice, and newer techniques are being evaluated for more efficiency, accuracy, and turnaround time.

ACG clinical guideline: genetic testing and management of hereditary gastrointestinal cancer syndromes. Syngal S, Brand RE, Church JM, Giardiello FM, Hampel HL, Burt RW. Am J Gastroenterol 2015; 110: 223–63.

A comprehensive document from the American College of Gastroenterology providing guidelines for evaluation, surveillance, and management of patients with a number of hereditary syndromes, including PJS. This review also provides recommendations for surveillance of associated internal malignancies.

Small bowel endoscopy and Peutz-Jeghers syndrome. Korsse SE, Dewint P, Kuipers EJ, van Leerdam ME. Best Pract Res Clin Gastroenterol 2012; 26: 263–78.

This article provides a systematic review of endoscopic techniques used to examine the small bowel in patients with PJS.

Small bowel surveillance is recommended in patients with PJS every 2 to 3 years from the age of 8 to 10 years. Visualization of the small bowel is technically challenging, and a gold standard method has not been established.

Peutz-Jeghers syndrome: a systematic review and recommendations for management. Beggs AD, Latchford AR, Vasen HF, Moslein G, Alonso A, Aretz S, et al. Gut 2010; 59: 975–86.

A review of current genotype–phenotype studies and an outline of consensus recommendations for screening and follow-up from a group of European experts who previously produced guidelines for the management of Lynch syndrome and familial adenomatous polyposis.

Surveillance in PJS aims to (1) reduce polyp burden and the incidence of intussusceptions in young patients and (2) reduce the burden of cancer. Capsule endoscopy allows for thorough, less invasive surveillance of the small bowel for polyposis. Evaluation of the small bowel with upper gastrointestinal (GI) endoscopy, colonoscopy, and double-balloon enteroscopy has been useful in preventing the need for subsequent surgical polypectomy; because double-balloon enteroscopy is often traumatic, it is reserved as a treatment modality.

Quality of life and psychological distress in patients with Peutz-Jeghers syndrome. Van Lier MG, Mathus-Vliegen EM, van Leerdam ME, Kuipers EJ, Looman CW, Wagner A, et al. Clin Genet 2010; 78: 219–26.

A cross-sectional study in order to assess the quality of life and psychological distress in PJS patients compared with the general population.

Compared with the general population, PJS patients reported a lower general health perception, more limitations due to emotional problems, and a lower mental well-being.

Genetics of the hamartomatous polyposis syndromes: a molecular review. Chen HM, Fang JY. Int J Colorectal Dis 2009; 24: 865–74.

A discussion of hamartoma syndromes, including clinical features and molecular diagnostic modalities, which help differentiate between them and identify at-risk patients.

Peutz–Jeghers syndrome. Heymann WR. J Am Acad Dermatol 2007; 57: 513–4.

A synopsis of the syndrome correlating molecular advances with the cutaneous, malignant, and endocrinologic features of the disorder.

Further observations on LKB1/STK11 status and cancer risk in Peutz-Jeghers syndrome. Lim W, Hearle N, Shah B, Murday V, Hodgson SV, Lucassen A, et al. Br J Cancer 2003; 89: 308–13.

A genotype–phenotype analysis demonstrating significant genetic heterogeneity in PJS.

The authors demonstrated an elevated relative risk of cancer development in patients with PJS. They also demonstrated that PJS may occur either as a result of several types of mutations within the mentioned gene or even in the absence of a mutation.

Peutz–Jeghers syndrome: confirmation of linkage to chromosome 19p13.3 and identification of a potential second locus, on 19q13.4. Mehenni H, Blouin JL, Radhakrishna U, Bhardwaj SS, Bhardwaj K, Dixit VB, et al. Am J Hum Genet 1997; 61: 1327–34.

The authors described the location of the most prevalent mutation in PJS, the LKB1/STK11 gene at location 19p13.3, and identified an additional locus.

Most patients with PJS have associated LKB1/STK11 mutations at location 19p13.3; however, a second disease locus at 19q13.4 has also

been demonstrated. Some patients have no mutation at either site, which serves as a limitation to genetic testing for diagnosis.

Harold Jeghers (1904–1990). Schwartz RA. In: Löser C, Plewig G, Burgdorf WHC, eds. Pantheon of Dermatology. Outstanding Historical Figures. Berlin: Springer Verlag, 2013; 553–6.

A biography of Harold Jeghers is presented with a review of this syndrome that carries his name.

First-Line Therapies	
• Q-switched Nd:YAG laser	C
• Ruby and alexandrite lasers	D

Q-switched Nd:YAG laser treatment for labial lentigines associated with Peutz-Jeghers syndrome. J Dtsch Dermatol Ges 2015; 13: 551–5.

Eleven patients with PJS received two to six treatments with Q-switched Nd:YAG laser (532 nm) with a spot size of 3 mm, fluence of 1.8 to 2.2 J/cm^2, and pulse duration ranging from 5 to 20 nm. Eight of 11 patients had greater than 75% clearance with minimal recurrence or complication after a mean follow-up of 41 months.

Q-switched alexandrite laser treatment of oral labial lentigines in Chinese subjects with Peutz-Jeghers syndrome. Xi Z, Hui Q, Zhong L. Dermatol Surg 2009; 35: 1084–8.

Fourteen cases of oral labial lentigines in patients with PJS were managed using a single treatment with Q-switched alexandrite laser with a 3-mm handpiece and a fluence of 4.0 to 9.0 J/cm^2. All exhibited successful elimination without scarring or recurrence at median 2-year follow-up.

Q-switched lasers, in particular the alexandrite laser, are preferred in the treatment of benign melanocytic lesions, including oral labial lentigines in PJS patients; acute side effects included edema, erythema, and occasional bleeding.

Q-switched ruby laser treatment of labial lentigos. Ashinoff R, Geronemus RG. J Am Acad Dermatol 1992; 27: 809–11.

The Q-switched ruby laser, with a wavelength of 694 nm and pulse duration of 40 ns, causes selective damage to pigmented cells. Three patients with labial lentigines treated with the Q-switched ruby laser noted dramatic clearing after one or two treatments with a fluence of 10 cm^2.

Ruby laser therapy for labial lentigines in Peutz–Jeghers syndrome. Kato S, Takeyama J, Tanita Y, Ebina K. Eur J Pediatr 1998; 157: 622–4.

Two children with PJS and labial lentigines were treated successfully without sequelae or recurrence.

Q-switched ruby laser treatment of tattoos and benign pigmented lesions: a critical review. Raulin C, Schrmark MP, Greve B, Werner S. Ann Plast Surg 1998; 41: 555–65.

This review discusses indications for the use of the Q-switched ruby laser. These include tattoos, café au lait macules, and lentigines, especially those on the lips and eyelids.

Second-Line Therapies	
• Other lasers	E
• Intense pulsed light	E
• Cryotherapy	E

Evidence Levels: **A** Double-blind study **B** Clinical trial ≥ 20 subjects **C** Clinical trial < 20 subjects **D** Series ≥ 5 subjects **E** Anecdotal case reports

Treatment of Peutz–Jeghers lentigines with the carbon dioxide laser. Benedict LM, Cohen B. J Dermatol Surg Oncol 1991; 17: 954–5.

One patient with PJS had successful treatment of perioral lentigines with a CO_2 laser.

Q-switched alexandrite laser in the treatment of pigmented macules in Laugier–Hunziker syndrome. Papadavid E, Walker NP. J Eur Acad Dermatol Venereol 2001; 15: 468–9.

Two patients with labial pigmented macules were treated with the Q-switched alexandrite laser. Recurrences were easily treated again.

Laugier–Hunziker syndrome, a disorder of mucocutaneous pigmentation similar to PJS, has no associated GI abnormalities. Treatment of pigmented lesions in this syndrome may provide insight into the treatment of those seen in PJS.

Treatment of pigmentation of the lips and oral mucosa in Peutz–Jeghers syndrome using ruby and argon lasers. Ohshiro T, Maruyama Y, Nakajima H, Mima M. Br J Plast Surg 1980; 33: 346–9.

Three PJS patients had successful treatment of pigmented oral macules with ruby and argon lasers.

Treatment of facial lentigines in Peutz–Jeghers syndrome with intense pulsed light source. Remington BK, Remington TK. Dermatol Surg 2002; 28: 1079–81.

A 10-year-old child had complete clearance of cosmetically concerning lentigines over the course of 12 treatment sessions to different facial regions. Most resolved with a single treatment.

This report demonstrated the first use of intense pulsed light in PJS and provided a viable alternative to laser treatment.

Simple cryosurgical treatment of the oral melanotic macule. Yeh CJ. Clin Oral Maxillofac Surg 2000; 90: 12–3.

Simple cryotherapy for labial melanotic macules is discussed; a specific protocol is provided.

Cryosurgery needs no sophisticated equipment and is inexpensive. Recurrence is common, and inadequate destruction may occur.

Chemopreventive efficacy of rapamycin on Peutz-Jeghers syndrome in a mouse model. Wei C, Amos CI, Zhang N, Zhu J, Wang X, Frazier ML. Cancer Lett 2009; 18: 149–54.

Rapamycin treatment of mice with LKB1 mutations led to a reduction in both polyp burden and polyp size, suggesting that rapamycin may be an option for chemoprevention in humans with PJS.

Suppression of Peutz-Jeghers polyposis by targeting mammalian target of rapamycin signaling. Wei C, Amos CI, Zhang N, Wang X, Rashid A, Walker CL, et al. Clin Cancer Res 2008; 14: 1167–71.

Mice with germline LKB1 mutations and polyposis were treated with rapamycin at the dose of 2 mg/kg/d for 2 months. Rapamycin decreased the tumor burden of large polyps (>8 mm).

Rapamycin effectively suppresses Peutz–Jeghers polyposis in a mouse model, suggesting that it and other inhibitors of the mammalian target of rapamycin (mTOR) may represent targeted therapy for this disorder.

Pinta and yaws

Omar Lupi, Daniela Martinez, Helena Camasmie

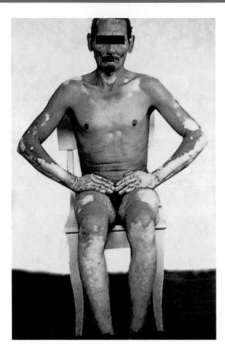

Pinta and yaws belong to the group of neglected, endemic, and nonvenereal treponematoses. These distinct and chronic diseases predominantly affect economically disadvantaged, isolated, rural areas of tropical and subtropical countries.

Yaws is currently thought to be endemic in 14 countries, mostly in West Africa, Southeast Asia and the Pacific, whereas pinta is restricted to Latin America, in particular Mexico and Colombia. Pinta is caused by *Treponema carateum*, and yaws is caused by *Treponema pallidum* ssp. *pertenue*. Both are gram-negative spirochetes, morphologically and antigenically identical to each other and to the etiologic agent of syphilis; therefore specification has to be based on clinical and epidemiologic aspects. The only known reservoir is humans.

MANAGEMENT STRATEGY

Both treponematoses are transmitted by direct skin contact through breaks in the skin from small cuts, scratches, or other skin damage. Most patients acquire the infection during childhood. Both diseases comprise multiple stages.

Pinta is considered the most benign among them, with skin-limited manifestations. It is classified into two different clinical stages. The primary stage is divided into two phases: an early phase (initial period) and a secondary phase (period of cutaneous dissemination). The primary lesions appear 7 to 10 days after inoculation and are characterized by erythematous papules on the face and upper and lower extremities. These lesions tend to grow, producing erythematosquamous or hyperpigmented asymptomatic plaques. Within 6 months to 2 to 3 years of the first appearance of lesions, erythematohypochromic patches appear, initiating the period of cutaneous dissemination. They

are polymorphic and referred to as *pintides*, affecting larger areas of the body with normal skin in the center.

The hallmark of the late stage, 2 to 5 years after the first lesion, is the appearance of achromic patches, especially over body prominences. Plantar hyperkeratosis is frequent. There is no evidence of involvement of other organs, even after many years.

The initial lesion of yaws is called *mother yaws*, arising at the site of entry of the organism, most commonly on the lower limbs, 21 days after inoculation. *Mother yaws* is an erythematous infiltrated papule or a group of papules on an erythematous base, which may ulcerate. They are painless and considered highly infectious. *Mother yaws* frequently heals spontaneously, leaving an atrophic and hypopigmented scar. Systemic symptoms such as fever and joint pain are sometimes present, as well as regional lymphadenopathy.

Disseminated cutaneous lesions appear in untreated cases after healing of the inicial lesion. Characterizing the secondary stage: a bilateral and symmetric eruption that may be present in two main clinical features: a large one that resembles the mother yaws and is called *daughter yaws* and a micropapular type, called *miniature yaws*. The mostly affected locations are the face and intertriginous moist surfaces. Usually the soles present hyperkeratotic plaques with fissures and pain, forcing the patients to walk with a peculiar gait known as *crab yaws*. Cutaneous lesions usually heal, leaving a hypochromic area. Painful osteoperiostitis and polydactylitis may occur, as well as systemic symptoms (fever, headache, generalized adenopathy, and nocturnal bone pain).

Late tertiary yaws appears in 10% of cases after several years, involving subcutaneous tissues, mucous membranes, bones, and joints. The presence of neurologic, cardiovascular, and ophthalmologic lesions is very controversial. The lesions of late yaws are characterized by nodular and tubercular pianides, gummatous lesions, palmar and plantar keratoderma, osteoarticular lesions, palate and nasal septum destruction (*gangosa*), exostoses of the nasal bridge (*goundou*), and juxtaarticular nodes.

Serologic tests, such as rapid plasma reagin (RPR), venereal disease research laboratory (VDRL), FTA-ABS and *Treponema pallidum* particle agglutination (TPPA) and hemagglutination (TPHA) assays remain the cornerstone of the diagnosis, although they cannot distinguish syphilis from any of the nonvenereal treponematoses. Dark-field microscopic examination, radiologic, and histopathologic studies have also been used. Pathogenic treponemes cannot be cultured in vitro. *T. pallidum* PCR assays can be applied to the diagnosis of endemic treponematoses as a direct method with high sensitivity. Access to these facilities may be difficult for the affected, isolated, rural communities, which brings difficulty to the diagnosis.

There is no proof of a spontaneous cure for the disease, and because cell-mediated immunity is not completely effective, the infection persists indefinitely. Patients may harbor subclinical disease and be contagious for a long time.

Intramuscular *benzathine penicillin* remains the mainstay of treatment for the endemic treponemal diseases for over 50 years. A single dose is effective, which ranges from 1.2 million units for patients over 10 years old, with half the dose necessary for patients aged under 10 and contacts.

World Health Organization (WHO) programs in the 1950s to 1960s successfully reduced the number of cases of yaws by administering single-dose penicillin, but failure to adequately identify and treat contacts and latent cases led to noneradication of the disease.

A study was conducted in infected children with a 30 mg/kg single oral dose of *azithromycin*, and it was proven to be noninferior to penicillin, with the benefit of avoiding the need for injection equipment and medically trained personnel. Changing to

Evidence Levels: **A** Double-blind study **B** Clinical trial ≥ 20 subjects **C** Clinical trial < 20 subjects **D** Series ≥ 5 subjects **E** Anecdotal case reports

the simpler azithromycin treatment regimen could enable yaws elimination through mass drug administration programs, renewing WHO efforts to eradicate the disease by 2020. Six-month follow-up includes clinical and serologic surveys to detect and treat remaining cases and their contacts. Awareness to the possibility of azithromycin resistance is important, as it has occurred in syphilis.

At present the WHO has not yet developed a specific strategy for the control or eradication of pinta.

Specific Investigations

- Serologic tests
- Dark-field microscopy
- Direct fluorescent antibody test
- Histopathology
- PCR

Yaws. Marks M, Mitjà O, Solomon AW, Asiedu KB, Mabey DC. Br Med Bull. 2015; 113: 91–100.

Dark field microscopy allows direct visualization of spirochaetes.

Genetic diversity in *Treponema pallidum*: implications for pathogenesis, evolution and molecular diagnostics of syphilis and yaws. Smajs D, Norris SJ, Weinstock GM. Infect Genet Evol 2012; 12: 191–202.

Genome analyses also shed light on treponemal evolution and on chromosomal targets for molecular diagnostics of treponemal infections.

A retrospective study on genetic heterogeneity within *Treponema* strains: subpopulations are genetically distinct in a limited number of positions. Čejková D, Strouhal M, Norris SJ, Weinstock GM, Šmajs D. PLoS Negl Trop 2015; 9: e0004110.

Heterogeneous sites likely represent both the selection of adaptive changes during infection of the host and an ongoing diversifying evolutionary process.

Advances in the diagnosis of endemic treponematoses: yaws, bejel, and pinta. Mitjà O, Šmajs D, Bassat Q. PLoS Negl Trop Dis 2013; 7: e2283.

Serologic tests are still considered standard laboratory methods for the diagnosis of endemic treponematoses, and new rapid point-of-care treponemal tests have become available. In the past 10 years, there has been an increasing effort to apply polymerase chain reaction to treponematoses, and whole genome fingerprinting techniques have identified genetic signatures that can differentiate the existing treponemal strains.

Histopathology is important in diagnosis. It is possible to demonstrate the presence of the treponeme in the epidermis through Warthin–Starry staining in all lesions, with the exception of achromic lesions.

First-Line Therapies

Penicillin G benzathine	B
Azithromycin (yaws)	B

Pinta: Latin America's forgotten disease? Stamm LV. Am J Trop Med Hyg 2015; 93: 901–3.

All stages of pinta are treatable with a single intramuscular injection of penicillin.

Serologic cross-reactivity of syphilis, yaws, and pinta. De Caprariis PJ, Della-Latta P. Am Fam Physician 2013; 15; 87: 80.

Penicillin G benzathine is the recommended treatment for all three treponemal diseases; a single dose is adequate for yaws, pinta, and primary syphilis, but inadequate for late latent and tertiary syphilis.

Endemic treponemal diseases. Marks M, Solomon AW, Mabey DC. Trans R Soc Trop Med Hyg 2014; 108: 601–7.

For endemic treponemal diseases a dose of 1.2 million units is recommended for patients aged 10 or over, whereas a dose of 0.6 million units is recommended for patients aged under 10 and for contacts.

Single-dose azithromycin versus benzathine benzylpenicillin for treatment of yaws in children in Papua New Guinea: an open-label, non-inferiority, randomised trial. Mitjà O, Hays R, Ipai A, Penias M, Paru R, de Lazzari E et al. Lancet 2012; 379: 342–47.

A single dose of oral azithromycin (30 mg/kg with a maximum of 2 g) is as effective as intramuscular benzathine penicillin for treatment of yaws in children in Papua New Guinea.

Yaws: renewed hope for eradication. Stamm LV. JAMA Dermatol 2014; 150: 933–34.

Although azithromycin is safer than penicillin and should make mass treatment significantly easier, its use will require monitoring for emergence of resistance due to 23S ribosomal RNA point mutations, as observed with the syphilis agent.

Second-Line Therapies

Tetracycline	E
Doxycycline	E
Erythromycin	E

Yaws in the Western Pacific region: a review of the literature. Capuano C, Ozaki M. J Trop Med 2011; 2011: 1–15.

Tetracycline, erythromycin, or doxycycline can be used for patients with penicillin hypersensitivity.

New treatment schemes for yaws: the path toward eradication. Mitjà O, Hays R, Rinaldi AC, McDermott R, Bassat Q. Clin Infect Dis 2012; 55: 406–12.

Oral tetracycline, doxycycline, or erythromycin for 15 days is also likely to be effective. These recommendations, however, are based solely upon known clinical efficacy in small series of patients and not upon the results of any clinical trials

Endemic treponematosis: review and update. Farnsworth N, Rosen T. Clin Dermatol 2006; 24: 181–90.

Penicillin remains the drug of choice, but the tetracycline class of antibiotics and erythromycin also appear to be effective.

Tropical dermatology: bacterial tropical diseases. Lupi O, Madkan V, Tyring SK. J Am Acad Dermatol 2006; 54: 559–78.

This is a large update on bacterial tropical diseases, including pinta and yaws. Alternative therapies such as tetracycline or erythromycin are discussed.

190

Pitted and ringed keratolysis (keratolysis plantare sulcatum)

Eunice Tan, John Berth-Jones

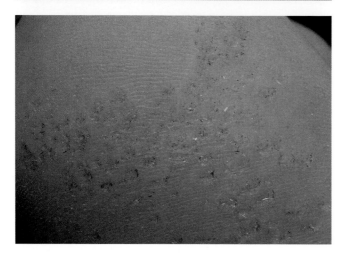

Pitted keratolysis (PK) manifests as shallow, punched-out, circular erosions, primarily on weight-bearing, sweaty areas of the feet, and less commonly on the non–weight-bearing areas of the feet and the palms of the hands. This superficial infection of the stratum corneum is caused by *Corynebacterium*, *Dermatophilus*, *Actinomyces*, or *Kytococcus* (formerly named *Micrococcus*). These organisms possess keratin-degrading enzymes and produce sulfur compounds, resulting in a foul odor. Hyperhidrosis and maceration often occur concurrently.

MANAGEMENT STRATEGY

Most patients experience little or mild irritation. Maceration, foul odor, and soreness are the main reasons for consultation. Hyperhidrosis, sweat retention, prolonged occlusion, immersion, and increases in the skin pH appear to be important causes of PK. Industrial workers wearing rubber shoes or soldiers whose feet are continually occluded or wet are at high risk of developing this infection. Initial management strategies should therefore include instruction on *foot hygiene* and *avoidance of occlusive footwear*.

Treatment involves use of topical or systemic antimicrobial agents and/or reduction of the hyperhidrosis.

The topical antibiotic most commonly used by the authors is *fusidic acid*, which can be prescribed as 2% fusidic acid cream or ointment three to four times daily for a week. Topical *1% clindamycin, benzoyl peroxide, 1% clindamycin with 5% benzoyl peroxide gel, 2% or 3% erythromycin, mupirocin ointment,* and *tetracycline and gentamicin sulfate* cream have been reported to be effective. Although 1% clindamycin hydrochloride can be made up with 660 mg dissolved in 55 mL of 70% isopropyl alcohol and 5% propylene glycol, we suggest Dalacin T topical solution may be used instead. This can be applied two or three times

daily. Erythromycin 2% cream or ointment has been reported to be effective if used twice daily. We suggest using 2% erythromycin gel, available as Eryacne, or 2% erythromycin solution, available as Stiemycin. Japanese dermatologists have had some success in treating PK with gentamicin sulfate cream, but this is unavailable in the UK. Mupirocin 2% ointment may be administered two to three times daily; 3% tetracycline hydrochloride ointment may be applied one to three times daily. PK has also responded to topical antifungals such as *clotrimazole* and *miconazole;* 1% clotrimazole cream or 2% miconazole cream or ointment may be applied twice daily. Topical antiseptics can be effective.

Systemic antibiotics can be reserved for severe and resistant cases. A 7-day course of oral erythromycin 250 mg four times a day is usually well tolerated. The use of penicillin or sulfonamides does not seem to be effective. Antibiotic resistance has been reported with *Micrococcus sedentarius* to penicillin, methicillin, ampicillin, oxacillin, and erythromycin.

Topical 20% *aluminum chloride hexahydrate* in absolute anhydrous ethyl alcohol, available as Driclor, may reduce hyperhidrosis and odor, but the pits remain. The solution is applied at night, allowed to dry, and washed off the next day. Initially it should be used daily until the condition is brought under control, when it can be used less frequently. The use of 20% aluminum chloride hexahydrate for palmoplantar hyperhidrosis has not been as successful as its use for axillary hyperhidrosis. Topical 4% *formaldehyde solution* applied with gauze soaks as the patient sits or stands with his or her feet on the gauze in a bowl for 10 to 15 minutes once or twice daily reduces the hyperhidrosis. Alternatively, immersion of the soles of the feet in *5% formaldehyde* may be utilized. Formalin ointment 40% has been used with some success but is not commercially available in the UK.

Topical 2% *glutaraldehyde* has been reported to have good therapeutic results in PK but sometimes the patient may require the 10% strength to reduce hyperhidrosis. Glutaraldehyde is available in the UK as Cidex (25% or 50% strength), which is used for instrument sterilization, and is somewhat hazardous to handle. Like formaldehyde, glutaraldehyde may cause contact sensitization, but it does not cross-react with formaldehyde.

Iontophoresis is frequently used in palmar and plantar hyperhidrosis and can be used in the treatment of PK. *Botulinum toxin* has also been used. Oral anticholinergics are perhaps excessive.

Various other agents have been tried topically but with limited success. These include 0.1% *triamcinolone acetonide* once or twice daily, *iodochlorhydroxyquin-hydrocortisone cream* (vioform-hydrocortisone) once or twice daily, *flexible collodion, Whitfield ointment* (6% benzoic and 3% salicylic acid ointment in a petrolatum base) twice daily, and Castellani paint. Water-repellent silicone ointment has been found not to significantly improve PK.

Specific Investigations

No investigation is routinely required
- Wood light examination may reveal a coral red fluorescence, but this is not consistently helpful
- Dermoscopy may reveal small black pits in a parallel pattern on the ridges of the stratum corneum
- Starch iodine test may identify areas of hyperhidrosis
- Shave biopsies processed with methenamine silver stain, Gram stain, or periodic acid–Schiff stains are more helpful than punch biopsies
- Swabs may be obtained for cultures of the organisms

Evidence Levels: **A** Double-blind study **B** Clinical trial ≥ 20 subjects **C** Clinical trial < 20 subjects **D** Series ≥ 5 subjects **E** Anecdotal case reports

Pitted keratolysis. The role of *Micrococcus sedentarius*. Nordstrom KM, McGinley KJ, Cappiello L, Zechman JM, Leyden JJ. Arch Dermatol 1987; 123: 1320–5.

Micrococcus sedentarius isolated from PK lesions on the feet of eight patients was tested for antibiotic sensitivities and found to be resistant to penicillin, ampicillin, methicillin, and oxacillin. PK lesions were reproduced in one volunteer inoculated with *M. sedentarius* after 6 weeks of occlusion.

Isolation and characterization of micrococci from human skin, including two new species: *Micrococcus lylae* and *Micrococcus kristinae*. Kloos WE, Torrabene TG, Schleifer KH. Int J Syst Bacteriol 1974; 24: 79–101.

M. sedentarius was observed to be resistant to penicillin, methicillin, and erythromycin, which is characteristic of the genus *Micrococcus*.

First-Line Therapies	
• Topical fusidic acid	E
• Topical aluminum chloride hexahydrate	E

Isolation of *Kytococcus sedentarius* from a case of pitted keratolysis. Ertam İ, Aytimur D, Yüksel SE. Ege Tip Dergisi 2005; 44: 117–8.

A case report of a patient with plantar PK in which *Kytococcus* was isolated, with complete response to 3 weeks of oral erythromycin and topical fusidic acid.

Second-Line Therapies	
• Topical mupirocin	E
• Topical tetracyclines	E
• Topical clindamycin	D
• Topical clotrimazole	E
• Topical benzoyl peroxide	D
• Topical erythromycin	C
• Topical miconazole	E
• Oral erythromycin	E
• Topical formaldehyde	E

Pitted keratolysis: successful management with mupirocin 2% ointment monotherapy. Greywal T, Cohen PR. Dermatol Online J 2015; 15: 21.

Complete resolution of a patient with pitted keratolysis occurred after monotherapy with twice-daily application of mupirocin 2% ointment for a duration of 3 weeks. There was no recurrence at a follow-up visit 8 weeks later.

P1606 *Kytococcus sedentarius* nail infection. Towerser L, Azulay RD, Filho PJS, Fischman-Gompertz O, Hay RJ. J Am Acad Dermatol Supplement 2008; 58: AB88.

A case report of a patient with *Kytococcus* PK and associated nail dystrophy responding to systemic amoxicillin and potassium clavulanate, topical mupirocin cream for feet lesions, and gentamicin sulfate solution for nail lesions.

Pitted keratolysis: a new form of treatment [Letter]. Burkhart CG. Arch Dermatol 1980; 116: 1104.

Three patients with PK were treated with topical 1% clindamycin hydrochloride solution (660 mg dissolved in 55 mL of 70%

isopropyl alcohol and 5% propylene glycol). The solution was applied to the plantar surface three times daily, and within 4 weeks there was complete resolution of the clinical lesions.

Road rash with a rotten odor. Schissel DJ, Aydelotte J, Keller R. Military Med 1999; 164: 65–7.

Case report of a soldier treated with topical clotrimazole cream twice a day, topical clindamycin solution twice a day, and topical ammonium chloride each evening. At his 2-week follow-up appointment, he reported resolution of the odor, tenderness, and interdigital pruritus, and at 8 weeks he had complete resolution.

The use of a clindamycin 1%-benzoyl peroxide 5% topical gel in the treatment of pitted keratolysis: a novel therapy. Vlahovic TC, Dunne SP, Kemp K. Adv Skin Wound Care 2009; 22: 564–6.

The combination topical gel of clindamycin 1% with benzoyl peroxide 5% was reported to be effective in four patients, but efficacy required the concurrent use of aluminum chloride hexahydrate solution.

Comparative study of benzoyl peroxide versus clindamycin phosphate in treatment of pitted keratolysis. Kim BJ, Park KU, Kim JY, Ahn JY, Won CH, Lee JH, et al. Korean J Med Mycol 2005; 10: 144–50.

A total of 44 patients with PK were reported in this study. Seventeen received benzoyl peroxide alone, 15 received clindamycin alone, and 12 received combination benzoyl peroxide and clindamycin therapy. There was no difference in treatment efficacy between monotherapy or combination therapy. Although not significant, the clindamycin group had a slightly higher recurrence rate. Four cases recurred within 3 months and all were related to hyperhidrosis.

Pitted keratolysis: a clinicopathologic review. Stanton RL, Schwartz RA, Aly R. J Am Podiatry Assoc 1982; 72: 436–9.

Topical 2% erythromycin applied twice daily resulted in resolution of PK in both feet within 4 weeks of treatment in one case.

Pitted keratolysis, erythromycin, and hyperhidrosis. Pranteda G, Carlesimo M, Pranteda G, Abruzzese C, Grimaldi M, De Micco S, et al. Dermatol Ther 2014; 27: 101–4.

Erythromycin 3% gel was applied twice daily in an uncontrolled study on 97 patients. Clinical manifestations regressed within 10 days.

Painful, plaque-like, pitted keratolysis occurring in childhood. Shah AS, Kamino H, Prose NS. Pediatr Dermatol 1992: 9: 251–4.

Two children were reported with these lesions; treatment with topical 2% erythromycin solution twice a day was curative in both patients within 3 weeks of commencing treatment.

Ultrastructure of pitted keratolysis. De Almeida Jr HL, De Castro LAS, Rocha NEM, Abrantes VL. Int J Dermatol 2000; 39: 698–709.

A case report of a patient who responded to topical erythromycin with good results.

Coexistent erythrasma, trichomycosis axillaris, and pitted keratolysis: an overlooked corynebacterial triad? Shelley WB, Shelley ED. J Am Acad Dermatol 1982; 7: 752–7.

A case report of two patients with this triad, one of whom was treated with oral erythromycin 250 mg four times daily and a solution of 20% aluminum chloride applied nightly to the soles.

Three weeks later the plantar hyperhidrosis and odor were significantly reduced, but the pits remained. The other patient declined treatment for PK.

Pitted and ringed keratolysis. A review and update. Zaias N. J Am Acad Dermatol 1982; 7: 787–91.

The author has personal observations (noncontrolled) that treatment of PK with topical clotrimazole, miconazole, erythromycin, tetracycline, clindamycin, glutaraldehyde, formaldehyde, and oral erythromycin are curative. Penicillin has not been useful.

Formaldehyde treatment for pitted keratolysis. Primary Care Dermatologic Society website. http://www.pcds.org.uk/patient-information-leaflets (accessed March 2016).

Patient information leaflet: 5% formaldehyde soaks for 10 minutes daily for 4 to 6 weeks for the treatment of PK.

Third-Line Therapies

• Topical glutaraldehyde	D
• Topical gentamicin	E
• Topical Whitfield ointment	E
• Topical triamcinolone	E
• Topical iodochlorhydroxyquin–hydrocortisone	E
• Topical flexible collodion	E
• Botulinum toxin injections	E

Pitted keratolysis: forme fruste old treatments. Gordon HH. Arch Dermatol 1981; 117: 608.

Buffered glutaraldehyde 2% used with beneficial therapeutic results on PK and hyperhidrosis (uncontrolled personal observations). The author also advises that proper instructions on foot hygiene be given and sandals worn as much as possible. He reports sensitization to glutaraldehyde in some cases.

Pitted keratolysis: forme fruste. A review and new therapies. Gordon HH. Cutis 1975; 15: 54–8.

Buffered glutaraldehyde 2% applied twice daily in five patients resulted in relief of signs and symptoms except in one patient addicted to wearing boots, who continued to have hyperhidrosis. Treatment with gentamicin cream resulted in improvement.

Hyperhidrosis: treatment with glutaraldehyde. Gordon HH. Cutis 1972; 9: 375–8.

Eight patients with a mixture of palmar and plantar hyperhidrosis were treated with varying strengths of 2%, 2.5%, 5%, and 10% aqueous glutaraldehyde with good results. Glutaraldehyde 10%, not alkalinized, was found to be rapidly effective but was associated with brown staining. Use of a 5% starting strength three times weekly minimized the tanning, and these patients were then placed on 2% or 2.5% strengths as required for maintenance treatment. None of these patients developed contact dermatitis.

Glutaraldehyde solution. Shah MK. Indian J Dermatol Venereol Leprol 2004; 70: 319–20.

Sometimes the patient with PK may require 10% glutaraldehyde to treat the hyperhidrosis. The 10% strength is likely to result in brown staining. Buffering with sodium bicarbonate may reduce the irritation but may also reduce its efficacy and stability. Glutaraldehyde 10% is prepared by mixing 15 mL of water with 10 mL of 25% glutaraldehyde. To buffer to pH 7.5, 1.65 g of sodium bicarbonate is added to 100 mL of 10% glutaraldehyde solution. The buffered solution should be used within half an hour. The author recommends thrice-weekly applications for 2 weeks then once weekly as needed.

Keratolysis plantare sulcatum. Higashi N. Jpn J Clin Dermatol 1972; 26: 321–5.

Two patients with KP were treated with topical gentamicin sulfate cream and reported to have good results.

Symptomatic pitted keratolysis. Lamberg SI. Arch Dermatol 1969; 100: 10–11.

Report of 12 military personnel with symptomatic PK treated with various topical agents. One foot was used for treatment, and the other was utilized as a control without treatment or compared with another topical agent. These included steroid creams, antibiotic creams, iodochlorhydroxyquin–hydrocortisone (vioform hydrocortisone) cream, flexible collodion, Whitfield ointment, and formalin in Aquaphor (20–40%). Formalin (40%) ointment appeared to be the most effective and was used for the remainder of both asymptomatic and symptomatic patients with PK. All cases returned to full duty with the ointment after a single outpatient visit, and on reexamination the PK had resolved.

Pitted keratolysis. Gill KA Jr, Buckels LJ. Arch Dermatol 1968; 98: 7–11.

Water-repellent *silicone ointment* has no effect on PK. Lesions resolved spontaneously without treatment after removal from the moist environment.

Plantar hyperhidrosis and pitted keratolysis treated with botulinum toxin injection. Tamura BM, Cucé LC, Souza RL, Levites J. Dermatol Surg 2004; 30: 1510–4.

Two patients resistant to topical and systemic treatments responded completely to one course of low-dose botulinum toxin injections to the plantar aspects of the feet.

Evidence Levels: **A** Double-blind study **B** Clinical trial ≥ 20 subjects **C** Clinical trial < 20 subjects **D** Series ≥ 5 subjects **E** Anecdotal case reports

191

Pityriasis rubra pilaris

Anne-Marie Tobin, Brian Kirby, Mark Lebwohl

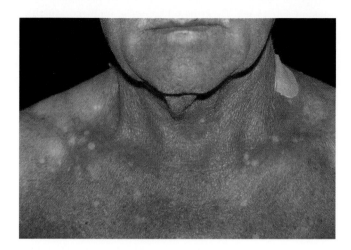

Pityriasis rubra pilaris (PRP) is a rare papulosquamous disorder characterized by erythroderma, orange-red keratoderma, and "islands of sparing." It can be divided into six subtypes based on morphologic phenotype, age of onset, and presence of HIV infection:

- Type I: classical adult; rapid-onset erythroderma, scale, and keratoderma in a craniocaudal pattern
- Type II: atypical adult pattern
- Type III: classical juvenile pattern
- Type IV: atypical juvenile pattern
- Type V: well-circumscribed pattern
- Type VI: HIV-associated PRP

More than 50% of cases are of the classical type I adult-onset PRP. The majority of cases of type I classical PRP go into spontaneous remission after 1 to 3 years.

As PRP is a rare condition, there are no randomized controlled trials assessing treatment efficacy. Treatment recommendations are based on case reports and small case series. PRP has been reported in association with malignancies, including cholangiocarcinoma, metastatic squamous cell carcinoma, colon cancer, and adenocarcinoma of the lung. It is unclear if these are simply chance associations or if they have a role in the development of PRP. There are reports of familial PRP, including rare autosomal-dominant forms of the disease. CARD14 mutations have been reported in familial and sporadic forms of PRP.

Development of PRP after Epstein-Barr virus (EBV) infection has been reported, and antiretroviral therapy has resulted in improvement of type VI PRP. Multiple drugs have also been associated with the development of PRP, including insulin, bevacizumab, sofosbuvir, imatinib, and ponatinib. PRP has also been reported after photodynamic therapy and after treatment with infliximab, a drug that has also been used to treat PRP. There is one report of PRP developing after exposure to dolomite. These reports have been inconsistent and suggest a chance occurrence rather than a true association.

MANAGEMENT STRATEGY

Topical therapies are primarily used as antipruritic agents. *Emollient* use should be encouraged in combination with emollient baths. *Topical steroids* may reduce pruritus but are often ineffective.

There are a few case reports of effective use of both *narrowband UVB and PUVA* for PRP. PRP can often be exacerbated by UV light, and we recommend that narrowband UVB and PUVA be only used cautiously and only when other treatments are contraindicated.

Oral retinoids have been the mainstay of therapy for classical type I and type III PRP. Doses of 0.5 mg/kg and upward of *acitretin* are required for adequate control. This often results in significant mucocutaneous side effects and hair loss. Skin fragility and pruritus are common side effects at these doses. It is our practice to initiate treatment with acitretin for rapid improvement but to add in a second agent if intolerable side effects ensue or if the response is inadequate. Recently a new retinoid, *alitretinoin*, has been used effectively to treat PRP, and it has fewer side effects.

Methotrexate has been reported in several case series as being effective in classical type I PRP. The long-term efficacy of methotrexate is well established. Doses of up to 30 mg weekly are necessary, and concomitant folic acid is recommended. Despite reservations of its use with acitretin regarding hepatotoxicity, it has been reported as a safe combination, and we would concur with that view.

Due to its similarity to psoriasis, PRP has been treated with *TNF-α inhibitors, ustekinumab, secukinumab,* and *apremilast*. When monotherapy doesn't work, combination therapy can be effective.

Specific Investigations

- Histology
- HIV testing
- Flow cytometry
- Chemistry screen and complete blood count (CBC)

Histology of the affected skin may be useful in aiding the diagnosis. It is important to obtain histology and flow cytometry to rule out other causes of erythroderma, especially cutaneous T-cell lymphoma.

Routine blood tests are recommended as markers of general health and as screening for the use of systemic agents. An HIV test should be done in all patients.

First-Line Therapies

Retinoids	**D**
Methotrexate	**D**

Late onset pityriasis rubra pilaris type IV treated with low-dose acitretin. Mota F, Carvalho S, Sanches M, Selores M. Acta Dermatovenerol Alp Pannonica Adriat 2016; 25: 15–7.

A 19-year-old with PRP cleared completely after acitretin 25 mg orally every other day for 6 months.

This and other publications advocate acitretin in doses of 0.5 to 0.75 mg/kg daily for PRP.

Alitretinoin (9-*cis* retinoic acid) is effective against pityriasis rubra pilaris: a retrospective clinical study. Amann PM, Susic M, Glüder F, Berger H, Krapf W, Löffler H. Acta Derm Venereol 2015; 95: 329–31.

Four of five patients with PRP responded to oral alitretinoin 30 mg daily for up to 22 weeks.

Where it is available, alitretinoin may be a good alternative retinoid to acitretin because it has fewer mucocutaneous side effects.

Pityriasis rubra pilaris. Griffiths WAD. Clin Exp Dermatol 1980; 5: 105–12.

Methotrexate treatment of PRP is discussed in these papers. In one series, methotrexate was effective in 17 of 42 patients only. This was a retrospective report where various doses and dosing regimens were used. It is the authors' view that doses up to 30 mg weekly may be needed for control.

Second-Line Therapies	
• Ciclosporin	E
• TNF-α inhibitors	D
• Ustekinumab	E
• Secukinumab	E
• Apremilast	E

Three cases of pityriasis rubra pilaris successfully treated with cyclosporin A. Usuki K, Sekiyama M, Shimada T, Shimada S, Kanzaki T. Dermatology 2000; 200: 324–7.

Three cases were successfully treated with 5 mg/kg daily and responded in 3 to 4 weeks. The ciclosporin dose was then gradually tapered.

Some patients require long-term low-dose ciclosporin to maintain remission. Because of the nephrotoxicity of ciclosporin and the malignancies associated with long-term use, switching to alternative therapies should be attempted.

Effectiveness of infliximab in pityriasis rubra pilaris is associated with pro-inflammatory cytokine inhibition. Adnot-Desanlis L, Antonicelli F, Tabary T, Bernard P, Reguiaï Z. Dermatology 2013; 226: 41–6.

Etanercept-induced clinical remission of type II pityriasis rubra pilaris with rheumatoid arthritis. Kim JH, Park MC, Kim SC. Acta Derm Venereol 2012; 92: 399–400.

Clinical remission of pityriasis rubra pilaris with adalimumab in an adolescent patient. Kim BR, Chae JB, Park JT, Byun SY, Youn SW. J Dermatol 2015; 42: 1122–3.

A systematic review of the literature on the treatment of pityriasis rubra pilaris type I with TNF-alpha antagonists. Petrof G, Almaani N, Archer CB, Griffiths WA, Smith CH. J Eur Acad Dermatol Venereol 2013; 27: e131–5.

Successful treatment of pityriasis rubra pilaris (type 1) under combination of infliximab and methotrexate. Barth D, Harth W, Treudler R, Simon JC. J Dtsch Dermatol 2009; 7: 1071–4.

Eighty-three percent of 15 patients achieved a complete response. In most of these cases the remission achieved was attributable to TNF inhibition. The majority of patients who have been treated with TNF inhibitors have type I classic adult PRP.

The same doses of TNF blockers used for psoriasis have been effective for PRP: etanercept at doses of 25 mg administered subcutaneously twice weekly or 50 mg one to two times per week; subcutaneous adalimumab 80 mg followed by 40 mg every other week; and infusions of

infliximab at doses of 5 mg per kg at weeks 0, 2, and 6 and every 6 to 8 weeks thereafter. Clearing occurs in weeks to months, but the condition can recur upon discontinuation of the drug.

Long-term ustekinumab treatment for refractory type I pityriasis rubra pilaris. Di Stefani A, Galluzzo M, Talamonti M, Chiricozzi A, Costanzo A, Chimenti S. J Dermatol Case Rep 2013; 7: 5–9.

A patient with PRP refractory to acitretin, methotrexate, and ciclosporin responded within 4 weeks of his first injection of ustekinumab 45 mg. He achieved complete remission after the third injection and maintained remission on treatment through 64 weeks.

Ustekinumab in psoriasis doses (i.e., 45 mg under 100 kg and 90 mg over 100 kg) at weeks 0 and 4 and every 12 weeks thereafter has been used successfully for PRP in several case reports.

Successful treatment of refractory pityriasis rubra pilaris with secukinumab. Schuster D, Pfister-Wartha A, Bruckner-Tuderman L, Schempp CM. JAMA Dermatol 2016; 152: 1278–80.

A patient with PRP refractory to acitretin responded to secukinumab in the same dose as is used for psoriasis: 300 mg subcutaneously weekly for 5 weeks followed by 300 mg per month. Response was noted in 3 weeks and complete clearing by 8 weeks.

Treatment of refractory pityriasis rubra pilaris with novel phosphodiesterase 4 (pde4) inhibitor apremilast. Krase IZ, Cavanaugh K, Curiel-Lewandrowski C. JAMA Dermatol 2016; 152: 348–50.

A 70-year-old male with PRP developed small cell lymphocytic leukemia shortly after starting infliximab for the PRP. He later responded to apremilast starting at 10 mg per day increased over 5 days to 30 mg twice daily (as is routine for psoriasis).

Third-Line Therapies	
• Acitretin and narrowband UVB	E
• Acitretin and UVA1	E
• Intravenous immunoglobulin	E
• Extracorporeal photochemotherapy	E
• Fumaric acid esters	E
• Anti-retroviral therapy	E
• Vitamin A	E

Pityriasis rubra pilaris treated with acitretin and narrow-band UVB (Re-TL-01). Kirby B, Watson R. Br J Dermatol 2000; 142: 376–7.

This is a single case report of juvenile classic PRP (type III).

Combination ultraviolet A1 radiation and acitretin therapy as a treatment option for pityriasis rubra pilaris. Herbst RA, Vogelbruch M, Ehnis A, Kapp A, Weiss J. Br J Dermatol 2000; 142: 574–5.

This is a case report of long-wave UVA and retinoid in combination for the treatment of classic type I PRP.

Photoaggravated pityriasis rubra pilaris. Evangelou G, Murdoch SR, Palamaras I, Rhodes LE. Photodermatol Photoimmunol Photomed 2005; 21: 272–4.

PRP may be aggravated by UV light, and these treatments should be considered only when other more effective therapies are ineffective or contraindicated.

Evidence Levels: **A** Double-blind study **B** Clinical trial ≥ 20 subjects **C** Clinical trial < 20 subjects **D** Series ≥ 5 subjects **E** Anecdotal case reports

Extracorporeal photochemotherapy for the treatment of erythrodermic pityriasis rubra pilaris. Hofer A, Mullegger R, Kerl H. Arch Dermatol 1999; 135: 475–6.

Extracorporeal photochemotherapy for the treatment of exanthemic pityriasis rubra pilaris. Haenssle HA, Bertsch HP, Wolf C, Zutt M. Clin Exp Dermatol 2004; 29: 244–6.

These are single case reports of the efficacy of extracorporeal photochemotherapy in PRP.

Type II adult-onset pityriasis rubra pilaris successfully treated with intravenous immunoglobulin. Kerr AC, Ferguson J. Br J Dermatol 2007; 156: 1055–6.

This is a report of the successful use of IVIG at a dose of 2 g/kg given over 3 days. The dose was repeated every 4 weeks. The patient had failed therapy with anti-TNF agents.

Successful treatment of type I pityriasis rubra pilaris with ustekinumab. Ruiz-Villavarde R, Sanchez-Cano D. Eur J Dermatol 2010; 20: 630–1.

Fumaric acid esters: a new treatment modality for pityriasis rubra pilaris. Coras B, Vogt TH, Ulrich H, Landthaler M, Hohenleutner U. Br J Dermatol 2005; 152: 388–99.

Despite their widespread use in psoriasis, we can find only one case report of fumaric acid ester use in PRP. This was the successful use of fumaric acid esters in a patient with atypical juvenile (type IV) PRP.

HIV-associated pityriasis rubra pilaris: response to triple anti-retroviral therapy. Gonzalez-Lopez A, Velasco E, Pozo T, Del Vilar A. Br J Dermatol 1999; 140: 931–4.

PRP associated with HIV infection may respond to antiretroviral therapy. The response appears to correlate with a reduction in viral load.

Successful treatment of pityriasis rubra pilaris with oral vitamin A in oil (Chocola A) for an 18-month-old child. Kan Y, Sumikawa Y, Yamashita T. J Dermatol 2015; 42: 1210–1.

An 18-month-old infant with PRP was treated with vitamin A 20,000 units daily without response until the dose was increased to 60,000 units daily. Skin lesions resolved after 2 months on that dose, but recurred 2 weeks after the vitamin A was discontinued. The vitamin A was continued intermittently to control the PRP.

Pityriasis lichenoides chronica

Matthew J. Scorer, Graham A. Johnston

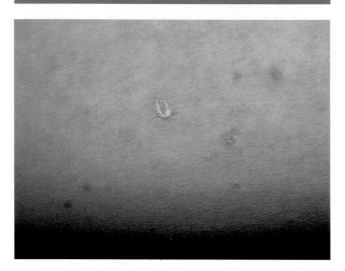

Pityriasis lichenoides chronica (PLC) typically consists of small erythematous papules, which may be purpuric. These develop a characteristic, shiny, micalike scale attached to the center. They occur predominantly over the trunk and proximal limbs. As the name implies, PLC may persist for many years, though spontaneous resolution does occur. Patients should be warned that relapse is common and that recurrent courses of therapy may be required.

Anecdotally, PLC was said to run a more benign, self-limiting course in children, but more recently it has been shown that in children it is more likely to run an unremitting course, with greater lesional distribution, more dyspigmentation, and a poorer response to treatment. Some authors argue that there is an overlap with cutaneous lymphoma.

Pityriasis lichenoides chronica: stratification by molecular and phenotypic profile. Crowson AN, Morrison C, Li J. Hum Pathol 2007; 38: 479–90.

A prospective study of 46 patients concluded that PLC is an indolent, cutaneous T-cell dyscrasia with a limited propensity for progression to mycosis fungoides.

MANAGEMENT STRATEGY

There are few therapeutic trials for this condition, and case series are only small. In many therapeutic trials PLC has been grouped together with pityriasis lichenoides et varioliformis acuta (PLEVA), and management strategies are therefore often similar or interchangeable.

Topical corticosteroids are only reported as effective anecdotally in textbooks rather than in studies. They are often used with *antihistamines* to reduce pruritus, but they are not reported to affect the course of the disease.

The majority of reports describe benefits with *UV therapy*, and therefore either UV alone or *psoralen plus UVA (PUVA)* therapy

is recommended for all patients. The response appears to be unpredictable, however, and the total dose required is extremely variable.

Antibiotics appear to be more helpful in children, sometimes used in combination therapy.

For severe or refractory cases *methotrexate, photochemotherapy,* and *etanercept* have all been described as effective in small numbers of patients.

For most treatment modalities, patients who have been described as improved have usually had fewer new lesions developing, a shortened disease course, and a greater time to relapse than untreated patients.

Specific Investigation
• Consider skin biopsy

Although a skin biopsy is usually unnecessary in clinically obvious cases, it may be useful before commencing systemic therapy with more potential adverse effects.

An infective etiology is often suggested, but no pathogen has yet been implicated, though associations with toxoplasmosis, human herpesvirus-8 (HHV8), and parvovirus B19 have been described. These reports tend to come from endemic areas, and so investigation for a triggering infection is unnecessary in cases without evidence of specific infection.

The relationship between toxoplasmosis and pityriasis lichenoides chronica. Nassef NE, Hamman MA. J Egypt Soc Parasitol 1997; 27: 93–9.

Twenty-two patients with PLC and 20 healthy controls were examined clinically and serologically for toxoplasmosis. Three (15%) of the controls had toxoplasmosis, compared with 8 (36%) of the patients with PLC. Five of the latter had subsidence of skin lesions after pyrimethamine and sulfapyrimidine treatment.

Pityriasis lichenoides et varioliformis acuta and pityriasis lichenoides chronica: comparison of lesional T-cell subsets and investigation of viral associations. Kim JE, Yun WJ, Mun SK, Yoon GS, Huh J, Choi JH, et al. J Cutan Pathol 2011; 38: 649–56.

Fifty-one patients with pityriasis lichenoides (not subdivided into PLEVA and PLC) were analyzed. HHV-8 was found in 11 (21%) of affected patients but in none of the 25 controls.

Pityriasis lichenoides: a cytotoxic T-cell-mediated skin disorder. Evidence of human parvovirus B19 DNA in nine cases. Tomasini D, Tomasini CF, Cerri A, Sangalli G, Palmedo G, Hantschke M, et al. J Cutan Pathol 2004; 31: 531–8.

Thirty tissue samples from cases of pityriasis lichenoides (both PLEVA and PLC) underwent molecular investigation for parvovirus B19 DNA, which was present in nine cases (30%).

First-Line Therapies	
• Ultraviolet B, Psoralen and UVA	C
• Combined UVA and UVB	D
• PUVA	D

Comparative studies of treatments for pityriasis lichenoides. Gritiyarangsan P, Pruenglampoo S, Ruangratanarote P. J Dermatol 1987; 14: 258–61.

Evidence Levels: **A** Double-blind study **B** Clinical trial ≥ 20 subjects **C** Clinical trial < 20 subjects **D** Series ≥ 5 subjects **E** Anecdotal case reports

In this open study 30 patients with pityriasis lichenoides were recruited, although the authors did not specify how many had PLEVA and how many PLC. The first group of 8 were given topical corticosteroid, and half had a partial or complete response. The second group were also given oral tetracycline, and the majority had a partial response. The third group of 8 chronic refractory cases were given oral methoxsalen 0.6 mg/kg with UVA three times per week for an average of 2 months; 5 were cleared and 2 had a partial response.

Is narrowband ultraviolet B monotherapy effective in the treatment of pityriasis lichenoides? Park JM, Jwa SW, Song M, Kim HS, Chin HW, Ko HC, et al. Int J Dermatol 2013; 52: 1013–8.

This retrospective study of 70 patients did not separate PLEVA from PLC but reported a 91.9% complete response rate with narrowband ultraviolet B (NB-UVB). This was not significantly different from the response rate to systemic immunosuppressive therapy or a combination of systemic therapy and NB-UVB.

Narrowband UVB (311 nm, TL01) phototherapy for pityriasis lichenoides. Aydogen K, Saricaoglu H, Turan H. Photodermatol Photoimmunol Photomed 2008; 24: 128–33.

TL-01 phototherapy led to clearance in seven out of eight PLC patients (87.5%) with a mean cumulative dose of 18.4 J/cm^2 after a mean of 45.8 exposures. Relapses occurred in four patients within a mean period of 6 months.

Phototherapy of pityriasis lichenoides. LeVine MJ. Arch Dermatol 1983; 119: 378–80.

PLC in 12 patients cleared completely after an average of 30 treatments of minimally erythemogenic doses of UVA/UVB from fluorescent sunlamps. The average UV dose required was 388 mJ/cm^2.

Phototherapy for pityriasis lichenoides: our experience. Macias VC, Marques-Pinto G, Cardoso J. Cutan Ocul Toxicol 2013; 32: 124–7.

This retrospective study reports the use of PUVA or UVA combined with UVB in 13 patients (11 with PLC, 2 with PLEVA). Complete response to PUVA was achieved in 5 patients, with partial response in 2. In the UVA/UVB group, 2 patients had complete response, and 2 had partial response. One patient in each treatment group did not have a therapeutic response.

Comparison of the therapeutic effects of narrowband UVB vs. PUVA in patients with pityriasis lichenoides. Farnaghi F, Seirafi H, Ehsani AH, Agdari ME, Noormohammadpour P. J Eur Acad Dermatol Venereol 2011; 25: 913–6.

This was a study of 15 patients (not stated how many were PLC or PLEVA) who were randomized to receive UVB (complete response 7 of 8, partial 1 of 8) or PUVA (complete 5 of 7, partial 2 of 7). The authors state that the difference in response is insignificant and that both options are acceptable.

Second-Line Therapy	
• Erythromycin	C

Pityriasis lichenoides: the differences between children and adults. Wahie S, Hiscutt E, Natarajan S, Taylor A. Br J Dermatol 2007; 157: 941–5.

In this retrospective study only two of eight children cleared with erythromycin, whereas three out of four adults cleared without relapse. Phototherapy was more effective in both groups.

Pityriasis lichenoides in childhood: a retrospective review of 124 patients. Ersoy-Evans S, Greco MF, Mancini AJ, Subasi N, Paller AS. J Am Acad Dermatol 2007; 56: 205–10.

This was a retrospective study of 124 children, of whom 46 had PLC. The median age of onset was 60 months and median duration was 20 months (range 3–132 months). Two thirds of children had at least a partial response to erythromycin.

Childhood pityriasis lichenoides and oral erythromycin. Hapa A, Ersoy-Evans S, Karaduman A. Pediatr Dermatol 2012; 29: 719–24.

The records of 24 children (age range 2–14), 15 with PLC, 6 with PLEVA, and 3 overlap started on erythromycin (30–50 mg/kg/day for 1–4 months), were reviewed. Sixty-four percent showed a good response at 1 month, rising to 83% at 3 months. Of 16 patients with follow-up, 3 relapsed (time not given).

Third-Line Therapies	
• Methotrexate	E
• Acitretin plus PUVA	E
• UVA1	E
• Topical tacrolimus	E
• Photodynamic therapy	E
• Etanercept	E

Methotrexate treatment of pityriasis lichenoides and lymphomatoid papulosis. Lynch PJ, Saied NK. Cutis 1979; 23: 635–6.

Three patients received methotrexate 25 mg/week intramuscularly or orally. All responded within weeks, but two relapsed on cessation of therapy.

Pityriasis lichenoides chronica induced by adalimumab therapy for Crohn's disease: report of 2 cases successfully treated with methotrexate. Said BB, Kanitakis J, Graber I, Nicolas JF, Saurin JC, Berard F. Inflamm Bowel Dis 2010; 16: 912–3.

Pityriasis lichenoides chronica induced by infliximab, with response to methotrexate. López-Ferrer A, Puig L, Moreno G, Camps-Fresneda A, Palou J, Alomar A. Eur J Dermatol 2010; 20: 511–2.

Adalimumab-induced pityriasis lichenoides chronica that responded well to methotrexate in a patient with psoriasis. Martínez-Peinado C, Galán-Gutiérrez M, Ruiz-Villaverde R, Solorzano-Mariscal R. Actas Dermosifiliogr 2016; 107: 167–9.

There are four reported cases of PLC, all thought to have been caused by anti-TNFα therapies, that responded well to methotrexate.

Photochemotherapy for pityriasis lichenoides: 3 cases. Panse I, Bourrat E, Rybojad M, Morel P. Ann Dermatol Venereol 2004; 131: 201–3.

One patient with pityriasis lichenoides and two patients with PLEVA unresponsive to other therapies, including topical corticosteroids, antibiotics, and UVB, responded within weeks to acitretin plus PUVA.

Medium-dose ultraviolet A1 therapy for pityriasis lichenoides varioliformis acuta and pityriasis lichenoides chronica. Pinton PC, Capezzera R, Zane C, De Panfilis G. J Am Acad Dermatol 2002; 47: 410–4.

Eight patients (five with PLC and three with PLEVA) were treated. Three patients with PLC showed complete clinical and histologic recovery. Two showed partial improvement.

Successful treatment of pityriasis lichenoides with topical tacrolimus. Simon D, Boudny C, Nievergelt H, Simon HU, Braathen LR. Br J Dermatol 2004; 150: 1033–5.

Two children with long-lasting refractory PLC were cleared of skin lesions after 14 and 18 weeks of treatment, respectively.

Pityriasis lichenoides chronica: good response to photodynamic therapy. Fernandez-Guarino M, Harto A, Reguero-Callerjas ME, Urrutia S, Jaen P. Br J Dermatol 2008; 158: 198–200.

A woman with 15 lesions of PLC had each occluded with methyl aminolevulinic acid for 3 hours followed by a 595-nm pulsed dye laser as a light source (one pulse for each lesion). Lesions cleared after only one treatment.

Etanercept in therapy multiresistant overlapping pityriasis lichenoides. Nikkels AF, Gillard P, Pierard GE. J Drugs Dermatol 2008; 7: 990–2.

A 65-year-old woman had a 5-year history of pityriasis lichenoides unhelped by UVB, PUVA, methotrexate, dapsone, and ciclosporin. She was commenced on etanercept with marked improvement in pruritus and inflammation after 2 months and no new lesions after 4 months when treatment was stopped. However, she relapsed after 1 month.

Conflictingly, there are reports of etanercept, infliximab, and adalimumab causing *pityriasis lichenoides.*

Evidence Levels: **A** Double-blind study **B** Clinical trial ≥ 20 subjects **C** Clinical trial < 20 subjects **D** Series ≥ 5 subjects **E** Anecdotal case reports

193

Pityriasis lichenoides et varioliformis acuta

David Veitch, Graham A. Johnston

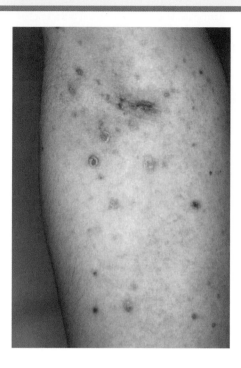

Pityriasis lichenoides et varioliformis acuta (PLEVA) is an eruption of small, erythematous papules that become vesicular and hemorrhagic. Some ulcerate and necrose, leaving pitted scars. The name refers to the morphology, not the duration of the condition, because a significant proportion of cases regress, with or without treatment, only to recur. Patients should be warned that relapse is common and that recurrent courses of therapy may be required. Febrile ulceronecrotic Mucha–Habermann disease is a rare and severe form of PLEVA characterized by an abrupt onset of an ulceronecrotic eruption associated with a high fever and systemic symptoms.

MANAGEMENT STRATEGY

There are only a handful of controlled trials for this condition, and large series are rare. Unfortunately, in many therapeutic trials PLEVA is often reported together with and alongside pityriasis lichenoides chronica, and management strategies are therefore often similar or interchangeable.

Although a "wait and see" approach is justifiable in infants, children should be given a 6-week course of *high-dose erythromycin*. Tetracycline should not be given because of its effects on dentition.

Topical corticosteroids are only reported anecdotally in textbooks rather than in studies. They are used with *antihistamines* to reduce pruritus but have no reported effect on disease course.

Second-line therapy in children, and possibly first-line in adults, is *UV light* or *psoralen plus ultraviolet A (UVA) (PUVA)*. The only comparative study has shown Psoralen and ultraviolet A (PUVA) to be more effective.

In more extensive or symptomatic disease *low-dose methotrexate* is useful, and *systemic corticosteroids* or *ciclosporin* have also been used.

In Mucha–Habermann disease, given its severe nature, *combination therapy* is often prescribed. Intravenous immunoglobulin (IVIG) has been utilized recently.

Specific Investigation

- Consider skin biopsy

A diagnostic skin biopsy is unnecessary in clinically obvious cases but may be useful to exclude lymphomatoid papulosis or before commencing aggressive systemic therapy. Classically a lichenoid infiltrate is seen in the superficial dermis with parakeratosis in the stratum corneum and keratinocyte necrosis in the epidermis. There may be red cell extravasation, including trapped red cells in the epidermis, and a lymphocytic infiltration around the dermal vascular plexus and the dermoepidermal junction.

An infective etiology for PLEVA is suggested by reports of clustering of cases, resolution after tonsillectomy, and occurrence in five members of a family. Varicella-zoster virus (VZV) has been isolated from lesional skin, and DNA from VZV has been demonstrated using polymerase chain reaction (PCR) in skin samples of patients with PLEVA. Case reports exist associating PLEVA with parvovirus, adenovirus in the urine, Staphylococci from throat cultures, Epstein–Barr virus, toxoplasmosis, and Human immunodeficiency virus (HIV) therefore investigation for an infective trigger may be useful.

Pityriasis lichenoides in childhood: a retrospective review of 124 patients. Ersoy-Evans S, Greco MF, Mancini AJ, Subaşi N, Paller AS. J Am Acad Dermatol 2007; 56: 205–10.

The clinical similarity between PLEVA and primary varicella infection and the appearance of cases after chickenpox pointed to the possibility of VZV involvement in this disorder.

Is varicella-zoster virus involved in the etiopathogeny of pityriasis lichenoides? Boralevi F, Cotto E, Baysse L, Jouvencel AC, Léauté-Labrèze C, Taïeb A. J Invest Dermatol 2003; 121: 647–8.

VZV PCR in skin samples was positive in 8/13 cases (61.5%) of histologically confirmed PLEVA.

Pityriasis lichenoides: a cytotoxic T-cell-mediated skin disorder. Evidence of human parvovirus B19 DNA in nine cases. Tomasini D, Tomasini CF, Cerri A, Sangalli G, Palmedo G, Hantschke M, et al. J Cutan Pathol 2004; 31: 531–8.

This study suggested that pityriasis lichenoides is mediated by a cytotoxic T-cell effector population.

The identification of parvovirus B19 DNA in nine cases may be interpreted ambiguously.

Febrile ulceronecrotic Mucha-Habermann disease: proposed diagnostic criteria and therapeutic evaluation. Nofal A, Assaf M, Alakad R, Amer H, Nofal E, Yosef A. Int J Dermatol 2016; 55: 729–38.

The authors propose constant features that must be present to secure a diagnosis of FUMHD (fever, acute onset of generalized ulceronecrotic papules and plaques, rapid and progressive course, histopathology consistent with PLEVA) and variable features that may help avoid missing cases (previous history of PLEVA, mucous membrane involvement, systemic involvement).

First-Line Therapies	
• Oral erythromycin	C
• Oral or IV aciclovir	C

Pityriasis lichenoides in childhood: a retrospective review of 124 patients. Ersoy-Evans S, Greco MF, Mancini AJ, Subasi N, Paller AS. J Am Acad Dermatol 2007; 56: 205–10.

This was a retrospective study of 124 children, 71 of whom had PLEVA. The disease was recurrent in 77%. Erythromycin was given to 79.7% of the affected children, and 66.6% of these showed at least a partial response.

Pityriasis lichenoides in children: therapeutic response to erythromycin. Truhan AP, Hebert AA, Esterly NB. J Am Acad Dermatol 1986; 15: 66–70.

In this retrospective uncontrolled study, 11 children aged 2 to 11 years with biopsy-proven PLEVA were given oral erythromycin 200 mg three or four times daily. Nine improved within a month, and 2 to 6 months after stopping the drug there was only one recurrence. One patient improved on an increased dose, and one failed to respond.

Further case reports describe response to roxithromycin and azithromycin.

Second-Line Therapies	
• Broadband ultraviolet B (UVB)	C
• Narrowband UVB	D
• PUVA	D
• Acitretin and PUVA	E

Pityriasis lichenoides in children: a long term follow-up of 89 cases. Gelmetti C, Rigoni C, Alessi E, Ermacora E, Berti E, Caputo R. J Am Acad Dermatol 1990; 23: 473–8.

In a retrospective review of 89 cases seen since 1974 the authors did not differentiate between the treatment of PLEVA and that of pityriasis lichenoides chronica (PLC). However, 77 of the children were treated with 4- to 8-week courses of (presumably broadband) UVB phototherapy, which seemed to alleviate symptoms and acute eruptions without modifying the course of the disease. The remaining 12 patients were given oral erythromycin 20 to 40 mg/kg daily for 1 to 2 weeks, and the response was described as "moderately effective."

Comparative studies of treatment for pityriasis lichenoides. Gritiyarangsan P, Pruenglampoo S, Ruangratanarote P. J Dermatol 1987; 14: 258–61.

In this open study 30 patients with pityriasis lichenoides were recruited, although the authors did not specify how many had PLEVA and how many PLC. The first group of eight patients were given topical corticosteroid, and half had a partial or complete response. The second group were given corticosteroid plus oral tetracycline, and the majority had a partial response. The third group of eight patients with chronic refractory pityriasis lichenoides were given oral methoxsalen 0.6 mg/kg with UVA three times a week for an average of 2 months; five cleared and two had a partial response.

Narrowband UVB (311 nm, TL01) phototherapy for pityriasis lichenoides. Aydogan K, Saricaoglu H, Turan H. Photoderatol Photoimmunol Photomed 2008; 24: 128–33.

TL01 treatment led to a complete response in 15 out of 23 PLEVA patients with a mean cumulative dose of 23 J/cm^2 after a mean of 43.4 exposures. There was a partial response in 8 patients (34.8%) with a cumulative dose of 15.6 J/cm^2 after a mean of 32.3 exposures.

Photochemotherapy for pityriasis lichenoides. Panse I, Bourrat E, Rybojad M, Morel P. Ann Dermatol Venereol 2004; 131: 201–3.

Two patients, aged 6 and 18 years, presented with a 1-month and 3-month history of PLEVA, respectively. They had received different treatments without significant effect: topical corticosteroids, antibiotic, UVB therapy, and dapsone. A combination of acitretin and PUVA was described as dramatically effective within a few weeks.

Third-Line Therapies	
• Methotrexate	E
• ciclosporin	E
• Systemic corticosteroids	E
• Intravenous immunoglobulin	E
• Azithromycin and topical tacrolimus	E

Febrile ulceronecrotic Mucha-Habermann disease: two cases with excellent response to methotrexate. Griffith-Bauer K, Leitenberger SL, Krol A. Pediatr Dermatol 2015; 32: 307–8.

Two biopsy-proven cases of this condition in 6- and 7-year-old boys. One was treated with clindamycin and corticosteroids with minimal benefit. The other was treated with corticosteroids and cefazolin without benefit. Both were then commenced on 7.5 mg/week of methotrexate, leading to clinical improvement within 4 weeks.

Methotrexate treatment in children with febrile ulceronecrotic Mucha-Habermann disease: case report and literature review. Bulur I, Kaya Erdoğan H, Nurhan Saracoglu Z, Arik D. Case Rep Dermatol Med 2015; 357973.

Eleven-year-old male with biopsy-proven Mucha–Habermann disease treated unsuccessfully with 10 days of 32 mg/day methylprednisolone. Marked improvement was seen after 6 weeks of 15 mg/week methotrexate.

Febrile ulceronecrotic Mucha-Habermann disease in a 34-month-old boy: a case report and review of the literature. Perrin BS, Yan AC, Treat JR. Pediatr Dermatol 2012; 29: 53–8.

Thirty-four-month-old boy treated with corticosteroids, IVIG, dapsone, and aciclovir, without complete resolution of disease. He was then commenced on methotrexate 15 mg/week with disease resolution at 6 weeks.

Resistant pityriasis lichenoides et varioliformis acuta in a 3-year-old boy: successful treatment with methotrexate. Lazaridou E, Fotiadou C, Tsorova C, Trachana M, Trigoni A, Patsatsi A, et al. Int J Dermatol 2010; 49: 215–7.

A 3-year-old boy was diagnosed with biopsy-proven PLEVA. The only therapeutic approach that eventually managed to cease the disease evolution was the combination of prednisolone (1 mg/kg for 8 weeks) and methotrexate (5 mg/week for 8 weeks).

Successful therapy of cyclosporin A in pityriasis lichenoides et varioliformis acuta preceded by hand, foot and

Evidence Levels: A Double-blind study B Clinical trial ≥ 20 subjects C Clinical trial < 20 subjects D Series ≥ 5 subjects E Anecdotal case reports

mouth disease. Lis-Święty A, Michalska-Bańkowska A, Zielonka-Kucharzewska A, Pypłacz-Gumprecht A. Antivir Ther 2015; 21(3): 273–5.

Enteroviral infection complicated by biopsy-proven PLEVA in a 30-year-old woman. Treatment with 3 mg/kg/day cyclosporin A resulted in rapid clinical improvement and discontinuation after 4 weeks.

Successful long-term use of cyclosporin A in HIV-induced pityriasis lichenoides chronica. Griffiths JK. J AIDS 1998; 18: 396.

A 42-year-old woman with AIDS developed biopsy-proven Pityriasis lichenoides chronica (PLC), which then developed into life-threatening, febrile, ulceronecrotic PLEVA. Treatment with ciclosporin 200 mg daily produced a rapid response, though prolonged maintenance treatment was required. Interestingly, the severity of symptoms appeared to parallel the viral load.

Pityriasis lichenoides et varioliformis acuta: case report and review of the literature. Pereira N, Brinca A, Manuel Brites M, José Julião M, Tellechea O, Gonçalo M. Case Rep Dermatol 2012; 4: 61–5.

A 63-year-old man with biopsy-proven PLEVA was treated with erythromycin (1 g/day) and methylprednisolone (32 mg/day) reduced gradually over 5 months, with a slow but complete response.

Transition of pityriasis lichenoides et varioliformis acuta to febrile ulceronecrotic Mucha–Habermann disease is associated with elevated serum tumor necrosis factor-alpha. Tsianakas A, Hoeger PH. Br J Dermatol 2005; 152: 794–9.

The authors describe a child whose progression from PLEVA to Mucha–Habermann disease was accompanied by a rapid rise in serum tumor necrosis factor (TNF)-α. She was treated successfully with methotrexate.

The authors postulate that therapy with TNF antagonists may be indicated in these cases.

Febrile ulceronecrotic Mucha-Habermann disease: treatment with infliximab and intravenous immunoglobulins and review of the literature. Meziane L, Caudron A, Dhaille F, Jourdan M, Dadban A, Lok C, et al. Dermatology 2012; 225: 344–8.

A 65-year-old woman with a resistant form of Mucha–Habermann disease was treated with the TNF-alpha inhibitor infliximab (5 mg/kg 6 weekly). However, despite every 6 weeks for 12 months of treatment the patient began to develop new lesions, and treatment became complicated by severe sepsis. The introduction of IVIG (2 mg/kg monthly) induced improvement after "several" months.

High dose immunoglobulins and extracorporeal photo-chemotherapy in the treatment of febrile ulceronecrotic Mucha–Habermann disease. Marenco F, Fava MT, Quaglino P, Bernengo G. Dermatol Ther 2010; 23: 419–22.

A 23-year-old man responded to IVIG (400 mg/kg/day for 5 days monthly) plus methotrexate 10 mg/m² weekly with remission after five courses. He was then started on extracorporeal chemotherapy as maintenance treatment.

Successful association in the treatment of pityriasis lichenoides et varioliformis acuta. Di Constanzo L, Balato N, La Bella S, Balato A. J Eur Acad Dermatol Venereol 2009; 23: 971–2.

A 9-year-old girl who failed on oral erythromycin showed "significant improvement" on oral azithromycin 500 mg/day for 3 consecutive days on alternate weeks and daily topical tacrolimus 0.1% ointment. Total duration of treatment was not stated, but there was no recurrence at 4 months.

Pityriasis rosea

Anna E. Muncaster

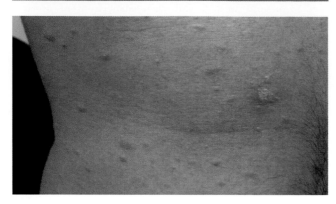

Pityriasis rosea is a common, acute, self-limiting, papulosquamous disorder affecting the trunk and limbs. It is usually seen in the 10- to 35-year age group and has a recorded incidence of between 0.39% and 4.8% in dermatology patients. It has a classical clinical appearance and is associated with little or no constitutional upset, but can have associated itching. Secondary syphilis and drug eruptions are diagnostic pitfalls.

MANAGEMENT STRATEGY

Pityriasis rosea usually resolves spontaneously after approximately 6 weeks, and, if asymptomatic, reassurance is all that is required. Epidemiologic and microbiologic studies have strongly suggested an infectious etiology, most likely viral. The most likely culprits are human herpesvirus-6 (HHV-6) and -7, and in fact reactivation of latent HHV-6 or -7 is postulated but as yet there is no definite proof of causality. Studies have also looked at, but failed to prove, an etiologic role for HHV-8, and there have been two case reports of a pityriasis rosea–like eruption occurring in patients with H1N1 influenza A virus. There have been case reports of pityriasis rosea–like eruptions after many drugs, including captopril, ketotifen, and more recently adalimumab, imatinib mesylate, and etanercept. However, there is no evidence that true pityriasis rosea is drug induced.

For patients who do require treatment, *topical corticosteroids* may be helpful, although evidence for this is purely anecdotal. *Emollients* and oral *antihistamines* have also been mentioned as being of some benefit, as has *ultraviolet light*.

Studies have shown that UVB can reduce itch and disease severity, and a study using low-dose UVA1 phototherapy showed significant reduction in the severity and extent of the disease but little impact on pruritus.

For patients with more extensive severe eruptions, *oral prednisolone* can be tried; however, this should be used with caution, as there are also reports that oral steroids can exacerbate the condition.

A trial of *oral erythromycin* produced complete clearance after 2 weeks in the majority of patients. The best results with all the treatments noted earlier have been obtained when treatment is started within the first 2 weeks of the appearance of the eruption. There has been one case report of vesicular pityriasis rosea responding to 10 days of oral erythromycin at a dose of 250 mg four times a day, but further trials using oral erythromycin, azithromycin, and clarithromycin have all failed to show any benefit.

Oral *acyclovir* has been used in pityriasis rosea at both high and low doses with positive results. One study compared high-dose acyclovir with erythromycin and found acyclovir to be more effective. There has also been one case report of pityriasis rosea clearing after oral acyclovir and one showing clearance with dapsone.

Specific Investigations

- Consider mycologic examination
- Consider syphilis serology

First-Line Therapies

• Topical corticosteroids	E
• Emollients	E
• Oral antihistamines	E

Pityriasis rosea update: 1986. Parsons JM. J Am Acad Dermatol 1986; 15: 159–67.

The author relates his own experience of using topical corticosteroids, emollients, and oral antihistamines in the treatment of pityriasis rosea. He claims all three treatments to have been of some benefit.

A comprehensive review article.

Interventions for pityriasis rosea. Chuh AAT, Dofitas BL, Comisel CG, Reveiz L, Sharma V, Garner SE, et al. Cochrane Database Syst Rev 2007; 2: CD005068.

The authors found that good evidence for the efficacy of most treatments for pityriasis rosea was lacking and suggest more research is needed to fully evaluate erythromycin and other treatments.

Second-Line Therapies

• UVB	B
• UVA1	C

Treatment of pityriasis rosea with UV radiation. Arndt KA, Paul BS, Stern RS, Parrish JA. Arch Dermatol 1983; 119: 381–2.

Twenty patients with symptomatic and extensive pityriasis rosea were treated with UVB phototherapy in a bilateral comparison study using the left side of their body as a control. Five consecutive daily erythemogenic exposures resulted in both clinical and subjective improvement in disease severity and pruritus in 50% of the patients.

UVB phototherapy for pityriasis rosea: a bilateral comparison study. Leenitaphong V, Jiamton S. J Am Acad Dermatol 1995; 33: 996–9.

Seventeen patients with extensive pityriasis rosea were treated unilaterally with 10 daily erythemogenic doses of UVB in a bilateral comparison study using 1 J of UVA to the other half of the body as a control. This resulted in a significant reduction in disease severity in 15 out of the 17 patients but no difference in pruritus.

UVB phototherapy for pityriasis rosea. Valkova S, Trashlieva M, Christova PJ. Eur Acad Dermatol Venereol 2004; 18: 111–2.

Evidence Levels: **A** Double-blind study **B** Clinical trial ≥ 20 subjects **C** Clinical trial < 20 subjects **D** Series ≥ 5 subjects **E** Anecdotal case reports

In a letter to the editor the authors describe a study of 101 patients (including children) who received broadband UVB either to half the body (24 patients), using UVA on the other half as a control, or to the whole body (77 patients). They showed clearance of the disease in both groups, with those patients having more severe disease requiring significantly more treatments.

Low-dose ultraviolet A1 phototherapy for treating pityriasis rosea. Lim SH, Kim SM, Oh BH, Ko JH, Lee YW, Choe YB, et al. Ann Dermatol 2009; 21: 230–6.

Fifteen patients were treated with UVA1 starting at doses of 10 to 20 J/cm² using 20% increments up to 30 J/cm² given two to three times a week until complete clearance was achieved. Twelve out of the 15 patients showed complete clearance, and the other 3 showed significant improvement with less than 25% of lesions persisting. The mean number of treatments was 6.5.

Third-Line Therapies	
• Oral prednisolone	D
• Oral erythromycin	B
• Oral acyclovir	A
• Dapsone	E

One year review of pityriasis rosea at the National Skin Centre, Singapore. Tay YK, Goh CL. Ann Acad Med Singapore 1999; 28: 829–31.

In this retrospective case note study of 368 patients, 20 with extensive pruritic disease were treated with short reducing courses of prednisolone over 2 to 3 weeks, with improvement.

Pityriasis rosea: exacerbation with corticosteroid treatment. Leonforte JF. Dermatologica 1981; 163: 480–1.

This was a case series of 18 patients, all of whom had received oral corticosteroids for pityriasis rosea. Five were observed while they received their corticosteroid course, and the other 13 were seen after completing their course. In those patients who did report an exacerbation, this was worse the higher the dose of corticosteroid received, the longer the course of treatment, and in those who were treated earlier on in their disease.

Erythromycin in pityriasis rosea: a double-blind, placebo-controlled clinical trial. Sharma PK, Yadav TP, Gautam RK, Taneja N, Satyanarayana L. J Am Acad Dermatol 2000; 42: 241–4.

Ninety patients, including children, were randomly assigned to a treatment or a control group. Those in the treatment group received 2 weeks of oral erythromycin 250 mg four times a day for adults or 25 to 40 mg/kg in four divided doses for children. Of patients in the treatment group, 73% had a complete response compared with none of the controls.

Vesicular pityriasis rosea: response to erythromycin treatment. Miranda SB, Lupi O, Lucas E. J Eur Acad Dermatol Venereol 2004; 18: 622–5.

A case report of a 32-year-old woman with a 6-week history of biopsy-proven vesicular pityriasis rosea who achieved almost complete clearance after 10 days of oral erythromycin at a dose of 250 mg four times a day. No recurrence was observed during a 4-month follow-up period.

The comparison between the efficacy of high dose acyclovir and erythromycin on the period and signs of pityriasis rosea. Eshani A, Esmaily N, Noormohammadpour P, Toosi S, Hosseinpour A, Hosseini M, et al. Indian J Dermatol 2010; 55: 246–8.

In this randomized controlled trial 15 patients with pityriasis rosea were treated with erythromycin 400 mg four times a day for 10 days and the other 15 with acyclovir 800 mg five times a day for 10 days. When evaluated at 8 weeks, 13 out of the 15 patients treated with acyclovir had complete response compared with only 6 of the patients on erythromycin, which was statistically significant. No patients achieved complete response within the first 2 weeks.

A randomized, double-blind, placebo-controlled study of efficacy of oral acyclovir in the treatment of pityriasis rosea. Ganguly S. J Clin Diag Res 2014; 8: YC01–4

In this randomized, double-blind, placebo-controlled trial 38 patients were started on high-dose acyclovir (800 mg five times daily for adults, 20 mg/kg for children four times daily) for 7 days, and 35 were assigned to the placebo group. Results from day 7 and 14 showed a statistically significant response in the treatment group over placebo with 53.33% complete response at day 7 compared with 10% placebo and 86.66% response at day 14 compared with 33.33% in the placebo group

Use of high-dose acyclovir in pityriasis rosea. Drago F, Veccio F, Rebora A. J Am Acad Dermatol 2006; 54: 82–5.

In this placebo-controlled trial, 87 consecutive patients were treated with either oral acyclovir (800 mg five times daily) or placebo for 1 week. At 14 days 78.6% of treated patients achieved complete regression, compared with only 4.4% of the placebo group.

Low dose acyclovir may be an effective treatment against pityriasis rosea: a random investigator-blind clinical trial on 64 patients. Rassai S, Feily A, Sina N, Abtahian SA. J Eur Acad Dermatol Venereal 2011; 25: 24–6.

Sixty-four patients with pityriasis rosea were enrolled in this randomized, comparative, investigator-blinded trial. Patients were randomized to receive acyclovir 400 mg five times a day for 1 week or control. Fifty-four patients completed the study. At the 4-week follow-up 92.8% of patients in the acyclovir group had significant reduction of erythema compared with 61.5% of patients in the control group.

Antivirals for pityriasis rosea. Castanedo-Cazares JP, Lepe V, Moncada B. Photodermatol Photoimmunol Photomed 2004; 20: 110.

In a letter to the editor the authors relate the successful treatment of a case of pityriasis rosea with a short course of oral acyclovir. Dosage and length of treatment were not stated.

Dapsone treatment in a case of vesicular pityriasis rosea. Anderson CR. Lancet 1971; 2: 493.

A case report of a 55-year-old man with histologically proven pityriasis rosea resistant to oral prednisolone responding to dapsone 100 mg twice daily for 1 month.

Polycystic ovary syndrome

Kristina J. Liu, Rachel V. Reynolds

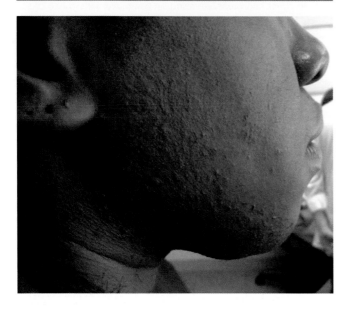

Polycystic ovary syndrome (PCOS) is a common endocrine disorder affecting 6% to 25% of reproductive-aged women. It is characterized by hyperandrogenism, menstrual irregularities, polycystic ovaries, and metabolic derangement.

MANAGEMENT STRATEGY

Several diagnostic criteria for PCOS exist, including definitions from the National Institutes of Health (NIH), the Rotterdam criteria, and the Androgen Excess & Polycystic Ovary Syndrome Society.

Polycystic ovary syndrome diagnostic criteria

1990 National Institutes of Health criteria (both criteria required)
- Chronic anovulation
- Clinical and/or biochemical signs of hyperandrogenism

2003 Rotterdam criteria (two out of three criteria required)
- Oligoovulation or anovulation
- Clinical and/or biochemical signs of hyperandrogenism
- Polycystic ovaries by ultrasound and exclusion of other etiologies (congenital adrenal hyperplasia, androgen-secreting tumors, Cushing's syndrome)

2009 Androgen Excess and Polycystic Ovary Syndrome Society (both criteria are required)
- Oligoovulation or anovulation or polycystic ovaries
- Clinical and/or biochemical signs of hyperandrogenism

Box adapted from Setji TL, Brown AJ. Polycystic ovary syndrome: update on diagnosis and treatment. Am J Med 2014; 127: 912–9.

Treatment of PCOS is targeted toward decreasing androgen excess, normalizing menses, and ameliorating metabolic syndrome and cardiovascular complications. Although treatment of the reproductive and metabolic complications decreases the risk of endometrial cancer and cardiovascular issues, treatment of cutaneous disease is also integral to the care of these patients and their quality of life.

Cutaneous manifestations resulting from androgen excess may include acne in 25% to 35%, hirsutism in 40% to 92%, female pattern alopecia, seborrhea, and, in some, acanthosis nigricans, a sign of hyperinsulinemia. Therefore as dermatologists, we are in a unique position to identify and treat patients early in the course of their disease.

Cutaneous manifestations, including acne and hirsutism, may be targeted using topical or oral retinoids and/or topical or systemic antibiotics. If the response is inadequate, combined oral contraceptives (OCPs) and/or antiandrogen therapy may be beneficial. Mechanical hair removal methods may be utilized. In patients with PCOS, lifestyle modification is the first-line treatment, and weight loss may correct all metabolic abnormalities. In those with inadequate response, insulin resistance may be treated with insulin-sensitizing agents, such as metformin.

PCOS is associated with several mental health problems, including depression and anxiety, body dissatisfaction and eating disorders, diminished sexual satisfaction, and lowered health-related quality of life. Patients should be evaluated for psychological issues and referred for appropriate counseling as needed.

Specific Investigations

- Ovary ultrasound imaging
- Serum androgen levels (testosterone, dehydroepiandrosterone sulfate (DHEA-S), 17-hydroxyprogesterone)
- Pregnancy (urine or serum hCG)
- Other hormone tests (follicle-stimulating hormone (FSH), luteinizing hormone (LH), thyroid stimulating hormone (TSH), prolactin, 24-hour urine free cortisol)
- Metabolic factors, diabetes (body mass index (BMI), fasting lipid panel, oral glucose-tolerance test)
- Blood pressure

Polycystic ovary syndrome: a review for dermatologists. Part I. Diagnosis and manifestations. Housman E, Reynolds RV. J Am Acad Dermatol 2014; 71: 847.e1–e10.

PCOS is a common disorder that affects up to 8% of women of reproductive age. Other etiologies of hyperandrogenism and anovulation should be ruled out before making a diagnosis of PCOS.

Metformin and lifestyle modification in polycystic ovary syndrome: systematic review and meta-analysis. Naderpoor N, Shorakae S, de Courten B, Misso ML, Moran LJ, Teede HJ. Hum Reprod Update 2015; 21: 560–74.

A meta-analysis comparing the effects of lifestyle modification, metformin, or the combination of these two therapies on metabolic, reproductive, anthropometric, and psychological outcomes.

Lifestyle modification together with metformin is associated with improved menstruation and lower BMI in women with PCOS compared with either therapy alone.

Impaired glucose tolerance, type 2 diabetes and metabolic syndrome in polycystic ovary syndrome: a systematic review and meta-analysis. Moran LJ, Misso ML, Wild RA, Norman RJ. Hum Reprod Update 2010; 16: 347–63.

Evidence Levels: **A** Double-blind study **B** Clinical trial ≥ 20 subjects **C** Clinical trial < 20 subjects **D** Series ≥ 5 subjects **E** Anecdotal case reports

Women with PCOS have increased glucose levels, type 2 diabetes, and metabolic syndrome.

PCOS is strongly linked with insulin resistance and glucose intolerance. Screening for impaired glucose tolerance requires an oral glucose-tolerance test (75 g, 0- and 2-hour values), as HbA_{1c} demonstrates lower sensitivity in comparison.

Meta-analysis of cardiovascular disease risk markers in women with polycystic ovary syndrome. Toulis KA, Goulis DG, Mintziori G, Kintiraki E, Eukarpidis E, Mouratoglou SA, et al. Hum Reprod Update 2011; 17: 741–60.

A meta-analysis of 130 studies revealed that women with PCOS have more coronary artery calcification, vascular endothelial dysfunction, and elevated C-reactive protein and homocysteine levels. Although women with PCOS have increased serum concentrations of cardiovascular disease (CVD) risk markers, an association with increased incidence of CVD is unclear.

Periodic assessment of diabetes, blood pressure, fasting lipid panel, and BMI is recommended in women with PCOS.

Risk of endometrial, ovarian and breast cancer in women with polycystic ovary syndrome: a systematic review and meta-analysis. Barry JA, Azizia MM, Hardiman PJ. Hum Reprod Update 2014; 20: 748–58.

Women of all ages with PCOS are three times more likely to develop endometrial cancer, but there is no evidence of increased risk of breast cancer or ovarian cancer.

First-Line Therapies

• Weight loss	A
• Topical and systemic therapy for acne	A
• Oral contraceptives	A
• Topical eflornithine	B
• IPL (intense pulsed light)/laser hair removal	B
• Minoxidil	B

Lifestyle changes in women with polycystic ovary syndrome. Moran LJ, Hutchison SK, Norman RJ, Teede HJ. Cochrane Database Syst Rev 2001; 7: CD007506.

Lifestyle intervention improves hyperandrogenism (based on clinical hirsutism and total testosterone level), waist circumference, and fasting insulin. Weight management is proposed as an initial treatment strategy.

Treatment of hirsutism and acne in hyperandrogenism. Moghetti P, Toscano V. Best Pract Res Clin Endocrinol Metab 2006; 20: 221–34.

Topical retinoids are the first-line therapy for comedonal acne and may be combined with a topical antibiotic. Azelaic acid demonstrates moderate antibacterial, antiinflammatory, and keratolytic activity. Topical benzoyl peroxide is weakly comedolytic, but is a potent antibiotic. Concomitant use of benzoyl peroxide decreases incidence of antibiotic resistance.

Topical treatments are first-line therapy in acne. In the presence of scarring acne or treatment failure, oral therapy is indicated.

Polycystic ovary syndrome: a review for dermatologists. Part II. Treatment. Buzney E, Sheu J, Buzney C, Reynolds RV. J Am Acad Dermatol 2014; 71: 859.e1–e15.

Combination OCPs are effective for hirsutism, with the addition of spironolactone (starting at 50 mg per day) when appropriate. Topical therapies remain first line for acne, and in patients who fail to respond, addition of combination OCPs are effective. Finasteride and flutamide lack sufficient data for recommendation of their use.

Combination OCPs have demonstrated efficacy for hirsutism and acne in patients with PCOS with low side effect profiles.

Combined oral contraceptive pills for treatment of acne. Arowojolu AO, Gallo MF, Lopez LM, Grimes DA. Cochrane Database Syst Rev 2012; 7: CD004425.

Combined oral contraceptives (COCs) reduced acne lesion counts, severity grades, and self-assessed acne. Those containing chlormadinone acetate or cyproterone acetate (CPA) were more effective than levonorgestrel. Overall, few differences in efficacy were found between the COC types in treatment of acne.

Food and Drug Administration (FDA)–approved OCPs for acne include norgestimate/EE (ethinyl estradiol), norethindrone acetate/EE, and drospirenone/EE.

Hirsutism: an evidence-based treatment update. Somani N, Turvy D. Am J Clin Dermatol 2014; 15: 247–66.

Physical modalities are recommended as first-line treatments, including the use of electrolysis for permanent hair removal and lasers for permanent hair reduction. Other recommended therapies include OCPs and antiandrogens.

Randomized, double-blind clinical evaluation of the efficacy and safety of topical eflornithine HCl 13.9% cream in the treatment of women with facial hair. Wolf JE Jr, Shander D, Huber F, Jackson J, Lin CS, Mathes BM, et al. Int J Dermatol 2007; 46: 94–8.

Topical eflornithine cream, applied twice daily for 24 weeks, significantly reduced hair length and mass.

A randomized controlled trial of laser treatment among hirsute women with polycystic ovary syndrome. Clayton WJ, Lipton M, Elford J, Rustin M, Sherr L. Br J Dermatol 2005; 152: 986–92.

Treatment with alexandrite laser reduced severity of facial hair and decreased depression and anxiety in patients with PCOS.

Evidence-based treatments for female pattern hair loss: a summary of a Cochrane systematic review. van Zuuren EJ, Fedorowicz Z, Carter B. Br J Dermatol 2012; 167: 995–1010.

Minoxidil induced a moderate increase in hair regrowth in patients with androgenic alopecia.

Second-Line Therapies

• Antiandrogens	B
• Metformin	B

Spironolactone versus placebo or in combination with steroids for hirsutism and/or acne. Brown J, Farquhar C, Lee O, Toomath R, Jepson RG. Cochrane Database Sys Rev 2009; 2: CD000194.

Spironolactone 100 mg daily resulted in subjective decrease in hair growth. There was no evidence for effectiveness in treating acne.

In general, spironolactone is considered the first choice in antiandrogen drugs in the treatment of hirsutism. Lower-grade evidence supports anecdotal efficacy in acne.

Comparison of spironolactone, flutamide, and finasteride efficacy in the treatment of hirsutism: a randomized, double blind, placebo-controlled trial. Moghetti P, Tosi F, Tosti A, Negri C, Misciali C, Perrone F, et al. J Clin Endocrinol Metab 2000; 85: 89–94.

Forty hirsute female subjects were randomized to receive spironolactone 100 mg daily, flutamide 250 mg daily, finasteride 5 mg daily, or placebo. All treatment groups revealed similar reduction in hair diameter.

Due to high cost and potential adverse liver effects, flutamide is rarely used.

Antiandrogens should not be used without effective contraception, given the potential risk for femininization of a male fetus.

Metformin use in women with polycystic ovary syndrome. Johnson NP. Ann Transl Med 2014; 2: 56.

Metformin improves insulin resistance and anovulatory infertility in women with PCOS.

Limited evidence suggests that metformin may improve hirsutism and acne in PCOS. Five hundred mg three times daily has been suggested in the literature.

Third-Line Therapies

• Pioglitazone	**D**
• Rosiglitazone	**D**

Thiazolidinediones for the therapeutic management of polycystic ovary syndrome: impact on metabolic and reproductive abnormalities. Elkind-Hirsch KE. Treat Endocrinol 2006; 5: 171–87.

Convincing data from appropriately powered randomized controlled trials are still needed to determine whether thiazolidinediones are safe and effective in PCOS.

When should an insulin sensitizing agent be used in the treatment of polycystic ovary syndrome? Frank S. Clin Endocrinol (Oxf) 2011; 74: 148–51.

Metformin has been shown to be safer than other insulin-sensitizing agents.

Evidence Levels: **A** Double-blind study   **B** Clinical trial ≥ 20 subjects   **C** Clinical trial < 20 subjects   **D** Series ≥ 5 subjects   **E** Anecdotal case reports

196

Polymorphic light eruption

Warwick L. Morison, Elisabeth G. Richard

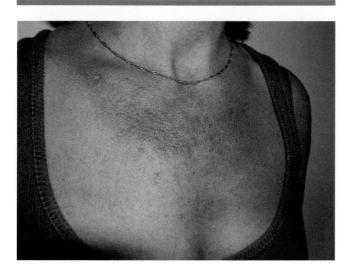

Polymorphic light eruption is the most common photodermatosis, with a prevalence of 10% to 20% in temperate climates, particularly among young women. It develops on sun-exposed body parts hours to a day or more after specific exposure to sunlight, usually in spring or early summer. The morphology varies, with papular or papulovesicular forms being most common, and the rash is always pruritic. Plaques, insect-bite type, and erythema multiforme variants are much less common. In most patients the tendency to develop polymorphic light eruption diminishes with repeated exposures to sunlight, a phenomenon called *hardening*.

MANAGEMENT STRATEGY

The treatment of polymorphic light eruption consists of two phases: treatment of established disease after the rash has appeared, and the prevention of the rash in patients known to have the disease. Application of a *midpotency* or *high-potency corticosteroid cream* or *ointment*, two or three times daily, is usually sufficient to reduce symptoms and clear the rash in most patients with established disease. Use of topical corticosteroids as treatment is based on historical clinical experience rather than formal clinical studies. A few patients with extensive disease and marked symptoms require *oral prednisone* in a dose of 60 to 80 mg for a few days, followed by rapid reduction of the dose over a week.

Preventive management is the best choice for patients diagnosed with the disease. The majority of patients with polymorphic light eruption have high-threshold disease, so they require prolonged exposure to sunlight or artificial sources of ultraviolet (UV) radiation to trigger the reaction. Most of these individuals do not seek medical advice but learn to limit their exposure to levels below their threshold or, in some cases, to prevent the disease by use of sunscreens. Patients seeking medical advice usually have low-threshold disease, often triggered by 15- to 30-minute exposures to sunlight, leading to marked limitation of outdoor activities.

The initial approach to the prevention of polymorphic light eruption is *avoidance of exposure to sunlight* using a combination of reduced time spent outdoors, restriction of exposure to early morning and late afternoon hours, wearing of protective clothing, and application of *broadband sunscreens* that protect against both UVA and UVB wavelengths. This strategy is most likely to be effective in patients with high-threshold disease and those triggered by UVB radiation.

The most effective approach for patients with low-threshold disease is desensitization using a course of *PUVA (psoralen–UVA), narrowband (311 nm) UVB phototherapy, or broadband UVB phototherapy* in spring, followed by regular exposures to sunlight during summer to maintain tolerance. Photo(chemo)therapy stimulates the hardening phenomenon and aims to induce photoadaption. This approach is successful in preventing polymorphic light eruption in up to 90% of patients, but requires planning, as treatment lasts for about a month. Patients who develop polymorphic light eruption while on treatment should continue therapy and may require topical or oral corticosteroids to control the rash.

Hydroxychloroquine, β-carotene, Polypodium leucotomos, and *nicotinamide* are reported to provide moderate and safe protection in polymorphic light eruption and may be considered in patients unable to undertake, or who are unresponsive to, desensitization therapy. Hydroxychloroquine is sometimes a useful preventive measure during a brief winter vacation in a warm climate. It should be started 3 days before the vacation in a dose of 400 mg daily and continued throughout the vacation.

Specific Investigations

- Skin biopsy
- Phototesting
- Lupus serologies

Marked papillary dermal edema – an unreliable discriminator between polymorphous light eruption and lupus erythematosus or dermatomyositis. Pincus LB, LeBoit PE, Goddard DS, Cho RJ, McCalmont TH. J Cutan Pathol 2010; 37: 416–25.

The histologic pattern of this subgroup is characteristic but not pathognomonic.

Clinical and therapeutic aspects of polymorphous light eruption. Dummer R, Ivanova K, Scheidegger EP, Burg G. Dermatology 2003; 207: 93–5.

Clinical aspects and photoprovocation testing are reviewed. Narrowband UVB is recommended as the first line for photohardening, with PUVA as second line.

An optimal method for experimental provocation of polymorphic light eruption. van de Pas CB, Hawk JLM, Young A, Walker SL. Arch Dermatol 2004; 140: 286–92.

Solar-simulated radiation was effective in inducing the rash in almost 70% of patients, and there was no difference in success rate between previously affected and previously unaffected skin.

Because 100% of patients have developed polymorphic light eruption from exposure to sunlight or an indoor source of UV radiation such as a suntan parlor, the most reliable method of reproducing the eruption is to request the patient to deliberately expose his or her skin to the source of light that produced his or her rash and to return for inspection and biopsy. Polymorphic light eruption can be induced by UVA and/or UVB.

The prevalence of antinuclear antibodies in patients with apparent polymorphic light eruption. Murphy GM, Hawk JLM. Br J Dermatol 1991; 125: 448–51.

Of 142 patients with a history consistent with polymorphic light eruption, 6% had a positive Ro antibody test or subsequently developed lupus erythematosus. A lupus panel of tests is essential in patients being considered for active desensitization treatment.

First-Line Therapies

• Restriction of sun exposure	E
• Sun screens	A
• Protective clothing	E
• Mid- to high-potency topical corticosteroids	E

A new ecamsule-containing SPF 40 sunscreen cream for the prevention of polymorphous light eruption: a double-blind, randomized, controlled study in maximized outdoor conditions. DeLeo VA, Clark S, Fowler J, Poncet M, Loesche C, Soto P. Cutis 2009; 83: 95–103.

A broad-spectrum sunscreen containing two UVA filters was significantly better at preventing flares of polymorphous light eruption than a similar product containing just one UVA filter.

Textiles and sun protection. Robson J, Diffey BL. Photodermatol Photoimmunol Photomed 1990; 7: 32–4.

Transmission of UV radiation through clothing varies greatly, providing an "SPF" in this study from 2 for a polyester blouse to 1571 for cotton denim jeans. The tightness of the weave is the main variable determining transmission of light. Transmission of UV radiation for all fabrics is increased when a fabric is wet.

Clothing and hats are now available specifically designed to provide protection from sunlight while maintaining a high level of comfort.

Second-Line Therapies

• PUVA therapy	C
• Narrowband (311 nm) phototherapy	C
• Broadband UVB phototherapy	C

UVB phototherapy and photochemotherapy (PUVA) in the treatment of polymorphic light eruption and solar urticaria. Addo HA, Sharma SC. Br J Dermatol 1987; 116: 539–47.

Patients were treated with a regular schedule of oral PUVA or high-dose (erythemogenic) broadband UVB phototherapy three times weekly for 5 weeks during the spring and were then instructed to maximize their exposure to sunlight during summer. Ninety percent of PUVA-treated patients and about 70% of UVB-treated patients were free of symptoms of polymorphic light eruption during the summer. Development of the eruption during the active treatment was common, usually mild, and did not interfere with treatment.

A comparison of narrowband (TL-01) and photochemotherapy (PUVA) in the management of polymorphic light eruption. Bilsland D, George SA, Gibbs NK, Aitchison T, Johnson BE, Ferguson J. Br J Dermatol 1993; 129: 708–12.

A regular schedule of oral PUVA therapy or narrowband (311 nm) phototherapy was given to patients three times a week for 5 weeks in the spring, resulting in about 85% of patients in each treatment group being adequately protected from developing polymorphic light eruption during the summer. The necessity for regular sun exposure every week during the summer may not have been emphasized.

Third-Line Therapies

• Prednisolone	A
• Hydroxychloroquine	A
• β-Carotene	C
• Nicotinamide	B
• Azathioprine	E
• Ciclosporin	E
• Flavonoid antioxidant	A
• Topical liposomal DNA repair enzymes	A
• *Polypodium leucotomos*	B
• LED photoprevention	C

Efficacy of short-course oral prednisolone in polymorphic light eruption: a randomized controlled trial. Patel DC, Bellaney GJ, Seed PT, McGregor JM, Hawk JLM. Br J Dermatol 2000; 143: 828–31.

A 7-day course of 25 mg prednisolone daily was superior to placebo when started at the onset of the rash. This low dose of steroid is suitable for managing patients who are on brief vacations in a sunny climate.

Prednisone would be a suitable alternative.

Hydroxychloroquine in polymorphic light eruption: a controlled trial with drug and visual sensitivity monitoring. Murphy GM, Hawk JLM, Magnus IA. Br J Dermatol 1987; 116: 379–86.

Hydroxychloroquine in a dose of 400 mg daily for 1 month, and 200 mg daily for 2 months, was superior to placebo in preventing development of the rash; however, almost all patients did have a rash and irritation during the trial. The degree of protection was judged to be moderate and was related to serum level of the drug; the dose of 400 mg daily provided better protection. No visual toxicity was observed.

Comparison of PUVA and beta-carotene in the treatment of polymorphous light eruption. Parrish JA, Le Vine MJ, Morison WL, Gonzalez E, Fitzpatrick TB. Br J Dermatol 1979; 100: 187–91.

β-Carotene (3.0 mg/kg) in a twice-daily divided dose given for the entire summer provided full protection for 30% of patients and partial protection for another 20%. There were no adverse effects.

Treatment of polymorphous light eruption with nicotinamide: a pilot study. Neumann R, Rappold E, Pohl-Markl H. Br J Dermatol 1986; 115: 77–80.

Nicotinamide given in a dose of 1 g orally three times daily starting 2 days before sun exposure provided complete protection in 60% of patients. The dose was reduced to 2 g daily after 1 week; about half of these patients developed polymorphic light eruption. A few patients had mild fatigue.

Successful treatment of severe polymorphous light eruption with azathioprine. Norris PG, Hawk JLM. Arch Dermatol 1989; 125: 1377–9.

Two patients with year-round photosensitivity triggered by as little as 1 to 2 minutes of sun exposure and unresponsive to all standard treatments were treated with 0.8 to 2.5 mg/kg of azathioprine daily for 3 months, with complete remission of symptoms and normal sun tolerance.

The erythemal responses to UVB radiation were reduced in both patients and to UVA radiation in one, which is an unusual finding in typical cases of polymorphic light eruption.

Evidence Levels: **A** Double-blind study **B** Clinical trial ≥ 20 subjects **C** Clinical trial < 20 subjects **D** Series ≥ 5 subjects **E** Anecdotal case reports

Prophylactic short-term use of cyclosporine in refractory polymorphic light eruption. Lasa O, Trebol I, Gardeazabal J, Diaz-Perez JL. J Eur Acad Dermatol Venereol 2004; 18: 747–8.

Ciclosporin in a dose of 3 to 4 mg/kg/day over 2 or 4 weeks was effective in preventing the development of an eruption in three patients during a short vacation in a sunny climate. The patients had not responded to other preventive measures. No adverse effects were observed, and this appears to have promise as a prophylactic treatment in patients resistant to other therapies.

Polymorphous light eruption (PLE) and a new potent antioxidant and UVA-protective formulation as prophylaxis. Hadshiew IM, Treder-Conrad C, Bülow RV, Klette E, Mann T, Stäb F, et al. Photodermatol Photoimmunol Photomed 2004; 20: 200–4.

A flavonoid antioxidant plus a broad-spectrum sunscreen was more effective in preventing PLE than sunscreen alone or placebo.

Topical liposomal DNA-repair enzymes in polymorphic light eruption. Hofer A, Legat FJ, Gruber-Wackernagel A, Quehenberger F, Wolf P. Photochem Photobiol Sci 2011; 10: 1118–28.

After-sun lotion containing liposomal DNA-repair enzymes decreased polymorphous light eruption symptoms. Of note, pretreatment with SPF30 sunscreen prevented polymorphous light eruption in this group of susceptible patients.

Oral administration of a hydrophilic extract of *Polypodium leucotomos* for the prevention of polymorphic light eruption. Tanew A, Radakovic S, Gonzalez S, Venturini M, Calzavara-Pinton P. J Am Acad Dermatol 2012; 66: 58–62.

Photoprovocation tests were administered to 35 polymorphic light eruption patients before and after an open label, 2-week course of *Polypodium leucotomos* 720 mg to 1200 mg daily depending on weight. Thirty percent of patients with UVA-induced polymorphic light eruption did not respond to the repeat exposure, and 28% of those induced by UVB did not respond to the second exposure. For the remaining patients, significantly more exposure was required to elicit polymorphic light eruption.

This study suggests that pretreatment with Polypodium leucotomos *for 2 weeks before sun exposure and during the period of sun exposure may be beneficial.*

Photoprotective activity of oral *Polypodium leucotomos* extract in 25 patients with idiopathic photodermatoses. Caccialanza M, Percivalle S, Piccinno R, Brambilla R. Photodermatol Photoimmunol Photomed 2007; 23: 46–7.

Daily oral administration of *Polypodium leucotomos* extract provided improvement in over 40% of patients in terms of tolerance to sun exposure without developing PLE.

LED photoprevention: reduced MED response following multiple LED exposures. Barolet D, Boucher A. Lasers Surg Med 2008; 40: 106–12.

In patients with and without history of PLE, pretreatment with 660 nM light power LED light source reduced redness at all MEDs tested.

197

Porokeratoses

Agustin Martin-Clavijo, John Berth-Jones

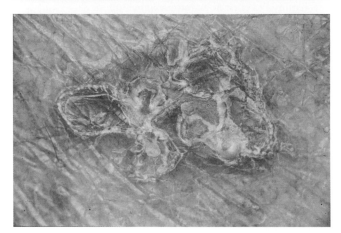

The porokeratoses are a group of disorders of keratinization characterized by lesions with a peripheral keratotic ridge, manifesting histologically as a cornoid lamella. Terminology and classification are debated, but the main recognized forms are (1) disseminated forms, of which disseminated superficial actinic porokeratosis (DSAP) is predominant; (2) porokeratosis of Mibelli (PM); (3) palmoplantar porokeratosis (porokeratosis palmaris, plantaris et disseminata – PPPD); and (4) linear porokeratosis (LP). An autosomal-dominant mode of inheritance has been reported in the disseminated form, which is not always "actinic" in origin. Overexpression of the p53 tumor suppression protein has been identified in the cornoid lamella. Porokeratotic lesions are progressive and carry malignant potential, especially large long-standing lesions and the linear variants. In addition, the lesions can cause pruritus and represent a cosmetic problem for some patients.

MANAGEMENT STRATEGY

The family history should be reviewed and the patient's immune function assessed, particularly with the disseminated forms. Discontinuation of immunosuppression has led to resolution of lesions in some patients.

The lesions are usually asymptomatic, but may be pruritic, and the palmoplantar variant may cause functional disability due to pain and discomfort.

Treatment is not always required, but may be indicated, not only for cosmetic benefit and symptomatic relief but also to reduce the risk of malignancy. Optimal therapy therefore depends on the type and extent of porokeratosis and the level of concern over malignant progression. Management should include avoidance of irradiation (UV or x-rays) and observation for signs of malignant transformation (squamous cell carcinoma, basal cell carcinoma, Bowen disease).

When present, pruritus associated with disseminated lesions is often responsive to *topical corticosteroids*. Localized disease responds to "surgical" methods such as *cryotherapy, CO_2 laser, curettage and cautery,* or *excision,* but these can result in significant scarring, especially when the lesions are numerous.

Topical 5-fluorouracil, imiquimod, and vitamin D analogs can be helpful, but only partial responses are likely in DSAP. Inflammatory reactions are likely when using 5-fluorouracil or imiquimod and indicate a greater likelihood of response. With some caution, these modalities can be used under occlusion, treating one area at a time. In the authors' experience results are inconsistent, even with occlusion.

Systemic retinoids have been effective in localized and systemic disease, but there have been reports of exacerbation of preexisting lesions. Recurrence is common on discontinuation of therapy, and a long-term maintenance dose may be required. This modality might also reduce the risk of malignant transformation.

A recent report of the use of topical ingenol mebutate may prove to be an advance if the results are found to be consistent.

There is one report of genital DSAP responding partially to *topical diclofenac,* but a subsequent case series demonstrated very limited benefit. There are also reports of the effectiveness of *topical retinoids, dermabrasion, various lasers and IPL, corticosteroids,* and *topical photodynamic therapy.* Treatments used in combination have included CO_2 *laser and tacalcitol,* CO_2 *laser and photodynamic therapy, 5-fluorouracil and imiquimod,* and *calcipotriol with adapalene.*

Specific Investigations

- Biopsy
- Dermoscopy
- Assessment of immune function

Dermoscopy for the diagnosis of porokeratosis. Delfino M, Argenziano G, Nino M. J Eur Acad Dermatol Venereol 2004; 18: 194–5.

Dermoscopic examination of DSAP showed a characteristic central scarlike area with a single or double "white track" structure at the margin. The histopathologic correlate of the linear structure was shown to be the cornoid lamella.

First-Line Therapy

• Cryotherapy	D

Porokeratosis of Mibelli: successful treatment with cryosurgery. Dereli T, Ozyurt S, Osturk G. J Dermatol 2004; 31: 223–7.

Eight patients with 20 lesions received treatment with 30-second cycles of cryospray followed by sharp dissection of the lesion border. Most lesions resolved after one treatment; two required one further treatment.

Cryosurgery of porokeratosis plantaris discreta. Limmer BL. Arch Dermatol 1979; 115: 582–3.

Twenty-one lesions of porokeratosis in 11 patients were treated with cryotherapy, resulting in a cure rate of 90.5%. The lesions were pared before treatment. There was no evidence of recurrence over an average follow-up period of 22 months.

Second-Line Therapies

• 5-Fluorouracil	D
• Imiquimod	E
• Vitamin D analogs	E

Evidence Levels: **A** Double-blind study **B** Clinical trial ≥ 20 subjects **C** Clinical trial < 20 subjects **D** Series ≥ 5 subjects **E** Anecdotal case reports

Fluorouracil ointment treatment of porokeratosis of Mibelli. Gonçalves JC. Arch Dermatol 1973; 108: 131–2.

Six patients with facial lesions were treated with 5% fluorouracil ointment three times daily. The treatment was maintained for 8 to 10 days after a strong inflammatory response occurred. There was no recurrence at 9-month follow-up.

Disseminated superficial porokeratosis: rapid therapeutic response to 5-fluorouracil. Shelley WB, Shelley ED. Cutis 1983; 32: 139–40.

Resolution of porokeratosis was observed after 3 weeks of daily application of 5% 5-fluorouracil cream. There was no recurrence at 5-month follow-up.

Porokeratosis of Mibelli: successful treatment with 5% imiquimod cream. Agarwal S, Berth-Jones J. Br J Dermatol 2002; 146: 338–9.

A 3-cm lesion of PM on the leg was initially treated with topical imiquimod 5% cream five times a week for 3 months, with no improvement. Subsequent treatment with imiquimod 5% cream five times a week under occlusion with an adhesive polythene dressing was successful. There was no recurrence at 1 year.

Disseminated superficial actinic porokeratosis treated effectively with topical imiquimod 5% cream. Arun B, Pearson J, Chalmers R. Clin Exp Dermatol 2011; 3: 509–11.

One patient with DSAP responded to imiquimod 5% cream five times a week for 6 weeks.

Disseminated superficial actinic porokeratosis: treatment with topical tacalcitol. Bohm M, Luger TA, Bonsmann G. J Am Acad Dermatol 1999; 40: 479–80.

DSAP responded to 5 months of topical daily treatment with 0.0004% tacalcitol and remained clear on alternate-day maintenance therapy.

Disseminated superficial actinic porokeratosis responding to calcipotriol. Harrison PV, Stollery N. Clin Exp Dermatol 1994; 19: 95.

Three patients were treated with topical calcipotriol daily for 6 to 8 weeks. An overall improvement of 50% to 75% was noted and maintained for up to 6 months in two patients.

Third-Line Therapies

• Systemic retinoids	D
• Topical retinoids	E
• CO$_2$ laser	D
• Nd:YAG laser	E
• Pulsed dye laser	E
• Ruby laser	E
• Fractional photothermolysis	E
• Intense pulse light (IPL)	D
• Photodynamic therapy	E
• Dermabrasion	E
• Fluor-hydroxy pulse peel	E
• Corticosteroids	E
• Diclofenac 3% gel	C
• Ingenol mebutate	E
• 5-Fluorouracil with imiquimod cream	E
• Photodynamic therapy with CO$_2$ laser	E
• Excision and skin graft	E
• Ciclosporin (for intense pruritus)	E
• Cantharidin	E

Generalized linear porokeratosis: a rare entity with excellent response to acitretin. Garg T, Ramchander Varghese B, Barara M, Nangia A. Dermatol Online J 2011; 17: 3.

A patient with generalized LP was treated with acitretin 0.5 mg/kg. There was marked flattening of the lesions after 6 weeks but not complete resolution after 5 months of treatment.

Disseminated porokeratosis Mibelli treated with Ro 10-9359. Bundino S, Zina AM. Dermatologica 1980; 160: 328–36.

Two patients with DSAP were treated with 50 to 75 mg daily of etretinate, with significant clinical improvement after 5 weeks; 25 mg daily was sufficient to maintain the results. Recurrence was observed 3 to 4 weeks after cessation of treatment.

Treatment of disseminated superficial actinic porokeratosis with a new aromatic retinoid (Ro 10-9359). Kariniemi A, Stubb S, Lassus A. Br J Dermatol 1980; 102: 213–4.

Treatment with 50 to 100 mg daily of etretinate led to significant clinical improvement and resolution of pruritus within 40 days. A dose of 25 mg on alternate days was required to maintain the results. After 6 months of treatment the patient developed follicular hyperkeratosis with tiny keratin horns on the skin of both forearms.

Porokeratosis plantaris, palmaris, et disseminata. Report of a case and treatment with isotretinoin. McCallister RE, Estes SA, Yarbrough CL. J Am Acad Dermatol 1985; 13: 598–603.

A patient with familial PPPD received treatment with 1 mg/kg daily of isotretinoin. Significant clinical improvement was noted after 3 months of treatment. Two months after discontinuation of treatment a gradual recurrence was observed.

A case of extensive linear porokeratosis with evaluation of topical tretinoin versus 5-fluorouracil as treatment modalities. Grover C, Goel A, Nanda S, Khurana N, Reddy BS. J Dermatol 2005; 32: 1000–4.

One patient with LP was treated with topical tretinoin and 5-fluorouracil. Both agents were efficacious, but tretinoin was better tolerated.

Calcipotriol and adapalene therapy for disseminated superficial actinic porokeratosis. Nakamura Y, Yamaguchi M, Nakamura A, Muto M. Indian J Dermatol Venereol Leprol 2014; 80: 373–4.

Calcipotriol 0.005% ointment was applied in the morning and adapalene (0.1%) gel at night. After 3 months the skin lesions improved substantially, leaving only slight hyperpigmentation.

Treatment of porokeratosis of Mibelli with CO$_2$ laser vaporization versus surgical excision with split-thickness skin graft. Rabbin PE, Baldwin HE. J Dermatol Surg Oncol 1993; 19: 199–202.

CO$_2$ vaporization resulted in better cosmetic and functional improvement than split-skin grafting in the same patient.

Treatment of lichen amyloidosis (LA) and disseminated superficial porokeratosis (DSP) with frequency-doubled Q-switched Nd:YAG laser. Liu HT. Dermatol Surg 2000; 26: 958–62.

A patient's face and arms were treated four times, 1 month apart, resulting in marked improvement, but not complete clearance, of the lesions.

Successful treatment of porokeratosis with 585 nm pulsed dye laser irradiation. Alster TS, Nanni CA. Cutis 1999; 63: 265–6.

This is a case of LP that responded to a series of 585-nm pulsed dye laser treatments.

Treatment of disseminated superficial actinic porokeratosis (DSAP) with the Q-switched ruby laser. Lolis MS, Marmur ES. J Cosmet Laser Ther 2008; 10: 124–7.

This patient received three treatments with Q-switched ruby laser (694 nm) with good improvement.

Fractional photothermolysis: a novel treatment for disseminated superficial actinic porokeratosis. Chrastil B, Glaich AS, Goldberg LH, Friedman PM. Arch Dermatol 2007; 143: 1450–2.

Two patients received three to six courses of fractionated photothermolysis (erbium-doped fiber laser). Both patients reported 50% improvement.

Disseminated superficial actinic porokeratosis improved with fractional 1927-nm laser treatments. Ross NA, Rosenbaum LE, Saedi N, Arndt KA, Dover JS. J Cosmet Laser Ther 2016; 18: 53–5.

Two patients were successfully treated with the 1927-nm thulium fiber fractional laser.

Unconventional use of intense pulsed light. Piccolo D, Di Marcantonio D, Crisman G, Cannarozzo G, Sannino M, Chiricozzi A, et al. Biomed Res Int 2014: 1–10.

Successful use of IPL in a series of 10 cases. Split 550-nm filter pulses, of 5 to 10 msec, with a 10-msec delay, and fluence of 10 to 12 J/cm^2 were applied up to four times at intervals of 20 to 30 days.

Topical photodynamic therapy in disseminated superficial actinic porokeratosis. Nayeemuddin FA, Wong M, Yell J, Rhodes LE. Clin Exp Dermatol 2002; 27: 703–6.

A report on three patients treated with 20% aminolevulinic acid cream under occlusion for 5 hours before illumination with 100 J/cm^2 of broadband red light (Waldmann 1200). Resolution of two lesions of DSAP was observed in one case, but the response could not be reproduced in this or two other cases.

Successful treatment of disseminated superficial actinic porokeratosis with methyl aminolevulinate-photodynamic therapy. Cavicchini S, Tourlaki A. J Dermatol Treat 2006; 17: 190–1.

This case demonstrated a striking improvement in response to two treatments, 1 week apart, using methyl aminolevulinate cream 160 mg/g applied with occlusion for 3 hours before illumination with a red light (Aktilite) 37 J/cm^2.

Response of linear porokeratosis to photodynamic therapy in an 11-year-old girl. Garrido-Colmenero C, Ruiz-Villaverde R, Martínez-García E, Aneiros-Fernández J, Tercedor-Sánchez J. J Dermatol Case Rep 2015; 9: 118–9.

Methyl aminolevulinate hydrochloride cream 160 mg/g (Metvix) was applied under occlusion for 2 hours and lesions illuminated with a dose of 37 J/cm^2 (Aktilite) over 8 minutes. Treatment was repeated 3 weeks later. The authors assessed the result as good.

Successful treatment of porokeratosis of Mibelli with diamond fraise dermabrasion. Spencer JM, Katz BE. Arch Dermatol 1992; 128: 1187–8.

No recurrence observed at 15-month follow-up, but the lesion healed with slight hyperpigmentation and mild hypertrophy in a 79-year-old Filipino woman.

Linear porokeratosis: successful treatment with diamond fraise dermabrasion. Cohen PR, Held JL, Katz BE. J Am Acad Dermatol 1990; 23: 975–7.

An excellent cosmetic result. No recurrence or scarring observed after 8 months.

The use of fluor-hydroxy pulse peel in actinic porokeratosis. Teixeira SP, de Nascimento MM, Bagatin E, Hassun KM, Talarico S, Michalany N. Dermatol Surg 2005; 31: 1145–8.

This is a case of DSAP treated with a combination of a 70% glycolic peel and a 5% 5-fluorouracil solution every 2 weeks for 4 months. The result was improvement in the appearance and texture of the treated areas and reduced dyskeratosis and epidermal atypia.

Dexamethasone pulse treatment in disseminated porokeratosis of Mibelli. Verma KK, Singh OP. J Dermatol Sci 1994; 7: 71–2.

A familial case of progressive porokeratosis received pulses of 100 mg dexamethasone in 5% dextrose intravenously on 3 consecutive days in a month. No new lesions appeared after the first pulse, and clinical improvement was noted after four pulses. There was an 80% improvement after 18 pulses. The patient was then lost to follow-up.

Diclofenac sodium 3% gel as a potential treatment for disseminated superficial actinic porokeratosis. Marks S, Varma R, Cantrell W, Chen SC, Gold M, Muellenhoff M, et al. J Eur Acad Dermatol Venereol 2009; 23: 42–5.

An open-label, multicenter trial; 17 patients were treated with 3% diclofenac applied twice daily for 3 to 6 months to a target area. The areas treated progressed less than the untreated areas.

Treatment of disseminated superficial actinic porokeratosis with topical diclofenac gel: a case series. Vlachou C, Kanelleas A, Martin-Clavijo A, Berth-Jones J. J Eur Acad Dermatol Venereol 2008; 22: 1343–5.

Eight patients with DSAP were treated with 3% diclofenac gel (Solaraze gel) twice daily for at least 6 months. At 6 months a partial improvement was seen in two cases but no improvement in the others.

Treatment of porokeratosis of Mibelli with ingenol mebutate: a possible new therapeutic option. Kindem S, Serra-Guillén C, Sorní G, Guillén C, Sanmartín O. JAMA Dermatol 2015; 151: 85–6.

A patient was treated with two courses, separated by a month, of ingenol mebutate 0.015% gel, applied once daily for 3 consecutive days. Resolution of the hyperkeratotic annular component was observed, although the treatment did not improve the central area of atrophy and hypopigmentation.

Porokeratosis of Mibelli: successful treatment with 5% topical imiquimod and topical 5% 5-fluorouracil. Venkatarajan S, LeLeux TM, Yang D, Rosen T, Orengo I. Dermatol Online J 2010; 16: 10.

A patient with PM was treated with 5-fluorouracil twice a day and 5% imiquimod cream once a day for 12 weeks, leading to resolution of the lesion.

Photodynamic therapy combined with CO$_2$ laser vaporization on disseminated superficial actinic porokeratosis: a report of 2 cases on the face. Kim HS, Baek JH, Park YM, Kim HO, Lee JY. Ann Dermatol 2011; 23: S211–3.

Evidence Levels: **A** Double-blind study   **B** Clinical trial ≥ 20 subjects   **C** Clinical trial < 20 subjects   **D** Series ≥ 5 subjects   **E** Anecdotal case reports

Two patients were treated with CO_2 laser to the cornoid lamella followed by photodynamic therapy. There was marked response after four treatments.

Recalcitrant digital porokeratosis of Mibelli: a successful surgical treatment. Shahmoradi Z, Sadeghiyan H, Pourazizi M, Saber M, Abtahi-Naeini B. N Am J Med Sci 2015; 7: 295–6.

A case successfully treated by excision and split-thickness skin graft.

Inflammatory disseminated pruritic porokeratosis with a good response to ciclosporin. Montes-Torres A, Camarero-Mulas C, de Argila D, Gordillo C, Daudén E. Actas Dermo-Sifiliogr 2016; 107: 261–2.

Intense distressing pruritus was improved by ciclosporin, initially at 4 mg/kg day. Dose reduction below 1 mg/kg/day resulted in recurrence of pruritus. This is proposed to be a subgroup of highly symptomatic, inflammatory porokeratosis with a low risk of malignant transformation.

Use of this immunosuppressant drug would be contraindicated in most cases of porokeratosis, as the danger of promoting malignancy outweighs the severity of the symptoms.

Treatment of porokeratosis of Mibelli with cantharidin. Levitt JO, Keeley BR, Phelps RG. J Am Acad Dermatol 2013; 69: e254–5.

Two cases of porokeratosis of Mibelli treated successfully with one application of a thin film of cantharidin to the circumference of the lesion.

Porphyria cutanea tarda

Maureen B. Poh-Fitzpatrick

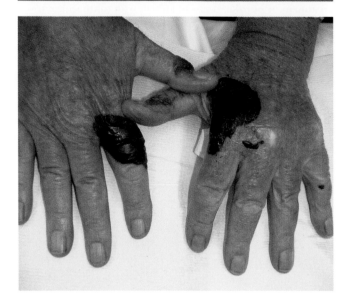

The term *porphyria cutanea tarda (PCT)* encompasses several related inherited or acquired disorders in which insufficient hepatic uroporphyrinogen decarboxylase enzyme activity causes overproduction of polycarboxylated porphyrins. These porphyrins mediate cutaneous photosensitivity manifested as fragility, bullae, hypertrichosis, dyspigmentation, sclerodermoid features, and scarring. PCT usually presents in adults but occasionally in children. Multiple factors may contribute to its expression: mutant uroporphyrinogen decarboxylase genes, hemochromatosis (HFE) genes, or other predisposing genetic determinants; ethanol abuse; smoking; medicinal estrogen; iron overload; hepatitis and/or human immunodeficiency viral infections (HIV); chronic dialysis treatment; toxic aromatic hydrocarbon exposure; and, rarely, hepatic tumors. Increased tissue iron, a common feature of alcoholism, hepatitis C infection, hemochromatosis, and end-stage renal disease, plays a central role in the pathogenesis of PCT. Iron-dependent partial oxidation of uroporphyrinogen to uroporphomethene, a competitive inhibitor of uroprophyrinogen decarboxylase, may be the mechanism by which its activity is reduced in PCT (Phillips et al. Proc Natl Acad Sci USA 2007; 104: 5079–84). Iron-enhanced complete oxidation of porphyrinogens accumulated due to inhibited enzyme activity yields photoactive porphyrins. Hepatic siderosis or porphyrin crystallization in hepatocytes may lead to hepatocellular carcinoma in long-standing active PCT. Ferrodepletion by serial phlebotomy is the preferred first-line therapy for PCT patients with iron overload.

MANAGEMENT STRATEGY

Precise diagnosis is essential because optimal management calls for remission induction using strategies inappropriate for other porphyrias or pseudoporphyrias. Associated disorders that may influence management (viral infections, hemochromatosis, or other causes of iron overload; lupus erythematosus; diabetes mellitus; anemias) should be identified. Sun exposure and mechanical

skin trauma should be minimized until full clinical remission is achieved. Eliminating contributory factors and pursuing ferrodepletion by *serial phlebotomy, iron chelation,* or *erythropoiesis stimulation,* or increasing porphyrin excretion with *chloroquine* or *hydroxychloroquine,* can reproducibly induce biochemical and clinical remissions. Phlebotomy and hydroxychloroquine protocols adjusted for pediatric parameters are available. Alternative therapies are less well established. Porphyrin excretion can also be increased by *enteric sorbents* or *metabolic alkalinization. Antiviral drugs* may benefit PCT coincident with hepatitis C or HIV infections. *Vitamins E and C, plasmapheresis or plasma exchange, high-flux hemodialysis,* and *cimetidine* have had limited use. Hepatoerythropoietic porphyria, caused by coinheritance of two uroporphyrinogen decarboxylase gene mutations, resists induction of remission and thus requires lifelong vigilant photoprotection. *Photothermolysis* using light with selected wavelengths may reduce persistent hypertrichosis.

Specific Investigations

- Porphyrin concentrations and types in erythrocytes, serum or urine, feces
- Hematologic and iron profiles, serum ferritin, hemochromatosis gene analysis
- Liver function profile; serum α-fetoprotein level, liver imaging, liver biopsy if clinically indicated
- Hepatitis A, B, and C and human immunodeficiency viral serologies
- Fasting blood glucose
- Serum antinuclear antibody
- Mutation analysis of the uroporphyrinogen decarboxylase gene

Hepatitis C, porphyria cutanea tarda and liver iron: an update. Ryan Caballes F, Sendi H, Bonkovsky HL. Liver Int 2012; 32: 880–93.

A review emphasizing pathophysiologic roles of hepatitis C virus, iron-facilitated oxidative stress, and hepcidin (a key regulator of iron absorption and metabolism that is downregulated in PCT). Treatment guidelines are offered.

Porphyria cutanea tarda, hepatitis C, and HFE gene mutations in North America. Bonkovsky HL, Poh-Fitzpatrick MB, Pimstone N, Obando J, Di Bisceglie A, Tattrie C, et al. Hepatology 1998; 27: 1661–9.

Of 70 American patients with PCT, 53% had evidence of hepatitis C infection, and 43% of 26 patients had HFE gene mutations associated with hereditary hemochromatosis.

Hepatocellular carcinoma risk in patients with porphyria cutanea tarda. Gisbert JP, Garcia-Buey L, Alonso A, Rubio S, Hernandez A, Pajares JM, et al. Eur J Gastroenterol Hepatol 2004; 16: 689–92.

Recommendations include viral hepatitis serologies and liver biopsy at initial evaluation. PCT patients with hepatitis C infection or advanced fibrosis/cirrhosis should be monitored with semiannual ultrasonography and serum α-fetoprotein testing.

The decision for liver biopsy should be weighed carefully. Patients without risk factors for hepatic siderosis or other liver pathology (e.g., women with estrogen use as the only PCT-inducing factor) may not need this invasive procedure.

First-Line Therapies

• Opaque sunscreens, physical sunlight barriers	C
• Serial phlebotomies	B
• Chloroquine, hydroxychloroquine	B

Evidence Levels: **A** Double-blind study **B** Clinical trial ≥ 20 subjects **C** Clinical trial < 20 subjects **D** Series ≥ 5 subjects **E** Anecdotal case reports

Efficiency of opaque photoprotective agents in the visible light range. Kaye ET, Levin JA, Blank IH, Arndt KA, Anderson RR. Arch Dermatol 1991; 127: 351–5.

Efficacy and quality of sunscreens containing zinc oxide, titanium dioxide, and iron oxide are described.

Minimizing sunlight exposure by lifestyle changes, opaque sunscreens, protective clothing, window glass barrier filters, etc., is essential until photosensitivity remits completely.

Treatment of porphyria cutanea tarda by phlebotomy. Ippen H. Semin Hematol 1977; 14: 253–9.

Repeated venesection resulted in reduction of porphyrins and serum iron, improvement of photocutaneous lesions, and normalization of liver function tests in the majority of 351 patients.

Phlebotomy schedules should be adjusted to the tolerance of individual patients, typically ranging from 200 to 500 mL of whole blood at twice-weekly to fortnightly or monthly intervals. Keeping hemoglobin over 10 to 11 g/dL minimizes symptoms of iatrogenic anemia.

Childhood-onset familial porphyria cutanea tarda: effects of therapeutic phlebotomy. Poh-Fitzpatrick MB, Honig PJ, Kim HC, Sassa S. J Am Acad Dermatol 1992; 27: 896–900.

Pediatric phlebotomy guidelines are described.

Plasma ferritin levels as a guide to the treatment of porphyria cutanea tarda by venesection. Ratnaike S, Blake D, Campbell D, Cowen P, Varigos G. Australas J Dermatol 1988; 29: 3–8.

Phlebotomy can be terminated when iron stores, as reflected by plasma ferritin concentration, have fallen to low-normal levels.

Reduction of porphyrins in plasma (or serum or urine) and clinical improvement typically begin during therapy and continue for weeks to months after venesection stops. Clinical improvement precedes full biochemical normalization.

Treatment of porphyria cutanea tarda with chloroquine. Kordać V, Semrádová M. Br J Dermatol 1974; 90: 95–100.

Twenty-one adults received oral chloroquine 125 mg twice weekly until cutaneous blistering and fragility ceased and urinary uroporphyrins fell below three times the normal limit. Mean duration of treatment was 8.5 months (range 4–11 months) in 19 patients. Serum transaminases and urinary uroporphyrins rose during initial weeks of therapy and then progressively diminished.

Chloroquine risks include irreversible retinopathy after large cumulative doses (>100–300 g), but this is infrequent at dose rates <4 mg/ kg daily (<6.5 mg/kg daily for hydroxychloroquine). Ophthalmologic examination is recommended at baseline; if normal, no further testing is needed unless treatment continues beyond 5 years (unlikely for PCT). The risk of hemolysis can be minimized by pretreatment testing for glucose-6-phosphate dehydrogenase deficiency and interval monitoring of hematologic profiles during therapy.

Childhood-onset porphyria cutanea tarda: successful therapy with low-dose hydroxychloroquine (Plaquenil). Bruce AJ, Ahmed I. J Am Acad Dermatol 1998; 38: 810–4.

A 4-year-old child given hydroxychloroquine 3 mg/kg twice weekly for 14 months, plus vitamin E 200 U/day, achieved remission without adverse side effects.

Choice of therapy in porphyria cutanea tarda. Adjarov D, Naydenova E, Ivanov E, Ivanova A. Clin Exp Dermatol 1996; 21: 461–2.

The effectiveness of phlebotomy (500 mL weekly for 4 weeks, then monthly) versus oral chloroquine 250 mg twice weekly alone versus combined phlebotomy/chloroquine therapies was retrospectively analyzed in unequal groups totaling 115 patients.

Remissions occurred more quickly and reliably with phlebotomy than with chloroquine. Combined therapy shortened the mean total treatment course by approximately 1.5 months only when initial urinary uroporphyrin levels exceeded 3000 nmol/24 hours.

Others found remissions more rapid with chloroquine than with venesection (10.2 months in 24 patients, 12.5 months in 15 patients, respectively). Combination therapy was quickest (3.5 months in 20 patients) (Seubert S, Seubert A, Stella AM, Guzman H, Battle A. Z Hautkr 1990; 65: 223–5). In another study, urinary porphyrin excretion significantly improved in 22 of 30 hydroxychloroquine-treated subjects (200 mg twice weekly), but in only eight of 31 phlebotomy-treated subjects (400 mL whole blood twice monthly) after 1 year, while clinical improvement was similar in both groups. (Cainelli T, Di Padova C, Marchesi L, Gori G, Rovagnati P, Podenzani SA, et al. Br J Dermatol 1983; 108: 593– 600). Low-dose hydroxychloroquine (13 subjects) was similarly effective as biweekly phlebotomy (17 subjects) in inducing normal plasma porphyrin levels (6.1 and 6.9 months, respectively). (Singal AK, Kormos-Hallenberg C, Lee C, Sadagoparamanujam VM, Grady JJ, Freeman DH, et al. Clin Gastroenterol Hepatol 2012; 10: 1402–9).

Hemochromatosis (HFE) gene mutations and response to chloroquine in porphyria cutanea tarda. Stolzel U, Kostler E, Schuppan D, Richter M, Wollina U, Doss MO, et al. Arch Dermatol 2003; 139: 379–80.

Chloroquine was effective in heterozygotes with one of the major HFE mutations (C282Y, H63D) or in compound heterozygotes, but C282Y homozygotes failed to improve; serum iron decreased only in patients with PCT and wild-type HFE. Phlebotomy was the recommended therapy for patients with PCT and HFE gene mutations.

Second-Line Therapies

• Iron chelation	B, C
• Erythropoietin	E

Liver iron overload and desferrioxamine treatment of porphyria cutanea tarda. Rocchi E, Cassanelli M, Borghi A, Paolillo F, Pradelli M, Pellizzardi S, et al. Dermatologica 1991; 182: 27–31.

Ferrodepletion by desferrioxamine 1.5 g subcutaneous pump infusions 5 days/week (18 patients) or 200 mg/kg infused intravenously once weekly (5 patients) or by serial phlebotomies (22 patients) led to clinical remission after nearly 6 months with all treatments. Normalization of serum ferritin and uroporphyrins occurred at approximately 11 months with chelation and approximately 13 months with venesection; liver function improved with both modalities.

Subcutaneous chelation is expensive and cumbersome and thus is best reserved for cases in which first-line therapies are inadequate or inappropriate.

Deferasirox for porphyria cutanea tarda. Pandya AG, Nezafati KA, Ashe-Randolph M, Yalamanchili R. Arch Dermtol 2012; 148: 898–901.

Among eight patients considered to have PCT treated with deferasirox 250 to 500 mg/day orally for 6 months, reductions in blistering (eight), urinary porphyrins (six), and serum ferritin levels (eight) resulted.

Although true PCT was questionable in two cases, these promising results encourage larger confirmatory trials.

Successful treatment of haemodialysis-related porphyria cutanea tarda with deferoxamine. Pitche P, Corrin E, Wolkenstein P, Revuz J, Bagot M. Ann Dermatol Venereol 2003; 130: 37–9.

Intravenous deferoxamine 40 mg/kg weekly for 6 weeks led to normalization of clinical and biological signs of PCT in one patient that persisted for 12 months in the setting of end-stage renal disease and chronic hemodialysis.

Successful treatment of hemodialysis-related porphyria cutanea tarda with deferoxamine. Stockenhuber F, Kurz R, Grimm G, Moser G, Balcke, P. Nephron 1990; 55: 321–4.

Erythropoietin for the treatment of porphyria cutanea tarda in a patient on long-term hemodialysis. Anderson KE, Goeger DE, Carson RW, Lee SM, Stead RB. N Engl J Med 1990; 322: 315–7.

An end-stage renal disease patient treated with chronic hemodialysis received erythropoietin 150 U/kg after every dialysis session, plus several low-volume phlebotomies. Reticulocytosis and lowered serum ferritin and plasma porphyrin levels followed, and blistering resolved.

Management of porphyria cutanea tarda in the setting of chronic renal failure: a case report and review. Shieh S, Cohen JL, Lim HW. J Am Acad Dermatol 2000; 42: 645–52.

High-dose erythropoietin (80–360 U/kg U thrice weekly) plus 100-mL phlebotomies weekly for several months was followed by clinical remission, normalized serum ferritin, and 10-fold lower plasma porphyrin levels in one patient. Positive and negative aspects of alternative treatment for PCT in the context of renal failure are reviewed, including several third-line therapies listed next.

Third-Line Therapies

• Antiviral therapies for hepatitis C virus or human immunodeficiency virus	E
• Vitamin E, vitamin C	D
• Plasmapheresis, plasma exchange	D
• High-flux hemodialysis	D
• Enteric sorbents (cholestyramine, activated charcoal)	D
• Metabolic alkalinization by oral sodium bicarbonate	D
• Cimetidine	E
• Photothermolysis	E

Highly active antiretroviral therapy leading to resolution of porphyria cutanea tarda in a patient with AIDS and hepatitis C. Rich JD, Mylonakis E, Nossa R, Chapnick RM. Dig Dis Sci 1999; 44: 1034–7.

The association between PCT and HIV infection is less well established than that of PCT with hepatitis C infection. Coinfection with hepatitis C virus may trigger PCT in patients with HIV infection.

Dramatic resolution of skin lesions associated with porphyria cutanea tarda – interferon-alpha therapy in a case of chronic hepatitis C. Shiekh MY, Wright RA, Burruss JB. Dig Dis Sci 1998; 43: 529–33.

Anecdotal reports of PCT improvement during interferon treatment of concurrent hepatitis C infection must be balanced against those of PCT appearing 1–4 months after initiation of interferon/ribavirin protocols (Thevenot T, Bachmeyer C, Hammi R, Dumouchel P, Ducamp-Posak I, Cadranel JF. J Hepatol 2005; 42: 607–8). Ribavirin-induced hemolysis may increase liver iron, thereby triggering PCT. Measures to reduce liver iron (e.g., phlebotomy) prior to initiation of interferon, especially when combined with ribavirin, are recommended in patients with viral hepatitis and coincident symptomatic PCT or indices of excess tissue iron stores.

Treatment of chronic hepatitis with boceprevir leads to remission of porphyria cutanea tarda. Aguilera M, Laguno M, To-Figueras J. Br J Dermatol 2014; 171: 1595-6.

A patient with both HIV and hepatitis C infections whose PCT had not improved with chloroquine and phlebotomy achieved biochemical and clinical remission 2 months after boceprevir was added to a pegylated interferon/ribavirin regimen to which he had been previously unresponsive.

High-dose vitamin E lowers urine porphyrin levels in patients affected by porphyria cutanea tarda. Pinelli A, Trivulzio S, Tomasoni L, Bertolini B, Pinelli G. Pharmacol Res 2002; 45: 355–9.

Oral vitamin E (1 g daily) reduced urinary uroporphyrin levels and attenuated skin lesions during a 4-week trial in five subjects, who continued to imbibe at least 1.5 L of red wine each day.

Although urinary porphyrin levels were lower during vitamin E treatment, they remained very abnormal. Convincing confirmatory studies are needed.

Porphyria cutanea tarda: a possible role for ascorbic acid. Anderson KE. Hepatology 2007; 45: 6–8.

Deficiencies of vitamin C (ascorbic acid) and perhaps other antioxidants may facilitate development of PCT. Adequate dietary or supplemental vitamin C and other nutrients should be ingested by patients with PCT but should not usually be used as primary therapy instead of phlebotomy or chloroquine/hydroxychloroquine.

Removal of plasma porphyrins with high-flux hemodialysis in porphyria cutanea tarda associated with end stage renal disease. Carson RW, Dunnigan EJ, DuBose TD Jr, Goeger DE, Anderson KE. J Am Soc Nephrol 1992; 2: 1445–50.

High-flux hemodialysis removes porphyrins more effectively than conventional techniques.

Treatment of hemodialysis related porphyria cutanea tarda with plasma exchange. Disler P, Day R, Burman N, Blekkenhorst G, Eales L. Am J Med 1982; 72: 989–93.

This may aid patients with PCT and chronic renal failure for whom other treatments are unavailable.

The adsorption of porphyrins and porphyria precursors by sorbents: a potential therapy for the porphyrias. Tishler PV, Gordon RJ, O'Connor JA. Meth Find Exp Clin Pharmacol 1982; 4: 125–31.

Metabolic alkalinization therapy in porphyria cutanea tarda. Perry HO, Mullanax MG, Weigand SE. Arch Dermatol 1970; 102: 359–67.

Cimetidine in the treatment of porphyria cutanea tarda. Horie Y, Tanaka K, Okano J, Ohgi N, Kawasaki H, Yamamoto S, et al. Intern Med 1996; 35: 717–9.

In this report cimetidine reduced porphyrin levels within 2 weeks. This benign treatment might be offered to patients unwilling or unable to try standard therapeutic approaches.

Convincing confirmatory reports are needed.

Successful and safe treatment of hypertrichosis by high-intensity pulses of noncoherent light in a patient with hepatoerythropoietic porphyria. Garcia-Bravo M, Lopez-Gomez S, Segurado-Rodriguez MA, Morán-Jimánez MJ, Méndez M, Enriquez de Salamanca R, et al. Arch Dermatol Res 2004; 296: 139–40.

Hypertrichosis was almost completely removed after seven sessions, without development of skin lesions.

Evidence Levels: **A** Double-blind study **B** Clinical trial ≥ 20 subjects **C** Clinical trial < 20 subjects **D** Series ≥ 5 subjects **E** Anecdotal case reports

199

Port wine stain ("nevus flammeus")

Dawn Z. Eichenfield, Lawrence F. Eichenfield

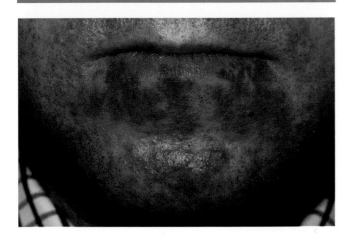

Port wine stains (PWS), also known as *nevus flammeus*, are benign capillary malformations of the superficial cutaneous vasculature. These lesions are almost always congenital, though they may be acquired secondary to trauma and, thus, may rarely develop in adolescence or adulthood. The head and neck are sites of predilection, but any part of the integument can be affected. Morphologically, these lesions present as light pink to red patches that typically grow proportionately with the child's somatic growth. Unlike the salmon patch (also known as *nevus simplex* or *angel kiss*), which usually disappears within 1 or 2 years, untreated PWS persist throughout a patient's life and tend to darken with time. Confusing this clinical picture is the fact that PWS may appear to lighten during the first 3 to 6 months of life; this is a physiologic change most likely due to the decrease in blood hemoglobin concentration (typically 15–17 g/dL at birth to a nadir of 8–10 g/dL by age 3 months) and should not be interpreted as a sign of clinical resolution. Skin thickening and the development of surface irregularities (nodules or "blebs") and soft tissue hypertrophy may also occur, especially in the V2 distribution. PWS may also present with an inflammatory component consisting of scaling, excoriations, oozing, and crusting, which resembles an eczematous dermatitis.

Although the exact molecular pathogenesis of these capillary malformations has yet to be elucidated, it is believed that complex, localized defects in pathways controlling embryogenesis and angiogenesis play crucial roles. Recent whole-genome sequencing of DNA from paired samples of affected and normal tissue from persons with Sturge–Weber syndrome (SWS) has shown that a nonsynonymous single-nucleotide–activating mutation in *GNAQ* (c.548G→A, p.Arg183Gln) encoding a $G\alpha_q$ protein responsible for the hydrolysis and inactivation of GTP and thus mediating increased downstream MAP kinase signaling is associated with both SWS-associated and nonsyndromic PWS. Mutations in RASA1 encoding the p120-rasGTPase-activating protein (p120-rasGAP) along the Ras/MAP kinase pathway have been identified in patients with atypical capillary malformations, with or without concurrent arteriovenous malformations or arteriovenous

fistulas. Evolving work using targeted next-generation sequencing has uncovered several somatic mutations seen with PWS in association with overgrowth syndromes (e.g., PIK3CA, GNA11). Further research is needed to elucidate how these genes influence PWS development, why certain PWS seem to follow specific anatomic distributions, and if therapies may be developed targeting specific genetic pathways.

In addition to being potentially cosmetically distressing and at risk for long-term deformation, PWS may be associated with serious physical, social, and psychological sequelae. The presentation of a PWS on the face in the V1 distribution, for example, has been classically linked to the development of ocular and/or neurologic complications in the form of glaucoma or SWS, especially with complete unilateral involvement of V1; bilateral involvement of V1; or a combination of V1, V2, and V3. Of note, anatomic variation in the distribution of V1 and V2 at the medial and lateral canthus (the so-called *watershed areas*) has resulted in considerable difficulty in definitively defining distribution of a PWS occurring in these areas. Several papers have posited alternative methods of characterizing facial PWS and risk of SWS, highlighting segmental patterns that differ from traditional dermatomal designations. Two papers show that the distribution of facial PWS appears to follow the embryonic vasculature of the face instead of following the traditional delineation of the trigeminal nerve, with hemifacial (upper quarter and cheek involvement) and median (forehead) patterns representing the strongest predictor of SWS and possible later neural and ophthalmologic complications.

PWS may also be associated with limb overgrowth and complex malformations (e.g., capillary–venous, capillary–venous–lymphatic, capillary–arteriovenous); evaluation of nonfacial PWS for limb overgrowth or evidence of complex malformations may warrant consideration of magnetic resonance imaging/magnetic resonance angiography (MRI/MRA) if symptomatic and/or referral to genetics or multidisciplinary vascular lesion clinics for diagnostic evaluation and management.

MANAGEMENT STRATEGY

Because of the well-recognized, predictable physical and psychosocial comorbidities associated with PWS, many specialists advocate treatment of PWS as soon as possible after birth. Support for early intervention is based on the fact that the lesions themselves are physically smaller in size and comprise vessels that are smaller in diameter and more superficial; thus early treatment may improve responsiveness, decrease the overall number of treatments, and reduce the likelihood of long-term adverse outcomes.

Many therapeutic modalities have been used to treat PWS, including surgical excision and grafting, dermabrasion, cryotherapy, sclerotherapy, radium implants, x-ray therapy, electrocautery, tattooing, and cosmetic camouflage. Vascular-targeted photodynamic therapy has also been used for patients with darker skin types, with long-term studies in the Chinese population demonstrating mixed results and several serious complications. These modalities have limited results, and many—if not all of them—have been associated with unfavorable outcomes.

Various *lasers* have been used, including CO_2, Nd:YAG, argon, and copper vapor lasers, but results have been unsatisfactory, with the risk of scarring unacceptably high. Consequently, the *flashlamp-pumped pulsed dye laser* (PDL) is considered by most authorities to be the gold standard of treatment for PWS. A lack of controlled studies with single parameter differences has made it difficult to optimize treatment settings. In general, wavelengths of 585 to 595 nm, fluences of 4 to 13 J/cm^2, spot sizes of 2 to

10 mm, and pulse durations of about 0.45 ms (short-pulse PDL characterized by the clinical end point of immediate purpura) to 1.5 ms (long-pulse PDL) are generally utilized, allowing for a deep, safe, and specific action that is confined to the targeted vasculature. Lightening and/or reduction in size of the stain is directly related to the number of treatments. Initial treatments usually give the highest percentage of improvement. Generally, the smaller, more superficial vessels are targeted first, and deeper, larger-caliber vessels may require longer pulse durations or longer wavelengths. Graying of tissue is an indication of possible over-treatment. Other modalities have been used for refractory PWS, including long-pulsed alexandrite and Nd:YAG lasers, intense-pulsed light, and photodynamic therapy.

Swelling, erythema, and pain are frequently present immediately after treatment with PDL. Other potential adverse events include postinflammatory dyspigmentation (especially in darker-skinned patients), immediate postlaser purpura, and recurrence of the lesion itself. Rarely, blistering, crusting, scarring, and infection may also occur. For these reasons, a test area may be performed before a full treatment session. Sun exposure can drastically affect pigmentary changes, and sun avoidance/protection should be optimized between treatment sessions. Before and after photos are a helpful tool for demonstrating clinical efficacy and for assuaging patient and family fears.

Cooling the skin via an attached device utilizing a targeted cryogenic spray or by application of a cool air machine is crucial to minimizing damage to surrounding tissues and reducing the risk of postoperative complications. Cold compresses and/or bags of ice applied immediately to the treated area are also useful for preventing postoperative complications.

Measures to overcome the pain and anxiety associated with laser use include topical anesthetics such as lidocaine 4% gel, eutectic mixture of 2.5% lidocaine and 2.5% prilocaine, local lidocaine infiltration, nerve block, sedation, and general anesthesia. Concerns about general anesthesia and potential neurotoxic effects in young children have been raised and should be considered in discussions about approaches to therapy, though not negating the utility and effectiveness of early laser therapy.

Topical daily treatment with 1% rapamycin cream after laser treatment may improve responsiveness to laser therapy through an unknown mechanism, possibly by decreasing vascular proliferation through the mTOR and HIF-1α pathway, resulting in statistically significant photographic improvements and patient-described subjective improvement of their lesions.

Specific Investigations

- Ophthalmologic examination in infants with V1 PWS (or equivalent facial pattern).
- MRI/MRA may be considered in infants with V1 PWS, hemifacial, or median patterns or suspected SWS to delineate the extent of central nervous system (CNS) abnormalities and in PWS that may be associated with complex vascular malformations or overgrowth syndromes. CT is an alternative, but not preferred, imaging method.
- Genetic testing for mutation analysis can be considered.

Facial port wine stain and Sturge–Weber syndrome. Enjolras O, Riche MC, Merland JJ. Pediatrics 1985; 76: 48–51.

SWS was present in 28.5% of patients with PWS covering the V1 trigeminal sensory area alone or in association with V2 and V3, and 9.5% had glaucoma. None of the patients with PWS

located in the V2 and/or the V3 areas had ocular or pial vascular abnormalities.

Sturge–Weber syndrome in patients with facial port-wine stain. Piram M, Lorette G, Sirinelli D, Herbreteau D, Giraudeau B, Maruani A. Pediatr Dermatol 2012; 29: 32–37.

This cross-sectional study of 259 patients with facial PWS included 15 patients with a diagnosis of SWS. All patients with SWS showed involvement of the V1 trigeminal cutaneous area. SWS was significantly associated with bilateral topography of the PWS, its extension to another territory, and involvement of the upper eyelid.

This study provides valuable data to support risk stratification of a facial PWS for SWS and glaucoma based on anatomic distribution.

Facial port-wine stain: when to worry? Melancon JM, Dohil MA, Eichenfield LF. Pediatr Dermatol 2012; 29: 131–3.

A "comment" on the aforementioned article by Piram et al. discussing the anatomic variations that have made direct comparison of the available literature difficult and providing insight in terms of management.

Location of port wine stains and the likelihood of ophthalmic and/or central nervous system complications. Tallman B, Tan OT, Morelli JG, Piepenbrink J, Stafford TJ, Trainor S, et al. Pediatrics 1991; 87: 323–7.

Among patients with trigeminal PWS, 8% had evidence of eye and/or CNS involvement. PWS of the eyelids, bilateral distribution, and unilateral PWS involving all three branches of the trigeminal nerve were associated with a significantly higher likelihood of having eye and/or CNS complications.

Patients with such presentations should be screened for glaucoma, and the risk of CNS involvement should be discussed with the family and appropriate testing considered.

New vascular classification of port-wine stains: improving prediction of Sturge-Weber risk. Waelchli R, Aylett SE, Robinson K, Chong WK, Martinez AE, Kinsler VA. Br J Dermatol 2014; 171: 861–7.

Of 192 children with facial PWS seen in 2011 to 2013, PWS involving any part of the forehead, which involves all three divisions of the trigeminal nerve, which corresponds well to the embryonic vascular development of the face, was the best predictor of adverse outcomes.

Children with PWS on any part of the forehead should undergo ophthalmologic evaluation and brain MRI.

A prospective study of risk for Sturge-Weber syndrome in children with upper facial port-wine stain. Dutkiewicz AS, Ezzedine K, Mazereeuw-Hautier J, Lacour JP, Barbarot S, Vabres P, et al. J Am Acad Dermatol 2015; 72: 473–80.

In this prospective multicenter study of 66 patients, 11 presented with SWS and 4 had suspected SWS without neurologic manifestations. These patients predominantly had hemifacial or median PWS patterns that were high risk for SWS.

Hemifacial or median PWS patterns conform to areas of somatic mosaicism and are high risk for SWS.

Sturge–Weber syndrome and dermatomal facial port wine stains: incidence, association with glaucoma, and pulsed tunable dye laser treatment effectiveness. Hennedige AA, Quaba AA, Al-Nikib K. Plast Reconstruct Surg 2008; 121: 1173–80.

In this study of 874 patients, SWS occurred in 3% of all patients with facial PWS and 10% of those whose PWS were in a dermatomal distribution. Although both SWS and glaucoma occurred in patients with only V1 involvement, the risk increased substantially with V1 + V2 and V1 + V2 + V3 involvement. No patients with only V3 involvement had eye or CNS findings.

Children at risk of SWS should have ophthalmologic examination in the neonatal period and require ophthalmologic follow-up because glaucoma may develop subsequent to initial presentation.

Sturge–Weber syndrome. The current neuroradiologic data. Boukobza M, Enjolras O, Cambra M, Merland J. J Radiol 2000; 81: 765–71.

Neonatal neuroimaging workup using CT or MRI may not demonstrate the pial anomaly and may be delayed or repeated after 6 to 12 months in an at-risk infant with V1 PWS.

First-Line Therapy

- Pulsed dye laser   **B**

Anatomic differences of port wine stains in response to treatment with pulsed dye laser. Renfro L, Geronemus RG. Arch Dermatol 1993; 129: 182–8.

Centrofacial lesions and lesions involving dermatome V2 responded less favorably than lesions located elsewhere on the head and neck.

Facial port wine stains in childhood: prediction of the rate of improvement as a function of the age of the patient, size and location of the port wine stain and the number of treatments with the pulsed dye (585 nm) laser. Nguyen CM, Yohn JJ, Huff C, Weston WL, Morelli JG. Br J Dermatol 1998; 138: 821–5.

Major determinants of treatment response, in order of decreasing importance, are PWS location, size, and patient age. The most successful responses are seen in young patients (under 1 year of age) with small PWS (<20 cm²) located over bony areas of the face, such as the central forehead. The greatest percentage of size reduction occurred after the first five treatments. There was less reduction in size with subsequent treatments.

Why do port-wine stains (PWS) on the lateral face respond better to pulsed dye laser (PDL) than those located on the central face? Yu W, Ma G, Qiu Y, Chen H, Jin Y, Yang X, et al. J Am Acad Dermatol 2016; 74: 527–35.

In 13 patients with PWS who underwent PDL treatments in both central and lateral areas of the face, lateral facial PWS responded better to PDL treatments than did PWS located in the central face.

Efficacy of early treatment of facial port wine stains in newborns: a review of 49 cases. Chapas AM, Eickhorst K, Geronemus RG. Lasers Surg Med 2007; 39: 563–8.

Patients who received treatment with the cryogen spray–cooled 595-nm PDL before 6 months of age achieved a mean 88.6% clearance after 1 year after an average of nine treatments. Higher clearance rates were observed for smaller lesions and V1 dermatome lesions.

Treatment of port wine stains (capillary malformations) with the flash lamp pumped pulsed dye laser. Goldman MP, Fitzpatrick RE, Ruiz-Esparza J. J Pediatr 1993; 122: 71–7.

Initial treatment in children with PWS results in approximately 40% improvement, and each subsequent treatment up to six adds a further increment of 10% improvement. Treatments should be continued as long as there is incremental improvement.

Double pass 595 nm pulsed dye laser at a 6 minute interval for the treatment of port-wine stains is not more effective than single pass. Peters MA, Drooge AM, Wolkerstorfer A, van Gemert MJ, van der Veen JP, Bos JD, et al. Lasers Surg Med 2012; 44: 199–204.

In each patient (*n* = 16), two similar PWS areas were randomly allocated to PDL with either a single pass (595 nm; 12 J/cm² fluence; 7-mm spot; 1.5-ms pulse duration) or, as a new treatment, a double pass (11 J/cm²). Test areas were treated two times, 8 weeks apart. At 3 months, follow-up, no significant difference was noted in any of the outcomes.

High-fluence modified pulsed dye laser photocoagulation with dynamic cooling of port wine stains in infancy. Geronemus RG, Quintana AT, Lou WW, Kauvar AN. Arch Dermatol 2000; 136: 942–3.

Early intervention using a modified PDL with a longer wavelength (595 nm), broader pulse width (1.5 ms), dynamic cooling spray, and high-energy fluences can result in lightening or clearing of PWS with minimal risk of adverse effects.

Redarkening of port-wine stains 10 years after pulsed-dye-laser treatment. Huikeshoven M, Koster PH, deBorgie CA, Beek JF, van Gemert MJ, van der Horst CM. N Engl J Med 2007; 356: 1235–40.

After follow-up for a median of 9.5 years, PWS, on average, were darker than when measured after the last of the five initial treatments, although still lighter than when measured before treatment.

Patients should be counseled that due to progressive ectasia of PWS vessels, "recurrence," or redarkening of the stain, is a possibility.

Effects of percutaneous local anaesthetics on pain reduction during pulse dye laser treatment of port wine stains. McCafferty DF, Woolfson AD, Handley J, Allen G. Br J Anaesth 1997; 78: 286–9.

Both EMLA and 4% tetracaine gel were statistically superior to placebo in reducing pain caused by the laser treatment.

Effect of the topical anesthetic EMLA on the efficacy of pulsed dye laser treatment of port wine stains. Ashinoff R, Geronemus RG. J Dermatol Surg Oncol 1990; 16: 1008–11.

The use of topical anesthetic creams or sedating agents has been shown not to interfere with laser therapy.

Cryogen spray cooling and higher fluence pulsed dye laser treatment improve port wine stain clearance while minimizing epidermal damage. Chang CJ, Nelson JS. Dermatol Surg 1999; 25: 767–72.

A retrospective study of 196 patients with head and neck PWS, indicating the statistically significant advantage of using a cryogen spray–cooling device with PDL by permitting higher light dosages and a subsequently higher clearance rate without increasing the rate of complications.

General anesthesia for pediatric dermatologic procedures: risks and complications. Cunningham BB, Gigler V, Wang K, Eichenfield LF, Friedlander SF, Garden JM, et al. Arch Dermatol 2005; 141: 573–6.

A review of 881 cases performed on 269 pediatric patients, 88% of which were PDL treatment of vascular lesions, including PWS. There were no life-threatening events, and the mortality rate was zero.

The use of general anesthesia for dermatologic procedures performed in a children's hospital setting is safe with a low rate of complications.

Anesthetic neurotoxicity—clinical implications of animal models. Rappaport BA, Suresh S, Hertz S, Evers AS, Orser BA. N Engl J Med 2015; 372: 796–7.

A perspective paper discussing possible animal studies and ongoing clinical studies in children undergoing prolonged or repeated general anesthesia.

While awaiting clinical studies that can definitively determine whether anesthetics cause injury in humans, surgeons, anesthesiologists, and parents should consider carefully how urgently surgery is needed, particularly in children under 3 years of age.

US Safety Warning: about using general anesthetics and sedation drugs in young children. https://www.fda.gov/downloads/Drugs/DrugSafety/UCM533197.pdf

The U.S. Food and Drug Administration (FDA) has communicated that repeated or lengthy use of general anesthetic and sedation drugs during surgeries or procedures in children younger than 3 years may affect the development of children's brains. Health care professionals should balance the benefits of appropriate anesthesia in young children against the potential risks. Discuss with parents, caregivers, and pregnant women the benefits, risks, and appropriate timing of surgery or procedures requiring anesthetic and sedation drugs. Anesthetic and sedation drugs are necessary for infants, children, and pregnant women who require surgery or other painful and stressful procedures, especially when they face life-threatening conditions requiring surgery that should not be delayed. In addition, untreated pain can be harmful to children and their developing nervous systems.

Second-Line Therapies	
• Alexandrite 755-nm laser	B
• Neodymium:yttrium–aluminum–garnet (Nd:YAG) laser	B
• Intense pulsed light source	B

Split-face comparison of intense pulsed light with short- and long-pulsed dye lasers for the treatment of port-wine stains. Babilas P, Schremi S, Eames T, Hohenleutner U, Szeimies RM, Landthaler M. Lasers Surg Med 2010; 42: 720–7.

This study evaluated the efficacy and side effects of intense pulsed light (IPL) treatment of PWS in a direct comparison to the short-pulsed dye laser (SPDL) and the long-pulsed dye laser (LPDL). Test spots were applied with IPL (555–950 nm; pulse duration 8–14 ms [single pulse]; fluence 11 to 17.3 J/cm²) versus SPDL (585 nm; pulse duration 0.45 ms; fluence 6 J/cm²) versus LPDL (585/590/595/600 nm; pulse duration 1.5 ms; fluence 12/14/16/18 J/cm²) in a side-by-side modus. Subjects included those with both untreated (n = 11) and previously treated (n = 14) PWS, and lesion clearance was evaluated by three blinded investigators based on follow-up photography 6 weeks after treatment. In both untreated and previously treated PWS, IPL treatments were rated significantly better than SPDL; in both groups, IPL and LPDL treatments did not differ significantly. Side effects were rare with all modalities.

Intense pulsed light source for the treatment of dye laser resistant port-wine stains. Bjerring P, Christiansen K, Troilius A. J Cosmet Laser Ther 2003; 5: 7–13.

A greater than 50% reduction was achieved after four treatments with IPL source in 46.7% of 15 patients with PWS previously treated by PDL. None of the lesions located in V2 responded.

There are several case reports of successful treatment of resistant PWS with IPL source. However, controlled studies are needed to confirm this observation.

Treatment of hypertrophic and resistant port wine stains with a 755 nm laser: a case series of 20 patients. Izikson L, Nelson JS, Anderson RR. Lasers Surg Med 2009; 41: 427–32.

Many PWS that respond well initially to PDL treatment may reach a response plateau, and many hypertrophic PWS are less responsive to PDL in general. Based on the theory of selective photothermolysis, the deoxyhemoglobin and oxyhemoglobin in the deeper vessels within these lesions may be targeted with a 755-nm laser. This retrospective case review of 20 patients demonstrated the utility of the 755-nm laser for improving hypertrophic and treatment-resistant PWS in both adult and pediatric patients. Most commonly encountered complications included pain, edema, bullae, crusting, and rare scarring.

Some scarring with the 755-nm laser is inevitable if one uses the laser enough; however, the technique for PWS is difficult enough that these authors recommend its use by experienced laser specialists only.

Treatment endpoints for resistant port wine stains with a 755 nm laser. Izikson L, Anderson RR. J Cosmet Laser Ther 2009; 11: 52–5.

Deeper vessels may be targeted with the near-infrared light from the 755-nm laser. It is more difficult to assess laser-induced changes within the deeper dermis, however, and adverse effects include deep dermal burns. The authors treated a resistant PWS with a 755-nm laser at high fluences (40–100 J/cm²; 1.5-ms pulse duration) with a dynamic cooling device. Mild-to-moderate lightening of the PWS was associated with the immediate clinical end point of a transient gray color that gradually evolved into persistent deep purpura within several minutes. The authors recommend judicious use of 755 nm for resistant PWS.

Long-pulsed neodymium:yttrium–aluminum–garnet laser treatment for port wine stains. Yang MU, Yaroslavsky AN, Farinelli WA, Flotte TJ, Rius-Diaz F, Tsao S, et al. J Am Acad Dermatol 2005; 52: 480–90.

Treatment achieved similar 50% to 75% clearing with both the PDL and the Nd:YAG laser at minimum purpura dose (MPD). The PDL performed significantly better than the Nd:YAG at fluences lower than 1 MPD, and scarring occurred in the only patient who was treated with the Nd:YAG laser at a fluence greater than 1 MPD.

Nd:YAG may be an alternative treatment option, although there is a narrow margin at which this laser is both safe and effective.

Combined 595 nm and 1064 nm laser irradiation of recalcitrant and hypertrophic port-wine stains in children and adults. Alster TS, Tanzi EL. Dermatol Surg 2009; 35: 914–9.

The purpose of this study was to evaluate the safety and efficacy of a novel device that delivers sequential pulses of 595-nm and 1064-nm wavelengths in the treatment of recalcitrant and hypertrophic PWS. Twenty-five subjects (aged 2–75) with skin types I to III were identified showing incomplete clearance after 10+ (mean = 16.9) prior PDL treatments. Nineteen had a PWS in a trigeminal location and six on the extremities. Subjects were treated at 6- to 8-week intervals. Continued improvement was noted in these resistant lesions. Side effects included transient erythema, edema, mild purpura, and rare vesicle formation.

A direct comparison of pulsed dye, alexandrite, KTP and Nd:YAG lasers and IPL in patients with previously treated capillary malformations. McGill DJ, MacLaren W, Mackay IR. Lasers Surg Med 2008; 40: 390–8.

Patients with PWS previously treated with PDL were treated using the alexandrite, KTP (potassium titanyl phosphate), and Nd:YAG lasers and IPL, with additional PDL patches as a control. Fifty-five percent of patients achieved some lightening with the alexandrite laser, although a high percentage also developed hyperpigmentation or scarring. Thirty-three percent achieved some lightening with IPL, 11% each for KTP and Nd:YAG, and 28% with further PDL pulses.

Third-Line Therapies

• Potassium titanyl phosphate laser	B
• Imiquimod (as antiangiogenic therapy)	B
• Photodynamic therapy	B
• Rapamycin (as antiangiogenic therapy)	B

Potassium titanyl phosphate laser treatment of resistant port-wine stains. Chowdhury MU, Harris S, Lanigan SW. Br J Dermatol 2001; 144: 814–7.

A greater than 50% reduction was seen in 17% of 30 patients with PWS previously treated by PDL; 20% of patients experienced side effects, including scarring or hyperpigmentation.

Treatment of PWS with KTP laser is advocated by some, although studies have shown it to have limited utility and an increased incidence of scarring.

Pilot study examining the combined use of pulsed dye laser and topical imiquimod versus laser alone for treatment of port wine stain birthmarks. Chang CJ, Hsiao YC, Mihm MC Jr, Nelson JS. Lasers Surg Med 2008; 40: 605–10.

This retrospective review of 20 Asian subjects (aged 3–56 years) with PWS used three test sites on each subject for treatment assignments to the following regimens: (1) PDL + imiquimod; (2) PDL alone; and (3) imiquimod alone. PDL sites were treated once with a 585-nm wavelength, 10 J/cm^2 fluence, 1.5-ms pulse duration, and 7-mm spot size, with cryogen spray cooling. For the PDL + imiquimod and imiquimod-alone test sites, subjects applied imiquimod topically once a day for 1 month after PDL exposure or alone. Subjects were followed at 1, 3, 6, and 12 months after PDL exposure to evaluate all three test sites. The primary efficacy measurement was the quantitative assessment of blanching responses as measured by a DermoSpectrometer to calculate the hemoglobin index of each site at follow-up visits after PDL exposure. The authors report statistically significant differences in blanching responses over time favoring PDL + imiquimod compared with either PDL alone or imiquimod alone. Some evidence of redarkening, thought to be related to revascularization of blood vessels, was noted at 12 months at test sites treated with PDL + imiquimod and PDL alone. Transient hyperpigmentation was noted but had resolved on all sites without medical intervention within 6 months. The authors note that clinical validation in larger patient samples is necessary.

Enhanced port-wine stain lightening achieved with combined treatment of selective photothermolysis and imiquimod. Tremaine AM, Armstrong J, Huang YC, Elkeeb L, Ortiz A, Harris R, et al. J Am Acad Dermatol 2012; 66: 634–41.

Twenty-four patients with PWS were treated with PDL and randomized to apply posttreatment placebo cream or imiquimod 5% cream for 8 weeks. Chromameter measurements were taken at baseline and compared with measurements taken 8 weeks posttreatment. The change in erythema and the change in color between normal-appearing skin and PWS skin were the primary end points. Greater reduction in erythema and greater color improvement were noted with imiquimod. The authors note that the true clinical duration of effect is unknown. Minor skin irritation and other adverse events were noted.

Photodynamic therapy of port-wine stains: long-term efficacy and complication in Chinese patients. Xiao Q, Li Q, Yuan KH, Cheng B. J Dermatol 2011; 38: 1146–52.

The authors profess that PDL is not suitable for PWS patients with Fitzpatrick skin type V or with nodular lesions. In this retrospective study, the authors studied 642 Chinese patients who had received PDT in a 5-year period (totaling 3066 treatment sessions; average of 2.6–8.2 sessions per patient). Seventy percent of patients had more than 25% clearing, and over 5% of patients had complete clearing. Ten percent of patients experienced complications that included hyperpigmentation (4.3%), scabbing (2.2%), blistering (1.4%), hypopigmentation (1.2%), prolonged blistering that persisted for >2 months (<0.7%), photoallergy (0.6%), and eczematous dermatitis (0.4%).

Topical rapamycin combined with pulse dye laser in the treatment of capillary vascular malformations in Sturge-Weber syndrome: phase II, randomized, double-blind, intraindividual placebo-controlled clinical trial. Marques L, Nunez-Cordoba JM, Aquado L, Pretel M, Boixeda P, Naqore E, et al. J Am Acad Dermatol 2014; 72: 151–8.

In 23 patients with SWS and facial PWS, four interventions were evaluated: placebo, PDL + placebo, rapamycin, and PDL + rapamycin. PDL + rapamycin showed a statistically significant improvement visually subjectively per patient and had a lower percentage of vessels in histologic analysis.

Topical daily treatment with 1% rapamycin cream after laser treatment may improve responsiveness to laser therapy by decreasing vascular proliferation.

Postinflammatory hyperpigmentation and other disorders of hyperpigmentation

Seemal Desai

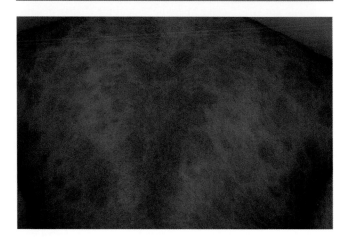

Pigmentary disorders are among the most common conditions encountered in dermatologic practice. They may be due to increased activity of melanocytes or proliferation of the latter. The spectrum includes both congenital and acquired conditions. The latter can further be divided into localized dermatoses such as postinflammatory hyperpigmentation, melasma, etc., or generalized dermatoses such as those seen secondary to malignancy, metabolic disorders, autoimmune diseases, etc. The conditions presenting with predominant epidermal hypermelanosis present clinically with brownish pigmentation, whereas those with dermal hypermelanosis present with slate gray–colored macules. This chapter describes some of these common acquired dermatoses and gives a brief overview of the treatment options available.

POSTINFLAMMATORY HYPERPIGMENTATION

It is a common acquired cause of hypermelanosis that results from cutaneous injury/inflammation. It is more commonly seen in patients with skin of color (Fitzpatrick skin type IV–VI) than Caucasians. The population with higher phototypes is believed to be more prone to postinflammatory hyperpigmentation due to higher epidermal melanin content. The resulting pigmentation is also more intense and prolonged. Overproduction of melanin after cutaneous inflammation has been suggested as the etiology of the pigmentation. Common disorders that lead to postinflammatory hyperpigmentation include acne, allergic reactions, insect bite, atopic dermatitis, cutaneous infection, hypersensitivity reaction, drug-induced cutaneous injury, papulosquamous disorders, etc. The increase in the activity of the melanocytes after the cutaneous insult is secondary to the release of cytokines, chemokines, and reactive oxygen species. These mediators of inflammation lead to increased activity of melanocytes and tyrosinase. After an

insult, the pigment can also be released into the dermis by the basal keratinocytes. This pigment when phagocytosed by the dermal macrophages imparts a slate blue color to the skin, in contrast to the brownish color seen after epidermal hypermelanosis.

FRECKLES

Freckles are pigmented, tan-colored, tiny macules present over the sun-exposed area of the face such as the nose and malar area. The pigmentation of the lesions varies according to the sun exposure. The lesions are more common among the light-skinned individuals. Light microscopy reveals increased pigmentation of the basal layer with normal number of melanocytes.

LENTIGINES

Lentigines present clinically similar to freckles but have a few differentiating features. The color of the lesion is unaffected by sun exposure in contrast to freckles (increased pigmentation noticed on sun exposure). The histopathology of the lesion reveals increased number of basal melanocytes. The most common type is lentigo simplex, also called a *simple lentigo*. The lesions present at birth or soon after. Sun exposure and medical diseases have no association with this type.

The "solar lentigo," "old age spot," or "senile freckles" present on sun-exposed parts of the body such as face, forearms, dorsa of hands, and bald scalp. With aging, basal cells containing lipofuscin bodies accumulate in the basal layer. With increased aging more and more aged cells accumulate and form a brown spot.

PUVA lentigo is commonly seen in patients undergoing PUVA therapy.

Ink spot lentigo, also called *sunburn lentigo*, is a result of sun exposure. The lesions are located over the shoulders and are indicators of increased risk of skin cancer.

Apart from the previously mentioned types, lentigines can be part of lentiginosis syndromes such as LEOPARD syndrome, Moynahan syndrome, Peutz–Jeghers syndrome, etc.

MELASMA

Melasma is a common acquired disorder of pigmentation that is encountered in females of child-bearing age. It is derived from the Greek word *melas* meaning black. Melasma appearing in pregnancy is referred to as *chloasma*. It has also been reported in men and constitutes less than 10% of the cases. Although all races are affected, the highest incidence is seen among populations living in regions where there is intense ultraviolet light exposure such as in Latinos of Caribbean origin, Asians, and African descendants. The etiology of melasma is multifactorial and includes both genetic factors and environmental influences. Exposure to sunlight, phototoxic drugs, pregnancy, oral contraceptives, thyroid dysfunction, and cosmetics are some of the environmental triggers that have been implicated in the pathogenesis. Ultraviolet light leads to melanocortin hormone stimulation in the melanocytes, which eventually leads to increase in melanogenesis. Recently the role of visible light has also been shown to play a role in the pathogenesis.

The lesions clinically consist of well-defined, brownish to tan-colored macules with irregular, serrated borders present over the facial convexities (forehead, cheek), neck, and forearm. Based on the clinical pattern three types have been described: the centrofacial pattern involving forehead, cheeks, chin, and upper lip;

Evidence Levels: **A** Double-blind study **B** Clinical trial ≥ 20 subjects **C** Clinical trial < 20 subjects **D** Series ≥ 5 subjects **E** Anecdotal case reports

the malar type involving cheeks and lip; and the mandibular pattern involving the ramus of the mandible. Histologic examination reveals increased pigmentation of the epidermis and dermis with perivascular lymphohistiocytic infiltrate.

PERIORBITAL HYPERPIGMENTATION

It is a common complaint affecting both sexes and all races. It presents clinically as homogeneous areas of hyperpigmentation present around the eyes. The condition gets worse with age due to thinning of skin and loss of subcutaneous fat around the eyes. Periorbital melanosis can be secondary to an inflammatory process such as atopic/allergic dermatitis, fixed drug eruption, erythema dyschromicum perstans, etc. Other etiologic factors include dermal melanin deposition, superficial placement of blood vessels, and anatomic factors such as prominent lacrimal sulcus, loss of periorbital fat, edema, and chronic photodamage.

RIEHL MELANOSIS

Riehl melanosis, also called *pigmented contact dermatitis,* is an acquired pigmentary anomaly presenting as grayish to brown areas of reticulate pigmentation over the forehead and temples. It is a photocontact dermatitis resulting from the use of photosensitizing chemicals such as coal tar, minoxidil, cosmetics, etc. Ultraviolet radiation plays an important role by inducing a photoallergic reaction. Other photoexposed sites such as neck, forearm, and dorsa of hands are also frequently involved. Histologic examination reveals degeneration of the basal cell layer with pigment incontinence in the dermis and lymphohistiocytic infiltrate.

PHOTOTOXIC DERMATITIS

It is a condition due to the reaction between a photosensitizing substance and ultraviolet radiation. The phototoxic substances implicated include systemic drugs, topically applied cosmetics, fragrances, and plants containing furocoumarins. The lesions may present as bullae and erythema in the acute stage and resolve to leave behind patches of hyperpigmentation. Berloque dermatitis is a condition resulting from the use of bergamot oil in fragrances and colognes. The pigmentation is present at the sites of application of perfumes such as the retroauricular area and sides of the neck. Histology of the lesions reveals increased melanin in the basal layer and dermal melanophages.

ERYTHEMA DYSCHROMICUM PERSTANS

Erythema dyschromicum perstans, also called *ashy dermatosis* or *gray dermatosis,* is an acquired cause of hyperpigmentation presenting as brownish macules situated over the trunk, face, and extremities. It was first described by Ramirez, and it has been more commonly reported among the Latin American population. Etiology is unknown. Possible causative factors that have been implicated include oral ingestion of x-ray contrast media, hepatitis C infection, and environmental contaminants. The disease is more common among Hispanics, and there is no sexual predilection. The lesions are oval grayish-colored macules over the trunk and proximal extremities. The initial lesions have a raised erythematous border that disappears later. Histopathologic examination of the initial lesion shows vacuolization of the basal layer with mononuclear infiltrate in the dermis. Older lesions show only pigment incontinence.

LICHEN PLANUS PIGMENTOSUS

It is a variant of lichen planus reported from the Indian subcontinent and the Middle East. It presents with coalescing grayish macules present over the sun-exposed parts. The lesions clinically resemble erythema dyschromicum perstans but can be distinguished by lack of inflammatory border and presence of lesions in sun-exposed parts. Histology reveals basal layer degeneration, bandlike lymphohistiocytic infiltrate present in the dermis, and Civatte bodies.

POIKIODERMA OF CIVATTE

Poikioderma is a term that clinically represents a triad of pigmentation, atrophy, and telangiectasia. It is mostly seen in fair-skinned middle-age to elderly females. Sun exposure has been implicated as one of the most important factors in its pathogenesis. The distribution of the lesions in sun-exposed areas also favors the role of actinic damage in its causation. Other causative factors include photosensitizing cosmetics and fragrances. Lesions clinically consist of reticulate pigmentation along with atrophy and telangiectasia present along the sides of the cheeks and neck. Sun-protected sites, such as below the chin, are often spared. Light microscopic examination of lesions reveals atrophy of the epidermis, degeneration of the basal layer, and pigment incontinence and lymphocytic infiltrate in the dermis.

MANAGEMENT STRATEGY

The diagnosis of these hyperpigmentary dermatoses is often clinical; the need for a thorough history and examination cannot be underestimated. The age at onset, progression of lesions, characteristics and distribution of the lesions, and any preceding cutaneous lesion should be noted. History of drug intake, any systemic disorder, and hormonal abnormality should be ruled out before beginning treatment. Detailed history regarding the use of fragrances and cosmetics is essential to reach a correct diagnosis. Histopathology and dermoscopy may aid when the diagnosis is unclear.

Many compounds are available for the treatment of hypermelanosis. The selection of a therapeutic option is dependent on a number of factors such as past treatment taken, the therapeutic response reported, sensitivity of skin, Fitzpatrick skin type, etc. The role of sun protection cannot be underestimated in the treatment of pigmentation disorders. Patients with Fitzpatrick skin types IV to V who are exposed to high ultraviolet radiation particularly benefit by the use of sunscreens. Sunscreen with a broad spectrum of sun protection is pivotal in the prevention and treatment of these disorders. Physical sunscreens containing zinc oxide and titanium oxide are preferred over the chemical sunscreens, which carry a risk of allergic contact dermatitis. Physical sunscreens are also cosmetically more acceptable as they cause less exothermic reaction and thus are more suitable for patients living in hot and humid conditions.

Evaluation of the effectiveness of a broad-spectrum sunscreen in the prevention of chloasma in pregnant women. Lakhdar H, Zouhair K, Khadir K, Essari A, Richard A, Seité S, et al. J Eur Acad Dermatol Venereol 2007; 21: 738–42.

Two hundred women older than 18 years and less than 3 months pregnant were included in the study. Patients were prescribed sunscreen (SPF 50+, UVA-PF 28) every 2 hours. Participants were advised to avoid sunlight, heat, scrubbing, rubbing, and use of photosensitizing products. Follow-up was done at 3, 6, and 9 months. A total of 185 patients completed the study. Evaluation was done by the patient and the dermatologist (colorimetric evaluation) at each follow-up visit. Among the 185 patients completing the study 38% finished with lighter skin, 21% with darker, and 41% unchanged. Only five new cases of chloasma were noted among the total 185 participants at the end of the study corresponding to 2.7%, and only two cases reported worsening of existing melasma. The study demonstrated an effective role of the use of broad-spectrum sunscreen in the prevention of chloasma during pregnancy.

Recently the role of visible light in the pathogenesis of melasma has been stressed. Wavelength in the visible spectrum interferes with the action of depigmenting agents and increases risk of relapses posttreatment. It has been shown to increase inflammatory response after sun exposure, increasing the neutrophil and macrophage infiltration. Visible light increases the sun-induced photodamage and induces cell vacuolization and melanocytic response. It also makes the cells more susceptible to damage by solar radiation.

The treatment of all hyperpigmentation disorders includes a common group of depigmenting agents (Table 200.1). The prototype drug is hydroquinone and is considered the gold standard, although it is not available everywhere. The efficacy of any new depigmenting agent is compared with hydroquinone.

First-Line Therapies

- 4% hydroquinone
- Hydroquinone plus other depigmenting agent
- Hydroquinone allergy/long-term use: arbutin, kojic acid, azelaic acid

A randomized controlled trial of the efficacy and safety of a fixed triple combination (fluocinolone acetonide 0.01%, hydroquinone 4%, tretinoin 0.05%) compared with hydroquinone 4% cream in Asian patients with moderate to severe melasma. Chan R, Park KC, Lee MH, Lee ES, Chang SE, Leow YH, et al. Br J Dermatol 2008; 159: 697–703.

This was a multicenter trial in nine centers (Korea, Philippines, Singapore, and Hong Kong) on 260 Southeast Asian patients with melasma. The study population was randomized into two groups: one group received triple combination (fluocinolone acetonide 0.01%, hydroquinone 4%, tretinoin 0.05%) and the other 4% hydroquinone for a total of 8 weeks. A questionnaire-based assessment for patient satisfaction was done. The participants in the triple combination group reported significantly more improvement (71%) compared with the hydroquinone group (50%) (p value = 0.005). Physician-reported improvement using static global assessment score confirmed those results. Significantly more patients in the triple combination group (87/125) reported a score of 0 (clear) or 1 (mild hyperpigmentation) compared with the 4% hydroquinone group (57/129). The triple combination group reported earlier onset of response with significant differences in score from 4 weeks onward. The cutaneous side effects reported such as erythema, itching, and discomfort were significantly more in the triple combination group compared with the hydroquinone group. An assessment was also made among the participants on how much they were bothered by the treatment side effects. A total of 43% of patients in the triple combination group were not bothered by treatment side effects compared with 77% (significantly more) in the hydroquinone group.

Efficacy and safety of a new triple-combination agent for the treatment of facial melasma. Taylor SC, Torok H, Jones T, Lowe N, Rich P, Tschen E, et al. Cutis 2003; 72: 67–72.

Table 200.1 Mechanism of action of commonly used hypopigmenting agents

Mechanism of action	Hypopigmenting agent
Tyrosinase inhibition	Hydroquinone
	Kojic acid
	Arbutin
	Azelaic acid
	Licorice
	Ellagic acid
	Flavonoids
Reactive oxygen scavengers	Ascorbic acid
Skin turnover acceleration	Retinoic acid
	Lactic acid
	Glycolic acid
	Salicylic acid
Inhibition of melanosome transfer	Niacinamide
	Soya/milk extracts
Prostaglandin inhibition	Tranexamic acid

Participants (641) were randomly divided into four groups: triple combination cream (4% hydroquinone, tretinoin 0.05%, and fluocinolone acetonide 0.01%; n = 161), dual combination agent (tretinoin 0.05% and 4% hydroquinone; n = 158), dual combination agent (tretinoin 0.05% and fluocinolone acetonide 0.01%; n = 161), or dual combination agent (4% hydroquinone and fluocinolone acetonide 0.01%; n = 161), each applied daily at night for 8 weeks. Of those receiving the triple combination cream, 26.1% had complete clearing of melasma compared with 9.5%, 1.9%, and 2.5%, respectively, in each of the dual combination creams. Side effects were more common in the tretinoin hydroquinone group (80%) followed by tretinoin fluocinolone acetonide (65%) group, triple combination (63%) group, and hydroquinone fluocinolone group (34%).

Hydroquinone has been extensively used to treat hypermelanosis. It is used in 2% to 4% concentration as either monotherapy or in combination with other agents. Effect becomes evident after 5 to 7 weeks; treatment can be continued for 1 year. Short-term side effects include erythema and burning, whereas long-term effects include ochronosis and confetti-like depigmentation. It is a strong oxidant and gets rapidly converted into melanocyte-toxic products, which are responsible for depigmentation caused by the product. Recently concern has been raised regarding the long-term use of hydroquinone after reports of its carcinogenicity potential in rodents that were fed high doses of hydroquinone. Regulatory agencies in Europe, Japan, and the United States have banned its use in cosmetic preparations and over-the-counter products. However, over the 40 to 50 years of experience with this product for medical purposes, not a single report of malignancy was documented.

Azelaic acid 20% cream in the treatment of facial hyperpigmentation in darker skinned patients. Lowe NJ, Rizk D, Grimes P, Billips M, Pincus S. Clin Ther 1998; 20: 945–59.

A double-blind, randomized, vehicle-controlled trial in which 52 patients (Fitzpatrick skin types IV–VI) of melasma and postinflammatory hyperpigmentation were evaluated to determine the efficacy and safety of 20% azelaic acid cream. Results were evaluated at the end of 24 weeks. The group receiving azelaic acid showed a greater decrease in pigment intensity versus the other group. Results were evaluated using investigators' subjective scale (p = 0.021) and chromometric analysis ($p < 0.039$). Side effects reported were mild.

There is a growing need for nonhydroquinone-based, natural, efficacious, and safe skin-lightening agents. These agents selectively target hyperactive melanocytes and inhibit key enzymes in the melanogenic pathway. A combination of multiple ingredients is often used to increase effectiveness. However, large-scale clinical trials are lacking for most of the botanical agents to substantiate their claims of effectiveness.

Second-Line Therapies

- Chemical peels
- Laser
- Light therapy
- Microdermabrasion

Comparison of 30% salicylic acid with Jessner's solution for superficial chemical peeling in epidermal melasma. Ejaz A, Raza N, Iftikhar N, Muzzafar F. J Coll Physicians Surg Pak 2008; 18: 205–8.

A trial conducted in Pakistan to compare Jessner peel (14% salicylic acid, 14% lactic acid and 14% resorcinol) to 30% salicylic acid peel after priming with 0.05% tretinoin for 2 weeks nightly. Sixty patients were randomized into two groups; each group underwent fortnightly peeling sessions with either Jessner or salicylic acid peel for a total duration of 12 weeks. Total contact time was 5 min. Participants were followed up for 12 weeks after treatment discontinuation. No significant difference in the reduction of melasma was noted at the end of 12 or 24 weeks. Eight of 34 participants in the Jessner group reported adverse events compared with 10/26 in the salicylic acid group. The side effects reported included crusting, pigmentation, sunburn, and acneiform eruption. Three patients did not follow up after 12 weeks, and 14 patients did not follow up after 24 weeks.

Chemical peels cause controlled exfoliation of the epidermis. Superficial and medium-depth peels are used for treatment of pigmentation. Prolonged use of medium-depth peels carries a risk of dyschromia, especially in dark-skinned individuals. Choosing the right patient with adequate priming, strict sun protection, and concomitant topical therapy forms the backbone of a good peeling regimen.

Successful treatment of melasma using a combination of microdermabrasion and Q-switched Nd:YAG lasers. Kauvar AN. Lasers Surg Med 2012; 44: 117–24.

In this study, 27 female patients with melasma refractory to conventional therapy were treated with Nd:YAG laser session after microdermabrasion. Low-fluence laser treatment was used with 5- to 6-mm spot size and energy of 1.6 to 2 J/cm^2. Postprocedure, patients were discharged on sunscreen and topical preparation containing hydroquinone with tretinoin or vitamin C. Treatment was repeated at monthly intervals. About 50% of the patients reported improvement after 1 month of starting the treatment. Remission was noted for 6 months. Side effects reported included mild postprocedural erythema and exacerbation of lesions, which resolved in a few weeks after topical treatment.

Q-switched, fractional, IPL, and combination lasers are used in the treatment of pigmentary dermatosis with variable results. Individuals with higher Fitzpatrick skin types carry a risk of postinflammatory hyperpigmentation after the procedure. Other side effects reported include rebound hyperpigmentation, physical urticaria, acneiform eruption, etc.

Pregnancy dermatoses

Lauren E. Wiznia, Miriam Keltz Pomeranz

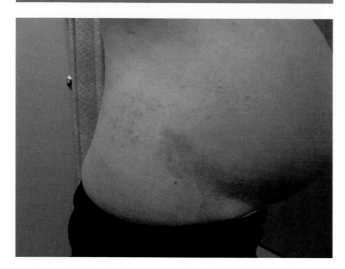

Dermatoses specifically associated with pregnancy and the puerperium include polymorphic eruption of pregnancy, pemphigoid gestationis (PG), intrahepatic cholestasis of pregnancy, and atopic eruption of pregnancy. In addition to these classic dermatoses of pregnancy, pregnant women can develop all of the same pruritic dermatoses as nonpregnant women. There are also many skin changes during pregnancy that are normal physiologic changes. Because some pregnancy-related dermatoses may adversely affect the fetus, it is important to correctly diagnose and treat these diseases. Pustular psoriasis of pregnancy (previously impetigo herpetiformis), which we will not address in this chapter as it is discussed elsewhere, can have a detrimental effect on pregnancy outcome as well.

POLYMORPHIC ERUPTION OF PREGNANCY

Polymorphic eruption of pregnancy (PEP), also known as *pruritic urticarial papules and plaques of pregnancy (PUPPP)*, is an intensely pruritic dermatosis that usually begins in the third trimester of first pregnancies or in the immediate postpartum period. Pruritic urticarial papules are often the initial lesions. The immediate periumbilical area, face, palms, and soles are commonly uninvolved. Many patients develop polymorphic lesions, including erythema, vesicles, target lesions, and eczematous plaques. PEP tends not to recur in subsequent pregnancies.

MANAGEMENT STRATEGY

PEP has no increased risk of fetal or maternal morbidity, and the eruption resolves over an average of 4 weeks or within a few days of delivery. Treatment is often required to provide relief from intense itching. If pemphigoid gestationis is in the clinical differential, then consider a perilesional biopsy for direct immunofluorescence microscopy, which has nonspecific patterns in PEP (but is pathognomonic in pemphigoid gestationis). Contact dermatitis, drug eruptions, erythema

multiforme, insect bites, and urticaria should be considered in the differential diagnosis.

In women with localized disease, application of *midstrength topical corticosteroids* provides symptomatic relief in most cases. Most patients benefit from emollients and topical antipruritics with additives such as menthol. Treatment should be initiated with lower strength corticosteroids and escalated to a higher strength if the patient is not responding adequately. Use of clobetasol should not exceed 300 grams during the course of a pregnancy. As the pregnancy continues, many patients require therapy only once a day or can stop treatment before delivery.

Oral first-generation H_1 antihistamines may offer some benefit in severely pruritic patients at bedtime. Hydroxyzine is avoided because of an increased risk (5.8%) of congenital anomalies.

In more widespread cases and those that do not respond adequately to topical corticosteroids, a systemic corticosteroid treatment may be considered. *Oral prednisone or prednisolone 40 mg daily* or less over a taper of 1 to 2 weeks is very effective. Currently, PEP is not considered an indication for early delivery.

Specific Investigations (only if PG is being considered)

- Biopsy for direct immunofluorescence (DIF)
- Serum for indirect immunofluorescence (IIF) or ELISA BP 180

A prospective study of 200 women with dermatoses of pregnancy correlating clinical findings with hormonal and immunopathological profiles. Vaughan Jones SA, Hern S, Nelson-Piercy C, Seed PT, Black MM. Br J Dermatol 1999; 141: 71–81.

A prospective study of 200 women with dermatoses of pregnancy, 44 of whom had PEP. IIF was negative in all 44 cases of PEP, and DIF showed nonspecific findings. The most common histopathologic features on lesional skin biopsy were papillary dermal edema and a perivascular infiltrate, often with numerous eosinophils. Epidermal changes were common, with focal spongiosus and, less frequently, parakeratosis or hyperkeratosis.

Usefulness of BP180 NC16a enzyme-linked immunosorbent assay in the serodiagnosis of pemphigoid gestationis and in differentiating between pemphigoid gestationis and pruritic urticarial papules and plaques of pregnancy. Powell AM, Sakuma-Oyama Y, Oyama N, Albert S, Bhogal B, Kaneko F, et al. Arch Dermatol 2006; 141: 705–10.

A study of 412 women, 82 with PG and 164 with PEP and 166 age- and sex-matched controls, demonstrated that the NC16a ELISA is 96% sensitive and specific in differentiating PG from PEP.

First-Line Therapies

• Topical corticosteroids	**D**
• Antihistamines	**D**

Pruritic urticarial papules and plaques of pregnancy. Clinical experience in 25 patients. Yancey KB, Hall RP, Lawley TJ. J Am Acad Dermatol 1984; 10: 473–80.

Of 25 patients, 22 were successfully treated with frequent applications of high-potency topical corticosteroids, providing relief from pruritus and controlling the eruption. Three patients were treated with brief courses of systemic corticosteroids, ranging from 10 to 40 mg daily. Seven patients self-administered antihistamines or received them from referring physicians; two used cocoa butter, one used calamine lotion, and one used emollients; the authors noted that these agents were unsuccessful in controlling pruritus and lesion formation.

Pruritic urticarial papules and plaques of pregnancy (PUPPP). A clinicopathologic study. Callen JP, Hanno R. J Am Acad Dermatol 1981; 5: 401–5.

Of 15 cases, PEP cleared before delivery (5 cases), within 1 week of delivery (9 cases), and at 6 weeks postpartum (1 case). Treatment included various potent topical corticosteroids and diphenhydramine in all cases except one.

Safety of topical corticosteroids in pregnancy. Chi CC, Wang SH, Wojnarowska F, Kirtschig G, Davies E, Bennett C. Cochrane Database Syst Rev 2015; 10: CD007346.

A Cochrane review that assessed the effects of topical corticosteroids in pregnant women on pregnancy outcomes identified a probable association between low birth weight and maternal use of potent to very potent topical steroids, especially with very large cumulative dosage. Maternal exposure to topical corticosteroids of any potency was not associated with an increase in adverse pregnancy outcomes, including mode of delivery, congenital abnormality, preterm delivery, fetal death, or low Apgar score.

Safety of dermatologic medications in pregnancy and lactation: part I. Pregnancy. Murase JE, Heller MM, Butler DC. J Am Acad Dermatol 2014; 70: 401.e1–14.

Fetal growth restriction has been reported with potent topical steroid use during the third trimester, particularly when using >300 grams. Guidelines recommend mild to moderate over potent corticosteroids, which should be used only for short periods. First-generation antihistamines are preferred over second-generation. Among second-generation antihistamines, loratadine remains first and cetirizine second choice. Hydroxyzine is avoided because of an increased risk (5.8%) of congenital anomalies. Antihistamine use within 2 weeks of delivery in neonates born prematurely has been reported to double the risk of retinopathy of prematurity (previously retrolental fibroplasia). Overdose and intravenous use of antihistamines can stimulate uterine contractions and increase the risk of fetal hypoxia.

Polymorphic eruption of pregnancy: clinicopathology and potential trigger factors in 181 patients. Rudolph CM, Al-Fares S, Vaughan-Jones SA, Müllegger RR, Kerl H, Black MM. Br J Dermatol 2006; 154: 54–60.

A retrospective analysis of 181 patients with PEP reported symptoms to be controlled in most patients with emollients and topical steroids. Systemic therapy with antihistamines was required in 25%. Systemic corticosteroids (prednisone and prednisolone) were required in 9%.

Second-Line Therapy

- Systemic corticosteroids   **D**

Pruritic urticarial papules and plaques of pregnancy. Clinical experience in twenty-five patients. Yancey KB, Hall RP, Lawley TJ. J Am Acad Dermatol 1984; 10: 473–80.

Please see previous section for discussion of systemic corticosteroid use.

Polymorphic eruption of pregnancy: clinicopathology and potential trigger factors in 181 patients. Rudolph CM, Al-Fares S, Vaughan-Jones SA, Müllegger RR, Kerl H, Black MM. Br J Dermatol 2006; 154: 54–60.

Please see previous section for discussion of systemic corticosteroid use.

Although only a limited number of severe cases of PEP that required oral corticosteroids are reported in the literature, it is generally accepted that this treatment is effective and safe if prednisone or prednisolone are chosen and used in the third trimester. However, larger series and prospective studies are lacking.

PEMPHIGOID GESTATIONIS

PG, previously herpes gestationis, is a rare dermatosis of pregnancy seen in 1 in 1700 to 1 in 50,000 pregnancies. It presents with urticarial followed by vesicular lesions on the trunk and extremities in mid- to late pregnancy or the early postpartum period. It occurs in the presence of paternally derived tissue (fetus, hydatidiform mole, or choriocarcinoma). Unlike PEP, PG involves periumbilical skin.

MANAGEMENT STRATEGY

An important part of managing PG is making the diagnosis. Patients in whom PG is suspected usually require biopsy for histology and DIF. DIF with C3 in a linear band at the dermal–epidermal junction is pathognomonic for PG. Circulating autoantibodies are directed against the same target antigens as in bullous pemphigoid, more commonly against BP180 than BP230. The ELISA can be sent (with specificity and sensitivity as high as 96%) or, if available, IIF studies for the BP180 antigen.

Treatment can begin with topical steroids and a systemic antihistamine. First-generation antihistamines are favored over second-generation (see also discussion earlier about the use of antihistamines in PEP). Most patients require *systemic corticosteroid* treatment. Initially doses of prednisolone or its equivalent in the range of ½ mg/kg body weight may be tried, but in severe cases, 1 mg/kg of prednisolone may be necessary.

Many women will improve and may decrease doses of or even discontinue steroids. In cases that do not respond satisfactorily to prednisolone alone or in cases where prolonged treatment with corticosteroids is contraindicated, plasmapheresis or intravenous immunoglobulins may be considered.

The maternal prognosis is very good, with most cases resolving within a few months postpartum; however, it may take weeks, months, or even years until complete remission; 75% of women flare postpartum, requiring treatment. Exacerbations may occur postpartum with oral contraceptives and during the menstrual cycle. PG often recurs and is commonly more severe in subsequent pregnancies.

Newborns of mothers with PG may develop bullous lesions, which are transient and require no therapy. PG is associated with premature delivery and a risk of low birth weight, and the risk of these fetal complications correlates with maternal disease severity. Therefore patients with PG should be followed more carefully by the obstetrician.

- Biopsy for histopathology and DIF
- Serum for enzyme-linked immunosorbent assay (immunoblot) and/or IIF

Clinical and immunologic profiles of 25 patients with pemphigoid gestationis. Tani N, Kimura Y, Koga H, Kawakami T, Ohata C, Ishii N, et al. Br J Derm 2015; 172: 120–9.

Clinical and immunologic profiles were performed on 25 patients with PG. DIF showed C3 deposition in the basement membrane zone in all patients, and IIF revealed circulating IgG anti-basement membrane zone autoantibodies in 92% of patients. Immunoblotting and ELISA of the NC16a domain of BP180 recombinant protein were positive in 96% and 92% of patients, respectively. Only 4 patients had a positive ELISA for BP230.

First-Line Therapies

Topical corticosteroids	D
Systemic corticosteroids	D
Antihistamines	D

Clinical features and management of 87 patients with pemphigoid gestationis. Jenkins RE, Hern S, Black MM. Clin Exp Dermatol 1999; 24: 255–9.

A review of 142 pregnancies in 87 patients with PG. Only 69 patients had documented treatment information. Thirteen of these 69 patients (18.8%) were treated with topical corticosteroids without systemic therapy. Chlorpheniramine suppressed pruritus in most patients. Fifty-six out of 69 (81.2%) required systemic corticosteroids with initial doses of prednisolone of 5 to 110 mg daily, with suppression of blistering in most patients. Two patients' eruptions were not controlled with high-dose systemic corticosteroids, with disease persistence for more than 10 years.

Pregnancy outcome after first trimester exposure to corticosteroids: a prospective controlled study. Gur C, Diav-Citrin O, Shechtman S, Arnon J, Ornoy A. Reprod Toxicol 2004; 18: 93–101.

This study, which was powered to find a 2.5-fold increase in teratogenicity, supports that glucocorticosteroids do not represent a major teratogenic risk in humans.

Second-Line Therapies

Plasmapheresis	E
High-dose intravenous immunoglobulin (IVIG)	E

Plasma exchange in herpes gestationis. Van de Wiel A, Hart HC, Flinterman J, Kerckhaert JA, Du Boeuff JA, Imhof JW. Br Med J 1980; 281: 1041–2.

A case report of a 40-year-old patient with PG initially treated with antihistamines and pyridoxine, both of which were ineffective. Systemic corticosteroid treatment was thought inadvisable, and the patient received three exchanges during the twenty-sixth week of pregnancy. Within 24 hours of the first exchange, the patient's pruritus subsided and no new lesions developed. After three exchanges, the lesions had largely resolved. After delivery, an exacerbation occurred that required four additional exchanges within 1 week. A flare 3 weeks postpartum required two more exchanges.

Successful treatment of a severe persistent case of pemphigoid gestationis with antepartum and postpartum intravenous immunoglobulin followed by azathioprine. Gan DC, Wels B, Webster M. Australas J Dermatol 2012; 53: 66–9.

A case of PG affecting a 37-year-old patient in both of her pregnancies. The patient failed to respond to high-dose oral prednisone in her second pregnancy. She was treated successfully with IVIG (2 g/kg each infusion cycle), both during the antepartum and postpartum period. After ceasing IVIG, azathioprine (up to 1 mg/kg/day) was initiated for control.

Antepartum intravenous immunoglobulin therapy in refractory pemphigoid gestationis: case report and literature review. Doiron P, Pratt M. J Cutan Med Surg 2010; 14: 189–92.

A case report of a 34-year-old woman who developed PG with three pregnancies. The PG in her first two pregnancies was managed with oral prednisone and topical agents. PG in the patient's third pregnancy was initially treated with prednisone but ultimately required monthly infusions of IVIG. A healthy baby was delivered at 37.5 weeks.

Third-Line Therapies

Azathioprine	E
Cyclophosphamide	E
Ciclosporin	E
Dapsone	D
Sulfapyridine	E
Pyridoxine	E
Rituximab	E

A severe persistent case of pemphigoid gestationis treated with intravenous immunoglobulin and cyclosporine. Hern S, Harman K, Bhogal BS, Black MM. Clin Exp Dermatol 1998; 23: 185–8.

A report of a patient with severe PG that persisted for 1.5 years postpartum. The patient was treated with prednisolone (initially at 80 mg daily) and two doses of IVIG (5-day course at 0.4 g/kg daily) and then required ciclosporin (initially at 100 mg and then tapered).

Chronic herpes gestationis and antiphospholipid antibody syndrome successfully treated with cyclophosphamide. Castle SP, Mather-Mondrey M, Bennion S, David-Bajar K, Huff C. J Am Acad Dermatol 1996; 34: 333–6.

A report of a patient with PG treated postpartum with pulse-dose intravenous cyclophosphamide (1.245 g, 0.75 g/m²). The patient was initially treated at 19 weeks of gestation with oral prednisone with no effect; increasing dosages of prednisone were administered (up to 120 mg/day) with no effect. The patient continued to have lesions postpartum, despite continued oral prednisone. Azathioprine treatment was initiated 8 months postpartum but was discontinued within 1 month secondary to increased liver enzyme values. Pulsed intravenous cyclophosphamide was administered 9 months postpartum. The patient received two doses during a 2-month period with resolution of skin lesions

Evidence Levels: **A** Double-blind study **B** Clinical trial ≥ 20 subjects **C** Clinical trial < 20 subjects **D** Series ≥ 5 subjects **E** Anecdotal case reports

and associated symptoms. A mild recurrence 5 months later was treated with an additional dose.

Cytotoxic agents such as cyclophosphamide for the treatment of PG can only be used in the postpartum period while the mother is not breastfeeding.

Clinical features and management of 87 patients with pemphigoid gestationis. Jenkins RE, Hern S, Black MM. Clin Exp Dermatol 1999; 24: 255–9.

A review of 142 pregnancies in 87 patients with PG. Azathioprine, dapsone, sulfapyridine, and pyridoxine were used as adjunctive therapy with oral corticosteroids (in 2, 6, 2, and 5 out of 56 patients, respectively).

Severe persistent pemphigoid gestationis: long-term remission with rituximab. Cianchini G, Masini C, Lupi F, Corona R, De Pita O, Puddu P. Br J Dermatol 2007; 157: 388–9.

A case report of a 31-year old woman who, during the fifth month of her third pregnancy, developed PG resistant to systemic corticosteroid therapy. A male infant was born at 32 weeks, 2 days, after which the patient flared. After 5 months of unsuccessful corticosteroid therapy with azathioprine daily, she was treated with dapsone for 3 months. IVIG was then initiated, followed by rituximab (375 mg/m^2 weekly for four consecutive weeks). Azathioprine was discontinued and prednisone tapered. Clinical remission lasted for 2 months, at which time another four infusions of rituximab (375 mg/m^2 at 2-month intervals) were given.

The benefit of these drugs on the course of the disease remains questionable.

INTRAHEPATIC CHOLESTASIS OF PREGNANCY

Intrahepatic cholestasis of pregnancy (ICP, previously pruritus gravidarum and prurigo gravidarum) is a rare, reversible cholestasis that typically occurs in late pregnancy. Patients present with dramatic pruritus that may initially involve the palms and soles; jaundice can occur in 10% of patients. ICP is the only pregnancy dermatosis that presents without primary skin lesions. A reduced excretion of bile acids likely contributes to severe maternal pruritus that typically resolves soon after delivery. More concerning are harmful effects on the fetus, including an increase in premature births, intrapartum fetal distress, and fetal death.

MANAGEMENT STRATEGY

ICP must be differentiated from other causes of pruritus during pregnancy. The differential diagnosis can include scabies, eczema, urticaria, and drug eruptions, as well as early cases of PEP and PG. Total serum bile acid levels greater than 11 μmol/L are consistent with ICP. Liver function tests may be abnormal as well, often with an elevated alkaline phosphatase. The maternal pruritus and cholestasis usually resolve within a few days of delivery. ICP may recur with subsequent pregnancies and oral contraceptive pill use.

First-line treatment includes *ursodeoxycholic acid* (either a dose of 15 mg/kg/day or, independent of body weight, 1 g/day is administered either as a single dose or divided into two or three doses until delivery), which is thought to correct the maternal serum bile acid profile, relieve symptoms, and improve fetal prognosis. Early delivery at 38 weeks or before is frequently advocated by obstetricians to reduce the risk of intrauterine fetal demise.

In mild disease, pruritus may improve with the adjuvant use of topical treatments such as *cooling lotions or creams* and antihistamines. *Phototherapy* may also be of benefit. These adjuvant treatments will not affect fetal outcome.

Specific Investigations

- Liver function tests, total serum bile acid
- Hepatitis C serologies

Specific pruritic disease of pregnancy. A prospective study of 3192 pregnant women. Roger D, Vaillant L, Fignon A, Pierre F, Bacq Y, Brechot JF, et al. Arch Dermatol 1994; 130: 734–9.

A prospective study of pregnant women presenting with pruritus identified 17 patients with ICP. The increase in mean values of alanine aminotransferase, aspartate aminotransferase, total serum bile salt, serum cholylglycine, serum 5′-nucleotidase, and total alkaline phosphatase was statistically significant compared with the control group.

Intrahepatic cholestasis of pregnancy: relationships between bile acid levels and fetal complication rates. Glantz A, Marschall HU, Mattsson LA. Hepatology 2004; 40: 287–8.

Prospective cohort study that identified 693 ICP cases. The probability of preterm delivery, asphyxia events, and green staining of placenta and membranes did not increase until bile acid levels exceeded 40 μmol/L, and the probability of meconium staining of amniotic fluid started to rise when bile acid levels exceeded 20 μmol/L.

The importance of serum bile acid level analysis and treatment with ursodeoxycholic acid in intrahepatic cholestasis of pregnancy: a case series from central Europe. Ambros-Rudolph CM, Glatz M, Trauner M, Kerl H, Müllegger RR. Arch Dermatol 2007; 143: 757–62.

A retrospective study of 13 patients with ICP reported elevated total serum bile acid levels in all patients. Pregnancies complicated by fetal distress or prematurity demonstrated higher total bile acid levels than those with normal fetal outcome. Other hepatic function test abnormalities were noted in 77% of patients, with elevated serum aspartate aminotransferase in 62%, alanine aminotransferase in 46%, gamma-glutamyl transferase in 23%, total serum bilirubin in 15%, and alkaline phosphatase in 100%.

Intrahepatic cholestasis of pregnancy in hepatitis C virus infection. Paternoster DM, Fabris F, Palu G, Santarossa C, Bracciante R, Snijders D, et al. Acta Obstet Gynecol Scand 2002; 81: 99–103.

A prospective study of the prevalence of hepatitis C virus infection and incidence of ICP reported 56 patients to have developed intrahepatic cholestasis of pregnancy (ICP), 12 of whom were HCV-RNA positive. ICP was observed more commonly in HCV-RNA–positive women than in HCV-RNA–negative women, leading the authors to conclude that ICP during the third trimester should prompt assessment of patients' HCV status.

Intrahepatic cholestasis of pregnancy: maternal and fetal outcomes associated with elevated bile acid levels. Brouwers L, Koster MP, Page-Christiaens GC, Kemperman H, Boon J, Evers IM, et al. Am J Obstet Gynecol 2015; 212: 100.e1.

A retrospective study of 215 ICP patients studied the correlation of bile acid levels and pregnancy outcome. The group was divided into mild (bile acid levels 10–39 μmol/L), moderate (40–99 μmol/L), and severe (≥100 μmol/L) ICP. Higher bile acid levels were significantly associated with spontaneous preterm birth, meconium-stained amniotic fluid, and perinatal death. Gestational age at diagnosis and delivery was significantly lower in the severe compared with the mild ICP group.

Fetal outcomes in pregnancies complicated by intrahepatic cholestasis of pregnancy in a Northern California cohort. Rook M, Vargas J, Caughey A, Bacchetti P, Rosenthal P, Bull L. PLoS One 2012; 7: e28343.

A study of 101 women with ICP reported fetal complications in 33% of deliveries, with respiratory distress accounting for the majority of complications. The study found no statistically significant clinical or biochemical predictors of increased risk of fetal complications.

First-Line Therapies	
• Ursodeoxycholic acid (UDCA)	A
• Early delivery	D

Ursodeoxycholic acid in the treatment of cholestasis of pregnancy: a randomized, double-blind study controlled with placebo. Palma J, Reyes H, Ribalta J, Hernández I, Sandoval L, Almuna R, et al. J Hepatol 1997; 27: 1022–8.

A study of 24 patients with ICP detected before week 33 of pregnancy randomly assigned patients to receive UDCA or placebo until delivery. Of the 15 patients who completed the study, 8 received UDCA and 7 placebo. After 3 weeks of treatment, patients receiving UDCA had statistically significant improvements in pruritus, serum bilirubin, aspartate aminotransferase, and alanine aminotransferase. A nonstatistically significant decrease in serum total bile salts was noted. Patients treated with UDCA delivered at or near term compared with five of the seven patients treated with placebo who delivered before week 36 of pregnancy, including one stillbirth.

Ursodeoxycholic acid in the treatment of intrahepatic cholestasis of pregnancy. A 12-year experience. Zapata R, Sandoval L, Palma J, Hernandez I, Ribalta J, Reyes H, et al. Liver Int 2005; 25: 548–54.

A retrospective analysis of 32 ICP patients who received UDCA for at least 3 weeks before delivery and were compared with 16 historical controls. UDCA treatment decreased pruritus, serum bilirubin, ALT, and bile salt levels. Term delivery occurred in 65.7% of UDCA-treated patients compared with only 12.5% of the control group. Infants born to mothers treated with UDCA weighed a mean of 500 g more than those born to controls.

Efficacy of ursodeoxycholic acid in treating intrahepatic cholestasis of pregnancy: a meta-analysis. Bacq Y, Sentilhes L, Reyes HB, Glantz A, Kondrackiene J, Binder T, et al. Gastroenterology 2012; 143: 1492–1501.

A meta-analysis of nine randomized controlled trials comprising data from 454 ICP patients compared the effects of UDCA to other drugs, placebo, or no specific treatment. UDCA was associated with reduced or resolved pruritus, normalization of liver function tests, fewer premature births, reduced fetal distress, less frequent respiratory distress syndrome, and fewer neonates in the intensive care unit in analyses of UDCA compared with all controls. In analyses of UDCA compared with placebo, UDCA reduced pruritus and normalized liver function tests.

Interventions for treating cholestasis in pregnancy. Gurung V, Middleton P, Milan SJ, Hague W, Thornton JG. Cochrane Database Syst Rev 2013; 6: CD000493.

A Cochrane review of randomized controlled trials compared intervention strategies for patients with ICP. Twenty-one trials involving 1197 women were included, with 11 different interventions resulting in 15 different comparisons. UDCA showed improvement in pruritus in 5 out of 7 trials. There were significantly fewer total preterm births with UDCA and fewer (although not statistically significant) instances of fetal distress/asphyxia events in the UDCA groups compared with placebo.

The risk of infant and fetal death by each additional week of expectant management in intrahepatic cholestasis of pregnancy by gestational age. Puljic A, Kim E, Page J, Esakoff T, Shaffer B, LaCoursiere DY, et al. Am J Obstet Gynecol 2015; 212: 667.e1.

A retrospective study of 1,604,386 singleton pregnancies of women between 34 and 40 weeks' gestation with and without ICP. Among women with ICP, the mortality risk of delivery is lower than the risk of expectant management at 36 weeks' gestation. The authors concluded that delivery at 36 weeks' gestation would reduce perinatal mortality risk compared with expectant management.

Primum non nocere: how active management became modus operandi for intrahepatic cholestasis of pregnancy. Henderson CE, Shah RR, Gottimukkala S, Ferreira KK, Hamaoui A, Mercado R. Am J Obstet Gynecol 2014; 211: 189–96.

To evaluate ICP as an indication for early term delivery, the authors divided 16 articles based on whether or not obstetric care included active management. They found no evidence to support active management for ICP, noting that the stillbirth rates in both groups were similar to their respective national stillbirth rate.

Second-Line Therapies	
• Phototherapy	E
• Emollients and topical antipruritic agents	D
• Antihistamines	D

Dermatoses of pregnancy. Shornick JK. Semin Cutan Med Surg 1998; 17: 172–81.

Review indicating that UVB phototherapy may be useful for symptomatic treatment of ICP.

Specific pruritic disease of pregnancy. A prospective study of 3192 pregnant women. Roger D, Vaillant L, Fignon A, Pierre F, Bacq Y, Brechot JF, et al. Arch Dermatol 1994; 130: 734–9.

A prospective study of pregnant women presenting with pruritus identified 17 patients with ICP. Thirteen patients received emollients and oral antihistamines. Pruritus resolved in all cases within 2 weeks of delivery.

ATOPIC ERUPTION OF PREGNANCY

Atopic eruption of pregnancy (AEP, previously prurigo of pregnancy, prurigo gestationis, early onset prurigo of pregnancy, pruritic folliculitis of pregnancy, and eczema in pregnancy) is the most common pregnancy dermatosis. It is a benign pruritic disorder that presents early in pregnancy (in 75% of patients before the third trimester) with eczematous and/or papular lesions in patients with an atopic diathesis. For approximately 80% of AEP patients, the eruption is the first occurrence of atopy, whereas it represents an exacerbation for the remaining 20%. AEP tends to recur in subsequent pregnancies.

MANAGEMENT STRATEGY

There are no fetal or maternal risks associated with AEP other than significant maternal pruritus. Topical corticosteroids with or without systemic antihistamines are often sufficient for resolution of lesions and improvement of pruritus. Emollients and topical antipruritic agents also play a role. Severe cases may require a short course of systemic corticosteroids and antihistamines, and secondary bacterial infections may require oral antibiotics. Phototherapy (UVB) is an additional option, particularly for severe cases in early pregnancy.

Specific Investigations

- None

The specific dermatoses of pregnancy revisited and reclassified: results of a retrospective two-center study on 505 pregnant patients. Ambros-Rudolph CM, Müllegger RR, Vaughan-Jones SA, Kerl H, Black MM. J Am Acad Dermatol 2006; 54: 395–404.

A retrospective study of 505 pregnant patients proposed a reclassification of eczema in pregnancy, prurigo of pregnancy, and pruritic folliculitis of pregnancy into the category of AEP.

First-Line Therapies

- Topical corticosteroids
- Antihistamines

For their use in pregnancy, see the discussion earlier in the section discussing PEP.

Second-Line Therapy

- UVB

The authors would like to acknowledge the work of the previous edition's contributor, Wolfgang Jurecka, MD.

Pretibial myxedema

Elizabeth R. Ghazi, Warren R. Heymann

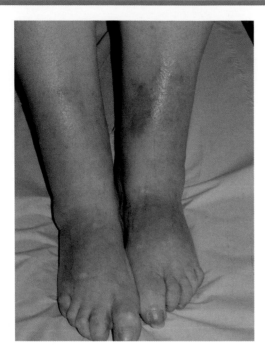

Pretibial myxedema, more accurately termed *thyroid dermopathy*, is characterized by nonpitting edema and skin-colored to violaceous nodules or plaques. These are most commonly distributed pretibially but can sometimes be seen over the arms, shoulders, head, and neck. The differential diagnosis of thyroid dermopathy includes lymphedema, lipodermatosclerosis, and the newly described *obesity-associated lymphedematous mucinosis*.

MANAGEMENT STRATEGY

Pretibial myxedema is an autoimmune phenomenon that tends to occur after treatment of patients with Graves disease. The condition can, however, develop in hypothyroid and euthyroid patients. It is helpful to look for other clinical signs of thyroid disease, including thyroid acropachy (characterized by clubbing of the fingers and toes, periosteal proliferation of the phalanges and long bones, and swelling of the soft tissue overlying bony structures) and the presence of a goiter. Pretibial myxedema typically follows the onset of ophthalmopathy, often years after the diagnosis of hyperthyroidism. Goals of treatment include cosmesis and the prevention of long-term side effects such as elephantiasis, decreased range of motion, or footdrop from neural entrapment. Resolution may occur without treatment.

Patients with significant thyroid dermopathy should be started on a trial of *high-potency topical corticosteroids*, alone or under occlusion, for at least 2 months. If symptoms persist, *intralesional corticosteroids* may be effective. A combination of these methods in conjunction with *compression bandages* can be beneficial when monotherapy proves inadequate. Both *oral* and *intravenous corticosteroids* have also been shown to improve lesions in several patients. However, their use is limited by systemic side effects.

Pentoxifylline, an analog of methylxanthine theobromine, has been shown to reduce the extent of lesions and can also be used in conjunction with topical and/or intralesional corticosteroids. Although there are conflicting data, the use of *intravenous immunoglobulin (IVIG)* may improve lesions of pretibial myxedema. Subcutaneous or intralesional *octreotide*, a somatostatin analog, yields conflicting results. *Plasmapheresis* has been reported to be beneficial in improving severe cases and has been successful when used in combination with rituximab.

Temporary improvement with *cytotoxic agents* has been observed. Pretibial myxedema is not a life-threatening condition, and so the use of such agents should be limited to severe, debilitating cases. *Surgical excision* has been shown to be effective in a minority of cases. The high risk of recurrence makes surgical intervention an infrequently used modality; however, postoperative intralesional steroids can minimize this risk. *Complete decongestive physiotherapy* has shown some success in treating the elephantiasic form of pretibial myxedema.

Pretibial ultrasonography, with or without digital infrared thermal imaging, to measure skin thickness may be useful in assessing treatment response. Measuring serum hyaluronic acid levels to follow therapeutic response may also be of value.

Specific Investigations

- Thyroid function tests
- Antithyroglobulin and antithyroid peroxidase antibodies
- Antithyroid-stimulating hormone receptor antibodies
- Pretibial ultrasound and/or digital infrared thermal imaging
- Serum hyaluronic acid

Pretibial myxedema. Fatourechi V. In: Heymann WR, ed. Thyroid Disorders with Cutaneous Manifestations. London: Springer Verlag 2008; 103–19.

Pretibial myxedema: case presentation and review of treatment options. Kim WB, Mistry N, Alavi A, Sibbald C, Sibbald RG. Int J Low Extrem Wounds 2014; 13: 152–4.

A classic case of pretibial myxedema in a 57-year-old woman treated for Graves disease is presented.

This article details how to differentiate pretibial myxedema from lymphedema and lipodermatosclerosis.

Pretibial myxedema as the initial manifestation of Graves' disease. Georgala S, Katoulis AC, Georgala C, Katoulis EC, Hatziolou E, Stavrianeas NG. J Eur Acad Dermatol Venereol 2002; 16: 380–3.

A 28-year-old Greek woman presented initially with asymptomatic pretibial myxedema, which ultimately led to a diagnosis of Graves disease. This patient had elevated anti-TSH-receptor antibodies.

An assessment of thyroid function is warranted because most patients with pretibial myxedema have clinical or laboratory evidence of autoimmune thyroid disease.

Observing pretibial myxedema in patients with Graves' disease using digital infrared thermal imaging and high-resolution ultrasonography: for better records, early detection and further investigation. Shih SR, Lin MS, Li HY, Yang HY, Hsiao YL, Chang MT, et al. Eur J Endocrinol 2011; 164: 605–11.

Digital infrared thermal imaging (DITI) detects surface temperature, and sonography reflects composition changes in soft tissue. Lower leg temperatures of normal volunteers decreased gradually from proximal to distal parts. In all patients with pretibial myxedema, DITI showed abnormally low focal temperatures over the lesions. In Graves disease patients with mild diffuse nonpitting edema and Graves disease patients with normal appearance of lower legs, DITI showed abnormally low focal temperature in 90.9% and 65.2% of the patients, respectively. Areas of clinically visible pretibial myxedema and low focal temperature detected by DITI were sonographically characterized with increased skin thickness, hypoechoic substance deposition in the cutaneous tissue, and blurred boundary lines between dermis and subcutaneous tissue.

The use of DITI and high-resolution ultrasonography to analyze pretibial skin of patients with Graves disease allows for early detection of pretibial myxedema in patients with and without visible dermopathy. We anticipate that newer technologies such as optical coherence tomography will also be utilized for assessing patients with thyroid dermopathy.

First-Line Therapies

• Topical corticosteroids with or without occlusion	C
• Intralesional corticosteroids	D
• Compression	D

Dermopathy of Graves disease (pretibial myxedema): review of 150 cases. Fatourechi V, Pajouhi M, Fransway AF. Medicine 1994; 73: 1–7.

Treatment with topical 0.05% to 0.1% triamcinolone acetonide cream under occlusion for 2 to 10 weeks led to partial remission in 29 of 76 patients in this retrospective study; 1% had complete remission.

Treatment of pretibial myxedema with topical steroid ointment application with sealing cover in Graves' patients. Takasu N, Higa H, Kinjou Y. Intern Med 2010; 49: 665–9.

The authors detail their experience of six patients with pretibial myxedema treated with triamcinolone 0.1% under occlusion. Only two patients responded to therapy; these patients had their treatments initiated within months of the appearance of pretibial myxedema.

A delay in treatment of 5 to 10 years or advanced Graves disease manifested by exophthalmos may be associated with refractory disease when treated with topical steroids under occlusion.

Intralesional triamcinolone therapy for pretibial myxedema. Lang PG, Sisson JC, Lynch PJ. Arch Dermatol 1975; 111: 197–202.

Seven of nine patients treated with monthly injections of 8 mL or less of intralesional triamcinolone acetonide solution (5 mg/mL, 1 mL per injection site) had complete remission of pretibial myxedema after a total of three to seven visits. The other two patients, despite withdrawing from the study prematurely for nonmedical reasons, showed a partial improvement.

Pretibial myxedema: a review of the literature and case report. Frisch DR, Roth I. J Am Podiatr Med Assoc 1985; 75: 147–52.

A 29-year-old woman with pretibial myxedema was treated with rest, elevation, and topical 0.05% fluocinonide cream under occlusion. Outpatient therapy included weekly intralesional Celestone Soluspan injections followed by topical 0.05% fluocinonide cream under occlusion. Compression dressings with an Unna boot were applied weekly. After 2 months the lesions were greatly improved.

Compression stockings may also be beneficial. Unless contraindicated, compression should be used in conjunction with any therapeutic approach for this disorder.

Pretibial myxoedema with autoimmunity and hyperplasia treated with glucocorticoids and surgery. Lan C, Li C, Yang M, Mei X, He Z, Chen W, et al. Br J Dermatol 2012; 166: 457–9.

A patient with pretibial myxedema presenting as verruciform plaques failed initial treatment with monthly intralesional injections of 1 mL betamethasone, 0.2 mL at each of five points, but responded when the injections were increased to every 2 weeks. A second patient with tumorous lesions responded to surgical removal of tumors with postoperative intralesional triamcinolone acetonide 10 mg at five points every 3 days as prophylaxis to prevent recurrence.

Second-Line Therapies

• Pentoxifylline	E
• Pentoxifylline with topical and/or intralesional steroid	E

Pentoxifylline inhibits the proliferation and glycosaminoglycan synthesis of cultured fibroblasts derived from patients with Graves' ophthalmopathy and pretibial myxedema. Chang CC, Chang TC, Kao SC, Kuo YF, Chien LF. Acta Endocrinol 1993; 129: 322–7.

Pentoxifylline caused an in vitro dose-dependent decrease in fibroblast proliferation and glycosaminoglycan synthesis in fibroblast cultures taken from pretibial sites. A preliminary trial with a dose of 400 mg intravenously and 800 mg orally daily of pentoxifylline reduced the size of pretibial myxedema lesions within 1 week.

Successful combined pentoxifylline and intralesional triamcinolone acetonide treatment of severe pretibial myxedema. Engin B, Gumusel M, Ozdemir M, Cakir M. Dermatol Online J 2007; 13: 16.

A 32-year-old man achieved partial remission with clobetasol under occlusion combined with pentoxifylline 400 mg three times daily and intralesional triamcinolone (5 mg/mL).

Third-Line Therapies

• Intravenous immunoglobulin	D
• Systemic corticosteroids (including pulse corticosteroid therapy)	D
• Octreotide	E
• Plasmapheresis	D
• Plasmapheresis with rituximab	E
• Cytotoxic therapy	E
• Surgery	E
• Complete decongestive physiotherapy	E
• UVA1 in combination with topical and intralesional steroids	D
• Radiotherapy	E

Pretibial myxedema and high-dose intravenous immunoglobulin treatment. Antonelli A, Navarranne A, Palla R, Alberti B, Saracino A, Mestre C, et al. Thyroid 1994; 4: 399–408.

Improvement of pretibial myxedema began after a few weeks in six patients treated with 400 mg/kg daily of high-dose IVIG given over 3 to 4 hours on 5 consecutive days. The cycle was repeated three times every 21 days. Maintenance therapy of 400 mg/kg for 1 day was then administered for 7 to 15 more cycles every 21 days. Total treatment ranged from 7 to 12 months, with maximum response occurring after an average of 6 months.

Lack of response of elephantiasic pretibial myxoedema to treatment with high-dose intravenous immunoglobulins. Terheydem P, Kahaly GJ, Zillikens D, Brocker EB. Clin Exp Dermatol 2003; 28: 224–6.

IVIG did not significantly improve the lesions of a patient with elephantiasic pretibial myxedema.

Corticoid therapy for pretibial myxedema: observations on the long-acting thyroid stimulator. Benoit FL, Greenspan FS. Ann Intern Med 1967; 66: 711–20.

Oral prednisolone, begun at 60 mg and then tapered, and methylprednisolone starting at 40 mg cleared the pretibial lesions of four patients and improved the lesions of two others. Of the various corticosteroid treatments studied, the best results were obtained with high-dose systemic corticosteroids for 2 weeks.

Refractory pretibial myxoedema with response to intralesional insulin-like growth factor 1 antagonist (octreotide): downregulation of hyaluronic acid production by the lesional fibroblasts. Shinohara M, Hamasaki Y, Katayana I. Br J Dermatol 2000; 143: 1083–6.

Intralesional octreotide 200 µg daily improved the lesions of pretibial myxedema in a male patient with Graves disease after 4 weeks of therapy.

Octreotide inhibits insulin-like growth factor-1–induced hyaluronic acid secretion by lesional fibroblasts, which may play a role in the pathogenesis of pretibial myxedema.

Octreotide and Graves' ophthalmopathy and pretibial myxoedema. Chang TC, Kao SC, Huang KM. Br Med J 1992; 304: 158.

Three patients with pretibial myxedema were successfully treated with 100 µg of octreotide three times daily.

The authors do not comment on the route of administration of the octreotide acetate. According to the Physicians' Desk Reference, the drug may be administered either by subcutaneous injection or intravenously.

Lack of effect of long-term octreotide therapy in severe thyroid-associated dermopathy. Rotman-Pikielny P, Brucker-Davis F, Turner ML, Sarlis NJ, Skarulis MC. Thyroid 2003; 13: 465–70.

Three women did not show a statistically significant benefit from octreotide 300 µg.

The conflicting results from these small studies regarding the use of octreotide for thyroid dermopathy mandates that only larger, controlled studies will verify whether it is a useful modality for this condition.

Effect of plasmapheresis and steroid treatment on thyrotropin binding inhibitory immunoglobulins in a patient with exophthalmos and a patient with pretibial myxedema. Kuzuya N, DeGroot LJ. J Endocrinol Invest 1982; 5: 373–8.

Two patients, one with elephantiasis-like lesions, were treated with 16 exchanges over 4 to 5 months with 1 to 2 L of the patient's plasma removed and replaced with 1300 mL of purified protein fraction and 700 mL 0.9% saline. Immunoglobulin G fraction was separated out, thereby reducing total thyrotropin-binding inhibitory immunoglobulin (TBII) activity per unit of serum. The pretibial myxedema was partially and temporarily improved with plasmapheresis, and abnormal antibodies were reduced.

Beneficial effects of plasmapheresis followed by immunosuppressive therapy in pretibial myxedema. Noppen M, Velkeniers B, Steenssens L, Vanhaelst L. Acta Clin Belg 1988; 43: 381–3.

A patient with pretibial myxedema unresponsive to topical corticosteroids was cured after 5 days of plasmapheresis followed by 100 mg of azathioprine twice daily for 3 months. Azathioprine was tapered to 50 mg twice daily and continued for a year, at which time no recurrence was noted.

Pretibial myxedema (elephantiasic form): treatment with cytotoxic therapy. Hanke CW, Bergfeld WF, Guirguis MN, Lewis LJ. Cleve Clin Q 1983; 50: 183–8.

Fibroblasts from pretibial myxedema sites of a 44-year-old man showed reduced DNA content in vitro with the use of cytotoxic agents. Melphalan, which reduced hyaluronic acid levels to the greatest extent, was given orally (8 mg daily) for 4 days and repeated monthly for 6 months. This regimen provided transient improvement, but the patient's condition then worsened.

Successful combined surgical and octreotide treatment of severe pretibial myxoedema reviewed after 9 years. Felton J, Derrick EK, Price ML. Br J Dermatol 2003; 148: 825–6.

A 56-year-old man with pretibial myxedema was treated with surgical shave removal followed by daily subcutaneous octreotide injections for 6 months. His lesions did not recur over a 9-year follow-up period.

Pretibial myxedema. Matsuoka LY, Wortsman J, Dietrich JG, Pearson R. Arch Dermatol 1981; 117: 250–1.

Pretibial myxedema recurred in a split-thickness skin graft 3 years after placement.

Treatment-resistant elephantiasic thyroid dermopathy responding to rituximab and plasmapheresis. Heyes C, Nolan R, Leahy M, Gebauer K. Australas J Dermatol 2012; 53: e1–4.

A 55-year-old woman underwent plasmapheresis once every 6 days and received rituximab infusions once per week for 1 to 7 weeks on seven occasions for a total of 29 doses of rituximab and 241 episodes of plasmapheresis over 3.5 years. She remained clear 6 months after completion of treatment.

Rituximab has been utilized successfully for an ever-expanding list of autoimmune disorders. Further study is warranted to determine whether rituximab without the concomitant use of plasmapheresis would be of value.

Elephantiasic pretibial myxedema: a novel treatment for an uncommon disorder. Susser WS, Heermans AG, Chapman MS, Baughman RD. J Am Acad Dermatol 2002; 46: 723–6.

A 67-year-old woman with elephantiasic pretibial myxedema had a 47% reduction of leg edema after 6 weeks of intensive complete decongestive physiotherapy. This response was sustained for 2 years after treatment.

Complete decongestive physiotherapy consists of manual massage of the lower extremities to promote lymphatic drainage, followed by compressive bandages, exercise, and skin care.

Efficacy of trimodality therapy for pretibial myxoedema: a case series of 20 patients. Chen X, Zhao X, Li X, Shi R, Zheng J. Acta Derm Venereol 2016; 96: 714–5.

Severe thyroid dermopathy was treated for 12 weeks. The triple therapy comprised intralesional injections of betamethasone dipropionate 5 mg and betamethasone disodium phosphate 2 mg for a total of 4 to 6 mL, topical 0.1% mometasone furoate

670

cream under occlusive dressing, and UVA1 at a dose of 80 J/cm^2 per treatment three times a week for 2 weeks, twice a week for 2 weeks, and once a week for 8 weeks. At the end of the trimodality treatment, 8 and 12 patients achieved complete and partial remission, respectively. Dermal thickness was decreased as detected by ultrasound.

Radiation therapy as part of the therapeutic regimen for extensive multilocular myxedema in a patient with exophthalmos, myxedema and osteoarthropathy syndrome: a case report. Elsayad K, Kriz J, Bauch J, Scobioala S, Haverkamp U, Sunderkötter C, et al. Oncol Lett 2015; 9: 2404–8.

A 48-year-old male patient was diagnosed with thyroid dermopathy in the setting of proptosis and acropathy. Radiation therapy was commenced to treat the lower left leg and foot at a total dose of 5 Gy. Simultaneously, radiotherapy of the lower right leg and foot was commenced, with the administration of ≤20 Gy. Radiotherapy was well tolerated, with the exception of skin edema and slight erythema. Results were maintained with follow-up excision, pentoxifylline, and repeat radiation.

Prurigo nodularis

Junie Li Chun Wong, Niall Wilson

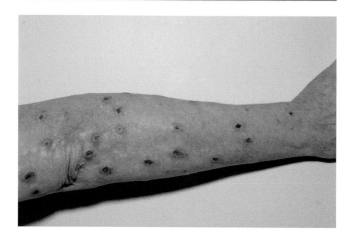

Nodular prurigo (NP, also known as *prurigo nodularis* or *prurigo nodularis of Hyde*) is a chronic condition characterized by the presence of highly pruritic, hyperkeratotic papules or nodules, ranging from a few to hundreds in numbers. Accompanying features include severe excoriation, crusting, and lichenification and the presence of postinflammatory hyperpigmentation or hypopigmentation. Lesions are often distributed symmetrically over the extensor surfaces of the limbs. However, any other part of the body, particularly the sacral area, abdomen, face, palms, and genitalia, may be affected.

NP may arise at any age but more commonly develops in middle age with a slight female preponderance. It is often regarded as a secondary reaction to chronic pruritus and scratching rather than as a primary cutaneous disease. In over 80% of patients, an underlying cause can be found. This is most commonly atopy, which is present in just under 50% of cases. Cutaneous disorders associated with the development of NP include atopic eczema, venous eczema, allergic contact eczema, dermatitis herpetiformis, Grover disease, lichen planus, and cutaneous lymphoma.

Metabolic diseases have been identified in up to 40% of cases. Diabetes mellitus, thyroid diseases, food (sorbitol, lactose, and fructose) intolerance and malabsorption, iron deficiency, and renal and hepatic failure have all been described. Infections with *Helicobacter pylori*, hepatitis C and human immunodeficiency virus (HIV), underlying malignancies, and neurologic causes such as neuropathy and chronic pain syndrome have also been reported. Concomitant psychosocial disorders can be found; anxiety and depression may be primary associations or secondary to the chronic pruritus of NP.

MANAGEMENT STRATEGY

Management should be holistic and directed toward treating the symptoms of pruritus and identifying and correcting any underlying cause. A thorough medical history and physical examination, in combination with a range of relevant investigations, are needed to determine any driver (or drivers) for the itching, whether cutaneous, systemic, or psychological.

General measures such as clipping the fingernails and recommending the use of gloves and mittens can help reduce excoriation. Patients should be encouraged to apply emollients regularly, as xerosis can worsen pruritus. Preparations containing menthol, camphor, or phenol can be useful.

Oral antihistamines are effective for symptom control, and the use of sedating antihistamines such as promethazine 25 to 75 mg may be helpful at night. Potent topical or intralesional corticosteroid injections (triamcinolone acetonide 40 mg/mL injected in amounts of 0.1 mL/nodule and repeated every 6 weeks) can be used to treat individual lesions. Topical calcineurin inhibitors or topical vitamin D_3 analogs may be used as adjuncts or substitutes for topical corticosteroids to ameliorate the risk of skin atrophy associated with prolonged use of the latter. The use of occlusive bandaging or dressings such as hydrocolloid pads, preferably in combination with a topical medication, can interrupt the itch–scratch cycle and facilitate the healing of lesions.

Other oral antipruritic agents include antiepileptic drugs, such as pregabalin 25 mg or gabapentin 300 mg three times a day, or tricyclic antidepressants, such as amitriptyline initially started at a low dose of 10 to 25 mg taken at night. Naltrexone, an opioid receptor antagonist, has been reported to have a potent antipruritic effect in patients with NP. These agents may be more useful for cases with underlying neurologic or psychological causes.

In cases with more widespread involvement, phototherapy with narrowband ultraviolet B (UVB), broadband UVB, psoralens and ultraviolet A (PUVA), or long-wavelength ultraviolet A (UVA1) may be helpful. In severe cases that have failed to respond to topical treatment or phototherapy, systemic immunosuppressive agents such as ciclosporin, azathioprine, and methotrexate can be considered. These may be particularly effective for NP associated with atopic eczema. Thalidomide, due to its side effect profile, should be reserved for patients with debilitating disease in whom all other conventional treatment options have failed.

In cases of NP with an identifiable underlying cause, treatment should be directed toward correcting this; for example, prescribing iron supplements in iron-deficiency anemia.

Specific Investigations

- Full blood count
- Blood urea, creatinine, and electrolytes
- Liver function tests
- Hematinics (iron studies, vitamin B_{12} and folate)
- Calcium
- Thyroid function tests
- Erythrocyte sedimentation rate
- Consider hepatitis B and C and HIV serology
- Consider chest x-ray
- Consider serum immunoglobulin levels and electrophoresis
- Consider total serum IgE
- Consider indirect immunofluorescence
- Consider biopsies for histopathology and direct immunofluorescence to exclude differential diagnoses such as pemphigoid nodularis and squamous cell carcinoma in cases with lone or a small number of lesions

Nodular prurigo: a clinicopathological study of 46 patients.
Rowland Payne CM, Wilkinson JD, McKee PH, Jurecka W, Black MM. Br J Dermatol 1985; 113: 431–44.

Evidence Levels: **A** Double-blind study **B** Clinical trial ≥ 20 subjects **C** Clinical trial < 20 subjects **D** Series ≥ 5 subjects **E** Anecdotal case reports

The clinical presentations; associated disorders; hematologic, renal, hepatic, and microbiologic results; and histologic findings of 46 patients are described in this study.

Prurigo as a symptom of atopic and nonatopic diseases: aetiologic survey in a consecutive cohort of 108 patients. Iking A, Grundmann S, Chatzigeorgakidis E, Phan NQ, Klein D, Stander S. J Eur Acad Dermatol Venereol 2013; 27: 550–7.

The distribution of coexisting diseases affecting NP patients is described in the largest cohort study of NP to date.

Nodular prurigo: metabolic diseases are a common association. Winhoven SM, Gawkrodger DJ. Clin Exp Dermatol 2007; 32: 224–5.

Psychosocial and metabolic disorders—in particular, diabetes mellitus—are commonly associated with NP, as demonstrated in this retrospective analysis of 72 patients.

First-Line Therapies

• Topical corticosteroid	A
• Topical calcineurin inhibitor	A
• Topical corticosteroids with occlusion	C
• Occlusion	E
• Antihistamines	D
• Intralesional corticosteroids	E

Prurigo nodularis. Rowland Payne CME. In: Bernhard JD, ed. Itch – Mechanisms and Management of Pruritus. New York: McGraw-Hill, 1994; 103–19.

Based on a series of 67 patients, the overall patient management of NP is discussed comprehensively.

Evaluation of the antipruritic effects of topical pimecrolimus in nonatopic prurigo nodularis: results of a randomized, hydrocortisone-controlled, doubled-blind phase II trial. Siepmann D, Lotts T, Blome C, Braeutigam M, Phan NQ, Butterfass-Bahloul T, et al. Dermatology 2013; 227: 353–60.

The antipruritic effects of 1% hydrocortisone and 1% pimecrolimus creams are compared in this within-participant, right-left, controlled trial involving 30 patients. A significant reduction in pruritus intensity was achieved on both pimecrolimus- and hydrocortisone-treated sites. No therapeutic difference between pimecrolimus and hydrocortisone was found. Dermatology Life Quality Index scores among subjects improved significantly after treatment.

This is one of very few comparative trials of topical therapies for NP. Although this study looked at the relative efficacy of hydrocortisone, other studies had employed the use of at least potent-strength topical corticosteroids. The highly pruritic nature of NP is such that the use of potent or superpotent topical corticosteroids is often necessary and should be used as first-line treatment.

Treatment of pruritic diseases with topical calcineurin inhibitors. Stander S, Schurmeyer-Horst F, Luger TA, Weisshaar E. Ther Clin Risk Manag 2006; 2: 213–8.

Eleven patients were treated with twice-daily application of topical pimecrolimus or tacrolimus. Five patients achieved 70% or greater reduction of itch with healing or major improvement of lesions.

Topical calcineurin inhibitors are known to have antipruritic and immunosuppressive effects in atopic eczema and, as demonstrated in this study, in nonatopic NP. They represent an effective and nonatrophogenic alternative to topical steroids and may potentially be a safer option for long-term use.

An occlusive dressing containing betamethasone valerate 0.1% for the treatment of prurigo nodularis. Saraceno R, Chiricozzi A, Nistico SP, Tiberti S, Chimenti S. J Dermatolog Treat 2010; 21: 363–6.

A bilateral-paired comparison study involving 12 patients comparing 0.1% betamethasone valerate tape against a moisturizing itch-relief cream containing feverfew. Occlusion enhanced the efficacy of treatment, preventing scratching, and the side treated with betamethasone valproate 0.1% tape demonstrated a higher clinical response.

Use of occlusive membrane in prurigo nodularis. Meyers LN. Int J Dermatol 1989; 28: 275–6.

Four patients with NP responded to weekly application of an occlusive hydrocolloid pad, which also served as a negative reinforcer of scratching.

The use of adhesive occlusive pads, dressings, or bandaging can serve as a deterrent to repetitive scratching of the skin that perpetuates the disease and can disrupt the itch–scratch cycle.

Second-Line Therapies

• Topical vitamin D_3 analog	A
• UVB phototherapy	D
• Narrowband UVB	C
• PUVA or bath PUVA	B
• UVA1 phototherapy	D
• Monochromatic excimer light	C
• Modified Goeckerman regimen	E

Double-blind, right/left comparison of calcipotriol ointment and betamethasone ointment in the treatment of prurigo nodularis. Wong SS, Goh CL. Arch Dermatol 2000; 136: 807–8.

A randomized, double-blind, right/left comparative study evaluating the efficacy of calcipotriol ointment versus 0.1% betamethasone valerate ointment. Calcipotriol was found to be more effective than betamethasone valerate after 8 weeks of treatment, with a greater reduction in number and size of nodules from baseline.

Topical vitamin D3 (tacalcitol) for steroid-resistant prurigo. Katayama I, Miyazaki Y, Nishioka K. Br J Dermatol 1996; 135: 237–40.

Nine of 11 patients treated with twice-daily application of topical tacalcitol showed a significant clinical response within 4 weeks.

Phototherapy in nodular prurigo. Divekar PM, Palmer RA, Keefe M. Clin Exp Dermatol 2003; 28: 99–100.

The responses of 14 patients treated with a total of 19 courses of phototherapy (8 courses of broadband UVB, 4 courses of bath PUVA, and 7 courses of oral PUVA) are reported. Partial resolution was achieved in 68% of treatment courses. Complete resolution occurred in three patients, but two relapsed within 1 year.

Narrow-band ultraviolet B phototherapy in patients with recalcitrant nodular prurigo. Tamagawa-Mineoka R, Katoh N, Ueda E, Kishimoto S. J Dermatol 2007; 34: 691–5.

Ten patients with recalcitrant NP received once-weekly narrowband UVB therapy. Complete or marked clearance was achieved in all patients after a mean cumulative dose of 23.88 J/cm^2 over a mean of 24 sessions. At 1-year follow up, only one patient had relapsed.

UV treatment of generalized prurigo nodularis. Hann SK, Cho MY, Park YK. Int J Dermatol 1990; 29: 436–7.

The treatment of two patients with UVB, followed by the use of topical PUVA for resistant lesions, is described.

Phototherapy of generalized prurigo nodularis. Bruni E, Caccialanza M, Piccinno R. Clin Exp Dermatol 2010; 35: 549–50.

Nineteen patients with generalized NP who had failed a range of previous therapies, including topical corticosteroids, coal tar, oral antihistamines, and ciclosporin, were treated with phototherapy mainly in the UVA range with a spike at 390 nm. A median number of 23 sessions, with a mean total dose of 6.07 J/cm^2, was required. Out of 15 patients who improved with treatment, 2 patients achieved complete remission, and 8 patients achieved marked improvement.

Long-term results of topical trioxsalen PUVA in lichen planus and nodular prurigo. Karoven J, Hannuksela M. Acta Derm Venereol 1985; 120: 53–5.

Bath and ointment trioxsalen PUVA (primary treatment episode of 2–4 weeks, with mean cumulative dose of 7 J/cm^2) was initiated in 63 patients with NP. Good results were achieved in 81% of patients. At follow-up over 1 to 6 years, 18% of patients were totally healed, although the majority of patients relapsed and further treatments were required to maintain results.

Efficacy of UVA1 phototherapy in 230 patients with various skin diseases. Rombold S, Lobisch K, Katzer K, Grazziotin TC, Ring J, Eberlein B. Photodermatol Photoimmunol Photomed 2008; 24: 19–23.

UVA1 was given to 17 patients with NP, with a mean cumulative dose of 650 J/cm^2 given over a mean of 13.9 irradiations. Improvement was observed in 82% of patients, with 41% of patients achieving a marked improvement.

Monochromatic excimer light (308 nm) in the treatment of prurigo nodularis. Saraceno R, Nistico SP, Capriotti E, de Felice C, Rhodes LE, Chimenti S. Photodermatol Photoimmunol Photomed 2008; 24: 43–5.

A study of 11 patients treated with weekly monochromatic excimer light (MEL). Partial or complete clinical and histologic remission was observed in all 9 patients who completed an average of eight treatment sessions.

UVB 308-nm excimer light and bath PUVA: combination therapy is very effective in the treatment of prurigo nodularis. Hammes S, Hermann J, Roos S, Ockenfels HM. J Eur Acad Dermatol Venereol 2011; 25: 799–803.

The efficacy of bath PUVA alone versus combination of PUVA and MEL was compared in this randomized, unblinded study involving 22 patients. Adding MEL sped up the healing process and required 30% less PUVA radiation. There was no significant difference in the proportion of patients achieving complete clearance.

Successful use of a modified Goeckerman regimen in the treatment of generalized prurigo nodularis. Sorenson E, Levin E, Koo J, Berger TG. J Am Acad Dermatol 2015; 72: 40–2.

Four patients were treated with an outpatient modified Goeckerman regimen consisting of 5 days per week broadband UVB therapy followed by application of crude coal tar and topical corticosteroids under occlusion for 4 hours. After a mean 45.5 sessions of modified Goeckerman therapy, patients continued with three sessions of broadband UVB per week with topical steroids

applied to recalcitrant nodules. Remission lengths between 2.5 and 8 months were observed.

Third-Line Therapies	
• Cryotherapy	E
• Capsaicin	B
• Pulsed dye laser	E
• Fexofenadine and montelukast	C
• Naltrexone	C
• Pregabalin	B
• Gabapentin	E
• Ciclosporin	C
• Azathioprine	E
• Methotrexate	C
• Thalidomide	C
• Lenalidomide	E
• Oral tacrolimus	E
• Intravenous immunoglobulin	E

Cryotherapy improves prurigo nodularis. Waldinger TP, Wong RC, Taylor WB, Voorhees JJ. Arch Dermatol 1984; 120: 1598–600.

A patient with corticosteroid and phototherapy-resistant NP was treated successfully with blistering cryotherapy.

Cryotherapy to the point of blistering may cause scarring and hypopigmentation, as it did in this patient.

Treatment of prurigo nodularis: use of cryosurgery and intralesional steroids plus lidocaine. Stoll DM, Fields JP, King LE Jr. J Dermatol Surg Oncol 1983; 9: 922–4.

Two patients were treated with liquid nitrogen applied with a cotton-tipped applicator for a freeze time of 10 seconds, followed by intralesional injection of triamcinolone acetonide (10 mg/mL) mixed with lidocaine (lignocaine) 0.75%. All lesions resolved after four to eight injections at 4- to 6-week intervals.

Treatment of prurigo nodularis with topical capsaicin. Stander S, Luger T, Metze D. J Am Acad Dermatol 2001; 44: 471–8.

Topical capsaicin (0.025%–0.3%) was administered to 33 patients four to six times daily, over periods ranging from 2 weeks to 10 months. Pruritus resolved in all patients within 12 days but returned in 16 of 33 patients within 2 months of discontinuation of therapy.

Nodular prurigo successfully treated with the pulsed dye laser. Woo PN, Finch TM, Hindson C, Foulds IS. Br J Dermatol 2000; 143: 215–6.

A patient with NP unresponsive to topical and intralesional steroids and PUVA improved after six sessions of treatment with pulsed dye laser (595 nm), spaced 6 weeks apart. He remained symptom free 18 months after discontinuation of treatment.

Combination therapy of fexofenadine and montelukast is effective in prurigo nodularis and pemphigoid nodularis. Shintani T, Ohata C, Koga H, Ohyama B, Hamada T, Nakama T, et al. Dermatol Ther 2014; 27: 135–9.

Nine of 12 patients with NP improved after 4 weeks of treatment with 10 mg montelukast once a day and 240 mg fexofenadine twice a day.

Efficacy and safety of naltrexone, an oral opiate receptor antagonist, in the treatment of pruritus in internal and dermatologic diseases. Metze D, Reimann S, Beissert S, Luger T. J Am Acad Dermatol 1999; 41: 533–9.

Evidence Levels: **A** Double-blind study **B** Clinical trial ≥ 20 subjects **C** Clinical trial < 20 subjects **D** Series ≥ 5 subjects **E** Anecdotal case reports

Naltrexone 50 mg once daily was initiated in 17 patients with NP. Nine patients achieved greater than 50% improvement in pruritus, which contributed to healing of skin lesions. Two of these patients experienced tachyphylaxis after 1 and 7 months but improved when the dose of naltrexone was doubled to 50 mg twice daily.

Treatment of prurigo nodularis with pregabalin. Mazza M, Guerriero G, Marano G, Janiri L, Bria P, Mazza S. J Clin Pharm Ther 2013; 38: 16–8.

Thirty patients were treated with pregabalin 25 mg three times a day for 3 months. In 23 patients, a complete resolution of pruritus with reduction of lesions was seen; only 1 patient failed to improve. Treatment was generally well tolerated, and only 6 patients reported side effects.

Therapeutic hotline: treatment of prurigo nodularis and lichen simplex chronicus with gabapentin. Gencoglan G, Inanir I, Gunduz K. Dermatol Ther 2010; 23: 194–8.

Four patients with NP were treated with gabapentin and achieved at least partial remission.

Antipruritic effect of ciclosporin microemulsion in prurigo nodularis: results of a case series. Siepmann D, Luger TA, Stander S. J Dtsch Dermatol Ges 2008; 6: 941–6.

Monotherapy with oral ciclosporin (3–5 mg per kg daily) was initiated in 14 patients. Ten patients experienced at least 80% reduction of pruritus and in 3 patients, pruritus reduced by 40% to 70%, with healing of prurigo nodules during treatment. Maximal antipruritic effect was observed after 2 weeks to 12 months. Fifty percent of patients described side effects. One patient developed angioedema, and another patient had to abort treatment after embolism of the popliteal artery.

Nodular prurigo responsive to azathioprine. Lear JT, English JS, Smith AG. Br J Dermatol 1996; 134: 1151.

The responses of two patients treated with azathioprine 50 mg twice daily for 6 and 12 months are described. After 2 to 3 months of treatment, pruritus improved and lesions became less prominent. Disease relapse occurred after 2 months of treatment cessation in one patient and after 3 years in another.

Prurigo nodularis: retrospective study of 13 cases managed with methotrexate. Spring P, Gschwind I, Gilliet M. Clin Exp Dermatol 2014; 39: 468–73.

Thirteen patients who failed to respond to topical steroids, phototherapy, and antipruritic agents were treated with subcutaneous injections of methotrexate 7.5 to 20 mg once weekly for a minimum of 6 months. In 10 cases, there was remission or marked improvement (greater than 75% improvement in both clinical assessment of disease activity and patient's perception of symptoms). A trend to improvement was observed in two other patients.

Thalidomide in 42 patients with prurigo nodularis Hyde. Anderson TP, Fogh K. Dermatology 2011; 223: 107–12.

A retrospective study of 42 patients treated with an average dose of thalidomide 100 mg daily over a mean period of 105 weeks. Clinical improvement was observed in 32 patients. Side effects, such as neuropathy and sedation, were the most common reason for discontinuation of treatment.

Efficacy of thalidomide in the treatment of prurigo nodularis. Taefehnorooz H, Truchetet F, Barbaud A, Schmutz JL, Bursztejn AC. Acta Derm Venereol 2011; 91: 344–5.

A retrospective study of 13 patients treated with thalidomide 50 to 200 mg once daily over 3 to 142 months. In 7 patients, pruritus resolved, and a reduction of nodules occurred after a mean treatment duration of 3 months.

Thalidomide is one of the most reported and studied treatments of NP. However, side effects are common and can be serious and unpredictable. These include fatigue, constipation, sedation, dizziness, and peripheral neuropathy, which may be irreversible. It is linked to severe birth defects and must be avoided in pregnant women. As such, thalidomide should be reserved for exceptional circumstances, in debilitating disease, and when other treatment options have been exhausted.

Treatment of refractory prurigo nodularis with lenalidomide. Kanavy H, Bahner K, Korman NJ. Arch Dermatol 2012; 148: 794–6.

A patient with refractory NP who had responded only to thalidomide developed peripheral neuropathy after 18 months of therapy. Lenalidomide was chosen as an alternative due to its similar mechanism of action but reduced risk of peripheral neuropathy. Near-complete resolution of pruritus and visible healing of nodules was achieved after 1 month of treatment with lenalidomide 5 mg/day, and the patient remained in remission during 2 years of treatment.

Oral tacrolimus treatment of pruritus in prurigo nodularis. Halvorsen JA, Aasebo W. Acta Derm Venereol 2015; 95: 866–7.

A patient with NP achieved good response to ciclosporin but experienced hypertrichosis as a side effect. She started periodic treatment with oral tacrolimus 10 to 20 mg daily, alternating with ciclosporin. Monotherapy with tacrolimus led to a reduction of itch but without the side effect of hypertrichosis.

Atopic prurigo nodularis responds to intravenous immunoglobulins. Feldmeyer L, Werner S, Kamarashev J, French LE, Hofbauer GF. Br J Dermatol 2012; 166: 461–2.

A patient with refractory NP achieved dramatic improvement with intravenous immunoglobulins (IVIG, 2 g/kg monthly, given intravenously over 3 days) in combination with methotrexate. After three therapy cycles with IVIG, she experienced sustained improvement on methotrexate and topical steroids.

Prurigo pigmentosa

Yukiko Tsuji-Abe, Hiroshi Shimizu

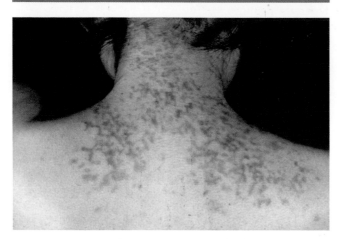

Prurigo pigmentosa is a pruritic eruption that begins with urticarial papules or papulovesicles on the neck, chest, and back, followed by reticular pigmentation. It most commonly affects women in their twenties and thirties. Most of the patients reported have been Japanese.

MANAGEMENT STRATEGY

Prurigo pigmentosa has a distinctive clinical course. Lesions initially start as pruritic, urticarial papules or papulovesicles. The lesions resolve spontaneously within a week, but repetition of the episode results in reticular pigmentation. The pathogenesis of prurigo pigmentosa remains unknown. Friction from clothing, especially in wet conditions such as sweating or swimming, can trigger the disease. In some cases, ketosis caused by diabetes mellitus, sudden weight loss from a low-carbohydrate diet, or anorexia nervosa precedes prurigo pigmentosa. Treatment of these conditions can lead to clinical resolution. Several case reports described individuals who developed this condition in association with other disorders, including contact allergic reactions to certain chemical agents, infection with *Helicobacter pylori* or spirochetes, an atopic diathesis, and pregnancy.

Minocycline (100–200 mg daily) and *dapsone* (25–100 mg daily) are usually very effective for prurigo pigmentosa. The effects are mostly observed within 3 to 7 days after treatment and lead to reductions in itching and papular lesions. Minocycline is regarded as the first-line therapy because it produces fewer adverse reactions, and the remission is reportedly longer than for dapsone. Topical or systemic corticosteroids and antihistamines are usually ineffective.

Specific Investigation

- Urinalysis for ketones

Unilateral prurigo pigmentosa: a report of two cases. Teraki Y, Hitomi K. J Dermatol 2016; 43: 846–7.

Prurigo pigmentosa: a clinicopathologic study of 16 cases. Oh YJ, Lee MH. J Eur Acad Dermal Venereol 2012; 26: 1149–53.

Prurigo pigmentosa on a patient with soft-drink ketosis. Mitsuhashi Y, Suzuki N, Kawaguchi M, Kondo S. J Dermatol 2005; 32: 767–8.

Prurigo pigmentosa (Nagashima) associated with anorexia nervosa. Nakada T, Sueki H, Iijima M. Clin Exp Dermatol 1998; 23: 25–7.

In all these reports, prurigo pigmentosa was associated with ketosis. Disease activity is sometimes correlated with urinary ketone concentration. In some cases, lesions resolved after treatment of the associated condition.

First-Line Therapies

• Minocycline	C
• Treatment of ketosis or any other potentially causative factors	D

Prurigo pigmentosa: clinicopathological study and analysis of 50 cases in Korea. Kim JK, Chung WK, Chang SE, Ko JY, Lee JH, Won CH, et al. J Dermatol 2012; 39: 891–7.

Among 50 patients, 28 patients were treated with minocycline (100–200 mg daily), 7 with dapsone (100 mg daily), and 4 with both minocycline and dapsone; all patients responded well to these therapies.

Bullous prurigo pigmentosa in a pregnant woman with hyperemesis gravidarum. Hanami Y, Yamamoto T. J Dermatol 2015; 42: 436–7.

A pregnant woman with severe hyperemesis gravidarum lost 7 kg in body weight. The urinary ketone concentration was positive. Her general condition improved with fluid therapy and bed rest, and the skin lesions disappeared after 1 month.

Prurigo pigmentosa associated with diabetic ketoacidosis. Ohnishi T, Kisa H, Ogata E, Watanabe S. Acuta Derm Venereol 2000; 80: 447–8.

Eighteen cases of prurigo pigmentosa were associated with diabetic ketoacidosis. Treatment of ketoacidosis improved eruptions in eight cases, and treatment with topical corticosteroid improved the rash in one case; progress was unknown in one case.

Minocycline (100–200 mg daily) is usually very effective. The effects—reductions in pruritic and papular lesions—are mostly observed within a few days after treatment. The therapeutic effects of minocycline and the antibiotics described next are likely attributable to the fact that leukocyte activation and inflammation are key pathologic features in prurigo pigmentosa.

Second-Line Therapies

• Dapsone	C
• Doxycycline	C E
• Roxithromycin	E E
• Clarithromycin	E

Prurigo pigmentosa in Korea: clinicopathological study. Shin JW, Lee SY, Lee JS, Whang KU, Park YL, Lee HK. Int J Dermal 2012; 51: 152–7.

Evidence Levels: **A** Double-blind study **B** Clinical trial ≥ 20 subjects **C** Clinical trial < 20 subjects **D** Series ≥ 5 subjects **E** Anecdotal case reports

Dapsone and minocycline were used alone or in combination to treat 37 of 49 patients. Lesions and pruritus rapidly resolved in all patients.

Prurigo pigmentosa: a clinical and histopathologic study of 11 cases. Lin SH, Ho JC, Cheng YW, Huang PH, Wang CY. Chang Gung Med J 2010; 33: 157–63.

Among 11 patients with prurigo pigmentosa, 10 patients were treated with doxycycline (200 mg daily) and exhibited a good response.

Prurigo pigmentosa: not an uncommon disease in the Turkish population. Baykal C, Buyukbabani N, Akinturk S, Saglik E. Int J Dermatol 2006; 45: 1164–8.

Three of six patients with prurigo pigmentosa responded well to doxycycline 100 mg daily; another three responded well to tetracycline 500 mg daily.

The successful treatment of prurigo pigmentosa with macrolide antibiotics. Yazawa N, Ihn H, Yamane K, Etoh T, Tamaki K. Dermatology 2001; 202: 67–9.

Two patients with prurigo pigmentosa responded well to roxithromycin 300 mg daily; another two responded well to clarithromycin 400 mg daily. In all patients, the effect was quick, and pruritus and papules disappeared within 1 week.

Prurigo pigmentosa. Gürses L, Gürbüz O, Demirçay Z, Kotiloglu E. Int J Dermatol 1999; 38: 924–5.

One of two patients responded well to doxycycline 200 mg daily; prurigo pigmentosa resolved spontaneously in the other patient.

Doxycycline—a member of the tetracycline antibiotics group—and macrolide antibiotics such as roxithromycin and clarithromycin are reported to be effective for prurigo pigmentosa. These drugs are recommended for patients who respond poorly to first-line treatment and those for whom dapsone and minocycline are contraindicated.

Third-Line Therapies	
• Isotretinoin	E
• Narrowband Ultraviolet B (UVB) therapy	E

Vesiculous prurigo pigmentosa in a 13-year-old girl: good response to isotretinoin. Requena Caballero C, Nagore E, Sanmartín O, Botella-Estrada R, Serra C, Guillén C. Int J Eur Acad Dermatol Venereol 2005; 19: 474–6.

The initial diagnosis was a vesiculobullous form of Darier disease, and the patient was started on isotretinoin 40 mg/day, which resulted in a good response in 10 days. The lesion relapsed 5 months later, and treatment with minocycline 100 mg/day resulted in resolution within 7 days.

Prurigo pigmentosa successfully treated with low-dose isotretinoin. Akoglu G, Boztepe G, Karaduman A. Dermatology 2006; 213: 331–3.

An 18-year-old woman was successfully treated with isotretinoin 20 mg daily (0.3 mg/kg/day). Pruritus and erythematous macules resolved within 1 month after the start of therapy.

Successful treatment with narrowband UVB phototherapy in prurigo pigmentosa associated with pregnancy. Jang MS, Baek JW, Kang DY, Kang JS, Kim ST, Suh KS. Eur J Dermatol 2011; 21: 634–5.

A woman in the thirteenth week of pregnancy was treated with narrowband UVB for prurigo pigmentosa. Pruritus decreased significantly after the first irradiation, and erythema resolved after the fifth session.

Most patients with prurigo pigmentosa respond well to first- or second-line therapies or achieve spontaneous remission, but these treatment alternatives might be useful in unusual cases.

Pruritus

Amit Garg, Jeffrey D. Bernhard

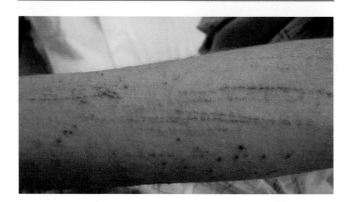

Pruritus is a cutaneous sensation (usually unpleasant) that evokes an urge to scratch, rub, pick, and, in extreme cases, mutilate the skin in an attempt to obtain relief. We use the terms *itch* and *pruritus* interchangeably. Itch occurs as a characteristic feature of many skin diseases, such as atopic dermatitis, bullous pemphigoid, lichen planus, and scabies. It can also occur as an unusual symptom of certain systemic disorders, such as hyperthyroidism, cholestasis, and uremia. Pruritus in the absence of a detectable rash, whether localized or generalized, poses both a diagnostic and therapeutic challenge to even the most seasoned dermatologist. To make matters even worse, secondary changes caused by rubbing and scratching may camouflage specific physical findings. New discoveries in the neurophysiology of itch have led to specific therapies that target particular pathways and receptors in the nervous system.

MANAGEMENT STRATEGY

Management of pruritus is directed toward its cause, which may not always be apparent. Many different dermatoses itch; it is beyond the scope of this chapter to discuss them all. Xerosis and scabies deserve special mention because both can have subtle findings with intense itching out of proportion to the rash. In xerosis, an adequate skin care regimen and emollients are indispensable. One of the more common and embarrassing errors is to miss the diagnosis of scabies; consideration of this diagnosis may avoid undue suffering and delays in treatment. Pre-bullous pemphigoid, dermatitis herpetiformis, adult-onset atopic dermatitis, cutaneous lymphoma, and drug reactions are among the other most difficult to diagnose diseases of the skin.

Failure to diagnose a primary skin disease does not rule out the possibility that one is present; time, repeated observation, and laboratory tests such as a skin biopsy may be required. When no rash is present, or when a rash is present but cannot be diagnosed, further evaluation is indicated. The evaluation should include a thorough medical history and physical examination, complete with a precise medication review and review of systems. The physical examination should include palpation for organomegaly and lymphadenopathy. The examiner should not be misled by nonspecific secondary changes caused by rubbing, scratching, or secondary infection. A "peculiar" eczematous dermatitis resistant to treatment may be a secondary phenomenon, not necessarily the

primary diagnosis. Laboratory investigations are often essential in the clinical assessment of chronic pruritus, whether a rash is present or not. The presence or absence of constitutional signs or symptoms should be determined at the initial and follow-up visits.

The most serious error is to miss the diagnosis of an underlying systemic disease associated with pruritus. Some of the systemic disorders that may cause pruritus include hematologic and solid malignancies, lymphoproliferative disorders, HIV, thyroid disease, iron deficiency, renal disease, hepatobiliary disease, connective tissue disease, neurologic disease, and drug hypersensitivity. Interval reevaluation for associated systemic disease should be undertaken because pruritus may precede the diagnosis of a systemic disease by many months (as in primary biliary cirrhosis and Hodgkin disease). A review of systems—with particular emphasis on the presence or absence of constitutional signs or symptoms—may be quite helpful.

For symptomatic relief, general skin hygiene measures (e.g., *moisturization*) and *elimination of exacerbating factors* (e.g., excessively dry air) are worthwhile but rarely sufficient. Tepid water baths using fragrance-free *moisturizing soaps, emollients, unscented bath oils* applied liberally after bathing, a cool moisture-rich environment, and loose-fitting clothing are helpful. In the management of pruritus that does not respond to simple measures, treatment should be individualized based on etiology, severity, and regard for safety.

Specific Investigations

Screening
- Complete medical history
- Careful medication history
- Thorough review of systems
- Complete physical examination
- Complete blood count with differential
- Blood urea nitrogen, creatinine
- Fasting glucose
- Hepatic function testing
- Thyroid function testing
- Chest radiograph (posteroanterior and lateral)
- Age-appropriate cancer screening

Additional testing to consider
- Scraping for scabies
- Hepatitis B and C profiles
- HIV testing
- Erythrocyte sedimentation rate
- Serum iron and ferritin
- Serum protein electrophoresis, urine protein electrophoresis
- Stool for ova and parasites
- Antimitochondrial antibody test
- Skin biopsy

Itch and pruritus: what are they and how should itches be classified? Bernhard JD. Dermatol Ther 2005; 18: 288–91.

Clinical classification of itch: a position paper of the International Forum for the Study of Itch. Ständer S, Weisshaar E, Mettang T, Szepietowski JC, Carstens E, Ikoma A, et al. Acta Derm Venereol 2007; 87: 291–4.

These two papers explain the terms used to signify different categories of pruritic disorders.

Neurophysiological and neurochemical basis of modern pruritus treatment. Ständer S, Weisshaar E, Luger TA. Exp Dermatol 2008; 17: 161–9.

This review highlights modern neurophysiologic and neurochemical therapeutic strategies on the basis of neuronal mechanisms underlying chronic pruritus.

Chronic pruritus. Yosipovitch G, Bernhard JD. N Engl J Med 2013; 368: 1625–34.

This review describes the evaluation and symptomatic treatment of patients without a clear diagnosis.

Ultraviolet phototherapy for pruritus. Rivard J, Lim HW. Dermatolog Ther 2005; 18: 344–54.

Ultraviolet therapy is used to treat a variety of pruritic conditions. In this review, mechanisms of action for phototherapy are discussed. Treatment limitations, side effects, and common dosing protocols are reviewed.

Pruritus in chronic liver disease: mechanisms and treatment. Bergasa NV. Curr Gastroenterol Rep 2004; 6: 10–6.

This is an excellent and succinct review of cholestatic pruritus. It presents what is known regarding the pathophysiology of itch and cholestasis, and it discusses targeted treatment strategies in cholestatic disorders.

NEUROPATHIC ITCH

Neuropathic itch arises as a consequence of pathology at one or more points along the afferent (sensory) pathway of the peripheral or central nervous system. Brachioradial pruritus (BRP) and notalgia paresthetica (NP) are the two best examples of the isolated sensory peripheral neuropathies seen by dermatologists. It is believed that dorsal spinal nerve radiculopathy, usually secondary to degenerative disease of cervical and thoracic vertebral bodies, leads to persistent itching, paresthesia, hypesthesia, or burning/stinging pain. The involved areas may also be hyperpigmented and excoriated. These forms of localized pruritus may go undiagnosed for quite some time. By the time a patient fails to respond to multiple treatments and a dermatology consultation is obtained, the itch has often been going on for months and may have become generalized, often with secondary changes that may be mistaken for a primary dermatosis. Several investigators have observed patients in whom BRP appears to have triggered generalization to areas beyond those normally involved in classic BRP.

Although evidence for the use of *gabapentin* in the treatment of BRP and NP is mostly anecdotal to date, it is being used increasingly with success for more widespread or otherwise recalcitrant neuropathic dysesthesias, including itch and pain. Doses as high as 3600 mg daily in three or four divided doses, as tolerated, may be necessary. *Pregabalin*, an analog of gabapentin, has also been effective in the treatment of neuropathic pain syndromes (such as postherpetic neuralgia and diabetic neuropathy); there is evidence that it is effective in treating neuropathic itch as well (e.g., BRP and postherpetic pruritus) in doses ranging from 150 to 450 mg in two to three divided doses. Repeated application of *capsaicin cream*, which depletes axonal stores of substance P, may be an effective approach to the treatment of localized areas of neuropathic pain or itch. Although there is evidence to support its use for neuropathic itch, in practice the application of capsaicin is limited by its low tolerability, its restriction to smaller application areas, and its unknown long-term safety risks.

First-Line Therapy

• Gabapentin or pregabalin	**D**

Gabapentin treatment for notalgia paresthetica, a common isolated peripheral sensory neuropathy. Loosemore MP, Bordeaux JS, Bernhard JD. J Eur Acad Dermatol Venereol 2007; 21: 1440–1.

An 82-year-old man with NP and BRP was treated with gabapentin 600 mg at night with resolution of symptoms. Symptoms recurred when gabapentin was stopped and then resolved with reinitiation of the medication.

Brachioradial pruritus: response to treatment with gabapentin. Winhoven SM, Coulson IH, Bottomley WW. Br J Dermatol 2004; 150: 786–7.

In this report, two patients with BRP resistant to other therapies responded to gabapentin 300 mg three times daily.

Brachioradial pruritus: report of a new case responding to gabapentin. Kanitakis J. Eur J Dermatol 2006; 16: 311–2.

A 54-year-old man with BRP noted significant (90%) improvement in pruritus with gabapentin 600 mg three times daily and the use of an antipruritic cream containing 8% calamine and essential fatty acids. He initially had diarrhea and sleepiness at this dose. Pruritus returned with discontinuation of gabapentin and again resolved with its reinitiation.

Gabapentin treatment for brachioradial pruritus. Bueller HA, Bernhard JD, Dubroff LM. J Eur Acad Dermatol Venereol 1999; 13: 227–8.

First report on the use of this class of drugs for the treatment of neuropathic itches such as BRP. BRP is probably more common than previously realized, and it can be unbearable.

Pregabalin in the treatment of chronic pruritus. Ehrchen J, Ständer S. J Am Acad Dermatol 2008; 58: S36–7.

Second-Line Therapy

• Capsaicin	**A**

Successful treatment of notalgia paresthetica with topical capsaicin: vehicle-controlled, double-blind, crossover study. Wallengren J, Klinker M. J Am Acad Dermatol 1995; 32: 287–9.

In this 10-week study, 20 patients with notalgia paresthetica were treated with capsaicin cream or placebo five times daily for 1 week and then three times daily for 3 weeks. Treatment was stopped for 2 weeks before all patients using capsaicin cream resumed the same schedule as before. Seventy percent of patients treated with capsaicin cream had improved symptoms compared with only 30% on placebo. Pruritus did not intensify during the washout period in patients who received capsaicin cream in the first 4 weeks.

Successful treatment of refractory neuropathic pruritus with capsaicin 8% patch: a bicentric retrospective study with long-term follow-up. Misery L, Erfan N, Castela E, Brenaut E, Lantéri-Minet M, Lacour JP, et al. Acta Derm Venereol 2015; 95: 864–5.

A retrospective case series in which seven patients with BRP and NP responded to treatment with a capsaicin 8% dermal patch

Solar (brachioradial) pruritus – response to capsaicin cream. Knight TE, Hayashi T. Int J Dermatol 1994; 33: 206–9.

In this open-label trial of capsaicin cream, 10 of 13 patients completing the study found significant relief (itching much improved or gone) from itch on the treated arm after 3 weeks compared with the untreated control arm.

CHOLESTATIC ITCH

Cholestasis, a reduction of bile flow, results from a variety of hepatic, as well as extrahepatic, diseases. Although the pathophysiologic link between cholestasis and pruritus is not fully understood, an increasing body of evidence supports the proposition that it occurs as a consequence of increased levels of endogenous opioids. Pruritus of cholestasis is typically widespread, characteristically involves the palms and soles, and may be accompanied by jaundice. Therapeutic interventions have focused on the removal of presumed pruritogens from the circulation (through the use of *ursodeoxycholic acid, cholestyramine*), induction of hepatic enzymes *(rifampin)*, antagonism of endogenous opioid receptors *(naltrexone, naloxone, nalmefene)*, modulation of serotonin neurotransmission *(sertraline)*, activation of cannabinoid receptors *(dronabinol)*, and clearing water-soluble and protein-bound pruritogens through albumin-based dialysis (Molecular Adsorbent Recycling System, Prometheus). *Ultraviolet B (UVB) phototherapy* and parenteral *lidocaine* are further therapeutic considerations.

First-Line Therapies	
• Rifampin	A
• Naltrexone, nalmefene, naloxone	A

Rifampin is safe for treatment of pruritus due to chronic cholestasis: a meta-analysis of prospective randomized-controlled trials. Khurana S, Singh P. Liver Int 2006; 26: 943–8.

This meta-analysis includes five prospective randomized controlled trials with 61 patients who had pruritus associated with chronic liver disease. Complete or partial resolution of symptoms occurred in 77% of patients taking rifampin 300 to 600 mg daily.

The efficacy and safety of bile acid binding agents, opioid antagonists, or rifampin in the treatment of cholestasis-associated pruritus. Tandon P, Rowe BH, Vandermeer B, Bain VG. Am J Gastroenterol 2007; 102: 1528–36.

In this review of 12 randomized controlled trials, both rifampin and opioid antagonists significantly reduced cholestasis-associated pruritus. There was insufficient data to assess the efficacy of cholestyramine.

Efficacy and safety of oral naltrexone treatment for pruritus of cholestasis, a crossover, double blind, placebo-controlled study. Terg R, Coronel E, Sordá J, Muñoz AE, Findor J. J Hepatol 2002; 37: 717–22.

In this double-blind, randomized, placebo-controlled crossover trial of 20 patients with cholestasis-associated pruritus, 9 of 20 patients taking naltrexone 50 mg daily experienced a greater than 50% reduction in symptoms relative to baseline, including 5 whose pruritus disappeared completely. Adverse effects included a short-lived opioid withdrawal–like phenomenon.

Oral nalmefene therapy reduces scratching activity due to the pruritus of cholestasis: a controlled study. Bergasa NV, Alling DW, Talbot TL, Wells MC, Jones EA. J Am Acad Dermatol 1999; 41: 431–4.

In a randomized, double-blind, placebo-controlled study with pruritus associated with chronic liver disease, nalmefene therapy was associated with a 75% reduction in the mean hourly scratching activity and a decrease in the mean visual analog scale (VAS) score of the perception of pruritus in all eight patients.

Effects of naloxone infusions in patients with the pruritus of cholestasis. A double-blind, randomized, controlled trial. Bergasa NV, Alling DW, Talbot TL, Swain MG, Yurdaydin C, Turner ML, et al. Ann Intern Med 1995; 123: 161–7.

In this double-blind, placebo-controlled, crossover trial in 29 patients with liver disease, naloxone infusions resulted in significantly improved VAS scores and hourly scratching activity compared with placebo.

The itch of liver disease. Bergasa NV. Semin Cutan Med Surg 2011; 30: 93–8.

Update on the treatment of the pruritus of cholestasis. Bergasa NV. Clin Liver Dis 2008; 12: 219–34.

Two relevant discussions on pruritus of cholestasis, its mechanism, and endogenous mediators, as well as the potential role of a behavioral component to disease manifestation.

Second-Line Therapies	
• Cholestyramine	A
• Ursodeoxycholic acid	A
• Sertraline	A

Double-blind placebo-controlled clinical trial of microporous cholestyramine in the treatment of intra- and extrahepatic cholestasis: relationship between itching and serum bile acids. Di Padova C, Tritapepe R, Rovagnati P, Rossetti S. Methods Find Exp Clin Pharmacol 1984; 6: 773–6.

In this double-blind, placebo-controlled trial in 10 patients, microporous cholestyramine 3 g three times daily over a 4-week period significantly reduced itch intensity and serum bile acids over placebo.

Randomised controlled trials of ursodeoxycholic-acid therapy for primary biliary cirrhosis: a meta-analysis. Goulis J, Leandro G, Burroughs AK. Lancet 1999; 354: 1053–60.

In this meta-analysis, ursodeoxycholic acid was effective in treating pruritus associated with primary biliary cirrhosis in 2 of 11 randomized controlled trials.

The potent bile acid sequestrant colesevelam is not effective in cholestatic pruritus: results of a double-blind, randomized, placebo-controlled trial. Kuiper EM, van Erpecum KJ, Beuers U, Hansen BE, Thio HB, de Man RA, et al. Hepatology 2010; 52: 1334–40.

In this randomized, double-blind, multicenter trial, 35 patients with cholestatic pruritus received 1875 mg of colesevelam, an anion-exchange resin with a sevenfold higher bile acid–binding capacity than cholestyramine, or an identical placebo twice daily for 3 weeks. Despite significantly lower mean serum bile acid levels in the colesevelam-treated group, there was no significant difference between groups with respect to the following: percent of patients with ≥40% reduction in pruritus VAS scores, quality-of-life scores, and severity of cutaneous scratch lesions.

Sertraline as a first-line treatment for cholestatic pruritus. Mayo MJ, Handem I, Saldana S, Jacobe H, Getachew Y, Rush AJ. Hepatology 2007; 45: 666–74.

In this randomized, double-blind, placebo-controlled trial, 21 patients with pruritus associated with chronic liver disease experienced significant improvements in perceived itch and in physical evidence of scratching while taking sertraline 75 to 100 mg daily.

Evidence Levels: **A** Double-blind study **B** Clinical trial ≥ 20 subjects **C** Clinical trial < 20 subjects **D** Series ≥ 5 subjects **E** Anecdotal case reports

Long-term efficacy of sertraline as a treatment for cholestatic pruritus in patients with primary biliary cirrhosis. Browning J, Combes B, Mayo MJ. Am J Gastroenterol 2003; 98: 2736–41.

A retrospective report of 40 patients enrolled in a prospective study to examine the efficacy of ursodeoxycholic acid in patients with primary biliary cirrhosis. These patients kept itch diaries during the study. Itch in six of seven patients started on sertraline for depression improved significantly, and these patients were able to discontinue other medications for itch.

Third-Line Therapies

- Albumin-based dialysis   E
- Ultraviolet B phototherapy   E
- Parenteral lidocaine   A
- Dronabinol   E

Treatment of severe refractory pruritus with fractionated plasma separation and adsorption (Prometheus). Rifai K, Hafer C, Rosenau J, Athmann C, Haller H, Peter Manns M, et al. Scand J Gastroenterol 2006; 41: 1212–7.

Seven patients with recalcitrant pruritus associated with liver disease were treated with Prometheus for three to five sessions. Six patients with bile acid elevations reported significant improvement in pruritus, which was also associated with a parallel decrease in serum bile acids. The patient with no initial bile acid elevation did not report an improvement in pruritus. In four of the six patients, improvement lasted at least 4 weeks.

Therapy of intractable pruritus with MARS. Acevedo Ribó M, Moreno Planas JM, Sanz Moreno C, Rubio González EE, Rubio González E, Boullosa Graña E, et al. Transplant Proc 2005; 37: 1480–1.

All three patients with intractable pruritus associated with primary biliary cirrhosis who underwent two to three sessions of the molecular adsorbent recirculating system had marked improvement of pruritus and decreased bilirubin levels. Improvement lasted only a few days in all cases.

Extracorporeal albumin dialysis: a procedure for prolonged relief of intractable pruritus in patients with primary biliary cirrhosis. Pares A, Cisneros L, Salmeron JM, Caballería L, Mas A, Torras A, et al. Am J Gastroenterol 2004; 99: 1105–10.

Four patients with recalcitrant pruritus associated with primary biliary cirrhosis were treated with two extracorporeal albumin dialysis sessions 1 day apart. Two patients reported resolution of itch, whereas the two other patients reported a marked decrease in pruritus. Scratching decreased in a parallel fashion to reduced pruritus. Pruritus eventually recurred over months in all four patients.

Treatment of intractable pruritus in drug induced cholestasis with albumin dialysis: a report of two cases. Bellmann R, Feistritzer C, Zoller H, Graziadei IW, Schwaighofer H, Propst A, et al. ASAIO J 2004; 50: 387–91.

Two patients with drug-induced cholestasis and severe pruritus who underwent three sessions of the molecular adsorbent recirculating system experienced sustained relief of pruritus as well as a decline in plasma bilirubin and serum 3α-hydroxy bile acid levels.

Phototherapy for primary biliary cirrhosis. Perlstein SM. Arch Dermatol 1981; 117: 608.

In this case report, two patients with pruritus treated with weekly UVB phototherapy improved.

Efficacy of lidocaine in the treatment of pruritus in patients with chronic cholestatic liver diseases. Villamil AG, Bandi JC, Galdame OA, Gerona S, Gadano AC. Am J Med 2005; 118: 1160–3.

In this double-blind trial, 18 patients were randomized (2:1) to receive parenteral lidocaine 100 mg or placebo. Patients receiving lidocaine reported significantly reduced severity of pruritus and fatigue compared with placebo.

Preliminary observation with dronabinol in patients with intractable pruritus secondary to cholestatic liver disease. Neff GW, O'Brien CB, Reddy KR, Bergasa NV, Regev A, Molina E, et al. Am J Gastroenterol 2002; 97: 2117–9.

In this report, three patients with intractable cholestatic-related pruritus were started on 5 mg of dronabinol (Δ^9-tetrahydrocannabinol) at bedtime with a decrease in pruritus, marked improvement in sleep, and eventual return to work. Resolution of depression occurred in two of three.

ITCH ASSOCIATED WITH CHOLESTASIS OF PREGNANCY

First-Line Therapy

- Ursodeoxycholic acid   A

Ursodeoxycholic acid and S-adenosylmethionine in the treatment of intrahepatic cholestasis of pregnancy: a multicentered randomized controlled trial. Zhang L, Liu XH, Qi HB, Li Z, Fu XD, Chen L, et al. Eur Rev Med Pharmacol Sci 2015; 19: 3770–6.

In this randomized controlled trial, ursodeoxycholic acid monotherapy, S-adenosylmethionine monotherapy, and both as combined therapy showed similar efficacies for intrahepatic cholestasis of pregnancy.

Intrahepatic cholestasis of pregnancy: amelioration of pruritus by UDCA is associated with decreased progesterone disulphates in urine. Glantz A, Reilly SJ, Benthin L, Lammert F, Mattsson LA, Marschall HU. Hepatology 2008; 47: 544–51.

In this randomized controlled trial, women with intrahepatic cholestasis of pregnancy treated with ursodeoxycholic acid (UDCA) experienced amelioration of pruritus, which was associated with increased hepatobiliary excretion of progesterone disulfates.

Intrahepatic cholestasis of pregnancy: a randomized controlled trial comparing dexamethasone and ursodeoxycholic acid. Glantz A, Marschall HU, Lammert F, Mattsson LA. Hepatology 2005; 42: 1399–405.

In this randomized, double-blind, placebo-controlled trial consisting of 130 women with intrahepatic cholestasis of pregnancy, 3 weeks of UDCA 1 g daily resulted in significant relief from pruritus and marked reduction of serum bile acids.

Second-Line Therapies

- S-adenosyl-L-methionine   B
- Cholestyramine   B

Randomized prospective comparative study of ursodeoxycholic acid and S-adenosyl-L-methionine in the treatment of intrahepatic cholestasis of pregnancy. Binder T, Salaj P, Zima T, Vítek L. J Perinat Med 2006; 34: 383–91.

In this study, 78 women with intrahepatic cholestasis of pregnancy treated with UDCA, S-adenosyl-L-methionine, or a combination of the two experienced a significant improvement in pruritus. Only UDCA monotherapy and combination therapy led to improvement in serum concentrations of bile acids and transaminases, with the combination therapy leading to faster results.

A randomised controlled trial of ursodeoxycholic acid and S-adenosyl-L-methionine in the treatment of gestational cholestasis. Roncaglia N, Locatelli A, Arreghini A, Assi F, Cameroni I, Pezzullo JC, et al. Br J Obstet Gynaecol 2004; 111: 17–21.

In this study, 46 women with intrahepatic cholestasis of pregnancy and pruritus were randomly assigned to receive oral S-adenosyl-L-methionine 500 mg twice daily or oral UDCA 300 mg twice daily. Both therapies significantly and equally improved pruritus. Women receiving UDCA had significantly greater improvements in serum bile acids, aspartate aminotransferase, alanine aminotransferase, and bilirubin.

Efficacy and safety of ursodeoxycholic acid versus cholestyramine in intrahepatic cholestasis of pregnancy. Kondrackiene J, Beuers U, Kupcinskas L. Gastroenterology 2005; 129: 894–901.

In this study, 84 women with intrahepatic cholestasis of pregnancy and pruritus were randomized to receive either UDCA 8 to 10 mg/kg body weight daily or cholestyramine 8 g daily for 14 days. The group receiving UDCA had greater improvement in pruritus, deliveries that were closer to term, greater reductions in serum alanine and aspartate aminotransferase activities, greater decrease in endogenous serum bile acid levels, and fewer adverse effects compared with the group receiving cholestyramine.

RENAL ITCH

Patients with renal itch tend to have dry skin, have increased numbers of dermal mast cells, and may have a variety of unidentified circulating pruritogens, possibly including opioid peptides. Pruritus associated with chronic renal failure is usually an unremitting generalized itch, which is more common among hemodialysis patients. Some dialysis patients experience itch localized to the shunt arm. Presence or intensity of pruritus does not correlate with blood urea or creatinine levels. The condition is difficult to manage, and the only reliably effective treatment remains kidney transplant. Fortunately, the incidence of uremic pruritus is decreasing as dialysis membranes with improved biocompatibility are being used. Optimizing general skin care measures with emollients to reduce xerosis should be a fundamental part of the treatment plan. Antihistamines are generally not helpful for uremic pruritus. However, the tricyclic antihistamine *doxepin*, whose use in renal itch is not described in the literature, may be helpful because of its sedating and antidepressant properties. Although *UVB phototherapy* is the mainstay of treatment, *gabapentin* and *naltrexone* have also shown efficacy in trials. A number of other less conventional therapeutic interventions have reported success.

First-Line Therapies	
• Emollients with high water content	A
• Narrowband UVB phototherapy	B
• Broadband UVB phototherapy	B
• Gabapentin	A
• Pregabalin	B
• Naltrexone	A
• Nalfurafine hydrochloride	B

Effect of skin care with an emollient containing a high water content on mild uremic pruritus. Okada K, Matsumoto K. Ther Apher Dial 2004; 8: 419–22.

In this placebo-controlled trial involving 20 hemodialysis patients with mild pruritus, twice-weekly application of an aqueous gel containing 80 g of water for 2 weeks significantly improved reported pruritus scores and xerosis compared with the control group.

Narrowband ultraviolet B phototherapy for patients with refractory uraemic pruritus: a randomized controlled trial. Ko MJ, Yang JY, Wu HY, Hu FC, Chen SI, Tsai PJ, et al. Br J Dermatol 2011; 165: 633–9.

In this single-blind, randomized, controlled trial patients with refractory uremic pruritus were randomized to receive NB-UVB phototherapy or time-matched long-wave UVA radiation as a control. NB-UVB was given three times per week for 6 weeks. The dose of NB-UVB was started at 210 mJ/cm^2 and was increased by 10% for each treatment. Both NB-UVB and control groups had significant and comparable improvement in the pruritus-intensity VAS scores during phototherapy and follow-up. Compared with the control group, the NB-UVB group showed a significant improvement in the affected body surface area ($p = 0.006$) but not in sleep quality. The authors concluded that NB-UVB phototherapy does not show a significant effect in reducing pruritus intensity compared with a control group for refractory uremic pruritus.

Treatment of uremic pruritus with narrowband ultraviolet B phototherapy: an open pilot study. Ada S, Seçkin D, Budakoğlu I, Ozdemir FN. J Am Acad Dermatol 2005; 53: 149–51.

In this study, 20 patients with uremic pruritus were treated with NB-UVB phototherapy for 6 weeks. Of the 10 who completed the study, 8 showed 50% or greater improvement in pruritus scores. Of the 10 patients who left the study before 6 weeks, 6 were satisfied with their response. In the 6-month follow-up period, 3 of 7 responders who could be examined were in remission, whereas in the remaining 4 responders, pruritus recurred within a mean time interval of 2.5 months.

Generalized pruritus treated with narrowband UVB. Seckin D, Demircay A, Akin O. Int J Dermatol 2007; 46: 367–70.

Fifteen patients with uremic pruritus included in the analysis of this open-label trial were treated with NB-UVB phototherapy three times weekly with a mean number of 22 treatments and a mean cumulative UVB dose of 24,540 mJ/cm^2. These patients showed greater than 50% improvement in visual analog and pruritus grading scores. Of the 6 patients who were followed up at a mean time of 5.3 months, 2 remained in remission.

Ultraviolet phototherapy of uremic pruritus. Long-term results and possible mechanism of action. Gilchrest BA, Rowe JW, Brown RS, Steinman TI, Arndt KA. Ann Intern Med 1979; 91: 17–21.

This is the classic study of 38 patients with uremic pruritus treated with UVB phototherapy. A comparison of three schedules varying from one to three treatments weekly showed that the percentage of patients responding was not influenced by frequency of UVB exposure, although patients treated more intensively improved faster. Patients receiving only half-body treatments improved as well, indicating a systemic rather than local effect. Overall, 32 of 38 patients improved after a course of six or eight UVB exposures.

Gabapentin: a promising drug for the treatment of uremic pruritus. Naini AE, Harandi AA, Khanbabapour S, Shahidi S, Seirafiyan S, Mohseni M. Saudi J Kidney Dis Transpl 2007; 18: 378–81.

Evidence Levels: A Double-blind study B Clinical trial ≥ 20 subjects C Clinical trial < 20 subjects D Series ≥ 5 subjects E Anecdotal case reports

In this double-blind, placebo-controlled trial of 34 hemodialysis patients, those who received gabapentin 400 mg twice weekly after hemodialysis sessions for 4 weeks reported significantly improved pruritus score compared with placebo.

Gabapentin therapy for pruritus in haemodialysis patients: a randomized, placebo-controlled, double-blind trial. Gunal AI, Ozalp G, Yoldas TK, Gunal SY, Kirciman E, Celiker H. Nephrol Dial Transplant 2004; 19: 3137–9.

In this double-blind, placebo-controlled, crossover study of 25 hemodialysis patients, those who received gabapentin 300 mg three times a week after each hemodialysis session for 4 weeks reported a significantly improved pruritus score compared with placebo.

Use of pregabalin in the management of chronic uremic pruritus. Shavit L, Grenader T, Lifschitz M, Slotki I. J Pain Symptom Manage 2013; 45: 776–81.

This prospective observational study in a cohort of 12 patients showed significant improvement in long-standing uremic pruritus as measured by mean VAS scores 1, 4, and 24 weeks after initiation of pregabalin.

Comparison of pregabalin with ondansetron in treatment of uraemic pruritus in dialysis patients: a prospective, randomized, double-blind study. Yue J, Jiao S, Xiao Y, Ren W, Zhao T, Meng J. Int Urol Nephrol 2015; 47: 161–7.

In this 12-week prospective, randomized, double-blind trial, patients in the pregabalin group experienced significantly reduced severity of pruritus compared with patients in the ondansetron and the placebo groups. Final pruritus scores were not different between the ondansetron and the placebo groups.

Pregabalin versus gabapentin in the treatment of neuropathic pruritus in maintenance hemodialysis patients: a prospective crossover study. Solak Y, Biyik Z, Atalay H, Gaipov A, Guney F, Turk S, et al. Nephrology 2012; 17: 710–7.

Randomised crossover trial of naltrexone in uraemic pruritus. Peer G, Kivity S, Agami O, Fireman E, Silverberg D, Blum M, et al. Lancet 1996; 348: 1552–4.

Naltrexone 50 mg daily was given to 15 hemodialysis patients with severe resistant pruritus. All 15 patients responded to treatment, and the median pruritus scores were significantly reduced compared with baseline values.

Naltrexone does not relieve uremic pruritus: results of a randomized placebo-controlled crossover study. Pauli-Magnus C, Mikus G, Alscher DM, Kirschner T, Nagel W, Gugeler N, et al. J Am Soc Nephrol 2000; 11: 514–9.

In this double-blind, placebo-controlled, crossover study, 23 patients taking naltrexone 50 mg daily showed no difference in reported pruritus and intensity of pruritus scores compared with placebo.

This study contradicts the previous one. Why is not clear.

Kappa-opioid system in uremic pruritus: multicenter, randomized, double-blind, placebo-controlled clinical studies. Wikström B, Gellert R, Ladefoged SD, Danda Y, Akai M, Ide K, et al. J Am Soc Nephrol 2005; 16: 3742–7.

In this multicenter, randomized, double-blind, placebo-controlled study involving 144 patients with uremic pruritus, those who received posthemodialysis intravenous nalfurafine for 2 to 4 weeks reported significant reductions in itch intensity, sleep disturbances, and excoriations compared with placebo.

Nalfurafine hydrochloride for the treatment of pruritus. Inui S. Expert Opin Pharmacother 2012; 13: 1507–13.

A review that describes the pharmacology, efficacy, and potential adverse effects of nalfurafine hydrochloride, a combined mu-opioid receptor antagonist and kappa-opioid agonist, in the treatment of pruritus. It is not yet available in the United States.

Second-Line Therapies	
• Zinc sulfate	A
• Capsaicin 0.03% cream	A
• Acupuncture: Quchi (LI11) acupoint	A
• Homeopathic treatment with verum	A

Zinc sulfate for relief of pruritus in patients on maintenance hemodialysis. Najafabadi MM, Faghihi G, Emami A, Monghad M, Moeenzadeh F, Sharif N, et al. Ther Apher Dial 2012; 16: 142–5.

In this double-blind, randomized, placebo-controlled trial, 40 adults with end-stage renal disease (ESRD) on maintenance hemodialysis in two Iranian university hospitals were randomized to receive either zinc sulfate (440 mg/day) or placebo for 2 consecutive months. Pruritus was assessed at baseline and then every 2 weeks using a numeric rating scale from 0 to 10 until 1 month after treatment. Pruritus was decreased in both groups after treatment, but there was a significantly greater decrease in the zinc sulfate group compared with placebo ($p = 0.018$).

Topical capsaicin therapy for uremic pruritus in patients on hemodialysis. Makhlough A, Ala S, Haj-Heydari Z, Kashi Z, Bari A. Iran J Kidney Dis 2010; 4: 137–40.

In this randomized, double-blind, crossover clinical trial, 34 patients on hemodialysis with uremic pruritus were randomized to receive capsaicin 0.03% cream or placebo for 4 weeks. After a 2-week washout period, subjects crossed over arms. After each week of treatment, pruritus scores in the capsaicin arm were significantly ($p < 0.001$) improved compared with the placebo group. A repeated measurement test showed that the decrease in pruritus severity in the capsaicin group was greater than in the placebo group during the treatment period ($p < 0.001$).

Acupuncture in haemodialysis patients at the Quchi (LI11) acupoint for refractory uraemic pruritus. Che-Yi C, Wen CY, Min-Tsung K, Chiu-Ching H. Nephrol Dial Transplant 2005; 20: 1912–5.

In this randomized controlled study involving 40 patients with refractory uremic pruritus, those who received acupuncture applied unilaterally at the Quchi (LI11) acupoint thrice weekly for 1 month reported significantly reduced pruritus scores after acupuncture and at 3-month follow-up compared with acupuncture applied at a nonacupoint.

Effects of homeopathic treatment on pruritus of haemodialysis patients: a randomised placebo-controlled double-blind trial. Cavalcanti AM, Rocha LM, Carillo R Jr, Lima LU, Lugon JR. Homeopathy 2003; 92: 177–81.

In this double-blind, placebo-controlled, randomized trial of 28 hemodialysis patients, those who received verum reported significantly reduced pruritus scores throughout the trial compared with placebo. Patients reported a 49% reduction in the pruritus score at the end of the study.

Third-Line Therapies

• Cholestyramine	A
• Activated charcoal	D
• Thalidomide	B
• Parathyroidectomy	B

Cholestyramine in uraemic pruritus. Silverberg DS, Iaina A, Reisin E, Rotzak R, Eliahou HE. Br Med J 1977; 1: 752–3.

This randomized, placebo-controlled, double-blind study showed cholestyramine 5 g twice daily for 4 weeks improved pruritus in four of five subjects.

Relief of idiopathic generalized pruritus in dialysis patients treated with activated oral charcoal. Pederson JA, Matter BJ, Czerwinski AW, Llach F. Ann Intern Med 1980; 93: 446–8.

Oral charcoal 6 g daily for 8 weeks improved pruritus in 10 of 11 hemodialysis patients in this double-blind, placebo-controlled, crossover study.

Thalidomide for the treatment of uremic pruritus: a crossover randomized double-blind trial. Silva SR, Viana PC, Lugon NV, Hoette M, Ruzany F, Lugon JR. Nephron 1994; 67: 270–3.

Twenty-nine patients in this study were assigned to receive thalidomide or placebo at bedtime for 7 days. After a washout period of 7 days, drugs were crossed over. Over half of the patients had a greater than 50% reduction in pruritus while on thalidomide.

A study on pruritus after parathyroidectomy for secondary hyperparathyroidism. Chou F, Ji-Chen H, Shun-Chen H, Shyr-Ming S. J Am Coll Surg 2000; 190: 65–70.

Thirty-seven dialysis patients with secondary hyperparathyroidism underwent parathyroidectomy. Twenty-two patients had pruritus before parathyroidectomy, and in those patients with itch, pruritus scores improved significantly. This was accompanied by improvement in the calcium–phosphorus product.

ITCH ASSOCIATED WITH MALIGNANCY

Pruritus associated with malignancy is a common occurrence among patients with lymphomas and advanced malignancy. It may be one of the most bothersome symptoms to a cancer patient, and its management is challenging. The best evidence to date in the treatment of pruritus associated with malignancy exists for *paroxetine.*

First-Line Therapy

• Paroxetine	A

Paroxetine in the treatment of severe nondermatologic pruritus: a randomized, controlled trial. Zylicz Z, Krajnik M, Sorge AA, Costantini M. J Pain Symptom Manage 2003; 26: 1105–12.

This is a prospective, randomized, double-blind, placebo-controlled, crossover study involving 26 patients, of whom 17 had solid tumors, 4 had hematologic malignancies, and 5 had various nonmalignant conditions associated with pruritus. Patients reported significantly reduced pruritus intensity scores during treatment with paroxetine 20 mg daily. Nine of 24

patients completing the study experienced at least 50% reduction of intensity of pruritus. Onset of antipruritic action was observed usually after 2 to 3 days.

Second-Line Therapies

• Mirtazapine	E
• Butorphanol	E

Mirtazapine for pruritus. Davis MP, Frandsen JL, Walsh D, Andresen S, Taylor S. Pain Symptom Manage 2003; 25: 288–91.

In this case series of four patients with cholestasis, lymphoma, and uremic pruritus, each patient showed improvement in pruritus with mirtazapine 15 to 30 daily.

Butorphanol for treatment of intractable pruritus. Dawn AG, Yosipovitch G. J Am Acad Dermatol 2006; 54: 527–31.

In a patient with non-Hodgkin lymphoma and intractable pruritus, butorphanol 1 mg daily improved itch and sleep after only one dose without improvement of daytime itch. After undergoing chemotherapy with concurrent butorphanol 3 mg daily, the patient's pruritus resolved as the cancer regressed. Butorphanol is currently unavailable in the United States.

ITCH ASSOCIATED WITH HEMATOLOGIC DISORDERS

Pruritus associated with hematologic diseases (e.g., polycythemia vera and myelodysplastic syndrome) is often severe and intractable to the limited therapies available. *Phototherapy* remains the primary line of therapy for these patients.

First-Line Therapies

• Narrowband UVB phototherapy	D
• Psoralen photochemotherapy	D

Narrowband (TL-01) ultraviolet B phototherapy for pruritus in polycythaemia vera. Baldo A, Sammarco E, Plaitano R, Martinelli V, Monfrecola. Br J Dermatol 2002; 147: 979–81.

In this series, 10 patients with pruritus associated with polycythemia vera were treated with NB-UVB phototherapy thrice weekly. In 8 of 10 patients, complete remission of pruritus occurred within 2 to 10 weeks of treatment and a median cumulative dose of 5371.46 mJ/cm^2.

Efficacy of photochemotherapy on severe pruritus in polycythemia vera. Jeanmougin M, Rain JD, Najean Y. Ann Hematol 1996; 73: 91–3.

In this series, 10 of 11 patients with polycythemia rubra vera improved with psoralen photochemotherapy, and maintenance therapy was generally necessary.

The efficacy of psoralen photochemotherapy in the treatment of aquagenic pruritus. Menagé HD, Norris PG, Hawk JLM, Greaves MW. Br J Dermatol 1993; 129: 163–5.

In this series of five patients with aquagenic pruritus, psoralen photochemotherapy was an effective treatment. One patient had associated polycythemia rubra vera, and another had myelodysplastic syndrome. Maintenance therapy or a further course of PUVA was necessary to maintain remission.

Second-Line Therapies

- Paroxetine   **D**
- Fluoxetine   **E**

Selective serotonin reuptake inhibitors are effective in the treatment of polycythemia vera-associated pruritus. Tefferi A, Fonseca R. Blood 2002; 99: 2627.

In this series of patients with polycythemia vera–associated intractable pruritus, nine were treated with paroxetine 20 mg daily and one received fluoxetine 10 mg daily. All patients had a favorable initial response, and eight patients experienced complete or near-complete resolution of pruritus. Response occurred within 48 hours in most patients.

Third-Line Therapy

- Pregabalin   **E**

Pregabalin in the treatment of chronic pruritus. Ehrchen J, Ständer S. J Am Acad Dermatol 2008; 58: S36–7.

Two patients with aquagenic pruritus and one with idiopathic pruritus who had severe generalized itch were all treated with pregabalin initially at 75 mg twice daily and increased to 150 mg twice daily. The patients reported greater than 70% reduction of symptoms 5 to 8 weeks after starting therapy. The longest follow-up period was 6 months, at which time the effects of pregabalin were stable. Weight gain, somnolence, dizziness, and peripheral edema were observed side effects.

MISCELLANEOUS DISEASES ASSOCIATED WITH ITCH

Miscellaneous diseases associated with itch include psychogenic pruritus, nocturnal itch, HIV, hydroxyethyl starch deposition–induced pruritus, and essential pruritus of the elderly (Willan itch).

Paroxetine in a case of psychogenic pruritus and neurotic excoriations. Biondi M, Arcangeli T, Petrucci RM. Psychother Psychosom 2000; 69: 165–6.

In this case 20 to 30 mg daily of paroxetine reduced the sensation of itch in a patient with psychogenic pruritus and neurotic excoriations.

Mirtazapine for reducing nocturnal itch in patients with chronic pruritus: a pilot study. Hundley JL, Yosipovitch G. J Am Acad Dermatol 2004; 50: 889–91.

In this open, uncontrolled pilot study of three patients with inflammatory skin diseases and severe nocturnal pruritus, mirtazapine, a noradrenergic and specific serotonergic antidepressant, improved symptoms.

UVB phototherapy is an effective treatment for pruritus in patients infected with HIV. Lim HW, Vallurupalli S, Meola T, Soter NA. J Am Acad Dermatol 1997; 37: 414–7.

Twenty-one HIV-positive patients with pruritus treated with UVB phototherapy three times weekly reported reduced pruritus scores. A mean number of 20.7 ± 2.3 treatments resulted in maximal improvement.

Oxatomide in the treatment of pruritus senilis. A double-blind placebo-controlled trial. Dupont C, de Maubeuge J, Kotlar W, Lays Y, Masson M. Dermatologica 1984; 169: 348–53.

In this double-blind, placebo-controlled study involving 35 patients with pruritus senilis, oxatomide 30 mg twice daily for 2 months resulted in complete suppression or marked improvement of symptoms in 79% of treated patients.

Efficacy and safety of naltrexone, an oral opiate receptor antagonist, in the treatment of pruritus in internal and dermatological diseases. Metze D, Reimann S, Beissert S, Luger TA. J Am Acad Dermatol 1999; 41: 533–9.

Fifty patients with itch of various causes were treated with naltrexone 50 milligrams daily; 70% of patients achieved a significant therapeutic response as demonstrated by improvement in a VAS for itch. Seventeen patients developed peripheral neuropathy.

Transnasal butorphanol for the treatment of opioid-induced pruritus unresponsive to antihistamines. Dunteman E, Karanikolas M, Filos KS. J Pain Symptom Manage 1996; 12: 255–60.

All six patients with opioid-induced pruritus who received 2 mg intranasal butorphanol every 4 to 6 hours reported significant relief from pruritus. Five patients noted an improvement within 15 minutes.

Butorphanol for treatment of intractable pruritus. Dawn AG, Yosipovitch G. J Am Acad Dermatol 2006; 54: 527–31.

Butorphanol, a kappa-opioid agonist and mu-opioid antagonist, resulted in rapid and marked improvement in five patients with intractable pruritus associated with inflammatory skin diseases or systemic diseases. The combination of a kappa-opioid agonist with a mu-opioid antagonist holds out much promise. Oral preparations are under investigation.

Antipruritic treatment with systemic μ opioid receptor antagonists: a review. Phan NQ, Bernhard JD, Luger TA, Ständer S. J Am Acad Dermatol 2010; 63: 680–8.

This review discusses the antipruritic action of systemic mu-opioid receptor antagonists, including naloxone, nalmefene, and naltrexone, which are used in the treatment of chronic cholestatic and several other types of pruritus.

Systemic kappa opioid receptor agonists in the treatment of chronic pruritus: a literature review. Phan NQ, Lotts T, Antal A, Bernhard JD, Ständer S. Acta Derm Venereol 2012; 92: 555–60.

An overview of the promising role of kappa-opioid receptor agonists in the pathophysiology and treatment of pruritus.

Pruritus ani

Michal Martinka, Gabriele Weichert

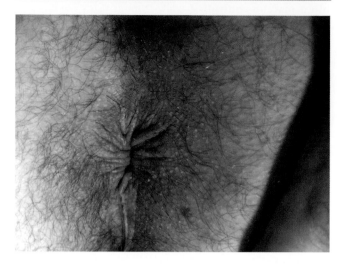

Pruritus ani is characterized by intensely pruritic perianal skin. It is classified into primary (idiopathic) and secondary (induced by an underlying cause). It is common, with incidence ranging from 1% to 5%. Chronic cases are associated with significant discomfort, embarrassment, and sleep disturbance.

MANAGEMENT STRATEGY

Diagnosis requires a detailed search for a potential cause. Categories include inflammatory (atopic dermatitis, psoriasis, or lichen sclerosus), infectious (bacterial, viral, fungal, parasitic, or infestations), systemic disease (diabetes, thyroid disorders, hepatic disorders, leukemia, and lymphoma), local irritants (fecal contamination, moisture, soaps, diet, topical or systemic medications), and colorectal and anal causes (hemorrhoids, anal fissures, diarrhea). A complete history, including diet, bowel movements, cleansing techniques, and treatments, is prudent, and patients should undergo a total body skin examination to identify other underlying etiologies. With this approach, most causes of secondary pruritus can be identified and treated. It is the patient in whom none of these factors are identified who suffers from idiopathic pruritus ani.

Overcleansing is not uncommon and may be irritating or sensitizing. Potential topical sensitizers should be stopped. *Avoidance of toilet paper* after bowel movements can be helpful, as this may be abrasive. Many patients suffer from low-grade fecal incontinence. This is often evident on examination of the underclothes or of the perianal skin.

Therapy is directed at the underlying cause. However, if secondary causes have been ruled out and a diagnosis of primary pruritus ani has been made, empiric treatment is directed toward proper anal hygiene, removal of common irritators, and protection of perianal skin. Advise patients to cleanse the perianal skin twice a day and after bowel movements using cotton balls or cotton squares (make-up removal pads) moistened with warm water or a liquid cleanser and then dried with a hair drier on "cool" setting. Patients with low-grade

fecal incontinence should perform this routine several times a day. *Cleansing* has been shown to be as effective as topical steroids. A short (few weeks) course of a *low- to midpotency topical steroid* is recommended. Caution must be taken with prolonged high-potency steroid use, as this area is prone to atrophy. *Topical tacrolimus* may be used in clearance or maintenance treatment. After cleansing, *topical zinc paste* can limit the degree of irritant dermatitis in patients with fecal incontinence. A *sedating antihistamine* may provide welcome sleep in the early weeks of treatment.

A *biopsy* should be performed if the diagnosis is in doubt or the condition is not responding to treatment. If a patient fails to improve, lower gastrointestinal investigations should be considered to rule out neoplastic disease. *Patch testing* should be performed in patients who fail to improve. Avoidance of caffeine and increased dietary fiber intake may be helpful. For a second-line therapy, *topical capsaicin* can be used. Capsaicin will initially cause perianal irritation in most patients during therapy. Finally, *intralesional steroid* injections to the perianal skin may be considered. *Intradermal methylene blue* injections are reported to damage dermal nerve endings and provide relief. *Injection with phenol in almond oil* has been reported to be beneficial.

Specific Investigations

- Bacterial swab
- Fungal microscopy and culture
- Biopsy
- Skin scrapings for scabies
- Patch testing
- Gastrointestinal investigations

Pruritus ani: diagnosis and treatment. Nasseri Y, Osborne M. Gastroenterol Clin North Am 2013; 42: 801–13.

Over 100 different etiologies have been reported to cause pruritus ani.

Allergic contact dermatitis in patients with anogenital complaints. Bauer A, Geier J, Elsner P. J Reprod Med 2000; 45: 649–54.

A 5-year collection of patients demonstrated an increased incidence of benzocaine and (chloro-)methyl-isothiazolinone allergy. A diagnosis of allergic contact dermatitis was made in 34.8%. The authors recommend using the standard tray plus dibucaine, propolis, bufexamac, and other ingredients gained from the patient's history.

Pruritus ani as a manifestation of systemic contact dermatitis: resolution with dietary nickel restriction. Silvestri D, Barmettler S. Dermatitis 2011; 22: 50–5.

A patient with recalcitrant pruritus ani was found to be highly nickel allergic on patch testing. A low-nickel diet led to resolution of his symptoms, and recurrence appeared with rechallenge.

Abnormal transient internal sphincter relaxation in idiopathic pruritus ani: physiological evidence from ambulatory monitoring. Farouk R, Duthie GS, Pryde A, Bartolo DC. Br J Surg 1994; 81: 603–6.

Abnormal rectal sphincter tone was demonstrated in patients with pruritus ani. This may well be the contributing factor in patients who have occult fecal leakage as a component of their itch.

Evidence Levels: **A** Double-blind study **B** Clinical trial ≥ 20 subjects **C** Clinical trial < 20 subjects **D** Series ≥ 5 subjects **E** Anecdotal case reports

Pruritus ani. Causes and concerns. Daniel GL, Longo WE, Vernava AM. Dis Colon Rectum 1994; 37: 670–4.

In this series of 104 patients, 52% had anorectal disease (including hemorrhoids, anal fissures, genital warts, and fistulas) and 23% had a colorectal neoplasm found with investigations. In those without neoplasia, there was a direct correlation between increased caffeine intake and severity of irritation. Patients with primary pruritus ani improved with dietary restrictions (not defined), dietary fiber, steroid creams, and drying agents.

First-Line Therapies

• Topical corticosteroids	A
• Topical tacrolimus	A
• Hygiene	B

1% hydrocortisone ointment is an effective treatment of pruritus ani: a pilot randomized control crossover trial. Al-Ghnaniem R, Short K, Pullen A, Fuller LC, Rennie JA, Leather AJ. Int J Colorectal Dis 2007; 22: 1463–7.

Nineteen patients were randomized to 1% hydrocortisone in paraffin twice daily or paraffin base for 2 weeks followed by crossover treatment for 2 weeks. Visual analog score (VAS) showed a 68% reduction with steroid treatment.

Randomized study of topical tacrolimus ointment as possible treatment for resistant idiopathic pruritus ani. Suys E. J Am Acad Dermatol 2012; 66: 327–8.

Twenty-one patients were randomized to 0.1% tacrolimus versus petrolatum twice daily for 4 weeks with a further 4-week crossover phase. There was improvement in itch intensity and frequency on tacrolimus, but Dermatology Life Quality Index (DLQI) was not significantly different compared with placebo. One patient had a temporary burning sensation.

Idiopathic perianal pruritus: washing compared with topical corticosteroids. Oztas MO, Oztas P, Onder M. Postgrad Med J 2004; 80: 295–7.

In this study, 28 patients applied topical methylprednisolone cream twice daily for 2 weeks. In a separate group, 32 patients were instructed to cleanse the perianal area twice daily with a liquid cleanser. Effectiveness was similar at 92.3% in the first and 90.6% in the second group.

Second-Line Therapies

• Topical capsaicin	A
• Topical acrylate barrier	D

Topical capsaicin: a novel and effective treatment for idiopathic intractable pruritus ani: a randomised, placebo controlled, crossover study. Lysy J, Sistiery-Ittah M, Israelit Y, Shmueli A, Strauss-Liviatan N, Mindrul V, et al. Gut 2003; 52: 1323–6.

Capsaicin 0.006% cream was applied three times a day for 1 month. The control treatment was 1% menthol cream. Of 44 patients, 31 experienced partial relief of symptoms ($p < 0.0001$). All patients experienced some degree of perianal burning. The menthol cream was not effective.

A liquid-forming acrylate cream for the treatment of anal pruritus. Tomi N, Weiser R, Strohal R, Mittlboeck M. Br J Nurs 2012; 21: 98–102.

Twenty-eight patients applied an acrylate protection cream (Cavilon Durable Barrier Cream, 3M) daily for 3 weeks. There was an 80% reduction in VAS.

Third-Line Therapies

• Intralesional corticosteroids	C
• Intradermal methylene blue	B
• Subcutaneous phenol injection	B

The use of intralesional triamcinolone hexacetonide in the treatment of idiopathic pruritus ani. Minvielle L, Hernandez VL. Dis Colon Rectum 1969; 12: 340–3.

Nineteen patients were treated weekly for 4 weeks at 5 to 20 mg/week. Nine of 19 (73.6%) patients had excellent progress, 2 of 19 reported fair improvement, and 3 failed to improve. No perianal atrophy was noted at the end of 4 weeks.

Long-term results of single intradermal 1% methylene blue injection for intractable idiopathic pruritus ani: a prospective study. Samalavicius N, Poskus T, Gupta R, Lunevicius R. Tech Coloproctol 2012; 16: 295–7.

Ten patients received 15 mL of 1% methylene blue intradermally; all had initial resolution of symptoms at 4 weeks. At 60-month follow-up, six patients felt better than baseline or had complete resolution of symptoms.

Methylene blue has been shown by electron microscopy to cause damage to dermal nerve endings. This is the proposed mechanism of action for this modality.

A new concept of the anatomy of the anal sphincter mechanism and the physiology of defecation. XXIII. An injection technique for the treatment of idiopathic pruritus ani. Shafik A. Int Surg 1990; 75: 43–6.

In this series, 67 patients were treated with an injection of 5% phenol in almond oil: 62/67 (92.4%) experienced complete relief. Five patients relapsed. Repeat injection led to cure.

Pruritus vulvae

Ginat W. Mirowski, Bethanee J. Schlosser

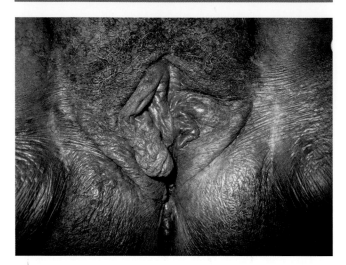

Pruritus vulvae is the external sensation of itching that results in a need to scratch or rub the vulva. Primary findings are representative of the underlying disease process and may include macular or papular erythema, cigarette-paper atrophy, dyspigmentation, and erosion; scale is rarely seen due to the inherently moist environment. Secondary findings include lichenification, erosions, fissures, and pigmentary changes from scratching. Vaginal discharge is normal. Pruritus vulvae may be primary (essential), secondary, or multifactorial. Essential pruritus vulvae is the condition in which no etiology can be identified. Regardless of etiology, long-standing pruritus vulvae may result in lichenification indistinguishable from lichen simplex chronicus.

MANAGEMENT STRATEGY

Pruritus vulvae describes a symptom that may be both psychologically distressing and socially embarrassing. An underlying etiology should be sought by obtaining a thorough history and performing a mucocutaneous physical examination. Examination findings may include both primary and secondary. A personal or family history of any inflammatory dermatosis may direct the differential diagnosis. Secondary pruritus vulvae may be caused by infections, dermatoses, systemic diseases, and malignant or premalignant lesions. Appropriate treatment should be instituted.

If no etiology is identified, then symptomatic relief is the goal of therapy. The tenets of treatment are to interrupt the itch–scratch cycle, restore the skin barrier, and minimize impact on quality of life.

The mainstay of treatment of pruritus vulvae is to *identify and remove all suspected local irritants and allergens*. The patient should be instructed to discontinue all local products, including soaps, personal hygiene products, sanitary pads, medications (complementary/alternative, nonprescription, and prescription), and occlusive/synthetic clothing. The patient should bathe with lukewarm (not hot) water, pat (not rub) dry, wipe from front to back, change underpants daily, and launder clothing using a double-rinse cycle. The patient may resist these measures, as they may believe in the need to have a "clean" vulva and that natural secretions and odors are offensive or the cause of their symptoms. The patient may develop elaborate hygiene regimens that contribute to local irritation and contact sensitivity and may confound or be the primary cause of persistent pruritus. Toilet (tissue) paper and commercial wipes may contribute to local irritation. Furthermore, both may contain allergens such as formaldehyde, benzalkonium chloride, and fragrance that could contribute to persistent pruritus. Talc and other powders may combine with sweat to cause mechanical irritation much like fine sandpaper. Furthermore, there is increasing evidence regarding an association between the use of talc in the genital area and ovarian cancer. Urine, stool, sweat, and cervical or vaginal secretions may contribute to local irritation. Urinary incontinence and contact with stool should be addressed. Cotton washcloths, cool Sitz baths, and use of fragrance-free feminine hygiene products should be advocated.

The use of *barrier petrolatum- and zinc-based ointments*, used to prevent diaper rash in both children and adults, helps to seal in moisture and protect the affected skin. In low-estrogen states (postpartum, lactation, perimenopause, and postmenopause), the use of topical or systemic estrogen helps restore vaginal and vulvar mucosal barrier function.

Systemic or topical corticosteroids are used to reduce inflammation. Ointment-based formulations are preferred for the following reasons: 1) ointments are water insoluble and will not be diluted in the naturally moist vulvar environment; 2) ointments serve as a barrier against further external chemical and physical insults; and 3) ointments generally contain fewer inactive ingredients, which may be potential irritants or allergens. Topical preparations may contribute to allergic or irritant contact dermatitis due either to inactive ingredients or, less commonly, due to the corticosteroid itself. Corticosteroid ointment, used sparingly, should be applied once or twice a day. Close clinical supervision is necessary to minimize adverse effects such as striae, folliculitis, and atrophy. Systemic agents are used to treat infections and to provide symptomatic relief of pruritus in order to limit complications of local agents. *Intralesional triamcinolone acetonide injection* and *systemic corticosteroids* may be effective for recalcitrant pruritus.

Although corticosteroids reduce pruritus, they are often not sufficient to interrupt the itch–scratch cycle. Nightly *sedating antihistamines* such as hydroxyzine or doxepin are recommended. For daytime pruritus, a low-dose *selective serotonin reuptake inhibitor (SSRI)* is advised.

Specific Investigations

- Visual and manual examination of the vulva, vagina, perianal skin, and the complete mucocutaneous integument, including the oral cavity, conjunctivae, total body skin, scalp, and nails
- Palpation of inguinal lymph nodes
- Sensory testing for light touch and Q-Tip evaluation of vulva and vaginal vestibule
- Saline wet mount of vaginal secretions (cytologic evaluation, presence of lactobacilli, *Trichomonas vaginalis*, bacterial vaginosis)
- Whiff test (bacterial vaginosis)
- KOH (fungi, scabies)
- Vaginal pH (bacterial vaginosis, atrophic vaginitis)
- Tape test (*Enterobius vermicularis*)
- Microbiologic tests (bacterial, fungal, viral)

Evidence Levels: **A** Double-blind study **B** Clinical trial ≥ 20 subjects **C** Clinical trial < 20 subjects **D** Series ≥ 5 subjects **E** Anecdotal case reports

- Laboratory tests (fasting blood glucose, liver/renal/thyroid function, complete blood count with differential, iron studies including ferritin)
- Biopsy (H&E, direct immunofluorescence, special stains)
- Wood lamp (erythrasma)
- Patch testing (allergic contact dermatitis)
- Colposcopy (in consultation with gynecology, vulvar intraepithelial neoplasia, anal intraepithelial neoplasia)
- Nerve conduction studies (neuropathy)

Anogenital pruritus – an overview. Swamiappan M. J Clin Diagn Res 2016; 10: WE10–3.

Excellent review of anogenital pruritus with emphasis on pathophysiology of itch.

Clinical care of vulvar pruritus, with emphasis on one cause, lichen simplex chronicus. Stewart KM. Dermatol Clin 2010; 28: 669–80.

An excellent review on the treatment of vulvar pruritus. Extensive clinical differential diagnosis is also discussed. The author focuses on lichen simplex chronicus as a primary etiology of vulvar itch.

An approach to the treatment of anogenital pruritus. Weichert GE. Dermatol Ther 2004; 17: 129–33.

Reviews the common causes of acute and chronic anogenital pruritus with a focus on vulvar pruritus. The therapeutic approach to the management of pruritus vulvae in the absence of a clear cause is discussed.

Recurrent vulvovaginal candidosis: focus on the vulva. Beikert FC, Le MT, Koeninger A, Technau K, Clad A. Mycoses 2011; 54: e807–10.

A prospective study of 139 women with recurrent vulvovaginal candidiasis revealed a positive correlation between pruritus and *Candida albicans*–positive vulvar fungal cultures (OR 5.4).

Pruritus in diabetes mellitus: investigation of prevalence and correlation with diabetes. Neilly JB, Martin A, Simpson N, MacCuish AC. Diabetes Care 1986; 9: 273–5.

Three hundred diabetic and 100 nondiabetic outpatients were evaluated for the presence of generalized and localized pruritus. Pruritus vulvae, the most common symptom, was noted in 18.4% of diabetic women. This was significant ($p < 0.05$), as only 5.6% of nondiabetic women had pruritus vulvae. Symptoms correlated with glycosylated hemoglobin.

Vulvar intraepithelial neoplasia (VIN) diagnostic and therapeutic challenges. Rodolakis A, Diakomanolis E, Vlachos G, Iconomou T, Protopappas A, Stefanidis C, et al. Eur J Gynaecol Oncol 2003; 24: 317–22.

A retrospective study of 113 women with VIN revealed that pruritus was the most common presenting symptom (60.1%). Diagnosis was made by colposcopy and biopsy.

Prospective study of patch testing in patients with vulval pruritus. Haverhoek E, Reid C, Gordon L, Marshman G, Wood J, Selva-Nayagam P. Australas J Dermatol 2008; 49: 80–5.

Forty-four percent of 43 women with vulval pruritus demonstrated one or more relevant contact allergens.

Patients with vulval pruritus: patch test results. Utas S, Ferahbas A, Yildiz S. Contact Dermatitis 2008; 58: 296–8.

Sixteen percent of 50 women with vulval pruritus exhibited one or more relevant allergen reactions. The most common relevant allergens included cosmetics, preservatives, and medications.

Neuropathic scrotal pruritus: anogenital pruritus is a symptom of lumbosacral radiculopathy. Cohen AD, Vander T, Medvendovsky E, Biton A, Naimer S, Shalev R, et al. J Am Acad Dermatol 2005; 52: 61–6.

The role of radiculopathies or pudendal nerve entrapment as a cause of vulvar pruritus is recognized but has not been studied.

Similarities between neuropathic pruritus sites and lichen simplex chronicus sites. Cohen AD, Andrews ID, Medvedovsky E, Peleg R, Vardy DA. Isr Med Assoc J 2014; 16: 88–90.

A large clinical study utilizing nerve conduction studies revealed neuropathy in more than 80% (29 of 36) of patients with anogenital pruritus.

First-Line Therapies

• Oral naltrexone	C
• Topical pimecrolimus	C
• Avoidance of irritants	E
• Hygiene	E
• Topical estrogen	E

Treatment of refractory vulvovaginal pruritus with naltrexone, a specific opiate antagonist. Bottcher B, Wildt L. Eur J Obstet Gynecol Reprod Biol 2014; 174: 115–6.

Initial report detailing the rapid and complete response to oral naltrexone 50 mg once daily in 5 women otherwise healthy with long-standing vulvovaginal pruritus.

Pimecrolimus 1% cream for pruritus in postmenopausal diabetic women with vulvar lichen simplex chronicus: a prospective non-controlled case series. Kelekci HK, Uncu HG, Yilmaz B, Ozdemir O, Sut N, Kelekci S. J Dermatolog Treat 2008; 19: 274–8.

A study of pimecrolimus 1% cream for vulvar lichen simplex chronicus in 12 postmenopausal diabetic women revealed significant improvement in patient-reported pruritus and clinical examination findings.

Efficacy of topical pimecrolimus in the treatment of chronic vulvar pruritus. A prospective case series: a non-controlled, open-label study. Sarifakioglu E, Gumus II. J Dermatol Treat 2006; 17: 276–8.

In 15 patients with chronic vulvar pruritus, pimecrolimus 1% cream applied twice daily for 1 month resulted in complete response in 10 patients and improvement in 3; 2 patients did not return for follow-up.

Contact dermatitis of the vulva. Schlosser BJ. Dermatol Clin 2010; 28: 697–706.

A comprehensive review of irritant and allergic contact dermatitis of the vulva. Avoidance of irritants and potential allergens and the importance of patient education are emphasized.

Lichen simplex chronicus (atopic/neurodermatitis) of the anogenital region. Lynch P. Dermatol Ther 2004; 17: 8–19.

This paper suggests diagnostic tips and a differential diagnosis for vulvar lichen simplex chronicus. The management of lichen simplex chronicus is divided into four categories: identification of any underlying disease, repair of the barrier layer function, reduction of inflammation, and breaking of the itch–scratch cycle. Treatment options for each category are discussed.

Pruritus vulvae in prepubertal children. Paek SC, Merritt DF, Mallory SB. J Am Acad Dermatol 2001; 44: 795–802.

This paper reviews the causes and treatments of pruritus vulvae in 44 prepubertal girls. Seventy-five percent had nonspecific pruritus. Lichen sclerosus, bacterial infections, yeast infection, and pinworm infestation were seen in a minority of patients. Poor hygiene and irritants are major contributors to pruritus vulvae in this population.

The common problem of vulvar pruritus. Bornstein J, Pascal B, Abramovici H. Obstet Gynecol Surv 1993; 48: 111–8.

The authors of this review article recommend stopping use of all soaps, douches, and perfumed deodorants, keeping the vulva dry, wearing cotton underpants, and avoiding tight pants as basic principles in the treatment of pruritus vulvae.

Vulvovaginal dryness and itching. Margesson LJ. Skin Ther Letter 2001; 6: 3–4.

Vulvar signs of estrogen deficiency and treatment options are discussed.

Second-Line Therapies

• Topical antihistamine	A
• Subcutaneous triamcinolone	B

Efficacy of topical oxatomide in women with pruritus vulva. Origoni M, Garsia S, Sideri M, Pifarotti G, Nicora M. Drugs Exp Clin Res 1990; 16: 591–6.

A double-blind, controlled study evaluated the efficacy of topical oxatomide, an antihistamine available in Europe but not in the United States, in 29 patients with pruritus vulvae. All patients reported improvement in both intensity and duration of itching. Seven patients experienced complete regression. Results were statistically significant ($p < 0.001$) compared with placebo.

No follow-up studies on the use of topical oxatomide in pruritus vulvae have been published.

Subcutaneous injection of triamcinolone acetonide in the treatment of chronic vulvar pruritus. Kelly RA, Foster DC, Woodruff JD. Am J Obstet Gynecol 1993; 169: 568–70.

A series of 45 patients with chronic pruritus vulvae were treated with subcutaneous intralesional injection of triamcinolone acetonide (total 15–20 mg) into the vulva. Thirty-five experienced relief of pruritus for more than 1 month (mean 5.8 months).

Third-Line Therapies

• Acupuncture	D
• Gonadotropin-releasing hormone	E
• Hypnosis	E

56 cases of chronic pruritus vulvae treated with acupuncture. Huang WY, Guo ZR, Yu J, Hu XL. J Trad Chin Med 1987; 7: 1–3.

Fifty-four of 56 patients with intractable pruritus vulvae experienced symptomatic and clinical improvement with up to seven sessions of acupuncture.

Chronic vulvovaginal pruritus treated successfully with GnRH analogue. Banerjee AK, de Chazal R. Postgrad Med J 2006; 82: e22.

A case report of a 35-year-old woman with intractable cyclical vulvovaginal itching. Suppression of ovulation and empiric treatment with intramuscular injection of leuprorelin acetate (a GnRH analog) for 4 weeks resulted in complete resolution of symptoms. Autoimmune progesterone dermatitis was hypothesized as the primary etiology. The patient declined a progesterone challenge test. Pruritus did not recur with resumption of normal menses.

Hypnosis in a case of long-standing idiopathic itch. Rucklidge JJ, Saunders D. Psychosom Med 1999; 61: 355–8.

A case report of long-standing pruritus vulvae and ani with complete relief of symptoms after training in self-hypnosis.

Effectiveness of treating non-specific pruritus vulvae with topical steroids: a randomized controlled trial. Lagro-Janssen AL, Sluis A. Eur J Gen Pract 2009; 15: 29–33.

A randomized, double-blind, placebo-controlled trial of 50 women with nonspecific vulvar pruritus showed no difference between triamcinolone acetonide 0.1% cream and placebo. Patients with infections and inflammatory dermatoses were excluded.

In contrast to the well-established effectiveness of topical corticosteroids for treating lichen sclerosus–associated pruritus, topical corticosteroids appear to have no benefit in the treatment of nonspecific pruritus vulvae.

Evidence Levels: **A** Double-blind study **B** Clinical trial ≥ 20 subjects **C** Clinical trial < 20 subjects **D** Series ≥ 5 subjects **E** Anecdotal case reports

208

Pseudofolliculitis barbae

Gary J. Brauner

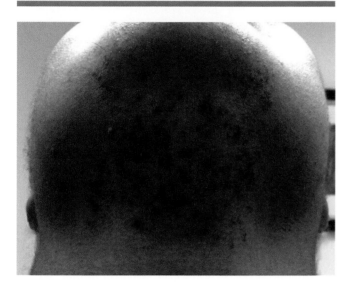

Pseudofolliculitis barbae (PFB) is a chronic inflammatory disease of hair-bearing areas induced by shaving or plucking of curved hairs, with resultant transepithelial or transfollicular penetration by the sharpened hair remnant and a foreign body reaction. It is characterized clinically by papules, papulopustules, focal or diffuse postinflammatory hyperpigmentation, growth grooves, and rarely hypertrophic or keloidal scarring.

MANAGEMENT STRATEGY

PFB is usually a straightforward clinical diagnosis. As it is induced by hair manipulation (i.e., shaving or plucking), it is not associated with other diseases. Differential diagnoses include true bacterial folliculitis requiring systemic antibiotics and, rarely, yeast folliculitis. Careful clinical inspection and possibly skin biopsy should be performed to rule out granulomatous disease such as sarcoidosis or dental sinusitis in the presence of apparently hypertrophic or keloidal scars. Rarely, ciclosporin therapy may induce a pseudofolliculitis-like condition. Recent French literature cites necrotic folliculitis–like lesions and pathergy as common cutaneous presentations of Behçet syndrome; this "pseudofolliculitis" is not the PFB of ingrowing hairs.

Because this process is induced by shaving, its cure is simple: by *not shaving* or plucking at all and allowing the hairs to grow to beyond 1 cm in length, the disease will spontaneously involute. If a clean-shaven appearance is preferred or deemed necessary by occupational or social demands, management involves three elements: *extraction of the foreign body* by lifting the embedded distal sharpened ends of hairs, *prevention of further embedding* by proper shaving technique or permanent disruption of the follicle's ability to produce new hair, and *treatment of postinflammatory hyperpigmentation or hypertrophic scarring*.

Embedded hairs should be *lifted*, not plucked, just before shaving. A safety razor set on its "gentlest" setting, or a preadjusted razor such as the PFB Bumpfighter, should be used but with the

opposite hand kept off the face to prevent skin stretching. Shaving is performed in the direction of hair growth, not against it, again to prevent too-close shaving and transfollicular penetration. A *long presoak* with a hot wet facecloth will allow hairs to swell and lift; a shaving cream that lathers and holds well will keep those hairs saturated and elevated. Shaving must be performed daily; by 2 to 3 days of no shaving, transepidermal reentry penetration will occur. If morning shaving is routine, the affected areas should be gently *buffed* or brushed the evening before with a toothbrush, a rough dry washcloth, or a Buf Puf to loosen hairs about to embed.

Hair clippers will cut hair closely but not so close as to allow transfollicular penetration. Because razor shaving is much closer, clippers should be used at least twice daily to avoid a permanent "5 o'clock shadow."

Powder chemical depilatories are not practical. They are messy to use, hard to mix accurately, difficult to remove rapidly, and, because they are so irritating, cannot be used more than every 3 days, which already allows PFB to recur. Lotion depilatories are much easier to apply and remove and, being less irritating, can be used every 2 days to produce a satisfactory cosmetic appearance.

Antibiotics are not necessary because this is a sterile foreign body reaction. Irritants such as *retinoic acid* or *glycolic acid* may enhance lifting of hairs and diminish hyperpigmentation.

Several longer wavelength long pulsed *lasers* (alexandrite, 810-nm diode, and Nd:YAG) or intense pulse light (IPL) sources combined with epidermal protective chilling devices can be used to produce dramatic long-lasting remission, even in Fitzpatrick types IV, V, and VI patients and represent a breakthrough treatment for recalcitrant disease. Caution must be employed in dosage selection based on the patient's underlying skin color, because the hyperpigmented papules themselves may act as highly absorbing hotspots not anticipated by overall lighter skin color and may develop visible burns. Hyperpigmentation may involute without specific bleaching agents as the inflammation subsides when hairs disappear. Otherwise strategies employing techniques for both epidermal and tattoolike dermal pigmentation need to be attempted.

Specific Investigation

- Skin biopsy in rare instances

Scar sarcoidosis in pseudofolliculitis barbae. Norton S, Chesser R, Fitzpatrick J. Military Med 1991; 156: 369–71.

A man with hilar adenopathy had smooth, firm, purplish papules (lupus pernio) on his face and PFB in his beard area. Biopsies of papules of both the lupus pernio and the PFB revealed noncaseating granulomas consistent with sarcoidosis.

Pseudofolliculitis barbae induced by oral minoxidil. Liew H, Morris-Jones R, Diaz-Cano S, Bashir S. Clin Exp Dermatol 2012; 37: 800–1.

A 61-year-old Afro-Caribbean man with chronic folliculitis of his face and scalp complicated by *Pseudomonas* and enterococcal infection and resulting in papules mimicking keloids, all of which appeared after institution of oral minoxidil (for hypertension) with accompanying increased growth of hair and ceasing only with termination of minoxidil therapy.

Pseudofolliculitis is not demonstrated clinically or histologically in this mistitled paper; folliculitis papillaris with pyoderma is a more appropriate diagnosis.

Disseminated cryptococcosis presenting as pseudofolliculitis in an AIDS patient. Coker L, Swain R, Morris R, McCall C. Cutis 2000; 66: 207–10.

A 42-year-old African American man with AIDS had countless dome-shaped excoriated papules on his trunk, arms, and face, initially diagnosed as folliculitis (not pseudofolliculitis of ingrowing hairs) with biopsy-proven disseminated cutaneous cryptococcosis.

Hyperplastic pseudofolliculitis barbae associated with cyclosporine. Lear J, Bourke JF, Burns DA. Br J Dermatol 1997; 136: 132–3.

A condition resembling keloid reactions in PFB is reported as an unusual reaction to ciclosporin.

Hypertrophic pseudofolliculitis in white renal transplant recipients. Lally A, Wojnarowska F. Clin Exp Dermatol 2007; 32: 268–71.

Five cases of hyperplastic PFB in white patients with renal transplants and ciclosporin immunosuppression are reported with chin involvement in all, but two also had involvement of the nose and occiput, which is otherwise never seen.

The photographs reveal folliculitis papillaris, not PFB.

First-Line Therapies	
• Beard growth	D
• Razor shaving technique	D
• Hair clippers	D
• Chemical depilatories	D
• Adjunctive hair extraction	D

Pseudofolliculitis of the beard. Strauss J, Kligman A. Arch Dermatol Syphilol 1956; 74: 533–42.

The first modern description of the pathogenesis of this disease and the rationale for allowing beard growth and spontaneous involution.

Pseudofolliculitis barbae. Medical consequences of interracial friction in the US Army. Brauner G, Flandermeyer K. Cutis 1979; 23: 61–6.

PFB is a minor disease affecting only, and almost all, black people who shave. Due to the continued requirement of the U.S. Army for clean-shaven faces, significant interracial turmoil and animosity have been aroused. Unclear standards of care of the disease and haphazard policing of shaving habits led to a chaotic process, with effective dermatologic care almost paralyzed by the hostile parties. During the Vietnam War era randomly approached lower ranking enlistees and draftees were much more likely to complain about their disease, even if minor, and were more likely to refuse to shave and be unkempt even without permission to grow a beard (in contravention of Army regulations). Career black enlistees are likely to underreport the severity of their disease and not seek medical help, possibly because of fear of continuous harassment and inability to be promoted by their superiors. Lotion depilatories or hair clippers, combined with routine lifting of ingrown hairs, are the most effective treatments, although complete cessation of shaving is required first.

Pseudofolliculitis barbae. 2. Treatment. Brauner G, Flandermeyer K. Int J Dermatol 1977; 16: 520–5.

The disease can be cured only by complete cessation of shaving, but it can be adequately controlled in most patients by carefully shaving the hairs neither too close nor too long and by meticulous lifting out of penetrating hairs.

A variety of practical methods of shaving are described in detail.

Comparative evaluation of men's depilatory composition versus razor in black men. Kindred C, Oresajo C, Yatskayer M, Halder R. Cutis 2011; 88: 98–103.

The authors studied 45 black men over a period of only 1 week with shaving on Saturday of the whole face and then shaving every 2 days on one side of the face and using one of two patient-mixed and applied depilatory pastes or a depilatory cream to the other side. The results confirmed observations by this author (see earlier) 45 years ago that pastes cannot be safely applied for shaving every 2 days without intolerable irritation, and only a depilatory cream can be so used. The depilatories improved tactile and visual roughness and unevenness better than every-other-day shaving, which is not surprising because nondaily shaving promotes the appearance and persistence of PFB.

Use of depilatory cream every 2 days and shaving daily on "virginal skin" after total clearance of PFB by beard growth for 1 month and follow-up for 1 month would have more accurately represented how proper shaving technique is done and provided an accurate comparison.

Pseudofolliculitis barbae and related disorders. Halder R. Dermatol Clin 1988; 6: 407–12.

Not all regimens will work for each patient. This thorough review discusses beards, triple "O" electric clippers, chemical depilatories, safety razors including the foil-guarded system to reduce cutting edge, electric razors including the adjustable three-headed rotary razor, manual lifting of hairs, tretinoin lotion, electrolysis, and surgical depilation.

Pseudofolliculitis barbae and acne keloidalis nuchae. Kelly A. Dermatol Clin 2003; 21: 645–53.

Concise review with good descriptions of various and specific shaving devices.

Second-Line Therapies	
• Retinoic acid	E
• Glycolic acid	B
• Topical clindamycin	A

Pseudofolliculitis of the beard and topically applied tretinoin. Kligman A, Mills O. Arch Dermatol 1973; 107: 5515–2.

Tretinoin solution is described as a useful adjunctive treatment.

Pseudofolliculitis: revised concepts of diagnosis and treatment. Report of three cases in women. Hall J, Goetz C, Bartholome C, Livingood C. Cutis 1979; 23: 798–800.

Three cases are described in black American women. Topical retinoic acid cream was useful in all three.

Twice-daily applications of benzoyl peroxide 5%/clindamycin 1% gel versus vehicle in the treatment of pseudofolliculitis barbae. Cook-Bolden F, Barba A, Halder R, Taylor S. Cutis 2004; 73: 18–24.

Seventy-seven men with 16 to 100 combined papules and pustules on the face and neck were randomized to receive twice-daily benzoyl peroxide 5%/clindamycin 1% (BP/C) gel or vehicle for 10 weeks; 77.3% of the participants were black. All patients were required to shave at least twice a week with a disposable Bumpfighter razor and to use a standardized shaving regimen. At weeks 2, 4, and 6, mean percentage reductions from baseline in combined papule and pustule counts were statistically significantly greater with BP/C gel than with vehicle, but for both were >50% by 10 weeks, particularly in black men. There was a

Evidence Levels: **A** Double-blind study **B** Clinical trial ≥ 20 subjects **C** Clinical trial < 20 subjects **D** Series ≥ 5 subjects **E** Anecdotal case reports

significant change in nonblack men but no difference between test and controls.

Although 77% of test patients thought they were much better compared with 47% in the control vehicle group, the authors do not explain the remarkable improvement in the control group nor why or how they assume their test product alone "worked."

Treatment of pseudofolliculitis barbae with topical glycolic acid: a report of two studies. Perricone N. Cutis 1993; 52: 232–5.

Two placebo-controlled trials in 35 adult men showed that glycolic acid lotion was significantly more effective than placebo in treating PFB. There was a reduction of over 60% in lesions on the treated side, which allowed daily shaving with little irritation.

Third-Line Therapies

• Laser depilation	A
• Surgical depilation	C

Comparative evaluation of long pulse alexandrite laser and intense pulsed light systems for pseudofolliculitis barbae treatment with one year of follow up. Leheta T. Indian J Dermatol 2009; 54: 364–8.

Twenty male patients, allegedly Fitzpatrick types II to IV with pseudofolliculitis, were treated in a double-blind, split-face study by alexandrite laser on one side and intense pulsed light (IPL) on the other while continuing to shave or clip the bearded face. The alexandrite was 755 nm with a 15-mm spot size and was operated at 3 ms eventually at 16 to 18 J/cm^2, whereas the IPL had a 610- to 1200-nm filter and a 50-mm × 15-mm spot size and was operated at 12 to 15 J/cm^2, both at 4- to 6-week intervals for four sessions and then 4- to 8-week intervals. Both techniques improved the condition, but the alexandrite laser required an average of seven sessions to reach about 80% improvement in papule count and hyperpigmentation, whereas the IPL-treated side needed 10 to 12 sessions to reach about 50% improvement. Both techniques, however, showed some relapse at 1 year after end of treatments, the IPL more so.

The differences seen may be due to the low settings for both devices; fluences of 20 to 30+ J/cm^2 are frequently required for effective laser- or IPL-induced follicular fatigue or destruction, especially in type II to IV skin.

Low-fluence 1064-nm laser hair reduction for pseudofolliculitis barbae in skin types IV, V, and VI. Schulze R, Meehan KJ, Lopez A, Sweeney KJ, Winstanley D, Apruzzese W, et al. Dermatol Surg 2009; 35: 98–107.

Twenty-two patients with PFB refractory to conservative therapy received five weekly treatments (unlike the customary every 5 weeks) over the anterior neck using a 1064-nm Nd:YAG laser with a 10-mm spot size set at 12 J/cm^2 and pulse duration 20 ms. Eleven patients demonstrated 83% improvement.

The study was an attempt to reduce energy levels because of high incidence of intolerance to pain in standard settings. The effects were clear, but only temporary, and worsening of PFB after switching to a razor blade as a shaving device suggests an imperfect solution because most blacks shave with razors.

Topical eflornithine hydrochloride improves the effectiveness of standard laser hair removal for treating pseudofolliculitis barbae: a randomized, double-blinded, placebo-controlled trial. Xia Y, Cho S, Howard R, Maggio K. J Am Acad Dermatol 2012; 67: 694–9.

Twenty-seven patients (24 black, 3 Caucasian) with Fitzpatrick type II to VI skin were enrolled in a split-neck study comparing four monthly treatments with Nd:YAG laser with 10-mm spot and at 25 to 30 J/cm^2 with 20- to 30-ms pulse duration with and without twice-daily application of 13.9% eflornithine cream. Shaving was continued. A very significant decrease in countable hairs and papules was evident after only two treatments, and almost no papules were evident at 16 weeks; the eflornithine side was moderately better at each stage. Pain measures were not discussed.

This promising study for shortening treatment course had much too short a follow-up period (i.e., immediately at the end of 16 weeks of treatment). Permanence was not ascertainable. It was peculiar that the eflornithine side responded more quickly when the medication should be causing a progressively smaller target for the laser, suggesting a more dramatic effect on hair production than just the caliber of hair.

Pseudofolliculitis barbae. Quarles F, Brody H, Johnson B, Badreshia S, Vause SE, Brauner G, et al. Dermatol Ther 2007; 20: 133–6.

Anecdotal comments by each member of a large panel of experts concerning useful approaches to the treatment of PFB.

Modified superlong pulse 810 nm diode laser in the treatment of pseudofolliculitis barbae in skin types V and VI. Smith E, Winstanley D, Ross E. Dermatol Surg 2005; 31: 297–301.

Ten of 13 patients with type V or VI skin treated with superlong-pulse 810-nm diode laser at 2-week intervals three times with a mean 29 J/cm^2 and 438 ms for type V and 26 J/cm^2 at 450 ms for type VI skin and then followed up to only 3 months showed clinical improvement of PFB papules, which was statistically significant. The authors note that the 26 J/cm^2 maximum tolerable dose may not be sufficient to cause long-term reduction in hair growth. The follow-up of the study was not long enough to determine such reduction either. The authors claim that the ratio of minimal damaging fluence to minimum effective fluence in very dark skin was 1.2:1, versus the safer 1.5 to 2:1 for long-pulse Nd:YAG laser for PFB.

Pseudofolliculitis of the neck and the shoulder: a new effective treatment with alexandrite laser. Valeriant M, Terracina F, Mezzana P. Plast Reconstruct Surg 2002; 110: 1195–6.

Two Caucasian men with chronic folliculitis and pseudofolliculitis of the neck and shoulders were treated with 790-nm alexandrite laser for 30 ms with a 10-mm spot size and 16 to 18 J/cm^2 for four sessions at 6-week intervals. They had a hair loss of 60% to 70% and 90% improvement in PFB, which persisted during 1-year follow-up.

Treatment of pseudofolliculitis with a pulsed infrared laser. Kauvar A. Arch Dermatol 2000; 136: 1343–6.

Ten women with Fitzpatrick skin types III to V and a history of pseudofolliculitis on the face, axilla, or groin for at least 1 year had three consecutive treatments at 6- to 8-week intervals with an 810-nm diode laser and a chill tip at 30 to 38 J/cm^2 and 20-ms pulse duration. After their last visit all showed more than 75% improvement in the pseudofolliculitis and had a 50% reduction in hair growth. No blistering occurred.

Laser-assisted hair removal for darker skin types. Battle E, Hobbs L. Dermatol Ther 2004; 17: 177–83.

The authors carefully review the rationale for use of diode, especially long-pulsed diode, and Nd:YAG lasers for highly pigmented patients, as well as testing, dosing, and cooling precautions to improve patient safety.

Treatment of pseudofolliculitis barbae in skin types IV, V, and VI with a long-pulsed neodymium:yttrium aluminum garnet laser. Ross E, Cooke L, Timko A, Overstreet KA, Graham BS, Barnette DJ. J Am Acad Dermatol 2002; 47: 263–70.

Thirty-seven patients with pseudofolliculitis and Fitzpatrick skin types IV, V, and VI were tested with Nd:YAG laser. There was 33%, 43%, and 40% hair reduction on the thigh for the 50-, 80-, and 100-J/cm^2 fluences, respectively, after 90 days. The highest doses tolerated by the epidermis were 50, 100, and 100 J/cm^2 for types VI, V, and IV skin, respectively. After testing on the face, mean papule counts after 90 days were 6.95 and 1.0 for the control vs. treatment sites, respectively.

Treatment of pseudofolliculitis barbae using the long-pulse Nd:YAG laser on skin types V and VI. Weaver S, Sagaral E. Dermatol Surg 2003; 29: 1187–91.

Twenty subjects with Fitzpatrick type V and VI skin and PFB on the neck or mandible were given two 2-cm × 2-cm treatments with Nd:YAG laser and 10-mm spot size at 40 to 50 ms and 24 to 40 J/cm^2 3 to 4 weeks apart, assessed by photographic papule/pustule and hair counts at 1, 2, and 3 months after the final treatment and compared with a neighboring untreated site. The 76% to 90% reduction in the number of papules/pustules was statistically significant. Hair reduction of 80% 1 month after testing diminished to 23% by 3 months.

Although side effects were noted as transient and without blistering, the two illustrated patients both show scarring.

Surgical depilation for the treatment of pseudofolliculitis or local hirsutism of the face: experience in the first 40 patients. Hage J, Bouman F. Plast Reconstruct Surg 1991; 88: 446–51.

Forty patients, all but three of whom were Caucasian, were operated on over a 15-year period for local hirsutism ($n = 24$), pseudofolliculitis ($n = 11$), and beard growth ($n = 12$) in transgender procedures. The skin of the affected areas was incised and everted in a dermal–subcutaneous plane, and the hair bulbs were excised. Marked diminution of hair numbers occurred, but 15 patients required further electrolysis. Side effects were significant, with wound edge necrosis in 8, seroma or hematoma in 8, and significant subcutaneous scar formation in 15, which was later preventable by postoperative long-term (at least 3 months) pressure bandages. See also Comments in Plast Reconstruct Surg 1992; 90: 332–3.

694

209

Pseudoxanthoma elasticum

Roselyn Kellen, Mark G. Lebwohl

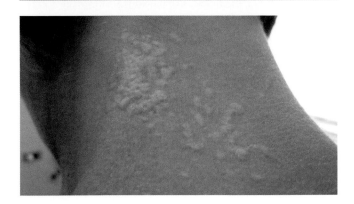

Pseudoxanthoma elasticum (PXE) is a rare autosomal recessive disorder causing abnormal fragmentation and calcification of the elastic fibers in the skin, retina, and cardiovascular system. The primary lesions are small, asymptomatic, yellow papules on the flexural surfaces of the skin. The papules gradually coalesce into plaques, and the skin begins to appear slightly thickened, inelastic, and leatherlike. Ophthalmologic complications include retinal angioid streaks, choroidal neovascularization, and subretinal hemorrhages with resultant scarring causing central vision loss. Cardiovascular complications include narrowing of the cerebral arteries, intracranial hemorrhage, intermittent leg claudication due to peripheral arterial disease, diminished peripheral pulses, hypertension, and angina pectoris. Gastrointestinal bleeding is reported in about 10% of patients, which may also be due to non-PXE–related factors. The prevalence of PXE in the population is approximately 1:50,000.

Most patients with PXE are found to harbor mutations in ATP-binding cassette sub-family C member 6 *(ABCC6) gene* on chromosome 16p13.1, which codes for an ATP-dependent transmembrane transporter. Hundreds of mutations have been identified, but approximately one third are premature termination mutations. More recently, patients with PXE-like skin changes have been found to have mutations in genes for ecto-nucleotide pyrophosphatase/phosphodiesterase 1 *(ENPP1)* and gamma-glutamyl carboxylase *(GGCX)* Certain mutations might be more commonly found in Caucasians compared with Asian patients.

MANAGEMENT STRATEGY

Establishing the diagnosis of PXE may be difficult during the early stages of the disorder. The initial clinical signs appear most commonly during the early teenage years in flexural skin sites on the neck, axillae, antecubital fossae, and groin as variably sized patches of slightly thickened, leathery-looking skin. The diagnosis is often missed during these early years. Larger patches gradually develop with age. Angioid streaks in the

retina usually appear later, beginning in the late teens or early twenties. Frank retinal hemorrhages begin most commonly in the fifth decade, causing central vision loss. Cardiovascular changes are rarely noted in children, although rare cases have been reported.

A heart-healthy lifestyle, including a low-cholesterol diet, aerobic exercises, and avoidance of smoking, should be encouraged. Because of the bleeding diathesis, patients should be advised to avoid aspirin and other blood thinners unless essential, as well as contact sports and other activities that increase the risk of eye trauma. There is some evidence that increased dietary calcium results in more rapid progression of the disease, so patients should be encouraged to avoid calcium supplementation and excessive ingestion of milk products. In contrast, experiments with animal models suggest that diets high in magnesium can inhibit tissue mineralization. An interdisciplinary approach involving dermatologists, retina specialists, and cardiologists is essential. Because this is a rare disease, it is important to provide patients with resources. The following two organizations are good references for patients:

Pseudoxanthoma elasticum (PXE) International: https://www.pxe.org
National Association for Pseudoxanthoma Elasticum (NAPE): www.napeusa.com

Specific Investigations

- Family history for evidence of similar problems
- Complete skin examination, with special reference to all flexural skin sites and oral mucosa
- General physical examination and routine laboratory tests, including lipid panel, with a focus on risk factors for cardiovascular disease
- A 3- to 4-mm punch biopsy of suspicious lesions and a von Kossa stain to detect calcified elastic fibers to establish a diagnosis
- Retinal examination and photographs for evidence of angioid streaks, neovascularization, and hemorrhages
- Genetic studies on blood may be used to verify the diagnosis of PXE in questionable cases. The tests are expensive and rarely essential to confirm the diagnosis
- Cardiology referral and echocardiogram. There are elastic fibers in cardiac valves so it should not be surprising that cardiac valvular abnormalities, such as mitral valve prolapse, are common in patients with PXE

First-Line Therapies

- Good nutrition; avoidance of trans fats; dietary calcium intake based on patient age and the current recommended dietary intake | **B**
- Regular exercise program, with care to avoid sports with potential for head or eye injury | **B**
- Vigorous control of hypertension, abnormal lipid profiles, and other risk factors for cardiovascular disease | **C**
- Avoid long-term use of anticoagulants (to minimize the risk of ocular, gastrointestinal, and other sources of bleeding) | **C**

- Retinal referral and follow-up on regular basis with a retinal specialist familiar with PXE. If early or threatened retinal hemorrhages, consider possible treatment with bevacizumab (Avastin) or ranibizumab (Lucentis)   C
- Cardiology referral; echocardiogram to look for cardiac and valvular abnormalities   C

Long-term effectiveness of intravitreal bevacizumab for choroidal neovascularization secondary to angioid streaks in pseudoxanthoma elasticum. Finger RP, Charbel IP, Schmitz-Valckenberg S, Holz FG, Scholl HN. Retina 2011; 31: 1268–78.

Intravitreal bevacizumab improved visual acuity, stabilized leakage from active choroidal neovascularizations, and reduced central retinal thickness. There was improvement of visual acuity in early disease and preservation of function in advanced disease. Initiation of therapy as early as possible is important to preservation of vision.

Intravitreal injection of vascular endothelial growth factor inhibitors has dramatically improved the prognosis of PXE eye disease.

Treatment with ranibizumab for choroidal neovascularization secondary to a pseudoxanthoma elasticum: results of the French observational study PIXEL. Ebran JM, Mimoun G, Cohen SY, Grenet T, Donati A, Jean-Pastor M-J, et al. J Fr Ophtalmol 2016; 39: 370–5.

Ranibizumab provided stable visual acuity for at least 2 years in patients with choroidal neovascularization and decreased the frequency of neovascularization relapses. The treatment was well tolerated.

In a different case report, a 54-year-old man with ophthalmologic complications from PXE did not improve after three injections (once a month) of bevacizumab. He received 21 ranibizumab injections (0.5 mg/50 μL), which helped maintain visual acuity over a 6-month period.

Second-Line Therapies

- Cosmetic surgery for removal of objectionable lesions if desired by patient for cosmetic reasons   B
- Observe pregnant women more carefully. Incidence of gastrointestinal hemorrhage is questionably increased during pregnancy   C

Third-Line Therapies

- Sevelamer hydrochloride 800 mg three times daily   A
- Increase in dietary magnesium   E
- Fractional CO$_2$ laser   E
- Injectable collagen   E

A randomized controlled trial of oral phosphate binders in the treatment of pseudoxanthoma elasticum. Yoo JY, Blum RR, Singer GK, Stern DR, Emanuel PO, Fuchs W, et al. J Am Acad Dermatol 2011; 65: 341–8.

Sevelamer hydrochloride 800 mg three times daily resulted in reduced calcification of elastic fibers on microscopy and improved clinical scores, but the benefit was not significant compared with placebo.

The placebo was discovered to contain magnesium, which may explain the benefit achieved by the placebo group.

Pseudoxanthoma elasticum, the paradigm of heritable ectopic mineralization disorders: can diet help? LaRusso J, Li Q, Uitto J. Dtsch Fermatol Ges 2011; 9: 586–93.

A fivefold increase in dietary magnesium inhibited tissue mineralization in a mouse model of PXE.

Animal studies have examined the relationship between magnesium in the diet and mineralization of the vasculature. Mice fed a diet with magnesium oxide supplementation for 2 months had a lower carotid intima-media thickness compared with mice fed a standard diet. In contrast, a low-magnesium diet accelerated calcium deposition.

Pseudoxanthoma elasticum treatment with fractional CO$_2$ laser. Salles AG, Remigio AF, Moraes LB, Varoni AC, Gemperli R, Ferreira MC. Plast Reconstr Surg Glob Open 2014; 2: e219.

A 32-year-old woman was treated with a fractional CO$_2$ laser applied to the anterior cervical region (four sessions) and posterior cervical region (five sessions). Significant improvement was noted 1 month after the first session. Two years after the last session, she had improvements in surface irregularities and distensibility.

Pseudoxanthoma elasticum: temporary treatment of chin folds and lines with injectable collagen. Galadari H, Lebwohl M. J Am Acad Dermatol 2003; 49: S265–6.

Two patients with horizontal mental creases received injectable collagen. The first patient received 0.5 mL of collagen (Zyderm II) and showed immediate improvement; however, rhytides and creases recurred 6 months later. The second patient received 1.0 mL of collagen (Zyderm) in 2 sessions (2 weeks apart), and improvement was noted for at least 6 months. Nine months later, she received 1.0 mL intradermal collagen with effects that lasted for only 1 month. A third injection (1.0 mL Zyplast) provided improvement for 4 weeks.

It is likely that any of the new fillers currently available would work as well as injectable collagen.

Acknowledgment

We would like to acknowledge Dr. Kenneth Neldner for his contributions to the previous edition of this chapter.

Evidence Levels: **A** Double-blind study **B** Clinical trial ≥ 20 subjects **C** Clinical trial < 20 subjects **D** Series ≥ 5 subjects **E** Anecdotal case reports

210

Psoriasis

Mark G. Lebwohl, Peter van de Kerkhof

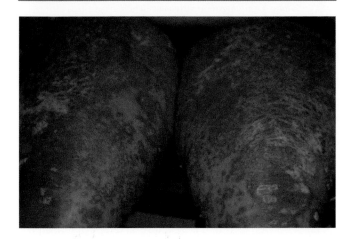

Plaque psoriasis is a common disorder in which environmental factors contribute to the development of sharply demarcated, erythematous, scaling plaques in genetically predisposed individuals. Because there is an overlap in treatments, guttate psoriasis, inverse psoriasis, and impetigo herpetiformis will be discussed under "Management Strategy" next. Erythrodermic psoriasis and pustular psoriasis will be discussed at the end of the chapter. Palmoplantar pustulosis is addressed in its own chapter. Patients should be questioned and examined for psoriatic arthritis, and because of recent evidence linking psoriasis to cardiovascular disease, risk factors should be addressed. Involvement of rheumatologists or cardiologists may be necessary.

MANAGEMENT STRATEGY

The treatment of psoriasis must take many factors into account, including the extent of involvement, areas of involvement, the patient's lifestyle, and other health problems and medications. For example, patients who live far from phototherapy centers may not have the option to be treated with psoralen and UVA (PUVA), but a home phototherapy unit can be ordered for patients who can be taught to administer their own UVB therapy. In sunny climates, sun exposure can be added to the therapeutic regimen. If patients are taking medications such as lithium that are known to exacerbate psoriasis, alternatives should be sought. In patients who have had multiple skin cancers, PUVA and ciclosporin should be avoided as they increase the tendency to develop skin cancers; acitretin, which suppresses the development of skin cancers, should be considered for these individuals.

The body surface area affected in patients with psoriasis is important in the selection of therapies. In individuals with less than 5% body surface area involvement, topical therapy is usually started unless the patient has previously failed topical therapy or the psoriasis is debilitating because of the site of involvement. In patients with mild localized plaques, *mild, midpotency, or potent topical corticosteroids* can be prescribed, or other topical agents such as *calcipotriol (calcipotriene)*, *calcitriol*, or *tazarotene* can be tried. *Anthralin preparations* have fallen into disfavor because they

are messy, but they still offer an effective alternative to corticosteroids. In Europe anthralin preparations are used in some daycare centers. Often patients have been using a topical medication that is inadequate as monotherapy, and in such cases combination therapy is warranted. The combination of a superpotent corticosteroid and calcipotriol or tazarotene is often effective when monotherapy with either of the agents does not work, and new formulations that combine betamethasone dipropionate with calcipotriol are available.

Some areas may be limited in extent, but require alternative treatments. For example, involvement of the palms and soles can be debilitating, and these areas are notoriously difficult to treat. Pustular psoriasis of the palms and soles, for example, only occasionally responds to topical therapy. Although the palms and soles involve only a small percentage of the body surface area, treatment with oral medications or injected medications or *phototherapy* may be warranted. The combination of *acitretin* 25 mg daily with *"bath-PUVA"*—applied by soaking the hands in a water-filled basin to which *methoxsalen* has been added, followed by UVA irradiation—has been used successfully. The *excimer* laser can also be effective for palm and sole psoriasis, as can *oral methotrexate, acitretin, apremilast,* and *ciclosporin*. Double-blind placebo-controlled trials have demonstrated the efficacy of adalimumab for palm and sole psoriasis, and it is likely that other biologic therapies are effective, though they are not as effective for palms and soles as they are for psoriasis on other parts of the body. Involvement of the scalp is common and requires gels, solutions, sprays, or foams that are not as messy as ointments and creams. *Shampoos containing tars, salicylic acid, or corticosteroids* are useful adjunctive therapies for the scalp. A new home device that delivers narrowband UVB to the scalp through fiber-optic filaments has recently been introduced.

The face and intertriginous sites are highly responsive to topical medications, but are particularly sensitive to the side effects of many topical agents. Topical corticosteroids cause cutaneous atrophy, telangiectasia, and striae. Therefore only milder, safer corticosteroids should be used on the face and intertriginous sites, and alternating with noncorticosteroids may be optimal if psoriasis recurs. The topical immunomodulators *tacrolimus 0.1% ointment* and *pimecrolimus 1% cream* are effective and safe for facial and intertriginous psoriasis, but not as effective on thick plaques on the rest of the body. *Calcipotriol* (50 μg/g) can be irritating on facial or intertriginous psoriasis, but alternative vitamin D analogs such as calcitriol and tacalcitol are less irritating and therefore particularly suited for facial or flexural psoriasis. *Tazarotene* may be too irritating to use on genital skin, but it can be used on the face. The irritation of tazarotene can also be minimized by using it in a regimen with topical corticosteroids.

With 5% to 10% body surface involvement, topical therapy is usually prescribed, but may require the addition of *phototherapy* or *oral medications*. In those with more than 10% body surface involvement, topical therapy may be impractical for all lesions but may provide a useful adjunct to phototherapy or systemic therapy.

Phototherapy with *UVB* has been in use in the treatment of psoriasis for a century and has a proven record of safety and efficacy. It is particularly useful in patients who have responded well to sun exposure. Patients who have failed UVB or have not done well with sun exposure often respond to *narrowband UVB*. PUVA is one of the most effective treatments for psoriasis and offers long remissions for many patients. Because of its increased risk of cutaneous malignancy, PUVA is usually reserved for those who do not achieve adequate remissions with UVB.

In patients who have not achieved satisfactory results with these treatments, *low-dose oral retinoids* can be added. *Acitretin* in doses of 10 to 25 mg daily dramatically improves the response to UVB and to PUVA. By keeping the dose at 25 mg or less, the side effects of acitretin can be minimized. For those who are not candidates for UVB phototherapy or PUVA, *oral methotrexate* is highly effective in combination with other treatments or as monotherapy. It is associated with hepatic fibrosis in some patients, and regular monitoring of liver function tests in addition to blood counts is necessary. Current guidelines in the United States call for periodic liver biopsies in selected patients treated with methotrexate. In parts of Europe, the serum level of the aminoterminal propeptide of type III procollagen has been used as a marker for hepatic fibrosis as an alternative to routine use of liver biopsy. *Ciclosporin* is also dramatically effective as monotherapy for psoriasis, but is associated with nephrotoxicity as well as hypertension and a theoretical risk of malignancy with long-term use. Consequently, current guidelines call for limiting use of ciclosporin to 1 or 2 years. The most recently approved oral medication for psoriasis, *apremilast*, is another moderately effective option. *Tofacitinib*, an oral agent approved in the United States for rheumatoid arthritis, has also been studied for psoriasis.

In recent years, the ability to create new drugs that target specific parts of the immune system has led to the development of biologic agents for psoriasis. These drugs are not associated with the nephrotoxicity of ciclosporin or the hepatotoxicity and bone marrow toxicity of methotrexate, but the cost of biologics is often prohibitive. Psoriasis experts are divided on the point at which biologics should be considered. Some consider them first-line therapy when the disease is too extensive for topical therapy. Because of their expense, biologics are used by others only after phototherapy or other systemic therapies have been tried.

Because of their efficacy and safety, use of biologics is growing for psoriasis and for psoriatic arthritis. Agents that block tumor necrosis factor-α (TNF-α), including *etanercept, infliximab, adalimumab, golimumab, and certolizumab,* are ideal for patients with psoriatic arthritis. TNF-blocking agents have unique side effects, including the reactivation of latent tuberculosis, exacerbation of multiple sclerosis, and the development of antinuclear antibodies. *Ustekinumab,* a drug that blocks the p40 component of interleukin (IL)-12 and IL-23, has been studied in 45-mg and 90-mg doses; dose elevation can be beneficial in overweight patients. The drug can be administered as infrequently as every 3 months. The recently approved drugs *ixekizumab and secukinumab,* which block IL-17, and *brodalumab,* an investigational drug that blocks the IL-17 receptor, are highly effective therapies that can achieve 100% clearing of psoriasis. Other biologic therapies targeting IL-23 are on the way. When all else fails, *combination therapy* using different medications is often effective. Because many of the treatments available are immunosuppressive, side effects of additive immunosuppression must be considered when combining different modalities.

GUTTATE PSORIASIS

Guttate psoriasis is characterized by widespread erythematous, scaling papules. The management of guttate psoriasis is very similar to that of extensive plaque psoriasis. Because streptococcal infection often precedes guttate psoriasis, underlying infection should be sought and treated. Lesions are usually too widespread for topical therapy, so most patients are started on *phototherapy with UVB or narrowband UVB.* If that is ineffective, *oral retinoids* can be added, or patients can be switched to *PUVA.* This form of psoriasis frequently responds to phototherapy, so it is only occasionally necessary to resort to more aggressive second-line or third-line therapies listed later.

INVERSE PSORIASIS

Patients with inverse psoriasis develop lesions in the axillae, between the buttocks, on the medial aspects of the thighs, and in the umbilicus. These sites are easily treated with *mild topical corticosteroids,* but are more susceptible to corticosteroid side effects such as atrophy and formation of striae. Consequently, nonsteroidal treatments can be attempted. *Calcipotriol* (50 μg/g) can be irritating on intertriginous sites but is nevertheless effective. *Other vitamin D analogs (calcitriol, tacalcitol)* cause less irritation. *Tazarotene* can be used on the face, but is usually too irritating to use in the axillae or groin. *Tars and anthralin* are likewise irritating in intertriginous sites. *Topical tacrolimus ointment and pimecrolimus cream,* albeit not approved for psoriasis, are highly effective for facial and intertriginous psoriasis, but less effective for thick plaques elsewhere on the body. Topical phosphodiesterase inhibitors and Janus kinase inhibitors are likely to be introduced for psoriasis, and these may be effective for facial and intertriginous psoriasis without the atrophogenicity of corticosteroids.

IMPETIGO HERPETIFORMIS

Impetigo herpetiformis is characterized by a generalized pustular eruption with fever and leukocytosis developing during pregnancy. Many consider this to be a variant of pustular psoriasis that occurs during pregnancy. If *bed rest, emollients, compresses,* and *mild topical corticosteroids* are ineffective, *systemic corticosteroids* have been used effectively in the past. More recently, *oral ciclosporin* has proved effective for impetigo herpetiformis. This drug, which has a pregnancy category C rating, is administered in two divided doses totaling 4 to 5 mg/kg daily. Concerns about cumulative toxicity, such as nephrotoxicity, are less worrisome in impetigo herpetiformis because the disorder may resolve at the end of pregnancy, limiting the amount of ciclosporin prescribed. Although there is not as much experience in the use of biologic agents for impetigo herpetiformis, the limited data available for these agents suggests that they are relatively safe during pregnancy. Most are rated as pregnancy category B, meaning that there is no evidence of fetal toxicity in animal studies; however, these drugs can affect the fetal immune system, and postnatal immune infection has occurred.

Specific Investigations

- Skin biopsy (if the clinical diagnosis of psoriasis is uncertain)
- Laboratory investigations
- Serum electrolytes and calcium for patients with pustular psoriasis
- ASO or bacterial cultures for patients with guttate psoriasis
- Appropriate drug-related monitoring for patients on systemic therapies

Investigation is not required in the majority of cases. Skin biopsy may be helpful if the diagnosis is in question, but is usually not needed.

As discussed later, a range of investigations are required for screening and monitoring when using systemic therapies.

Routine screening for tuberculosis has been advised for patients treated with biologic therapies. Because methotrexate and ciclosporin are also immunosuppressive, testing for tuberculosis and, if positive, chest radiography have been suggested before

Evidence Levels: **A** Double-blind study   **B** Clinical trial ≥ 20 subjects   **C** Clinical trial < 20 subjects   **D** Series ≥ 5 subjects   **E** Anecdotal case reports

treatment with these agents. Ciclosporin guidelines call for frequent monitoring of blood pressure and chemistry screening, with particular attention to serum creatinine and magnesium. Methotrexate guidelines call for periodic monitoring of complete blood count (CBC) and platelet counts and chemistry screening with liver function tests. Assays·for hepatic fibrosis such as the serum aminoterminal propeptide of type III procollagen or liver biopsies are advised in certain patients. Monitoring for viral hepatitis or HIV infection should be considered in populations at risk for those disorders, and many advocate routine hepatitis screening in any patient before biologic therapy, methotrexate, or ciclosporin. Serum cholesterol and triglycerides are particularly important in patients treated with oral acitretin.

From the Medical Board of the National Psoriasis Foundation: monitoring and vaccinations in patients treated with biologics for psoriasis. Lebwohl M, Bagel J, Gelfand JM, Gladman D, Gordon KB, Hsu S, et al. J Am Acad Dermatol 2008; 58: 94–105.

Apart from history, physical examination, routine chemistry screening, CBC, and platelet counts, testing for tuberculosis is advised for patients treated with all of the biologics. Liver function tests should be monitored more frequently in patients treated with infliximab; testing for hepatitis B and C is now advocated before starting biologic therapy.

Cyclosporine and psoriasis: 2008 National Psoriasis Foundation Consensus Conference. Rosmarin DM, Lebwohl M, Elewski BE, Gottlieb AB; National Psoriasis Foundation. J Am Acad Dermatol 2010; 62: 838–53.

Oral ciclosporin in doses up to 5 mg/kg daily is dramatically effective for psoriasis, but is limited by the development of nephrotoxicity.

This article presents guidelines regarding dosage and monitoring, drug interactions, and complications of ciclosporin.

In patients treated with ciclosporin, blood and platelet counts as well as comprehensive serum chemistries are warranted, including blood urea nitrogen, creatinine, potassium, magnesium, uric acid, liver function tests, and lipids. Two baseline serum creatinine levels and two baseline blood pressure measurements should be obtained before starting ciclosporin therapy. Baseline testing for hepatitis B and C is advocated. Tuberculosis testing should be performed at baseline and annually thereafter.

Methotrexate and psoriasis: 2009. National Psoriasis Foundation Consensus Conference. Kalb R, Strober B, Weinstein G, Lebwohl M. J Am Acad Dermatol 2009; 60: 824–37.

Methotrexate in psoriasis: consensus conference. Roenigk HH Jr, Auerbach R, Maibach H, Weinstein G, Lebwohl M. J Am Acad Dermatol 1998; 38: 478–85.

Methotrexate remains one of the most effective systemic agents for psoriasis. After an initial test dose of 2.5 to 7.5 mg, weekly doses ranging from 15 to 30 mg can be used to clear psoriasis in most patients. The most worrisome side effects are hepatotoxicity and bone marrow suppression.

These articles review many of the publications on methotrexate and cover laboratory monitoring guidelines, including blood work and liver biopsy, dosage guidelines, drug interactions, and side effects.

Patients treated with methotrexate should have baseline blood and platelet counts as well as liver function tests and creatinine. Many advocate baseline serologic studies for hepatitis B and hepatitis C, and new guidelines require baseline and annual testing for tuberculosis. In Europe, assays for the aminoterminal propeptide

of type III procollagen are obtained. In patients without risk factors for hepatic fibrosis (such as obesity), liver biopsies may not be required or their frequency markedly reduced. Many dermatologists in the United States still obtain periodic liver biopsies to monitor hepatic fibrosis.

First-Line Therapies	
• Anthralin (dithranol)	B
• Coal tar	A
• Salicylic acid	C
• Topical corticosteroids	A
• Vitamin D analogs	A
• Tazarotene	A
• Sun exposure	B
• Tacrolimus ointment	A
• Pimecrolimus cream	A

A randomized, double-blind, vehicle-controlled study of a novel liposomal dithranol formulation in psoriasis. Saraswat A, Agarwal R, Katare OP, Kaur I, Kumar B. J Dermatol Treat 2007; 18: 40–5.

Twenty patients were enrolled in a bilateral comparison controlled trial of 0.5% dithranol entrapped in phospholipid liposomes on one side of the body compared with the vehicle (10 patients) or a conventional 1.15% dithranol, 1.15% salicylic acid, and 5.3% coal tar preparation (10 patients) applied daily, using a 30-minute short-contact regimen for 6 weeks. Both active preparations resulted in significant improvement in psoriasis, but there was less perilesional erythema and skin staining on the side treated with the liposome preparation than with the conventional cream.

Anthralin preparations have been used successfully for psoriasis for decades, but staining and irritation have limited their acceptance by both patients and physicians. Attempts to formulate nonstaining, nonirritating versions of anthralin have had limited success.

Efficacy of topical 5% liquor carbonis detergens vs. its emollient base in the treatment of psoriasis. Kanzler MH, Gorsulowsky DC. Br J Dermatol 1993; 129: 310–4.

Liquor carbonis detergens 5% resulted in more improvement in psoriasis than its vehicle emollient base in a bilateral-paired comparison study.

Tars are available in gels, creams, emollient creams, and ointments and are also available in emulsions that are added to the bath. There is a general belief that more cosmetically elegant preparations are better tolerated by patients but less effective. Crude coal tar is quite effective, but quite messy.

The role of salicylic acid in the treatment of psoriasis. Lebwohl M. Int J Dermatol 1999; 38: 16–24.

Salicylic acid is a keratolytic agent that removes scale and allows other topical medications to penetrate. There is a marked increase in penetration of topical corticosteroids when combined with 2% to 10% salicylic acid. Combinations of salicylic acid and tar or anthralin have also been used successfully, but salicylic acid inactivates calcipotriol. Moreover, salicylic acid blocks UVB and should therefore not be applied before phototherapy.

Evaluation of the efficacy and safety of clobetasol propionate spray in the treatment of plaque-type psoriasis. Jarratt MT, Clark SD, Savin RC, Swinyer LJ, Safley CF, Brodell RT, et al. Cutis 2006; 78: 348–54.

The efficacy and tolerability of clobetasol propionate foam 0.05% in the treatment of mild to moderate plaque-type psoriasis of nonscalp regions. Gottlieb AB, Ford RO, Spellman MC. J Cutan Med Surg 2003; 7: 185–92.

Clobetasol propionate shampoo 0.05%: a new option to treat patients with moderate to severe scalp psoriasis. Jarratt M, Breneman D, Gottlieb AB, Poulin Y, Liu Y, Foley V. J Drugs Dermatol 2004; 3: 367–73.

The efficacy of topical corticosteroids for psoriasis has been demonstrated in numerous double-blind, placebo-controlled trials of large numbers of patients. Topical corticosteroids are available in many vehicles, including foams, emollient foams, sprays, shampoos, solutions, lotions, creams, emollient creams, ointments, tapes, and gels.

Superpotent corticosteroids such as clobetasol can be associated with cutaneous and systemic side effects. Clinically significant adrenal suppression is seldom considered, and tests for adrenal function are virtually never performed. Practicing dermatologists are more concerned with the side effects of atrophy, telangiectasia, striae, and tachyphylaxis. For all these reasons, superpotent corticosteroid use should be limited to 2 to 4 weeks and less than 50 g/week. Superpotent corticosteroids should not be occluded and should not be used on the face or intertriginous sites. If at all possible, they should be avoided in children.

An investigator-masked comparison of the efficacy and safety of twice daily applications of calcitriol 3 μg/g ointment vs. calcipotriol 50 μg/g ointment in subjects with mild to moderate chronic plaque-type psoriasis. Zhu X, Wang B, Zhao G, Gu J, Chen Z, Briantais P, et al. J Eur Acad Dermatol Venereol 2007; 21: 466–72.

In this investigator-blinded study, 250 subjects were treated twice daily for 12 weeks with either calcitriol or calcipotriol ointments. Both agents were comparably effective, but there were more local cutaneous adverse events in patients treated with calcipotriol than those treated with calcitriol.

Because local irritation occurs in up to 20% of patients treated with calcipotriol on facial or intertriginous skin, calcitriol may be a better therapeutic option for those sites.

Once daily treatment of psoriasis with tacalcitol compared with twice daily treatment with calcipotriol. A double-blind trial. Veien NK, Bjerke JR, Rossmann-Ringdahl I, Jakobsen HB. Br J Dermatol 1997; 137: 581–6.

Tacalcitol ointment applied once daily proved to be slightly less effective than calcipotriol ointment twice daily in this 8-week, double-blind study conducted in 287 patients.

A 52-week randomized safety study of a calcipotriol/betamethasone dipropionate two-compound product (Dovobet/Daivobet/Taclonex) in the treatment of psoriasis vulgaris. Kragballe K, Austad J, Barnes L, Bibby A, de la Brassinne M, Cambazard F, et al. Br J Dermatol 2006; 154: 1155–60.

Six hundred and thirty-four patients were treated once daily for 4 weeks with a combination ointment containing calcipotriol and betamethasone dipropionate. After 4 weeks they were randomized to receive either the combination product or the combination product alternating with calcipotriol ointment at 4-week intervals or calcipotriol ointment alone as needed for 48 weeks in this double-blind trial. The combination product was consistently more effective than calcipotriol, and patients treated throughout with the combination product had the fewest side effects. Cutaneous atrophy occurred in four (1.9%) of those randomized to receive the combination ointment for 52 weeks.

Calcipotriol is a relatively unstable molecule that is inactivated upon mixing with many other topical agents, so the availability of a stable combination ointment of calcipotriol with a corticosteroid is desirable. Long-term therapy with any product containing a topical corticosteroid should be done with caution to avoid cutaneous atrophy and especially the development of striae. To minimize local cutaneous side effects, avoid strong corticosteroids on the face and intertriginous sites. Use intermittent dosing such as weekend therapy for maintenance of therapeutic effect.

Tazarotene cream in the treatment of psoriasis: two multicenter, double-blind, randomized, vehicle-controlled studies of the safety and efficacy of tazarotene creams 0.05% and 0.1% applied once daily for 12 weeks. Weinstein GD, Koo JY, Krueger GG, Lebwohl M, Love NJ, Menter MA, et al; Tazarotene Cream Clinical Study Group. J Am Acad Dermatol 2003; 48: 760–7.

Tazarotene creams 0.1% and 0.05% were compared with vehicle once daily for 12 weeks in this double-blind study. Tazarotene 0.1% was more effective, but also more irritating, than the 0.05% cream, and both were superior in efficacy to vehicle.

Tazarotene creams are slightly less effective, but also less irritating, than tazarotene 0.1% and 0.05% gels.

Tacrolimus ointment is effective for facial and intertriginous psoriasis. Lebwohl M, Freeman AK, Chapman MS, Feldman SR, Hartle JE, Henning A; Tacrolimus Ointment Study Group. J Am Acad Dermatol 2004; 51: 723–30.

One hundred and sixty-seven patients were treated in this double-blind, placebo-controlled trial of tacrolimus 0.1% ointment applied twice daily for 8 weeks for facial and intertriginous psoriasis. At the end of 8 weeks 65.2% of tacrolimus ointment–treated patients and 31.5% of vehicle-treated patients were clear or almost clear.

Pimecrolimus cream 1% in the treatment of intertriginous psoriasis: a double-blind, randomized study. Gribetz C, Ling M, Lebwohl M, Pariser D, Draelos Z, Gottlieb AB, et al. J Am Acad Dermatol 2004; 51: 731–8.

In this double-blind study 57 patients were treated with 1% pimecrolimus cream or placebo. At the end of week 8, 71% of pimecrolimus-treated patients were clear or almost clear, compared with 41% of vehicle-treated patients.

Topical calcineurin inhibitors are valuable alternatives for psoriasis in facial and intertriginous sites, which are particularly susceptible to corticosteroid side effects and easily irritated by calcipotriol or tazarotene.

The percentage of patients achieving PASI 75 after 1 month and remission time after climatotherapy at the Dead Sea. Harari M, Novack L, Barth J, David M, Friger M, Moses SW. Int J Dermatol 2007; 46: 1087–91.

Sixty-four patients were treated with climatotherapy at the Dead Sea, which included bathing in Dead Sea water and gradually increasing sun exposure. All patients achieved PASI 50, and 75.9% achieved PASI 75. The median time to recurrence of a lesion of psoriasis was 23.1 weeks, and the median duration of effect, defined as the time to 50% relapse in the PASI improvement, was 33.6 weeks.

The Dead Sea is the lowest point on earth and has the highest concentration of minerals of any body of water on the earth. The mineral haze in the atmosphere through which sunlight passes results in a unique spectrum of sunlight that accounts for the exceptional therapeutic responses. Two to four weeks of Dead Sea sun exposure and bathing are required to achieve significant benefit.

Evidence Levels: **A** Double-blind study **B** Clinical trial ≥ 20 subjects **C** Clinical trial < 20 subjects **D** Series ≥ 5 subjects **E** Anecdotal case reports

Second-Line Therapies	
• UVB	A
• Narrowband UVB	A
• PUVA	A
• Acitretin	A
• Apremilast	A
• Adalimumab	A
• Etanercept	A
• Infliximab	A
• Ustekinumab	A
• Secukinumab	A
• Ixekizumab	A
• Methotrexate	A
• Ciclosporin	A

Components of the Goeckerman regimen. Le Vine MJ, White HA, Parrish JA. J Invest Dermatol 1979; 73: 170–3.

The efficacy of UVB phototherapy is improved by the addition of a topical tar preparation or lubricating base; 5% crude coal tar is no more effective than lubricating base when combined with a phototherapy regimen.

The original Goeckerman regimen involved inpatient application of crude coal tar, which was removed before daily UVB phototherapy. Most current phototherapy regimens involve outpatient treatment three times per week with topical application of mineral oil or petrolatum.

Narrowband UV-B produces superior clinical and histopathological resolution of moderate-to-severe psoriasis in patients compared with broadband UV-B. Coven TR, Burack LH, Gilleaudeau R, Keogh M, Ozawa M, Krueger JG. Arch Dermatol 1997; 133: 1514–22.

Twenty-two patients were treated in a bilateral comparison study with narrowband UVB on one side and broadband UVB on the other. The side treated with narrowband UVB cleared more quickly and more completely than the side treated with broadband UVB.

Randomized double-blind trial of the treatment of chronic plaque psoriasis: efficacy of psoralen-UV-A therapy vs. narrowband UV-B therapy. Yones SS, Palmer RA, Garibaldinos TT, Hawk JL. Arch Dermatol 2006; 142: 836–42.

In this double-blind study 93 patients were treated twice weekly with either narrowband UVB or PUVA until clearance or up to a maximum of 30 sessions. In patients with skin types 1 to 4, PUVA was significantly more effective than UVB, with 84% of PUVA-treated patients clearing compared with 65% of narrowband UVB-treated patients. PUVA cleared patients after a median of 17 treatments, compared with 28.5 treatments for narrowband UVB. Six months after the last treatment 68% of patients treated with PUVA remained clear, compared with 35% of patients treated with narrowband UVB.

Although PUVA is more effective than narrowband UVB, it is more difficult to administer and has an increased risk of phototoxicity and carcinogenicity. Baseline and annual eye examinations have been suggested for patients treated with oral PUVA, but initial concerns about the development of cataracts in these patients have not been borne out over time. Baseline serologies for lupus were once recommended before starting patients on PUVA, but are now only obtained in patients who have other signs or symptoms of the disease.

PUVA therapy for psoriasis: comparison of oral and bath-water delivery of 8-methoxypsoralen. Lowe NJ, Weingarten D, Bourget T, Moy LS. J Am Acad Dermatol 1986; 14: 754–60.

Bath-water delivery of methoxsalen (bath-PUVA) 3.7 mg/L (approximately 60 mg dissolved in a tub of water) is as effective as oral PUVA, but requires less UVA and is not associated with systemic side effects such as nausea. Phototoxicity may be increased.

Side effects of burning, sun sensitivity, and, especially, photocarcinogenicity are of concern. Topically applied methoxsalen has also been shown to be effective for psoriasis, but is associated with more phototoxicity.

Efficacy and safety results from the randomized controlled comparative study of adalimumab vs. methotrexate vs. placebo in patients with psoriasis (CHAMPION). Saurat JH, Stingl G, Dubertret L, Papp K, Langley RG, Ortonne JP, et al. Br J Dermatol 2008; 158: 558–66.

Adalimumab 40 mg every other week after an 80-mg loading dose was compared with methotrexate 7.5 mg orally, increased according to clinical response up to 25 mg per week or placebo for 16 weeks. Of adalimumab-treated patients, 79.6% achieved PASI 75, compared with 35.5% of those patients treated with methotrexate and 18.9% of those treated with placebo. Methotrexate patients suffered the most adverse events leading to study discontinuation, mostly related to hepatic complications.

This was the first placebo-controlled trial of methotrexate for psoriasis. The trial design has been criticized for starting methotrexate at a low dose. Nevertheless, the clear efficacy of adalimumab and the side effects of methotrexate were demonstrated by this study.

A double-blind, placebo-controlled trial of acitretin for the treatment of psoriasis. Olsen EA, Weed WW, Meyer CJ, Cobo LM. J Am Acad Dermatol 1989; 21: 681–6.

In a double-blind study 15 patients were treated with a daily acitretin dose of 25 or 50 mg or placebo for 8 weeks. All were then treated in an open-label study with either 25 or 75 mg of acitretin daily. Improvement in psoriasis was only moderate.

Acitretin plus UVB therapy for psoriasis. Comparisons with placebo plus UVB and acitretin alone. Lowe NJ, Prystowsky JH, Bourget T, Edelstein J, Nychay S, Armstrong R. J Am Acad Dermatol 1991; 24: 591–4.

Photochemotherapy for severe psoriasis without or in combination with acitretin: a randomized, double-blind comparison study. Tanew A, Guggenbichler A, Hönigsmann H, Geiger JM, Fritsch P. J Am Acad Dermatol 1991; 25: 682–4.

This was a double-blind study of 60 patients treated with either PUVA alone or PUVA in combination with acitretin. Ninety-six percent of patients treated with acitretin and PUVA achieved marked or complete clearing, compared with 80% of patients treated with PUVA alone. The cumulative UVA dose used for the acitretin + PUVA group was 42% lower than for the patients treated with PUVA alone.

Acitretin monotherapy has limited benefit for psoriasis, partly because of its limited efficacy and partly because higher dosing results in more mucocutaneous side effects, such as hair loss and cheilitis. In combination with other treatments such as UVB or PUVA, even low doses of acitretin result in dramatically enhanced efficacy. It is also useful in combination or monotherapy for palm and sole psoriasis.

Methotrexate versus cyclosporine in moderate-to-severe chronic plaque psoriasis. Heydendael VM, Spuls PI, Opmeer BC, de Borgie CA, Reitsma JB, Goldschmidt WF, et al. N Engl J Med 2003; 349: 658–65.

Eighty-eight patients were randomized to treatment with either methotrexate starting at 15 mg and adjusted according to clinical response or ciclosporin starting at 3 mg/kg and adjusted according to clinical response. Psoriasis improved in both groups, with a slightly greater response in the ciclosporin group. Twelve of 44 patients in the methotrexate group had to discontinue treatment because of liver function test abnormalities.

Apremilast, an oral phosphodiesterase 4 (PDE4) inhibitor, in patients with moderate to severe plaque psoriasis: results of a phase III, randomized, controlled trial (Efficacy and Safety Trial Evaluating the Effects of Apremilast in Psoriasis [ESTEEM] 1). Papp K, Reich K, Leonardi CL, Kircik L, Chimenti S, Langley RG, et al. J Am Acad Dermatol 2015; 73: 37–49.

Patients were treated with either apremilast 30 mg twice daily or placebo for the first 12 weeks of this study. At week 16, 33.1% of patients achieved PASI 75 compared with 5.3% of placebo-treated patients. *Although these results are modest compared with newer biologic therapies, the advantage of an oral formulation is clear. The safety profile, at least in the short term, appears to be good, with the main adverse events being gastrointestinal symptoms and weight loss.*

Etanercept treatment for children and adolescents with plaque psoriasis. Paller AS, Siegfried EC, Langley RG, Gottlieb AB, Pariser D, Landells I, et al.; Etanercept Pediatric Psoriasis Study Group. N Engl J Med 2008; 358: 241–51.

Two hundred and eleven patients age 4 to 17 years participated in this double-blind trial of weekly injections of placebo or 0.8 mg/kg of etanercept. Fifty-seven percent of etanercept-treated children achieved PASI 75, compared with 11% of those treated with placebo.

In adults etanercept can be administered in doses of 50 mg twice weekly. In the United States, after 3 months the dosage is lowered to 50 mg administered subcutaneously once weekly, but in other countries the twice-weekly dosing can continue. As in adults, the pediatric dose of 0.8 mg/kg is effective in children with psoriasis and psoriatic arthritis.

Adalimumab therapy for moderate to severe psoriasis: a randomized, controlled phase III trial. Menter A, Tyring SK, Gordon K, Kimball AB, Leonardi CL, Langley RG, et al. J Am Acad Dermatol 2008; 58: 106–15.

In this 1212-patient, double-blind, placebo-controlled trial of adalimumab 40 mg every other week for 15 weeks, 71% of adalimumab-treated patients achieved PASI 75, compared with 7% of placebo-treated patients.

Even higher response rates were achieved in patients treated with adalimumab 40 mg subcutaneously every week. A loading dose of 80 mg of adalimumab results in much faster clinical responses.

A randomized comparison of continuous vs. intermittent infliximab maintenance regimens over 1 year in the treatment of moderate-to-severe plaque psoriasis. Menter A, Feldman SR, Weinstein GD, Papp K, Evans R, Guzzo C, et al. J Am Acad Dermatol 2007; 56: 31.e1–15.

In this double-blind study 835 patients with moderate to severe psoriasis were treated with either infliximab 3 mg/kg or 5 mg/kg or placebo at weeks 0, 2, and 6. PASI 75 was achieved by 75.5% of patients in the 5 mg/kg group, compared with 70.3% in the 3 mg/kg group. At week 14, infliximab-treated patients were rerandomized to continuous or intermittent maintenance regimens. Greater improvements in psoriasis occurred with continuous rather than intermittent treatment and with the 5 mg/kg dose.

Continuous infliximab therapy may suppress the development of human antichimeric antibodies, which have been associated with more infusion reactions and reduced responsiveness to the drug.

Efficacy and safety of ustekinumab, a human interleukin-12/23 monoclonal antibody, in patients with psoriasis: 52-week results from a randomised, double-blind, placebo-controlled trial (PHOENIX 2). Papp KA, Langley RG, Lebwohl M, Krueger GG, Szapary P, Yeilding N, et al. Lancet 2008; 371: 1675–84.

In this double-blind study 1230 patients were treated with ustekinumab 45 mg or 90 mg or placebo. The drug was administered subcutaneously at weeks 0 and 4 and every 12 weeks thereafter. Of those treated with 45 mg, 66.7% achieved PASI 75 compared with 75.7% of those treated with 90 mg and 3.7% of those treated with placebo. At week 28 partial responders (i.e., those who achieved PASI 50 but not PASI 75) were rerandomized to increase dosing to every 8 weeks or to continue every 12 weeks. Of those who increased to 90 mg of ustekinumab every 8 weeks, 68.8% achieved PASI 75 by week 52, compared with only 33.3% of those who continued dosing every 12 weeks.

Ustekinumab is highly effective for psoriasis, and safety data up to 8 years are promising with regard to infection, malignancy, and cardiovascular disease. Because of the duration of its effect, ustekinumab can be administered as infrequently as every 12 weeks, although many patients need injections every 8 weeks to maintain clearing.

Secukinumab in plaque psoriasis—results of two phase 3 trials. Langley RG, Elewski BE, Lebwohl M, Reich K, Griffiths CE, Papp K, et al. N Engl J Med 2014; 371: 326–38.

Subcutaneous secukinumab 300 mg, 150 mg, or placebo was administered once weekly for 5 weeks and then every 4 weeks and compared with placebo or etanercept 50 mg twice weekly in this double-blind study. Up to 81.6% of patients achieved PASI 75 with the 300-mg dose of secukinumab and up to 71.6% with the 150-mg dose, which were superior to etanercept and to placebo.

Secukinumab 300 mg (two 150-mg subcutaneous injections) is the preferred dose and results in rapid and sustained clearing of psoriasis. Significant numbers of patients achieved PASI 90 and even PASI 100. The only side effect clearly linked to the drug was an increase in monilial infections.

Comparison of ixekizumab with etanercept or placebo in moderate-to-severe psoriasis (UNCOVER-2 and UNCOVER-3): results from two phase 3 randomised trials. Griffiths CE, Reich K, Lebwohl M, van de Kerkhof P, Paul C, Menter A, et al. Lancet 2015; 386: 541–51.

Subcutaneous 160 mg of ixekizumab followed by 80 mg every 2 weeks or every 4 weeks was compared with etanercept 50 mg every 2 weeks or placebo in this double-blind, double-dummy study. PASI 75 was achieved by up to 89.7% of patients treated with ixekizumab every 2 weeks and up to 77.5% in those treated every 4 weeks. Both regimens were superior to etanercept and to placebo.

After a loading dose of 160 mg (two 80-mg subcutaneous injections), 80 mg of ixekizumab every 2 weeks is the approved dose for up to 12 weeks. Thereafter, 80 mg every 4 weeks is approved for maintenance, although every-2-week maintenance is being studied. Rapid, sustained clearing of psoriasis can be expected, and significant numbers of patients achieve PASI 90 and PASI 100. Monilial infections can occur.

Evidence Levels: **A** Double-blind study **B** Clinical trial ≥ 20 subjects **C** Clinical trial < 20 subjects **D** Series ≥ 5 subjects **E** Anecdotal case reports

Third-Line Therapies

• Combination therapy	A
• Topical 5-fluorouracil	C
• Indigo naturalis	A
• Sulfasalazine (sulphasalazine)	A
• Mycophenolate mofetil	B
• Hydroxycarbamide (hydroxyurea)	B
• Azathioprine	C
• FK-506	A
• Fumaric acid esters	B
• Antibiotics	C
• Colchicine	C
• Laser (excimer, pulsed dye)	C
• Cryotherapy	C
• Grenz rays	B
• Leflunomide	A
• Golimumab	A
• Certolizumab	A
• Brodalumab	A
• Tofacitinib	A
• Topical Janus kinase inhibitors	A

Combination treatments for psoriasis: a systematic review and meta-analysis. Bailey EE, Ference EH, Alikhan A, Hession MT, Armstrong AW. Arch Dermatol 2012; 148: 511–22.

The side effects of psoriasis treatments can be minimized and efficacy enhanced by combining low doses of different therapies. Rotational therapy refers to a method in which patients cleared with one psoriasis therapy are subsequently treated with different therapies to minimize the cumulative toxicity of any given treatment. Thus the hepatotoxicity of cumulative doses of methotrexate, the nephrotoxicity of ciclosporin, and the carcinogenicity of PUVA can be minimized.

The most commonly used combinations involve retinoids and UVB and retinoids and PUVA. UVB and PUVA have been used in combination with one another as well as with methotrexate. Retinoids are among the safest systemic agents for psoriasis and have been combined with methotrexate and ciclosporin, although liver function tests should be watched carefully when methotrexate and acitretin are used together. The combination of methotrexate and ciclosporin is a dramatically effective therapy, as is the combination of ciclosporin and hydroxycarbamide. Methotrexate has also been used with hydroxycarbamide, but blood counts must be watched very carefully.

Although this conference predated the introduction of biologic therapies for psoriasis, all of the currently approved biologics have been administered with methotrexate, acitretin, ciclosporin, and phototherapy. Because methotrexate and ciclosporin are immunosuppressive, they should be used cautiously with biologics and for as short a period of combination as possible. An exception may be the combination of methotrexate with infliximab, as concomitant methotrexate has been shown to reduce the development of antichimeric antibodies.

Clinical efficacy of a 308 nm excimer laser for treatment of psoriasis vulgaris. He YL, Zhang XY, Dong J, Xu JZ, Wang J. Photodermatol Photoimmunol Photomed 2007; 23: 238–41.

In this open-label study 40 patients were treated twice weekly for up to 15 treatments. PASI scores improved by approximately 90%.

The excimer laser is a useful therapy for localized plaques of psoriasis. Its main side effect is local cutaneous burning.

Targeted UVB phototherapy for psoriasis: a preliminary study. Lapidoth M, Adatto M, David M. Clin Exp Dermatol 2007; 32: 642–5.

This high-intensity targeted UVB lamp (290–320 nm; Be Clear) resulted in significant improvement in localized plaques without treating normal surrounding skin.

Efficacy of the pulsed dye laser in the treatment of localized recalcitrant plaque psoriasis: a comparative study. Erceg A, Bovenschen HJ, van de Kerkhof PC, Seyger MM. Br J Dermatol 2006; 155: 110–4.

Pulsed dye laser (PDL) was compared with the combination calcipotriol/betamethasone dipropionate ointment in an open-label, bilateral comparison study. Twelve weeks after treatment there was 62% improvement in psoriasis severity scores on the PDL-treated side, compared with 19% reduction on the combination calcipotriol/betamethasone dipropionate side.

Weekly pulse dosing schedule of fluorouracil: a new topical therapy for psoriasis. Pearlman DL, Youngberg B, Engelhard C. J Am Acad Dermatol 1986; 15: 1247–52.

Fourteen patients were treated with topical 5-fluorouracil with occlusion 2 to 3 days per week for a mean of 15.7 weeks. Eleven patients achieved 90% clearing of treated lesions, compared with 6% for placebo.

Because of concern about absorption, topical 5-fluorouracil should only be used on isolated plaques. Irritation is the main side effect.

Clinical assessment of patients with recalcitrant psoriasis in a randomized, observer-blind, vehicle-controlled trial using indigo naturalis. Lin YK, Chang CJ, Chang YC, Wong WR, Chang SC, Pang JH. Arch Dermatol 2008; 144: 1457–64.

Indigo naturalis proved to be an effective topical therapy for psoriasis with clearance or near clearance in 31 of 42 subjects (74%). Staining of skin and clothing is a drawback.

Sulfasalazine improves psoriasis. A double-blind analysis. Gupta AK, Ellis CN, Siegel MT, Duell EA, Griffiths CE, Hamilton TA, et al. Arch Dermatol 1990; 126: 487–93.

Fifty patients participated in this double-blind, placebo-controlled trial. Marked improvement was reported in 41% of the sulfasalazine-treated patients and moderate improvement in another 41%. Over one quarter of the sulfasalazine-treated patients discontinued the study because of side effects of rash or nausea.

Mycophenolate mofetil (CellCept) for psoriasis: a two- center, prospective, open-label clinical trial. Zhou Y, Rosenthal D, Dutz J, Ho V. J Cutan Med Surg 2003; 7: 193–7.

Twenty-three patients were treated in an open-label study of mycophenolate mofetil 2 to 3 g daily for 12 weeks. At the end of 12 weeks PASI scores improved by 47%. Only 22% of patients did not have a significant response. Five patients developed nausea, and one developed transient leukopenia.

Mycophenolate mofetil is highly effective in a subset of psoriasis patients. Gastrointestinal side effects can be limited by administering the drug in four divided daily doses instead of the twice-daily dosing recommended in the package insert. An enteric-coated form is also helpful in reducing nausea.

Hydroxyurea in the management of therapy resistant psoriasis. Layton AM, Sheehan-Dare RA, Goodfield MJ, Cotterill JA. Br J Dermatol 1989; 121: 647–53.

Eighty-five patients with psoriasis were treated with long-term hydroxycarbamide in doses of 0.5 to 1.5 g daily. Remissions occurred in 61%. Reversible bone marrow suppression occurred in 35% of patients. Four patients developed cutaneous side effects.

Azathioprine in psoriasis. Greaves MW, Dawber R. Br Med J 1970; 2: 237–8.

Azathioprine can be effective monotherapy for psoriasis, but its use is limited by bone marrow toxicity.

As with 6-thioguanine and hydroxycarbamide, the therapeutically effective dose of azathioprine is close to doses that are toxic to the bone marrow. With all three of these drugs, frequent blood counts are essential.

Systemic tacrolimus (FK 506) is effective for the treatment of psoriasis in a double-blind, placebo-controlled study. European FK 506 Multicentre Psoriasis Study Group. Arch Dermatol 1996; 132: 419–23.

Fifty patients with psoriasis were treated for 9 weeks in this double-blind, placebo-controlled study. Starting doses were 0.05 mg/kg daily and could be increased up to 0.15 mg/kg daily. Tacrolimus-treated patients had significantly greater improvements in PASI scores than those receiving placebo. Diarrhea, paresthesias, and insomnia were the most commonly reported side effects.

Treatment of psoriasis with fumaric acid esters: results of a prospective multicentre study: German Multicentre Study. Mrowietz U, Christophers E, Altmeyer P. Br J Dermatol 1998; 138: 456–60.

Of 101 patients who started this prospective study, 70 completed 4 months of treatment. There was an 80% reduction in PASI scores. Side effects consisted of lymphocytopenia, gastrointestinal complaints, and flushing.

Although not noted in this study, nephrotoxicity has been a recognized side effect of fumaric acid therapy.

Use of rifampin with penicillin and erythromycin in the treatment of psoriasis. Preliminary report. Rosenberg EW, Noah PW, Zanolli MD, Skinner RB Jr, Bond MJ, Crutcher N. J Am Acad Dermatol 1986; 14: 761–4.

All nine patients with streptococcal-associated psoriasis responded to a 5-day course of rifampin (rifampicin) combined with 10 to 14 days of oral penicillin or erythromycin.

The use of oral antibiotics has been championed by Rosenberg and colleagues. Although supported by sound theories and numerous anecdotes, the use of antibiotics for psoriasis has not been supported by controlled clinical trials. Other infections have been linked to psoriasis flares, and other agents that have been used include oral nystatin and oral fluconazole; even tonsillectomy has been advocated.

Therapeutic trials with oral colchicine in psoriasis. Wahba A, Cohen H. Acta Dermatol Venereol 1980; 60: 515–20.

Twenty-two patients were treated in an open trial of colchicine 0.02 mg/kg daily for 2 to 4 months. Of the nine patients with thin papules and plaques, eight noted marked improvement or clearing, but there was little improvement in patients with thick plaques.

Cryotherapy for psoriasis. Nouri K, Chartier TK, Eaglstein WH, Taylor JR. Arch Dermatol 1997; 133: 1608–9.

Target plaques of psoriasis were treated with cryotherapy, resulting in improvement. Local reactions, including pain and vesiculation, were the only side effects other than discoloration.

As with lasers, cryotherapy is only practical for isolated, localized plaques. Despite the Koebner phenomenon, psoriasis does not commonly occur in frozen plaques, but scarring or discoloration can occur.

Psoriasis of the scalp treated with Grenz rays or topical corticosteroid combined with Grenz rays. A comparative randomized trial. Lindelof B, Johannesson A. Br J Dermatol 1988; 119: 241–4.

Forty patients were treated with either Grenz rays or Grenz rays plus topical corticosteroids for scalp psoriasis. Grenz rays were administered at a dosage of 4 Gy at weekly intervals for six treatments; 84% of the Grenz ray–treated patients and 72% of the Grenz ray plus corticosteroid group healed. The addition of topical corticosteroids offered little benefit.

The association between x-ray therapy and squamous cell carcinomas, particularly in patients subsequently treated with PUVA, has led to less use of this valuable modality.

Efficacy and safety of leflunomide in the treatment of psoriatic arthritis and psoriasis: a multinational, double-blind, randomized, placebo-controlled clinical trial. Kaltwasser JP, Nash P, Gladman D, Rosen CF, Behrens F, Jones P, et al.; Treatment of Psoriatic Arthritis Study Group. Arthritis Rheum 2004; 50: 1939–50.

One hundred and ninety patients with psoriasis and psoriatic arthritis were treated in this double-blind, placebo-controlled trial.

Leflunomide proved to be effective for psoriatic arthritis but only modestly effective for psoriasis.

Golimumab, a human TNF-alpha antibody, administered every 4 weeks as a subcutaneous injection in psoriatic arthritis: clinical efficacy, radiographic, and safety findings through 1 year of the randomized, placebo-controlled, GO-REVEAL study. Kavanaugh A, van der Heijde D, McInnes I, Krueger GG, Gladman D, Gómez-Reino J, et al. Arthritis Rheum 2012; 64: 2504–17.

Golimumab 50 mg or 100 mg administered subcutaneously every 4 weeks resulted in significant improvement in symptoms of psoriatic arthritis. Prevention of x-ray progression of disease was documented.

Although golimumab is approved for psoriatic arthritis, this TNF antagonist also benefits skin lesions of psoriasis.

Successful treatment of moderate to severe plaque psoriasis with the PEGylated Fab' certolizumab pegol: results of a phase II randomised, placebo-controlled trial with a re-treatment extension. Reich K, Ortonne JP, Gottlieb AB, Terpstra IJ, Coteur G, Tasset C, et al. Br J Dermatol 2012; 167: 180–90.

After a loading dose of certolizumab pegol 400 mg, subjects were treated with subcutaneous injections of 200 mg, 400 mg, or placebo every other week; 75%, 83%, and 7% of subjects achieved PASI 75, respectively.

Although certolizumab is approved for Crohn disease and for rheumatoid arthritis in the United States, this TNF antagonist is highly effective for psoriasis.

Phase 3 studies comparing brodalumab with ustekinumab in psoriasis. Lebwohl M, Strober B, Menter A, Gordon K, Weglowska J, Puig L, et al. N Engl J Med 2015; 373: 1318–28.

Psoriasis patients were treated with brodalumab (210 mg or 140 mg every 2 weeks), ustekinumab (45 mg for patients with a body weight ≤100 kg and 90 mg for patients >100 kg at weeks 0 and 4), or placebo for the first 12 weeks of these double-blind trials. Up to 86% of patients achieved PASI 75 and up to 44% achieved PASI 100 with the 210-mg dose of brodalumab, which was superior in several outcomes to 140-mg brodalumab, ustekinumab, and placebo. *A low frequency of monilial infections occurred in brodalumab-treated subjects in these early trials. In later phases of this study and in other studies there were a small number of suicides, which may not be related to the drug, but which did not occur with other treatments blocking IL-17. As a result brodalumab is being scrutinized more closely.*

Evidence Levels: **A** Double-blind study   **B** Clinical trial ≥ 20 subjects   **C** Clinical trial < 20 subjects   **D** Series ≥ 5 subjects   **E** Anecdotal case reports

ERYTHRODERMIC PSORIASIS

Erythrodermic psoriasis is characterized by marked erythema and scaling affecting the entire cutaneous surface. All the protective functions of the skin are lost, including protection against infection, temperature control, and prevention of fluid loss. Loss of nutrients through the skin leads to anemia and electrolyte imbalance. The most common precipitating cause of erythrodermic psoriasis is the withdrawal of systemic corticosteroids; this should be avoided in patients with psoriasis. Excessive use of topical superpotent corticosteroids, phototherapy burns, and infections have also been implicated as causes of erythrodermic psoriasis.

Patients may require hospitalization with bed rest, emollients, and application of *mild topical corticosteroids*. Because sepsis and shock are complications of erythrodermic psoriasis, monitoring of temperature, blood pressure, urine output, and weight may be important, depending on the severity of the condition. In males and in females not of childbearing potential, *oral retinoids* are among the safest treatments for erythrodermic psoriasis, but are not as reliably effective as *biologics, ciclosporin, or methotrexate*. *Acitretin* can be started in doses of 25 mg daily and can be increased to 50 mg or higher. *Ciclosporin* in doses of 4 to 5 mg/kg daily results in rapid improvement. *Oral methotrexate* starting at 15 mg per week and gradually increasing up to 30 mg/week is effective within a few weeks. Once erythema has cleared with topical or systemic agents, patients can occasionally be switched to phototherapy or PUVA or to other long-term therapies, including the biologics. Many of the available biologic agents, including *infliximab, adalimumab, etanercept, ustekinumab, and ixekizumab*, have been used to treat erythrodermic psoriasis When these agents either do not work or cannot be used, many of the third-line therapies listed for psoriasis are effective. For example, there are anecdotal reports of *mycophenolate mofetil, azathioprine, and hydroxycarbamide* working for erythrodermic psoriasis. Combination therapy such as the *combination of methotrexate and ciclosporin* in low doses, or the combination of *methotrexate and infliximab*, can also be effective. There are also anecdotal reports of *carbamazepine* clearing erythrodermic psoriasis.

First-Line Therapies

• Emollients	D
• Topical corticosteroids	D

Second-Line Therapies

• Retinoids	B
• Ciclosporin	B
• Infliximab	D
• Etanercept	D
• Adalimumab	D
• Ustekinumab	D
• Anti-IL-17 antibodies	D
• Methotrexate	B

Third-Line Therapies

• Combination therapy	D
• Mycophenolate mofetil	E
• Hydroxycarbamide (hydroxyurea)	E
• Azathioprine	E
• Carbamazepine	E

Use of short-course class 1 topical glucocorticoid under occlusion for the rapid control of erythrodermic psoriasis. Arbiser JL, Grossman K, Kaye E, Arndt KA. Arch Dermatol 1994; 130: 704–6.

Erythrodermic psoriasis will respond rapidly to oral corticosteroids or to superpotent corticosteroids with occlusion, but withdrawal of these agents often results in a more severe flare. Consequently, these treatments are avoided in patients with erythrodermic psoriasis.

Management of erythrodermic psoriasis with low-dose cyclosporine. Studio Italiano Muticentrico nella Psoriasi (SIMPSO). Dermatology 1993; 187: 30–7.

Thirty-three patients with erythrodermic psoriasis were treated with ciclosporin, starting with up to 5 mg/kg daily; 67% achieved complete remission in a median of 2 to 4 months, and another 27% noted substantial improvement.

Treatment of erythrodermic psoriasis with etanercept. Esposito M, Mazzotta A, de Felice C, Papoutsaki M, Chimenti S. Br J Dermatol 2006; 155: 156–9.

Ten patients were treated with open-label etanercept 25 mg subcutaneously twice weekly. By week 12, 50% had achieved at least 75% improvement in psoriasis severity scores, and that number increased by week 24.

Erythrodermic psoriasis can be a life-threatening condition requiring more rapid-acting agents than etanercept. The latter biologic can be useful in more chronic and stable forms of the disease.

Efficacy and safety of biologics in erythrodermic psoriasis: a multicentre, retrospective study. Viguier M, Pagès C, Aubin F, Delaporte E, Descamps V, Lok C, et al. Br J Dermatol 2012; 167: 417–23.

Twenty eight patients with 42 flares of erythrodermic psoriasis were treated with infliximab (n = 24), adalimumab (n = 7), etanercept (n = 6), ustekinumab (n = 3), or efalizumab (n = 2).

The authors point out that short-term control is good with these agents but because of a lack of efficacy or side effects, only one third of patients are on the same biologic at the end of a year.

Efficacy and safety of open-label ixekizumab treatment in Japanese patients with moderate-to-severe plaque psoriasis, erythrodermic psoriasis and generalized pustular psoriasis. Saeki H, Nakagawa H, Ishii T, Morisaki Y, Aoki T, Berclaz PY, et al. J Eur Acad Dermatol Venereol 2015; 29: 1148–55.

This study included eight patients with erythrodermic psoriasis and five with generalized pustular psoriasis. All erythrodermic psoriasis patients and four of five pustular psoriasis patients improved. *It is likely that secukinumab and brodalumab, which work by similar mechanisms, will be effective for erythrodermic psoriasis as well.*

Treatment of pustulous and erythrodermic psoriasis with PUVA therapy and methotrexate. Lekovic B, Dostanic I, Konstantinovic K, Kneitner I. Hautarzt 1982; 33: 284–5.

The combination of PUVA and methotrexate successfully treated five patients with erythrodermic psoriasis and two with pustular psoriasis. According to the authors, annual methotrexate doses could be reduced by 50% by adding PUVA to the regimen.

It is difficult to distinguish a PUVA burn from erythrodermic psoriasis. Nevertheless, some patients with erythrodermic psoriasis are successfully controlled with PUVA. Monotherapy with methotrexate is used more typically.

The treatment of psoriasis with etretinate and acitretin: a follow-up of actual use. Magis NL, Blummel JJ, Kerkhof PC, Gerritsen RM. Eur J Dermatol 2000; 10: 517–21.

In a retrospective review of 94 patients treated with retinoids, there were no serious side effects after 10 years of follow-up. The efficacy of retinoids for pustular and erythrodermic psoriasis was stressed.

Accidental success with carbamazepine for psoriatic erythroderma. Smith KJ, Skelton HG. N Engl J Med 1996; 335: 1999–2000.

A patient with HIV infection and erythrodermic psoriasis was inadvertently treated with carbamazepine instead of etretinate. The patient's erythroderma cleared.

Carbamazepine in doses of 200 to 400 mg daily has been reported to clear erythrodermic psoriasis in some, but not all, patients. Further controlled clinical studies are warranted.

PUSTULAR PSORIASIS

Management of pustular psoriasis begins with the *removal of precipitating causes*. Lithium, antimalarials, diltiazem, propranolol, and irritating topical therapy with tar have all been implicated, but the most common cause is the withdrawal of systemic corticosteroids. As in erythrodermic psoriasis, all the protective functions of skin are compromised, and patients are susceptible to infection, fluid loss, electrolyte imbalance, loss of nutrients through the skin, and loss of temperature control. Supportive care and treatment of infection are mandatory. *Oral acitretin* results in rapid improvement. In women of childbearing potential *isotretinoin* may be preferred because the period of teratogenicity of this drug is shorter than that of acitretin. *Ciclosporin, infliximab, adalimumab*, and *methotrexate* are also highly effective for this life-threatening condition. TNF blockers have been used to treat pustular psoriasis, but caution should be exercised as there have been rare cases of pustular psoriasis caused by their use. *Hydroxycarbamide (hydroxyurea), 6-thioguanine, mycophenolate mofetil, azathioprine, dapsone*, and *colchicine* have also been used in isolated patients.

First-Line Therapies	
• Topical corticosteroids	E
• Retinoids	B
• Ciclosporin	E
• Infliximab	E
• Adalimumab	E
• Ustekinumab	E
• Ixekizumab and other anti-IL-17 antibodies (see reference under erythrodermic psoriasis)	D
• Methotrexate	B

Second-Line Therapies	
• Topical calcipotriol	E
• Etanercept	E
• 6-Thioguanine	E
• Hydroxycarbamide (hydroxyurea)	E
• Mycophenolate mofetil	E
• Azathioprine	E

Isotretinoin vs. etretinate therapy in generalized pustular and chronic psoriasis. Moy RL, Kingston TP, Lowe NJ. Arch Dermatol 1985; 121: 1297–301.

Although isotretinoin was less effective than etretinate for plaque psoriasis, 10 of 11 patients with pustular psoriasis responded.

Many consider acitretin or isotretinoin to be the treatment of choice for patients with pustular psoriasis. Apart from the shorter period of teratogenicity of isotretinoin, it also causes less hair loss than acitretin.

Generalized pustular psoriasis (von Zumbusch) responding to cyclosporine A. Meinardi MM, Westerhof W, Bos JD. Br J Dermatol 1987; 116: 269–70.

This is one of numerous case reports documenting the dramatic response of pustular psoriasis to ciclosporin.

Ciclosporin in doses of 4 to 5 mg/kg daily is usually effective in the treatment of pustular psoriasis.

Infliximab in recalcitrant generalized pustular arthropatic psoriasis. Vieira Serrão V, Martins A, Lopes MJ. Eur J Dermatol 2008; 18: 71–3.

This is a case report of a patient with psoriatic arthritis and acute generalized pustular psoriasis refractory to acitretin, methotrexate, and corticosteroids that responded rapidly to treatment with infliximab, with complete clearing of lesions by week 12, along with improvement in psoriatic arthritis.

Pustular psoriasis induced by infliximab. Thurber M, Feasel A, Stroehlein J, Hymes SR. J Drugs Dermatol 2004; 3: 439–40.

Despite several reports describing the efficacy of infliximab in pustular psoriasis, there are a small number of reports of pustular psoriasis developing in patients treated with infliximab for other indications.

Several reports of psoriasis, and specifically pustular psoriasis, developing after treatment with TNF-α blockers have emerged. Nevertheless, these agents can be highly useful for the treatment of pustular psoriasis.

Long-term efficacy of adalimumab in generalized pustular psoriasis. Zangrilli A, Papoutsaki M, Talamonti M, Chimenti S. J Dermatol Treat 2008; 19: 185–7.

Adalimumab 40 mg subcutaneously once weekly resulted in rapid remission of chronic pustular psoriasis. The remission persisted throughout 72 weeks of treatment.

Ustekinumab: effective in a patient with severe recalcitrant generalized pustular psoriasis. Daudén E, Santiago-et-Sánchez-Mateos D, Sotomayor-López E, García-Díez A. Br J Dermatol 2010; 163: 1346–7.

There have been paradoxic cases of pustular psoriasis induced by ustekinumab.

Etanercept at different dosages in the treatment of generalized pustular psoriasis: a case series. Esposito M, Mazzotta A, Casciello C, Chimenti S. Dermatology 2008; 216: 355–60.

Six patients with generalized pustular psoriasis who failed to respond to conventional treatments were treated with etanercept 25 to 50 mg twice weekly for 48 weeks, with good efficacy.

Because etanercept can be slower acting than other systemic or biologic agents, and because generalized pustular psoriasis can be life threatening, a more rapid-acting agent should be considered for severe disease.

Generalised pustular psoriasis: response to topical calcipotriol. Berth-Jones J, Bourke J, Bailey K, Graham-Brown RA, Hutchinson PE. Br Med J 1992; 305: 868–9.

Three cases of pustular psoriasis responded to topical application of calcipotriol, and the treatment was well tolerated.

Evidence Levels: **A** Double-blind study **B** Clinical trial ≥ 20 subjects **C** Clinical trial < 20 subjects **D** Series ≥ 5 subjects **E** Anecdotal case reports

It is important to monitor serum calcium when using calcipotriol in this way. Although irritation was not a problem in the reported cases, some care is required in case this develops.

Systemic corticosteroids and folic acid antagonists in the treatment of generalized pustular psoriasis. Evaluation and prognosis based on the study of 104 cases. Ryan TJ, Baker H. Br J Dermatol 1969; 81: 134–45.

Despite the short-term benefit of systemic corticosteroids for pustular psoriasis, once the dose is reduced, rebound flares occur. In this study a significant proportion of patients treated with systemic corticosteroids died.

Methotrexate remains a highly effective modality for the treatment of pustular psoriasis. Doses beginning at 15 mg per week (after an initial test dose) are used.

Third-Line Therapy

• Colchicine   E

Colchicine in generalized pustular psoriasis: clinical response and antibody-dependent cytotoxicity by monocytes and neutrophils. Zachariae H, Kragballe K, Herlin T. Arch Dermatol Res 1982; 274: 327–33.

Three of four patients with pustular psoriasis cleared within 2 weeks of starting oral colchicine.

Colchicine 0.6 mg twice daily can be effective for pustular psoriasis. The dose can be increased by one pill daily, but side effects of diarrhea frequently intervene.

211
Psychogenic excoriation

*Michael E. Abrouk, Jillian W. Wong Millsop,
John Y.M. Koo*

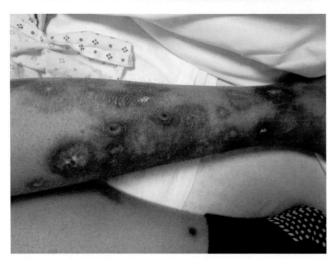

Psychogenic excoriation is a psychodermatologic condition in which patients participate in destructive scratching and picking of normal skin or skin with minor surface irregularities. Such behaviors may cause self-inflicted ulcers, abscesses, or scars that can ultimately become disfiguring. Although traditionally called *neurotic excoriation*, the authors prefer the term *psychogenic excoriation* because the underlying psychopathology may not be neurosis and may range from depression to obsessive-compulsive disease to even psychosis. The traditional term *neurotic excoriation* does our specialty a disservice, making dermatologists feel as if we know what is going on with the patient psychologically when the reality is that there is no way we can know what the underlying psychopathology is without carefully interviewing the patient regarding his or her mental status. Therefore the authors recommend the following approach:

First, do not be fooled by the term *neurotic excoriation*; go beyond the skin to clearly ascertain the nature of the underlying psychopathology. Patient behavior may be associated with underlying depression, anxiety, obsessive-compulsive disorder, psychosis, or borderline personality disorder. Psychogenic excoriations may also be precipitated by emotional stress.

Second, before diagnosing a patient with psychogenic excoriation, it is important to rule out other psychodermatologic disorders, such as dermatitis artefacta (often associated with damage done with sharp objects rather than just fingernails, characteristic secrecy about the etiology of lesions, and often associated with demanding and manipulative personality), or delusions of parasitosis (associated with delusional ideation, particularly the strongly held belief of organisms infesting the skin).

Finally, the appropriate treatment strategy can be determined based on the nature of the underlying psychopathology.

MANAGEMENT STRATEGY

Because psychogenic excoriation is primarily a psychiatric disorder, for a dermatologist without time or training for psychotherapy, psychopharmacology could be the most feasible line of therapy.

If depression or anxiety is the underlying psychopathology, antidepressants and antianxiolytics are considered first-line treatment. One of the author's (J.K.) preferred medications is the tricyclic antidepressant *doxepin*. There is an insufficient number of clinical trials demonstrating its efficacy in this condition, but doxepin is often useful due to its combined antidepressant and antihistaminic/antipruritic activity, which may be critical in disrupting the itch–scratch cycle. Doxepin is usually started at 10 to 25 mg at bedtime, with a gradual increase in dose of 10 to 25 mg every 2 to 4 weeks until the patient is taking up to 100 mg every evening, which is the typical effective antidepressant dose, particularly if the underlying psychopathology is major depression. If the patient requires even higher dosages, a maximum of up to 300 mg daily may be used, provided there are no side effects. Because doxepin can prolong the QT interval, a screening electrocardiogram (ECG) is recommended for patients over age 55 or any patient with a past history of cardiac dysrhythmia. Sedation, syncope, seizures, weight gain, and orthostatic hypotension are other potential side effects.

Selective serotonin reuptake inhibitors (SSRIs) also have been shown in several reports to be effective in patients with psychogenic excoriation. These antidepressant drugs have better safety profiles than doxepin, as they are less associated with sedation and cardiac conduction abnormalities. Other *tricyclic* antidepressants, such as *clomipramine* and *amitriptyline*, and various *benzodiazepines* are third-line therapies that should only be considered if the patient does not respond to more conventional treatments or cannot tolerate the side effects.

For treatment of underlying psychosis, antipsychotics can be effective. *Pimozide*, a traditional antipsychotic; *olanzapine*, an atypical antipsychotic; *aripiprazole*, a second-generation antipsychotic; and *naltrexone*, an opioid antagonist, may have a role for these patients with psychogenic excoriation.

As for borderline personality as the underlying psychopathology, *psychotherapy* is recommended. *Psychotherapy* and *cognitive behavioral techniques*, including aversion therapy and habit reversal treatments, have been reported in certain cases to be effective for this disorder and can be used as adjunctive therapy for other underlying psychopathologies, including those discussed earlier. There are two case reports of the efficacy of *cognitive psychotherapy with laser irradiation* of disfiguring skin lesions, as well as a case report on the efficacy of *hypnosis* to alleviate psychogenic excoriation.

Other strategies for treatment may further enhance systemic pharmacologic treatments and psychotherapy. Treating associated infection and pruritus through the prudent use of *antibiotics* and *antihistamines (oral or topical)*, respectively, and using *topical corticosteroids* may provide additional symptomatic benefit for patients with psychogenic excoriation. Last, a recent study demonstrated *narrowband ultraviolet (NB-UVB) phototherapy* may be helpful for psychogenic excoriation.

Specific Investigation

- Close follow-up with a primary care physician or psychiatrist is recommended because of the high incidence of comorbid psychiatric conditions

Psychogenic excoriation. Clinical features, proposed diagnostic criteria, epidemiology and approaches to treatment. Arnold LM, Auchenbach MB, McElroy SL. CNS Drugs 2001; 15: 351–9.

Evidence Levels: **A** Double-blind study **B** Clinical trial ≥ 20 subjects **C** Clinical trial < 20 subjects **D** Series ≥ 5 subjects **E** Anecdotal case reports

A review article that outlines the clinical features of psychogenic excoriation, comorbid psychiatric conditions, therapies, and potential criteria for diagnosis.

Characteristics of 34 adults with psychogenic excoriation. Arnold LM, McElroy SL, Mutasim DF, Dwight MM, Lamerson CL, Morris EM. J Clin Psychiatry 1998; 59: 509–15.

Patients with psychogenic excoriations have a high prevalence of concurrent psychiatric illnesses such as mood disorders (68%), anxiety disorders (41%), somatoform disorders (21%), substance abuse (12%), and eating disorders (12%).

Neurotic excoriations and dermatitis artefacta. Koblenzer CS. Dermatol Clin 1996; 14: 447–55.

A good review article.

The psychiatric profile of patients with psychogenic excoriations. Mutasim DF, Adams BB. J Am Acad Dermatol 2009; 61: 611–3.

In a study of 50 patients with psychogenic excoriations compared with controls, the most significantly associated psychiatric comorbidities are depression and bipolar disorder.

Dermatology and conditions related to obsessive–compulsive disorder. Stein DJ, Hollander E. J Am Acad Dermatol 1992; 26: 237–42.

Patients with psychogenic excoriations often have obsessive-compulsive symptoms and may therefore respond to specific therapies aimed at this type of disorder.

Neurotic excoriations: a diagnosis of exclusion. Anetakis Poulos G, Algothani L, Bendo S, Zirwas MJ. J Clin Aesthet Dermatol 2012; 5: 63–4.

A 53-year-old woman with a history of schizophrenia, depression, hepatitis C, and diabetes was clinically misdiagnosed with neurotic excoriations instead of her true diagnosis: bullous pemphigoid.

It is essential that the diagnosis of psychogenic excoriations be made when other dermatologic diagnoses are definitively ruled out.

Psychogenic excoriation in a systemic lupus erythematosus patient. Silva BS, Bonin CC, Carvalho JF. Acta Rheumatol Port 2010; 35: 396.

A 37-year-old woman with systemic lupus erythematosus was referred to dermatology due to persistence of lesions refractory to therapy. She was diagnosed with psychogenic excoriation and started on sertraline with complete healing of her dermatologic disease.

The reconstructive challenges and approach to patients with excoriation disorder. Galdyn IA, Chidester J, Martin MC. J Craniofac Surg 2015; 26: 824–5.

Treating patients with psychogenic excoriation requires a multidisciplinary approach. Before any surgical repair or treatment can be rendered, the patient must be stabilized from a psychiatric standpoint.

First-Line Therapy

• Doxepin	E

Psychopharmacology for dermatologic patients. Koo J, Gambla C. Dermatol Clin 1996; 14: 509–24.

Describes in further detail the use of doxepin in psychogenic excoriations.

Improvement of chronic neurotic excoriations with oral doxepin therapy. Harris BA, Sherertz EF, Flowers FP. Int J Dermatol 1987; 26: 541–3.

Case report of two patients who responded to doxepin 30 mg and 75 mg daily.

Second-Line Therapies

• Sertraline	B
• Paroxetine	E

Sertraline in the treatment of neurotic excoriations and related disorders. Kalivas J, Kalivas L, Gilman D, Hayden CT. Arch Dermatol 1996; 132: 589–90.

Sertraline was started at 25 to 50 mg daily and titrated upward to 100 to 200 mg daily as necessary, with improvements seen in 19 of 28 patients (68%) at an average of 4 weeks.

Paroxetine in a case of psychogenic pruritus and neurotic excoriations. Biondi M, Arcangeli T, Petrucci RM. Psychother Psychosom 2000; 69: 165–6.

This is one case report demonstrating success with the SSRI paroxetine, which was thought to work secondary to its anticompulsive activity.

Third-Line Therapies

• Fluoxetine	A
• Fluvoxamine	C
• Venlafaxine	E
• Escitalopram	D
• Clomipramine	E
• Amitriptyline	E
• Benzodiazepines	E
• Pimozide	E
• Olanzapine	D
• Aripiprazole	E
• Naltrexone	E
• Psychotherapy	D
• Cognitive behavioral therapy	E
• Hypnosis	E
• Narrowband ultraviolet light	C

A double-blind trial of fluoxetine in pathologic skin picking. Simeon D, Stein DJ, Gross S, Islam N, Schmeidler J, Hollander E. J Clin Psychiatry 1997; 58: 341–7.

Fluoxetine was started at 20 mg daily and increased by 20 mg/week up to a maximum of 80 mg daily. Improvements in the treatment arm were statistically significant (based on an intent-to-treat analysis) at 6 weeks, with an average dose of 55 mg daily.

This trial is limited by a small sample (10 patients in the study arm and 11 in the placebo arm), a high dropout rate (40% in the fluoxetine group), and a study period of only 10 weeks, but the study substantiated earlier case reports.

An open clinical trial of fluvoxamine treatment of psychogenic excoriation. Arnold LM, Mutasim DF, Dwight MM, Lamerson CL, Morris EM, McElroy SL. J Clin Psychopharmacol 1999; 19: 15–8.

Fluvoxamine was started at 25 to 50 mg daily and increased by up to 50 mg/week to a maximum of 300 mg daily for 12 weeks.

Although all 14 participants demonstrated significant improvement in six of eight self-reported scales, the 7 subjects who completed the study (50%) had improvement in only two of eight self-reported scales.

Use of escitalopram in psychogenic excoriation. Pukadan D, Antony J, Mohandas E, Cyriac M, Smith G, Elias A. Aust NZ J Psychiatry 2008; 42: 435–6.

Escitalopram was administered at 10 mg/day to two patients: a 63-year-old woman with a 1-month history of diffuse pruritus and excessive excoriation, as well as major depressive disorder; and a 24-year-old man with a 10-year history of repeated nail biting and features of major depressive disorder. In both patients, scratching abated within 2 weeks.

Neurotic excoriations: a review and some new perspectives. Gupta MA, Gupta AK, Haberman HF. Compr Psychiatry 1986; 27: 381–6.

A case report of successful treatment using clomipramine 50 mg every evening for 6 months.

Neurotic excoriations: a personality evaluation. Fisher BK, Pearce KI. Cutis 1974; 14: 251–4.

Successful treatment with amitriptyline 50 to 75 mg daily was reported.

Neurotic excoriations. Fisher BK. Can Med Assoc J 1971; 105: 937–9.

This is a case report of the success of benzodiazepines before the availability of SSRIs. In general, benzodiazepines may be useful only if anxiety is the primary cause of psychogenic excoriations.

Clinical experience with pimozide: emphasis on its use in postherpetic neuralgia. Duke EE. J Am Acad Dermatol 1983; 8: 845–50.

This case report primarily demonstrates the efficacy of pimozide (2 mg two or three times daily) in the treatment of postherpetic neuralgia (eight patients) and psychogenic excoriations (two patients).

Efficacy of olanzapine in the treatment of psychogenic excoriation. Blanch J, Grimalt F, Massana G, Navarro V. Br J Dermatol 2004; 151: 714–6.

This article describes a series of six patients with psychogenic excoriation who improved dramatically after treatment with olanzapine 2.5 to 10 mg daily.

The treatment of psychogenic excoriation and obsessive compulsive disorder using aripiprazole and fluoxetine. Curtis AR, Richards RW. Ann Clin Psychiatry 2007; 19: 199–200.

This is a case report on the success of aripiprazole, a second-generation antipsychotic, and fluoxetine in an 18-year-old woman with psychogenic excoriations and obsessive–compulsive disorder.

Aripiprazole augmentation of venlafaxine in the treatment of psychogenic excoriation. Carter WG, 3rd, Shillcutt SD. J Clin Psychiatry 2006; 67: 1311.

This case report discusses the success of aripiprazole and venlafaxine in a 50-year-old woman with psychogenic excoriation, major depressive disorder, and generalized anxiety disorder who had been unresponsive to a serotonin–norepinephrine reuptake inhibitor alone.

Naltrexone for neurotic excoriations. Smith KC, Pittelkow MR. J Am Acad Dermatol 1989; 20: 860–1.

This article discusses the reported efficacy of naltrexone for psychogenic excoriations.

Psychotherapeutic strategy and neurotic excoriations. Fruensgaard K. Int J Dermatol 1991; 30: 198–203.

This article reports a positive impact of goal-directed psychotherapy in 22 patients followed over a period of approximately 5 years for psychogenic excoriations.

Treatment of facial scarring and ulceration resulting from acne excoriée with 585-nm pulsed dye laser irradiation and cognitive psychotherapy. Bowes LE, Alster TS. Dermatol Surg 2004; 30: 934–8.

Two case reports of successful treatment of acne excoriée with a pulsed dye laser to improve the appearance of scars and ulcers, as well as cognitive psychotherapy to maintain improvement.

Acne excoriée: a case report of treatment using habit reversal. Kent A, Drummond LM. Clin Exp Dermatol 1989; 14: 163–4.

This is a case report on the success of habit reversal, a cognitive behavioral technique, for psychogenic excoriations.

The behavioral treatment of neurodermatitis through habit reversal. Rosenbaum MS, Ayllon J. Behav Res Ther 1981; 19: 313–8.

This article reports a response to habit reversal therapy for neurodermatitis in three patients.

Treatment of neurodermatitis by behavior therapy: a case study. Ratcliffe R, Stein N. Behav Res Ther 1968; 6: 397–9.

This is a case report in which neurodermatitis secondary to psychogenic excoriation improved after aversion therapy, a cognitive behavioral technique.

Using hypnosis to facilitate resolution of psychogenic excoriations in acne excoriée. Shenefelt PD. Am J Clin Hypn 2004; 46: 239–45.

In this case report, the acne excoriée in a pregnant woman was successfully alleviated through hypnotic suggestion.

Narrow-band ultraviolet B as a potential alternative treatment for resistant psychogenic excoriation: an open-label study. Ozden MG, Aydin F, Senturk N, Bek Y, Canturk T, Turanli A. Photodermatol Photoimmunol Photomed 2010; 26: 162–4.

A prospective study assessing the effectiveness of phototherapy for psychogenic excoriation. Of the seven patients who completed the study and received NB-UVB, 50% or more reduction in clinical improvement scale scores was found in 71.4% (five of seven) of patients. The only side effects were xerosis and moderate erythema.

Evidence Levels: **A** Double-blind study **B** Clinical trial ≥ 20 subjects **C** Clinical trial < 20 subjects **D** Series ≥ 5 subjects **E** Anecdotal case reports

212

Pyoderma gangrenosum

John Berth-Jones

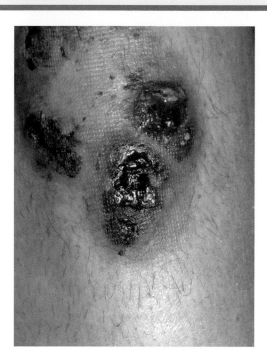

Pyoderma gangrenosum (PG) is a clinically diagnosed entity presenting as pustules that enlarge, forming ulcers with a dark, necrotic, and undermined margin. Any skin site may be affected. Although PG is usually self-limiting, there is a danger of disfiguring scarring.

MANAGEMENT STRATEGY

No treatment is always effective. The most consistent results are reported with *systemic corticosteroids* and *ciclosporin*, and these effective but potentially toxic modalities can be employed when the severity of the disease justifies the risks (e.g., when there is facial involvement, extensive disease, or rapid progression). *Infliximab* has been shown to be beneficial in a controlled trial. The evidence regarding other modalities is less conclusive. PG tends to resolve spontaneously, so some of the reports of therapeutic success may simply be the result of the disease following its natural course.

In cases where scarring is not a major concern, consideration should be given to conservative treatment with *wound dressing* only, as most lesions resolve spontaneously. The relatively safe first-line treatments can be tried first. A wide variety of other treatments have been reported to be effective at a more anecdotal level, some are potentially hazardous, some are not universally available, and some are costly, and these third-line modalities can be considered when others are ineffective.

PG may demonstrate the Koebner phenomenon; care should be taken to avoid trauma to the skin. When surgery is unavoidable in patients with a history of PG, the surgeon should be made aware of this risk. Surgical incisions should be kept as short as possible. Careful wound closure may be helpful. *Prophylactic systemic corticosteroids or ciclosporin* may be indicated perioperatively.

Effective management of associated systemic diseases such as ulcerative colitis often seems to result in improvement of the PG.

Specific Investigations

- Hematology
- Plasma protein electrophoresis
- Rheumatoid factor
- Antineutrophil cytoplasmic antibodies (ANCA) in selected patients where clinically indicated
- Gastrointestinal workup for inflammatory bowel disease

The many recognized associations with PG include rheumatoid disease, inflammatory bowel disease, myeloproliferative disease such as acute myeloblastic leukemia, plasma cell dyscrasias, and Wegener granulomatosis. These may warrant investigation and may also influence the choice of treatment.

First-Line Therapies

• Topical tacrolimus	C
• Topical corticosteroids	C
• Dapsone	D
• Intralesional corticosteroids	D
• Minocycline	D
• Nicotine	D
• Topical pimecrolimus	E
• Sodium cromoglycate	D
• Sulfasalazine	D

Topical tacrolimus for pyoderma gangrenosum. Reich K, Vente C, Neumann C. Br J Dermatol 1998; 139: 755–7.

Tacrolimus ointment 0.1% proved effective when used in combination with systemic ciclosporin and also when used alone.

Topical tacrolimus in the management of peristomal pyoderma gangrenosum. Lyon CC, Stapleton M, Smith AJ, Mendelsohn S, Beck MH, Griffiths CEM. J Dermatol Treat 2001; 12: 13–7.

Seven out of 11 cases of peristomal PG healed completely after 2 to 10 weeks of applying tacrolimus 0.3% in carmellose sodium paste (Orabase). Serum levels of tacrolimus were undetectable in all cases. In this open study the results were at least as good as those from clobetasol propionate.

Caution: A case of systemic absorption and acute nephrotoxicity has been reported in a patient who applied 60 mg of tacrolimus ointment (i.e., presumably 60 g of 0.1% ointment) daily to PG.

Pyoderma gangrenosum of the scalp. Peachey RDG. Br J Dermatol 1974; 90: 106.

A case showed slow but steady improvement on 0.1% betamethasone valerate lotion applied under polythene occlusion at night.

Beclomethasone inhaler used to treat pyoderma gangrenosum. Chriba M, Skellett AM, Levell NJ. Clin Exp Dermatol 2010; 35: 337–8.

A case of peristomal PG healed over 4 weeks using beclomethasone dipropionate 200 µg, four puffs daily.

The accepted efficacy of systemic corticosteroids would suggest that topical application might also be beneficial. However, there are only anecdotal reports, often in conjunction with other treatments, to support their efficacy. Potent compounds are generally used, applied once daily, under an occlusive dressing.

Sulfapyridine and sulphone-type drugs in dermatology. Lorincz AL, Pearson RW. Arch Dermatol 1962; 85: 42–56.

Dapsone was successfully employed in the treatment of PG at doses of up to 400 mg daily.

Low cost and familiarity of dermatologists with this drug probably contribute to its popularity. Dapsone has often been used in combination with other modalities, especially systemic corticosteroids. There are also many published cases in which this drug has proved ineffective. Dapsone has been successfully used in children with PG. The mechanism of action is believed to be inhibition of neutrophil migration and the myeloperoxidase system. Crushed dapsone applied topically is reported as effective in a case of peristomal PG.

Triamcinolone and pyoderma gangrenosum. Gardner LW, Acker DW. Arch Dermatol 1972; 106: 599–600.

A case of multifocal PG responded to intralesional triamcinolone acetonide 10 mg/mL. Doses ranging from 40 mg to 200 mg were injected at any one time.

Intralesional or perilesional injection of corticosteroids appears to be very helpful in some cases. The corticosteroid is usually injected into the skin around the active margins of lesions.

The successful use of minocycline in pyoderma gangrenosum – a report of seven cases and review of the literature. Berth-Jones J, Tan SV, Graham-Brown RAC, Pembroke AC. J Dermatol Treat 1989; 1: 23–5.

Seven cases improved on minocycline at doses of 100 mg twice daily or 200 mg twice daily. Improvement was often observed within a few days.

Successful treatment of pyoderma gangrenosum with topical 0.5% nicotine cream. Patel GK, Rhodes JR, Evans B, Holt PJ. J Dermatol Treat 2004; 15: 122–5.

Two cases responded to nicotine in cetomacrogol cream.

There are also reports of PG responding to nicotine chewing gum, application of nicotine patches to lesions, and application of Swedish moist snuff containing nicotine.

Successful treatment of severe pyoderma gangrenosum with pimecrolimus cream 1%. Bellini V, Simonetti S, Lisi P. J Eur Acad Dermatol Venereol 2008; 22: 113–5.

A patient was cleared of PG lesions within 8 weeks using pimecrolimus cream twice daily.

Pyoderma gangrenosum. A study of 19 cases. Perry HO, Brunsting LA. Arch Dermatol 1957; 75: 380–6.

Six out of seven patients with PG associated with colitis demonstrated a good response to sulfasalazine 0.5 g every 3 hours. A good response was also seen in three of four cases of PG when colitis was not present.

This drug may be particularly useful in cases of PG associated with inflammatory bowel disease, and it can also be effective in those that are not. The initial dose ranges from 0.5 to 2 g four times daily. Doses at the upper end of this range are usually reduced for maintenance therapy.

The treatment of pyoderma gangrenosum with sodium cromoglycate. De Cock KM, Thorne MG. Br J Dermatol 1980; 102: 231–3.

Two cases responded to sodium cromoglycate aqueous solution (2% w/v, Rynacrom nasal spray). In one patient, healing occurred within 3 weeks.

This is a remarkably safe treatment. Solutions have been applied to lesions in concentrations from 1% to 4%. Various nasal sprays and nebulizer solutions have proved suitable for application. The solution can be sprayed on to the ulcer or applied on gauze or under occlusion with a hydrocolloid dressing. This drug may act by inhibiting neutrophil migration or cytotoxicity.

Second-Line Therapies	
• Ciclosporin	B
• Systemic corticosteroids	B

Treatment of pyoderma gangrenosum with ciclosporin: results in seven patients. Elgart G, Stover P, Larson K, Sutter C, Scheibner S, Davis B, et al. J Am Acad Dermatol 1991; 24: 83–6.

Six of seven patients, including cases associated with rheumatoid disease and cryoglobulinemia, improved on ciclosporin, with four healing completely.

The response to ciclosporin seems to be fairly consistent. Because the toxicity of this drug is largely related to prolonged use, it can be a reasonably safe approach to gaining control of PG, which is often a brief, self-limiting illness. High doses have been used (5–10 mg/kg/day) and are probably safe for a few days in an urgent situation. However, it is likely that lower doses of 5 mg/kg/day will often be adequate.

Pyoderma gangrenosum. Clinical and laboratory findings in 15 patients with special reference to polyarthritis. Holt PJA, Davies MG, Saunders KC, Nuki G. Medicine 1980; 59: 114–33.

Twelve of these patients received, and responded to, corticosteroid treatment. Doses of up to 100 mg daily were required to induce remission.

Therapeutic efficacy in the treatment of pyoderma gangrenosum. Johnson RB, Lazarus GS. Arch Dermatol 1982; 118: 76–84.

Intravenous doses of methylprednisolone 1 g daily for 5 days induced prompt responses in three cases.

Systemic corticosteroids (prednisone/prednisolone) have been one of the most frequently used treatments for PG, and extensive published experience indicates that they are generally considered highly effective. High doses of 40 to 100 mg/day may be required, and the morbidity may be considerable. Lower doses of 7.5 to 20 mg daily are sometimes adequate for maintenance. Other systemic and topical agents are usually employed simultaneously in order to minimize the dose.

Comparison of the two most commonly used treatments for pyoderma gangrenosum: results of the STOP GAP randomised controlled trial. Ormerod AD, Thomas KS, Craig FE, Mitchell E, Greenlaw N, Norris J, et al. BMJ 2015; 350: h2956.

In this study with 112 randomized patients, prednisolone 0.75 mg/kg/day was compared with ciclosporin 4 mg/kg/day to a maximum dose of 75 and 400 mg/day, respectively. The treatments did not differ across a range of objective and patient-reported outcomes. At 6 months, 47% of ulcers had healed in each group. Infections were more common serious adverse events in the group receiving prednisolone.

Evidence Levels: **A** Double-blind study **B** Clinical trial ≥ 20 subjects **C** Clinical trial < 20 subjects **D** Series ≥ 5 subjects **E** Anecdotal case reports

Third-Line Therapies

• Infliximab	A
• Other TNFα-antagonists	C
• Alkylating agents (cyclophosphamide, chlorambucil)	D
• Plasmapheresis (plasma exchange)	E
• Leukocytapheresis	D
• Intravenous immunoglobulin	C
• Intralesional ciclosporin	E
• Tacrolimus (FK506)	D
• Azathioprine or mercaptopurine	D
• Colchicine	D
• Thalidomide	D
• Potassium iodide	E
• Topical nitrogen mustard (mechlorethamine)	E
• Mycophenolate mofetil	D
• GM-CSF	E
• Methotrexate	E
• Topical platelet-derived growth factor	E
• Platelet-rich plasma	E
• Recombinant human epidermal growth factor	E
• Clofazimine	D
• Hyperbaric oxygen	D
• Isotretinoin	E
• Anakinra	E
• Ustekinumab	E
• Imiquimod	E
• Visilizumab	E
• Topical phenytoin	D
• Surgical debridement, closure, graft, or flap	E

Infliximab for the treatment of pyoderma gangrenosum: a randomised, double blind, placebo controlled trial. Brooklyn TN, Dunnill MG, Shetty A, Bowden JJ, Williams JD, Griffiths CE, et al. Gut 2006; 55: 505–9.

A placebo-controlled trial with 30 subjects. Two weeks after an infusion of infliximab 5 mg/kg or placebo, significantly more patients in the infliximab group had improved. In a later, open-label phase, 29 patients received infliximab with 20 demonstrating a response.

Improvement of pyoderma gangrenosum and psoriasis associated with Crohn's disease with anti-tumor necrosis factor alpha monoclonal antibody. Tan MH, Gordon M, Lebwohl O, George J, Lebwohl MG. Arch Dermatol 2001; 137: 930–3.

Numerous case reports have further established the response to infliximab.

Treatment of pyoderma gangrenosum with etanercept. McGowan JW 4th, Johnson CA, Lynn A. J Drugs Dermatol 2004; 3: 441–4.

The first of several cases reported to respond to etanercept 25 to 50 mg twice weekly.

Adalimumab therapy for recalcitrant pyoderma gangrenosum. Fonder MA, Cummins DL, Ehst BD, Anhalt GJ, Meyerle JH. J Burns Wounds 2006; 5: e8.

In this case improvement occurred on treatment with adalimumab after infliximab had failed to improve the pyoderma.

Adalimumab for treatment of pyoderma gangrenosum. Pomerantz RG, Husni ME, Mody E, Qureshi AA. Br J Dermatol 2007; 157: 1274–5.

Improvement occurred in a case that had failed to respond to etanercept.

Conventional dosing regimens have been employed: 40 to 80 mg fortnightly with and without an initial loading dose of 80 mg.

Pyoderma gangrenosum. Response to cyclophosphamide therapy. Newell LM, Malkinson FD. Arch Dermatol 1983; 119: 495–7.

A very refractory case of PG responded to cyclophosphamide 150 mg daily. Healing was evident after 14 days and almost complete after 109 days.

Intravenous cyclophosphamide pulses in the treatment of pyoderma gangrenosum associated with rheumatoid arthritis. Report of 2 cases and review of the literature. Zonana-Nacach A, Jimenez-Balderas FJ, Martinez-Osuna P, Mintz G. J Rheumatol 1994; 21: 1352–6.

Two patients improved on pulsed intravenous cyclophosphamide at doses of 500 mg/m² combined with oral corticosteroid. The first received three pulses over 5 weeks and the second seven pulses over 14 weeks. In both cases remission was subsequently maintained using oral cyclophosphamide 100 mg daily.

Chlorambucil is an effective corticosteroid-sparing agent for recalcitrant pyoderma gangrenosum. Burruss JB, Farmer ER, Callen JP. J Am Acad Dermatol 1996; 35: 720–4.

Chlorambucil, 2 mg to 4 mg daily, was successfully used in six cases, both alone and in combination with systemic corticosteroids.

Pyoderma gangrenosum – response to topical nitrogen mustard. Tsele E, Yu RCH, Chu AC. Clin Exp Dermatol 1992; 17: 437–40.

The application of nitrogen mustard 20 mg/100 mL in aqueous solution on gauze swabs proved helpful in a single case associated with IgA paraprotein that had resisted many other treatment modalities. Patients can prepare this solution at home using tap water. Plasmapheresis was also helpful in this case. This was performed weekly for 2 years, successfully controlling the PG during this time.

Plasmapheresis is a relatively safe treatment involving removal of plasma while returning the blood cells to the circulation. Exchanges have generally been performed once to three times weekly, and prompt responses have been reported.

Leukocytapheresis treatment for pyoderma gangrenosum. Fujimoto E, Fujimoto N, Kuroda K, Tajima S. Br J Dermatol 2004; 151: 1090–2.

Efficacy of granulocyte and monocyte adsorption apheresis for three cases of refractory pyoderma gangrenosum. Seishima M, Mizutani Y, Shibuya Y, Nagasawa C, Aoki T. Ther Apher Dial 2007; 11: 177–82.

Three patients improved after weekly treatments for 10 or 11 weeks.

Extracorporeal removal of leukocytes is reported to have been effective in several cases of PG occurring both in isolation and in association with ulcerative colitis and rheumatoid disease.

Intravenous immunoglobulin for pyoderma gangrenosum. Kreuter A, Reich-Schupke S, Stucker M, Altmeyer P, Gambichler T. Br J Dermatol 2008; 158: 856–7.

A series of seven cases successfully treated with 0.5 g/kg body weight per day over 2 or 3 consecutive days in combination with systemic steroids and other drugs.

Clearing of pyoderma gangrenosum by intralesional cyclosporin A. Mrowietz U, Christophers E. Br J Dermatol 1991; 125: 498–9.

A lesion on the shoulder improved after two injections in 1 week of 35 mg ciclosporin into the active edges and beneath the lesion. The injection was formulated by diluting Sandimmune with normal saline in a ratio of 1:3.

Recalcitrant pyoderma gangrenosum treated with systemic tacrolimus. Lyon CC, Kirby B, Griffiths CE. Br J Dermatol 1999; 140: 562–4.

A refractory case of periostomal PG responded to tacrolimus 0.15 mg/kg/day.

Successful therapy of refractory pyoderma gangrenosum and periorbital phlegmona with tacrolimus (FK506) in ulcerative colitis. Baumgart DC, Wiedenmann B, Dignass AU. Inflamm Bowel Dis 2004; 10: 421–4.

Two cases associated with ulcerative colitis responded to tacrolimus 0.1 mg/kg/day.

Crohn's disease with cutaneous involvement. Parks AG, Morson BC, Pegum JS. Proc R Soc Med 1965; 58: 241.

Mercaptopurine was used at the dose of 75 mg/day with prednisone 20 mg/day.

Mercaptopurine is the active metabolite of azathioprine. Azathioprine has often been employed for PG, both alone and as a steroid-sparing agent. Doses have generally ranged from 100 to 150 mg daily. Less often, higher doses of up to 2.5 mg/kg/day are used. This drug seems useful in some cases, but results are not consistent.

Treatment of pyoderma gangrenosum with colchicine. Paolini O, Hebuterne X, Flory P, Charles F, Rampal P. Lancet 1995; 345: 1057–8.

Colchicine, 1 mg daily, was effective and well tolerated in PG associated with Crohn colitis.

Case report. Severe pyoderma associated with familial Mediterranean fever: favorable response to colchicine in three patients. Lugassy G, Ronnen M. Am J Med Sci 1992; 304: 29–31.

Treatment was commenced at 2 mg/day and reduced to 1 mg/day for maintenance.

Pyoderma gangrenosum with severe pharyngeal involvement. Buckley C, Bayoumi AHM, Sarkany I. J R Soc Med 1990; 83: 590–1.

A refractory case responded to thalidomide 100 mg daily.

Pyoderma gangrenosum chez un enfant: traitement par la thalidomide. Venencie PY, Saurat J-H. Ann Pediatr 1982; 1: 67–9.

A 3-year-old child refractory to other treatments responded well to thalidomide 150 mg daily.

Pyoderma gangrenosum associated with Behçet's syndrome – response to thalidomide. Munro CS, Cox NH. Clin Exp Dermatol 1988; 13: 408–10.

A case refractory to prednisolone 100 mg daily combined with dapsone 100 mg daily responded within 48 hours to thalidomide 400 mg daily.

This drug may be of particular value in cases associated with Behçet disease, as it is also reportedly effective in severe aphthous ulceration.

Successful treatment of pyoderma gangrenosum with potassium iodide. Akihiko A, Yohei M, Yayoi T, Hiroshi M, Kunihiko T. Acta Derm Venereol 2006; 86: 84–5.

Oral KI 900 mg/day was added to prednisolone 17.5 mg, dapsone 50 mg, and minocycline 200 mg daily, which had not been effective. Improvement was observed within a few days. The dose of potassium iodide was increased to 1200 mg/day after 2 weeks, and the PG had disappeared almost completely after 1 month.

Potassium iodide has also been used to treat Sweet syndrome.

Mycophenolate mofetil in pyoderma gangrenosum. Lee MR, Cooper AJ. J Dermatol Treat 2004; 15: 303–7.

Mycophenolate 1 to 2.5 g daily was used in combination with prednisolone in three cases and as monotherapy (with 500 mg twice daily) in one.

Mycophenolate has most often been used in combination with other agents, such as ciclosporin and corticosteroids.

Pyoderma gangrenosum in myelodysplasia responding to granulocyte macrophage-colony stimulating factor (GM-CSF). Bulvic S, Jacobs P. Br J Dermatol 1997; 136: 637–8.

A case responded to subcutaneous GM-CSF in a dose of 400 mg daily.

Pyoderma gangrenosum successfully treated with perilesional GM-CSF. Shpiro D, Gilat D, Fisher-Feld L, Shemer A, Gold I, Trau H. Br J Dermatol 1998; 138: 368–9.

In this case the GM-CSF was injected perilesionally at a weekly dose of 400 mg for 4 weeks.

The use of this agent has also been reported to aggravate PG. A variety of hypersensitivity reactions, including anaphylaxis, have occasionally occurred.

Treatment of pyoderma gangrenosum with methotrexate. Teitel AD. Cutis 1996; 57: 326–8.

A case failing to respond to prednisone 60 mg daily improved within 2 weeks of adding methotrexate 15 mg weekly.

Topical platelet-derived growth factor accelerates healing of myelodysplastic syndrome-associated pyoderma gangrenosum. Braun-Falco M, Stock K, Ring J, Hein R. Br J Dermatol 2002; 147: 829–31.

Complete healing occurred over 9 weeks in this case after becaplermin was added to the treatment regimen.

Autologous platelet rich plasma in pyoderma gangrenosum – two case reports. Budamakuntla L, Suryanarayan S, Sarvajnamurthy SS, Hurkudli SD. Indian J Dermatol 2015; 60: 204–5.

These cases improved after 20 days and 5 weeks of once-weekly applications.

Recombinant human epidermal growth factor enhances wound healing of pyoderma gangrenosum in a patient with ulcerative colitis. Kim TY, Han DS, Eun CS, Chung YW. Inflamm Bowel Dis 2008; 14: 725–7.

Another case reported to improve in response to topical application of a growth factor.

Clofazimine. A new agent for treatment of pyoderma gangrenosum. Michaelsson G, Molin L, Ohman S, Gip L, Lindstrom B, Skogh M. Arch Dermatol 1976; 112: 344–9.

A good response was observed in eight cases using 300 to 400 mg daily.

Pyoderma gangrenosum treated with hyperbaric oxygen therapy. Wasserteil V, Bruce S, Sessoms SL, Guntupalli KK. Int J Dermatol 1992; 31: 594–6.

Hyperbaric oxygen has been reported as beneficial in several cases of PG. However, like all other treatments, it is not effective in all cases. This treatment may be worth trying when facilities are available.

Superficial pyoderma gangrenosum responding to treatment with isotretinoin. Proudfoot LE, Singh S, Staughton RC. Br J Dermatol 2008; 159: 1377–8.

A previously refractory case of PG responding to isotretinoin 0.25 mg/kg/day.

Do not forget there are reports of isotretinoin therapy inducing exacerbations of inflammatory bowel disease and PG-like eruptions.

Targeted treatment of pyoderma gangrenosum in PAPA (pyogenic arthritis, pyoderma gangrenosum and acne) syndrome with the recombinant human interleukin-1 receptor antagonist anakinra. Brenner M, Ruzicka T, Plewig G, Thomas P, Herzer P. Br J Dermatol 2009; 161: 1199–201.

A single case of PG associated with an autosomal dominant genodermatosis.

A case of PG associated with inflammatory bowel disease has been reported not to respond.

Interleukin 23 expression in pyoderma gangrenosum and targeted therapy with ustekinumab. Guenova E, Teske A, Fehrenbacher B, Hoerber S, Adamczyk A, Schaller M, et al. Arch Dermatol 2011; 147: 1203–5.

A case healed on 45 mg subcutaneous ustekinumab, repeated after 4 weeks, in combination with topical tacrolimus.

Experience of using this drug for PG remains limited to a further couple of case reports.

Penile pyoderma gangrenosum successfully treated with topical imiquimod. Rathod SP, Padhiar BB, Karia UK, Shah BJ. Indian J Sex Transm Dis 2011; 32: 114–7.

A case of refractory penile ulceration of 18 months' duration was treated with imiquimod 5% cream once a day for 4 weeks. The lesion healed after 3 weeks.

Monoclonal gammopathy of undetermined significance related pyoderma gangrenosum successfully treated with autologous peripheral blood stem cell transplantation. Chang CM, Hwang WL, Hsieh ZY, Wang RC, Teng CL. Ann Hematol 2010; 89: 823–4.

Refractory PG, and the paraprotein, resolved after autologous stem cell transplant.

Pyoderma gangrenosum treated successfully with visilizumab in patients with ulcerative colitis. Lorincz M, Kleszky M, Szalóki T Jr, Szalóki T. Orv Hetil 2010; 151: 144–7.

A long-standing case of PG resolved 6 months after administration of visilizumab, two doses of 5 μg/kg intravenously. This is a T-cell–suppressing monoclonal antibody to CD3.

Two percent topical phenytoin sodium solution in treating pyoderma gangrenosum: a cohort study. Fonseka HF, Ekanayake SM, Dissanayake M. Int Wound J 2010; 7: 519–23.

A 2% suspension, prepared by mixing phenytoin sodium powder from capsules with normal saline, was applied to the lesions daily on gauze. Four cases of varied etiology healed, and two improved within 4 weeks—an inexpensive therapy.

Split skin grafts in the treatment of pyoderma gangrenosum: a report of four cases. Cliff S. Dermatol Surg 1999; 25: 299–302.

Free flap coverage of pyoderma gangrenosum leg ulcers. Classen DA, Thomson C. J Cutan Med Surg 2002; 6: 327–31.

Extensive abdominal wall and genital pyoderma gangrenosum: combination therapy in unusual presentations. Shahmoradi Z, Mokhtari F, Pourazizi M, Abtahi-Naeini B, Saffaei A. J Cutan Aesthet Surg 2014; 7: 238–40.

In this case surgical debridement and closure of the lesions by suturing were undertaken successfully in combination with corticosteroid therapy.

Surgical techniques can successfully accelerate healing when the PG is no longer active or is effectively suppressed by medical treatment. However, caution is required, because active PG often demonstrates the Koebner phenomenon.

Pyogenic granuloma

Danielle M. DeHoratius

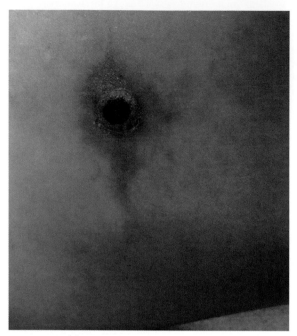

Pyogenic granuloma (PG), also known as a *lobular capillary hemangioma*, is a common benign vascular growth. It often develops rapidly into a solitary erythematous papule or polyp. PGs are often friable and hemorrhagic and frequently ulcerate. They most commonly occur in children and young adults. The etiology is unclear, although reactive neovascularization is suspected because of their occurrence at sites of previous trauma. They have also been reported as a cutaneous adverse effect of various medications. There is no gender or racial predominance. The most common locations are the head and neck region (including the oral mucosa, especially in pregnant women, known as *granuloma gravidarum*) and digits. Occasionally, PGs have been found in subcutaneous or intravascular locations. The term *PG* is a misnomer—there is no infectious or granulomatous component to these lesions.

MANAGEMENT STRATEGY

Histologic confirmation is beneficial, as other disorders may clinically mimic PGs, examples being amelanotic melanoma, Kaposi sarcoma, and bacillary angiomatosis. Dermoscopy of these lesions can be useful but should not substitute for histology. The most sensitive and specific pattern is a reddish homogeneous area, white collarette, and white rail lines.

Although they can eventually resolve spontaneously, treatment is usually required. Because this is a benign growth, it is important to consider the cosmetic outcome of the therapeutic intervention. PGs are most commonly treated by destruction using *shave excision with electrocautery* to the base, *curettage with electrodesiccation,* or *cryotherapy*. There is a possibility of recurrence and/or the development of satellite lesions, but these options are less invasive than excision and do not result in significant scarring.

Complete *excision* requiring sutures may lower the recurrence rate and reduce the possibility of bleeding; however, a linear scar will be present. Hemostasis can be obtained by electrocautery, silver nitrate, or argon laser photocoagulation.

Vascular *lasers* also destroy these lesions, although multiple treatments are usually required, and there is no histologic confirmation. *Pulsed dye laser* has proved to be more successful with smaller lesions. For larger lesions the *Nd:YAG laser* has been efficacious. *Sclerotherapy* destroys these vascular lesions and has been reported to have a very high cure rate in experienced hands. Various application schedules of *imiquimod* 5% have resolved these lesions, presumably due to its antiangiogenic properties. Recently success has been reported using topical *timolol* 0.05% ophthalmic gel. *Photodynamic therapy* has been shown to be effective with very few adverse events.

Specific Investigation

- Histology

First-Line Therapies

Simple shave excision/curettage with electrocautery of the base	A
Full-thickness skin excision	A
Cryotherapy	A
Silver nitrate cautery	D

Pyogenic granuloma in children. Pagliai KA, Cohen BA. Pediatr Dermatol 2004; 21: 10–3.

A retrospective study of 128 children, including follow-up phone interviews of 76. Of these, 72.3% underwent a shave excision with electrocautery. The second most common treatment was laser therapy (16.9%). Fifty-five percent of the children in the first group reported a subtle scar, and 33% of the CO_2 laser group and 44% of the pulsed dye laser group reported a similar scar. All patients were pleased with the cosmetic result.

Comparison of cryotherapy and curettage for the treatment of pyogenic granuloma: a randomized trial. Ghodsi SZ, Raziel M, Taheri A, Karami M, Mansoori P, Farnaghi F. Br J Dermatol 2006; 154: 671–5.

Eighty-nine patients were treated with either liquid nitrogen cryotherapy or curettage followed by electrodesiccation. Of the 86 patients who completed the study, all had complete resolution of the lesions after one to three sessions (mean 1.42) in the cryotherapy group and after one to two sessions (mean 1.03) in the curettage group. No scar or residual pigmentation was reported in 57% of the cryotherapy group or in 69% of the curettage group. The authors concluded that curettage should be a first-line therapy as fewer treatment sessions were necessary and cosmesis was better.

Treatment of pyogenic granuloma by shave excision and laser photocoagulation. Kirschner R, Low D. Plast Reconstruct Surg 1999; 104: 1346–9.

Shave excision was performed on the exophytic portion and photocoagulation of the base through a glass slide. The lasers used were an argon, argon-pumped tunable yellow dye, or KTP laser. All treatments were performed until complete hemostasis

Evidence Levels: A Double-blind study **B** Clinical trial ≥ 20 subjects **C** Clinical trial < 20 subjects **D** Series ≥ 5 subjects **E** Anecdotal case reports

was achieved. Complete resolution was seen in 18 of the 19 patients after a single treatment. Of note, the preoperative diagnosis was erroneous in 18.8% of the cases.

The efficacy of silver nitrate cauterization for pyogenic granuloma of the hand. Quitkin HM, Rosenwasser MP, Strauch RJ. J Hand Surg Am 2003; 28: 435–8.

Thirteen lesions were treated with simple removal and cautery of the base using silver nitrate. Eighty-five percent of the lesions resolved with an average of 1.6 treatments. The average time to complete healing was 3.5 weeks. There was no need for expensive equipment, and this was simple and cost effective.

Pyogenic granuloma – the quest for optimum treatment. Audit of treatment of 408 cases. Giblin AV, Clover AJ, Athanassopoulos A, Budny PG. Plast Reconstruct Aesthet Surg 2007; 60: 1030–5.

A retrospective study of 408 cases analyzed between 1994 and 2004. The excision and direct closure group had the fewest recurrences.

Cryotherapy in the treatment of pyogenic granuloma. Mirshams M, Daneshpazhooh M, Mirshekari A, Taheri A, Mansoori P, Hekmat S. J Eur Acad Dermatol Venereol 2006; 20: 788–90.

A prospective study of 135 patients treated with liquid nitrogen cryotherapy using a cotton-tipped applicator. Patients required anywhere from one to four treatments (mean 1.58). All patients had complete resolution, with 96.2% occurring after three treatments. Minor scars were reported in 11.8%, and 5.1% had hypopigmentation.

These authors report that cryotherapy should be considered first-line therapy as it is an easy and inexpensive technique; however, the main limitation is that no tissue is obtained for histology.

Second-Line Therapies	
• Pulsed dye	B
• CO$_2$ laser	B
• Nd:YAG laser	B

Treatment of pyogenic granuloma in children with the flash-lamp-pumped pulsed dye laser. Tay YK, Weston WL, Morelli JG. Pediatrics 1997; 99: 368–70.

Twenty-two children with solitary lesions were treated with a vascular-specific (585 nm), pulsed (450 ms) dye laser using a 5-mm spot size with energy of 6 to 7 J/cm^2 without anesthesia. This treatment was successful in 91%, and all healed without scarring. Fifteen patients required from two to six treatments at 2-week intervals, and seven required three or more. The two patients who did not respond had larger lesions (0.5–1 cm). No recurrences were reported during the follow-up period (6 months to 3 years). The limitation of this laser modality was that the depth of penetration was only 1 mm.

This can be a useful modality in children, as no anesthesia is required and there is minimal scarring. The drawback is that no tissue is obtained for histology.

The combined continuous-wave/pulsed carbon dioxide laser for treatment of pyogenic granuloma. Raulin C, Greve B, Hammes S. Arch Dermatol 2002; 138: 33–7.

One hundred patients were treated. The laser was first used in the continuous mode (power 15 W) and then in the pulsed mode (pulse length 0.6–0.9 ms; energy fluence 500 mJ/pulse). Follow-up was 6 weeks and 6 months, and 98 of 100 patients had complete resolution after one treatment. In 88 patients there were no visible scars, and 10 had only slight textural changes. No erythema or pigmentary changes were observed.

Pyogenic granulomas: treatment with the 1064-nm long-pulsed neodymium-doped yttrium aluminum garnet laser in 20 patients. Hammes S, Kaiser K, Pohl L, Metelmann HR, Enk A, Raulin C. Dermatol Surg 2012; 38: 918–23.

Twenty patients required one to four treatment sessions (settings used: fluences 60–180 J/cm^2, spot size of 7 mm, and a pulse duration of 40 ms). Nineteen had recurrence-free healing (follow-up duration 6–22 months) with good cosmetic results. Only slight textural changes were noted. This can be a satisfactory laser modality, especially when the diameter of the lesion is larger.

Third-Line Therapies	
• Ligation	E
• Imiquimod 5%	C
• Sclerotherapy	D
• Photodynamic therapy	D
• Intralesional corticosteroids	E
• Intralesional bleomycin	E
• Topical phenol	E
• Topical timolol, ophthalmic gel	E

Surgical pearl: ligation of the base of a pyogenic granuloma – an atraumatic, simple, and cost-effective procedure. Holbe HC, Frosch PJ, Herbst RA. J Am Acad Dermatol 2003; 49: 509–10.

A pedunculated PG was ligated using an absorbable suture tightly tied at the base. Over a few days the lesion became necrotic and fell off.

This was atraumatic and required no anesthesia, but there was also no histologic confirmation.

Pyogenic granuloma in ten children treated with topical imiquimod. Tritton SM, Smith A, Wong LC, Zagarella S, Fischer G. Pediatr Dermatol 2009; 26: 269–72.

Children with a mean age of 2.5 years were instructed to apply imiquimod 5% once a day, twice a day, or three times per week, depending on the clinical response. They were assessed either weekly or biweekly. All lesions were located on the face (3–6 mm), and local erythema was unanimously observed. Three had no residual disease, whereas five had either small hypopigmented or erythematous lesions, which were continuing to improve at the completion of the study. No systemic side effects were reported.

The authors suggest a trial of three times per week initially, increasing to daily if tolerated, for up to 2 months. Treatment should be discontinued 1 week after complete disappearance of the lesion. This appears a reasonable alternative to surgical excision.

Treatment of pyogenic granuloma by sodium tetradecyl sulfate sclerotherapy. Moon SE, Hwang EJ, Cho KH. Arch Dermatol 2005; 141: 644–6.

Fifteen PGs were injected with 0.5% sodium tetradecyl sulfate until blanching appeared. Follow-up was every 1 to 2 weeks, and at 6 weeks 80% showed complete resolution. In two patients a small shallow vascular area remained, which responded to the CO$_2$ laser.

The authors felt that this treatment can be an alternative to excision because of its simplicity and lack of scarring; however, multiple treatments may be necessary to achieve resolution. There is no tissue for histologic sampling.

Photodynamic therapy with 5-aminolevulinic acid intralesional injection for pyogenic granuloma. Lee DJ, Kim EH, Jang YH, Kim YC. Arch Dermatol 2012; 148: 126–8.

Fourteen lesions were injected (26-gauge needle) with 0.3 mL/cm³ of 5-aminolevulinic acid, 20% solution, followed by occlusion with polyurethane film. The lesions were then illuminated with red light (600–720 nm, light dose 100 J/cm², and fluence 100 mW/cm²). Eleven patients showed a marked response and had no recurrence at 1-year follow-up. One patient showed moderate response (lesion was on the lip), and two did not respond (lesions large >1 cm). Only three patients complained of perilesional swelling.

The authors felt that this treatment can be an alternative to standard therapy, especially in patients with small lesions who refuse surgery. It is important to consider the location and size of the lesion. Intralesional was suggested to be more effective than topical application of the photosensitizer.

Pyogenic granuloma that responded to local injection of steroid. Niiyama S, Amoh Y, Katsuoka K. J Plast Reconstr Aesthet Surg 2009; 62: 153–4.

Two lesions were injected with triamcinolone acetonide 2 mg weekly for a total of seven to eight times. The lesions became smaller and were subsequently excised.

This can be used when the lesion is in an unfavorable location for simple excision.

Complete resolution of recurrent giant pyogenic granuloma on the palm of the hand following single dose of intralesional bleomycin injection. Daya M. J Plast Reconstr Aesthet Surg 2010; 63: e331–3.

A 63-year-old woman presented with a recurrent giant PG (5 cm × 6 cm). Previous treatments included surgical excision and intralesional steroids. The lesion was injected with a total of 8 mL of 0.5 mg/mL of bleomycin given under general anesthesia with tourniquet control. The lesion regressed after 2 months and did not recur. The patient reported only mild hypersensitivity within the scar.

Topical phenol as a conservative treatment for periungual pyogenic granuloma. Losa Iglesias ME, Becerro de Bengoa Vallejo R. Dermatol Surg 2010; 36: 675–8.

A report of 18 patients treated with a 98% phenol solution, three applications of 1 minute each consecutively. The entire tumor and a small surrounding area turned white. The areas were then treated with 10% silver sulfadiazine and 10% povidone iodine and wrapped in sterile gauze. The frequency of additional treatments varied based on size. At 14 weeks all lesions had resolved. The treatments were well tolerated with no scarring or adverse events.

This approach is simple to perform, fairly inexpensive, and relatively pain free; however, recurrence is possible, and treatment may necessitate frequent office visits.

Pyogenic granuloma in a 5-month-old treated with topical timolol. Khorsand K, Maier M, Branding-Bennett HA. Ped Dermatol 2015; 32: 650–1.

An infant treated with topical 0.5% gel-forming solution. Regression was noted after 1 month, and there was no recurrence at 8 months.

This treatment can be very useful, especially in areas of significant scarring; however, the limitation would be a lack of histology.

Evidence Levels: **A** Double-blind study **B** Clinical trial ≥ 20 subjects **C** Clinical trial < 20 subjects **D** Series ≥ 5 subjects **E** Anecdotal case reports

214

Radiation dermatitis

Megan Rogge, Joshua A. Zeichner

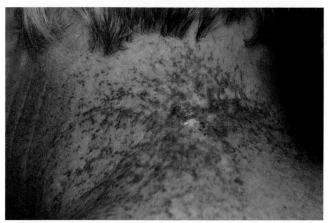

Courtesy of Mark Lebwohl, MD.

Radiation dermatitis is a common complication of cutaneous radiation exposure, most frequently from interventional radiologic procedures or treatment of malignancies. Acute radiation dermatitis typically occurs within 2 to 3 weeks of radiation exposure and is caused by damage to appendageal structures and basal keratinocytes. Acute radiation dermatitis manifests as erythema, edema, epilation, dry or wet desquamation, and blistering. Pain and pruritus often accompany these changes. The most widely used tools for assessment are the National Cancer Institute's Common Terminology Criteria for Adverse Events and the Radiation Therapy Oncology Group, which both grade acute radiation dermatitis from 1 to 4. Chronic radiation dermatitis is defined as skin changes persisting 90 days after radiation exposure, and these changes result from radiation-induced dermal and vascular damage leading to atrophy, dyspigmentation, telangiectasia, fibrosis, ulceration, and necrosis (see figure). Radiation recall is a dermatitis developing at sites of prior radiation exposure, usually induced by chemotherapeutic drugs such as doxorubicin or dactinomycin.

MANAGEMENT STRATEGY

Despite advances in radiation technology aimed at reducing side effects, skin toxicity is still a significant problem. The goals of treatment consist of maintaining skin integrity, minimizing patient discomfort, and preventing trauma and infection. *Bland emollients* treat dry desquamation (painless peeling of the skin), whereas moist desquamation (painful, full-thickness loss of the epidermis) should be treated with *occlusive dressings to prevent infections*. *Topical corticosteroids* control pruritus and reduce inflammation. Patients should also avoid friction from tight-fitting clothing. *Topical silver sulfadiazine* (SSD) may provide prophylaxis against bacterial infection and aid in the healing process. Patients may gently wash the skin with water and mild soap and use antiperspirants.

Chronic radiation dermatitis is also treated symptomatically. Topical emollient creams and corticosteroids can be employed as needed. Skin necrosis or ulceration must be carefully monitored for signs of infection. For reduction of skin fibrosis, some recommend physical *massage* of the skin or oral supplements such as *pentoxifylline* and *vitamin E*. Telangiectasias can be treated with *pulse dye laser.*

Specific Investigations

- History of previous radiation exposure and chemotherapeutic drugs
- Evaluation of affected skin for development of malignancy

Radio-induced malignancies of the scalp about 98 patients with 150 lesions and literature review. Maalej M, Frikha H, Kochbati L, Bouaouina N, Sellami D, Benna F, et al. Cancer Radiother 2004; 8: 81–7.

Basal cell carcinomas are the most common malignancies to develop in the skin at sites of previous radiation exposure, especially on the head and the neck.

First-Line Therapies

Acute radiation dermatitis

Topical corticosteroids	A
Emollients	B
Topical silver sulfadiazine	B

Chronic radiation dermatitis

Pentoxifylline	B
Vitamin E	B
Pulsed dye laser (PDL)	C

Clinical practice guidelines for the prevention and treatment of acute and late radiation reactions from the MASCC Skin Toxicity Study Group. Wong RK, Bensadoun RJ, Boers-Doets CB, Bryce J, Chan A, Epstein JB, et al. Support Care Cancer 2013; 21: 2933–48.

This article provides evidence-based recommendations from randomized controlled trials (RCTs) with standardized measurement of outcomes. Washing with water, with or without a mild soap, and allowing use of antiperspirants are supported by RCT, as well as topical prophylactic corticosteroids to reduce pain and pruritus. There is some evidence that SSD cream can reduce dermatitis score. For chronic radiation dermatitis, the panel suggests use of PDL, pentoxifylline, and vitamin E.

A potent steroid cream is superior to emollients in reducing acute radiation dermatitis in breast cancer patients treated with adjuvant radiotherapy. A randomised study of betamethasone versus two moisturizing creams. Ulff E, Maroti M, Serup J, Falkmer U. Radiother Oncol 2013; 108: 287–92.

Betamethasone-17-valerate cream was compared with a moisturizer with and without 5% urea in this double-blinded RCT of 102 patients who underwent 5 weeks of radiation therapy (RT). The creams were applied twice per day for 7 weeks beginning with the start of RT. Radiation dermatitis scores were significantly improved in the topical betamethasone group at week 4 and 5. Itch, burning, and irritation were significantly improved in the betamethasone group at week 6.

Topical silver sulfadiazine for the prevention of acute dermatitis during irradiation for breast cancer. Hemati S, Asnaashari O, Sarvizadeh M, Motlagh BN, Akbari M, Tajvidi M, et al. Support Care Cancer 2012; 20: 1613–8.

Topical SSD 1% cream was applied three times a day for the 3 consecutive days after weekly radiation treatment for 5 weeks and 1 week thereafter in women receiving radiation for breast cancer. Patients using the SSD cream developed significantly less severe dermatitis as scored by a blinded observer compared with a control group who were treated with general skin care alone.

Striking regression of chronic radiotherapy damage in a clinical trial of combined pentoxifylline and tocopherol. Delanian S, Balla-Mekias S, Lefaix JL. J Clin Oncol 1999; 17: 3283–90.

Patients with radiation-induced fibrosis (RIF) for a mean period of 8.5 ± 6.5 years were treated with a combination of oral pentoxifylline 800 mg/day and vitamin E 1000 IU/day for at least 6 months and had mean RIF surface area, and subjective objective medical management and analytic injury evaluation scores improved significantly at 3, 6, and 12 months.

Intense pulsed light vs. long-pulsed dye laser treatment of telangiectasia after radiotherapy for breast cancer: a randomized split-lesion trial of 2 different treatments. Nymann P, Hedelund L, Haedersdal M. Brit J Dermatol 2009; 160: 1237–41.

Thirteen patients with Fitzpatrick skin types II-III received a series of three treatments at 6-week intervals with long-pulsed dye (LPDL) (V-beam Perfecta, 595 nm) and intense pulsed light (Ellipse Flex). LPDL was superior in telangiectasia clearance, pain scores and patient satisfaction.

Second-Line Therapies	
Acute radiation dermatitis	
• Oral zinc supplement	A
• Hyaluronic acid cream	A
• Topical calendula	B
• Silver nylon dressing	B
• Film dressing	B
• Hydrogel or hydrocolloid dressing	B
• Topical trolamine	B
• Oral curcumin	A

Zinc supplementation to improve mucositis and dermatitis in patients after radiotherapy for head-and-neck cancers: a double-blind, randomized study. Lin LC, Que J, Lin LK, Lin FC. Int J Radiat Oncol Biol Phys 2006; 65: 745–50.

This double-blind, placebo-controlled RCT in patients with head-and-neck cancers receiving RT found that patients on an oral zinc supplement (25 mg Pro-Z), 3 tablets per day for approximately 2 months during RT, had a delayed grade 2 dermatitis, decreased development of grade 3 dermatitis, and overall milder dermatitis than those taking the placebo.

Double-blind, randomised clinical study comparing hyaluronic acid cream to placebo in patients treated with radiotherapy. Liguori V, Guillemin C, Pesce GF, Mirimanoff RO, Bernier J. Radiother Oncol 1997; 42: 155–61.

Patients who used hyaluronic acid 0.2% cream (Lalugenâ) twice per day for six weeks during RT had a delayed onset of acute dermatitis and significantly improved irradiated skin scores. This effect started at week 3 and continued through week 7, with no significant differences found between the groups in weeks 8 through 10.

Phase III randomized trial of *Calendula officinalis* compared with trolamine for the prevention of acute dermatitis during irradiation for breast cancer. Pommier P, Gomez F, Sunyach MP, D'Hombres A, Carrie C, Montbarbon X. J Clin Oncol 2004; 22: 1447–53.

At the onset of radiotherapy, Calendula or trolamine ointment were applied at least twice per day, by 254 women. Incidence of grade 2 to 3 acute skin toxicity and mean maximal pain scores were significantly less in the calendula treated group. Trolamine ointment was considered easier to apply.

Silver clear nylon dressing is effective in preventing radiation-induced dermatitis in patients with lower gastrointestinal cancer: results from a phase III study. Niazi TM, Vuong T, Azoulay L, Marijnen C, Bujko K, Nasr E, et al. Int J Radiat Oncol Biol Phys 2012; 84: e305–10.

Rectal or anal cancer patients undergoing RT were randomized to either use a silver clear nylon dressing (SCND) applied on day 1 of RT and worn continuously until 2 weeks after treatment completion or standard skin care comprising sulfadiazine cream applied at the time of skin dermatitis with photographs scored by blinded observers. On the last day of RT, the mean dermatitis scores were significantly lower in the SCND-treated group compared with the standard group.

Effect of film dressing on acute radiation dermatitis secondary to proton beam therapy. Arimura T, Ogino T, Yoshiura T, Toi Y, Kawabata M, Chuman I, et al. Int J Radiat Oncol Biol Phys 2016; 95: 472–6.

In this trial of 271 patients undergoing proton beam therapy for prostate cancer, patients self-randomized to using a continuously applied film dressing (FD) with no medical ingredients, Airwall, or to standard treatment. Patients using the FD showed a significantly decreased grade 2 radiation dermatitis. Side effects of FD use included itching sensation, redness, and folliculitis.

RCT on gentian violet versus a hydrogel dressing for radiotherapy-induced moist skin desquamation. Gollins S, Gaffney C, Slade S, Swindell R. J Wound Care 2008; 17: 268–75.

Patients who used a hydrogel dressing (2nd Skin) continuously had a significantly increased area of healing with shortened healing time (12 days) as opposed to those who treated their skin with 0.5% aqueous gentian violet (GV) several times per day (30 days to heal on average). Furthermore, several of the GV patients dropped out of the study due to failure to heal and stinging upon application.

Curcumin for radiation dermatitis: a randomized, double-blind, placebo-controlled clinical trial of thirty breast cancer patients. Ryan JL, Heckler CE, Ling M, Katz A, Williams JP, Pentland AP, et al. Radiat Res 2013; 180: 34–43.

Patients taking the antioxidant, antiinflammatory curcumin (C3 Complexâ 2000 mg) three times daily during their RT were compared with a placebo group. The curcumin group had significantly decreased radiation dermatitis severity scores, and fewer patients had moist desquamation.

Third-Line Therapy	
• Skin grafting	E

Evidence Levels: **A** Double-blind study **B** Clinical trial ≥ 20 subjects **C** Clinical trial < 20 subjects **D** Series ≥ 5 subjects **E** Anecdotal case reports

Chronic radiodermatitis injury after cardiac catheterization.
Barnea Y, Amir A, Shafir R, Weiss J, Gur E. Ann Plast Surg 2002;
49: 668–72.

Two patients with painful, nonhealing wounds at the site of
chronic radiation dermatitis underwent wound excision with
grafting. The skin healed completely, but the pain was only partially relieved.

Raynaud disease and phenomenon

Dina Ismail, Ian Coulson

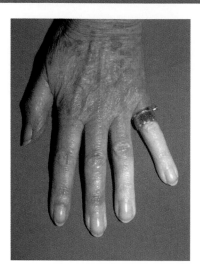

Raynaud phenomenon (RP) is characterized by intermittent peripheral vasoconstriction leading to pallor, cyanosis, and reactive vasodilatation of the arterioles of the fingers and toes. It is caused by vasospasm in response to cold, emotion, hormones, and certain vasospastic drugs. Primary Raynaud disease is a milder, idiopathic form, whereas secondary RP coexists with autoimmune connective tissue disorders such as systemic lupus erythematosus and systemic sclerosis (SSc) or other conditions that reduce blood flow, such as localized structural abnormalities. The pathogenesis and pathophysiology vary between the primary (idiopathic) and the secondary forms, but are still not fully understood.

Primary Raynaud disease is often mild and may not require treatment; the vasospasm is entirely reversible. However, secondary Raynaud disease often involves fixed blood vessel damage in addition to vasospasm; therefore the ischemia can be more severe. Complications include digital ulcers and gangrene, which can lead to amputation.

MANAGEMENT STRATEGY

Treatment is often nonpharmacologic, including avoiding cold (especially sudden drops in temperature) and smoking cessation. The use of *warming devices* such as hand or toe warmers is beneficial. Avoidance of triggers should be stressed (e.g., use of vibratory equipment). Drugs that may exacerbate the condition include β-blockers, bleomycin, caffeine, cisplatin, ergot preparations, interferon, methysergide, nicotine, oral contraceptives, reboxetine, tegaserod, and vinblastine and should be avoided.

Calcium channel antagonists, such as *nifedipine* (10–60 mg daily), are considered first-line treatment. The side effect profile includes hypotension, vasodilatation, peripheral edema, and headaches. Other treatments that have been studied in randomized, controlled trials include *phosphodiesterase-5*

inhibitors (PDE-5) (e.g., *sildenafil*, 25–50 mg up to four times a day) and *nitrates (topical or oral), angiotensin II inhibitors, and selective serotonin reuptake inhibitor (fluoxetine 20–60 mg daily)*. PDE-5 inhibitors are effective in patients who respond poorly to calcium channel antagonists as an alternative or adjunct and in patients with severe SSc-related RP. For more serious Raynaud disease or its complications, *prostacyclin* agonists may be used. This may be particularly useful for RP associated with connective tissue disease. Endothelin receptor blockade with *bosentan* (62.5 mg twice a day) has been demonstrated to reduce the number of new digital ulcers in scleroderma patients. However, it does not affect the healing period and has no effect on the number and severity of attacks of RP in those without ulcers.

Specific Investigations

- Nail fold capillaroscopy
- Screening serology: ANF estimation
- Anticentromere and anti-Scl-70 antibodies
- Rheumatoid factor
- Cryoglobulins
- Chest x-ray
- Pulmonary function tests
- Echocardiography

Careful history taking and clinical examination followed by investigation to detect potential underlying disease are essential: capillaroscopy and specific autoantibody tests are the most productive in aiding diagnosis.

Assessment of nailfold capillaroscopy by × 30 digital epiluminescence (dermoscopy) in patients with Raynaud phenomenon. Beltran E, Toll A, Pros A, Carbonell J, Pujol RM. Br J Dermatol 2007; 156: 892–8.

The sclerodermic pattern showed a sensitivity of 76.9% and a specificity of 90.9% in Sjögren syndrome (SS). A typical capillaroscopic pattern of SS was observed in 73% of cases of limited SS and in 82% of cases of diffuse SS. Patients with SS and dermatopolymyositis SS showed a nonspecific capillaroscopic pattern. All patients with primary RP presented a normal capillaroscopic pattern. A normal capillaroscopic pattern was also observed in 11 of 12 patients with pre-SS. This technical variation allows the identification of specific capillaroscopic patterns associated with connective tissue diseases. It also permits us to differentiate primary RP from secondary RP.

First-Line Therapies

Calcium channel blockers	A
Glyceryl trinitrate	A
Prostacyclin analogs	A
Phosphodiesterase-5 inhibitors	A

Calcium channel blockers for primary Raynaud's phenomenon. Ennis H, Hughes M, Anderson ME, Wilkinson J, Herrick AL. Cochrane Database Syst Rev 2016; 25: CD002069.

A meta-analysis of seven randomized trials with 296 patients evaluating the effects of nifedipine and nicardipine in the treatment of primary RP only. A decrease in the frequency of attacks was reported for patients on a calcium channel blocker (CCB). Doses of nifedipine used included 10 to 20 mg three times daily and 30 to 60 mg sustained-release daily. Nicardipine doses ranged between 20 to 30 mg thrice daily and 50 mg long-acting preparation twice daily. Trials included were of moderate quality.

Head-to-head comparison of udenafil vs. amlodipine in the treatment of secondary Raynaud's phenomenon: a double-blind, randomized, cross-over study. Lee EY, Park JK, Lee W, Kim YK, Park CS-Y, Giles JT, et al. Rheumatology 2014; 53: 658–64.

Twenty-nine patients with secondary RP associated with connective tissue diseases received udenafil 100 mg daily or amlodipine 10 mg daily for 4 weeks. Both decreased the rate of RP attacks with comparable efficacy.

Comparison of sustained-release nifedipine and temperature biofeedback for treatment of primary Raynaud phenomenon. Results from a randomized clinical trial with 1-year follow-up. Raynaud's Treatment Study Investigators. Arch Intern Med 2000; 160: 1101.

Patients with primary RP received sustained-release nifedipine (30 or 60 mg daily), placebo, or two different forms of biofeedback therapy for 1 year (n = 313). Nifedipine was the superior intervention and led to a 66% reduction in attacks compared with placebo.

A double-blind placebo controlled crossover randomized trial of diltiazem in Raynaud's phenomenon. Rhedda A, McCans J, Willan AR, Ford PM. J Rheumatol 1985; 12: 724–7.

The results showed a significant reduction in both frequency and duration of attacks of vasospasm in the hands using diltiazem 60 to 240 mg daily. There was no detectable difference in response between patients with primary and those with secondary RP.

Phosphodiesterase-5 inhibitors for the treatment of secondary Raynaud's phenomenon: systematic review and meta-analysis of randomised trials. Herrick AL, van den Hoogen F, Gabrielli A. Ann Rheum Dis 2013; 72: 1696.

Six randomized controlled trials (RCTs) were included: one with sildenafil (50 mg twice daily), one with modified-release sildenafil (200 mg once daily), three with tadalafil (20 mg on alternate days when used as add-on therapy), and 20 mg once daily. One study looked at vardenafil 10 mg twice daily. A meta-analysis showed PDE-5 inhibitors significantly decreased frequency and duration of RP attacks compared with placebo in secondary RP.

Comparison of intravenous infusions of iloprost and oral nifedipine in treatment of Raynaud's phenomenon in patients with systemic sclerosis: a double blind randomised study. Rademaker M, Cooke ED, Almond NE, Beacham JA, Smith RE, Mant TG, et al. Br Med J 1989; 298: 561–4.

This study compared the long-term effects of short-term intravenous infusions of iloprost (0.5–2 ng/kg/minute) with those of oral nifedipine in patients with SSc-associated RP. It was concluded that both iloprost and nifedipine are beneficial in the treatment of RP. However, side effects are common with nifedipine. Short-term infusions of iloprost provide long-lasting relief of symptoms. Side effects occur only during the infusions and are dose dependent.

A multi-centre, blinded, randomised, placebo-controlled, laboratory-based study of MQX-503, a novel topical gel formulation of nitroglycerine, in patients with Raynaud phenomenon. Hummers LK, Dugowson CE, Dechow FJ, Wise RA, Gregory J, Michalek J, et al. Ann Rheum Dis 2013; 72: 62–7.

In this multicenter, double-blind, randomized, placebo-controlled, cross-over study, 37 subjects were treated with 0.5% or 1.25% nitroglycerine or placebo gel. There was significant improvement in skin blood flow compared with placebo.

MQX-503, a novel formulation of nitroglycerin, improves the severity of Raynaud's phenomenon. Chung L, Shapiro L, Fiorentino D, Baron M, Shanahan J, Sule S, et al. Arthritis Rheum 2009; 60: 870–7.

Patients with a clinical diagnosis of primary or secondary RP received 0.9% MQX-503 gel or matching placebo during the treatment period (n = 219). There was a 2-week, single-blind, run-in period to determine baseline severity, followed by a 4-week double-blind treatment. The intervention was well tolerated and more effective than placebo for the treatment of RP.

Sustained-release transdermal glyceryl trinitrate patches as a treatment for primary and secondary Raynaud's phenomenon. Teh LS, Manning J, Moore T, Tully MP, O'Reilly D, Jayson MI. Br J Rheumatol 1995; 34: 636–41.

In this randomized, double-blind, placebo-controlled, crossover study patients with primary Raynaud disease and patients with RP secondary to SSc (n = 21) were included. Glyceryl trinitrate patches (0.2 mg/h) were found to be effective in reducing the number and severity of Raynaud attacks in both groups of patients.

Iloprost treatment in patients with Raynaud's phenomenon secondary to systemic sclerosis and the quality of life: a new therapeutic protocol. Milio G, Corrado E, Genova C, Amato C, Raimondi F, Almasio PL, et al. Rheumatology 2006; 45: 999–1004.

In this randomized study 30 patients were treated with iloprost given by intravenous infusion at progressively increasing doses (from 0.5–2 ng/kg/minute) over a period of 6 hours each day for 10 days in 2 consecutive weeks, with repeated cycles at regular intervals of 3 months for 18 months. The results were compared with those obtained in 30 other patients who received the same drug but with different dosing regimens. The total average daily duration of the attacks, the average duration of a single attack, and the average daily frequency of the attacks were reduced significantly in all treatment groups, but the comparison between the groups demonstrated significant differences between patients treated with the new protocol and the others at later times (12 and 18 months).

Oral iloprost in Raynaud's phenomenon secondary to systemic sclerosis: a multicentre, placebo-controlled, dose-comparison study. Black CM, Halkier-Sorensen L, Belch JJ, Ullman S, Madhok R, Smit AJ, et al. Br J Rheumatol 1998; 37: 952–60.

Oral iloprost 50 μg or 100 μg twice a day was effective in reducing the duration of attacks, but not the severity or frequency. In this study of 103 patients the 50-μg dose was better tolerated.

Negative reports about beraprost (another oral prostacyclin analog) and oral iloprost also exist.

Effects of long-term cyclic iloprost therapy in systemic sclerosis with Raynaud's phenomenon: a randomized controlled study. Scorza R, Caronni M, Mascagni B, Berruti V, Bazzi S, Micallef E, et al. Clin Exp Rheumatol 2001; 19: 503.

A 12-month prospective, randomized, parallel-group, blind-observer trial to compare the effects of intravenously infused iloprost (2 ng/kg/min on 5 consecutive days over a period of 8 hours/day and subsequently for 8 hours on 1 day every 6 weeks) with those of conventional vasodilating therapy with nifedipine (40 mg/day orally) in 46 patients with SSc and RP. Both iloprost and nifedipine were able to significantly reduce RP symptoms, with no differences between treatments.

Second-Line Therapies

- Selective serotonin reuptake inhibitors (fluoxetine) — **B**
- Endothelin receptor antagonist (bosentan) — **B**
- Angiotensin II receptor type I antagonist (losartan) — **B**
- Oral vasodilators — **B**
- Alpha-1-adrenergic receptor antagonist (prazosin) — **A**
- Hexopal — **A**

Treatment of Raynaud's phenomenon with the selective serotonin reuptake inhibitor fluoxetine. Coleiro B, Marshall SE, Denton CP, Howell K, Blann A, Welsh KI, et al. Rheumatology 2001; 40: 1038–43.

This pilot study compared fluoxetine, a selective serotonin reuptake inhibitor (20–60 mg/day), with nifedipine as treatment for primary or secondary RP. The results confirmed the tolerability of fluoxetine and suggest that it would be effective as a novel treatment for RP.

Bosentan treatment of digital ulcers related to systemic sclerosis: results from the RAPIDS-2 randomised, double-blind placebo-controlled trial. Matucci-Cerinic M, Denton CP, Furst DE, Mayes MD, Hsu VM, Carpentier P, et al. Ann Rheum Dis 2011; 70: 32–8.

This double-blind, placebo-controlled, multicenter trial randomized 188 patients with SSc with at least one active digital ulcer (DU) to bosentan 62.5 mg twice daily for 4 weeks and 125 mg twice daily thereafter for 20 weeks or placebo. Bosentan was found to reduce the occurrence of new DUs compared with placebo in patients with SSc but had no effect on DU healing.

Losartan therapy for Raynaud's phenomenon and scleroderma: clinical and biochemical findings in a fifteen-week, randomized, parallel group, controlled trial. Dziadzio M, Denton CP, Smith R, Howell K, Blann A, Bowers E, et al. Arthritis Rheum 1999; 42: 2646–55.

Treatment with losartan (50 mg daily) was shown to reduce the severity and frequency of attacks in primary and scleroderma RP at 12 weeks.

Double-blind, placebo-controlled study of prazosin in Raynaud's phenomenon. Wollersheim H, Thien T, Fennis J, van Elteren P, van 't Laar A. Clin Pharmacol Ther 1986; 40: 219–25.

In this study, prazosin 1 mg thrice daily was compared with placebo and showed a moderate subjective improvement with a reduction in daily number and duration of attacks. No differences in treatment response were identified between patients with Raynaud disease and secondary RP.

Dose-response study of prazosin in Raynaud's phenomenon: clinical effectiveness versus side effects. Wollersheim H, Thien T. J. Clin Pharmacol 1988; 28: 1089–93.

In a dose-response study of prazosin in 24 patients with RP, the clinical effectiveness and side effects of 3, 6, and 12 mg prazosin administered daily were compared. No major differences among these three dose regimens were identified.

Oral vasodilators for primary Raynaud's phenomenon. Vinjar B, Stewart M. Cochrane Database Syst Rev 2008; 2: CD006687.

Two trials examined the effects of captopril; the rest were single trials of single drugs. For captopril, beraprost, dazoxiben, and ketanserin there was no evidence of an effect on the frequency, severity, or duration of attacks. Beraprost and moxisylyte gave significantly more adverse effects than placebo.

A double-blind randomized placebo controlled trial of Hexopal in primary Raynaud's disease. Sunderland GT, Belch JJ, Sturrock RD, Forbes CD, McKay AJ. Clin Rheumatol 1988; 7: 46–9.

Hexopal (hexanicotinate inositol) (2–4 g daily) is safe and effective in reducing the vasospasm of primary Raynaud disease during the winter months.

Third-Line Therapies

- Prostaglandin E$_1$ (alprostadil) — **B**
- Dipyridamole and low-dose acetylsalicylic acid — **B**
- Calcitonin gene-related peptide — **C**
- L-Arginine — **D**
- Heating, Ozonation, UV (HOU) therapy — **C**
- Triiodothyronine — **C**
- *Helicobacter pylori* treatment — **B**
- Sympathectomy — **C**
- Low-level laser therapy — **C**
- Acupuncture — **C**
- Evening primrose oil supplementation — **C**
- Fish oil supplementation — **B**
- Botulinum toxin — **A**
- Spinal cord stimulation — **E**
- Rituximab — **E**
- Statins — **A**
- Low-molecular-weight heparin — **B**

Efficacy evaluation of prostaglandin E1 against placebo in patients with progressive systemic sclerosis and significant Raynaud's phenomenon. Bartolone S, Trifilatti A, De Nuzzo G, Scamardi R, Larosa D, Sottilotta G, et al. Minerva Cardioangiol 1999; 47: 137–43.

Alprostadil infusions at 60 µg in 250 mL for 6 days reduced the frequency and severity of attacks in patients with secondary RP.

A double-blind controlled trial of low dose acetylsalicylic acid and dipyridamole in the treatment of Raynaud's phenomenon. Van der Meer J, Wouda AA, Kallenberg CG, Wesseling H. Vasa 1987; 18: 71–5.

This analgesic and antithrombotic combination (aspirin 50–100 mg/day, dipyridamole 200 mg twice a day) is safe and helpful in treating patients with RP who have severe digital ulceration.

Calcitonin gene-related peptide in treatment of severe peripheral vascular insufficiency in Raynaud's phenomenon. Bunker CB, Reavley C, O'Shaugnessy DJ, Dowd PM. Lancet 1993; 342: 80–3.

Calcitonin gene-related peptide, a potent vasodilator, given intravenously (0.6 µg/minute for 3 hours a day for 5 days) resulted in an increase in blood flow, ulcer healing, and effective vascular dilation in patients with severe RP.

Oral L-arginine can reverse digital necrosis in Raynaud's phenomenon. Rembold CM, Ayers CR. Mol Cell Biochem 2003; 244: 139–41.

The authors demonstrate a beneficial response to oral L-arginine therapy (up to 8 g daily), which reversed digital necrosis and improved the symptoms of severe RP. This evidence suggests that a defect in nitric oxide synthesis or metabolism is associated with RP and demonstrates the potential effectiveness of L-arginine therapy.

Treatment of severe Raynaud's syndrome by injection of autologous blood pretreated by heating, ozonation, and exposure to ultraviolet light (H-O-U) therapy. Cooke ED, Pockley AG, Tucker AT, Kirby JD, Bolton AE. Int Angiol 1997; 16: 250–4.

Treatment was successful in patients with severe RP. Results included reduction of attacks for at least 3 months and, for some, no attacks at all.

Triiodothyronine treatment for Raynaud's phenomenon: a controlled trial. Dessin PH, Morrison RC, Lamparelli RD, van der Merwe CA. J Rheumatol 1990; 17: 1025–8.

In this trial T_3 80 μg/day increased finger skin temperature and reduced recovery times after cold exposure. Treatment is recommended for patients with severe RP and digital ulcers.

***Helicobacter pylori* eradication ameliorates primary Raynaud's phenomenon.** Gasbarrini A, Massari I, Serrichio M, Tondi P, De Luca A, Franceschi F, et al. Dig Dis Sci 1998; 43: 1641–5.

Of 46 RP patients, 36 were infected with *H. pylori*. After treatment to eradicate *H. pylori*, RP disappeared in 17% of patients; 72% of the remaining patients noticed a reduction in frequency and duration of their vasospastic attacks.

The use of digital artery sympathectomy as a salvage procedure for severe ischemia of Raynaud's disease and phenomenon. McCall TE, Petersen DPM, Wong LB. J Hand Surg [Am] 1999; 24: 173–7.

In six of seven patients the use of digital artery sympathectomy was effective; the patients' digital ulcers healed and amputation was avoided.

Double-blind, randomised, placebo controlled low laser therapy study in patients with primary Reynaud's phenomenon. Hirschl M, Katzenschlager R, Ammer K, Melnizky P, Rathkolb O, Kundi M, et al. Vasa 2002; 31: 91–4.

This study examined 15 patients with primary RP and demonstrated that low-level laser therapy reduced the intensity of the attacks during laser irradiation without significantly affecting the frequency of attacks. Additionally, after laser irradiation the temperature gradient after cold exposure was reduced, but there was no effect on the number of fingers showing prolonged rewarming.

Treatment of primary Raynaud's syndrome with traditional Chinese acupuncture. Appiah R, Hiller S, Caspary L, Alexander K, Creutzig A. J Intern Med 1997; 241: 119–24.

Thirty-three patients with primary Raynaud disease (16 controls, 17 treatment) were studied. Overall, attacks were reduced by 63%.

Evening primrose oil (Efamol) in the treatment of Raynaud's phenomenon: a double-blind study. Belch JJ, Shaw B, O'Dowd A, Saniabadi A, Leiberman P, Sturrock RD, et al. Thromb Haemost 1985; 54: 490–4.

Twenty-one patients were studied. Evening primrose oil (12 capsules daily) provided symptomatic improvement.

Fish-oil dietary supplementation in patients with Raynaud's phenomenon: a double blind controlled, prospective study. DiGiacomo RA, Kremer JM, Shah DM. Am J Med 1989; 86: 158–64.

In this trial involving 32 patients supplementation with omega-3 fatty acids (3.96 g eicosapentaenoic acid and 2.64 g docosahexaenoic acid) was shown to be of benefit in patients with primary, but not secondary, RP.

A 28-day prospective, randomized, double-blind, placebo controlled clinical trial of botulinum toxin type A for Raynaud's phenomenon. Webb KN, Berry NN, Bueno RA, Neumeister MW. Plast Reconstr Surg 2014; 133: 13.

Thirty-five patients were treated with either placebo or botulinum toxin type A (Btx-A) 100 U into the palm around involved digital neuromuscular bundles. Ten percent of placebo patients reported pain relief compared with 62% of Btx-A–treated patients (p = 0.0288). Average pain relief duration was 127 days, and 60% of patients with digital ulcers healed after Btx-A injection.

Clinical and objective data on spinal cord stimulation for the treatment of severe Raynaud's phenomenon. Neuhauser B, Perkmann R, Klingler PJ, Giacomuzzi S, Kofler A, Fraedrich G, et al. Am Surg 2001; 67: 1096–7.

Spinal cord stimulation was shown to effectively improve red blood cell velocity, capillary density, and capillary permeability in a 77-year-old woman with severe RP.

Severe primary Raynaud's disease treated with rituximab. Shabrawishi M, Albeity A, Almoallim H. Case Rep Rheumatol 2016; 2016: 2053804.

A case of a 55-year-old female with primary RP who failed first-line therapies. Due to persistent symptoms, rituximab therapy was initiated (1 g 2 weeks apart) with complete resolution of digital ischemia. Recurrence of symptoms resolved after a second cycle of rituximab (375 mg/m² weekly for 4 weeks). Full remission was achieved.

Statins: potentially useful in therapy of systemic sclerosis-related Raynaud's phenomenon and digital ulcers. Abou-Raya A, Abou-Raya S, Helmii M. J Rheumatol 2008; 35: 1801.

This randomized trial involving 84 patients demonstrated that atorvastatin 40 mg daily for 4 months reduced overall number of digital ulcers, severity, and pain in SSc-related RP.

Long-term beneficial effects of statins on vascular manifestations in patients with systemic sclerosis. Kuwana M, Okazaki Y, Kaburaki J. Mod Rheumatol 2009; 19: 530.

A 24-month, open-label trial where patients received atorvastatin 10 mg daily. RP improved during treatment, with significant reductions in the Raynaud's Condition Score and patient visual analog scale.

Long-term low molecular weight heparin therapy for severe Raynaud's phenomenon: a pilot study. Denton CP, Howell K, Stratton RJ, Black CM. Clin Exp Rheumatol 2000; 18: 499.

Low-molecular-weight heparin was used as an add-on therapy for patients with primary or secondary RP already receiving at least one oral anti-Raynaud agent. There was an improvement in attack severity after 4 weeks of heparin therapy, maximal by 20 weeks, compared with the control group.

216

Reactive arthritis

Clinton W. Enos, Sara Samimi, Abby S. Van Voorhees

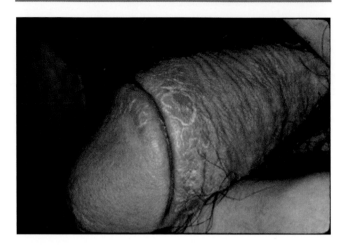

Reactive arthritis (ReA), formerly known as *Reiter syndrome*, is one of the reactive forms of seronegative spondyloarthropathies. It is both a genetically determined and immune-mediated disease that primarily affects the skin and joints 2 to 4 weeks after an enteric or urogenital infection. Commonly implicated gastrointestinal pathogens include *Yersinia*, *Salmonella*, *Shigella*, *Campylobacter*, and *Clostridium difficile*; common urogenital pathogens include *Chlamydia trachomatis*, *Neisseria gonorrhea*, and *Ureaplasma urealyticum*. Rarely, ReA can manifest after a respiratory infection with *Chlamydia pneumoniae* or group A β-hemolytic streptococcus. ReA is relatively rare condition that is more common in young adults ages 20 to 40. There is no predilection for either sex when a gastrointestinal pathogen is the inciting agent; however, males have a greater incidence after *Chlamydia trachomatis* infection. The HLA-B27 allele has been associated with ReA, although it is not a diagnostic criterion.

ReA is a clinical diagnosis characterized by a triad of urethritis, conjunctivitis, and oligoarthritis; however, only roughly one third of patients present with a complete triad, making the diagnosis largely dependent on patient history. General guidelines set forth by the American College of Rheumatology (ACR) proposed major and minor criteria to aid in a definite diagnosis (see later). Similarly, European guidelines for sexually acquired ReA incorporate the recognition of a monoarthritis or oligoarthritis preceded by a symptomatic urethritis. Additional extraarticular findings can include enthesitis, tendinitis, bursitis, conjunctivitis, anterior uveitis, and keratitis. The classic skin manifestations include keratoderma blennorrhagica and circinate balanitis. Nail changes, oral lesions, and ulcerative vulvitis may also be seen. Erythema nodosum can also occur and is more common in the setting of a *Yersinia* infection. The differential diagnosis may include atopic dermatitis, Behçet disease, contact dermatitis, and pustular psoriasis.

MANAGEMENT STRATEGY

The mucocutaneous lesions of uncomplicated ReA are usually self-limited and clear within a few months. Severe, extensive, and chronic cutaneous presentations, which are more common in the setting of human immunodeficiency virus (HIV) infection, are generally treated in the same manner as pustular psoriasis. Initial therapy for limited skin disease includes *topical steroids, topical vitamin D preparations, tacrolimus,* and *tazarotene*. Second-line agents include *UVB* and *systemic retinoids*. Severe disease can be treated with *psoralen plus UVA (PUVA)* and *immunosuppressive agents such as methotrexate and ciclosporin*. Anti–tumor necrosis factor (TNF) agents have also been used successfully in patients with refractory disease as well as those with HIV, but data from randomized, placebo-controlled trials are lacking.

In most patients, the symptoms of arthritis and inflammation of the peripheral ligamentous or muscular attachments (entheses) dictate the focus of treatment. *Nonsteroidal antiinflammatory drugs (NSAIDs)* are the first-line therapy. *Corticosteroid injections* can provide temporary relief of the pain caused by arthritis or bursitis, and oral corticosteroids may also be beneficial when severe. *Sulfasalazine* and *methotrexate* have been shown to be effective and well tolerated in cases refractory to both NSAIDs and steroids. *TNF inhibitors* have also shown efficacy in treating severe disease. Of note, emerging biologics such as ustekinumab, apremilast, and secukinumab have not been investigated in the treatment of ReA.

Transient and mild conjunctivitis does not require specific therapeutic intervention. Symptoms of eye pain or blurry vision require immediate referral to ophthalmology to determine whether these symptoms are due to conjunctivitis or a more serious eye problem such as uveitis, iritis, or keratitis. Treatment often involves topical and/or systemic corticosteroids and immunosuppressive medications such as methotrexate.

The effects of short-term and long-term *antibiotic therapy* for ReA are controversial. Although there is some evidence that antibiotics may be beneficial during the infectious phase before arthritis has developed, it is not clear whether the introduction of antibiotics after the development of arthritis will modify the disease course. A meta-analysis of 10 trials indicated that there is no significant benefit for the use of antibiotics in ReA. However, due to the heterogeneity of trials included in this analysis, the possible benefit of antibiotics in certain subgroups or at certain time points cannot be completely excluded. For example, a double-blind, placebo-controlled study suggested no advantage of combination antibiotics (roxithromycin and ofloxacin) over placebo in the treatment of recent-onset ReA, but another small study reports a beneficial effect of combination treatment with *doxycycline* and *rifampin* for chronic spondyloarthritis. If the inciting organism is documented by culture or polymerase chain reaction (PCR), antibiotics are indicated. The true benefits of antibiotics, their dosage, and their duration remain to be clarified. However, when evaluating a patient with ReA after a urogenital infection, it is also important to consider treatment of the patient's partner for further disease prevention.

ReA in HIV-infected individuals may be more prevalent, severe, and progressive because it is more refractory to treatment. However, one report describes ReA as part of an immune reconstitution syndrome that is rapidly responsive to a 2-week course of doxycycline. Another case report describes the resolution of ReA symptoms upon initiating antiretroviral therapy.

Evidence Levels: **A** Double-blind study **B** Clinical trial ≥ 20 subjects **C** Clinical trial < 20 subjects **D** Series ≥ 5 subjects **E** Anecdotal case reports

The pathogenic link between HIV and ReA is not completely understood; however, case reports highlight the benefit of closely comanaging HIV-1 infection and the symptoms of ReA.

Specific Investigations

- Recent history of gastrointestinal or genitourinary infection or symptoms
- Skin biopsy
- Urinalysis
- Urethral, cervical, and stool cultures
- Serum antibodies to chlamydia
- Erythrocyte sedimentation rate (ESR), C-reactive protein (CRP), complete blood count
- HIV testing/status
- Rheumatoid factor and antinuclear antibody (ANA) (negative in reactive arthritis)
- Synovial fluid analysis
- Radiographic imaging
- HLA-B27 typing
- Ophthalmologic slit lamp examination
- Electrocardiogram (ECG) in chronic disease

Proposed Diagnostic Criteria by the ACR (1999). Major criteria:

1. Arthritis with at least two of the following: asymmetry, monoarthritis or oligoarthritis, lower limb involvement
2. Preceding symptomatic infection
   a. Enteritis that consists of diarrhea for at least 1 day, 3 days to 6 weeks before onset of arthritis
   b. Urethritis that consists of dysuria for at least 1 day, 3 days to 6 weeks before onset of arthritis

   Minor criteria:

1. Evidence of a triggering infection via one or both of the following:
   a. Urine ligase reaction or urethral/cervical swab positive for *Chlamydia trachomatis*
   b. Positive stool cultures for pathogens associated with ReA.
2. Evidence of persistent synovial infection via immunohistochemical or PCR studies for *Chlamydia*

A definite diagnosis includes both major criteria and a relevant minor criterion. A probable diagnosis consists of both major criteria with no minor criteria, or one major criterion and one or more relevant minor criteria.

First-Line Therapies

Cutaneous disease

Topical steroids	C
Calcipotriene (calcipotriol)	E
Tazarotene	E
Tacrolimus	E

Reiter syndrome. Rothe MJ, Kerdel FA. Int J Dermatol 1991; 30: 173–80.

Mucocutaneous lesions may necessitate only local care for mucosal erosions and topical steroids for psoriasiform lesions.

Because treatment in ReA is typically directed toward the musculoskeletal component and urethritis, there is a paucity of studies designed for the treatment of cutaneous disease. However, despite the lack of controlled studies, topical steroids are accepted as first-line therapy for mild cutaneous lesions.

Successful treatment of chronic skin disease with clobetasol propionate and a hydrocolloid dressing. Volden G. Acta Derm Venereol 1992; 72: 69–71.

Two patients with skin lesions of reactive arthritis and 19 patients with palmoplantar pustulosis responded to clobetasol propionate lotion once weekly under occlusion. The mean interval to remission was 3 weeks for the skin lesions of ReA and 2.2 weeks for palmoplantar pustulosis.

Reiter's disease in a homosexual HIV-positive male. Vaughan Jones SA, McGibbon DH. Clin Exp Dermatol 1994; 19: 430–3.

A case report of a 32-year-old male with AIDS whose psoriasiform lesions improved after 2 weeks of topical corticosteroids and a course of flucloxacillin.

Tacrolimus therapy for circinate balanitis associated with reactive arthritis. Herrera-Esparza R, Medina F, Avalos-Diaz E. J Clin Rheumatol 2009; 15: 377–9.

A report of three patients with evidence of circinate balanitis refractory to systemic therapy with corticosteroids and sulfasalazine but responsive to treatment with topical tacrolimus 0.1%.

Reiter's disease in a 6-year-old girl. Arora S, Arora G. Indian J Dermatol Venereol Leprol 2005; 71: 285–6.

A case report of a 6-year-old child with ReA whose primary keratoderma blennorrhagicum lesions were treated with topical salicylic acid and hydrocortisone with complete resolution in 3 weeks.

The use of topical calcipotriene/calcipotriol in conditions other than plaque-type psoriasis. Thiers BH. J Am Acad Dermatol 1997; 37: S69–71.

A 47-year-old man with relapsing ReA, with pustules and hyperkeratotic plaques on his palms and soles, as well as circinate balanitis, responded to 14 days of doxycycline (100 mg twice a day) and topical calcipotriene.

Treatment of keratoderma blenorrhagicum with tazarotene gel 0.1%. Lewis A, Nigro M, Rosen T. J Am Acad Dermatol 2000; 43: 400–2.

A case report of a 64-year-old man with ReA who responded to daily application of tazarotene gel 0.1% to his soles.

Second-Line Therapies

Cutaneous disease

Systemic retinoids	D
UVB/PUVA	D
Antiretroviral therapy	E

Acitretin and AIDS-related Reiter's disease. Blanche P. Clin Exp Rheum 1999; 17: 105–6.

A case report of a 46-year-old patient with AIDS and ReA whose arthritis and skin lesions responded to 2 weeks of acitretin

(25 mg daily). Therapy was continued for 5 months; a recurrence occurred several months after the acitretin was stopped despite maintenance on antiretroviral therapy. Acitretin was resumed, resulting in prompt resolution of disease, and continued for 6 months. No recurrence was observed after 13 months.

Reiter's syndrome-like pattern in AIDS-associated psoriasiform dermatitis. Romani J, Puig L, Baselga E, De Moragas JM. Int J Dermatol 1996; 35: 484–8.

A retrospective review of seven HIV-positive patients with Reiter-like psoriasiform dermatitis. Etretinate alone and RePUVA (etretinate 1 mg/kg daily, 8-methoxypsoralen 0.6 mg/kg followed by UVA) were safe and effective in controlling skin disease. Methotrexate (15 mg weekly in three divided doses) was effective, but was complicated by hematologic toxicity in two patients. Ciclosporin (2.5 mg/kg daily) was moderately effective and was not associated with progression of AIDS.

Successful treatment of severe Reiter's syndrome associated with human immunodeficiency virus infection with etretinate. Report of 2 cases. Louthrenoo W. J Rheumatol 1993; 20: 1243–6.

A report of two cases of HIV-related ReA responding dramatically to 4 weeks of etretinate (0.5–1.0 mg/kg daily).

Reactive arthritis responding to antiretroviral therapy in an HIV-1-infected individual. Scott C, Brand A, Natha M. Int J STD AIDS 2012; 23: 373–4.

A report of an HIV-1 infected patient with severe ReA who failed conventional therapy with steroids, disease-modifying antirheumatic agents, and nonsteroidal antiinflammatory drugs but experienced resolution of ReA symptoms after initiation of antiretroviral therapy. Antiretroviral use may be beneficial for symptomatic relief, suggesting that patients should be managed closely by both rheumatology and infectious disease.

Human immunodeficiency virus associated spondyloarthropathy: pathogenic insights based on imaging findings and response to highly active antiretroviral treatment. McGonagle D, Reade S, Emery P. Ann Rheum Dis 2001; 60: 696–8.

Case report of a 31-year-old HIV-positive man with ReA with extensive polyenthesitis and osteitis. The patient's arthritis worsened despite treatment, including indomethacin, tramadol, and sulfasalazine, but improved dramatically after antiretroviral treatment (lamivudine, ritonavir, and stavudine). Improvement was accompanied by a significant rise in CD4 T-lymphocyte counts.

Clinical improvement of HIV-associated psoriasis parallels a reduction of HIV viral load induced by effective antiretroviral therapy. Fischer T, Ramadori G. AIDS 1999; 13: 628–9.

Case report of a 38-year-old HIV-positive male with viremia and psoriasis. The patient was started on multiple antiretroviral agents in addition to topical steroids and vitamin D_3 analogs. Despite antiretroviral therapy, his viral load remained high and his psoriasis persisted. It was not until his viral load decreased below 400 that his skin lesions started to improve.

Third-Line Therapies

Cutaneous disease

• Methotrexate	C
• Ciclosporin	E
• TNF inhibitors	C

A review of methotrexate therapy in Reiter syndrome. Lally EV, Ho G Jr. Semin Arthritis Rheum 1985; 15: 139–45.

A case report and review of the literature. Eighteen of 20 patients noted dramatic improvement in skin lesions within 2 weeks of receiving methotrexate; 15 of 20 patients had significant improvement in arthritis, although the response was generally slower. Methotrexate was generally well tolerated, but the drug had to be discontinued in three cases due to adverse effects. Methotrexate was used for exacerbations and was then discontinued after clinical improvement. The usual dosage was 10 to 50 mg/week administered either orally or parenterally.

Successful treatment of Reiter's syndrome in a patient with AIDS with methotrexate and corticosteroids. Berenbaum F, Duvivier C, Prier A, Kaplan G. Br J Rheumatol 1996; 35: 295.

A case report of a 37-year-old man with AIDS and severe ReA who responded to prednisone 20 mg daily and methotrexate 20 mg/week. This was combined with antiretroviral therapy, chemoprophylaxis of infection, and aggressive therapy of Kaposi sarcoma without exacerbation of his AIDS.

Successful treatment of severe recurrent Reiter's syndrome with cyclosporine. Kiyohara A, Ogawa H. J Am Acad Dermatol 1997; 36: 482–3.

A case report of a 48-year-old man with postchlamydia ReA not responsive to topical steroids and etretinate treated successfully with 5 mg/kg daily ciclosporin that was slowly tapered. No recurrence of the disease was noted at 18 months.

Infliximab in the treatment of an HIV positive patient with Reiter's syndrome. Gaylis N. J Rheumatol 2003; 30: 2.

A case report of a 41-year-old man with ReA who responded to infliximab, methotrexate, and systemic corticosteroid treatment regimens. During therapy his arthritis resolved, as did the onycholysis and keratoderma blennorrhagica of the soles. The patient was able to discontinue systemic corticosteroids and was maintained on intravenous infliximab at a dose of 300 mg (3 mg/kg) every 6 to 7 weeks and intramuscular methotrexate at a dose of 15 mg/week for 18 months without a decrease in his CD4 cells or a rise in his viral load.

Decreased pain and synovial inflammation after etanercept therapy in patients with reactive and undifferentiated arthritis: an open-label trial. Flagg S, Meador R, Schumacher HR. Arthritis Rheum 2005; 53: 613–7.

Describes a 6-month open-label trial of 16 patients with undifferentiated or reactive arthritis treated with etanercept (25 mg subcutaneous twice weekly). Seven patients met the criteria for ReA, and 9 had a similar pattern of arthritis without evidence for infection. Ten patients completed the trial. Three patients tested positive for HLA-B27. All patients had been on NSAIDs, and 11 had been treated with sulfasalazine and/or methotrexate. Of the 10 completers, 9 were classified as responders with less tender joints and decreased swelling of joints. The tenth had improvement in pain but no change in the number of tender or swollen joints.

Successful use of infliximab in the treatment of Reiter's syndrome: a case report and discussion. Gill H, Majithia V. Clin Rheumatol 2008; 27: 121–3.

A case report of a 28-year-old man with HIV with ReA complicated by circinate balanitis and arthritis, as well as onycholysis and keratoderma blennorrhagica who did not respond to aggressive treatment with NSAIDs, prednisone (60–20 mg/day), and methotrexate (15 mg/week) for 3 months. He was treated with

Evidence Levels: **A** Double-blind study **B** Clinical trial ≥ 20 subjects **C** Clinical trial < 20 subjects **D** Series ≥ 5 subjects **E** Anecdotal case reports

infliximab 200 mg (3 mg/kg) intravenously with rapid improvement of skin lesions and arthritis. This regimen was well tolerated. The patient was subsequently lost to follow-up.

Use of adalimumab in poststreptococcal reactive arthritis.
Sanchez-Cano D, Callejas-Rubio JL, Ortego-Centeno N. J Clin Rheum 2007; 13: 176.

A case report describing a 21-year-old female with oligoarthritis affecting the lower extremities after pharyngitis 2 weeks before the onset of arthritis. NSAIDs, prednisone (1 mg/kg/day), hydroxychloroquine (6 mg/kg/day), and methotrexate (25 mg/weekly) were not effective. Clinical response was achieved 8 weeks after introduction of adalimumab (40 mg subcutaneously every 2 weeks) and was maintained. Steroids and methotrexate were discontinued; no side effects were observed after 1 year of treatment with adalimumab.

The use of antitumor necrosis factor therapy in HIV-positive individuals with rheumatic disease.
Cepeda E, William F, Ishimori M, Weisman M, Reveille J. Ann Rheum Dis 2008; 67: 710–2.

Eight HIV-positive patients with rheumatic diseases (two with rheumatoid arthritis, three with psoriatic arthritis, one with ReA, one with undifferentiated spondyloarthritis, and one with ankylosing spondyloarthritis) refractory to disease-modifying antirheumatic drugs who have a CD4 count >200 mm^3 and an HIV viral load of <60,000 copies/mm^3 and no active concurrent infections were treated with TNF blockers. No significant clinical adverse effect was noted over 28 months. CD4 counts and HIV viral loads remained stable. Three patients on etanercept and two on infliximab had sustained improvement in their rheumatic disease.

Prolonged remission of chronic reactive arthritis treated with three infusions of infliximab.
Wechalekar M, Rischmueller M, Whittle S, Burnet S, Hill C. J Clin Rheumatol 2010; 16: 79–80.

A case report of a 25-year-old female with an 11-month history of progressive oligoarthritis and increasing CRP after *Chlamydia trachomatis* infection. She failed treatment with azithromycin, NSAIDs, corticosteroid injections, methotrexate, sulfasalazine, and hydroxychloroquine. Subsequently, infliximab at a dose of 6 mg/kg was given. After the first two doses her symptoms resolved with normalization of her CRP. Methotrexate, sulfasalazine, and hydroxychloroquine were tapered without evidence of recurrent disease.

Safety and efficacy of antitumor necrosis factor α therapy in ten patients with recent-onset refractory reactive arthritis.
Meyer A, Chatelus E, Wendling D, Berthelot JM, Dernis E, Houvenagel E, et al. Arthritis Rheum 2011; 63: 1274–80.

A retrospective review of anti-TNF-α therapy in 10 patients with evidence of new-onset ReA. Five patients were given infliximab (4 received 5 mg/kg and 1 received 3 mg/kg), 4 etanercept (50 mg/week), and 1 adalimumab (40 mg every 2 weeks). Concomitant therapies included NSAIDs (7 patients), oral corticosteroids (8 patients), methotrexate (7 patients), and sulfasalazine (3 patients). No severe adverse events were reported during the median 20.6 months. Nine of 10 patients had improvement in their rheumatic symptoms with a median of 15 days for >30% improvement in their pain score and tender joint count, and a median of 33 days for >30% improvement in their swollen joint count. Improvement of anterior uveitis (in 5 patients after 6 months) and cutaneous manifestations were also noted.

Spectacular evolution of reactive arthritis after early treatment with infliximab.
Thomas-Pohl M, Tissot A, Banal F, Lechevalier D. Joint Bone Spine 2012; 79: 524.

A case report describing a 32-year-old male with acute febrile polyarthritis 1 month after gastrointestinal infection. After failing NSAIDs, ofloxacin (200 mg twice daily for 16 days), rifampin (300 mg twice daily for 4 days), and methylprednisone, he was given infliximab (5 mg/kg). Immediately after the infusion, he reported a decrease in pain with improvement of inflammatory markers.

Antibiotics

Antibiotics for treatment of reactive arthritis: a systematic review and meta-analysis.
Barber CE, Kim J, Inman RD, Esdalle JM, James MT. J Rheumatol 2013; 40: 916–28.

A meta-analysis of 10 out of 12 eligible trials. There was no significant benefit comparing antibiotic use and disease remission. The authors also report substantial heterogeneity in the results and attributed this to differences in study design. Ultimately, the efficacy of antibiotics remains uncertain.

Combination antibiotics as a treatment for chronic *Chlamydia*-induced reactive arthritis: a double-blind, placebo controlled, prospective trial.
Carter JD, Espinoza LR, Inman RD, Sneed KB, Ricca LR, Vasey FB, et al. Arthritis Rheum 2010; 62: 1298–307.

A prospective randomized trial with 42 patients who had evidence of chronic postchlamydial reactive arthritis. Patients were randomized to receive either doxycycline and rifampin (12 patients), azithromycin and rifampin (15 patients), or matching oral placebos (15 patients) for 6 months; 22% of subjects on combination antibiotic therapy achieved complete resolution of their symptoms in comparison to 0% of those receiving placebo. An increased number of patients in the antibiotic group became PCR negative for *Chlamydia* compared with the placebo group.

Regional pain and complex regional pain

David Rosenfeld, Kristen Heins Fernandez

COMPLEX REGIONAL PAIN SYNDROME

Complex regional pain syndrome (CRPS) is a disorder characterized by spontaneous pain and signs of sympathetic dysfunction localized to a specific body region, often the distal limbs. It typically begins after trauma, such as a fracture, soft tissue injury, or surgery, and the associated pain is usually disproportionate to the expected course of injury. Although the pain in CRPS is regional, it does not tend to follow a specific dermatome or nerve territory. In addition to pain, if untreated, patients will suffer from swelling, limited range of motion, patchy bone demineralization, and skin changes.

CRPS is often referred to by its older alternative names, including reflex sympathetic dystrophy and causalagia. Currently, two subtypes of CRPS have been recognized: type I and type II. Type I (formerly reflex sympathetic dystrophy) refers to patients with CRPS who lack evidence of peripheral nerve injury. This occurs in 90% of clinical presentations. Type II (formerly causalgia) refers to cases in which evidence of peripheral nerve injury is present. Currently, the pathophysiology of CRPS is unclear, but there appears to be involvement of both proinflammatory cytokines and the sympathetic nervous system.

CRPS typically presents in three stages. Acutely, it begins with throbbing or burning pain and is associated with localized edema. During this phase, bone demineralization can occur. Stage two begins a few months later, when the disease progresses to soft tissue damage, and is characterized by brawny, thickened skin and muscle wasting. Finally, the third, or atrophic, phase involves ridged nails, atrophic skin changes, and limitations of movement.

Early management of CRPS is critical, and therefore identification during the first stage is extremely important. Early diagnosis, however, can be quite challenging as the localized edema is often mistaken for other skin conditions. As a result, dermatologists can play a crucial role in its diagnosis and management.

MANAGEMENT STRATEGY

Managing CRPS is dependent on an accurate and timely diagnosis, which is based upon clinical features, history, and physical examination. Symptoms tend to affect a distal limb, and the patient will describe a history of trauma. The majority of patients will complain of impairment in motor function, which may involve paresis and clumsiness. Muscle spasms can be seen, often in patients with longer durations of CRPS type I. These can present as tremor, myoclonus, or dystonic postures. About 70% of patients will describe hypoesthesia, most frequently in a stockinglike or glovelike distribution. Other dysesthetic symptoms include allodynia (pain to touch), hyperpathia (exaggerated response to painful stimuli), and anesthesia dolorosa, when an area has lost its sensitivity to touch but demonstrates severe pain. Physical examination findings, particularly in the earlier stages, include edema, which is secondary to autonomic

dysfunction. Atrophy and skin discoloration can occur during the later phases, along with atrophy of the soft tissues, bones, and muscles. Another hallmark of CRPS is altered skin temperature, which is a reflection of vasomotor instability. Many investigators have recognized "warm" and "cold" subtypes of CRPS, with the warm subtype being more associated with an inflammatory etiology. Later-stage disease may present with a limited range of motion. This is a result of a variety of skin and connective tissue changes, including increased hair growth, changes in nail growth, skin atrophy, and contraction and fibrosis of joints and fascia.

The diagnosis of CRPS is a clinical one based on the Budapest consensus criteria. First, the patient must have continuing pain that is disproportionate to the inciting event. The patient must also have at least one *sign* in two or more of the categories, as well as report at least one *symptom* in three or more of the categories. Lastly, no other diagnosis should better explain the signs and symptoms. The categories of signs and symptoms are as follows:

Sensory –
   allodynia
   hyperesthesia
Vasomotor –
   temperature asymmetry (>1°C)
   skin color changes
   skin color asymmetry
Sudomotor/edema –
   edema
   sweating changes and/or sweating asymmetry
Motor/trophic –
   decreased range of motion
   motor dysfunction (weakness, tremor, dystonia)
   trophic changes (hair, nail, skin)

On initial presentation, it is important to rule out several other conditions that may mirror CRPS. The differential diagnoses include infection, compartment syndrome, peripheral vascular disease, peripheral neuropathy, rheumatoid arthritis, deep vein thrombosis, Raynaud phenomenon, vascular thoracic outlet syndrome, conversion disorder, and factitious disorder.

Based on the presenting symptoms, it is reasonable to suspect an inflammatory arthropathy or vasculitis. Therefore blood work (complete blood count [CBC], erythrocyte sedimentation rate [ESR], C-reactive protein) and bone scan should be considered. Nerve conduction studies and electromyography (EMG) may be helpful in determining nerve damage, as seen in diabetes or nerve root avulsions. These can also be used to distinguish between CRPS type I and II, as in type II, EMG will confirm the presence of nerve injury, whereas in type I, nerve conduction studies will be normal.

Currently, the best treatment for CRPS is prevention. After a fracture or surgery, *vitamin C* supplementation has been shown to reduce the risk of developing CRPS. Early mobilization may also reduce the risk. When it comes to management of CRPS, earlier therapy results in better outcomes. First-line treatment involves physical and occupational therapy with adjuvant pharmacologic pain management, including *nonsteroidal antiinflammatory drugs (NSAIDs), anticonvulsants, and topical anesthetics.* The efficacies of a pain management specialist are largely unknown, although referral is a reasonable option. Second-line treatment involves interventional therapies, including *sympathetic nerve blockade and spinal cord stimulation.* The evidence for these in reducing pain in CRPS

Evidence Levels: **A** Double-blind study **B** Clinical trial ≥ 20 subjects **C** Clinical trial < 20 subjects **D** Series ≥ 5 subjects **E** Anecdotal case reports

patients is currently unsupported, although many physicians anecdotally support them. Early interventional nerve blocks may help reduce pain, allowing patients to complete more rigorous physical therapy and therefore allowing for more rapid improvement.

Specific Investigations

- Plain radiography
- Bone scans
- Bone densitometry
- Thermography
- Sympathetic blocks
- CBC, ESR, C-reactive protein when vasculitis or arthritis suspected

---

Several investigations have been shown to be complementary to the clinical diagnostic criteria for CRPS. They can also help to objectively identify abnormal characteristics of the disease. Plain radiography can monitor significant changes over time, especially if normal at baseline. Patchy osteoporosis and periarticular osteopenia is often seen in plain radiographs as early as 2 weeks after onset of symptoms. Bone scans are extremely sensitive, although nonspecific, and can often detect osseous changes before plain radiography. Findings characteristic of CRPS include increased periarticular uptake in the third phase and vasomotor instability and abnormal patterns of flow distribution. As disease duration progresses, studies have shown the sensitivity of bone scans decreases, whereas specificity increases.

Bone densitometry is a useful tool in assessing efficacy of CRPS treatment. Densitometry will often reveal lowered bone mineral density early in the disease course, but as therapy progresses, density should improve. Thermography can be helpful in the diagnostic phase and allows the measurement of several symmetric points on the affected and contralateral extremity. Temperature differences can allude to the extent of CRPS—a difference in $0.5\,^\circ$C is considered mildly asymmetric, whereas a difference of $1.0\,^\circ$C is considered significant.

When determining treatment options for patients with CRPS, it is important to establish whether or not their pain is sympathetically dependent or independent. Sympathetically maintained pain (SMP) will respond favorably to an IV injection of phentolamine, resulting in transient pain relief. This is in contrast to patients with sympathetically independent pain (SIP), in which pain is not resolved by nerve blockade. Another option besides phentolamine is the use of local anesthetics—cervicothoracic blocks for upper extremity symptoms and lumbar paravertebral blocks for lower extremity symptoms. Results of sympathetic blockade help to guide further therapy.

PREVENTION

• Vitamin C	A

Can vitamin C prevent complex regional pain syndrome in patients with wrist fractures? Zollinger PE, Tuinebreijer WE, Breederveld RS, Kreis RW. J Bone Joint Surg Am 2007; 89: 1424.

In a meta-analysis of 416 older women with risk factures, CRPS was less prevalent in those who received vitamin C vs. placebo (any dose versus placebo, 2.4% versus 10.1%). Some women in the study received 200, 500, and 1500 mg of vitamin C, and the

higher doses (500 and 1500 mg/day) had greater mean reductions in the relative risk of CRPS than did the lower dose (RR of 0.13, 0.17, and 0.41, respectively).

First-Line Therapies

• Anticonvulsant	**A**
• Physical and occupational therapy	**B**
• NSAID	**B**
• Bisphosphonate	**B**
• Tricyclic antidepressant	**B**
• Topical local anesthetic	**E**

The primary goal of therapy is to reduce pain and increase limb mobility and function. If treatment in these areas is successful, associated abnormalities will often improve. Physical therapy helps reduce edema and decrease guarding. It will also assist in improving daily activities. Physical therapy includes a range of active and passive movement exercise, as well as bandaging and desensitization techniques. Stress loading and functional therapy are important to help regain range of motion and dexterity. Early on, physical therapy may be required as often as three to five times a week. These activities and requirements vary from patient to patient. If a dermatologist is consulted on a diagnosis of CRPS, it is important to make quick referrals to physical and occupational therapy. Ultimately, a multidisciplinary approach is required, including patient education and addressing psychosocial contributing factors. In addition to these therapies, pharmacologic pain management is recommended for adjuvant treatment. Pain relief is an important part in allowing patients to adequately complete the necessary physical therapy, and therefore, analgesics such as NSAIDs and topical local anesthetics are recommended.

Physiotherapy for pain and disability in adults with complex regional pain syndrome (CRPS) types I and II. Smart KM, Wand BM, O'Connell NE. Cochrane Database Syst Rev 2016; 2: CD010853.

Some newer therapies involve graded motor imagery and mirrors—these help to reduce the pain of CRPS and consist of imagined movement and mirror movement phases over a 6-week period. The best available data show that mirror therapy may provide meaningful improvements in pain and function in people with CRPS (type I), although the quality of supporting evidence is currently low.

Evidence based guidelines for complex regional pain syndrome type 1. Perez RS, Zollinger PE, Dijkstra PU, Thomassen-Hilgersom IL, Zuurmond WW, Rosenbrand KC, et al; CRPS I Task Force. BMC Neurol 2010; 10: 20.

NSAIDs are a great adjuvant treatment to physical therapy, although they are not well studied for CRPS. A typical regimen may include ibuprofen 400 to 800 mg three times a day or naproxen 240 to 500 mg twice daily. Antidepressants, particularly tricyclic antidepressants, have also been shown to reduce pain and are a valuable addition to physical therapy.

Randomised controlled trial of gabapentin in complex regional pain syndrome type 1. van de Vusse AC, Stomp-van den Berg SG, Kessels AH, Weber WE. BMC Neurol 2004; 4: 13.

Anticonvulsants such as gabapentin may also be beneficial for patients with CRPS, particularly if it is related to neuropathic pain. However, its efficacy in CRPS is currently not proven. In a randomized trial of 58 patients with CRPS, gabapentin produced no significant improvement in pain. However, clinical experience by physicians suggests that gabapentin and pregabalin may actually be helpful.

Bisphosphonate therapy of reflex sympathetic dystrophy syndrome. Adami S, Fossaluzza V, Gatti D, Fracassi E, Braga V. Ann Rheum Dis 1997; 56: 201.

Bisphosphonates have been shown to produce consistent and rapid remission of CRPS. In a study of 82 subjects with CRPS of the hand or foot who had disease duration of 4 months or less *and* abnormal uptake in bone scan, there was a significant decrease in visual analog pain scale for those in the neridronate group in comparison to the placebo group (−47 mm vs. −22.6 mm). There were no significant adverse events reported.

Early adjunct treatment with topical lidocaine results in improved pain and function in a patient with complex regional pain syndrome. Hanlan AK, Mah-Jones D, Mills PB. Pain Physician 2014; 17: E629–35.

Topical 5% lidocaine ointment is a great noninvasive, inexpensive, and effective adjuvant therapy to CRPS treatment. Topical lidocaine is valuable in early CRPS and has been shown to reduce severe allodynia, allowing patients to participate more readily in rehabilitation strategies.

Second-Line Therapies	
• Sympathectomy	A
• Glucocorticoids	B
• Sympathetic nerve block	B
• Spinal cord stimulation	B

Glucocorticoids are considered a viable option only if previous pharmacologic therapies have failed. In addition, interventional procedures may also be considered, including regional sympathetic nerve block, spinal cord stimulation, and sympathectomy. Although their efficacies are still unclear, many physicians recommend increasingly invasive interventions, particularly in patients receiving noninvasive therapy without improvement. The effectiveness of sympathetic nerve block in particular is dependent on whether or not the patient was responsive to diagnostic sympathetic blockade. When starting interventional therapy, it is generally recommended to allow 2 weeks for improvement before progressing to another form of treatment. Many care centers consider spinal cord stimulation the most invasive therapy, and therefore, it should only be considered 12 to 16 weeks from the start of CRPS treatment.

Comparison of prednisolone with piroxicam in complex regional pain syndrome following stroke: a randomized controlled trial. Kalita J, Vajpayee A, Misra UK. QJM 2006; 99: 89.

In a study of patients with CRPS poststroke, corticosteroids were shown to be more effective than NSAIDs. The mean change in CRPS pain score in the prednisolone group was 6.47 compared with 0.47 in the piroxicam group. However, it is recommended to use NSAIDs and use glucocorticoids only when patients are unresponsive to other medications.

Local anaesthetic sympathetic blockade for complex regional pain syndrome. Stanton TR, Wand BM, Carr DB, Birklein F, Wasner GL, O'Connell NE. Cochrane Database Syst Rev 2013; 8: CD004598.

In an analysis of 12 studies, including 386 patients, most of them found no difference in pain outcomes between sympathetic block and other active treatments. The current evidence on the efficacy and safety of local anesthetics is very limited, but thus far, the data do not suggest that local anesthetics are effective in reducing pain in CRPS.

Spinal cord stimulation in patients with chronic reflex sympathetic dystrophy. Kemler MA, Barendse GA, van Kleef M, de Vet HC, Rijks CP, Furnée CA, et al. N Engl J Med 2000; 343: 618.

Spinal cord stimulation may be considered when other treatment modalities have failed. In a study of 36 patients with CRPS, 24 received implanted spinal cord stimulators plus physical therapy, whereas the remaining 12 patients received physical therapy only. The intensity of pain was measured on a visual analog scale from 0 cm (no pain) to 10 cm (very severe pain). In the group that received spinal cord stimulation, there was a mean reduction of 2.4 cm in the intensity of pain at 6 months compared with an increase of 0.2 cm in the group that received physical therapy only. It is reasonable to conclude that in patients with chronic CRPS, electrical spinal cord stimulation can reduce pain and improve quality of life.

Cervico-thoracic or lumbar sympathectomy for neuropathic pain and complex regional pain syndrome. Straube S, Derry S, Moore RA, Cole P. Cochrane Database Syst Rev 2013; 9: CD002918.

The only study that met their criteria was one that compared lumbar sympathectomy with lumbar sympathetic neurolysis with phenol in 20 participants with CRPS. There was no comparison of sympathectomy versus sham or placebo. There was no significant difference in pain scoring between the two groups initially and over 4 months. However, patients who received radiofrequency ablation sympathectomy complained of an "unpleasant sensation."

Sympathectomy should only be considered in patients with a positive pain response to diagnostic sympathetic blockade and when all other treatment modalities have failed. Patients must also be informed of the high rates of adverse effects, including increased pain, new neuropathic pain, and bothersome sweating.

Evidence Levels: **A** Double-blind study **B** Clinical trial ≥ 20 subjects **C** Clinical trial < 20 subjects **D** Series ≥ 5 subjects **E** Anecdotal case reports

218

Relapsing polychondritis

David P. D'Cruz

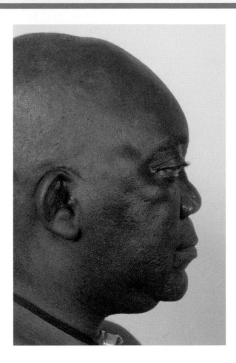

Relapsing polychondritis is an autoimmune rheumatic disorder characterized by cartilage inflammation. Characteristic features include nasal bridge, auricular and ocular inflammation, and major airway disease. It is rare with an incidence of 0.71/million/year, with an increased mortality rate, and there is often a delay in establishing a diagnosis.

The diagnosis is established by the presence of chondritis in two of three characteristic anatomic sites: auricular, nasal, laryngotracheal, or one of these sites and two other features, including ocular inflammation, audiovestibular damage, or seronegative inflammatory arthritis. In most patients, histologic confirmation is not necessary for diagnosis.

Auricular chondritis manifests as ear pain, redness, and swelling with sparing of the noncartilaginous lobule. After repeated relapses, the pinnae may be floppy and distorted or have a cauliflower-like appearance. The ear may become rigid after extensive calcification. Recurrent nasal chondritis results in a saddle-nose deformity.

Skin manifestations include oral ulceration, sometimes with genital ulceration, nodules, purpura, papules, sterile pustules, superficial phlebitis, livedo reticularis, skin ulcers, and distal necrosis.

Laryngeal chondritis presents with hoarseness, tracheal ring tenderness, cough, breathlessness, and stridor. All patients with suspected pulmonary disease should undergo computed tomography (CT) imaging, including end-inspiratory and dynamic expiratory volumetric imaging. End-inspiratory scanning may reveal tracheal and bronchial stenosis, wall thickening, and calcification. Expiratory scans may demonstrate tracheobronchial malacia with airway collapse and air trapping.

Cardiovascular complications eventually occur in half of all patients and are the second most frequent cause of mortality. Aortic valve inflammation, the most common cardiac manifestation (10% of patients), may occur in asymptomatic patients and can silently progress during seemingly effective systemic corticosteroid therapy. Atrioventricular block, mitral regurgitation, and acute pericarditis may also occur.

Central and peripheral nerve involvement is rare. Cranial nerve lesions are the most common, but other complications include seizures, cerebral dysfunction, confusion, headaches, cerebral aneurysm, and rhomboencephalitis.

All patients should be monitored for the development of renal disease with routine urine dip testing for blood and protein.

Disease activity is assessed clinically by standard methods. There is an objective scoring system, the Relapsing Polychondritis Disease Activity Index (RPDAI), that provides objective disease assessment for use in clinical studies.

Otologic manifestations of relapsing polychondritis. Review of literature and report of nine cases. Bachor E, Blevins NH, Karmody C, Kühnel T. Auris Nasus Larynx 2006; 33: 135–41.

A good description of the broad spectrum of ear manifestations. No patients died, suggesting patients with limited disease have a good prognosis.

Up to 46% of patients have impaired hearing, and inadequately treated patients can suffer permanent hearing loss. Screening audiometry is highlighted. Ocular, neurologic, and renal disease can also occur in relapsing polychondritis. Cardiac manifestations include aortic regurgitation, aortic aneurysm, atrioventricular block, mitral regurgitation, and acute pericarditis, making periodic cardiac examination mandatory.

Relapsing polychondritis: prevalence of expiratory CT airway abnormalities. Lee KS, Ernst A, Trentham DE, Lunn W, Feller-Kopman DJ, Boiselle PM. Radiology 2006; 240: 565–73.

Dynamic expiratory CT scans demonstrated abnormalities such as tracheomalacia and air trapping in 94% of relapsing polychondritis patients who had pulmonary symptoms, yet only half the patients demonstrated abnormalities on routine inspiratory CT scans. The most common findings were air trapping (94%), malacia (72%), and calcification (39%).

Expiratory CT scans show clinically relevant bronchopulmonary abnormalities earlier than standard inspiratory CT scans, allowing earlier institution of aggressive therapy to prevent disease progression.

Airway manifestations are ultimately present in over 50% of patients and are the leading cause of death. Airway obstruction may be asymptomatic in the earlier stages, detected only on pulmonary function testing. Other sources stress the importance of plain radiography, CT, and Magnetic resonance imaging (MRI) for early detection of tracheal narrowing and upper airway disease.

Dermatologic manifestations of relapsing polychondritis. A study of 200 cases at a single center. Francés C, el Rassi R, Laporte JL, Rybojad M, Papo T, Piette JC. Medicine (Baltimore) 2001; 80: 173–9.

Cutaneous manifestations of patients with relapsing polychondritis: an association with extracutaneous complications. Shimizu J, Oka H, Yamano Y, Yudoh K, Suzuki N. Clin Rheumatol 2016; 35: 781–3.

Two of the largest series in the literature of >200 patients described a variety of skin manifestations, including oral ulceration sometimes with genital ulceration, nodules, purpura, papules, sterile pustules, superficial phlebitis, livedo reticularis, neutrophilic dermatoses including Sweet syndrome, skin ulcers, and distal necrosis. In Francés et al.'s paper, oral ulceration was the most common finding in patients with relapsing polychondritis who did not have any other disease, and in seven patients genital ulcers were also seen. The acronym MAGIC (mouth and genital ulceration with inflamed cartilage) has previously been coined to describe patients who appear to have relapsing polychondritis with oral and genital ulceration. However, this syndrome is controversial, and these patients are more likely to be an overlap of Behçet disease with relapsing polychondritis, especially as relapsing polychondritis may occur in association with other autoimmune rheumatic diseases.

Nodules on the limbs were the most common skin lesions and have been described as erythema nodosum–like lesions with septal panniculitis. Histologic findings included vasculitis in 19 patients (leukocytoclastic in 17 and lymphocytic in 2), neutrophil infiltrates in 6, thrombosis of skin vessels in 4, septal panniculitis in 3, and minor nonspecific changes in 2 patients. Both these studies described patients with myelodysplastic syndromes and relapsing polychondritis, and these patients were much more likely to have dermatologic manifestations, most commonly limb nodules, purpura, papules, and livedo reticularis, as well as neutrophilic dermatoses including Sweet syndrome. They recommend that elderly patients with relapsing polychondritis and skin lesions be investigated for an underlying myelodysplastic syndrome. This confirmed previous data from Hebbar et al. from 1995 (see next).

Association of myelodysplastic syndrome and relapsing polychondritis: further evidence. Hebbar M, Brouillard M, Wattel E, Decoulx M, Hatron PY, Devulder B, et al. Leukemia 1995; 9: 731–3.

Twenty-eight percent (5 of 18) of relapsing polychondritis patients over a period of 13 years were found to have myelodysplastic syndromes.

Anemia is a poor prognostic sign in patients with relapsing polychondritis; those with concurrent myelodysplasia often develop refractory anemia requiring transfusions. Several patients have progressed to leukemia.

MANAGEMENT STRATEGY

Treatment of relapsing polychondritis is aimed at reducing inflammation, which may progressively destroy the ears, nose, eyes, joints, respiratory tract, and cardiovascular system. The most common cause of mortality is laryngotracheal involvement. A multidisciplinary approach, including referral to specialist centers, is crucial to evaluate and treat multiple organ involvement. There are no controlled trials: treatment is empiric and should be tailored to the severity of disease.

Mildly affected patients may be managed using *nonsteroidal anti-inflammatory agents*. They should be used sparingly and for short periods given the long-term risks of gastrointestinal, renal, and cardiovascular complications. *Colchicine* 0.5 mg twice daily and *dapsone* 50 to 100 mg daily have also provided benefit, but toxicity may occur, especially with dapsone and G6PD (glucose-6-phosphate dehydrogenase) deficiency.

Corticosteroids are widely used for more severe disease. Life-threatening airway obstruction may be treated with pulsed intravenous methylprednisolone (500 mg to 1 g/day for 3 days). The traditional dose of 1 mg/kg/day is completely non–evidence based, is excessive, and should be abandoned. High-dose corticosteroids contribute significantly to long-term damage, which is associated with premature mortality. Most patients with moderate disease will benefit from doses of prednisolone between 10 and 20 mg daily in a tapering dose irrespective of body weight. The lowest possible maintenance dose should be used, and some patients may be able to use intermittent short courses of prednisolone 20 mg daily for 1 to 2 weeks. Bone prophylaxis with calcium and vitamin D supplementation should be considered in corticosteroid-dependent patients.

Second-line therapies should be considered for patients unable to taper corticosteroid doses. The most commonly used agents are methotrexate (considered first line by most experts) 5 to 25 mg weekly, azathioprine 1.5–2 mg/kg/day, ciclosporin 5 mg/kg/day, mycophenolate mofetil 2 to 3 g/day, leflunomide, and chlorambucil. Intravenous cyclophosphamide has been used for severe rapidly progressive and life-threatening disease, especially for aortitis or glomerulonephritis. Plasma exchange and intravenous immunoglobulin (IVIG) therapy are usually not successful, but isolated case reports have described clinical benefit.

Biologic agents are increasingly being used off label for treatment-resistant patients with some success. Infliximab, adalimumab, etanercept, tocilizumab, and anakinra have all been reported to improve disease control in isolated case reports.

Topical steroids may be used to treat skin manifestations and are standard therapy for ocular inflammation. Inhaled steroids may be useful in mild airway inflammation, and nebulized ephedrine has been used occasionally.

Respiratory support with continuous positive airway pressure and other noninvasive ventilation devices may improve quality of life for patients where surgical intervention or stenting is not feasible.

Surgical intervention may be needed acutely when tracheostomy is needed for tracheal stenosis. Other surgical interventions to manage fibrotic or stenotic complications should only be considered electively when the disease is in remission. Tracheal surgery, including reconstruction procedures, may be needed for localized stenosis. Balloon dilatation may be used either alone or in combination with other surgical procedures. Large airway stenting has been successfully used, although metallic stents, usually used for malignant disease, may erode the airways over time. Silicon stents are more likely to migrate or be expectorated. Endobronchial ultrasound has been used to identify localized stenotic lesions and to measure airway size before positioning of stents.

Cardiac valve replacement and aortic surgery are associated with significant surgical morbidity and mortality, but several case reports describe successful outcomes. Any general anesthetic that requires intubation and ventilation before surgery requires careful preoperative anesthetic review.

Specific Investigations

- Otolaryngologic evaluation
- Audiometry
- Pulmonary evaluation
- Chest radiograph and/or CT/MRI
- Dynamic expiratory CT examination
- Pulmonary function tests (especially flow/volume loops)
- Endobronchial ultrasonography
- Cardiovascular examination
- Electrocardiogram and/or echocardiogram (CT/MRI may also be useful)
- Ophthalmologic examination
- Urinalysis

First-Line Therapies

• NSAIDs	D
• Colchicine	C
• Dapsone	C
• Systemic corticosteroids	C

Treatment of relapsing polychondritis with dapsone. Barranco VP, Monor DB, Solomon H. Arch Dermatol 1976; 112: 1268–88.

Three patients were successfully treated with dapsone (100–200 mg daily), each showing complete resolution of an acute attack of relapsing polychondritis within 2 weeks of starting therapy.

Although not all patients respond to dapsone, those who do may improve dramatically within 1 to 2 weeks. The effectiveness of dapsone seems to be dose dependent, with 200 mg daily being the most commonly reported effective dose. G6PD levels should be measured before treatment to avoid the risk of dapsone-induced hemolytic anemia.

Relapsing polychondritis. Kent PD, Michet CJ Jr, Luthra HS. Curr Opin Rheumatol 2004; 16: 56–61.

A well-written and comprehensive review of the clinical features, assessment, and management of relapsing polychondritis. Recommendations for corticosteroid doses are given ranging from 10 to 20 mg daily of prednisolone for mild to moderate disease up to high-dose prednisolone and intravenous methylprednisolone 500 mg to 1 g/day for 3 days.

Second-Line Therapies

• Azathioprine	D
• Ciclosporin	D
• Methotrexate	D
• Mycophenolate mofetil	D
• Leflunomide	D
• Cyclophosphamide	E
• Intravenous immunoglobulin	E
• Infliximab	D
• Adalimumab	E
• Etanercept	E
• Inhaled fluticasone	E
• Continuous positive airway pressure	E
• Tracheobronchial stents	E

Relapsing polychondritis. Trentham DE, Le CH. Ann Intern Med 1998; 129: 114–22.

In this review, 23 of 31 patients were able to reduce their prednisone dose from an average of 19 mg daily to 5 mg daily by adding methotrexate (average weekly methotrexate dose 15.5 mg).

A good review article.

Relapsing polychondritis: a clinical update. Longo L, Greco A, Rea A, Lo Vasco VR, De Virgilio A, De Vincentiis M. Autoimmun Rev 2016; 15: 539–43.

An excellent clinical review of relapsing polychondritis and its treatment, covering the use of corticosteroids, immunosuppressive agents, and biologics in some depth.

Successful treatment of relapsing polychondritis with mycophenolate mofetil. Goldenberg G, Sangueza OP, Jorizzo JL. J Dermatol Treat 2006; 17: 158–9.

A 50-year-old man with bilateral ear pain was successfully treated with a prednisone taper and mycophenolate 3 g/day (increased from an initial dose of 2 g/day). At 17 months' follow-up the patient maintained his improvement on prednisone 5 mg daily and mycophenolate 3 g/day.

Successful treatment of relapsing polychondritis with infliximab. Richez C, Dumoulin C, Coutoly X, Schaeverbeke T. Clin Exp Rheumatol 2004; 22: 629–31.

One patient had marked improvement in symptoms 4 days after an infusion of 4 mg/kg infliximab. Control was maintained with repeat treatments every 6 to 8 weeks.

Infliximab seems to be an effective therapy for relapsing polychondritis unresponsive to conventional therapy, as well as a steroid-sparing agent.

Sustained response to etanercept after failing infliximab, in a patient with relapsing polychondritis with tracheomalacia. Subrahmanyam P, Balakrishnan C, Dasgupta B. Scand J Rheumatol 2008; 37: 239–40.

A 54-year-old woman with relapsing polychondritis complicated by tracheomalacia experienced a dramatic improvement in her symptoms and an 18-month sustained response after etanercept was substituted for infliximab.

Prolonged response to antitumor necrosis factor treatment with adalimumab (Humira) in relapsing polychondritis complicated by aortitis. Seymour MW, Home DM, Williams RO, Allard SA. Rheumatology 2007; 46: 1739–41.

A 43-year-old woman who had undergone aortic valve replacement continued to experience aortitis despite a variety of immunosuppressive drugs and cytotoxic agents. Despite an initial good response to infliximab, after 10 months her symptoms returned. Switching her anti–tumor necrosis factor (TNF) agent to adalimumab and continuing methotrexate and corticosteroids resulted in improvement; she has subsequently been maintained on adalimumab and low-dose corticosteroids.

These two reports suggest that switching anti-TNF agents may benefit patients with recalcitrant relapsing polychondritis.

Complete remission in refractory relapsing polychondritis with intravenous immunoglobulins. Terrier B, Aouba A, Bienvenu B, Bloch-Queyrat C, Delair E, Mallet J, et al. Clin Exp Rheumatol 2007; 25: 136–8.

A young woman with relapsing episodes of nasal chondritis and severe scleritis with scleromalacia received IVIG every 3 then every 4 weeks (2 g/kg on 2 days) in association with 25 mg/day of prednisone after treatment with corticosteroids, infliximab, methotrexate, mycophenolate, and cyclophosphamide failed to control her symptoms. Dramatic improvement of symptoms was sustained for 11 months, but when IVIG treatments were spaced every 6 weeks hearing loss and episcleritis recurred. Reinstitution treatment every fourth week brought her symptoms under control.

Use of inhaled fluticasone propionate to control respiratory manifestations of relapsing polychondritis. Tsuburai T, Suzuki M, Tsurikisawa N, Ono E, Oshikata C, Taniguchi M, et al. Respirology 2009; 14: 299–301.

A 19-year-old patient with relapsing polychondritis used high-dose fluticasone propionate, which reduced oral corticosteroid requirements and dramatically decreased the patient's obstructive airway impairment.

Treatment of diffuse tracheomalacia secondary to relapsing polychondritis with continuous positive airway pressure.

Adliff M, Ngato D, Keshavjee S, Brenaman S, Granton JT. Chest 1997; 112: 1701–4.

A patient with relapsing polychondritis of the trachea and bronchi was treated with nasal continuous positive airway pressure. This approach is now widely used.

Management of airway manifestations of relapsing polychondritis: case reports and review of the literature. Sarodia SD, Dasgupta A, Mehta AC. Chest 1999; 116: 1669–75.

Five patients with severe respiratory involvement (three of whom required continuous mechanical ventilation due to airway collapse) benefited from placement of self-expandable metallic tracheobronchial stents. A total of 17 stents of varying sizes were placed in these patients over a period of 3 years, with favorable outcomes in four patients.

When severe, progressive disease leads to extensive destruction of the tracheobronchial tree despite maximal medical therapy, and tracheostomy or tracheobronchial stent placement may preserve or improve respiratory function and reduce patients' reliance on mechanical ventilation.

Endobronchial ultrasonography in the diagnosis and treatment of relapsing polychondritis with tracheobronchial malacia. Miyazu Y, Miyazawa T, Kurimoto N, Iwamoto Y, Ishida A, Kanoh K, et al. Chest 2003; 124: 2393–5.

Endobronchial ultrasonography revealed poorly defined bronchial wall structure with two patterns of cartilaginous damage: fragmentation and edema. Successful treatment was achieved by the implantation of nitinol stents, the sizes of which were determined by endobronchial ultrasonography.

Surgical treatment of the cardiac manifestations of relapsing polychondritis: overview of 33 patients identified through literature review and the Mayo Clinic records. Dib C, Moustafa SE, Mookadam M, Zehr KJ, Michet CJ Jr, Mookadam F. Mayo Clin Proc 2006; 81: 772–6.

Clinically important aortic or mitral regurgitation occurs in about 10% of relapsing polychondritis patients, with aortic regurgitation being the more common and more urgent. In this retrospective series and literature review the mean time between initial onset of relapsing polychondritis and surgery was about 5 years. In contrast to previous reports of 70% 1-year mortality after valve replacement, in this analysis 50% of patients were alive 1 year after surgery.

Aortic regurgitation is a serious complication of relapsing polychondritis. Baseline chest CT, MRI, or transesophageal echocardiography should be performed upon diagnosis and repeated every 6 months. All aortic segments should be regularly evaluated because involvement of multiple thoracic and abdominal aneurysms has been reported in several patients.

Anesthesia in a patient with acute respiratory insufficiency due to relapsing polychondritis. Biro P, Rohling R, Schmid S, Matter C, Lang M. J Clin Anaesth 1994; 6: 59–62.

This case report highlights the need for careful preoperative evaluation of vital organ functions, with particular reference to airway management, so that the anesthetic approach can be tailored to the individual needs of the patient.

Relapsing polychondritis can be characterized by 3 different clinical phenotypes: analysis of a recent series of 142 patients. Dion J, Costedoat-Chalumeau N, Séne D, Cohen-Bittan J, Leroux G, Dion C, et al. Arthritis Rheumatol 2016; 68: 2992–3001.

This study used cluster analysis to define three groups that were clinically relevant in terms of prognosis: cluster 1, which had the highest mortality, included more men who were older at diagnosis, with myelodysplasia, general symptoms, and cutaneous and cardiac disease; cluster 2 had younger patients with predominant large airway disease; and cluster 3 had patients with mild disease and long-lasting remissions.

Evidence Levels: **A** Double-blind study   **B** Clinical trial ≥ 20 subjects   **C** Clinical trial < 20 subjects   **D** Series ≥ 5 subjects   **E** Anecdotal case reports

219

Rhinophyma

Surod Qazaz, John Berth-Jones

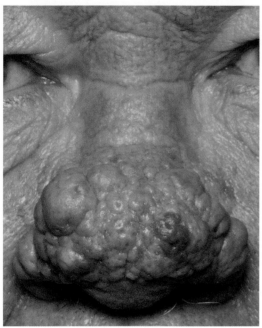

Phymas, of which rhinophyma is the most common, are localized swellings of facial soft tissues due to a variable combination of fibrosis, sebaceous hyperplasia, and lymphedema. They occur on the nose (rhinophyma) and, less often, the ears, forehead, or chin. They are seen much more frequently in males than in females. Rhinophyma may develop in patients with a long history of rosacea, when it is often regarded as a complication or "end stage" of the disease. However, rhinophyma is also seen in patients who have no history of rosacea. Occasionally rhinophyma is complicated by the development of a malignancy.

MANAGEMENT STRATEGY

Phymas require *physical ablation* or removal, usually by *surgery*. Remodeling is most often achieved simply by paring off the excess tissue with a scalpel. Other techniques that can be useful in the hands of those with the necessary expertise include electrosurgery, excision/vaporization with argon, CO_2, Nd:YAG or Er:YAG lasers, and cryotherapy. Ionizing radiation has been used in cases with coexisting malignancy. Systemic *isotretinoin* can significantly reduce the bulk of rhinophyma, although it does not restore normal skin contours. It is possible, but not established, that treatment of rosacea may inhibit the development of rhinophyma.

Specific Investigation

- Biopsy is occasionally indicated to exclude malignancy

Rhinophyma and coexisting occult skin cancers. Lutz ME, Otley CC. Dermatol Surg 2001; 27: 201–2.

Rhinophyma can be complicated by the development of a malignancy, which can be difficult to recognize.

Rhinophyma and nonmelanoma skin cancer: an update. Lazzeri D, Agostini T, Pantaloni M, Spinelli G. Ann Chir Plast Esthet 2012; 57: 183–4.

In addition to basal cell, squamous cell, and basosquamous carcinomas, rarely, angiosarcoma and sebaceous carcinoma may occur.

First-Line Therapy

• Surgical paring	C

Triple approach to rhinophyma. Curnier A, Choudhary S. Ann Plast Surg 2002; 49: 211–4.

The authors report pleasing results in six patients treated by tangential excision for debulking, the use of scissors for sculpting, and mild dermabrasion for final contouring.

Second-Line Therapies

• Electrosurgery	C
• Argon laser	C
• CO_2 laser	C
• Nd:YAG laser	E
• Er:YAG laser	D
• Cryotherapy	D
• Isotretinoin	C
• Microdebrider	E
• Shaw scalpel	E
• Radiotherapy	E
• Hydrosurgery	D

Electrosurgical treatment of rhinophyma. Clark DP, Hanke CW. J Am Acad Dermatol 1990; 22: 831–7.

This treatment was inexpensive and associated with few complications and gave good or excellent cosmetic results in 13 cases.

Surgical management of rhinophyma: report of eight patients treated with electrosection. Rex J, Ribera M, Bielsa I, Paradelo C, Ferrándiz C. Dermatol Surg 2002; 28: 347–9.

Eight male patients were treated using radiofrequency electrosurgery to remove thin layers of tissue until the nose shape was re-created. All patients achieved acceptable cosmetic results.

Rhinophyma treated by argon laser. Halsbergen-Henning JP, van Gemert MJ. Lasers Surg Med 1983; 2: 211–5.

Thirteen cases were treated. This laser is believed to work by selectively coagulating capillaries that cause redness of the nose and that feed the hypertrophic regions, as well as by directly causing coagulation shrinkage of the hypertrophic connective tissue. The result was a smooth and more natural appearance of the nose without redness. Pustulosis was also reduced.

Comparison of CO_2 laser and electrosurgery in the treatment of rhinophyma. Greenbaum SS, Krull EA, Watnick K. J Am Acad Dermatol 1988; 18: 363–8.

The results from the CO_2 laser and electrosurgery were compared in three patients by treating one side of the nose by each method. There was little to choose between them in terms of results, but electrosurgery was more cost effective.

Carbon dioxide laser treatment of rhinophyma: a review of 124 patients. Madan V, Ferguson JE, August PJ. Br J Dermatol 2009; 161: 814–8.

Exuberant sebaceous tissue was ablated using the Sharplan 40C CO_2 laser under local anesthesia. The laser was used in a continuous mode to debulk the larger rhinophymas and in a resurfacing mode (Silk Touch scanner; Sharplan, 4–7 mm spot at 20–40 W) or continuous mode (10–20 W using a defocused 2–3-mm beam) to reshape the nasal contours. Results were classified as good to excellent in 118 and poor in 6 patients.

Spectrum of results after treatment of rhinophyma with the carbon dioxide laser. El Azhary RA, Roenigk RK, Wang TD. Mayo Clin Proc 1991; 66: 899–905.

A review of 30 patients treated with the CO_2 laser and followed up for 1 to 4 years. Milder cases were treated with laser vaporization, more severe cases with CO_2 laser excision and then vaporization. Dilated pores developed in many patients. Leukoderma, unilateral alar lift, and mild hypertrophic scarring developed in single cases.

Surgical correction of rhinophyma: comparison of two methods in a 15-year-long experience. Lazzeri D, Larcher L, Huemer GM, Riml S, Grassetti L, Pantaloni M, et al. J Craniomaxillofac Surg 2013; 41: 429–36.

Long-term results in 45 cases treated with tangential excision and 22 treated with the CO_2 laser. Minor complications, including scarring and hypopigmentation, were seen in six patients. All patients were satisfied with their outcomes at the follow-up visit, and no major complications were detected. The authors did not consider the extra cost of laser treatment to be justified.

Excision of rhinophyma with Nd:YAG laser: a new technique. Wenig BL, Weingarten RT. Laryngoscope 1993; 103: 101–6.

Treatment of rhinophyma with Er:YAG laser. Orenstein A, Haik J, Tamir J, Winkler E, Frand J, Zilinsky I, et al. Lasers Surg Med 2001; 29: 230–5.

Use of a dual-mode erbium:YAG laser for the surgical correction of rhinophyma. Fincher EF, Gladstone HB. Arch Facial Plast Surg 2004; 6: 267–71.

In each of these reports six cases of rhinophyma were treated with satisfactory outcomes. The Er:YAG laser provides both controlled ablation of tissue and hemostasis.

Rhinophyma treated by liquid nitrogen spray cryosurgery. Sonnex TS, Dawber RPR. Clin Exp Dermatol 1986; 11: 284–8.

Five cases were treated using two freeze–thaw cycles, each freeze lasting 30 seconds after the ice field was established, with a 4-minute intervening thaw. A pethidine and diazepam premedication was used. In three cases small residual prominent areas responded to further treatment after 2 months. The final result was satisfactory in each case, with no scarring.

Isotretinoin in the treatment of rosacea and rhinophyma. Irvine C, Kumar P, Marks R. In: Marks R, Plewig G, eds. Acne and Related Disorders. London: Martin Dunitz, 1989; 311–5.

A study in which nine men with rhinophyma were treated with isotretinoin 1 mg/kg daily for up to 18 weeks. Isotretinoin reduced the volume of rhinophyma (assessed objectively using molds of the noses) by 9% to 23% but did not restore normal skin contours in advanced cases.

The authors report good results in five cases and consider this their treatment of choice.

New surgical adjuncts in the treatment of rhinophyma: the microdebrider and FloSeal. Kaushik V, Tahery J, Malik TH, Jones PH. J Laryngol Otol 2003; 117: 551–2.

This is a report of a single case treated using this approach. The microdebrider is a powered rotary shaving device. FloSeal is a hemostatic mixture of thrombin and gelatin applied topically after the surgery. The use of these adjuncts allowed precise sculpting and immediate hemostasis.

Surgical treatment of rhinophyma with the Shaw scalpel. Eisen RF, Katz AE, Bohigian RK, Grande DJ. Arch Dermatol 1986; 122: 307–9.

The Shaw scalpel is a device in which a scalpel blade can be heated. A rhinophyma was treated using a temperature of 150°C to achieve hemostasis while paring. Contours were then refined using a CO_2 laser and light dermabrasion.

Rhinophyma, associated with carcinoma, treated successfully with radiation. Plenk HP. Plast Reconstruct Surg 1995; 95: 559–62.

Two patients with basal cell carcinoma complicating rhinophyma had complete control of both conditions by radiotherapy using orthovoltage x-radiation. The authors suggest that this modality might be useful for rhinophyma alone.

Rhinophyma treated with kilovoltage photons. Skala M, Delaney G, Towell V, Vladica N. Australas J Dermatol 2005; 46: 88–9.

A rhinophyma was successfully treated with 90-kV photons to a total dose of 40 Gy in 20 daily fractions.

Treatment of rhinophyma with the Versajet Hydrosurgery System. Taghizadeh R, Mackay SP, Gilbert PM. J Plast Reconstruct Aesthet Surg 2008; 61: 330–3.

Six patients were treated successfully.

The Versajet Hydrosurgery System is a novel surgical device that uses a high-velocity jet of water for excision and vacuum aspiration of water and debris.

A new surgical technique of rhinophyma (gull-wing technique). Karacor-Altuntas Z, Dadaci M, Ince B, Altuntas M. J Craniofac Surg 2015; 26: e28–30.

A severe rhinophyma underwent full-thickness excision using gull-wing elevation of the nasal tip and dorsal skin. The patient was very satisfied with the result.

Evidence Levels: **A** Double-blind study **B** Clinical trial ≥ 20 subjects **C** Clinical trial < 20 subjects **D** Series ≥ 5 subjects **E** Anecdotal case reports

Rocky Mountain spotted fever and other rickettsial infections

Amer Ali Almohssen, George G Kihiczak, Robert A. Schwartz

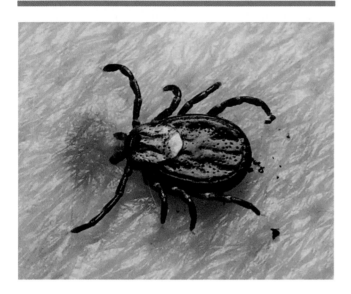

The Rickettsiae are a family of obligate intracellular gram-negative bacteria that cause infections with a diverse array of clinical presentations. They are vectorborne diseases that may be divided into the spotted fevers (including Rocky Mountain spotted fever), the typhus group, rickettsialpox, Q fever, and ehrlichiosis.

RICKETTSIAL SPOTTED FEVERS

These infections include African tick bite fever *(Rickettsia africae)*, Astrakhan fever *(R. conorii)*, Flinders Island spotted fever *(R. honei)*, Indian tick typhus *(R. conorii)*, Israeli spotted fever *(R. conorii)*, Japanese spotted fever *(R. japonica)*, Mediterranean spotted fever *(R. conorii)*, Queensland tick typhus *(R. australis)*, Siberian tick typhus *(R. sibirica)*, and Rocky Mountain spotted fever *(R. rickettsii)*.

Rocky Mountain spotted fever (RMSF) is caused by *Rickettsia rickettsii* and is endemic to almost all areas of the United States with a high degree of prevalence in North Carolina, Tennessee, and Oklahoma. RMSF is transmitted by *Demacentor andersoni* in the western United States and by *D. variabilis* (pictured on the back of a patient in the figure above) in the eastern United States. The classic triad seen early in the course of the disease consists of a tick bite, rash, and fever. The characteristic rash is composed of pink macules that appear on the wrists and ankles; become petechial and purpuric; and then progress to the palms, soles, extremities, and trunk, sparing the face.

This macular rash does not appear until the third day after the onset of symptoms and is seen in more than 90% of cases. A petechial rash is usually not evident until the sixth day and only occurs in 35% to 60% of patients. Atypical rashes, confined to one region of the body, may be evident.

Fever, myalgias, and severe headaches are present in most cases, with bilateral calf pain being the most common presenting complaint. Gastrointestinal symptoms such as abdominal pain, diarrhea, nausea, and vomiting occur in nearly half of patients, usually early in the course of the illness. These findings often lead to a misdiagnosis or delay in therapy. Vascular injury to the small intestine, appendix, and gallbladder may occur, in some cases mimicking acute cholecystitis.

Prognosis is related to the timely diagnosis and initiation of effective treatment. Prevention is achieved by avoiding areas with ticks. Covering skin with long protective clothing reduces the risk of exposure. Clothing may be impregnated with acaricidal compounds for added protection. Any uncovered skin should be treated with a topical insect repellent before activities in high-risk areas. Unfortunately, most insect repellents are effective for only short periods and need to be reapplied frequently. Thorough skin examinations should be conducted on a regular basis, at least twice daily in endemic areas, and any ticks removed. The scalp, axillary, and pubic hair require particularly careful examination. There is currently no effective vaccine, although immunogenic surface protein antigens have been cloned and sequenced.

MANAGEMENT STRATEGY

Clinical suspicion of a spotted fever is sufficient to warrant treatment. Serologic confirmation should not delay the initiation of appropriate therapy. Diagnosis is difficult, as the characteristic rash is not a reliable sign of disease, and the classic triad of tick bite, rash, and fever is often not evident.

The spotted fevers progress rapidly and, therefore, immediate treatment is required, ideally in the first 3 to 4 days. Doxycycline is the best first-line agent for treating RMSF and other spotted fevers, as shown by extensive data and clinical experience. Doxycycline is administered at a dose of 100 mg twice daily orally in adults. Children under 45.4 kg should receive 2.2 mg/kg per dose twice daily orally. The therapeutic benefit provided by doxycycline in the treatment of RMSF is thought to outweigh the potential risk for tooth discoloration in children receiving doxycycline. These oral antibiotics are taken for a minimum of 7 days and are continued until the patient is afebrile for 72 hours. Within 24 hours of the initiation of treatment, a response may be observed. Within the first 48 hours considerable clinical improvement is seen; apyrexia is often achieved by 72 hours. In severe cases requiring hospitalization, intravenous doxycycline every 12 hours is the recommended treatment.

Tetracycline (500 mg every 6 hours, maximum dose 2 g) is efficacious, but is contraindicated in patients with renal failure, during pregnancy, and in children under 8 years of age.

Chloramphenicol (50–75 mg/kg daily, divided into four doses, for 7 days) is the recommended treatment for pregnant women. When using chloramphenicol, close monitoring is prudent due to the limited data on treatment as well as the increased risk of gray baby syndrome in pregnant women and aplastic anemia in children.

Death occurs at a higher rate in those untreated beyond 5 days of illness onset. Of note, early discontinuation of therapy may result in relapse. RMSF has a case-fatality rate as high as 30% in certain untreated patients. Even with treatment, hospitalization rates of 72% and case fatality rates of 4% are seen.

Supportive care is also an important component in successful treatment. A high-protein diet, adequate hydration, and continuous monitoring of blood volume are critical. In cases in which renal, pulmonary, or cardiac complications occur, other specialized therapies may be required.

Specific Investigations

- Skin biopsy, direct immunofluorescence/
  immunoperoxidase
- Serologic testing for antirickettsial antibodies
- Polymerase chain reaction (PCR)

Diagnosis is most often based on clinical presentation, as patients may have a history of a tick bite after spending time in an endemic area. Clinical suspicion requires the rapid initiation of therapy even when confirmatory tests are pending, as mortality increases when treatment is delayed. Direct immunofluorescence or immunoperoxidase staining of skin biopsy specimens is a relatively rapid way of diagnosing RMSF. Serologic tests, including indirect immunofluorescence, latex agglutination, and enzyme immunoassay, that detect antirickettsial antibodies are available. However, these tests usually yield negative readings in the critical first days of the disease, as antibodies are not detectable until 7 to 10 days after the onset of the illness. Confirmation of the diagnosis using acute- and convalescent-phase serum samples is possible with these tests. The indirect hemagglutination antibody and immunofluorescent antibody tests are most useful because of their high sensitivity and specificity. The immunofluorescent test is especially beneficial because of its capacity to assess IgG and IgM levels. A highly specific and sensitive PCR assay for the detection of the spotted fever and typhus group of Rickettsiae was recently developed to provide rapid confirmation of the diagnosis when rickettsial loads are low. A complete blood count and liver function tests should be obtained. Most patients will have some degree of anemia or leukopenia, though in some cases the white blood count may be elevated. Thrombocytopenia may occur in severe cases. Hepatic enzymes, bilirubin, and lactate dehydrogenase are often elevated. Blood cultures or a skin biopsy specimen may be used to confirm the diagnosis, but are not helpful in the initial diagnosis of spotted fevers due to the length of time they require for results. Rickettsiae do not stain well with Gram stain, and instead should be stained with Giemsa, Machiavello, or Castaneda stains.

Clinical and laboratory features, hospital course, and outcome of Rocky Mountain spotted fever in children. Buckingham SC, Marshall GS, Schutze GE, Woods CR, Jackson MA, Patterson LE, et al. J Pediatr 2007; 150: 180–4.

A retrospective chart review of 92 children with laboratory-diagnosed RMSF from 1990 to 2002 was performed. Results revealed the most common presenting symptoms were fever (98%), rash (97%), and nausea/vomiting (73%). Only four patients received antirickettsial therapy upon initial presentation. Three patients ultimately died, and 13 survivors had neurologic deficits at the time of discharge. These results demonstrate the commonness of delayed diagnosis and underscore the importance of the rapid initiation of appropriate therapy.

Laboratory diagnosis of Rocky Mountain spotted fever. Walker DH, Burday MS, Folds JD. South Med J 1980; 73: 1143–6.

Immunofluorescence staining of 16 skin biopsies proved this test to be the best for early diagnosis of RMSF. A specificity of 100% and sensitivity of 70% were reported.

Immunofluorescence must be conducted within 48 hours after initiating antirickettsial therapy.

A highly sensitive and specific real-time PCR assay for the detection of spotted fever and typhus group Rickettsiae. Stenos J, Graves SR, Unsworth NB. Am J Trop Hyg 2005; 73: 1083–5.

PCR was developed to target the citrate synthase gene of rickettsiae. This quantitative assay can confirm the diagnosis of a spotted disease when rickettsial numbers are low and makes possible the enumeration of rickettsiae in clinical specimens as well. *R. akari, R. australis, R. conorii, R. honei, R. marmionii, R. sibirica, R. rickettsii, R. typhus,* and *R. prowazekii* all were detectable by this PCR.

Identification of rickettsial infections by using cutaneous swab specimens and PCR. Bechah Y, Socolovschi C, Raoult D. Emerg Infect Dis 2011; 17: 83–6.

A study using noninvasive diagnostic cutaneous swabs was performed on nine human patients with suspected rickettsial infection. Eschars were swabbed in each of the nine patients, followed by DNA extraction from the swab. The DNA was tested by quantitative PCR for a specific gene sequence found in the Rickettsiae group. Spotted fever group rickettsial DNA was detected in eight of nine swab samples, thus demonstrating an effective noninvasive diagnostic test.

First-Line Therapies

- Doxycycline (in adults and children)   C
- Tetracycline (in adults)   C
- Azithromycin (in pregnant patients)   D

Rickettsia rickettsii is sensitive to tetracyclines, chloramphenicol, and rifampicin. Doxycycline is the therapy of choice and should be administered early in the illness. Adults and children weighing 45 kg or more should take 100 doses of doxycycline at 12-hour intervals either orally or intravenously. Children weighing less than 45.4 kg should receive 2.2 mg/kg body weight per dose administered twice daily.

No visible dental staining in children treated with doxycycline for suspected Rocky Mountain spotted fever. Todd SR, Dahlgren FS, Traeger MS, Beltrán-Aguilar ED, Marianos DW, Hamilton C, et al. J Pediatr 2015; 166: 1246–51.

This study failed to demonstrate enamel hypoplasia, dental staining, or tooth color changes in children <8 years of age who received short-term courses of doxycycline. Confidence in the use of doxycycline for children suspected of RMSF may be improved if the drug's label was changed to reflect these findings.

Fatal Rocky Mountain spotted fever in the United States, 1999–2007. Dahlgren FS, Holman RC, Paddock CD, Callinan LS, McQuiston JH. Am J Trop Med Hyg 2012; 86: 713–9.

The study highlights several risk groups more likely of dying of RMSF: children 5 to 9 years of age, American Indians, immunosuppressed patients, and severe cases experiencing delayed diagnosis and/or treatment. Doxycycline should be used as the first-line drug against RMSF for all ages, even in children less than 8 years old.

Rocky Mountain spotted fever in children. Woods CR. Pediatr Clin North Am 2013; 60: 455–70.

RMSF is often undifferentiated from many infections during the first days of illness. Accordingly, doxycycline should not be delayed pending confirmation even in children under the age of 8 years.

Risk factors for fatal outcome from Rocky Mountain spotted fever in a highly endemic area—Arizona, 2002–2011. Regan JJ, Traeger MS, Humpherys D, Mahoney DL, Martinez M, Emerson GL, et al. Clin Infect Dis 2015; 60: 1659–66.

Evidence Levels: **A** Double-blind study   **B** Clinical trial ≥ 20 subjects   **C** Clinical trial < 20 subjects   **D** Series ≥ 5 subjects   **E** Anecdotal case reports

Treatment with doxycycline during the first 3 days of the disease can decrease morbidity and mortality from RMSF in this region. Risk factors associated with doxycycline delay and fatal outcome include 1) gastrointestinal symptoms, 2) alcoholism, and 3) chronic lung disease. There should be a low threshold for initiating doxycycline, especially in endemic areas like tribal lands in Arizona.

Revisiting doxycycline in pregnancy and early childhood – time to rebuild its reputation?. Cross R, Ling C, Day NP, McGready R, Paris DH. Expert Opin Drug Saf 2016; 15: 367–82.

A systematic review of the literature on the use of doxycycline during pregnancy and in children revealed that there is no correlation between the use of doxycycline and teratogenic effects during pregnancy or dental staining in children.

Mediterranean spotted fever during pregnancy: case presentation and literature review. Bentov Y, Sheiner E, Kenigsberg S, Mazor M. Eur J Obstet Gynecol Reprod Biol 2003; 107: 214–6.

Although the treatment of choice for Mediterranean spotted fever during pregnancy is chloramphenicol, azithromycin may be a viable alternative because of its effectiveness, safety in pregnancy and in children, high placental penetration, and increased compliance due to single daily dose.

Second-Line Therapies

• Tetracycline (in children)	C
• Azithromycin (adults and children)	B
• Clarithromycin (adults and children)	B

Analysis of risk factors for fatal Rocky Mountain spotted fever: evidence for superiority of tetracyclines for therapy. Holman RC, Paddock CD, Curns AT, Krebs JW, McQuiston JH, Childs JE. J Infect Dis 2001; 184: 1437–44.

A study of RMSF derived from reports received by the Centers for Disease Control and Prevention by state health departments and private physicians consisting of 5600 confirmed and probable cases occurring from 1981 to 1998. Age, race, and time of treatment with respect to onset of illness were used to stratify the patient population. Four treatments groups were studied: tetracycline without chloramphenicol, chloramphenicol without tetracycline, chloramphenicol with tetracycline, and neither chloramphenicol nor tetracycline. Patients with RMSF who did not receive tetracycline had an increased risk of death.

Clarithromycin versus azithromycin in the treatment of Mediterranean spotted fever in children: a randomized controlled trial. Cascio A, Colomba C, Antinori S, Paterson DL, Titone L. Clin Infect Dis 2002; 34: 154–8.

This open-label randomized controlled trial compared azithromycin (10 mg/kg daily in one dose for 3 days) and clarithromycin (15 mg/kg daily in two divided doses for 7 days) in the treatment of Mediterranean spotted fever in children. Both of these agents may be suitable for children 8 years old and under.

Third-Line Therapy

• Chloramphenicol (pregnant and nonpregnant adults)	C

Analysis of risk factors for malignant Mediterranean spotted fever indicates that fluoroquinolone treatment has a deleterious effect. Botelho-Nevers E, Rovery C, Richet H, Raoult D. J Antimicrob Chemother 2011; 66: 1821–30.

Fluoroquinolones have been previously associated with failure in the treatment of typhus and scrub typhus, and fluoroquinolones are not recommended to treat any rickettsial diseases.

TYPHUS GROUP

Epidemic typhus

Epidemic typhus is caused by *R. prowazekii*, transmitted via the body louse. Recommended treatment is doxycycline taken orally (200 mg daily for 5 days), or intravenously in more severe cases. Chloramphenicol is effective also. Prevention is crucial and can be achieved through bathing, washing clothes, and the use of insecticides.

Murine typhus

Murine typhus (or endemic typhus) is due to *R. typhi*, transmitted via the rat flea and the rat louse. Doxycycline, taken orally at 200 mg daily for 7 to 15 days or until 3 days of defervescence, is recommended. Chloramphenicol may also be effective, though relapses may occur. Prevention is achieved using insecticides and by controlling the rat population.

Scrub typhus

Scrub typhus is caused by *R. tsutsugamushi*, transmitted via larval mites. Tetracyclines are recommended in adults: doxycycline (200 mg daily) or tetracycline (2 g daily) for 2 to 14 days. Chloramphenicol, although effective, does not act as quickly as the tetracyclines.

MANAGEMENT STRATEGY

Specific Investigations

Epidemic typhus
- Serology: microimmunofluorescent and plate microagglutination tests

Murine typhus
- Serology: indirect fluorescent antibody, latex agglutination, solid-phase immunoassay

Scrub typhus
- Serology: indirect fluorescent antibody test

First-Line Therapies

Epidemic typhus	
• Doxycycline	A
Murine typhus	
• Doxycycline	A
Scrub typhus	
• Doxycycline	A
• Azithromycin	A

Rickettsioses and Q fever in travelers (2004–2013). Delord M, Socolovschi C, Parola P. Travel Med Infect Dis 2014; 12: 443–58.

Doxycycline remains the standard treatment for all spotted fever group rickettsioses. Doxycycline is also the standard of treatment for scrub, murine, and epidemic typhus infections.

Doxycycline and rifampicin for mild scrub-typhus infections in northern Thailand: a randomized trial. Watt G, Kantipong P, Jongaskul K, Watcharapichat P, Phulsuksombati D, Strickman D. Lancet 2000; 356: 1057–61.

A randomized study of adults with mild scrub typhus in which patients received oral doxycycline 200 mg daily (*n* = 28), oral rifampicin 600 mg daily (*n* = 26), or oral rifampicin 900 mg daily (*n* = 24). Patients treated with rifampicin at either dosage demonstrated a significantly shorter median duration of pyrexia than did the doxycycline patients.

Doxycycline versus azithromycin for treatment of leptospirosis and scrub typhus. Phimda K, Hoontrakul S, Suttinont C, Chareonwat S, Losuwanaluk K, Chueasuwanchai S, et al. Antimicrob Agents Chemother 2007; 51: 3259–63.

A randomized controlled trial in which 296 patients were allocated to receive either a 7-day course of doxycycline or a 3-day course of azithromycin. The group studied included 57 patients (19.3%) with scrub typhus, 14 (4.7%) with murine typhus, 69 (23.3%) with leptospirosis, and 11 (3.7%) with both leptospirosis and a rickettsial infection. Both regimens demonstrated similar effectiveness and fever clearance times. Azithromycin has fewer adverse effects, but is more expensive.

Second-Line Therapies	
All typhus groups	
• Rifampicin	A
• Chloramphenicol	D

Comparison of the effectiveness of five different antibiotic regimens on infection with *Rickettsia typhi*: therapeutic data from 87 cases. Gikas A, Doukakis S, Pediaditis J, Kastanakis S, Manios A, Tselentis Y. Am J Trop Med Hyg 2004; 70: 576–9.

A retrospective study of five different antibiotic regimens used in 87 patients with endemic typhus. Mean time to defervescence was 2.9 days for doxycycline, 4 days for chloramphenicol, and 4.2 days for ciprofloxacin.

Murine typhus in central Greece: epidemiological, clinical, laboratory, and therapeutic-response features of 90 cases. Chaliotis G, Kritsotakis EI, Psaroulaki A, Tselentis Y, Gikas A. Int J Infect Dis 2012; 16: e591–6.

A 5-year prospective study of 90 adult patients with murine typhus revealed a shorter time to defervescence using doxycycline in comparison to ofloxacin alone or doxycycline plus ofloxacin.

RICKETTSIALPOX

Rickettsialpox is due to *R. akari*. The house mouse is the reservoir; mites transmit the bacteria to humans. This disease is self-limited. It manifests as headache, fever, papulovesicular rash over the trunk and extremities, and an eschar in 80% of cases. Treatment in adults is doxycycline (200 mg daily) for 10 days.

MANAGEMENT STRATEGY

Specific Investigation	
• Serology: complement fixation	

First-Line Therapy	
• Doxycycline	A

A case of rickettsialpox in Northern Europe. Renvoisé A, van't Wout JW, van der Schroeff JG, Beersma MF, Raoult D. Int J Infect Dis 2012; 16: e221–2.

A patient was cured using doxycycline 200 mg per day for 10 days. Due to international interest in anthrax and bioterrorism, there has been a noticeable increase in the reported cases of rickettsialpox, as both diseases are eschar associated.

Q FEVER

Q fever is caused by *Coxiella burnetti*. Transmission to humans occurs via aerosolized urine, feces, or birth products of ungulates (hoofed mammals). This disease usually has no skin findings. Patients often present with febrile illness, severe headache, and with or without pneumonia, hepatitis, or endocarditis. Vaccines for this occupational disease of sheep and dairy workers are not available in the United States.

MANAGEMENT STRATEGY

Acute Q fever

The primary treatment of choice in adults is doxycycline (100 mg orally twice a day for 14 days). Moxifloxacin (400 mg daily for 14 days) may be used as an alternative. In vitro the disease has been susceptible to fluoroquinolones, chloramphenicol, rifampin, and trimethoprim–sulfamethoxazole.

Chronic Q fever

The most common chronic manifestation is endocarditis, which is often resistant to treatment, due to the bacteriostatic rather than the bactericidal effects of antibiotics on *C. burnetii*. Currently, combination therapy with doxycycline (100 mg twice daily) and hydroxychloroquine (200 mg three times daily) is the mainstay of treatment given their bactericidal activity. Treatment must be carried out for a minimum of 18 months. The duration must further be tailored to the individual clinical response.

Specific Investigations	
Acute Q fever	
• Serology: complement fixation, immunofluorescent antibody	
• PCR	
Chronic Q fever	
• Echocardiography	
• Serology	

Evidence Levels: **A** Double-blind study **B** Clinical trial ≥ 20 subjects **C** Clinical trial < 20 subjects **D** Series ≥ 5 subjects **E** Anecdotal case reports

High throughput detection of *Coxiella burnetii* by real-time PCR with internal control system and automated DNA preparation. Panning M, Kilwinski J, Greiner-Fischer S, Peters M, Kramme S, Frangoulidis D, et al. BMC Microbiol 2008; 8: 77.

A sensitive real-time PCR was established for the rapid screening of *C. burnetii* in local outbreaks. Although serology is the gold standard for diagnosis, it is inadequate for early case detection.

Evaluation of commonly used serological tests for the detection of *Coxiella burnetti* antibodies in well-defined acute and follow-up sera. Wegdam-Blans MC, Wielders CC, Meekelenkamp J, Korbeeck JM, Herremans T, Tjhie HT, et al. Clin Vaccine Immunol 2012; 19: 1105–10.

In this study of 126 patients with acute Q fever, detection of *Coxiella burnetii* antibodies during IgG phase I, IgG phase II, and IgM phase II was compared among enzyme-linked immunosorbent assay (ELISA), indirect fluorescent antibody test (IFAT), and complement fixation. Results demonstrated equal efficacy among the three serologic tests in diagnosing acute Q fever (within 3 months); however, IFAT was more sensitive in follow-up serology (12 months) and thus more beneficial for prevaccination screening programs.

First-Line Therapies	
Acute Q fever	
• β-Lactams	B
• Doxycycline	B
• Macrolides	B
• Quinolones	B
Chronic Q fever	
• Doxycycline and hydroxychloroquine	B

Second-Line Therapy	
Chronic Q fever	
• Quinolone and doxycycline	B

The natural history of acute Q fever: a prospective Australian cohort. Hopper B, Cameron B, Li H, Graves S, Stenos J, Hickie I, et al. QJM 2016; 109: 661–8.

Q fever is a worldwide zoonotic infection that can vary widely in severity and duration.

EHRLICHIOSIS

The ehrlichioses consists of two tickborne diseases: human monocytic ehrlichiosis due to *Ehrlichia chaffeensis* (the most common form in the United States) and human granulocytic ehrlichiosis due to *E. equi*. Both are found in mammalian reservoirs such as deer, dogs, and horses and are transmitted via ticks. Commonly encountered symptoms include fever, headaches, lack of appetite, and a highly variable exanthema. If inappropriately treated, ehrlichioses can progress to life-threatening respiratory failure and meningoencephalitis.

MANAGEMENT STRATEGY

Doxycycline (100 mg orally twice daily for adults, or 4 mg/kg daily in children 8 years of age and older) is the treatment of choice. The treatment ought to be continued for a minimum of 7 days and for 3 days after defervescence.

Specific Investigation
• Serology: immunofluorescent antibody

First-Line Therapy	
• Doxycycline	A

Fatal ehrlichial myocarditis in a healthy adolescent: a case report and review of the literature. Havens NS, Kinnear BR, Mató S. Clin Infect Dis 2012; 54: e113–4.

Doctors should have a low threshold for treatment with doxycycline during the peak season in endemic areas, as a delay of antibiotics has been shown to increase both morbidity and mortality. Therapy becomes even less effective if delayed beyond 1 week.

Second-Line Therapy	
• Rifampin (rifampicin)	D

Successful treatment of human monocytic ehrlichiosis with rifampin. Abusaada K, Ajmal S, Hughes L. Cureus 2016; 8: e444.

Rifampin (rifampicin) was successfully used in the treatment of a patient who had doxycycline allergy.

Clinical determinants of Lyme borreliosis, babesiosis, bartonellosis, anaplasmosis, and ehrlichiosis in an Australian cohort. Mayne PJ. Int J Gen Med 2014; 8:15–26.

In a study of 500 Lyme disease patients, 317 had coinfection with babesiosis, ehrlichiosis coinfection was noted in 3, and 30 patients had a positive rickettsial serology.

Rosacea

John Berth-Jones

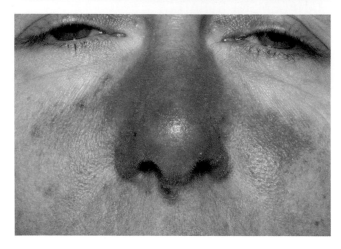

Rosacea is a common inflammatory skin disease, generally confined to the face, principally the cheeks, forehead, nose, and chin. In some cases lesions may extend onto the scalp and occasionally also onto the neck and the upper part of the body. A common early feature is flushing, often accompanied by a burning sensation. Inflammatory lesions (papulation and pustulation) are characteristic and may become florid. Vascular changes (telangiectasia and erythema) are also frequently observed. These are initially mild, but may later become very conspicuous. Other later features are the development of lymphedema, thickening, and induration. On the nose and, less often, the ears, forehead, or chin, hypertrophy and lymphedema of subcutaneous tissue may develop into distinct swellings known as *phymas*, of which rhinophyma is most familiar. Ocular involvement is frequent and manifests as a sensation of grittiness, which may be accompanied by conjunctivitis, blepharitis, episcleritis, chalazion, hordeolum, iritis, and occasionally severe keratitis.

MANAGEMENT STRATEGY

Rosacea is a clinical diagnosis. It should be noted that the classical progression described earlier is far from consistent, and features of rosacea may develop in isolation or in any combination or sequence.

Patients may find it beneficial to *avoid "triggers"*—*alcohol, spicy food, hot drinks*, etc., which may induce flushing and promote the development of telangiectasia. Exposure to irritants should be avoided, and emollients can be helpful. *Cosmetic camouflage* of the erythema and telangiectasia may be worthwhile. *Facial massage* may promote lymphatic drainage and reduce the development of lymphedema. Papulation and pustulation can be effectively suppressed using a variety of *topical and systemic antibiotics, topical ivermectin, retinoids,* and other agents described later. Controlling inflammation with these modalities may also reduce erythema, but does not usually prove very helpful for suppressing flushing and has little effect on established telangiectasia. Erythema can be treated more

specifically with topical application of vasoconstrictors, of which *brimonidine* is best established. Telangiectasia can be effectively treated by physical measures to ablate the vessels, such as *intense pulsed light or vascular lasers*. Flushing is usually the most difficult feature to treat, but sometimes improves during treatment of erythema and telangiectasia. Ocular rosacea is often treated symptomatically with a range of *"artificial tears"* (the ophthalmic equivalent of emollients). *Systemic tetracyclines*, used as for cutaneous rosacea, are also helpful. The use of *retinoids* for rosacea requires special care in patients with eye involvement and may be poorly tolerated. Treatments are discussed later in sections focused on inflammatory rosacea, erythematotelangiectatic rosacea, flushing, lymphedema, ocular rosacea, and rosacea fulminans. Treatments for rhinophyma and perioral dermatitis are described in separate chapters.

Specific Investigations

In selected cases

- Exclude carcinoid syndrome; urine 5-HIAA, plasma serotonin, chromogranin-A
- Exclude lupus; serology, histology

INFLAMMATORY ROSACEA

First-Line Treatments

• Topical metronidazole	A
• Topical ivermectin	A
• Topical azelaic acid	A
• Oral tetracyclines	A
• Oral erythromycin	C
• Emollients	C

The efficacy of metronidazole 1% cream once daily compared with metronidazole cream twice daily and their vehicles in rosacea: a double-blind clinical trial. Jorizzo JL, Lebwohl M, Tobey RE. J Am Acad Dermatol 1998; 39: 502–4.

This study confirmed improvements in numbers of inflammatory lesions and in erythema relative to placebo. However, there was no apparent difference between once-daily and twice-daily application.

Topical metronidazole maintains remissions of rosacea. Dahl MV, Katz HI, Krueger GG, Millikan LE, Odom RB, Parker F, et al. Arch Dermatol 1998; 134: 679–83.

Eighty-eight subjects who had responded to treatment with systemic tetracycline and topical metronidazole were randomized to receive 0.75% metronidazole gel or placebo gel for 6 months. In those applying the metronidazole, 23% developed a relapse of papulopustular lesions and 55% a worsening of erythema, compared with 42% and 74% of subjects, respectively, in the placebo gel group.

Efficacy and safety of ivermectin 1% cream in treatment of papulopustular rosacea: results of two randomized, double-blind, vehicle-controlled pivotal studies. Stein L, Kircik L, Fowler J, Tan J, Draelos Z, Fleischer A, et al. J Drugs Dermatol 2014; 13: 316–23.

Each study recruited nearly 700 subjects. Treatments were applied once daily. At 12 weeks assessments of "clear" or "almost

Evidence Levels: **A** Double-blind study **B** Clinical trial ≥ 20 subjects **C** Clinical trial < 20 subjects **D** Series ≥ 5 subjects **E** Anecdotal case reports

clear" were seen in 38.4% and 40.1% of the ivermectin group and 11.6% and 18.8% of the vehicle group ($p < 0.001$).

Superiority of ivermectin 1% cream over metronidazole 0.75% cream in treating inflammatory lesions of rosacea: a randomized, investigator-blinded trial. Taieb A, Ortonne JP, Ruzicka T, Roszkiewicz J, Berth-Jones J, Peirone MH, et al. Br J Dermatol 2015; 172: 1103–10.

A 16-week study with 962 subjects. Subjects receiving ivermectin cream experienced an 83% reduction in inflammatory lesion count (the primary end point), compared with a reduction of 74% in the metronidazole group ($p < 0.001$).

In separate reports from this trial, topical ivermectin has also been shown to improve quality of life more than metronidazole and to induce longer remissions (median 115 vs. 85 days).

A randomized, double-blind, placebo-controlled trial of the combined effect of doxycycline hyclate 20 mg tablets and metronidazole 0.75% topical lotion in the treatment of rosacea. Sanchez J, Somolinos AL, Almodovar PI, Webster G, Bradshaw M, Powala C. J Am Acad Dermatol 2005; 53: 791–7.

Combinations of topical and systemic treatment are often used and seem likely to be more effective than either used alone. In this study the addition of low-dose (20 mg) doxycycline improved the response to topical metronidazole.

Double-blind comparison of azelaic acid 20% cream and its vehicle in treatment of papulo-pustular rosacea. Bjerke R, Fyrand O, Graupe K. Acta Derm Venereol 1999; 79: 456–9.

A 3-month randomized, double-blind study compared the efficacy and safety of azelaic acid 20% cream, applied twice daily, with its vehicle in 116 patients. Azelaic acid cream produced significantly greater mean reductions in total inflammatory lesions than did vehicle: 73.4% vs. 50.6%, respectively. Erythema also responded.

A clinical trial of tetracycline in rosacea. Sneddon IB. Br J Dermatol 1966; 78: 649–52.

A double-blind trial with 78 evaluable subjects comparing tetracycline 250 mg twice daily with placebo after 4 weeks of treatment. There was a significantly superior response to active treatment, even though a pronounced placebo effect was observed. During subsequent follow-up it was found that some patients could be completely controlled using only 100 mg daily.

Two randomized phase III clinical trials evaluating anti-inflammatory dose doxycycline (40-mg doxycycline, USP capsules) administered once daily for treatment of rosacea. Del Rosso JQ, Webster GF, Jackson M, Rendon M, Rich P, Torok H, et al. J Am Acad Dermatol 2007; 56: 791–802.

Doxycycline appears effective even at low doses.

A double-blind study of 1% metronidazole cream versus systemic oxytetracycline therapy for rosacea. Nielsen PG. Br J Dermatol 1983; 109: 63–65.

Improvement occurred in 90% of the patients. There was no significant difference between the treatments.

Both tetracycline and oxytetracycline are generally used at the dose of 250 to 500 mg twice daily. Other systemic tetracyclines, such as minocycline 100 mg daily, doxycycline 40 mg or 100 mg daily, and lymecycline 408 mg daily, are also often prescribed. These offer the advantage of once-daily administration, and their absorption is less influenced by dietary calcium, so they can be taken with food. Erythromycin 250 to 500 mg twice daily is also often prescribed and widely held to be effective and can be

useful when rosacea occurs in children, for whom tetracyclines are contraindicated.

Beneficial use of Cetaphil moisturizing cream as part of a daily skin care regimen for individuals with rosacea. Laquieze S, Czernielewski J, Baltas E. J Dermatol Treat 2007; 18: 158–62.

Twice-daily application of a moisturizer appeared beneficial in this open study on 20 patients.

Second-Line Treatments	
• Topical erythromycin	C
• Topical clindamycin	C
• Oral metronidazole	A
• Topical benzoyl peroxide	A
• Ampicillin	A
• Azithromycin	B

Topically applied erythromycin in rosacea. Mills OH, Kligman AM. Arch Dermatol 1976; 112: 553–4.

A 2% solution applied twice daily to 15 patients produced a 50% to 100% improvement in 87% of cases, and treatment was effective by 4 weeks. Once-daily application was sufficient once the disease was controlled.

Treatment of rosacea: topical clindamycin versus oral tetracycline. Wilkin JK, DeWitt S. Int J Dermatol 1993; 32: 65–67.

A randomized, blinded trial comparing topical clindamycin lotion twice daily with oral tetracycline in 43 patients evaluated over 12 weeks. Similar improvements were found in both groups, although clindamycin was superior in eradication of pustules.

Double-blind, randomized, vehicle-controlled clinical trial of once-daily benzoyl peroxide/clindamycin topical gel in the treatment of patients with moderate to severe rosacea. Breneman D, Savin R, VandePol C, Vamvakias G, Levy S, Leyden J. Int J Dermatol 2004; 43: 381–7.

This combination of 5% benzoyl peroxide and 1% clindamycin was effective and well tolerated.

Treatment of rosacea by metronidazole. Pye RJ, Burton JL. Lancet 1976; 1: 1211–2.

A double-blind, placebo-controlled, parallel-group trial demonstrating the efficacy of oral metronidazole 200 mg twice daily after 6 weeks of treatment. Ten out of 14 patients treated with metronidazole showed a good response.

A double-blinded trial of metronidazole versus oxytetracycline therapy for rosacea. Saihan EM, Burton JL. Br J Dermatol 1980; 102: 443–5.

Forty patients were treated for 12 weeks with oxytetracycline 250 mg twice daily or metronidazole 200 mg twice daily. On both drugs the degree of improvement was greater after 12 weeks than after 6 weeks. There was no significant difference between them.

Although metronidazole is generally well tolerated and it has been used long term, there is a risk of peripheral neuropathy if it is used for longer than 3 months.

Topical treatment of acne rosacea with benzoyl peroxide acetone gel. Montes LF, Cordero AA, Kriner J. Cutis 1983; 32: 185–90.

Benzoyl peroxide gel (5% increasing to 10%) was significantly superior to vehicle, although it was poorly tolerated and there was a high dropout rate.

Comparative effectiveness of tetracycline and ampicillin in rosacea. A controlled trial. Marks R, Ellis J. Lancet 1971; 2: 1049–52.

A double-blind, placebo-controlled trial lasting 6 weeks and completed by 56 patients. Both antibiotics were significantly more effective than placebo. Tetracycline was apparently (but not significantly) more effective than ampicillin.

A novel treatment for acne vulgaris and rosacea. Elewski BE. J Eur Acad Dermatol Venereol 2000; 14: 423–4.

Ten patients were treated in an open study of azithromycin, 500 mg on day 1, followed by 250 mg/day for 4 consecutive days beginning on the first and fifteenth days of each month for 3 months. All patients improved, and nine were clear by 3 months.

Oral use of azithromycin for the treatment of acne rosacea. Fernandez-Obregon A. Arch Dermatol 2004; 140: 489–90.

Ten patients responded well to azithromycin 250 mg/day for 3 days each week (Monday, Wednesday, and Friday) within 4 weeks. Ocular symptoms also improved.

Azithromycin has a relatively long half-life and is therefore suited to this sort of regimen.

Third-Line Treatments

• Systemic isotretinoin	B
• Topical tretinoin	C
• Topical adapalene	B
• Topical sulfur ± sulfacetamide	B
• Topical corticosteroids	D
• Topical bifonazole	D
• Photodynamic therapy	D
• Spironolactone	D
• *Demodex* eradication	B
• Praziquantel 3% ointment	B
• *Helicobacter pylori* eradication	D
• Sunscreens	E
• Topical tacrolimus	C
• Topical pimecrolimus	D
• Octreotide	C
• Inhibition of ovulation	C
• Topical 1-methylnicotinamide	C
• Oral nicotinamide with zinc	C
• Zinc sulfate	B
• Long-pulsed, 1064-nm, Nd:YAG laser	C
• Kanuka honey	B

A randomized-controlled trial of oral low-dose isotretinoin for difficult-to-treat papulopustular rosacea. Sbidian E, Vicaut É, Chidiack H, Anselin E, Cribier B, Dréno B, et al. J Invest Dermatol 2016; 136: 1124–9.

One hundred and fifty-six subjects used isotretinoin 0.25 mg/kg/day or placebo over a 4-month treatment period. Response (90% reduction in inflammatory lesions) was observed in 57% on isotretinoin vs. 10% on placebo ($p < 0.0001$). The proportions of patients discontinuing therapy due to adverse events were similar in the two groups.

There have been several reports of the use of isotretinoin at doses of 10 to 60 mg/day or 0.5 to 1 mg/kg/day. Variable relapse rates have been reported after discontinuing the drug, there being a trend toward more frequent relapse in those given lower total doses. However, doses often need to be kept low to avoid aggravating ocular symptoms. Partly for this reason, some investigators have advocated the use of continuous low-dose therapy with isotretinoin.

Topical tretinoin for rosacea: a preliminary report. Kligman AM. J Dermatol Treat 1993; 4: 71–3.

Topical tretinoin 0.025% for 6 to 12 months improved rosacea in about 70% of cases in this open study with 19 patients. Improvement was seen in telangiectasia as well as inflammatory lesions.

Adapalene vs. metronidazole gel for the treatment of rosacea. Altinyazar HC, Koca R, Tekin NS, Estürk E. Int J Dermatol 2005; 44: 252–5.

In an investigator-blinded, parallel-group trial with 55 patients, adapalene 0.1% gel produced results similar to those of metronidazole 0.75% gel.

Topical treatment with sulfur 10% for rosacea. Blom I, Hornmark A-M. Acta Derm Venereol 1984; 64: 358–9.

A randomized study with 40 patients. Treatment duration was 4 weeks. Topical sulfur 10% in a cream base (Diprobase) was as effective as oral lymecycline 150 mg/day. A greater reduction in inflammatory lesions was observed in the group treated with sulfur, although there were a greater number of lesions at baseline in this group.

The treatment of rosacea: the safety and efficacy of sodium sulfacetamide 10% and sulfur 5% lotion (Novacet) is demonstrated in a double-blind study. Saunder DN, Miller R, Gratton D, Danby W, Griffiths C, Phillips S. J Dermatol Treat 1997; 8: 79–85.

Efficacy of 10% sodium sulfacetamide and 5% sulfur was demonstrated in an 8-week randomized, vehicle-controlled, multicenter study with 103 patients.

Comparative study of triamcinolone acetonide and hydrocortisone 17-butyrate in rosacea with special regard to the rebound phenomenon. Go MJ, Wuite J. Dermatologica 1976; 152: 239–46.

In this study with 19 subjects, topical steroids given in conjunction with tetracycline did not cause a rebound phenomenon when the steroids were discontinued.

The place of steroids in rosacea is ill defined and probably very limited, although their use has been reported in conjunction with standard treatments.

Treatment of rosacea with bifonazole cream: a preliminary report. Veraldi S, Schianchi-Veraldi R. Ann Ital Derm Clin Sper 1990; 44: 169–71.

Topical bifonazole 1% cream was used successfully in eight cases of rosacea, with no recurrence at 3 months.

Photodynamic therapy in a series of rosacea patients. Bryld LE, Jemec GB. J Eur Acad Dermatol Venereol 2007; 21: 1199–202.

A series of 17 patients with rosacea refractory to previous therapy were treated with photodynamic therapy using 16% methyl aminolevulinic acid (Metvix) cream applied for 3 hours, followed by 37 J/cm² of red light. Initially patients received one or two treatments at an interval of 1 week, and up to four treatments were used on each treated area if required. A good response was observed in 10 cases.

Oral spironolactone therapy in male patients with rosacea. Aizawa H, Niimura M. J Dermatol 1992; 19: 293–7.

Spironolactone at a dose of 50 mg/day for 4 weeks was reported to benefit 7 of 13 male patients with rosacea. Two of the patients did not tolerate the drug.

Evidence Levels: **A** Double-blind study **B** Clinical trial ≥ 20 subjects **C** Clinical trial < 20 subjects **D** Series ≥ 5 subjects **E** Anecdotal case reports

Demodex folliculorum **and topical treatment: action evaluated by standardized skin surface biopsy.** Forton F, Seys B, Marchal JL, Song AM. Br J Dermatol 1998; 138: 461–6.

This study of 34 patients with high *Demodex* carriage compared the miticidal effect of topical metronidazole, permethrin, sulfur, lindane, crotamiton, and benzyl benzoate. Benzyl benzoate and crotamiton had particular effects on the mite population, suggesting that they may be appropriate treatment for some cases of rosacea and "rosacea-like demodecosis."

Permethrin 5% cream versus metronidazole 0.75% gel for the treatment of papulopustular rosacea. A randomized double-blind placebo-controlled study. Koçak M, Yagli S, Vahapoglu G, Eksioglu M. Dermatology 2002; 205: 265–70.

Treatments were applied twice daily for 2 months. Permethrin was more effective in improving erythema and papules than placebo and as effective as metronidazole 0.75% gel, but had no effect on telangiectasia, rhinophyma, or pustules. Reduction of *Demodex* counts was significantly greater with permethrin than with metronidazole or placebo.

Treatment of rosacea-like demodicidosis with oral ivermectin and topical permethrin cream. Forstinger C, Kittler H, Binder M. J Am Acad Dermatol 1999; 41: 775–7.

A patient suffering from a follicular, papulopustular facial eruption with a long history of unsuccessful treatment responded to ivermectin 200 µg/kg. This was followed by once-weekly application of 5% permethrin cream to prevent reinfestation.

Clinical and experimental assessment of the effects of a new topical treatment with praziquantel in the management of rosacea. Bribeche MR, Fedotov VP, Gladichev VV, Pukhalskaya DM, Kolitcheva NL. Int J Dermatol 2015; 54: 481–7.

A single-blind, randomized study with 65 subjects treated with 3% praziquantel ointment or vehicle ointment applied twice daily for 16 weeks. Significant benefit was observed relative to placebo in investigators' global assessments, erythema assessment scale, and Dermatology Life Quality Index (DLQI).

Praziquantel is a broad-spectrum antiparasitic agent that has been proposed to act by suppressing Demodex.

There are increased numbers of Demodex mites in rosacea, suggesting that they are implicated in the pathogenesis. This has provided a rationale for the use of a range of therapies aimed at eradication of the mites, including topical ivermectin, which also has antiinflammatory properties and is now regarded as a first-line therapy.

Helicobacter pylori **eradication treatment reduces the severity of rosacea.** Utas S, Ozbakir O, Turasan A, Utas C. J Am Acad Dermatol 1999; 40: 433–5.

Thirteen patients with rosacea having evidence of *H. pylori* infection received a course of amoxicillin 500 mg three times daily for 2 weeks, metronidazole 500 mg three times daily for 2 weeks, and bismuth subcitrate 300 mg four times daily for 4 weeks. There was a significant reduction in the severity of the rosacea at the end of treatment.

The effect of the treatment of *Helicobacter pylori* infection on rosacea. Bamford JL, Tilden RL, Blankush JL, Gangeness DE. Arch Dermatol 1999; 135: 659–63.

A randomized, double-blind, placebo-controlled trial of *H. pylori* eradication with clarithromycin and omeprazole or placebo. There was no difference in the rosacea between the two groups at 60 days.

Several investigators have proposed an association between H. pylori *and rosacea, although this remains highly controversial.*

Effective sunscreen ingredients and cutaneous irritation in patients with rosacea. Nichols K, Desai N, Lebwohl MG. Cutis 1998; 61: 344–6.

Patients with rosacea are particularly susceptible to the irritation caused by sunscreen ingredients. Formulations with protective constituents, such as dimethicone and cyclomethicone, may be preferable.

Tacrolimus effect on rosacea. Bamford JTM, Elliott BA, Haller IV. J Am Acad Dermatol 2004; 50: 107–8.

Topical tacrolimus 0.1% reduced erythema but not papulopustular lesions in this open study with 24 subjects.

Pimecrolimus for treatment of acne rosacea. Crawford KM, Russ B, Bostrom P. Skinmed 2005; 4: 147–50.

An open-label study on 12 patients. Improvements were seen in erythema and papulopustular lesions.

Pimecrolimus cream 1% for papulopustular rosacea: a randomized vehicle-controlled double-blind trial. Weissenbacher S, Merkl J, Hildebrandt B, Wollenberg A, Braeutigem M, Ring J, et al. Br J Dermatol 2007: 156: 728–32.

Pimecrolimus was no more effective than placebo.

Topical tacrolimus and pimecrolimus have both been reported to induce rosacea-like eruptions. If there is a role for these topical agents in the management of rosacea, this remains to be clarified.

Incidental control of rosacea by somatostatin. Piérard-Franchimont C, Quatresooz P, Piérard GE. Dermatology 2003; 206: 249–51.

Four cases improved during incidental treatment of diabetic retinopathy with a long-acting octreotide injection (Sandostatin 20 mg) monthly.

Octreotide is a somatostatin analog known to be highly active in suppressing the secretion of vasoactive hormones by carcinoid tumors and reduces the flushing associated with the carcinoid syndrome.

Effect of oral inhibitors of ovulation in treatment of rosacea and dermatitis perioralis in women. Spirov G, Berova N, Vassilev D. Aust J Dermatol 1971; 12: 149–54.

An oral contraceptive was associated with improvement of rosacea in 90% of 30 women. An open, uncontrolled study.

Topical application of 1-methylnicotinamide in the treatment of rosacea: a pilot study. Wozniacka A, Sysa-Jedrzejowska A, Adamus J, Gebicki J. Clin Exp Dermatol 2005; 30: 632–5.

This compound is a metabolite of nicotinamide with antiinflammatory properties. Thirty-four patients were treated twice daily with a gel containing 0.25% methylnicotinamide in this open-label pilot study. Improvement was good in 9 cases and moderate in 17.

The Nicomide Improvement in Clinical Outcomes Study (NICOS): results of an 8-week trial. Niren NM, Torok HM. Cutis 2006; 77: 17–28.

This compound formulation (Nicomide), comprising nicotinamide 750 mg, zinc 25 mg, copper 1.5 mg, and folic acid 500 µg, was reported as effective in an open-label study on 198 patients with acne vulgaris and/or rosacea.

Oral zinc sulfate in the treatment of rosacea: a double-blind, placebo-controlled study. Sharquie KE, Najim RA, Al-Salman HN. Int J Dermatol 2006; 45: 857–61.

Zinc sulfate 100 mg/day proved more effective than placebo in this crossover trial with 25 patients.

Efficacy of the long-pulsed 1064-nm neodymium:yttrium-aluminum-garnet laser (LPND) (rejuvenation mode) in the treatment of papulopustular rosacea (PPR): a pilot study of clinical outcomes and patient satisfaction in 30 cases. Lee JH, Kim M, Bae JM, Cho BK, Park HJ. J Am Acad Dermatol 2015; 73: 333–6.

Improvement was reported after three treatment sessions at 4-week intervals. This was an uncontrolled study in which subjects also applied moisturizer and sunscreen and avoided known triggers.

Randomised controlled trial of topical kanuka honey for the treatment of rosacea. Braithwaite I, Hunt A, Riley J, Fingleton J, Kocks J, Corin A, et al. BMJ Open 2015; 5: e007651.

An assessor-blinded study. Honey or cetomacrogol cream (control) were applied twice daily. At 8 weeks 24/68 in the honey group and 12/69 in the control group had a ≥2 point improvement in global assessment compared with baseline (p = 0.02).

Kanuka is a tree species related to manuka.

ERYTHEMATOTELANGIECTATIC ROSACEA

First-Line Therapies

• Cosmetic camouflage	C
• Brimonidine tartrate	A
• Intense pulsed light	B
• Vascular lasers	B

Decorative cosmetics improve the quality of life in patients with disfiguring skin diseases. Boehncke WH, Ochsendorf F, Paeslack I, Kaufmann R, Zollner TM. Eur J Dermatol 2002; 12: 577–80.

Twenty women with a range of dermatoses, including nine with rosacea, completed the DLQI questionnaire before and after instruction by a cosmetician. The mean score improved from 9.2 to 5.5.

Once-daily topical brimonidine tartrate gel 0.5% is a novel treatment for moderate to severe facial erythema of rosacea: results of two multicentre, randomized and vehicle-controlled studies. Fowler J, Jarratt M, Moore A, Meadows K, Pollack A, Steinhoff M, et al. Br J Dermatol 2012; 166: 633–41.

Two placebo-controlled trials. One study examined response to a single application using a range of concentrations. The other examined results from 4 weeks of treatment once or twice daily and followed by 4 weeks washout. Reduced redness was apparent at 30 minutes and persisted for 12 hours. There was no evidence of tachyphylaxis or rebound.

Although not an ideal formulation, brimonidine ophthalmic drops can also be effective. Additionally, there have been several reports of rebound erythema secondary to brimonidine.

Objective and quantitative improvement of rosacea-associated erythema after intense pulsed light treatment. Mark KA, Sparacio RM, Voigt A, Marenus K, Sarnoff DS. Dermatol Surg 2003; 29: 600–4.

Objective assessments were performed on four subjects before and after intense pulsed light (IPL) therapy for rosacea. Five treatments at 3-week intervals were undertaken using the Photoderm VL machine, with a 515-nm filter, a single pulse of 3 ms duration, and various fluences. Facial blood flow was reduced by 30%, the area of the cheek occupied by telangiectasia was reduced by 29%, and erythema intensity was reduced by 21%.

Treatment of rosacea with intense pulsed light. Taub AF. J Drugs Dermatol 2003; 2: 254–9.

Thirty-two patients underwent one to seven treatments. Eighty-three percent had reduced redness, 75% noted reduced flushing, and 64% noted fewer acneiform breakouts. The treatment was well tolerated.

IPL can improve not only telangiectasia, but also erythema and flushing, and is generally better tolerated than lasers. Some expertise is required for optimal results.

Neodymium-yttrium aluminum garnet laser versus pulsed dye laser in erythemato-telangiectatic rosacea: comparison of clinical efficacy and effect on cutaneous substance (P) expression. Salem SA, Abdel Fattah NS, Tantawy SM, El-Badawy NM, Abd El-Aziz YA. J Cosmet Dermatol 2013; 12: 187–94.

A split-face study on 15 patients treated on three occasions at 4-week intervals. Excellent response was achieved in 73.3% of patients after Nd-YAG and in 53.3% of patients after PDL.

Comparative effectiveness of nonpurpuragenic 595-nm pulsed dye laser and microsecond 1064-nm neodymium:yttrium-aluminum-garnet laser for treatment of diffuse facial erythema: a double-blind randomized controlled trial. Alam M, Voravutinon N, Warycha M, Whiting D, Nodzenski M, Yoo S, et al. J Am Acad Dermatol 2013; 69: 438–43.

A split-face study in which 14 patients completed four treatments at 1-month intervals. Subjects rated redness as improved by 52% as a result of PDL and 34% as a result of Nd:YAG. Nd:YAG was somewhat less painful.

The effect of pulsed dye laser on the Dermatology Life Quality Index in erythematotelangiectatic rosacea patients: an assessment. Shim TN, Abdullah A. J Clin Aesthet Dermatol 2013; 6: 30–2.

Mean DLQI improved from 17.3 to 4.3 ($p < 0.0001$) in this study of 20 patients.

How laser surgery can help your rosacea patients. West T. Skin Aging 1998; 43–6.

A review of the use of lasers and IPL for rosacea telangiectasia. IPL is considered to require more operator skill than the KTP or pulsed dye lasers. This article includes recommended parameters for the use of lasers and IPL.

Hair dryer use to optimize pulsed dye laser treatment in rosacea patients. Kashlan L, Graber EM, Arndt KA. J Clin Aesthet Dermatol 2012; 5: 41–4.

This reviews a range of physical and pharmacologic approaches to increasing efficacy of photothermolysis by inducing vasodilation, including exercising, overdressing, consuming trigger foods and beverages, inverting the head, and topical nicotinic acid. Possible agents not yet reported in the literature might include topical nitroglycerin, tetracaine, and lidocaine.

Evidence Levels: A Double-blind study B Clinical trial ≥ 20 subjects C Clinical trial < 20 subjects D Series ≥ 5 subjects E Anecdotal case reports

Second-Line Therapies	
• Oxymetazoline	E
• Ondansetron	E
• Botulinum toxin	D
• Cromolyn sodium	D
• Rifaximin	D

First-Line Therapies	
• Clonidine	D
• Rilmenidine	D
• β-Blockers	D
• Naloxone	D
• Cosmesis	C
• Pulsed dye laser	D
• Intense pulsed light	D
• Hypnosis	E
• Granisetron	D
• Botulinum toxin	D

Successful treatment of the erythema and flushing of rosacea using a topically applied selective alpha1-adrenergic receptor agonist, oxymetazoline. Shanler SD, Ondo AL. Arch Dermatol 2007; 143: 1369–71.

Two cases of erythematotelangiectatic rosacea were treated with a commercially available 0.05% solution of oxymetazoline hydrochloride applied once daily to the face. Redness and flushing were markedly improved.

A 1% cream formulation of oxymetazoline is now commercially available.

The response of erythematous rosacea to ondansetron. Wollina U. Br J Dermatol 1999; 140: 561–2.

Two cases responded to the serotonin receptor antagonist ondansetron. This drug is used mainly as an antiemetic during chemotherapy. It was initially given intravenously at a dose of 12 mg daily and later orally at doses of 4 to 8 mg twice daily. Erythema and ocular symptoms also improved.

Improvement of erythema and flushing has also been reported with granisetron (see later).

Botulinum toxin for the treatment of refractory erythema and flushing of rosacea. Park KY, Hyun MY, Jeong SY, Kim BJ, Kim MN, Hong CK. Dermatology 2015; 230: 299–301.

Impact of intradermal abobotulinumtoxinA on facial erythema of rosacea. Bloom BS, Payongayong L, Mourin A, Goldberg DJ. Dermatol Surg 2015; 41 (Suppl 1): S9–16.

Two reports of facial erythema (and probably also flushing) responding to facial intradermal botulinum toxin in 2 and 15 cases, respectively.

Mast cells are key mediators of cathelicidin initiated skin inflammation in rosacea. Muto Y, Wang Z, Vandenberghe M, Two A, Gallo RL, DiNardo A. J Invest Dermatol 2014; 134: 2728–36.

A randomized, vehicle-controlled trial. Ten subjects with erythematotelangiectatic rosacea applied cromolyn sodium 4% solution or placebo twice daily for 8 weeks. Erythema was reduced in the treatment group.

Rosacea and small intestinal bacterial overgrowth: prevalence and response to rifaximin. Weinstock LB, Steinhoff M. J Am Acad Dermatol 2013; 68: 875–76.

Clearing or marked improvement of rosacea was reported in 46% of a group of 28 patients treated for small intestinal bacterial overgrowth with this nonabsorbed antibiotic. Most patients had vascular rosacea, but ocular disease also improved.

ROSACEA FLUSHING

The flushing associated with rosacea is often the most difficult symptom to treat. This often persists even when the inflammatory component is effectively treated. However, some improvement of flushing is not uncommon when erythematotelangiectatic disease is treated with the various modalities described earlier. Additional approaches are described here.

Clonidine and facial flushing in rosacea. Cunliffe WJ, Dodman B, Binner JG. Br Med J 1977; 1: 105.

Clonidine 0.05 mg twice daily was compared with placebo in a crossover trial with 17 subjects. Five reported improvement in severity and frequency of flushing while on clonidine.

Flushing in rosacea: a possible mechanism. Guarrera M, Parodi A, Cipriani C, Divano C, Rebora A. Arch Dermatol Res 1982; 272: 311–6.

A study of possible pharmacologic inhibitors of rosacea flushing. A single 0.15-mg dose of clonidine inhibited the flushing induced by ingestion of 100 mL of beer in all five patients tested. The testing was undertaken 1 hour after the oral dose so that the blood level of clonidine was at its peak during the investigation.

Effect of subdepressor clonidine on flushing reactions in rosacea. Change in malar thermal circulation index during provoked flushing reactions. Wilkin JK. Arch Dermatol 1983; 119: 211–4.

Clonidine can reduce menopausal flushing. In this study clonidine 0.05 mg given orally twice daily did not suppress the flushing reactions provoked by water at 60°C, red wine, and chocolate. Clonidine did reduce the temperature of malar skin, suggesting a vasoconstrictor effect.

Rilmenidine has also been assessed in a small trial with a suggestion of benefit.

Effect of nadolol on flushing reactions in rosacea. Wilkin JK. J Am Acad Dermatol 1989; 20: 202–5.

A placebo-controlled trial of nadolol 40 mg daily. Spontaneous flushing and flushing provoked in the laboratory by challenges with hot drinks, alcohol, and nicotinic acid were evaluated in 15 subjects. Nadolol had no effect on objective measurements of provoked flushing. There was a trend toward improvement in patient-reported spontaneous flushing.

Alcohol-induced rosacea flushing blocked by naloxone. Bernstein JE, Soltani K. Br J Dermatol 1982; 107: 59–61.

In an experimental setting five subjects with rosacea were investigated to determine whether alcohol-induced rosacea flushing could be inhibited by naloxone 0.8 mg subcutaneously, placebo injection, or chlorpheniramine 12 mg orally. Naloxone effectively prevented alcohol-induced rosacea flushing. Chlorpheniramine or placebo had no consistent effect. This suggests that there may be a role for opioid antagonists in inhibition of this reaction.

Hypnosis in dermatology. Shenefelt PD. Arch Dermatol 2000; 136: 393–9.

Hypnosis has been reported to improve the blushing associated with rosacea.

This is a comprehensive review of the many potential applications for hypnosis in dermatology.

Influence of the 5-HT3 receptor antagonist granisetron on erythema and flushing tendency in rosacea patients. Jansen T. Kosmet Med 2005; 26: 22–4.

Both symptoms improved in a series of 10 patients treated with this antiemetic agent.

ROSACEA LYMPHEDEMA (MORBIHAN DISEASE)

This is a particularly refractory chronic form of rosacea that has received little attention in the literature. Indurated edema develops mainly over the upper half of the face. Treatment is difficult, and the evidence base is very limited. Measures that are generally employed include control of underlying inflammatory rosacea using broad-spectrum antibiotics and facial massage to improve lymphatic drainage.

First-Line Therapies

• Broad-spectrum antibiotics	E
• Facial massage	E
• Isotretinoin	D
• Prednisolone with metronidazole	E
• Prednisolone and doxycycline	E
• CO_2 laser blepharoplasty	E
• Surgical debulking of the eyelids	E

Successful long-term use of oral isotretinoin for the management of Morbihan disease: a case series report and review of the literature. Smith LA, Cohen DE. Arch Dermatol 2012; 148: 1395–8.

Five cases were treated with doses from 40 to 80 mg/day for 10 to 24 months. Treatment was successful, with disease-free follow-up of 1 to 24 months. However, substantial improvement was not seen until 6 months.

Persistent facial swelling in a patient with rosacea. Scerri L, Saihan EM. Arch Dermatol 1995; 131: 1069–74.

A marked reduction in facial swelling was reported in one case from a reducing course of prednisolone, starting at 30 mg daily, and metronidazole 400 mg/day over a 4-month period, followed by metronidazole 200 mg/day.

Successful treatment of Morbihan's disease with oral prednisolone and doxycycline. Ranu H, Lee J, Hee TH. Dermatolog Ther 2010; 23: 682–5.

A single case responded to doxycycline 100 mg daily when after 6 weeks this was combined with prednisolone at the dose of 20 mg daily for 2 weeks, then 10 mg for 1 week.

Morbihan's disease: treatment with CO_2 laser blepharoplasty. Bechara FG, Jansen T, Losch R, Altmeyer P, Hoffmann K. J Dermatol 2004; 31: 113–5.

CO_2 laser blepharoplasty led to good cosmetic results and reduced visual impairment.

Chronic eyelid lymphedema and acne rosacea. Report of two cases. Bernardini FP, Kersten RC, Khouri LM, Moin M, Kulwin DR, Mutasin DF. Ophthalmology 2000; 107: 2220–3.

Surgical debulking of the affected soft tissue resulted in very satisfactory cosmetic and functional improvement in both patients.

OCULAR ROSACEA

Ocular involvement in rosacea is very common and may even be seen in isolation or before the onset of cutaneous features. Many patients complain simply of "dry eyes," often a manifestation of meibomian gland dysfunction. Reduced meibomian lipid secretion is thought to result in rapid evaporation of the aqueous component of the tear film. Additional symptoms are related to the occurrence of blepharitis, episcleritis, chalazion, or hordeolum. Rosacea keratitis can be a serious complication and may occur in adults and children. Severe or refractory cases of ocular disease require specialist ophthalmologic supervision. Particular care is required if systemic retinoids are to be used for inflammatory rosacea when ocular features are present, as retinoids impair meibomian gland secretion.

First-Line Therapies

• "Artificial tears" and lubricants (e.g. phospholipid liposomal eye sprays, carbomers, liquid paraffin, hypromellose)	B
• Warm compresses	B
• Eyelid cleansing/hygiene	B
• Oral tetracyclines	A
• Topical ciclosporin	A
• Topical antibiotics	C
• Omega-3 fatty acid supplementation	A
• *H. pylori* eradication	D
• Ondansetron	E

Meibomian gland dysfunction: report of the subcommittee on management and treatment of meibomian gland dysfunction. Geerling G, Tauber J, Baudouin C, Goto E, Matsumoto Y, O'Brien T, et al. Invest Ophthalmol Vis Sci 2011; 52: 2050–64.

This is a helpful review of current practice and the evidence base supporting it. A wide range of artificial tears and lubricants (eye drops, sprays, and ointments) are employed. More viscous compounds may be more effective, but less well tolerated due to visual disturbance. Warm compresses are commonly recommended but poorly standardized. Mechanical lid hygiene (scrubs, mechanical expression of meibomian glands, cleansing of the eyelashes and lid margins with various solutions, eyelid massage) is often recommended in conjunction with warming. Commonly used topical antibiotics include bacitracin, fusidic acid, metronidazole, fluoroquinolones, and macrolides. Some of these may act through antiinflammatory properties. Scrubs with tea tree oil and tea tree shampoo have been reported as beneficial, possibly by reducing *Demodex* infestation. Systemic tetracyclines may reduce bacterial colonization, but also exert antiinflammatory effects, including suppression of microbial lipases, which release deleterious free fatty acids. Topical and intralesional corticosteroids can be useful for acute inflammatory episodes, but carry significant risks if use is prolonged. Topical ciclosporin appears to be helpful, but takes 2 months or more to obtain optimal benefit. The authors provide a useful treatment algorithm.

Comparative investigation of treatments for evaporative dry eye. Khaireddin R, Schmidt KG. Klin Monbl Augenheilkd 2010; 227: 128–34.

A randomized, controlled trial with 216 subjects of 3 months' duration. A liposomal phospholipid spray was superior to hyaluronate artificial tears, producing double the increase in tear film break-up time.

Evidence Levels: **A** Double-blind study **B** Clinical trial ≥ 20 subjects **C** Clinical trial < 20 subjects **D** Series ≥ 5 subjects **E** Anecdotal case reports

Comparative study of treatment of the dry eye syndrome due to disturbances of the tear film lipid layer with lipid-containing tear substitutes. Dausch D, Lee S, Dausch S, Kim JC, Schwert G, Michelson W. Klin Monbl Augenheilkd 2006; 223: 974–83.

A crossover study on 74 subjects with 6-week treatment periods comparing an eye gel containing triglycerides with a liposomal phospholipid eye spray. Seventy-five percent of the patients favored the spray. Eyelid inflammation and tear film breakup time were also improved more by the liposomal spray.

Oxytetracycline in the treatment of ocular rosacea: a double-blind trial. Bartholomew RS, Reid BJ, Cheesbrough MJ, Macdonald M, Galloway NR. Br J Ophthalmol 1982; 66: 386–8.

Thirty-five patients were investigated in a trial of systemic oxytetracycline, 250 mg twice daily for 6 weeks. Oxytetracycline produced a significantly higher number of remissions than placebo.

Efficacy of doxycycline and tetracycline in ocular rosacea. Frucht-Pery J, Sagi E, Hemo I, Ever-Hadani P. Am J Ophthalmol 1993; 116: 88–92.

Twenty-four patients were randomized to receive doxycycline 100 mg/day or tetracycline 1 g/day. Both groups improved. At 6 weeks all patients except one had symptomatic improvement.

Treatment of ocular rosacea: comparative study of topical ciclosporin and oral doxycycline. Arman A, Demirseren DD, Takmaz T. Int J Ophthalmol 2015; 8: 544–9.

Thirty-eight patients with rosacea-associated eyelid and ocular surface changes and dry eye complaints were randomized to receive 3 months' topical ciclosporin twice daily or oral doxycycline 100 mg twice daily for 1 month, then once daily for 2 months. Both drugs were found to be effective on rosacea-associated ocular changes. ciclosporin was more effective in symptomatic relief and in the treatment of eyelid signs ($p = 0.01$). There was a statistically significant increase in the mean Schirmer score and tear breakup time scores in the ciclosporin group compared with the doxycycline group ($p < 0.05$). The authors conclude that ciclosporin is more effective in ocular rosacea complications and avoids long-term side effects of doxycycline, such as gastrointestinal upset and photosensitivity.

Efficacy of topical ciclosporin for the treatment of ocular rosacea. Schechter BA, Katz RS, Friedman LS. Adv Ther 2009; 26: 651–9.

A double-masked, randomized, 3-month clinical trial on 37 patients comparing twice-daily instillation of ciclosporin ophthalmic emulsion 0.05% with an artificial tear solution. There was significant improvement relative to the control in objective parameters (Schirmer scores, tear breakup time, corneal staining) and quality of life (Ocular Surface Disease Index).

Placebo controlled trial of fusidic acid gel and oxytetracycline for recurrent blepharitis and rosacea. Seal DV, Wright P, Ficker L, Hagan K, Troski M, Menday P. Br J Ophthalmol 1995; 79: 42–5.

Seventy-five percent of patients with blepharitis and associated rosacea were symptomatically improved by fusidic acid gel and 50% by oxytetracycline, but fewer (35%) appeared to benefit from combined treatment.

A randomized controlled trial of omega 3 fatty acids in rosacea patients with dry eye symptoms. Bhargava R, Chandra M, Bansal U, Singh D, Ranjan S, Sharma S. Curr Eye Res 2016; 6: 1–7.

One hundred and thirty patients were treated with the omega-3 fatty acid (O3FA) supplement or placebo (olive oil) for 6 months. Symptoms, Schirmer test, and tear film breakup time improved significantly on O3FA compared with placebo.

Ocular rosacea and treatment of symptomatic *Helicobacter pylori* infection: a case series. Dakovic Z, Vesic S, Vukovic J, Milenkovic S, Jankovic-Terzic K, Dukic S, et al. Acta Dermatovenerol Alp Panonica Adriat 2007; 16: 83–6.

Ocular disease responded better than cutaneous rosacea to eradication of *H. pylori* in this series of seven patients.

The response of erythematous rosacea to ondansetron. Wollina U. Br J Dermatol 1999; 140: 561–2.

Two cases of resistant rosacea responded to the serotonin receptor antagonist ondansetron. This drug is used mainly as an antiemetic during chemotherapy. It was initially given intravenously at a dose of 12 mg daily and later orally at doses of 4 to 8 mg twice daily. Erythema and also ocular symptoms improved.

ROSACEA FULMINANS

Rosacea fulminans (pyoderma faciale) is a very severe facial eruption of sudden onset with prominent pustulation and abscess formation. In addition to conventional treatment modalities for rosacea, a short course of systemic steroids is often indicated to reduce the acute inflammation. Isotretinoin seems to be useful in this condition.

First-Line Therapies	
• Systemic corticosteroids	C
• Topical corticosteroids	D
• Isotretinoin	C
• Systemic antibiotics	C

Pyoderma faciale: a review and report of 20 additional cases: is it rosacea? Plewig G, Jansen T, Kligman AM. Arch Dermatol 1992; 128: 1611–7.

Ten of these 20 patients were hospitalized to commence treatment. Prednisolone was commenced at 1 mg/kg/day for 1 to 2 weeks before adding isotretinoin 0.2 to 0.5 mg/kg/day. The corticosteroid was then tapered off over 2 to 3 weeks and the isotretinoin continued for 3 to 4 months.

Treatment of rosacea fulminans with isotretinoin and topical alclometasone dipropionate. Veraldi S, Scarabelli G, Rizzitelli G, Caputo R. Eur J Dermatol 1996; 6: 94–6.

Five cases were treated successfully with this combination. Alclometasone dipropionate cream (a moderate-potency corticosteroid) was applied twice daily for 10 days then daily for 10 days. The initial dose of isotretinoin was 0.5 mg/kg/day for 1 month followed by 0.7 mg/kg/day for 3 months. Combined cyproterone acetate/ethinylestradiol was used as a contraceptive. Marked improvement was observed after a month and complete resolution after 4 months.

Pyoderma faciale: a clinical study of 29 patients. Massa MC, Su WP. J Am Acad Dermatol 1982; 6: 84–91.

Thirteen of these patients were hospitalized. All were treated with antibiotics, most frequently tetracycline, minocycline, or erythromycin. Vleminckx packs (containing sulfur, calcium polysulfide, and calcium thiosulfate) were used for 21 cases and were considered the most effective topical treatment. Other modalities employed included benzoyl peroxide and UVB.

Sarcoidosis

Niraj Butala, Brittany Scarpato, Warren R. Heymann

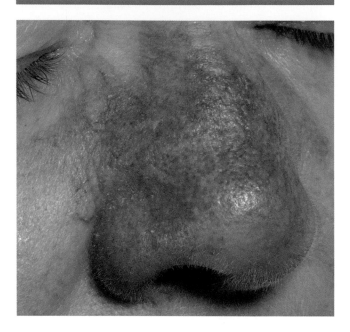

Sarcoidosis is a multisystem disease of unknown etiology characterized histologically by noncaseating granulomas. It is considered to be immune mediated, with a Th1-predominant cytokine profile. Skin manifestations are observed in approximately 25% of cases. Sarcoidosis has been reported to develop after exposure to inorganic particles in the environment. The use of polymerase chain reaction (PCR) techniques has also led to the identification of mycobacterial and propionibacterial DNA and RNA in sarcoidal tissue. Sarcoidosis may be the end result of immune responses to those or other specific triggers. Therapy for erythema nodosum associated with sarcoidosis is addressed in the chapter on erythema nodosum.

MANAGEMENT STRATEGY

The treatment of cutaneous sarcoidosis depends on the types and extent of lesions present and is directed at suppressing the formation of granulomas. Guidelines for treating extracutaneous involvement can be found elsewhere, but it should be recognized that therapy for internal involvement may take precedence over skin disease and that response to treatment may be variable, depending on the type of tissue involved.

In small papular or extremely localized sarcoidosis, treatment with *potent topical corticosteroids* or *intralesional triamcinolone acetonide (3.3–10 mg/mL)* is reasonable. If this is ineffective or involvement is more diffuse, *oral chloroquine (up to 3.5 mg/kg/day)* or *hydroxychloroquine (up to 6.5 mg/kg/day)*, methotrexate, or tetracyclines may be effective. If no response is seen or disfiguring lesions are present, *oral prednisone* can be used at a dose of 1 mg/kg daily (maximum 60 mg) for up to 3 months and then tapered if improvement or a stable level is reached, to a maintenance dose of 5 to 10 mg on alternate days for several months. Periodic escalations in dose are necessary with flares of the disease.

Methotrexate may be used as a corticosteroid-sparing agent or as monotherapy in those patients with lupus pernio, ulcerative sarcoidosis, or severe disease that has not responded to prednisone. Initial doses of 15 to 20 mg weekly are favored. *Mycophenolate mofetil* has also shown promise as a steroid-sparing agent. *Thalidomide, azathioprine, chlorambucil, isotretinoin,* or *allopurinol* could be considered if methotrexate or mycophenolate mofetil fails in this subset of patients. Azathioprine and chlorambucil are better studied in patients with pulmonary sarcoidosis. Thalidomide seems to be more effective than isotretinoin and allopurinol in cutaneous disease. Reported failures are described with etretinate and allopurinol.

Biologic agents that inhibit tumor necrosis factor (TNF)-α are therapeutic modalities that should be considered in patients with lupus pernio or cutaneous sarcoidosis recalcitrant to systemic steroids or steroid-sparing agents. *Infliximab* may be more effective than *adalimumab* but may be associated with a higher rate of infection and autoimmune disease. Etanercept does not appear to be useful for the treatment of sarcoidosis; indeed, some studies have reported on its potential role in patients developing sarcoidosis or in relapse of preexisting sarcoidosis.

Leflunomide and *apremilast* have shown promise in the treatment of cutaneous sarcoidosis unresponsive to other therapies, but further studies are needed to establish long-term usefulness.

Localized disease that does not respond to topical or intralesional corticosteroids, or in those cases in which the use of systemic antimalarial drugs or corticosteroids is undesirable, may represent a niche for other modalities, such as *excision, laser, photodynamic therapy, PUVA, surgery* (lupus pernio), or *intralesional chloroquine.*

Specific Investigations

- Special stains, cultures, and polarization of biopsy specimens
- Electrolytes, blood urea nitrogen, creatinine, serum calcium, liver function tests, complete blood count, 24-hour urine calcium, and serum angiotensin-converting enzyme
- Ophthalmologic evaluation, including slit-lamp examination
- Chest radiograph, pulmonary function tests
- Electrocardiogram
- FDG PET (18-fluoro-deoxyglucose positron-emission tomography) is useful in identifying sites for diagnostic biopsy (for patients without apparent lung involvement)
- MRI with gadolinium (neurologic sarcoidosis may occur without any other internal organ involvement)
- DEXA (dual x-ray absorptiometry) bone density scans in patients on long-term oral corticosteroids

---

Cutaneous sarcoidosis. Wanat KA, Rosenbach M. Clin Chest Med 2015; 36: 685–702.

A thorough review of the literature that discusses advances in the diagnosis and treatment of sarcoidosis and the challenges that clinicians may encounter.

Sarcoidosis: a comprehensive review and update for the dermatologist – part I. Cutaneous disease. Haimovic BA, Sanchez M, Judson MA, Prytowsky S. J Am Acad Dermatol 2012; 66: 699, e1–18.

An extensive review of cutaneous sarcoid, including epidemiology, pathogenesis including the Th1 pathway, morphologies, and treatment. The discussion includes a proposed treatment algorithm.

First-Line Therapies	
• Topical corticosteroids	C
• Intralesional corticosteroids	C
• Oral corticosteroids	C
• Chloroquine	B
• Hydroxychloroquine	C
• Methotrexate	B

Verrucous cutaneous sarcoidosis in an adolescent with dark skin. Corradin MT, Forcione M, Fiorentino R, Bordignon M, Alaibac M, Belloni-Fortina A. Eur J Dermatol 2010; 20: 659–60.

A 16-year-old African boy presented with violaceous, verrucous nodules on his forehead, right pectoral region, right arm, and left elbow. The patient was treated with topical mometasone furoate 0.1% cream daily with clearance of lesions in 3 weeks.

Potent topical corticosteroid use is reported to be of some value in anecdotal reports. Most authors believe that intralesional corticosteroids are more effective, yet this, too, is anecdotal. Small lesions are optimal candidates; however, lupus pernio has also been reported to respond.

A case of scar sarcoidosis of the eyelid. Kim YJ, Kim YD. Korean J Ophthalmol 2006; 20: 238–40.

A 29-year-old man presented with cutaneous sarcoid on his right eyelid. The patient had no other findings of systemic sarcoidosis. A total of 0.6 mL of intralesional triamcinolone 40 mg/mL was injected at 1-cm intervals along the eyelid. Dramatic improvement of the lesion had occurred when he returned for his 1-month follow-up: he received an additional 1 mL of triamcinolone at the same site, which resolved the lesion completely.

Anecdotal reports suggest small, papular sarcoid responds best. The strength of triamcinolone acetonide varies from 2 to 40 mg/mL, and frequency varies from weekly to monthly.

Evidence-based therapy for cutaneous sarcoidosis. Baughman RP, Lower EE. Clin Dermatol 2007; 25: 334–40.

Whereas the recommended starting dose of prednisone for pulmonary sarcoidosis is suggested to be 20 to 40 mg daily, the dose and duration of treatment for cutaneous sarcoidosis have not been established. The authors suggest using this as a benchmark and tapering the steroid dose after 1 or 2 months to one that controls the disease while avoiding toxicity. The authors report that the need for long-term systemic corticosteroids for treatment of chronic sarcoidosis occurs in about a quarter of patients.

Another suggested regimen for prednisone in cutaneous sarcoidosis is 30 mg orally on alternate days until the granulomas fade. The dose is then tapered over several months to 15 mg orally on alternate days. Other protocols report a good response with prednisone 30 to 40 mg orally daily, with a gradual taper to 10 to 20 mg orally on alternate days for 1 year, or prednisone 1 mg/kg orally daily (maximum 60 mg) for 8 to 12 weeks, with a taper to 0.25 mg/kg daily continued for 6 months.

With long-term treatment, prevention of corticosteroid-induced osteoporosis with bisphosphonates and Pneumocystis pneumonia prophylaxis with trimethoprim–sulfamethoxazole should be considered.

Treatment of cutaneous sarcoidosis with chloroquine: review of the literature. Zic JA, Horowitz DH, Arzubiaga C, King LE. Arch Dermatol 1991; 127: 1034–40.

A review of the efficacy and safety of chloroquine in the treatment of cutaneous sarcoidosis. The article cites four studies (three open clinical trials and one case series) that support the use of chloroquine. The authors recommend an initial dose of 250 mg twice daily for 14 days, then 250 mg daily for long-term suppression, though most studies have used 500 mg daily for several months. Relapses after discontinuation of treatment are frequent.

Hydroxychloroquine is effective therapy for control of cutaneous sarcoidal granulomas. Jones EJ, Callen JP. J Am Acad Dermatol 1990; 23: 487–9.

Seventeen patients were treated with 200 mg or 400 mg daily of hydroxychloroquine. Cutaneous lesions regressed in 12 patients within 4 to 12 weeks, and 3 patients had a partial response. Of the 12 patients with the best response, 6 had a recurrence after a dosage reduction or discontinuation.

Hydroxychloroquine may have a better safety profile than chloroquine; however, chloroquine has been better studied in sarcoidosis. Although retinal toxicity is rare, in order to prevent this complication, doses of chloroquine should not exceed 3.5 mg/kg/day, and hydroxychloroquine should not exceed 6.5 mg/kg/day.

Methotrexate is steroid sparing in acute sarcoidosis: results of a double blind, randomized trial. Baughman RP, Winget DB, Lower EE. Sarcoidosis Vasc Diffuse Lung Dis 2000; 17: 60–6.

Twenty-four patients with new-onset symptomatic pulmonary disease were randomized to receive either methotrexate or placebo in addition to their prednisone. Although only 15 patients received at least 6 months of therapy, the methotrexate group required less prednisone than the placebo group. There was no difference in toxicity between the methotrexate and the placebo groups.

A favorable response is usually expected after several months of therapy, and the dose can be tapered weekly after 4 to 6 months. Some studies indicate that methotrexate may be particularly useful for those with ulcerative sarcoidosis.

Prolonged use of methotrexate for sarcoidosis. Lower EE, Baughman RP. Arch Intern Med 1995; 155: 846–51.

Fifty patients were treated with methotrexate, 10 mg weekly, for a minimum of 2 years. Most patients did not have cutaneous involvement, but in those who did a good response was seen. In many patients methotrexate was used in conjunction with prednisone with favorable results.

Second-Line Therapies	
• Mycophenolate mofetil	D
• Infliximab	B
• Minocycline, doxycycline	D

Mycophenolate mofetil may serve as a steroid-sparing agent for sarcoidosis. Kouba DJ, Mimouni D, Rencic A, Nousari HC. Br J Dermatol 2003; 148: 147–8.

A 53-year-old African American with extensive mucocutaneous disease and pulmonary involvement was recalcitrant to standard first-line treatments. He was given oral treatments with prednisone 60 mg tapered to 5 mg every other day over 5 months, hydroxychloroquine 6 mg/kg daily, and mycophenolate mofetil 45 mg/kg daily for 12 months. Significant improvement was noted at 6 weeks and remained at 18 months follow-up with significant reduction of systemic disease.

Treatment of lupus pernio: the results of 116 treatment courses in 54 patients. Stagaki E, Mountford WK, Lackland DT, Judson MA. Chest 2009; 135: 468–76.

This retrospective study of 54 patients with cutaneous sarcoid undergoing 116 treatment regimens showed infliximab-containing regimens to have a high likelihood of complete or near-complete resolution compared with those containing corticosteroids, methotrexate, and hydroxychloroquine. Additionally, when systemic steroids were combined with a second agent there was a significant reduction in prednisone dose requirement.

Infliximab has become a second-line agent, particularly in cases of lupus pernio and neurocutaneous lupus. Studies suggest that infliximab can be used as an induction agent with long-term methotrexate. Superiority to etanercept has been demonstrated.

Recently a double-blind randomized trial for treatment of ocular sarcoidosis with etanercept showed no comparative improvement in the sarcoidal lesions. Also, sarcoidosis was reported to develop in a patient with ankylosing spondylitis after being treated with etanercept. Therefore etanercept does not appear to be useful for the treatment of sarcoidosis.

Infliximab for chronic cutaneous sarcoidosis: a subset analysis from a double-blind randomized clinical trial. Baughman RP, Judson MA, Lower EE, Drent M, Costabel U, Flavin S, et al. Sarcoidosis Vasc Diffuse Lung Dis 2016; 15; 32: 289–95.

A subset analysis of 17 patients with chronic cutaneous sarcoidosis from a larger study of 138 patients with pulmonary disease reviewed their response to infliximab (3 or 5 mg/kg) versus placebo over 24 weeks. The Sarcoidosis Activity and Severity Index (SASI) scoring system found significant improvement in desquamation and induration at week 24, but erythema, percentage of area involved, and evaluation of paired photographs did not show a significant difference.

Infliximab, although effective, has been shown to increase the risk of tuberculosis reactivation, the risk of other granulomatous infections, lymphomas, and autoimmune disease. Therapy is expensive, costing up to thousands of dollars per infusion. One must be aware of the side effects and cost.

The use of tetracyclines for the treatment of sarcoidosis. Bachelez H, Senet P, Cadranel J, Kaoukhov A, Dubertret L. Arch Dermatol 2001; 137: 69–73.

Twelve patients with cutaneous sarcoidosis, three of whom had systemic involvement, were treated with minocycline at a daily dose of 200 mg orally for a median duration of 12 months. Ten patients showed a response, eight complete and two partial; one patient's symptoms remained stable and one patient's disease progressed. Four patients experienced relapse after discontinuation of minocycline; doxycycline was then utilized, resulting in remission.

Due to the safety profile and moderate success, tetracyclines can be considered a second-line therapy in limited cutaneous disease.

Third-Line Therapies

• Thalidomide	D
• Allopurinol	D
• Isotretinoin	E
• Azathioprine	E
• Chlorambucil	B
• Quinacrine	D
• Topical tacrolimus	E
• Intralesional chloroquine	E
• Excision	D
• Laser	E
• Melatonin	D
• Pentoxifylline	E
• Apremilast	C
• Leflunomide	D
• Adalimumab	E
• Medium-dose ultraviolet A1 (UVA1)	E
• PUVA	D
• Photodynamic therapy	D
• Dapsone	E
• Intralesional 5-fluorouracil	E

Treatment of cutaneous sarcoidosis with thalidomide. Nguyen YT, Dupuy A, Cordoliani F, Vignon-Pennamen MD, Lebbé C, Morel P, et al. J Am Acad Dermatol 2004; 50: 235–41.

A retrospective evaluation of 12 patients with cutaneous sarcoidosis, 2 with systemic involvement and 10 of whom were treated successfully with a treatment duration of 2 to more than 16 months, with a daily dose of thalidomide ranging from 50 to 200 mg orally daily. Two patients received combined therapy with oral corticosteroids (dose ranging from 7.5–30 mg daily), one patient used potent topical corticosteroids, and one received combined therapy with methotrexate (dose 25 mg weekly). The average response time was 2 to 3 months. The main adverse effect noted in this series was deep venous thrombosis in one patient.

A case of cutaneous acral sarcoidosis with response to allopurinol. Antony F, Layton AM. Br J Dermatol 2000; 142: 1052–3.

A 38-year-old Afro-Caribbean man with painful sarcoidal nodules around the ends of his fingers (but no evidence of sarcoidal arthritis) had a partial response to oral and intralesional steroids with subsequent recurrence of his lesions. He had no improvement with hydroxychloroquine, methotrexate, or azathioprine. He was started on allopurinol 100 mg twice daily, which was increased to 300 mg daily after 3 weeks. This resulted in sustained objective clinical improvement.

A few case reports demonstrate resolution of truncal and extremity plaques of sarcoidosis after 12 weeks of allopurinol.

Cutaneous sarcoidosis: complete remission after oral isotretinoin therapy. Georgiou S, Monastirli A, Pasmatzi E, Tsambaos D. Acta Derm Venereol 1998; 78: 457–9.

A 31-year-old woman with nodules and plaques on the trunk and extremities showed a complete remission with 8 months of isotretinoin at 1 mg/kg daily; 15-month follow-up revealed continuing remission.

Two other cases report improvement with a 30-week course (0.67–1.34 mg/kg daily) and a 6-month course (0.4–1 mg/kg daily), respectively, of isotretinoin.

Long-term use of azathioprine as a steroid-sparing treatment. Hof DG, Hof PC, Godfrey WA. Am J Respir Crit Care Med 1996; 153: 870A.

Of the 21 patients in this study, 8 had "multisystem" involvement and 1 had skin-only involvement. All patients with extrapulmonary disease achieved a complete remission with azathioprine and a tapering dose of prednisone.

Chlorambucil treatment of sarcoidosis. Israel HL, McComb BL. Sarcoidosis 1991; 8: 35–41.

In this study, 31 patients received chlorambucil, either because complicating diseases prevented them from receiving corticosteroids or they did not respond to them. Marked improvement was noted in 15 patients and moderate improvement in 13 patients, but relapses were very common upon discontinuation. No immune suppression–related side effects were noted.

Scar sarcoidosis following tattooing of the lips treated with mepacrine. Yesudian PD, Azurdia RM. Clin Exp Dermatol 2004; 29: 552–4.

A 50-year-old woman with disfiguring scar sarcoidosis of the lips responded poorly to steroids and was unable to tolerate hydroxychloroquine; she was started on mepacrine 100 mg daily with significant remission to practically normal lip margins. She has had no flares in 10 months of follow-up visits.

The yellow discoloration of the skin and sclera observed with quinacrine (one third of patients) makes chloroquine and hydroxychloroquine better alternatives.

Successful treatment of recalcitrant cutaneous sarcoidosis with fumaric acid esters. Nowack U, Gambichler T, Hanefeld C, Kastner U, Altmeyer P. BMC Dermatol 2002; 24: 215.

Report of three patients with cutaneous sarcoidosis treated with fumaric acid esters for 4 to 12 months, resulting in complete clearance of cutaneous lesions.

Lichenoid type of cutaneous sarcoidosis: great response to topical tacrolimus. Vano-Galvan S, Fernandez-Guarino M, Carmona LP, Harto A, Carrillo R, Jaen P. Eur J Dermatol 2008; 18: 89–90.

A 33-year-old female with lichenoid-type cutaneous sarcoidosis was treated with 0.1% tacrolimus ointment twice daily. Near-complete resolution was noted at 2 months, and the patient remained free of disease at 4 months.

Topical pimecrolimus as a new optional treatment in cutaneous sarcoidosis of lichenoid type. Tammaro A, Abruzzese C, Narcisi A, Cortesi G, Parisella FR, DiRusso PP, et al. Case Rep Dermatol Med 2014; 2014: 976851.

A 66-year-old woman with violaceous, lichenoid sarcoidosis previously unresponsive to clobetasol resolved with topical tacrolimus.

Intralesional chloroquine for the treatment of cutaneous sarcoidosis. Liedtka JE. Int J Dermatol 1996; 35: 682–3.

Multiple injections of intralesional chloroquine hydrochloride (50 mg/mL) were effective in treating five lesions in a single patient, with minimal side effects.

Cutaneous nasal sarcoidosis: treatment by excision and split-skin grafting. Goldin JH, Jawad SMA, Reis AP. J Laryngol Otol 1983; 97: 1053–6.

Split-thickness and full-thickness skin grafts, dermabrasion, and primary closure have been attempted, with mixed results. Surgery has been used in ulcerative and nonulcerative sarcoidosis.

Several recent reports utilizing primary closure, a paramedian forehead flap, and a full-thickness graft continue to show mixed long-term results.

CO_2 laser vaporization for disfiguring lupus pernio. Young HS, Chalmers RJ, Griffiths CE, August PJ. J Cosmet Laser Ther 2002; 4: 87–90.

CO_2 laser resurfacing was used in two patients with lupus pernio with a favorable cosmetic result.

Flashlamp pulsed dye laser and Q-switched ruby laser were beneficial in one case report of lupus pernio. However, exacerbations of lupus pernio—namely, generalized ulceration in treated and untreated lesions—have been reported after this therapy.

Scar sarcoidosis in a child: case report of successful treatment with the pulsed dye laser. Holzmann RD, Astner S, Forschner T, Sterry G. Dermatol Surg 2008; 34: 393–6.

A 10-year-old boy with a 1-cm lesion of varicella zoster–induced scar sarcoidosis on the left cheek had not responded to systemic antibiotics or systemic steroids. Clinical remission occurred after three pulsed dye laser treatments at 6-week intervals, which consisted of two to four pulses using a 595-nm wavelength and a 0.5-ms pulse duration. At 12 months' follow-up there was no evidence of recurrence, although the varicella scar became more visible once the sarcoidosis disappeared.

Successful treatment of cutaneous sarcoidosis lesions with the flashlamp pumped pulsed dye laser: a case report. Roos S, Raulin C, Ockenfels H, Karsai S. Dermatol Surg 2009; 35: 1139–40.

A 63-year-old Caucasian female with nodular sarcoid on her back was treated with flashlamp pumped pulsed dye laser at 6 J/cm^2 (585 nm, 0.5 ms, 12 mm) with complete resolution in 4 weeks. Prednisone was utilized for iridocyclitis after the laser treatments were completed. She remained clear 13 months after discontinuation of systemic steroids.

Melatonin is a safe and effective treatment for chronic pulmonary and extrapulmonary sarcoidosis. Pignone AM, Rosso AD, Fiori G, Matucci-Cerinic M, Becucci A, Tempestini A, et al. J Pineal Res 2006; 41: 95–100.

Melatonin was given to 18 chronic sarcoid patients for 2 years at a dose of 20 mg/day during the first year and 10 mg/day during the second year. Skin lesions, present in three patients, completely disappeared after 24 months of treatment. No side effects were reported.

Melatonin may increase drowsiness and has been associated with hypothermia, hypotension, and bradycardia.

Efficacy and safety of apremilast in chronic cutaneous sarcoidosis. Baughman RP, Judson MA, Ingledue R, Craft NL, Lower EE. Arch Dermatol 2012; 148: 262–4.

A study of 15 patients on systemic steroids treated with 20 mg twice-daily (once daily if not tolerated) apremilast (a novel phosphodiesterase type 4 inhibitor). A significant reduction in SASI induration score was observed at 4 and 12 weeks. Relapse was noted in three patients at the 3-month follow-up. Pentoxifylline has been reported as an effective treatment for pulmonary sarcoidosis; however, efficacy in cutaneous sarcoidosis needs further investigation.

Leflunomide for chronic sarcoidosis. Baughman RP, Lower EE. Sarcoidosis Vasc Diffuse Lung Dis 2004; 21: 43–8.

In a case series study, 32 patients with sarcoidosis involving the eye, lung, and/or skin were treated with leflunomide. Remission (complete and partial) was seen in 12 of 17 patients treated with leflunomide and 13 of 15 patients treated with leflunomide and methotrexate. An initial dose of leflunomide 100 mg/day for 3 days was followed by 20 mg daily after that.

Adverse events, including gastrointestinal problems, and hypersensitivity reactions, including erythema multiforme and Stevens–Johnson syndrome, have been reported.

Adalimumab for treatment of cutaneous sarcoidosis. Heffernan MP, Smith DI. Arch Dermatol 2006; 142: 17–9.

A 46-year-old black woman with sarcoid papules on the nose and ulcerating nodules on the legs had failed local therapy with topical clobetasol and intralesional triamcinolone, hydroxychloroquine, and pentoxifylline. She did not tolerate minocycline. Adalimumab was administered at a dose of 40 mg subcutaneously once weekly. After 10 weeks the nodules on her legs were completely healed and the lesions on her nose were significantly improved.

According to Au et al. (Adalimumab induced subcutaneous nodular sarcoidosis: a rare side effect of tumor necrosis factor-α inhibitor. Sarcoidosis Vasc Diffuse Lung Dis 2014; 31: 249–51), "Adalimumab and other tumor necrosis factor-α inhibitors have been shown in the recent years to successfully treat sarcoidosis refractory to systemic corticosteroids and other agents. However, there have been an increasing number of cases of sarcoidosis paradoxically induced by these agents. It is hypothesized that this is due to the disruption of the fine balance of cytokines involved in granuloma formation."

Cutaneous sarcoidosis treated with medium-dose UVA1. Mahnke N, Medve-Koenigs K, Berneburg M, Ruzicka T, Neumann NJ. J Am Acad Dermatol 2004; 50: 978–9.

An 82-year-old woman with cutaneous sarcoidosis affecting 80% of her body surface was treated with medium-dose UVA1 radiation four times weekly. She received 20 J/cm^2 for the first three treatment sessions, 40 J/cm^2 for the next 12 sessions, and then 60 J/cm^2 for the next 35 sessions. After 50 sessions, nearly all lesions had resolved.

Treatment of cutaneous sarcoid with topical gel psoralen and ultraviolet A. Gleeson CM, Morar N, Staveley I, Bunker CB. Br J Dermatol 2011; 164: 892–4.

A series of six patients with recalcitrant cutaneous sarcoidosis were treated with topical gel psoralen and UVA twice weekly at 0.2 J/cm^2. Patients were placed on oral prednisolone; five patients were tapered at the start of therapy, and one remained on long-term oral prednisolone. In follow-up at 4 months to 3 years, three patients had complete resolution, and three patients had greater than 50% improvement.

Photodynamic therapy for the treatment of cutaneous sarcoidosis. Penrose C, Mercer SE, Shim-Chang H. J Am Acad Dermatol 2011; 65: e12–4.

A 52-year-old African American female with topical and systemic steroid-resistant cutaneous sarcoidosis (likely lupus pernio) had significant improvement after 10 sessions of aminolevulinic acid and photodynamic therapy at 2-week intervals.

Photodynamic therapy utilizing intense pulsed light has also been beneficial in a patient with facial cutaneous sarcoidosis (Hasegawa T, Suga Y, Mizuno Y, Haruna K, Ikeda S. Photodynamic therapy using intense pulsed light for cutaneous sarcoidosis. J Dermatol 2012; 39: 564–5).

Cutaneous sarcoidosis successfully treated with intralesional 5-fluorouracil. Gharavi N, Diehl J, Soriano T. Dermatol Surg 2015; 41: 1082–5.

A 48-year-old Caucasian male with large periorbital sarcoidal nodules significantly improved with three monthly treatments of 0.5 to 1.0 mL of 50 mg/mL of intralesional 5-fluorouracil. The exact mechanism by which 5-fluorouracil resolves granulomas remains unclear.

Resolution of cutaneous sarcoidosis following topical application of *Ganoderma lucidum* (reishi mushroom). Saylam Kurtipek G, Ataseven A, Kurtipek E, Kucukosmanoglu I, Toksoz MR. Dermatol Ther (Heidelb) 2016; 6: 105–9.

Ganoderma lucidum (reishi mushroom) has been used in traditional Chinese and Japanese medicine as an herbal remedy for over 2000 years. Studies have shown that *G. lucidum* has antiallergic, antioxidant, antitumor, antiviral, and antiinflammatory properties. A review of the literature revealed that there were no studies examining the use of *G. lucidum* for the treatment of skin diseases. A 44-year-old male patient who used soap enriched with G. lucidum and goat's milk for 3 days to treat annular cutaneous sarcoidosis, showed almost complete regression of the lesions.

Cutaneous sarcoid mimicking tinea imbricata. Reddy R, Vitiello M, Kerdel F. Int J Dermatol 2011; 50: 1132–4.

A 67-year-old Hispanic male with biopsy-proven cutaneous sarcoidosis who failed treatment with topical and intralesional steroids, topical tacrolimus, and oral ciclosporin showed improvement after starting oral prednisone and 100 mg dapsone daily.

Sarcoidosis is a great masquerader of other dermatoses. This case affirms the need for both diagnostic suspicion and combination therapy for patients with the disease.

Evidence Levels: **A** Double-blind study **B** Clinical trial ≥ 20 subjects **C** Clinical trial < 20 subjects **D** Series ≥ 5 subjects **E** Anecdotal case reports

223

Scabies

James B. Powell, William F.G. Tucker

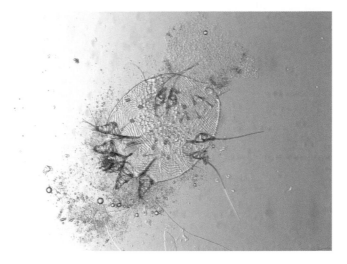

Scabies is an intensely pruritic skin condition due to infestation by the obligate skin parasite "itch mite" *Sarcoptes scabiei*. Endemic in many impoverished communities worldwide, with a global prevalence of 300 million, scabies is a common public health concern, especially in less developed countries. Of concern is the emergence of resistance to classical scabicides, meaning that already limited treatment options may be further diminished.

Prevalence of scabies and impetigo worldwide: a systematic review. Romani L, Steer AC, Whitfeld MJ, Kaldor JM. Lancet Infect Dis 2015; 15: 960–7.

Scabies and global control of neglected tropical diseases. Currie BJ. N Engl J Med 2015; 373: 2371–2.

The literature continues to be littered with cases of delayed diagnosis but unfortunately less so with systematic evidence regarding the efficacy of the multiple treatments used and their safety upon which to base treatment decisions. Multiple small and variable studies (regarding quality, treatment protocols, and measured outcomes) mostly from resource-poor settings have been analyzed in a Cochrane review originally conducted in 1997 with an update in 2007 and BMJ "Clinical Evidence" article by the same authors in 2013. These conclude that topical permethrin is the most effective treatment for scabies (including at reducing itch persistence), with oral ivermectin an effective (although less so than topical permethrin) oral alternative. This means that when considering treatment options apart from permethrin, the safety, side effects, and cost of such treatments should be strongly considered.

MANAGEMENT STRATEGY

Suspicion is the prerequisite for disease control, with scabies infestation coming to mind in any case of (unexplained) pruritus. Initial treatment failure should be expected, especially in heavy infestation and crusted scabies. Treatments may need to be repeated on a number of occasions and even combined. No agent seems greatly effective against the inflammatory skin reaction, and the difference between postscabetic itch and ongoing infestation can be difficult to decipher.

It is generally accepted that the face and scalp do not need treatment except in infants and the immunocompromised individual: topicals are therefore usually applied from the neck down. Reservoirs of infestation include the subungual areas, which must therefore be addressed when applying topical therapy. What is essential is that all intimates of the patient, whether apparently affected or not, are treated at about the same time. Many clinicians find an explanatory leaflet helpful, detailing exactly how to apply a prescribed antiscabetic and also the need to launder clothes and bedding. The skills and patience of the physician are often rigorously tested throughout this process!

Oral ivermectin in single doses of 200 µg/kg has been shown to be very effective in a number of studies, although it is not more effective than properly applied *permethrin*. It is unlicensed for this indication in humans but is used in animal "mange" and is widely and safely used in onchocerciasis. Its safety in children under 15 kg in weight is unknown. Oral ivermectin should therefore be reserved for when appropriate application of a topical antiscabetic is not possible or practicable—for example, compliance, severe eczematization, or as a part of a treatment regimen in crusted/hyperkeratotic and resistant cases. However, randomized controlled trials examining oral ivermectin in crusted scabies are lacking. Treatment with permethrin is repeated after 1 week, as it may not be effective against scabies mite eggs. This repeat treatment allows time for any such eggs not destroyed by the first treatment to hatch so the hatchlings may then be killed. Similarly oral ivermectin may not be effective against the ova, hence the reason why repeat dosing is often needed in practice and shows improved cure rates in studies.

Regarding other topical treatments, controversy exists in the literature over *lindane*, an organochloride insecticide, regarding safety and specifically neurotoxicity—hence, its demotion here to third-line therapies. In many settings its use need not be considered as other more or equally effective treatment options will be available. However, due to its low cost (and efficacy), lindane is still used in some countries. *Crotamiton* 10% is a safe topical antipruritic that may be most useful as an "add-on" therapy, for example, between or after other topical or oral agents where its emollient, antipruritic, and antiscabetic properties can be called into use. *Benzyl benzoate*, although effective, can be very irritating. *Sulfur* is another safe, low-cost (but smelly and also irritating) treatment.

When treating crusted scabies in practice combined topical and oral therapy may have to be considered and repeated to achieve a cure. Additional keratolytic therapy such as *emollients*, *salicylic acid*, and *bathing* may be needed to remove hyperkeratotic plaques, which harbor and protect the mites. There is, however, very little systematic evidence in this area. Recently a report of acitretin being used has emerged.

Specific Investigation

• Visualization of mites and burrows

The one specific investigation for scabies is to isolate the mite and/or its burrow; nothing is more guaranteed to ensure compliance than to show a patient his or her codweller under the bench microscope. These will not be found in all cases, however. Dermatologists take great delight in capturing their quarry, and each will be an advocate of one particular method. With standard scabies, burrows are generally easiest to find around the hands, and the mite can often be seen as a dark dot at one end. Using a dermatoscope to visualize the mite in situ revealing the characteristic triangle or "delta wing" appearance at the mite's head is a simple and quick way of confirming the diagnosis

Epiluminescence microscopy. A new approach to in vivo detection of *Sarcoptes scabiei*. Argenziano G, Fabbrocini G, Delfino M. Arch Dermatol 1997; 133: 751–73.

With the aid of a blunt needle or sewing pin, the mite can be out and placed on a glass slide. Alternatively, the burrow is carefully scraped or shaved with a 15 Bard–Parker blade, and the slice of stratum corneum placed on a glass slide with some immersion oil. Skin biopsy is often illuminating, particularly as the mite may be a surprise finding.

"Wake sign": an important clue for the diagnosis of scabies. Yoshizumi J, Harada T. Clin Exp Dermatol 2009; 34: 711–4.

The "wake sign" reported here refers to the scale that may be seen at the edges of scabies burrows, being reminiscent of the "wake" left behind, somewhat momentarily, on the surface of water by an object moving through it (e.g., a ship).

The burrow ink test and the scabies mite. Woodley D, Saurat JH. J Am Acad Dermatol 1981; 4: 715–22.

A fountain pen (or felt-tip pen/surgical marker, if none available) can be used to conduct the "burrow ink test." A blob of ink is carefully applied to a suspected burrow, left for a minute or so, and wiped off with an isopropyl alcohol swab. If a burrow is present, then capillary action will have led to tracking of the ink into the burrow, leaving a wiggly line.

Laboratory testing will frequently show a mild eosinophilia in peripheral blood. Serologic investigations may in the future become more accurate and therefore useful in certain cases.

A diagnostic test for scabies: IgE specificity for a recombinant allergen of *Sarcoptes scabiei*. Jayaraj R, Hales B, Viberg L, Pizzuto S, Holt D, Rolland JM, et al. Diagn Microbiol Infect Dis 2011; 71: 403–7.

In this study specific IgE antibodies to a major scabies antigen were measured in 140 plasma samples from currently infested and uninfested (control) subjects. Reported results showed 100% sensitivity and 93.75% specificity.

First-Line Therapies

• Permethrin 5% cream	A
• Oral ivermectin	A

Interventions for treating scabies. Strong M, Johnstone PW. Cochrane Database Syst Rev 2007; 3: CD000320.

A new search for studies and content was performed in 2010, but no changes to the conclusions were made. Authors identified 22 small trials for inclusion (19 from resource-poor countries) containing 2676 patients in total. No herbal or traditional medicine trials were identified for inclusion. Permethrin was identified as the most effective topical treatment for scabies, with ivermectin appearing to be an effective oral treatment.

Scabies. Johnstone PW, Strong M. BMJ Clin Evid 2014; 12: 1707.

In this more recent review of the evidence the authors of the Cochrane review class permethrin as "beneficial"; crotamiton

and oral ivermectin as "likely to be beneficial"; and benzyl benzoate, malathion, and sulfur compounds to be of "unknown effectiveness."

Topical permethrin and oral ivermectin in the management of scabies: a prospective, randomized, double blind controlled study. Sharma R, Singla A. Indian J Dermatol Venereol Leprol 2011; 77: 581–6.

One hundred twenty cases of scabies were included in this study from Delhi, India. Cure rates ("defined as >50% improvement in lesion count and pruritus and negative microscopy") of around 90% were seen at 4 weeks in those treated with either a single dose of 5% permethrin topically or ivermectin (200 µg/kg/dose) or "double dose regimen repeated at 2 weeks interval."

The efficacy of oral ivermectin vs. sulfur 10% ointment for the treatment of scabies. Alipour H, Goldust M. Ann Parasitol 2015; 61: 79–84.

This randomized study in Iran compared one dose of oral ivermectin (200 µg/kg) versus sulfur 10% ointment (applied for 3 consecutive days) in 420 patients. Treatment was assessed at 2 and 4 weeks. If there was treatment failure at 2 weeks, treatment was repeated. A single dose of ivermectin provided a cure rate of 61.9% at the 2-week follow-up, which increased to 78.5% at the 4-week follow-up after repeating the treatment. Treatment with sulfur 10% ointment was effective in 45.2% of patients at the 2-week follow-up, which increased to 59.5% at the 4-week follow-up after treatment was repeated.

Tratamiento de la escabiasis con ivermectina por vía oral. Macotela-Ruiz E, Pena-Gonzalez G. Gac Med Mex 1993; 129: 201–5.

This randomized trial compared the treatment of 55 patients with a clinical diagnosis of scabies with either a single dose of ivermectin 200 µg/kg or placebo. After 7 days the code was broken because there was such a significant improvement in the treated group: 23 of 29 versus 4 of 26.

A comparative trial of oral ivermectin and topical permethrin in the treatment of scabies. Usha V, Gopalakrishnan Nair TV. J Am Acad Dermatol 2000; 42: 236–40.

In this trial in 88 patients, permethrin came out better for cure at 2 weeks.

Safety of and compliance with community-based ivermectin therapy. Pacque M, Munoz B, Greene BM, White AT, Dukuly Z, Taylor HR. Lancet 1990; 335: 1377–80.

Adverse reactions after large-scale treatment of onchocerciasis with ivermectin: combined results from eight community trials. De Sole G, Remme J, Awadzi K, Accorsi S, Alley ES, Ba O, et al. J WHO 1989; 67: 707–19.

In both studies ivermectin was remarkably well tolerated, even in repeated courses.

Deaths associated with ivermectin treatment of scabies. Barkwell R, Shields S. Lancet 1997; 349: 1144–5.

This is the only "fly in the ointment" with ivermectin: the authors report on the treatment of 47 elderly, mentally disadvantaged residents of an institution with a single dose of ivermectin at 150 to 200 µg/kg body weight. All had failed to respond to multiple earlier courses of lindane and crotamiton. All were cured, but over the next 6 months 15 died from a number of causes, whereas only 5 died in an equivalent matched population within the same unit. Many patients were taking other drugs, raising the possibility of interactions. *The possibility that patients who are debilitated are more susceptible to scabies may have contributed to the increase in deaths in ivermectin-treated individuals.*

Difficult-to-treat scabies: oral ivermectin. National Institute for Health and Care Excellence. March 2014; nice.org.uk/guidance/esuom29.

Randomized controlled trials using oral ivermectin in scabies show either mild side effects (including transient worsening of itch) or report no adverse events.

Second-Line Therapies	
• Crotamiton	A
• Topical ivermectin	B
• Malathion 0.5% lotion	B
• Benzyl benzoate	B
• Sulfur	B

Comparison of oral ivermectin versus crotamiton 10% cream in the treatment of scabies. Goldust M, Rezaee E, Raghifar R. Cutan Ocul Toxicol 2014; 33: 333–6.

In this study from Iran 320 patients were randomized to receive a single dose of oral ivermectin 200 µg/kg or crotamiton 10% cream (topically twice daily for 5 consecutive days). Treatment was evaluated at 2 and 4 weeks and repeated if evidence of treatment failure. Ivermectin provided a cure rate of 62.5% at 2 weeks, which increased to 87.5% at the 4-week follow-up after repeating treatment. Treatment with crotamiton was effective in 46.8% of patients at the 2-week follow-up, which increased to 62.5% at the 4-week follow-up after repeating treatment.

Comparison of crotamiton 10% cream (Eurax) and permethrin 5% cream (Elimite) for the treatment of scabies in children. Taplin D, Meinking TL, Chen JA, Sanchez R. Pediatr Dermatol 1990; 7: 67–73.

This double-blind randomized study compared these drugs in children from 2 months to 5 years of age. A single overnight application was used. Cure rates were superior with permethrin at 2 weeks (30% vs. 13%) and at 4 weeks (89% vs. 60%).

A family based study on the treatment of scabies with benzyl benzoate and sulfur ointment. Gulati PV, Singh KP. Indian J Dermatol Venereol Leprol 1978; 44: 269–73.

One hundred fifty-eight clinically diagnosed patients were randomly allocated to use either 25% benzyl benzoate emulsion or 5% sulfur ointment. Treatment was applied at least three times over 24 hours. The sulfur seems to have been marginally more effective.

Treatment of scabies using 8% and 10% topical sulfur ointment in different regimens of application. Sharquie KE, Al-Rawi JR, Noaimi AA, Al-Hassany HM. J Drugs Dermatol 2012; 11: 357–64.

This single-blinded study from Iraq included 97 patients with scabies. Treatment for 3 days (e.g., washing off and reapplying every 24 hours) resulted in over 90% responding to treatment. A once-only application was much less effective but resulted in fewer side effects (irritant dermatitis, mild burning sensation).

Ivermectin versus benzyl benzoate applied once or twice to treat human scabies in Dakar, Senegal: a randomized controlled trial. Fatimata LY, Caumes E, Ndaw CAT, Ndiaye B, Mahe A. Bull WHO 2009; 87: 424–30.

In this study, which excluded those with crusted scabies, topical benzyl benzoate 12.5% was more effective than oral ivermectin in treating scabies infestation.

Comparison of ivermectin and benzyl benzoate for treatment of scabies. Glaziou P, Cartel JL, Alzieu P, Briot C, Moulia-Pelat JP, Martin PM. Trop Med Parasitol 1993; 44: 331–2.

A randomized study in French Polynesia compared a single dose of 100 µg/kg ivermectin with 10% benzyl benzoate lotion applied below the neck and repeated 12 hours later. Both were equally effective.

Treatment of scabies: topical ivermectin vs. permethrin 2.5% cream. Goldust M, Rezaee E, Raghifar R, Hemayat S. Ann Parasitol 2013; 59: 79–84.

In another study from Iran 380 patients with scabies were randomized into two groups: the first received 1% ivermectin topically, the second permethrin 2.5%. Both were applied twice over a week and treatment repeated at 2 weeks if there was evidence of treatment failure. Ivermectin provided a cure rate of 63.1% at the 2-week follow-up, which increased to 84.2% at the 4-week follow-up after repeating the treatment. Permethrin 2.5% was effective in 65.8% of patients at the 2-week follow-up, which increased to 89.5% at the 4-week follow-up.

***Sarcoptes scabiei* infestation treated with malathion liquid.** Hanna NF, Clay JC, Harris JRW. Br J Venereol Dis 1978; 54: 354.

An uncontrolled study using 0.5% malathion liquid in 30 patients, yielding an 83% cure rate at 4 weeks.

Third-Line Therapies	
• Lindane	B
• Monosulfiram soap	B
• Natural pyrethrins	B
• Thiabendazole	B
• Tea tree oil	E

Control of scabies by use of soap impregnated with "Tetmosol." Gordon RM, Davey TH, Unsworth K, Hellier FF, Parry SC, Alexander JR. Br Med J 1944; 2: 803–6.

A bath a day for 6 days using 20% Tetmosol (monosulfiram) soap cured all six patients; three baths cured 88 of 110 patients; the relapse rate was 20%.

Presumably the limiting factor in wartime Britain was the lack of hot bathwater!

Topically applied thiabendazole in the treatment of scabies. Hernandez-Perez E. Arch Dermatol 1976; 112: 1400–1.

A 10% suspension used to treat 40 patients achieved a "satisfactory response" in 80%.

Efficacy and tolerability of natural synergised pyrethrins in a new thermolabile foam formulation in topical treatment of scabies: a prospective randomized, investigator-blinded, comparative trial vs. permethrin cream. Amerio P, Capizzi R, Milan M. Eur J Dermatol 2003; 13: 69–71.

This trial included 40 patients, and the pyrethrin foam was reported to be "at least as effective" as permethrin.

Efficacy and tolerability of a new synergized pyrethrins thermophobic foam in comparison with benzyl benzoate in the treatment of scabies in convicts: the ISAC study. Biele M,

Campori G, Colombo R, De Giorgio G, Frascione P, Sali R, et al; ISAC Investigator Group. J Eur Acad Dermatol Venereol 2006; 20: 717–20.

In this multicenter, randomized, investigator-blinded trial synergized pyrethrins (over 3 consecutive days) and benzyl benzoate (over 5 consecutive days) both achieved a cure rate of over 90% at 4 weeks, but the pyrethrin foam was better tolerated by the convicts.

Therapeutic potential of tea tree oil for scabies. Thomas J, Carson CF, Peterson GM, Walton SF, Hammer KA, Naunton M, et al. Am J Trop Med Hyg 2016; 94: 258–66.

In the face of emerging resistance to ivermectin and permethrin, new cost-effective, safe treatments are needed. Tea tree oil has shown some promising effects, but randomized controlled studies are needed.

Efficacy and safety of a lindane 1% treatment regimen for scabies, confirmed by dermoscopy-guided skin scraping with microscopic examination. Park SE, Her Y, Kim SS, Kim CW. Clin Exp Dermatol 2015; 40: 611–6.

This retrospective study from Seoul, Korea, evaluated the efficacy of 1% lindane cream in treating microscopically confirmed scabies in 50 cases. Patients were treated with 1% lindane cream twice weekly. The cumulative efficacy of lindane 1% cream was 40% after 1 week, 88% after 2 weeks, and 98% after 3 weeks of treatment.

Comparison of oral ivermectin vs. lindane lotion 1% for the treatment of scabies. Mohebbipour A, Saleh P, Goldust M, Amirnia M, Zadeh YJ, Mohamad RM, et al. Clin Exp Dermatol 2013; 38: 719–23.

In this study from Iran including 148 patients a single dose of oral ivermectin was more effective than two applications of lindane lotion 1% 1 week apart (61% vs. 47%) after 2 weeks. After repeat treatment if evidence of infestation remained at 2 weeks, ivermectin was superior to lindane lotion 1% (89% vs. 73%).

Treatment of scabies: comparison of lindane 1% vs. permethrin 5%. Rezaee E, Goldust M, Alipour H. Skinmed 2015; 13: 283–6.

Superior efficacy for permethrin shown.

Lindane toxicity: a comprehensive review of the medical literature. Nolan K, Kamrath J, Levitt J. Pediatr Rev 2012; 29: 141–6.

This review describes 67 cases of adverse reactions and deaths associated with lindane use, where even "labeled" usage caused 43% of the "serious adverse reactions."

Treatment of crusted scabies with acitretin. Veraldi S, Nazzaro G, Serini SM. Br J of Dermatol 2015; 173: 862–3.

Here two cases of crusted scabies were treated with acitretin 30 mg daily and a 15% glycerine cream that achieved "complete remission after 6 weeks."

Evidence Levels: **A** Double-blind study **B** Clinical trial ≥ 20 subjects **C** Clinical trial < 20 subjects **D** Series ≥ 5 subjects **E** Anecdotal case reports

224

Scleredema

Amy E. Flischel, Stephen E. Helms, Robert T. Brodell

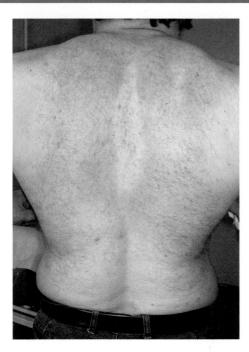

Scleredema (scleredema adultorum or scleredema of Buschke) is a connective tissue disorder characterized by progressive, symmetric induration and thickening of the skin secondary to increased amounts of collagen and glycosaminoglycans. Clinically, scleredema most commonly involves the posterior neck, shoulders, trunk, face, and arms. Three clinical categories are recognized: type I, postinfectious, accounts for 55% of cases—this usually resolves spontaneously within 6 months to 2 years; type II, malignancy-associated, accounts for 25% of cases, including paraproteinemias and monoclonal gammopathy with or without multiple myeloma; and type III, scleredema diabeticorum, which is seen in 20% of cases and is associated with poorly controlled insulin-dependent diabetes and persists indefinitely.

MANAGEMENT STRATEGY

Treatment of scleredema is difficult and usually unsatisfactory. However, there are case-based data to support the effectiveness of several therapies. In many cases, a candid discussion with the patient regarding limitations of treatment, cost, and side effects will lead to a decision to withhold treatment. This is particularly appropriate in patients with the postinfectious form, which can resolve spontaneously without any specific therapy. Of course, identification of a specific etiology, such as streptococcal pharyngitis, should lead to appropriate antibiotic treatment, even in the absence of evidence that antibiotics would alter the rate of clearing in this self-limited form of scleredema. In the forms associated with diabetes mellitus and monoclonal gammopathy, progressive involvement can lead to discomfort, unsightly

thickening, and even systemic complications such as restrictive pulmonary function, dysphagia secondary to tongue swelling, and cardiac arrhythmias. In these cases, patients will demand treatment.

Bath or cream PUVA has been recommended as initial therapy in moderately severe disease. More recently, narrowband UVB and UVA1 have been shown to be moderately effective. *Electron beam therapy* has been proposed as the leading recommendation for patients with severe disease, especially cases with restrictive pulmonary function. Alternative therapies have included *ciclosporin, allopurinol, tamoxifen,* and *high-dose penicillin.* Antidiabetic therapy has no effect on the evolution of scleredema in diabetics, as the progression of scleredema has been found to be unrelated to control of serum glucose levels.

Specific Investigations

- Fasting blood sugar, glucose tolerance test, hemoglobin A_{1c} (glycosylated hemoglobin)
- Serum protein electrophoresis, immunoelectrophoresis
- Antistreptolysin O, bacterial culture, C-reactive protein (CRP), erythrocyte sedimentation rate (ESR)

Scleredema adultorum due to streptococcal infection. Alp H, Orbak Z, Aktas A. Pediatr Int 2003; 45: 101–3.

In 65% to 95% of cases, scleredema occurs within a few days to 6 weeks after an acute febrile illness. Of these infections, 58% are streptococcal. These infections may present as tonsillitis, pharyngitis, scarlet fever, erysipelas, cervical adenitis, pneumonia, otitis media, pyoderma, impetigo, or rheumatic fever. Appropriate studies will rapidly determine whether an underlying infection is associated with scleredema.

Monoclonal gammopathy in scleredema: observations in three cases. Kovary PM, Vakilzadeh F, Macher E, Zaun H, Merk H, Goerz G. Arch Dermatol 1981; 117: 536–9.

Many subsequent reports have confirmed this association. Skin manifestations often precede the development of the gammopathy.

Scleredema associated with carcinoma of the gall bladder. Manchanda Y, Das S, Sharma VK, Srivastava DN. Br J Dermatol 2005; 152: 1373–4.

Scleredema has been associated with various internal malignancies. When clinically indicated, an evaluation for internal malignancies may be appropriate.

First-Line Therapies

- Identify and treat underlying disease   D
- Conservative management   D

Scleredema: a review of 33 cases. Venencie PY, Powell FC, Su D, Perry HO. J Am Acad Dermatol 1984; 11: 128–34.

Systemic corticosteroids, methotrexate, and D-penicillamine demonstrated no effect on the disease course. Both diabetic and nondiabetic patients were studied, and although some patients in both groups suffered from mild complications such as dysphagia and electrocardiogram (ECG) changes, the authors emphasize that scleredema is generally a mild disease that poses no threat to overall health.

Scleredema adultorum. Not always a benign self-limited disease. Curtis AC, Shulak BM. Arch Dermatol 1965; 92: 526–41.

A review of 223 scleredema patients revealed that 25% have had symptoms for more than 2 years. The following treatments demonstrated no therapeutic benefit: calcium gluconate, estradiol, fever, hot baths, hyaluronidase, nicotinic acid, ovarian extract, p-aminobenzoate, penicillin, pituitary extract, corticosteroids, thyroid hormone, and vitamin D.

Fulminans in dermatology: a call to action: a recommendation for consideration of the term scleredema fulminans. Sommer LL, Heymann WR. J Clin Aesthet Dermatol 2014; 7: 42–5.

A 43-year-old man with an 11-year history of human immunodeficiency virus presented with a 3-month history of abrupt-onset progressive neck, shoulder, and back swelling shortly after the patient was diagnosed with type 2 diabetes. Though generally considered a chronic disease, this case demonstrates the rapidity of onset seen in some patients.

Second-Line Therapies	
• Narrowband UVB phototherapy	E
• UVA1 phototherapy	D
• Electron beam therapy	E
• Bath PUVA and cream PUVA	E
• Physical therapy	E
• Tamoxifen	E
• High-dose penicillin	E
• Ciclosporin	E
• Extracorporeal photopheresis	E
• Chemotherapy (melphalan)	E
• Frequency-modulated electromagnetic neural stimulation	E
• Allopurinol	E
• Intravenous Immunoglobulin	E

Scleredema adultorum treated with narrow-band ultraviolet B phototherapy. Xiao T, Yang Z, He C, Chen H. J Dermatol 2007; 34: 270–2.

A 56-year-old Chinese man was treated with NB-UVB at an initial dose of 0.2 J/cm², three times weekly, increased by 25% per treatment. Significant improvement occurred after 10 treatments, and the patient received a total of 54 exposures (33.8 J/cm² dose). Beneficial effects were still evident 14 months after treatment was discontinued. NB-UVB phototherapy has several advantages over PUVA. It has shorter irradiation times, no need for protective glasses after treatment, and reduced risk of photocarcinogenesis. Further large-scale studies are needed to define the role of NB-UVB in scleredema.

UVA1 phototherapy for cutaneous diseases: an experience of 92 cases in the United States. Tuchinda C, Kerr H, Taylor C, Jacobe H, Bergamo B, Elmets C, et al. Photodermatol Photoimmunol Photomed 2006; 22: 247–53.

Six patients with scleredema were treated with UVA1 phototherapy (five received low-dose regimens and one a medium-dose regimen). One patient developed polymorphous light eruption and therapy was discontinued. Moderate-to-good responses were seen in four out of five patients treated. In recalcitrant cases UVA1 phototherapy should be considered as a therapeutic option.

Scleredema diabeticorum case series: successful treatment with UV-A1. Kroft EB, de Jong EM. Arch Dermatol 2008; 144: 947–8.

Three cases showed substantial clinical improvement after UVA1 therapy. Two patients were treated with 35 J/cm² per session and the third patient with 60 J/cm² per session.

Scleredema treated with broad-band ultraviolet A phototherapy plus colchicine. Yüksek J, Sezer E, Köseoğlu D, Markoç F, Yildiz H. Photodermatol Photoimmunol Photomed 2010; 26: 257–60.

A 23-year-old female with biopsy-confirmed scleredema was treated with low-dose broadband UVA phototherapy 15 J/cm², three times weekly for 40 sessions (total cumulative dose of 600 J/cm²) and colchicine 1800 mg/day for 1 year. Histopathologic and clinical improvement was noted. The authors conclude that more long-term follow-up studies in a larger series are needed.

Scleredema of Buschke successfully treated with electron beam therapy. Tamburin LM, Pena JR, Meredith R. Arch Dermatol 1998; 134: 419–22.

A patient with scleredema and insulin-dependent diabetes mellitus experienced complete resolution of skin induration after receiving electron beam therapy twice weekly for 36 days. Prior treatment with topical, intralesional, and systemic corticosteroids had failed. This patient also suffered significant restrictive pulmonary disease thought to be secondary to scleredema, and pulmonary function tests after electron beam therapy revealed marked improvement in lung function. This treatment should be considered in patients with severe persistent disease and systemic complications.

Electron-beam therapy in scleredema adultorum with associated monoclonal hypergammaglobulinaemia. Angeli-Besson C, Koeppel M, Jacquet P, Andrac L, Sayag J. Br J Dermatol 1994; 130: 394–7.

Ten sessions of electron beam therapy produced significant clinical improvement in the skin lesions of a patient with IgAκ monoclonal gammopathy. A trial of factor XIII and cyclofenil had proved unsuccessful. Although the patient had initially responded to systemic corticosteroids, she subsequently became resistant and the condition progressed. At that point, electron beam therapy was begun.

Paraproteinemia-associated scleredema treated successfully with intravenous immunoglobulin. Eastham AB, Femia AN, Velez NF, Smith HP, Vleugels RA. JAMA Dermatol 2014; 150: 788–9.

A woman in her forties with a 2-year history of progressive erythema and induration of the face, neck, and upper trunk denied recent infection or history of diabetes. There was significant limitation in range of motion of shoulders. After 2 cycles of IVIG given monthly, the patient noted significant improvement.

Bath-PUVA therapy in three patients with scleredema adultorum. Hager CM, Sobhi HA, Humzelmann N, Wickenhauser C, Scharenberg R, Krieg T, et al. J Am Acad Dermatol 1998; 38: 240–2.

Bath PUVA therapy (median of 59 treatments) produced substantial clinical improvement. One patient did not have a history of diabetes mellitus or preceding infection; the remaining two had diabetes. Diabetic patients with scleredema tend to have a long unremitting course without treatment.

Evidence Levels: **A** Double-blind study **B** Clinical trial ≥ 20 subjects **C** Clinical trial < 20 subjects **D** Series ≥ 5 subjects **E** Anecdotal case reports

Cream PUVA therapy for scleredema adultorum. Grundmann-Kollmann M, Ochsendorf F, Zollner TM, Spieth K, Kaufmann R, Podda M. Br J Dermatol 2000; 142: 1058–9.

Cream PUVA therapy (35 irradiations) produced marked clinical improvement and softening of the skin in a patient with a 10-year history of scleredema who also suffered non–insulin-dependent diabetes mellitus. Cream PUVA therapy is easier to administer than bath PUVA and may become an important treatment option for scleredema.

Ultrasonic massage and physical therapy for scleredema: improving activities of daily living. Bray SM, Varghese S, English JC 3rd. Arch Dermatol 2010; 146: 453–4.

A 42-year-old man with diabetes-associated scleredema was treated with hydroxychloroquine and psoralen UVA without clinical improvement. Physical therapy with ultrasonic massage, active range-of-motion exercises, and flexibility exercises three times a week was initiated. Ultrasonic massage therapy was performed using a Dynatron 709 series machine with the following parameters: 100%, 1 MHz, and 1.5 W/cm^2 for 10 minutes per session. The patient showed objective improvement in 9 of 10 range-of-motion parameters measured after 1 year of physical therapy.

Treatment of scleredema diabeticorum with tamoxifen. Alsaeedi SH, Lee P. J Rheumatol 2010; 37: 2636–7.

A 61-year-old woman with diabetic scleredema was treated with tamoxifen 20 mg twice daily after failing to improve after treatment with methotrexate and D-penicillamine. After 2 months, her symptoms improved, and after 48 months there was clinical evidence of softening of the skin on her back as well as improvement of shoulder flexibility. A 54-year-old female with diabetic scleredema was also treated with tamoxifen 20 mg twice daily and demonstrated similar improvement. Tamoxifen's antifibrotic effect may be an effective treatment for scleredema.

Persistent scleredema of Buschke in a diabetic: improvement with high-dose penicillin. Krasagakis K, Hettmannsperger U, Trautmann C, Tebbe B, Garbe C. Br J Dermatol 1996; 134: 597–8.

High-dose (3×10^6 IU daily) intravenous penicillin for 7 days led to a reduction in the severity of scleredema. Rather than acting as an antibiotic, penicillin appears to be effective because of its antifibrotic actions. This may explain why other antibiotics such as erythromycin are ineffective.

Cyclosporine in scleredema. Mattheou-Vakali G, Ioannides D, Thomas T, Lazaridou E, Tsogas P, Minas A. J Am Acad Dermatol 1996; 35: 990–1.

Ciclosporin at a dose of 5 mg/kg daily for 5 weeks was effective in completely clearing scleredema in two patients. Both presented with postinfectious scleredema and thus would have likely experienced resolution of their symptoms even without treatment.

Scleredema associated with paraproteinemia treated by extracorporeal photopheresis. Stables GI, Taylor PC, Highet AS. Br J Dermatol 2000; 142: 781–3.

Significant improvement in skin lesions followed treatment with extracorporeal photopheresis. When the treatment sessions were reduced from two per month to one, the patient's condition deteriorated, suggesting that the improvement was due to therapy rather than spontaneous resolution. Because scleredema associated with paraproteinemia usually has a progressive course, this treatment should be considered in patients with a similar presentation.

Beneficial effect of aggressive low-density lipoprotein apheresis in a familial hypercholesterolemic patient with severe diabetic scleredema. Koga N. Ther Apher 2001; 5: 506–12.

A 59-year-old woman with diabetic scleredema treated with weekly low-density lipoprotein (LDL) apheresis over a period of 3 years had significant improvement in her scleredema when her lipid levels were normalized. Histopathologic as well as clinical improvement was noted.

Treatment with chemotherapy of scleredema associated with IgA myeloma. Santos-Juanes J, Osuna CG, Iglesias JR, De Quiros JF, del Rio JS. Int J Dermatol 2001; 40: 720–1.

A 70-year-old woman with IgA myeloma and scleredema was treated with oral melphalan and prednisone over a 6-month period. During the 18 months she was followed, clinical evidence of softening of the indurated and taut skin was observed. Similar cases were cited in which chemotherapy for myeloma resulted in significant improvement of associated scleredema.

Treatment of acquired reactive perforating collagenosis with allopurinol incidentally improves scleredema diabeticorum. Lee FY, Chiu HY, Chiu HC. J Am Acad Dermatol 2011; 65: e115–7.

A 51-year-old man presented with acquired reactive perforating collagenosis associated with diabetes and scleredema of the upper back for over 20 years. Allopurinol 100 mg a day for 14 months proved effective for both conditions. Allopurinol is thought to improve endothelial function by profoundly reducing vascular oxidative stress.

Successful treatment of poststreptococcal scleredema adultorum Buschke with intravenous immunoglobulins. Aichelburg MC, Loewe R, Schicher N, Sator PG, Karlhofer FM, Stingl G, et al. Arch Dermatol 2012; 148: 1126–8.

A 38-year-old woman with a 3-week history of rapidly progressing scleredema of the upper trunk 7 weeks after pharyngitis. After failure of initial treatment with penicillin, UVA-1 therapy, and methylprednisolone, IVIG was initiated at a dosage of 2 g/kg over 2 consecutive days every 4 weeks for five cycles. Initial improvement was noted 10 days after the first administration.

Improvement in clinical symptoms of scleredema diabeticorum by frequency-modulated electromagnetic neural stimulation: a case report. Gandolfi A, Pontara A, Di Terlizzi G, Rizzo N, Nicoletti R, Scavini M, et al. Diabetes Care 2014; 37: e233–4.

Scleredema associated with type 1 diabetes was treated with frequency-modulated electromagnetic neural stimulation (FREMS), transcutaneous electrotherapy, a safe and effective therapy commonly used for diabetic neuropathy. Ten to 15 sessions of FREMS were given at 3-month intervals over 15 months. Initial improvement in both mobility and the Barthel Index of activities of daily living was seen after two series. Despite the clinical improvement, no histologic changes could be identified.

225

Scleroderma

Mark J.D. Goodfield, Ian H. Coulson

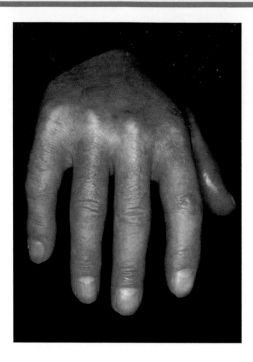

Systemic sclerosis (SSc), often called *scleroderma*, is a rare multisystem disease characterized by skin fibrosis, autoantibody production, and vascular abnormalities often leading to visceral disease. It can affect any organ system, particularly the gastrointestinal tract, kidney, heart, and lungs. Patients typically present with cutaneous sclerosis or Raynaud phenomenon (RP). The degree of skin involvement defines the clinical subset of the disease. Diffuse cutaneous SSc (dcSSc) involves the skin proximal to the neck, elbows, or knees, whereas involvement distal to these sites is known as *limited cutaneous SSc (lcSSc)*; some authors include an intermediate group. Localized scleroderma, or morphea, is a different condition.

MANAGEMENT STRATEGY

Limited cutaneous and dcSSc, with different severities and survivals, have been recognized as distinct subsets. Some authors have suggested an intermediate cutaneous form with intermediate survival.

In most cases cutaneous lesions and RP precede systemic involvement. The face and hands are typically involved, with patients displaying a characteristic shiny appearance of the skin and complaining of increased skin stiffness or rigidity. To date, no treatment has proved uniformly effective in modifying the course of the disease, and there is no specific therapy for the skin, although dry skin should be cared for daily using *emollient creams*. *Topical 0.025% to 0.05% tretinoin* may improve the perioral radial furrows and facial tightening. *Antihistamines* may help itch. Calcinosis cutis may require surgical removal of deposits, and *parenteral or intralesional sodium thiosulfate* is occasionally justified.

UVA phototherapy, Psoralens and Ultraviolet A, Ultraviolet A (PUVA and UVA1) has been reported to be effective in reducing skin thickness. *Vasodilators* such as *nifedipine* reduce vasospasm and improve peripheral blood flow. Also, *losartan*, an antagonist of angiotensin II receptor type I, has been found to be effective in reducing the severity and frequency of attacks of RP. Digital ulcers are a frequent problem in SSc—they may require antibiotics if they are infected, and recalcitrant ulcers may respond to a *PDE-5 antagonist* such as *sildenafil. Endothelin receptor antagonists* such as *bosentan* may improve digital perfusion. *Palmar sympathectomy* and *botulinum toxin injection* to digital nerves may be valuable. *Parenteral prostacyclin* analogs such as *iloprost* also improve both the severity and frequency of RP. Both *low-dose prednisolone* 20 mg/day and *methotrexate* 15 to 25 mg/week have been shown to reduce skin thickness scores. *ciclosporin* 3 to 4 mg/kg/day may improve skin induration, but has no effect on internal organ involvement. It should be used with caution as renal involvement with SSc is not uncommon. *Mycophenolate* (0.5–1.5 g twice daily) is of value for both skin and lung involvement. *Cyclophosphamide* 1 to 2 mg/kg/day is of proven value in reducing skin scores and preventing the development of lung fibrosis and other complications, and *pulsed therapy with cyclophosphamide* is also effective and possibly safer.

Biologics, including *rituximab, infliximab, basiliximab, and imatinib*, have all been investigated with varying success. Trials of *stem cell transplantation* show promising efficacy in progressive dcSSc with a poor prognosis, but have significant side effects and a mortality of 5%; timing needs to be judged depending on significant renal, lung, or cardiac disease contraindications. Respiratory complications of SSc develop in roughly 30% of patients. Pulmonary hypertension (PAH) may occur and should be confirmed by appropriate investigation, including right heart catheterization. Iloprost infusions have also been shown to reduce PAH. *Angiotensin-converting enzyme (ACE) inhibitors* are particularly effective in reducing the renal complications of the disease, and early treatment may prevent the onset of renal crisis. *Proton pump inhibitors* treat esophageal disease effectively. Prokinetic dopamine agonists may help dysphagia and reflux. Intermittent broad-spectrum antibiotics (e.g., ciprofloxacin) may diminish bacterial overgrowth and blind loop syndrome. Recent randomized controlled trials have suggested that oral minocycline and D-penicillamine are not effective in SSc. Although SSc carries a high case-specific mortality, there have been significant advances in the management of skin, renal, and pulmonary complications. The identification of novel signaling pathways and mediators that are altered in SSc and contribute to tissue damage allows their selective targeting. This in turn opens the door for therapeutic strategies using novel compounds or innovative ways of using already approved drugs.

Rarely, older patients with late-onset disease and associated antipolymerase 3 antibodies may have scleroderma as a paraneoplastic phenomenon.

Specific Investigations

- Skin biopsy
- Renal function tests
- Blood pressure
- Anticentromere and anti–Scl-70 antibodies
- Chest x-ray
- Pulmonary function tests
- Echocardiography, natriuretic peptide
- Consider paraneoplastic disease and evaluation

Evidence Levels: **A** Double-blind study   **B** Clinical trial ≥ 20 subjects   **C** Clinical trial < 20 subjects   **D** Series ≥ 5 subjects   **E** Anecdotal case reports

Evidence-based guidelines for the use of immunologic tests: anticentromere, Scl-70, and nucleolar antibodies. Basu D, Reveille JD. Autoimmunity 2005; 38: 65–72.

Anti–Scl-70 antibodies are very useful in distinguishing SSc patients from healthy controls, from patients with other connective tissue diseases, and from unaffected family members. Among patients with SSc, anti–Scl-70 positivity is useful in predicting those at higher risk for diffuse cutaneous involvement and interstitial fibrosis/restrictive lung disease, though the latter has not been universally observed.

Once a patient is determined as being anti–Scl-70 positive or negative, there is little justification for serial determinations.

Cancer and scleroderma: a paraneoplastic disease with implications for malignancy screening. Shah AA, Casciola-Rosen L. Curr Opin Rheumatol 2015; 27: 563–70.

Emerging data have demonstrated that patients with scleroderma and RNA polymerase III autoantibodies have a significantly increased risk of cancer within a few years of scleroderma onset. Genetic alterations in the gene encoding RNA polymerase III (*POLR3A*) have been identified, and patients with somatic mutations in *POLR3A* have evidence of mutation-specific T-cell immune responses with generation of cross-reactive RNA polymerase III autoantibodies. These data strongly suggest that scleroderma is a by-product of antitumor immune responses in some patients. Additional epidemiologic data demonstrate that patients developing scleroderma at older ages may also have a short cancer–scleroderma interval, suggestive of paraneoplastic disease.

First-Line Therapies

• Nifedipine	A
• Iloprost	A
• ACE inhibitors	B
• Sildenafil	C

Iloprost for the treatment of systemic sclerosis. Hachulla E, Launay D, Hatron P-Y. Presse Med 2008; 37: 831–9.

An imbalance between prostacyclin (PGI$_2$) and thromboxane A$_2$ is observed in patients with scleroderma. Iloprost is a stable analog of PGI$_2$ with a plasma half-life of 20 to 30 minutes. Intravenous iloprost is effective in the treatment of RP related to scleroderma, reducing the frequency and severity of attacks. It also appears useful for the treatment of digital ulcers. Intravenous iloprost improves kidney vasospasm in patients with scleroderma. The possible benefits of sequential intravenous iloprost on the natural course of scleroderma require further investigation.

Calcium channel blockers for Raynaud's phenomenon. Thompson AE, Pope JE. Rheumatology 2005; 44: 145–50.

Calcium channel blockers yield moderate clinical improvement in the severity and frequency of Raynaud attacks, with an average decrease of 2.8 to 5.0 attacks per week and a 33% improvement in the severity of attacks compared with placebo.

Outcome of renal crisis in systemic sclerosis: relation to availability of angiotensin converting enzyme (ACE) inhibitors. Steen VD, Costantino JP, Shapiro AP, Medsger TA Jr. Ann Intern Med 1990; 113: 352–7.

Patients with SSc who develop hypertension should be treated with an ACE inhibitor. Improved survival and successful discontinuation of dialysis are possible when ACE inhibitors are used to treat scleroderma-related renal crisis.

Prospective, open-label, uncontrolled pilot study to study safety and efficacy of sildenafil in systemic sclerosis-related pulmonary artery hypertension and cutaneous vascular complications. Kumar U, Sankalp G, Sreenivas V, Kaur S, Misra D. Rheumatol Int 2013; 33: 1047–52.

A prospective, open-label, uncontrolled pilot study to examine the safety and efficacy of oral sildenafil in PAH, RP, digital infarcts, and ulcers in SSc. Seventeen patients fulfilling American College of Rheumatology (ACR) classification criteria for scleroderma and who had PAH were recruited. All patients were treated with oral sildenafil 25 mg three times a day for a period of 3 months. The pretreatment and posttreatment values of mean pulmonary artery pressure (mPAP), 6-min walk test, World Health Organization (WHO) class of dyspnea, and severity of RP were compared to look for any significant change. Sixteen patients who completed the 3-month follow-up had shown statistically significant improvement in 6-min walk test, WHO class of dyspnea, severity of RP, and mPAP. Also, there was no occurrence of new digital infarcts or ulcers, and existing ulcers showed signs of healing. Sildenafil is highly efficacious, cheaper, and a safe alternative to other available therapies for SSc-associated PAH, RP, and digital infarcts/ulcers.

Second-Line Therapies

• Methotrexate	A
• Cyclophosphamide	B
• Prednisolone	B
• Losartan	B
• Acitretin	C
• Colchicine	C
• UVA	C
• Mycophenolate	C

Treatment outcome in early diffuse cutaneous systemic sclerosis: the European Scleroderma Observational Study (ESOS). Herrick AL, Pan X, Peytrignet S, Lunt M, Hesselstrand R, Mouthon L, et al. Ann Rheum Dis 2017; 76: 1207–18.

A prospective, observational cohort study of early dcSSc (within 3 years of onset of skin thickening) over 2 years. Clinicians selected one of four protocols for each patient: methotrexate, mycophenolate mofetil (MMF), cyclophosphamide, or "no immunosuppressant." The primary outcome was the change in modified Rodnan skin score (mRSS). As a secondary outcome, an Inverse Probability of Treatment (IPT)-weighted Cox model was used to test for differences in survival. Of 326 patients, 65 were prescribed methotrexate, 118 MMF, 87 cyclophosphamide, and 56 no immunosuppressant. A reported 276 (84.7%) patients completed 12 months and 234 (71.7%) 24 months' follow-up (or reached the last visit date). There were statistically significant reductions in mRSS at 12 months in all groups: –4.0 (–5.2 to –2.7) units for methotrexate, –4.1 (–5.3 to –2.9) for MMF, –3.3 (–4.9 to –1.7) for cyclophosphamide, and –2.2 (–4.0 to –0.3) for no immunosuppressant (p value for between-group differences = 0.346).

There were no statistically significant differences in survival between protocols before ($p = 0.389$) or after weighting ($p = 0.440$), but survival was poorest in the no immunosuppressant group (84.0%) at 24 months.

Randomized placebo controlled trial of methotrexate in systemic sclerosis. Das SN, Alam MR, Islam N, Rahman MH, Sutradhar SR, Rahman S, et al. Mymensingh Med J 2005; 14: 71–4.

Clinical improvement after treatment was observed in a third of patients in the methotrexate (MTX) group but none in the placebo group, but this difference was not statistically significant. Anorexia, nausea, and occasional vomiting were common side effects in the MTX group and subsided in most cases with the passage of time, despite the continuation of therapy.

The efficacy of oral cyclophosphamide plus prednisolone in early diffuse systemic sclerosis. Calguneri M, Apras S, Ozbalkan Z, Ertenli I, Kiraz S, Ozturk MA, et al. Clin Rheumatol 2003; 22: 289–94.

In this study 27 patients with early diffuse SSc were treated with oral cyclophosphamide (1–2 mg/kg/day) plus oral prednisolone (40 mg every other day) between the years 1995 and 1998. The results regarding the efficacy and toxicity of cyclophosphamide were compared with those of 22 early SSc patients who had been treated with oral D-penicillamine between 1992 and 1995. There was a significant improvement in the skin score, maximal oral opening, flexion index, predicted forced vital capacity, and carbon monoxide diffusing capacity in the cyclophosphamide group. The decrease in skin score in the cyclophosphamide group started earlier than in the D-penicillamine group.

Randomized unblinded trial of cyclophosphamide versus azathioprine in the treatment of systemic sclerosis. Nadashkevich O, Davis P, Fritzler M, Kovalenko W. Clin Rheumatol 2006; 25: 205–12.

Thirty patients were assigned to receive oral cyclophosphamide (2 mg/kg daily for 12 months and then maintained on 1 mg/kg daily), and 30 patients were assigned to receive oral azathioprine (2.5 mg/kg daily for 12 months and then maintained on 2 mg/kg daily). During the first 6 months of the trial the patients also received prednisolone, which was started at a dosage of 15 mg daily and tapered to zero by the end of the sixth month. This study showed that cyclophosphamide is a promising disease-modifying medication for SSc, as it exhibited a positive influence on the evolution of disease.

Efficacy and safety of intravenous cyclophosphamide pulse therapy with oral prednisolone in the treatment of interstitial lung disease with systemic sclerosis: 4-year follow-up. Tochimoto A, Kawaguchi Y, Hara M, Tateishi M, Fukasawa C, Takagi K, et al. Mod Rheumatol 2011; 21: 296–301.

This open-label study of pulsed cyclophosphamide ($0.49/m^2$) with oral prednisolone concluded that the regimen was effective in producing improvement in interstitial lung disease (and skin disease), but that relapse was common, occurring in 5 of 13 patients, so maintenance therapy should be investigated.

Treatment of early diffuse cutaneous systemic sclerosis patients in Japan by low-dose corticosteroids for skin involvement. Takehara K. Clin Exp Rheumatol 2004; 22: S87–9.

Twenty-three patients with early dcSSc were treated with 20 mg/kg of prednisolone, with a significant reduction in skin scores.

Retinoic acid for treatment of systemic sclerosis and morphea: a literature review. Thomas RM, Worswick S, Aleshin M. Dermatol Ther 2017; 30: e12455.

A review of the current status of utilizing retinoids for scleroderma and morphea.

Losartan therapy for Raynaud's phenomenon and scleroderma: clinical and biochemical findings in a fifteen-week, randomized, parallel-group, controlled trial. Dziadzio M, Denton CP, Smith R, Blann HK, Bowers E, Black CM. Arthritis Rheum 1999; 42: 2646–55.

Losartan is an antagonist of angiotensin II receptor type I. In this randomized controlled trial 25 patients with primary RP and 27 with RP secondary to SSc were treated with either losartan (50 mg/day) or nifedipine (40 mg/day). Losartan reduced the frequency and severity of RP.

Therapeutic management of acral manifestations of systemic sclerosis. Meyer MF, Daigeler A, Lehnhardt M, Steinau H-U, Klein HH. Med Klin 2007; 102: 209–18.

Patients with acral manifestations of SSc are ideally treated by a team that includes a rheumatologist, dermatologist, hand surgeon, physiotherapist, and, eventually, a psychologist. Calcium channel antagonists, α_1-adrenergic blockade with prazosin, and prostacyclin analogs proved to be effective in the treatment of scleroderma-related RP. Losartan, an angiotensin II receptor inhibitor, and fluoxetine, a selective serotonin reuptake inhibitor, have been beneficial for SSc-associated RP in pilot studies.

Long-term evaluation of colchicine in the treatment of scleroderma. Alarcon-Segovia D, Ramos-Niembro F, Ibanez de Kasep G, Alcocer J, Perez-Tamayo R. J Rheumatol 1979; 6: 705–12.

In this early uncontrolled study, 19 patients with dcSSc were treated with colchicine 10.1 mg/week with a follow-up of 19 to 57 months. They reported improvement in skin elasticity, mouth opening, and finger mobility and a reduction in dysphagia.

Different low doses of broad-band UVA in the treatment of morphea and systemic sclerosis. El-Mofty M, Mostafa W, El-Darouty M, Bosseila M, Nada H, Yousef R, et al. Photodermatol Photoimmunol Photomed 2004; 20: 148–56.

Fifteen patients complaining of SSc received 20 sessions of UVA (320–400 nm); all improved clinically.

UVA is well tolerated, and there is experimental evidence that UVA1 may be beneficial. Further trials are required to confirm efficacy.

Effect of mycophenolate sodium in scleroderma-related interstitial lung disease. Simeón-Aznar CP, Fonollosa-Plá V, Tolosa-Vilella C, Selva-O'Callaghan A, Solans-Laqué R, Vilardell-Tarrés M. Clin Rheumatol 2011; 30: 1393–8.

An open-label study in 14 patients (dose 0.5–1.5 g twice a day) showed stabilization of pulmonary diffusion capacity.

A prospective open-label study of mycophenolate mofetil for the treatment of diffuse systemic sclerosis. Derk CT, Grace E, Shenin M, Naik M, Schulz S, Xiong W. Rheumatology (Oxford) 2009; 48: 1595–9.

Fifteen patients with dcSSc took part in an open-label study using MMF to treat their disease over a 12-month period. The mRSS significantly improved in those patients who tolerated the medication for longer than 3 months, as did severity scores of the general, peripheral vascular involvement, and skin. Pulmonary function studies showed a trend toward improvement, though not of statistical significance. The mPAP by two-dimensional echocardiography did not change.

Third-Line Therapies

• Extracorporeal photochemotherapy	B
• Imatinib	B
• Ciclosporin	C
• Rituximab	C
• Autologous nonmyeloablative hemopoietic stem cell transplantation	C
• Etanercept	D

Evidence Levels: **A** Double-blind study **B** Clinical trial ≥ 20 subjects **C** Clinical trial < 20 subjects **D** Series ≥ 5 subjects **E** Anecdotal case reports

Systemic Sclerosis Study Group. A randomized, double-blind, placebo-controlled trial of photopheresis in systemic sclerosis. Knobler RM, French LE, Kim Y, Bisaccia E, Graninger W, Nahavandi H, et al. J Am Acad Dermatol 2006; 54: 793–9.

This randomized, double-blind, placebo-controlled clinical trial was conducted at 16 investigational sites in the United States, Canada, and Europe. Sixty-four patients with typical clinical and histologic findings of scleroderma of less than 2 years' duration were studied to evaluate the efficacy of photopheresis in the treatment of patients with SSc. Photopheresis induced significant improvement of skin and joint involvement in patients with scleroderma of recent onset.

Imatinib mesylate (Gleevec) in the treatment of diffuse cutaneous systemic sclerosis: results of a 1-year, phase IIa, single-arm, open-label clinical trial. Spiera RF, Gordon JK, Mersten JN, Magro CM, Mehta M, Wildman H, et al. Ann Rheum Dis 2011; 70: 1003–9.

Twenty-four of 30 patients showed an improved modified Rodnan skin score of more than 20% after 12 months of 400 mg daily of imatinib. Pulmonary diffusing capacity was stabilized. Unfortunately, adverse events were common and often severe.

Ciclosporin in systemic sclerosis. Clements PJ, Lachenbruch PA, Sterz M, Danovitch G, Hawkins R, Ippoliti A, et al. Arthritis Rheum 1993; 36: 75–83.

ciclosporin is an immunosuppressive drug that selectively inhibits the release of interleukin-2 (IL-2), which has been shown to be increased in SSc serum. This study showed that ciclosporin may improve skin induration, but had no effect on internal organ involvement.

The high incidence of nephrotoxicity with ciclosporin therapy reduces its use in SSc where renal crisis may occur.

B cell depletion in diffuse progressive systemic sclerosis: safety, skin score modification and IL-6 modulation in an up to thirty-six months follow-up open-label trial. Bosello S, De Santis M, Lama G, Spanò C, Angelucci C, Tolusso B, et al. Arthritis Res Ther 2010; 12: R54.

Rituximab (1 g by infusion twice at an interval of 2 weeks) improved the modified Rodnan skin score by a median of 43.3% in nine patients with diffuse type SSc. Treatment was well tolerated and appeared safe after 36 months follow-up. Retreatment was necessary in two patients to treat joint disease.

Autologous hematopoietic stem cell transplantation has better outcomes than conventional therapies in patients with rapidly progressive systemic sclerosis. Del Papa N, Onida F, Zaccara E, Saporiti G, Maglione W, Tagliaferri E, et al. Bone Marrow Transplant 2017; 52: 53–8.

A retrospective evaluation of the efficacy of autologous hematopoietic stem cell transplantation (AHSCT) in 18 patients with rapidly progressive diffuse cutaneous systemic sclerosis (rp-dcSSc), comparing their disease outcomes with those of 36 demographically and clinically matched patients treated with conventional therapies. Cutaneous involvement, measured by a modified Rodnan skin score (mRss), lung diffusion capacity measured by diffusing capacity of lung for carbon monoxide (DLCO), and disease activity utilizing the European Scleroderma Study Group (ESSG) scoring system, were the outcome variables measured at the baseline time and then every 12 months for the following 60 months in both the AHSCT-treated patients and the control group. In the AHSCT group, treatment-related mortality was 5.6%. In this group, both mRss and ESSG scores showed a

significant reduction 1 year after AHSCT ($p < 0.002$); these results were maintained until the end of follow-up. Conversely, DLCO values remained stable during the whole period of follow-up. Survival rate of the AHSCT group was much higher than that observed in the whole control group ($p = 0.0005$).

This study confirms that the AHSCT is effective in prolonging survival, as well as in inducing a rapid reduction of skin involvement and disease activity, and preserving lung function in patients with rp-dcSSc.

Etanercept as treatment for diffuse scleroderma: a pilot study. Ellman MH, McDonald PA, Hayes FA. Arthritis Rheum 2000; 43: s392.

This targeted fusion protein blocks TNF-α. Four out of 10 patients treated with etanercept 25 mg subcutaneously twice weekly had improvements of skin scores and healing of digital ulcers.

OTHER: INTERNAL ORGAN INVOLVEMENT

Prostacyclin for pulmonary hypertension in adults. Paramothayan NS, Lasserson TJ, Wells AU, Walters EH. Cochrane Database Syst Rev 2005; 2: CD002994.

There is evidence that intravenous prostacyclin, in addition to conventional therapy at tolerable doses optimized by titration, can confer some short-term benefits (up to 12 weeks of treatment) in exercise capacity, New York Heart Association (NYHA) functional class, and cardiopulmonary hemodynamics. There is also some evidence that patients with more severe disease based on NYHA functional class showed a greater response to treatment.

Review of bosentan in the management of pulmonary arterial hypertension. Gabbay E, Fraser J, McNeil K. Vasc Health Risk Manage 2007; 3: 887–900.

Bosentan was the first endothelin receptor antagonist approved for use in PAH. Clinical studies have shown that in PAH the use of bosentan is associated with improved exercise capacity, WHO functional class, cardiopulmonary hemodynamics, and quality of life and delayed time to clinical worsening compared with placebo. Further, long-term studies have demonstrated improved survival with the use of bosentan compared with historical controls, although there are no placebo-controlled data confirming a survival benefit.

Bosentan therapy for pulmonary arterial hypertension. Rubin LJ, Badesch DB, Barst RJ, Galie N, Black CM, Keogh A, et al. N Engl J Med 2002; 346: 896–903.

In this randomized control trial of patients with PAH, the dual endothelin receptor antagonist bosentan improved exercise capacity. SSc patients with PAH were shown to have improved exercise capacity on subgroup analysis.

Interstitial lung disease associated with systemic sclerosis: what is the evidence for efficacy of cyclophosphamide?. Berezne A, Valeyre D, Ranque B, Guillevin L, Mouthon L. Ann NY Acad Sci 2007; 1110: 271–84.

Since 1993, the beneficial effect of oral or intravenous cyclophosphamide in the treatment of SSc-related ILD has been reported in retrospective studies, with one showing improvement of pulmonary function test scores and/or chest CT at 1 year and improvement of survival at 16 months. The results of two controlled trials were recently reported. The Scleroderma Lung Study, a prospective, randomized, placebo-controlled trial, included 158 patients, of which 145 completed at least 6 months of treatment. The course of forced vital capacity (primary outcome) adjusted at 1 year was significantly better in the group treated with oral cyclophosphamide ($p < 0.03$), although the effect of cyclophosphamide was minor.

Cyclophosphamide is associated with pulmonary function and survival benefit in patients with scleroderma and alveolitis. White B, Moore WC, Wigley FM, Xiai HQ, Wise RA. Ann Intern Med 2000; 132: 947–54.

This retrospective cohort study involving 103 patients with SSc showed that lung inflammation (alveolitis) treated with cyclophosphamide improves lung function outcome and survival.

Renal transplantation in scleroderma. Chang YJ, Spiera H. Medicine 1999; 78: 382–5.

A retrospective study from data collected by the United Network for Organ Sharing (UNOS) Scientific Renal Transplant Registry. Between 1987 and 1997, 86 patients with SSc had renal transplantation. At 5-year follow-up, 47% of the patients were still alive. Patients whose renal function does not improve with ACE inhibitors should be considered for transplantation.

Evidence Levels: **A** Double-blind study **B** Clinical trial ≥ 20 subjects **C** Clinical trial < 20 subjects **D** Series ≥ 5 subjects **E** Anecdotal case reports

226

Sebaceous hyperplasia

Surod Qazaz, John Berth-Jones

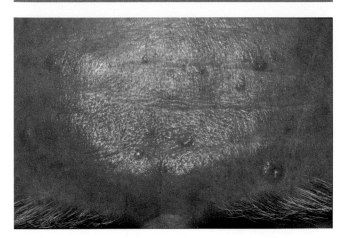

Sebaceous hyperplasia is a common benign condition mainly affecting adults of middle age and older, but it may occur at any time or even be present at birth. Lesions can be single or multiple and manifest as soft yellow papules, often with central umbilication, typically measuring 1 to 4 mm, mainly on the face (commonly the nose, cheeks, and forehead). Sebaceous hyperplasia occasionally appears in other areas such as the chest, areola, mouth, and genitalia. There are occasional reports of giant lesions or arrangement in linear or zosteriform patterns. They appear more frequently in immunocompromised patients, especially after transplantation in patients on ciclosporin and corticosteroids.

MANAGEMENT STRATEGY

Sebaceous hyperplasia is a completely benign condition that does not require treatment; however, lesions can be cosmetically unfavorable. There may also be concern over differential diagnoses, which include basal cell carcinoma, rhinophyma, angiofibroma, trichoepithelioma, nevus sebaceous, dermal nevus, plane warts, lupus miliaris disseminatus faciei, and syringoma.

We normally use *cautery (electrodesiccation)* or *cryotherapy* first line. It can be helpful to treat one or two test lesions to assess patient satisfaction before treating the rest. Cryotherapy can be fairly gentle in view of the benign nature of the lesions, and it can be helpful to protect surrounding skin using an auriscope speculum. Other treatments include *surgical excision, photodynamic therapy, laser, isotretinoin,* and *chemical peels.* Because the objective is cosmetic improvement, it is important to inform the patient about the risk of scarring with these techniques. Occasionally, sebaceous hyperplasia is treated surgically. This has the advantage of providing tissue for histology when there is any doubt about the diagnosis. Shave excision or curettage is usually sufficient, both to obtain histologic confirmation and to achieve removal with minimal scarring.

Specific Investigation

- No specific investigations are usually required, as the diagnosis is clinical.

Biopsy is occasionally indicated, mainly to exclude basal cell carcinoma; histology will show enlargement of individual glands with increased numbers of fully mature sebaceous lobules with no atypia or dysplasia.

Alta prevalencia de hiperplasias sebaceas en transplantados renales. Perez-Espana L, Prats I, Sanz A, Mayor M. Nefrologia 2003; 23: 179–80.

The authors looked at 163 renal transplant patients, of whom 26% had sebaceous hyperplasia. This was greatest in patients on ciclosporin. Other immunosuppressants (azathioprine, mycophenolate mofetil, and tacrolimus) showed no significant increase in the incidence of sebaceous hyperplasia.

First-Line Therapies

- Conservative management/cosmetic camouflage   **E**
- Electrodesiccation/cautery   **C**
- Cryotherapy   **E**

Surgical pearl: intralesional electrodesiccation of sebaceous hyperplasia. Bader RS, Scarborough DA. J Am Acad Dermatol 2000; 42: 127–8.

The authors describe a nice technique for intralesional electrodesiccation using a fine epilating needle. They report no recurrence in more than 30 lesions followed up to 7 months.

Guidelines of care for cryosurgery. American Academy of Dermatology Committee on Guidelines of Care. J Am Acad Dermatol 1994; 31: 648–53.

The authors include sebaceous hyperplasia as a condition treatable with cryotherapy.

Second-Line Therapies

- Surgery/curettage   **E**
- Isotretinoin   **B**
- Photodynamic therapy   **C**
- Topical retinoids   **E**

Successful treatment of ciclosporin-induced sebaceous hyperplasia with oral isotretinoin in two renal transplant recipients. McDonald SK, Goh MS, Chong AH. Australas J Dermatol 2011; 52: 227–30.

Treatment was effective and well tolerated.

Presenile diffuse familial sebaceous hyperplasia successfully treated with low-dose isotretinoin: a report of two cases and review of the published work. Liu YS, Cheng YP, Liu CI, Yang CY, Yang CY. J Dermatol 2016; 43: 1205–8.

Two cases of presenile diffuse familial sebaceous hyperplasia were successfully treated without recurrence with prolonged low-dose isotretinoin (0.2 mg/kg per day, a cumulative dose of 41 and 64 mg/kg, respectively).

Sebaceous hyperplasia: systemic treatment with isotretinoin. Tagliolatto S, Santos Neto Ode O, Alchorne MM, Enokihara MY. An Bras Dermatol 2015; 90: 211–5.

Twenty patients were treated with isotretinoin in a prospective study. Each received 1 mg/kg per day for 2 months. The number of the lesions decreased significantly, with benefit persisting after 2 years.

Treatment of sebaceous gland hyperplasia by photodynamic therapy with 5-aminolevulinic acid and a blue light source or intense pulsed light source. Gold MH, Bradshaw VL, Boring MM, Bridges TM, Biron JA, Lewis TL. J Drugs Dermatol 2004; 3: S6–9.

Twelve patients were randomized to topical aminolevulinic acid and either blue light or intense pulsed light. They had four treatments at 1-month intervals. Both treatment arms had more than 50% reduction in the number of the lesions without recurrence at 12 weeks' follow-up.

Third-Line Therapies

• Topical aminolevulinic acid and pulsed dye laser	D
• Pulsed dye laser	D
• Diode laser	D
• Argon laser	E
• Carbon dioxide laser	E
• Erbium:YAG laser	E
• 1720-nm laser	E
• Bichloroacetic acid	C
• Pin hole with squeezing technique	E

Photodynamic therapy with topical aminolevulinic acid and pulsed dye laser irradiation for sebaceous hyperplasia. Alster TS, Tanzi EL. J Drugs Dermatol 2003; 2: 501–4.

Ten patients were treated with topical 5-ALA followed 1 hour later by the 595-nm pulsed dye laser. They were compared with untreated lesions and laser-only–treated lesions. Laser photodynamic therapy yielded the best results; 70% of lesions had total clearing after one treatment, the remaining 30% after two treatments.

Elucidating the pulsed-dye laser treatment of sebaceous hyperplasia in vivo with real-time confocal scanning laser microscopy. Aghassi D, Gonzalez E, Anderson RR, Rajadhyaksha M, Gonzalez S. J Am Acad Dermatol 2000; 43: 49–53.

The authors treated 29 lesions on seven different patients with pulsed dye laser. There was improvement in 93% of lesions and complete clearance in 28%. No scarring or hyperpigmentation was noted. However, 28% of the lesions reappeared and 7% returned to their original size.

Pulsed-dye laser for treatment of sebaceous hyperplasia. Tsai T-H, Chang Y-J. J Am Acad Dermatol 2012; 664 (Suppl 1): AB215.

In this randomized, controlled, split-face trial, Asian (skin types 3–5) patients received two treatments separated by a 4-week interval, with one half of the face treated with long-pulsed dye laser (5 mm, 595-nm pulsed dye laser at pulse duration of 10 ms), and the other half of the face with short-pulsed dye laser (5-mm pulses of the 595-nm pulsed dye laser at pulse duration of 0.45 ms). Fluences ranged from 7 to 10 J/cm². The short pulse

achieved more obvious improvement of sebaceous hyperplasia than the long-pulsed dye laser, but adverse effects after short pulse included obvious purpura, which lasted about 1 to 2 weeks, and a few cases of crusts and postinflammatory hyperpigmentation. After long-pulsed dye laser, mild erythema and swelling lasted a few days without purpura.

Sebaceous hyperplasia treated with a 1450-nm diode laser. No D, McLaren M, Chotzen V, Kilmer SL. Dermatol Surg 2004; 30: 382–4.

The authors treated 10 patients. Both objective and subjective improvement was noted in the majority of patients, with very few side effects.

A 3 year experience with the argon laser in dermatotherapy. Landthaler M, Haina D, Waidelich W, Braun-Falco O. J Dermatol Surg Oncol 1984; 10: 456–61.

The authors report on 477 patients with different cutaneous lesions treated with an argon laser, including sebaceous hyperplasia.

Sebaceous gland hyperplasia as a side effect of cyclosporin A. Treatment with the CO₂ laser. Walther T, Hohenleutner U, Landthaler M. Dtsch Med Wochenschr 1998; 123: 798–800.

This article reports the treatment of a patient with CO₂ laser. The lesions cleared without scarring.

Controlled cosmetic dermal ablation in the facial region with the erbium:YAG laser. Riedel F, Bergler W, Baker-Schreyer A, Stein E, Hormann K. HNO 1999; 47: 101–6.

This article reports on 216 patients with different facial lesions. The authors report good to excellent results with sebaceous hyperplasia.

Treatment of sebaceous hyperplasia with a novel 1720-nm laser. Winstanley D, Blalock T, Houghton N, Ross EV. J Drugs Dermatol 2012; 11: 1323–6.

Four patients were treated with a test treatment followed by two full treatment sessions. At 3 months post treatment, there was nearly complete clearance without residual scarring.

The treatment of benign sebaceous hyperplasia with the topical application of bichloroacetic acid. Rosian R, Goslen JB, Brodell RT. J Dermatol Surg Oncol 1991; 17: 876–9.

The authors treated 67 lesions in 20 patients: 66 cleared after one application of 100% bichloroacetic acid, with minimal scarring.

Sebaceous hyperplasia effectively improved by the pin-hole technique with squeezing. Jae-Hong K, Hwa-Young P, Won-Soo L, Jin-Soo K. Ann Dermatol 2013; 25: 257–8.

The authors describe a technique of creating a 1-mm pinhole into the lesion with a carbon dioxide laser followed by squeezing the lesion with a comedo extractor. The procedure was performed with topical anesthetic cream. Most of the lesions were flattened after the treatment. There was no recurrence of any of the lesions 3 months after the treatment.

Evidence Levels: **A** Double-blind study **B** Clinical trial ≥ 20 subjects **C** Clinical trial < 20 subjects **D** Series ≥ 5 subjects **E** Anecdotal case reports

227

Seborrheic eczema

Anja K. Weidmann, Jason D.L. Williams,
Ian Coulson

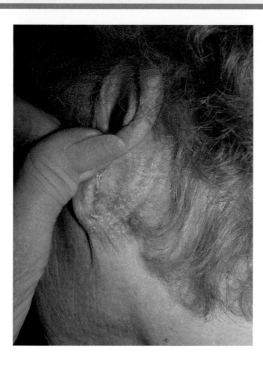

Seborrheic eczema (seborrheic dermatitis) is a chronic dermatitis affecting between 3% and 10% of adults, becoming more prevalent with age. It is more common in patients with both idiopathic and neuroleptic-induced Parkinson disease, HIV, AIDS, and chronic alcoholics and accounts for up to 3.5% of dermatology specialist outpatient consultations.

The signs and symptoms comprise erythema, greasy scaling, pruritus, burning, and dryness in a typical distribution pattern affecting the scalp and the face (particularly the nasolabial folds, eyebrows, and ears). Blepharoconjunctivitis may occur alone or in conjunction with skin lesions.

Seborrheic eczema can also affect infants up to the age of 3 to 4 months in the diaper area.

Although the etiology has yet to be fully elucidated, important factors are *Malassezia* yeasts, immune status, and individual susceptibility.

MANAGEMENT STRATEGY

Seborrheic eczema is a chronic relapsing dermatitis that responds to a variety of immunosuppressive and antifungal therapies, but there is no cure.

Seborrheic eczema of the face is dry and flaky, so that soap avoidance and substitution with a *light emollient cleanser* will help. Facial and flexural disease responds to *mild topical corticosteroids*, alone or in combination with a variety of *topical antipityrosporal agents* such as *miconazole, ketoconazole, bifonazole, itraconazole,* or *ciclopir oxolamine*. An ointment containing *lithium gluconate/succinate* may also be helpful.

Studies have demonstrated short-term efficacy with the topical calcineurin inhibitors *tacrolimus* and *pimecrolimus*. *Terbinafine cream* and *metronidazole gel* may also be beneficial, whereas resistant cases may respond to short courses of *oral itraconazole* or *terbinafine*.

Scalp seborrheic dermatitis can be helped with *topical ketoconazole, zinc pyrithione, selenium sulfide, corticosteroid* and *tar* shampoos, or a *propylene glycol* preparation formulated for scalp use. Severe cases with marked hyperkeratosis or pityriasis amiantacea may require topical keratolytics such as *salicylic acid ointment* or *coconut compound ointment*.

Specific Investigations

- Dermoscopy
- Tests for HIV infection
- Zinc levels

In neonates and children consider acrodermatitis enteropathica or transient neonatal zinc deficiency, which can mimic recalcitrant seborrheic dermatitis. A similar eruption in parenterally fed adults also can occur due to zinc deficiency.

Seborrheic dermatitis may represent a marker for HIV infection and should prompt consideration of testing.

Dermoscopy can be useful in differentiating scalp psoriasis from seborrhoeic dermatitis. Kim GW, Jung HJ, Ko HC, Kim MB, Lee WJ, Lee SJ, et al. Br J Dermatol 2011; 164: 652–6.

Dermoscopy features on the scalp include arborizing vessels and comma vessels.

These findings appear to have been replicated in several later studies. It may be of value to readers as a means of differentiating from scalp psoriasis.

New insights into HIV-1-primary skin disorders. Cedeno-Laurent F, Gömez-Flores M, Mendez N, Ancer-Rodríguez J, Bryant JL, Gaspari AA, et al. Int AIDS Soc 2011; 24: 14–5.

This article reports seborrheic dermatitis in up to 40% of patients with HIV with worsening severity as lymphocyte counts decline. Incidence in patients with AIDS is up to 80%.

Seborrheic dermatitis in neuroleptic induced parkinsonism. Binder RL, Jonelis FJ. Arch Dermatol 1983; 119: 473–5.

Comparison of 42 hospitalized patients with drug-induced parkinsonism using psychiatric patients as controls showed an incidence of seborrheic dermatitis of 59.5% in those with parkinsonism, compared with 15% in the control group.

Cutaneous changes in chronic alcoholics. Rao GS. Indian J Dermatol Venereol Leprol 2004; 70: 79–81.

In this study of 200 alcoholic patients attending for alcohol detoxification, seborrheic dermatitis was the second most common skin disorder (11.5% of cases).

NONSCALP DISEASE

First-Line Therapies

• Topical ketoconazole	A
• Mild to moderate topical corticosteroids	A
• Emollients and soap substitutes	D

Ketoconazole 2% cream versus hydrocortisone 1% cream in the treatment of seborrhoeic dermatitis. A double-blind comparative study. Stratigos JD, Antoniou C, Katsambas A, Böhler K, Fritsch P, Schmölz A, et al. J Am Acad Dermatol 1988; 19: 850–3.

In this double-blind study, 72 patients were treated daily for 4 weeks with either ketoconazole 2% cream or hydrocortisone 1% cream; 80.5% of the ketoconazole group showed a significant improvement in all symptoms compared with 94.4% of the hydrocortisone group. There was no significant difference in relapse rates between the two groups.

Topical antifungals for seborrhoeic dermatitis. Okokon EO, Verbeek JH, Ruotsalainen JH, Ojo OO, Bakhoya VN. Cochrane Database Syst Rev 2015; 5: CD008138.

This review included 51 studies with a total of 9052 participants examining a wide range of treatments. Eight trials compared use of topical 2% ketoconazole with placebo or vehicle. Active treatment was associated with a 31% lower risk of failure of clearance. Six trials compared topical ketoconazole with topical steroids. Remission rates were similar (RR 1.17, 95% confidence interval [CI] 0.58–1.64), but occurrence of side effects was 44% lower in the ketoconazole group. Quality of data was limited by study duration and heterogeneity between studies.

Second-Line Therapies	
• Lithium succinate/lithium gluconate	A
• Ciclopirox olamine cream	A
• Topical calcineurin inhibitors	A
• Topical azoles (miconazole/clotrimazole)	A

Lithium gluconate 8% vs. ketoconazole 2% in the treatment of seborrhoeic dermatitis: a multicenter, randomized study. Dreno B, Chosidow O, Revuz J, Moyse D. Br J Dermatol 2003; 148: 1230–6.

This randomized, noninferiority study compared 8% lithium gluconate twice daily for 8 weeks with ketoconazole 2% twice weekly for 4 weeks then once weekly for a further 4 weeks in moderate-to-severe seborrheic dermatitis. Two hundred and sixty-nine patients were treated, and complete response was achieved in 52.0% and 30.1%, respectively.

Randomized, placebo-controlled, double-blind study on clinical efficacy of ciclopirox olamine 1% cream in facial seborrhoeic dermatitis. Dupuy P, Maurette C, Amoric JC, Chosidow O. Br J Dermatol 2001; 144: 1033–7.

One hundred and twenty-nine patients were randomized to receive either 1% ciclopirox olamine cream twice daily for 28 days, followed by once-daily application for a further 28 days, or placebo. At 8 weeks, 63% of patients in the ciclopirox olamine group achieved clearance of their test lesions versus 34% of placebo patients (p < 0.007).

An open, randomized, prospective, comparative study of topical pimecrolimus 1% cream and topical ketoconazole 2% cream in the treatment of seborrheic dermatitis. Koc E, Arca E, Kose O, Akar A. J Dermatolog Treat 2009; 20: 4–9.

In this open-label, randomized comparison study, 48 patients received either pimecrolimus 1% cream or ketoconazole 2% cream twice daily for 6 weeks. At 12 weeks both groups achieved statistically significant reductions in clinical

severity scores, with an average decrease of 86.2% and 86.1%, respectively (p < 0.05). There was no significant difference between the two groups.

Single-blind, randomized controlled trial evaluating the treatment of facial seborrheic dermatitis with hydrocortisone 1% ointment compared with tacrolimus 0.1% ointment in adults. Papp KA, Papp A, Dahmer B, Clark CS. J Am Acad Dermatol 2012; 67: e11–5.

Thirty patients received either hydrocortisone 1% cream or tacrolimus 0.1% ointment twice daily to symptomatic areas for 12 weeks. Both groups showed improvement in clinical severity, with patients using tacrolimus needing fewer applications of treatment.

Proactive treatment of adult facial seborrhoeic dermatitis with 0.1% tacrolimus ointment: randomized, double-blind, vehicle-controlled, multicenter trial. Kim TW, Mun JH, Jwa SW, Song M, Kim HS, Ko HC, et al. Acta Derm Venereol 2013; 93: 557–61.

In this double-blind, placebo-controlled trial, 75 patients used tacrolimus 0.1% ointment twice daily to stabilize their facial seborrheic dermatitis. They were then randomized to use tacrolimus 0.1% once a week, twice a week, or vehicle twice a week, for 10 weeks. Both treatment groups showed significant improvements in erythema, scaling, and pruritus compared with baseline (p < 0.001) with lower recurrence rates compared with vehicle (p < 0.005).

Third-Line Therapies	
• Oral terbinafine	A
• Oral itraconazole	B
• Metronidazole gel	B
• Phototherapy	C
• Benzoyl peroxide	C
• Topical terbinafine	C

Oral terbinafine in the treatment of multisite seborrheic dermatitis: a multicenter, double-blind placebo-controlled study. Vena GA, Micala G, Santoianni P, Cassano N, Peruzzi E. Int J Immunopathol Pharmacol 2005; 18: 745–53.

One hundred and seventy-four patients with seborrheic dermatitis were randomized to receive either terbinafine 250 mg once daily or placebo for 6 weeks. Terbinafine was statistically more effective at achieving 50% improvement than placebo in nonexposed sites (70% vs. 45%) and in achieving patient satisfaction (66% vs. 40%). There was no statistical difference in patients with lesions on exposed sites.

Efficacy of oral itraconazole in the treatment and relapse prevention of moderate to severe seborrheic dermatitis: a randomized, placebo-controlled trial. Ghodsi SZ, Abbas Z, Abedeni R. Am J Clin Dermatol 2015; 16: 431–7.

In this double-blind, placebo-controlled trial, 68 patients with moderate/severe seborrheic eczema received itraconazole 200 mg once daily or placebo daily for 1 week and then for the first 2 days of the month for 3 months. The treatment group showed a more significant clinical improvement (p < 0.023) and lower relapse rates compared with placebo (p = 0.003) with response rates of 93.8%, 87.5%, and 93.1% at the end of 2 weeks, 1 month, and 4 months.

Evidence Levels: **A** Double-blind study **B** Clinical trial ≥ 20 subjects **C** Clinical trial < 20 subjects **D** Series ≥ 5 subjects **E** Anecdotal case reports

Metronidazole 0.75% gel vs. ketoconazole 2% cream in the treatment of facial seborrheic dermatitis: a randomized, double blind study. Seckin D, Gurbuz O, Akin O. J Eur Acad Dermatol Venereol 2007; 21: 345–50.

Sixty patients with facial seborrheic dermatitis used either 0.75% metronidazole gel (with ketoconazole cream as vehicle) or 2% ketoconazole cream (with metronidazole gel as vehicle) for 4 weeks. Around 80% improvement was noted in both groups, with no statistical difference.

Narrow-band ultraviolet B (TL-01) phototherapy is an effective and safe treatment option for patients with severe seborrhoeic dermatitis. Pirkhammer D, Seeber A, Honigsmann H, Tanew A. Br J Dermatol 2000; 143: 964–8.

Eighteen patients were treated three times weekly until complete clearing or to a maximum of 8 weeks. Six showed complete clearance and 12 marked improvement.

Benzoyl peroxide in seborrheic dermatitis. Bonnetblanc JM, Bernard P. Arch Dermatol 1986; 122: 752.

Twenty-eight of 30 patients showed improvement with 1 week's use of 2.5% benzoyl peroxide preparation. All relapsed within 2 to 12 weeks of stopping treatment.

Efficiency of terbinafine 1% cream in comparison with ketoconazole 2% cream and placebo in patients with facial seborrheic dermatitis. Azimi H, Golforoushan F, Jaberian M, Talghini S, Goldust M. J Dermatolog Treat 2013 [Epub ahead of print].

Ninety patients were randomized to use terbinafine 1% cream, ketoconazole 2% cream, or vehicle twice daily for 4 weeks. Both treatment groups showed a significant improvement in clinical severity scores compared with vehicle ($p = 0.003$). No significant difference was found between the two active treatments ($p > 0.05$).

SCALP DISEASE

First-Line Therapies

• Ketoconazole shampoo	A
• Ciclopirox shampoo	A
• Zinc pyrithione shampoo	A

Topical antiinflammatory agents for seborrhoeic dermatitis of the face or scalp. Kastarinen H, Oksanen T, Okokon EO, Kiviniemi VV, Airola K, Jyrkkä J, et al. Cochrane Database Syst Rev 2014; 5: CD009446.

Successful treatment and prophylaxis of scalp seborrhoeic dermatitis and dandruff with 2% ketoconazole shampoo: results of a multicenter, double-blind, placebo-controlled trial. Peter RU, Richarz-Barthauer U. Br J Dermatol 1995; 132: 441–5.

Five hundred seventy-five patients with moderate to severe scalp seborrheic dermatitis and dandruff were treated with ketoconazole 2% shampoo twice weekly for 2 months, producing clearance in 88%. Three hundred twelve responders were then randomized to active treatment or placebo once weekly. There were fewer relapses in the ketoconazole prophylactic treatment group after 6 months (47% vs. 19%).

Treatment and prophylaxis of seborrheic dermatitis of the scalp with antipityrosporal 1% ciclopirox shampoo. Shuster S, Meynadier J, Kerl H, Nolting S. Arch Dermatol 2005; 141: 47–52.

In this double-blind, vehicle-control trial, 949 patients received ciclopirox 1% shampoo either twice or once weekly or vehicle. After 4 weeks responders were randomized for maintenance therapy with one of the three regimens for a further 12 weeks. At 4 weeks both ciclopirox regimens were statistically more effective than placebo (response rates 57.9% vs. 45.4% vs. 31.6%). During the maintenance phase relapse rates were significantly lower for both active regimens compared with placebo (14.9% vs. 22.1% vs. 35.5%).

A multicenter randomized trial of ketoconazole 2% and zinc pyrithione 1% shampoos in severe dandruff and seborrheic dermatitis. Piérard-Franchimont C, Goffin V, Decroix J, Piérard GE. Skin Pharmacol Appl Skin Physiol 2002; 15: 434–41.

In this 4-week, open-label, randomized trial, 331 patients with either seborrheic dermatitis or dandruff were randomized to either twice-weekly ketoconazole 2% shampoo or at least twice-weekly zinc pyrithione 1% shampoo. Both groups showed clinical benefit with reductions in dandruff severity of 73% and 61%, respectively.

Second-Line Therapies

• Propylene glycol lotion	A
• Potent/super potent topical corticosteroids	A
• Miconazole	A
• Selenium sulfide shampoo	C

Propylene glycol in the treatment of seborrhoeic dermatitis of the scalp: a double-blind study. Faergemann J. Cutis 1988; 42: 69–71.

Thirty-nine patients with scalp seborrheic dermatitis were treated in a double-blind controlled study with 15% propylene glycol in a base of 50% ethanol and 35% water or vehicle alone: 89% in the group treated with propylene glycol showed healing, compared with 32% in the control group.

A randomized, double-blind, placebo-controlled trial of ketoconazole 2% shampoo versus selenium sulfide 2.5% shampoo in the treatment of moderate to severe dandruff. Danby FW, Maddin WS, Margeson LJ, Rosenthal D. J Am Acad Dermatol 1993; 29: 1008–12.

A total of 236 patients were included in the study. Both medicated shampoos were statistically better than placebo in treating scaling and itching. However, ketoconazole was superior to selenium shampoo.

Seborrhoeic dermatitis and *Pityrosporum orbiculare*: treatment of seborrhoeic dermatitis of the scalp with miconazole-hydrocortisone (Daktacort), miconazole and hydrocortisone. Faergemann J. Br J Dermatol 1986; 114: 695–700.

In this double-blind, randomized, controlled study, 70 patients received 2% miconazole base and 1% hydrocortisone (Daktacort), 2% miconazole base, or 1% hydrocortisone daily for 3 weeks. The drugs were incorporated into a solution of 60% ethyl alcohol, 10% propylene glycol, and purified water. After 3 weeks responders moved to maintenance therapy with the same agent for a further 3 weeks. Nonresponders continued with daily application.

All three groups showed reduced organism culture and clinical improvement with 82.6%, 65.2%, and 29.1% deemed clear in each group.

Multicenter, double-blind, parallel group study investigating the noninferiority of efficacy and safety of a 2% miconazole nitrate shampoo in comparison with a 2% ketoconazole shampoo in the treatment of seborrhoeic dermatitis of the scalp. Buechner SA. J Dermatolog Treat 2014; 25: 226–31.

In this randomized, double-blind, comparative, parallel-group, multicenter study, 274 patients used either miconazole nitrate 2% shampoo or ketoconazole 2% shampoo twice weekly for 4 weeks. Miconazole was found to be noninferior to ketoconazole.

Efficacy of betamethasone valerate 0.1% thermophobic foam in seborrhoeic dermatitis of the scalp: an open-label, multicenter, prospective trial on 180 patients. Milani M, Antonio Di Molfetta S, Gramazio R, Fiorella C, Frisario C, Fuzio E, et al. Curr Med Res Opin 2003; 19: 342–5.

In this open-label trial, 180 patients were treated with 2 g of betamethasone 17-valerate 0.1% foam daily for 15 days and then every other day for 15 days. At 4 weeks there was a statistically significant clinical improvement. Eighty-five percent of patients preferred the betamethasone foam to previous treatments.

Efficacious and safe management of moderate to severe scalp seborrhoeic dermatitis using clobetasol propionate shampoo 0.05% combined with ketoconazole shampoo 2%: a randomized, controlled study. Ortonne JP, Nikkels AF, Reich K, Ponce Olivera RM, Lee JH, Kerrouche N, et al. Br J Dermatol 2011; 165: 171–6.

This investigator-blind, randomized, controlled trial had four arms of treatment: ketoconazole 2% shampoo twice weekly, clobetasol propionate 0.05% shampoo twice weekly, alternating ketoconazole and clobetasol twice weekly, or ketoconazole four times weekly alternating with clobetasol twice weekly for 4 weeks. This was followed by a 4-week maintenance phase where all patients received weekly ketoconazole and a further 4-week follow-up phase. In total 326 patients were included. All groups demonstrated clinical improvement, and all three clobetasol-containing regimens were significantly more effective than ketoconazole alone. Of these the twice weekly alternating clobetasol and ketoconazole regimen was the most effective.

The authors would like to stress that potent and superpotent steroids may not be considered suitable for long-term use.

Evidence Levels: **A** Double-blind study   **B** Clinical trial ≥ 20 subjects   **C** Clinical trial < 20 subjects   **D** Series ≥ 5 subjects   **E** Anecdotal case reports

Seborrheic keratosis

Richard J. Motley

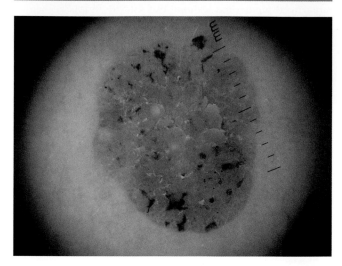

Seborrheic keratosis is a benign, exophytic, warty, pigmented growth of the skin surface that becomes increasingly common with age, with the degree of pigmentation varying with skin type from light gray to intense black. Found on all areas of the body, but mainly on the trunk, often at sites of pressure, it is a cosmetic nuisance and rarely a cause for diagnostic confusion. Several variants exist and are described later. Caution should be exercised, however, when considering this diagnosis for lesions around the genitalia where genital warts are a more likely diagnosis and appear morphologically similar.

MANAGEMENT STRATEGY

Many patients present with seborrheic keratoses because of concern about possible melanoma, and reassurance may be all that is required. Occasionally the lesion can become "irritated" and show erythema, crusting, and itching. In this case the appearance may resemble squamous cell carcinoma. Any significant change in a lesion previously diagnosed as seborrheic keratosis—such as the development of several colors, rapid increase in size, or bleeding—should prompt a reconsideration of the diagnosis, as true melanocytic nevi and even malignant melanoma may occasionally have a seborrheic keratosis–like appearance

Where treatment is requested there are several options, and the choice will depend on patient and physician preference. *Surgical excision*, although effective, is never the treatment of choice unless there is real concern about the possibility of a malignant melanoma. When the diagnosis is in doubt, material should be taken for histologic examination, preferably by a *shave* or *tangential biopsy* technique or by *sharp curettage*. Blunt curettage provides poor material for histologic assessment. *Electrodesiccation* or *cautery* is very effective at softening the lesion and separating it at the dermoepidermal junction, allowing it to be wiped away with cotton gauze. Electrodesiccation may also be used after shave excision to treat any tissue remnants. With all these treatments the aim is to remove the lesion but little of the underlying skin surface.

Cryotherapy using a liquid nitrogen spray is an alternative treatment. Liquid nitrogen is sprayed onto the lesion until it is frozen and then continued for 5 to 10 seconds. It is done without local anesthesia because freezing reduces sensation of pain, and this can be an advantage when treating multiple lesions. After a day or two the treated lesion blisters and crumbles away. The underlying wound heals over several days and is often quite exudative, requiring daily cleansing by the patient. Overall the recovery period is longer and the wound slower to heal than after curettage and cautery. After cryotherapy, hypopigmentation may occur, and for this reason it is not recommended in black people.

Seborrheic Keratosis Variants

Senile or "solar" lentigines can be considered flat versions of the seborrheic keratosis. Sometimes referred to as *age or liver spots*, these small pigmented papules and plaques are more commonly seen on areas of frequent sun exposure, such as the face and dorsa of the hands. Their true nature can be recognized by the slight velvety texture to the lesional surface, which is best seen with tangential lighting. This indicates that the lesion is not a true lentigo but a superficial keratosis. These lesions are amenable to very minor treatments. Topical *tretinoin* cream can be effective. Other treatments include light abrasion with an *exfoliating cream*, *light dermabrasion* or *laser resurfacing*, *cryotherapy*, or *chemical peels* using trichloroacetic acid or phenol. A favorite treatment is minimal cautery followed by curettage with a cotton gauze swab. This leaves an erythematous superficial wound that heals rapidly.

Dermatosis papulosa nigra is commonly seen on the cheeks of black adults. These small seborrheic warts are easily treated by light cautery or electrodesiccation followed by cotton gauze curettage, but patients should be warned about the possibility of hyperpigmentation.

Stucco keratoses are small, grayish-white seborrheic keratoses that are typically found on the forearms and lower legs and are easily removed with curettage without bleeding. The edge of these lesions is often curled up away from the skin surface.

Giant seborrheic keratoses are large lesions, usually found on the scalp, and are often several centimeters in diameter.

Multiple Seborrheic Keratoses

Seborrheic keratoses may have a familial tendency, especially when multiple. It is these patients who are often the most challenging to treat and also the most affected by their condition. Patients often present with multiple lesions and request their complete removal.

The sudden onset of multiple seborrheic keratoses may be associated with underlying malignancy (the sign of Leser–Trélat) and should prompt a full clinical examination for underlying malignancy. Eruptive seborrheic keratoses may also occur after widespread eczema (so-called *Williams warts*) and have been associated with adalimumab use.

Specific Investigation

- Consider the sign of Leser–Trélat and investigate for underlying malignancy

Sign and pseudosign of Leser–Trélat: case reports and a review of the literature. Husain Z, Ho IK, Hantash BM. J Drugs Dermatol 2013; 12: 79–87.

The sign of Leser–Trélat is a rare paraneoplastic sign characterized by a sudden eruption of multiple seborrheic keratoses or their rapid increase in size. Its association with malignant acanthosis nigricans, seen in 35% of patients, is one of several of its features that support its legitimacy as a true paraneoplastic disorder. Gastric adenocarcinoma was the most frequently associated malignancy. In over 68% of cases the sign preceded the diagnosis of malignancy. Similar, nonmalignancy-associated eruptions are referred to as the *pseudosign of Leser–Trélat*.

Eruptive seborrheic keratoses associated with adalimumab use. Eastman KL, Knezevich SR, Raugi GJ. J Dermatol Case Rep 2013; 7: 60–3.

Eruptive seborrheic keratoses were associated with adalimumab therapy for rheumatoid arthritis and resolved when the drug was discontinued.

First-Line Therapies	
• Reassurance	E
• Curettage and cautery	B
• Cryotherapy	B

Effectiveness of cryosurgery vs. curettage in the treatment of seborrheic keratoses. Wood LD, Stucki JK, Hollenbeak CS, Miller JJ. JAMA Dermatol 2013; 149: 108–9.

This pilot study showed that the majority of patients preferred cryotherapy over curettage at both the 6-week and greater-than-12-month survey points.

Treatment of dermatosis papulosa nigra in 10 patients: a comparison trial of electrodesiccation, pulsed dye laser, and curettage. Garcia MK, Azari R, Eisent DB. Dermatol Surg 2010; 36: 1967–72.

Pulsed dye laser treatment offered no advantage compared with electrodesiccation or curettage for dermatosis papulosa nigra. Goetze S, Ziemer M, Lipman RD, Elsner P. Dermatol Surg 2006; 32: 661–8.

Hydrocolloid dressings produced superior healing of superficial wounds after curettage of seborrhoeic keratoses.

Second-Line Therapies	
• Chemical peels for smaller, superficial lesions and dermatosis papulosa nigrans	C
• Lasers (pulsed CO_2, erbium:YAG)	C

Focal trichloroacetic acid peel method for benign pigmented lesions in dark-skinned patients. Chun EY, Lee JB, Lee KH. Dermatol Surg 2004; 30; 512–16.

After cleansing the skin with alcohol, 65% trichloroacetic acid was applied focally to seborrheic keratoses using a sharpened wooden applicator to create evenly frosted spots on each lesion. Crusts separated from the skin with gentle washing after 4 to 7 days, and healing was complete 10 to 14 days later. Twenty-three patients required a mean of 1.5 treatments, and in 57% of these the results were rated as excellent.

Use of a long-pulse alexandrite laser in the treatment of superficial pigmented lesions. Trafeli JP, Kwan JM, Meehan KJ, Domankevitz Y, Gilbert S, Malomo K, et al. Dermatol Surg 2007; 33: 1477–82.

Patients with solar lentigines were treated with a long-pulse alexandrite laser (755-nm wavelength). Optimal settings were spot size 10 mm, pulse duration 3 ms, and fluence 22 J/cm^2 (without skin cooling). The authors advocate undertaking some initial test spots and observing the result after 10 minutes before proceeding to treat an entire area. The desired end point is a slight darkening of each lesion and/or perilesional erythema. Treated lesions darken and crust and fall off within about 10 days.

Treatment of verruca vulgaris, seborrheic keratoses, lentigines, and actinic cheilitis. Clinical advantage of the CO_2 laser superpulsed mode. Fitzpatrick RE, Goldman MP, Ruiz-Esparza J. J Dermatol Surg Oncol 1994; 20: 449–56.

Continuous and superpulsed CO_2 lasers were compared in their effect on a variety of lesions, including seborrheic keratoses. Ideal parameters prevent unwanted thermal damage.

Ablation of cutaneous lesions using an erbium:YAG laser. Khatri KA. J Cosmet Laser Ther 2003; 5: 150–3.

Erbium:YAG laser was used to remove multiple benign skin lesions and found to be safe and effective for this purpose.

532-nm diode laser treatment of seborrhoeic keratoses with color enhancement. Gulbertson GR. Dermatol Surg 2008; 34: 525–8.

A red color marker was applied to seborrheic keratoses to enhance the laser absorption before treatment with a 532-nm diode laser; 93% of lesions responded completely.

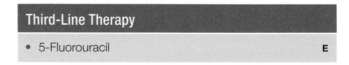

Third-Line Therapy	
• 5-Fluorouracil	E

Giant seborrhoeic keratosis on the frontal scalp treated with topical fluorouracil. Tsuji T, Morita A. J Dermatol 1995; 22: 74–5.

An unusual giant scalp seborrheic keratosis was successfully treated with topical fluorouracil.

Use of a keratolytic agent with occlusion for topical treatment of hyperkeratotic seborrhoeic keratoses. Burkhart CG, Burkhart CN. Skinmed 2008; 1: 15–8.

A topical 50% urea-containing product applied under occlusion was combined with superficial scraping to remove hyperkeratotic seborrheic keratoses on the trunk and extremities.

Evidence Levels: **A** Double-blind study **B** Clinical trial ≥ 20 subjects **C** Clinical trial < 20 subjects **D** Series ≥ 5 subjects **E** Anecdotal case reports

229

Sporotrichosis

Mahreen Ameen, Wanda Sonia Robles

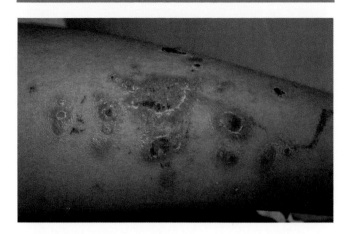

Sporotrichosis is a deep, cutaneous fungal infection caused by *Sporothrix schenckii*, a rapidly growing, dimorphic, saprophytic fungus found in soil and plant matter. It can affect both humans and animals and is prevalent worldwide, but is more common in the tropics. Disseminated infection, particularly to osteoarticular structures and viscera, is a risk in the immunocompromised and an emerging problem in those with advanced HIV infection. Infection is usually sporadic, but outbreaks may occur due to contaminated soil and wood. Cutaneous lesions develop after traumatic inoculation of *S. schenckii*. Infection is therefore more common in some occupations such as horticulturists, carpenters, and miners. Fifteen percent of cases occur in children less than 10 years of age. The initial lesion appears at the site of injury as an erythematous, ulcerated, or verrucous nodule. Lesions can be localized and are known as *fixed-type sporotrichosis*. The more common presentation is the lymphocutaneous form, where there is nodular lymphangitic spread.

MANAGEMENT STRATEGY

Although there have been cases describing the spontaneous remission of sporotrichosis, it is common practice to treat. Treatment includes local measures (thermotherapy), saturated solution of potassium iodide (SSKI), azoles, terbinafine, and amphotericin B. Historically, uncomplicated lymphangitic and fixed forms of sporotrichosis have been treated with high-dose SSKI initiated with 5 drops three times daily and increased as tolerated to 10 to 50 drops three times daily (equivalent to 250 mg to 1 g three times daily). Treatment is continued for 3 to 4 weeks after clinical cure. The mechanism of action of potassium iodide is not known, but it is highly effective, with reported cure rates ranging from 80% to 100%. It is also inexpensive and is the first-line treatment for sporotrichosis in most developing countries. However, it is inconvenient to administer, and side effects are common, although not serious, and include metallic taste, nausea, abdominal pain, and salivary gland enlargement.

Itraconazole is first-line therapy in countries where it is affordable. It should be initiated at a loading dose of 200 mg three times daily for 3 days followed by 100 to 400 mg daily. Cure rates

for cutaneous and lymphocutaneous infection are high, generally 90% to 100%. Terbinafine (250–1000 mg daily) produces similar efficacy. Fluconazole (400–800 mg daily) therapy gives response rates of 63% to 71% and therefore is recommended for second-line therapy only. Ketoconazole is ineffective for the treatment of sporotrichosis.

There are no clinical trials to guide therapy for disseminated or meningeal sporotrichosis, which can occur with immunosuppression. On the basis of case reports, parenteral amphotericin B (AmB) is the preferred treatment (AmB deoxycholate 0.7 mg/kg daily, or as a lipid formulation 3.0–5.0 mg/kg daily). A lipid formulation of AmB is recommended for meningeal infection. After AmB induction therapy, itraconazole (200 mg twice daily) is given as maintenance therapy. Thermotherapy (using infrared and far infrared wavelengths to heat tissues to 42°–43°C) is known to be effective, although there are few reports of its use. It has a useful role when systemic therapies are contraindicated. Clinical data demonstrating the potential of cryotherapy as an adjuvant to systemic therapy are limited.

Specific Investigations

- Culture
- Histology
- Serology for HIV infection (where relevant)

Direct microscopy of infected material is futile because the infective organisms are scarce in tissue. Culture is the most sensitive means of diagnosis and is characteristically rapid, with growth usually seen within 1 week in 90% of cases. In the remaining 10% it may take up to 4 weeks to achieve a positive result on Sabouraud agar culture. The diagnosis is confirmed by demonstrating dimorphism, or conversion to the yeast phase. Suitable material for culture may include lesion swab, aspirate, or biopsy. Data for polymerase chain reaction (PCR) are limited, and this technique requires further clinical validation.

The impact of sporotrichosis in HIV-infected patients: a systematic review. Moreira JA, Freitas DF, Lamas CC. Infection 2015, 43: 267–76.

This is a systematic review of reported cases of HIV-associated sporotrichosis found via PubMed (1984–2013). A total of 39 papers were included and 58 patients' data analyzed. A reported 56.9% cases were from Brazil and 31% from the United States. The median CD4 cell count was 97 cells/mm.[3] The most common clinical forms were disseminated and disseminated cutaneous, affecting 56.9% and 17.5% of patients, respectively. Mortality was 30% and significantly higher in those with central nervous system involvement and death.

In this group of patients amphotericin B was usually the drug of choice, and itraconazole was used as maintenance therapy.

Immune reconstitution inflammatory syndrome in HIV and sporotrichosis coinfection: report of two cases and review of the literature. Lyra MR, Nascimento ML, Varon AG, Pimentel MI, Antonio Lde F, Saheki MN, et al. Rev Soc Bras Med Trop 2014; 47: 806–9.

This is a report of two cases of patients with immune reconstitution inflammatory syndrome (IRIS) associated with cutaneous disseminated sporotrichosis and HIV coinfection. The patients received amphotericin and itraconazole combination treatment for sporotrichosis. However, 4 and 5 weeks after commencing antiretroviral therapy (ART), both patients experienced clinical exacerbation of skin lesions, despite increased T CD4+ cells and decreased viral load. They required treatment with several-month courses of systemic corticosteroids together with continued antifungal therapy. The authors noted that disease relapsed when corticosteroids were discontinued prematurely.

The risk of IRIS is higher in HIV-infected patients with low baseline CD4 counts before initiation of ART. In this group of patients the authors recommend close follow-up of patients at risk of IRIS and recommend prolonged corticosteroid treatment if necessary.

Sporotrichosis: an overview and therapeutic options. Mahajan VK. Dermatol Res Pract 2014; 2014: 272376.

This review reports that saturated solution of potassium iodide is generally used as a first-line treatment choice for uncomplicated cutaneous sporotrichosis in resource-limited countries. Itraconazole has very good efficacy and is recommended for the treatment of all forms of sporotrichosis. Terbinafine has demonstrated lower efficacy compared with itraconazole. Amphotericin B is used initially for the treatment of severe or systemic disease, during pregnancy, and in immunosuppressed patients followed by itraconazole prophylaxis if indicated.

Potassium iodide in dermatology: a 19th century drug for the 21st century: uses, pharmacology, adverse effects, and contraindications. Sterling JB, Heymann WR. J Am Acad Dermatol 2000; 43: 691–7.

This article reviews the pharmacology and adverse effects of potassium iodide as a therapeutic agent. It discusses contraindications to its use, which include a history of thyroid or kidney disease and pregnancy.

Disseminated sporotrichosis associated with treatment with immunosuppressants and tumor necrosis factor-alpha antagonists. Gottlieb GS, Lesser CF, Holmes KK, Wald A. Clin Infect Dis 2003; 37: 838–40.

A male adult patient developed disseminated infection after treatment with multiple immunosuppressants, including etanercept and infliximab for inflammatory arthritis. He was subsequently treated with a lipid formulation of amphotericin B.

With the increasing availability and use of anti–TNF-α agents, there is an increased risk of sporotrichosis presenting with disseminated infection rather than indolent cutaneous lesions only.

First-Line Therapies

• Itraconazole	A
• Terbinafine	A
• Potassium iodide	B
• Amphotericin B (for disseminated sporotrichosis)	E

Treatment of cutaneous sporotrichosis with itraconazole: study of 645 patients. de Lima Barros MB, Schubach AO, de Vasconcellos Carvalhaes de Oliveira R, Martins EB, Teixeira JL, Wanke B. Clin Infect Dis 2011; 52: e200–6.

This is the largest study of sporotrichosis (68.1% with lymphocutaneous form and 23.1% with fixed form) treated with itraconazole 50 to 400 mg/day. There was a 94.6% cure rate in the 619 patients who completed treatment (547 with 100 mg/day, 59 with 200–400 mg/day, and 4 children with 50 mg/day). Treatment was given until cure, and the median treatment duration was 12 weeks (range 2–64 weeks). Lymphocutaneous and disseminated forms required approximately 2 weeks longer to achieve cure than did the fixed form. The most frequent clinical

adverse effect was nausea. A reported 12.4% required further courses of treatment because of relapse. These were mainly those treated with the lower dose of 100 mg/day. One patient, despite dose escalation of itraconazole to 400 mg/day, failed and was cured only after switching to potassium hydroxide.

This study demonstrated that a dose of 100 mg daily is highly effective in the vast majority of patients with fixed or lymphocutaneous disease, although it was sometimes associated with a higher risk of relapse. This is important as it makes itraconazole a more affordable option in resource-poor regions. This report has also demonstrated that potassium iodide can be more efficacious than itraconazole, although there have been no comparative studies.

Efficacy and safety of itraconazole pulses vs. continuous regimen in cutaneous sporotrichosis. Song Y, Zhong SX, Yao L, Cai Q, Zhou JF, Liu YY et al. J Eur Acad Dermatol Venereol 2011; 25: 302–5.

This randomized controlled trial comparing pulse itraconazole 200 mg twice daily for 1 week every month (*n* = 25, mean course of treatment 2.65 ± 0.81 pulses) with continuous itraconazole 100 mg twice daily (*n* = 25, mean course of treatment 2.8 ± 2.33 months) demonstrated cure rates at 48 weeks of 81.8% and 95.8%, respectively. Side effects in the pulse therapy and continuous therapy groups were 4.5% versus 16.7%, respectively.

Pulse therapy has the advantages of lower cost and fewer adverse effects, although this small trial demonstrates higher efficacy with the continuous itraconazole regimen.

Cutaneous sporotrichosis in Himachal Pradesh, India. Mahajan VK, Sharma NL, Sharma RC, Gupta ML, Garg G, Kanga AK. Mycoses 2005; 48: 25–31.

One hundred and three cases of the lymphocutaneous and fixed cutaneous varieties of sporotrichosis are described during the period 1990 to 2002. Potassium iodide was used as first-line treatment, and in 93% of patients healing of lesions occurred in 4 to 32 weeks (average 8.7 weeks) without significant side effects. Itraconazole was used in 12 patients and was also highly effective.

This study demonstrates that the efficacy of potassium iodide is comparable to itraconazole.

Terbinafine (250 mg/day): an effective and safe treatment of cutaneous sporotrichosis. Francesconi G, Valle AC, Passos S, Reis R, Galhardo MC. J Eur Acad Dermatol Venereol 2009; 23: 1273–6.

Of 50 cases of sporotrichosis treated with terbinafine 250 mg daily, 96% (*n* = 48) were cured after a mean treatment period of 14 weeks with no recurrence after a mean follow-up period of 37 weeks. One patient discontinued drug therapy because of the development of a skin rash.

This study demonstrates that standard doses of terbinafine have adequate efficacy and that sporotrichosis does not generally require high-dose terbinafine therapy. The authors also point out that one of the advantages of terbinafine is that it has fewer drug–drug interactions than does itraconazole.

Comparative study of 250 mg/day terbinafine and 100 mg/day itraconazole for the treatment of cutaneous sporotrichosis. Francesconi G, Francesconi do Valle AC, Passos SL, de Lima Barros MB, de Almeida Paes R, Curi AL, et al. Mycopathologia 2011; 171: 349–54.

Itraconazole 100 mg daily and terbinafine 250 mg given to 249 and 55 patients, respectively, with culture-proven sporotrichosis demonstrated almost equal cure rates in both groups of 92% to 93% within a similar mean period (11.5–11.8 weeks). Adverse effects were equally frequent with both drugs, occurring in approximately 7% of those treated and were generally mild except in two patients receiving itraconazole who had to discontinue treatment.

This study provides further evidence for the efficacy of lower doses of itraconazole or terbinafine therapy. It also demonstrates that terbinafine is perhaps better tolerated.

Second-Line Therapies

• Fluconazole	**B**
• Thermotherapy	**D**
• Cryotherapy	**D**

Treatment of lymphocutaneous and visceral sporotrichosis with fluconazole. Kauffman CA, Pappas PG, McKinsey DS, Greenfield RA, Perfect JR, Cloud GA, et al. Clin Infect Dis 1996; 22: 46–50.

This clinical trial involved 14 patients with lymphocutaneous infection and 16 with osteoarticular or visceral sporotrichosis. Eleven of the 30 patients had previously been treated with other forms of antifungal therapy without success. Most patients were treated with fluconazole 400 mg/day. Four patients received fluconazole 200 mg/day, and another four received 800 mg/day. Seventy-one percent of patients (10/14) with lymphocutaneous sporotrichosis were cured. However, only 31% (5/16) with osteoarticular or visceral sporotrichosis responded to treatment.

This paper concluded that fluconazole is only modestly effective for the treatment of sporotrichosis and perhaps should be considered second-line therapy in patients who are unable to take itraconazole.

Hyperthermic treatment of sporotrichosis: experimental use of infrared and far infrared rays. Hiruma M, Kawada A, Noguchi H, Ishibashi A, Conti Díaz IA. Mycoses 1992; 35: 293–9.

Pocket warmers and infrared and far infrared rays were used to treat 14 cases of sporotrichosis, 7 in children and 7 in adults. Heat was applied daily to the lesions, and the devices warmed tissues to 42°C to 43°C. All lesions treated with pocket warmers were facial lesions in children. Infrared and far infrared rays generated more heat than pocket warmers, allowing the length of a single treatment to be reduced by three quarters to only a single 15-minute treatment daily. The overall cure rate was 71%.

The efficacy for this form of treatment has not been satisfactorily evaluated. However, it has an important role in the treatment of infection in those who are unable to take systemic therapy.

Cryosurgery as adjuvant therapy in cutaneous sporotrichosis. Ferreira CP, Galhardo MC, Valle AC. Braz J Infect Dis 2011; 15: 181–3.

Nine patients with one or two lesions of sporotrichosis that persisted despite completing drug therapy with either itraconazole, potassium iodide, or terbinafine were then treated with cryotherapy given monthly as two cycles of 15 seconds with a halo of 5 mm. The patients required one to four cryotherapy sessions to achieve cure.

The study has demonstrated the efficacy of cryotherapy and its ability to speed up disease resolution. By acting as an adjunctive therapy, it has the potential to decrease the duration of chemotherapy.

GUIDELINES

Clinical Practice Guidelines for the Management of Sporotrichosis: 2007 Update by the Infectious Diseases Society of America. Kauffman CA, Bustamante B, Chapman SW, Pappas PG. Clin Infect Dis 2007; 45: 1255–65.

For cutaneous and lymphocutaneous infection in developed countries, first-line recommended therapy is with itraconazole 200 mg daily, which is continued for 2 to 4 weeks after all lesions have resolved. Usually a 3- to 6-month course of treatment is recommended. Patients who fail to respond can be given either high-dose itraconazole 200 mg twice daily, terbinafine 500 mg twice daily, or SSKI initiated at a dose of 5 drops three times daily and increased as tolerated to 40 to 50 drops thrice daily. Children can be treated with the same drugs at a dose of 6 to 10 mg/kg for itraconazole (maximum 400 mg daily) and a maximum of 1 drop/kg of SSKI. Fluconazole should only be used in patients who cannot tolerate any of these treatments. Thermotherapy can be used for fixed lesions in those in whom oral therapy is contraindicated, such as pregnant women. Amphotericin B is the recommended first-line therapy for severe pulmonary or osteoarticular infection, disseminated, and meningeal sporotrichosis. After the initial response, itraconazole is recommended as step-down therapy and should be given to complete a total of at least 12 months of therapy. Amphotericin B is also the drug of choice for severe infection in pregnancy.

Future updated guidelines will need to incorporate recent data demonstrating the efficacy of lower doses of itraconazole and terbinafine for sporotrichosis.

Squamous cell carcinoma

Bassel H. Mahmoud, Suzanne M. Olbricht

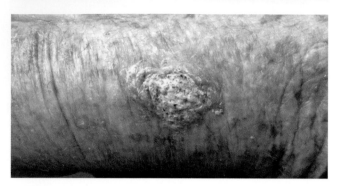

Cutaneous squamous cell carcinoma (SCC) originates from keratinizing cells of the epidermis or its appendages. Most commonly it presents as an erythematous papule or nodule with scale and crust, but it may also be ulcerated, hyperpigmented, or surmounted by a cutaneous horn.

SCC is not only the second most common type of skin cancer, but also the second most common malignancy of any kind in the United States. Incidence varies geographically, with higher rates at lower latitudes. The lifetime risk for SCC is increasing worldwide, escalating 50% to 300% in the last 3 decades. Cumulative ultraviolet light (UVL) exposure is the most common cause of SCC of the skin, which explains why the majority of SCCs occur on the head, neck, and extremities, areas of maximum sun exposure. Depletion of atmospheric ozone and longer life expectancy contribute to larger cumulative exposures. Other risk factors include use of tanning beds, chemical carcinogens, and immunosuppressive drug therapy; chronic scar; chronic dermatoses such as epidermolysis bullosa; human papilloma virus (HPV) infection; and genodermatoses such as xeroderma pigmentosum. A person with one SCC is at high risk for developing more SCCs as well as other skin cancers.

MANAGEMENT STRATEGY

The importance of prevention by educating everyone from an early age about this hazard of solar UV exposure cannot be overemphasized.

The goals of treatment of primary cutaneous SCC are to completely remove the tumor, to minimize the risk of metastasis and recurrence, to restore normal function after treatment, and to provide the best possible cosmetic outcome. Preoperative workup includes history of prior treatment, clinical size of the lesion, and an accurate histopathologic diagnosis. Physical examination should include regional lymph node palpation. A shave biopsy is generally sufficient for epidermal and deep dermal inspection, but punch biopsy to subcutaneous fat or an incisional or excisional biopsy can sometimes provide additional information. For reasons of prognostication, the pathology report should comment on depth of tumor invasion, histologic differentiation, and the presence or absence of sclerosis, single cell infiltration, and

neurotropism. Additional laboratory and imaging studies are not generally helpful, although they may be performed when an aggressive high-risk tumor is suspected.

High-risk tumors are recurrent; have a diameter of more than 2 cm; are present on the ear, temple, lip, or anogenital region; or have poor histologic differentiation or other histologic features noted earlier. The most recent American Joint Committee on Cancer (AJCC) and National Comprehensive Cancer Network (NCCN) Guidelines identified criteria for "high-risk" factors for local recurrence or metastases, which included poor differentiation, perineural invasion, and depth of tumor. Immunosuppression also increases risk, notably in transplant recipients.

When choosing therapy, the main consideration is the cure rate; however, every patient should be assessed individually with regard to site and size of the lesion, functional and cosmetic implications of treatment, the patient's general medical condition, ability to return for additional treatment, and the patient's preferences.

Mohs micrographic surgery (MMS) provides the best long-term cure rate and is the treatment of choice for large lesions in critical sites, as well as for high-risk and recurrent SCC, because of its unique method of margin control as well as its tissue-sparing benefits. In this technique marginal, normal-appearing skin is removed as a thin tangential layer around and under the clinically apparent tumor, precisely oriented, horizontally sectioned, and immediately processed as a frozen section for histologic evaluation. This is repeated until all margins are histologically clear. Based on the appropriate use criteria (AUC) developed by the American Academy of Dermatology, American College of Mohs Surgery, American Society for Dermatologic Surgery, and the American Society for Mohs Surgery, MMS is appropriate for all SCCs in the high-risk and intermediate-risk areas; for SCCs 11 mm in diameter or greater in any site; for SCC in situ in areas of chronic inflammation, osteomyelitis, prior radiation, or scar; for locally recurrent and incompletely excised SCC; and for all SCCs in immunosuppressed patients or in patients with genetic syndromes. MMS is also indicated in SCC with aggressive histologic features and those with perineural or perivascular invasion.

Standard surgical excision may be performed for well-circumscribed tumors with diameters less than 2 cm that do not occur on the ears, lips, eyelids, nose, or scalp and do not invade the fat. Surgical margins of 4 to 6 mm are usually adequate to achieve a 95% chance of a cure. Lesions with diameters of 2 cm or greater in low-risk locations may be excised with 10-mm margins, but tissue rearrangement should not be performed until there is pathologic verification of tumor-free margins. The main advantage of excisional surgery over destructive therapy is that there is histologic analysis of the excised tissue specimen.

Electrodesiccation and curettage (ED&C) is considered for the treatment of low-risk, well-differentiated primary SCC and SCC in situ <1 cm in diameter. It involves a sequence of three curette scrapings and electrodesiccations. A margin of 3 to 4 mm around the tumor should be included in the treatment area to ensure complete removal of the tumor. Treated lesions often require several weeks to heal and may leave a white atrophic or hypertrophic scar that can be cosmetically unappealing. Cosmetically sensitive areas, concave surfaces, and skin prone to keloid formation or poor wound healing should be avoided. Cure rates are highly technique dependent, but range from 80% to 95%.

Cryosurgery is another destructive technique that can be considered for small (<1 cm), low-risk SCC and SCC in situ with cure rates similar to treatment by ED&C if performed properly. Cryosurgery destroys a tumor if it is frozen to −60°C, achievable

Evidence Levels: A Double-blind study B Clinical trial ≥ 20 subjects C Clinical trial < 20 subjects D Series ≥ 5 subjects E Anecdotal case reports

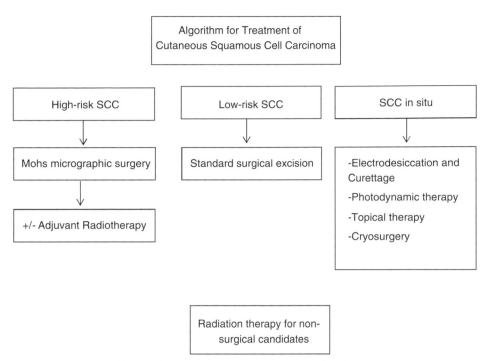

Algorithm for treatment of cutaneous squamous cell carcinoma.

with timed stages or the use of thermocouples. It leaves a wound that may blister and drain but otherwise heals without complication to a porcelain white atrophic scar. It has the advantage of being fast, simple, and inexpensive, but the success of the procedure is very much operator dependent.

Photodynamic therapy (PDT) involves the application of a photosensitizing agent onto the skin followed by irradiation with a light source. It is approved by the Food and Drug Administration (FDA) for the treatment of actinic keratosis, but other studies using different treatment regimens have documented some success for the treatment of nonmelanoma skin cancers.

Radiation therapy as a primary treatment modality for SCC is best reserved for those situations in which surgical risk is not acceptable. Because of the potential long-term sequelae, it is not advisable in patients under 60 years old. Treatment is given sequentially over several weeks. Complications include hypopigmentation, telangiectasia, loss of adnexae, radiation dermatitis, and the appearance of a new primary tumor 10 to 20 years later. Radiation therapy is also recommended as adjuvant therapy for SCC with substantial perineural involvement, especially when the involved nerves are 0.1 mm or greater in caliber. Brachytherapy has recently been widely used because of the ability to deliver energy at a high-dose rate, leading to fewer patient visits.

Other options may be useful for specific patients. *Topical therapy* has a low cure rate and is therefore reserved mainly for patients with SCC not amenable to surgical treatment or radiation due to either advanced disease stage or large number of lesions or both; topical therapy includes *imiquimod* or *5-fluorouracil (5-FU) cream*. Some patients with many lesions, particularly on the legs, may be successfully treated with *intralesional methotrexate, 5-FU, bleomycin, or interferon (IFN)*. For patients with many lesions who are immunosuppressed, systemic therapy with *retinoids* or *IFN* may be tried, but the results are mixed and there is usually only suppression of growth, not cure.

Systemic treatment for SCC includes *chemotherapy* for metastatic disease. *Cisplatin* has been used alone or in combination with *5-FU, methotrexate, bleomycin,* or *doxorubicin*. Epidermal growth factor receptor inhibitors, including *cetuximab* and *gefitinib*, have been used off-label to treat metastatic SCC because of the overexpression of epidermal growth factor (EGFR) in some tumors.

Patients with a history of SCC need continued lifelong cutaneous surveillance to monitor for tumor recurrence and metastasis, as well as for new developing lesions, as they are at higher risk of another skin cancer even within 5 years of the first tumor.

Specific Investigations

- Biopsy
- Radiologic examination (PET, MRI, CT, ultrasound) if high-risk tumor
- Sentinel lymph node biopsy (controversial) may be considered for very high-risk tumors

Cutaneous squamous cell carcinoma: a comprehensive clinicopathologic classification: part two. Cassarino DS, Derienzo DP, Barr RJ. J Cutan Pathol 2006; 33: 261–79.

SCC is one of the few cancers where progression from focal nests of atypical cells to in situ disease to invasive carcinoma can be surmised, both clinically and histologically. Invasive SCCs can be categorized into well-, moderately well-, moderately, and poorly differentiated subtypes. Poorly differentiated SCCs have a higher risk of recurrence and metastasis. Invasive SCC may exhibit mixed cell inflammation around the tumor, sclerotic stroma, and perineural infiltration. Histologic subtypes that have an increased risk of recurrence or metastasis are adenoid (acantholytic), desmoplastic spindle cell SCCs, and invasive Bowen disease carcinoma.

Reliability of the histopathologic diagnosis of keratinocyte carcinomas. Jagdeo J, Weinstock MA, Piepkorn M, Bingham S. J Am Acad Dermatol 2007; 57: 279–84.

A prospective blinded study of 3926 specimens reviewed by both pathologists and dermatopathologists showed highest intraobserver agreement for basal cell carcinoma (BCC) and lowest in the categories of invasive SCC, SCC in situ, and actinic keratosis, suggesting the boundaries of these diagnoses are imprecisely defined.

MR imaging of perineural tumor spread. Ginsberg LE. Magn Reson Imaging Clin N Am 2002; 10: 511–25.

Preoperative imaging studies should be obtained when there is suspicion of metastases, bone invasion, or perineural infiltration. Controversy remains regarding the choice of radiologic examination. Computed tomography (CT) is used to image extracapsular spread, central nodal necrosis, skull base, and cartilage invasion. Magnetic resonance imaging (MRI) provides improved imaging of tissue planes and neurotropic tumors. Positron emission tomography (PET) scans can detect metastases in areas of necrosis, dense fibrosis, or scarring from radiation therapy, whereas CT and MRI can identify soft tissue infiltration and bony erosion.

Impact of radiographic findings on prognosis for skin carcinoma with clinical perineural invasion. Galloway TJ, Morris CG, Mancuso AA, Amdur RJ, Mendenhall WM. Cancer 2005; 103: 1254–7.

When involvement of a large nerve is suspected, an MRI and CT scan should be obtained to evaluate the extent of disease and rule out intracranial involvement.

Evaluation of American Joint Committee on Cancer, International Union Against Cancer, and Brigham and Women's Hospital tumor staging for cutaneous squamous cell carcinoma. Karia PS, Jambusaria-Pahlajani A, Harrington DP, Murphy GF, Qureshi AA, Schmults CD. J Clin Oncol 2014; 32: 327–34.

A comparative evaluation of three tumor (T) staging systems. AJCC and UICC showed that most poor outcomes occurred in low stages (T1/T2), whereas at BWH, incidences of poor outcomes were low for low-stage tumors (T1/T2a) and higher for higher-stage tumors (T2b/T3).

High-risk cutaneous squamous cell carcinoma and the emerging role of sentinel lymph node biopsy: a literature review. Navarrete-Dechent C, Veness MJ, Droppelmann N, Uribe P. J Am Acad Dermatol 2015; 73: 127–37.

Evidence supports considering sentinel lymph node biopsy (SLNB) in SCC classified as AJCC-7 T2 larger than 2 cm in diameter. Patients with other high-risk factors such as recurrent SCC and immunosuppressed patients should also be included in clinical trials evaluating the utility of SLNB in SCC.

First-Line Therapies	
• Mohs micrographic surgery	B
• Standard excision	B
• Curettage and electrodesiccation	B
• Cryosurgery	B
• Radiation therapy	B

Mohs surgery for squamous cell carcinoma. Belkin D, Carucci JA. Dermatol Clin 2011; 29: 161–74.

MMS provides the highest cure rates for both primary and recurrent tumors. The 5-year recurrence rates for primary tumors of the skin were 7.9% for non-Mohs modalities and 3.1% for MMS. For primary SCC of the lip, 5-year recurrence rates were 10.5% for non-Mohs modalities and 2.3% for MMS. For primary SCC of the ear, 5-year recurrence rates were 18.7% for non-Mohs modalities and 5.3% for MMS.

High recurrence rates of squamous cell carcinoma after Mohs' surgery in patients with chronic lymphocytic leukemia. Mehrany K, Weenig RH, Pittelkow MR, Roenigk RK, Otley CC. Dermatol Surg 2005; 31: 38–42.

Patients with immunosuppression can have a higher recurrence rate and require close surveillance.

Surgical margins for excision of primary squamous cell carcinoma. Brodland DG, Zitelli JA. J Am Acad Dermatol 1992; 27: 241–8.

Based on a prospective study of subclinical microscopic tumor extension, it was recommended that minimal margins of 4 mm be taken around clinical borders of SCC. Margins of at least 6 mm were proposed for tumors ≥2 cm, histologic grade ≥2, with invasion of subcutaneous tissue, and/or location in high-risk areas.

The treatment of skin cancer. A statistical study of 1341 skin tumors comparing results obtained with irradiation, surgery, and curettage followed by electrodesiccation. Freeman RG, Knox JM, Heaton CL. Cancer 1964; 17: 535–8.

Low-risk SCCs have a high cure rate when treated with excision with standard surgical excision, ED&C, and cryosurgery.

Controversies in skin surgery: electrodessication and curettage versus excision for low-risk, small, well-differentiated squamous cell carcinomas. Reschly MJ, Shenefelt PD. J Drugs Dermatol 2010; 9: 773–6.

Two retrospective studies. One was a small controlled study in a Veterans Administration teaching hospital dermatology clinic that compared cure rates of low-risk SCCs at 1 year by curettage and electrodesiccation to those of surgical excision. A second study examined the cure rate of low-risk SCCs treated by curettage and electrodesiccation alone in a private practice. The first study found no significant difference in cure rates between curettage and electrodesiccation (14 of 14 cases successfully treated) and excision (15 of 16 successfully treated and 1 recurrence). The second study found the curettage and electrodesiccation cure rate (106 of 106 successfully treated) to be significantly greater than an arbitrary cure rate of 95%.

Prospective trial of curettage and cryosurgery in the management of non-facial, superficial, and minimally invasive basal and squamous cell carcinoma. Peikert JM. Int J Dermatol 2011; 50: 1135–8.

Sixty-nine patients with 100 nonfacial tumors, ≤2 cm in diameter, consisting of superficial BCC, superficial nodular BCC with papillary dermal invasion, SCC in situ, and SCC with papillary dermal invasion, were prospectively treated with curettage and cryotherapy and subsequently evaluated at 1- and 5-year intervals. No tumor recurred after 1 year of follow-up, and one recurrence occurred within the 5-year interval, for a 99% recurrence-free end point.

It is important to emphasize that because the more aggressive, high-risk tumors are treated with MMS, the reported recurrence rates for some non-Mohs modalities, particularly for electrodesiccation and curettage, reserved for low-risk skin cancers, are likely to be underestimated compared with those for MMS.

Statistical analysis in cryosurgery of skin cancer. Graham GF, Clark LC. Clin Dermatol 1990; 8: 101–7.

Evidence Levels: **A** Double-blind study **B** Clinical trial ≥ 20 subjects **C** Clinical trial < 20 subjects **D** Series ≥ 5 subjects **E** Anecdotal case reports

Cryosurgery should be considered only for small (<1 cm), low-risk SCC and SCC in situ because of the low cure rates achieved when the technique is used for higher-risk tumors. Permanent pigment loss, atrophy, and hypertrophic scarring are common.

Office-based radiation therapy for cutaneous carcinoma: evaluation of 710 treatments. Hernandez-Machin B, Borrego L, Gil-Garcia M, Hernandez BH. Int J Dermatol 2007; 46: 453–9.

A retrospective study of 604 BCCs and 106 SCCs irradiated between 1971 and 1996 revealed cure rates for SCC of 92.7% at 5 years and 78.6% at 15 years, suggesting that radiation therapy is an effective first option in many cases.

Management of nonmelanoma skin cancer in 2007. Neville JA, Welch E, Leffell DJ. Nat Clin Pract Oncol 2007; 4: 462–9.

Radiation therapy as a primary treatment modality for SCC is best reserved for those situations in which surgical risk is not acceptable. Radiation therapy is generally reserved for patients over 50 years of age because of the potential long-term sequelae.

The use of brachytherapy in the treatment of nonmelanoma skin cancer: a review. Alam M, Nanda S, Mittal BB, Kim NA, Yoo S. J Am Acad Dermatol 2011; 65: 377–88.

Recurrence after treatment of nonmelanoma skin cancer: a prospective cohort study. Chren MM, Torres JS, Stuart SE, Bertenthal D, Labrador RJ, Boscardin WJ. Arch Dermatol 2011; 147: 540–6.

This was a prospective, long-term study (median 6.6 years after treatment) to determine tumor recurrence rates after treatment. Consecutive samples were taken from all 495 patients with 616 primary nonmelanoma skin cancers diagnosed in 1999 and 2000. A total of 127 tumors were treated with curettage and electrodesiccation (20.9%), 309 with excision (50.8%), and 172 with Mohs surgery (28.3%). Over the course of the study, 21 tumors recurred (3.5%): 2 (2 BCC) after curettage and electrodesiccation (1.6%), 13 (9 BCC, 4 SCC) after excision (4.2%), and 6 (4 BCC, 2 SCC) after Mohs surgery (3.5%). Recurrent tumors were detected earliest after curettage and electrodesiccation (1.5 years) and latest after Mohs surgery (6.0 years). Median time to detection of recurrence after excision was 3.8 years.

High-risk cutaneous squamous cell carcinoma without palpable lymphadenopathy: is there a therapeutic role for elective neck dissection? Marinez JC, Cook JL. Dermatol Surg 2007; 33: 410–20.

A literature review suggested that patients with cutaneous SCC who underwent elective node dissection had no proven survival benefit over those who are initially staged as node negative and undergo therapeutic neck dissection after the development of apparent regional disease.

Second-Line Therapies

• Topical imiquimod	A
• Topical 5-fluorouracil	B
• Photodynamic therapy	B
• Intralesional interferon-α	B
• Intralesional methotrexate	D
• Intralesional 5-fluorouracil	B
• Electrochemotherapy with bleomycin	B
• Intralesional bleomycin	E

Imiquimod 5% cream in the treatment of Bowen's disease and invasive squamous cell carcinoma. Peris K, Micantonio T, Fargnoli MC, Lozzi GP, Chimenti S. J Am Acad Dermatol 2006; 55: 324–7.

This open-label clinical trial used imiquimod 5% cream five times a week for up to 16 weeks to treat seven invasive SCC lesions on 10 patients. Five sites (71.4%) showed complete clinicopathologic regression and two (28.6%) partial regression at 16 weeks. There were no recurrences at a mean of 31 months, follow-up.

Topical imiquimod or fluorouracil therapy for basal and squamous cell carcinoma: a systematic review. Love WE, Bernhard JD, Bordeaux JS. Arch Dermatol 2009; 145: 1431–8.

Clearance rates varied by drug regimen, and most of the studies lacked long-term follow-up. Imiquimod produced clearance rates of 73% to 88% for SCC in situ and 71% for invasive SCC. FU use produced 27% to 85% clearance for SCC in situ. Up to 100% and 97% of patients applying imiquimod and FU, respectively, experienced at least one adverse event such as erythema, pruritus, and pain.

Methyl-aminolevulinate photodynamic therapy for the treatment of actinic keratoses and non-melanoma skin cancers: a retrospective analysis of response in 462 patients. Fai D, Arpaia N, Romano I, Vestita M, Cassano N, Vena GA. G Ital Dermatol Venereol 2009; 144: 281–5.

This case series included 210 patients with actinic keratosis, 228 subjects with 348 BCCs, 17 patients with Bowen disease, and 7 patients with SCC. Bowen disease is very responsive to methyl-aminolevulinate photodynamic therapy, unlike microinvasive or invasive SCC.

Intralesional interferon alpha-2b in the treatment of basal cell carcinoma and squamous cell carcinoma: revisited. Kim KH, Yavel RM, Gross VL, Brody N. Dermatol Surg 2004; 30: 116–20.

Five BCCs and three SCCs were treated with a series of 1.0 to 2.5 million units IFN-α_{2b} intralesional injections administered over a 3- to 5-week period, for a total dosage of 9 to 30 million units. The mean follow-up period after treatment was 33 months. There were no clinically evident recurrences.

Intralesional methotrexate treatment for keratoacanthoma tumors: a retrospective study and review of the literature. Annest NM, VanBeek MJ, Arpey CJ, Whitaker DC. J Am Acad Dermatol 2007; 56: 989–93.

Cases of keratoacanthoma (KA) treated with intralesional methotrexate (MTX) were identified from the authors' institution ($n = 18$) and literature search ($n = 20$). Intralesional MTX achieved resolution in 92%, requiring an average of 2.1 injections an average of 18 days apart. Adverse events were rare, with two reports of pancytopenia in patients with chronic renal failure. The authors concluded that intralesional MTX is a useful nonsurgical therapy for KA, that histologic diagnosis before initiation of treatment is preferred, and a complete blood cell count at baseline and during treatment should be considered.

Intralesional chemotherapy for nonmelanoma skin cancer: a practical review. Kirby JS, Miller CJ. J Am Acad Dermatol 2010; 63: 689–702.

A review article with guidelines for the treatment of SCC, KA, and BCC with the most widely available intralesional agents (methotrexate, 5-FU, bleomycin, and IFN).

Intralesional agents in the management of cutaneous malignancy: a review. Good LM, Miller MD, High WA. J Am Acad Dermatol 2011; 64: 413–22.

A comprehensive review on intralesional agents and their role in cutaneous neoplasms.

Third-Line Therapies

• Systemic retinoids	B
• Chemotherapy	B
• Amputation	D

Acitretin suppression of squamous cell carcinoma: case report and literature review. Lebwohl M, Tannis C, Carrasco D. J Dermatol Treat 2003; 14: 3–6.

A patient with psoriasis who developed multiple SCCs after being previously treated with psoralen and ultraviolet A for 4.5 years was started on 25 mg daily of acitretin, which resulted in a reduction in the number of SCCs. The mechanism of action is reviewed.

Oral retinoid use reduces cutaneous squamous cell carcinoma risk in patients with psoriasis treated with psoralen-UVA: a nested cohort study. Nijsten TEC, Stern RS. J Am Acad Dermatol 2003; 49: 644–50.

A cohort of 135 patients participating in the PUVA follow-up study with at least 1 year of substantial retinoid use was identified. Each patient's tumor incidence during retinoid therapy was compared with the incidence of SCC development in periods of no use. Overall, a 30% reduction in SCC incidence was noted when patients were on oral retinoid therapy. Retinoids (isotretinoin, acitretin) may play a role in the treatment of patients with SCC not amenable to surgical extirpation due to advanced stage of disease or large number of lesions, with an overall response rate of about 70%.

Systemic retinoids for chemoprevention of non-melanoma skin cancer in high-risk patients. Marquez C, Bair SM, Smithberger E, Cherpelis BS, Glass LF. J Drugs Dermatol 2010; 9: 753–58.

A review of the literature on susceptible individuals, such as organ transplant recipients and those with xeroderma pigmentosum.

Update on the management of high-risk squamous cell carcinoma. LeBoeuf NR, Schmults CD. Semin Cutan Med Surg 2011; 30: 26–34.

Cisplatin alone or in combination with 5-FU, methotrexate, bleomycin, or doxorubicin. Capecitabine is an oral prodrug of 5-FU that is metabolized to 5-FU within tumor cells and has fewer adverse effects than systemically administered 5-FU. EGFR inhibitors, including cetuximab and gefitinib, have been used off-label to treat metastatic SCC because of the overexpression of EGFR in some tumors.

Squamous cell carcinoma arising in osteomyelitis and chronic wounds. Treatment with Mohs micrographic surgery vs. amputation. Kirsner RS, Spencer J, Falanga V, Garland LE, Kerdel FA. Dermatol Surg 1996; 22: 1015–8.

Patients with extensive local or metastatic SCC of the leg involving bone may require amputation if MMS would render the remaining limb unstable.

Evidence Levels: **A** Double-blind study **B** Clinical trial ≥ 20 subjects **C** Clinical trial < 20 subjects **D** Series ≥ 5 subjects **E** Anecdotal case reports

231

Staphylococcal scalded skin syndrome

Dimitra Koch, Saleem M. Taibjee

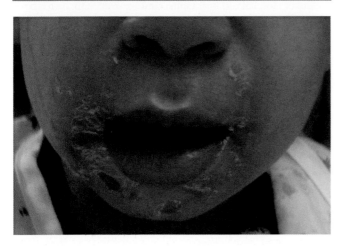

Staphylococcal scalded skin syndrome (SSSS) is a highly contagious, blistering condition triggered by exfoliative, toxin-producing *Staphylococcus aureus*, most commonly affecting neonates and children under the age of 6 years. It rarely presents in adults, usually in association with renal failure, immunocompromis, and possibly nonsteroidal antiinflammatory drugs (NSAIDs). SSSS can develop after viral illnesses such as respiratory tract infections and varicella and after skin-penetrating procedures such as heel prick and vitamin K injections in neonates, intraarticular injections, and peritoneal dialysis.

The estimated incidence in Western countries ranges from 0.56 to 2.51 cases/year/million inhabitants with a reported seasonal peak in summer/autumn. In healthy infants mortality is uncommon, with reported rates up to 3%, contrasting with up to 50% to 60% in adults with comorbidity. Death occurs due to complications such as pneumonia, hypovolemia, electrolyte imbalance, and sepsis.

SSSS is caused by hematogenous spread of exfoliative toxin (ET), mainly ET-A and/or B, produced by *S. aureus*, including methicillin-sensitive (MSSA), methicillin-resistant (MRSA), and multidrug resistant strains. Approximately 5% of all *S. aureus* produce ET. ET-producing MRSA strains appear more prevalent in Japan. ETs are serine proteases specifically cleaving desmosomal protein desmoglein-1, disrupting keratinocyte adhesion in the superficial epidermis. Increased susceptibility may reflect impaired renal clearance of ET in neonates and adults with renal failure or low titers of ET-specific antibodies in immunocompromised individuals.

Clinical features include a prodrome of malaise, irritability, and fever. Skin manifestations develop within 24 to 48 hours. Tender erythema is followed by superficial, flaccid blistering, most pronounced in flexural and periorificial areas, sparing mucosal surfaces, and ranging from localized blisters to widespread exfoliation. This leads to impaired thermoregulation and fluid balance and susceptibility to sepsis and secondary infection. Nikolsky sign is positive. With successful treatment SSSS resolves

over 10 to 14 days. Bullae rupture to leave denuded skin, followed by reepithelialization without scarring.

The causative organism cannot usually be cultured from affected skin, because this is a circulating toxin-mediated process. The infection may be acquired by skin-to-skin contact from another individual with either a symptomatic infection or who is an asymptomatic carrier. It may be possible to culture ET-producing *S. aureus* from extracutaneous sites, most commonly the nasopharynx, but also the rectum, conjunctiva, urinary tract, umbilicus, and blood. Polymerase chain reaction (PCR) or random amplified polymorphic DNA analysis may identify the toxin-encoding genes. Histology of affected skin typically shows a superficial subcorneal blister; absence of epidermal necrosis and minimal inflammation. A frozen section of blister roof can confirm the superficial level of cleavage, facilitating a more rapid diagnosis.

The main differential diagnosis is the Stevens–Johnson syndrome–toxic epidermal necrolysis spectrum, in which distinguishing features include targetoid skin lesions, mucosal involvement, and subepidermal level of blistering with full-thickness epidermal necrosis. Additional differential diagnoses in infants include hereditary conditions such as epidermolysis bullosa, epidermolytic ichthyosis, and bullous mastocytosis.

MANAGEMENT STRATEGY

Treatment includes antibiotic therapy in combination with supportive measures addressing electrolyte and fluid balance, temperature regulation, nutrition, analgesia, and skin care. Bland *emollients* such as 50:50 white soft paraffin/liquid paraffin should be applied regularly to reduce friction and insensible fluid losses. Nonadherent dressings are used to cover denuded areas, with avoidance of adhesive tapes directly on skin. *Systemic β-lactamase–resistant antibiotics* are necessary to eradicate the causative *S. aureus* strain. Patients with extensive SSSS require intravenous antibiotics and in-hospital care provided by a multidisciplinary team experienced in delivering optimal skin care (e.g., on a burns unit). In view of the growing emergence of resistant ET-producing *S. aureus* strains, in particular MRSA and fusidic acid–resistant strains, antibiotic choice should be guided by local protocols/microbiology advice.

SSSS outbreaks on maternity and neonatal units are reported. Strict infection control measures are advisable, including patient isolation, barrier nursing, and scrupulous handwashing. Screening programs may identify *S. aureus* carriers among contacts, including health care workers. Colonized individuals require treatment with topical antiseptics (e.g., *chlorhexidine*) with nasal carriage eradicated by topical antibiotics such as *mupirocin*.

Nosocomial staphylococcal scalded skin syndrome caused by intraarticular injection. Emberger M, Koller J, Laimer M, Hell M, Oender K, Trost A, et al. J Eur Acad Dermatol Venereol 2011; 25: 227–31.

Nosocomial outbreak of SSSS in three patients on NSAIDs who received intraarticular injections by an orthopedic surgeon with confirmed ET-producing *S. aureus* nasal colonization.

Nosocomial outbreak of staphylococcal scalded skin syndrome in neonates: epidemiologic investigation and control. El Helali N, Carbonne A, Naas T, Kerneis S, Fresco O, Giovangrandi YP, et al. J Hosp Infect 2005; 61: 130–8.

SSSS outbreak affecting 13 neonates in a maternity unit; temporary removal from duty of a nurse with chronic hand dermatitis confirmed as a carrier of the causative ET-producing *S. aureus*. Infection control measures (patient isolation, barrier-nursing, chlorhexidine handwashing, treatment of carriers with nasal mupirocin, and chlorhexidine showers) controlled the outbreak. All affected neonates were successfully treated with oxacillin.

Health care workers are an important potential source in outbreaks.

Specific Investigations

- Nose, throat, conjunctival, umbilical, rectal, and skin swabs for bacterial culture and sensitivities
- Culture from suspected site of primary infection
- Polymerase chain reaction (PCR) for rapid detection and characterization of SSSS-associated *S. aureus*
- Blood cultures
- Full blood count
- Serum urea, creatinine, and electrolytes
- Skin biopsy or frozen section of blister roof
- Dermoscopy
- Screening contacts for *S. aureus* carriage

Isolating *Staphylococcus aureus* from children with suspected staphylococcal scalded skin syndrome is not clinically useful. Ladhani S, Robbie S, Chapple DS, Joannou CL, Evans RW. Pediatr Infect Dis J 2003; 22: 284–6.

Polymerase chain reaction for *ETA* and *ETB* genes and Western blotting confirmed ET-producing strains in only 17 of 54 (31%) isolates over a 4-year study period.

Failure to isolate ET-producing S. aureus *from affected skin does not exclude the diagnosis of SSSS.*

Staphylococcal scalded skin syndrome in an extremely low-birth-weight neonate: molecular characterization and rapid detection by multiplex and real-time PCR of methicillin-resistant *Staphylococcus aureus*. Shi D, Ishii S, Sato T, Yamazaki H, Matsunaga M, Higuchi W, et al. Pediatr Int 2011; 53: 211–7.

Multiplex and PCR assays were developed to target five virulence genes (*ETA, ETB, ETD, PVL, CNA*), aiming at rapid detection of SSSS-associated MRSA.

Adult case of staphylococcal scalded skin syndrome differentiated from toxic epidermal necrolysis with the aid of dermoscopy. Miyashita K, Ogawa K, Iioka H, Miyagawa F, Okazaki A, Kobayashi N, et al. J Dermatol 2016; 43: 842–3.

Dermoscopy as a diagnostic tool was utilized to demonstrate superficial level of cleavage at a fresh exfoliation site; subcorneal detachment was subsequently confirmed histologically.

Nosocomial outbreak of staphylococcal scalded skin syndrome in neonates in England, December 2012 to March 2013. Paranthaman K, Bentley A, Milne LM, Kearns A, Loader S, Thomas A, et al. Euro Surveill 2014; 19: 1–7.

A health care worker with chronic hand dermatitis was identified as the source of the outbreak after mass screening involving multisite swabbing and pooled, enrichment culture.

First-Line Therapy

- β-Lactamase–resistant penicillins (e.g., flucloxacillin, oxacillin) **D**

Epidemiological data of staphylococcal scalded skin syndrome in France from 1997 to 2007 and microbiological characteristics of *Staphylococcus aureus* associated strains.

Lamand V, Dauwalder O, Tristan A, Casalegno JS, Meugnier H, Bes M, et al. Clin Microbiol Infect 2012; 18: E514–21.

This retrospective study reports 349 cases of SSSS, including bullous impetigo and generalized exfoliative exanthema. All cases were MSSA-induced except one MRSA-associated case.

Antibiotic sensitivity and resistance patterns in pediatric staphylococcal scalded skin syndrome. Braunstein I, Wanat KA, Abuabara K, McGowan KL, Yan AC, Treat JR. Pediatr Dermatol 2014; 31: 305–8.

This retrospective study of 21 culture-confirmed SSSS cases at the Children's Hospital of Philadelphia between 2005 and 2011 reports 86% oxacillin-susceptible and 52% clindamycin-resistant SSSS cases.

Mild staphylococcal scalded skin syndrome: an underdiagnosed clinical disorder. Hubiche T, Bes M, Roudiere L, Langlaude F, Etienne J, Del Giudice P. Br J Dermatol 2012; 166: 213–5.

Five children, age range 7 to 48 months, with a mild form of SSSS devoid of systemic symptoms, were successfully treated with intravenous oxacillin (100 mg/kg daily); one patient had additional gentamicin.

Second-Line Therapy

- Glycopeptide antibiotic (e.g., vancomycin) **E**

Emergence of *Staphylococcus aureus* carrying multiple drug resistance genes on a plasmid encoding exfoliative toxin B. Hisatsune J, Hirakawa H, Yamaguchi T, Fudaba Y, Oshima K, Hattori M et al. Antimicrob Agents Chemother 2013; 57: 6131–40.

ETB-producing *S. aureus*, including MRSA strains, causing impetigo/SSSS is more prevalent in Japan than in Western countries. Reports indicate a significant increase in strains resistant to beta-lactams, erythromycin, and gentamicin in Japan.

Staphylococcal scalded skin syndrome in the course of lupus nephritis. Rydzewska-Rosolowska A, Brzosko S, Borawski J, Mysliwiec M. Nephrology 2008; 13: 265–6.

An adult with systemic lupus erythematosus, antiphospholipid syndrome, and chronic renal failure receiving pulsed cyclophosphamide and prednisolone developed SSSS due to MRSA. She recovered with intravenous vancomycin therapy (750 mg every 48 hours).

A reduced vancomycin dosage is required in renal failure.

Staphylococcal scalded skin syndrome in an adult due to methicillin-resistant *Staphylococcus aureus*. Ito Y, Yoh MF, Toda K, Shimazaki M, Nakamura T, Morita E. J Infect Chemother 2002; 8: 256–61.

An adult with diabetes mellitus and metastatic renal cell carcinoma who developed cholecystitis and SSSS due to ET-producing MRSA was successfully treated with a combination of intravenous vancomycin and teicoplanin and percutaneous transhepatic gallbladder drainage.

Third-Line Therapies

- Cephalosporins **D**
- Aminoglycosides **D**
- Pooled human immunoglobulin **E**
- Fresh-frozen plasma **E**
- Skin substitute dressings **E**
- Plasma exchange **E**

Evidence Levels: **A** Double-blind study **B** Clinical trial ≥ 20 subjects **C** Clinical trial < 20 subjects **D** Series ≥ 5 subjects **E** Anecdotal case reports

Staphylococcal scalded skin syndrome in neonates: an 8-year retrospective study in a single institution. Li MY, Wei GH, Qiu L. Pediatr Dermatol 2014; 31: 43–7.

Thirty-nine neonates were successfully treated at a southwest Chinese neonatal unit between 2004 and 2012 for clinically diagnosed SSSS. Four received a cephalosporin (50–100 mg/kg/day), 2 a β-lactam (50–100 mg/kg/day), 24 both cephalosporin and β-lactam (50–100 mg/kg/day), 5 vancomycin (20 mg/kg/day), and 4 gamma globulin in addition to cephalosporin and β-lactam. Median days of hospitalization were longer for immunoglobulin therapy.

Staphylococcal scalded skin syndrome as a harbinger of late-onset staphylococcal septicaemia in a premature infant of very low birth weight. Hütten M, Heimann K, Baron JM, Wenzl TG, Merk H, Ott H. Acta Derm Venereol 2008; 88: 416–7.

A preterm (29 weeks of gestation), extremely low-birth-weight (985 g) male infant developed SSSS (ETA- and B-producing MSSA strain) at 37 days with systemic symptoms and was successfully treated with intravenous cefuroxime (100 mg/kg body weight) in an incubator with high air humidity, minimal handling, and 100% maintenance fluid plus the Parkland correction for a 15% epidermal loss.

Neonatal staphylococcal scalded skin syndrome: clinical and outbreak containment review. Neylon O, O'Connell NH, Slevin B, Powell J, Monahan R, Boyle L, et al. Eur J Pediatr 2010; 169: 1503–9.

Five neonates were successfully treated for MSSA ET-A–mediated SSSS with flucloxacillin and gentamicin given intravenously for a mean of 5.8 days followed by a mean of 3.8 days, oral flucloxacillin.

Adult staphylococcus scalded skin syndrome in a peritoneal dialysis patient. Suzuki R, Iwasaki S, Ito Y, Hasegawa T, Yamamoto T, Ideura T, et al. Clin Exp Nephrol 2003; 7: 77–80.

An adult undergoing peritoneal dialysis developed acute peritonitis initially treated with intraperitoneal and intravenous vancomycin (0.5 g/day each, 1 g/day total). He subsequently developed SSSS with septic shock and was successfully treated with intravenous amikacin (100 mg/day) for 1 day followed by cefoperazone with sulbactam.

Staphylococcal scalded skin syndrome in an extremely premature neonate: a case report with a brief review of the literature. Kapoor V, Travadi J, Braye S. J Pediatr Child Health 2008; 44: 374–6.

A premature neonate with SSSS was successfully treated with intravenous flucloxacillin and a single dose of intravenous immunoglobulin 1 g/kg in view of transient low IgG levels.

Severe staphylococcal scalded skin syndrome in children. Blyth M, Estela C, Young ER. Burns 2008; 34: 98–103.

Four children with severe SSSS were successfully treated with a regimen including intravenous penicillinase-resistant penicillin and fresh-frozen plasma, postulated to possess antitoxin properties.

An innovative local treatment for staphylococcal scalded skin syndrome. Mueller E, Haim M, Petnehazy T, Acham-Roschitz B, Trop M. Eur J Clin Microbiol Infect Dis 2010; 29: 893–7.

The benefits of a synthetic copolymer wound dressing (Suprathel, based on DL-lactic acid) are illustrated in a 14-month-old boy with whole-body skin denudation secondary to severe SSSS. The dressing reportedly relieves pain, prevents heat loss and secondary infection, and accelerates wound healing. It is transparent, allowing wound inspection without removal of the dressing, and is cost effective.

Use of skin substitute dressings in the treatment of staphylococcal scalded skin syndrome in neonates and young infants. Baartmans MGA, Docter J, den Hollander JC, Kroon AA, Oranje AP. Neonatology 2011; 100: 9–13.

The use of skin substitutes such as Omiderm, a water vapor–permeable polyurethane membrane, and Suprathel as valuable adjuvant treatments in severe SSSS is described in seven infants.

Optimal skin care with supportive topical treatments provided by an experienced multidisciplinary team is essential (e.g., on a burns unit).

Adult staphylococcal scalded skin syndrome successfully treated with plasma exchange. Kato T, Fujimoto N, Nakanishi G, Tsujita Y, Matsumura K, Eguchi Y, et al. Acta Derm Venereol 2015; 95: 612–3.

A 68-year-old-man with infective endocarditis and MRSA sepsis was initially treated with intravenous immunoglobulin, methylprednisolone, and daptomycin for presumed toxic epidermal necrolysis. The skin desquamation improved after plasma exchange therapy. SSSS was diagnosed retrospectively upon skin histology and bacterial culture results.

232

Steatocystoma multiplex

Ian Coulson

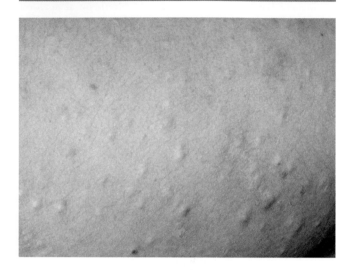

Although probably genetically heterogeneous, steatocystoma multiplex often demonstrates an autosomal-dominant pattern of inheritance. Some pedigrees have demonstrable keratin 17 abnormalities. It is characterized by the development in adolescence or early adulthood of cysts on the trunk and proximal limbs, or in some patients on the face and scalp. These are true sebaceous cysts: they contain sebum, and sebaceous gland lobules are present in the their walls. Overlap with eruptive vellus hair cysts and association with pachyonychia congenita type II have been reported. Some cases may be associated with persistent primary dentition.

MANAGEMENT STRATEGY

The cysts persist indefinitely. Although usually a minor cosmetic problem, they can be highly disfiguring. Paradoxically, those patients who would benefit the most from treatment are sometimes regarded as being unsuitable for surgery because they have too many cysts to excise. The *surgical* technique described later is quick and so can be used on large numbers of lesions in one session. It produces good cosmetic results.

Lesions can become inflamed due to rupture of the cyst wall, with leakage of the contents into the dermis, or because of secondary bacterial infection. Suppuration and scarring may follow. The clinical picture then resembles cystic acne and is called *steatocystoma multiplex suppurativum*. Oral *isotretinoin* is an effective treatment for inflammatory lesions but not for noninflamed cysts. This suggests it operates by a direct antiinflammatory effect rather than by reducing the sebum excretion rate. Alternatively, inflamed cysts can be treated with *incision and drainage*, *intralesional triamcinolone*, *tetracycline* 1 g/day, or *minocycline* 100 to 200 mg/day.

Topical treatment is largely ineffective because it does not penetrate to reach the cyst wall.

Specific Investigations

* Skin biopsy if diagnosis is in doubt
* Keratin gene testing

A novel mutation (p.Arg94Gly) of keratin 17 in a Chinese family with steatocystoma multiplex. Zang D, Zhou C, He M, Ma X, Zhang J. Eur J Dermatol 2011; 21: 142–4.

Steatocystoma multiplex, oligodontia and partial persistent primary dentition associated with a novel keratin 17 mutation. Gass JK, Wilson NJ, Smith FJ, Lane EB, McLean WH, Rytina E, et al. Br J Dermatol 2009; 161: 1396–8.

First-Line Therapies	
Lesions not inflamed	
• Surgical incision and extraction of cyst wall	D
Inflamed lesions	
• Isotretinoin	D
• Antibiotics	E
• Incision and drainage	E

Steatocystoma multiplex suppurativum: treatment with isotretinoin. Schwartz JL, Goldsmith LA. Cutis 1984; 34: 149–53.

The treatment of steatocystoma multiplex suppurativum with isotretinoin. Statham BN, Cunliffe WJ. Br J Dermatol 1984; 111: 246.

Isotretinoin in the treatment of steatocystoma multiplex: a possible adverse reaction. Rosen BL, Broadkin RH. Cutis 1986; 115: 115–20.

Steatocystoma multiplex treated with isotretinoin: a delayed response. Mortiz DL, Silverman RA. Cutis 1988; 42: 437–9.

Treatment of steatocystoma multiplex and pseudofolliculitis barbae with isotretinoin. Friedman SJ. Cutis 1987; 39: 506–7.

These five papers report a total of seven patients treated with oral isotretinoin at a dose of approximately 1 mg/kg/day for about 20 weeks. Inflammation of cysts was greatly reduced. Noninflammatory lesions were unaffected and in one patient appeared to increase in size and number. One successfully treated patient relapsed 10 weeks after ceasing therapy, but other patients did not relapse during a follow-up period of up to 8 months.

Successful treatment of steatocystoma multiplex by simple surgery. Keefe M, Leppard BJ, Royle G. Br J Dermatol 1992; 127: 41–4.

Five generations with steatocystoma multiplex congenita: a treatment regimen. Pamoukian VN, Westreich M. Plast Reconstruct Surg 1997; 99: 1142–6.

Surgical pearl: mini-incisions for the extraction of steatocystoma multiplex. Schmook T, Burg G, Hafner J. J Am Acad Dermatol 2001; 44: 1041–2.

Evidence Levels: **A** Double-blind study **B** Clinical trial ≥ 20 subjects **C** Clinical trial < 20 subjects **D** Series ≥ 5 subjects **E** Anecdotal case reports

A simple surgical technique for the treatment of steato-cystoma multiplex. Kaya TI, Ikizoglu G, Kokturk A, Tursen U. Int J Dermatol 2001; 40: 785–8.

Suggestion for the treatment of steatocystoma multiplex located exclusively on the face. Duzova AN, Senturk GB. Int J Dermatol 2004; 43: 60–2.

The vein hook successfully used for eradication of steato-cystoma multiplex. Lee SJ, Choe YS, Park BC, Lee WJ, Kim DW. Dermatol Surg 2007; 33: 82–4.

Perforation and extirpation of steatocystoma multiplex. Madan V, August PJ. Int J Dermatol 2009; 48: 329–30.

These seven reports describe variants of a simple surgical technique for noninflamed cysts. Local, regional, general, or no anesthesia is used, depending on the exact technique and the number of cysts being treated. In most cases a 1- to 10-mm incision is made with a surgical blade, and the contents of the cyst are expressed; fine artery forceps are then passed through the opening to grasp the base of the cyst, which is pulled out. The incisions heal by secondary intention. Good cosmetic results and a very low recurrence rate are reported.

Excision of cysts and aspiration have also been described.

Second-Line Therapies

- CO_2 laser therapy   **E**
- Combination laser therapy   **E**

CO_2 laser therapy for steatocystoma multiplex. Krahenbuhl A, Eichmann A, Pfaltz M. Dermatologica 1991; 183: 294–6.

"Fairly good" results were reported.

1450-nm diode laser in combination with the 1550-nm fractionated erbium-doped fiber laser for the treatment of steatocystoma multiplex: a case report. Moody MN, Landau JM, Goldberg LH, Friedman PM. Dermatol Surg 2012: 38; 1104–6.

A single case report showing substantial clearance of chest and abdominal steatocystoma after two laser treatment sessions using two complementary lasers: a 1450-nm diode laser to target the abnormal sebaceous glands and a 1550-nm fractionated erbium-doped fiber laser to target the dermal cysts.

Carbon dioxide laser perforation and extirpation of steato-cystoma multiplex. Bakkour W, Madan V. Dermatol Surg 2014; 40: 658–62.

A series of eight patients with multiple lesions treated by CO_2 laser puncturing of the cysts, followed by enucleation of the cyst contents with a Volkmann spoon. This resulted in high patient satisfaction and low recurrence rates, with minimal scarring.

Fractionated ablative carbon dioxide laser treatment of steatocystoma multiplex. Kassira S, Korta DZ, de Feraudy S, Zachary CB. J Cosmet Laser Ther 2016; 16: 1–12.

A 51-year-old woman with steatocystoma limited to the face, who after two treatments with a fractionated ablative carbon dioxide laser remained free of cysts for 3 years.

Third-Line Therapy

- Cryotherapy   **E**

Treatment of lesions of steatocystoma multiplex and other epidermal cysts by cryosurgery. Notowicz A. J Dermatol Surg Oncol 1980; 6: 98–9.

Three or 4 days after cryotherapy, the necrotic skin overlying the cyst was removed and the intact cyst expressed through the opening.

Stoma care

Calum C. Lyon

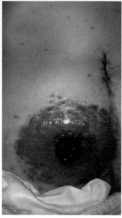
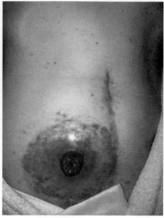
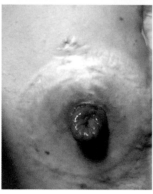

Stomas are artificial openings created to maintain proper drainage from internal structures. The most common are colostomies, ileostomies, and urostomies (ileal conduits), formed as either a temporary or a permanent measure. They are ideally produced electively, having been correctly sited by a stoma nurse specialist, but may be created under emergency conditions. Even with the best of preventative measures dermatologic problems will occur in over 50% of patients at some time. These are mostly irritant reactions to body fluids, particularly in the higher-output stomas (ileostomy and urostomy), but a range of common skin disorders, infections, or any dermatosis exacerbated by trauma or irritation may also be seen (Table 233.1 online).

MANAGEMENT STRATEGY

Although all irritant reactions share similar histologic features, the clinical appearance depends on the type of stoma and the source of irritation. Ileostomies have a high output containing degradative enzymes and irritant bile acids, so severe dermatitis and erosions may be seen. Irritated colostomies generally have a milder dermatitis, often due to occlusion, but sizeable hypergranulating polyps and acanthomas can occur where there are leaks. Urostomy dermatitis may also be erosive because of the high output and ileal mucus production, predisposing to leaks. Chronic papillomatous dermatitis is a distinct eruption comprising aggregating hyperplastic papulonodules that usually affects leaking urostomies. It responds to appliance modifications and acidification of the urine.

Input from an expert stoma nurse is essential when managing irritant reactions. He or she can advise on the most appropriate appliance so that mechanical trauma to the skin or stoma and exposure of normal skin to effluent can be avoided. Patients anxious to avoid leaks, smells, etc., sometimes wear bags too tightly or change them excessively, frequently resulting in skin damage and irritation. The stoma nurse specialist is trained to identify and resolve such issues.

It is appropriate to treat symptomatic irritant inflammation with antiinflammatory preparations such as *topical corticosteroids*, *tacrolimus*, or *pimecrolimus*. The choice of vehicle is very important, as oily creams, etc., will prevent proper adhesion and cause leaks. Products useful on peristomal skin include a range of foams, lotions, and gels formulated for scalp, ear, or eye disorders, and corticosteroid asthma inhalers (Table 233.2 and online). *Flurandrenolide tape*, an occlusive corticosteroid therapy, is particularly useful because the stoma device can be applied over the tape. Leaks and inflammation are sometimes inevitable despite appliance changes. It may be necessary to use topical antiinflammatories intermittently, with care taken to avoid steroid atrophy. Hypergranulation can be treated with *silver nitrate*, *cryotherapy*, or *cautery ± shave or curettage*.

Allergic contact dermatitis is rare, as ostomy manufacturers strive to minimize allergens in their products. When it occurs it is mostly due to perfumed deodorizers and excipients in topical products (e.g., biocides in wet wipes). Usage tests are particularly helpful in identifying the offending product, even if patch testing fails to identify the precise allergen. Treatment is as for irritant reactions.

Skin infection is not uncommon in the moist and warm environment under a stoma bag, especially folliculitis in those who shave their abdomens. All rashes should be swabbed for culture and sensitivity, because bacterial infection can present as a nonspecific dermatitis under occlusion, and preexisting rashes can become secondarily infected. Treatment involves careful hygiene and the use of specific antimicrobials.

Preexisting skin diseases that particularly affect stomas are psoriasis, seborrheic dermatitis, cutaneous Crohn disease, pyoderma gangrenosum, lichen sclerosus, and eczema.

Specific Investigations

- Skin biopsy
- Wound culture
- Patch testing and usage test

The spectrum of skin disorders in abdominal stoma patients. Lyon CC, Smith AJ, Griffiths CEM, Beck MH. Br J Dermatol 2000; 143: 1248–60.

This large cohort study documented the many different types of skin disorders that can occur around a stoma. Initial evaluations for patients presenting with inflammation include a bacterial swab because infections are relatively common and easy to treat. Allergic contact hypersensitivity should be suspected in any patient with persistent disease that is unresponsive to treatment. A biopsy should be performed for any peristomal skin disorder with ulceration or a papular component.

This is a comprehensive review discussing the various different pathologies that can occur with a stoma and how to evaluate them.

Evidence Levels: **A** Double-blind study **B** Clinical trial ≥ 20 subjects **C** Clinical trial < 20 subjects **D** Series ≥ 5 subjects **E** Anecdotal case reports

Table 233.1 Peristomal skin disorders according to primary source

Source of skin problems	Examples	Effects on skin
Appliance (pouch)	Chronic occlusion (common) Potential allergens or irritants (very rare) in appliances such as adhesives and tackifiers	Damage to skin barrier function resulting in dermatitis
Accessories: (1) pastes (fillers); (2) wet cleansing wipes; (3) deodorizing sprays; (4) skin barrier wipes/lotions; (5) adhesive removers	Irritant contact dermatitis (ICD) Allergic contact dermatitis (ACD)	ICD, e.g., alcohol in pastes and wipes, karaya (powder and pastes) ACD, especially fragrances or preservatives
Stoma effluent where there are leaks	Urine, especially if infection is present Stool, particularly where the consistency is more liquid or volume produced is high. More proximal stomas will produce larger volume with greater enzymic content. *Measures to thicken the stool should be considered, including diet advice and antimotility drugs, e.g., loperamide.*	Irritant reactions, including dermatitis, granulomas, and chronic papillomatous dermatitis
Stoma	Type: loop stomas are associated with more skin complications Structural integrity: short, buried, or prolapsed stomas are more prone to leaks	As earlier
Skin	Genetic problems (rare), e.g., ichthyotic or bullous disorders Common acquired disorders such as eczema or psoriasis can present atypically under occlusion. Rarer disorders may be more frequent than expected because of the population affected, e.g., pemphigoid in older patients with colostomies and pyoderma gangrenosum in young adults with ileostomies for inflammatory bowel disease.	Any inflammatory or scaly skin disease may impair bag adhesion and cause leaks that precipitate irritant reactions that in turn can worsen the primary skin problem
Infections	Dermatophyte, *Candida,* and viral infections present typically. Bacterial infections may mimic or secondarily affect common disorders such as eczema	Eroded dermatitis, folliculitis, and occasionally ulceration

Table 233.2 Available topical corticosteroid preparations for inflammatory peristomal disorders

Preparation	Trade name	Other ingredients
Betamethasone valerate 0.1% scalp lotion[1]	Betnovate	Carbomer, sodium hydroxide, and water
Betamethasone dipropionate 0.05% scalp lotion	Diprosone	Carbomer, sodium hydroxide, and water
Clobetasol propionate 0.05% scalp lotion	Dermovate	Carbomer, sodium hydroxide, and water
Clobetasol propionate 0.05% spray scalp foam	Clarelux	Cetyl alcohol, propylene glycol, stearyl alcohol
Fluocinolone 0.025% scalp gel	Synalar	Benzoates and propylene glycol
Betamethasone and calcipotriol scalp gel to treat psoriasis	Dovobet gel	Paraffin, liquid, polyoxypropylene-15 stearyl ether, castor oil, butylhydroxytoluene (E321)
Beclomethasone dipropionate 200 mcg/metered dose asthma inhaler[2]	Clenil Modulite	None
Crushed prednisone tablets to treat pyoderma gangrenosum[3]		
Fludroxycortide 4 mcg/cm² tape	Haelan	None

The incidence of stoma and peristomal complications during the first 3 months after ostomy creation. Salvadalena GD. J Wound Ostomy Continence Nurs 2013; 40: 400–6.

A prospective case series showing irritation and infection to be the most common problems.

A prospective audit of stomas – analysis of risk factors and complications and their management. Arumugam PJ, Bevan L, Macdonald L, Watkins AJ, Morgan AR, Beynon J, et al. Colorectal Dis 2003; 5: 49–52.

Healthy peristomal skin is dependent on good surgical technique, with more problems being associated with short stomas (ileostomies <20 mm and colostomies <5 mm) and after emergency procedures. Body mass index and diabetes are significantly associated with skin problems. Bleeding hypergranulation is more common in colostomies. Careful postoperative stoma nurse follow-up helps prevent skin problems.

The relevance of patch testing in peristomal dermatitis. Al-Niaimi F, Beck M, Almaani N, Samarasinghe V, Williams J, Lyon C. Br J Dermatol 2012; 167: 103–9.

A subset of 149 patients from a cohort of 850 were patch-tested to a comprehensive series of potential allergens. Only seven of these had reactions of current relevance, and most of these were to common fragrances and preservatives in stoma accessories rather than pouching systems.

First-Line Therapies	
• Change appliance	D
• Absorbent powders	D
• Antibiotics	D
• Topical corticosteroids	B

Dermatologic considerations of stoma care. Rothstein MS. J Am Acad Dermatol 1986; 15: 411–32.

Ill-fitting devices can cause stoma and skin irritation. The chemical irritation caused from the stomal effluent, mechanical irritation, and contact dermatitis can all be alleviated by replacing the stoma device at the earliest sign of irritation. Additionally, careful drying of the skin after washing and the use of absorbent powders will alleviate irritation caused by intertrigo and ill-fitting devices.

Peristomal dermatoses: a novel indication for topical steroid lotions. Lyon CC, Smith AJ, Griffiths CEM, Beck MH. J Am Acad Dermatol 2000; 43: 679–82.

This large clinical study demonstrated the benefits of treating inflammatory peristomal skin diseases with topical corticosteroids formulated in an aqueous alcohol lotion. This formulation was found advantageous because it did not interfere with adhesion of the ostomy bag to the skin.

Topical therapy for peristomal pyoderma gangrenosum (PPG). Nybaek H, Olsen AG, Karslmark T, Jemec G. J Cutan Med Surg 2004; 8: 220–3.

Most cases of PPG respond to topical therapy, usually corticosteroids.

Second-Line Therapies	
• Sucralfate	C
• Tacrolimus ointment or pimecrolimus cream	E
• Intralesional corticosteroids	C

Topical sucralfate in the management of peristomal skin disease: an open study. Lyon CC, Stapelton M, Smith AJ, Griffiths CE, Beck MH. Clin Exp Dermatol 2000; 25: 584–8.

The authors demonstrated the ability of sucralfate to help treat peristomal erosions. Sucralfate is a basic aluminum salt of sucrose octasulfate that polymerizes in acidic environments providing a viscous barrier on mucosal surfaces. Sucralfate was effective for erosions and irritation caused by either feces or urine. However, it was ineffective for peristomal pyoderma gangrenosum (PPG).

Peristomal pyoderma gangrenosum. Keltz M, Lebwohl M, Bishop S. J Am Acad Dermatol 1992; 27: 360–4.

A patient with PPG is described who responded well to intralesional corticosteroids.

This article also discusses the difficulties in diagnosing PPG.

Peristomal lichen sclerosus (LS): the role of occlusion and urine exposure? Al-Niaimi F, Lyon C. Br J Dermatol 2013; 168: 643–6.

Nine of 12 patients required intralesional corticosteroids to achieve complete resolution of active lichen sclerosus.

Topical tacrolimus in the management of peristomal pyoderma gangrenosum. Lyon CC, Stapelton M, Smith AJ, Mendelsohn S, Beck MH, Griffiths CE. J Dermatol Treat 2001; 12: 13–7.

Topical tacrolimus (0.3% in carmellose sodium paste) in conjunction with other treatments was found to rapidly heal pyoderma gangrenosum.

Third-Line Therapies	
• Botulinum toxin	C
• Oral dapsone	E
• Ciclosporin	D
• Tumor necrosis factor–blocking drugs	E
• Collagen injections	E
• Lipectomy	E
• Stoma revision surgery	E

Management of peristomal pyoderma gangrenosum. Poritz LS, Lebo MA, Bobb AD, Ardell CM, Koltun WA. J Am Coll Surg 2008; 206: 311–5.

PPG is a difficult and frequently misdiagnosed condition. Dapsone, topical cromolyn sodium, ciclosporin, mycophenolate mofetil, or infliximab can be beneficial in treating PPG. PPG will resolve if the stoma can be closed, but resizing a stoma to treat PPG is not indicated, as it will recur at the new stoma site.

Paraileostomy recontouring by collagen sealant injection: a novel approach to one aspect of ileostomy morbidity. Report of a case. Smith GH, Skipworth RJ, Terrace JD, Helal B, Stewart KJ, Anderson DN. Dis Colon Rectum 2007; 50: 1719–23.

Peristomal dermal deformity such as skin creasing impairs appliance placement. A dermal contour defect was successfully treated with intradermal injections of collagen.

A novel use for botulinum toxin A (BoNT-A) in the management of ileostomy and urostomy leaks. Smith VM, Lyon CC. J Wound Ostomy Continence Nurs 2015; 42: 83–8.

Seven of 10 consecutive patients presenting with actively contractile stomas, which shortened spasmodically, resulting in leaks, responded to BoNT-A injected into stoma musculature.

Troublesome colostomies and urinary stomas treated with suction assisted lipectomy. Samdal F, Amlamd PF, Bakka A, Aasen AO. Eur J Surg 1995; 161: 361–4.

Synchronous panniculectomy with stomal revision for obese patients with stomal stenosis and retraction. Katkoori D, Samavedi S, Kava B, Soloway MS, Manoharan M. BJU Int 2009; 105: 1586–9.

Suction lipectomy or surgical panniculectomy can correct leakage problems, particularly in morbidly obese patients with retracted stomas and without the need for laparotomy.

There is no ideal topical preparation applicable to stomas that is available "off the shelf." The table details some corticosteroid preparations that can be used. Lotions containing oils should be avoided, and the patient should be warned that gel preparations containing propylene glycol should be left to dry for 10 minutes before placing their bag. Alcoholic scalp lotions can sting when applied to broken skin and can be applied to the bag directly and left to dry before fitting. Some patients, particularly those with longer stomas, are able to use creams or ointments applied to the peristomal skin for 30 to 60 minutes during which time the patient is inactive and a stoma bag is held in place over the stoma using a waist belt. The greasy medicament can then be cleaned from the skin and a bag applied normally. The potency of steroid is increased under occlusion. Continuous daily treatment should be for no more than 4 weeks and thereafter no more than three times per week to avoid skin atrophy.

Striae

Adam S. Nabatian, Hooman Khorasani

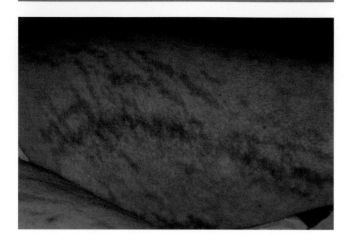

Striae distensae are extremely common lesions that do not cause medical problems. Early striae (striae rubra) are linear, red-to-violaceous patches or plaques that may be pruritic. Gradually, they become white, atrophic, linear, depressed patches along lines of skin tension. They are considered to be linear dermal scars with epidermal atrophy as evidenced by a finely wrinkled appearance and telangiectasias. Common locations include the breasts and abdomen of pregnant women and the shoulders of body builders. Striae are common in teenagers undergoing their growth spurts and in overweight individuals. Extensive striae that are deeper and wider, and include facial skin, are seen with long-term systemic corticosteroid use. Striae are likely the result of a combination of factors, including genetics, mechanical stress (e.g., growth spurt, bodybuilding, pregnancy), and hormones (e.g., cortisol, estrogen). Although striae will generally fade and become inconspicuous, patients frequently request cosmetic treatments.

MANAGEMENT STRATEGY

The goal of treatment is a gradual, incremental improvement. In general, the "older" the lesion (striae alba), the less dramatic and more slowly the treatment response will be. The best results are achieved by combining multiple treatment modalities early in the course of evolution. Currently, no "gold standard" treatment modality has been determined.

Several studies have shown that *topical tretinoin* improves the appearance of striae. Based on these reports, striae rubra respond better to this therapy. Although not formally investigated, it is expected that *other topical retinoids (e.g., tazarotene, adapalene)* may also provide some improvement.

Nonablative lasers produce improvement by stimulating an increase in dermal collagen and elastin. The *pulsed dye laser* has been most studied. Recent studies suggest that improvement is more common in early striae that are pink to red in color. *Ablative lasers* may be more useful than the nonablative counterparts, but have more significant downtime and an increased risk of complications. *Radiofrequency devices* may work by a similar mechanism of dermal heating. Platelet-rich

plasma (PRP) is a new treatment used alone or in combination with other treatment modalities such as fractionated lasers or microneedling with good results. PRP is an autologous concentrate of platelets in a small volume of plasma containing high concentrations of growth factors and cytokines that stimulate the production of collagen and proliferation of fibroblasts and keratinocytes. The *excimer laser, intense pulsed light,* and *glycolic acid products* appear to be the most promising treatments for mature striae.

Specific Investigations

- Thorough history and physical examination
- Skin biopsy (not generally necessary)
- Serum adrenocorticotropin levels, 24-hour urine free cortisol level, plasma cortisol levels (if no history of growth spurt, bodybuilding, or pregnancy)

The diagnosis and cause of striae are usually straightforward to elucidate. When the lesions are particularly severe and the cause is unknown, laboratory testing to exclude Cushing syndrome is advised. In Cushing syndrome, striae are characterized by their excessive size, depth, and striking red-to-purple color. Occasionally, striae may be confused with linear focal elastosis, which are striae-like, asymptomatic, slightly palpable, yellow bands commonly found on the lower back of older adults. Histologic evaluation, with specific attention given to the elastic fiber content, will clearly differentiate these two entities.

First-Line Therapy

- Observation   D

It is well known that striae tend to become less conspicuous with time. Thus reassurance may be all that is required for the patient who is not overly concerned about his or her striae.

Adolescent striae. Ammar NM, Roa B, Schwartz RA, Janniger CK. Cutis 2000; 65: 69–70.

Striae cutis distensae. Nigam PK. Int J Dermatol 1989; 28: 426–7.

Second-Line Therapies

- Ablative fractional photothermolysis 10,600-nm laser   B
- Nonablative fractional photothermolysis 1550-nm laser   B
- Pulsed dye laser (PDL) (585 nm)   B
- Intense pulsed light (IPL)   B
- Topical tretinoin   B

Treatment of striae distensae using an ablative 10,600-nm carbon dioxide fractional laser: a retrospective review of 27 participants. Lee SE, Kim JH, Lee SJ, Lee JE, Kang JM, Kim YK, et al. Dermatol Surg 2010; 36: 1683–90.

Evidence Levels: **A** Double-blind study   **B** Clinical trial ≥ 20 subjects   **C** Clinical trial < 20 subjects   **D** Series ≥ 5 subjects   **E** Anecdotal case reports

Twenty-seven women with striae were treated with fractional CO_2 (DeepFX, Lumenis Esthetic, Inc., Santa Clara, CA) at pulse energy of 10 mJ and density of 2 (percentage coverage of 10%). Three months after treatment 2 of the 27 participants (7.4%) had grade 4 clinical improvement, 14 (51.9%) had grade 3 improvement, 9 (33.3%) had grade 2 improvement, and 2 (7.4%) had grade 1 improvement. None of the participants showed worsening.

Treatment of striae distensae with nonablative fractional laser versus ablative CO_2 fractional laser: a randomized controlled trial. Yang YJ, Lee GY. Ann Dermatol 2011; 23: 481–9.

Twenty-four patients with varying degrees of atrophic striae alba in the abdomen were enrolled in a randomized, blind, split study. The patients were treated with 1550-nm fractional Er:glass laser (Mosaic, Lutronic Co., Seoul, Korea; pulse energy of 50 mJ, a spot density of 100 spots/cm², using a scan area of 5 mm × 10 mm in a static mode with one pass administered per treatment site without overlapping) and ablative fractional CO_2 laser resurfacing (eCO₂, Lutronic Co., Seoul, Korea; pulse energy of 40–50 mJ, a spot density of 75–100 spots/cm², using a scan area of 8 mm × 8 mm in a static mode). Each half of the abdominal lesion was randomly selected and treated three times at intervals of 4 weeks using the same parameters. Posttreatment pruritus, redness, and hyperpigmentation were reported side effects for both modalities. Clinical improvements were not found to be statistically significant between treatments, although both showed a significant clinical and histopathologic improvement over pretreatment sites.

Treatment of striae distensae with fractional photothermolysis. Bak H, Kim BJ, Lee WJ, Bang JS, Lee SY, Choi JH, et al. Dermatol Surg 2009; 35: 1215–20.

Twenty-two Asian women were treated with two laser treatments (Fraxel SR1500) separated by 4 weeks at pulse energy 30 mJ, density level of 6, and eight passes. Six of 22 (27%) demonstrated marked improvement in striae, with the other 16 showing mild improvement. Outcomes were better in patients with white rather than red striae.

Efficacy of pulsed dye laser versus intense pulsed light in the treatment of striae distensae. Shokeir H, El Bedewi A, Sayed S, El Khalafawy G. Dermatol Surg 2014; 40: 632–40.

Sixteen patients with striae rubra and four with striae alba had treatment with PDL for striae on one side of their bodies and treatment with IPL for striae on the other side for five sessions with a 4-week interval between the sessions. 595-nm PDL (Cynosure, Chelmsford, MA) was used with a spot size of 10 mm, pulse duration of 0.5 milliseconds, energy density of 2.5 J/cm², and pulse rate of 1 Hz. Fluorescence IPL (Medical Bio Care, Gothenburg, Sweden) was used with a wavelength of 565 nm, spot size of 10 × 20 mm, pulse duration of 50 to 70 milliseconds, and energy density of 17.5 J/cm². Striae width was decreased, skin texture was improved, and collagen expression was increased significantly after both PDL and IPL. However, PDL induced the expression of collagen I in a significant manner compared with IPL. Striae rubra gave a superior response with either PDL or IPL compared with striae alba.

Topical tretinoin 0.1% for pregnancy-related abdominal striae: an open-label, multicenter, prospective study. Rangel O, Aries I, García E, Lopez-Padilla S. Adv Ther 2001; 18: 181–6.

One week post delivery, 20 patients applied tretinoin cream 0.1% once a day for 3 months to half of the abdomen. Eighty percent noted a marked or moderate improvement. Measured striae decreased by 20% in length and by 23% in width.

Third-Line Therapies

• Excimer laser (308 nm)	C
• Copper bromide laser (577–511 nm)	C
• 1064-nm Nd:YAG laser	C
• Radiofrequency and 585-nm PDL	B
• Radiofrequency device	C
• Needling therapy	B
• Platelet-rich plasma (PRP) and microdermabrasion	B
• 20% glycolic acid/0.05% tretinoin	C
• 20% glycolic acid/10% L-ascorbic acid	C
• 70% glycolic acid lotion	A
• 70% glycolic acid gel/40% trichloroacetic acid chemical peel	D

The 308-nm excimer laser in the darkening of the white lines of striae alba. Ostovari N, Saadat N, Nasiri S, Moravvej H, Toossi P. J Dermatolog Treat 2010; 21: 229–31.

Ten subjects were treated using excimer laser on the white lines of striae, whereas the normal skin near to and between the lines was treated with zinc oxide cream. Some repigmentation was noted, and therapy with excimer laser was described as "weakly effective." Before and after photographs demonstrated that 80% of patients had poor or moderate results.

Two-year follow-up results of copper bromide laser treatment of striae. Longo L, Postigli MG, Marangoni O, Melato M. J Clin Laser Med Surg 2003; 21: 157–60.

Thirteen of 15 patients experienced improvement in their striae that remained after 1 to 2 years. One third of the patients had total disappearance of selected striae.

Stretch marks: treatment using the 1064-nm Nd:YAG laser. Goldman A, Rossato F, Prati C. Dermatol Surg 2008; 34: 686–91.

Twenty patients with striae rubra were treated with the 1064-nm Nd:YAG laser; all considered the results satisfactory, and a majority (55%) found the results to be excellent.

Radiofrequency and 585-nm pulsed dye laser treatment of striae distensae: a report of 37 Asian patients. Suh DH, Chang KY, Son HC, Ryu JH, Lee SJ, Song KY. Dermatol Surg 2007; 33: 29–34.

Thirty-seven patients were treated with one session of radiofrequency (Thermage) and three monthly sessions of the 585-nm PDL. A majority of patients (89.2%) showed "good" or "very good" improvement.

Treatment of striae distensae with a TriPollar radiofrequency device: a pilot study. Manuskiatti W, Boonthaweeyuwat E, Varothai S. J Dermatolog Treat 2009; 20: 359–64.

Seventeen females with skin phototypes IV to V and striae received six weekly treatments with a TriPollar radiofrequency device. At 1 week after the final treatment, 38.2% and 11.8% of the subjects were assessed to have 25% to 50% and 51% to 75% improvement of their striae, respectively. No adverse effects were noted.

Treatment of striae distensae with needling therapy versus CO_2 fractional laser. Khater MH, Khattab FM, Abdelhaleem MR. J Cosmet Laser Ther 2016; 28: 1–5.

Ten female patients with striae were treated with needling therapy, and another 10 were treated with fractional CO_2 (Deka,

Italy) every 1 month for three sessions. The CO_2 settings were spot diameter of 1 to 10 mm according to lesion width, pulse energy of 100 watts, repetition rate of 20 Hz, using a single pass. Nine of 10 needle-treated patients showed improvement, whereas only 5 of 10 CO_2-treated patients showed clinical improvement.

Comparison between the efficacy and safety of platelet-rich plasma vs. microdermabrasion in the treatment of striae distensae: clinical and histopathological study. Ibrahim ZA, El-Tatawy RA, El-Samongy MA, Ali DA. J Cosmet Dermatol 2015; 14: 336–46.

Forty patients with striae rubra and 28 patients with striae alba were treated by intradermal injection of PRP alone, microdermabrasion (aluminum oxide/sodium chloride–based system [deep clean (EME-Italy) apparatus]) alone, or combination of PRP and microdermabrasion in the same session every 2 weeks for a maximum of six sessions or until the patients' satisfaction was achieved. PRP alone was more effective than microdermabrasion alone, but it was better to use the combination of both for more and rapid efficacy. With PRP alone or PRP plus microdermabrasion, both striae alba and rubra improved after repeated treatments, but striae rubra improved less than alba. In the microdermabrasion group, striae rubra showed more clinical improvement than alba.

A superficial texture analysis of 70% glycolic acid topical therapy and striae distensae. Mazzarello V, Farace F, Ena P, Fenu G, Mulas P, Piu L, et al. Plast Reconstr Surg 2012; 129: 589e–90e.

Double-blind, placebo-controlled trial on 40 patients with both striae rubra and striae alba treated with 70% glycolic acid lotion in a bilateral comparison study. In both types, a significant decrease in furrow width was noted after 6 months. Skin texture parameters analyzed were anisotropy, number of skin furrows, and furrow width, using the silicone replica technique, where silicone casts were analyzed by scanning electron microscopy and imaging software.

Comparison of topical therapy for striae alba (20% glycolic acid/0.05% tretinoin versus 20% glycolic acid/10% L-ascorbic acid). Ash K, Lord J, Zukowski M, McDaniel DH. Dermatol Surg 1998; 24: 849–56.

Ten patients with skin types I to V and abdominal and thigh striae associated with childbirth applied glycolic acid in the morning and either tretinoin or L-ascorbic acid in the evening for a total of 12 weeks. All patients felt that they had improvement of their striae.

Chemical peel of nonfacial skin using glycolic acid gel augmented with TCA and neutralized based on visual staging. Cook KK, Cook WR. Dermatol Surg 2000; 26: 994–9.

The authors comment on their experience treating over 3100 patients with nonfacial peels using a combination of 70% glycolic acid gel combined with 40% trichloroacetic acid. It is reported that striae, including atrophic hypopigmented striae, can be improved with this treatment.

Evidence Levels: **A** Double-blind study   **B** Clinical trial ≥ 20 subjects   **C** Clinical trial < 20 subjects   **D** Series ≥ 5 subjects   **E** Anecdotal case reports

235

Subacute cutaneous lupus erythematosus

Lisa Pappas-Taffer, Jeffrey P. Callen

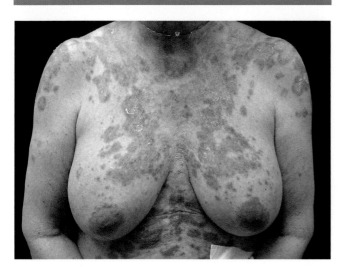

Subacute cutaneous lupus erythematosus (SCLE) is a nonscarring, photosensitive variant of cutaneous lupus erythematosus (CLE). Patients can have annular or papulosquamous plaques, or a morphologic combination, that is characteristically in a sun-exposed distribution. Although SCLE does not scar, it can result in significant dyspigmentation.

MANAGEMENT STRATEGY

SCLE can be diagnosed clinically, but should be confirmed with skin biopsy. The patient should have a careful history, physical examination, and laboratory studies directed at uncovering systemic manifestations of systemic lupus erythematosus (SLE). Historical details that could help uncover exacerbating factors or that could affect therapeutic choice should be obtained. There are few double-blind, placebo-controlled trials of drugs used in the treatment of SCLE. The goals of management are to treat current lesions and symptoms and to prevent lesion formation. This is done through a combination of patient education, sun protection, and topical and systemic therapies.

The cornerstone of treatment of CLE includes using the most benign drugs possible to achieve disease control. The most common therapies utilized include *photoprotection, topical corticosteroids, calcineurin inhibitors,* and oral *antimalarials.* Although systemic corticosteroids can be effective, steroid-sparing systemic agents (e.g. *methotrexate, mycophenolate mofetil, azathioprine*) are preferred to avoid corticosteroid-associated side effects. CLE can affect quality of life. In addition to increased disease control, cosmetic agents used to camouflage lesions or dyspigmentation are important adjuncts.

SCLE can have numerous associations that need to be addressed, including more recalcitrant disease in the setting of tobacco use and a potential risk for neonatal lupus during pregnancy.

Up to 50% of patients with SCLE meet four or more of the criteria of the American College of Rheumatology for classification of SLE. However, they do so by fulfilling the criteria involving skin lesions, photosensitivity, and positive serologies. As a result, those classified as SLE typically only have mild systemic symptoms with major end organ damage occurring in <10%.

Up to 30% of SCLE is induced or exacerbated by a medication. Over 100 different agents have been reported, including antihypertensive agents, statins, antifungals, tumor necrosis factor (TNF) inhibitors, antiepileptics, and proton pump inhibitors. A complete list of the patient's medications will assist in the exclusion of drug-induced SCLE. In the setting of treatment for cancer, SCLE can occur as a result of chemotherapy exposure, radiation exposure, or as a paraneoplastic syndrome itself.

There are controversial data regarding whether tobacco affects the effectiveness of antimalarial agents. However, multiple studies have reported that cigarette smokers have more severe disease and that a subset of these patients is more refractory to therapies. Hence, patients should be counseled on smoking cessation for the benefit of their skin as well as the increased risk of cardiovascular disease with SLE and possibly CLE.

Specific Investigations

- Ro/SSA antibody
- Exclude systemic disease
- Medication review
- Smoking status

First-Line Therapies

Local therapy

• Cosmetics	E
• Sunscreens, protective clothing, and sun avoidance	A
• High-potency corticosteroids	B
• Topical tacrolimus or pimecrolimus	A
• Topical retinoids	E

Systemic therapy

• Antimalarials (hydroxychloroquine, chloroquine, ± the addition of quinacrine)	A

Photoprotective effects of a broad-spectrum sunscreen in ultraviolet-induced cutaneous lupus erythematosus: a randomized, vehicle-controlled, double-blind study. Kuhn A, Gensch K, Haust M, Meuth AM, Boyer F, Dupuy P, et al. J Am Acad Dermatol 2010; 64: 37–48.

Of the 16 CLE patients who had positive provocation study results to UVA or UVB, 88% developed CLE lesions in the vehicle control area, whereas none developed lesions in the broad-spectrum, SPF 60, sunscreen-applied areas.

Discoid lupus erythematosus. Diagnostic features and evaluation of topical corticosteroid therapy. Roenigk HH Jr, Martin JS, Eichorn P, Gilliam JN. Cutis 1980; 25: 281–5.

Despite the long-standing use of high-potency topical corticosteroids as first-line therapy, this is the only randomized, controlled trial examining the efficacy in CLE.

Intralesional triamcinolone is effective for discoid lupus erythematosus of the palms and soles. Callen JP. J Rheumatol 1985; 12: 630–3.

The use of topical calcineurin inhibitors in lupus erythematosus: an overview. Wollina U, Hansel G. J Eur Acad Dermatol Venereol 2008; 22: 1–6.

A good summary of the literature up until 2008 regarding calcineurin inhibitors in CLE, with each table corresponding to all the reported literature for tacrolimus or pimecrolimus response divided by CLE subtype.

Efficacy of tacrolimus 0.1% ointment in cutaneous lupus erythematosus: a multicenter, randomized, double-blind, vehicle-controlled trial. Kuhn A, Gensch K, Haust M, Schneider SW, Bonsmann G, Gaebelein-Wissing N, et al. J Am Acad Dermatol 2011; 65: 54–64.

Significant improvement in all end points was noted in all CLE subtypes after 4 and 8 weeks, but not after 12 weeks. The four patients with SCLE in this study improved, but this was not statistically significant compared with placebo.

Although there are case reports documenting the use of topical retinoids for chronic CLE, there are no reports of using these agents in the setting of SCLE.

Treatment of cutaneous lupus erythematosus with acitretin and hydroxychloroquine. Ruzicka T, Sommerburg C, Goerz G, Kind P, Mensing H. Br J Dermatol 1992; 127: 513–8.

In this multicenter, randomized controlled trial, 50% of patients treated with hydroxychloroquine (HCQ) improved at 8 weeks.

Low blood concentrations of hydroxychloroquine in patients with refractory cutaneous lupus erythematosus: a French multicenter prospective study. Francès C, Cosnes A, Duhaut P, Zahr N, Soutou B, Ingen-Housz-Oro S, et al. Arch Dermatol 2012; 148: 479–84.

In this study of 300 patients with CLE, blood HCQ concentrations greater than 755 ng/mL were associated with a better clinical efficacy.

Monitoring HCQ blood concentrations may be an alternative to the use of a fixed dose of HCQ or to prescribing based on the patient's weight.

The effect of increasing the dose of hydroxychloroquine (HCQ) in patients with refractory cutaneous lupus erythematosus (CLE): an open-label prospective pilot study. Chasset F, Arnaud L, Costedoat-Chalumeau N, Zahr N, Bessis D, Francès C. J Am Acad Dermatol 2016; 74: 693–9.

Of 34 patients (11 with SCLE) who didn't respond clinically to weight-based HCQ after 3 months, with HCQ blood level <750 ng/mL, increasing the dose to 600 mg/day resulted in clinical response in 26/34 (81%) of patients. This clinical response corresponded to HCQ levels of >750 ng/mL. Among responders, the daily dose of HCQ could be decreased back to 400 mg/day in 73% of responders, with one third of responders having sustained cutaneous improvement despite dose reduction, but the remaining two thirds of the responders experiencing a relapse of CLE.

In patients on weight-based HCQ without response, one could attempt a short-term dose increase of HCQ if low HCQ blood levels are present, with the goal of reducing the dose. The former may increase the likelihood of eye toxicity if therapy at higher doses is prolonged. This study also suggests one might consider checking HCQ levels in recalcitrant patients.

Response to antimalarial agents in cutaneous lupus erythematosus: a prospective analysis. Chang AY, Piette EW, Foering KP, Tenhave TR, Okawa J, Werth VP. Arch Dermatol 2011; 147: 1261–7.

Of 11 patients started on HCQ, 55% were responders. Of 15 patients who were nonresponders to HCQ monotherapy, 67% gained response with the addition of quinacrine, as measured via cutaneous lupus erythematosus disease area and severity index (CLASI).

This report demonstrates the efficacy of combination therapy. The authors use the same algorithmic clinical approach to antimalarial treatment as outlined in this study. HCQ was dosed at 200 to 400 mg/day, and chloroquine was dosed at 250 mg/day for 5 to 7 days per week, both determined by ideal body weight. Quinacrine was dosed at 100 mg/day. If first-line HCQ treatment fails after 3 to 6 months, we add quinacrine. If HCQ–quinacrine treatment fails after 3 to 6 months (or the patient doesn't have access to a compounding pharmacy for quinacrine), we replace HCQ with chloroquine (± quinacrine). Of note, HCQ is first-line due to less eye toxicity than chloroquine (but it is also less efficacious). Quinacrine is a great adjunct to either HCQ or chloroquine, as it does not add to eye toxicity. Use of the HCQ and chloroquine combination is contraindicated due to compounded eye toxicity. Quinacrine must be compounded, and chloroquine is becoming much harder to obtain.

Hydroxychloroquine sulfate treatment is associated with later onset of systemic lupus erythematosus. James JA, Kim-Howard XR, Bruner BF, Jonsson MK, McClain MT, Arbuckle MR, et al. Lupus 2007; 16: 401–9.

Second-Line Therapies	
Immunosuppressive Agents	
• Mycophenolate mofetil, enteric-coated mycophenolate sodium*	B
• Methotrexate	D
• Azathioprine	D
Immunomodulators	
• Dapsone	D
• Thalidomide, lenalidomide	B, C
• Oral retinoids	B

*Double-blind study in SLE population evaluating mucocutaneous (CLE) change, but without the use of a CLE-specific assessment tool.

Mycophenolate sodium for subacute cutaneous lupus erythematosus resistant to standard therapy. Kreuter A, Tomi NS, Weiner SM, Huger M, Altmeyer P, Gambichler T. Br J Dermatol 2007; 156: 1321–7.

In this prospective, open-label pilot study, 10 patients with recalcitrant SCLE were treated with enteric-coated mycophenolate sodium as monotherapy. They had statistically significant reductions in CLASI after 3 months of treatment (1440 mg/day). No serious side effects were noted.

This is the equivalent of 1000 mg twice daily of mycophenolate mofetil (MMF). Table 3 is a good summary of MMF (1–3 g/day) and enteric-coated mycophenolate sodium (720–2160 mg/day) efficacy in treating SCLE in multiple case reports and small studies. Pisoni et al. (2005) is the only report of a lack of MMF response in seven SLE/CLE patients (one of which had SCLE); however, patients failed to respond to a median of 4 (range 2–10) different CLE drugs, and treatment efficacy was determined after only 2 months of MMF therapy in 3/7 patients.

Typically MMF in the treatment of CLE is done in combination with antimalarials and topical therapies, with the goal of tapering to the lowest-needed dose/therapies. Authors typically have good response with MMF in patients who fail first-line therapies.

Evidence Levels: **A** Double-blind study **B** Clinical trial ≥ 20 subjects **C** Clinical trial < 20 subjects **D** Series ≥ 5 subjects **E** Anecdotal case reports

Methotrexate treatment for refractory subacute cutaneous lupus erythematosus. Kuhn A, Specker C, Ruzicka T, Lehmann P. J Am Acad Dermatol 2002; 46: 600–3.

Contains a summary of retrospective studies and reports from the literature of treatment with methotrexate (MTX), including 19 CLE patients (8 SCLE patients), with doses ranging from 10 to 25 mg/week.

In patients who fail antimalarials, MTX orally or subcutaneously once weekly is an option.

Efficacy and safety of methotrexate in recalcitrant cutaneous lupus erythematosus: results of a retrospective study in 43 patients. Wenzel J, Brähler S, Bauer R, Bieber T, Tüting T. Br J Dermatol 2005; 153: 157–62.

A retrospective analysis of 43 treatment-refractory CLE patients (15 SCLE) treated with methotrexate 15 to 25 mg weekly. Improvement of CLE occurred in nearly all patients (42/43). *This is a large number of patients with excellent improvement. This agent has not been as successful in the patients the authors have treated, often necessitating the addition of combined antimalarial therapy, or transitioning to MMF, when MTX therapy fails.*

Azathioprine: an effective, corticosteroid-sparing therapy for patients with recalcitrant cutaneous lupus erythematosus or with recalcitrant cutaneous leukocytoclastic vasculitis. Callen JP, Spencer LV, Burruss JB, Holtman J. Arch Dermatol 1991; 127: 515–22.

Report of six patients with refractory CLE (five SCLE) treated with azathioprine 100 to 150 mg/day. Three of six patients had near clearing within 3 months, one of which had palmoplantar ulceration that healed after 6 weeks.

Case series from the 1980s and 1990s have shown successful treatment of CLE (mainly generalized and palmoplantar discoid lupus erythematosus [DLE], but also a series including SCLE) with azathioprine 100 to 150 mg daily.

Dapsone as second-line treatment for cutaneous lupus erythematosus? A retrospective analysis of 34 patients and a review of the literature. Klebes M, Wutte N, Aberer E. Dermatology 2016; 232: 91–6.

This is a retrospective analysis of 34 CLE patients (8 with SCLE) treated with dapsone, most in combination with antimalarials, over a 7-year period. The median dose of dapsone was 100 mg/day (50–125 mg/day) for a mean duration of 16 months (ranging 1–82 months). Forty-one percent of patients improved after 2 months, with 18% showing complete remission within 7 months. The best effect was seen in SCLE patients, with disease remission or improvement in six of eight patients. *Of note, no validated activity measurement tools were used. The authors also summarized the literature (case reports and retrospective analyses that include 137 CLE patients, of which 7 are SCLE) in table 1. Of seven SCLE cases in the literature, all had improvement or clearance with 25 to 150 mg/day dosing.*

Dapsone, given in doses of 25 to 200 mg daily, is especially effective in the treatment of bullous lupus, but case reports and case series have also shown usefulness in the treatment of CLE, especially SCLE lesions and the vasculitic lesions that may accompany SCLE.

Thalidomide in cutaneous lupus erythematosus. Pelle MT, Werth VP. Am J Clin Dermatol 2003; 4: 379–87.

This is a summary of reports of the use of thalidomide for CLE through 2003, specifically the Knop et al. 1983 study of 60 patients showing 90% complete or partial response with 25% peripheral polyneuropathy and the 200 Ordi-Ros et al. prospective study of 22 refractory CLE patients (including 7 SCLE), in which 100 mg daily then reduction to 25 to 50 mg/day was used as maintenance. Initial improvement was noted after 2 weeks and maximum benefit within 3 months, complete remission in 75%, and partial in 25%. Of the 7 SCLE patients, 6/7 cleared with low-dose thalidomide in an average of 2.2 months. After 2013, there are >3 retrospective studies confirming these earlier results. Many demonstrate low-dose thalidomide (50 mg daily) is as effective as higher doses, but does not reduce neurotoxicity (Cuadrado et al. 2005).

Thalidomide in the treatment of refractory cutaneous lupus erythematosus: prognostic factors of clinical outcome. Cortes-Hernandez J, Torres-Salido M, Castro-Marrero J, Vilardell-Tarres M, Ordi-Ros J. Br J Dermatol 2012; 166: 616–23.

In this prospective observational study, 60 patients with refractory CLE (18 SCLE) on prednisone and antimalarials were treated with thalidomide 100 mg/day and followed for a mean of 8 years (range 2–18). Once complete clinical improvement was achieved, dose reduction to 50 mg daily then 50 mg alternating days occurred. Ninety-eight percent achieved response, with 85% achieving complete response, typically within a mean of 8 weeks (range 3–16). Mean duration of therapy was 6 months (3–36 months). By the end of the 8 years, 70% who had attained complete remission had at least one relapse, whereas the rest (30%) remained in remission despite medication withdrawal after at least 8 years of follow-up. Neurologic symptoms occurred in 18% of patients (reported as high as 45% in retrospective studies) with nerve conduction studies being positive in half of the cases. Neurologic symptoms and signs on electromyography (EMG) resolved after 12 months (range 6–18) status postwithdrawal.

This is the first prospective thalidomide study utilizing CLASI to measure clinical response. Patients with SCLE had a lower relapse rate and required a lower cumulative dose and duration of therapy of thalidomide compared with other CLE subtypes.

Thalidomide (50–100 mg/day) has been shown to be highly efficacious in the treatment of CLE, including SCLE, and much less effective for SLE (can induce SLE flare). Numerous retrospective studies, and the previously mentioned prospective study, show on average 80% of patients achieving complete response. CLE responds quickly, beginning at 2 to 4 weeks, and doses can often be tapered lower after improvement. Thalidomide should only be used to treat severe, refractory CLE at the lowest dose possible. Studies have shown that starting with a low dose is as effective as higher doses, but unfortunately has not been shown to reduce the incidence of neurotoxicity. Although highly efficacious, it is reserved as second-line therapy because of its cost, the degree of monitoring by the System for Thalidomide Education and Prescribing Safety (STEPS) protocol, its teratogenicity, and adverse effects, including peripheral neuropathy. Thalidomide works well as a rescue medication or for maintenance at low or intermittent dosing (e.g., 25 mg every 2–3 days) to try and minimize toxicity.

Lenalidomide treatment of cutaneous lupus erythematosus: the Mayo Clinic experience. Kindle SA, Wetter DA, Davis MD, Pittelkow MR, Sciallis GF. Int J Dermatol 2016; 55(8): e431–9. http://dx.doi.org/10.1111/ijd.13226. PMID: 26873674.

This is a retrospective analysis of nine patients with treatment-refractory CLE (six DLE, one SCLE) treated with lenalidomide 5 to 10 mg/day. Patients were refractory to at least one antimalarial and one immunosuppressive agent. Patients with lupus panniculitis (two) did not respond. Seven of nine DLE and SCLE patients achieved either complete or partial response, with the initial response occurring within 2 to 3 months.

Kindle et al. includes a review of prior studies (one case report and three prospective studies), which included five SCLE patients treated with lenalidomide 5 to 10 mg/day. Collectively, two cases of complete response and two cases of partial response in SCLE patients treated with lenalidomide. Braunstein et al. (2012) found four of five highly recalcitrant CLE patients (two with SCLE) treated with 5 mg/day lenalidomide had clinical improvement. One responder developed SLE, suggesting there might be an increased risk of developing a severe SLE flare with lenalidomide. Cortes-Hernandez et al. (2012) treated 15 CLE patients (2 with SCLE) prospectively with 5 to 10 mg/day lenalidomide, then tapered to clinical response. Eighty-six percent achieved complete response (CLASI 0), but clinical response was frequent (75%), occurring 2 to 8 weeks after drug withdrawal. Only two patients, those with SCLE, obtained a sustained remission after withdrawing medication. Okon et al. (2014) reported the results of a 52-week prospective trial of five treatment-refractory CLE patients treated with 5 mg daily for 6 weeks followed by 6 mg every other day in those who responded, or increased to 10 mg/day in nonresponders. All five patients had significant reductions in CLASI-measured disease activity at 12 weeks.

Lenalidomide is a thalidomide derivative with a better side effect profile than thalidomide. Lenalidomide is helpful in treating refractory CLE, similar to thalidomide, but with less associated sedation, constipation, peripheral neuropathy, and thrombophilic effects than with thalidomide. Similar to thalidomide, it does not work well in the treatment of SLE. Lenalidomide is currently being evaluated in a randomized controlled trial for the treatment of refractory CLE.

Treatment of cutaneous lupus erythematosus with acitretin and hydroxychloroquine. Ruzicka T, Sommerburg C, Goerz G, Kind P, Mensing H. Br J Dermatol 1992; 127: 513–8.

In this randomized, double-blind, multicenter study, overall improvement was noticed in 13/28 (46%) of patients treated with acitretin 50 mg/day and hydroxychloroquine 400 mg/day, with five of the six SCLE patients having complete clearance. The median duration of treatment was 56.5 days.

Subacute cutaneous lupus erythematosus: report of a patient who subsequently developed a meningioma and whose skin lesions were treated with isotretinoin. Richardson TI, Cohen PR. Cutis 2000; 66: 183–8.

This is a good review of the literature regarding malignancy-associated SCLE (table 1), as well as the use of acitretin and isotretinoin for CLE. Acitretin has been shown to be effective in 50% of CLE patients in a randomized controlled trial, whereas isotretinoin's efficacy has been seen in multiple case reports of three SCLE patients treated with 0.7 to 1 mg/kg with great response (D'Erme et al; 2012. Farner et al. 1990; Newtown et al. 1998). The response is often not durable, and low-dose maintenance therapy is needed. *Although use in SCLE is limited, it is still a valid option with the advantage of a shorter half-life than acitretin for women of child-bearing age.*

Alitretinoin for cutaneous lupus erythematosus. Kuhn A, Patsinakidis N, Luger T. J Am Acad Dermatol 2012; 67: e123–6.

The patient with SCLE showed total clearance after 2 months of therapy with 30 mg/day.

Third-Line Therapies	
• Intravenous immunoglobulin	D
• Cyclophosphamide*	D
• Rituximab (anti-CD20 chimeric antibody)*	E
• Belimumab (anti-BLys monoclonal antibody)*	E
• Antiinterferon alpha monoclonal antibody (investigational)	A
• Pulsed dye laser	D
Historical and/or experimental therapies without proven efficacy and/or therapies with unfavorable risk–benefit ratio	
• Clofazimine	A
• Phenytoin	B
• Gold	B
• Cytokine therapy (interferon, CD4 monoclonal antibody)	D
• TNF inhibitors	D
• Ustekinumab	E
• Leflunomide	E

*Double-blind study in SLE population evaluating mucocutaneous (CLE) change, but without the use of a CLE-specific assessment tool

Efficacy of intravenous immunoglobulin monotherapy in patients with cutaneous lupus erythematosus: results of proof-of-concept study. Ky C, Swasdibutra B, Khademi S, Desai S, Laquer V, Grando SA. Dermatol Reports 2015; 7: 5804.

In this open-label prospective study, 16 treatment-refractory CLE patients (subtypes not listed) were treated as monotherapy with IVIG 2g/kg/month for 3 months and followed for 6 months off the drug. The study showed rapid and persistent decreases in disease activity within a few weeks (as measured by CLASI). Three treatment cycles (3 months) were sufficient to achieve clinical response, but three patients had mild relapses.

In general, one could consider IVIG a bridge therapy while waiting for another systemic medication to take effect or to abort an acute flare. There have been a handful of prospective studies with positive results; however, De Pita et al. (1997) showed no improvement of refractory CLE with IVIG 1.5 g/kg/day (a lower dose) monthly for 1 year.

Pulse cyclophosphamide treatment for severe refractory cutaneous lupus erythematosus. Raptopoulou A, Linardakis C, Sidiropoulos P, Kritikos HD, Boumpas DT. Lupus 2010; 19: 744–7.

Six patients with severe, refractory SCLE were treated with monthly cyclophosphamide pulses, followed by azathioprine 100 to 200 mg/day as maintenance therapy. HCQ was continued as well. Significant improvement in CLASI was seen in all patients, with complete remission in four and partial remission in two patients. The authors report no relapses and no major adverse events in more than 3 years' follow-up.

Refractory subacute cutaneous lupus erythematosus successfully treated with rituximab. Kieu V, O'Brien T, Yap LM, Baker C, Foley P, Mason G, et al. Australas J Dermatol 2009; 50: 2002–6.

This is a case report of a patient with treatment-refractory SCLE. After IV rituximab (375 mg/m^2) weekly for 4 weeks, she had regression of skin lesions at 16 weeks. At 11-month follow-up, SCLE recurred, and the same rituximab regimen was repeated with maintenance therapy every 8 weeks for 2 years, with ongoing disease remission.

Brief report: responses to rituximab suggest B cell-independent inflammation in cutaneous systemic lupus erythematosus. Vital EM, Wittmann M, Edward S, Yusof MY, MacIver H, Pease CT, et al. Arthritis Rheumatol 2015; 67: 1586–91.

In this report, 82 patients with SLE who were receiving rituximab were prospectively studied. Among patients with SLE, one of two patients with baseline SCLE responded to rituximab. Flares of new SCLE and DLE occurred in 12 patients who either had no skin disease at baseline or had acute CLE only at baseline (i.e., a switch in subtype) at the time of near-complete or complete B-cell depletion.

This study suggests that rituximab does not work well for CLE, with the exception of acute CLE, and patients with SLE can have CLE flares despite a lack of skin involvement at baseline.

Evidence Levels: **A** Double-blind study   **B** Clinical trial ≥ 20 subjects   **C** Clinical trial < 20 subjects   **D** Series ≥ 5 subjects   **E** Anecdotal case reports

Effects of belimumab, a B lymphocyte stimulator-specific inhibitor, on disease activity across multiple organ domains in patients with systemic lupus erythematosus: combined results from two phase III trials. Manzi S, Sanchez-Guerrero J, Merrill JT, Furie R, Gladman D, Navarra SV, et al. Ann Rheum Dis 2012; 71: 1833–8.

In phase III trials, belimumab (approved for SLE) plus standard therapy showed improvement in mucocutaneous parameters, specifically rash, mucosal ulcers, and alopecia.

It is unclear how well belimumab works for CLE, as these studies employed SLE-specific rather than CLE-specific tools to assess activity and monitor outcomes. It is thought to work better for SLE than for CLE.

Safety and efficacy of sifilmumab, an anti IFN-alpha monoclonal antibody, in a phase 2b study of moderate to severe systemic lupus erythematosus (SLE). Khamashta MMJ, Werth VP, Furie R, Kalunian K, Illeis GG, Drappas J, et al. Arthritis Rheum 2014; 66: 3530–1.

Anifrolumab, an anti-Interferon-α receptor monoclonal antibody, in moderate-to-severe systemic lupus erythematosus. Furie R, Kahamashta M, Merrill JT, Werth VP, Kalunian K, Brohawn P, et al. Arthritis Rheumatol 2017; 69: 376–86.

Recently, phase II trials demonstrated reduced mucocutaneous activity and are promising regarding SCLE therapy.

Pulsed dye laser treatment of subacute cutaneous lupus erythematosus. Gupta G, Roberts DT. Clin Exp Dermatol 1999; 24: 498–9.

A recalcitrant SCLE patient was successfully treated with pulsed dye laser (PDL) (585 nm, 450-ms pulse duration, 5-mm spot size, and fluence 5.3 J/cm^2) on four occasions, 1 month apart, resulting in marked improvement of the erythema.

236

Subcorneal pustular dermatosis

Gorav N. Wali, Vanessa Venning

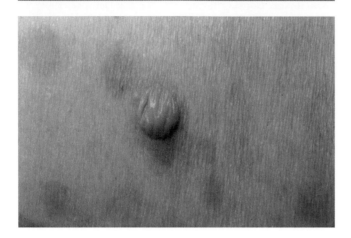

Subcorneal pustular dermatosis is a rare, chronic, neutrophilic dermatosis of unknown etiology, in which flaccid pustules and vesicopustules, classically resembling a hypopyon, arise in crops on truncal and flexural skin. The condition can occur at any age, more commonly in females. It usually follows a relapsing and remitting course, but generally the patient remains systemically well.

The condition may be difficult to differentiate from other vesiculopustular dermatoses. Some cases may be a variant of pustular psoriasis, whereas others appear to overlap with the subcorneal pustular variant of IgA pemphigus. In "classical" subcorneal pustular dermatosis, immunofluorescence studies are negative; however, there are patients with identical clinical and histologic features that have intercellular IgA deposition in the upper epidermis targeting desmosal components, most commonly desmocollins.

Subcorneal pustular dermatosis is associated with monoclonal IgA paraproteinemia and myeloma, which may occur many years after presentation. Other reported associations are pyoderma gangrenosum, inflammatory bowel disease, rheumatoid arthritis, infections (in particular *Mycoplasma pneumoniae*), and drugs.

MANAGEMENT STRATEGY

Dapsone is the treatment of choice (25–200 mg daily) and normally results in resolution of the rash within 4 weeks; the drug usually needs to be continued long term because relapse is common on withdrawal of therapy. After control is gained, the dose should be tapered to the lowest dose required to maintain remission. Other sulfones (*sulfapyridine, salazosulfapyridine*) have also been found to be beneficial in isolated reports.

In a proportion of cases the response to dapsone is poor; *retinoids* (formerly etretinate, now replaced by acitretin) have been substituted with success, using an initial dose of 0.5 to 1.0 mg/kg daily and then reducing to the lowest dose that will maintain

control. Alternatively, for those unable to tolerate dapsone in the dose required, retinoids have been added to dapsone; this has enabled lower doses of each to be used. There are a few case reports detailing good response to *phototherapy—psoralen and UVA (PUVA), narrowband UVB, or broadband UVB—*in combination with dapsone or retinoids.

Both *topical* and *systemic corticosteroids* have been reported in isolated cases to provide some degree of control. Unacceptably high doses of systemic corticosteroids may be required, but combination with other treatments may allow control with lower doses.

A number of *dapsone*-resistant cases have been treated with novel therapies such as *anti-TNFα inhibitors,* but experience with these newer agents is limited.

Subcorneal pustular dermatosis tends to run a chronic course. Maintenance of a continuing beneficial response may be difficult, as may be inferred from the extensive range of treatment options described. Although *dapsone* appears to offer the best chance of a good therapeutic response, treatment regimens for this condition have not been formally evaluated.

Specific Investigations

- Full blood count
- Immunoglobulin levels
- Serum protein electrophoresis
- Bence–Jones protein
- Autoantibodies
- Skin biopsy with immunofluorescence

Subcorneal pustular dermatosis: 50 years on. Cheng S, Edmonds E, Ben-Gashir M, Yu RC. Clin Exp Dermatol 2008; 33: 229–33.

A useful review of the literature. The authors discuss the relationship between subcorneal IgA pemphigus and classical subcorneal pustular dermatosis and accept that several authorities now consider this former subgroup to be a rare variant of pemphigus.

Subcorneal pustular dermatosis: a clinical study of ten patients. Lutz ME, Daoud MS, McEvoy MT, Gibson LE. Cutis 1998; 61: 203–8.

Four of the seven patients in whom immunoglobulins were checked had paraproteinemia: three of IgA and one of IgG type; none of these patients had IgA deposits on direct immunofluorescence.

Subcorneal pustular dermatosis and IgA λ myeloma: an uncommon association but probably not coincidental. Vaccaro M, Cannavó SP, Guarneri F. Eur J Dermatol 1999; 9: 644–6.

A case report of IgA λ myeloma associated with subcorneal pustular dermatosis. Treatment of the underlying myeloma had no effect on the skin disease.

A case of subcorneal pustular dermatosis with IgG monoclonal gammopathy of undetermined significance: a rare association. Kavala M, Karadag AS, Zindanci I, Turkoglu Z, Ozturk E, Zemheri E, et al. Int J Dermatol 2015; 54: 551–3.

A case of subcorneal pustular dermatosis associated with IgG kappa monoclonal gammopathy of uncertain significance.

Sneddon–Wilkinson disease in association with rheumatoid arthritis. Butt A, Burge SM. Br J Dermatol 1995; 132: 313–5.

Useful overview of all reported cases associated with either seronegative or seropositive arthritis.

Subcorneal pustular dermatosis triggered by *Mycoplasma pneumonia*: a rare clinical association. Bohelay G, Duong TA, Ortonne N, Chosidow O, Valeyrie-Allanore L. J Eur Acad Dermatol Venereol 2015; 29:1022–5.

A case of subcorneal pustular dermatosis in association with *Mycoplasma pneumoniae* pneumonitis. Literature review identified seven cases associated with *M. pneumoniae*.

Sneddon-Wilkinson disease induced by sorafenib in a patient with advanced hepatocellular carcinoma. Tajiri K, Nakajima T, Kawai K, Minemura M, Sugiyama T. Intern Med 2015; 54: 597–600.

A case of subcorneal pustular dermatosis that developed after sorafenib administration. It improved after cessation of sorafenib and worsened by its readministration.

First-Line Therapy	
• Dapsone	C

Subcorneal pustular dermatosis. Sneddon IB, Wilkinson DS. Br J Dermatol 1956; 68: 385–93.

Three of six patients responded to dapsone 50 to 100 mg daily.

Sneddon–Wilkinson disease in association with rheumatoid arthritis. Butt A, Burge SM. Br J Dermatol 1995; 132: 313–5.

A further five patients who responded to dapsone.

Subcorneal pustular dermatosis and IgA gammopathy. Burrows D, Bingham EA. Br J Dermatol 1984; 111: 91–3.

The addition of etretinate enabled control in a patient intolerant of higher-dose dapsone.

Sneddon–Wilkinson disease. Four case reports. Launay F, Albes B, Bayle P, Carriere M, Lamant L, Bazex J. Rev Med Interne 2004; 25: 154–9.

Three of four patients responded to dapsone.

Subcorneal pustular dermatosis in a young boy. Garg BR, Sait MA, Baruah MC. Indian J Dermatol 1985; 30: 21–3.

Subcorneal pustular dermatosis in childhood: a case report and review of the literature. Scalvenzi M, Palmisano F, Annunziata MC, Mezza E, Cozzolino I, Costa C. Case Rep Dermatol Med 2013; 2013: 5. http://dx.doi.org/10.1155/2013/424797. Article ID 424797.

Two reports of successful response to dapsone in children.

Second-Line Therapies	
• Sulfones	D
• Corticosteroids	D
• Etretinate (no longer marketed)	D
• Acitretin	E
• PUVA	D
• Narrowband UVB	E
• Broadband UVB	E

Subcorneal pustular dermatosis. Sneddon IB, Wilkinson DS. Br J Dermatol 1956; 68: 385–93.

Two patients were controlled on sulfapyridine 1 g twice daily.

Subcorneal pustular dermatosis in children. Johnson SAM, Cripps DJ. Arch Dermatol 1974; 109: 73–7.

Two children were controlled, but not cleared, with topical and systemic corticosteroids.

Role of tumor necrosis factor-α in Sneddon–Wilkinson subcorneal pustular dermatosis. Grob JJ, Mege JL, Capo C, Jancovicci E, Fournerie JR, Bongrand P, et al. J Am Acad Dermatol 1991; 25: 944–7.

Methylprednisolone induced remission in this patient who failed to respond to dapsone, etretinate, or plasma exchange. A maintenance dose of 12 mg daily was required.

An unusual severe case of subcorneal pustular dermatosis treated with cyclosporine and prednisolone. Zachariae CO, Rossen K, Weismann K. Acta Derm Venereol 2000; 80: 386–7.

After failure with dapsone and prednisolone (because of abnormal liver enzymes), ciclosporin (400 mg daily) was substituted for dapsone; onset of resolution was swift, and ciclosporin was stopped after 3 weeks; prednisolone was slowly withdrawn over 2 months with no recurrence.

Treatment of subcorneal pustulosis by etretinate. Iandoli R, Monfrecola G. Dermatologica 1987; 175: 235–8.

A patient who failed to respond to dapsone 300 mg daily and topical corticosteroids responded well to etretinate 1 mg/kg daily. A maintenance dose of 0.75 mg/kg daily was required.

A case of subcorneal pustular dermatosis in association with monoclonal IgA gammopathy successfully treated with acitretin. Canpolat F, Akipınar H, Çevirgen C, Eskıoğlu F, Öztürk E. J Dermatol Treat 2010; 21: 114–6.

A patient who failed to respond to dapsone and topical corticosteroids subsequently responded to acitretin 25 mg daily within 2 weeks. This was reduced to 10 mg daily after 3 months and stopped after 4 months with no subsequent relapse.

Successful treatment of subcorneal pustular dermatosis (Sneddon–Wilkinson disease) by acitretin: report of a case. Marliére V, Beylot-Barry M, Beylot C, Doutre M-S. Dermatology 1999; 199: 153–5.

This paper reviews the use of retinoids for subcorneal pustular dermatosis.

Subcorneal pustular dermatosis treated with PUVA therapy. Bauwens M, De Coninck A, Roseeuw D. Dermatology 1999; 198: 203–5.

A patient resistant to dapsone alone responded well to combination with PUVA. This paper contains a useful overview of PUVA therapy.

Subcorneal pustular dermatosis (Sneddon–Wilkinson disease) treated with narrowband (TL-01) UVB phototherapy. Cameron H, Dawe RS. Br J Dermatol 1997; 137: 150–1.

This patient was initially controlled with minocycline 200 mg daily and topical corticosteroids, but suffered a flare that was poorly responsive. Narrowband UVB phototherapy enabled corticosteroids to be withdrawn and control to be maintained with minocycline alone.

Subcorneal pustular dermatosis responsive to narrowband (TL-01) UVB phototherapy. Orton DI, George SA. Br J Dermatol 1997; 137: 149–50.

After long-term PUVA treatment this patient achieved a satisfactory response with narrowband UVB phototherapy.

Third-Line Therapies	
• Etanercept	E
• Infliximab	E
• Tacalcitol (1-α,24-dihydroxyvitamin D₃)	E
• Maxacalcitol (1-α,25-dihydroxy-22-oxacalcitriol)	E
• Mizoribine	E
• Ketoconazole	E
• Tetracycline, minocycline	E
• Benzylpenicillin	E
• Vitamin E	E
• Mebhydrolin	E
• Intravenous immunoglobulins	E
• Ciclosporin	E

Sneddon–Wilkinson disease treated with etanercept: report of two cases. Berk DR, Hurt MA, Mann C, Sheinbein D. Clin Exp Dermatol 2009; 34: 347–51.

Two patients with refractory disease responded to etanercept 50 mg twice weekly (in combination with low-dose acitretin in one case).

Early but not lasting improvement of recalcitrant subcorneal pustular dermatosis (Sneddon–Wilkinson disease) after infliximab therapy: relationships with variations in cytokine levels in suction blister fluids. Bonifati C, Trento E, Cordiali Fei P, Muscardin L, Amantea A, Carducci M. Clin Exp Dermatol 2005; 30: 662–5.

Infliximab (antitumor necrosis factor alpha antibody): a novel, highly effective treatment of recalcitrant subcorneal pustular dermatosis (Sneddon–Wilkinson disease). Voigtlander C, Luftl M, Schuler G, Hertl M. Arch Dermatol 2001; 137: 1571–4.

The case of SLE associated Sneddon-Wilkinson pustular disease successfully and safely treated with infliximab. Naretto C, Baldovino S, Rossi E, Spriano M, Roccatello D. Lupus 2009; 18: 856–7.

Three reports of initial, but in one case not sustained, benefit of infliximab given at standard doses.

Recalcitrant subcorneal pustular dermatosis and bullous pemphigoid treated with mizoribine, an immunosuppressive purine biosynthesis inhibitor. Kono T, Terashima T, Oura H, Ishii M, Taniguchi S, Muramatsu T. Br J Dermatol 2000; 143: 1328–30.

Two patients responded to mizoribine (Bredinin) 150 mg daily, one to mizoribine alone, the other with combined prednisolone 50 mg and mizoribine 150 mg daily.

A case of subcorneal pustular dermatosis treated with tacalcitol (1-alpha,24-dihydroxyvitamin D₃). Kawaguchi M, Mitsuhashi Y, Kondo S. J Dermatol 2000; 27: 669–72.

Therapie der pustulosis subcornealis Sneddon Wilkinson mit tacalcitol. Muhlhoff C, Megahed M. Hautarzt 2009; 60: 360–70.

Two cases of topical vitamin D₃ leading to sustained resolution of lesions.

Successful treatment of subcorneal pustular dermatosis with maxacalcitol. Hoshina D, Tsujiwaki M, Furuya K. Clin Exp Dermatol 2016; 41: 102–3.

A case controlled with topical maxacalcitol (1-α,25-dihydroxy-22-oxacalcitriol), a vitamin D₃ analog.

Ketoconazole as a therapeutic modality in subcorneal pustular dermatosis. Verma KK, Pasricha JS. Acta Derm Venereol 1977; 77: 407–8.

After failing to respond to dapsone, a patient achieved remission using ketoconazole 200 mg daily. Although this was initially started in conjunction with dapsone, withdrawal of ketoconazole led to a disease flare; the patient was subsequently satisfactorily controlled on ketoconazole alone.

Subcorneal pustular dermatosis (Sneddon–Wilkinson). Mandel EH, Gonzales V. Arch Dermatol 1969; 99: 246–7.

Tetracycline 250 mg four times daily controlled new pustule formation.

Subcorneal pustular dermatosis controlled by vitamin E. Ayres S, Mihan R. Arch Dermatol 1974; 109: 74.

Vitamin E (400 IU D-α-tocopheryl acetate), when added to prednisolone 40 mg daily, enabled the dosage of prednisolone to be reduced to 5 mg daily.

Subcorneale pustulose Sneddon–Wilkinson: therapie mit mebhydrolin. Dorittke P, Wassilew SW. Z Hautkr 1988; 63: 1025–7.

Treatment with mebhydrolin 50 mg three times daily was successful.

Subcorneal pustulosis with combined lack of IgG/IgM and monoclonal gammopathy type IgA/kappa. Rasch A, Schimmer M, Sander CA. J Dtsch Dermatol Ges 2009; 7: 693–6.

Intravenous immunoglobulins 0.2g/kg in a patient with IgG/IgM deficiency resulted in complete resolution of lesions, with three weekly cycles maintaining remission.

Evidence Levels: **A** Double-blind study **B** Clinical trial ≥ 20 subjects **C** Clinical trial < 20 subjects **D** Series ≥ 5 subjects **E** Anecdotal case reports

Subcutaneous fat necrosis of the newborn

Bernice Krafchik

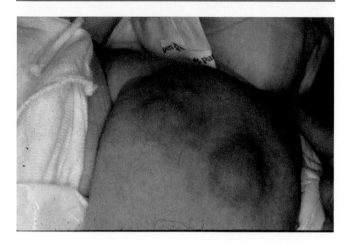

Subcutaneous fat necrosis of the newborn (SFN) is a rare, self-limited, lobular panniculitis of the skin that occurs in the first few weeks of life. The eruption affects areas where fat tissue is found and usually presents with a clinical picture of erythema and induration over the back of the proximal extremities, the upper back, buttocks, and thighs. Individual lesions vary from a few millimeters to several centimeters and may coalesce. The etiology/pathogenesis is unknown, but most infants suffer from some form of perinatal difficulty that includes asphyxia, peripheral hypoxia (tissue) or hypoxemia (blood), meconium aspiration, and maternal diabetes. A number of recent articles have described infants who have developed SFN after being treated with total body cooling for hypoxic ischemic encephalopathy (HIE). It is unlikely that the HIE is the cause of the SFN as SFN has also been described in patients receiving hypothermia for cardiac surgery. Most infants with SFN have been delivered by cesarean section, making birth trauma an unlikely cause.

The most important complication seen with SFN is hypercalcemia; it occurred in one third of patients admitted to a hospital for evaluation and treatment. The cause of the hypercalcemia is unknown; one theory postulates that increased calcium absorption occurs as a result of unregulated extrarenal 1,25-dihydroxyvitamin D. In severe cases of hypercalcemia, hypercalciuria and nephrocalcinosis may occur, increasing the possibility of seizures and death. Other symptoms of hypercalcemia are nonspecific; they include fever, vomiting, lethargy, constipation, feeding difficulties, and failure to thrive. Very rarely thrombocytopenia, hypoglycemia, anemia, hypervitaminosis D, and hypertriglyceridemia may occur.

SFN resolves spontaneously within 3 to 6 months leaving normal skin or small pitted scars and occasionally an absence of fat tissue in the affected area. Treatment of the lesions is seldom necessary, except in the rare instances when liquefaction of the fat tissue occurs or when hypercalcemia or other blood chemistry abnormalities develop.

MANAGEMENT STRATEGY

Biopsy, with its typical pathology, is usually not warranted as the clinical picture is typical. Aspiration biopsy can be helpful in establishing the diagnosis. It is a simple alternative to a punch biopsy in lesions that are not clinically diagnostic. Magnetic resonance imaging (MRI) and ultrasound investigation demonstrate characteristic features and highlight nephrocalcinosis and other areas of calcification if present. Patients should have blood work to ascertain whether blood calcium is high. It is important to recognize that serum calcium in both normal patients and those with SFN may be low in the first 2 weeks of life. Infants with SFN should be monitored weekly to see if there is any increase in blood calcium values, and if levels of calcium increase, blood should be checked biweekly for up to 6 months. If the infant is sick, tests for other abnormal indices should be performed.

Treatment is determined by the levels of hypercalcemia and hypercalciuria. If levels are marginally raised, monitoring the serum and urine levels of calcium may be all that is necessary, and a spontaneous return to normal levels often occurs. If there are mildly increased levels that persist or a further rise occurs, treatment should be instigated. Mild hypercalcemia is treated by the *withdrawal of vitamin D* and by using a *low-calcium diet.* This is best accomplished by breastfeeding as breast milk is low in calcium and vitamin D, and if this strategy produces no benefit or calcium continues to rise, *intravenous saline* is used to promote the normal excretion of calcium. *Furosemide* promotes further excretion. Other options for nonresponders include *calcitonin,* oral *corticosteroids* (hydrocortisone and prednisone), and *bisphosphonate* (pamidronate and others). Pamidronate works by interfering with bone resorption. It is more potent than saline and calcitonin and starts working in 2 days. The latter treatments should be instituted with the help of a pediatric endocrinologist.

The rare occurrence of liquefaction in the lesions should be removed with a large-bore needle.

Specific Investigations

- Biopsy or fine needle aspiration for diagnosis (if required)
- Renal ultrasound for nephrocalcinosis, nephrolithiasis
- MRI of torso if indicated by high calcium levels
- Serum and urine calcium weekly for 6 months, biweekly if elevated
- Monitor urine calcium/creatinine ratio

Fine-needle aspiration as a method of diagnosis of subcutaneous fat necrosis of the newborn. Schubert PT, Razak R, Vermaak A, Jordaan HF. Pediatr Dermatol 2016; 33: e220–1.

The article reviews previous findings by the same authors, emphasizing the advantages of fine needle aspiration: it is thought to be as helpful as punch biopsy. The typical pathologic picture includes clumped lobules of fat with opaque cytoplasm and/or necrotic aspirates of dispersed fat cells with opaque cytoplasm, foamy macrophages, multinucleated giant cells, lymphocytes and neutrophils, and the characteristic radially oriented and loose refractile needle-shaped crystals in the cytoplasm of the fat cells lying in the necrotic background.

Subcutaneous fat necrosis in a newborn after brief therapeutic cooling hypothermia: ultrasonagraphic examination. Tognetti L, Fillippou G, Bertrando S, Picerno V, Buornocore G, Frediani B, et al. Pediatr Dermatol 2015; 32: 427–9.

The authors describe the cutaneous and subcutaneous features of ultrasounds performed on patients who had developed SFN after the use of therapeutic hypothermia to treat HIE. The ultrasound procedures were easy to perform. Newborn adipose tissue is mainly composed of high-melting-point saturated fatty acids. Low temperatures can induce fat crystallization and necrosis. Increased local pressure, hypoperfusion of fat cells, and tissue hypoxia stimulate saturated fatty acid deposition and are thought to be mechanisms of the SFN. These changes appears as hypoechoic shadows on ultrasound.

Subcutaneous fat necrosis of the newborn: a review of eleven cases. Burden AD, Krafchik BR. Pediatr Dermatol 1999; 16: 384–7.

Ten of the patients had been delivered by cesarean section for fetal distress: four developed hypercalcemia. Patients should be monitored for 6 months even if the SFN lesions have disappeared, as hypercalcemia can still occur without clinical lesions.

First-Line Therapies	
• No treatment for the majority of patients	C
• Low-calcium and low–vitamin D diet (either breast milk or formula)	C

Severe hypercalcemia due to subcutaneous fat necrosis: presentation, management and complications. Shumer DE, Thaker V, Taylor GA, Wassner AJ. Arch Dis Child Fetal Neonatal Ed 2014; 99: F419–21.

The authors of this article followed seven children with severe hypercalcemia associated with SFN described in the past literature as an unusual event with an estimated incidence of between 36% and 56%; the hypercalcemia and follow-up were short. The hypercalcemia in this study occurred within 6 weeks of birth, and nephrocalcinosis, found on ultrasonography, was the most frequent complication occurring in 83%. In their 4-year follow-up the nephrocalcinosis persisted, unlike the information in prior reports. No associated renal problems were reported. Other findings were fevers without infection and mild eosinophilia. Treatments varied; all were treated with intravenous hydration and formula that has low calcium. Glucocorticoids (prednisone and methyl prednisolone) were used (1 to 2 mg/mg/kg/dose). Calcitonin was not helpful.

Extensive subcutaneous fat necrosis of the newborn associated with therapeutic hypothermia. Hogeling M, Meddles K, Berk DR, Bruckner A, Shimotake T, Frieden I. Pediatr Dermatol 2012; 29: 59–63.

The authors of this article reviewed the increased occurrence of SFN associated with the treatment of HIE with hypothermia. The SFN usually develops from 1 to 4 weeks, but can occur as early as 72 hours. Hypercalcemia occurred in a third of the patients studied. Control of hypercalcemia may prevent cardiac and renal complications and metastatic calcification.

Second-Line Therapies	
• Intravenous saline at 1.5 times the normal maintenance dose	D
• Furosemide 1 to 1.5 mg/kg every 6 to 12 hours for 5 days	D

Third-Line Therapies	
• Oral or IV steroids (prednisone and methyl prednisone, 1–2 mg/kg/per dose for 5 days)	C
• Subcutaneous calcitonin (4–8 IU/kg every 6–12 hours for 2–3 days)	E
• Bisphosphonates (pamidronate 0.25–0.5 mg/kg/dose for 2–4 days)	D

Neonatal hypercalcemia secondary to subcutaneous fat necrosis successfully treated with pamidronate. A case series and literature review. Samedi VM, Yusuf K, Yee W, Obiad H, Al Awad EH. AJP Report 2014; 4: e93–6.

The authors stress that with increasing use of therapeutic cooling for the treatment of HIE with or without symptoms, patients who develop SFN should be monitored for the development of hypercalcemia, which may be very severe, and treatment should be instigated as soon as needed. They include hyperhydration, diuretics, corticosteroids, and bisphosphonates.

Most of the articles regarding the use of bisphosphonates for the treatment of patients with SFN have been single case studies. In one article, after adding calcitonin to the pamidronate, which had already been started, the effect of the combination was immediate. The authors suggest that calcitonin works faster (12–48 hours) than pamidronate, that it takes 2–4 days to work, and that both medications are more efficacious when used together.

Evidence Levels: **A** Double-blind study **B** Clinical trial ≥ 20 subjects **C** Clinical trial < 20 subjects **D** Series ≥ 5 subjects **E** Anecdotal case reports

238

Sweet syndrome

Asha Gowda, Karolyn A. Wanat, William D. James

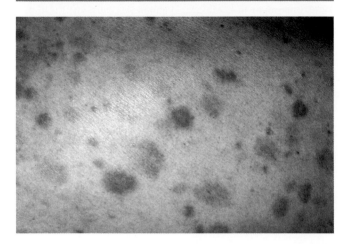

Sweet syndrome is a neutrophilic dermatosis characterized clinically by multiple painful, well-demarcated, nonscarring, erythematous plaques or pustules on the face, neck, upper trunk, and extremities. There can be a pseudovesicular appearance. Fever, leukocytosis, arthralgias, myalgias, headaches, and general malaise may occur. Oral, ocular, and internal organ involvement is rare. On histopathology, there is a diffuse neutrophilic infiltrate in the upper dermis without evidence of primary leukocytoclastic vasculitis. Neutrophilic dermatosis of the dorsal hands (NDDH) is classified as an anatomically limited subset of Sweet syndrome.

MANAGEMENT STRATEGY

Sweet syndrome is often idiopathic, but may be associated with malignancy (most commonly acute myelogenous leukemia, but also lymphomas, dysproteinemias, and carcinomas), inflammatory bowel disease, infection (commonly *Streptococcus* or *Yersinia*), medication, radiation, and pregnancy. Workup includes skin biopsy, complete physical examination, and laboratory studies. Treatment of the underlying associated condition or discontinuation of the causative medication may lead to resolution of skin lesions. The standard treatment is *corticosteroids*. For patients with contraindications to corticosteroids, or for therapeutic failures, second-line therapies may be used.

Specific Investigations

- Complete blood count with differential
- Erythrocyte sedimentation rate (ESR) or C-reactive protein (CRP)
- Cultures as indicated by history and physical examination
- Malignancy screening: age-appropriate screening, evaluation if hematologic abnormalities exist, and consideration of serum protein/serum immunofixation electrophoresis; bone marrow biopsy may be considered

- Pregnancy test (in women of childbearing potential)
- Medication history

First-Line Therapies

• Oral corticosteroids	C
• Topical and intralesional corticosteroids	C

Sweet's syndrome: a review of current treatment options. Cohen PR, Kurzrock R. Am J Clin Dermatol 2002; 3: 117–31.

A review of the literature regarding treatment for Sweet syndrome.

Corticosteroid therapy (oral prednisone 0.5–1.5 mg/kg daily tapered over 4–6 weeks) results in rapid relief of systemic symptoms (within 1–2 days) and skin lesions within 3 to 9 days. Up to one third of patients will relapse.

High-potency topical corticosteroids and intralesional corticosteroids may be useful as monotherapy for patients with limited or mild disease or as adjuvant treatment.

Second-Line Therapies

• Potassium iodide	C
• Colchicine	C
• Indometacin	C
• Pulse intravenous corticosteroids	D
• Dapsone	D
• Clofazimine	D
• Doxycycline	E
• Metronidazole	E

Potassium iodide in dermatology: a 19th century drug for the 21st century - uses, pharmacology, adverse effects, and contraindications. Sterling JB, Heymann WR. J Am Acad Dermatol 2000; 43: 691–7.

The usual dosage of potassium iodide is 40 to 60 mg orally three times a day up to 300 mg three times a day. A supersaturated solution of potassium iodide (SSKI) may also be used. Start at 3 drops orally three times daily and increase by 1 drop per dose up to 10 drops (500 mg) three times daily until clear, then taper. SSKI is contraindicated in pregnancy, in hyperkalemia, and in patients with renal disease. Baseline thyroid function tests and periodic monitoring are required for patients on SSKI.

Long-term suppression of chronic Sweet's syndrome with colchicine. Ritter S, George R, Serwatka LM, Elston DM. J Am Acad Dermatol 2002; 47: 323–4.

A case report of successful long-term treatment using 0.6 mg colchicine twice daily.

Indomethacin treatment of eighteen patients with Sweet's syndrome. Jeanfils S, Joly P, Young P, Le Corvaisier-Pieto C, Thomine E, Lauret P. J Am Acad Dermatol 1997; 36: 436–9.

A prospective open-label, uncontrolled study of 18 patients treated with indometacin 150 mg daily for 7 days, followed by 100 mg daily from days 7 to 21. Seventeen of 18 patients responded within 48 hours, and no relapses occurred.

Association of acute neutrophilic dermatosis and myelodysplastic syndrome with (6;9) chromosome translocation: a case report and review of the literature. Megarbane B, Bodemer C, Valensi F, Radford-Weiss I, Fraitag S, MacIntyre E, et al. Br J Dermatol 2000; 143: 1322–4.

Pulse corticosteroid therapy was successful for refractory and/or recurrent Sweet syndrome. Intravenous methylprednisolone up to 1000 mg daily for 3 to 5 days was used, followed by a low-dose taper of an oral corticosteroid with or without another immunosuppressant.

Treatment of giant cellulitis-like Sweet syndrome with dapsone. Koketsu H, Ricotti C, Kerdel FA. JAMA Dermatol 2014; 150: 457–9.

A case report of a patient with giant inflammatory Sweet syndrome lesions treated with dapsone 100 mg daily, allowing for complete resolution of symptoms.

Sulfapyridine may be used as an alternative to dapsone in doses from 1 to 4 g per day.

Sweet's syndrome in association with generalized granuloma annulare in a patient with previous breast cancer. Anthony F, Holden CA. Clin Exp Dermatol 2001; 26: 668–70.

A report of Sweet syndrome successfully treated with clofazimine.

Clofazimine 200 mg daily for 4 weeks followed by 100 mg daily for 4 weeks has been reported to be an effective dosage regimen in six patients.

Successful treatment of Sweet's syndrome with doxycycline. Joshi RK, Atukorala DN, Abanmi A, Al Khamis O, Haleem A. Br J Dermatol 1993; 128: 584–6.

Two patients with Sweet syndrome reported resolution of skin lesions after treatment with 100 mg doxycycline twice daily.

Sweet's syndrome in association with Crohn's disease: report of a case and review of the literature. Rappaport A, Shaked M, Landau M, Dolev E. Dis Colon Rectum 2001; 44: 1526–9.

A patient successfully treated with metronidazole and prednisone.

> ### Third-Line Therapies
>
> - Ciclosporin — E
> - Interferon — E
> - Cyclophosphamide — E
> - Chlorambucil — E
> - Etretinate — E
> - Etanercept — E
> - Thalidomide — E
> - Anakinra — E
> - Intravenous immunoglobulin (IVIG) — E
> - Sulfapyridine — E
> - Azathioprine — E
> - Azacitidine — E
> - Lenalidomide — E
> - Rituximab — E

Peripheral ulcerative keratitis: an extracutaneous neutrophilic disorder. Report of a patient with rheumatoid arthritis, pustular vasculitis, pyoderma gangrenosum, and Sweet's

syndrome with an excellent response to cyclosporine therapy. Wilson DM, John GR, Callen JP. J Am Acad Dermatol 1999; 40: 331–4.

One patient with Sweet syndrome responded to ciclosporin.

Initial doses of 2 to 10 mg/kg daily have been used successfully and should generally be limited to short-term use given its potential renal toxicity when used chronically.

Systemic interferon-alpha treatment for idiopathic Sweet's syndrome. Bianchi L, Masi M, Hagman JH, Piemonte P, Orlandi A. Clin Exp Dermatol 1999; 24: 443–5.

One patient responded to interferon-α 3 million units intramuscularly three times weekly plus hydroxyurea 500 mg twice daily for 30 days, tapered to 500 mg daily for an additional 30 days. The patient maintained remission for 2 years with intramuscular interferon-α as monotherapy.

Cyclophosphamide therapy in Sweet's syndrome complicating refractory Crohn's disease: efficacy and mechanism of action. Meinhardt C, Buning J, Fellermann K, Lehnert H, Schmidt KJ. J Crohns Colitis 2011; 5: 633–7.

Cyclophosphamide pulse therapy at a dose of 15 mg/kg in a patient with Crohn-associated Sweet syndrome yielded rapid response with significant relief of clinical symptoms. Thereafter, treatment was given three times at 4-week intervals.

Etanercept treatment in Sweet's syndrome with inflammatory arthritis. Ambrose NL, Tobin AM, Howard D. J Rheumatol 2009; 36: 6.

A patient with concurrent inflammatory arthritis experienced remarkable improvement upon treatment with etanercept 50 mg/week subcutaneously.

Thalidomide in the treatment of recalcitrant Sweet's syndrome associated with myelodysplasia. Browning C, Dixon J, Malone J, Callen J. J Am Acad Dermatol 2005; 53: S135–8.

A patient cleared completely with thalidomide 100 mg daily.

The use of pulse methylprednisolone and chlorambucil in the treatment of Sweet's syndrome. Case JD, Smith SZ, Callen JP. Cutis 1989; 44: 125–9.

Chronic and relapsing Sweet syndrome successfully treated with pulsed intravenous methylprednisolone. Remission was maintained with oral chlorambucil 4 mg daily.

Efficacy of antiinterleukin-1 receptor antagonist anakinra (Kineret) in a case of refractory Sweet's syndrome. Kluger N, Gil-Bistes D, Guillot B, Bessis D. Dermatology 2011; 222: 123–7.

One of three case reports of Sweet syndrome refractory to multiple medications with a rapid and sustained response to anakinra 100 mg/day as monotherapy.

Favorable outcome of severe, extensive granulocyte colony-stimulating factor-induced, corticosteroid-resistant Sweet's syndrome treated with high-dose intravenous immunoglobulin. Calixto R, Menezes Y, Ostronoff M, Sucupira A, Botelho LF, Florencio R, et al. J Clin Oncol 2014; 32: e1–2.

A case report of granulocyte colony-stimulating factor (G-CSF)–induced Sweet syndrome in a patient with underlying multiple myeloma that did not resolve upon discontinuation of G-CSF or institution of steroids. The patient responded to IVIG within hours. A 2-day course of IVIG 1 g/kg per day led to complete resolution of skin lesions in 7 days.

Evidence Levels: **A** Double-blind study **B** Clinical trial ≥ 20 subjects **C** Clinical trial < 20 subjects **D** Series ≥ 5 subjects **E** Anecdotal case reports

Histiocytoid Sweet syndrome treated with azathioprine: a case report. Miller J, Lee N, Sami N. Dermatol Online J 2015; 21: 13.

A patient treated with 50 mg of azathioprine daily reported excellent control of cutaneous and systemic symptoms. Studies describe the potential of azathioprine to induce Sweet syndrome and other neutrophilic dermatoses, and thus, this therapy may be beneficial exclusively in this rare variant.

Complete remission of Sweet's syndrome after azacytidine treatment for concomitant myelodysplastic syndrome. Martinelli S, Rigolin GM, Leo G, Gafa R, Lista E, Cibien F, et al. Int J Hematol 2014; 99: 663–7.

A patient successfully treated with subcutaneous azacitidine (75 mg/m²/day). Medication was administered for 5 days, followed by a 2-day intermission, and an additional 2-day course of treatment. Multiple reports also describe the drug's tendency to induce Sweet syndrome.

Lenalidomide as a steroid sparing agent in a myelodysplastic syndrome patient with refractory Sweet syndrome. Chaulagain CP, Miller KB. Int J Blood Res Disord 2014; 1: 1–3.

A patient with Sweet syndrome and concurrent myelodysplastic syndrome reported resolution of cutaneous lesions with 5 mg lenalidomide three times weekly. On the contrary, there are a few reports indicating the drug's association with Sweet syndrome.

Rituximab for refractory subcutaneous Sweet's syndrome in chronic lymphocytic leukemia: a case report. Hashemi SM, Fazeli SA, Vahedi A, Golabchifard R. Mol Clin Oncol 2016; 4: 436–40.

A case report of a patient with chronic lymphocytic leukemia treated for refractory Sweet syndrome with rituximab (375 mg/m² body surface).

Syphilis

Eavan G. Muldoon, Derek Freedman

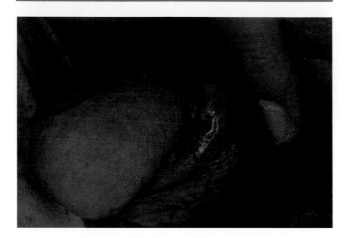

Syphilis is an ancient disease that many mistakenly believe to be on the decline. Caused by the spirochete *Treponema pallidum*, syphilis is an indicator disease for human immunodeficiency virus (HIV). A syphilis diagnosis provides opportunities for screening and early diagnosis of HIV, which will have a significant impact on patients' prognosis and further infection transmission. *T. pallidum* facilitates the transmission of HIV by increasing viral load, disrupting the mucous membrane barrier, and increasing HIV shedding. Prompt recognition and treatment of syphilis have significant public and personal health benefits, particularly for "risk takers," who are afforded an opportunity to make lifestyle choices.

Men who have sex with men (MSM), commercial sex workers, or patients from areas with a high prevalence of syphilis have a higher risk of syphilis acquisition. A thorough history is essential and may uncover past potential risks that may not be immediately evident, such as woman with past partners who are MSM. However, most are unaware of their risk status, and routine testing is always required.

Transmission of syphilis is by direct contact with an infectious individual. Sexual contact is the most common mode of transmission. However, in the current era of so-called *safer sex practices* transmission by close contact with an active lesion, such as oral sex, biting, and even kissing, has become more common. Transplacental transmission, blood transfusion, or accidental inoculation can also rarely occur.

MANAGEMENT STRATEGY

The appropriate management is determined by the stage of syphilis infection. Infection is divided into:

- Incubation period
- Primary syphilis characterized by a primary sore or chancre(s)
- Secondary syphilis
- A period of subclinical infection or latent syphilis
- Tertiary syphilis, which does not occur in every patient

The patient is most infectious in the early stages of disease, particularly when the primary chancre, mucous patch, or condyloma lata are present. An immunologically intact person cannot spread syphilis after 4 years of infection.

Incubation Period

T. pallidum penetrates the intact mucous membrane or gains access through abraded skin. Within hours to days it enters the lymphatic system and/or bloodstream and disseminates throughout the body. This occurs soon after contact; patients have been infected by blood transfusions from donors with negative serology who are in the incubation period. The incubation period is directly proportional to the size of the inoculum. The median incubation period is 3 weeks, but can vary from 3 to 90 days.

Primary Syphilis

Classically, a primary chancre is described as a single painless papule that occurs at the site of inoculation. This is not limited to the genital region. Any area where contact with an infectious lesion has occurred can be involved. The mouth and anal area are common extragenital sites.

The chancre appears after the incubation period, erodes, ulcerates, and becomes indurated with a cellular infiltration—this is a reflection of the immune response. The base is usually smooth, and the borders are raised and firm with a cartilaginous consistency. It is painless and has a clean appearance with no exudate unless it is superinfected. Regional lymphadenopathy with moderately enlarged, firm, nonsuppurative, and painless lymph nodes frequently accompanies the primary lesion.

The differential diagnosis of a primary chancre is *Herpes simplex*, chancroid, and traumatic superinfected lesions. Other diagnoses that should be considered are early warts caused by human papilloma virus, granuloma inguinale, tuberculosis, or atypical mycobacterial infections. Perianal lesions may be dismissed as hemorrhoids. The area should always be visualized and examined.

Secondary Syphilis

Secondary syphilis is when the spirochete multiplies and disseminates throughout the body. It lasts until a sufficient host response develops to control the organism. It begins 2 to 8 weeks after the appearance of the chancre; however, this is highly variable and the signs of primary and secondary infection may overlap. Many patients presenting with secondary syphilis do not recall a primary chancre. The manifestations of secondary syphilis are protean and varied.

Dermatologic manifestations are the most commonly recognized signs of secondary syphilis. The rash of secondary syphilis may be macular, maculopapular, papular, pustular, or a combination of these and is generally nonpruritic. Vesicular lesions occur only in congenital syphilis. Skin lesions usually begin on the trunk and proximal extremities. Classically, they are pink-red macular lesions 3 to 10 mm in diameter. Any surface area can become involved. The rash can last from a few days up to 8 weeks. The lesions may evolve into papules and in some patients into pustules, known as *pustular syphilids*. All types of rash may be present at the same time, and the rash can involve any body surface. Palmar and plantar rashes are highly suggestive of syphilis. Fever can accompany the rash, and the clinical syndrome can be mistaken for acute HIV infection, infectious mononucleosis, or a nonspecific viral syndrome.

Evidence Levels: **A** Double-blind study **B** Clinical trial ≥ 20 subjects **C** Clinical trial < 20 subjects **D** Series ≥ 5 subjects **E** Anecdotal case reports

Alopecia occurs with hair follicle involvement. In warm, moist areas, such as the genital and perianal areas, inner aspects of the thighs, the skin under breasts, nasolabial folds, axillae, antecubital fossae, and webs of fingers and toes, the papules can coalesce and erode, resulting in painless, broad, gray-white, highly infectious plaques called *condylomata lata*. They can be easily mistaken for warts or hemorrhoids. Lesions may also develop on mucous membranes—so-called *mucous patches*. Enlargement of the epitrochlear lymph nodes is a unique finding that should always suggest the diagnosis of syphilis.

Neurologic Syphilis

Neurosyphilis—that is, syphilitic infection of the central nervous system—can present at any time after infection. It can be classified into early and late disease. Early neurosyphilis will involve the cerebrospinal fluid (CSF), meninges, and vasculature, whereas later tertiary disease syphilis tends to affect the brain parenchyma and spinal cord. Currently neurosyphilis is most commonly seen in patients with HIV infection, and these patients often present with eye disease. An unsuspecting ophthalmologist may be the first physician to encounter the patient with ocular syphilis. Ocular involvement varies with the most common presentation being uveitis. Any unexpected ocular condition, particularly in a man, should prompt the thought of ocular syphilis, which should be ruled out by serology. Auditory syphilis is less common, but should not be forgotten.

Latent Syphilis

Latent syphilis is the asymptomatic period after infection. It is usually divided into early latent disease, within 2 years of infection, and late latent disease, after 2 years of infection. Careful history is required to attempt to stage asymptomatic disease. Sexual history, obstetric history, and travel history will all offer valuable clues, but are frequently elusive.

Tertiary Syphilis

Progression to tertiary syphilis is only seen in approximately 25% of untreated patients. It takes the form of neurologic disease, cardiovascular disease, and gummatous disease. It is rarely seen today due to antibiotic therapy; however, it may be more prevalent in certain immigrant populations.

DIAGNOSTICS AND TREATMENT

The diagnosis of syphilis depends on the stage of the disease. *T. pallidum* is too slender to be visualized by direct microscopy, and the bacterium cannot be cultured. Dark-field or dark-ground microscopy, a specialized technique that utilizes an oblique light to visualize the organism, is classically used in cases when patients have demonstrable clinical lesions; it has a sensitivity of 50% in experienced hands. Moist lesions containing large numbers of treponemes, such as primary chancres, condyloma lata, or mucous patches, are particularly amenable to dark-field microscopy. It is not recommended for oral lesions, as commensal oral spirochetes are indistinguishable from *T. pallidum*. Although no *T. pallidum* detection tests are commercially available, some laboratories provide locally developed and validated polymerase chain reaction (PCR) tests for the detection of *T. pallidum* DNA. These provide a more sensitive tool and will identify *T. pallidum* from oral lesions. The vast majority of cases of syphilis are diagnosed by serology, an indirect diagnostic method.

Serologic tests fall into two categories: nontreponemal tests and treponemal tests. Nontreponemal tests such as rapid plasma reagin (RPR) or venereal disease research laboratory (VDRL) tests have traditionally been used for screening and may still be used in resource-limited settings. Automated enzyme immunoassay (EIA) is now recommended for screening before nontreponemal and treponemal tests. Positive tests are then confirmed with a treponemal test such as *Treponema pallidum* particle agglutination (TPPA) or fluorescent treponemal antibody absorbed (FTA-ABS). False-positive reactions may be seen with the nontreponemal tests in autoimmune conditions and various other infections, including HIV. Quantitative nontreponemal tests are useful for providing a baseline from which change can be measured. Reinfection can be demonstrated by a fourfold rise in titer, for example. The reactivity of the test can differ depending on variation in antigen preparation, and for this reason it is recommended that sequential tests be performed using the same laboratory method and preferably performed by the same laboratory. If the clinical suspicion for syphilis is high and the nontreponemal tests are negative, a "prozone" phenomenon caused by very high antibody titers should be considered. Dilution of the serum unmasks the test to positive.

Guidelines on treatment differ; however, the basic principles are the same. *Long-acting penicillin* is the treatment of choice in all patients. Patients with neurologic or ocular involvement will need daily treatment for a minimum of 10 to 14 days with parenteral penicillin. For those allergic to penicillin, *doxycycline* is an alternative to penicillin; but in the case of neurologic disease and pregnant patients, penicillin desensitization is preferred. Patients need to be followed with regular serology after treatment to ensure adequate response to therapy.

The Jarisch–Herxheimer reaction may occur within hours of treatment, manifested by fever, chills, headache, myalgias, exacerbation of skin lesions, and other systemic symptoms. Treatment with nonsteroidal antiinflammatory agents or, in more severe cases, systemic steroids may be necessary.

Syphilis is an easily treatable disease with diverse manifestations. It is an indicator disease for HIV; consequently, all patients diagnosed with syphilis must be screened for HIV and all other sexually transmitted infections. Careful history taking regarding risks factors for the acquisition of the infection, possible chancrous lesions, systemic illness, and rash may offer vital clues in making the diagnosis of this curable disease, but routine serologic testing of all patients is a mandatory safeguard to avoid missing the diagnosis.

Tracing and management of sex partners forms part of the management of patients with syphilis. Sexual transmission is thought to be limited to the time when mucocutaneous lesions are present and is unusual after the first year of infection. Persons who have had sexual contact within 90 days with a person who has primary, secondary, or early latent syphilis should be treated presumptively. Long-term partners should be evaluated in all cases. In areas of high endemicity, partners of late latent patients with a high nontreponemal titer (RPR >1:32) may also be treated presumptively, as these titers may be indicative of reinfection.

Referral to a genitourinary or infectious disease consultant is often appropriate

Specific Investigations

- Dark-field microscopy for primary chancre
- Enzyme immunoassay
- VDRL or RPR + FTA-ABS or TPPA
- PCR (not routinely used)
- HIV
- Sexually transmitted infection screen

Sexually transmitted diseases treatment guidelines, 2015. Workowski KA, Bolan G, Centers for Disease Control and Prevention (CDC). MMWR Recomm Rep 2015; 64: 1–137.

The definitive diagnostic test is dark-field microscopy; however, this is obviously limited to those patients who have a lesion amenable to dark-field microscopy, such as a genital lesion. Most diagnoses are made using serologic methods. An alternative is PCR; however, there are no commercial tests, and availability of PCR will depend on the individual laboratory. The combination of a nontreponemal test (e.g., VDRL or RPR) and a treponemal test (e.g., FTA-ABS or TPPA) should be used to confirm the diagnosis. Nontreponemal antibody titers correlate with disease activity: a fourfold rise in titer is necessary to demonstrate a clinically significant difference. Tests should be performed using the same method and preferably the same laboratory. VDRL and RPR are equally valid assays; however, quantitative results from the two tests cannot be compared directly. Nontreponemal titers should decline after treatment and may become nonreactive with time, particularly in patients treated for primary syphilis. Follow-up serology should be performed at 6 and 12 months after treatment. All patients diagnosed with syphilis should have a HIV test and a full sexually transmitted infection (STI) screen.

If the patient has clinical signs of neurosyphilis (e.g., cranial nerve dysfunction, meningitis, stroke, altered mental status, loss of vibration sensation, or hearing or visual changes), further investigation with lumbar puncture and treatment is warranted.

Direct comparison of the traditional and reverse syphilis screening algorithms in a population with a low prevalence of syphilis. Binnicker MJ, Jespersen DJ, Rollins LO. J Clin Microbiol 2012; 50: 148–50.

Traditionally, serum for syphilis serology was screened by use of a nontreponemal test such as the RPR and positives confirmed with a treponemal test. However, more recently laboratories have been using automated treponemal tests such as an EIA to deal with the large volumes of samples that need to be screened. Direct comparison of this method indicates that it will pick up more false positives by EIA (0.6%); however, additional cases are also likely to be detected.

High annual syphilis testing rates among gay men in Australia, but insufficient retesting. Guy R, Wand H, Holt M, Mao L, Wilson DP, Bourne C, et al. Sex Transm Dis 2012; 39: 268–75.

Testing for syphilis is now recommended every 3 months in HIV-positive MSM and every 6 months for MSM not infected with HIV. In this survey of 6329 MSM, 14% had never tested for syphilis. Risks for not having tested were older age, lower number of sexual partners, and not being aware that syphilis may be asymptomatic. In men that were deemed high risk, not living in a metropolitan area and not being aware that syphilis could be spread through oral sex were additional risks.

First-Line Therapies	
• Benzathine penicillin	A
• Procaine plus probenecid	A

Sexually transmitted diseases treatment guidelines, 2015. Workowski KA, Bolan G, Centers for Disease Control and Prevention (CDC). MMWR Recomm Rep 2015; 64: 1–137.

UK national guidelines on the management of syphilis 2015. Kingston M, French P, Higgins S, McQuillan O, Sukthankar A, Stott C, et al. Int J STD AIDS 2016; 27: 421–46.

Penicillin is the first-line therapy recommended in international guidelines for all stages of syphilis infection. Penicillin desensitization is recommended for pregnant patients or those diagnosed with neurosyphilis who have a penicillin allergy.

T. pallidum penicillin resistance has never been reported, despite >60 years of use.

Relapse of secondary syphilis after benzathine penicillin G: molecular analysis. Myint M, Bashiri H, Harrington RD, Marra CM. Sex Transm Dis 2004; 31: 196–9.

Relapse of infectious syphilis after treatment with the recommended dose of penicillin is rare, but does occur. For this reason, it is important to follow treated patients both clinically and serologically. These patients respond to higher and more prolonged doses of penicillin.

Second-Line Therapy	
• Doxycycline	B
• Tetracycline	B
• Amoxicillin plus probenecid	B
• Ceftriaxone	B

All patients not receiving penicillin require close follow-up to ensure response to therapy. Pregnant patients and patients diagnosed with neurosyphilis should be treated with penicillin and desensitized if they report a penicillin allergy.

Management of adult syphilis. Ghanem KG, Workowski KA. Clin Infect Dis 2011; 53: S110–28.

The data for using alternative agents for the treatment of neurosyphilis are limited. There are two retrospective trials looking at doxycycline in early disease; however, no patients with late syphilis infection were included, and there were few HIV-positive patients. Careful follow-up of HIV-positive patients to ensure serologic response is essential if these agents are used.

Ceftriaxone therapy for syphilis: report from the emerging infections network. Augenbraun M, Workowski K. Clin Infect Dis 1999; 29: 1337–8.

A single injection of 1 g ceftriaxone is not effective for treating infectious syphilis. Daily or alternate-day injections for 8 to 10 days appear to be efficacious, but more data are needed to evaluate late failures.

Response of HIV-infected patients with syphilis to therapy with penicillin or intravenous ceftriaxone. Spornraft-Ragaller P, Abraham S, Lueck C, Meurer M. Eur J Med Res 2011; 16: 47–51.

In a retrospective study, 24 consecutive HIV-positive patients with early syphilis infection treated with either benzathine penicillin or ceftriaxone were compared. After 20 months of follow-up, 23 of 24 patients had a serologic response to therapy, suggesting that ceftriaxone may have comparable efficacy in HIV-positive patients with higher CD4 counts.

Third-Line Therapies	
• Azithromycin	C
• Erythromycin	C

Evidence Levels: A Double-blind study B Clinical trial ≥ 20 subjects C Clinical trial < 20 subjects D Series ≥ 5 subjects E Anecdotal case reports

Azithromycin should not be used for the treatment of pregnant patients or MSM due to high rates of resistance.

Macrolide resistance in *Treponema pallidum* in the United States and Ireland. Lukehart SA, Godornes C, Molini BJ, Sonnett P, Hopkins S, Mulcahy F, et al. N Engl J Med 2004; 351: 154–8.

A mutation that makes *T. pallidum* resistant to azithromycin was identified with the use of a restriction-digestion assay in 15 of 17 samples (88%) from Dublin, 12 of 55 samples (22%) from San Francisco, 3 of 23 samples (13%) from Seattle, and 2 of 19 samples (11%) from Baltimore. The study suggests that a mutated strain was either introduced into a sexual network or has been selected for among persons who engage in high-risk behavior.

Azithromycin resistance in *Treponema pallidum*. Katz KA, Klausner JD. Curr Opin Infect Dis 2008; 21: 83–91.

Azithromycin resistance in *T. pallidum* is increasing in the United States, Canada, and Ireland. Closer observation for treatment failures is needed in patients treated with azithromycin.

Macrolide resistance in *Treponema pallidum* correlates with 23S rDNA mutations in recently isolated clinical strains. Molini BJ, Tantalo LC, Sahi SK, Rodriguez VI, Brandt SL, Fernandez MC, et al. Sex Transm Dis 2016; 43: 579–83.

In a rabbit model, using clinical isolates with the 23S rDNA mutations, azithromycin uniformly failed to cure the infection; benzathine penicillin was effective.

Stages of Syphilis Infection

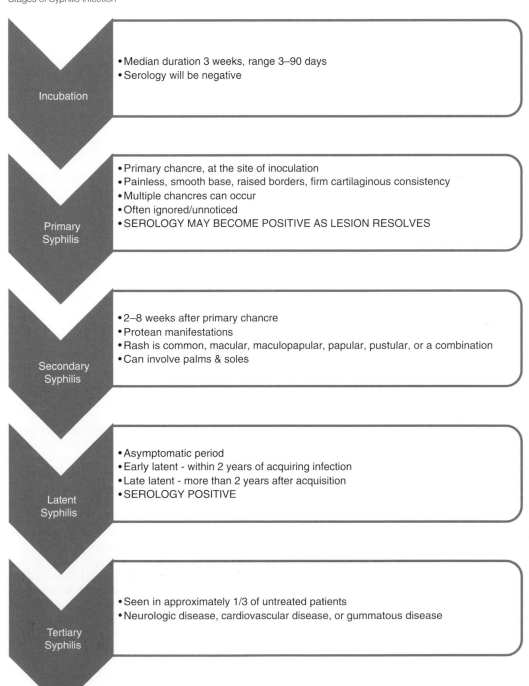

Incubation
- Median duration 3 weeks, range 3–90 days
- Serology will be negative

Primary Syphilis
- Primary chancre, at the site of inoculation
- Painless, smooth base, raised borders, firm cartilaginous consistency
- Multiple chancres can occur
- Often ignored/unnoticed
- SEROLOGY MAY BECOME POSITIVE AS LESION RESOLVES

Secondary Syphilis
- 2–8 weeks after primary chancre
- Protean manifestations
- Rash is common, macular, maculopapular, papular, pustular, or a combination
- Can involve palms & soles

Latent Syphilis
- Asymptomatic period
- Early latent - within 2 years of acquiring infection
- Late latent - more than 2 years after acquisition
- SEROLOGY POSITIVE

Tertiary Syphilis
- Seen in approximately 1/3 of untreated patients
- Neurologic disease, cardiovascular disease, or gummatous disease

Syringomata

James A.A. Langtry

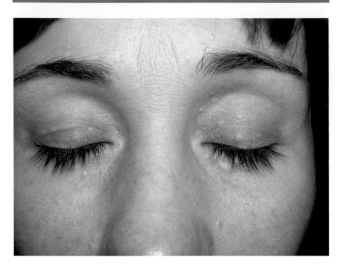

Syringomata are benign appendageal tumors of the intraepidermal eccrine sweat duct that have a characteristic histologic appearance. The typical clinical presentation is of individual skin- or tan-colored papules, with a rounded or flat surface, 1 to 5 mm in diameter. Single tumors can occur, but more commonly they are multiple and symmetric, more common in females, and from adolescence onward. Syringomata most often involve the lower eyelids, although they may occur at other sites, including the cheeks, axillae, abdomen, and vulva. A linear distribution, familial occurrence, a variant associated with Down syndrome, and generalized forms have all been described. Frequent onset around puberty and reports of symptoms during pregnancy or menstruation have led to immunohistochemical studies of estrogen and progesterone receptors, with varying results and uncertain relevance.

MANAGEMENT STRATEGY

Syringomata of the eyelids and cheeks are in a prominent site and may appear conspicuous, and treatment may be sought to improve appearance. The syringomata are situated in the upper to mid-dermis. Available treatments aim to remove or flatten the papule produced by each syringoma. The majority of treatments are ablative in nature. Some patients may be troubled by only a few individual lesions, whereby *excision* of these is an option. Ablative modalities include scissor excision with secondary-intention healing, surgical excision of the entire cosmetic unit of the lower eyelids in patients who would also benefit from lower eyelid blepharoplasty, *electrocautery, electrodesiccation, intralesional electrodesiccation, dermabrasion, cryotherapy,* ablation with *CO_2 or erbium:YAG laser,* and *radiofrequency* ablation.

Local anesthesia is needed before treatment, and this may be topical or by local injections, with or without nerve blocks. Local anesthetic injections producing a field block are most commonly employed, as good anesthesia is helpful when using ablative treatments near the eye. Patients should be warned about the

possibility of postoperative bruising. Eye protection is of paramount importance, and specific precautions relevant to the use of lasers must be taken if laser treatment is used.

Ablative treatments will produce some degree of scarring and the aim is to make this imperceptible and produce an excellent cosmetic result. Possible sequelae, including scarring and hypo- or hyperpigmentation (especially with increasing skin pigmentation), should always be discussed before treatment.

There are no studies comparing different treatment modalities for syringomata and a dearth of long-term follow-up data on which to base recommendations for treatment. On the basis of experience and the limited evidence available, it is not necessary to have the latest and most expensive technology to achieve good results. Expertise and good outcomes with simple, "low-tech" methods are as important as with "high-tech" modalities. Each has benefits as well as pitfalls for the novice or unwary. It is more important to be expert in the use and application of one or more modalities than to "have a go" at them all.

Specific Investigations

> The clinical features of periorbital syringomata are usually diagnostic, and a skin biopsy may be undertaken for confirmation or when there is uncertainty.

First-Line Therapies

• Surgical excision	E
• Snip excision and secondary intention healing	E
• Electrocautery	E
• Intralesional electrodesiccation	D
• CO_2 laser	D

Cosmetic dermatologic surgery, 2nd edn. Stegman SS, Tromovitch TA, Glogau RG, eds. Chicago: Year Book Medical, 1992; 32.

A commonsense approach to treatment of syringomata, advocating the use of surgical excision, electrosurgery, or laser.

An easy method for removal of syringoma. Maloney ME. J Dermatol Surg Oncol 1982; 8: 973–5.

A single case is reported with a good outcome after removal of four to six lesions per session in 12 sessions over 5 months.

A good photographic demonstration of the removal of periorbital syringomata with fine ophthalmic spring-action scissors.

True electrocautery in the treatment of syringomas and other benign cutaneous lesions. Langtry JAA, Carruthers JA. J Cutan Med Surg 1997; 2: 60–3.

The technique of electrocautery is described and good results reported in a number of benign skin lesions, including syringomata.

Intralesional electrodesiccation of syringomas. Karma P, Benedetto AV. Dermatol Surg 1997; 23: 921–4.

Twelve patients were treated with electrodesiccation via a fine electrode into the center of the syringoma with the aim of localizing the effect and minimizing scarring. All reported excellent results and no recurrence after a follow-up of 18 to 48 months. Two patients with Fitzpatrick skin type IV had focal hyperpigmentation, which cleared in 2 to 3 months.

Evidence Levels: **A** Double-blind study **B** Clinical trial ≥ 20 subjects **C** Clinical trial < 20 subjects **D** Series ≥ 5 subjects **E** Anecdotal case reports

Syringomas treated by intralesional insulated needles without epidermal damage. Hong S-W, Lee H-J, Cho S-H, Soe J-K, Lee D, Sung H-S. Ann Dermatol 2010; 22: 367–96.

Favorable outcome reported in two patients treated by intralesional electrosurgery with insulated needles.

Treatment of multiple facial syringomas with the carbon dioxide (CO₂) laser. Wang JJ, Roenigk Jr HH. Dermatol Surg 1999; 25: 136–9.

A description of 10 patients treated with CO_2 laser reporting excellent results. Patients with more lesions needed more treatment sessions. The median follow-up was 16 months, and one patient had new syringomata at other periorbital sites 18 months after treatment. Erythema lasted 6 to 12 weeks in all patients. One patient with Fitzpatrick type IV skin had minimal focal areas of hyperpigmentation, which cleared after 2 to 3 months.

Treatment of syringoma using an ablative 10,600-nm carbon dioxide fractional laser. Cho SB, Kim HJ, Lee SJ, Kim YK, Lee JH. Dermatol Surg 2011; 37: 433–8.

Thirty-five patients with periorbital syringomata were treated with two sessions of fractional CO_2 laser at 10-month intervals. At 2 months' follow-up clinical improvement (pretreatment and posttreatment clinical photographs and patient satisfaction rates) was total in 9%, marked in 43%, moderate in 34%, and minimal in 14%.

Periorbital syringoma treated with radiofrequency and carbon dioxide (CO₂) laser in five patients. Hasson A, Farias MM, Nicklas C, Navarrete C. J Drugs Dermatol 2012; 11: 879–80.

Good cosmetic results reported in five patients with periorbital syringomata treated with the combination of radiofrequency and CO_2 laser.

Second-Line Therapies	
• Electrodesiccation and curettage	E
• Cryotherapy	E
• Combination of CO_2 laser and trichloroacetic acid	D

Syringoma: removal by electrodesiccation and curettage. Stevenson TR, Swanson SA. Am Plast Surg 1985; 15: 151–4.

The technique is described and well illustrated. Good results are reported, but there is no description of numbers of patients treated, clinical details, or follow-up data using this technique.

Cryosurgery. Dawber RPR. In: Lask GP, Moy RL, eds. Principles and Techniques of Cutaneous Surgery. New York: McGraw-Hill, 1996; 154.

Syringoma is listed as a condition treatable by cryotherapy.
Details are not given, and periorbital syringomata are not specifically mentioned.

A new treatment for syringoma. Combination of carbon dioxide laser and trichloroacetic acid. Kang H, Kim NS, Kim YB, Shim WC. Dermatol Surg 1998; 24: 1370–4.

This study evaluates the histopathology and efficacy of combined CO_2 laser and 50% trichloroacetic acid treatment in 20 Korean patients with periorbital syringomata. Results were reported as excellent (11 patients), good (6), and fair (3), without complications such as scarring, infection, or textural change, using the technique detailed.

Erbium YAG laser treatment of periorbital syringomas by using the multiple ovoid-shape ablation method. Kitano Y. J Cosmet Laser Ther 2016; 18: 280–5.

Forty-nine patients with syringomata were treated every 2 months with an erbium:YAG laser, ablating multiple 2- to 4-mm egg-shaped fields. More than 75% of syringomata disappeared in 43 of 49 patients after an average of 3.77 treatments.

Third-Line Therapies	
• Dermabrasion	E
• Trichloroacetic acid	E E
• Topical atropine	E E
• Topical tretinoin	E

Dermabrasion by diamond fraises revolving at 85000 revolutions per minute. Fulton JE. J Dermatol Surg Oncol 1978; 4: 777–9.

High-speed dermabrasion is described and good results are reported in 65 patients with acne scarring, actinic damage, adenoma sebaceum, and syringomata.

The treatment of eruptive syringomas in an African American patient with a combination of trichloroacetic acid and CO₂ laser destruction. Frazier CC, Camacho AP, Cockerell CJ. Dermatol Surg 2001; 27: 489–92.

A single case report of eruptive facial syringomata in an African American woman treated by 35% trichloroacetic acid peel, followed 2 weeks later by CO_2 laser, with acceptable cosmetic results and without significant side effects.

Eruptive pruritic syringomas: treatment with topical atropine. Sanchez TS, Dauden E, Casas AP, Garcia-Diez A. J Am Acad Dermatol 2001; 44: 148–9.

A single case report of pruritic syringomata of the chest and neck improving with topical 1% atropine.

Eruptive syringoma: treatment with topical tretinoin. Gomez MI, Perez B, Azana JM, Nunez M, Ledo A. Dermatology 1994; 189: 105–6

A 23 year old woman with asymptomatic eruptive syringoma treated with 0.1% tretinoin cream daily for 4 months, resulting in flattening of the lesions in the areas treated.

Tinea capitis

Elisabeth M. Higgins[†]

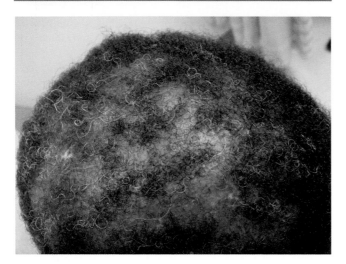

Tinea capitis (scalp ringworm) is the term used to describe a fungal infection of the scalp caused by dermatophyte species. Infections may be passed from person to person (anthropophilic, in which man is the primary host) or acquired from animals (zoophilic). Several different species of fungi may be responsible, predominantly *Microsporum* and *Trichophyton* species, and can be identified by their varied characteristics on microscopy and culture. Species that invade only the inside of the hair shaft are termed *endothrix infections,* whereas those that invade both the inside and the outside of the hair shaft are responsible for ectothrix infections. The disease is most prevalent in children and usually presents with areas of scaling and alopecia, with a varying degree of inflammation. There may be associated cervical lymphadenopathy. Some species of dermatophyte induce a very inflammatory, pustular reaction, which may lead to scarring and permanent alopecia. However, this is fortunately relatively rare with modern treatment regimens, in which full regrowth of hair is the norm.

A transient pruritic, papular dermatophytid ("id") reaction, characteristically involving the ear, but often more widespread, may occur either before or on initiation of treatment, particularly in kerion infections, but should not be confused with a drug hypersensitivity.

MANAGEMENT STRATEGY

Treatment of tinea capitis is aimed at eradicating the organism to prevent the spread of infection and minimize scarring. Established infections cannot be treated topically, and oral therapy is required. Although *griseofulvin* remains the only licensed oral antifungal agent for use in tinea capitis in children in the UK, many countries have adopted newer treatment protocols. Although only weakly fungistatic, griseofulvin is effective in the treatment of most varieties of tinea capitis, but may need to be given in high doses over a prolonged period. Each case should

be monitored to ensure adequate treatment and eradication of the organism. Traditionally this has been done using Wood light examination, but this is only viable in cases due to species that fluoresce (e.g., *Microsporum* infections). An increasing number of cases in the UK and North America today are due to the emergence of *Trichophyton tonsurans,* a nonfluorescent endothrix species. Treatment response therefore has to be followed mycologically by sending specimens to the laboratory. Mycologic cure should be the gold standard of treatment. However, evidence is emerging that dermoscopy may provide a rapid diagnostic tool for initiation of treatment.

In recent years the azoles *itraconazole, ketoconazole,* and *fluconazole* and the allylamine *terbinafine* have become available for systemic use. Many studies have demonstrated that these agents have at least equal efficacy to *griseofulvin* in a variety of types of tinea capitis, and treatment times are often shorter. Although more expensive, shorter treatment regimens may help compliance and reduce the spread of infection.

Over the past decade, the use of intermittent or pulsed treatment regimens using *fluconazole* or *itraconazole* has been explored. This treatment strategy is based on the long half-life of the drugs in keratin. Such regimens do not appear to confer any benefit in terms of cure rates, but may reduce the total cost of treatment.

There are variations in the response of different dermatophyte species to the different antifungal agents, and treatment should be tailored accordingly. Overall, *griseofulvin* appears superior in the clearance of *Microsporum* infections, but newer agents appear more effective against *Trichophyton.* Itraconazole probably has the broadest spectrum of action. However, so far no agent has been shown to achieve a 100% cure rate. Ectothrix infections are generally caused by *Microsporum* species, most notably the zoophilic *M. canis* or the anthropophilic *M. audouinii,* and almost always occur in children. Historically, *griseofulvin* has been the standard treatment at a dose of 10 to 20 mg/kg/day, but clearance may be slow, and treatment should be continued for as long as necessary, which is at least 6 weeks, but may be 12 to 16 weeks, and monitored as outlined earlier. Itraconazole may be considered an alternative. Although there are licensing restrictions in some countries, it has now superseded griseofulvin as the treatment of choice in parts of Europe.

Endothrix infections, most commonly with *T. tonsurans* or *T. violaceum,* are more prevalent in children, but may occasionally occur in adults (usually the contacts/carers of children). Higher-dose regimens of *griseofulvin* tend to be required to achieve cure. The newer *azoles* and *terbinafine* appear to achieve clearance more rapidly (usually in 4 weeks). In adults with tinea capitis due to *Trichophyton* species, *terbinafine* 250 mg/day for 4 weeks is the treatment of choice. Although unlicensed in children, the current British Association of Dermatology guidelines and *British National Formulary* give the dosing schedule for *terbinafine* in children, in recognition of its widespread use in tinea capitis in this age group (<20 kg, 62.5 mg/day; 20–40 kg, 125 mg/day; >40 kg, 250 mg/day). Current evidence suggests that either this or *itraconazole* should become the treatment of choice in children with *Trichophyton* infections. Both drugs are now licensed for use in children in many countries and have replaced *griseofulvin,* which has now been withdrawn from some countries. Topical antifungal creams and shampoos are sometimes used in conjunction with oral therapy, with the aim of reducing patient infectivity, but have no role in prophylaxis.

In the current urban epidemics of *T. tonsurans,* asymptomatic infection in household contacts is posing a significant problem in reinfection/relapse, and there is merit in screening all family members (including adults), where practical, to reduce reinfection rates.

† deceased

Evidence Levels: **A** Double-blind study **B** Clinical trial ≥ 20 subjects **C** Clinical trial < 20 subjects **D** Series ≥ 5 subjects **E** Anecdotal case reports

Specific investigations

- Examination of hair and scalp scale by direct microscopy and culture
- Direct observation under Wood light for fluorescence
- Dermoscopy/trichoscopy
- Screen contacts, especially siblings, where possible

Fungal Infection: Diagnosis and Management. Richardson MD, Warnock DW. Oxford: Blackwell, 2003; 21, 87.

Scalp hairs infected by *M. audouinii*, *M. canis*, and *T. schoenleinii* fluoresce bright green under Wood light. Direct microscopic examination of hairs reveals arthrospores of the fungus either inside (endothrix) or on the outside of the hair shaft. Individual dermatophyte species can be identified by specific appearances in culture.

Trends in tinea capitis in an Irish population and a comparison of scalp brushings versus scalp scrapings as methods of investigation. Nasir S, Ralph N, O'Neill C, Cunney R, Lenane P, O'Donnell B. Pediatr Dermatol 2014; 31: 622–3.

A study of 391 children with tinea capitis showed hairbrush sampling was superior to scalp scrapings in confirming mycologic diagnosis, but using both methods increases the diagnostic yield ($p < 0.001$).

Screening for asymptomatic carriage of *Trichophyton tonsurans* in household contacts of patients with tinea capitis: results of 209 patients from south London. White JM, Higgins EM, Fuller LC. J Eur Acad Dermatol Venereol 2007; 21: 1061–4.

More than 50% of household contacts in this study had positive fungal cultures (7.1% overt infection and 44.5% silent fungal carriage). Children under 16 were most likely to be affected ($p < 0.001$), especially girls ($p < 0.01$).

Tinea capitis: predictive value of symptoms and time to cure with griseofulvin treatment. Lorch-Dauk KC, Comrov E, Blumer JL, O'Riordan MA, Furman LM. Clin Pediatr 2010; 49: 280–6.

In a prospective, nonblind intervention study of 99 children, the predictive value of any one of four cardinal signs/symptoms of tinea capitis (scalp scaling, alopecia, pruritus, lymphadenopathy) was shown to be 88%.

Treatment of tinea capitis often needs to be started before laboratory confirmation is obtained. Treatment should be started on the basis of clinical evidence, but appropriate mycology samples should always be sent before initiation of therapy.

Trichoscopy in pediatric patients with tinea capitis: a useful method to differentiate from alopecia areata. Ekiz O, Sen BB, Rifaioğlu EN, Balta I. J Eur Acad Dermatol Venereol. 2014; 28: 1255–8.

A study of 25 children (15 with tinea capitis and 10 with alopecia areata) identified distinctive features on dermoscopy of the hair and scalp in children with fungal infections, including broken, dystrophic, corkscrew, barcode, and comma hairs, as well as black dots.

The use of handheld magnification is a cheap technique and is proving increasingly valuable in confirming the diagnosis of tinea capitis and differentiating from other causes of alopecia.

Are dermatophytid reactions in patients with kerion celsi much more common than previously thought? A prospective study. Topaloğlu Demir E, Karadag AS. Pediatr Dermatol 2015; 32: 635–40.

A prospective study identified dermatophytid reactions in 13 of 19 children (68%) being treated for kerion.

Dermatophytid reactions in children with tinea capitis are probably underrecognized and underreported.

First-Line Therapies

• Griseofulvin	A
• Terbinafine	A
• Itraconazole	A

Meta-analysis of randomized controlled studies comparing griseofulvin and terbinafine in the treatment of tinea capitis. Tey HL, Tan AS, Chan YC. J Am Acad Dermatol 2011; 64: 663–70.

A pooled analysis of seven studies, involving 2163 subjects, revealed no overall difference in efficacy between 8 weeks' (range 6–12 weeks) griseofulvin and 4 weeks' (range 2–6 weeks) terbinafine, but the latter had shorter treatment regimens (odds ratio = 1.22 in favor of terbinafine; 95% CI = 0.785–1.919; $p = 0.37$). However, subanalysis by species shows terbinafine has significantly greater efficacy against *T. tonsurans* (odds ratio = 1.49; 95% CI = 1.274–2.051; $p < 0.001$). In contrast, griseofulvin was superior in the treatment of *Microsporum* species (odds ratio in favor of griseofulvin = 0.48, 95% CI, 0.254–0.656; $p < 0.001$).

Terbinafine is superior in the treatment of T. tonsurans; *griseofulvin is more effective in the treatment of* Microsporum *species, but the treatment course is longer. Both drugs are well tolerated in children.*

Terbinafine hydrochloride oral granules versus oral griseofulvin suspension in children with tinea capitis: results of two randomised investigator-blinded, multicenter, international, controlled trials. Elewski BE, Cáceres HW, Deleon L, El Shimy S, Hunter JA, Korotkiy N, et al. J Am Acad Dermatol 2008; 59: 41–54.

A multicenter, investigator-blinded, randomized controlled study comparing 6 weeks' treatment with griseofulvin 10 to 20 mg/kg/day ($n = 509$) with terbinafine 5 to 8 mg/kg/day ($n = 1040$) in children with microscopy-proven tinea capitis. Complete cure rates (45.1% vs. 33.01%) and mycologic cure (61.55% vs. 55.5%) were significantly higher for terbinafine than for griseofulvin ($p < 0.05$), even at higher doses (>20 mg/kg/day). Subgroup analysis revealed that terbinafine was significantly better than griseofulvin for all cure rates (clinical, mycologic, and complete) in *T. tonsurans* infection but not for *M. canis* ($p < 0.001$). In contrast, for *M. canis*, mycologic and clinical cure rates were significantly better with griseofulvin ($p < 0.05$). Fifty percent of patients in each group reported mild side effects with treatment, but there was no significant effect on liver transaminases.

This largest pediatric study to date highlights the safety and efficacy of a new formulation of terbinafine in the treatment of tinea capitis in children. However, limitations of the study included not using a standard dose of griseofulvin in each center, inconsistency in the use of adjuvant topical therapy, and the inclusion of more than one causal species. Subanalysis shows a clear differentiation in response rates between organisms, and therapy should probably be tailored, with terbinafine being the treatment of choice in T. tonsurans *infection, whereas griseofulvin is superior in* Microsporum *infections.*

Systemic antifungal therapy for tinea capitis in children. González U, Seaton T, Bergus G, Jacobson J, Martínez-Mónzon C. Cochrane Database Syst Rev 2007; 4: CD004685.

An analysis of 21 randomized control trials involving 1812 subjects under the age of 18 years, in which systemic antifungal therapy was used in mycologically proven tinea capitis. In view of varying susceptibilities, studies were evaluated according to the causal organism. For *Trichophyton* species, *terbinafine* given on a weight-related dosage schedule for 4 weeks showed similar efficacy to *griseofulvin* given for 8 weeks in three studies involving 382 subjects (RR 1.09; 95% CI, 0.95–1.26). Itraconazole and griseofulvin given for 6 weeks showed similar cure rates in a study of 35 children (RR 1.06; 95% CI, 0.81–1.39). However, *itraconazole* given for short periods may also be as effective as griseofulvin given for 6 weeks (RR 0.89; 95% CI, 0.76–1.04), and both itraconazole and terbinafine given for 2 to 3 weeks were equally effective in two studies involving 160 participants (RR 0.93; 95% CI, 0.72–1.19). For *Microsporum* species, overall, no difference was found between the efficacy of griseofulvin and that of terbinafine in clearance of *Microsporum* infections, but there was little evidence on the use of systemic agents in this species that met the study inclusion criteria.

The authors conclude that terbinafine and itraconazole are probably preferable to griseofulvin in the treatment of Trichophyton *tinea capitis because of the shorter treatment duration, even though these agents are more expensive and may not always be available in a pediatric formulation.*

Tinea capitis in early infancy treated with itraconazole. Binder B, Richtig E, Weger W, Ginter-Hanselmayer G. J Eur Acad Dermatol Venereol 2009; 23: 1161–3.

In a pilot study of seven infants <1 year of age with *M. canis* tinea capitis, itraconazole was found to be effective and well tolerated.

Itraconazole has been shown to be safe in the treatment of young infants, including neonates, although study numbers were inevitably small.

Second-Line Therapies	
• Fluconazole	B
• Short-duration terbinafine	B
• Short-duration itraconazole	B

Comparative evaluation of griseofulvin, terbinafine and fluconazole in the treatment of tinea capitis. Grover C, Arora P, Manchanda V. Int J Dermatol 2012; 51: 455–8.

A prospective, nonblinded, cross-sectional study of 75 children comparing griseofulvin, terbinafine, and fluconazole in the treatment of tinea capitis (predominantly *T. violaceum*) revealed cure rates of 96%, 88%, and 84%, respectively. Seven patients required more prolonged therapy, but all three drugs were well tolerated.

Although well tolerated, fluconazole had comparatively lower cure rates in this population, and therefore appears to confer no advantage over standard protocols using griseofulvin. However, some patients required prolonged treatment, and these may have been due to infections with other species, but full subanalysis by drug and organism was not undertaken due to the small numbers involved.

Once weekly fluconazole is effective in children in the treatment of tinea capitis: a prospective multicenter study. Gupta AK, Dlova N, Taborda P, Morar N, Taborda V, Lynde CW, et al. Br J Dermatol 2000; 142: 965–8.

An open, multicenter assessment of 61 children treated with oral fluconazole 8 mg/kg once weekly for 8 weeks (extended for a further 4 weeks if clinically indicated). Causal organisms were *T. violaceum* (n = 33), *T. tonsurans* (n = 11), and *M. canis* (n = 17). All 44 children with *Trichophyton* infections had mycologic and clinical cure at 16 weeks after the start of treatment; the majority (35/44) only required 8 weeks of therapy, but 9 out of 33 of the *T. violaceum* group required treatment for 12 weeks. Twelve out of 17 of the *M. canis* group were clinically clear after 8 weeks. Treatment

was extended for a total of 12 weeks in one and 16 weeks in 3 patients, but overall 16 of 17 children in this group had complete cure 2 months after the end of therapy. One child had asymptomatic and reversible elevation of liver function tests.

Short duration treatment with terbinafine for tinea capitis caused by *Trichophyton* or *Microsporum* species. Hamm H, Schwinn A, Brautigan M, Weidinger G. Br J Dermatol 1999; 140: 480–2.

A double-blind study of 35 children comparing the efficacy of 1 or 2 weeks of oral terbinafine, 62.5 to 250 mg/day according to weight. Patients were followed up for 12 weeks, and nonresponders were given an additional 4 weeks of therapy. Twenty-three children had *Trichophyton* infections (n = 12 with *T. tonsurans* infection), and 12 had *M. canis* infection; cure rates after 1 and 2 weeks of therapy were 86% and 56%, respectively. However, only 1 of the 12 children with *Microsporum* infection responded initially, although a further 4 cleared with 4 more weeks of treatment.

Short-duration (2 weeks) and intermittent treatment regimens show remarkable clearance rates, particularly in infections with Trichophyton *species, and may offer a significant cost savings.*

Third-Line Therapies	
• 2% ketoconazole	B
• Selenium sulfide shampoo	B
• Prednisolone	B

A retrospective study of the management of pediatric kerion in *T. tonsurans* infection. Proudfoot LE, Higgins EM, Morris-Jones R. Pediatr Dermatol 2011; 78: 655–7.

A retrospective study of all children less than 10 years of age presenting with kerion infection to a single unit over a 6-year period revealed no advantage in concomitant use of oral or intralesional steroids compared with oral antifungal therapy alone.

A randomised comparative trial of treatment of kerion celsi with griseofulvin plus oral prednisolone vs. griseofulvin alone. Hussain I, Muzzafar F, Rashid T, Jahangir M, Haroon TS. Med Mycol 1999; 37: 97–9.

A randomized study of 30 patients with scalp kerion comparing treatment with griseofulvin and prednisolone to griseofulvin alone. Evaluation at 12 weeks revealed similar cure rates in both groups.

Although traditionally many clinicians have used prednisolone to reduce the inflammation of kerions in an effort to minimize scarring and hence the possibility of permanent alopecia, the limited evidence that exists does not support its use. Kerion formation is not uncommon in the current spate of T. tonsurans *infections in the UK. However, scarring is exceptionally rare, and full regrowth of hair can be expected after appropriate oral antifungal therapy alone.*

Successful treatment of tinea capitis with 2% ketoconazole shampoo. Greer DL. Int J Dermatol 2000; 39: 302–4.

Sixteen children aged 3 to 6 years with *T. tonsurans* tinea capitis were treated with 2% ketoconazole shampoo daily for 8 weeks. All showed clinical improvement, some as early as 2 weeks. Six of 15 (40%) had negative cultures at 8 weeks, and 5 (33%) remained clear 1 year later.

Comparison of 1% and 2.5% selenium sulphide in the treatment of tinea capitis. Gibbens TG, Murray MM, Baker RC. Arch Pediatr Adolesc Med 1995; 149: 808–11.

Evidence Levels: A Double-blind study B Clinical trial ≥ 20 subjects C Clinical trial < 20 subjects D Series ≥ 5 subjects E Anecdotal case reports

A randomized controlled trial of 54 patients showing that selenium sulfide, as either a lotion or a shampoo, reduces surface counts of dermatophytes in children being treated with griseofulvin 15 mg/kg/day.

Prophylactic ketoconazole shampoo for tinea capitis in a high risk pediatric population. Bookstaver PB, Watson HJ, Winters SD, Carlson AL, Schulz RM. J Pediatr Pharmacol Ther 2011; 16: 199–203.

A retrospective analysis of 97 vulnerable children considered at high risk of tinea capitis showed no benefit from twice-weekly use of 2% ketoconazole shampoo in the prevention of infection.

These small studies support the use of an antifungal shampoo to reduce surface counts of the organism, and therefore aid clearance and possibly reduce the risk of transmission. If systemic therapy is contraindicated or unavailable, there may be a limited benefit in using 2% ketoconazole shampoo alone. However, shampoos have not been shown to prevent infection, even in vulnerable children, and have no place in prophylaxis.

Tinea pedis and skin dermatophytosis

Aditya K. Gupta, Kelly A. Foley, Sarah G. Versteeg

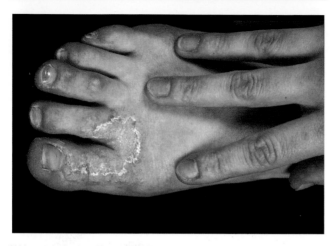

(With permission from Tinea pedis. Busam Klaus J, ed. Dermatopathology: A Volume in the Series: Foundations in Diagnostic Pathology, 2nd edn. Philadelphia, PA: Elsevier, 2010.)

Dermatophytosis is a cutaneous fungal infection commonly caused by *Epidermophyton*, *Trichophyton*, and *Microsporum*, affecting the soles of the feet and interdigital spaces (tinea pedis), groin (tinea cruris), face (tinea faciei), and skin (tinea corporis). Cutaneous fungal infections have a worldwide prevalence of 20% to 25%; with an increase in urbanization, communal sports, and an aging population, prevalence of dermatophyte infections may be on the rise. Additionally, due to extreme humidity and high temperatures, skin dermatophytoses frequently occur in tropical and subtropical regions.

Epidemiologic trends in skin mycoses worldwide. Havlickova B, Czailka VA, Friedrich M. Mycoses 2008; 51: 2–15.

This review is a summary of the geographic prevalence of skin dermatophytoses and the causative fungal organisms. In addition to already established risk factors (e.g., gender, foot trauma), an increase in public sporting events, diabetes, and travel has increased the prevalence of tinea pedis in developed countries, whereas in developing parts of the world, tinea capitis may be more abundant.

Epidemiology of dermatophytoses: retrospective analysis from 2005 to 2010 and comparison with previous data from 1975. Garofalo A, Bosco A, Cassano N. New Microbiol 2012; 35: 207–13.

This is a retrospective analysis of all cases of dermatophytoses (6133 patients) presenting to an Italian dermatology clinic from 2005 to 2010. Tinea corporis (22.7%) and tinea pedis (20.4%) were the most common skin dermatophytoses observed. Cases of tinea pedis showed a male predominance with trends of an increase in occurrence.

Tinea pedis: the etiology and global epidemiology of a common fungal infection. *Ilkit* M, Durdu M. Crit Rev Microbiol 2015; 41: 374–88.

Tinea pedis is commonly found in adult males (31–60 years old) with a higher prevalence in high-risk occupations (e.g., miners, soldiers, runners). Complications associated with tinea pedis include cellulitis, id reaction, and Majocchi granuloma.

MANAGEMENT STRATEGY

Topical therapies (e.g., azoles, allylamines) are the first line of defense when treating tinea pedis, localized tinea corporis, and tinea cruris. Many topical treatments do not require a prescription, and treatment durations ranging from 2 to 4 weeks are usually sufficient for successful management of most dermatophytoses. Where infection is serious or more extensive (i.e., covers a large surface area of the body) or is recurrent, oral antifungal treatments may be needed. High mycological cure rates have been found with oral treatments such as terbinafine (75%–85%), itraconazole (79%), and fluconazole (93%). Treatments with additional antibacterial capabilities (e.g., ciclopirox olamine, miconazole nitrate, ketoconazole, etc.) can also be beneficial as bacterial superinfections can co-occur with tinea infections. Some preventative measures, including educational programs, maintaining proper hygiene, avoiding communal areas, and using antimicrobial fabrics, may help limit relapse and prevent transmission.

Management of tinea corporis, tinea cruris, and tinea pedis: a comprehensive review. Sahoo AK, Mahajan R. Indian Dermatol Online J 2016; 7: 77–86.

Topical therapies (e.g., antifungals) are effective at treating tinea infections (e.g., tinea corporis, tinea cruris, tinea faciei, tinea pedis), and nonpharmacologic management (e.g., loose-fitting socks) can help to reduce moisture. Oral therapy is suggested for extensive or nonresponsive infections.

Specific investigations

- Direct microscopy on KOH specimens
- Fungal culture

In order to successfully treat dermatophytosis, accurately diagnosing the infection is paramount, as tinea infections can mimic other lesional conditions. The two main test methods used to diagnose dermatophyte infections include direct microscopy and fungal culture. Lesional scrapings can be obtained with a blade (no. 15) or banana-shaped knife, and blisters/pustule tops can be ruptured to allow for adequate sampling.

Identifying signs of tinea pedis: a key to understanding clinical variables. Canavan TN, Elewski BE. J Drugs Dermatol 2015; 14: 42–7.

T. rubrum, *T. mentagrophytes*, and *E. floccosum* are the most common causes of tinea pedis. Tinea pedis can be found worldwide and is endemic to Southeast Asia and Western Africa. Interdigital (e.g., macerated skin), moccasin (e.g., dry, hyperkeratotic scales), vesicular (e.g., small vesicles, erythema), and acute ulcerative (e.g., ulcers, erosions) are four clinical patterns of tinea pedis.

The sensitivity and specificity of potassium hydroxide smear and fungal culture relative to clinical assessment in the evaluation of tinea pedis: a pooled analysis. Levitt JO, Levitt BH, Akhavan A, Yanofsky H. Dermatol Res Pract 2010; 2010: 1–8.

Sensitivity and specificity of KOH smears and fungal culture were determined through a pooled analysis of vehicle-treated

Evidence Levels: **A** Double-blind study **B** Clinical trial ≥ 20 subjects **C** Clinical trial < 20 subjects **D** Series ≥ 5 subjects **E** Anecdotal case reports

participants from five randomized, double-blind clinical studies (n = 460). KOH smears (73.3%) are more sensitive than fungal cultures (41.7%) when confirming clinical assessment (negative or positive); fungal cultures (77.7%) are more specific than KOH smears (42.5%, p < 0.0001 and p < 0.0001, respectively).

Inflammatory tinea pedis/manuum masquerading as bacterial cellulitis. Sweeney SM, Wiss K, Mallory SB. Arch Pediatr Adolesc Med 2002; 156: 1149–52.

Four cases of children with tinea pedis or tinea manuum initially diagnosed with bacterial cellulitis are described. Infections in children may mimic bacterial infections. KOH examination produced positive results and may help in diagnosis.

First-Line Therapies

Topical

• Clotrimazole	A
• Miconazole	A
• Luliconazole	A
• Econazole nitrate	A
• Naftifine hydrochloride	A
• Sertaconazole nitrate	A

Efficacy of topical antifungal drugs in different dermatomycoses: a systematic review with meta-analysis. Rotta I, Otuki MF, Sanches AC, Correr CJ. Rev Assoc Med Bras 2012; 58: 308–18.

A meta-analysis of 49 studies revealed allylamines to be more effective than azoles when evaluating sustained cure rates for treatment of dermatomycoses. Azoles and allylamines showed higher efficacy rates (e.g., mycological cure, sustained cure) for treatment of tinea pedis, tinea cruris, and tinea corporis compared with placebo.

Efficacy and safety of once-daily luliconazole 1% cream in patients ≥ 12 years of age with interdigital tinea pedis: a phase 3, randomized, double-blind, vehicle-controlled study. Jarratt M, Jones T, Adelglass J, Bucko A, Pollak R, Roman-Miranda A, et al. J Drugs Dermatol 2014; 13: 838–46.

A phase III, vehicle-controlled study was conducted on interdigital tinea pedis patients with daily application of luliconazole for 14 days (n = 321). Clinical cure, mycological cure, and complete clearance rates 28 days posttreatment were significantly higher with luliconazole treatment (29.2%, 62.3%, and 26.4%, respectively) compared with vehicle treatment (7.8%, 17.5%, and 1.9%, respectively) (p < 0.001, p < 0.001, and p < 0.001, respectively).

Econazole nitrate foam 1% for the treatment of tinea pedis: results from two double-blind, vehicle-controlled, phase 3 clinical trials. Elewski BE, Vlahovic TC. J Drugs Dermatol 2014; 13: 803–8.

Two vehicle-controlled, 4-week, double-blind, multicenter studies were conducted with econazole nitrate (1%) for treatment of interdigital tinea pedis (n = 505). Complete cure and mycological cure rates were higher with econazole nitrate foam (24.3% and 67.6%, respectively) compared with vehicle (3.6% and 16.9%, respectively) (p < 0.001 and p < 00001, respectively).

Naftifine hydrochloride gel 2%: an effective topical treatment for moccasin-type tinea pedis. Stein Gold LF, Vlahovic T, Verma A, Olayinka B, Fleischer AB Jr. J Drugs Dermatol 2015; 14: 1138–44.

A posthoc analysis of two pooled, 6-week, double-blind, vehicle-controlled, multicenter clinical trials was conducted to evaluate naftifine hydrochloride for treatment of moccasin-type tinea pedis (n = 380). Complete cure, mycological cure, and treatment effectiveness were higher with naftifine gel (19.2%, 65.8%, and 51.4%, respectively) compared with vehicle (0.9%, 7.8%, and 4.4%) 4 weeks posttreatment (p < 0.0001, p < 0.0001, and p < 0.0001, respectively).

Sertaconazole: a review of its use in the management of superficial mycoses in dermatology and gynecology. Croxtall JD, Plosker G. Drugs 2009; 69: 339–59.

Sertaconazole 2% cream was found to be more effective compared with miconazole 2% cream for treatment of tinea pedis in a placebo-controlled trial. Mycological cure was found with once-a-day and twice-a-day sertaconazole application. This antifungal is effective in both solution and cream formation.

Second-Line Therapies

Topical

• Terbinafine 1% as cream, solution, gel, or film-forming solution	A
• Ciclopirox (hydroxypyridone)	A
• Ketoconazole	D

Comparable efficacy and safety of various topical formulations of terbinafine in tinea pedis irrespective of the treatment regimen: results of a meta-analysis. Korting HC, Kiencke P, Nelles S, Rychlik R. Am J Clin Dermatol 2007; 8: 357–64.

A meta-analysis of 19 randomized controlled trials revealed that terbinafine is three times more likely to produce clinical cure in tinea pedis patients compared with placebo. Cure rates found with terbinafine are comparable to other antifungal therapies used to treat tinea pedis. The efficacy and safety of terbinafine are not influenced by treatment formulation, duration of therapy, or frequency of application.

Ciclopirox gel in the treatment of patients with interdigital tinea pedis. Aly R, Fisher G, Katz I, Levine N, Lookingbill DP, Lowe N, et al. Int J Dermatol 2003; 42: 29–35.

Two multicenter, double-blind, vehicle-controlled, clinical trials evaluated the efficacy of ciclopirox (0.77%) to treat mild-to-moderate interdigital tinea pedis with twice-daily application for 28 days (n = 374). Treatment success (mycological cure and ≥75% clinical improvement) was found in 60% of ciclopirox-treated participants and 19% of vehicle-treated participants. Mycological cure was found in 85% of participants treated with ciclopirox and 16% of participants treated with vehicle.

Ketoconazole 2% cream in the treatment of tinea pedis, tinea cruris, and tinea corporis. Lester M. Cutis 1995; 55: 181–3.

A large study of 232 patients were evaluated after 4 and 8 weeks of treatment with once-daily ketoconazole 2% cream. Forty-nine percent of patients had total symptom scores of absent or mild at the end of treatment, and 82% responded to the treatment.

Third-Line Therapies	
Topical	
• 40% urea cream	D
• Photodynamic therapy	D
Systemic	
• Terbinafine	A
• Itraconazole	A
• Fluconazole	A
• Griseofulvin	A

Urea: a comprehensive review of the clinical literature. Pan M, Heinecke G, Bernardo S, Tsui C, Levitt J. Dermatol Online J 2013; 19: 20392.

Eighty-one studies met inclusion criteria, with four studies specifically evaluating urea for treatment of tinea pedis. Urea showed antibacterial properties and enhanced the efficacy of topical treatments (e.g., lanoconazole, bifonazole, ciclopirox, butenafine hydrochloride).

Photodynamic therapy in the treatment of superficial mycoses: an evidence-based evaluation. Qiao J, Li R, Ding Y, Fang H. Mycopathologia 2010; 170: 339–43.

An evidence-based review found seven studies that used phototherapy for treatment of superficial mycoses that met inclusion criteria. After phototherapy sessions, 80% of tinea cruris patients (n = 10) and 60% of tinea pedis patients (n = 10) were mycologically cured.

Oral treatments for fungal infections of the skin of the foot. Bell-Syer SEM, Khan SM, Torgerson DJ. Cochrane Database Syst Rev 2012; 10: CD003584.

Terbinafine was a more effective tinea pedis treatment than griseofulvin as evaluated across 15 selected randomized, controlled trials. No significant differences in efficacy rates were found between fluconazole and itraconazole or between terbinafine and itraconazole.

A comparison of the efficacy of oral fluconazole, 150 mg/ week versus 50 mg/day, in the treatment of tinea corporis, tinea cruris, tinea pedis and cutaneous candidosis. Nozickova M, Koudelkova V, Kulikova Z, Malina L, Urbanowski S, Silny W. Int J Dermatol 1998; 37: 703–5.

To determine the efficacy of fluconazole, patients with dermatophytoses and cutaneous candidosis were treated for 4 to 6 weeks (n = 245). Positive clinical responses (cure and marked improvement) were found in 79% to 88% of non–pedis-infected patients and in 79% to 93% of pedis-infected patients.

Efficacy and safety of short-term itraconazole in tinea pedis: a double-blind, randomized, placebo-controlled trial. Svejgaard E, Avnstorp C, Wanscher B, Nilsson J, Heremans A. Dermatology 1998; 197: 368–72.

Seventy-two patients with plantar or moccasin type tinea pedis received itraconazole 200 mg twice daily or placebo for 1 week. Efficacy was evaluated after an 8-week follow-up period. Itraconazole was significantly more effective than placebo in treating tinea pedis. The success rate (clinical response and mycological cure) was 53% for itraconazole compared with 3% for placebo (p < 0.001), and the mycological cure rate was 56% for itraconazole compared with 8% for placebo (p < 0.001).

Safety and efficacy of tinea pedis and onychomycosis treatment in people with diabetes: a systematic review. Matricciani L, Talbot K, Jones S. J Foot Ankle Res 2011; 4: 26.

Continuous oral therapy (e.g., terbinafine) is the suggested treatment for patients with tinea pedis and/or toenail onychomycosis and who have been diagnosed with diabetes (type 1 or 2).

Evidence Levels: **A** Double-blind study **B** Clinical trial ≥ 20 subjects **C** Clinical trial < 20 subjects **D** Series ≥ 5 subjects **E** Anecdotal case reports

243

Tinea unguium

Antonella Tosti

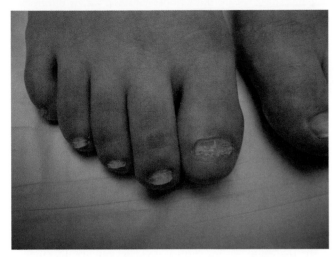

Onychomycosis accounts for about half of all nail abnormalities and a third of all fungal infections of the skin. It affects about 10% of the general population, with figures that vary in different areas of the world. About 85% of cases of onychomycosis are due to dermatophytes, the most common being *Trichophyton rubrum*, followed by *Trichophyton interdigitale*. The prevalence of onychomycosis increases with age, and the toenails are most frequently affected. Tinea pedis *is* associated with onychomycosis in most patients. Predisposing factors for onychomycosis include old age, diabetes, HIV infection, peripheral vascular impairment, peripheral neuropathies, podiatric abnormalities, sports activities, and traumatic nail disorders.

MANAGEMENT STRATEGY

Different clinical patterns of nail infection result from the way in which fungi colonize the nail. In distal subungual onychomycosis (DSO), the most common type, fungi reach the nail from the hyponychium and colonize the nail bed, producing onycholysis and subungual hyperkeratosis. In proximal subungual onychomycosis (PSO), fungi penetrate the nail matrix via the proximal nail fold and colonize the deep portion of the proximal nail plate, resulting in a subungual white patch located in the lunula area. In white superficial onychomycosis (WSO), fungi are localized on the nail plate surface and produce whitish, opaque, friable areas on the nail plate. The type of nail invasion depends on both the causative fungus and host susceptibility.

The goals for antifungal therapy are mycologic cure and a normal-looking nail. Clinical cure, which requires several months due to slow nail growth, can be impossible to achieve when onychomycosis is associated with traumatic nail dystrophies. Immediately after treatment with systemic agents, which usually lasts 3 months, it is common to observe a still-abnormal nail; signs of a good response are no proximal progression and a proximal area of normal-appearing nail.

Treatment of onychomycosis depends on the clinical type of the onychomycosis, the number of affected nails, and the severity of involvement. A systemic treatment with *terbinafine, itraconazole, or fluconazole* is always required in PSO and in DSO involving the lunula region. WSO and DSO limited to the distal nail can be treated with a topical agent such as *efinaconazole, tavaborole, amorolfine, or ciclopirox. Combined systemic and topical treatment* increases the cure rate.

In recent years, the number of patients with AIDS-related or iatrogenic immunosuppression has substantially increased, leading to the appearance of new patterns of nail invasion by fungi. There is now evidence that some clinical varieties of superficial onychomycosis (i.e., in transverse lines) may be due to fungal invasion of the nail plate under the ventral nail fold: this substantially changes treatment options, because topical therapy does not cure these cases. New types of PSO have also been described. These include nondermatophyte PSO, usually due to *Fusarium* or *Aspergillus* species, which is typically associated with acute periungual inflammation.

Terbinafine is an allylamine with fungicidal properties. Interactions of terbinafine with other drugs are extremely rare. Adverse effects may involve gastrointestinal function and the skin. Patients with known lupus erythematosus or photosensitivity are predisposed to drug-induced or drug-exacerbated disease. Liver toxicity can occasionally occur. Terbinafine is administered at a dose of 250 mg daily; treatment duration is 6 weeks for fingernails and 12 weeks for toenails. Clinical trials have repeatedly demonstrated a higher efficacy of terbinafine compared with other antifungal treatments. A meta-analysis of 18 studies on terbinafine for onychomycosis showed a mycologic cure rate of 76%.

Terbinafine persists in the nail for at least 30 weeks after the completion of treatment and is effective also when administered as a pulse regimen at a dose of 250 mg for 1 week per month every 2 or 3 months.

Itraconazole is a synthetic triazole with fungistatic activity and a broad spectrum of action. It is approved at a daily 200-mg dose. It can also be administered as pulse therapy at a dose of 400 mg daily for 1 week a month. Treatment duration is 6 weeks for fingernails and 12 weeks for toenails. The drug should be administered with a high-fat meal and/or an acidic beverage to improve its absorption. It is now not widely prescribed due to safety profile and drug interactions. A meta-analysis of six studies on pulse itraconazole for onychomycosis showed a mycologic cure rate of 63%.

Fluconazole is a bis-triazole, broad-spectrum, fungistatic drug with high oral bioavailability that is widely utilized but not approved for this indication. It is administered as a pulse treatment, with regimens ranging from 150 to 450 mg once a week for 6 (fingernails) to 9 (toenails) months. A meta-analysis of three studies on fluconazole for onychomycosis showed a mycologic cure rate of 48%.

Posaconazole is a new azole that has been evaluated in onychomycosis, and its use is likely to be limited to second-line treatment in terbinafine-refractory infections, those with nondermatophyte mold infections, or those sensitive to or intolerant of terbinafine. It showed a mycologic cure rate of 48%.

Topical treatment can be an option in cases of mild-to-moderate onychomycosis not involving the lunula region and white superficial onychomycosis. Two new topical antifungals, efinaconazole 10% nail solution and tavaborole 5% nail solution, have recently been approved by the Food and Drug Administration (FDA) for treatment of mild-to-moderate onychomycosis of the toenails. Efinaconazole 10% solution is a topical triazole antifungal solution with a broad spectrum of activity. It should be applied daily, and results from clinical studies indicate that 25% of patients achieve complete or almost complete cure, defined as ≤5% affected target nail area and mycologic cure after for 48 weeks of treatment. Tavaborole is a novel, broad-spectrum, oxaborole antifungal agent with strong antifungal activity against *T. rubrum* and *T. mentagrophytes*. It should be applied daily, and results from clinical studies show that 16.6% of patients achieve almost complete cure, defined as ≤5% affected target nail area and mycologic cure after 48 weeks of therapy

Other topical antifungals include *amorolfine* 5% nail lacquer (not approved in the United States) and *ciclopirox olamine* 8% nail lacquer. Amorolfine is applied once a week, whereas ciclopirox olamine is applied daily. The clinical efficacy of monotherapy with nail lacquers is low.

Topical antifungals combined with oral treatment may increase cure rates. Numerous new topical formulations are currently being evaluated.

A new systemic antifungal, VT-1161, a potent and selective inhibitor of fungal CYP51, showed promising results in a phase IIb clinical trial.

Surgical or chemical debridement of the thickened nail plate increases cure rate.

Photodynamic therapy after application of a solution of ALA methyl ester in aqueous cream on the nails has recently been reported to be effective in *T. rubrum* onychomycosis. Several laser devices have been marketed to treat onychomycosis, including Nd:YAG lasers and diode lasers. Evidence-based data on efficacy of these different lasers are still poor.

Poor prognostic factors of onychomycosis include areas of nail involvement >50%, involvement of the lateral portion of the nail, subungual hyperkeratosis thicker than 2 mm, white/yellow or orange/brown streaks in the nail (including dermatophytoma), diffuse nail involvement that includes the matrix, and immunosuppression.

Recurrence (relapse or reinfection) of onychomycosis is not uncommon, with reported rates ranging from 10% to 53%.

Specific Investigations

- Nail clipping microscopy
- Nail clipping culture
- Direct microscopy of 40% KOH preparations of subungual scales
- Cultures of nail scrapings in Sabouraud-agar-chloramphenicol and Sabouraud-agar-chloramphenicol + actidione media
- Histopathology of PAS-stained nail clippings
- Dermatophyte test strip
- Polymerase chain reaction (PCR)

The diagnosis of onychomycosis always requires laboratory confirmation, as differential diagnosis from psoriasis or traumatic onychodystrophy is often impossible on a clinical basis.

Fungal elements in the affected nails can be detected using KOH preparations of the nail samples or histopathology of PAS-stained nail clippings. An immunochromatography test, the Dermatophyte Test Strip, can also be used. It detects dermatophytes by visualizing mycotic antigens. PCR assays have high sensitivity, provide fast results, and are now not very expensive. They might, however, be too sensitive and produce false-positive results.

Cost-effectiveness of diagnostic tests for toenail onychomycosis: a repeated-measure, single-blinded, cross-sectional evaluation of 7 diagnostic tests. Lilly KK, Koshnick RL, Grill JP,

Khalil ZM, Nelson DB, Warshaw EM. J Am Acad Dermatol 2006; 55: 620–6.

This study compared the cost effectiveness of diagnostic tests for onychomycosis. KOH and PAS were equally sensitive. Identification of the responsible fungus can, however, only be done using cultures. A negative mycologic result does not rule out onychomycosis, as direct microscopy is negative in up to 10% of cases and culture in up to 30%.

Correct sampling of nail debris is mandatory for obtaining reliable mycologic results. In the most common variety of onychomycosis, DSO, culture sensitivity improves the more proximal the location of the sample.

Optimising the diagnostic strategy for onychomycosis from sample collection to fungal identification: evaluation of a diagnostic kit for real-time PCR. Petinataud D, Berger S, Ferdynus C, Debourgogne A, Contet-Audonneau N, Machouart M. Mycoses 2016; 59: 304–11.

This study evaluates a commercial real-time PCR kit on 180 nail samples, showing that the kit has high specificity and sensitivity in detecting dermatophytes, regardless of sample quality.

Clinical study of Dermatophyte Test Strip, an immunochromatographic method, to detect tinea unguium dermatophytes. Tsunemi Y, Hiruma M. J Dermatol 2016; 43: 1417–23.

The Dermatophyte Test Strip allows easy and fast detection of dermatophytes by visualizing mycotic antigens by immunochromatography. This test only identifies dermatophyte infections and in this study was positive in 90.5% of specimens.

A new classification system for grading the severity of onychomycosis: Onychomycosis Severity Index. Carney C, Tosti A, Daniel R, Scher R, Rich P, DeCoster J, et al. Arch Dermatol 2011; 147: 1277–82.

The Onychomycosis Severity Index (OSI) has recently been proposed to grade the severity of DSO. The OSI score is obtained by multiplying the score for the area of involvement (range, 0–5) by the score for the proximity of disease to the matrix (range, 1–5). Ten points are added for the presence of a longitudinal streaking or a patch (dermatophytoma) or for a subungual hyperkeratosis greater than 2 mm. Mild onychomycosis corresponds to a score of 1 to 5; moderate, 6 to 15; and severe, 16 to 35.

First-Line Therapy

- Systemic terbinafine 250 mg/day (for 6 weeks for fingernails and 12 weeks for toenails)

Onychomycosis: diagnosis and definition of cure. Scher RK, Tavakkol A, Sigurgeirsson B, Hay RJ, Joseph WS, Tosti A, et al. J Am Acad Dermatol 2007; 56: 939–44.

This article promotes guidelines for the correct management of onychomycosis, including criteria for diagnosis of dermatophyte onychomycosis, list of poor prognostic factors, criteria for assessing cure, and risk of relapses.

Oral therapy for onychomycosis: an evidence-based review. de Sá DC, Lamas AP, Tosti A. Am J Clin Dermatol 2014; 15: 17–36.

Evidence Levels: A Double-blind study B Clinical trial ≥ 20 subjects C Clinical trial < 20 subjects D Series ≥ 5 subjects E Anecdotal case reports

Terbinafine 250 mg daily is the most effective oral treatment of onychomycosis.

Cost-effectiveness of confirmatory testing before treatment of onychomycosis. Mikailov A, Cohen J, Joyce C, Mostaghimi A. JAMA Dermatol 2016; 152: 276–81.

Reevaluating the need for laboratory testing in the treatment of onychomycosis. Safety and cost-effectiveness considerations. Kanzler MH. JAMA Dermatol 2016; 152: 263–4.

Liver injury from terbinafine treatment is extremely rare (1 case per 50,000–120,000 treatments), and evaluating liver enzymes before starting treatment is not cost effective.

This article also discusses that confirming diagnosis is not cost effective in the case of terbinafine, as this medication is now very inexpensive.

Second-Line Therapies

- Systemic itraconazole — A
- Systemic fluconazole — A
- Systemic posaconazole — A
- Systemic itraconazole 200 mg/day or 400 mg/day for 1 week a month (for 2 months for fingernails and 3 months for toenails). A novel 200-mg formulation of itraconazole was recently introduced in the market.
- Systemic fluconazole 300 to 450 mg/week (for 6 months for fingernails and 9 months for toenails)
- Systemic posaconazole

Evidence-based optimal fluconazole dosing regimen for onychomycosis treatment. Gupta AK, Drummond-Main C, Paquet M. J Dermatolog Treat 2013; 24: 75–80.

Duration of treatment is more important than weekly fluconazole doses for cure of toenail, and possibly fingernail, onychomycosis.

The safety of oral antifungal treatments for superficial dermatophytosis and onychomycosis: a meta-analysis. Chang CH, Young-Xu Y, Kurth T, Orav JE, Chan AK. Am J Med 2007; 120: 791–8.

Treatment discontinuation due to adverse events was 3.44% for continuous terbinafine, 2.58% for pulse itraconazole, and 5.76% for intermittent fluconazole 300 to 450 mg/week. The risk of asymptomatic elevation of serum transaminase not requiring treatment discontinuation was less than 2.0% for all treatment regimens evaluated.

Third-Line Therapy

- Photodynamic therapy (PDT)

Usefulness of photodynamic therapy in the management of onychomycosis. Robres P, Aspiroz C, Rezusta A, Gilaberte Y. Actas Dermosifiliogr 2015; 106: 795–805.

According to their own experience and review of previous studies, the authors propose a protocol of three PDT sessions, separated by an interval of 1 or 2 weeks, using methyl aminolevulinate

16% and red light. Treatment should be preceded by nail plate avulsion using 40% urea. Clinical trials are needed to optimize PDT protocols and to identify those patients who will benefit most from this treatment.

Laser therapies for onychomycosis—critical evaluation of methods and effectiveness. Franczik W, Fritz K, Salavastru C. J Eur Acad Dermatol Venereol 2016; 30: 936–42.

The authors review the available studies on lasers in onychomycosis. The majority of studies used an Nd:YAG laser device. Methodology was not homogeneous, and data are not evidence based. Efficacy is still not determined.

Topical Therapies

- Topical amorolfine — A
- Topical ciclopirox olamine — A
- Topical efinaconazole — A
- Topical tavaborole — A

Two new topical antifungals, efinaconazole 10% nail solution and tavaborole 5% nail solution, have been recently approved by the FDA for treatment of mild-to-moderate onychomycosis of the toenails. They should be applied daily on the affected nail, periungual tissues, and hyponychium. The area of infection is in fact also reached through the subungual space. Old topical antifungals include the transungual delivery systems *amorolfine* 5% nail lacquer (not approved in the United States) and *ciclopirox olamine* 8% nail lacquer. Amorolfine is applied once a week, whereas ciclopirox olamine is applied daily.

Treatment duration is long and clinical efficacy moderate to low.

There are no data on association of new topical antifungals with oral treatment. Some data show that the association of *amorolfine* with oral terbinafine may increase cure rates. Several other new topical formulations are currently undergoing clinical trials.

Efinaconazole 10% solution in the treatment of toenail onychomycosis: two phase III multicenter, randomized, double-blind studies. Elewski BE, Rich P, Pollak R, Pariser DM, Watanabe S, Senda H, et al. J Am Acad Dermatol 2013; 68: 600–8; Erratum in: J Am Acad Dermatol 2014; 70: 399.

Efficacy of efinaconazole 10% solution was evaluated in two 52-week, prospective, multicenter, randomized, double-blind studies in patients 18 years and older (18–70 years of age) with mild-to-moderate DLSO, without dermatophytoma or lunula (matrix) involvement. These studies enrolled 1655 subjects, who were treated for 48 weeks, with a 4-week follow-up.

Pooled data from the two studies show that at the end of study, 54.4% of subjects treated with efinaconazole 10% solution obtained mycologic cure compared with 16.9% with vehicle, and 16.5% achieved clinical cure compared with 4.4% with vehicle.

A complete or almost complete cure, defined as ≤5% affected target nail area and mycologic cure, was achieved in 25% of patients on efinaconazole and 7.2% of patients on vehicle.

Treatment success, defined as affected target toenail area of ≤10%, was obtained in 42.6% of patients treated with efinaconazole 10% solution compared with 16.1% with vehicle.

Efficacy and safety of tavaborole topical solution, 5%, a novel boron-based antifungal agent, for the treatment of toenail onychomycosis: results from 2 randomized phase-III studies. Elewski BE, Aly R, Baldwin SL, González Soto RF, Rich P, Weisfeld M, et al. J Am Acad Dermatol 2015; 73: 62–9.

Efficacy of tavaborole 5% solution was evaluated in two 52-week prospective, multicenter, randomized, double-blind studies in patients 18 years and older (18–70 years of age) with mild-to-moderate DLSO (20%–60% nail involvement), without dermatophytoma or lunula (matrix) involvement. These studies enrolled 1198 subjects, who were treated for 48 weeks, with a 4-week follow-up.

Pooled data from the two studies show that at the end of study, 33.5% of subjects treated with tavaborole 5% solution obtained mycologic cure compared with 9.7% with vehicle, and 7.8% achieved clinical cure compared with 1% with vehicle.

A complete or almost complete cure, defined as ≤5% affected target nail area and mycologic cure, was achieved in 16.6% of patients on tavaborole and 2.7% of patients on vehicle.

A multicenter, randomized, controlled study of the efficacy, safety and cost-effectiveness of a combination therapy with amorolfine nail lacquer and oral terbinafine compared with oral terbinafine alone for the treatment of onychomycosis with matrix involvement. Baran R, Sigurgeirsson B, de Berker D, Kaufmann R, Lecha M, Faergemann J, et al. Br J Dermatol 2007; 157: 149–57.

Two hundred and forty-nine patients were randomized to receive either a combination of amorolfine hydrochloride 5% nail lacquer once weekly for 12 months plus terbinafine 250 mg once daily for 3 months, or terbinafine alone once daily for 3 months. A significantly higher success rate was observed for patients in the combination group relative to those in the terbinafine monotherapy group at 18 months (59.2% vs. 45.0%).

Evidence Levels: **A** Double-blind study **B** Clinical trial ≥ 20 subjects **C** Clinical trial < 20 subjects **D** Series ≥ 5 subjects **E** Anecdotal case reports

Tinea versicolor (pityriasis versicolor)

Aditya K. Gupta, Elizabeth A. Cooper, Kelly A. Foley

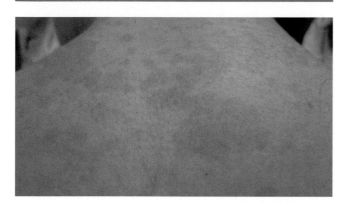

Pityriasis (tinea) versicolor (PV) has a worldwide distribution, though the prevalence is higher in tropical climates than in temperate ones (30%–40% vs. 1%–4%, respectively). PV is caused by the lipophilic yeast species *Malassezia*. *Malassezia* organisms are a normal part of human commensal skin flora, and PV results when they are converted from the yeast phase to a mycelial phase, which is able to infect the stratum corneum, producing the characteristic hypopigmented or hyperpigmented lesions.

Infection is associated with sebaceous gland activity; hence infection is most often seen in adults and postpubescent adolescents and rarely in prepubescent children. An equal prevalence between the sexes has been noted. Predisposing factors include high temperature and humidity, malnutrition, the use of oral contraceptives, hyperhidrosis, genetic susceptibility, increased plasma cortisol levels, and immunodeficiency.

Initially only two species under the genus name *Pityrosporum* were described. Genetic research in the 1990s confirmed at least seven species of *Malassezia*, and more have since been discovered. The most common species contributing to PV lesions are *M. globosa* (50%–60%), *M. sympodialis* (3%–59%), *M. furfur*, and *M. slooffiae* (each 1%–10%). It is not currently known whether the clinical pattern of infection or antifungal susceptibility vary between the different infecting species.

MANAGEMENT STRATEGY

Topical treatment is the first-line therapy in most cases. *Topical azoles* formulated as gels, creams, solutions, or shampoos (ketoconazole, fluconazole, bifonazole, clotrimazole, miconazole, etc.) have demonstrated efficacy for PV. The allylamine *terbinafine* has several topical formulations (solution, cream, gel, or spray) that have been used effectively, as have formulations of the benzylamine *butenafine*. *Topical ciclopirox* provides both antifungal and antiinflammatory activity against *Malassezia*.

Systemic antifungal therapies may be warranted in severe cases or cases with widespread body involvement, patients with recurrent disease, or those who are immunocompromised. Patients may also prefer a short-duration oral therapy to frequent application of a topical agent.

Second-line therapy for cases refractory to topical therapy may be treated with oral antifungals. *Itraconazole, fluconazole,* and *ketoconazole* show high efficacy in the literature; however, it is now recommended by the U.S. Food and Drug Administration (FDA) and Health Canada that oral ketoconazole not be used for superficial fungal infections when less hepatotoxic alternatives are available.[1,2] In contrast to topical terbinafine, oral terbinafine is not effective; nor is griseofulvin.

Treatment does not vary with hyperpigmented versus hypopigmented disease. Although fungal organisms may be eradicated after 2 to 4 weeks of therapy, it may take significantly longer before the skin's normal pigmentation is restored, particularly with hypopigmented lesions.

Relapse of PV is common due to endogenous host factors: recurrence rates have been reported as high as 60% to 90% 2 years after treatment. Both ketoconazole (a single 400-mg dose or 200 mg daily for 3 days once monthly) and itraconazole (a single 400-mg dose once monthly for 6 months) have been used in prophylactic regimens for PV, though ketoconazole is not recommended because of its potential for hepatotoxicity.

Specific Investigations

- Direct microscopy on KOH specimens
- Wood light

Malassezia organisms should be identified by skin scrapings for definitive diagnosis and are easily identified, where microscopic examination of skin scrapings reveals fungal hyphae in a typical "spaghetti and meatball" pattern. PV lesions fluoresce yellow/green or gold under Wood light; however, the examination is positive in only one third of all PV cases, most likely when the causative organism is *M. furfur*.

First-Line Therapies

Topical antifungal agents

Ketoconazole	A
Bifonazole	A
Terbinafine	A
Clotrimazole	A
Econazole	A
Oxiconazole	A
Butenafine	A
Ciclopirox	A
Fluconazole shampoo	A
Selenium sulfide 2.5%	B
Tioconazole	B
Zinc pyrithione shampoo	B

Pityriasis versicolor: a review of pharmacological treatment options. Gupta AK, Kogan N, Batra R. Exp Opin Pharmacother 2005; 6: 165–78.

This is a thorough summary of peer-reviewed studies of topical and oral therapies in the treatment of tinea versicolor until 2005. Azole topical agents have shown good mycologic cure, clinical cure, and complete cure in many double-blind, randomized clinical trials, as have the nonspecific topical agents (zinc pyrithione shampoo, selenium sulfide, etc.) and terbinafine.

Terbinafine 1% cream and ketoconazole 2% cream in the treatment of pityriasis versicolor: a randomized comparative clinical trial. Rad F, Nik-Khoo B, Yaghmaee R, Gharibi F. Pak J Med Sci 2014; 30: 1273–6.

A randomized, single-blind trial with terbinafine 1% cream or ketoconazole 2% cream applied twice daily for 2 weeks. Cure rates (negative KOH microscopy with clinical cure) at 2 weeks (terbinafine: 72.1%; ketoconazole: 64.3%) and 8 weeks (terbinafine: 70.8%; ketoconazole: 61.9%) were not significantly different between treatments.

Can pityriasis versicolor be treated with 2% ketoconazole foam? Cantrell WC, Elewski BE. J Drugs Dermatol 2014; 13: 855–9.

Eleven patients in this pilot study applied ketoconazole 2% foam twice daily for 2 weeks. Clinical improvement was observed over 4 weeks, and seven patients showed negative KOH microscopy.

A randomized controlled trial of combination treatment with ketoconazole 2% cream and adapalene 0.1% gel in pityriasis versicolor. Shi T-W, Zhang J-A, Tang Y-B, Yu H-X, Li Z-G, Yu J-B. J Dermatol Treat 2015; 26: 143–6.

A double-blind trial comparing combination once-daily ketoconazole cream and adapalene gel with twice-daily ketoconazole cream for 2 weeks. Total improvement rate (clinical improvement with negative microscopy) at 4 weeks was 92% in the combination group and 72% in the ketoconazole group ($p = 0.009$).

Second-Line Therapies

Oral antifungal agents

• Itraconazole	A
• Fluconazole	A

Oral prophylaxis

• Itraconazole	A

Systematic review of systemic treatments for tinea versicolor and evidence-based dosing regimen recommendations. Gupta AK, Lane D, Paquet M. J Cutan Med Surg 2014; 18: 79–90.

This is an extensive evidence-based review of clinical trials published up to mid-2013 that reported mycologic cure for PV. The literature supports regimens for itraconazole (200 mg/day for 5 or 7 days) and fluconazole (150 or 300 mg weekly for 2 or 4 weeks).

Efficacy of itraconazole in the prophylactic treatment of pityriasis (tinea) versicolor. Faergemann J, Gupta AK, Al Mofadi A, Abanami A, Shareaah AA, Marynissen G. Arch Dermatol 2002; 138: 69–73.

Patients achieving mycologic cure after open treatment with itraconazole 200 mg once daily for 7 days entered a double-blind, placebo-controlled trial of itraconazole prophylaxis (itraconazole or placebo: 200 mg twice daily 1 day per month for 6 consecutive months). At the end of prophylaxis, 88% of itraconazole patients remained mycologically negative, compared with only 57% of placebo-treated patients ($p < 0.001$).

Single-dose oral fluconazole versus topical clotrimazole in patients with pityriasis versicolor: a double-blind randomized controlled trial. Dehghan M, Akbari N, Alborzi N, Sadani S, Keshtkar AA. J Dermatol 2010; 37: 699–702.

Patients were randomized to receive a single 400-mg dose of oral fluconazole with placebo cream or a placebo capsule with 1% clotrimazole cream, each applied twice daily for 2 weeks. At 12 weeks, 92% of the fluconazole group achieved complete cure, whereas 81.8% of the clotrimazole group achieved complete cure ($p = 0.77$).

Third-Line Therapies

• Pramiconazole (oral triazole)	A
• Adapalene	A
• Naftifine (topical allylamine)	B
• Dapaconazole tosylate (topical imidazole)	B
• *Cymbopogon citratus* (DC) *Stapf* essential oil	B
• Isotretinoin	E

A double-blind, randomized, placebo-controlled, dose-finding study of oral pramiconazole in the treatment of pityriasis versicolor. Faergemann J, Todd G, Pather S, Vawda ZFA, Gillies JD, Walford T, et al. J Am Acad Dermatol 2009; 61: 971–6.

Participants were randomized into six pramiconazole treatment groups: (1) 100 mg taken once; (2) 200 mg taken once; (3) 200 mg taken once daily for 2 days; (4) 200 mg taken once daily for 3 days; (5) 400 mg taken once; (6) placebo taken once daily for 3 days. The primary efficacy outcome was effective treatment (negative KOH microscopy and resolution or minimal residual of clinical signs for participants with severe baseline scores). At day 28, the highest proportion of participants with an effective cure received 200 mg daily for 2 days, 84.0% (95% confidence interval [CI], 69.6–98.4) and 200 mg daily for 3 days, 84.6% (95% CI, 70.7–98.5).

Pramiconazole is not currently approved or marketed. As more data accumulate, the level of evidence may alter.

Role of adapalene in the treatment of pityriasis versicolor. Shi T, Ren X, Yu H, Tang Y. Dermatol 2012; 224: 184–8.

A prospective, randomized, double-blind clinical trial compared adapalene cream and 2% ketoconazole cream applied to the torso twice daily for 2 weeks. No significant difference between treatments was found at 4 weeks. Participants experienced 75% and 70% mycologic cure in the adapalene and ketoconazole groups, respectively.

Adapalene is not an antifungal drug; results are based on alterations in the skin's properties.

An open-label study of naftifine hydrochloride 1% gel in the treatment of tinea versicolor. Gold MH, Bridges T, Avakian E, Plaum S, Pappert EJ, Fleischer AB, et al. Skinmed 2011; 9: 283–6.

Participants received 1% naftifine gel twice daily for 2 weeks. At 6 weeks posttreatment, 50% of the participants had achieved a mycologic cure.

A randomized double-blind, non-inferiority phase II trial, comparing dapaconazole tosylate 2% cream with ketoconazole 2% cream in the treatment of pityriasis versicolor. Gobbato AA, Babadopulos T, Gobbato CA, Ilha Jde O, Gagliano-Juca T, De Nucci G. Expert Opin Investig Drugs 2015; 24: 1399–407.

Treatment once daily for 28 days with dapaconazole tosylate 2% cream was noninferior to ketoconazole 2% cream for clinical and mycologic cure.

Evidence Levels: **A** Double-blind study **B** Clinical trial ≥ 20 subjects **C** Clinical trial < 20 subjects **D** Series ≥ 5 subjects **E** Anecdotal case reports

Treatment of pityriasis versicolor with topical application of essential oil of *Cymbopogon citratus* (DC) *Stapf*—therapeutic pilot study. Carmo ES, de Oliveira Pereira F, Cavalcante NM, Gayoso CW, de Oliveira Lima E. An Bras Dermatol 2013; 88: 381–5.

A phase I and phase II study of essential oil formulations compared with ketoconazole cream. Improvement was seen in both groups, with significantly more patients achieving mycologic cure in the ketoconazole cream group ($p < 0.05$).

Tinea versicolor clearance with oral isotretinoin therapy. Bartell H, Ransdell BL, Ali A. J Drugs Dermatol 2006; 5: 74–5.

This is a single case report of a 14-year-old boy presenting with acne vulgaris recalcitrant to oral antibiotic therapy, who also presented with PV infection on the upper back and shoulders. One month after starting oral isotretinoin 40 mg twice daily, the PV lesions had completely resolved. Resolution was attributed to the sebum-altering properties of isotretinoin.

The use of isotretinoin cannot be advocated because of the potential for serious side effects, particularly in females. In cases of concomitant PV and acne, no additional medication may be required for the PV infection.

References

1. Health Canada. Ketoconazole - Risk of Potentially Fatal Liver Toxicity - For Health Professionals. [Internet]. 2013. Available from: http://healthycanadians.gc.ca/recall-alert-rappel-avis/hc-sc/2013/34173a-eng.php.
2. The U.S. Food and Drug Administration (FDA). FDA Drug Safety Communication: FDA limits usage of Nizoral (ketoconazole) oral tablets due to potentially fatal liver injury and risk of drug interactions and adrenal gland problems [Internet]. Available from: http://www.fda.gov/Drugs/DrugSafety/ucm362415.htm.

Toxic epidermal necrolysis and Stevens–Johnson syndrome

Nicholas M. Craven, Daniel Creamer

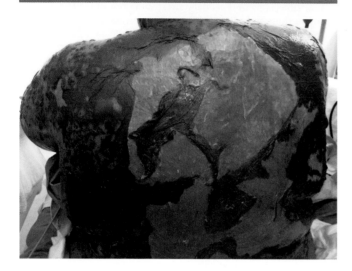

Toxic epidermal necrolysis (TEN) and Stevens–Johnson syndrome (SJS) form a spectrum of rare, potentially life-threatening conditions manifesting widespread erythematous macules or atypical target lesions and severe erosions of mucous membranes. The epithelial changes are caused by extensive apoptosis, a process initiated by drug-induced cytotoxic T lymphocytes. A number of proapoptotic molecules, including TNF-α and IFN-γ, link drug-induced immune responses to keratinocyte damage. Ultimately, keratinocyte death is caused by directly acting apoptosis mediators, with the major trigger being granulysin. Confluence of cutaneous lesions leads to epidermal loss, which by definition involves less than 10% of total body surface area in SJS, 10% to 30% in overlap cases, and more than 30% in TEN. Complications develop similarly to those seen after burns. In the majority of cases, SJS and TEN (SJS/TEN) can be attributed to a drug reaction.

MANAGEMENT STRATEGY

The causative drug should be identified and discontinued. In general, drugs introduced in the 4 weeks before the onset of symptoms are usually responsible. The most common drugs causing SJS/TEN are allopurinol, carbamazepine, lamotrigine, nevirapine, oxicam nonsteroidal antiinflammatory drugs (NSAIDs), phenobarbital, phenytoin, sulfasalazine, sulfamethoxazole, and other sulfur antibiotics.

Extensive epidermal loss in SJS/TEN is accompanied by numerous systemic sequelae, many of which are life threatening. Therefore the patient should be managed in a specialist intensive care unit or burn unit for the delivery of critical care management and specialist nursing. Supportive therapy is directed at fluid replacement, maintaining a warm environment, nutritional support, analgesia, organ support (when necessary), surveillance for infection, and appropriate dressings. *Fluid replacement* requirements depend on the extent of involvement of the skin and may be 5 to 7 L in the first 24 hours. *The ambient temperature* should be raised to 25°C. *Nutritional support* may require nasogastric tube feeding until the oral mucosa has healed. *Analgesia* with opiates is often necessary. *Infection surveillance* includes taking skin swabs from lesional skin throughout the acute phase and sending these for bacteriology. Administration of prophylactic antibiotics is not recommended, as this increases skin colonization (particularly with *Candida albicans*) and promotes resistance. All lines should be checked daily for signs of infection, changed at least every 3 days, and the tips of all discarded lines and catheters sent for culture. If signs of sepsis develop (rising or falling temperature, rigors, hypotension, fall in urine output, or deterioration of respiratory status, diabetic control, or level of consciousness), initial antibiotic therapy can be guided by the results of swabs taken from the skin and mucous membranes. Blisters should be decompressed by piercing and expression of tissue fluid. Blister roofs and detached epidermis can be left in situ to act as a biologic dressing. Folded, necrosed epidermis should be removed gently.

Ophthalmologic review should be obtained as soon as possible after diagnosis to minimize the risk of conjunctival scarring and blindness. Regular instillation of an ocular lubricant, topical antibiotic, and corticosteroid drops is recommended. Separation of conjunctival adhesions must be carried out by an ophthalmologist or ophthalmically trained nurse. Oral and nasal debris should be removed regularly. Antiinflammatory and antiseptic mouthwashes must be used frequently. Tracheal and bronchial involvement is an underappreciated manifestation of SJS/TEN and may be a marker of disease severity and mortality. Respiratory failure can occur, requiring ventilation.

The use of *systemic corticosteroids* in the management of TEN and SJS remains controversial (see later). Several reports suggest that the use of corticosteroids increases morbidity and mortality, usually by increasing the risk of sepsis. Conversely, a number of case reports and short studies advocate the use of high-dose corticosteroids in the early stages of the evolution of these conditions. It is therefore possible that high-dose corticosteroids may prove beneficial in aborting further epithelial loss in patients with evolving SJS/TEN, but this has not yet been tested in a randomized controlled trial. Nevertheless, it is generally accepted that continuing administration of corticosteroids is counterproductive once extensive skin loss has occurred.

Several other potential disease-modifying treatments (*intravenous immunoglobulin* [IVIG], *cyclosporin, pentoxifylline, plasmapheresis, anti-TNF agents*) have been reported in small numbers of patients, but there is currently no strong evidence base for recommending any specific intervention other than supportive care.

Survivors of SJS/TEN should avoid exposure to the culprit drug and related compounds.

Specific Investigations

- Histology of a skin biopsy
- Hematologic and biochemical monitoring, including glucose and bicarbonate
- Chest x-ray

Established TEN can usually be diagnosed clinically. Biopsy and immunofluorescence of an affected area of skin can exclude conditions such as staphylococcal scalded skin syndrome and paraneoplastic pemphigus.

Evidence Levels: **A** Double-blind study **B** Clinical trial ≥ 20 subjects **C** Clinical trial < 20 subjects **D** Series ≥ 5 subjects **E** Anecdotal case reports

Stevens–Johnson syndrome and toxic epidermal necrolysis: assessment of medication risks with emphasis on recently marketed drugs. The EuroSCAR study. Mockenhaupt M, Viboud C, Dunant A, Naldi L, Halevy S, Bouwes Bavinck JN, et al. J Invest Dermatol 2008; 128: 35–44.

The results of a multinational case-control study of risk for developing SJS and TEN from various drugs, showing a strong association for nevirapine and lamotrigine; a weaker association for sertraline, pantoprazole, and tramadol; and confirming a strong association for previously recognized culprit drugs: sulfonamide antibiotics, allopurinol, carbamazepine, phenobarbital, phenytoin, and oxicam NSAIDs.

SCORTEN: a severity-of-illness score for toxic epidermal necrolysis. Bastuji-Garin S, Fouchard N, Bertocchi M, Roujeau JC, Revuz J, Wolkenstein P. J Invest Dermatol 2000; 115: 149–53.

Assessment of seven clinical parameters within the first 24 hours of admission (age over 40 years; history of malignancy; tachycardia >120 bpm; skin loss >10%; urea >10 mmol/L; glucose >14 mmol/L; bicarbonate <20 mmol/L) can be used to predict risk of mortality (score 0 or 1: 3% risk of death; 2: 12%; 3: 35%; 4: 58%; 5+: 90%).

Comprehensive survival analysis of a cohort of patients with Stevens-Johnson syndrome and toxic epidermal necrolysis. Sekula P, Dunant A, Mockenhaupt M, Naldi L, Bouwes Bavinck JN, Halevy S, et al. for the RegiSCAR study group. J Invest Dermatol 2013; 133: 1197–204.

All-cause mortality rates at 6 weeks in this cohort of 460 patients (recruited between 2003 and 2007) were 12%, 29%, and 46% for SJS, SJS/TEN overlap, and TEN, respectively.

First-Line Therapies	
• Supportive measures	E
• Withdrawal of culprit drug	E
• Transfer to a specialist unit	E

UK guidelines for the management of Stevens-Johnson syndrome/toxic epidermal necrolysis in adults 2016. Creamer D, Walsh SA, Dziewulski P, Exton LS, Lee HY, Dart JK, et al. Br J Dermatol 2016; 174: 1194–227.

This guideline is a review of all aspects of SJS/TEN management in adults, concentrating on the details of supportive care. Recommendations for practical use are highlighted.

Toxic epidermal necrolysis and Stevens–Johnson syndrome: does early withdrawal of causative drugs decrease the risk of death? Garcia-Doval I, LeCleach L, Bocquet H, Otero XL, Roujeau JC. Arch Dermatol 2000; 136: 323–7.

Early discontinuation of the causative drug improved prognosis in this study of 113 patients.

ALDEN, an algorithm for assessment of drug causality in Stevens–Johnson syndrome and toxic epidermal necrolysis: comparison with case-control analysis. Sassolas B, Haddad C, Mockenhaupt M, Dunant A, Liss Y, Bork K, et al. Clin Pharmacol Ther 2010; 88: 60–8.

Seventy percent to 80% of cases of SJS, TEN, and SJS/TEN overlap are attributable to drugs. This paper describes a validated algorithm for assessing the likelihood of causality of drugs in such cases.

A multicenter review of toxic epidermal necrolysis treated in U.S. burn centers at the end of the twentieth century. Palmieri TL, Greenhalgh DG, Saffle JR, Spence RJ, Peck MD, Jeng JC, et al. J Burn Care Rehab 2002; 23: 87–96.

A retrospective multicenter study of 199 patients admitted with TEN to 15 burn centers from 1995 to 2000. Overall mortality was 32%, increasing to 51% for patients transferred to a burn center more than 1 week after the onset of TEN.

There are several studies (but no controlled trials) showing benefit from early transfer of TEN patients to specialist units.

Second-Line Therapies	
• Ciclosporin	B
• Systemic corticosteroids	B
• Intravenous immunoglobulin	B

Open trial of cyclosporin treatment for Stevens–Johnson syndrome and toxic epidermal necrolysis. Valeyrie-Allanore L, Wolkenstein P, Brochard L, Ortonne N, Maître B, Revuz J, et al. Br J Dermatol 2010; 163: 847–53.

Twenty-nine patients with SJS ($n = 10$), SJS/TEN overlap ($n = 12$), and TEN ($n = 7$) were treated with cyclosporin via a nasogastric catheter at a dose of 3 mg/kg for 10 days, then 2 mg/kg for 10 days, and finally 1 mg/kg for 10 days. Treatment was tolerated well in most patients, and although the prognostic score predicted 2.75 deaths, none occurred. In addition, the progression of detachment of epidermis seemed lower than expected.

Retrospective review of Stevens-Johnson syndrome/toxic epidermal necrolysis treatment comparing intravenous immunoglobulin with cyclosporine. Kirchhof MG, Miliszewski MA, Sikora S, Papp A, Dutz JP. J Am Acad Dermatol 2014; 71: 941–7.

Single-center retrospective study of 64 patients with SJS/TEN. Predicted mortality based on SCORTEN was compared with actual mortality for patients treated with either cyclosporin (3–5 mg/kg/day for up to 7 days) or IVIG (2–5 g/kg total dose). The results showed an apparently improved mortality with ciclosporin over that predicted by SCORTEN (standardized mortality ratio [SMR] 0.43) compared with an apparently increased mortality with IVIG (SMR 1.43). Although aware of the limitations of the study, the authors concluded that the results suggested a possible benefit from using ciclosporin in the treatment of TEN and SJS.

Treatment of toxic epidermal necrolysis with cyclosporin A. Arévalo JM, Lorente JA, González-Herrada C, Jiménez-Reyes J. J Trauma 2000; 48: 473–8.

An improved outcome was reported in 11 consecutive patients with TEN treated with cyclosporin 3 mg/kg daily, compared with six historical controls treated with cyclophosphamide and corticosteroids. Both groups were of comparable age, with similar extent of skin loss and delay between onset of TEN and admission. Patients treated with cyclosporin had more rapid reepithelialization, were less likely to suffer multiorgan failure, and had a lower mortality (0 of 11 vs. 3 of 6).

There are now several reports of the successful use of cyclosporin in SJS/TEN. Because most of the hazards of this drug are associated with long-term use, it seems logical to use this drug in SJS/TEN, as treatment will only be needed for a few days.

Effects of treatments on the mortality of Stevens–Johnson syndrome and toxic epidermal necrolysis: a retrospective study on patients included in the prospective EuroSCAR study. Schneck J, Fagot JP, Sekula P, Sassolas B, Roujeau JC, Mockenhaupt M. J Am Acad Dermatol 2008; 58: 33–40.

A large, multicenter, retrospective study of treatment of 281 patients with TEN enrolled in EuroSCAR (a case-control study of risk factors for severe cutaneous adverse reactions) showed no significant effect on mortality with the administration of IVIG, but a trend for beneficial effect of corticosteroids was considered worthy of further exploration.

Corticosteroids in Stevens-Johnson Syndrome/toxic epidermal necrolysis: current evidence and implications for future research. Law EH, Leung M. Ann Pharmacother 2015; 49: 335–42.

Six studies that used steroids for SJS, TEN, and/or overlap were included in this review. All were retrospective cohort studies with no case-control or cross-sectional studies. Only one reported a statistically significant mortality benefit with steroid use (odds ratio = 0.4; 95% confidence interval [CI] = 0.2–0.9). None of the studies reported adverse event rates. The authors concluded that there is a need for prospective, randomized controlled trials to provide more definitive evidence supporting steroid use in patients with SJS, TEN, and/or overlap.

Systematic review of treatments for Stevens-Johnson syndrome and toxic epidermal necrolysis using the SCORTEN score as a tool for evaluating mortality. Roujeau JC, Bastuji-Garin S. Ther Adv Drug Saf 2011; 2: 87–94.

A pooled analysis of published series addressing treatment efficacy by comparing the mortality observed to the mortality predicted by the SCORTEN score. The analyzed series comprised a total of 439 patients. Supportive care was used only in 199 patients with a pooled mortality ratio (MR) of 0.89 (CI, 0.67–1.16; $p = 0.43$), corticosteroids were administered to 78 patients with a pooled MR of 0.92 (CI, 0.53–1.48; $p = 0.84$), and IVIG in 162 with a pooled MR of 0.82 (CI 0.58–1.12, $p = 0.23$). In conclusion, even though this analysis had some limitations, it strongly suggested that neither corticosteroids nor IVIG provide any important improvement in mortality over that predicted by SCORTEN in SJS and TEN.

The efficacy of intravenous immunoglobulin for the treatment of toxic epidermal necrolysis: a systematic review and meta-analysis. Huang YC, Li YC, Chen TJ BJ. Dermatol 2012; 167: 424–32.

A meta-analysis evidence-based examination of IVIG efficacy in TEN compared the clinical differences between (1) high-dose (≥2g/kg) and low-dose (<2g/kg) IVIG treatment in adult patients and (2) pediatric and adult patients treated with IVIG.

Although high-dose IVIG exhibited a trend toward improved mortality and children treated with IVIG had a good prognosis, the authors concluded that the evidence overall did not support a clinical benefit of IVIG and stated that randomized controlled trials are necessary.

The role of intravenous immunoglobulin in toxic epidermal necrolysis: a retrospective analysis of 64 patients managed in a specialized center. Lee HY, Lim YL, Thirumoorthy T, Pang SM. Br J Dermatol 2013; 169: 1304–9.

This single-center study of use of IVIG in the management of 64 patients with SJS/TEN overlap and TEN demonstrated no survival benefit even when corrected for IVIG dosages.

Intravenous immunoglobulin in the treatment of Stevens-Johnson syndrome and toxic epidermal necrolysis: a meta-analysis with metaregression of observational studies. Barron SJ, Del Vecchio MT, Aronoff SC. Int J Dermatol 2015; 54: 108–15.

Thirteen studies met the inclusion criteria for this meta-analysis, eight of which included a control group. Although there was no significant overall benefit of using IVIG in SJS or TEN (overall standardized MR 0.814, 95% CI 0.617–1.076), the metaregression found a strong inverse correlation between IVIG dosage and mortality, and the authors concluded that IVIG at dosages of ≥2 g/kg appears to significantly decrease mortality in patients with SJS or TEN.

A systematic review of treatment of drug-induced Stevens-Johnson syndrome and toxic epidermal necrolysis in children. Del Pozzo-Magana BR, Lazo-Langner A, Carleton B, Castro-Pastrana LI, Rieder MJ. J Popul Ther Clin Pharmacol 2011; 18: e121–33.

The four main treatment modalities in the included studies were IVIG, steroids (prednisolone, methylprednisolone, dexamethasone), dressings with or without surgical debridement, and supportive treatment alone. A number of miscellaneous treatments were reported: of 12 patients, 3 received ulinastatin, 4 received plasmapheresis, 2 received IV pentoxifylline, and the last 3 patients received a different treatment each (cyclosporine, methylprednisone/G-CSF, and methylprednisolone/IVIG). Steroids and IVIG seem to improve the outcome of SJS and TEN in pediatric patients, but results from different reports are variable. Patients treated only with care support seem to have higher morbidity and mortality. The authors conclude that further studies are necessary to define optimal management of TEN and SJS in children.

As with all data on treatment of SJS/TEN, interpretation of the available literature is limited by lack of uniformity in the treatment regimens used, by the lack of adequate control data, and/or by the relatively small size of the studies. Systematic reviews and meta-analyses are helpful in this respect, but mainly serve to confirm the lack of strong evidence of benefit for any intervention other than best supportive care delivered in a suitable setting.

Third-Line Therapies

• Plasmapheresis	C
• Pentoxifylline	E
• Anti-TNF therapy	E

Plasmapheresis as an adjunct treatment in toxic epidermal necrolysis. Egan CA, Grant WJ, Morris SE, Saffle JR, Zone JJ. J Am Acad Dermatol 1999; 40: 458–61.

A retrospective study of 16 patients, 6 of whom were selected for plasmapheresis (one to four treatments) based on rapid progression of disease in the 24 hours after admission. None of the patients treated with plasmapheresis died, whereas 4 of the other 10 patients did die.

Lack of significant treatment effect of plasma exchange in the treatment of drug-induced toxic epidermal necrolysis? Furubacke A, Berlin G, Anderson C, Sjoberg F. Intens Care Med 1999; 25: 1307–10.

The outcomes in eight patients with SJS/TEN who received one to eight plasma exchange treatments was compared with

Evidence Levels: **A** Double-blind study **B** Clinical trial ≥ 20 subjects **C** Clinical trial < 20 subjects **D** Series ≥ 5 subjects **E** Anecdotal case reports

outcomes in patients from two other centers that used almost identical treatment protocols but without plasma exchange. The results showed no benefit in terms of mortality (12.5%), time to reepithelialization, or duration of stay in the burn intensive care unit. The authors concluded that the results did not support the use of plasma exchange in the treatment of SJS/TEN.

Pentoxifylline in toxic epidermal necrolysis and Stevens–Johnson syndrome. Sanclemente G, De La Roche CA, Escobar CE, Falabella R. Int J Dermatol 1999; 38: 878–9.

Two children with SJS and SJS/TEN overlap were treated with intravenous pentoxifylline 12 mg/kg daily. In both cases skin loss stopped on commencement of treatment; in one child the skin deteriorated when pentoxifylline was temporarily discontinued.

Toxic epidermal necrolysis successfully treated with infliximab. Zárate-Correa LC, Carrillo-Gómez DC, Ramírez-Escobar AF, Serrano-Reyes C. J Investig Allergol Clin Immunol 2013; 23: 61–3.

This report describes the use of infliximab (single infusion of 300 mg) in four patients with TEN. The infusions were given between 2 and 8 days after onset of symptoms due to progression of skin loss. All four patients recovered, although three developed bacteremia, which responded to antibiotic therapy.

Etanercept therapy for toxic epidermal necrolysis. Paradisi A, Abeni D, Bergamo F, Ricci F, Didona D, Didona B. J Am Acad Dermatol 2014; 71: 278–83.

Ten patients with SJS/TEN were treated with a single dose of etanercept. There was no control group. None of the patients died, despite a mean predicted mortality rate of 50%.

Randomised comparison of thalidomide versus placebo in toxic epidermal necrolysis. Wolkenstein P, Latarjet J, Roujeau J-C, Duguet C, Boudeau S, Vaillant L, et al. Lancet 1998; 352: 1586–9.

Patients with TEN were randomized to either a 5-day course of thalidomide 400 mg daily (12 patients) or placebo (10 patients). The study was stopped early because of excess mortality in the treatment arm.

Transient acantholytic dermatosis (Grover disease)

Murtaza Khan, John Berth-Jones

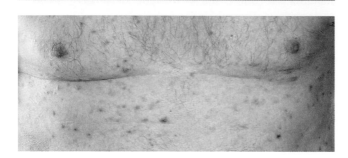

Grover disease is an uncommon disorder characterized clinically by discrete erythematous, edematous papulovesicles or keratotic papules, which are usually pruritic, and histologically focal acantholytic dyskeratosis. It can be self-limiting or chronic. It is more common in middle-aged and elderly people, especially men, and involves mainly the trunk. The evolution is acute or chronic, lasting weeks to months, and it may be persistent or recurrent. The etiology is unknown, but excessive UV exposure, heat, sweating, and ionizing radiation are linked to the disease. Drugs, chemotherapeutic agents, dialysis, and cancers are also reported triggers. Other skin disorders such as psoriasis or eczema of various types may coexist.

MANAGEMENT STRATEGY

Histology is helpful, but immunofluorescence does not aid in diagnosis.

Treatment is difficult, and the evidence base is anecdotal. Patients should be advised to avoid excessive sun exposure, strenuous exercise, heat, and occlusive fabrics. In mild cases, simple antipruritic measures such as avoidance of soap, simple emollients, and soothing baths with bath oils or colloidal oatmeal may be of benefit. Wet compresses with zinc oxide, calamine, or topical corticosteroids may help relieve the itching.

Topical calcipotriol (ointment) twice daily 50 µg/g may be helpful after 3 to 4 weeks of treatment.

Systemic therapy may be indicated in more extensive and persistent disease. *Oral vitamin A* has been recommended in the past. The aromatic retinoid *acitretin* has been used successfully in doses of 0.5 mg/kg daily. *Isotretinoin* 40 mg daily has been used for periods ranging from 2 to 12 weeks. It may be administered on a reducing regimen if the initial response is rapid, with a maintenance dose of 10 mg daily.

Systemic corticosteroids have been used to suppress inflammation and pruritus, but relapses frequently occur on drug withdrawal.

Psoralen with UVA (PUVA) may be useful, but an initial exacerbation may occur. There are reports of the success of narrowband UVB and of medium-dose UVA1 phototherapy.

Topical 5-fluorouracil, dapsone, antibiotics, and cryotherapy are ineffective. Recently rituximab and etanercept have been reported to be useful.

Specific Investigation

- Skin biopsy

First-Line Therapies

• Emollients	D
• Avoid heat/sweating	D
• Topical corticosteroids	D

Transient acantholytic dermatosis. Heenan PJ, Quirk CJ. Br J Dermatol 1980; 102: 515–20.

This study looked at a series of 24 cases of transient acantholytic dermatosis. Most of them required topical fluorinated corticosteroids to control the pruritus, and two required intermittent courses of oral corticosteroids.

Incidence of transient acantholytic dermatosis (Grover's disease) in a hospital setting. French LE, Piletta PA, Etienne A, Salomon D, Saurat JH. Dermatology 1999; 198: 410–1.

A prospective study of 28 hospital inpatients diagnosed with Grover disease. In over 80% of cases the duration of hospitalization exceeded 2 weeks and was associated with strict bed rest. The authors suggested a sweat-related pathogenesis.

Second-Line Therapies

• Calcipotriol	E
• Tacalcitol	E
• Systemic corticosteroids	D
• Vitamin A	D

Treatment of Grover's disease with calcipotriol (Dovonex). Keohane SG, Cork MJ. Br J Dermatol 1995; 132: 832–3.

A 50-year-old man had a 13-month history of Grover disease that responded poorly to oxytetracycline, topical corticosteroids, dapsone, and etretinate. Lesions cleared after hospitalization and prednisone 100 mg daily, but he relapsed with any reduction in dose. Oral corticosteroids were stopped, and he was commenced on an alternating regimen of calcipotriol ointment at night and 0.025% betamethasone valerate ointment (we presume in the morning). There was complete clearance of lesions after 1 month of treatment, but the disease relapsed when treatment was stopped.

Successful treatment of Grover's disease with calcipotriol. Mota AV, Correia TM, Lopes JM, Guimaraes JM. Eur J Dermatol 1998; 8: 33–5.

An 84-year-old man with a 2-year history of Grover disease improved significantly, despite initial moderate irritation, after a 3-week course of calcipotriol 50 µg/g twice daily. Lesions did not recur during a 6-month follow-up.

Treatment of Grover's disease with tacalcitol. Hayashi H. Clin Exp Dermatol 2002; 27: 160–1.

Evidence Levels: **A** Double-blind study **B** Clinical trial ≥ 20 subjects **C** Clinical trial < 20 subjects **D** Series ≥ 5 subjects **E** Anecdotal case reports

A 31-year-old man with a 2-month history of Grover disease who failed to respond to topical corticosteroid was commenced on tacalcitol ointment twice daily. He improved dramatically within 1 week and was in remission after 1 month.

Treatment of transient acantholytic dermatosis. Rohr JR, Quirk CJ. Arch Dermatol 1979; 115: 1033–4.

Eight patients were treated with vitamin A 50,000 units three times a day for up to 2 weeks; all patients responded. Once initial improvement was noted the dose was reduced to 50,000 units daily as maintenance or for several weeks. No signs of toxicity were noted. One patient required reinstitution of the drug due to recurrence on cessation of treatment.

Third-Line Therapies

• Systemic retinoids (acitretin/etretinate/isotretinoin)	E
• PUVA	E
• UVA1	E
• Photodynamic therapy	E
• Trichloroacetic acid	E
• Etanercept	E
• Rituximab	E

Persistent acantholytic dermatosis. Dodd HJ, Sarkany I. Clin Exp Dermatol 1984; 9: 431–4.

A case report of a 41-year-old man with a 5-year history of an itchy truncal and lower limb rash consistent with persistent acantholytic dermatosis. Bath emollients and aqueous cream British pharmacopoeia afforded minor relief. Etretinate (50 mg daily) cleared the skin lesions and reduced the itching.

Etretinate has been replaced by its active metabolite acitretin. Lower doses of the latter may be effective.

Grover's disease treated with isotretinoin. Helfman RJ, Gables C. J Am Acad Dermatol 1985; 12: 981–4.

Four patients with biopsy-proven Grover disease responded to 40 mg daily of isotretinoin for 2 to 4 months. In two patients most lesions had cleared after 3 to 4 weeks of treatment. Their dose was reduced by 10 mg daily for a further 8 weeks. One patient required 40 mg daily for 8 weeks. These patients remained in remission for up to 10 months after treatment. The final patient obtained partial relief and then discontinued treatment because of elevated triglycerides.

Response of transient acantholytic dermatosis to photochemotherapy. Paul BS, Arndt KA. Arch Dermatol 1984; 120: 121–2.

A 59-year-old man with persistent Grover disease was unresponsive to oral prednisone and vitamin A (300,000 units daily). PUVA was initiated with 50 mg (0.6 mg/kg) methoxsalen and 2 J/cm^2 of UVA. Treatment was twice weekly, and the UVA dosage was increased by 0.5 J/cm^2 with each treatment. The patient experienced a flare after four treatments, but improved by week 6, with maximal improvement by week 8. Therapy was then tapered off over the next 4 weeks, with complete clearing. No recurrence had occurred 25 months after therapy.

Reports show that approximately 10 treatments are required for resolution of pruritus, and 20 to 30 treatments may be needed to clear the eruption.

Medium-dose ultraviolet A1 phototherapy in transient acantholytic dermatosis (Grover's disease). Breuckmann F, Appelhans C, Altmeyer P, Kreuter A. J Am Acad Dermatol 2005; 52: 169–70.

A 78-year-old man with persistent Grover disease had failed to respond to topical and oral corticosteroids. He was treated with a medium-dose UVA1 cold light monophototherapy containing a special filtering and cooling system (21°C). Irradiation (50 J/cm^2, 1.9 J/cm^2/minute; 26 minutes), six times weekly for 3 weeks, then three times weekly for 3 weeks. A total of 24 treatments was given with a cumulative dose of 1200 J/cm^2. Complete remission was achieved after 4 weeks, with no subsequent relapse.

Successful novel treatment of recalcitrant transient acantholytic dermatosis (Grover disease) using red light 5-aminolevulinic acid photodynamic therapy. Liu S, Letada PR. Dermatol Surg 2013; 39: 960–1.

This appeared helpful in one case.

Effective treatment of persistent Grover's disease with trichloroacetic acid peeling. Kouba DJ, Dasgeb B, Deng AC, Gaspari AA. Dermatol Surg 2006; 32: 1083–8.

A 46-year-old woman had a 6-month history of progressive Grover disease with intractable pruritus. She failed to respond to topical calcipotriene (Dovonex). She was treated with an even, light application of 40% (w/v) trichloroacetic acid (TCA)—single-pass strokes with TCA-dampened gauze. Individual lesions of Grover disease were identified and were re-treated with 40% TCA using a cotton-tipped applicator. Three weeks postprocedure she had reepithelialized, was disease free, and was still in remission 8 months later.

The authors stress that practitioners not accustomed to using TCA in office applications should use low-strength formulations such as 20% to 30% to avoid scarring.

Use of etanercept in treating pruritus and preventing new lesions in Grover disease. Norman R, Chau V. J Am Acad Dermatol 2011; 64: 796–8.

A 55-year-old man had a 2-year history of Grover disease that did not respond to topical or oral steroids and antihistamines. Isotretinoin given for 2 months resulted in improvement of his pruritus but was discontinued after he had a myocardial infarction. He was prescribed etanercept 50 mg subcutaneously twice weekly for 6 weeks, which reduced the pruritus by 98%. Over the next 4 months he had very mild symptoms and did not develop any new lesions.

Remission of transient acantholytic dermatosis after the treatment with rituximab for follicular lymphoma. Ishibashi M, Nagasaka T, Chen KR. Clin Exp Dermatol 2008; 33: 206–7.

An 80-year-old woman developed Grover disease simultaneously with a relapse of follicular lymphoma. Six years before this episode her lymphoma had been treated with rituximab. She was given rituximab again, and her skin lesions cleared within a week. The lymphoma improved initially, but after nine cycles of treatment she suffered another relapse. Her skin lesions did not recur.

Trichotillomania

Mio Nakamura, John Koo

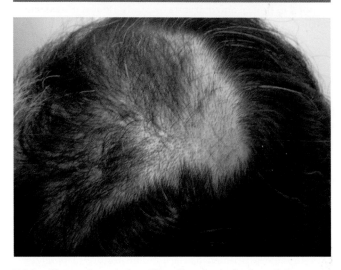

Trichotillomania, or hair-pulling disorder, is the impulsive, repetitive action of pulling out hair, resulting in significant hair loss. Any region of the body with hair can be involved, with the eyebrows, eyelashes, and scalp comprising the most common sites. The reported prevalence of trichotillomania is approximately 0.6% in the general population. It is predominantly observed in females, with an early age of onset averaging between 11 and 13 years.

The *Diagnostic and Statistical Manual of Mental Disorders*, 5th edition (DSM-V), categorizes trichotillomania under "obsessive-compulsive disorder," which is a change from the previous editions of DSM, which categorized trichotillomania under "impulse disorders." Obsessive-compulsive disorders include intrusive thoughts or urges that are experienced as unwanted (obsession), often necessitating repetitive behaviors or rituals to help alleviate the otherwise intolerable anxiety (compulsion). The following are the DSM-V diagnostic criteria for trichotillomania:

A. Recurrent pulling out of one's hair resulting in noticeable hair loss.
B. An increasing sense of tension immediately before pulling out the hair or when attempting to resist the behavior.
C. Pleasure, gratification, or relief when pulling out the hair.
D. The disturbance is not better accounted for by another mental disorder and is not due to general medical conditions.
E. The disturbance causes clinically significant distress or impairment in social, occupational, or other important areas of functioning.

Patients with trichotillomania often admit to hair pulling; however, some patients are unwilling or ashamed to acknowledge the self-inflicted nature of their skin findings, whereas others are not conscious of their hair pulling. Some patients practice specific rituals after hair pulling including rolling the hair between the fingers, running the hair over the lips or through the teeth, and biting the hair. In rare cases, the patient may also eat the hair root (trichorhizophagia) as a secretive activity, and in even rarer cases the whole hair is eaten (trichophagia). It is possible to develop gastrointestinal hairballs (trichobezoars), which have a high morbidity and can be fatal. Children with trichotillomania who present with episodes of obscure abdominal pain, weight loss, nausea, vomiting, anorexia, and foul breath should be investigated for gastric trichobezoars.

Many patients with trichotillomania have underlying psychiatric disease. It is estimated that up to 80% of patients with trichotillomania have comorbid psychiatric disease, most commonly anxiety and depression. Patients with trichotillomania may have other types of obsessive-compulsive disorders, specifically body-focused repetitive behavioral disorders (BFRBD), such as skin picking and nail biting. The patient may be delusional in cases such as trichophobia, in which an individual has an irrational fear of hair.

DIAGNOSIS

Patients with trichotillomania present with alopecia that is generally irregular and nonscarring. Broken, sparse hair on a background of excoriations is often observed. Hairs are broken at different lengths on the scalp. The diagnosis of trichotillomania can be made on a clinical basis with careful examination of the scalp. Dermatologic differential diagnoses that should be ruled out include alopecia areata, androgenic alopecia, alopecia mucinosa, tinea capitis, lichen planopilaris, folliculitis decalvans, and discoid lupus erythematosus. Tinea capitis may be ruled out by the absence of scaling and negative fungal culture. Laboratory investigations such as complete blood count, thyroid function tests, and iron levels may also be indicated. Dermoscopy can be useful to detect black dots (exclamation points) or broken hairs, as well as curled hairs, suggestive of trichotillomania. However, because the dermoscopy findings of trichotillomania can overlap with other causes of hair loss such as alopecia areata, a skin biopsy may be indicated in some cases. Trichotillomania presents histologically as an increased number of catagen hairs, traumatized hair bulbs in the absence of perifollicular inflammation (trichomalacia), empty follicles, follicular keratin debris, and melanin pigment casts.

MANAGEMENT STRATEGY

Trichotillomania can cause significant social isolation and psychological disability; therefore treatment of this disorder is important to restore the patient's quality of life. Treatments that have been shown to be effective for trichotillomania are largely psychological in nature and include behavioral therapy, including habit-reversal therapy, in both pediatric and adult populations. Habit-reversal training is a form of behavioral therapy that focuses on four key aspects: awareness (increase awareness of hair-pulling behavior), competing response training (perform a specific action when there is an urge to pull hair), social support or contingency management (a person who reinforces the former), and stimulus control (minimize the influence of environmental factors on pulling behavior). Habit-reversal training has been shown to decrease repetitive, self-inflicted behaviors. Children can benefit from behavioral therapy to prevent worsening of their disease into adulthood.

Effective pharmacologic treatments involve treating the underlying psychiatric disease. The first-line pharmaceutical approach depends on the nature of the involved underlying psychopathology; the underlying causes of trichotillomania such as anxiety, depression, substance abuse, and eating disorders should be treated accordingly.

Evidence Levels: **A** Double-blind study **B** Clinical trial ≥ 20 subjects **C** Clinical trial < 20 subjects **D** Series ≥ 5 subjects **E** Anecdotal case reports

Studies of pharmacologic therapy for the treatment of trichotillomania have been limited. The tricyclic antidepressant clomipramine (Anafranil), indicated for obsessive-compulsive disorder, is the most studied medication for trichotillomania, and it has been shown to reduce the frequency of hair-pulling urges. Clomipramine is started at a dose of 25 mg per day and is titrated up to 125 to 250 mg per day. Side effects include headache, orthostatic hypotension, anticholinergic effects, QT prolongation, and seizures.

High-dose selective-serotonin reuptake inhibitors (SSRIs), such as paroxetine (Paxil), fluoxetine (Prozac), or sertraline (Zoloft), can also be used to treat trichotillomania. Paxil is typically started at 20 mg daily initially and then increased by 10 mg weekly to up to 50 to 60 mg per day. Fluoxetine is started at a dose of 10 mg per day and titrated up to an effective dose, which usually ranges from 20 to 80 mg per day. The usual starting dose of sertraline is 50 mg per day, with an effective dose ranging typically from 50 to 200 mg per day. Side effects of SSRIs include gastrointestinal upset, headache, sexual dysfunction, and suicidality. Although SSRIs alone have not shown significant evidence to effectively treat trichotillomania, the combination of pharmacotherapy and habit-reversal training has been shown to be effective in decreasing the frequency of hair pulling. Atypical antipsychotics such as olanzapine (Zyprexa) and aripiprazole (Abilify) have been reported to successfully treat trichotillomania in case reports.

Specific Investigations

- Hair microscopy
- Dermoscopy
- Scalp biopsy
- Laboratory testing (complete blood count, thyroid stimulating hormone, ferritin)

Trichotillomania. Presentation, etiology, diagnosis and therapy. Walsh KH, McDougle CJ. Am J Clin Dermatol 2001; 2: 327–33.

This is a comprehensive and detailed review of trichotillomania.

First-Line Therapies

Behavioral therapy/habit-reversal therapy	A

Behavior therapy for pediatric trichotillomania: a randomized controlled trial. Franklin ME, Edson AL, Ledley DA, Cahill SP. J Am Acad Child Adolesc Psychiatry 2011; 50: 763–71.

Behavioral therapy produced superior outcomes compared to a control group in a randomized controlled trial of pediatric patients with trichotillomania.

Psychological treatments for trichotillomania. Rehm I, Moulding R, Nedelikovic M. Australas Psychiatry 2015; 23: 365–8.

Advances in the understanding of the phenomenology of trichotillomania have led to the augmentation of behavioral treatments with dialectical behavior therapy and acceptance and commitment therapy. Further studies of treatment component efficacy and cognitive behavioral models are needed.

Behavioral treatment of trichotillomania: 2-year follow-up results. Keijsers GP, van Minnen A, Hoogduin CA, Klaassen BN, Hendriks MJ, Tanis-Jacobs J. Behav Res Ther 2006; 44: 359–70.

The manual-based behavioral therapy consisted of self-control procedures offered in six sessions. The area of the patch of trichotillomania was assessed and was reduced by 49% and 70% at 3 months and 2 years. Better 2-year follow-up results were associated with lower pretreatment levels of depressive symptoms and with complete abstinence from hair pulling immediately after treatment.

Second-Line Therapies

Clomipramine	B
SSRI	B
Combination of habit-reversal therapy and pharmacotherapy	C

Pharmacotherapy of trichotillomania (hair pulling disorder): an updated systematic review. Rothbart R, Stein DJ. Expert Opin Pharmacother 2014; 15: 2709–19.

A systematic review of clinical trials of pharmacotherapeutic agents for the treatment of trichotillomania. Although limited, various clinical trials overall have shown modest benefit of pharmacotherapy such as clomipramine and SSRIs.

Single modality versus dual modality treatment for trichotillomania. Dougherty D. J Clin Psychiatry 2006; 67: 1086–92.

Habit reversal and SSRI drug therapy together was better than either alone.

Third-Line Therapy

Antipsychotics	A

Systematic review. Pharmacologic and behavioral treatment for trichotillomania. Block M, Landeros-Weisenberger A, Dombrowski P, Kelmendi B, Wegner R, Nudel J, et al. Biol Psychiatry 2007; 62: 839–46.

There are multiple case reports and case series reporting favorable responses to antipsychotics as monotherapy and augmentation agents in the literature. Controlled trials are necessary.

Tuberculosis and tuberculids

Yasaman Mansouri, John Berth-Jones

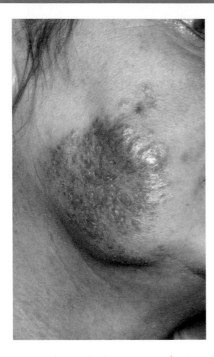

Cutaneous tuberculosis (TB) is an infection caused by *Mycobacterium tuberculosis*, and occasionally by *M. bovis* and bacillus Calmette-Guérin (BCG), an attenuated strain of *M. bovis*. The spectrum of clinical manifestations varies depending on the host's immunity, the route of infection, the infectious load, and virulence factors. Cutaneous disease can occur by direct inoculation from an exogenous source (tuberculous chancre and tuberculosis verrucosa cutis/warty TB; rarely lupus vulgaris) or from an endogenous source, via lymphatic, hematogenous, or contiguous spread and causes periorificial TB, lupus vulgaris (LV), scrofuloderma, acute miliary TB, and tuberculous gumma. Scrofuloderma is the most common variant worldwide. The tuberculids are a group of "hypersensitivity" reactions to extracutaneous sources of *M. tuberculosis* (tuberculous antigen) in individuals with high immunity. These include erythema induratum of Bazin, erythema nodosum, lichen scrofulosorum, papulonecrotic tuberculid, and nodular tuberculid.

MANAGEMENT STRATEGY

The diversity of clinical findings, the relatively rare occurrence of cutaneous disease, and the difficulty in demonstrating acid-fast bacilli (AFB) on histology specimens often lead to misdiagnosis or significant delays in correctly identifying cutaneous TB, so a high index of suspicion is required for prompt diagnosis. Initially this is based on the correlation of clinical findings with histopathologic identification of granulomatous inflammation with or without caseous necrosis on tissue

samples. The gold standard for TB diagnosis remains the identification of *M. tuberculosis* in tissue culture, but this is time consuming and often fails. Polymerase chain reaction (PCR) is being used more frequently because of its high sensitivity and specificity.

The tuberculin skin test (TST) can be false positive as a result of previous BCG vaccination or sensitization to nontuberculous mycobacteria (such as *M. avium* and *M. scrofulaceum*) and false negative in patients with reduced cellular immunity and the elderly.

Interferon-γ release assays (IGRAs) such as T-SPOT Assay TB test (T-SPOT) and QuantiFERON-TB Gold test (QTF-G) have low false-positive rates, regardless of BCG vaccination, and high specificity for identification of *M. tuberculosis* infection. These blood tests require only one patient visit and are therefore preferred over TST.

It is imperative to search for an extracutaneous focus of infection. Contact tracing is an important component of efficient TB management. HIV testing is recommended in all patients with diagnosed or suspected TB.

The aims of treatment are to rapidly cure the patient, to reduce transmission of TB to others, and to prevent the development and transmission of drug resistance. A past history of tuberculosis should be determined, as these patients are more likely to be infected with a strain of mycobacterium that is resistant to anti-tuberculosis drugs.

Treatment of cutaneous tuberculosis does not differ from conventional antituberculous therapy, and tuberculids generally resolve after treatment of the underlying infection. Regimens are based on controlled trials on pulmonary TB. The standard 6-month regimen for adults comprises rifampicin (10 mg/kg), isoniazid (INH) (5 mg/kg), pyrazinamide (35 mg/kg), and ethambutol (15 mg/kg) for the initial 2 months of intensive phase treatment, followed by rifampicin and INH for a further 4 months in the continuation phase, ideally in fixed-dose combinations. Daily dosing throughout treatment is preferred. Occasionally longer treatment regimens may be necessary (e.g., in HIV-positive cases). Multidrug-resistant tuberculosis should be managed at specialist centers.

Specific Investigations

- Skin biopsy for histopathology
- Culture of tissue or pus for *M. tuberculosis*
- Interferon-γ–based assays
- PCR for *M. tuberculosis* DNA in skin
- Screening for tuberculosis at other sites: chest x-ray, cultures of sputum, early morning urine, etc.
- TST
- HIV screen

Usefulness of interferon-γ release assays in the diagnosis of erythema induratum. Vera-Kellet C, Peters L, Elwood K, Dutz JP. Arch Dermatol 2011; 147: 949–52.

IGRAs confirmed the diagnosis in five patients and supported initiation of anti-TB treatment in four of five patients who had positive TST with a history of prior BCG vaccination.

Interferon-γ release assay and reverse blot hybridization assay: diagnostic role in cutaneous tuberculosis. Chung HC, Kim BK, Hong H, Wang HY, Kim Y, Lee H, et al. Acta Derm Venereol 2016; 96: 126–7.

Evidence Levels: A Double-blind study **B** Clinical trial ≥ 20 subjects **C** Clinical trial < 20 subjects **D** Series ≥ 5 subjects **E** Anecdotal case reports

IGRAs and the reverse blot hybridization assay (REBA) confirmed the diagnosis in seven patients, six of whom had been diagnostically challenging, with negative staining or culture from skin samples. These patients were successfully treated.

PCR based detection of mycobacteria in paraffin wax embedded material routinely processed for morphologic examination. Frevel T, Schäfer KL, Tötsch M, Böcker W, Dockhorn-Dworniczak B. Mol Pathol 1999; 52: 283–8.

PCR-based techniques are sensitive, specific, and rapid methods for the detection of mycobacteria in routinely processed, formalin-fixed, paraffin wax–embedded, histologic samples.

Papulcrotic tuberculid. Identification of *Mycobacterium tuberculosis* DNA by polymerase chain reaction. Victor T, Jordaans HF, van Niekerk DJ, Louw M, Jordaan A, Van Helden PD. Am J Dermatopathol 1992; 14: 491–5.

Mycobacterial antigens may also be detected in tuberculids using PCR.

Cutaneous tuberculosis with nonreactive PPD skin test: a diagnostic challenge. Nassif PW, Rosa AP, Gurgel AC, Campanerut PA, Fillus Neto J, Cardoso RF. An Bras Dermatol 2015; 90: 128–30.

A 63-year-old female patient with cutaneous chancre had a negative PPD despite being immunocompetent. Diagnosis was confirmed by PCR.

First-Line Therapy

- Antituberculous drugs **A**

Treatment of Tuberculosis: Guidelines for National Programmes, 4th ed. Geneva: World Health Organization, 2009. New patients with pulmonary TB should receive a regimen containing 6 months of rifampicin. The essential anti-TB drugs recommended are isoniazid (H) (5 mg/kg), rifampicin (R) (10 mg/kg), pyrazinamide (Z) (25 mg/kg), streptomycin (S) (15 mg/kg), and ethambutol (E) (15 mg/kg). The recommended regimen is 2 months of HRZE followed by 4 months of HR. The WHO recommends that daily dosing throughout the duration of therapy (2HRZE/4HR) is optimal for all newly diagnosed patients with TB.

The WHO no longer recommends omission of ethambutol during the intensive phase of treatment for patients with a low risk of resistance to INH. In tuberculous meningitis, ethambutol should be replaced by streptomycin.

Comparative efficacy of drug regimens in skin tuberculosis. Ramesh V, Misra RS, Saxena U, Mukherjee A. Clin Exp Dermatol 1991; 16: 106–9.

Three antituberculous drug regimens were employed to study the response in 90 cases. The first two regimens contained rifampicin (adults 450 mg, children 15 mg/kg), INH (adults 300 mg, children 5 mg/kg), and either pyrazinamide (adults 1500 mg, children 30 mg/kg) or thiacetazone (adults 150 mg, children 4 mg/kg); the third regimen had rifampicin and INH only. The patients with lupus vulgaris and warty tuberculosis cleared with all three regimens in 4 and 5 months for localized and generalized disease, respectively. Patients with scrofuloderma responded well to both triple-drug regimens, with the skin lesions subsiding completely within 5 months in the localized and 6 months in

the widespread forms of the disease. However, 9 to 10 months of treatment were necessary in the group receiving isoniazid and rifampicin.

Atypical cutaneous tuberculosis in a patient with rheumatoid arthritis treated with infliximab. Asano Y, Kano Y, Shiohara T. Acta Derm Venereol 2008; 88: 183–4.

A 73-year-old woman developed cellulitis-like cutaneous TB after infliximab initiation for rheumatoid arthritis. Quadruple therapy was started, and the lesion resolved after 5 months of treatment.

Plaques on a butcher's fingers. Arunachalam M, Scarfi F, Galeone M, Maio V, Bellandi S, Difonzo E. Arch Dermatol 2012; 148: 531–6.

A 63-year-old butcher presented with tuberculosis verrucosa cutis of two fingers of the left hand. This was successfully treated with rifampicin (450 mg/d) and isoniazid (300 mg/d) for 4 months.

Tuberculous granuloma: a rare cause of a non-healing ulcer. Graham GE, Jones R, Derry D. BMJ Case Rep 2014; pii: bcr2014205899.

A 78-year-old immunosuppressed woman presented cutaneous TB manifesting as a cystic swelling of the forehead. Because she was unable to swallow tablets, she received liquid rifampicin and liquid isoniazid for 9 months, which resulted in successful clearance.

Second-Line Therapies

- Excision **D**
- Calcipotriol **E**

Scrofuloderma of the lower extremity treated with wide resection: a case report and review of the literature. Connolly B, Pitcher JD Jr, Roth B, Youngberg RA, Devine J. Am J Orthop 1999; 28: 417–20.

A report of an immunocompromised patient presenting with scrofuloderma of the lower extremity. This failed to resolve with the standard antituberculous regimen consisting of four drugs: INH, rifampicin, pyrazinamide, and ethambutol for 2 months, followed by INH and rifampicin for 3 months, but was then successfully treated with wide resection under spinal anesthesia.

Lupus vulgaris of the ear lobe. Okazaki M, Sakurai A. Ann Plast Surg 1997; 39: 643–6.

A 59-year-old woman with an initial diagnosis of hemangioma had surgical treatment followed by antituberculous therapy (INH, rifampicin, and pyridoxine for 9 months) for lupus vulgaris of the earlobe.

Lupus vulgaris responding to calcipotriol. Moriarty B, Kennedy C, Bourke JF, Fitzgibbon J. J Am Acad Dermatol 2009; 60: AB106.

A 73-year-old male with plaque form lupus vulgaris of the buttock developed drug-induced hepatitis and fulminant hepatic failure due to antituberculous medication. A 6-month trial of topical calcipotriol 50 µg/g ointment then led to resolution of the lesion without recurrence.

Urticaria and angioedema

Marcus Maurer, Torsten Zuberbier

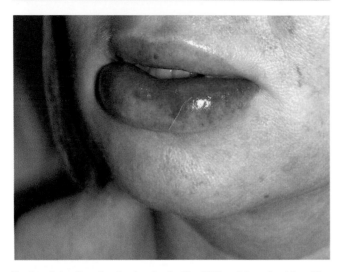

Treatment algorithms for chronic urticaria. The 2013 update and revision of the EAACI/GA²LEN/EDF/WAO guideline for urticaria (1) recommends following a three-step algorithm for the treatment of patients with chronic urticaria *(panel a)*. During the guideline consensus conference URTICARIA2016 on December 1, 2016, in Berlin, an update and revision of this guideline was proposed, discussed and consented *(panel b)*. This takes new data on safety and efficacy into consideration and that licensed products should be preferred. The algorithm shown in panel b is pending final approval by the urticaria guideline expert panel members and the endorsing societies.

Urticaria is a frequent disease affecting up to 20% of us at least once during our lifetimes. The hallmark feature of urticaria is the wheal, which is caused by mast cell–derived mediators such as histamine that produce transient increases in the vasopermeability of cutaneous blood vessels resulting in a short-lived, superficial skin swelling. In addition to these wheals (sometimes called *hives*), many urticaria patients develop deep swellings of the dermis and subcutis, known as *angioedema*. Some urticaria patients exclusively experience angioedema, and they never have wheals. Wheals and angioedema are not pathognomonic for urticaria, that is, patients with other diseases may experience whealing or angioedema. For example, angioedema without wheals can be mediated by bradykinin independently of mast cell degranulation and histamine, and wheals also occur in patients with urticarial vasculitis or autoinflammatory syndromes, which are mediated by interleukin-1 rather than mast cell–derived histamine or bradykinin.

URTICARIA

INTRODUCTION

The signs and symptoms of urticaria are brought about by the degranulation of cutaneous mast cells. Skin mast cells are preferentially localized in the vicinity of sensory nerves and small blood vessels. Their activation by certain signals, such as IgE crosslinking, can lead to their degranulation and the release of de novo synthesized and preformed mediators (e.g., histamine). These mediators induce sensory nerve stimulation (itch, burning pain); vasodilatation (flare); edema (wheal, angioedema); and the recruitment of immune cells such as neutrophils, eosinophils, and basophils.

Clinically, urticaria is characterized by the rapid development of wheals, angioedema, or both. Wheals are associated with itching or burning as well as a flare reaction. They resolve spontaneously, usually within a few hours. In contrast, angioedemas are deeper, pronounced, and sometimes painful swellings of the lower dermis and subcutis and can also affect the mucous membranes. They are of longer duration and slower resolution than are wheals and can last for several hours to a few days.

Urticaria is either acute (less than 6 weeks' duration) or chronic. Urticaria patients develop wheals and/or angioedema spontaneously (spontaneous urticaria) or in response to a specific trigger (inducible urticaria). The specific triggers of whealing and angioedema formation in chronic inducible urticaria can be physical, for example, contact with cold or heat (cold urticaria, heat urticaria), irradiation with UV light or visible light (solar urticaria), friction (symptomatic dermographism), pressure (pressure urticaria), or vibration (vibratory angioedema). In contrast to these so-called *physical forms* of inducible urticaria, the development of signs and symptoms in the other types of inducible urticaria is triggered by skin contact with urticariogenic substances, including water (contact urticaria, aquagenic urticaria), or by active or passive overheating (cholinergic urticaria).

In chronic spontaneous urticaria, wheals occur most often at the legs and arms, whereas angioedema is most commonly localized in the face (e.g., the lips and eyes). In contrast, chronic inducible urticaria is characterized by whealing and/or angioedema formation at the skin sites that are exposed to the eliciting trigger. Disease activity and control in chronic spontaneous urticaria are assessed by the use of the urticaria activity score (UAS7), which relies on patient documentation of daily wheal numbers and itch intensity, and the urticaria control test (UCT), respectively. The UCT is a validated and reliable four-item retrospective tool to assess disease control in patients with chronic urticaria (spontaneous and inducible). Disease activity in inducible urticarias is measured by assessing trigger thresholds via provocation testing.

Important differential diagnoses of urticaria are severe allergic reactions (e.g., anaphylactic shock), where wheals and/or angioedema co-occur with systemic manifestations, urticarial vasculitis, autoinflammatory syndromes, and bradykinin-mediated angioedema (e.g., hereditary or acquired C1 inhibitor deficiency).

MANAGEMENT STRATEGY

The aim of the treatment of patients with urticaria is the elimination of signs and symptoms. This may be achieved by treating an underlying cause or condition, by avoiding eliciting triggers, by preventing mast cell degranulation, or by blocking the effects of histamine or other mast cell mediators. For the inducible urticarias, causes are largely unknown, and their triggers of wheal and/or angioedema development may be difficult or impossible for patients to avoid. All urticarias are self-limited, and very effective and safe symptomatic treatment options are available. The prevention of recurring urticaria signs and symptoms by medication that protects patients from the effects of relevant mast cell degranulating signals or of the mediators released by mast cells is, therefore, the most common approach for the management of urticaria.

Evidence Levels: **A** Double-blind study **B** Clinical trial ≥ 20 subjects **C** Clinical trial < 20 subjects **D** Series ≥ 5 subjects **E** Anecdotal case reports

Acute urticaria

Acute urticaria in most patients can be managed with oral second-generation H_1 antihistamines (sgAHs). Add-on oral glucocorticosteroids may be used for a few days for severe cases, and they can reduce disease activity and duration when given at the onset of the disease. sgAHs used in the treatment of chronic urticaria include the following:

Second-generation antihistamine	Daily standard dose
Bilastine	20 mg
Cetirizine	10 mg
Desloratadine	5 mg
Fexofenadine	180 mg
Levocetirizine	5 mg
Loratadine	10 mg
Mizolastine	10 mg
Rupatadine	10 mg

Chronic spontaneous urticaria

By taking a good history and asking the patient to keep a diary, it is often possible to identify exacerbating factors that increase disease activity, for example, stress or the intake of nonsteroidal antiinflammatory drugs. Avoiding these triggers can help to reduce disease activity. Other nonpharmacologic interventions include the avoidance of foods that contain pseudoallergens by keeping a specific diet for 3 weeks.

Current guidelines recommend a step-up approach for the pharmacologic treatment of patients with chronic spontaneous urticaria, with standard-dosed and up-to-fourfold-dosed sgAHs followed by add-on omalizumab or ciclosporin in treatment-resistant patients. Based on the available evidence and experience, these treatment options work in most patients and should be explored before moving to other therapies.

The signs and symptoms of chronic spontaneous urticaria are largely driven by mediators released from activated skin mast cells. The most prominent one is histamine, which exerts its action via H_1 receptors on cutaneous blood vessels and nerves. The first-line pharmacologic approach for the treatment of all patients with chronic spontaneous urticaria is, therefore, the use of sgAHs at licensed doses. All sgAHs are inverse agonists that promote the inactivate state of the H_1 receptor and prevent its binding of histamine. sgAHs should, therefore, be taken regularly (i.e., every day) to prevent histamine-mediated extravasation and to protect from the development of skin lesions rather than as on-demand medication after skin lesions have already developed. sgAHs are highly selective for the H_1 receptor and are minimally or nonsedating because of their low penetration of the blood–brain barrier, an important difference to first-generation antihistamines. The use of standard-dosed sgAHs as first-line therapy of chronic spontaneous urticaria is supported by a large body of high-quality evidence for their efficacy and safety from numerous randomized controlled trials. Current guidelines recommend not using first-generation AHs routinely in the management of chronic spontaneous urticaria, as they can have anticholinergic effects, cause sedation, impair the quality of sleep, affect cognitive and psychomotor functions, and exhibit interactions with other drugs.

In patients with chronic spontaneous urticaria who continue to show signs and symptoms after 2 weeks of standard-dosed sgAH treatment, updosing of the sgAH to up to fourfold the licensed dose should be considered. This second-line therapy, with one sgAH at a higher-than-standard dose, is preferable to combining different H_1 antihistamines at the same time in the same patient. The recommendation to updose sgAHs in treatment-resistant patients is based on several randomized controlled trials (RCTs), numerous real-life surveys, and long-standing and broad experience, all of which support the notion that updosed sgAHs show higher efficacy in chronic spontaneous urticaria compared with standard-dose sgAH treatment. In general, higher-than-standard doses of sgAHs are held to be safe and well tolerated, even with long-term use. Most modern sgAHs have been described to also have antiinflammatory effects, often only at high doses. However, individual sgAHs exhibit differences in the strength of the evidence in support of their safety and efficacy when used at higher-than-standard doses. Thus responses to treatment both in terms of disease control and sedation or other possible side effects need to be monitored continuously.

Most patients with chronic spontaneous urticaria benefit from sgAH treatment, but many do not show complete control. In patients who exhibit continued recurrence of urticaria signs and symptoms after a few weeks of high-dose sgAH therapy, add-on treatment with omalizumab should be considered. The long-term use of systemic glucocorticosteroids is to be avoided, but a short course may be tried to control acute exacerbation. Omalizumab is a humanized antibody against IgE licensed for the treatment of asthma and chronic spontaneous urticaria. Recently a meta-analysis of its use in seven RCTs found omalizumab to be very safe and effective in patients with chronic spontaneous urticaria who were treatment resistant to H_1 antihistamine treatment in licensed doses or up to four times the licensed dose (Zhao et al., 2016). The first RCT performed in chronic spontaneous urticaria used the omalizumab dosing regimen established for severe asthma, but subsequent trials revealed that urticaria symptoms and quality of life improved significantly with a standard dose of 150 mg or 300 mg/4 weeks omalizumab, independent of body weight or IgE serum levels. The largest decrease of disease activity and the highest number of patients with complete response were found in the 300-mg group. Similar to antihistamines, omalizumab is a symptomatic rather than a curative treatment, and the adaptation of dosing and treatment intervals to fluctuations in disease activity should be considered, based on continued monitoring of disease control and impact on patients.

The treatment of patients with chronic spontaneous urticaria with omalizumab during the past years confirms the good risk/benefit profile of this therapy seen in clinical trials. It also indicates that the onset of action of omalizumab in most patients is fast, often within a few days after the first administration, but that up to five treatments may be needed for some patients to respond. Most omalizumab-treated patients with chronic spontaneous urticaria are able to stop all concomitant therapies and remain free of symptoms with omalizumab alone. Omalizumab appears to also be effective in chronic spontaneous urticaria patients with both wheals and angioedema, as well as in those suffering from isolated angioedema.

The use of ciclosporin as in a back-up treatment option in treatment-resistant patients is supported by the long-standing experience and evidence that this drug is effective in up to two thirds of patients. Ciclosporin is usually given over 3 to 4 months at a starting dose of 4 mg/kg/day with a fast onset of action, usually within a week, in most patients. When working with ciclosporin, its known side effects, including hypertension, hypertrichosis, increase of creatinine levels up to renal failure, and dyslipidemia, need to be considered and checked for in treated patients. Patients treated with ciclosporin should be examined and monitored before and during treatment.

Many other treatments have been used in chronic spontaneous urticaria, but either their effects have not been studied in controlled settings or the strength of the evidence in support of their use is low. Treatments that may be used in chronic spontaneous urticaria patients who are treatment resistant to sgAHs, omalizumab, and/ or ciclosporin include, but are not limited to, autologous whole blood or serum therapy, azathioprine, cyclophosphamide, colchicine, dapsone, H_2 antagonists, intravenous immunoglobulins, leukotriene antagonists, methotrexate, and mycophenolate mofetil.

Chronic inducible urticaria

The treatment approaches and medications used for chronic inducible urticarias are, by and large, similar to those for chronic spontaneous urticaria. Patients can benefit from knowing what triggers their urticaria and knowing their individual trigger threshold, as this can help them to avoid situations associated with disease exacerbation. For many forms of chronic inducible urticaria, however, it is very difficult or impossible for patients to completely avoid any exposure to the eliciting trigger, for example, mechanical irritation of the skin in symptomatic dermographism. Because of this, pharmacologic treatment is very important and needed for most patients with chronic inducible urticaria. sgAHs are the first-line treatment of choice, and doses should be increased up to fourfold in patients who do not respond. All sgAHs are licensed for use in chronic inducible urticarias. Moreover, based on clinical experience and some studies, they are effective and safe in all forms of chronic inducible urticaria. However, for most forms of chronic inducible urticaria, no controlled studies have been performed with standard-dosed and/or higher-than-standard doses of sgAHs. Several case series and reports indicate that omalizumab is effective and safe for the treatment of patients with inducible forms of chronic urticaria, but it is not licensed for this. Treatment suggestions that are specific for individual forms or groups of chronic inducible urticaria are, in general, backed only by weak evidence or no evidence (Magerl et al., 2016). For example, in some forms of chronic inducible urticaria such as cold urticaria, solar urticaria, and cholinergic urticaria, tolerance can be induced by desensitization protocols using repeated exposure to the relevant trigger with gradually increasing strength. However, this tolerance is transient, patients usually require daily maintenance exposure, and severe side effects have been described.

Specific Investigations

Acute urticaria
- None

Chronic spontaneous urticaria
- Exclude differential diagnoses
- Check for systemic inflammation (C-reactive protein [CRP], erythrocyte sedimentation rate [ESR], differential blood count)
- Assess disease activity and control, for example, by use of the urticaria activity score (UAS7) and the urticaria control test (UCT), respectively
- In patients with uncontrolled or long-standing disease, consider underlying causes based on history and physical examination
- Consideration of histamine release assays (when available) in cases of suspected autoimmunity

Chronic inducible urticaria
- Exclude differential diagnoses
- Confirm relevance of trigger(s) by provocation testing
- Determine disease activity by assessing trigger threshold and use of the UCT

The EAACI/GA²LEN/EDF/WAO Guideline for the definition, classification, diagnosis and management of urticaria. The 2013 revision and update. Zuberbier T, Aberer W, Asero R, Bindslev-Jensen C, Brzoza Z, Canonica GW, et al. Allergy 2014; 69: 868–87.

The definition, diagnostic testing and management of chronic inducible urticarias – update and revision of the EAACI/GA²LEN/EDF/UNEV 2016 consensus panel recommendations. Magerl M, Altrichter S, Borzova E, Giménez-Arnau A, Grattan CEH, Lawlor F, et al. Allergy 2016; 71: 780–802.

First-Line Therapy
- Second-generation H_1 antihistamines   **A**

Second-Line Therapy
- Up to fourfold standard dose second-generation H_1 antihistamines   **A**

Third-Line Therapy
- Omalizumab   **A**

Omalizumab for the treatment of chronic spontaneous urticaria: a meta-analysis of randomized clinical trials. Zhao Z, Ji C, Yu W, Meng L, Hawro T, Wei JF, et al. J Allergy Clin Immunol 2016; 137: 1742–50.

This meta-analysis of seven RCTs with omalizumab in CSU demonstrates that this treatment is safe and effective and that 300 mg of omalizumab every 4 weeks is the preferred dose.

Fourth-Line Therapy
- Ciclosporin   **A**

Cyclosporine in chronic idiopathic urticaria: a double blind, randomized, placebo-controlled trial. Vena GA, Cassano N, Colombo D, Peruzzi E, Pigatto P; NEO-I-30 Study Group. J Am Acad Dermatol 2006; 55: 705–9.

Ninety-nine patients with severe chronic urticaria were treated with ciclosporin for 16 weeks or for 8 weeks followed by 8 weeks placebo, or placebo for 16 weeks. Ciclosporin was started at a dose of 5 mg/kg and reduced in two steps to 3 mg/kg by day 28. Symptom scores improved significantly in both ciclosporin groups.

ANGIOEDEMA

INTRODUCTION

In contrast to mast cell–mediated angioedema, which is a frequent feature and sign of chronic urticaria, non-mast cell–mediated angioedema is a group of diseases. These include hereditary angioedema (HAE) with or without C1 inhibitor (C1INH) deficiency, acquired C1INH deficiency, and drug-induced angioedema such as angiotensin-converting enzyme inhibitor (ACEI)–associated angioedema. Patients with these angioedema diseases, all of which are held to be bradykinin mediated, usually do not exhibit wheals.

Evidence Levels: **A** Double-blind study   **B** Clinical trial ≥ 20 subjects   **C** Clinical trial < 20 subjects   **D** Series ≥ 5 subjects   **E** Anecdotal case reports

Two major forms of HAE, both of them rare, have been described: HAE with C1INH deficiency, subclassified as type I and type II based on low antigenic and functional C1INH levels, respectively, and HAE with normal C1INH levels, with or without mutations in Hageman factor (coagulation factor XII). Angioedema attacks in all HAE patients are held to be due to the enhanced generation of bradykinin. The group of acquired forms of non-mast cell mediator–mediated angioedema includes those that are due to acquired C1INH deficiency (e.g., increased catabolism of C1INH) and angioedema due to certain drugs, mainly ACEIs. As in HAE, attacks of patients with these forms of angioedema are linked to elevated bradykinin levels.

In patients with HAE due to C1INH deficiency, recurrent angioedema attacks primarily involve the hands and feet, the abdomen, the face, the oropharynx, or a combination of these. HAE patients often experience prodromal symptoms (e.g., erythema marginatum). Typical HAE attacks progress for several hours and then slowly resolve over many hours to several days. Attacks involving the extremities and abdomen are the most common, and attacks of the oropharynx are the most dangerous, with a significant risk of mortality due to suffocation. In comparison, HAE with normal C1INH is more likely to affect females, to first occur after puberty, and to come with fewer attacks. Triggers of attacks are common and similar in all forms of HAE and include trauma, increased estrogen levels, and stress.

Attacks in patients with angioedema due to acquired C1INH deficiency are similar to those of HAE patients, but the former show a later age of onset and no family history. Attacks in patients with ACEI-induced angioedema typically affect the face, especially the lips and tongue. The time to onset of angioedema attacks after the start of ACEI treatment is usually less than 1 month, but in one of four affected patients it is greater than 6 months, and up to 10 years in some patients.

The diagnosis of bradykinin-mediated angioedema requires a thorough history, exclusion of differential diagnoses (especially chronic urticaria), and laboratory testing for C1INH deficiency. Angioedema in patients taking an ACEI is due to the ACEI until or unless proven otherwise.

MANAGEMENT STRATEGY FOR BRADYKININ-MEDIATED ANGIOEDEMA

The management of HAE with C1INH deficiency consists of the avoidance of known triggers of attacks and pharmacotherapy, that is, the use of on-demand treatment for attacks, their prevention by prophylactic treatment, or both. Today, five highly effective and safe drugs are available for the on-demand treatment of attacks: three different C1INHs (two plasma-derived and one recombinant), as well as icatibant, a selective bradykinin B2 receptor antagonist, and ecallantide, which inhibits plasma kallikrein, the protease that cleaves kininogen and generates bradykinin. Patients with HAE due to C1INH deficiency may also require prophylaxis. Preprocedural prophylaxis is usually done with C1INH with the aim to protect patients from attacks that occur in response to unavoidable triggers such as dental work or surgery. Long-term prophylaxis, that is, the regular use of medication to prevent angioedema attacks, should be considered in all HAE patients with C1INH deficiency, especially in those with high attack frequency and severity or limited access or response to on-demand treatment. C1INH is the preferred medication for long-term prophylaxis. Patients with HAE and normal C1INH, as well as patients with acquired bradykinin-mediated angioedema, can also benefit from on-demand treatment with C1INH or icatibant. Importantly, the standard treatment for attacks in patients with mast cell mediator–mediated angioedema such as glucocorticosteroids or H_1 antihistamines does not have any beneficial effect on HAE attacks and should not be used as on-demand medication for the treatment of bradykinin-mediated angioedema attacks.

Specific Investigation

- C4, C1INH level and function

Guideline for the management of hereditary angioedema: World Allergy Organization consensus document. Craig T, Aygören Pürsün E, Bork K, Bowen T, Boysen H, Farkas H, et al. WAO J 2012; 5: 182–99.

First-Line Therapies

On demand

• C1INH	A
• Ecallantide	A
• Icatibant	A

Prophylaxis

• C1INH	A

An evidence based therapeutic approach to hereditary and acquired angioedema. Bork K. Curr Opin Allergy Clin Immunol 2014; 14: 354–62.

Varicella

John Berth-Jones

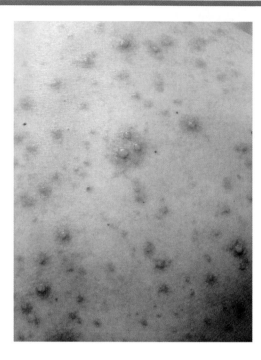

Varicella, or chickenpox, is the exanthematic illness caused by infection with the herpesvirus varicella zoster (VZV). Varicella has a typical incubation period of 10 to 14 days, spreading by direct person-to-person contact or by airborne droplets. The disease is infectious from 48 hours before the rash appears until the vesicles crust.

Varicella occurs most commonly in young children. Systemic symptoms are usually mild, although complications may occur. In adolescents, adults, and immunocompromised individuals of any age it is a more severe disease with a higher complication rate. Treatment is most commonly recommended in this group of individuals. Potential complications include secondary bacterial infection of the skin, bacterial pneumonia, and varicella pneumonitis. Rare complications of varicella include aseptic meningitis, encephalitis, cerebellar ataxia, myocarditis, corneal lesions, nephritis, arthritis, acute glomerulonephritis, Reye syndrome, bleeding diathesis, and hepatitis. Delayed complications include vasculopathy, which may resemble giant cell arteritis, and herpes zoster (shingles). The latter is the subject of a separate chapter.

MANAGEMENT STRATEGY

In the United States, a two-dose live attenuated *vaccine* is recommended for all healthy persons who have not had varicella. The first dose is administered at age 12 to 15 months and the second at 4 to 6 years. A second dose catch-up vaccination is recommended for individuals of all ages who have previously received one dose. Postexposure immunization may also be effective for household contacts if given within 3 days of the appearance of the rash in the index case. In the UK, routine vaccination is not recommended, except for nonimmune health care workers and other carers who are in frequent contact with individuals (mainly immunocompromised patients) who would be especially vulnerable to the infection, the purpose being to protect these vulnerable individuals.

In **healthy children** below the age of 12 years, *symptomatic treatment* is all that is generally required. *Acetaminophen (paracetamol)* is suitable. Aspirin should be avoided because of the risk of Reye syndrome. If a child is the second affected case in a family the illness can run a more severe course, and antiviral therapy should be considered. Oral *aciclovir* is the antiviral of choice and should be started within 24 hours of the rash developing.

In **healthy adolescents and adults**, *oral aciclovir* commenced within 24 hours of development of the rash has been shown to be beneficial. Heavy smokers and people with chronic lung disease are at greater risk of developing complications, particularly varicella pneumonitis. Treatment with aciclovir should be given if they are seen within 24 hours of the rash developing. There is no evidence confirming significant benefit if treatment is started after 24 hours in cases where infection is following the normal course and there are no complications. These patients should be treated symptomatically and advised to return promptly if they deteriorate. Patients with complications require hospital assessment.

Pregnant women are more likely to develop severe or complicated disease. Those who are not immune to varicella should avoid contact with varicella and zoster, and if this occurs they should report the contact immediately. Nonimmune pregnant women who have had contact with a person with varicella should receive specific *varicella zoster immune globulin (VZIG)*. VZIG is effective up to 10 days after contact. This has been shown to prevent varicella or modify disease severity. It also reduces the risk of fetal transmission if disease develops. Fetal infection between 3 and 28 weeks' gestation may cause the fetal varicella syndrome (including developmental abnormalities of the eyes and central nervous system). This occurs in an estimated 0.91% of pregnancies complicated by chickenpox during the first 20 weeks of gestation. The risk is probably greatest when infection occurs between 13 and 20 weeks. During the first trimester the use of *aciclovir* carries a theoretical risk of possible teratogenesis, although it is not a recognized teratogen. Beyond 20 weeks' gestation, oral aciclovir can be unequivocally recommended if the patient is seen within 24 hours of the onset of the rash. Pregnant women who are smokers, have chronic lung disease, are taking steroids, or are in the latter half of pregnancy are at greater risk of developing systemic symptoms. *Hospitalization* should be considered in late pregnancy and in women with chest or neurologic symptoms, a hemorrhagic rash, bleeding, or very severe disease with a dense rash and mucosal lesions.

Neonates whose mothers had varicella 7 days before to 7 days after delivery should be given prophylaxis with *VZIG*. Neonates with varicella whose mothers developed varicella within 7 days before delivery may develop severe disease and should be treated with intravenous *aciclovir*. Treatment should also be considered within 48 hours of development of the rash in other infants with congenital varicella (rash within 16 days of delivery) and severe clinical disease.

Immunocompromised individuals exposed to varicella should be given *prophylactic VZIG*. It is most effective when given within 72 hours but may still modify the disease if given up to 10 days after exposure. Those who develop varicella, including those on oral corticosteroids or with a history of oral corticosteroid intake for more than 3 weeks in the preceding 3 months, should be admitted to the the hospital and treated with *intravenous aciclovir*, as they are at risk of severe disease and complications. Resistance

Evidence Levels: **A** Double-blind study   **B** Clinical trial ≥ 20 subjects   **C** Clinical trial < 20 subjects   **D** Series ≥ 5 subjects   **E** Anecdotal case reports

to aciclovir can occur in immunocompromised individuals after long-term aciclovir therapy. In patients with proven aciclovir-resistant VZV strains, intravenous *foscarnet* provides an alternative.

Newer anti-VZV drugs have been developed. These include *valaciclovir, famciclovir,* and *brivudin,* although they are currently only licensed for use in herpes zoster.

Specific Investigations

- Virology on vesicle fluid
- Serology on acute and convalescent sera

The virus can be identified by electron microscopy, immune electron microscopy, tissue culture or shell viral culture, immunofluorescence, immunostaining, or detection of viral DNA by PCR.

First-Line Therapies

• Symptomatic therapy	C
• Aciclovir	A

Aciclovir for treating varicella in otherwise healthy children and adolescents. Klassen TP, Belseck EM, Wiebe N, Hartling L. Cochrane Database Syst Rev 2004; CD002980.

Aciclovir initiated within 24 hours after rash onset shows a therapeutic benefit in reducing the length of time with fever and the maximum number of lesions in immunocompetent children. Symptomatic treatment with analgesics and topical agents such as calamine lotion or crotamiton cream and daily baths are all that is required in most children.

When required, aciclovir is the antiviral of choice. It is usually given orally. In children up to 12 years of age it is given at a dose of 20 mg/kg 6-hourly (to a maximum of 800 mg/dose) for 5 days. In adolescents and adults the dose is 800 mg five times daily for 7 days. Aciclovir is given intravenously in severe disease and in immunocompromised individuals.

Treatment of adult varicella with oral acyclovir: a randomized, placebo-controlled trial. Wallace MR, Bowler WA, Murray NB, Brodine SK, Oldfield EC III. Ann Intern Med 1992; 117: 358–63.

A study of 148 evaluable military personnel hospitalized for varicella and treated with either aciclovir 800 mg orally five times per day for 7 days or placebo. Patients treated within 24 hours of onset of the rash had fewer lesions and shorter time to crusting. Treatment after 24 hours had no effect.

Combining corticosteroids and acyclovir in the management of varicella pneumonia: a prospective study. Anwar SK, Masoodi I, Alfaifi A, Hussain S, Sirwal IA. Antivir Ther 2014; 19: 221–4.

A prospective study of 32 adult cases treated with an intravenous injection of aciclovir (10 mg/kg) every 8 hours for 4 to 10 days and of corticosteroids (100 mg hydrocortisone) every 8 hours for 5 days, supporting the use of this treatment combination. Resolution was achieved in 31 cases, and a single fatality occurred.

Second-Line Therapies

• Foscarnet	D
• Famciclovir	C
• Valaciclovir	D
• Valganciclovir	E

Foscarnet therapy in five patients with AIDS and acyclovir resistant varicella zoster virus infection. Safrin S, Berger TG, Wolfe PR, Wosby CB, Mills J, Biron KK. Ann Intern Med 1991; 115: 19–21.

Five patients with AIDS and aciclovir-resistant VZV were treated with foscarnet. Four had healing of the lesions and negative cultures during therapy. Fluorescent antigen testing remained positive in two patients: one healed completely, but the other had concomitant clinical failure of therapy.

Foscarnet is used in patients who have developed resistance to aciclovir. The dose is 40 mg/kg 8-hourly in 1-hour transfusions for 10 days.

Pharmacokinetics and safety of famciclovir in children with herpes simplex or varicella-zoster virus infection. Sáez-Llorens X, Yogev R, Arguedas A, Rodriguez A, Spigarelli MG, De León Castrejón T, et al. Antimicrob Agents Chemother 2009; 53: 1912–20.

After 7 days on an oral regimen VZV disease had resolved in 49 of 53 children. Doses were adjusted according to body weight (BW) using a nonlinear 8-point scale. The mean BW-adjusted daily dose was 40.8 mg/kg for 1- to <2-year-olds, 40.6 mg/kg for 2- to <6-year-olds, and 35.5 mg/kg for 6- to ≤12-year-olds, divided into three doses.

Varicella in a pediatric heart transplant population on non-steroid maintenance immunosuppression. Dodd DA, Burger J, Edwards KM, Dummer JS. Pediatrics 2001; 108: E80.

Six of 14 pediatric heart transplant patients with varicella were treated with oral valaciclovir, dose range 61 to 88 mg/kg/day, for 7 days.

Complete remission of VZV reactivation treated with valganciclovir in a patient with total lymphocyte depletion and acute kidney injury after allogeneic bone marrow transplantation. Maximova N, Antonio P, Marilena G, Rovere F, Tamaro P. APMIS 2015; 123: 77–80.

PREGNANCY

Chickenpox in pregnancy. Green-top Guideline No. 13. Royal College of Obstetricians and Gynecologists. January 2015. https://www.rcog.org.uk/globalassets/documents/guidelines/gtg13.pdf.

VZIG is recommended for postexposure prophylaxis. Oral aciclovir is recommended if patients present within 24 hours of the rash and are at more than 20 weeks' gestation. Use of aciclovir before 20 weeks should also be considered.

Management of varicella infection (chickenpox) in pregnancy. Shrim A, Koren G, Yudin MH, Farine D; Maternal Fetal Medicine Committee. J Obstet Gynaecol Can 2012; 34: 287–92.

Varicella immunization is recommended for all nonimmune women as part of prepregnancy and postpartum care. Varicella vaccination should not be administered in pregnancy. However, termination of pregnancy should not be advised because of inadvertent vaccination during pregnancy. The antenatal varicella immunity status of all pregnant women should be documented by history of previous infection, varicella vaccination, or serology. All nonimmune pregnant women should be informed of the risk of varicella infection to themselves and their fetuses. They should be instructed to seek medical help after any contact with a person who may have been contagious. In the case of a possible exposure to varicella in a pregnant woman with unknown immune status, serum testing should be performed. If results are negative or unavailable within 96 hours from exposure, VZIG should be administered. Women who develop varicella infection in pregnancy need to be made aware of the potential adverse maternal and fetal sequelae, the risk of transmission to the fetus, and the options available for prenatal diagnosis. Detailed ultrasound and appropriate follow-up are recommended for all women who develop varicella in pregnancy to screen for fetal harm. Women with significant (e.g., pneumonitis) varicella infection in pregnancy should be treated with oral antiviral agents (e.g., aciclovir 800 mg five times daily). In cases of progression to varicella pneumonitis, maternal admission to hospital should be seriously considered. Intravenous aciclovir can be considered for severe complications in pregnancy (oral forms have poor bioavailability). The dose is usually 10 to 15 mg/kg or 500 mg/m^2 IV every 8 hours for 5 to 10 days for varicella pneumonitis, and it should be started within 24 to 72 hours of the onset of rash. Neonatal health care providers should be informed of peripartum varicella exposure in order to optimize early neonatal care with VZIG and immunization. VZIG should be administered to neonates whenever the onset of maternal disease is between 5 days before and 2 days after delivery.

PROPHYLAXIS

• Vaccines	A
• Varicella zoster immune globulin	B
• Intravenous immunoglobulin	C
• Aciclovir	B

SAGE working group on varicella and herpes zoster vaccines: background paper on varicella vaccine SAGE review 2015. http://www.who.int/immunization/sage/meetings/2014/april/1_SAGE_varicella_background_paper_FINAL.pdf.

The review concludes "There is strong scientific evidence that varicella vaccine is safe and effective in preventing varicella related morbidity and mortality in immunocompetent individuals."

Introduction of varicella vaccination in the United States and elsewhere has been followed by reduced incidence and morbidity in all age groups, apparently indicating significant benefits from "herd immunity."

Use of combination measles, mumps, rubella, and varicella vaccine: recommendations of the Advisory Committee on Immunization Practices (ACIP). Marin M, Broder KR, Temte JL, Snider DE, Seward JF; Centers for Disease Control and Prevention (CDC). MMWR Recomm Rep 2010; 59: 1-12.

Combined vaccination with measles, mumps, and rubella vaccine (MMRV) is generally preferred, except for initial dosing before 48 months of age (as there appears to be a slightly increased risk of febrile seizure in this age group associated with the use of quadruple vaccine for the first dose).

A varicella outbreak in a school with high one-dose vaccination coverage, Beijing, China. Lu L, Suo L, Li J, Zhai L, Zheng Q, Pang X, et al. Vaccine 2012; 30: 5094–8.

Of the 951 students, 916 had received one dose of varicella vaccine, and only 2 had received two doses before the outbreak. A total of 87 cases occurred, but 95% had mild disease. Single-dose varicella vaccination was 89% effective in preventing any varicella and 99% in preventing moderate/severe varicella.

Single-dose vaccination does not prevent outbreaks but probably protects against severe disease.

Vaccines for postexposure prophylaxis against varicella (chickenpox) in children and adults. Macartney K, Heywood A, McIntyre P. Cochrane Database Syst Rev 2014; 6: CD001833.

Three small studies suggest vaccines administered within 3 days of household exposure reduce infection rates and severity.

Varicella vaccination in the immunocompromised. Malaiya R, Patel S, Snowden N, Leventis P. Rheumatology 2015; 54: 567–9.

A review of the risks from varicella in patients receiving immunosuppressive medication and the diverse recommendations regarding vaccination of this group. The authors recommend that the immune status of patients be established, and nonimmune (varicella naïve) patients should be vaccinated at least 2 weeks before commencing immunosuppressive treatment if the delay is considered tolerable. Use of varicella or zoster vaccines is not recommended in naïve patients who are already immunosuppressed.

Updated recommendations for use of VariZIG—United States, 2013. Centers for Disease Control and Prevention (CDC). Morb Mortal Wkly Rep 2013; 62: 574–6.

The CDC recommends administration of VZIG as soon as possible after exposure to VZV and within 10 days for people without evidence of immunity to varicella who are at high risk from varicella, who have been exposed to varicella or zoster, and for whom varicella vaccine is contraindicated. High-risk groups include immunocompromised patients, newborn infants whose mothers have signs and symptoms of varicella around the time of delivery (i.e., 5 days before to 2 days after), hospitalized premature infants born at ≥28 weeks of gestation whose mothers do not have evidence of immunity to varicella, hospitalized premature infants born at <28 weeks of gestation or who weigh ≤1000 g at birth, regardless of their mothers' evidence of immunity to varicella, and pregnant women without evidence of immunity.

Intravenous immunoglobulin prophylaxis in children with acute leukemia following exposure to varicella. Chen SH, Liang DC. Pediatr Hematol Oncol 1992; 9: 347–51.

Five children with leukemia received a single dose (200 mg/kg) of IVIG within 3 days of exposure to varicella. None developed the infection.

IVIG appears to be an effective and safe alternative when VZIG is unavailable.

Postexposure prophylaxis of varicella in family contact by oral acyclovir. Asano Y, Yoshikawa T, Suga S, Kobayashi I, Nakashima T, Yazaki T, et al. J Pediatr 1993; 92: 219–22.

Twenty-five children were treated with oral aciclovir 40 or 80 mg/kg daily in four divided doses, 7 to 9 days after household exposure to varicella. Twenty-five age-matched control subjects who had been exposed but did not receive treatment were also followed. Twenty of the 25 treated subjects were protected from disease, but 4 of them failed to seroconvert. All 25 controls developed varicella.

Although its efficacy is not as well established as that of VZIG, oral aciclovir also seems likely to be effective in postexposure prophylaxis. It is given approximately 9 days after exposure for 1 week and may abort the disease or reduce its severity.

Evidence Levels: **A** Double-blind study **B** Clinical trial ≥ 20 subjects **C** Clinical trial < 20 subjects **D** Series ≥ 5 subjects **E** Anecdotal case reports

Antiviral prophylaxis and treatment in chickenpox. A review prepared for the UK Advisory Group on Chickenpox on behalf of the British Society for the Study of Infection. Ogilvie MM. J Infect 1998; 36: 31–8.

A review of the use of VZIG, live attenuated varicella vaccine, and aciclovir. Oral aciclovir is only considered effective if begun within 24 hours of rash onset. It is recommended for treatment of varicella in otherwise healthy adults and adolescents but not for routine use in children under 13 years of age unless they are sibling contacts or have other medical conditions. Aciclovir has a high therapeutic index and good safety profile, but caution is advised with use in pregnancy.

Prophylactic role of long-term ultralow-dose acyclovir for varicella zoster virus disease after allogeneic hematopoietic stem cell transplantation. Kawamura K, Wada H, Yamasaki R, Ishihara Y, Sakamoto K, Ashizawa M, et al. Int J Infect Dis 2014; 19: 26–32.

A study of 141 patients treated prophylactically with aciclovir 200 mg daily for up to a year. Discontinuation of the drug was followed by a pronounced increase in frequency of VZV disease.

251

Viral exanthems: rubella, roseola, rubeola, and enteroviruses

Julia A. Siegel, Julia O. Baltz, Karen Wiss

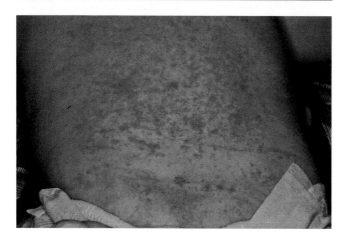

RUBELLA

Rubella (German measles, 3-day measles) is usually a mild disease of low-grade fever, generalized erythematous macules and papules, and generalized lymphadenopathy. It is caused by an enveloped RNA virus of the *Togaviridae* family.

MANAGEMENT STRATEGY

In children, there is typically no prodrome. In adolescents and adults, a prodrome of fever, malaise, sore throat, nausea, anorexia, and generalized lymphadenopathy is common. The erythematous pink macules and papules start on the face and neck and spread down and out in a centrifugal fashion over 1 to 2 days, disappearing in 2 to 3 days. Forchheimer spots, an enanthem consisting of petechiae on the hard palate, may accompany the rash.

Rubella is a self-limited illness. The treatment is generally *supportive*. Teenagers and adults may experience transient polyarthralgia and polyarthritis. Thrombocytopenia and encephalitis are extremely rare complications. During the first trimester of pregnancy, maternal rubella can result in fetal death or congenital rubella syndrome. The main fetal anomalies include ophthalmic disease (cataracts, glaucoma, microphthalmia, and chorioretinitis), sensorineural deafness, cardiac abnormalities (patent ductus arteriosus, atrial septal defects, ventricular septal defects), pulmonic stenosis, and blueberry muffin lesions (extramedullary hematopoiesis). Survivors of congenital rubella have a higher risk of developmental delay, including autism.

It can be difficult to distinguish rubella from other viral exanthems, in particular enteroviruses. Rubella also mimics measles, parvovirus B19, human herpes virus (HHV)-6, and arboviruses. It

is essential to differentiate infection among these viruses during pregnancy. Virus identification by culture is available. In congenital infections, rubella can be isolated from the blood, urine, cerebrospinal fluid, and the posterior pharynx. In postnatal infections, the virus is harbored in the nasopharynx, and the timing of specimen collection is crucial, as samples are only virus positive on the first day of rash through 7 to 10 days afterward. Amplification is accomplished by reverse transcription polymerase chain reaction (RT-PCR). Viral serology is also available for diagnosis, but IgM is only present in 50% of samples on the first day of rash, with levels peaking 5 days later. Both serum IgM and seroconversion of convalescent IgG with a fourfold increase in titer suggest recent infection. A more reliable diagnosis is obtained by both RT-PCR and serology, which can detect virus on day 0 of rash eruption. Avidity tests may help determine timing of infection, as low-avidity antirubella IgG is associated with recent infection. Microarray technology is a cheap and promising future methodology for diagnosis of acute infection. Children with rubella should be *excluded from school for 7 days after onset of the rash*. Rubella vaccine is recommended in combination with the measles and mumps vaccine, with or without the varicella vaccine (MMR or MMRV), at 12 to 15 months of age with a second dose at 4 to 6 years. However, an increased risk of febrile seizures has been reported with the combination MMRV vaccine. Postpubertal females can be tested for rubella IgG and vaccinated if necessary. The vaccine contains live virus and should not be given to pregnant women.

Specific Investigations

- Viral culture
- Serology (acute IgM or acute and convalescent IgG)
- PCR

Diagnosis of recent primary rubella virus infections: significance of glycoprotein-based IgM serology, IgG avidity and immunoblot analysis. Wandinger KP, Saschenbrecker S, Steinhagen K, Scheper T, Meyer W, Bartelt U, et al. J Virol Methods 2011; 174: 85–93.

The rubella IgM positive predictive value has decreased with high vaccination and seroprevalence rates in the United States. It is important to distinguish IgM reactivity due to primary rubella infection from IgM reactivity due to persistence, reinfection, polyclonal B-cell stimulation, and cross-reactivity. This may be done using specific IgG avidity and immunoblot analyses.

First-Line Therapies

• Antipyretics: acetaminophen (paracetamol), ibuprofen	E
• Analgesics: nonsteroidal antiinflammatory drugs	E
• School avoidance for 7 days	A
• Immunization	A

Rubella. Lambert N, Strebel P, Orenstein W, Icenogle J, Poland GA. Lancet 2015; 385: 2297–307.

Since the advent of the national rubella vaccination program, rubella virus is no longer endemic in the United States. From 2000 to 2012, rubella cases decreased by 99.9% in the Americas, from 39,228 to only 21.

Post-exposure passive immunisation for preventing rubella and congenital rubella syndrome. Young MK, Cripps AW, Nimmo GR, van Driel ML. Cochrane Database Syst Rev 2015.

Evidence Levels: **A** Double-blind study **B** Clinical trial ≥ 20 subjects **C** Clinical trial < 20 subjects **D** Series ≥ 5 subjects **E** Anecdotal case reports

Polyclonal immunoglobulins may prevent rubella up to 5 days after exposure, with dose-dependent effectiveness. Evidence of congenital rubella prevention with polyclonal immunoglobulins is inconclusive.

ROSEOLA

Roseola infantum (exanthem subitum, sixth disease) is a disease of high fever in a well-appearing child with eruption of pink macules and papules upon defervescence. It is caused by infection with HHV-6 (which includes HHV-6A and HHV-6B species) or HHV-7.

MANAGEMENT STRATEGY

Roseola is an illness of children between 6 and 36 months of age. The first sign of illness is a high fever (>39.5°C) that persists for 3 to 7 days, followed by an exanthem that spreads centrifugally from the neck, lasting hours to days. Typically, no treatment is necessary and the illness resolves in a few days. Febrile seizures are common in infants during the febrile phase, often requiring emergency room care.

Identification of HHV-6 or -7 is difficult because most infections are asymptomatic. Culture from peripheral blood is available in specialized facilities, but is of limited use due to slow turnover. High population seroprevalence (~95%) also renders serology less useful. Seroconversion of convalescent IgG with a fourfold increase in titer is more indicative of acute infection; however, there is considerable antibody cross-reactivity between HHV-6, -7, and cytomegalovirus (CMV). Viral DNA detection by nucleic acid amplification of whole blood, serum, or plasma is the current method of diagnosis, though standardized methods of measurement are yet to be determined. PCR alone cannot reliably distinguish between active and latent infection; a multiple assay approach is more sensitive and specific. Antibody avidity can help clarify timing, as high avidity indicates at least 6 weeks since infection. Additionally, two new RT-qPCR assays have been developed to detect specific viral transcripts expressed during multiplication, allowing for better differentiation between active and latent infection. Digital droplet PCR is useful for viral quantification and identification of chromosomally integrated HHV-6.

Most individuals harbor HHV-6 and -7 in their saliva, whereas only 1% of the population carries chromosomally integrated viral DNA. In the immunocompromised, viral reactivation frequently causes severe disease such as fever, bone marrow suppression, hepatitis, pneumonia, lymphoproliferative disorders, and encephalitis. In these patients, *ganciclovir* and *foscarnet* are first-line treatments, although conflicting evidence exists regarding survival benefit. Foscarnet has shown prophylactic efficacy in stem cell transplant patients. In vitro studies show that ganciclovir, cidofovir, and foscarnet inhibit HHV-6 and -7 replication. Individual case reports have suggested benefit from these agents in immunocompetent patients with end organ disease. Infection with HHV-6 can be associated with a severe course of drug-induced hypersensitivity syndrome (DIHS), also known as drug reaction with eosinophilia and systemic symptoms (DRESS).

Specific Investigations

* No investigation is required routinely
* HHV-6 serology (acute IgM or acute and convalescent IgG)
* PCR

First-Line Therapy

• Antipyretics (acetaminophen, ibuprofen)	E

Second-Line Therapies

• Ganciclovir	D
• Foscarnet	D

High-dose ganciclovir in HHV-6 encephalitis of an immunocompetent child. Olli-Lähdesmäki T, Haataja L, Parkkola R, Waris M, Bleyzac N, Ruuskanen O. Pediatr Neurol 2010; 43: 53–6.

Though antiviral treatment is usually reserved for immunocompromised patients, high-dose ganciclovir (18 mg/kg/day) was safe and efficacious in this 15-month-old with HHV-6 encephalitis.

Human herpesvirus type 6 and human herpesvirus type 7 infections of the central nervous system. Dewhurst S. Herpes 2004; 11: 105A–11A.

Ganciclovir and foscarnet may be used for managing HHV-6–related disease. Ganciclovir, but not foscarnet, may be useful for HHV-7–related illness.

Safety of pre-engraftment prophylactic foscarnet administration after allogeneic stem cell transplantation. Ishiyama K, Katagiri T, Ohata K, Hosokawa K, Kondo Y, Yamazaki H, et al. Transpl Infect Dis 2012; 14: 33–9.

In 10 stem cell transplant patients, prophylactic foscarnet reduced the risk of HHV-6 or -7–associated encephalitis but was unable to prevent HHV-6 reactivation.

Diagnostic clues to human herpesvirus 6 encephalitis and Wernicke encephalopathy after pediatric hematopoietic cell transplantation. Sadighi Z, Sabin ND, Hayden R, Stewart E, Pillai A. J Child Neurol 2015; 30: 1307–14.

Rapid treatment with intravenous foscarnet or ganciclovir in HHV-6 encephalitis after hematopoietic cell transplantation may optimize neurologic recovery. Foscarnet has been shown to be effective against both HHV-6A and HHV-6B, whereas ganciclovir has only been shown to work against HHV-6B.

Human herpesvirus types 6 and 7 infection in pediatric hematopoietic stem cell transplant recipients. Fule Robles JD, Cheuk DK, Ha SY, Chiang AK, Chan GC. Ann Transplant 2014; 19: 269–76.

Multiple studies have shown that ganciclovir and foscarnet resolve viremia, but may not improve survival. If these medications fail in severe HHV-6 or -7 infections, cidofovir may be tried. However, cidofovir has poor cerebrospinal fluid (CSF) penetration and may not be effective in treating herpes virus encephalopathy.

RUBEOLA

Rubeola (measles) is a systemic illness with fever, cough, coryza, conjunctivitis, erythematous macules and papules, and Koplik spots. It is caused by infection with the measles virus, an enveloped RNA virus of the *Paramyxoviridae* family.

MANAGEMENT STRATEGY

The measles rash begins along the hairline and behind the ears and spreads down the body. It is the prototype of the "morbilliform eruption." Koplik spots, the pathognomonic enanthem of clustered white dots on the buccal mucosa, precede the rash by approximately 2 days. It is important to distinguish the measles rash from drug eruptions, Kawasaki disease, and other viral infections, in particular exanthems from enteroviruses and adenoviruses. Complications include pneumonia, croup, diarrhea, encephalitis, and death. Subacute sclerosing panencephalitis due to persistent measles infection is a rare degenerative neurologic disease that can occur years after original infection.

Rapid diagnosis by immunofluorescence of desquamated nasal mucosal cells is available. Both serum IgM at the onset of rash and seroconversion of convalescent IgG with a fourfold increase in titer suggest recent infection. RT-PCR of nasopharyngeal secretions, oral fluids, or serum provides the most reliable diagnostic method of acute infection. Oral fluid assays may represent the future of measles detection, as sampling is painless and cost effective.

Children with measles should be *isolated for 4 days after rash eruption*, and physicians should *notify* the appropriate monitoring authorities. Measles *vaccine* contains live virus and is recommended as part of the MMR or MMRV regimen at 12 to 15 months with a second dose at 4 to 6 years of age. It can also be given as a measles-only formulation.

Individuals with poor nutritional status are at greatest risk for complications from measles. *Dietary supplementation with vitamin A* may reduce the morbidity and mortality of the disease. Supplementation should be given to children 6 to 24 months of age who are hospitalized for measles complications. Any child with measles and compromised immune function, malnutrition, vitamin A deficiency, or recent travel to high-measles-mortality areas is also a candidate for treatment. The World Health Organization recommends two doses of 50,000 IU for infants <6 months, 100,000 IU for children 6 to 12 months, and 200,000 IU for individuals >1 year. A recent meta-analysis demonstrated that at least two doses of 200,000 IU for children >1 year and 100,000 IU for infants were found to reduce measles mortality by approximately 60%. *Immunoglobulin prophylaxis* can prevent or modify disease within 7 days of exposure. It is recommended for susceptible household contacts, especially for infants, pregnant women, or immunocompromised individuals.

Measles virus is susceptible to *ribavirin* in vitro, although its clinical efficacy is questionable. It has been given intravenously and intranasally to treat immunocompromised children with severe illness. Novel nonnucleoside inhibitors of measles RNA polymerase, such as ERDRP-0519, which targets morbillivirus RNA-dependent RNA polymerase, are in development and show promise.

Measles is a notifiable disease in many jurisdictions, including the UK and United States.

Specific Investigations

- Immunofluorescence of nasal mucosal cells
- Serology (acute IgM or acute and convalescent IgG)
- Viral culture
- PCR

Assessment of measles diagnostic from gingival fluid in Côte d'Ivoir. Bénié BVJ, Attoh-Touré H, Aka LN, Fofana N, Tiembré I, Dagnan NS. Bull Soc Pathol Exot 2015; 108: 262–4.

Oral fluid demonstrates equal diagnostic ability compared with the gold standards of serum enzyme-linked immunosorbent assay (ELISA). In addition, oral fluid collection is painless, cost effective, and does not require complicated technical skills.

First-Line Therapies

• Antipyretics: acetaminophen, ibuprofen	E
• Measles vaccine (prevention and after exposure)	A

Progress toward regional measles elimination worldwide, 2000–2013. Centers for Disease Control and Prevention. MMWR 2014; 63: 1034–8.

From 2000 to 2012, an increase in routine vaccination and supplementary immunization activities led to a 77% decrease in reported annual measles incidence worldwide and a 78% decrease in measles mortality (from 562,400 to 122,000), preventing an estimated 13.8 million deaths.

Measles cases exceed 100 in US outbreak. McCarthy M. BMJ 2015; 350: h622.

In 2014, 644 measles cases were reported in the United States, a record high since measles elimination in 2000, and over 100 cases were reported in 2015. The majority of infected individuals have not been vaccinated. High rates of vaccine refusal cluster geographically, where parents are concerned about the safety of vaccines.

Effectiveness of measles vaccination for control of exposed children. Barrabeig I, Rovira A, Rius C, Muñoz P, Soldevila N, Batalla J, et al. Pediatr Infect Dis J 2011; 30: 78–80.

There is considerable debate about the efficacy of postexposure prophylaxis with measles vaccine. This study demonstrated that vaccination within 72 hours of exposure prevented 90.5% of disease cases.

Second-Line Therapies

• Oral vitamin A	A
• Immunoglobulin prophylaxis	A
• Ribavirin and IFN-α	D

Effectiveness of measles vaccination and vitamin A treatment. Sudfeld CR, Navar AM, Halsey NA. Int J Epidemiol 2010; 39: i48–55.

One dose of measles vaccine is 85% effective in preventing measles disease, whereas a second dose is estimated to be 98.1% to 100% effective. Vitamin A treatment demonstrated a 62% reduction in measles mortality with two doses of 200,000 IU in children >1 year and 100,000 IU for infants.

An assessment of measles vaccine effectiveness, Australia, 2006–2012. Pillsbury A, Quinn H. WPSAR 2015; 6: 43–50.

One dose of measles vaccine is 96.7% effective in preventing measles disease, whereas a second dose is estimated to be 99.7% effective.

Post-exposure passive immunisation for preventing measles. Young MK, Nimmo GR, Cripps AW, Jones MA. Cochrane Database Syst Rev 2014: CD010056.

Passive immunization with immunoglobulins in nonimmune individuals decreases the risk of measles by 83% and decreases mortality by 76% when administered within 7 days of exposure.

Measles control—can measles virus inhibitors make a difference? Plemper RK, Snyder JP. Curr Opin Investig Drugs 2009; 10: 811–20.

Evidence Levels: **A** Double-blind study **B** Clinical trial ≥ 20 subjects **C** Clinical trial < 20 subjects **D** Series ≥ 5 subjects **E** Anecdotal case reports

Ribavirin and IFN-α are used clinically for severe cases of measles infection, though their efficacy and side effect profiles are unfavorable. A novel antiviral agent is greatly needed, and novel nonnucleoside inhibitors of measles RNA polymerase show potential.

An orally available, small-molecule polymerase inhibitor shows efficacy against a lethal morbillivirus infection in a large animal model. Krumm SA, Yan D, Hovingh ES, Evers TJ, Enkirch T, Reddy GP, et al. Sci Transl Med 2014; 6: 232ra52.

A novel, orally available, antimorbillivirus drug, ERDRP-0519, which targets morbillivirus RNA-dependent RNA polymerase, has recently been reported as capable of curing a lethal morbillivirus infection when administered at the first onset of viremia. This drug was efficacious against measles virus in vitro and against the closely related canine distemper virus (CDV) in vivo in ferrets.

ENTEROVIRUSES

Enteroviruses are a group of nonenveloped RNA viruses that include coxsackieviruses A and B, enteroviruses 68 to 71, echoviruses, and polioviruses. As polio has been eliminated in the United States, nonpolioviruses are the main concern. There is a wide spectrum of clinical disease, including mild fever, upper respiratory tract infections, aseptic meningitis, myocarditis, and encephalitis. Enteroviruses also cause more specific syndromes, such as hand, foot, and mouth disease; herpangina; hemorrhagic conjunctivitis; and pleurodynia.

MANAGEMENT STRATEGY

The majority of enterovirus infections are mild and self-limited, peaking in summer and fall seasons. The viruses are transmitted by the orofecal route, and distribution is worldwide. Young children are most frequently affected and commonly present with fever, malaise, diarrhea, vomiting, and upper respiratory symptoms. The exanthem is typically a nonpruritic, morbilliform eruption, often with a petechial component.

Hand, foot, and mouth disease is typically caused by coxsackievirus A16. There is a prodrome of fever, malaise, and sore throat followed by painful red macules, which become vesicles, on the tongue, soft palate, uvula, and tonsillar pillars. Ovoid, opaque vesicles with a surrounding rim of erythema may be noted on the hands, feet, and buttocks. The disease is usually self-limited. Epidemics in Taiwan, caused by enterovirus 71, led to deaths due to pulmonary hemorrhage/edema, meningitis, encephalitis, myocarditis, and flaccid paralysis.

Herpangina may present with a similar prodrome. White-gray vesicles with a rim of erythema are later observed on the soft palate, uvula, and tonsillar pillars. Typically fewer than 20 lesions are noted.

Enteroviral infections may be diagnosed by rapid or traditional viral culture of the oropharynx or stool and occasionally of the

blood, CSF, urine, or tissue. The specific serotype can usually be identified. Disadvantages to viral culture include low sensitivity and slow turnover. Serology is not routinely used but is commercially available. Because all enteroviruses share common genomic sequences, PCR detects almost all enterovirus serotypes and is particularly reliable in the CSF.

Treatment of most enteroviral infections, including hand, foot, and mouth disease and herpangina, consists of *hydration* and *pain control*. These infections are of particular concern in newborns and immunosuppressed patients who have been treated with *immunoglobulin* for severe life-threatening illness. *Pleconaril* is an antiviral drug that prevents viral attachment and fusion and has the potential to improve morbidity and mortality. Presently, its use is limited to severe life-threatening infections, specifically meningitis and neonatal sepsis. Small interfering RNA (siRNA) shows promise as a future treatment option.

Specific Investigations
- Viral culture
- Enteroviral PCR

First-Line Therapies
Antipyretics such as acetaminophen or ibuprofen	E
Analgesics	E
Hydration	E

Second-Line Therapies
Immunoglobulin	C
Pleconaril	B

Enteroviral encephalitis in children: clinical features, pathophysiology, and treatment advances. Jain S, Patel B, Bhatt GC. Pathog Glob Health 2014; 108: 216–22.

Specific antiviral therapy is currently not available for enteroviral infections, but pleconaril and immunoglobulin are used to treat enteroviral infections of the central nervous system (CNS). Of note, immunoglobulin therapy has not been properly validated in clinical trials. Bovine lactoferrin, shRNA (small hairpin RNA), siRNA, rupintrivir, ribavirin, and 17-AAG have been tested in vivo and may become future therapeutic options.

A randomized, double-blind, placebo-controlled trial of pleconaril for the treatment of neonates with enterovirus sepsis. Abzug MJ, Michaels MG, Wald E, Jacobs RF, Romero JR, Sánchez PJ, et al. J Pediatric Infect Dis Soc 2016; 5: 53–62.

Those treated with pleconaril had greater survival and earlier negative cultures and PCR tests compared with the placebo group.

Viral warts

Rabia S. Rashid, Imtiaz Ahmed

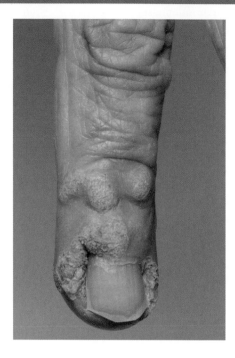

Warts are a common disease caused by infection with various strains of the human papillomavirus (HPV). They appear on different sites of the body and in various forms, including common, flat, filiform, periungual, plantar, mosaic, and genital warts. Children most commonly present with common or periungual warts on hands and feet, whereas adults often present with common warts on the back of hands or filiform warts on the face and neck. Genital warts are discussed in another chapter.

MANAGEMENT STRATEGY

Most warts resolve spontaneously with time. However, patients and children's parents often ask for treatment because of pain, social stigma, or concern over infectivity. In some cases warts cause ridicule, distorted self-image, impaired dexterity, worry over loss of employment, or a health and safety issue. Immunosuppressed patients may have extensive and resistant warts.

Most patients will treat themselves with over-the-counter preparations containing *keratolytics* before presenting to the dermatologist. Salicylic acid has the best evidence base and is the most commonly used therapy. It can be applied in various concentrations, with or without occlusion, and is suitable for any cutaneous site except the face. However, it requires frequent application, and it may cause irritation of the surrounding skin. *Cryotherapy* with dimethyl ether and propane applicator, silver nitrate pencils, and occlusive "duct tape" are also available over the counter.

When a dermatologist sees patients with warts, the diagnosis and the possibility of *spontaneous resolution* and watchful waiting should be explained. The patient should be educated on how to apply topical preparations accurately. Keeping the warts well pared down with the use of a file or pumice stone after

soaking is especially important for plantar warts. Young and healthy individuals with short duration of infection have the highest clearance rate. Cryotherapy with liquid nitrogen is one of the most common treatments used by the dermatologist. Liquid nitrogen is applied with a cryospray or a cotton bud. The wart should be frozen outward from the center to include a 2-mm rim of normal skin and the freeze maintained for 5 seconds. Cryotherapy is best repeated at 2- to 3-week intervals. Hyperkeratotic warts should be pared before cryotherapy and plantar warts treated by two freeze–thaw cycles. This treatment is painful and not always well tolerated by young children. The treated warts are sore and may blister. In pigmented skin, posttreatment hypopigmentation and hyperpigmentation can be a problem. Cryotherapy with liquid nitrogen can be combined with other topical preparations such as salicylic acid. Cryotherapy with carbon dioxide snow or dimethyl ether applicators does not produce temperatures as low as liquid nitrogen and is less effective.

If cryotherapy is not successful then various other options are available, including *immunotherapy* with diphencyprone (DCP), squaric acid, and intralesional mumps or *Candida* antigen. *Intralesional bleomycin* may be injected into the wart or the solution applied to the wart and then repeatedly pricked through with a lancet. Laser ablation, hyperthermia, curettage and cautery, or even surgical excision of troublesome and resistant warts can be attempted, but the risk of scarring and recurrence of the warts in the scar can be a problem. The *pulsed dye laser* (PDL), thought to target the rich capillary network in warts, can be effective. *Photodynamic therapy* (PDT) is another option; however, pain during and after ALA (aminolevulinic acid)-PDT is well recognized. *Other treatments* used occasionally include 5-fluorouracil, zinc, levamisole, cimetidine, topical and oral retinoids, and imiquimod.

First–Line Therapies	
• Salicylic acid preparations	A
• Silver nitrate	B
• Cryotherapy with dimethyl ether and propane	C

An assessment of methods of treating viral warts by comparative treatment trials based on a standard design. Bunney MH, Nolan MW, Williams DA. Br J Dermatol 1976; 94: 667–79.

This paper looked into 11 trials with over 1800 patients. In a randomized blind trial involving 389 patients, salicylic acid with lactic acid paint was as effective as cryotherapy with liquid nitrogen, with cure rates of 67% and 69%, respectively. The salicylic acid with lactic acid paint comprised 17% salicylic acid, 17% lactic acid, and 66% flexible collodion. In another study of 382 warts, 84% of patients were cured after 12 weeks of salicylic acid with lactic acid paint application. A separate study showed a 44% clearance with salicylic acid and lactic acid paint versus 47% of patients applying 10% glutaraldehyde.

Topical treatments for cutaneous warts. Kwok CS, Gibbs S, Bennett C, Holland R, Abbott R. Cochrane Database Syst Rev 2013; 9: CD001781.

This updated review contained 26 new studies. According to 85 trials meeting the criteria for inclusion, the best evidenced therapy for cutaneous warts is for salicylic acid. Data pooled from six placebo-controlled trials showed a statistically significant result favoring the topical application of salicylic acid for warts at all

Evidence Levels: **A** Double-blind study **B** Clinical trial ≥ 20 subjects **C** Clinical trial < 20 subjects **D** Series ≥ 5 subjects **E** Anecdotal case reports

sites (response rate [RR] 1.56, 95% confidence interval, 1.20–2.03). On the contrary, no benefit was found between cryotherapy and placebo in three studies.

Efficacy of 10% silver nitrate solution in the treatment of common warts: a placebo-controlled, randomized, clinical trial. Ebrahimi S, Dabiri N, Jamshidnejad E, Sarkari B. Int J Dermatol 2007; 46: 215–7.

A topical solution of 10% silver nitrate applied to the warts on alternate days for 3 weeks in 30 patients resulted in complete clearance in 63% of patients after 6 weeks in the treatment group versus no healing in the placebo group.

Cryosurgical treatment of warts: dimethyl ether and propane versus liquid nitrogen: case report and review of the literature. Nguyen NV, Burkhart CG. J Drugs Dermatol 2011; 10: 1174–6.

Other coolants are probably less effective than liquid nitrogen.

Second-Line Therapies

• Cryotherapy with liquid nitrogen	B
• Cryotherapy in combination with salicylic acid	B

Cryotherapy versus salicylic acid for the treatment of plantar warts: a randomised controlled trial. Cockayne S, Hewitt C, Hicks K, Jayakody S, Kang'ombe AR, Stamuli E, et al. BMJ 2011; 342: d3271.

A study of 240 patients treated by health care professionals with liquid nitrogen, for up to four treatments, 2 to 3 weeks apart, was compared with patient self-treatment with 50% salicylic acid daily, for up to 8 weeks. Overall, 14% had complete clearance at 12 weeks, with no significant difference between the two groups.

A two-week interval is better than a three-week interval for reducing the recurrence rate of hand–foot viral warts after cryotherapy: a retrospective review of 560 hand–foot viral warts patients. Youn SH, Kwon IH, Park EJ, Kim KH, Kim KJ. Ann Dermatol 2011; 23: 53–60.

In a retrospective study with 560 patients, a 2-week interval was compared with a 3-week interval between cryotherapy with liquid nitrogen. For the 2- and 3-week groups, cure rates were 77% and 75%, respectively. Recurrence rates were 13% and 25%, and mean time to recurrence was 9.8 months and 6.9 months, respectively.

Two-week cryotherapy is optimal not only because of the rapid cure but also because of the lower recurrence rate.

Cryotherapy of common viral warts at intervals of 1, 2 and 3 weeks. Bourke JF, Berth-Jones J, Hutchinson PE. Br J Dermatol 1995; 132: 433–6.

This study carried out on 225 patients showed a 45% cure rate for warts treated with liquid nitrogen. The mean times to clearance of warts in each group were 5.5, 9.5, and 15 weeks in the weekly, 2- and 3-weekly groups, respectively. The mean numbers of treatments needed to achieve clearance were similar in each group (5.5, 4.75, and 5 treatments). The study showed that clearance of the warts was related to the number of treatments received, and it was independent of the interval between treatments.

Value of a second freeze–thaw cycle in cryotherapy of common warts. Berth-Jones J, Bourke J, Eglitis H, Harper C, Kirk P, Pavord S, et al. Br J Dermatol 1994; 131: 883–6.

In a randomized trial 300 patients received cryotherapy with either one or two freeze–thaw cycles at a 3-week interval. In addition, all subjects used keratolytic wart paints, and plantar warts were pared before freezing. At 3 months, the cure rate was 57% from the single freeze technique versus 62% from the double freeze technique. In plantar warts, the cure rate was 41% from single freezing and 65% for double freezing, whereas in the hand warts there was no additional benefit from the second freeze.

Liquid nitrogen and salicylic/lactic acid paint in the treatment of cutaneous warts in general practice. Steele K, Irwim WG. J R Coll Gen Pract 1988; 38: 256–8.

In this randomized study 207 patients with common hand warts and simple plantar warts were assigned to one of three treatment groups: cotton wool bud cryotherapy applied weekly, daily application of wart paint (lactic acid one part, salicylic acid one part, collodion four parts), or a combination of the two. Combination therapy cured 87% of common hand warts over a 6-week period and was significantly more effective than either agent used separately ($p < 0.05$). The results for simple plantar warts were disappointing, and no treatment regimen proved to be significantly better than any other.

Third-Line Therapies

Immunologic therapy

• Imiquimod	B
• Contact immunotherapy	
• Diphencyprone	B
• Squaric acid	D
• Topical BCG	D
• Intralesional immunotherapy	
• Candida	D
• MMR	D
• Cimetidine	D
• Zinc	
• Zinc oxide (topical)	A
• Zinc sulfate (intralesional)	B
• Zinc (oral)	B
• Interferon	B

Destructive therapies

• Cantharidin	D
• Glycolic acid	D
• Formic acid	B
• Monochloroacetic acid	B
• Trichloroacetic acid	B
• Hyperthermia	B
• Electrosurgery	B
• Pulsed dye laser	B
• Photodynamic therapy	A
• CO_2 laser	D
• Nd:YAG laser	D
• Er:YAG laser	D

Virucidal agents

• Formaldehyde	D
• Glutaraldehyde	B

Immunologic Therapy

Topical treatment of warts and mollusca with imiquimod. Hengge UR, Goos M. Ann Intern Med 2000; 132: 95.

In this trial, 65 patients with warts and molluscum were treated with 5% topical imiquimod and achieved 56% clearance of recalcitrant warts after 9.5 weeks of treatments. The frequency of imiquimod treatment was not stated by the authors.

Topical 5% imiquimod long-term treatment of cutaneous warts resistant to standard therapy modalities. Grussendorf-Conen EI, Jacobs S, Rübben A, Dethlefsen U. Dermatology 2002; 205: 139–45.

In this study, 10 of 37 (27%) patients cleared with imiquimod self-applied twice daily with mean duration of 19 weeks.

Investigations of the efficacy of diphenylcyclopropenone immunotherapy for the treatment of warts. Suh DW, Lew BL, Sim WY. Int J Dermatol 2014; 53: e567–71.

Patients were sensitized with 0.1% diphenylcyclopropenone (DPCP), and 2 weeks after sensitization, DPCP was applied to warts weekly. High clearance rates of 141/170 patients (82.9%) were achieved and 434/511 lesions (84.9%). Immunotherapy proved more effective in patients <20 years of age and for hand warts. The mean ± standard deviation number of applications was 9.02 ± 2.59. Side effects occurred in 36 patients, with blistering at the sensitized site being the most common. No serious adverse events occurred.

Diphencyprone immunotherapy for viral warts in immuno-suppressed patients. Audrain H, Siddiqui H, Buckley DA. Br J Dermatol 2013; 168: 1138–9.

Ten immunosuppressed patients and 28 immunocompetent patients with refractory warts were sensitized with 1% DCP, with a repeat application at 1 week. DCP was then applied to all warts at 2- to 4-week intervals. In the immunocompetent group, 27 patients (96%) cleared completely with a median of six treatments over 7 months. In the immunosuppressed group, six patients (60%) cleared completely with a median of 9.5 treatments over 9 months, and the remaining four also improved.

Does immunotherapy of viral warts provide beneficial effects when it is combined with conventional therapy? Choi JW, Cho S, Lee JH. Ann Dermatol 2011; 23: 282–7.

This study assessed the efficacy DCP as an adjunctive to cryotherapy. Retrospective chart review of 124 patients with warts showed that DCP may be a successful adjuvant to cryotherapy in reducing the number of cryotherapy sessions.

Squaric acid immunotherapy for warts in children. Silverberg NB, Lim JK, Paller AS, Mancini AJ. J Am Acad Dermatol 2000; 42: 803–8.

In this retrospective study, 61 children had their warts treated with home application of 0.2% squaric acid, 3 to 7 nights per week, for at least 3 months, after initial sensitization with 2% squaric acid on the forearm. Complete clearance after 7 weeks of this treatment occurred in 58% of patients, partial clearance occurred in 18%, and no response in 24%.

Treatment of common and plane warts in children with topical viable bacillus Calmette-Guerin. Salem A, Nofal A, Hosny D. Pediatr Dermatol 2013; 30: 60–3.

Topical BCG paste (containing 3 mg of salicylic acid, dissolved in 3 mL of glycerin) was applied to all warts in 40 children, weekly for maximum of 12 weeks. A control group of 40 children were treated with saline once weekly for same duration. Complete response occurred in 65% of children with common warts and 45% of plane warts with no response in the control group. A statistically significant difference was found between the active and control groups.

Intralesional *Candida* antigen immunotherapy for the treatment of recalcitrant and multiple warts in children. Muñoz Garza FZ, Roé Crespo E, Torres Pradilla M, Aguilera Peiró P, Baltá Cruz S, Hernández Ruiz ME, et al. Pediatr Dermatol 2015; 32: 797–801.

In this retrospective review, 220 children with refractory warts received three intralesional injections of 0.2 mL of *Candida albicans* antigen, one per visit, at 3-week intervals. Results showed that 156 (70.9%) had a complete response, 37 (16.8%) had a partial response, and 27 (12.2%) had no response. An average of 2.7 injections were required.

Two-year experience of using the measles, mumps and rubella vaccine as intralesional immunotherapy for warts. Na CH, Choi H, Song SH, Kim MS, Shin BS. Clin and Exp Dermatol 2014; 39: 583–9.

A retrospective study of 136 patients with various types of warts were treated for a total of six times at 2-week intervals. Thirty-six patients (26.5%) experienced complete resolution with an average of five treatments; 51.5% experienced >50% reduction in size and number of warts. Common warts showed statistically higher treatment response than other types of warts.

Cimetidine therapy for recalcitrant warts in adults: is it any better than placebo? Rogers CJ, Gibney MD, Siegfried EC, Harrison BR, Glaser DA. J Am Acad Dermatol 1999; 41: 123–7.

In this double-blind, placebo-controlled study, 70 patients with multiple viral warts were randomized to cimetidine 25 to 40 mg/kg daily or placebo for 3 months. Cimetidine was found to be no more effective than placebo.

Cimetidine therapy for recalcitrant warts in adults. Glass AT, Solomon BA. Arch Dermatol 1996; 132: 680–2.

In this prospective study, 20 patients received cimetidine 30 to 40 mg/kg/day. Complete resolution or a dramatic improvement was achieved in 84% of the 18 patients after 3 months.

Topical zinc oxide vs. salicylic acid-lactic acid combination in the treatment of warts. Khattar JA, Musharrafieh UM, Tamim H, Hamadeh GN. Int J Dermatol 2007; 46: 427–30.

Evidence Levels: **A** Double-blind study   **B** Clinical trial ≥ 20 subjects   **C** Clinical trial < 20 subjects   **D** Series ≥ 5 subjects   **E** Anecdotal case reports

In this double-blind trial, 44 patients were treated with either 20% zinc oxide ointment or 15% salicylic acid ointment + 15% lactic acid ointment combination, twice daily for 3 months. In the zinc oxide group, 50% patients were cured versus 42% with salicylic acid–lactic acid.

Topical zinc sulfate solution for treatment of viral warts. Sharqie KE, Khorhseed AA, Al-Nuaimy AA. Saudi Med J 2007; 28: 1418–21.

Topical zinc sulfate solution used three times daily for 4 weeks led to a higher cure rate than water placebo in a double-blind trial of 40 patients with plane warts and 50 patients with common warts. The cure rate appeared to be dependent on the concentration of zinc solution used and was better for plane than common warts. For plane warts, cure rates were 85.7% for 10% zinc sulfate (6/7 patients), 42.8% for 5% zinc sulfate (3/7 patients), and 10% for placebo 10% (1/10 patients). For common warts, cure rates were 11%, 5%, and 0%, respectively.

Treatment of viral warts by intralesional injection of zinc sulphate. Sharquie KA, Al-Nuaimy AA. Ann Saudi Med 2002; 22: 26–8.

One hundred patients with 623 warts were divided into two groups. In the treatment group, 53 patients had 173 warts treated with 2% zinc sulfate intralesionally, whereas 176 warts were left untreated as control. Within 6 weeks in the treatment group 98% of the warts cleared versus none in the control group.

Evaluation of oral zinc sulfate effect on recalcitrant multiple viral warts: a randomized placebo-controlled clinical trial. Yeghoobi R, Sadighha A, Baktash D. J Am Acad Dermatol 2009; 60: 706–8.

After 2 months of treatment with oral zinc sulfate (10 mg/kg to a maximum of 600 mg daily), 78% of patients cleared their warts (25/32) compared with 13% in the placebo group (3/23). The baseline serum zinc levels did not differ significantly between the two groups, but mean levels in both groups were low pretreatment.

Oral zinc sulfate for unresponsive cutaneous viral warts: too good to be true? A double-blind, randomized, placebo-controlled trial. López-Garcia DR, Gómez-Flores M, Arc-Mendoza AY, de la Fuente-Guarcia A, Ocampo-Candiani J. Clin Exp Dermatol 2009; 34: e984–5.

This double-blind randomized controlled trial (RCT) showed no difference between oral zinc sulfate and placebo.

Successful treatment of verruca plantaris with a single sublesional injection of interferon-α2a. Aksakal AA, Ozden MG, Atahan C, Onder M. Clin Exp Dermatol 2009; 34: 16–9.

In this placebo-controlled, single-blind study, 45 patients with a variety of hand or foot warts were treated with single-dose 4.5 MU IFN-α2a (three study arms) versus 8 controls treated with normal saline. As local anesthesia, liquid nitrogen was sprayed onto the injection site of the IFN group for 3 to 4 seconds. At 12-month follow-up 19/24 patients (79.2%) with single verruca plantaris cleared completely, whereas only 2/8 patients (25%) had partial response in the control group.

Destructive Therapies

Cantharidin treatment for recalcitrant facial flat warts: a preliminary study. Kartal Durmazlar SP, Atacan D, Eskioglu F. J Dermatolog Treat 2009; 20: 114–9.

A study of 15 patients with plane facial warts who were treated with cantharidin 0.7% solution applied for 4 to 6 hours, washed off, and repeated every 3 weeks. All 15 patients achieved clearance within 16 weeks with one to four treatments.

Glycolic acid 15% plus salicylic acid 2%: a new therapeutic pearl for facial flat warts. Rodríguez-Cerdeira C, Sánchez-Blanco E. Clin Aesthet Dermatol 2011; 4: 62–4.

All 20 patients who applied a fine layer of glycolic acid 15% and salicylic acid 2% gel to their warts once daily clinically were cured within 8 weeks.

A double blind, randomized trial of local formic acid puncture technique in the treatment of common warts. Faghihi G, Vali A, Radan M, Eslamieh G, Tajammoli S. Skinmed 2010; 8: 70–1.

In this trial, 34 patients applied 85% formic acid in distilled water solution on their warts on one side of the body and distilled water as placebo on the other side of the body every other day using a needle puncture technique. Follow-up occurred every 2 weeks for 3 months. Complete clearance was achieved in 91% of patients who received formic acid versus 10% in the placebo group.

Monochloroacetic acid application is an effective alternative to cryotherapy for common and plantar warts in primary care: a randomized controlled trial. Bruggink SC, Gussekloo J, Egberts PF, Bavinck JN, de Waal MW, Assendelft WJ, et al. J Invest Dermatol 2015; 135: 1261–7.

Patients were randomly allocated to monochloroacetic acid (MCA) versus liquid nitrogen cryotherapy every 2 weeks for common warts ($n = 188$) and MCA versus cryotherapy combined with daily salicylic acid (SA) self-application for patients with plantar warts ($n = 227$). MCA was found to be an effective alternative to cryotherapy for both types of warts with cure rates at 13 weeks comparable in all treatment groups. In the common wart group, cure rates were 43% for MCA and 54% for cryotherapy, and in the plantar wart group, cure rates were 46% for MCA and 39% for cryotherapy combined with SA.

Comparative study of topical 80% trichloroacetic acid with 35% trichloroacetic acid in the treatment of the common wart. Pezeshkpoor F, Banihashemi M, Yazdanpanah MJ, Yousefzadeh H, Sharghi M, Hoseinzadeh H. J Drugs Dermatol 2012; 11: e66–9.

In this single-blind study, 62 patients were randomly assigned to weekly treatment with TCA in two different concentrations until complete clearance for a maximum of 6 weeks. Fifty-five patients were included in the final analysis. With the higher concentration of TCA, 46.7% of patients cleared >75% warts versus 12% for the lower concentration.

Local hyperthermia at 44°C for the treatment of plantar warts: a randomized, patient-blinded, placebo-controlled trial. Huo W, Gao XH, Sun XP, Qi RQ, Hong Y, Mchepange UO, et al. J Infect Dis 2010; 201: 1169–72.

In this study, 54 patients had their warts treated with local hyperthermia of 44°C with an infrared-emitting source for 30 minutes a day for three consecutive days plus two additional days 2 weeks later. Within 3 months, 54% of patients in the treatment group were cured versus 12% in the control group.

Controlled localized heat therapy in cutaneous warts. Stern P, Levine N. Arch Dermatol 1992; 128: 945–8.

In this placebo-controlled, randomized trial, 13 patients had their 29 warts treated by a handheld radiofrequency heat generator device between one and four times for 30 to 60 seconds so that a temperature of 50°C was achieved in the warts. Complete clearance was achieved in 86% in the heat therapy group versus 41% in the control group.

Electrosurgery vs. 40% salicylic acid in the treatment of warts. Sudhakar Rao KM, Ankad BS, Naidu V, Sampaghavi VV, Unni MM, Aruna MS. J Clin Diagn Res 2012; 6: 81–4.

In this prospective randomized comparative study, 60 patients with viral warts received either electrosurgery or 40% salicylic acid (protocol or equipment not specified) and were followed up monthly for 6 months. Clearance rate with electrosurgery was 90% (27 out of 30 patients) versus 16.7% with salicylic acid (5 out of 30 patients).

Pulsed dye laser treatment for facial flat warts. Grilo W, Boixeda P, Ballester A, Miguel-Morrondo A, Truchuelo T, Jaén P. Dermatol Ther 2014; 27: 31–5.

In this prospective study, 32 patients were treated with pulsed dye laser (PDL) at 595-nm wavelength, a laser energy density of 9 or 14 J/cm^2 with a spot size of 7 or 5 mm, respectively, with air cooling and a pulse duration of 0.5 millisecond. Patients were treated in one to two sessions, 3 weeks apart, with one to three passes for each session. A complete response was noted in 14 patients (44%) and an excellent response in 18 patients (56%). There were only four recurrences at 1-year follow-up.

Pulsed-dye laser for recalcitrant viral warts: a retrospective case series of 227 patients. Sparreboom EE, Luijks HG, Luiting-Welkenhuyzen HA, Willems PW, Groeneveld CP, Bovenschen HJ. Br J Dermatol 2014; 171: 1270–3.

A retrospective study of 227 consecutive patients with recalcitrant warts (those that failed all available topical therapy and repetitive cryotherapy). Overall efficacy for PDL treatment was 86%. This was achieved with generally more powerful laser settings than in the previous literature. Up to six treatments with fluences of 12.5 to 15.0 J/cm^2 and treatment intervals of 3 to 4 weeks were recommended to achieve maximal treatment success.

Photodynamic therapy with 5-aminolaevulinic acid or placebo for recalcitrant foot and hand warts: randomized double-blind trial. Stender IM, Na R, Fogh H, Gluud C, Wulf HC. Lancet 2000; 335: 963–6.

Forty-five adults with refractory warts received ALA-PDT or placebo PDT and showed cure rates of 64/114 (56% of warts) and 47/113 (42% of warts), respectively, which was statistically significant ($p < 0.05$). All warts were also treated with paring and topical salicylic acid (Verucid).

Is the step-up therapy of topical 5-aminolevulinic acid photodynamic therapy effective and safe for the patients with recalcitrant facial flat wart? Quian G, Wang S, Deng D, Yang G. Dermatolog Ther 2014; 27: 83–8.

Step-up therapy of ALA-PDT was used on 30 patients in a maximum of three treatment sessions. Concentrations of ALA used were 5%, 10%, and 20%, and the treatment was increased at 2-weekly intervals if clearance was not achieved, to a maximum of three treatment sessions. The treatment response was good with 12 patients clearing completely after one session, 3 by two sessions, and 10 by the third session. Tolerance to ALA-PDT could improve with step-up therapy.

Successful treatment of recalcitrant warts in pediatric patients with carbon dioxide laser. Serour F, Somekh E. Eur J Pediatr Surg 2003; 13: 219–23.

In this case series, 40 children with 54 warts were treated with CO_2 laser ablation under local anesthesia. Healing time was 4 to 5 weeks, and there was no recurrence at 12 months. Hypopigmentation was noticed in 11 cases.

Combination of carbon dioxide laser therapy and artificial dermis application in plantar warts: human papilloma virus DNA analysis after treatment. Mitsuishi T, Sasagawa T, Kato T, Iida K, Ueno T, Ikeda M, et al. Dermatol Surg 2010; 36: 1401–5.

In 31 patients, CO_2 laser was used for ablation of 35 warts, and the defects were covered with artificial dermis. Follow-up periods ranged from 3 to 12 months. Complete clearance was achieved in 31/35 warts after one treatment. After complete remission, HPV DNA was not detected in the upper epidermis of the postoperative site.

Long-pulsed Nd:YAG laser treatment of warts: report on a series of 369 cases. Han TY, Lee JH, Lee CK, Ahn JY, Seo SJ, Hong CK. J Korean Med Sci 2009; 24: 889–93.

A 96% clearance rate of recalcitrant common, palmoplantar, and periungual warts was achieved in 369 patients treated with Nd:YAG laser over the course of a year.

Pulsed dye laser versus Nd:YAG in the treatment of plantar warts: a comparative study. El-Mohamady Ael-S, Mearag I, El-Khalawany M, Elshahed A, Shokeir H, Mahmoud A. Lasers Med Sci 2014; 29: 1111–6.

Forty-six subjects with multiple plantar warts were included in the study. In each patient, half the lesions were treated with Nd:YAG laser and half with PDL fortnightly for a maximum of six sessions. There was no significant difference between cure rates for PDL (73.9%) and Nd:YAG (78.3%), but Nd:YAG was more painful and associated with more complications.

Er:YAG laser followed by topical podophyllotoxin for hard to treat palmoplantar warts. Wollina U. J Cosmet Laser Ther 2003; 5: 35–7.

Complete resolution of warts was observed in 31/35 patients after treatment with Er:YAG laser, followed with topical podophyllotoxin for 3 days on, 4 days off, for up to six cycles.

Virucidal Treatments

Treatment of plantar warts in children. Vickers CF. BMJ 1961; 2: 743–5.

A study of 646 children with plantar warts showed that 3% formalin foot soaks to pared plantar warts for 15 to 20 minutes each night for 6 to 8 weeks cured 80% of the warts.

The U.S. National Toxicology Program (on June 10, 2011) described formaldehyde as "known to be a human carcinogen."

An assessment of methods of treating viral warts by comparative treatment trials based on a standard design. Bunney MH, Nolan MW, Williams DA. Br J Dermatol 1976; 94: 667–79.

In a study of 81 patients with mosaic plantar warts, buffered 10% glutaraldehyde solution was compared with salicylic acid (SA) paint. There was no significant difference between the efficacies for SA paint (44% cure) and glutaraldehyde (47% cure) at 12 weeks.

Topical treatment of resistant warts with glutaraldehyde. Hirose R, Hiro M, Shakuwa T, Udano M, Yamada M, Koide T, et al. J Dermatol 1994; 21: 248–53.

Evidence Levels: **A** Double-blind study **B** Clinical trial ≥ 20 subjects **C** Clinical trial < 20 subjects **D** Series ≥ 5 subjects **E** Anecdotal case reports

A cure rate of 72% was achieved in 25 patients treated topically with 20% glutaraldehyde solution. The treatment did not cause pain or permanent pigmented change.

Glutaraldehyde is suitable for home treatment, as there is no need for special instruments or special technique, and the cure rates are almost equal to those with cryotherapy.

Cutaneous necrosis secondary to topical treatment of wart with 20 p. 100 glutaraldehyde solution. Prigent F, Iborra C, Meslay C. Ann Dermatol Venereol 1996; 123: 644–6.

Case reports like this led to the withdrawal of a glutaraldehyde product from the market in France in December 1995.

Antiproliferative Agents

Wart treatment with anthralin. Flindt-Hansen H, Tikjob G, Brandrup F. Acta Derm Venereol 1984; 64: 177–9.

An RCT of dithranol 2% cream versus Verucid (11% SA, 4% lactic acid with copper) showed a higher cure rate for dithranol: 56% (15/27) versus 26% (8/31).

Treatment of plantar warts with elastoplast and podophyllin. Duthie DA, McCallum DI. BMJ 1951; 2: 216–8.

Forty patients with plantar warts were treated with podophyllin 25% in liquid paraffin under prolonged adhesive plaster occlusion, repeated at intervals of 1 to 2 weeks, and reported a clearance rate of 72.5% at 3 months.

A controlled trial on the use of topical 5-fluorouracil on viral warts. Hursthouse MW. Br J Dermatol 1975; 92: 93–5.

In this double-blind trial of 60 patients, 5-fluorouracil 5% cream was applied daily to hand or foot warts on one side of the body, whereas a placebo cream was applied on the other side of the body for 4 weeks. In the active group, 60% of patients cleared versus 17% in the placebo group.

Topical 5% 5-fluorouracil cream in the treatment of plantar warts: a prospective randomized and controlled clinical study. Salk RS, Grogan KA, Chang TJ. J Drugs Dermatol 2006; 5: 418–24.

In this study, 40 patients were treated either with 5-fluorouracil 5% with tape occlusion or tape occlusion alone with regular debridement for 12 weeks. In the active group 19/20 patients achieved complete cure versus 2 of 20 in the tape occlusion group.

Treatment of common warts with an intralesional mixture of 5-fluorouracil, lidocaine, and epinephrine: a prospective placebo-controlled, double-blind randomized trial. Yazdanafar A, Farshchian M, Fereydoonnejad M. Dermatol Surg 2008; 34: 656–9.

Forty patients were included in the study. A pair of warts on each subject was randomized to receive weekly intralesional 5-fluorouracil 4% (in combination with 2% lidocaine and 0.0125 mg/mL of epinephrine) or normal saline placebo. Sixty-five percent of warts cleared up with four injections compared with 35% in the placebo group.

Efficacy of intralesional bleomycin in palmo-plantar and periungual warts. Soni P, Khandelwal K, Aara N, Ghiya BC, Mehta RD, Bumb RA. J Cutan Aesthet Surg 2011; 4: 188–91.

Twenty-five patients were allocated to 0.1% intralesional bleomycin (1-mg/mL solution) or normal saline placebo fortnightly for maximum of two injections; 96% (82/85) of warts treated with

bleomycin cleared, whereas only 11% of warts (8/72) treated with placebo showed clearance at 3 months. Moderate pain was observed in both groups, and no patients experienced systemic toxicity.

Intralesional bleomycin in the treatment of cutaneous warts: a randomized clinical trial comparing it with cryotherapy. Dhar SB, Rashid MM, Islam A, Bhuiyan M. Indian J Dermatol Venereol Leprol 2009; 75: 262–7.

Eighty participants were randomized to cryotherapy (one to four sessions) versus 0.1% intralesional bleomycin injection. Treatments were 3-weekly, using one body side for each treatment and a maximum of four treatments. The clearance rates in context of number of patients and number of warts were 94.9% and 97% for bleomycin and 76.5% and 82% for cryotherapy respectively ($p < 0.05$ by x(2) analysis and RR = 7.67).

Recalcitrant warts and topical cidofovir: predictive factors of good response. Padilla España L, Del Boz J, Fernández-Morano T, Escudero-Santos I, Arenas-Villafranca J, de Troya M. J Eur Acad Dermatol Venereol 2016; 30: 1218–20.

A retrospective study of 126 immunocompetent patients treated with 3% or 1% cidofovir cream, with or without occlusion and once or twice a day, showed complete response in 67 (53.2%) and partial response in 35 (27.8%). Median duration of treatment was 12 weeks and median follow-up 7 months. Based on their results, the authors recommended using cidofovir 3% cream initially twice daily with occlusion for a period of 12 weeks.

Intralesional cidofovir for the treatment of multiple and recalcitrant cutaneous viral warts. Broganelli P, Chiaretta A, Fragnelli B, Bernengo MG. Dermatol Ther 2012; 25: 468–71.

In an open study, 288 patients were treated with monthly intralesional injections of cidofovir (15 mg/mL). Resolution of warts occurred in 98% of patients, with an average of 3.2 injections required.

The efficacy of duct tape vs. cryotherapy in the treatment of verruca vulgaris (the common wart). Focht DR, Spicer C, Fairchok MP. Arch Pediatr Adolesc Med 2002; 156: 971–4.

In this randomized study, 61 children and young adults received treatment with either cryotherapy with a 10-second freeze for a maximum of six treatments every 2 to 3 weeks or duct tape occlusion applied for 6.5 days every 7 days followed by debridement of the wart upon removal of tape for a maximum of 2 months. Complete resolution was achieved in 22/30 patients (71%) in the duct tape arm versus 15/31 (46%) in the cryotherapy group.

Efficacy of duct tape vs. placebo in the treatment of verruca vulgaris (warts) in primary school children. de Haen M, Spigt MG, van Uden CJT, van Neer P, Feron FJM, Knottnerus A. Arch Paediatr Adolesc Med 2006; 160: 1121–5.

No significant effect of duct tape occlusion.

Duct tape for the treatment of common warts in adults: a double blind randomized controlled trial. Wenner R, Askari SK, Cham PMH, Kedrowski DA, Liu A, Warshaw EM. Arch Dermatol 2007; 143: 309–13.

No difference between duct tape and moleskin occlusion.

Plantar warts treated with topical adapalene. Gupta R. Indian J Dermatol 2011; 56: 513–4.

All 118 warts cleared within 8 weeks in 10 patients treated with topical 0.1% adapalene gel after paring of warts. This was followed by occlusive dressing with a polythene sheet for 1 week and continued until the clearance of all the warts.

Treatment of extensive and recalcitrant viral warts with acitretin. Choi YL, Lee KJ, Kim WS, Lee DY, Lee JH, Lee ES, et al. Int J Dermatol 2006; 45: 480–2.

In one case report, oral acitretin 1 mg/kg/day achieved almost complete clearance of recalcitrant warts on the hands after 2 months, but relapse occurred after cessation of therapy at 1 month, which promptly improved with resumption of acitretin.

A double-blind, randomized, placebo-controlled trial of oral isotretinoin in the treatment of recalcitrant facial flat warts. Olguin-Garcia MG, Jurado-Santa Cruz F, Peralta-Pedrero ML, Morales-Sánchez MA. J Dermatol Treat 2015; 26: 78–82.

Isotretinoin 30 mg/day or placebo was administered to 16 and 15 patients, respectively, for 12 weeks. All patients in the active treatment group showed complete resolution of warts versus no improvement in the placebo group ($p = 0.0001$). The most frequent adverse event was cheilitis. The patients did not undergo follow-up to assess for recurrence after the study ended.

Treatment of plane warts with a low-dose oral isotretinoin. Al-Hammy HR, Salman HA, Abdulsattar NA. ISRN Dermatol 2012; 2012:163929.

An open study of 26 child and adult patients with facial plane flat warts reported 73% clearance after 2 months of treatment with isotretinoin 0.5 mg/kg/day.

Complementary and Alternative Therapies

Effects of hypnotic, placebo, and salicylic acid treatments on wart regression. Spanos NP, Williams V, Gwynn MI. Psychosom Med 1990; 52: 109–14.

A randomized study comparing hypnosis with salicylic acid, control (no treatment), and placebo (base carrier from SA) showed a greater effect with hypnosis at 6-week follow-up, but the numbers were small (only 10 patients per group).

The successful treatment of flat warts with auricular acupuncture. Ning S, Li F, Qian L, Xu D, Huang Y, Xiao M, et al. Int J Dermatol 2012; 51: 211–5.

This single-blind, randomized study compared weekly auricular acupuncture with tretinoin 0.1% ointment nightly for 10 weeks. Overall, 53% (16/30) of patients treated with acupuncture cleared, compared with 3% (1 of 30) in the tretinoin group.

Oral supplementation with a nutraceutical containing echinacea, methionine and antioxidant/immunostimulating compounds in patients with cutaneous viral warts. Cassano N, Ferrari A, Fai D, Pettinato M, Pellé S, Del Brocco L, et al. G Ital Dermatol Venereol 2011; 146: 191–5.

The aim of this open-label study was to determine the effects of nutraceutical oral supplementation containing methionine, echinacea, zinc, and probiotics on the response of cutaneous warts to conventional standard therapy with salicylic and lactic acids or cryotherapy with liquid nitrogen. All 172 eligible patients were allocated to conventional standard therapy alone or combined conventional standard therapy with nutraceutical oral supplementation for 4 months. Complete remission was achieved in 55% of patients in the conventional standard therapy group versus 86% in the conventional standard therapy and oral supplementation group at 6 months' follow-up.

Evidence Levels: **A** Double-blind study **B** Clinical trial ≥ 20 subjects **C** Clinical trial < 20 subjects **D** Series ≥ 5 subjects **E** Anecdotal case reports

253

Vitiligo

John Harris, Mehdi Rashighi

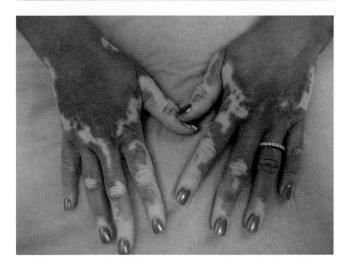

Vitiligo is a common autoimmune disease of the skin resulting from the destruction of epidermal melanocytes by cytotoxic CD8+ T cells. It presents with multiple white macules and patches, which can significantly affect patients' self-esteem and quality of life.

Vitiligo is estimated to affect about 1% to 2% of the population, regardless of gender and ethnicity (more than 3 million individuals in the United States). Existing treatments are non-targeted, time consuming, and offer moderate efficacy. With the exception of *monobenzone cream* (monobenzyl ether of hydroquinone), which is used to permanently depigment unaffected skin in patients with widespread vitiligo, there are currently no Food and Drug Administration (FDA)–approved medical treatments, and so management is primarily through the use of off-label therapies.

MANAGEMENT STRATEGY

The mainstay of treatment in vitiligo is *topical immunosuppressives* and *phototherapy*. Multiple factors, including disease extent, activity, and distribution, should be considered when developing a management strategy in each patient. These treatments may be less effective in patients with the segmental variant of vitiligo, which is characterized by rapid progression of depigmentation in a unilateral distribution, which then stabilizes and remains confined to this focal area.

Vitiligo is not a life-threatening condition; patients may therefore decline treatment. However, early and aggressive treatment is associated with better outcomes, which should be addressed with each patient. Regardless, education about the disease and psychological support should be offered to all patients. For treatment purposes, vitiligo patients are generally classified into two groups: patients with limited body surface area (BSA) involvement and patients with more widespread disease.

Segmental Vitiligo and Limited Vitiligo

First-line treatment in patients with limited body involvement, including segmental vitiligo, is treatment with *potent topical steroids* (clobetasol propionate 0.05%) and/or *calcineurin inhibitors* (tacrolimus 0.3%–0.1% or pimecrolimus 1%). Weaker steroids have not demonstrated efficacy in clinical trials, and thus potent steroids are preferred. Steroids are slightly more effective than calcineurin inhibitors in head-to-head studies; however, the potential side effects limit prolonged use, especially in areas such as the face, genitals, axillae and breasts. One common strategy is to use both steroids and topical calcineurin inhibitors in an alternating schedule. This can be achieved by application of steroids twice daily for 1 week, followed by calcineurin inhibitors twice daily for the next week, and continued in this way through an alternating weekly schedule. For sensitive areas like the face, genitals, axillae, and breasts, use of calcineurin inhibitors without steroids is preferred.

Targeted *phototherapy devices* (excimer laser or monochromatic lamp), which deliver light in the UVB range (peak at 308 nm), can be considered a second-line option in patients who do not respond to topical treatments. Sessions are typically administered two or three times per week and continued for at least 3 months before deciding whether the patient is responsive to the treatment or not.

Surgical procedures can be considered in a minority of carefully selected patients with highly stable disease (at least 6 months without worsening of the existing lesions or development of new lesions) and have the best outcome in patients with the segmental variant. The main concept of this treatment is to transfer healthy melanocytes from nonlesional skin to the affected area within the same patient (autologous transplant). There are multiple different techniques to achieve this, including punch grafting, epidermal blister grafting, and cellular grafts, each with advantages and disadvantages. Epidermal cellular suspension transplant, however, is usually considered to provide the best outcome. Regardless of the technique being used, surgical procedures are contraindicated in patients with unstable disease or evidence of the Koebner phenomenon.

Widespread Disease (>3% BSA)

Phototherapy with *narrowband UVB* (NB-UVB) is considered the first-line treatment in patients with widespread disease and has largely replaced older phototherapy protocols. NB-UVB has been shown to be at least as effective as PUVA therapy with better color match, less risk of burning, and lower risk of skin cancer. Treatment should be delivered two or three sessions per week for at least 3 months and then continued for several additional months in patients who respond.

The decision to deliver two or three phototherapy sessions per week is usually based on patient compliance and personal preference. A three-session-per-week schedule induces a more rapid response; however, there is probably no significant difference between the two schedules in terms of the extent of repigmentation achieved after a prolonged period. NB-UVB therapy can be combined with topical steroids or calcineurin inhibitors to improve the treatment efficacy, especially in limited areas that might be cosmetically more important to patients.

Systemic corticosteroids may be indicated to arrest disease activity in patients with highly progressive disease, before other therapies have time to demonstrate efficacy. This is usually delivered as pulse therapy (4 mg dexamethasone on Saturday and Sunday or alternate-day doses of 20 mg prednisone, e.g.) to reduce the risk of side effects.

Surgical procedures may be considered to treat selected areas with high cosmetic impact that do not respond to medical treatment. However, this should be reserved for stable lesions, particularly in those with segmental vitiligo, and only in patients with no evidence of koebnerization.

Maintenance Therapy

Relapse of disease is common after discontinuation of treatment. Tacrolimus 0.1% applied twice weekly may prevent relapse in patients and thus be a reasonable approach to maintenance therapy.

Emerging Treatments

Afamelanotide is a potent synthetic analog of α-melanocyte stimulating hormone (α-MSH), a naturally occurring neuropeptide that stimulates melanogenesis. Recently a small trial reported that a combination of afamelanotide with NB-UVB therapy may promote faster and more extensive repigmentation compared with phototherapy alone.

Janus kinase (JAK) inhibitors comprise a new class of drugs that selectively inhibit enzymes involved in signal transduction of several cytokines, including IFN-γ. Recently two patients with widespread vitiligo were reported to demonstrate significant repigmentation after being treated with two different oral JAK inhibitors, tofacitinib and ruxolitinib. Further studies are needed to determine whether this class of drugs is a safe and effective option in vitiligo treatment.

Pseudocatalase is a cream that is proposed to work as a topical oxygen radical scavenger in the skin. Consistent with a proposed role for elevated levels of melanocyte stress in vitiligo pathogenesis, studies have shown that there is an increased level of hydrogen peroxide (H_2O_2) in lesional skin of vitiligo patients. A small number of studies from a single investigator have reported that pseudocatalase may enhance repigmentation when combined with NB-UVB phototherapy; however, others have been unable to reproduce these results, and larger independent studies are needed to confirm these observations.

> ### Specific Investigation
>
> - Screening for associated autoimmune diseases

Vitiligo is a clinical diagnosis, and a skin biopsy is rarely necessary. Patients with vitiligo generally have a higher incidence of other autoimmune diseases, including thyroiditis, type 1 diabetes, lupus, alopecia areata, Addison disease, and pernicious anemia. However, the majority of patients do not have any accompanying autoimmune disease, and directed medical history and physical examination are sufficient to identify high-risk individuals who require further evaluation.

Low yield of routine screening for thyroid dysfunction in asymptomatic patients with vitiligo. Kroon MW, Joore IC, Wind BS, Leloup MA, Wolkerstorfer A, Luiten RM, et al. Br J Dermatol 2012; 166: 532–8.

Thyroid function tests and anti-TPO antibody titers were assessed in 434 patients with nonsegmental vitiligo. The overall

prevalence of thyroid dysfunction was higher than reported in the general population. However, most patients had symptoms indicative of thyroid dysfunction and had been already diagnosed by their general practitioners. Moreover, in the majority of these patients thyroid involvement preceded the onset of vitiligo. Thyroid disease was found mostly among older women and in subjects with a positive family history of thyroid disease. Thus a thorough review of systems for signs of thyroid disease is sufficient, and routine screening is not necessary.

> ### First-Line Therapies
>
> #### Segmental vitiligo or limited vitiligo
> - Topical corticosteroids and/or calcineurin inhibitors   **A**
>
> #### Widespread vitiligo (>3% BSA)
> - NB-UVB ± topical corticosteroids or calcineurin inhibitors   **A**

Effectiveness of 0.1% topical tacrolimus in adult and children patients with vitiligo. Udompataikul M, Boonsupthip P, Siriwattanagate R. J Dermatol 2011; 38: 536–40.

Forty-two patients (22 adults and 20 children) were enrolled. Tacrolimus 0.1% ointment was given twice daily for 6 months. The response rate was 76%. Children had approximately nine times better response than adults. Better response was found in patients with disease duration of 5 years or less.

A double-blind randomized trial of 0.1% tacrolimus vs. 0.05% clobetasol for the treatment of childhood vitiligo. Lepe V, Moncada B, Castanedo-Cazares JP, Torres-Alvarez MB, Ortiz CA, Torres-Rubalcava AB. Arch Dermatol 2003; 139: 581–5.

Twenty patients with vitiligo were treated for 2 months: 90% experienced some repigmentation. Repigmentation was 49.3% for clobetasol and 41.3% for tacrolimus. Tacrolimus is almost as effective as clobetasol and is better for sensitive areas (eyelids) because it does not cause skin atrophy.

Randomized double-blind trial of treatment of vitiligo: efficacy of psoralen-UV-A therapy vs. narrowband-UV-B therapy. Yones SS, Palmer RA, Garibaldinos TM, Hawk JL. Arch Dermatol 2007; 143: 643–6.

Fifty-six patients with nonsegmental vitiligo were enrolled into this randomized, double-blind, comparative trial. At the end of therapy, 64% of patients in the NB-UVB group showed greater than 50% improvement in BSA affected compared with 36% in the PUVA group. The color match of the repigmented skin was excellent in all patients in the NB-UVB group but in only 44% of those in the PUVA group ($p < 0.001$). In patients who completed 48 sessions, the improvement in BSA affected by vitiligo was greater with NB-UVB therapy than with PUVA therapy ($p = 0.007$). Twelve months after the cessation of therapy, the superiority of NB-UVB tended to be maintained.

Treatment of vitiligo with narrowband-UVB (TL01) combined with tacrolimus ointment (0.1%) vs. placebo ointment, a randomized right/left double-blind comparative study. Nordal EJ, Guleng GE, Rönnevig JR. J Eur Acad Dermatol Venereol 2011; 25: 1440–3.

Evidence Levels: **A** Double-blind study **B** Clinical trial ≥ 20 subjects **C** Clinical trial < 20 subjects **D** Series ≥ 5 subjects **E** Anecdotal case reports

Whole-body NB-UVB was given twice or thrice weekly for at least 3 months. Forty patients were studied. Twenty-seven patients had a better effect on the tacrolimus side. Combination of NB-UVB and tacrolimus ointment (0.1%) was more effective than UV treatment alone.

The efficacy of pimecrolimus 1% cream plus narrow-band ultraviolet B in the treatment of vitiligo: a double-blind, placebo-controlled clinical trial. Esfandiarpour I, Ekhlasi A, Farajzadeh S, Shamsadini S. J Dermatol Treat 2008; 16: 1–5.

This study involved 68 patients. A combination of NB-UVB with pimecrolimus induced better pigmentation of facial lesions than did NB-UVB alone (64.3% vs. 25.1%).

Combining UV phototherapies with topical immunosuppressants carries a theoretical risk of enhancing carcinogenesis.

Maintenance therapy of adult vitiligo with 0.1% tacrolimus ointment: a randomized, double blind, placebo-controlled study. Cavalie M, Ezzedine K, Fontas E, Montaudie H, Castela E, Bahadoran P, et al. J Invest Dermatol 2015; 135: 970–4.

Thirty-five vitiligo patients with 71 therapeutically repigmented lesions were enrolled in a controlled trial. Patients were randomly assigned to receive placebo or treatment. Twice-weekly application of 0.1% tacrolimus ointment was found to be effective in preventing relapse in previously successfully repigmented lesions.

Second-Line Therapies	
Segmental vitiligo or limited vitiligo	
• Targeted phototherapy devices (excimer laser or monochromatic lamp)	A
Widespread vitiligo (>3% BSA)	
• Systemic corticosteroids (oral minipulse therapy)	B

Vitiligo treatment with monochromatic excimer light (MEL) and tacrolimus: results of an open randomized controlled study. Nisticó S, Chiricozzi A, Saraceno R, Schipani C, Chimenti S. Photomed Laser Surg 2012; 30: 26–30.

Fifty-three patients with vitiligo were enrolled. Combination treatment of 0.1% tacrolimus ointment (once daily) plus 308-nm MEL (twice per week) and 308-nm MEL monotherapy for 12 weeks are both effective and safe for the treatment of vitiligo. The combination of topical immunomodulators could enhance the clinical response in vitiligo, especially in resistant sites.

The efficacy of 308-nm excimer laser/light (EL) and topical agent combination therapy versus EL monotherapy for vitiligo: a systematic review and meta-analysis of randomized controlled trials (RCTs). Bae JM, Hong BY, Lee JH, Lee JH, Kim GM. J Am Acad Dermatol 2016; 74: 907–15.

Eight randomized controlled trials comprising a total of 425 patches/patients that assessed the efficacy of EL alone or in combination with topical treatments were analyzed. Topical calcineurin inhibitors in conjunction with EL were found to be more effective in treating vitiligo compared with EL alone.

Efficacy and safety of 308-nm monochromatic excimer lamp versus other phototherapy devices for vitiligo: a systematic

review with meta-analysis. Lopes C, Trevisani VF, Melnik T. Am J Clin Dermatol 2016; 17: 23–32.

Six randomized controlled trials comprising a total of 411 patients/764 lesions that compared the efficacy of monochromatic excimer lamp versus excimer laser and NB-UVB were analyzed. These three modalities were all found to be safe and effective in treating vitiligo, and no significant differences were found among them.

Combination therapy with 308-nm excimer laser, topical tacrolimus, and short-term systemic corticosteroids for segmental vitiligo: a retrospective study of 159 patients. Bae JM, Yoo HJ, Kim H, Lee JH, Kim GM. J Am Acad Dermatol 2015; 73: 76–82.

A retrospective interventional case-series study was performed on 159 patients with segmental vitiligo to assess the effectiveness of combination therapy with 308-nm excimer laser, topical tacrolimus, and short-term systemic corticosteroids. The combination therapy was found to be effective, and prolonged disease duration, poliosis, and plurisegmental subtype were shown to be independent prognostic factors of poor response to the treatment.

Randomized controlled trial comparing the effectiveness of 308-nm excimer laser alone or in combination with topical hydrocortisone 17-butyrate cream in the treatment of vitiligo of the face and neck. Sassi F, Cazzaniga S, Tessari G, Chatenoud L, Reseghetti A, Marchesi L, et al. Br J Dermatol 2008; 159: 1186–91.

Eighty-four patients were treated with 308-nm excimer laser twice weekly alone or in combination with topical hydrocortisone 17-butyrate cream twice daily for 3 weeks. A total of 16.6% patients in the excimer monotherapy group and 42.8% in the combination group showed 75% or more reduction of vitiligo lesions at 12 weeks.

Randomized, parallel group trial comparing home-based phototherapy with institution-based 308 excimer lamp for the treatment of focal vitiligo vulgaris. Tien Guan ST, Theng C, Chang A. J Am Acad Dermatol 2015; 72: 733–5.

Forty-four patients with stable focal vitiligo were randomized to receive either three-times-a-week, home-based phototherapy or twice-a-week excimer laser in the clinic. Patients who received the home-based phototherapy were found to have a better response, primarily due to a higher compliance to the treatment.

Intrapatient comparison of 308-nm monochromatic excimer light and localized narrow-band UVB phototherapy in the treatment of vitiligo: a randomized controlled trial. Verhaeghe E, Lodewick E, van Geel N, Lambert J. Dermatology 2011; 223: 343–8.

Eleven patients participated in this prospective, intrapatient, placebo-controlled, randomized trial. In each patient, three lesions were selected and treated with 308-nm excimer light, localized 311-nm NB-UVB, or placebo during 24 sessions. NB-UVB efficacy was found to be superior to excimer laser in inducing repigmentation.

A randomized comparative study of oral corticosteroid minipulse and low-dose oral methotrexate in the treatment of unstable vitiligo. Singh H, Kumaran MS, Bains A, Parsad D. Dermatology 2015; 231: 286–90.

Fifty-two patients with unstable vitiligo were enrolled in a prospective open-label noninferiority study and randomly assigned to oral methotrexate (10 mg weekly) or oral minipulse dexamethasone (2.5 mg on two consecutive days in a week) for 24 weeks. Both drugs were found to be equally effective in controlling the disease activity.

Third-Line Therapies

Segmental vitiligo or limited vitiligo

- Surgical treatment (autologous melanocyte transplant)   **A**

Widespread vitiligo (>3% BSA)

- Surgical treatment (autologous melanocyte transplant)   **A**
- Monobenzyl ether of hydroquinone   **C**

A systematic review of autologous transplantation methods in vitiligo. Njoo MD, Westerhof W, Bos JD, Bossuyt PM. Arch Dermatol 1998; 134: 1543–9.

Sixty-three studies were analyzed: 16 on minigrafting, 13 on split-thickness grafting, 15 on grafting of epidermal blisters, 17 on grafting of cultured melanocytes, and 2 on grafting of noncultured epidermal suspension. The highest success rates were achieved with split-skin grafting and epidermal blister grafting.

Treatment of vitiligo by transplantation of cultured pure melanocyte suspension: analysis of 120 cases. Chen YF, Yang PY, Hu DN, Kuo FS, Hung CS, Hung CM. J Am Acad Dermatol 2004; 51: 68–74.

A total of 120 patients were treated with transplantation of autologous cultured pure melanocyte suspension after CO_2 laser abrasion. Overall, 90% to 100% coverage was achieved in 84% of patients with stable localized vitiligo and in 54% of patients with stable generalized vitiligo, but only 14% of patients with active generalized vitiligo achieved good repigmentation.

Repigmentation of vitiligo with punch grafting and narrow-band UV-B (311 nm) – a prospective study. Lahiri K, Malakar S, Sarma N, Banerjee U. Int J Dermatol 2006; 45: 649–55.

Punch grafts were used to treat 66 patients with stable refractory vitiligo in different regions, followed by NB-UVB. Successful pigmentation was achieved in 86.36% of cases.

Comparison of minipunch grafting versus split-skin grafting in chronic stable vitiligo. Khandpur S, Sharma VK, Manchanda Y. Dermatol Surg 2005; 31: 436–41.

Sixty-four patients with stable vitiligo were involved. Grafting was followed by PUVAsol. Split-skin grafting gave much better repigmentation and cosmetic matching than minipunch grafting (83.3% of patients vs. 44.1%).

Subjective and objective evaluation of noncultured epidermal cellular grafting for repigmenting vitiligo. van Geel N, Vander Haeghen Y, Vervaet C, Naeyaert JM, Ongenae K. Dermatology 2006; 213: 23–9.

Noncultured autologous melanocytes and keratinocytes were used to treat 40 patients with stable refractory vitiligo: 70% or more repigmentation was noted in 62% of patients.

Epidermal grafting in vitiligo: influence of age, site of lesion, and type of disease on outcome. Gupta S, Kumar B. J Am Acad Dermatol 2003; 49: 99–104.

This was a retrospective, uncontrolled case series and literature review of suction blister epidermal grafting in patients with stable and recalcitrant vitiligo. The procedure outcome was found to be significantly better in segmental/focal vitiligo than in the generalized type and in individuals <20 years of age. However, unlike in medical therapies, localization of the vitiligo patch did not appear to influence the treatment outcome significantly.

The additive effect of excimer laser on noncultured melanocyte-keratinocyte transplantation for the treatment of vitiligo: a clinical trial in an Iranian population. Ebadi A, Rad MM, Nazari S, Fesharaki RJ, Ghalamkarpour F, Younespour S. J Eur Acad Dermatol Venereol 2015; 29: 745–51.

Thirty-nine patches from 10 patients with stable generalized vitiligo were enrolled in a nonrandomized comparative trial. Application of two to three times weekly excimer laser (308 nm) for 24 sessions, starting 2 weeks after transplant procedure, significantly increased the pigmentation rate in the treated areas.

Surgical interventions for vitiligo: an evidence-based review. Mulekar SV, Isedeh P. Br J Dermatol 2013; 169 (Suppl 3): 57–66.

A systematic literature review of studies reporting on vitiligo surgical therapies found that the split-thickness skin grafts had the highest repigmentation success rate compared with the other surgical methods, including punch/minigraft, blister roof grafting, cultured, and noncultured cellular transplantation. Overall, postoperative complications included milia, scarring, cobblestone appearance, or hyperpigmentation of treated areas.

A randomized comparison of excimer laser versus narrow-band ultraviolet B phototherapy after punch grafting in stable vitiligo patients. Linthorst Homan MW, Spuls PI, Nieuweboer-Krobotova L, de Korte J, Sprangers MA, Bos JD, et al. J Eur Acad Dermatol Venereol 2012; 26: 690–5.

Fourteen patients were treated with the punch-grafting technique on two symmetric vitiligo patches. Starting 1 week after the punch grafting, the vitiligo patches were treated twice weekly with either 308-nm excimer laser or NB-UVB. No difference was found in repigmentation rate between the two methods, but patients were significantly more satisfied with NB-UVB, primarily due to a more rapid response.

Comparison between autologous noncultured epidermal cell suspension and suction blister epidermal grafting in stable vitiligo: a randomized study. Budania A, Parsad D, Kanwar AJ, Dogra S. Br J Dermatol 2012; 167: 1295–1301.

Forty-one patients with 54 stable vitiligo lesions were randomized to receive either autologous noncultured epidermal cell suspension (NCES) or suction blister epidermal grafting (SBEG). The follow-up evaluation 16 weeks after surgery indicated that NCES was superior to SBEG in terms of the extent of repigmentation and improvement in the Dermatology Life Quality Index.

A randomized controlled study of the effects of different modalities of narrow-band ultraviolet B therapy on the outcome of cultured autologous melanocytes transplantation in treating vitiligo. Zhang DM, Hong WS, Fu LF, Wei XD, Xu AE. Dermatol Surg 2014; 40: 420–6.

Four hundred thirty-seven patients undergoing cultured autologous melanocyte transplantation were randomly assigned to receive NB-UVB therapy before and/or after the procedure. Combination

Evidence Levels: **A** Double-blind study   **B** Clinical trial ≥ 20 subjects   **C** Clinical trial < 20 subjects   **D** Series ≥ 5 subjects   **E** Anecdotal case reports

of transplantation with NB-UVB therapy both before and after the procedure resulted in the best treatment response.

Comparison between autologous noncultured extracted hair follicle outer root sheath cell suspension and autologous noncultured epidermal cell suspension in the treatment of stable vitiligo: a randomized study. Singh C, Parsad D, Kanwar AJ, Dogra S, Kumar R. Br J Dermatol 2013; 169: 287–93.

Thirty patients with 47 stable vitiligo lesions were randomized to receive either autologous noncultured "epidermal cell suspension" or "extracted hair follicle outer root sheath cell suspension." Both techniques were found to be safe and effective in inducing repigmentation with comparable efficacy.

Monobenzyl ether of hydroquinone. Moser D, Parrish J, Fitzpatrick T. Br J Dermatol 1977; 97: 669–79.

In eighteen patients treated with monobenzyl ether of hydroquinone therapy twice daily over a 1-year period, eight achieved complete depigmentation and three had marked depigmentation. The depigmentation was permanent. Side effects were erythema, pruritus, and contact dermatitis.

Emerging Treatments

Tofacitinib citrate for the treatment of vitiligo: a pathogenesis-directed therapy. Craiglow BG, King BA. JAMA Dermatol 2015; 151: 1110–2.

This is the first report of a vitiligo patient being successfully treated by an oral JAK inhibitor. The patient was initiated on oral tofacitinib, a JAK 1/3 inhibitor, 5 mg every other day for 3 weeks, which was later increased to 5 mg daily. Five months after starting the treatment the patient showed significant repigmentation on her forehead and hands.

Rapid skin repigmentation on oral ruxolitinib in a patient with coexistent vitiligo and alopecia areata (AA). Harris JE, Rashighi M, Nguyen N, Jabbari A, Ulerio G, Clynes R, et al. J Am Acad Dermatol 2016; 74: 370–1.

A patient with coexistent vitiligo and AA was initiated on 20 mg twice daily of oral ruxolitinib, a JAK 1/2 inhibitor. Twelve weeks after starting the treatment, the patient noted some repigmentation on his face in addition to scalp hair regrowth. At week 20, the patient exhibited substantial repigmentation on his face and other areas. Twelve weeks after discontinuing ruxolitinib, although his hair regrowth was maintained, much of the regained pigment had regressed.

Afamelanotide and narrowband UV-B phototherapy for the treatment of vitiligo: a randomized multicenter trial. Lim HW, Grimes PE, Agbai O, Hamzavi I, Henderson M, Haddican M, et al. JAMA Dermatol 2015; 151: 42–50.

Fifty-five patients with generalized vitiligo were randomized to NB-UVB therapy or NB-UVB in combination with afamelanotide, an analog of α–melanocyte-stimulating hormone. Monthly subcutaneous implantation of 16 mg of afamelanotide resulted in a significantly superior and faster repigmentation compared with NB-UVB monotherapy, especially in patients with darker skin type.

From basic research to the bedside: efficacy of topical treatment with pseudocatalase PC-KUS in 71 children with vitiligo. Schallreuter KU, Krüger C, Würfel BA, Panske A, Wood JM. Int J Dermatol 2008; 47: 743–53.

This was an uncontrolled retrospective study to assess the efficacy of topical NB-UVB–activated pseudocatalase. Seventy-one children with vitiligo were included. The majority of patients exhibited at least 75% repigmentation on their face, neck, and trunk, but the treatment was not effective on the hands or feet.

Vulvodynia

Yasaman Mansouri

Vulvodynia is defined as "vulvar pain of at least 3 months' duration, without clear identifiable cause, which may have potential associated factors." This new terminology was formed in 2015 by a consensus among international expert societies. Typical symptoms are burning, stinging, rawness, irritation, and associated dyspareunia. Vulvodynia can be further described as localized (e.g., vestibulodynia, clitorodynia) or generalized, provoked (elicited by contact), spontaneous, or mixed. Onset may be primary (present since the patient's first episode of vaginal penetration) or secondary (after a period of pain-free activities). Localized provoked vulvodynia is the most common subtype. Vulvodynia is a common condition that is poorly understood. The pathogenesis is likely multifactorial and may involve genetic predisposition, hormonal factors, pelvic floor muscle dysfunction, inflammation, and immune factors. Other pain conditions such as interstitial cystitis, fibromyalgia, temporomandibular joint disorder, or irritable bowel syndrome may occur in the same patient.

Vulvodynia can be distressing to patients, and clinicians are often not familiar and comfortable in managing this disease.

MANAGEMENT STRATEGY

Vulvodynia is a diagnosis of exclusion. Thorough physical examination and appropriate laboratory testing should be performed to exclude other etiologies of pain, including infections, dermatoses, endometriosis, and neurologic conditions (e.g., herpes neuralgia, spinal nerve compression). A complete evaluation should include detailed pain, medical, surgical, and sexual histories and psychological assessment.

Treatment is challenging, and despite its prevalence, most treatments for vulvodynia are not well studied and are largely based on expert opinion and uncontrolled studies. The therapeutic approach should be individualized and multidisciplinary, including dermatology, gynecology, physical therapy, and psychology. No single treatment is effective in all women, and many therapies are often tried before relief is achieved. Noninvasive treatments are often tried first, including topical lidocaine, pelvic floor physical therapy, antidepressants, and anticonvulsants. Combining treatments may be beneficial. Surgical interventions are reserved for women refractory to other modalities and are not considered first-line due to their invasive nature. However, high success rates have been reported with vestibulectomy, which can be considered in patients with localized disease.

Specific Investigations

- Visual and manual examination of the vulva, vagina, oral cavity, skin, scalp, and nails
- Assessment of pelvic floor musculature
- Palpation of inguinal lymph nodes
- Cotton swab testing of entire genital region, including vulval vestibule for point tenderness
- Tampon test
- Wet mount of vaginal secretions (*Trichomonas vaginalis*, bacterial vaginosis)
- pH assessment of vaginal secretions (bacterial vaginosis, atrophic vaginitis, inflammatory vaginitis)
- KOH microscopic examination (fungi, scabies)
- Microbiologic cultures (bacterial, yeast, viral)
- Papanicolaou smear (in select cases)
- Colposcopy of vulva (in select cases)
- Biopsy, if lesion present
- Patch testing (allergic contact dermatitis)
- Psychological evaluation

Current concepts in vulvodynia with a focus on pathogenesis and pain mechanisms. Thornton AM, Drummond C. Australas J Dermatol 2016; 57: 253–63.

This review article discusses the possible pathogenesis of vulvodynia and assessment of patients and proposes a therapeutic ladder.

Vulvodynia: assessment and treatment. Goldstein AT, Pukall CF, Brown C, Bergeron S, Stein A, Kellogg-Spadt S. J Sex Med 2016; 13: 572–90.

Comprehensive review of evaluation of vulvodynia patients with suggested treatment options.

2013 vulvodynia guideline update. Stockdale CK, Lawson HW. J Low Genit Tract Dis 2014; 18: 93–100.

This article reviews clinical diagnosis and therapeutic approaches.

Impact of a multidisciplinary vulvodynia program on sexual functioning and dyspareunia. Brotto LA, Yong P, Smith KB, Sadownik LA. J Sex Med 2015; 12: 238–47.

This study evaluated the efficacy of a multidisciplinary program in 132 patients. Treatments included educational seminars, psychological skills training, pelvic floor physiotherapy, and gynecologic management. Results showed significant reduction in dyspareunia and sex-related distress.

Women with provoked vestibulodynia experience clinically significant reductions in pain regardless of treatment: results from a 2-year follow-up study. Davis SN, Bergeron S, Binik YM, Lambert B. J Sex Med 2013; 10: 3080–7.

In this secondary analysis of a prospective study, 239 women completed a questionnaire at study initiation and after 2 years. Patients had received various therapies, although 41% did not undergo any treatment. At 2 years, there was significant improvement in pain, sexual function, and depression for the group as a whole. Women not receiving any treatment also improved significantly. The authors conclude that no single treatment is superior and that spontaneous resolution may occur.

First-Line Therapies

Antidepressants (oral or topical amitriptyline, oral desipramine, oral milnacipran, etc.)	A
Topical lidocaine	B
Anticonvulsants (oral or topical gabapentin, oral pregabalin, oral lamotrigine)	C
Pelvic floor physical therapy	C

Evidence Levels: **A** Double-blind study   **B** Clinical trial ≥ 20 subjects   **C** Clinical trial < 20 subjects   **D** Series ≥ 5 subjects   **E** Anecdotal case reports

Oral desipramine and topical lidocaine for vulvodynia: a randomized controlled trial. Foster DC, Kotok MB, Huang LS, Watts A, Oakes D, Howard FM, et al. Obstet Gynecol 2010; 116: 583–93.

This study consisted of four treatment arms. One hundred and thirty-three women with vulvodynia were randomly assigned to 12 weeks of oral desipramine, topical lidocaine, oral desipramine plus topical lidocaine, or placebo. There was no statistically significant benefit in pain reduction of the treatment arms compared with placebo. However, there was significant improvement in sexual functioning in the desipramine group. The authors discuss the importance of including a placebo arm in vulvodynia studies.

Self-management, amitriptyline, and amitriptyline plus triamcinolone in the management of vulvodynia. Brown CS, Wan J, Bachmann G, Rosen R. J Womens Health 2009; 18: 163–9.

In this open-label trial, 53 women were randomized to self-management, oral amitriptyline (10–20 mg/day), or topical triamcinolone plus oral amitriptyline. The treatment groups were not superior to self-management with regard to pain reduction. There were significant within-group differences in the amitriptyline group, but the authors state that these may not have been clinically meaningful.

Treatment of vulvodynia with tricyclic antidepressants: efficacy and associated factors. Reed BD, Caron AM, Gorenflo DW, Haefner HK. J Low Genit Tract Dis 2006; 10: 245–51.

A prospective cohort study of 209 women initially treated with a tricyclic antidepressant (TCA). One hundred and eighty-three were given amitriptyline, 23 received desipramine, and 3 were treated with another TCA. The dose was titrated up to a maximum of 225 mg if required. Of 83 women taking a TCA at first follow-up (median 3.2 months), 59.3% improved by more than 50% compared with 38% of women not taking a TCA.

Milnacipran in provoked vestibulodynia: efficacy and predictors of treatment success. Brown C, Bachmann G, Foster D, Rawlinson L, Wan J, Ling F. J Low Genit Tract Dis 2015; 19: 140–4.

In this 12-week open-label trial, 22 women were treated with milnacipran, a serotonin–norepinephrine reuptake inhibitor. Milnacipran significantly reduced pain severity. The authors note that treatment success was predicted by pretreatment sexual satisfaction.

Use of amitriptyline cream in the management of entry dyspareunia due to provoked vestibulodynia. Pagano R, Wong S. J Low Genit Tract Dis 2012; 16: 394–7.

A prospective study of 150 patients treated with amitriptyline 2% cream twice daily for 3 months. Fifty-six percent reported symptom reduction, and 10% were completely pain free.

Overnight 5% lidocaine ointment for treatment of vulvar vestibulitis. Zolnoun DA, Hartmann KE, Steege JF. Obstet Gynecol 2003; 102: 84–7.

An open-label trial of 61 women treated with nightly application of 5% lidocaine ointment. Dyspareunia decreased by at least 50% in 57% of women. Seventy-six percent of patients were able to have intercourse after treatment compared with 36% before drug initiation.

Pregabalin-induced remission in a 62-year-old woman with a 20-year history of vulvodynia. Jerome L. Pain Res Manage 2007; 12: 212–4.

Case report of a 62-year-old woman with long-standing vulvodynia who reported 80% pain reduction after a 12-week course of oral pregabalin.

A retrospective study of the management of vulvodynia. Jeon Y, Kim Y, Shim B, Yoon H, Park Y, Shim, B, et al. Korean J Urol 2013; 54: 48–52.

Retrospective study of vulvodynia patients treated with either oral gabapentin or botulinum toxin A injections. Sixty-two women received gabapentin 300 to 900 mg/day for a period of 0.5 to 6 months. Eleven patients received intralesional botulinum toxin A injections. Significant pain reduction was reported in both groups, and both treatments were well tolerated.

Open-label trial of lamotrigine focusing on efficacy in vulvodynia. Meltzer-Brody SE, Zolnoun D, Steege JF, Rinaldi KL, Leserman J. J Reprod Med 2009; 54: 171–8.

Marked reductions in pain were noted at weeks 8 and 12 in this series involving 17 patients with generalized vulvodynia.

Topical gabapentin in the treatment of localized and generalized vulvodynia. Boardman LA, Cooper AS, Blais LR, Raker CA. Obstet Gynecol 2008; 112: 579–85.

Of 51 women included in this retrospective study, 35 patients had evaluable responses. Treatment with 2% to 6% gabapentin cream three times daily was well tolerated and led to at least 50% pain reduction in 28 of the 35 women.

Effectiveness of cognitive-behavioral therapy and physical therapy for provoked vestibulodynia: a randomized pilot study. Goldfinger C, Pukall CF, Thibault-Gagnon S, McLean L, Chamberlain S. J Sex Med 2016; 13: 88–94.

Twenty women were randomized to cognitive behavior therapy (CBT) or comprehensive physical therapy. The majority of patients in both groups reported at least 30% pain reduction, whereas improved sexual functioning was only seen in the CBT group.

Does physiotherapy treatment improve the self-reported pain levels and quality of life in women with vulvodynia? A pilot study. Forth HL, Cramp MC, Drechsler WI. J Obstet Gynaecol 2009; 29: 423–9.

A 3-month course of physiotherapy led to pain reduction in 14 women.

Second-Line Therapies	
• Electromyographic (EMG) biofeedback	B
• Nitroglycerin cream	B
• Acupuncture	B
• CBT	B
• Botulinum toxin	D

EMG biofeedback versus topical lidocaine gel: a randomized study for the treatment of women with vulvar vestibulitis. Danielsson I, Torstensson T, Brodda-Jansen G, Bohm-Starke N. Acta Obstet Gynecol Scand 2006; 85: 1360–7.

Four months of treatment with EMG biofeedback or 5% lidocaine ointment led to significant improvements in pain, sexual functioning, and psychosocial adjustments in both groups. Women in the EMG biofeedback group reported low compliance and did not complete all planned practice sessions.

Safety and efficacy of topical nitroglycerin for treatment of vulvar pain in women with vulvodynia: a pilot study. Walsh

KE, Berman JR, Berman LA, Vierregger K. J Gend Specif Med 2002; 5: 21–7.

This is the only report of the use of topical nitroglycerin 0.2% for the management of vulvodynia. The majority of the 21 women, who applied the cream before intercourse and completed all questionnaires, reported significant pain reduction.

Acupuncture for the treatment of vulvodynia: a randomized wait-list controlled pilot study. Schlaeger JM, Xu N, Mejta CL, Park CG, Wilkie DJ. J Sex Med 2015; 12: 1019–27.

Thirty-six women were randomly assigned to either acupuncture twice per week for 5 weeks or the control group, which consisted of continuing their usual treatment. Vulvar pain and dyspareunia reduced significantly and sexual functioning improved in the acupuncture group.

A randomized clinical trial comparing group cognitive-behavioral therapy and a topical steroid for women with dyspareunia. Bergeron S, Khalifé S, Dupuis MJ, McDuff P. J Consult Clin Psychol 2016; 84: 259–68.

This 13-week trial included 97 women with provoked vestibulodynia. Fifty-two were randomized to group CBT and 45 to hydrocortisone 1% cream. Both groups reported significant improvements in pain and sexual functioning after treatment and at 6-month follow-up; however, these effects were significantly greater in the CBT group.

Botulinum toxin type A: a novel treatment for provoked vestibulodynia? Results from a randomized, placebo controlled, double blinded study. Petersen CD, Giraldi A, Lundvall L, Kristensen E. J Sex Med 2009; 6: 2523–37.

Sixty-four women were randomized to receive 20 units botulinum toxin A or placebo injections; 60 completed the 6 months, follow-up. Significant pain reduction was reported in both groups, but there were no statistically significant differences.

The nonsuperiority of botulinum toxin A in this study may be due to the low dose used, compared with the next study.

Long-term assessment of effectiveness and quality of life of OnabotulinumtoxinA injections in provoked vestibulodynia. Pelletier F, Girardin M, Humbert P, Puyraveau M, Aubin F, Parratte B. J Eur Acad Dermatol Venereol 2016; 30: 106–11.

Nineteen patients who had received bilateral onabotulinumtoxinA injections (total of 100 units) into the bulbospongiosus muscles completed questionnaires 2 years after treatment. Pain, sexual function, and quality of life improved significantly, and 37% were pain free at 24 months. Eighteen of the 19 women had avoided intercourse before the treatment and were able to resume intercourse after treatment.

Third-Line Therapies	
• Enoxaparin	A
• Transcutaneous electrical nerve stimulation (TENS)	A
• Cultured fibroblasts	A
• Surgery	B
• Capsaicin	D
• Fractional CO$_2$ laser	D
• Multilevel local anesthetic nerve blockade	D
• Hypnosis	E
• Spinal cord stimulator	E
• Nutrition therapy	E
• Radiofrequency therapy	E
• Peripheral subcutaneous vulvar stimulation	E

Enoxaparin treatment for vulvodynia: a randomized controlled trial. Farajun Y, Zarfati D, Abramov L, Livoff A, Bornstein J. Obstet Gynecol 2012; 120: 565–72.

In this randomized, double-blind study, 40 women with localized, provoked vulvodynia self-administered enoxaparin, a low-molecular-weight heparin, or placebo via subcutaneous injection once daily for 90 days. Reduction of pain and dyspareunia were greater in the enoxaparin group.

Vestibulodynia: synergy between palmitoylethanolamide + transpolydatin and transcutaneous electrical nerve stimulation. Murina F, Graziottin A, Felice R, Radici G, Tognocchi C. J Low Genit Tract Dis 2013; 17: 111–6.

In a double-blind, placebo-controlled study, 20 patients were randomized to oral palmitoylethanolamide (PEA) 400 mg and polydatin 40 mg or placebo twice daily for 60 days. All patients also self-administered TENS therapy three times weekly. There was significant improvement in both groups.

Transcutaneous electrical nerve stimulation as an additional treatment for women suffering from therapy-resistant provoked vestibulodynia: a feasibility study. Vallinga MS, Spoelstra SK, Hemel IL, van de Wiel HB, Weijmar Schultz WC. J Sex Med 2015; 12: 228–37.

Thirty-nine women applied domiciliary TENS three times daily. There were significant reductions in vulvar pain directly after treatment and at follow-up (between 2 and 32 months), with improvements in sexual functioning.

Cream with cutaneous fibroblast lysate for the treatment of provoked vestibulodynia: a double-blind randomized placebo-controlled crossover study. Donders GG, Bellen G. J Low Genit Tract Dis 2012; 16: 427–36.

In this crossover study, 30 patients were randomized 1:1 to a topical lysate of cultured human fibroblasts or placebo. There was statistically significant reduction in dyspareunia with treatment, with no improvement with placebo use.

A randomized comparison of group cognitive-behavioral therapy, surface electromyographic biofeedback, and vestibulectomy in the treatment of dyspareunia resulting from vulvar vestibulitis. Bergeron S, Binik YM, Khalife S, Pagidas K, Glazer HI, Meana M, et al. Pain 2001; 91: 297–306.

In this study comparing group CBT, EMG biofeedback, and vestibulectomy, 78 women were randomly assigned to a treatment. Significant improvements in pain measures were reported in all three groups. Although pain reduction was more significant in the vestibulectomy group, seven women assigned to this treatment declined the intervention.

Localized provoked vestibulodynia: outcomes after modified vestibulectomy. Swanson CL, Rueter JA, Olson JE, Weaver AL, Stanhope CR. J Reprod Med 2014; 59: 121–6.

A total of 202 women treated with modified vestibulectomy at the Mayo Clinic were sent a questionnaire. A total of 90.4% of the 52 patients who reported pain with tampon insertion before surgery reported moderate to substantial pain reduction after surgery, and 84.1% of the 107 women who complained of dyspareunia noted significant improvement.

Capsaicin and the treatment of vulvar vestibulitis syndrome: a valuable alternative? Murina F, Radici G, Bianco V. MedGenMed 2004; 6: 48.

Thirty-three women applied capsaicin cream 0.05% twice daily for 30 days, then daily for 30 days, followed by twice weekly for

Evidence Levels: **A** Double-blind study **B** Clinical trial ≥ 20 subjects **C** Clinical trial < 20 subjects **D** Series ≥ 5 subjects **E** Anecdotal case reports

4 months. Fifty-nine percent reported a partial response, with relapse after cessation. All patients complained of severe burning as a side effect.

Before the application of capsaicin, patients applied topical lidocaine to avoid irritation. It is therefore unclear how much of the effect can be attributed to capsaicin.

Fractional CO$_2$ laser treatment of the vestibule for patients with vestibulodynia and genitourinary syndrome of menopause: a pilot study. Murina F, Karram M, Salvatore S, Felice R. J Sex Med 2016; 13: 1915-7.

This study included 37 patients who underwent three sessions of fractional microablative CO$_2$ laser treatment. Pain scores and dyspareunia improved significantly over 4 months, and the treatments were well tolerated.

Multilevel local anesthetic nerve blockade for the treatment of generalized vulvodynia: a pilot study. McDonald JS, Rapkin AJ. J Sex Med 2012; 9: 2919-26.

Twenty-six women completed all five multilevel local anesthetic nerve blocks at 2-week intervals. At follow-up 2 to 3 months later, there was significant improvement in vulvar pain and depression, but no changes in sexual functioning. Women with more severe pain at baseline had less improvement.

Effectiveness of hypnosis for the treatment of vulvar vestibulitis syndrome: a preliminary investigation. Pukall C, Kandyba K, Amsel R, Khalife S, Binik Y. J Sex Med 2007; 4: 417-25.

Six hypnotherapy sessions led to significant improvements in pain and sexual functioning in eight women.

Spinal cord stimulator for the treatment of a woman with vulvovaginal burning and deep pelvic pain. Nair AR, Klapper A, Kushnerik V, Margulis I, Del Priore G. Obstet Gynecol 2008; 111: 545-7.

Implantation of a spinal cord stimulator led to significant improvement in vulvodynia in a 57-year-old woman.

Vulvodynia and irritable bowel syndrome treated with an elimination diet: a case report. Drummond J, Ford D, Daniel S, Meyerink T. Integr Med (Encinitas) 2016; 15: 42-7.

A young woman with refractory vulvodynia and irritable bowel syndrome was treated with an elimination diet. During the 6 months of nutrition therapy, her pelvic pain decreased markedly.

Radiofrequency therapy for severe idiopathic vulvodynia. Kestřánek J, Špaček J, Ryška P, Adamkov J, Matula V, Buchta V. J Low Genit Tract Dis 2013; 17: e1-4.

Report of patient who responded to pulsed radiofrequency treatment of the hypogastric ganglion. Her pain reduced significantly for a period of around 6 months.

Peripheral subcutaneous vulvar stimulation in the management of severe and refractory vulvodynia. De Andres J, Sanchis-Lopez N, Asensio-Samper JM, Fabregat-Cid G, Dolz VM. Obstet Gynecol 2013; 121: 495-8.

Two vulvar subcutaneous electrodes were implanted in a young woman with refractory vulvodynia who underwent peripheral subcutaneous vulvar field stimulation. Pain scores reduced significantly posttreatment and at 12 months, follow-up.

Wells syndrome

Wisam Alwan, Emma Benton, Ian Coulson

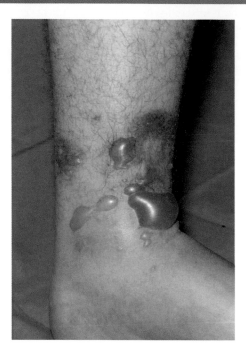

Wells syndrome (eosinophilic cellulitis) is a rare condition resembling a bacterial cellulitis. Patients are often treated with antibiotics and fail to respond before the diagnosis of Wells syndrome is considered and then confirmed on skin biopsy. Although the precise etiology is unknown, there are several disease associations, including drug-induced disease. It is postulated that Wells syndrome represents a hypersensitivity reaction to a variety of stimuli, both endogenous and exogenous. The condition can be recurrent, and although thought to be sporadic, familial patterns have been reported. The most common clinical manifestations are erythematous patches and plaques, but papulonodular and bullous types of Wells syndrome have been described. Characteristic histologic features include dermal edema with a marked eosinophilic infiltrate and flame figures (representing deposition of eosinophilic proteins and degradation products onto collagen fibers), although this is not specific to the condition. The usual course is of a pruritic sensation, followed rapidly by indurated, erythematous plaques of edema with violaceous edges that can form blisters. The lesions progress over a few days, resolving without scarring within 8 weeks. There is no anatomic predilection for plaques, and they may be solitary or multiple.

MANAGEMENT STRATEGY

Although there is no known cause, several precipitating factors have been suggested (Table 255.1). Some of the associations are well reported, others anecdotal. Injection site skin lesions have been associated with the tumor necrosis factor antagonists etanercept and adalimumab and also with interferon-beta. Interestingly, adalimumab has also been successfully used to treat refractory

Wells syndrome in two cases. Minocycline can also induce a Wells syndrome–like disorder.

Suspect culprit drugs should be withdrawn. If an underlying systemic disease is identified, this will require treatment in its own right. Many cases of Wells syndrome associated with internal malignancy resolved with treatment of the initial tumor.

The most frequently reported therapy is with *systemic (oral) corticosteroids*, used at moderate doses to gain control of symptoms, followed by tapering. Cases may resolve spontaneously. As with bullous pemphigoid, localized disease may respond to *superpotent topical steroids*. Topical *tacrolimus* has also been used successfully. The H_1 antihistamine with antieosinophil action *cetirizine* has been effective; levocetirizine and hydroxyzine in combination have also proven successful. *Minocycline, dapsone, antimalarials, griseofulvin, adalimumab,* and *ciclosporin* are anecdotally beneficial.

Specific Investigations

- Peripheral blood eosinophil count
- Skin biopsy
- Look for known associations of the disease

Wells syndrome: a clinical and histopathologic review of seven cases. Moossavi M, Mehregan DR. Int J Dermatol 2003; 42: 62–7.

Eosinophilic cellulitis-like reaction to subcutaneous etanercept injection. Winfield H, Lain E, Horn T, Hoskyn J. Arch Dermatol 2006; 142: 218–20.

Eosinophilic cellulitis (Wells syndrome) as a cutaneous reaction to the administration of adalimumab. Boura P, Sarantopoulos A, Lefaki I, Skendros P, Papadopoulos P. Ann Rheum Dis 2006; 65: 839–40.

Systemic lupus erythematosus associated with Wells syndrome. Yin G, Xie Q. Rheumatol Int 2012; 32: 1087–9.

Wells syndrome associated with Churg–Strauss syndrome. Fujimoto N, Wakabayashi M, Kato T, Nishio C, Tanaka T. Clin Exp Dermatol 2011; 36: 46–8.

Wells' syndrome associated with chronic myeloid leukemia. Nakazato S, Fujita Y, Hamade Y, Nemoto-Hasebe I, Sugita J, Nishie W, et al. Acta Derm Venereol 2013; 93: 375–6.

Bullous eosinophilic cellulitis associated with giardiasis. Aslam A, Salman W, Chaudhry IH, Coulson IH, Owen CM. Clin Exp Dermatol 2014; 39: 264–5.

Eosinophilic cellulitis (Wells syndrome) caused by a temporary henna tattoo. Nacaroglu HT, Celegen M, Karkiner CS, Günay I, Diniz G, Can D. Postepy Dermatol Alergol 2014; 31: 322–4.

Influenza vaccination as a novel trigger of Wells syndrome in a child. Simpson JK, Patalay R, Francis N, Roberts N. Pediatr Dermatol 2015; 32: e171–2.

Other conditions anecdotally associated with Wells syndrome include chronic lymphocytic leukemia, angioimmunoblastic lymphadenopathy, adenocarcinoma of the lung, gastric cancer, renal (clear cell) cancer, colon cancer, botryomycosis, molluscum contagiosum, celiac disease, and ulcerative colitis. Some

Evidence Levels: **A** Double-blind study **B** Clinical trial ≥ 20 subjects **C** Clinical trial < 20 subjects **D** Series ≥ 5 subjects **E** Anecdotal case reports

Table 255.1 Reported associations with eosinophilic cellulitis

Infections: bacterial, viral (HIV, herpes simplex, parvovirus, varicella, molluscum contagiosum), parasitic (*Ascaris,* toxocariasis, giardiasis)
Insect bite reactions
Ulcerative colitis
Leukemia
Lymphoma
Solid cancers (lung, colon, gastric, renal)
Angioimmunoblastic lymphadenopathy
Hypereosinophilic syndrome
Drugs (including vaccines, particularly those containing thimerosal)
Churg–Strauss syndrome
Allergic asthma exacerbation
Systemic lupus erythematosus
Metallic alloy implants
Celiac disease
Allergic contact dermatitis (paraphenylenediamine [PPD] and black rubber in temporary henna tattoo)
IgG4-related disease

of the associations are based on single case reports and may be coincidental.

First-Line Therapy

• Oral corticosteroids	C

Recurrent granulomatous dermatitis with eosinophilia. Wells GC. Trans St Johns Hosp Dermatol Soc 1971; 57: 46–56.

Eosinophilic cellulitis. Wells GC, Smith NP. Br J Dermatol 1979; 100: 101–9.

Wells' first publications on the disease. Oral prednisolone, ranging in doses of 20 to 40 mg/day, is a reasonable starting point, tapering the dose until control and hopefully resolution. One month of tapering prednisolone has been used successfully in patients.

Second-Line Therapies

• Cetirizine	E
• Levocetirizine/hydroxyzine	E
• Ciclosporin	E
• Dapsone	E
• Interferon-α	E
• Minocycline	E
• Sulfasalazine	E
• Griseofulvin	E
• Tacrolimus	E
• Adalimumab	E

Eosinophilic cellulitis in a child successfully treated with cetirizine. Aroni K, Aivaliotis M, Liossi A, Davaris P. Acta Derm Venereol 1999; 79: 332.

Treatment of Wells syndrome in children with corticosteroids risks concerns regarding growth retardation, and the authors described a child successfully treated with cetirizine 10 mg daily.

Cetirizine 10 to 30 mg daily is a reasonable consideration in adults.

Eosinophilic cellulitis (Wells syndrome) successfully treated with low-dose ciclosporin. Herr H, Koh JK. J Korean Med Sci 2001; 16: 664–8.

A report of ciclosporin use in an adult with Wells syndrome; 2.5 to 5 mg/kg/day was used.

Eosinophilic cellulitis case report: treatment options. Lee MW, Nixon RL. Australas J Dermatol 1994; 35: 95–7.

Dapsone was added to oral steroids and antihistamines as a steroid-sparing agent as monotherapy with steroids alone gained inadequate control.

Doses of 50 to 150 mg/day would be an appropriate trial.

Interferon alfa treatment of a patient with eosinophilic cellulitis and HIV infection. Husak R, Goerdt S, Orfanos CE. N Engl J Med 1997; 337: 641–2.

Failure to control HIV-associated Wells syndrome with steroids prompted a successful trial of interferon-α treatment.

Eosinophilic cellulitis (Wells syndrome): treatment with minocycline. Stam-Westerveld EB, Daenen S, Van der Meer JB, Jonkman MF. Acta Derm Venereol 1998; 78: 157.

Minocycline 200 mg daily was used to control disease, and 100 mg daily was used as maintenance.

Oral tacrolimus treatment for refractory eosinophilic cellulitis. Ohtsuka T. Clin Exp Dermatol 2009; 34: 597–8.

The authors report a case of eosinophilic cellulitis that previously had been responsive to oral corticosteroids (prednisolone 15 mg/day). The patient failed to respond to this treatment on recurrence and was successfully treated with oral tacrolimus (1 mg/day).

Wells' syndrome mimicking facial cellulitis: a report of two cases. Cormerais M, Poizeau F, Darrieux L, Tisseau L, Safa G. Case Rep Dermatol. 2015; 9: 117–22.

The authors highlighted two patients who experienced no relapse during follow-up of between 3 and 12 months using levocetirizine 10 mg daily and hydroxyzine 50 mg daily.

Treatment of recalcitrant eosinophilic cellulitis with adalimumab. Sarin KY, Fiorentino D. Arch Dermatol 2012; 148: 990–2.

A 45-year-old woman with a 10-year history of Wells syndrome was unable to tolerate full-dose oral prednisolone and did not respond to systemic agents, including antihistamines, azathioprine, dapsone, and colchicine. The patient responded to fortnightly adalimumab.

Off-label use of TNF-alpha inhibitors in a dermatologic university department: retrospective evaluation of 118 patients. Sand FL, Thomsen SF. Dermatol Ther 2015; 28: 158–65.

The authors reported an elderly female patient with total clearance of disease on 6 months of adalimumab.

Xanthomas

*Lucile E. White, Marcelo G. Horenstein,
Christopher R. Shea*

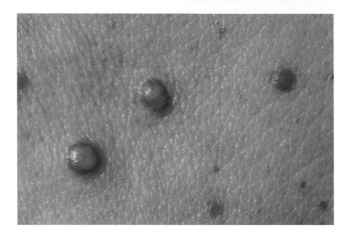

Xanthomas are flat, yellow plaques or nodules consisting of abnormal lipid deposits. Clinically, xanthomas can be classified as eruptive, tuberoeruptive, tuberous, tendinous, verruciform, or plane. Plane xanthomas are the most common and include xanthelasma palpebrarum, xanthoma striatum palmare, and intertriginous xanthomas. Verruciform xanthomas typically affect genital skin and may be a consequence of lymphedema. Necrobiotic xanthogranulomas are scarring, commonly ulcerated nodules with a predilection for the periorbital areas and are associated with paraproteinemia.

MANAGEMENT STRATEGY

Xanthomas may be idiopathic or a sign of underlying hyperlipidemia. *Diagnosing and treating the underlying disease* are necessary not only to decrease the size of the xanthomas but also to reduce the risk of atherosclerosis associated with lipoprotein disorders. Treatment of the hyperlipidemia initially consists of *diet and lipid-lowering agents* such as statins, fibrates, bile acid–binding resins, probucol, or nicotinic acid. The lipid-lowering effects of these agents have been well documented, but few studies document the efficacy of these drugs at resolving xanthomas. Anecdotally, eruptive xanthomas typically appear to resolve within weeks of initiating systemic treatment, and tuberous xanthomas after some months, but tendinous xanthomas may take years to resolve or even persist indefinitely. *Surgery or locally destructive modalities* can be used for idiopathic or unresponsive xanthomas.

Specific Investigations

- Serum lipid panel of cholesterol, triglycerides, VLDL, LDL, and HDL
- Gas–liquid and high-performance liquid chromatography to diagnose sitosterolemia
- Capillary gas chromatography of urine to diagnose cerebrotendinous xanthomatosis
- Serum protein electrophoresis, immunoelectrophoresis, or immunofixation to detect M proteins

Excluding an underlying condition is essential in the management of most clinical forms of xanthomas. Eruptive xanthomas typically occur in the setting of hypertriglyceridemia. Hypertriglyceridemia can be the result of lipoprotein lipase deficiency, familial hyperlipoproteinemia, or secondary causes such as diabetes mellitus, alcohol ingestion, or exogenous estrogens. Tuberoeruptive and tuberous xanthomas represent parts of a spectrum and are seen most commonly in the setting of familial dysbetalipoproteinemia. Tuberous xanthomas may also be a presentation of homozygous familial hypercholesterolemia, cerebrotendinous xanthomatosis (associated with neuropsychiatric symptoms), or sitosterolemia. Patients with sitosterolemia and cerebrotendinous xanthomatosis may have normal serum lipid panels; therefore diagnosis may require liquid chromatography for plant sterols or urinary gas chromatography. Tendinous xanthomas may also occur with cerebrotendinous xanthomatosis, sitosterolemia or, more commonly, heterozygous familial hypercholesterolemia. Certain xanthomas are diagnostic for an inherited hyperlipidemia: xanthoma striatum palmare for familial dysbetalipoproteinemia and intertriginous xanthomas for homozygous familial hypercholesterolemia. Even in the presence of these classic presentations, a serum lipid panel is still indicated to confirm the diagnosis.

Regarding xanthelasma palpebrarum, a type of plane xanthoma, levels of total cholesterol are elevated in only about half of patients; however, patients with xanthelasma may have elevated apolipoprotein B and decreased apolipoprotein A1 levels, as well as subclinical increases in carotid intima-media thickness. Moreover, xanthelasma is a risk factor for myocardial infarction, ischemic heart disease, severe atherosclerosis, and death, independently of plasma cholesterol and triglyceride concentrations. Less commonly, plane xanthomas can signal a monoclonal gammopathy. In this situation, the differential diagnosis of necrobiotic xanthogranuloma with paraproteinemia, a condition usually associated with lymphoproliferative disorders, should be considered.

First-Line Therapies

- Low-fat diet and systemic lipid-lowering therapy   **B**

Opposite effects on serum cholesteryl ester transfer protein levels between long-term treatments with pravastatin and probucol in patients with primary hypercholesterolemia. Inazu A, Koizumi J, Kajinami K, Kiyohar T, Chichibu K, Mabuchi H. Atherosclerosis 1999; 145: 405–13.

This prospective study examined whether pravastatin or probucol was better at regressing tendon xanthomas and xanthelasma in patients with primary hypercholesterolemia. In both the pravastatin and probucol groups, xanthelasma regressed in two of four patients. Achilles tendon xanthoma regressed in four of five patients treated with pravastatin and two of five patients on probucol.

A comparative study of the therapeutic effect of probucol and pravastatin on xanthelasma. Fujita M, Shirai K. J Dermatol 1996; 23: 598–602.

Fifty-four patients were treated with probucol or pravastatin. Xanthelasmas regressed in 13 of 36 patients treated with probucol and 1 of 18 patients treated with pravastatin.

Evidence Levels: **A** Double-blind study   **B** Clinical trial ≥ 20 subjects   **C** Clinical trial < 20 subjects   **D** Series ≥ 5 subjects   **E** Anecdotal case reports

Effects of probucol on xanthomata regression in familial hypercholesterolemia. Yamamoto A, Matsuzawa Y, Yokoyama S, Funahashi T, Yamamura T, Kishino B. Am J Cardiol 1986; 57: H29–35.

Fifty one patients, including eight homozygotes, were treated with combinations of probucol, cholestyramine, clofibrate, and compactin. Achilles tendon xanthomas shrank in all patients who received probucol. Probucol possibly reduces the size of HDL particles, increasing reverse cholesterol transport.

Successful treatment of xanthoma disseminatum with combined lipid lowering agents. Kim WJ, Ko HC, Kim BS, Kim MB. Ann Dermatol 2012; 24: 380–2.

Combination therapy with rosiglitazone 4 mg daily, simvastatin 10 mg daily, and fenofibrate 200 mg daily resulted in notable reduction of the skin lesions persisting 2 years later.

Second-Line Therapies	
• Surgery	B
• CO_2 laser	B
• Erbium:YAG laser	C
• Pulsed dye laser	B
• Argon laser	B
• Q-switched Nd:YAG laser	D
• KTP laser	D
• 1450-nm diode laser	C
• Low-voltage radiofrequency	C

Treatment of xanthelasma by excision with secondary intention healing. Eedy DJ. Clin Exp Dermatol 1996; 21: 273–5.

Xanthelasmas were removed in 28 patients by scissor excision. After 18 months, two patients, one with hypercholesterolemia and one with primary biliary cirrhosis, had recurrence. One patient developed scarring. No ectropion developed.

Upper and lower eyelid reconstruction for severe disfiguring necrobiotic xanthogranuloma. Schaudig U, Al-Samir K. Orbit 2004; 23: 65–76.

Severe cicatricial eyelid deformation caused by necrobiotic xanthogranuloma can be treated successfully by excision and free skin grafting.

Successful treatment of scrotal verruciform xanthoma with shave debulking and fractionated carbon dioxide laser therapy. Joo J, Fung MA, Jagdeo J. Dermatol Surg 2014; 40: 214–7.

A patient treated with combined shave debulking and fractionated CO_2 laser ablation. The procedure was well tolerated, and no recurrence was noted at 18 months.

Xanthelasma palpebrarum: treatment with the ultrapulsed CO_2 laser. Raulin C, Schoenermark MP, Werner S, Greve B. Lasers Surg Med 1999; 24: 122–7.

Ultrapulsed CO_2 laser delivers high energy in short pulses and reduces the risk of scarring and hyperpigmentation seen with continuous-mode CO_2 lasers. Twenty-three patients with 52 xanthelasmas were treated. All xanthelasmas were removed completely. No permanent hyperpigmentation or ectropion developed.

Xanthelasma palpebrarum: treatment with the erbium:YAG laser. Borelli C, Kaudewitz P. Lasers Surg Med 2001; 29: 260–4.

Fifteen patients with 33 xanthelasmas were treated with an Er:YAG laser at settings between of 300 mJ, 2 Hz for a 2-mm

spot size and 1200 mJ, 6 Hz for a 10-mm spot size. All xanthelasmas were removed completely. Postoperative erythema resolved within 2 weeks. No scarring or ectropion developed. No lesions recurred over a 7- to 12-month follow-up period.

New operative technique for treatment of xanthelasma palpebrarum: laser-inverted resurfacing. Preliminary report. Levy JL, Trelles MA. Ann Plast Surg 2003; 50: 339–43.

The authors propose use of pulsed Er:YAG vaporization of the lipomatous tissue off the inner surface of the eyelid after incision and eversion of the incised tissue to expose the xanthelasma. In two patients treated by this technique no recurrence was seen in up to 1 year of follow-up.

Treatment of xanthelasma palpebrarum by 1064-nm Q-switched Nd:YAG laser: a study of 11 cases. Fusade T. Br J Dermatol 2008; 158: 84–7.

Results after even a single treatment were reported to be good or excellent in 8 of 11 patients (in 26 of 38 lesions), and healing was rapid.

Is Q-switched neodymium-doped yttrium aluminium garnet laser an effective approach to treat xanthelasma palpebrarum? Results from a clinical study of 76 cases. Karsai S, Schmitt L, Raulin C. Dermatol Surg 2009; 35: 1962–9.

Most lesions failed to respond.

Treatment of xanthelasma palpebrarum with argon laser photocoagulation. Basar E, Oguz H, Oxdemir H, Ozkan S, Uslu H. Int Ophthalmol 2004; 25: 9–11.

Twenty-four patients with 40 xanthelasmas were treated with an argon laser at settings of 500 μm, 0.1 to 0.2 s, and 900 mW. Complete removal of all lesions occurred with one to four sessions at intervals of 2 or 3 weeks. Six lesions recurred over 8 to 12 months and required retreatment. Erythema persisted for 1 month in 8 lesions. Hyperpigmentation occurred in one patient and persisted for 3 months, whereas hypopigmentation occurred in 2 lesions.

Histopathological study of xanthelasma palpebrarum after pulsed dye laser. Soliman M. J Eur Acad Dermatol Venereol 2004; 18 (Suppl): 19–33.

Twenty-six patients were treated with fluences ranging from 6.5 to 8 J/cm^2, a spot size of 5 mm, and a pulse width of 450 ms. All experienced very good to excellent clinical improvement with one to three treatments at 3- or 4-week intervals.

KTP laser coagulation for xanthelasma palpebrarum. Berger C, Kopera D. J Dtsch Dermatol Ges 2005; 3: 775–9.

The authors employed the KTP laser (532 nm) to treat 14 patients. Over 70% tolerated laser irradiation without analgesia; 85.7% showed reduction of lesions after one to three treatment sessions, without reported side effects.

Xanthelasma palpebrarum treatment with a 1450-nm-diode laser. Park EJ, Youn SH, Cho EB, Lee GS, Hann SK, Kim KH, et al. Dermatol Surg 2011; 37: 791–6.

Sixteen patients received one to four treatments using a 1450-nm diode laser at 12 J/cm^2, 6-mm spot size, and 20 to 30 ms. Twelve patients experienced moderate to marked improvement. The treatment was well tolerated.

Effectiveness of low-voltage radiofrequency in the treatment of xanthelasma palpebrarum: a pilot study of 15 cases. Dincer D, Koc E, Erbil AH, Kose O. Dermatol Surg 2010; 36: 1973–8.

Fifteen patients were treated by superficial application of electrodes from a dual-frequency 4.0-MHz radiofrequency machine. All subjects completed the study; excellent results were achieved in 9 patients and good results in 5 patients.

Third-Line Therapies	
• Di- or trichloroacetic acid	C
• Cryotherapy	E
• Bleomycin	B
• Intralesional triamcinolone acetonide	D
• Chlorambucil	E
• Prednisolone	E
• Intravenous immunoglobulin	E
• Anakinra	E
• 2-chlorodeoxyadenosine (cladribine)	E
• Topical imiquimod	E
• Bexarotene	E

Evaluation of three different strengths of trichloroacetic acid in xanthelasma palpebrarum. Haque MU, Ramesh V. J Dermatolog Treat 2006; 17: 48–50.

Three strengths of trichloroacetic acid (TCA) were tested on 51 patients. For papulonodular lesions, on average approximately two applications were required with 100% or 70% TCA versus approximately four applications with 50% TCA. For flat plaques an average of approximately 1.5 applications of 100% or 70% TCA sufficed, versus approximately 3 applications with 50% TCA. Macular lesions responded to a single application of all strengths of TCA studied.

Cryotherapy may be effective for eyelid xanthoma. Hawk JL. Clin Exp Dermatol 2000; 25: 351.

One patient was treated with liquid nitrogen applied for 0.5 to 1 s. Treatment was carefully limited to only the yellow areas. Previous treatment with TCA had been unsuccessful.

Treatment of xanthelasma palpebrarum with intralesional pingyangmycin. Wang H, Shi Y, Guan H, Liu C, Zhang W, Zhang Y, et al. Dermatol Surg 2016; 42: 368–76.

Twelve patients with xanthelasma palpebrarum had a total of 21 lesions injected with intralesional pingyangmycin (bleomycin A5). All patients except one received satisfactory results, and only one patient experienced a local recurrence, 1 year after the treatment. No severe complications were identified.

Local corticosteroid treatment of eyelid and orbital xanthogranuloma. Elner VM, Mintz R, Demirci H, Hassan AS. Trans Am Ophthalmol Soc 2005; 103: 69–73.

Six patients received two intralesional injections of triamcinolone acetonide (40 mg/mL) for eyelid and orbital necrobiotic xanthogranuloma (four patients) or adult-onset xanthogranuloma (two patients). Local control was obtained in all six cases with no complications noted.

Necrobiotic xanthogranuloma treated with chlorambucil. Torabian SZ, Fazel N, Knuttle R. Dermatol Online J 2006; 12: 11.

A 56-year-old man with a 5-year history of multiple necrobiotic xanthogranulomas involving the periorbital area, extremities, and trunk was treated with chlorambucil at 2 mg/day, later increased to 4 mg/day, which resulted in complete resolution of the lesions.

Necrobiotic xanthogranuloma of extremities in an elderly patient successfully treated with low-dose prednisolone. Kawakami Y, Yamamoto T. Dermatol Online J 2011; 17: 13.

A 93-year-old woman with an IgG λ paraproteinemia and ulcerated, tender necrobiotic xanthogranulomas involving the left lower leg experienced resolution 4 weeks after starting treatment with oral prednisolone, 20 mg daily (0.5 mg/kg).

Successful treatment of necrobiotic xanthogranuloma with intravenous immunoglobulin. Hallermann C, Tittelbach J, Norgauer J, Ziemer M. Arch Dermatol 2010; 146: 957–60.

Two patients with necrobiotic xanthogranuloma and monoclonal gammopathy responded well to intravenous immunoglobulin, 0.5 g/kg/day, administered for 4 consecutive days at 4-week intervals.

Cerebral and cutaneous involvements of xanthoma disseminatum successfully treated with an interleukin-1 receptor antagonist: a case report and minireview. Campero M, Campero S, Guerrero J, Aouba A, Castro A. Dermatology 2016; 232: 171–6.

One patient with xanthoma disseminatum, including skin and brain lesions, received anakinra 100 mg subcutaneously daily, continued on a weekly dose for 2 years, and then as a monthly dose for 1 year. All skin lesions disappeared within 15 months, and there was a notable reduction in lesions of the brainstem, temporal lobes, and caudate nucleus; the patient remained asymptomatic at 5-year follow-up.

Xanthoma disseminatum: effective therapy with 2-chlorodeoxyadenosine in a case series. Khezri F, Gibson LE, Tefferi A. Arch Dermatol 2011; 147: 459–64.

Five patients received 2-chlorodeoxyadenosine at 0.14 mg/kg/day for 5 days, repeated monthly for five to eight treatment cycles. After three to five cycles, new mucocutaneous lesions stopped developing in all patients, and all patients had substantial improvement in established lesions. No serious adverse effects were reported. At follow-up ranging from 3 months to 8 years, all patients had achieved remission.

Successful treatment of verruciform xanthoma with imiquimod. Guo Y, Dang Y, Toyohara JP, Geng S. J Am Acad Dermatol 2013; 69: e184–6.

A 2-year-old girl with verruciform xanthoma on the vulva and around the anus received topical imiquimod cream 5% twice a week; the lesions almost entirely cleared 4 months later and remained in remission 9 months later.

Treatment of mycosis fungoides with bexarotene results in remission of diffuse plane xanthomas. Gregoriou S, Rigopoulos D, Stamou C, Nikolaou V, Kontochristopoulos G. J Cutan Med Surg 2013; 17: 52–4.

A patient with mycosis fungoides (MF) and plane xanthomas was treated with bexarotene for MF. Complete clinical remission of both the MF and the xanthomas was noted after 6 months, and the patient remained free of xanthomas after 3 years.

Evidence Levels: **A** Double-blind study **B** Clinical trial ≥ 20 subjects **C** Clinical trial < 20 subjects **D** Series ≥ 5 subjects **E** Anecdotal case reports

257

Xeroderma pigmentosum

*Deborah Tamura, Kenneth H. Kraemer,
John J. DiGiovanna*

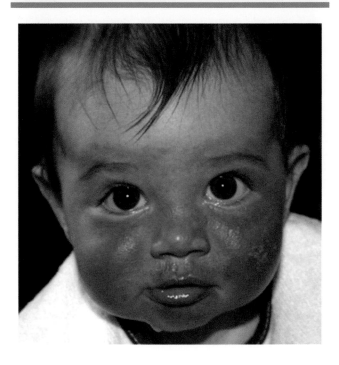

Xeroderma pigmentosum (XP) is a rare autosomal recessive disorder characterized by cellular hypersensitivity to the damaging effects of ultraviolet (UV) radiation, resulting in a 10,000-fold increased risk of skin cancers that often develop in the first decade of life. About half of patients present with acute photosensitivity to minimal sun exposure, resulting in severe erythema and blistering. Burns can be so severe that child abuse or neglect is suspected. The other half of the patients do not have these acute reactions and often develop early frecklelike pigmentation before age 2 years. This may be accompanied by a dry "aged" appearance to the skin, cheilitis, and photophobia. The eyes are particularly vulnerable, and damage may include dry eye, ectropion, pterygia, pinguecula, corneal clouding, and scarring leading to blindness; in addition they can develop cancer of the lids, sclera, or cornea. Cancers can also occur on the lips and tip of the tongue. Approximately 25% of XP patients develop a progressive neurodegeneration with loss of deep tendon reflexes, progressive sensorineural hearing loss, dysphagia and dysarthria, ataxia, and early demise.

The progressive skin and eye damage is due to an inability to repair UV-induced DNA damage in sun-exposed tissues. XP patients have mutations in one of eight genes. Seven (*XPA, XPB, XPC, XPD, XPE, XPF,* or *XPG*) are in the nucleotide excision repair (NER) pathway, and the other is DNA polymerase eta (XP variant). The NER pathway is critical for the identification, removal, and repair of UV-induced DNA damage, and polymerase eta bypasses unrepaired DNA damage.

MANAGEMENT STRATEGY

The diagnosis of XP is based on clinical features, and once suspected UV protection should be initiated immediately. XP should be suspected in a child with a history of freckling on sun-exposed skin before age 2 years, severe sunburn after minimal sun exposure, photophobia, or cancer of the skin or eye. Disorders that should be excluded include porphyria, lupus, LEOPARD syndrome, Carney complex, familial melanoma, and nevoid basal cell carcinoma syndrome.

DNA testing for mutations in several XP genes is available (www.genetests.org). Because XP is foremost a clinical diagnosis and mutation testing may not identify all XP gene mutations, failure to identify a mutation does not rule out the diagnosis of XP. The cells of XP patients in culture are extremely sensitive to the killing effects of UV, but there are currently no Clinical Laboratory Improvement Amendments (CLIA)-certified laboratories in the United States performing this type of cell survival XP test.

The most critical management goal for XP is UV protection. Although XP patients do not repair damage from UV exposure of tissues, they react normally to visible light. Eradicating all exposure to UV radiation may not be attainable; efforts should be directed toward providing a safer environment. Environments with high UV levels, such as outdoors during daylight hours, require the most rigorous protection and avoidance. However, long periods of lower levels of exposure also cause the accumulation of UV damage. We can sense differences in the intensity of visible light (e.g., less during a hazy day); however, our senses do not perceive UV and can be misled without the assistance of a UV meter. Patients and their families can be taught to recognize and avoid UV sources and to institute protective measures in their home, school, and other areas where the patient will spend long periods.

Protective measures should be a daily routine for XP patients. These include topically applied broad-spectrum sun preparations with an SPF (sun protection factor) of at least 30 or higher that protect against both UVB (short-wavelength UV 290–320 nm) and UVA (long-wavelength UV 320–400 nm) and sun-protective lip balms and/or makeup. The first application of the day should cover all exposed skin surface areas, and applications should be reapplied to uncovered skin (usually face, ears, neck, and hands) several times during the day. Finding the most acceptable sun block may take trial and error.

Clothing should cover as much skin surface as possible including long pants, long-sleeved shirts, socks and closed-toe shoes, hats that cover the ears or UV-blocking face shields and hoods, and UV-blocking sunglasses with side shields. For daytime outdoor exposure gloves or mittens can be worn to protect hands. Clothing material should be tightly woven (e.g., denim) or double layered. A simple test of effective UV protection by clothing is to hold the material up to a bright light. Material that permits visible light to pass will not block UV. Commercially available clothing made from sun-blocking material is available but may be expensive. One alternative is a laundry additive called SunGuard (https://sunguardsunprotection.com/index.php), which is advertised to increase the ability of clothing to block UV. They recommend regular washing of outer clothing (pants, shirts, jackets, socks, gloves, and hats) to increase UV protection. Because the cornea, sclera, and supporting tissues are also at risk, XP patients should wear UV-blocking sunglasses when in areas of potential exposure. The glasses should "wrap around" the eyes to protect the sides of the eyes and be large enough to fully protect both lids. Rigorous use of these measures should be initiated as soon as the diagnosis of XP is suspected and need to be the mainstay of lifelong protection.

The major source of UV is the sun. Although window glass blocks most UVB wavelengths, UVA can pass through glass (along with visible light). Extremely sensitive XP patients have burned through window glass. The Americans with Disability Act and other laws and regulations mandate that children and adults with XP be provided *safe educational and working environments*. Windows in rooms where XP patients will be spending substantial amounts of time, such as at home, in a car, in day care, school, and work, should be shielded from UV radiation. This can be done with clear UV protective film or, in some cases, by creating a consistently safe distance from windows. Schools should make accommodations during fire drills and physical education activities, because leaving the building during these activities is not safe for children with XP. An Individualized Educational Plan (IEP) should be developed to keep them protected from UV sources while encouraging interaction with other students.

Medical alert bracelets (http://www.medicalert.org/home/Home-gradient.aspx) and carrying an information card about the condition in a purse or wallet can be helpful in emergencies when affected individuals may not be able to communicate their UV sensitivity.

Unshielded fluorescent lighting and bare halogen bulbs are potential UV hazards. Replacing unshielded fluorescent bulbs with light-emitting diode (LED) lights or placing plastic shielding over fluorescent bulbs can substantially reduce environmental UV exposure. Halogen lights emit substantial levels of UVB and should be avoided.

Relatively inexpensive handheld UV meters can measure UVB and UVA. Although the UVB radiation is more damaging, UVA radiation can also produce DNA damage, so protection from all wavelengths of UV is desirable. Meters can be effective learning tools; because the level of UV cannot be easily estimated, directly measuring UV in the environment provides patients and families greater ability to assess the safety of surroundings.

Vitamin D is produced in the skin by UV exposure. Rigorous sun protection may lead to low levels of vitamin D in the blood and can eventually lead to increased risk of bone fracture. *Vitamin D–rich foods* such as "fatty" fish and vitamin D supplemented milk can help maintain normal vitamin D levels; however, patients should have periodic monitoring of vitamin D levels and oral supplementation if the serum levels of 25-OH vitamin D are low.

XP patients should not use any type of tobacco product and should be protected from second-hand smoke. The benzo[a]pyrene derivatives and other carcinogens found in tobacco products and smoke induce DNA damage repaired by the NER pathway, putting the XP patient at high risk for oral and respiratory tract cancers.

The substantial *lifestyle adjustment* necessary to provide a safer UV environment can be a challenge for the family. Outdoor activities should be avoided during daylight hours, particularly between 10 AM and 2 PM. Identifying appropriate indoor play and sports activities for the affected XP child, while continuing to meet the needs of the unaffected family members, can be difficult.

The diagnosis of XP necessitates the need for *adjustment in the entire family's activities*. Outdoor events will need to be adjusted. There will be a need for increased medical services that can place significant stressors on the family and developing child. The need for frequent painful procedures (surgeries, use of topical field agents, etc.) and hospitalizations for more extensive surgeries can lead in some instances to posttraumatic stress disorder–type symptoms in some patients and families. This type of reaction occurs in patients of all ages and can result in avoidance of care. It is important to consider pain management and stress reduction appropriate for the developmental level of the XP patient when planning care. In addition, physical changes such as scarring from surgeries or progressive neurodegeneration, with the resulting disruption of normal childhood and adolescent psychosocial development, can adversely affect self-esteem. The emotional and economic stability of the family is often affected and, as with any chronic illness, the family and patient will need to go through a period of adjustment to the lifestyle changes.

Obtaining health insurance and workplace accommodations may require considerable effort. The patients may be eligible for Social Security Disability Insurance or other medical assistance. XP support groups help patients connect with other affected families and minimize social isolation; these groups also sponsor UV-safe family activities. These include the XP Family Support Group, http://www.xpfamilysupport.org; the Xeroderma Pigmentosum Support Group UK, http://xpsupportgroup.org.uk; and the Xeroderma Pigmentosum Society, http://www.xps.org. There are also support groups in Germany, Japan, and the Middle East. In families with psychosocial pathologies (e.g., substance abuse or domestic violence), or if the family is having extreme difficulty coping with the diagnosis, referral to social services or a therapist may be advisable.

XP is a recessive disorder, with affecteds having two mutated alleles, and clinically normal parents (heterozygotes) carrying one mutated allele. The risk of having another affected child is 1 in 4 for each subsequent pregnancy. *Prenatal diagnosis* may be possible, and consultation with a genetic counselor can address genetic risks in future pregnancies.

For optimal management, the XP patient and family should partner with a dermatologist. Teaching patients and families to look for premalignant and malignant lesions can enable earlier identification and removal of small tumors. Depending on the rate of new tumor development, full skin examinations should be scheduled regularly (every 3–6 months). For rapidly evolving lesions more frequent visits may be necessary. Baseline whole-body photographs and close-up photos of lesions with a ruler in the image for size comparison can help track changes. Photos can be digitalized and given to the family for use at home and also kept in the medical record.

Premalignant lesions including actinic keratoses can be treated with *cryotherapy, topical 5-fluorouracil (5-FU), or topical imiquimod*. Care needs to be taken to ensure that existing skin cancers are adequately treated. When using topical 5-FU or imiquimod as field treatments there is a risk of treating the superficial areas of skin cancer but leaving deeper areas of tumor untreated. Well-controlled studies of topical field treatments in XP patients have not been published.

Dermabrasion or *dermatome shaving* has been used to remove the superficial photodamaged epidermal layers. Theoretically, these procedures allow replacement of severely damaged epidermal cells with cells arising from the deeper, less UV-damaged adnexal structures. Newer techniques using *laser methodology for resurfacing* have also been used in a few XP patients. For patients developing many new lesions chemoprevention with *oral retinoids* (isotretinoin or acitretin) has been used. A longitudinal study of a small number of XP patients performed at the National Institutes of Health found oral isotretinoin was effective in decreasing the number of new nonmelanoma skin cancers. However, there were many side effects in these patients, especially at the higher drug dosages. Vismodegib (Erivedge) has also been used in a few XP patients who were experiencing multiple basal cell carcinomas. There was a good response while on treatment; however, the

874

patients experienced multiple side effects requiring discontinuing the drug for varying amounts of time.

Early and adequate *treatment of skin cancers* is extremely important. All suspected tumors should be biopsied and removed. Standard techniques, including curettage and desiccation, surgical excision, or cryosurgical ablation, can be used for small superficial lesions. Due to the extensive poikilodermatous changes and scarring in XP patients, it can be difficult to differentiate recurrent from new lesions. Mohs micrographic surgery is optimal for combining effective tumor removal with tissue sparing, which should be highly considered in the surgical plan. Several factors complicate skin cancer treatment in XP patients. Cancers may develop in a "field" of extreme actinic damage, often with little normal-appearing skin either visibly or histologically. This complicates the goal of clear margins. A more practical goal would be a tumor-free margin. In addition, the quality of actinically damaged skin in XP differs from the non-XP skin cancer patient. The non-XP cancer patient typically has damage to both epidermal cellular DNA and dermal connective tissue (collagen, elastic tissue, etc.) from high doses of UV exposure that result in lax, wrinkled skin. In contrast, damage in XP patients is caused by unrepaired epidermal cellular DNA, and the total dose of UV they have received is generally insufficient to cause typical solar elastosis, lax skin, and wrinkling. Because they develop skin atrophy, XP patients may have very tight skin, which limits tissue movement for surgical repair. In addition, movement of tissue with flaps can be complicated because of the presence of precancers or small skin cancers in the severely damaged surrounding skin. Skin cancer removal with minimal margins is also necessary to preserve tissue for future surgeries, which are to be expected in these patients.

Despite their hypersensitivity to UV, many XP patients have demonstrated a normal response to x-ray therapy when it is used to treat recurrent skin and eye cancers or brain and spinal cord neoplasms.

XP patients have a significantly increased risk for developing cancers of the lips and squamous cell carcinoma of the tip of the tongue, and these areas should be regularly evaluated. Telangiectasia on the tip of the tongue is an early UV-induced change.

Ophthalmologic care is extremely important. Most ophthalmologic problems in XP patients occur in the surface structures of the eye and may begin in childhood as photophobia and conjunctivitis. Precancerous and cancerous lesions can arise on the cornea, sclera, lids, conjunctiva, and supporting tissues. UV damage on the cornea can lead to "dry eye," keratitis, and conjunctival inflammation. Ectropion of the lids, resulting in defects of eye closure, can occur secondary to eyelid atrophy and surgical removal of malignancies from the periocular skin. Ectropion exacerbates eye dryness and, if left untreated, can lead to corneal ulceration, scarring and opacification of the cornea, and blindness. Corneal transplants have been performed but frequently have led to rejection from vascularization of the area. A thorough ophthalmologic examination at least yearly can include the Schirmer test for dry eye and assessment of lid closure. Eye lubricants are recommended along with lubricating ointments at night, especially if lid closure is poor.

In the United States and Europe approximately 25% of XP patients develop progressive neurologic disease. The rate of symptom progression varies greatly among patients, with the most severe patients developing symptoms in early childhood (De Santis–Cacchione syndrome). Routinely testing reflexes during skin examinations can help identify XP patients at risk for neurologic disease. Loss of deep tendon reflexes, most notably in the lower extremities, may be the first manifestation of neurodegeneration and may be the only symptom for years. Some patients may

have microcephaly. Progression includes hearing loss, cognitive decline, dysarthria, dysphagia, mobility difficulties with ataxia, and falls; eventually a wheelchair may be needed. Magnetic resonance imaging (MRI) shows progressive dilation of the ventricles and loss of gray matter of the brain. Death may occur from aspiration pneumonia or other complications of severe debilitation. In a National Institutes of Health (NIH) study of 106 XP patients, the median age at death in XP patients with neurodegeneration (29 years) was significantly younger than those XP patients without neurodegeneration (37 years).

Progressive sensorineural hearing loss in XP patients may be diagnosed early, in the first decade of life, and may first be suspected secondary to inattentiveness in school. Audiology examinations provide a sensitive method for early detection. The hearing loss can be helped with hearing aids, and assisted hearing systems may be used in the classroom.

Some XP patients appear to have an increased risk for developing internal malignancies, including an approximately 50-fold increased risk of developing primary central nervous system tumors. These may respond to full-dose x-ray therapy with normal skin reaction. However, because some XP cell lines have increased sensitivity to x-radiation, a small test dose might be advised before full-dose exposure. In addition, XP patients have been reported with myelodysplasia, acute lymphoblastic leukemia, and thyroid cancer.

With improved health care and better protective measures, XP patients are living longer, more active lives, marrying, and having children. However, some adult women with XP have developed premature menopause in their twenties and thirties. When contemplating a pregnancy, referral for preconceptual genetic counseling is recommended.

Optimal management of XP patients is a multidisciplinary process involving several medical specialties and active cooperation and input from the patient and family. With early diagnosis, rigorous UV protection, and management of skin cancers, people with XP are living well into adulthood, working in the community and raising families.

Specific Investigations

- Regular, frequent skin examination, which may include dermoscopy, to monitor for skin cancers
- Clinical photography
- High index of suspicion and low threshold for biopsy to identify possible skin cancers
- Regular ophthalmologic examinations
- Regular neurologic examinations
- Regular audiologic examinations
- Regular overall history and physical examination for early detection of internal malignancy and thyroid abnormality
- UV sensitivity testing on cultured fibroblasts, if available
- DNA testing for XP gene mutations
- Exclusion of other photosensitive, pigmentary, or cancer-prone disorders (lupus, porphyria, LEOPARD syndrome, Carney complex, familial melanoma, nevoid basal cell carcinoma syndrome)

Total-body cutaneous examination, total-body photography, and dermoscopy in the care of a patient with xeroderma pigmentosum and multiple melanomas. Green WH, Wang SQ, Cognetta AB, Jr. Arch Dermatol 2009; 145: 910–5.

Case report describing the use of regular skin examination, photography, and dermoscopy in the management of an XP patient.

Unexpected extradermatological findings in 31 patients with xeroderma pigmentosum type C. Hadj-Rabia S, Oriot D, Soufir N, Dufresne H, Bourrat E, Mallet S, et al. Br J Dermatol 2013; 168: 1109–13.

Report on the phenotypes of a group of *XP-C* patients in France who demonstrate neoplasms of internal organs, short stature, and thyroid nodules in addition to skin cancer.

Deep phenotyping of 89 xeroderma pigmentosum patients reveals unexpected heterogeneity dependent on the precise molecular defect. Fassihi H, Sethi M, Fawcett H, Wing J, Chandler N, Mohammed S, et al. Proc Natl Acad Sci USA 2016; 113: E1236–45.

Cancer and neurologic degeneration in xeroderma pigmentosum: long term follow-up characterises the role of DNA repair. Bradford PT, Goldstein AM, Tamura D, Khan SG, Ueda T, Boyle J, et al. J Med Genet 2011; 48: 168–76.

Shining a light on xeroderma pigmentosum. DiGiovanna JJ, Kraemer KH. J Invest Dermatol 2012; 132: 785–96.

Xeroderma pigmentosum. Webb S. BMJ 2008; 336: 444–6.

Auditory analysis of xeroderma pigmentosum 1971 to 2012: hearing function, sun sensitivity and DNA repair predict neurologic degeneration. Totonchy MB, Tamura D, Pantell MS, Zalewski C, Bradford PT, Merchant SN, et al. Brain 2013; 136: 194–208.

First-Line Therapies	
• UV protection	C
• Removal of skin cancers	C

Living with xeroderma pigmentosum: comprehensive photoprotection for highly photosensitive patients. Tamura D, DiGiovanna JJ, Khan SG, Kraemer KH. Photodermatol Photoimmunol Photomed 2014; 30: 146–52.

Understanding xeroderma pigmentosum. Clinical Center, National Cancer Institute: http://clinicalcenter.nih.gov/ccc/patient_education/pepubs/xp7_17.pdf.

A patient information booklet written in lay terms for patients, family members, and health care providers.

Growing up in the hospital. Pao M, Ballard ED, Rosenstein DL. JAMA 2007; 297: 2752–5.

Strict sun protection results in minimal skin changes in a patient with xeroderma pigmentosum and a novel c.2009delG mutation in XPD (ERCC2). Emmert S, Ueda T, Zumsteg U, Weber P, Khan SG, Oh KS, et al. Exp Dermatol 2009; 18: 64–8.

A case report describing strict UV protection in an XP child with neurologic degeneration. The UV protection did not affect the neurodegeneration; however, there were only very mild skin manifestations and no skin cancer.

Second-Line Therapies	
• Topical imiquimod	B
• Topical 5-fluorouracil	B
• Oral retinoid therapy	C

Therapeutic response of a brother and sister with xeroderma pigmentosum to imiquimod 5% cream. Weisberg NK, Varghese M. Dermatol Surg 2002; 28: 518–23.

Siblings diagnosed with XP failed chemoprophylaxis for dozens of tumors with oral retinoids. Treatment with imiquimod 5% cream was initiated three times per week for several months. Both patients experienced reduction of new tumor development and resolution of multiple existing basal cell carcinomas. One sibling demonstrated a robust inflammatory response, and the other had little visible reaction.

5% 5-fluorouracil cream for the treatment of small superficial basal cell carcinoma: efficacy, tolerability, cosmetic outcome, and patient satisfaction. Gross K, Kircik L, Kricorian G. Dermatol Surg 2007; 33: 433–9.

Evaluated the efficacy, tolerability, cosmetic outcome, and patient satisfaction of 5% FU treatment for superficial basal cell carcinomas in 29 patients. Histologic cure rate was 90%, and patients were generally very satisfied with the treatment. These were not XP patients.

Prevention of skin cancer in xeroderma pigmentosum with the use of oral isotretinoin. Kraemer KH, DiGiovanna JJ, Moshell AN, Tarone RE, Peck GL. N Engl J Med 1988; 318: 1633–7.

Five XP patients were treated for a total of 2 years with high-dose (2 mg/kg/day) isotretinoin. The patients had a total of 121 tumors before treatment, and only 25 tumors occurred during treatment. The tumor frequency increased 8.5-fold after the drug was discontinued. However, there were significant side effects on the drug, including cutaneous, triglyceride, liver function, or skeletal problems.

Xeroderma pigmentosum: spinal cord astrocytoma with 9-year survival after radiation and isotretinoin therapy. DiGiovanna JJ, Patronas N, Katz D, Abangan D, Kraemer KH. J Cutan Med Surg 1998; 2: 153–8.

Case report of an XP patient who received radiation therapy for a spinal cord astrocytoma with normal cutaneous response to standard dosages.

Topical imiquimod or fluorouracil therapy for basal and squamous cell carcinoma: a systematic review. Love WE, Bernhard JD, Bordeaux JS. Arch Dermatol 2009; 145: 1431–8.

A systematic review of topical imiquimod or FU therapy in the treatment of basal cell and squamous cell carcinomas in the general population.

Topical imiquimod or fluorouracil therapy for basal and squamous cell carcinoma: a systematic review. Love WE, Bernhard JD, Bordeaux JS. Arch Dermatol 2009; 145: 1431–8.

A case report of an XP patient who had multiple skin grafts and experienced tumor recurrence, which originated under the skin graft.

Third-Line Therapy	
• Resurfacing and dermabrasion and chemical peels	E

Evidence Levels: A Double-blind study B Clinical trial ≥ 20 subjects C Clinical trial < 20 subjects D Series ≥ 5 subjects E Anecdotal case reports

The role of dermabrasion and chemical peels in the treatment of patients with xeroderma pigmentosum. Nelson BR, Fader DJ, Gillard M, Baker SR, Johnson TM. J Am Acad Dermatol 1995; 32: 623–6.

A case report of two XP patients treated periodically with trichloroacetic acid chemical peels; one also underwent dermabrasion. Both procedures provided some prophylactic effects, with the dermabrasion having better results. Before and after pictures are presented.

Acknowledgment

This research was supported by the Intramural Research Program of the NIH, National Cancer Institute, Center for Cancer Research.

Xerosis

Ian Coulson

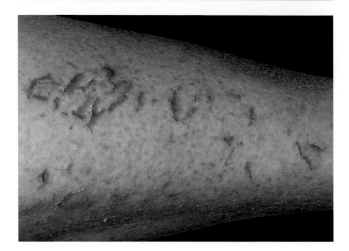

Xerosis is the term used to describe a condition where there is a rough, dry textural feel to the skin, accompanied by fine scaling and sometimes fine fissuring. Increasing xerosis is usually accompanied by increasing itch. It may result from a combination of environmental conditions (low humidity, degreasing of the skin by excessive bathing, soap, or detergent use); genetic disorders of keratinization (ichthyoses); atopic eczema (where it may be a manifestation of a filaggrin mutation); endocrine disease states (hypothyroidism); diabetes mellitus (39% of patients); and a host of underlying disease states such as chronic renal failure, liver disease (including 69% of patients with primary biliary cirrhosis), malnutrition, anorexia nervosa (58% of patients), essential fatty acid deficiency, Sjögren syndrome (56% of patients), HIV infection, lymphoma (where it may result in an acquired ichthyosis), and carcinomatosis (especially hematologic). It is more common in the elderly. Drugs (statins and targeted chemotherapeutic agents such as EGRF and BRAF inhibitors) are occasionally implicated. It is reported to be more frequent in the winter.

MANAGEMENT STRATEGY

Initial evaluation should seek to distinguish simple xerosis from a genetic ichthyosis, although management is similar for both conditions. Family history, distribution, and morphology will help to differentiate the two. A history of weight loss, diarrhea, dietary history, and body mass index may give clues toward an underlying metabolic or malabsorptive disorder. Dry eyes and mouth may indicate underlying Sjögren syndrome. History and clinical examination should seek symptoms and signs of hypothyroidism, diabetes mellitus, and chronic renal disease. Drug use and sexual contact history may reveal HIV infection. Xerosis is an almost universal accompaniment of atopic eczema.

The mainstay of therapy for xerosis after any underlying disorders (if possible) are corrected is *improvement of the humidity* in the patient's environment, *avoidance of exacerbating factors* such as soap and detergents, and the use of *emollients or humectants*.

Low environmental humidity both at home and work will exacerbate xerosis of any cause. Arid air is a problem in

air-conditioned homes, offices, and vehicles. Hot dry air directed to the lower legs during the winter in the front of automobiles is a common cause of lower leg xerosis. In the home or workplace humidifiers can be fitted over radiators; alternatively, placing wet towels or containers of water over them will increase air humidity.

Soaps and detergents degrease the skin, reduce epidermal thickness, and increase scale and itch, and so are best avoided, and light emollient cleansers (soap substitutes) are suggested in their place. Bathing in tepid water is often preferred by patients, and patting the skin dry will produce less scale and dryness than vigorous toweling.

Emollients (which simply produce an impervious film over the epidermis and prevent "transpiration") and humectants (such as lactic acid, urea, or glycerine that hold water in the epidermis osmotically) are the mainstays of therapy. Few good comparative studies exist for the most common type of xerosis, which is surprising because they are the most frequently used dermatologic products. They should be used liberally and as frequently as possible and applied in the direction of hair growth; emollients are particularly valuable after bathing or showering to hold water in the epidermis. Light emollients for use in the shower or bath may be preferred to *bath oils* by some. Choice of emollient is entirely personal to the patient. A pack with small amounts of a variety of products for home trial or a self-selection "tub tray" for the clinic is likely to enhance compliance. The best emollient is the one the patient likes; the most expensive is the one where 499 g remains in the tub!

Agents containing *α-hydroxy acids (AHAs)* may offer some advantages over conventional paraffin-based emollients, but this may be at the expense of irritation in some people. Low-concentration *salicylic acid* may help reduce scale in more severe xerosis, but it is essential to remember that systemic absorption and salicylism can occur.

Topical retinoids have only been used in the more severe ichthyoses and are too irritating for use in xerosis. Systemic therapies have little part to play in most patients.

Specific Investigations

- Thyroid function tests
- Renal function tests
- Random glucose
- Consider tests for Sjögren syndrome, HIV infection, malignancies, and malabsorption, if clinically indicated
- Drug history

Sjogren's syndrome: a retrospective review of the cutaneous features of 93 patients by the Italian Group of Immunodermatology. Bernacchi E, Amato L, Parodi A, Cottoni F, Rubegni P, De Pità O, et al. Clin Exp Rheumatol 2004; 22: 55–62.

Over half of 93 patients with Sjögren syndrome had xerosis, and its presence correlated with the presence of SSA and SSB antibodies.

HIV-associated pruritus: etiology and management. Singh F, Rudikoff D. Am J Clin Dermatol 2003; 4: 177–88.

Xerosis is one of the more common causes of itch in HIV infection and AIDS.

Noninfectious skin conditions associated with diabetes mellitus: a prospective study of 308 cases. Diris N, Colomb M,

Evidence Levels: **A** Double-blind study **B** Clinical trial ≥ 20 subjects **C** Clinical trial < 20 subjects **D** Series ≥ 5 subjects **E** Anecdotal case reports

Leymarie F, Durlach V, Caron J, Bernard P. Ann Dermatol Venereol 2003; 130: 1009–14.

Xerosis was noted in 39% of 309 patients.

Eating disorders and the skin. Strumia R. Clin Dermatol 2013; 31: 80–5.

Xerosis is a common feature of anorexia.

Xerosis from lithium carbonate. Hoxtell E, Dahl MV. Arch Dermatol 1975; 111: 1073–4.

Incidence and risk of xerosis with targeted anticancer therapies. Valentine J, Belum VR, Duran J, Ciccolini K, Schindler K, Wu S, et al. J Am Acad Dermatol 2015; 72: 656–72.

About 20% of patients receiving targeted therapies develop significant xerosis.

Litt's Drug Eruption Reference and Database lists in excess of 150 drugs (from acebutolol to zonisamide) that have been implicated in causing xerosis. Retinoids, cimetidine, protease inhibitors, statins, and nicotinamide are perhaps the best known. Epidermal growth factors and targeted chemotherapy agents are new agents that have xerosis among their protean dermatologic side effects.

First-Line Therapies	
• Soap avoidance	A
• Humidification	C
• Emollients	B
• Bath oils	B

Moisturizers are effective in the treatment of xerosis irrespectively from their particular formulation: results from a prospective, randomized, double-blind controlled trial. Shim JH, Park JH, Lee J, Lee DY, Lee JH, Yang JM. J Eur Acad Dermatol Venereol 2016; 30: 276–81.

A double-blind trial evaluating the effect of four conventional popular emollients, as well as a new cream containing recombinant epidermal growth factor and its control vehicle. All of the evaluated agents improved the clinical symptoms of xerosis. Consistent and regular moisturization was more important than the emollients' particular formulation. This reinforces the dogma that the best emollient is the one the patient likes and uses.

Emollients improve treatment results with topical corticosteroids in childhood atopic dermatitis: a randomized comparative study. Szczepanowska J, Reich A, Szepietowski JC. Pediatr Allergy Immunol 2008; 19: 614–8.

In a study of 52 children with atopic dermatitis, those applying emollients concurrently with topical corticosteroids had significantly improved xerosis.

How useful are soap substitutes? Berth-Jones J, Graham-Brown RAC. J Dermatol Treat 1992; 3: 9–11.

Thirty-eight subjects with atopic dermatitis, psoriasis, or senile xerosis were treated with emulsifying ointment BP or Wash E45 as soap substitutes. Dryness and itching improved in both groups. Wash E45 was considered more effective as a cleanser.

The value of oil baths for adjuvant basic therapy of inflammatory dermatoses with dry, barrier-disrupted skin. Melnik B, Braun-Falco O. Hautarzt 1996; 47: 665–72.

The use of oil baths with emollients is an integral and indispensable constituent of maintenance therapy in dry skin conditions, atopic eczema, and inflammatory dermatoses.

Second-Line Therapies	
• Urea-containing creams	A
• Lactic acid–containing creams	A
• Ammonium lactate creams	A
• Colloidal oatmeal	A
• AHA creams	B
• Thyroxine cream	D
• Glycerol containing creams	B
• Chia oil	D

A double blind comparison of two creams containing urea as the active ingredient. Assessment of efficacy and side effects by noninvasive techniques and a clinical scoring scheme. Serup J. Acta Derm Venereol 1992; 177: 34–43.

A comparison of 3% and 10% urea cream showed that both were effective at reducing scale, dryness, and laboratory parameters (transepidermal water loss and colorimetric changes). The 10% cream was better at restoring the skin's water barrier function.

Clinical evaluation of 40% urea and 12% ammonium lactate in the treatment of xerosis. Ademola J, Frazier C, Kim SJ, Theaux C, Saudez X. Am J Clin Dermatol 2002; 3: 217–22.

A double-blind study comparing 40% urea cream with 12% ammonium lactate cream showing superiority of the urea cream. Flexural irritation was a problem.

Many urea-containing products contain lower concentrations than used in this study.

Use of a urea, arginine and carnosine cream versus a standard emollient glycerol cream for treatment of severe xerosis of the feet in patients with type 2 diabetes: a randomized, 8 month, assessor-blinded, controlled trial. Federici A, Federici G, Milani M. Curr Med Res Opin 2015; 31: 1063–9.

Fifty diabetics with severe foot xerosis fared better with the combination cream in comparison to a simple glycerine-containing emollient.

A controlled two-center study of lactate 12% lotion and a petrolatum-based creme in patients with xerosis. Wehr R, Krochmal L, Bagatell F, Ragsdale W. Cutis 1986; 37: 205–7.

Lactate lotion 12% was significantly more effective than a petrolatum-based cream in reducing the severity of xerosis during treatment and posttreatment phases.

Comparative efficacy of 12% ammonium lactate lotion and 5% lactic acid lotion in the treatment of moderate to severe xerosis. Rogers RS III, Callen J, Wehr R, Krochmal L. J Am Acad Dermatol 1989; 21: 714–6.

This comparative study of twice-daily application of 5% lactic acid vs. 12% ammonium lactate lotion showed superiority of 12% ammonium lactate in reducing the severity of xerosis.

A double-blind clinical trial comparing the efficacy and safety of pure lanolin versus ammonium lactate 12% cream for the treatment of moderate to severe foot xerosis. Jennings MB, Alfieri DM, Parker ER, Jackman L, Goodwin S, Lesczczynski C. Cutis 2003; 71: 78–82.

A study showing equivalence of a petrolatum compound and 12% ammonium lactate cream for foot xerosis.

A randomized controlled clinical study to evaluate the effectiveness of an active moisturizing lotion with colloidal oatmeal skin protectant versus its vehicle for the relief of xerosis. Kalaaji AN, Wallo W. J Drugs Dermatol 2014; 13: 1265–8.

A randomized, double-blind, controlled clinical study to objectively compare a commercially available moisturizing product against its own vehicle. The active colloidal oatmeal moisturizer used in this study showed significant benefits versus its vehicle control in several dermatologic parameters used to measure skin dryness.

An evaluation of the effect of an alpha hydroxy acid-blend skin cream in the cosmetic improvement of symptoms of moderate to severe xerosis, epidermolytic hyperkeratosis, and ichthyosis. Kempers S, Katz HI, Wildnauer R, Green B. Cutis 1998; 61: 347–50.

Twenty subjects completed a course of treatment with either regular or extra-strength AHA-blend cream on a test site compared with a currently marketed, non-AHA moisturizing lotion on a control site. Improvements were significant compared with baseline and compared with sites treated with the control lotion, but the AHA cream did cause some local mild to moderate adverse effects; all subjects were able to continue using the test product for the duration of the study.

Randomized, double-blind study with glycerol and paraffin in uremic xerosis. Balaskas E, Szepietowski JC, Bessis D, Ioannides D, Ponticelli C, Ghienne C, et al. Clin J Am Soc Nephrol 2011; 6: 748–52.

An emollient containing glycerol and paraffin compared side to side with an emulsion devoid of these agents. The active treatment helped reduce the physical signs of xerosis as well as the pruritus.

Effectiveness of topical chia seed oil on pruritus of end-stage renal disease (ESRD) patients and healthy volunteers. Jeong SK, Park HJ, Park BD, Kim IH. Ann Dermatol 2010; 22: 143–8.

A small study demonstrating effectiveness using this *n*-3 fatty acid–containing oil in normal people and renal failure sufferers with xerosis.

Evidence Levels: **A** Double-blind study **B** Clinical trial ≥ 20 subjects **C** Clinical trial < 20 subjects **D** Series ≥ 5 subjects **E** Anecdotal case reports

Yellow nail syndrome

Robert Baran

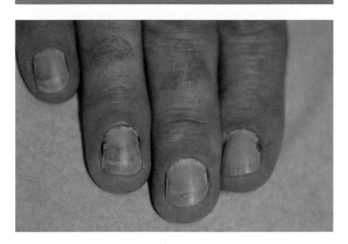

Table 259.1 Systemic causes possibly associated with yellow nail syndrome

Adenocarcinoma of the endometrium	Drugs: bucillamine, penicillamine, thiol, gold
Anaplastic undifferentiated tumor	Hodgkin disease
Arteriovenous fistula	Laryngeal carcinoma
Autoimmune hypothyroidism	Membranous glomerulonephritis
Breast carcinoma	Metastatic malignant melanoma
Common variable immunodeficiency	

(After Gupta AK. Cutis 1986; 37: 371–4 and Lotfolollhai L, et al. Tanaffos 2015; 14: 57–1.)

The yellow nail syndrome (YNS) is an uncommon disorder of unknown etiology characterized by the triad of yellow nails, lymphedema, and respiratory tract involvement. This term was originally used to describe the association of slow-growing yellow nails with primary lymphedema. Pleural effusion was later recognized to be an additional sign of the syndrome. Since then, other respiratory conditions, such as bronchiectasis, sinusitis, bronchitis, and chronic respiratory infections, have been associated with the disorder. Although all three signs that classically characterize the triad of YNS do not occur in every patient, the presence of typical nail alterations should be considered an absolute requirement for the diagnosis. The complete triad is seen in 25% of patients, lymphedema in 40%, and pleural effusions in only 2% of patients with yellow nails. A variant of yellow nails can also be seen in HIV infection.

MANAGEMENT STRATEGY

Although YNS may resolve spontaneously, treatment is often sought by sufferers. The nails are unsightly, discolored (yellowish or greenish), hard, show transverse overcurvature with a hump, and are very slow growing. Paronychia and onycholysis can be observed.

Underlying diseases such as respiratory disorders, malignancy (Table 259.1), infections, immunologic and hematologic abnormalities, endocrine, connective tissue, renal abnormalities, and miscellaneous disorders, including drug-induced YNS, *dental amalgams*, and *titanium exposure* (Box 259.1), should be sought. Improvement of any underlying disorder (e.g., lymphedema) may also result in improvement of the nail plate.

There are no large series or randomized trials in the treatment of yellow nail syndrome. *Oral vitamin E* has been used as monotherapy. The oral azole antifungals *itraconazole* and *fluconazole* have also been reported to be effective, alone or in combination with vitamin E. *The combination of fluconazole and vitamin E is certainly the best treatment for curing the nail unit.* This was confirmed by some anecdotal reports that supplement our own statistics. Repeated nail *matrix steroid injections* have been

successfully employed. *Octreotide, zinc,* and *medium-chain fatty acid triglyceride supplements* as well as *clarithromycin* have been used in anecdotal reports. *Treatment of underlying disease (or concomitant disorder) is mandatory but does not always bring resolution of the YNS, and cure of the nail is not always accompanied by disappearance of the other signs.*

Specific Investigations

- Rule out fungal or *Pseudomonas* infection
- Serum rheumatoid factors
- Complete blood count
- Chemistry profile with blood creatinine
- Urinalysis, proteinuria
- Sinus and chest radiography
- Immunoelectrophoresis
- Ear/nose/throat (ENT) and pulmonary investigations
- Thyroid-stimulating hormone (TSH)
- Liver enzymes, alkaline phosphatases
- Cone beam computed tomography (CBCT)
- Search for titanium dioxide in the nail

Box 259.1 Exposure to Titanium Dioxide

- Foods such as candy, chewing gum, and chocolate
- Personal care items, such as shampoo, sunscreen, and toothpaste
- Drugs such as multivitamins

(Modified from Decker A, et al. Skin Appendage Disord 2015; 1: 28–30.)

First-Line Therapies

• α-Tocopherol + fluconazole	**B**
• Treatment of the concomitant disorder	**E**

Combination of fluconazole and α-tocopherol in the treatment of yellow-nail syndrome. Baran R, Thomas L. J Drugs Dermatol 2009; 8: 276–8.

Daily treatment with 500 mg oral vitamin E morning and evening associated with weekly 300 mg fluconazole should be taken as long as needed.

Usually complete cure has been obtained in 18 to 24 months. However, there is still a wide discrepancy between the response of the nail to treatment and the remaining signs, which are usually unimproved.

T and B cell deficiency associated with yellow nail syndrome. Gupta S, Samra D, Yel L, Agrawal S. Scand J Immunol 2012; 75: 329–35.

Immunoglobulin administration resulted in the decreased frequency and severity of infections, and an impressive effect was observed on lymphedema and on the recurrence of pleural effusion.

Second-Line Therapies

- Intradermal triamcinolone injections in the proximal nail matrix **B**
- Clarithromycin **E**
- Physiotherapy **E**

Yellow nail syndrome treated by intralesional triamcinolone acetonide. Abell E, Samman PD. Br J Dermatol 1973; 88: 200–1.

Repeated intradermal triamcinolone injections in the proximal nail matrix might be effective on the nail unit, but they are no longer in use.

A case of yellow nail syndrome with dramatically improved nail discoloration by oral clarithromycin. Suzuki M, Yoshizawa A, Sugiyama H, Ichimura Y, Morita A, Takasaki J, et al. Case Rep Dermatol 2011; 3: 251–8.

Dramatic improvement of the yellow nail discoloration and growth of nails in one patient treated daily with 400 mg clarithromycin.

Syndrome des ongles jaunes d'évolution favorable: role de la kinésithérapie respiratoire?. Fournier C, Just N, Leroy S, Wallaert B. Rev Mal Resp 2003; 20: 969–72.

Besides the nail manifestations, the patient had bilateral bronchiectasis. Daily physiotherapy with bronchial drainage led to a progressive improvement in the respiratory signs. The nail abnormalities disappeared after 2 years of treatment.

Improvement in lymphatic function and partial resolution of nails, after complete decongestive physiotherapy in yellow nail syndrome. Szolnoky G, Lakatos B, Husz S, Dobozy A. Int J Dermatol 2005; 44: 501–3.

Manual lymphatic drainage was performed on each leg for 45 minutes, and multilayered compression bandaging was subsequently applied. This was repeated daily for 2 weeks, except at weekends, when the compression was not accompanied by massage. The edema reduction and the increase in lymph flow were associated with an improvement in the appearance of the toenail plates. Fingernails failed to show any change.

Third-Line Therapies

- Oral zinc supplementation **E**
- Dietary treatment **E**
- Octreotide treatment **E**

Improvement of yellow nail syndrome with oral zinc supplementation. Arroyo JF, Cohen ML. Clin Exp Dermatol 1993; 18: 62–4.

Total resolution of yellow nails and lymphedema was observed after oral zinc supplementation for 2 years.

Yellow nail syndrome in a 10-year-old girl. Göçmen A, Küçükosmanoğlu O, Kiper N, Karaduman A, Ozçelik U. J Pediatr 1997; 39: 105–9.

Low-fat diet supplemented with medium-chain triglycerides brought moderate improvement in the lymphedema of the lower extremities.

Successful octreotide treatment of chylous pleural effusion and lymphedema in the yellow nail syndrome. Makrilakis K, Pavlatos S, Giannikopoulos G, Toubanakis C, Katsilambros N. Ann Intern Med 2004; 141: 246–7.

Octreotide, a somatostatin analog, was effective in a classic case of YNS with yellow nails, lymphedema of lower extremities, and recurrent chylous pleural effusion.

Yellow nail syndrome: report of a case successfully treated with octreotide. Lotfollahi L, Abedini A, Alavi Darazam I, Kiani A, Fadaii A. Tanaffos 2015; 14: 67–71.

Evidence Levels: **A** Double-blind study **B** Clinical trial ≥ 20 subjects **C** Clinical trial < 20 subjects **D** Series ≥ 5 subjects **E** Anecdotal case reports

Index

Page numbers followed by b, t, and f indicate boxes, tables, and figures, respectively.

883

884

Blanchable erythema, in decubitus ulcers, 182
Blastomyces dermatitidis, 105
Blastomycosis, 105–107, 105f
Bleach (hypochlorite), for MRSA, 287
Bleaching, for hirsutism, 358
Bleomycin
    for basal cell carcinoma, 564
    for hemangiomas, 324
    for keloids, 401
    for keratoacanthoma, 403
    for pyogenic granuloma, 718
    for squamous cell carcinoma, 781, 783
    for warts, 852, 857
Blister management, for epidermolysis
    bullosa, 226
Blistering distal dactylitis (BDD), 108–109,
    108f
Blue light phototherapy, for acne vulgaris,
    10
Bluebottle stings, 381
Boceprevir, for porphyria cutanea tarda, 652
Body dysmorphic disorder (BDD), 110–113,
    110f
    screening questions for, 111t
Body louse (*Pediculus humanus*), 606, 609
Boils (furunculosis), 286, 286f
Bone marrow failure, in human parvovirus
    B19 infection, 605
Bone marrow transplantation
    for cytophagic histiocytic panniculitis,
      588
    for epidermolysis bullosa, 228
    for erythropoietic protoporphyria, 264
    for graft-*versus*-host disease, 298
    for papular urticaria, 592
Bone mineral density, in erythropoietic
    protoporphyria, 262
Borrelia afzelii, 464
Borrelia burgdorferi, lymphocytoma cutis
    from, 472
Borrelia garinii, 464
Borrelial lymphocytoma, 464
Bortezomib, for scleromyxedema, 434
Bosentan
    for digital ulcers related to systemic
      sclerosis, 724
    for pulmonary hypertension, 767
    for Raynaud's phenomenon, 722
Botox *see* Botulinum toxin A
Botulinum toxin
    for Hailey-Hailey disease, 317
    for hyperhidrosis, 355
    for notalgia paresthetica, 570
    for pitted and ringed keratolysis, 628
    for rosacea, 749
    for vulvodynia, 866
Botulinum toxin A
    for Darier disease, 180
    for dyshidrotic eczema, 320
    for Fox-Fordyce disease, 285
    for leiomyoma, 417
    for Raynaud's phenomenon, 725
Bowen's disease, 114–115, 114f
Box jellyfish (*Chironex fleckeri*), 381
Brachioradial pruritus (BRP), 679
Brachytherapy
    for keloids, 400
    for squamous cell carcinoma, 783
Bradykinin, for hereditary angioedema, 325
Bradykinin-mediated angioedema,
    management strategy for, 843

BRAF inhibitor, for melanoma, 484–485,
    488
BRAF mutation, in melanoma, 484
Breast cancer, in polycystic ovary syndrome,
    641
Breastfeeding, for subcutaneous fat necrosis
    of newborn, 805
Breathable backsheets, for diaper dermatitis,
    204
Brentuximab vedotin, for lymphomatoid
    papulosis, 477, 480
Brimonidine tartrate, for rosacea, 748
Brincidofovir, for rabbitpox virus infection,
    96
Brivudin, for varicella, 845
Brodalumab
    for generalized pustular psoriasis and
      psoriatic erythroderma, 254
    for psoriasis, 704
Buboes, in lymphogranuloma venereum,
    475
Bug Buster kit, for pediculosis capitis, 608
Bullous congenital ichthyosiform
    erythroderma, 253
Bullous dermatosis, linear IgA, 451–453,
    451f
Bullous impetigo, 371
Bullous pemphigoid, 116–119, 116f
    erythrodermic, 251
Bupivacaine, for postherpetic neuralgia, 342
Burning mouth syndrome (glossodynia),
    120–123, 120f
    consultations for, 121t
    laboratory evaluation of, 121t
    specific investigations of, 121t
Burns, xeroderma pigmentosum and, 873
Burrow ink test, for scabies mite, 758
Buruli ulcer (*Mycobacterium ulcerans*), 528
Butenafine, for pityriasis versicolor, 827
3-Butenyl 5-aminolevulinate gel, for acne
    vulgaris, 10
Butorphanol, for pruritus
    intractable, 684
    opioid-induced, 685

C

C1-esterase inhibitor (C1INH), for
    hereditary angioedema, 326–327
C1 inhibitor deficiency, 326
C4, for hereditary angioedema, 326
Caffeine
    for cellulite, 138
    pruritus ani and, 687
Calcineurin inhibitors
    for atopic dermatitis, 59
    for cutaneous lupus erythematosus, 210
    for discoid eczema, 206
    for irritant contact dermatitis, 379
    for Jessner lymphocytic infiltrate, 385
    for lichen sclerosus, 446
    for lichen simplex chronicus, 448
    for lupus erythematosus, 798
    perioral dermatitis induction with, 620
    for psoriasis, 700
    for vitiligo, 859
Calcinosis, associated with dermatomyositis,
    124, 198, 201
Calcinosis cutis, 124–127, 124f
Calciphylaxis, 128–130, 128f, 585

Calcipotriol/calcipotriene
    for acanthosis nigricans, 2
    for bullous congenital ichthyosiform
      erythroderma, 253
    for confluent and reticulated
      papillomatosis, 162
    for epidermolytic palmoplantar
      keratoderma of Vorner, 581
    for erosive pustular dermatosis, 234
    for erythema annulare centrifugum, 237
    for Grover disease, 834
    for inflammatory linear verrucous
      epidermal nevus, 222
    for lupus vulgaris, 839
    for morphea, 514
    for nail psoriasis, 544
    for porokeratosis, 647
    for progressive symmetric
      erythrokeratoderma, 256
    for prurigo nodularis, 673
    for psoriasis, 697, 700
      facial and intertriginous, 697
      pustular, 706–707
    for reactive arthritis, 727
Calcitonin, for subcutaneous fat necrosis of
    newborn, 805
Calcitonin gene-related peptide, for
    Raynaud's phenomenon, 724
Calcitriol
    for granuloma annulare, 305
    for Hailey-Hailey disease, 317
    for psoriasis, 700
Calcium
    for palmoplantar pustulosis, 582
    for pemphigus, 612
    for pseudoxanthoma elasticum
      progression, 695
    for relapsing polychondritis, 734
    serum, for subcutaneous fat necrosis of
      newborn, 805
Calcium channel blockers
    for chilblains, 145
    for erythromelalgia, 260
    for Raynaud's phenomenon, 722–723
Calcium dobesilate, for capillaritis, 133
Calendula officinalis, for radiation dermatitis,
    720
Campath-1H *see* Alemtuzumab
Canakinumab, for cryopyrin associated
    periodic syndromes, 165
Cancer/malignancy
    acanthosis nigricans and, 2
    dermatomyositis and, 198–199
    erythema annulare centrifugum and, 236
    erythema nodosum and, 245
    lymphomatoid papulosis and, 477
    nevus sebaceus and, 567
    Peutz-Jeghers syndrome and, 621
    porokeratoses and, 646
    scleroderma and, 765
    xeroderma pigmentosum and, 873, 875
    see also individual cancers
Candida, paronychia from, 601
Candida albicans
    cutaneous candidiasis from, 171
    diaper dermatitis and, 203
    erythema annulare centrifugum and,
      236
Candida antigen immunotherapy
    for molluscum contagiosum, 511
    for warts, 854